ENDOCRINOLOGY OF WOMAN

JOSÉ BOTELLA-LLUSIÁ, M.D., F.I.A.C.

Professor and Chairman,
Department of Obstetrics and Gynecology,
University of Madrid, Spain

Translated by
EDWARD A. MOSCOVIC, M.D.

Assistant Professor of Pathology,
College of Physicians and Surgeons,
Columbia University, New York

W. B. SAUNDERS COMPANY – 1973
PHILADELPHIA – LONDON – TORONTO

W. B. Saunders Company: West Washington Square
Philadelphia, Pa. 19105

12 Dyott Street
London, WC1A 1DB

833 Oxford Street
Toronto 18, Ontario

Endocrinology of Woman   ISBN 0-7216-1890-1

© 1973 by W. B. Saunders Company. Copyright under the International Copyright Union. All rights reserved. This book is protected by copyright. No part of it may be reproduced, stored in a retrieval system, or transmitted in any form or by any means, electronic, mechanical, photocopying, recording, or otherwise, without written permission from the publisher. Made in the United States of America. Press of W. B. Saunders Company. Library of Congress Catalog card number 74-183446.

Print No.:   9   8   7   6   5   4   3   2   1

FOREWORD

I made José Botella-Llusiá's acquaintance during a Gynecologic Congress in Paris in 1951. He had just been appointed Professor and Chairman of the Department of Gynecology of the University of Madrid. Europe was coming to life again and Spain strove to overcome its isolation. From the first moment of our meeting I was surprised by the new conception of Obstetrics and Gynecology of this young (in those days) Professor who was then only 39 years old. He not only considered both branches closely linked together in the American tradition, transcending thereby the old French and Latin-American distinction between Obstetrics and Gynecology, but also he thought that both specialties formed a single science to which he gave the name "Biology and Reproductive Pathology." Since 1949, Botella and his associates in his Department of Research, in Madrid, have been making important contributions to the study of the physiopathology of human reproduction. I should like to point out that this small and modest department was probably one of the very first dedicated to these investigations, which are now being carried out in many other modern institutions.

From that time on, and according to his physiological approach to Gynecology, Botella-Llusiá called special attention to the endocrinology of woman. He brought out in 1942 the first edition of the present book, with a preface written by his teacher, Gregorio Marañón.

Therefore, it antedated Hoffman and Hamblen's publications and appeared only 11 years after the first edition of Allen's *Sex and Internal Secretions*. Consequently we may say that this work is a pioneer in gynecologic endocrinology. This book is the fifth edition of *Endocrinología de la Mujer*.

Since 1942 knowledge of the female internal secretions has changed considerably. The present edition has been brought up to date to the end of 1970 and is a comprehensive summary of our present-day knowledge. The endocrinology of woman, just as knowledge of the other branches of internal secretion, has made great strides during the last years and it is very difficult for one man to cover in a single book all the biochemical, physiological and clinical aspects. It is for this reason that the modern trend is to publish comprehensive studies that require a separate specialist author for each chapter. This book by Botella-Llusiá is an unusual exception because he is the sole writer of the book. Aside from my admiration for this comprehensive work, I wondered if this decision was the right one or whether Botella-Llusiá should have had associated with him various specialists from Spain and other countries. I dare say the book, if multi-authored, might have been more precise but, on the other hand, books written by many authors usually lack unity, and not infrequently what is affirmed in one chapter is doubted or even denied in another. The reader who wants to have a comprehensive view of the subject is often bewildered. The advantage of a book written by only one author from his personal perspective is that the whole book maintains its unity of ideas and all the chapters are interdependent in relation to one another. This is especially praiseworthy because the chapters on physiology and the clinical chapters are in close relationship with one another. The book is structured in such a way that the first half, which is concerned with physiology, corresponds nearly always, chapter by chapter, with the second half, which is dedicated to the pathological and clinical aspects. It is for this reason that Botella-Llusiá's book is now unique among all the books on internal secretions of the female and, in introducing it to American readers, I consider it necessary and interesting to emphasize this important aspect — its unity.

There is another genuine merit of a book with this individual concept of feminine endocrinology. The author has, in some aspects, very special idea of reproductive physiology and the book is written with a certain degree of imagination. Some of the author's opinions are probably not in agreement with those of many readers. Nevertheless, his interesting way of presenting problems largely aids in clarifying them and this book is an excellent summary of woman's biology.

In addition to the fact that he has dedicated his life to a study of feminine endocrinology and to human reproduction, Botella-Llusiá is Professor of Obstetrics and Gynecology at the School of Medicine of the University of Madrid. His teachings have been collected in a very original and popular textbook in the Spanish-speaking countries, as proved by the fact that between 1946 and 1972 there have been 10 editions. In 1967 he published, in collaboration with other authors (Caballero, Clavero and Vilar), a book on Human Sterility and Infertility, which was revised in 1971. All this seems to make it impossible for Botella-Llusiá to have time enough to be, at present, Rector of the University of Madrid, a 60,000 student University with 9 Schools, various Institutes and more than 50 Colleges. At this University, there is presently great strife, as is occurring in other universities all over the world. Botella-Llusiá, now 60 years old, still works 14 hours a day to accomplish all he does.

The author of this book modestly apologizes in each edition for writing it, since he thinks it is too ambitious to presume to write a complete textbook on so difficult a subject. The first edition, which was quickly exhausted, was not followed by a second one for 13 years (until 1956). In his preface to this second edition Botella-Llusiá explained that he had decided to rewrite the book, hoping the second edition would incite young gynecologists and endocrinologists to work harder. I should like to express the wish that this American edition will encourage our young gynecologists and endocrinologists to continue (and with more fervor) their studies of endocrinology of women.

J. P. GREENHILL

PREFACE TO THE ENGLISH EDITION

To physicians in the Spanish-speaking world, the author certainly needs no introduction. Dr. Botella's comprehensive volumes on Obstetrics and Gynecology have been very popular and have been used as standard textbooks in Spain as well as in most countries of South America for many years. In contrast, only a few of his lectures have been translated into English. *Endocrinology of Woman*, now in its fifth Spanish edition, is the first complete, unabridged translation of one of Dr. Botella's major works.

The first edition of *Endocrinology of Woman*, published in 1942, was prefaced and warmly endorsed by the eminent endocrinologist Dr. Gregorio Marañón, at that time still living in exile as an aftermath of the Spanish Civil War. Several passages in Dr. Marañón's preface are just as relevant today as they were 30 years ago:

> Spain is a wonderful country but without much scientific atmosphere. True, she always had plenty of men of genius, aristocrats of the spirit, if you wish, and undoubtedly also has them now.... But she has lacked the bourgeoisie, the middle class of research . . . those well-disciplined and routine-geared parts in the huge machine presently required to unravel truth. Less and less, the times ahead of us shall be determined by individual greatness. Not because human thought is going into a decline, but because truth is bound to be less and less accessible to the spark of genius and instead, more and more so, to a concerted effort by many.
>
> Therefore, I am pleased to endorse a book as tempered, condensed and suggestive as that written by Dr. Botella-Llusiá, son and grandson of eminent physicians. During his initiation by my side, he had shown that restless, fiery, insatiable inquisitiveness of mind which is the unequivocal sign of a future man of science....
>
> A modern investigator must be equipped to endure the tension of every minute of his day lest he overlook something that might prove essential. Above all, he must be able to apply objective criteria in assigning the proper place to every new event and to every different point of view. Without achieving at least that much, a new book has no reason to exist. However, in questions as complex and as subtle as those Dr. Botella is concerned with, this is no easy task to accomplish. Both the resolve with which the author tackles the problems and the confidence with which he unravels them assure in him a great future master.

Dr. Marañón eventually returned to Spain and resumed teaching at the University of Madrid. There, during the early ninteeenfifties, I had the rare privilege of attending both his and Dr. Botella's courses. Dr. Marañón was a man endowed with uncanny eloquence and unrivaled clinical acumen. His lectures, delivered to a hushed, spellbound audience, were a memorable experience, fully measuring up to his fame as an outstanding endocrinologist, teacher, thinker, artist and humanist writer.

At this time, Dr. Botella was a young, dynamic scholar who represented a kind of transition to that new generation of scientists alluded to by Dr. Marañón. An indefatigable, eminently practical worker with a vigorous sense of discipline and organization, invariably well informed about the latest developments in his field, Dr. Botella translated the same qualities into his lectures and books.

While Dr. Botella's style has not changed perceptibly over the years, his personal experience and knowledge have grown immeasurably, enabling him to add the weight of his own authoritative opinion to almost any controversial issue under discussion today. From edition to edition, *Endocrinology of Woman* has grown commensurately in order to accommodate the ever-increasing flow of new information concerning the many facets of female reproductive function. This edition has incorporated the latest advances in the knowledge on lactation, the ovarian and uterine cycles, placental function, fetal steroidogenesis, immunochemistry of pituitary hormones, releasing factors and suppressors of pituitary function, and contraception, to mention just a few.

There is no doubt that the translation of a textbook is not the kind of after-hours occupation to be recommended for the busy pathologist. Nevertheless, if for no reason other than the personal allegiance we all believe we owe to our former teachers and professional peers, I could only welcome the suggestion, when it was made, that I translate this book which had been written by one of my former professors. For the initial encouragement necessary to commit myself to the backbreaking job, particular thanks are due to Dr. Sheldon C. Sommers, Director of Laboratories, Lenox Hill Hospital, New York, N.Y. I also wish to thank Mr. Robert B. Rowan, Vice President of W. B. Saunders Company, without whose understanding and unswerving support in the face of many unforeseen delays this work could not have been completed. I am deeply indebted to Dr. J. Botella-Llusiá for his manifold assistance kindly rendered during all phases of translation and proofreading. I further wish to acknowledge the excellent technical aid furnished by my former secretary, Miss D. B. Harris, who, at the sacrifice of leisure, assumed the heavy burden of typing the manuscript for endless hours. Finally, to all members of the Pathology Department of the College of Physicians and Surgeons of Columbia University, and those of the Harlem Hospital Division in particular, who for long months on end were unable to reach me for the full measure of accustomed cooperation, I owe my special gratitude for the way they have borne with me.

EDWARD A. MOSCOVIC

CONTENTS

Chapter 1
INTRODUCTION TO THE
ENDOCRINOLOGY OF WOMAN 1

Reproductive System and Sex Hormones 1

  1.1 Causality and Conditionality in Biology 1
  1.2 Function of Biocatalysts in Development and Reproduction 2
  1.3 Reproduction and Growth 3
  1.4 Forms of Reproduction 5
  1.5 Endocrine Characteristics of Gestation 6
  1.6 Importance of Effectors in Reproductive Physiology 7
  1.7 Interrelationship of Hormones and Nervous System 8
  1.8 Vegetative Sphere, Relational Sphere and Sexual Sphere 9
  1.9 The Vegetative Sphere, Relational Sphere and Sexual Sphere in the Female 9
  References 10

Part One
THE SEX HORMONES

Nomenclature of the Most Important Steroids 11

Chapter 2
ESTROGENS 13

  2.1 Definition, Nomenclature, History 13
    2.1.1 Definition 13
    2.1.2 Nomenclature 13
    2.1.3 History 13
  2.2 Chemistry 16
    2.2.1 Naturally Occurring Estrogens (Estrogen Hormones) 16
    2.2.2 Artificial Estrogens (Estrogen Drugs) 16
  2.3 Physiologic Action 17
    2.3.1 Effects of Estrogens upon the Gonads 17
    2.3.2 Effects upon Müllerian Organs 17
    2.3.3 Effects upon the Vulva and the Sex Characters 24
    2.3.4 Effects upon the Breast 24
    2.3.5 Effects of Estrogens upon Endocrine Glands 25
    2.3.6 Metabolic Effects of Estrogens 26
    2.3.7 Other Actions of Estrogens 26
    2.3.8 Differences of Action Between Estradiol and Estriol 26
    2.3.9 Mechanism of Action of Estrogens 27

  2.4 Biological Assay and Chemical Determination 27
    2.4.1 Bioassay of Estrogens 27
    2.4.2 Methods of Chemical Determination 27
    2.4.3 Units of Estrogens 28
  2.5 Formation, Metabolism and Excretion 28
    2.5.1 Formation 28
    2.5.2 Conversion and Inactivation 30
    2.5.3 Reactivation 31
    2.5.4 Beta-Glucuronidase 31
    2.5.5 Estrinase 31
    2.5.6 Circulation and Excretion of Estrogens 31
    2.5.7 The True Follicular Hormone 32
  2.6 Pharmacology 32
    2.6.1 Therapeutic Preparations 32
    2.6.2 Routes of Administration 32
    2.6.3 Antiestrogens 33
    2.6.4 Toxic Effects 33
  References 34

Chapter 3
PROGESTOGENS 38

  3.1 Definition, Nomenclature, History 38
    3.1.1 Definition 38
    3.1.2 Nomenclature 38
    3.1.3 History 39
  3.2 Chemistry 39
  3.3 Physiologic Action 42
    3.3.1 Effects on the Ovary 42
    3.3.2 Effects on the Fallopian Tubes 42
    3.3.3 Effects on the Endometrium 42
    3.3.4 Effects on the Myometrium 45
    3.3.5 Effects on the Uterine Cervix 45
    3.3.6 Effects on the Endometrial Mucosa in Nidation of the Ovum 46
    3.3.7 Effects on the Vagina 46
    3.3.8 Effects on the Glands of Internal Secretion 47
    3.3.9 Other Effects 47
  3.4 Biological Assay and Chemical Determination 48
    3.4.1 Bioassay 49
    3.4.2 Chemical Methods of Determination 49
  3.5 Formation, Metabolism and Excretion 49
    3.5.1 Sites of Biogenesis 49
    3.5.2 Biogenesis of Progesterone 51
    3.5.3 Ultimate Conversions of Progesterone 52
    3.5.4 Catabolites of Progesterone 53
    3.5.5 Circulation During the Cycle 53
    3.5.6 Transport 53
    3.5.7 Disintegration and Elimination 53
  3.6 Pharmacology 54
    3.6.1 Units of Progestogens 54

3.6.2 Modes of Administration................ 55
3.6.3 Dosage... 55
3.6.4 Toxic Effects................................ 55
3.6.5 Antigestagens: Ergocornine............ 55
3.7 Special Properties of Synthetic Progestogens....................................... 55
3.7.1 Actions Shared with Progesterone..... 56
3.7.2 Actions Differing from Those of Progesterone............................. 56
References... 58

Chapter 4
ANDROGENS IN THE FEMALE BODY.. 62

4.1 Definition, Nomenclature, History........... 62
4.1.1 Definition..................................... 62
4.1.2 Nomenclature............................... 62
4.1.3 History.. 63
4.2 Chemistry.. 63
4.3 Activity in the Male................................ 64
4.4 Activity in the Female Body.................... 65
4.4.1 Effects on the Ovary...................... 65
4.4.2 Effects on the Uterus..................... 66
4.4.3 Effects on the Vagina.................... 66
4.4.4 Effects on the Vulva..................... 66
4.4.5 Effects on the Somatic Features of Femininity............................... 66
4.4.6 Effects on the Feminine Psyche and on Libido............................... 67
4.4.7 Effects on Embryonal Male Genital Tract Rests.................................. 67
4.4.8 Effects of Androgens on the Prepubertal Female....................... 68
4.4.9 Other Effects................................ 68
4.5 Assay... 69
4.5.1 Bioassay...................................... 69
4.5.2 Chemical Determination................. 69
4.6 Formation, Metabolism, Excretion........... 70
4.6.1 Andropoiesis................................ 70
4.6.2 Metabolism of Androgens............... 75
4.6.3 Androgen Transport...................... 76
4.6.4 Excretion..................................... 76
4.7 Pharmacology....................................... 78
4.7.1 Androgen Units............................. 78
4.7.2 Uses and Mode of Administration..... 78
4.7.3 Dosages....................................... 79
4.7.4 Toxicity....................................... 79
4.7.5 Antiandrogens, Cyproterone........... 79
4.8 Significance of Androgens in the Female Body....................................... 80
References... 80

Chapter 5
NONSTEROID OVARIAN HORMONES RELAXIN— UTERORELAXING FACTOR............ 82

5.1 The Fourth Ovarian Hormone................. 82
5.2 History... 82
5.3 Physiologic Actions in Animals............... 83
5.3.1 Relaxation of Symphysis Pubis........ 83
5.3.2 Relaxation of Uterine Musculature with Paralyzing Effect on Contractility................................ 83
5.3.3 Cervical Softening and Dilatation...... 84
5.3.4 Increase in Weight of Uterus and in Its Water and Glycogen Content....................................... 84
5.3.5 Synergism with Both Estrogens and Progesterone.......................... 86

5.3.6 One, Two or Several Substances?...... 86
5.4 Clinical Actions..................................... 87
5.4.1 Effects on Uterine Motility............. 87
5.4.2 Cervix-Dilating Effects................... 87
5.4.3 Uterine Sedative and Pain-relieving Effects......................... 87
5.4.4 Progestational Type of Activity........ 87
5.5 Chemical Composition........................... 88
5.6 Estimation and Units of Measurement..... 89
5.7 Origin, Circulation, and Elimination......... 90
5.8 Clinical Uses.. 90
5.8.1 Commercial Preparations............... 90
5.8.2 Indications................................... 90
5.9 Critical Evaluation of Relaxin.................. 91
References... 92

Part Two
EXTRAGONADAL FACTORS GOVERNING SEXUALITY

Chapter 6
ADENOHYPOPHYSIS....................... 97

6.1 History of Pituitary Physiology................ 97
6.1.1 Anterior Lobe............................... 97
6.2 Hypothalamus and Pituitary.................... 98
6.3 Adenohypophysial Hormones.................. 99
6.4 Morphology of Adenohypophysis............ 100
6.4.1 Embryology................................. 100
6.4.2 Anatomy..................................... 100
6.4.3 Histology of Adenohypophysis........ 101
6.4.4 Cytology of Adenohypophysis......... 101
6.4.5 Pituitary Blood Supply.................. 103
6.4.6 Innervation.................................. 104
6.4.7 Interrelationships of Pituitary and Telencephalon by Way of the Hypothalamus............................. 104
6.5 Physiology of Adenohypophysis............. 105
6.5.1 Histophysiology............................ 105
6.5.2 Pituitary Variations Related to Sex...... 106
6.5.3 Physiology of Pituitary Hormones, with the Exception of Gonadotropins and Prolactin............................... 106
6.5.4 What Is Meant by Pituitary Hormones?.................................. 109
6.6 Chemistry of Anterior Lobe Hormones...... 109
6.6.1 Somatotropic Hormone.................. 109
6.6.2 Follicle-stimulating Hormone (FSH)... 110
6.6.3 Luteinizing Hormone (LH).............. 110
6.6.4 Prolactin..................................... 110
6.6.5 ACTH... 110
6.6.6 Thyrotropic Hormone.................... 111
6.7 Immunologic Properties of Anterior Lobe Hormones................................. 112
6.7.1 Somatotropin............................... 112
6.7.2 Prolactin..................................... 112
6.7.3 Thyrotropin and ACTH.................. 112
6.7.4 Gonadotropins............................. 112
References... 113

Chapter 7
GONADOTROPIC HORMONES......... 115

7.1 Physiologic Action................................. 115
7.1.1 Effect of Pituitary Extracts upon the Ovary................................... 115

Contents

7.1.2 Action of Pituitary Extracts upon the Testis.................... 118
7.1.3 Effect of Gonadotropins on Hypophysectomized Animals............ 120
7.1.4 Effects of Gonadotropins on Pregnancy......................... 120
7.1.5 Nomenclature of Gonadotropins......... 120
7.1.6 Effect of Gonadotropins on Ovulation....................... 121
7.1.7 Luteotropic Effect.......................... 122
7.1.8 Feedback Effect............................. 122
7.2 Secretion, Metabolism and Excretion of Gonadotropins.. 122
7.2.1 Secretion..................................... 122
7.2.2 Factors Influencing Gonadotropin Secretion..................................... 123
7.2.3 Metabolism of Gonadotropins........... 124
7.2.4 Criculation and Excretion of Gonadotropins............................... 124
7.2.5 Cyclic Fluctuations in Gonadotropin Plasma Levels............................... 125
7.3 Natural and Artificial Antigonadotropins...... 126
7.3.1 Antibodies to Gonadotropins............ 126
7.3.2 Antigonadotropic Drugs................... 127
7.4 Bioassay, Immunoassay and Radioimmunoassay of Gonadotropins......... 127
7.4.1 Bioassay of Chorionic Gonadotropin (HCG)....................... 127
7.4.2 Bioassay of FSH.............................. 128
7.4.3 Bioassay of LH................................ 128
7.4.4 Effects of FSH and LH on Batrachia... 130
7.4.5 Units of Gonadotropins..................... 130
7.5 Therapeutic Applications of Gonadotropins...................................... 131
7.6 Lactotropic Hormone or Prolactin............... 131
7.6.1 Definition, Nomenclature, History... 131
7.6.2 Chemistry of Prolactin...................... 133
7.6.3 Physiology...................................... 133
7.6.4 Estimation....................................... 134
7.6.5 Therapeutic Application................... 134
7.7 Synopsis of Pituitary Hormones.................. 134
References... 135

Chapter 8
NERVOUS SYSTEM AND ENDOCRINE GLANDS...................... 138

8.1 New Concept in Endocrine Physiology...... 138
8.2 Innervation of Female Genital Tract........... 138
8.2.1 Ovary.. 139
8.2.2 Fallopian Tube................................ 139
8.2.3 Uterus.. 140
8.2.4 Uterine Cervix................................ 140
8.3 The Releasing Factors of the Hypothalamus.. 140
8.3.1 Generalities.................................... 140
8.3.2 LHRF (Luteinizing Hormone Releasing Factor)............................. 143
8.3.3 FSHRF (Follicle-stimulating Hormone Releasing Factor)............... 144
8.3.4 PIF (Prolactin-inhibiting Factor)...... 144
8.3.5 TRF (Thyrotropin Releasing Factor)... 145
8.3.6 CRF (Corticotropin Releasing Factor) 146
8.3.7 GHRF (Growth Hormone Releasing Factor)............................. 146
8.3.8 MSHRF (Melanocyte-stimulating Hormone Releasing Factor).............. 147
8.3.9 Chemistry of Releasing Factors......... 147

8.4 Relationship of Hypothalamus to the Rest of the Brain..................................... 147
8.5 Effect of Steroids on the Median Eminence.. 148
8.5.1 Estrogens.. 148
8.5.2 Progestogens................................... 149
8.5.3 Androgens...................................... 149
8.6 General Significance of the Neurohormones of the Median Eminence... 150
8.6.1 Effect of Light on the Pituitary......... 150
8.6.2 Effect of Catecholamines on the Hypothalamic Sexual Center............ 150
8.7 Oxytocin and Vasopressin.......................... 151
8.7.1 Site of Origin of the So-Called Retrohypophysial Hormones............ 151
8.7.2 Physiopathology of Neurohormonal Reflexes... 155
8.7.3 Role of Oxytocin in Inducing and Maintaining Uterine Contractions.................................. 155
8.7.4 Effect of Oxytocin on Milk Ejection... 156
8.7.5 Chemistry of Oxytocin..................... 156
8.7.6 Actions by Pure Oxytocin................. 159
8.7.7 Vasopressin..................................... 160
8.7.8 Analogues of Oxytocin and Other Neurohormones............................... 160
8.8 Conclusion... 161
References... 161

Chapter 9
ADRENALS AND SEXUAL FUNCTION....................................... 165

9.1 Introduction... 165
9.2 Embryology... 165
9.3 Postnatal Development and Regeneration... 169
9.4 Effect of Sex Hormones on the Cortex......... 169
9.4.1 Changes in the Adrenal Cortex Resulting from Castration.................. 169
9.4.2 Structural Changes in the Cortex under the Effect of Sex Hormones...... 169
9.4.3 Effect of Sex Hormones on Corticoid Blood Levels..................... 170
9.5 Hormone Metabolism of the Adrenal Cortex... 170
9.5.1 Demonstration of Sex Hormones in the Adrenal Cortex....................... 170
9.5.2 Urinary Excretion of Steroids in Castrated Animals and Women...... 172
9.5.3 Metabolism of Cortical C-21 Steroids 173
9.5.4 Biosynthesis of Adrenocortical Steroids... 173
9.5.5 Urinary Excretion of Adrenocortical Steroids... 173
9.6 The Sexual Zone of the Adrenal Cortex...... 174
9.7 Effect of Pituitary on the Adrenal Cortex...... 176
9.7.1 ACTH and the Adrenal Cortex......... 176
9.7.2 LH and the Adrenal Cortex.............. 176
9.7.3 STH and the Adrenal Cortex............ 178
9.8 Place of the "Sexual Zone" in the Endocrine System..................................... 178
9.9 Other Sexual Aspects of Adrenal Physiology... 179
9.9.1 Unity or Plurality of Adrenal Function.. 179
9.9.2 The Third Gonad............................. 181
9.9.3 Sexual Actions by Corticoids............ 181
References... 185

Chapter 10
INFLUENCE OF OTHER ENDOCRINE GLANDS ON SEX......... 187

10.1 Thyroid Gland and Sexual Function......... 187
    10.1.1 The Normal Thyroid..................... 187
    10.1.2 Thyroid Changes Related to Sexual Function.......................... 188
    10.1.3 Effects of Thyroid Hormone on the Ovary................................ 189
    10.1.4 Effect of Thyroid on the Female Genital Tract...................... 190
    10.1.5 Effect of Thyroxine on the Breast... 191
    10.1.6 Effect of Thyroxine on the Male Genital Tract........................ 191
    10.1.7 Effect of Ovary on the Thyroid...... 191
    10.1.8 Thyroid and Gonadotropins............ 193
    10.1.9 Synopsis of Thyroid-Ovarian Interactions................................. 193
10.2 Pancreas and Sexual Function................. 194
10.3 Parathyroid Glands and Sexual Function... 196
10.4 Effect of Thymus on Sexual Function...... 197
10.5 Pineal Gland and Sexual Function........... 198
    10.5.1 Extragenital Effects of the Pineal... 198
    10.5.2 The Pineal and the Optic System... 200
    10.5.3 Sexual Effects of the Pineal........... 200
    10.5.4 Pineal Incretion: Melatonin............ 200
    10.5.5 Biosynthesis of Melatonin.............. 201
    10.5.6 The Pineal and Environmental Lighting....................................... 201
References... 202

Chapter 11
VITAMINS AND SEXUAL FUNCTION...................................... 205

11.1 Generalities... 205
11.2 Mode of Action of Vitamins..................... 206
    11.2.1 Vitamins as Biocatalysts................ 206
    11.2.2 Vitamins and Metabolism.............. 207
    11.2.3 Vitamins and Reproduction............ 207
11.3 Vitamins and Hormones.......................... 207
    11.3.1 Chemical Relationship Between Hormones and Vitamins... 208
    11.3.2 Similarities Between Vitamin and Hormone Synthesis.................. 208
11.4 Vitamin A and Sexual Function............... 208
    11.4.1 Effect of Vitamin A on the Ovary...... 209
    11.4.2 Effect of Vitamin A on the Testis...... 209
    11.4.3 Effect of Vitamin A on the Uterus and Vagina............................ 210
    11.4.4 Vitamin A and Pregnancy............. 210
    11.4.5 Effect of Vitamin A on Fetal Development................................ 211
    11.4.6 Hypervitaminosis A...................... 211
11.5 The Vitamin B Complex.......................... 212
    11.5.1 Vitamin B_1 (Aneurin, Thiamine)...... 212
    11.5.2 Other Vitamins of the B Complex..................................... 214
    11.5.3 Influence of B Complex on Hepatic Estrogenolysis.................. 217
11.6 Vitamin C (Ascorbic Acid)....................... 217
    11.6.1 Vitamin C and the Ovary.............. 218
    11.6.2 Ascorbemia, Ascorburia and Sexual Function........................... 219
    11.6.3 Pregnancy.................................... 219
    11.6.4 Vitamin C and the Adrenal........... 220
    11.6.5 Significance of Vitamin C in Genital Hormonopoiesis................ 220
    11.6.6 Effect of Ascorbic Acid Deficiency on Pregnancy............... 221
    11.6.7 Effect of Vitamin C Deficiency on Menstruation.......................... 221
11.7 Vitamin D... 221
    11.7.1 Effect of Vitamin D on the Genital Tract................................ 222
    11.7.2 Significance of Vitamin D in Pregnancy.................................... 222
11.8 Vitamin E... 223
    11.8.1 Effect of Vitamin E on the Female Sex................................. 223
    11.8.2 Effect of Vitamin E on the Testis.. 224
    11.8.3 Effect of Vitamin E on Pregnancy.................................... 224
    11.8.4 Placental Storage of Vitamin E...... 224
    11.8.5 Mode of Action of Tocopherol........ 225
11.9 Global Deficiency................................... 225
References... 226

Part Three
THE SEXUAL CYCLE

Chapter 12
ESTABLISHMENT OF THE SEXUAL CYCLE: THE OVARIAN CYCLE............................. 231

12.1 Establishment of the Sexual Cycle............ 231
    12.1.1 Sexual Life, Vegetative Life and Relational Life............................. 231
    12.1.2 The Phenomenon of Estrus........... 232
    12.1.3 Influence of Hypothalamus on Estrus... 232
    12.1.4 Estrus and Relational Life............. 233
    12.1.5 Estrus in Rodents......................... 233
12.2 The Sexual Cycle in Primates and in Woman... 235
    12.2.1 Internal "Rhythm" in the Cycle of Primates.................................. 235
    12.2.2 Differences Between the Male and Female Cycle......................... 236
    12.2.3 Exogenous Influences on the Cycle of Primates......................... 236
12.3 The Ovarian Cycle.................................. 236
    12.3.1 Histologic Features...................... 237
    12.3.2 Histochemical Modifications in the Ovarian Cycle........................ 242
    12.3.3 Cyclic Evolution of the Female Gamete....................................... 244
    12.3.4 Ovular Death Rate in the Course of the Cycle..................... 245
12.4 Regulation of the Ovarian Cycle............... 246
    12.4.1 The Role of Gonadotropins in the Regulation of the Menstrual Cycle... 246
    12.4.2 The Role of the Ovary in Gonadotropic Regulation, the Feedback Mechanism.................. 246
    12.4.3 Role of Hypothalamus in Regulating the Ovarian Cycle......... 247
12.5 Ovulation.. 247
    12.5.1 Description of Ovulation............... 247

12.5.2 Causes of Ovulation...................... 248
12.6 The Ovarian Hormonal Cycle.................. 249
    12.6.1 Cyclic Secretion of Estrogens......... 249
    12.6.2 Progesterone 250
12.7 Synopsis of the Ovarian Cycle and Its Effects... 254
References.. 254

Chapter 13
SEXUAL CYCLE IN TARGET ORGANS.. 257

13.1 Tubal Cycle.. 257
13.2 Uterine Cycle.. 258
    13.2.1 Endometrial Cycle......................... 258
    13.2.2 Vascular Cycle of the Endometrium............................... 262
    13.2.3 Relationships Between Stroma, Glands and Vessels........................ 264
    13.2.4 Histochemical Changes During the Endometrial Cycle.................... 265
    13.2.5 Biochemical Changes in the Endometrium in the Course of the Cycle................................. 268
13.3 Menstruation and Its Mechanism............... 269
    13.3.1 Definition of Menstruation............. 269
    13.3.2 Endocrine Causes of Menstruation................................ 270
    13.3.3 Vascular Causes Involved in Menstruation................................ 273
    13.3.4 Humoral Factors Involved in Vasospasm................................... 274
    13.3.5 Neural Factors Involved in Angiospasm.................................. 276
    13.3.6 Mechanism of Endometrial Shedding and Regeneration............ 277
    13.3.7 Menstruation as a Passive Event... 279
    13.3.8 Menstruation as an Active Event... 280
13.4 Myometrial Cycle.................................. 280
13.5 The Cervical Cycle................................ 281
    13.5.1 Cycle of Cervical Secretion............ 282
    13.5.2 The Cycle in the Endocervical Mucosa....................................... 284
    13.5.3 The Cycle of the Cervical and Isthmic Musculature................ 284
13.6 The Vaginal Cycle................................. 285
    13.6.1 Cell Types Found in the Exudate... 285
    13.6.2 Relation of Glycogen to the Vaginal Cycle............................... 287
13.7 The Cycle in the Breast and in Endocrine Glands.................................. 287
    13.7.1 Mammary Cycle............................ 288
    13.7.2 Pituitary Cycle............................. 288
    13.7.3 Thyroid Cycle.............................. 288
    13.7.4 Adrenal Cycle.............................. 288
    13.7.5 Changes Occurring in Other Glands of Internal Secretion......... 288
13.8 Systemic Changes During the Cycle......... 288
    13.8.1 Cyclic Changes in Body Temperature................................ 289
    13.8.2 Metabolic Changes....................... 290
    13.8.3 Hematologic Changes................... 290
    13.8.4 Allergic and Immunologic Changes During the Cycle........... 290
13.9 Summary of Cyclic Events in the Female Body... 291
References.. 291

Part Four
THE EVOLUTION OF SEX

Chapter 14
ORIGIN OF SEX: GENETIC SEX...... 297

14.1 Reproduction: the Gametes..................... 297
14.2 Sexual Differentiation............................. 297
14.3 Hermaphroditism.................................. 298
14.4 True Sexual Dimorphism........................ 299
14.5 Gametogenesis in Each Sex..................... 299
14.6 The Chromosomes................................. 301
14.7 Determination of Sex............................. 302
    14.7.1 The Germinal Route..................... 302
    14.7.2 Spermatic Dimorphism.................. 302
    14.7.3 The Active X Chromosome 304
    14.7.4 Sexual Differentiation Among Different Species........................... 304
    14.7.5 Characterization of X and Y Chromosomes................................ 305
    14.7.6 Experimentally Induced Determination of Sex..................... 305
14.8 Diagnosis of Sex: Chromatinic Sex and Chromosomal Sex 305
    14.8.1 The Sex Chromatin....................... 306
14.9 The Normal Karyotype.......................... 309
    14.9.1 Bone Marrow Cultures.................. 311
    14.9.2 Tissue Cultures............................ 311
    14.9.3 Leukocyte Cultures....................... 311
    14.9.4 The Denver System...................... 311
References.. 313

Chapter 15
DEVELOPMENT, EMBRYOGENESIS AND EMBRYOMECHANICS OF SEX......... 315

15.1 Embryologic Development of the Genital Tract.. 315
    15.1.1 Development of the Gonad............ 315
    15.1.2 Development of the Female Genital Tract, the Müllerian Duct... 322
    15.1.3 Development of the Wolffian Duct... 323
15.2 Embryomechanics of Sex and of Sexual Determination....................................... 324
    15.2.1 Goldschmidt's Theory and Protoplasmic Inheritance of Sex...... 324
    15.2.2 The Chemical Basis for the Determination of Sex..................... 326
    15.2.3 Summary.................................... 329
15.3 Sexual Differentiation............................. 330
    15.3.1 Substances Stimulating Müllerian Duct Development....................... 330
    15.3.2 Effects of Androgens..................... 331
    15.3.3 Autonomy of Differentiation of the Ducts of Wolff and Ducts of Müller..................................... 332
    15.3.4 Origin of Sexual Incretions During Embryonic Life................ 332
    15.3.5 Effects of Embryonic Castration on Sexual Differentiation 333
    15.3.6 Products of Extraction from the Embryonal Gonad.................. 334

15.3.7 Effects of Parabiosis and
Transplantation of the Gonad......... 334
15.4 Synopsis of Sexual Differentiation and
Embryomechanics of Sex........................ 336
  15.4.1 Theories of Sexual Differentiation... 336
  15.4.2 Influence of Genetic Sex and
  Target Organ Response in Sexual
  Differentiation............................. 337
  15.4.3 Basis Sex and Evolution of
  Sexuality.................................. 338
References.. 338

Chapter 16
PUBERTY.. 340

16.1 Generalities.................................... 340
  16.1.1 Definition................................. 340
  16.1.2 Age of Puberty........................... 340
  16.1.3 Chronology of Puberty................... 341
  16.1.4 Puberty and Nubility..................... 342
16.2 Clinical Aspects of Puberty.................... 343
  16.2.1 Local Changes in the Genital
  Apparatus.................................. 343
  16.2.2 Systemic Changes at Puberty........ 348
  16.2.3 Psychic Changes of Puberty......... 350
16.3 Endocrinology of Puberty....................... 351
  16.3.1 Ovarian Function During Puberty... 351
  16.3.2 Pituitary................................. 352
  16.3.3 Thyroid................................... 353
  16.3.4 Adrenals.................................. 353
  16.3.5 Factors Inhibiting Puberty............ 354
  16.3.6 Hypothalamic Influence on the
  Onset of Puberty.......................... 355
  16.3.7 Illumination and Puberty............... 355
16.4 Summary of Puberty............................. 356
References.. 356

Chapter 17
THE CLIMACTERIUM........................ 358

17.1 Concept... 358
  17.1.1 Menopause................................ 358
  17.1.2 The Climacterium........................ 358
17.2 Evolution....................................... 358
  17.2.1 Premenopausal Phase.................... 358
  17.2.2 Menopausal Phase........................ 360
  17.2.3 Mechanism Involved in the
  Cessation of Periodic Bleeding........ 360
  17.2.4 Postmenopausal Phase................... 362
17.3 Endocrinology of the Climacterium......... 363
  17.3.1 The Ovary................................ 363
  17.3.2 Estrogen Excretion at
  Menopause................................ 363
  17.3.3 Increased Gonadotropin Activity ... 363
17.4 The Postclimacteric and Senile Phase...... 364
  17.4.1 Postclimacteric Estrogenic
  Activity................................... 364
  17.4.2 Demonstration of Androgenic
  Activity During and After
  the Climacterium........................ 368
  17.4.3 The Pituitary and
  Gonadotropins........................... 368
  17.4.4 Belated Luteal Activity................ 369
  17.4.5 Demonstration of Adrenal
  Hyperactivity During the
  Climacterium............................. 369
  17.4.6 Gonadotropins and Sexual
  Cortex..................................... 369
  17.4.7 Are Postmenopausal Estrogens
  of Adrenal or of Gonadal Origin?... 370
  17.4.8 Liver Function in Relation to
  Sex Hormones............................ 371
  17.4.9 Hepatic Insufficiency in the
  Climacterium............................. 372
17.5 Clinical Effects of Sexual Secretion
in Women After the Climacterium........... 372
  17.5.1 Senile Metropathy....................... 373
  17.5.2 Malignant Degeneration of the
  Uterus and Breast....................... 373
References.. 373

Chapter 18
FEMALE CONSTITUTION, EVOLUTION OF SEXUALITY AND SEX CHARACTERS.................. 375

18.1 Introduction 375
18.2 Biotypological Classification of
Woman... 375
  18.2.1 The Two Phases in Female Life...... 376
  18.2.2 The Follicular System.................. 376
  18.2.3 The Luteinic System.................... 377
  18.2.4 Asthenic Habitus and Pyknic
  Habitus.................................... 377
18.3 Constitutional Forms of Development...... 381
  18.3.1 Characteristics of the Hypoplastic
  Biotype.................................... 381
  18.3.2 Characteristics of Intersexual
  Woman..................................... 382
  18.3.3 Integration of the Female
  Biotypes.................................. 382
18.4 The Doctrine of "Sexual Evolution"......... 383
  18.4.1 Generalities............................. 383
  18.4.2 Premature and Delayed Sexual
  Differentiation........................... 383
  18.4.3 The Theory of Maráñon................ 384
18.5 Genetic Explanation of the Theory
of Sexual Evolution............................. 385
18.6 Evolution of Sex in Lower Vertebrates...... 385
18.7 Protogyny and Protandry....................... 386
18.8 Male Dominance in Mammals.................. 387
18.9 Sex Characters.................................. 388
  18.9.1 Time Table for Sex Character
  Development............................. 388
  18.9.2 Determinism of Sex Characters...... 388
References.. 389

Part Five
GESTATION, LABOR AND THE PUERPERIUM FROM THE ENDOCRINE POINT OF VIEW

Chapter 19
ENDOCRINE PROTECTION OF PREGNANCY; TROPHOBLAST AND PLACENTA AS ENDOCRINE ORGANS... 393

19.1 Adaptation to Viviparity....................... 393
19.2 Nutrition Prior to Implantation............... 393
19.3 Endocrinology of Implantation................ 394
  19.3.1 Hormonal Control of
  Implantation.............................. 394

Contents

19.3.2 Deferred Implantation.................. 395
19.3.3 Endometrial Histochemistry
         and Implantation........................... 396
19.4 Establishment of Gravidic Correlations... 397
   19.4.1 Progestational Reaction of
          Hyperplasia................................. 397
   19.4.2 The Gestational Corpus Luteum... 397
19.5 The Placental Hormones......................... 400
   19.5.1 Chorionic Gonadotropin (CG)...... 400
   19.5.2 Placental Lactogen (HPL)............ 401
   19.5.3 Estrogens.................................... 401
   19.5.4 Progesterone.............................. 402
   19.5.5 Corticoids................................... 402
   19.5.6 Hormones Not Conclusively
          Demonstrated in the Placenta...... 403
19.6 Site of Hormone Synthesis in the
     Placenta... 403
19.7 Hormone Excretion During Pregnancy...... 407
   19.7.1 Chorionic Gonadotropin............... 407
   19.7.2 Estrogens.................................... 407
   19.7.3 Progesterone.............................. 408
   19.7.4 Feto-Placental Steroidogenic
          Unit... 408
   19.7.5 Corticoids................................... 409
19.8 Biogenesis of Placental Steroids............. 409
   19.8.1 Estrogens.................................... 409
   19.8.2 Progesterone.............................. 410
   19.8.3 Corticoids................................... 410
19.9 Summary... 410
     References... 415

Chapter 20
INCRETORY SYSTEMS OF THE
MOTHER AND FETUS DURING
GESTATION....................................... 419

20.1 The Maternal Incretory System................ 419
   20.1.1 Ovarian Function......................... 419
   20.1.2 The Pituitary in Pregnancy............ 423
   20.1.3 Thyroid and Pregnancy................ 425
   20.1.4 The Parathyroids in Pregnancy...... 426
   20.1.5 Pancreas in Pregnancy................. 427
   20.1.6 Adrenals and Pregnancy.............. 427
20.2 Fetal Incretory System........................... 428
   20.2.1 The Gonads During Fetal Life...... 430
   20.2.2 The Adrenal During Fetal Life...... 432
   20.2.3 Feto-placental Steroid Metabolism 434
   20.2.4 Fetal Thyroid.............................. 434
   20.2.5 Pancreas..................................... 436
   20.2.6 Pituitary...................................... 436
   20.2.7 Parathyroid................................. 437
   20.2.8 Fetal Thymus.............................. 437
   20.2.9 Endocrine Role of Fetal Liver...... 437
20.3 Maternal-Fetal Endocrine
     Interrelationships................................... 437
   20.3.1 Law of Compensatory Atrophy...... 438
   20.3.2 Maturity of the Target Organs......... 438
   20.3.3 Placental Permeability.................. 438
   20.3.4 Fetal Endocrinopathies................. 438
     References... 438

Chapter 21
MAINTENANCE AND
INTERRUPTION OF
GESTATION....................................... 442

21.1 Factors Responsible for Maintaining
     Gestation.. 442

21.1.1 Nutrition of the Implanted Egg...... 442
21.1.2 Active Uterine Growth During
       Gestation.................................... 442
21.1.3 Uterine-Sedating Action by
       Progesterone............................... 443
21.2 Factors Causing Interruption of
     Gestation.. 444
   21.2.1 Estrogens.................................... 444
   21.2.2 Neurohormones........................... 446
   21.2.3 The Placenta............................... 446
21.3 Evolution of the Placenta........................ 448
   21.3.1 Morphologic Evolution of the
          Placenta...................................... 448
   21.3.2 Uterine Irrigation During
          Gestation.................................... 452
   21.3.3 Placental Senescence and the
          Materno-fetal Conflict................... 453
21.4 Initiation of Labor.................................. 453
   21.4.1 "Timing" in Pregnancy.................. 453
   21.4.2 Hyperdistention of the
          Myometrium................................ 453
   21.4.3 Endocrine Causes of Labor........... 453
   21.4.4 Role of Oxytocin in Initiating
          Labor.. 455
   21.4.5 Mode of Action of Oxytocin........... 455
   21.4.6 Role of Hypothalamus in
          Controlling Oxytocin Secretion...... 457
   21.4.7 Other Neurohormones in Labor..... 458
   21.4.8 Histamine.................................... 458
   21.4.9 Antioxytocic Substances............... 459
21.5 Summary of Intrapartum Correlations...... 459
21.6 Regression of Gravidic Changes............... 460
     References... 460

Chapter 22
ENDOCRINE PHYSIOLOGY OF
THE BREAST..................................... 463

22.1 Introduction... 463
22.2 Mammogenesis...................................... 463
   22.2.1 Fetal Development of the Breast... 464
   22.2.2 Mammary Development After
          Birth... 464
   22.2.3 Effects of Castration on the
          Breast... 465
   22.2.4 Action of Estrogens..................... 465
   22.2.5 Action of Progesterone................. 466
   22.2.6 Pituitary and Mammary Growth...... 466
   22.2.7 Action of Androgens on the
          Mammary Gland............................ 467
   22.2.8 Other Hormones.......................... 467
   22.2.9 Mammogenesis at Term and
          During the Lactational Period...... 468
22.3 Induction of Milk Secretion (Lactogenesis) 468
   22.3.1 Hormones That Control
          Lactogenesis............................... 468
   22.3.2 Dynamics of Lactogenesis............ 470
22.4 Maintenance of Lactation (Lactopoiesis)... 473
   22.4.1 Endocrine Factors of Lactopoiesis... 473
   22.4.2 Neural Factors Involved in
          Lactopoiesis 475
22.5 Milk Ejection 475
22.6 Influence of Lactation on the Endocrine
     System and on the Reproductive Cycle..... 478
   22.6.1 Pituitary and Lactation................. 478
   22.6.2 Thyroid and Lactation 479
   22.6.3 Ovarian Changes During Lactation 479
     References 480

Part Six

EXPLORATION OF THE ENDOCRINE PATIENT

Chapter 23
CLINICAL EXPLORATION IN FEMALE ENDOCRINOLOGY 485

23.1 Clinical History 485
23.2 Physical Examination of the Endocrine Patient 487
    23.2.1 Inspection........................ 487
    23.2.2 Weight and Measurements 490
    23.2.3 Palpation 490
    23.2.4 Vaginal Examination 490
    23.2.5 Vaginoscopy 491
23.3 Routine Laboratory Tests 491
    23.3.1 Morphologic Examination of the Blood............................. 491
    23.3.2 Blood Chemistry 492
    23.3.3 Urinalysis.................. 492
    23.3.4 Basal Metabolism 492
    23.3.5 The Thorn Test 492
23.4 Study of Cervical Mucus 492
23.5 Basal Body Temperature 494
23.6 Peritoneoscopy or Culdoscopy................. 496
    23.6.1 Culdoscopy 496
    23.6.2 Transabdominal Celioscopy 500
23.7 Radiographic Exploration........................ 500
    23.7.1 Hysterosalpingography 500
    23.7.2 Gynecography 501
    23.7.3 Pneumokidney.................. 501
    23.7.4 Roentgenographic Exploration of the Sella Turcica......................... 501
    23.7.5 Radiologic Signs in Some Forms of Endocrine Gynecopathy............ 503
References.. 505

Chapter 24
HORMONE ASSAY 506

24.1 Chemical Methods of Estimating Urinary Steroids 506
    24.1.1 Introduction 506
    24.1.2 Determination of Urinary Estrogens, According to Brown...... 507
    24.1.3 Determination of Urinary Estrogens, According to Ittrich 510
    24.1.4 Estimation of Urinary Pregnanediol: Old Methods 511
    24.1.5 Chromatographic Determination of Pregnanediol, According to Toller and Carda 512
    24.1.6 Paper Chromatography for Urinary Pregnanediol, According to Elberlein and Bongiovanni 513
    24.1.7 Micromethod of Zander and Simmer for the Determination of Progesterone in Blood and Tissues 515
    24.1.8 Determination of Neutral 17-Ketosteroids in Urine, Based on the Principle of Zimmermann and Its Modifications 516
    24.1.9 Micromodification of the Preceding Method, by Vestergaard 517
24.2 Bioassay Methods for Sex Hormones in Blood and Urine 518
    24.2.1 Fundamentals of Bioassay of Estrogens................................. 518
    24.2.2 Modification by Lloyd, Rogers and Williams of the Preceding Method, Using Rats..................... 520
    24.2.3 Bioassay of Estrogens by the Chick Oviduct Method, According to Dorfman 520
    24.2.4 Bioassay for Minute Amounts of Progesterone, by Hooker and Forbes 521
    24.2.5 Measurement of Steroids by Means of Saturation Analysis......... 522
    24.2.6 Other Modern Methods for the Estimation of Steroids 522
    24.2.7 Method of Philpot and Philpot, Modified by Miyake and Pincus, for the Estimation of Carbonic Anhydrase in Endometrial Extracts 522
24.3 Estimation of Gonadotropins 523
    24.3.1 Estimation of Chorionic Gonadotropin, Using the Male of Rana Esculenta 523
    24.3.2 Technique................................. 524
    24.3.3 Standardization 525
    24.3.4 Bioassay of FSH, According to Heinrichs and Eulenfeld............... 526
    24.3.5 Bioassay of Luteinizing Gonadotropin (LH) by the Ovarian Ascorbic Depletion Method of Parlow 527
    24.3.6 Immunoassay of Protein Hormones 527
    24.3.7 Radioimmunoassay....................... 530
24.4 Functional or "Dynamic" Tests in Exploring the Endocrine System 531
    24.4.1 Introduction 531
    24.4.2 Adrenal Dynamic Tests 532
    24.4.3 Testicular Function Tests 535
    24.4.4 Ovarian Function Tests 535
References... 539

Chapter 25
ENDOCRINE CYTOLOGY 542

25.1 Vaginal Cytology 542
    25.1.1 History 542
25.2 Staining of Smears 543
    25.2.1 The Papanicolaou Staining Procedure 543
    25.2.2 Shorr's Staining Procedure............ 544
    25.2.3 Phase Contrast Microscopy 544
    25.2.4 Fluorescent Microscopy 546
25.3 Changes Observed in Vaginal Cytology ... 546
    25.3.1 Vaginal Cytology at Birth and During Childhood...................... 546
    25.3.2 Vaginal Cytology at Puberty 546
    25.3.3 Vaginal Cytology in the Course of the Menstrual Cycle..................... 546
    25.3.4 Vaginal Cytology in the Course of Pregnancy 547
    25.3.5 Vaginal Cytology at Menopause and Following Castration 549
25.4 Effects of Sex Hormones on Vaginal Cytology.. 549
    25.4.1 Estrogens................................... 549
    25.4.2 Progestogens 550
    25.4.3 Androgens................................. 550
    25.4.4 Corticoids, Pituitary Hormones....... 551
25.5 Endocrine Cytology of the Urinary Bladder, Endometrium and Oral Mucosa... 551
    25.5.1 Bladder Cytology 551
    25.5.2 Endometrial Cytology 551
    25.5.3 Oral Cytology 551
25.6 Other Endocrine Indications for Cytology 551
References... 551

Chapter 26
ENDOMETRIAL BIOPSY AND ITS DIAGNOSTIC VALUE 553

- 26.1 Introduction 553
  - 26.1.1 History 553
  - 26.1.2 General Principles of Endometrial Biopsy as a Means of Functional Diagnosis 553
- 26.2 Technique of Microcurettage 553
  - 26.2.1 Types of Microcurettage 553
  - 26.2.2 Preparation of Instruments 554
  - 26.2.3 Appropriate Time for Doing the Procedure 554
  - 26.2.4 Preparation of Patient and Surgeon 554
  - 26.2.5 Technique 555
  - 26.2.6 Microcurettage in Virgins 556
  - 26.2.7 Collection of Specimens 556
  - 26.2.8 Indications 556
- 26.3 Interpretation 556
  - 26.3.1 Secretory Phase 556
  - 26.3.2 Anovulatory Cycle........................ 559
  - 26.3.3 Conditions of Hyperestrinism......... 560
  - 26.3.4 Hypoestrinism............................. 560
  - 26.3.5 Irregularities in the Endometrial Cycle... 563
  - 26.3.6 Endometritis 563
  - 26.3.7 Diagnosis of Neoplasia, Especially of Adenocarcinoma of the Body 563
  - 26.3.8 Diagnosis of Abortive Rests and of Ectopic Pregnancy 564
- 26.4 Endometrial Histochemistry.................... 565
  - 26.4.1 Alkaline Glycerophosphatase......... 565
  - 26.4.2 Glycogen 565
  - 26.4.3 Mucopolysaccharides.................... 567
  - 26.4.4 Other Histochemical Reactions...... 568
- References 568

Part Seven
OVARIAN SYNDROMES

Chapter 27
HYPOESTRINISM................................... 570

- 27.1 Classification of Ovarian Functional Disorders 570
- 27.2 Hypoestrinism....................................... 571
  - 27.2.1 Definition 571
  - 27.2.2 Classification of Hypoestrinism...... 571
- 27.3 Primitive Hypoestrinism 573
  - 27.3.1 Primitive Ovarian Hypoestrinism... 573
  - 27.3.2 Symptomatology: General Signs ... 576
  - 27.3.3 Local Symptoms Confined to the Genital Tract 579
  - 27.3.4 Sex Reversal............................... 582
  - 27.3.5 Disorders of Receptivity to Estrogens..................................... 583
  - 27.3.6 Disorders of Receptivity to Gonadotropins 583
  - 27.3.7 Primitive Hypoestrinism of Pituitary Origin 583
  - 27.3.8 False Primitive Hypoestrinism 586
  - 27.3.9 Hypoestrinism of Thyroid and Adrenal Origin............................. 586
- 27.4 Secondary Hypoestrinism 587
  - 27.4.1 Pathogenesis of Secondary Hypoestrinism............................. 587
  - 27.4.2 Symptomatology 590
- 27.5 Treatment of Hypoestrinism.................... 592
  - 27.5.1 Primitive Hypoestrinism of Ovarian Origin............................. 592
  - 27.5.2 Treatment of Hypoestrinism of Pituitary Origin 594
  - 27.5.3 Induced Pseudopregnancy 594
  - 27.5.4 Treatment of Secondary Hypoestrinism............................. 594
- References 595

Chapter 28
HYPERESTRINISM 597

- 28.1 Definition, Incidence, Classification........ 597
  - 28.1.1 Incidence.................................... 597
  - 28.1.2 Classification 598
- 28.2 Pathogenic Forms; Ovarian Hyperestrinism..................................... 598
  - 28.2.1 Follicular Persistence 599
  - 28.2.2 Polymicrocystic Ovaries 600
  - 28.2.3 Thecal Hyperplasia and Fibrothecal Masses 601
  - 28.2.4 Follicle-Lutein Cysts.................... 603
  - 28.2.5 Adnexitic Ovary.......................... 605
  - 28.2.6 Syndrome of "The Remaining Ovary" 605
  - 28.2.7 The Ovarian Substrate of Acute Hyperestrinism 606
  - 28.2.8 Etiology of Ovarian Disorders Leading to Hyperestrinism............ 607
  - 28.2.9 Functioning Ovarian Tumors......... 608
- 28.3 Extraovarian Hyperestrinism 608
  - 28.3.1 Hyperestrinism of Adrenocortical Origin... 608
  - 28.3.2 Hepatic Hyperestrinism 609
  - 28.3.3 Iatrogenic Hyperestrinism 610
- 28.4 Clinical Forms of Hyperestrinism............ 610
  - 28.4.1 Acute Hyperestrinism 610
  - 28.4.2 Hemorrhagic Metropathy 611
  - 28.4.3 Hyperestrogenic Amenorrhea........ 614
  - 28.4.4 Functional Bleeding Associated with Atypical Hyperplasia 615
  - 28.4.5 Adenoma, Myoma, Endometriosis . 616
  - 28.4.6 Estrogens and Carcinoma............. 618
  - 28.4.7 Mammary Dysplasia.................... 618
- 28.5 Diagnosis of Hyperestrinism 620
  - 28.5.1 Vaginal Cytology......................... 621
  - 28.5.2 Endometrial Biopsy 621
  - 28.5.3 Assay of Estrogens 621
- 28.6 Treatment of Hyperestrinism 621
  - 28.6.1 Treatment with Progestogens 621
  - 28.6.2 Androgens 622
  - 28.6.3 Treatment with Estrogens 623
  - 28.6.4 Combinations of Hormones........... 623
  - 28.6.5 Treatment of Hyperhormonal Amenorrhea................................ 623
  - 28.6.6 Estrogen Antagonists.................... 624
  - 28.6.7 Radiotherapy and Surgery 625
- References 625

Chapter 29
CORPUS LUTEUM SYNDROMES, OVARIAN HYPERANDROGENISM ... 628

- 29.1 Luteal Insufficiency............................... 628
  - 29.1.1 Introduction 628
  - 29.1.2 Concept of Luteal Insufficiency 628

29.1.3	Incidence of Progestational Insufficiency	631
29.1.4	Anatomic Basis of Progestational Insufficiency	633
29.1.5	Mechanism of Infertility Due to Progestational Insufficiency	633
29.1.6	Diagnosis of Progestational Insufficiency	623
29.1.7	Progestational Insufficiency and Early Abortion	635
29.1.8	Progestational Insufficiency and Late Abortion	637
29.1.9	Etiology and Treatment of Progestational Insufficiency	638

29.2 Hyperluteinism and Dysluteinism 638
    29.2.1 Follicle-Lutein Cyst 639
    29.2.2 Corpus Luteum Persistence 639
    29.2.3 Luteinized Granulosa Cell Tumors and Luteomas 643

29.3 Ovarian Hyperandrogenism 643
    29.3.1 Physiopathology of Ovarian Androgen Biogenesis 643
    29.3.2 Syndrome of Masculinization Due to Ovarian Hilus Cell Activity 645
    29.3.3 Hyperthecosis 646
    29.3.4 "Essential" Ovarian Virilization 647
    29.3.5 Stein-Leventhal Syndrome 647
    29.3.6 Treatment 653
    29.3.7 The Stein-Leventhal Syndrome and Its Boundaries 654
References 654

Chapter 30
FUNCTIONAL TUMORS OF THE OVARY FROM THE ENDOCRINE POINT OF VIEW 657

30.1 General Considerations and Classification 657
30.2 Feminizing Tumors 658
    30.2.1 Histogenesis 658
    30.2.2 Relationship Between Tumors of the Granulosa and Those of the Theca 659
    30.2.3 Granulosa Cell Tumors 659
    30.2.4 Thecomas 662
    30.2.5 Endocrine Properties 664
    30.2.6 Luteinization of Granulosa and Theca Cell Tumors 664
    30.2.7 Tumors with Occasional Feminizing Effects 665
30.3 Masculinizing Tumors 665
    30.3.1 Arrhenoblastoma 665
    30.3.2 Adrenal Tumors of the Ovary, Ovarian Hypernephromas or Interrenomesenchymomas 668
    30.3.3 Masculinovoblastoma 669
    30.3.4 Leydig Cell Tumors of the Ovary... 671
    30.3.5 Gynandroblastoma of the Ovary 672
    30.3.6 Luteoma 672
    30.3.7 Tumors Occasionally Associated with Virilization 674
30.4 Other Tumors with Hormonal Activity 675
    30.4.1 Ovarian Chorioepithelioma (Chorioteratoblastoma) 675
    30.4.2 Struma Ovarii 675
References 676

Part Eight
ENDOCRINE SYNDROMES INVOLVING SEXUAL FUNCTION

Chapter 31
PITUITARY ENDOCRINOPATHY IN RELATION TO SEX 681

31.1 Classification 681
31.2 Hypopituitarism: Absolute Hypopituitarism 682
    31.2.1 Simmond's Disease 682
    31.2.2 Postpartum Necrosis of the Pituitary, or Sheehan's Syndrome... 684
31.3 Relative Hypopituitarism 686
    31.3.1 Gonadotropic Hypopituitarism 686
    31.3.2 Other Forms of Relative Hypopituitarism 689
31.4 Hyperpituitarism 690
    31.4.1 Somatotropic Hyperpituitarism (Gigantism and Acromegaly) 692
    31.4.2 Corticotropic Hyperpituitarism (Cushing's Syndrome) 694
    31.4.3 Gonadotropic Hyperpituitarism 698
    31.4.4 Galactotropic Hyperpituitarism 700
References 701

Chapter 32
SEXUAL SYNDROMES OF NEUROGENIC ORIGIN 703

32.1 Hypothalamic Syndromes 703
    32.1.1 Adiposogenital Syndrome of Froehlich 703
    32.1.2 Lawrence-Moon-Biedl Syndrome... 706
    32.1.3 Hypothalamic Obesity 707
    32.1.4 Hypothalamic Sexual Precocity 708
    32.1.5 Hypothalamic Syndrome 708
    32.1.6 Olfactogenital Syndrome 709
    32.1.7 Diabetes Insipidus 709
    32.1.8 Pituitary Tumors and the Hypothalamic Syndrome 710
    32.1.9 Synopsis of Sexual Hypothalamic Syndromes 710
32.2 Sexual Syndromes of Psychogenic Origin 712
    32.2.1 Psychogenic Amenorrhea 712
    32.2.2 Anorexia Nervosa 713
    32.2.3 Psychogenic Obesity and Froehlich's Syndrome of Psychogenic Origin 715
    32.2.4 Psychogenic Chiari-Frommell Syndrome 715
32.3 Central Influences on the Sexual Cycle and Its Anomalies 715
    32.3.1 Neural Influences in Syndromes of Hypoestrinism 716
    32.3.2 Hyperestrinism 716
    32.3.3 Anomalies in the Menstrual Rhythm from Neurogenic Causes... 717
    32.3.4 Syndrome of Pelvic Congestion 724
    32.3.5 Effects of Drugs on Hypothalamic Sex Regulation 725
References 725

Chapter 33
ADRENAL ENDOCRINOPATHIES IN RELATION TO SEX ... 727

33.1 General Considerations ... 727
    33.1.1 Bisexual Character of Adrenal Sexual Syndromes ... 727
    33.1.2 Dependency on Pituitary Pathology ... 728
    33.1.3 Coexistence with Other Adrenal Syndromes ... 728
33.2 Adrenogenital Syndrome ... 728
    33.2.1 Incidence ... 728
    33.2.2 Etiology ... 729
    33.2.3 Genetics of Adrenogenital Syndrome ... 733
    33.2.4 Anatomic Pathology ... 735
    33.2.5 Endocrinology ... 737
    33.2.6 Clinical Forms of Adrenogenital Syndrome ... 742
    33.2.7 Adrenal Carcinoma ... 746
    33.2.8 Diagnosis ... 747
    33.2.9 Treatment of Adrenogenital Syndrome ... 748
33.3 Other Syndromes of Hypercorticism Related to Adrenogenital Syndrome ... 749
    33.3.1 Cushing's Syndrome ... 749
    33.3.2 Achard-Thiers Syndrome ... 750
    33.3.3 Adrenogenital Syndrome and Addison's Disease ... 750
    33.3.4 False Congenital Adrenogenital Syndrome ... 751
33.4 Cortical Insufficiency of the Sexual Zone ... 753
    33.4.1 Syndrome of Congenital Cortical Insufficiency ... 753
    33.4.2 Sexual Cortical Insufficiency During Puberty ... 754
    33.4.3 During Pregnancy ... 755
    33.4.4 During the Climacterium and in Castration ... 755
References ... 755

Chapter 34
ENDOCRINE SYNDROMES OF OTHER GLANDS IN RELATION TO SEX ... 758

34.1 Thyroid Syndromes ... 758
    34.1.1 Generalities ... 758
    34.1.2 Hypothyroid Syndromes ... 759
    34.1.3 Hyperthyroidism ... 762
    34.1.4 Thyroidopathies and Gestation ... 763
34.2 Pineal Syndromes ... 763
    34.2.1 General Considerations ... 764
    34.2.2 Pineal Tumors ... 765
34.3 Thymic Syndromes ... 765
    34.3.1 Generalities ... 765
    34.3.2 Anatomic Pathology ... 766
    34.3.3 Thymic Hyperplasia and Status Thymicolymphaticus ... 767
    34.3.4 Myasthenia Gravis ... 767
34.4 Pancreatic Syndromes ... 767
    34.4.1 General Considerations ... 767
    34.4.2 Diabetes Mellitus ... 768
34.5 Parathyroid Syndromes ... 769
34.6 Alterations in Sexual Function in Deficiency Syndromes ... 769
References ... 770

Part Nine
PATHOLOGY OF THE EVOLUTION OF SEX

Chapter 35
PATHOLOGY OF SEXUAL DETERMINATION: CYTOGENETIC MECHANISM ... 775

by Prof. J. A. Clavero-Nuñez

35.1 Determination and Differentiation of Sex ... 775
35.2 Chromosomopathies and Endocrinopathies ... 775
    35.2.1 Anomalies of the Germinal Route ... 776
35.3 Cytogenetics of Chromosomopathies ... 777
    35.3.1 Numerical Aberrations ... 777
    35.3.2 Nondisjunction in Oogenesis ... 779
    35.3.3 Nondisjunction in Spermatogenesis ... 780
    35.3.4 The Resulting Zygotes ... 780
35.4 Numerical Aberrations of Autosomes ... 780
35.5 Qualitative Alterations ... 784
    35.5.1 Within the Same Chromosome ... 784
    35.5.2 Qualitative Alterations Involving Two Chromosomes: Translocations 788
    35.5.3 Mixed Alterations ... 790
    35.5.4 Mosaicism ... 790
35.6 Variations in the Occurrence of the Sex Chromatin ... 791
References ... 791

Chapter 36
PATHOLOGY OF SEX DETERMINATION: MAJOR GYNECOLOGIC SYNDROMES ... 793

by Prof. J. A. Clavero-Nuñez

36.1 Generalities ... 793
36.2 Gonadal Dysgenesis: Concept ... 794
36.3 Karyotype in Gonadal Dysgenesis ... 795
    36.3.1 XX Constitution ... 796
    36.3.2 XY Constitution ... 796
    36.3.3 XO Constitution ... 796
    36.3.4 Mosaicism and "Mixed" Types of Dysgenesis ... 797
    36.3.5 Xx Constitution ... 797
    36.3.6 X Isochromosome ... 797
    36.3.7 Poly-X Females ... 797
    36.3.8 Mosaicism ... 798
36.4 Clinical Picture of the Various Types of Gonadal Dysgenesis ... 798
    36.4.1 Turner's Syndrome ... 799
    36.4.2 Bonnevie-Ullrich Syndrome ... 804
    36.4.3 Rössle's Syndrome ... 804
    36.4.4 Swyer's Syndrome ... 804
36.5 Pseudohermaphroditism: Syndrome of Testicular Feminization ... 805
    36.5.1 Concept ... 805
    36.5.2 The Karyotype in Testicular Feminization ... 806
    36.5.3 Clinical Picture of Testicular Feminization ... 808
    36.5.4 Symptomatology ... 812
    36.5.5 Testicular Feminization as a Disorder Involving Target Organs ... 813

36.5.6 Summary.................................... 813
36.6 True Hermaphroditism........................... 813
    36.6.1 Concept...................................... 813
    36.6.2 Etiology..................................... 814
    36.6.3 Karyotype in True
           Hermaphroditism...................... 814
    36.6.4 Clinical Picture............................ 815
    36.6.5 Psychology and Therapeutic
           Management............................. 821
    References... 822

Chapter 37
ANOMALIES IN SEXUAL DIFFERENTIATION......................... 824

37.1 Generalities.. 824
37.2 Endocrine Basis of Congenital
     Anomalies Affecting the Female
     Genital Tract... 824
37.3 Isosexual Congenital Anomalies of the
     Female Genital Tract............................... 825
    37.3.1 Lack of Differentiation and
           Development of the Müllerian
           System..................................... 825
    37.3.2 Anomalies in Differentiation of
           the Urogenital Sinus.................... 828
37.4 Pseudohermaphroditism (Heterosexual
     Aberrations in Genital
     Differentiation)...................................... 831
    37.4.1 Male Pseudohermaphroditism...... 831
    37.4.2 Female Pseudohermaphroditism... 832
37.5 Pseudohermaphroditism in the Newborn
     Induced by Treatment of the
     Mother with Androgenic Substances
     During Gestation................................... 833
    37.5.1 Androgens................................ 834
    37.5.2 Progestogens............................. 834
    37.5.3 Estrogens.................................. 835
    References... 835

Chapter 38
ENDOCRINE PATHOLOGY OF PUBERTY............................ 837

38.1 General Considerations........................... 837
38.2 Precocious Puberty................................ 837
    38.2.1 Etiology and Classification........... 837
    38.2.2 Constitutional Precocious Puberty 838
    38.2.3 Precocious Puberty of Gonadal
           Origin...................................... 838
    38.2.4 Precocious Puberty of Adrenal
           Origin...................................... 840
    38.2.5 Hypothalamic Precocious
           Puberty.................................... 842
    38.2.6 Precocious Puberty of
           Pineal Origin............................ 843
    38.2.7 Albright's Syndrome.................... 844
    38.2.8 Cerebral Type of Precocious
           Puberty.................................... 844
    38.2.9 Hormonal Mechanism Involved
           in Precocious Puberty................ 844
38.3 Delayed Puberty................................... 844
    38.3.1 Constitutional Delayed Puberty...... 845
    38.3.2 Delayed Puberty of Uterine
           Origin...................................... 846
    38.3.3 Ovarian Type of Delayed Puberty... 846
    38.3.4 Pituitary Type of Delayed Puberty 846
    38.3.5 Hypothalamic Type of Delayed
           Puberty.................................... 848
    38.3.6 Cerebral Type of Delayed Puberty 848
    38.3.7 Adrenal Factors in Delayed Puberty 848
    38.3.8 Androgenic Type of Delayed
           Puberty.................................... 849
    38.3.9 Other Forms of Delayed Puberty... 849
38.4 Menstrual Disorders of Puberty and
     Adolescence; Juvenile Metropathy............. 850
    38.4.1 Etiology................................... 850
    38.4.2 Clinical Picture......................... 850
    38.4.3 Diagnosis................................. 851
    38.4.4 Treatment................................ 851
38.5 Dysmenorrhea or Menstrual Molimen......... 851
    38.5.1 Symptomatology........................ 852
    38.5.2 Etiology................................... 852
    38.5.3 Treatment................................ 854
    References... 854

Chapter 39
PATHOLOGY OF THE FEMALE CLIMACTERIC................... 857

39.1 Generalities.. 857
    39.1.1 The Climacteric Age.................... 857
    39.1.2 Constitution and Menopause........ 857
    39.1.3 Ovarian Factors......................... 858
    39.1.4 Pituitary Factors........................ 858
    39.1.5 Thyroid and Adrenal Factors........ 859
    39.1.6 History of Past Pregnancies.......... 859
    39.1.7 Other Factors Influencing the
           Chronology of Menopause........... 860
39.2 Endocrine Changes of Pathologic
     Climacterium....................................... 860
    39.2.1 Ovarian Pathology of the
           Climacteric............................... 860
    39.2.2 Pituitary Pathology in the
           Climacterium............................ 865
    39.2.3 Climacteric Hypercorticism.......... 866
    39.2.4 Climacteric Hyperthyroidism........ 867
    39.2.5 Pancreatic Disturbances and
           the Climacterium...................... 867
39.3 Symptomatology of the Pathologic
     Climacteric.. 867
    39.3.1 Sexual Symptoms; Climacteric
           and Postclimacteric Metropathy...... 867
    39.3.2 Circulatory Symptoms................. 868
    39.3.3 Digestive and Metabolic Symptoms 869
    39.3.4 Nervous Symptoms..................... 870
    39.3.5 Obesity................................... 870
    39.3.6 Climacteric Virilism.................... 871
    39.3.7 Climacteric Osteoporosis............. 872
39.4 Treatment... 874
    39.4.1 Pituitary Suppression.................. 874
    39.4.2 Treatment of Climacteric
           Hyperestrinism.......................... 875
    39.4.3 Outline of Treatment.................. 875
    39.4.4 Summary................................. 876
    References... 876

Chapter 40
VIRILISM... 878

40.1 Definition.. 878
40.2 Androgens in Female Physiology............... 879
    40.2.1 Effects of Androgens................... 879
    40.2.2 Androgen Synthesis by the Female
           Body Under Normal Conditions...... 879
40.3 "Physiologic Virilization"......................... 879
40.4 Classification and Clinical Forms
     of Virilization 880

40.4.1 Minor Forms of Virilism............ 881	42.4 "Unrecognized Habitual Abortion" as a Syndrome...................... 920
40.4.2 Virilization of Adrenal Origin........ 881	42.5 Repeated Abortion and Its Endocrine Aspects................................ 922
40.4.3 Ovarian Virilism........................ 882	42.6 Other Endocrine Causes of Abortion......... 925
40.4.4 Pituitary Virilism....................... 884	42.6.1 Hypothyroidism and Abortion...... 925
40.4.5 Constitutional Virilism................ 885	42.6.2 Adrenal Insufficiency as a Cause of Abortion.................... 926
40.5 Exploration of Virilism......................... 885	42.6.3 Diabetes and Abortion................ 926
40.5.1 Direct Diagnosis....................... 885	42.7 Diagnosis and Prognosis of Abortion......... 926
40.5.2 Differential Diagnosis of Virilism................................. 887	42.7.1 Pregnanediol Determinations....... 927
40.6 Androgenic Amenorrhea and Infertility... 887	42.7.2 Estriol..................................... 927
40.7 Treatment.. 888	42.7.3 Gonadotropinuria and Gonadotropinemia.................... 927
40.7.1 Treatment of Adrenal Virilism...... 888	42.7.4 Prognostic Value of Lactogen (HPL) 927
40.7.2 Treatment of Ovarian Forms of Virilism................................. 889	42.7.5 Vaginal Cytology as a Diagnostic and Prognostic Element in Abortion................................ 929
40.7.3 Treatment with Antiandrogens...... 889	42.7.6 Crystallization of Cervical Mucus... 930
References... 889	42.7.7 Sex of the Embryo and Prognosis of Abortion.................. 930
	42.8 Postabortive Metropathy...................... 930
	42.9 Treatment of Abortion of Endocrine Origin.. 933
	42.9.1 Treatment of Endocrine Abortion from Maternal Causes................ 934
	42.9.2 Oral Progestogens in the Treatment of Abortion................ 934
	References... 934

Part Ten
ENDOCRINE PATHOLOGY OF GESTATION

Chapter 41
ENDOCRINE FACTORS IN FEMALE STERILITY.................. 893

41.1 Ovarian Factors................................. 893	
41.1.1 Anovulatory Cycle..................... 893	
41.1.2 Luteal Insufficiency................... 904	
41.1.3 Other Ovarian Factors Causing Infertility.................... 906	
41.1.4 Sterility Due to Ovular Lethality..... 906	
41.2 Extraovarian Factors in Infertility............ 906	
41.2.1 Thyroid.................................. 906	
41.2.2 Pancreas................................. 907	
41.2.3 Adrenal.................................. 907	
41.3 Endocrine Causes Affecting the Fallopian Tubes................................ 907	
41.4 Endocrine Factors in Endometrial Sterility... 908	
41.5 Cervical Endocrine Disorders Causing Infertility............................. 908	
41.5.1 Hormonal Determination of the Cyclic Changes of Cervical Mucus 909	
41.5.2 Cervical Form of Sterility Resulting from Hypoestrinism...... 909	
41.5.3 Treatment............................... 909	
41.5.4 Prostaglandins......................... 910	
References... 910	

Chapter 42
ENDOCRINE ASPECTS OF ABORTION.................................... 913

42.1 Endocrine Abortion; Definition and Limits... 913	
42.2 Abortion from Luteal Insufficiency........... 913	
42.3 Abortion of Trophoblastic Origin............ 914	
42.3.1 Chorionic and Adrenal Progestopoiesis....................... 914	
42.3.2 Endocrinology of Abortion........... 915	
42.3.3 Abortive Eggs.......................... 917	
42.3.4 Histochemistry of Abortive Eggs... 919	
42.3.5 Chromosomal Aberrations in Abortive Eggs......................... 920	
42.3.6 Sporadic Abortion and Repeated Abortion................................ 920	

Chapter 43
ENDOCRINE ASPECTS OF HYDATIDIFORM MOLE AND CHORIOEPITHELIOMA.................. 937

43.1 Definition.. 937	
43.2 Hydatidiform Mole: Incidence................ 937	
43.3 Etiology of Hydatidiform Mole................ 938	
43.3.1 Genetic Factors........................ 938	
43.3.2 Environmental Factors............... 941	
43.4 Histopathology of Mole........................ 942	
43.5 Histochemistry of Mole........................ 944	
43.6 Hormone Biosynthesis by Molar Tissue... 946	
43.6.1 Gonadotropins......................... 946	
43.6.2 Estrogens................................ 946	
43.6.3 Pregnanediol........................... 947	
43.6.4 17-Ketosteroids........................ 947	
43.6.5 Mole and Thyroid Function.......... 947	
43.6.6 Placental Lactogen.................... 947	
43.7 Clinical Features of Mole...................... 948	
43.7.1 Concurrence of Mole and Toxemia................................. 948	
43.7.2 Polycystic Ovaries..................... 948	
43.7.3 Molar Metastases...................... 948	
43.7.4 Treatment............................... 948	
43.8 Chorioepithelioma.............................. 949	
43.8.1 Incidence................................ 949	
43.8.2 Etiology.................................. 949	
43.8.3 Biology of Trophoblastic Cells...... 950	
43.8.4 Chorioepithelioma as an "Inoculation" Tumor.................. 951	
43.8.5 Immunity to Chorionic Invasion... 952	
43.8.6 Hormone Synthesis by Chorioepithelioma.................... 952	
43.9 Evolution, Prognosis and Treatment......... 953	
43.9.1 Evolution................................ 953	
43.9.2 Prognosis................................ 953	
43.9.3 Treatment............................... 954	
References... 954	

Chapter 44
ENDOCRINE ASPECTS OF GRAVIDIC TOXEMIAS..................... 957

44.1 General Considerations......................... 957
44.2 Toxemias of the First Trimester of Gestation......................... 957
    44.2.1 Clinical and Metabolic Similarities..................... 957
    44.2.2 Endocrine Changes in Hyperemesis..................... 958
    44.2.3 Stress and Hyperemesis............. 959
    44.2.4 Treatment 960
44.3 Eclamptic Toxemia 960
    44.3.1 Pressor Substances..................... 961
    44.3.2 Uteroplacental Ischemia............. 962
    44.3.3 Hypercorticism............................ 963
    44.3.4 Placental Alterations.................... 965
44.4 Toxemia and the General Adaptation Syndrome (G.A.S.).................. 966
44.5 Syndrome of Placental Insufficiency and Its Endocrine Effects........................ 966
    44.5.1 Histologic and Histometric Aspects of Placental Senescence... 966
    44.5.2 Clinical Aspects of Placental Senescence................................ 967
    44.5.3 Repercussions of Placental Senescence on Estrogen Biosynthesis................................ 967
    44.5.4 Determination of Estriol in the Diagnosis of Placental Senescence and in the Prognosis of Fetal Viability............................ 968
    44.5.5 Other Methods for the Diagnosis of Placental Insufficiency................................ 969
    References... 971

Chapter 45
ENDOCRINE PATHOLOGY OF GESTATION... 974

45.1 Pituitary Pathology in Gestation................. 974
    45.1.1 Hypophysectomy and Gestation... 974
    45.1.2 Sheehan's Syndrome..................... 974
    45.1.3 Chiari-Frommel Syndrome............. 975
    45.1.4 Acromegaly and Pregnancy............ 976
    45.1.5 Diabetes Insipidus......................... 977
45.2 Thyroid Pathology and Gestation............. 977
    45.2.1 Hypothyroidism and Gestation...... 978
    45.2.2 Basedow's Disease........................ 978
45.3 Parathyroid Pathology in Gestation......... 978
45.4 Diseases of the Pancreas: Diabetes and Prediabetes in Gestation................... 979
    45.4.1 Endocrine Pathophysiology of Diabetes and Prediabetes............. 979
    45.4.2 Diabetes Mellitus Complicating Gestation..................... 984
    45.4.3 Prediabetes and Gestation............ 986
    45.4.4 Diabetes and Prediabetes: Two Distinct Syndromes...................... 989
45.5 Diseases of the Adrenal and Gestation...... 989
    45.5.1 Pheochromocytoma and Pregnancy 989
    45.5.2 Diseases of the Adrenal Cortex...... 989
45.6 Pathophysiology of the Hypophysioadrenal System in Pregnancy; Gestation and Labor as "Stressors".. 991
    45.6.1 Definition...................................... 991
    45.6.2 Endocrine Phenomena in Stress... 992
    45.6.3 The Hypophysioadrenal System in Pregnancy................................ 994
    45.6.4 Pregnancy as a "Stressor"............ 994
    45.6.5 Evolution of the Condition of Stress in the Course of Pregnancy..................................... 995
    45.6.6 Labor as a Stressor....................... 997
    45.6.7 Stress and Gravidic Toxemias......... 998
References... 999

Part Eleven
MISCELLANEOUS ASPECTS OF THE ENDOCRINOLOGY OF WOMAN

Chapter 46
ENDOCRINE BASES OF GENITAL TUMORIGENESIS......... 1005

46.1 Introduction.. 1005
46.2 Morphogenetic Factors: Determinants and Realizers...................................... 1005
46.3 Hereditary Factors in the Genesis of Uterine and Mammary Tumors................ 1006
    46.3.1 Nongenetic Factors...................... 1007
    46.3.2 Genetic Factors............................ 1007
    46.3.3 The Karyotype in Cases of Uterine and Breast Cancer............ 1007
46.4 Biocatalysts in the Genesis of Genital Neoplasia.................................. 1008
    46.4.1 Carcinogenesis from Aromatic Hydrocarbons............................ 1008
46.5. Estrogens and Endometrial Carcinoma... 1010
    46.5.1 Compounds with Both Estrogenic and Cancerogenic Properties................................... 1010
    46.5.2 Estrogens as Growth-Promoting Substances................................. 1011
    46.5.3 Clinical Arguments Favoring the Hormonal Origin of Endometrial Carcinoma............... 1011
    46.5.4 Arguments Against the Hormonal Origin of Endometrial Carcinoma................ 1014
    46.5.5 Diabetes and Endometrial Cancer 1015
46.6 Estrogens and Mammary Cancer............ 1015
    46.6.1 Evidence in Favor of Hyperestrinism............................ 1015
    46.6.2 Origin of the Estrogens in Breast Cancer........................ 1017
    46.6.3 Estrogen Receptivity in Mammary Tumor Tissue................ 1017
46.7 Estrogens and Benign Uterine Tumors... 1018
46.8 Other Endocrine Tumors........................ 1018
    46.8.1 Ovarian Tumors........................... 1018
    46.8.2 Pituitary and Adrenal Tumors....... 1018
    46.8.3 Mammogenic Factor and Mammary Cancer........................ 1018
46.9 Neoplasms in Time; Kinetics of Their Development................................ 1020
    46.9.1 Latency in Uterine Carcinoma...... 1020
    46.9.2 Acceleration of Tumorigenesis...... 1021
    46.9.3 Delay of Tumorigenesis................ 1021
    46.9.4 Conclusion.................................. 1022
References... 1023

Chapter 47
ORAL CONTRACEPTIVES 1026

- 47.1 Introduction 1026
- 47.2 Chemistry of Contraceptive Steroids 1026
  - 47.2.1 Synthetic Progestogens 1027
  - 47.2.2 Estrogens 1032
- 47.3 Effects of Contraceptive Steroids on the Animal and Human Genital Tracts 1032
  - 47.3.1 Action on the Ovary 1032
  - 47.3.2 Action on the Fallopian Tube 1033
  - 47.3.3 Action on the Endometrium 1036
  - 47.3.4 Action on the Uterine Cervix and on the Migration of Sperm 1038
  - 47.3.5 Action on Spermatic Capacitation 1038
  - 47.3.6 Action on the Vagina 1038
  - 47.3.7 Effects on Male Animals 1039
- 47.4 Effects of Ovulation Inhibitors on Hormone Elimination 1039
  - 47.4.1 Estrogens 1039
  - 47.4.2 Pregnanediol 1039
  - 47.4.3 Gonadotropins 1039
- 47.5 Basal Body Temperatures 1040
- 47.6 Mode of Action of Oral Contraceptives 1041
  - 47.6.1 Suspension of Ovulation 1041
  - 47.6.2 Paralysis of Tubal Ovitransport 1042
  - 47.6.3 Lack of Implantation 1042
  - 47.6.4 Paralysis of Spermatic Ascent 1042
  - 47.6.5 Synopsis of Contraceptive Mechanisms 1042
- 47.7 Modes of Administration of Contraceptives 1043
  - 47.7.1 Classical or Combined Therapy ... 1043
  - 47.7.2 Sequential Therapy 1043
  - 47.7.3 Continuous or Nonstop Therapy ... 1043
- 47.8 Harmful Effects of Oral Contraceptives ... 1043
  - 47.8.1 Circulatory Phenomena 1044
  - 47.8.2 Changes in Blood Coagulation 1044
  - 47.8.3 Digestive Changes 1044
  - 47.8.4 Psychological Disturbances 1044
  - 47.8.5 Thyroid 1044
  - 47.8.6 Risks of Causing Fetal Virilization 1044
  - 47.8.7 Risks of Inducing Malignancy 1045
  - 47.8.8 Hazards of Diabetes 1045
  - 47.8.9 Urinary Disturbances 1046
- 47.9 Long-Term Effects of Anovulation 1046
- References 1046

INDEX 1049

Chapter 1

INTRODUCTION TO THE ENDOCRINOLOGY OF WOMAN

REPRODUCTIVE SYSTEM AND SEX HORMONES

1.1. CAUSALITY AND CONDITIONALITY IN BIOLOGY

A phenomenon that gives rise to another is said to be the *cause* producing an effect. In biology there are two modalities of *causal relationship*: a *simple* one, in which there is a *proportion between the magnitude of the cause and its effect*, and a *catalytic* one, in which, through a chain of causes, effects multiply so that very small causative agents are capable of producing great effects. The circumstances which modify a response of this nature, by amplifying it, are known as *conditioning factors*. These, then, determine conditionality in the face of biologic causality.

The fact that events should take place in such a manner within the concrete terms of reproductive physiology is of extraordinary importance. Thus, we can see that, at the very moment of fertilization, the fusion of the gametes engenders a zygote, a tiny being, in whose nucleus is a highly complicated series—comparable to a mosaic—of established hereditary tendencies. It is bewildering to realize how these tendencies, enshrined within a micromosaic, can become magnified to the extent of affecting the development of the form and the functional characteristics of the adult individual. Considering how minimal the cause may be, the development of these hereditary tendencies would not be possible without "environmental" elements to *condition*, in the sense which we have just stated, the progress from cause to effect. Thus, in every morphogenetic process, whether embryonal development, growth of the young individual or reproduction in the adult, we must distinguish between two fundamental elements: one, *causality*, determined directly by the genetic combinations of heredity, and the other, *conditionality*, determined by the humoral environment in which primitive causality unfolds.

It follows that, in accordance with the ancient doctrines of Roux,[6] two types of factors must be distinguished in all morphogenetic phenomena: *factors of determination*, which are genetic and here represent biologic causality, and *factors of realization*, which are humoral and represent conditionality as determined by the biologic environment. The elements conditioning these responses may be of diverse nature. Some act by virtue of their mass, providing physical or chemical conditions necessary for development. For instance, a certain *temperature* range is an environmental condition necessary for the morphogenesis of homothermal animals. So is a given pH or a given redox potential, both of which are necessary for the first stages of embryonal development to take place.[3] Such environmental elements may also operate in a fashion similar to chemical substrates in reactions of growth, acting as "food" for morphogenesis. In this sense, action is exerted by the chemical principles and the salts involved. There are also specific needs for certain other chemical principles, certain proteins, and various lipids or carbohydrates; it is likewise known that certain salts are necessary for morphogenesis.[3] But, setting aside factors of conditionality that act through considerable mass, let us now consider a group of conditioning factors that activate hereditary tendencies by means of very little mass, i.e., in a manner analogous to what in chemistry is known as *catalysis*. Within the context of biologic conditionality, there exists a vast group of catalysts which have been called biologic catalysts or *biocatalysts*.

1.2. FUNCTION OF BIOCATALYSTS IN DEVELOPMENT AND REPRODUCTION

The biocatalysts are various substances that have the common characteristic of conditioning biologic phenomena by acting in very small quantities. They can be divided into four fundamental groups:

(1) Biocatalysts that regulate cellular metabolism. Originating in the interior of the cell itself, these so-called *enzymes*, or fermenta, act in regulating intracellular processes.

(2) Biocatalysts that act at a distance upon certain organs or tissues, or upon certain types of chemical or physiological phenomena. These biocatalysts, called *hormones*, are produced in certain tissues, or *glands*, of multicellular animals — the *glands of internal secretion* or incretory tissues.

(3) Another group of catalytic substances, the *vitamins*, although similar to the hormones in the significance of their action — i.e., they regulate an entire set of biochemical reactions or morphogenic processes oriented in the same direction — originate outside of the organism and, except for unusual circumstances, are not synthesized by the organism itself. The majority of the vitamins are derived from the vegetable kingdom.

(4) Embryonal organisms have a group of biocatalysts which are responsible for promoting embryonal development and organ differentiation. Exerting an effect quite similar to that of the morphogenetic hormones, these biocatalysts or hormones of embryonal development are called *evocators* or *organizers*. As we shall see, they are closely related to the hormones during the fetal period.

Though of different origin and endowed with different chemistry and metabolism, the modes of action of these four biocatalysts within the confines of the cell are fundamentally the same. For this reason, many attempts have been made to find a common designation for them. Von Euler[2] grouped together the vitamins and hormones under the common name of *ergones*, whereas Ammon and Dirscherl[1] have combined the hormones, vitamins and enzymes under the name of *ergines*. Seitz,[7] on the other hand, designated these components as *hormovitenzymes*.

It seems of little practical value to have a common generic term for these four groups of substances. In fact, they have little in common other than their biocatalytic action, which can just as well be performed by simple immediate principles, mineral elements or physical factors. The term "biocatalysts" is too broad to cover all of them. Their mission and biologic significance are sufficiently different from each other to preclude a pointless search for a group denominator.

The higher the phylogenetic and ontogenetic development of a species, the greater the number and complexity of substances present and the greater the differences between these distinct groups of substances. The protozoa, in a strict sense, lack both hormones and vitamins; in them, the function of hormones and vitamins is accomplished instead by the enzymes. With increasing organic complexity, the differences between the various groups become more distinguishable, becoming most distinct in the mammals. For instance, as we shall discuss later, the estrogenic substances behave as growth factors of a more or less enzymatic nature in all lower forms of life, and they eventually acquire their hormonal character only in the higher animals.

The relationship between enzymes and hormones has grown closer and closer in modern endocrine physiology. It is common knowledge today that many endocrinopathies, such as the adrenogenital syndrome (see Chapter 29) and the Stein-Leventhal syndrome (see Chapter 33), are largely the result of enzymatic alterations that hinder or modify the formation of some hormones.

At the same time, it seems probable that

Introduction to the Endocrinology of Woman

such enzymatic alterations result from *inborn errors of metabolism*,[8] which, in turn, arise from chromosomal abnormalities. Thus, the profound and unequivocal influence heredity exerts upon endocrine function can, at present, best be grasped by understanding the interrelationships of enzymes and hormones.

1.3. REPRODUCTION AND GROWTH

Reproduction is but a modality of growth. This is difficult to understand in higher animals, but is easy to see in protozoa. A protozoon, growing by progressive nourishment, eventually reaches a size which is incompatible with the preservation of a specific shape. The unicellular protozoa, as well as the cells in metazoa, cannot grow indefinitely without losing their characteristic, defining morphology. Once a certain size has been reached, a protozoon will divide into two progeny cells. By virtue of this phenomenon, the individual, growing to an excessive size, has disappeared but in doing so has engendered two equal successors. Both, in turn, will continue to grow and to divide, and to carry on the process initiated by the parent cell. Seen in this light, reproduction is but the continuation of growth in the form of "extra-individual growth" (Fig. 1–1).

In the metazoa, reproduction is also a form of growth. All cells of the organism can be classified into two kinds: *somatic* and *germ cells*. The soma, which comprises the large majority of the cells of the organisms, is bound to die, and undergoes mass death when the individual dies. The germ cell, whose function is to reproduce its kind and to continue its own survival over many generations, is the "immortal" part of the species. It is transmitted from parents to offspring, thus maintaining the physical continuity of inheritance and consequently also maintaining the characteristics of the species, which thereby perdures and does not become extinct. Hence, reproduction in the higher animals is likewise *extra-individual growth*, organized by nature so as to safeguard the survival of the species. It can be said, therefore, that *reproduction is to the species what growth is to the individual*, that is, the scheme that nature resorts to in order to prevent extinction (Fig. 1–2).

In considering reproduction as a modality of growth, it is evident that the biocatalytic regulation of reproductive processes is essentially the same as that involved in the processes of growth, and it is also evident that morphogenesis — i.e., the development of form at the expense of preestablished and "controlled" features — may be equally divided into *morphogenesis of growth and morphogenesis of reproduction*.

The lower animals do not require any biocatalysis for reproduction at all. Substances exciting cellular growth also trigger cell cleavage. The more complex the reproductive mechanism, the more intricate becomes the biocatalysis of reproduction. In the next section the manner in which the different reproductive processes take place is described briefly, in order to illustrate the basis of endocrine regulation, with special emphasis on the mammals.

All individual cells arising from protozoal cell division are equal to all the others, since they are derived from the same hereditary mass. They may be compared to the cells of a metazoon, or — perhaps more adequately — to the cells of a single type of tissue. Just as in the metazoa the cells of the soma are liable to undergo a process of senescence and eventual death, so too these cells, all equal and derived from a common progenitor cell by direct or indirect division, are subject to a "thanatotopic impulse," inexorably leading them toward degeneration and extinction. This is why the colonies of protozoa, known as biologic

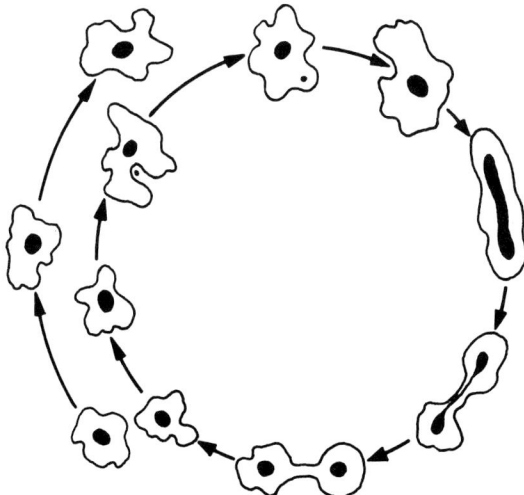

Figure 1–1. The reproductive cycle of the amoeba.

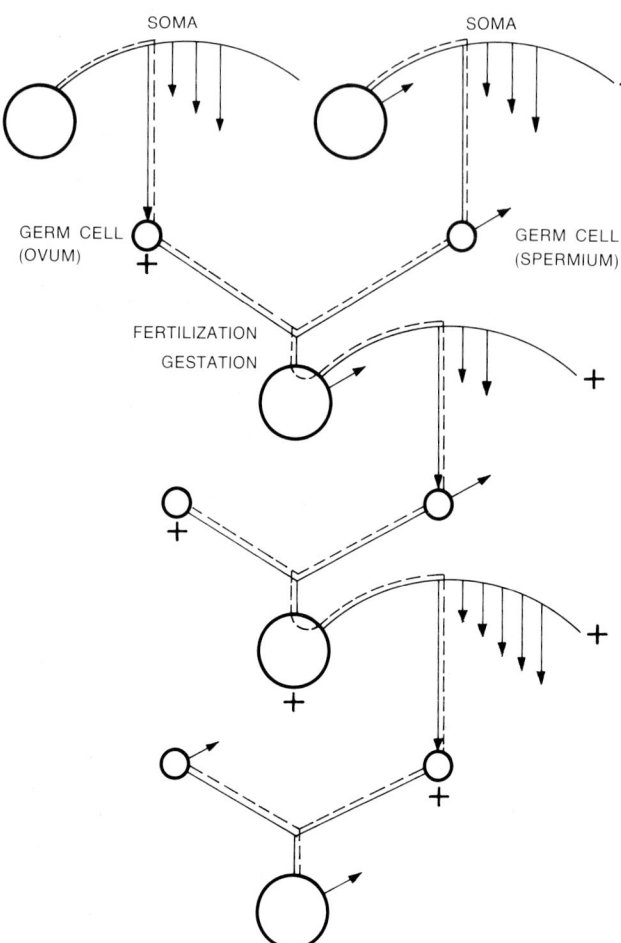

Figure 1-2. The germinal route in metazoa.

clones, are fatally doomed unless they can, in some way, regenerate their protoplasmic and nuclear mass. Comparable to an injection of a new sap, this necessary regeneration, which by modifying heredity lends new vitality to the species, is the origin of sexuality. Thus, for instance, in colonies of the Flagellata (e.g., of the genus *Scytomona*) it may be observed that, after many generations have been produced by direct division, two individuals belonging to different *clones*, with different nuclear characteristics as demonstrated by the investigations of some biologists, will unite in a given moment to fuse their chromatin masses in a kind of rudimentary fertilization and thus constitute a new being (Fig. 1-3). This is the basis of sexual reproduction. *Sexual reproduction is tantamount to an artifice of nature which, through the mingling of different genes, modifies the biologic conditions of the progeny toward greater efficacy by means of a fortuitous hereditary interbreeding.* Thus, sex means genetic cross fertilization; endocrinology, on the other hand, in the sexual sphere is but the *biocatalysis of that cross fertilization.*

The unicellular organisms are believed to have appeared on earth some 500 million years ago. The first reproduction must have been an asexual one and must have led to the degeneration and death of myriads of clones of unicellular beings. The first mingling of two different chromatin masses, that is, the first instance of *sexual reproduction*, probably occurred in the course of phagocytosis, in which the engulfed cell withstood destruction and strengthened the hereditary mechanism of the phagocytizing species, which thus survived and was spared the fate of its sibling clones.

Although it might be assumed that the phagocytized cell would have been smaller than the phagocytic cell and would, therefore, from the very first instance, have

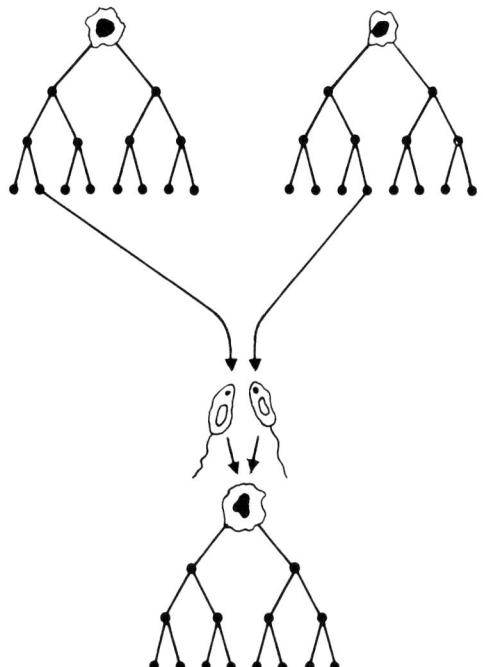

Figure 1-3. Diagram of sexual reproduction between individual protozoa belonging to different clones.

established the difference between the *microgamete* (male) and the *macrogamete* (female), the gametic differentiation giving rise to digametism in the species must have developed as a result of the emergence of the metazoa and, therefore, as an outgrowth of embryonal development. In unicellular beings, the engendered cell, or zygote, is already an adult organism in itself. In multicellular animals the zygote must first develop during an *ontogenic period*, which is brief in the lower species and often very long in the higher ones. All through this developmental period the embryo is a being dependent on nutrition called *embryonal nutrition*, to be provided by either one of the progenitors. With the exception of a few Amphibia (the toad *Alytes obstetricans*), and even among these with some exceptions, the care and nutrition of the embryo has been assigned to the *female sex*. For this reason, the female cell (i.e., the *ovum*) grows large and nutrient. For exactly the opposite reasons, the male cell or spermatozoid (antherozoid of fungi) is small and devoid of nutrient, and instead is endowed with active motion, enabling it to seek out and to fertilize the egg. *Sex is an artifice of nature designed to conjugate two different chromatin masses and, at the same time, facilitate the nutrition of the embryo.* The emergence of sex is secondary to the basic properties of living cells, and the specific sexual action of hormones is also an effect relatively subordinate to the fundamental physiologic actions of the hormones. *Sexuality is a late event in both the ontogeny and the phylogeny of the species.*

1.4. FORMS OF REPRODUCTION

The development of increasingly complex reproductive systems, culminating in the intricate forms that occur in the mammals, is related to the nutritional requirements of the embryo. In this respect, animal eggs can be divided into three types (Fig. 1-4): *aquatic eggs*, which absorb their nutrition from the surrounding environment; *cleidoic eggs*, which feed on a nutritional reserve, or yolk, deposited in the ovum before fertilization; and *placental eggs*, whose nutrition is mediated by an organ called the placenta at the expense of substances circulating in the maternal blood. The needs arising from the various types of nutrition in different species are also quite variable. In animals with aquatic eggs, for example, it is sufficient if the female is equipped with an egg-bearing organ (i.e., an *ovary*) and surrounded by an appropriate environment into which the eggs may be extruded.

A great step forward is made if the embryo is afforded care and protection during the precarious first stage of its life. In the Amphibia, the care of the egg may sometimes be assumed by the male (*Alytes obstetricans*). Some fishes possess paired oviducts in which the embryo may be retained for a brief gestational period, this being *the simplest rudimentary form of a uterus and gestation known.* However, a true uterus does not evolve except in the mammals.

In the lower mammalian forms that move on four legs in a horizontal position, a double or bicornuate uterus is a satisfactory solution for the protection of various types of embryos. In the primates, however, a double uterus with multiple fetuses would be liable to abortion. Hence the necessity for a central and single uterus with a single

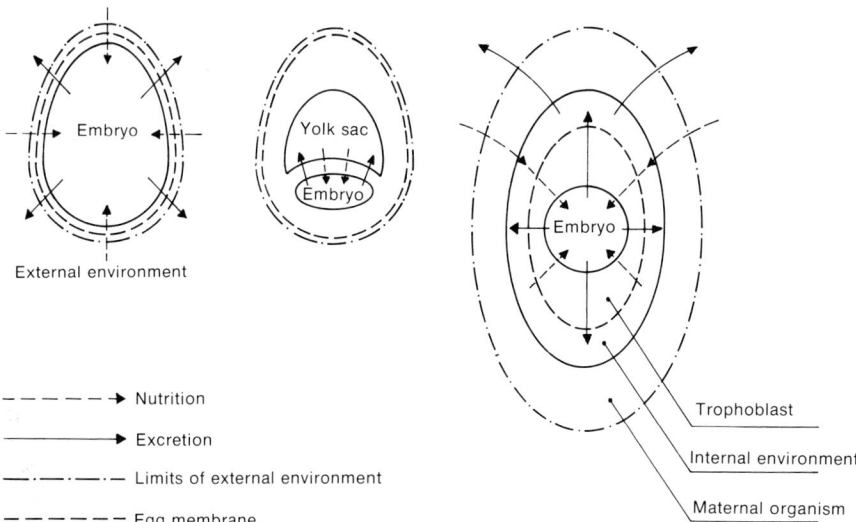

Figure 1-4. Types of eggs. *A*, Aquatic egg absorbing nutrition from aqueous environment. Egg membrane and limits of external environment are in contact. Interchange takes place freely at the level of egg membrane. *B*, In cleidoic eggs there is no exchange with external environment. Free and independent, the egg is completely "walled off". *C*, Placental egg is isolated from external environment. Its "environment" is mother's internal environment.

embryo. Arboreal life habits in the monkeys, just as *two-footedness* in man, determines the need for an *occlusive safety mechanism* in the uterus, which is provided in both forms by the uterine *cervix*.

The *placenta* appears only in the placental mammals (eutheria). The monotremes (prototheria) lay eggs, whereas the marsupials (metatheria) are ovoviviparous, passing the fetus into the brood-pouch, where it can be in firm contact with the nipple.

The placenta of the primates is not invariably hemochorial.[5] It is so in man and in the anthropoid apes, but in the lemurs it is epitheliochorial, and in the American monkeys it is endotheliochorial. Again, insectivorous animals, which are at a level of the animal scale lower than the American monkeys, have a hemochorial placenta. Grosser's classification therefore does not appear to be clear as far as evolution and perfection of the placenta are concerned.

The allantois in the *reptiles* develops underneath the chorion and this constitutes a rudiment of placenta not found in the birds, a fact which places the reptiles closer than any other species to the placental mammals.

Few living beings are more helpless than the newborn human infant. A human being matures both physically and mentally during the entire first quarter of his life. He depends on familial protection throughout this period. The reason for this lies in the great development of the cerebrum—so large it necessarily demands a longer learning process. The human hand is much more imperfect than its counterpart among most animals and is, for that manner, evolutionally less specialized than the hoof of a cow or that of a horse. And yet, the great capability and dexterity of that hand does not in itself depend on its anatomic constitution but on the cerebrum. A distinction must thus be drawn between *anatomic man* and *social man*. The latter has educated himself and has learned from others how to perform a series of acts which are those characterizing the human species ecologically. These constitute the reasons responsible for both the disproportionate helplessness and period of apprenticeship of the newborn and young human being respectively.

1.5. ENDOCRINE CHARACTERISTICS OF GESTATION

We have seen how the eventual endocrine structure in the mammals became subordinated to the absolute priorities of a highly complicated mechanism of reproduction and, in the ultimate instance, to the all-important *requisite of providing food for a delicate though more differentiated embryo over an extended period of time.* During pregnancy specific endocrine requirements must be met, and the organism strives not only to maintain the sheltered condition of the embryo but also to modify and mobilize effectively its own nutrition so that it may be used by the embryo. The corpus luteum, or its characteristic hormone, carries out an important function first by acting directly upon the uterus and second by exerting an indirect action upon the rest of the incretory apparatus and upon metabolism. The corpus luteum in the mammals persists longer than usually if pregnancy has taken place. In the primates it persists for the first trimester; in rodents the corpus luteum controls the endocrine functional state and the metabolism of the mother up to the very moment of delivery. For the corpus luteum to persist over a period of time, prolonging, to whatever extent, the span of its otherwise ephemeral cyclic existence, some specific stimulus in pregnancy must necessarily exist. This stimulus is found to be the internal secretions of the placenta. This organ, which developed, so to speak, from the outermost portion of the embryo, not only serves as a filter of substances and as a metabolic regulator but it also transiently plays the part of a most important endocrine gland, which takes over a large share of the endocrine and metabolic controls of pregnancy. The placenta begins to secrete a gonadotropic hormone equivalent to LH of the pituitary, which maintains the activity of the corpus luteum. The first act of the placenta in its capacity as endocrine organ is thus to *supplant* pituitary activity. However, the placenta of the primates—whether woman or monkey—whose corpus luteum remains functioning for only part of the gestational term, eventually acquires the capacity to secrete the hormone of the corpus luteum in addition to gonadotropic hormone. The placenta must then be conceived as an *endocrine organ of fetal origin designed to direct the processes of the maternal endocrine functional state.*

Knowledge of the latter fact has introduced a new concept into endocrine physiology. Insofar as the endocrinology of other glands and hormones is concerned, we are not aware of any other instance in which an endocrine regulatory mechanism originates outside the body which it affects, with the sole exception, perhaps, of artificially induced phenomena of parabiosis. From the standpoint of endocrinology, pregnancy may be qualified as a kind of *physiologic parabiosis.*

1.6. IMPORTANCE OF EFFECTORS IN REPRODUCTIVE PHYSIOLOGY

Disregarding momentarily what takes place in the female, and turning our attention towards the reproductive phenomena of the male, it is interesting to discover that the differentiation between the sexes with regard to their hormones is much more apparent than real. Considering the true significance of sex, it is easy to understand why sexuality in the biologic scale is a relatively late accident. The species appear to be divided into male and female along immutable and fixed lines, though this is the case only with the higher animals. Sufficiently well known are the *hermaphrodites* which constitute an important group of living beings both in the animal and vegetable kingdoms. While in their anatomic makeup, man and woman are independent and absolute entities, in the endocrinologic domain this independence is only relative. It is customary to say that ontogeny is a reduced replica of phylogeny. It is therefore not surprising that, whereas hermaphroditism and sexual undifferentiation in the lower species is the rule, there should also exist a stage of *sexual undifferentiation* in the mammalian embryo. The sexes, as we shall see later, are not yet defined during the first month or so of human embryonal development. This embryonal hermaphroditism disappears in its anatomical features quite early, but persists in its chemical character throughout life. Even though the ovary and the testis start quite early differentiating along divergent morphologic pathways, both of them do retain a common chemical constitution for the rest of their lives. So we can see that, just as the ovarian theca in the female elaborates the male sex hormone which is eliminated in the urine, so the Sertoli cell of the male testis produces folliculin which eventually also is excreted in the urine. Urine of both female and male thus contains both estrogens and androgens. Quantitatively, neither hormone is present in great enough excess over the other to justify the development of feminine or masculine characteristics, so that on the basis of a hormone assay it cannot be determined whether or not a given urine specimen pertains to a male or to a female.

This being the case, it is hard to understand why the development of the female gonads proceeds in one direction while that of the male develops in a diametrically opposed one. In face of an endocrine equilibrium that is nearly identical, this sexual dimorphism and sexual divergence can only be explained by assuming a *special way of reacting of the effector organs*. In this context, *that which characterizes what we generally consider to be hormonal action is largely the type of organ response*. The idea that the *effector organ* or *target organ* rather than the hormone itself conditions the response is a relatively recent one, but one that has today gained wide acceptance in the entire field of endocrinology. It might be said that masculinity is not so much the result of the type of hormones being secreted as rather the result of a "masculine" response on part of the organs and tissues. In the same way, it takes a "female" type of tissue response for the actions of the ovarian hormones to be exerted. This phenomenon must be explained, as recently pointed out by Pincus,[4] by accepting the idea that the hormones act on the cells in the same manner as would the substrate of a cellular enzymatic reaction.

The concept of a *variable cellular response to a constant hormonal stimulus* has thus found its way into endocrine physiology. It must be admitted that the hormones are most likely merely the *substrates* of cellular activity.

The recent findings regarding the *sex chromosome* have substantiated this concept (see Chapter 14). A pair of sex chromosomes, of different types in the male and in the female, are present in each somatic cell. Hence, not only the cells of the gonads but also those of the entire body are either male or female and have a special way of reacting owing to this pair of chromosomes, which from within the nucleus directs and creates a whole series of "sexual responses" particular to each cell.

It seems logical to assume that a cell tagged "female" would be responsive to the action of the estrogens and, on the contrary, would be more refractory to androgenic stimuli than a cell tagged "male," in which one would expect the opposite effect to be elicited. It must then be admitted that *sex does not exist only in the gonads and their incretions but is inherent down to the last cell of the metazoal organism.*

1.7. INTERRELATIONSHIP OF HORMONES AND NERVOUS SYSTEM

For many years, the regulation of organic functions had been attributed solely to the nerve endings. The "neurogenic era" in physiology prevailed during the latter part of the nineteenth century and the early years of the present century. Subsequent endocrine discoveries reoriented those ideas toward a new "humoral" physiology. However, both positions, when carried to the extreme, appear to be fallacious. Regulation is neither exclusively neural nor exclusively endocrine. We now know that sexual phenomena have an important bearing on neural physiology and are subordinate to it, and that, in turn, the secretion of the sex hormone is largely dependent on hypothalamic control. A significant advance has been made in recent years by gaining an understanding that the barriers between the humoral and nervous systems are not as rigid as they were once believed to be. In large part the effects of the vegetative nervous system take place through "chemical mediators," which are but hormones. Similarly, the neural system decisively influences the mode of regulation and propagation of hormonal impulses. Until recently it was believed to be axiomatic that the brain barrier was impermeable to the hormones and that none of these acted directly upon the nerve centers. This concept has been totally rebutted;[4] hormones are known to reach the nerve centers and to exert a manifest effect there, and this is particularly true for the sex hormones. An effect upon the hypothalamus by the ovarian hormones is beyond any doubt. Therefore, a "neuroendocrine" entity functioning as a whole in the regulation of sexual processes must be taken into account. The central nervous system, as well as psychogenic factors, will play a dominant part in the comprehension of sexual phenomena in the female.

1.8. VEGETATIVE SPHERE, RELATIONAL SPHERE AND SEXUAL SPHERE

It is customary to divide the functions of the organism into *vegetative functions* and *functions pertaining to external relations*. If sexual acts were to be included into such a classification they would be hard to place in either category; certainly, on one hand, sexual life is part of one's vegetative life but, on the other hand, it is also intimately connected with a person's relational life, since the choosing of mates and the procreation of the species will ultimately depend on the external world. Hence, because of its character of extraindividual growth, as was stated at the outset, reproductive life transcends the confines of vegetative life, which is merely concerned with the growth and preservation of the individual. The vegetative sphere, the reproductive sphere and the relational sphere are thus interrelated. Vegetative control is necessary for embryonal nutrition to be carried out, but some automatism in the phenomena of relational life is required if fertilization, without which reproduction is impossible, is to take place. These three spheres are distinct and may be represented by three intersecting circles (Fig. 1-5). The common area at which the three spheres overlap represents not the endocrine but the *neuroendocrine* system. Only by considering the control of vegetative life, relational life and sexual life as a function of the neurohormonal system can we fully comprehend the gearing of these three spheres in the life of the human individual.

Finally, it might be said that, while neurohormonal control is the coordinator between vegetative life, sexual life and relational life, this neuroendocrine unity provides also the basis and scaffolding for *biologic individuality*.

1.9. THE VEGETATIVE SPHERE, RELATIONAL SPHERE AND SEXUAL SPHERE IN THE FEMALE

Although the three circles in Figure 1-5 have been drawn with equal diameters, in general the extent of the activities involved on a quantitative scale differs markedly in the female and in the male. The duality of the sexes does not appear until phylogenetic differentiation has been reached. Many lower animals and the majority of the plants are hermaphrodites, each individual being the carrier of both sexes. The *allotment of physiologic workload emerged* when the species were divided into two kinds of individuals, some carrying the male gametes (males), the others carrying the female gametes (females). The male, whose minute gamete is designed to fertilize, soon also is converted into a fertilizing and active agent that seeks out the female, but who, once fertilization has been achieved, partakes little in the remainder of the processes of reproduction.

On the contrary, the female instead must meet the nutritional requirements of the fertilized egg, which entails a great amount of effort in those higher animals with a lengthy period of gestation. Pregnancy, particularly parturition, has increased this effort manifold. *The surcharge placed upon the female sex reaches its maximum in the human species.* The female's share in the workload of reproduction is incommensurably larger than that of the male.

A schematic representation of this is shown in the diagram of Figure 1-6 in which the three circles of sexual life, vegetative life and relational life have been drawn with consideration to the different roles they play in the two sexes. In general, the *male's share is greatest in the realm of external relations, while the female's is greatest in the sexual sphere,* the vegetative sphere retaining similar dimensions in both.

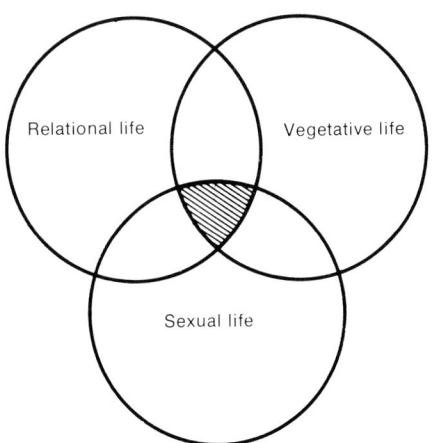

Figure 1-5. Reciprocal relationships among the spheres of relational life, vegetative life and sexual life.

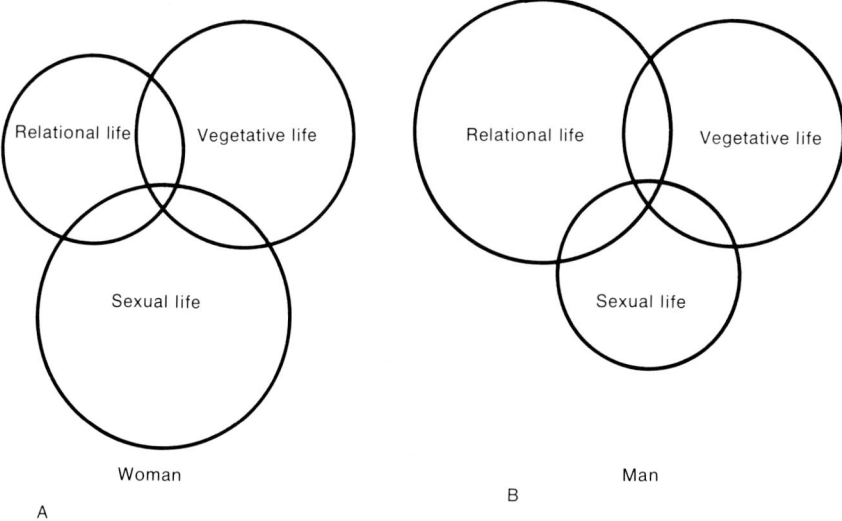

Figure 1-6. Diagram of woman's (A) and man's (B) traditional respective participation in sexual life and relational life. Because woman contributes more toward sexual life she is less burdened by the environmental struggle. The male, who hardly partakes in the reproductive effort, is obliged to put up a major contribution on behalf of the defense of both woman and kin (relational life). However, if these are compared, total areas of the two diagrams may be seen to be identical, conforming with the fact that effort put up by either man or woman is identical, though applied toward different ends. A woman who combines a career with raising a family contributes a share equal to that of man to relational life, but in addition has also to realize the more elevated contribution, proper of her sex, to sexual life. The total area of the three circles would in this instance be much greater than that in either A or B, which is a point in evidence that woman engaging in outside occupation renders a far greater effort than that of either man or traditional woman.

This *distinct mode of being* of the two sexes has most important implications in physiology and in pathology. The female organism is oriented towards itself and is, by nature, introverted, whereas the male is extroverted towards the external world. It is mainly in the terrain of physiology and sociology where this traditional *sexual dimorphism* and *bifunctionalism* is given its utmost prominence.

In ancient times, woman was the center of the family. Taking refuge in her household, she would partake neither in external life nor in the world's struggles. That was the man's duty, as it also was to provide for the defense and support of his kin. The greater share in relational life by the male was fully compensated by the wife's stronger contribution to reproductive life, so that their combined areas, as shown in Figure 1-6, remained balanced.

The ever increasing participation of modern woman in what up to the time were male forms of occupations has more and more enlarged the area of her relational sphere. Modern woman, in addition to her duties as a mother, has been shouldering more and more of the burdens that in the past befell the man exclusively. We have witnessed in the modern world the emergence of a vital anxiety in the woman, side by side with the vital anxiety in the man.

Many female endocrinopathies are but the expression of a conflict between these two spheres; they are psychosomatic endocrinopathies which we shall have an opportunity to analyze in the course of this book.

REFERENCES

1. Ammon, R., and Dirscherl, W.: *Fermente, Hormone und Vitamine.* Stuttgart, G. Thieme, 1957.
2. Euler, H. von: *Chemie der Enzyme.* Munich, J. F. Bergmann, 1934.
3. Needham, J.: *Biochemistry and Morphogenesis.* Cambridge, England, Cambridge University Press, 1942.
4. Pincus, G.: *J. Clin. Endocr.,* 12:1187, 1952.
5. Rhodes, P.: *Lancet,* 1:389, 1962.
6. Roux, W.: *W. Roux, Arch.,* 1:25, 1895.
7. Seitz, L.: *Wachstum, Geschlecht u. Fortpflanzung.* Berlin, J. Springer, 1939.
8. Zander, J.: *J. d'Endocr. Clin.,* 4:411, 1963.

Part One
THE SEX HORMONES

Reproductive life is controlled directly by the gonadal hormones in both the male and the female. Part One will be concerned with the study of the hormones that are elaborated by the female gonad. These are not two, as we have believed for many years, but actually four, since to the estrogens and progestogens have eventually been added both the androgens, the elaboration of which by the ovary even under physiologic conditions seems to be unquestionable, and relaxin, a not altogether well known hormone but one whose existence is certain and of a well defined individuality.

Estrogens, progestogens (gestagens) and androgens, together with the adrenal corticoids, are *steroid hormones*. These all possess the same aromatic ring, the cyclopentanophenanthrene, and all are linked by a *common metabolism*. Relaxin belongs to another vast group of hormones, the *protein hormones*, whose composition has not yet been completely elucidated. There is a third group of hormones, the *polypeptide hormones*, but none of these is known to be formed in the gonads.

In this introduction, it will be convenient to indicate the main steroids by their most commonly used name, conjointly with their correct chemical nomenclature.

NOMENCLATURE OF THE MOST IMPORTANT STEROIDS

Cholesterol	$\Delta 5$-Cholestene-3βol
Estrone	$\Delta 1,3,5(10)$-Estratriene-3-ol-17-one
17β-Estradiol	$\Delta 1,3,5(10)$-Estratriene-$3,17\beta$-diol
Estriol	$\Delta 1,3,5(10)$-Estratriene-$3,16\alpha,17\beta$-triol
Aldosterone	$\Delta 4$-Pregnene-$11\beta,21$-diol-3,20-dione-18-al
Androsterone	Androstane-3α-ol-17-one
Etiocholanolone	Etiocholane-3α-ol-17-one
	(or also 3α-hydroxy-5β-androstane-17-one)
Testosterone	$\Delta 4$-Androstene-17β-ol-3-one
Progesterone	$\Delta 4$-Pregnene-3,20-dione
Corticosterone	$\Delta 4$-Pregnene-$11\beta,21$-diol-3,20-dione
Deoxycorticosterone	$\Delta 4$-Pregnene-21-ol-3,20-dione
	(or also 21-hydroxyprogesterone)
Cortisone	$\Delta 4$-Pregnene-$17\alpha,21$-diol-3,11,20-trione
Cortisol	$\Delta 4$-Pregnene-$11\beta,17\alpha,21$-triol-3,20-dione

Chapter 2
ESTROGENS

2.1. DEFINITION, NOMENCLATURE, HISTORY

2.1.1. DEFINITION

The category of "estrogens" is not a chemical but a biologic one. It comprises those compounds which are capable of provoking estrus or vaginal shedding in the rat (see Chapter 12) and of producing proliferative changes in the female genital tract of mammals and, in general, of all vertebrates. As might be expected, this pharmacologically well definable action does not belong exclusively to any single structural entity. Essentially, two large groups possess such activity: the naturally occurring estrogens, or estrogenic hormones, and the artificial estrogens, or estrogenic drugs. These concepts will be discussed in detail in Section 2.2.

2.1.2. NOMENCLATURE

All estrogenic compounds are alcoholic derivatives of aromatic hydrocarbons, the nature of the hydrocarbon skeleton varying according to whether the estrogen is a naturally occurring one or an artificial one. The natural estrogens are all derived from the hydrocarbon *estrane* (Fig. 2–1). So inclusively is this the case that there is no known naturally occurring estrogen that is not derived from this basic hydrocarbon.

All estrane-derived natural estrogens have 18 carbon atoms, which distinguishes them from the androgens (see Chapter 4), which have 19 ring carbons, and from the progestogens (see Chapter 3), which have 21 carbon atoms. The corticoids (see Chapter 9) likewise have 21 carbon atoms. The estrogens are therefore also called C-18 steroids, the androgens C-19 steroids, and both the progestogens and corticoids the C-21 steroids. There are, nevertheless, some minor exceptions to this structural guideline.

2.1.3. HISTORY

Our knowledge of the estrogens is a relatively recent development. The consequences of castration from the resulting lack of estrogens were recognized mainly by Knauer at the end of the nineteenth century. In 1906, Marshall and Jolly dis-

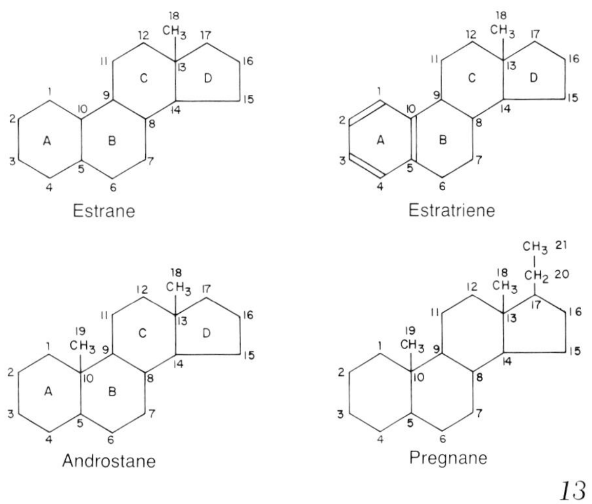

Figure 2–1. Structural formula of parent hydrocarbons giving rise to sex hormones. Estrane (saturated cyclopentanophenanthrene) is the parent hydrocarbon of all these compounds. Notice the manner of numbering the ring carbons and the use of letters for the different rings in the nomenclature. Estratriene is an estrane with three double bonds on ring A. Both androstane and estrane differ only from it because of a lateral chain (19). Finally, pregnane has two carbon atoms (20 and 21) more than androstane and three more than estrane. Pregnane is also the structural source of all adrenocortical steroids.

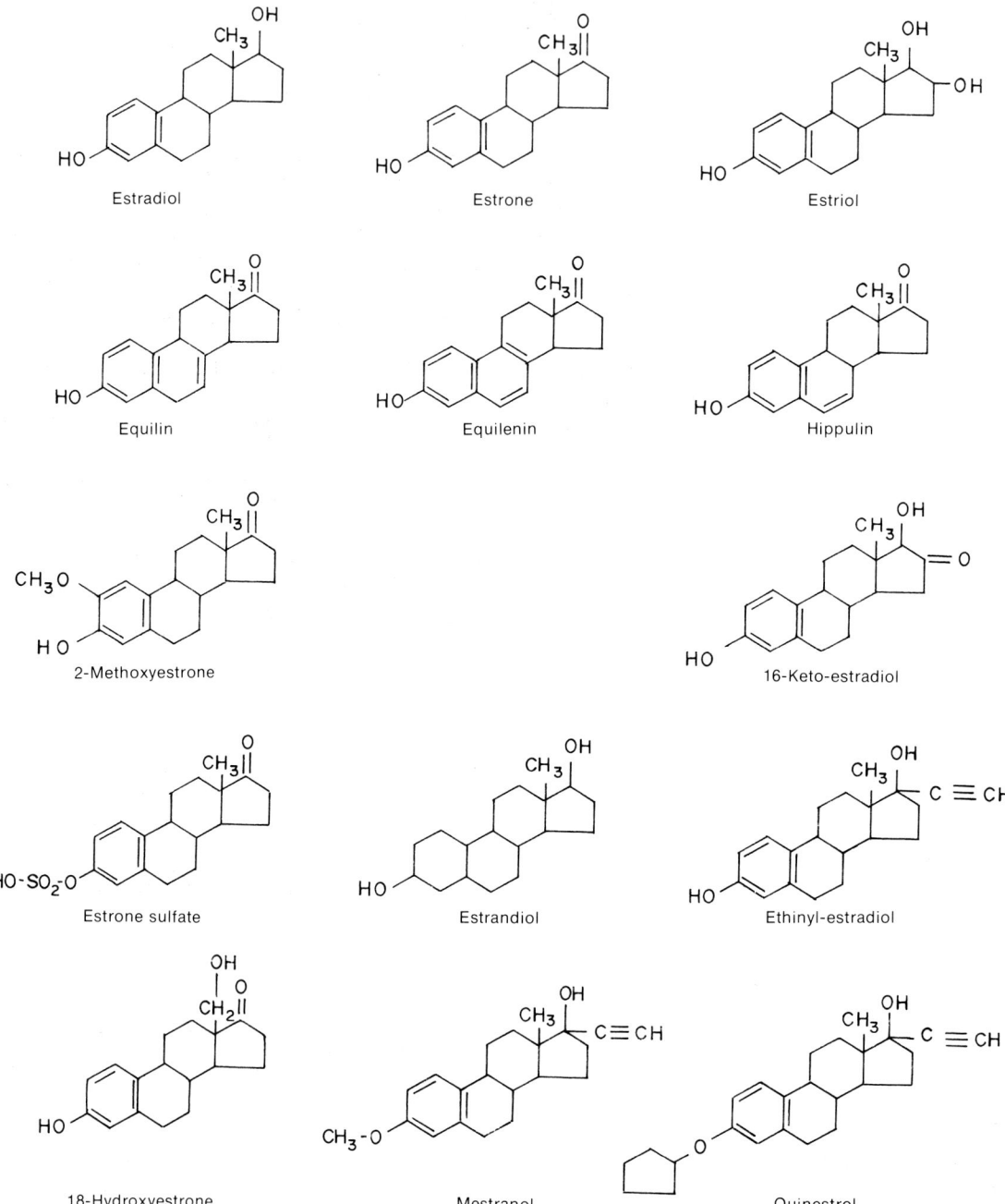

Figure 2-2. Natural estrogens. Estrone, estradiol and estriol occur in the human species and in the primates. Equilin, equilenin and hippulin are found in the mare. Ethinyl-estradiol, Mestranol and Quinestrol are synthetic compounds.

Estrogens

covered that the effects of castration could be reversed by injecting ovarian extracts. A few years later, Halban demonstrated that all the phenomena produced by castration, including atrophy of the genital organs, could be prevented by injecting ovarian and follicular fluid extracts. In 1922, Allen and Doisy made a meritorious contribution by creating a biologic test for the demonstration of the effects of ovarian extracts upon castrated rats. With their method, they were able to demonstrate the existence of an active ovarian principle which they called *estrin* (and which others subsequently renamed *folliculin*), the main source of which was follicular fluid.

. The same authors succeeded in isolating that substance in a nearly pure state in 1928, and a year later Doisy and Butenandt, working simultaneously but independently, successfully obtained folliculin in a pure crystallized form. That advance enabled Butenandt at Danzig and Marrian at Edinburgh three years later to elucidate the structural formula of *estrone*. Subsequently, a second substance was discovered in the ovary of women and of animals, which was also estrogenic but which differed from the one characterized by Butenandt and Doisy. This substance was *estradiol* (Fig. 2-2). Still later, Marrian found a third similar compound, *estriol*, in the urine of pregnant women. In 1933, Girard discovered a series of compounds similar to estrone, estriol and estradiol in the urine of the mare. Those were *equilin* and *equilenin*.

In the following years, between 1934 and 1939, Dodds and his collaborators synthesized most of the artificial estrogens, of which the first to be discovered was *stilbestrol*. Synthetic estrogens have since been described in ever increasing numbers (Fig. 2-3).

More recently, valuable contributions have been made through the studies of Pincus and his colleagues, which have

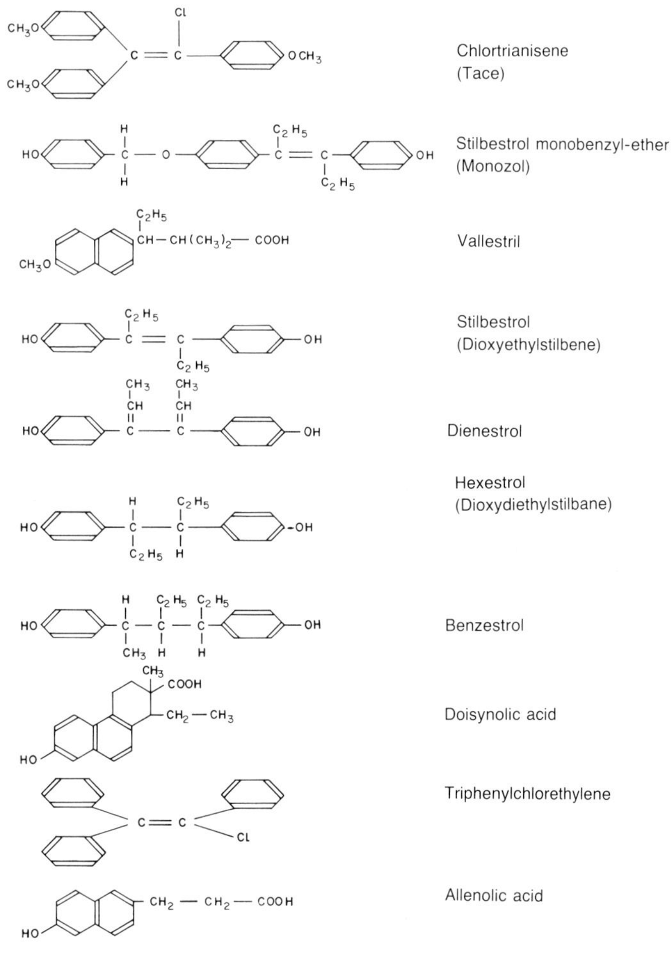

Figure 2-3. Artificial estrogens.

clarified the intermediary metabolism of estrogens; those of Diczfalusy, which comprise countless contributions, above all concerning the synthesis of estrogens in the fetus and during pregnancy; and those of Ryan, which appear to have shed some light on the manner in which these compounds are being elaborated in the ovary.

2.2. CHEMISTRY

A detailed description of the chemistry of estrogens is beyond the scope of this book. A distinction shall be made between the *naturally occurring estrogens* and the *artificial estrogens*, the latter, being quite heterogeneous compounds. So marked is the chemical difference between the two groups that, in a report we published earlier,[20] we suggested the terms *estrogen hormones* for the former and *estrogen drugs* for the latter.

2.2.1. NATURALLY OCCURRING ESTROGENS (ESTROGEN HORMONES)

The naturally occurring estrogens are so abundant that recently Diczfalusy and colleagues[46-48] listed as many as 75 substances, all with an estrane skeleton, capable of estrogenic activity. The most important ones are shown in Figure 2-2.

Another substance in this group, ethinylestradiol, is also an estrane-derived estrogen; however, this does not occur in nature and has been obtained only synthetically (Fig. 2-2). Similarly, doisynolic acid, which has an estrane skeleton with an open cyclopentane (Fig. 2-3), must not be considered as a natural estrogen. In spite of the estrane nucleus of these two estrogens, neither occurs naturally and both belong to a group intermediate between the estrogen hormones and estrogen drugs. The structural formula of their common parent hydrocarbon, estrane, and the manner of numbering the ring carbons were shown in Figure 2-1. Estrone is a 17-ketone, that is, an alcoholic ketone derived from estrane. Estradiol is a 3,17 dialcohol derivative of the same parent compound; estriol is a 3,16,17 trialcoholic derivative of estrane, and equilin, equilenin and hippulin are similar to estrone, from which they differ only by the position of the additional double bonds.

Up to 1954, it was generally believed that the only urinary estrogens were estrone, estradiol and estriol. Since then, however, the investigations of Brown and co-workers,[27] Diczfalusy and Lauritzen[46] and Smith and Ryan[189] have led to the isolation of seven additional catabolites: (1) 18-hydroxyestrone; (2) 16α-hydroxyestrone; (3) 17-epiestrol; (4) 16-ketoestrone; (5) 16-ketoestradiol-17β; (6) 16-epiestrol; and (7) 16β-hydroxyestrone. It is beyond the scope of this discussion to allow a detailed consideration of the stereoisomeric conditions in which these compounds may be found.

Ethinylestradiol, which has been included here despite the fact that it is an artificial estrogen, is a 17β-ethinyl-3,17α-diol of estrane.

2.2.2. ARTIFICIAL ESTROGENS (ESTROGEN DRUGS)

The chemical composition of this group of estrogens is much more heterogeneous. At their head are the derivatives of stilbene, which is the hydrocarbon resulting from the union of two benzene rings and an unsaturated ethylene chain (Fig. 2-3). The derivatives of stilbene are dioxydiethylstilbene or stilbestrol, and stilbestrol monobenzyl-ether (Monozol), which was introduced by Laberge and Rock.[127] Very similar to them, though derived not from stilbene but from other mixed aromatic-alkyl groups, are Dienestrol (a dioxydiethylenestilbane), and Hexestrol (a dioxydiethylstilbane). To the same group also belongs diphenyldiethylpropane, or Benzestrol, which differs from stilbestrol merely by having one more carbon on the intermediate chain. It has a comparable estrogenic effect.

Another group is formed by the derivatives of allenolic acid, which is a hydroxynaphthyl-β propionic acid. The most genuine representative of this group is dimethyl-ethyl-allenolic acid. Finally, a group of artificial estrogens is derived from doisynolic acid (Fig. 2-3), of which the most important ones are bisdehydrodoisynolic acid and methylbisdehydrodoisynolic acid. Also included in Figure 2-3 are *triphenylchlorethylene* and *trianisene* (TACE). Among the synthetic estrogens that have lately gained widespread acceptance is *Quinestrol* (see Fig. 2-3), which becomes deposited in the adipose tissue and therefore is endowed with markedly prolonged activity.[3, 144] Because it is not degraded in the liver, it is specially applicable in those cases in which a sustained, long-term effect is sought.

2.3. PHYSIOLOGIC ACTION

Estrogens show a wide range of activity. They can be summarized as being fundamentally *morphogenetic* hormones, with stimulatory proliferative effects upon the genital apparatus and the organs concerned with reproduction, as well as upon other systems. While this definition expresses the essential actions of estrogens, it does not cover them all, since there are, as will be seen later, certain estrogen effects that are not essentially morphogenetic.

2.3.1. EFFECTS OF ESTROGENS UPON THE GONADS

OVARY. Most of the estrogen effects upon the ovary of animals that have been described[103, 104, 151, 157] are attributable to intermediary actions by way of the pituitary gland and the hypothalamus (see Section 2.3.5.). Nevertheless, Bradbury[23] reports that ovarian tissue cultures subjected to the influence of estrogenic substances exhibit faster rates of growth. Bogdanove,[18] along with Keyes and Nalbandov,[121] points out that estrogens tend to prolong the life of the corpus luteum even in hypophysectomized animals.

TESTIS. Balze[7] has demonstrated that estrogens may cause the arrest of testicular descent and subsequent atrophy of the ectopic testis in infant animals. Bacon and Kirkman[6] also demonstrated, shortly thereafter, a *direct* effect of large doses of estrogens in producing atrophy of the seminiferous epithelium in adult animals.

2.3.2. EFFECTS UPON MÜLLERIAN ORGANS

FALLOPIAN TUBES. Until a few years ago, there had been doubt as to whether estrogens exerted any effects upon the mammalian fallopian tubes. It was known that in birds estrogens promote tubal growth,[133] and that radioactive estrogens are selectively trapped by the oviducts.[111] It could also be shown that ovitransportation in the rabbit,[96] in the rat[37] and in the mouse[97] was accelerated by the injection of estrogens. Similarly, in the rat[8] and the rabbit,[95] estrogens increase tubal motility both in vivo and in vitro. The studies conducted by de la Fuente (Fig. 2–4) on human fallopian tubes in our laboratory would make us assume a similar effect. The more recent investigations by Terragno and associates,[209, 210] also conducted at our school, have quite positively demonstrated the accelerating effects of estrogens upon tubal motility.

ENDOMETRIUM. While in the primates the most important effects of estrogens are seen in the endometrium, in mice and rats their prime action is exerted upon the vagina. Estrogens produce the characteristic *proliferative phase* in the endometrium of all mammals. This becomes noticeable by an increase in thickness of the mucosa in all three of its constituent elements, i.e., the glands, the stroma and the vessels. The proliferative effect on the endometrium has been demonstrated in different mammals: in the rat,[1] the rabbit,[9] the monkey[222] and the human[151] (Fig. 2–5). The dosage necessary to produce the proliferative reaction of the human endometrium has been esti-

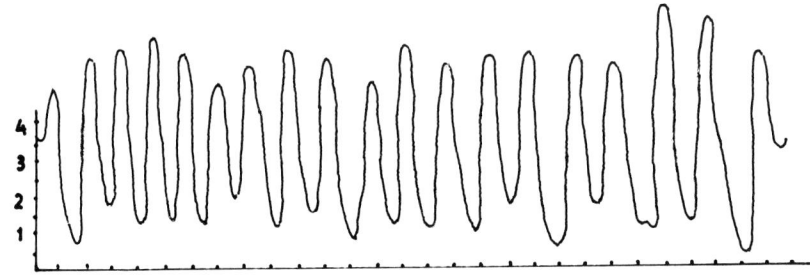

Figure 2–4. Tubal peristalsis under estrogenic influence. (From de la Fuente: Thesis, University of Madrid, 1948.)

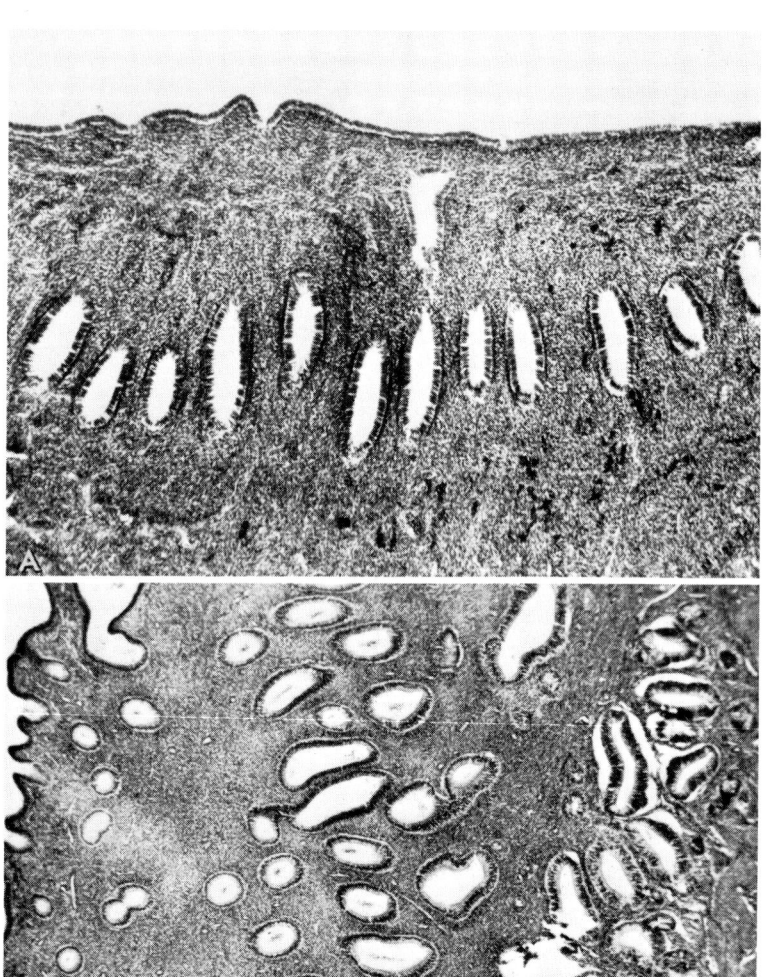

Figure 2–5. Effect of estrogens on endometrium of castrated monkey. A, Female *Macaca mulatta*, one month after castration. Atrophic endometrium with single row of glands. B, Same monkey 14 days following injection of 0.8 mg per kg body weight of estradiol valerianate. Note endometrial thickening, stromal proliferation and increase in number of glands.

mated, on the basis of amenorrheic women with ovarian insufficiency, to be 20 to 30 mg of estradiol. Subsequently, the required dose was found to be slightly higher for castrated women. It may be stated that the amount of 30 to 50 mg of estradiol is capable of provoking the complete regenerative growth of the human uterine mucosa.

The effects of estrogens upon the individual components of the endometrium can best be observed in histologic preparations. The *glands* increase in length and, owing to their elongation, tend to become tortuous; their epithelium increases in height and the nuclei become arranged in multiple rows, resembling pseudostratification (Fig. 2–6). Gomori's stain for alkaline phosphatase is strongly positive (Fig. 2–7), the most intense phosphatase activity being observed in the basilar portion of the cellular protoplasm. The estrogenic effects upon the *stroma* are noticeable in the cellular growth of its elements, which increase in size and number (Fainstat[65]). Finally, estrogens affect the *vessels* by promoting the growth of the spiral arterioles of the endometrium (Kao and Gam[115]). An interesting observation is the reported increase in imbibition of water of the endometrial

Estrogens

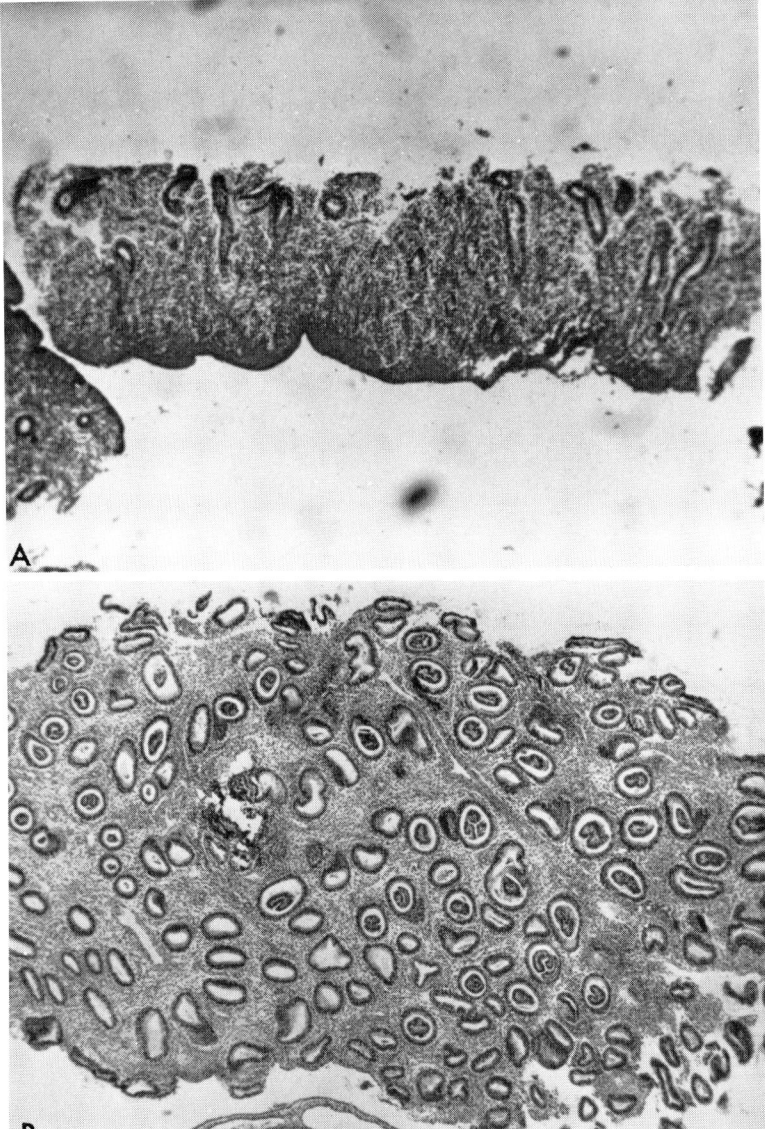

Figure 2-6. Effect of estrogens on endometrium of castrated woman. *A*, Endometrial aspiration biopsy 15 days after surgical castration, showing endometrial atrophy. *B*, Aspiration biopsy 14 days following injection of 0.8 mg per kg body weight of estradiol valerianate; note proliferative activity in mucosa.

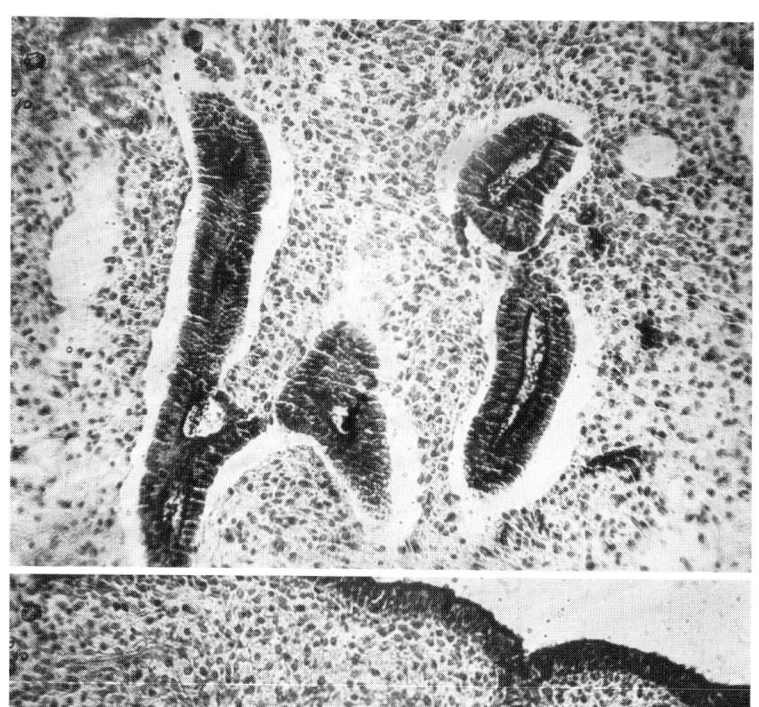

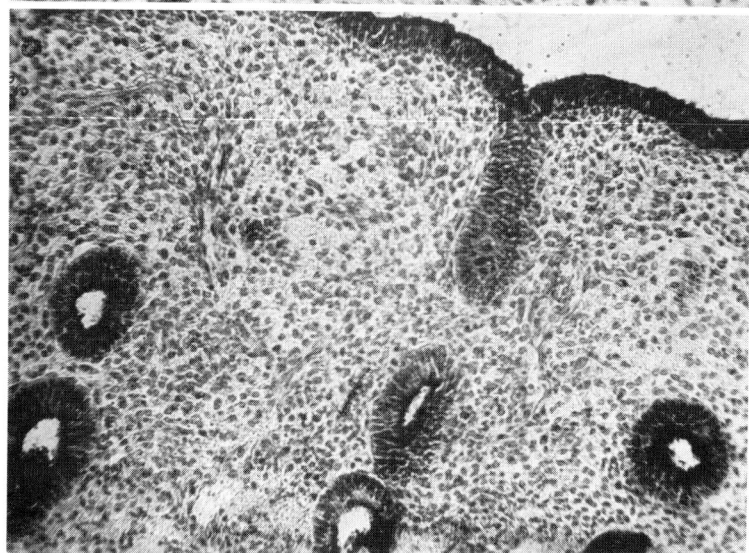

Figure 2-7. Alkaline phosphatase activity within endometrial glands under the influence of estrogens (Gomori stain).

tissues, as well as the demonstration that estrogens significantly increase endometrial oxygen consumption.[212]

EFFECTS UPON THE MYOMETRIUM. The mode of action of the ovarian hormones upon the myometrium of the rabbit was studied by Csapo and Corner.[41, 42] The muscular contraction of the myometrium is dependent on a contractile protein, actomyosin, which in association with adenosine triphosphate, under conditions of high intracellular potassium and high extracellular sodium concentrations, is able to effect the contraction and the release of energy. The contractile protein contained within the myocyte is the source of the energy of contraction.

The effects of estrogens upon uterine motility in animals has been known since antiquity. Bo and his colleagues[16] have studied the question at the ultrastructural level of the uterine muscle, reporting the finding of significant changes indicative of enhanced contractile activity. Spratto and Miller[196] have found an increase of catecholamines in the uterine muscle under estrogenic influence. Sol,[191] at our laboratory, has demonstrated the effect of estrogens on the oxytocic response of the isolated human uterus, and more recently, various authors[112, 124, 143] have confirmed these findings (Fig. 2-8).

METABOLIC EFFECTS OF ESTROGENS UPON THE UTERUS. The effects upon acto-

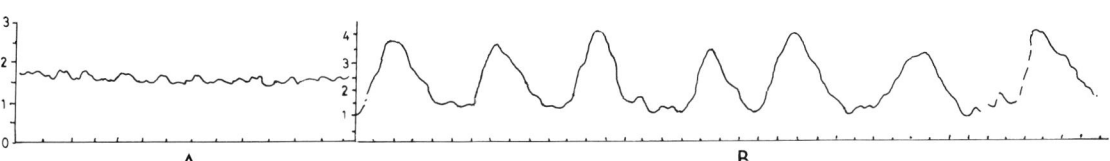

Figure 2–8. Action of estrogens upon spontaneous motility of an in vitro isolated strip of uterus. *A*, Spontaneous motility of postmenopausal uterus; *B*, in woman previously treated with estrogens (50 mg).

myosin were mentioned in the preceding paragraph. Currently, a great many of the actions of estrogens are being envisioned as resulting from their enzymatic and metabolic interactions at the uterine level. Increased uterine blood flow in both animals and women,[89, 195] as well as an elevation of intrauterine oxygen tension in rats,[149] has been shown to be associated with estrogenic activity. Estrogens induce an increased water[84] and glucose[15] content in the uterine space, the latter effects, it was noted,[174] resulting from an increased liberation of histamine. Estrogen activity is likewise responsible for an increased storage of nucleic acids in the endometrium[83, 92] as well as in the remainder of the entire uterus.[156, 157] The injected radioactive phosphorus (^{32}P) deposition in the rat is greater when accompanied by injections of estrogens;[92] phosphatase[140] and phosphoamidase activity in the myometrium similarly is enhanced under the effect of estradiol,[2, 101] and the protein composition of the uterine muscle, as determined by electrophoresis, equally undergoes modification.[152]

Special mention must be made of the effect of estradiol on the enzyme system of glycogen synthesis. There seems to be increased activity of the phosphorylases[14, 217] and of uridine phosphate.[14] The problem is presently still being debated owing to the views of some authors (see Chapter 3) who do not accept the role of estradiol in promoting glycogen synthesis. In this regard, Eckstein and Villee[55] report failure to notice any increased activity of these enzymes.

CERVIX. One of the most important targets of estrogens is the uterine cervix. Under the influence of estrogens,[53, 62] cervical mucus increases in amount, in viscosity and in its capacity for crystallization. The content of polysaccharides and SH groups in cervical mucus also increases.[184] In Chapter 41, the important part this effect plays in facilitating the ascent of spermatozoa through the cervix will be pointed out. Botella and Nogales[21] have also studied the effects that estrogens exert upon the morphology of the cervical mucosa. Finally, it must be said that while the amount of collagen in the cervical stroma decreases in response to progestogenic activity, it increases under the influence of estrogens.

CLINICAL EFFECTS OF ESTROGENS UPON THE HUMAN UTERUS. Even though the clinical effects of estrogens upon the uterus are to be discussed at a later stage it seems convenient to mention that what is generally observed is an increase in size of the uterus and the disappearance of flexures and distorted positions (such as forced anteflexion, sinistroposition, etc.). As a result, a so-called "infantile uterus" can be expected to acquire a more juvenile or even normal appearance. Just as scanty or irregular menstruation may be normalized under the action of these hormones, estrogenic activity often accounts for the correction of amenorrheas and reappearance of menstruation. Finally, it is not unusual to observe beneficial modifying effects of estrogens upon dysmenorrheas, too. All these effects, which shall be discussed later in detail, justify the wide therapeutic use of estrogens in certain functional disorders of the uterus.

EFFECTS OF ESTROGENS UPON THE IMPLANTATION OF THE EGG. In the rat, a small amount of estrogens must be present for implantation to take place successfully.[49] Should the dosage of estrogens be increased above a certain level, the blastocyst dies before implantation can take place effectively.[120, 136] This is partly due to an accelerated rate of tubal motility (see Chapter 44), which obliges the conceptus to enter the endometrial cavity prematurely, before it has reached a sufficient degree of development and the capacity for implantation.

EFFECTS OF ESTROGENS UPON THE DEVELOPMENT OF REPRODUCTIVE ORGANS. In embryos of batrachia[218] and of birds,[163]

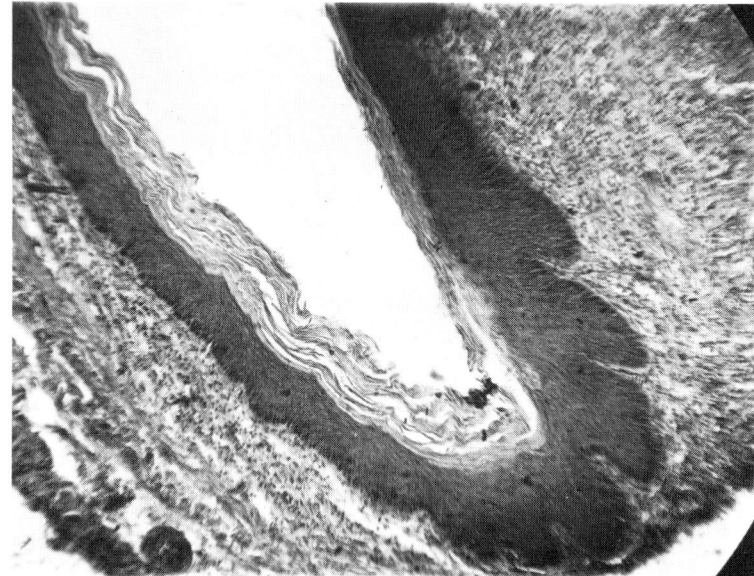

Figure 2-9. Phenomenon of estrus in vaginal wall of rat, seen in histologic section.

estrogens provoke rapid development of the oviducts. Similar effects have been demonstrated by Liu[131] in rodents. In cultures of tubal tissue, Kohler and Malley[125] made the observation that the addition of estrogens accelerated cellular differentiation. Clark and Gorski[40] found that the estrogen binding protein (see Section 2.5.6) was already present in the uteri of rat embryos on the tenth day of development.

EFFECTS OF ESTROGENS UPON THE VAGINA. We have already mentioned that the effects of estrogenic activity were first discovered in the vagina of rodents by Allen and Doisy in 1922. These changes become apparent with the cornification of the superficial cells (Fig. 2-10), which are eventually shed and show up in the vaginal exudate of the animals as flat, polyhedral, enucleate elements that are completely cornified. Cells of this description have been known as "squames" (or German

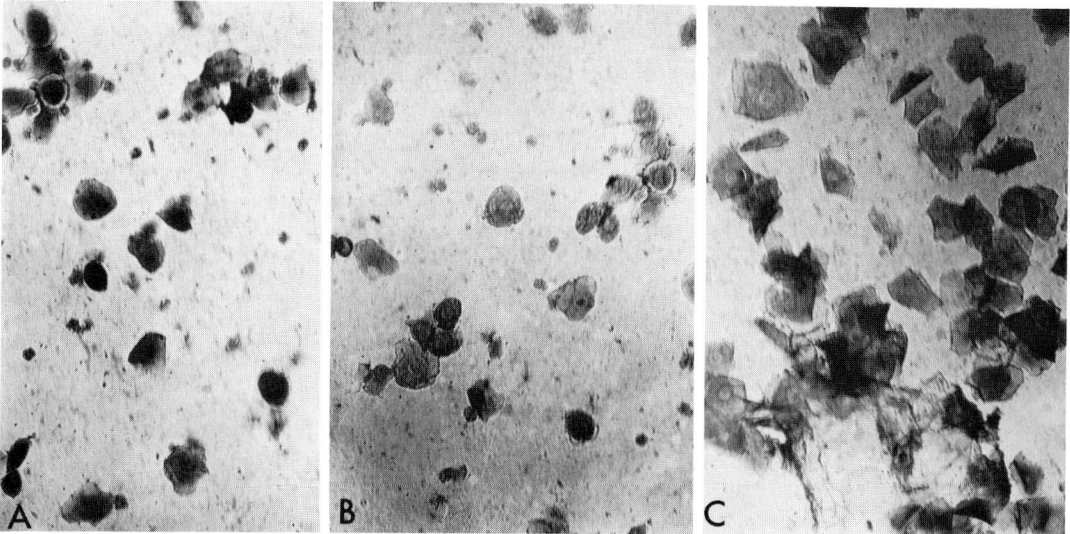

Figure 2-10. Phenomenon of estrus in rat vagina, seen in smears: A, Resting state (diestrus). B, Beginning of reaction (proestrus). C, Reaction of estrous activity (estrus).

Estrogens

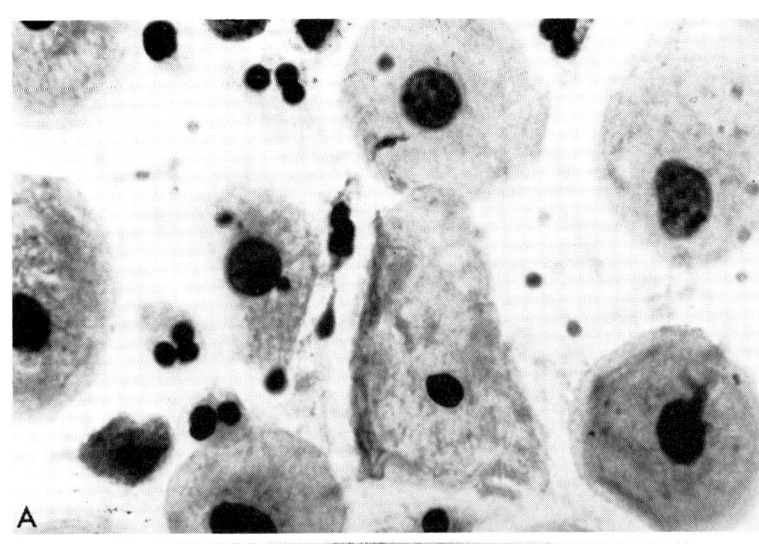

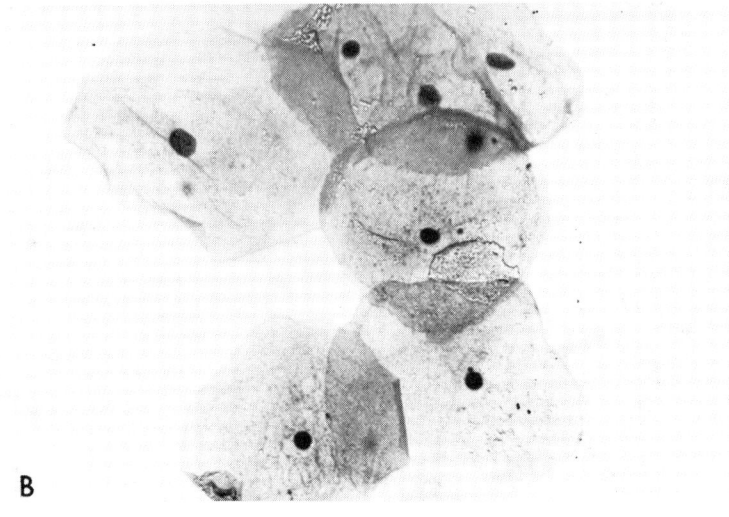

Figure 2–11. A, Regressive vaginal smear from surgically castrated patient, 15 days following castration (smear corresponds to top half of Fig. 2–6). Note hypoproliferative features of cells. B, Same patient, 14 days following injection of 0.8 mg per kg body weight of estradiol valerianate. Large polygonal cells with karyopyknotic nuclei appear.

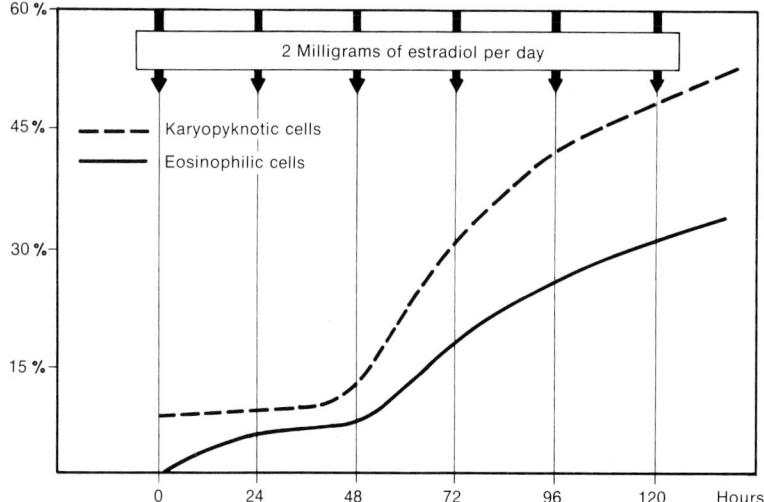

Figure 2-12. Effect of estrogen injections on female vaginal cytology. Estrogens produce: (a) elevation of the karyopyknotic index, characterized by an increase in the number of superficial cells with tiny, pyknotic nuclei, and (b) an increase in the number of "eosinophilic" or "acidophilic" cells, with distinctly pink staining cytoplasm by the Papanicolaou method. The karyopyknotic index expresses estrogenic activity more faithfully than does the acidophilic index, the latter being subject to modification by staining and particularly fixation artifacts.

"Schollen"). They have been used for the biologic estimation of estrogenic activity and have served as the basis for the bioassay or quantitation of estrogen activity. These effects have been confirmed by a large number of authors.

The effects of estrogenic activity are considerably less pronounced in the vagina of primates. Nevertheless, the marked increase in the number of karyopyknotic cells[155] in the vaginal cytology of both woman and the monkey has been well established as the expression of estrogenic activity (Figs. 2-11 and 2-12). An increased number of mitotic figures in the basal layer of the human vagina has also been observed.[159, 215] Another effect of estrogens upon the vaginal wall is increased storage of glycogen.[17, 21, 219] Moreover, recent studies with tritium labeled estradiol made it possible to observe selective accumulation of the hormone within the vaginal basal cell layer of both rodents and primates.

2.3.3. EFFECTS UPON THE VULVA AND THE SEX CHARACTERS

In some animals, such as rats, mice,[28] guinea pigs[194] and monkeys,[102] estrogens exert a quite manifest effect upon the vulva. In rats and mice, they provoke vaginal canalization and vulvar patency; in guinea pigs, they produce analogous effects but of such intensity that a method for the evaluation of minimal amounts of estrogens has been based on the resulting vulvar patency and edema (see Chapter 24). The changes of the sexual skin of the vulvoperineal region and in the face of monkeys are the most marked and conspicuous effects of the period of estrus. In woman, vulvar changes are minimal. However, under the influence of estrogens, the development of the labia majora and minora, as well as the greater turgescence and elasticity of their mucosa, can be clearly demonstrated. Increased piliation of the mons pubis and of the vulva has not been conclusively proved to be the result of purely estrogenic action. It would appear to be due instead to a combined action of estrogens and the secretions of the adrenal cortex (see Chapter 16).

Estrogens are also known to be instrumental in molding the female sex characters (see Chapter 18). Indeed, Davis,[44] who for 19 years treated with estrogens a young woman suffering from ovarian agenesis, was able to demonstrate the gradual acquiring of the characteristic features of femininity under this regimen.

2.3.4. EFFECTS UPON THE BREAST

The morphogenetic effects of estrogens upon the breast are unquestionable.[72, 74] Recently, Sander[181] has shown that estradiol-H^3 is selectively trapped by mammary tissue. This subject is treated in more detail in Chapter 22.

2.3.5. EFFECTS OF ESTROGENS UPON ENDOCRINE GLANDS

Whether directly or indirectly, estrogens act upon the entire endocrine system. However, the pituitary, the adrenal and the thyroid are most susceptible to estrogenic secretions.

HYPOTHALAMUS AND PITUITARY. Estrogens become concentrated in the hypothalamus[4, 99] If tritiated estradiol is injected, it will show up in great concentration in the region of the sex center. If, however, this region is first destroyed,[50] this selective concentration fails to take place. Kato and Villee[116] have shown that the accumulated amount of estrogens is related to the functional activity of the sex center. The *estrogen receptors*, to which so much significance is at present being attached (see Section 2.3.9), have been found to be particularly concentrated in the hypothalamic median eminence.[114]

Experimental studies in rats,[13, 168] rabbits[45] and hamsters,[88] as well as in the human species,[134, 154] furnished evidence to the effect that small amounts of injected estrogens stimulate LH release, probably by way of the hypothalamus, in which they produce an increase of LH releasing factor (LHRF) (see Chapter 8). Recent studies[32, 205] have helped to determine the amount necessary to produce such an effect in rats, which is equivalent to 0.6 micrograms per kilogram of body weight. Goldzieher and Fariss[82] estimate this amount to be 30 to 40 mcg for an adult woman—that is, if one uses the same kilogram per weight equivalent. Thus, at the end of the first phase of the human cycle, the gradually rising level of circulating estrogens would seem to determine the ovulatory peak of LH and to precipitate ovulation (see Chapter 12).

Nevertheless, the mode of action of the antiovulatory steroids (see Chapter 47) demonstrates the fact that estrogens may also act to induce inhibition of the LH peak[174] and cause the cessation of ovulation in the human ovary.[22] There is no contradiction between these two modes of action. One, according to Goldzieher and Fariss,[82] was seen to work with amounts of 30 to 50 mcg, whereas our own investigations[22] have proved that the minimal dosage of estrogens that is necessary to inhibit ovulation in a woman weighing 60 kg is 80 mcg or more. Recent work on rats[93] and women[119] has confirmed this biphasic character of estrogenic action on the hypothalamus.

Thus, while LH release is stimulated by small amounts of estrogens, it is inhibited by larger doses of over 80 mcg.

The early literature described a direct stimulatory effect of estrogens upon the adenohypophysis. Those studies also considered the effects that estrogens exerted on the hypothalamus as merely intermediary effects. This is not so. Modern investigations[73, 129, 214] demonstrate stimulatory effects irrespective of whether estrogens are injected into tissue cultures of the anterior lobe or into animals whose hypothalamus had been destroyed. Until recently, oxytocin secretion had not been thought to be influenced by estrogens, but Roberts and Share[171] have demonstrated that oxytocin secretion in the hypothalamic nuclei of the ewe increased following estrogen therapy.

As has been shown in newborn rats with injections of estradiol,[122] the sexual sensitivity of the hypothalamus is susceptible to one other facet of estrogenic activity—puberty. This mode of action will be discussed in Chapters 16 and 38.

ADRENAL. It has been many years since we demonstrated that the zona reticularis of the adrenal cortex was stimulated by the action of estrogens,[20] an effect that was subsequently confirmed.[5, 43] The explanation of this action unquestionably lies with the pituitary. It is believed that, by acting upon the latter, estrogens provoke a release of LH, which stimulates the adrenal zona reticularis specifically (see Chapter 9).

THYROID. Earlier observations of our own had demonstrated that estrogenic hormones stimulated thyroid function in the rat. Subsequently, protein bound iodine (PBI)[70] as well as thyroid binding globulin (TBG)[139] have been found to rise under the influence of estrogenic activity. In the same manner, ^{131}I is more readily trapped by the thyroid glands of both animals[60] and man[75] following treatment with estrogens. Estrogenic compounds intensify TSH release which, in experimental animals, is responsible for histologically detectable thyrotropic effects.[61, 62, 66] *Hence, modern investigations have come to substantiate the early hypothesis, held by both Marañón and ourselves, which postulated a stimulative effect of estrogens upon thyroid function.*

OTHER ENDOCRINE GLANDS. Pereira-Luz and co-workers[160] noted that estradiol valerianate induced thymic atrophy. A great many authors, among them Basabe and his colleagues,[11] have reported evidence of a diabetogenic effect, which will be analyzed in more detail later (Section 34.4).

2.3.6. METABOLIC EFFECTS OF ESTROGENS

Several metabolic effects of estrogens have so far been demonstrated. We shall cite four: (1) effects on water and mineral metabolism, (2) on carbohydrate metabolism, (3) on lipid metabolism and (4) on calcium metabolism.

EFFECTS ON WATER AND MINERAL METABOLISM. Estrogens cause *water retention by the tissues*.[188] *Premenstrual hyperestronism* produces edema. Similarly, estrogens increase storage of water in the uterine muscle. By and large, this water retaining effect must undoubtedly result from the increase of sodium in the intercellular spaces of the uterus, which has already been mentioned in discussing the mechanism of estrogenic action on the uterus (see page 21).

CARBOHYDRATE METABOLISM. Our earlier investigations had demonstrated that estrogens, to a certain degree, produced a diabetogenic effect. On the basis of recent studies,[76, 87] this action may be interpreted as resulting from an intermediary effect which is brought about by increasing activity of the growth hormone (STH).

EFFECTS ON LIPID METABOLISM. Recent studies have revealed that estradiol tends to cause increased lipemia[60] and cholesterolemia[71, 198] and to stimulate the production of cholesterol by the reticuloendothelial system. The apparent ketonemic response to estrogen activity has already been mentioned above.

CALCIUM METABOLISM AND OSSIFICATION. The appearance of osteoporosis following castration was an early observation (Edgren et al.[56]). By means of radioactive calcium, Govaerts and his co-workers[86] have demonstrated that estradiol favors increased osseous calcium deposition. A similar phenomenon was subsequently observed by Ranney[169] using radioactive phosphorus.

2.3.7. OTHER ACTIONS OF ESTROGENS

By virtue of their morphogenetic action, estrogens stimulate the development of the skin and mucosa.[126] They thus promote the regeneration of the skin and of the gastric mucosa. They also stimulate the development of the bladder epithelium in both the male and the female. An effect on the buccal mucosa has likewise been shown.

Aside from these, estrogens increase the peripheral circulation through the extremities, thus improving certain circulatory disturbances in adolescent females, by way of the neurovegetative system. An important action, which has only recently been described, is one that inhibits hematopoiesis[54, 148] and which, it would seem, results from the inhibition of iron uptake by the erythrocytes.[110] It would be beyond the scope of this work to examine the great many actions of estrogens in invertebrates.[85]

2.3.8. DIFFERENCES OF ACTION BETWEEN ESTRADIOL AND ESTRIOL

Since the discovery of estriol more than 30 years ago, the majority of investigators have considered it as a mere catabolite of estradiol and as a physiologically unimportant breakdown product. Smith[188] and Stone and Bagget[201] have called attention to the fact that in the presence of progesterone, both during the second half of the cycle and in pregnancy, estriol is always the estrogen that is eliminated in largest quantity, which is suggestive of a synergistic action. More detailed studies concerning the physiologic action of estriol upon the genital tract[56, 79, 167, 222] have shown that its mode of action differs significantly from that of estradiol. In the first place, estriol lacks antiprogestational activity; estradiol, on the contrary, has very intense antiprogestational activity, particularly on the gravid uterus of some animals. In the second place, estriol exerts its action upon the vagina and the uterine cervix with greater potency than upon the uterus itself and, in the uterus, the effect is more pronounced on the myometrium than on the endometrium (Claringbold,[39] Edgren et al.[56]).

Owing to their competitive action upon the vagina, estradiol and estriol are viewed as antagonists by Brecher and Wotiz.[24]

The inference one would draw from all this is that estriol is just the logical estrogen to synergize progesterone activity during the second half of the cycle and, *above all, during pregnancy* (Merrill,[146]

Everett[64]). During the latter, it would carry out the following functions: first, it will act without antagonizing progesterone activity and, hence, without provoking abortion; second, it will stimulate the gestational development of the vagina, cervix and uterus; and third, it will "prime" these three organs to render them more responsive to the influence of progesterone.

2.3.9. MECHANISM OF ACTION OF ESTROGENS

The investigations of the last few years have focused their attention particularly on the study of the *mechanism of action of estrogens*. Special attention has been devoted to the question of the *incorporation of estrogens* by certain tissues, specifically those on which estrogens act and whose estrogenic activity has been found to be proportional to the degree of incorporation.[165, 208] Injections into animals of tritiated estradiol (estradiol-H³) revealed uptake of the substance in those sites on which estrogens exert their effects: uterus,[25, 150] vagina,[58] hypothalamus in rats.[59] The same holds true in rabbits and women[165, 172] and, as pointed out earlier, also applies to the breast.[197] In spayed rats, the rates of uterine uptake are even greater, denoting an avidity for estrogens on the part of the uterus,[164] whereas such an uptake has not been observed to take place in testosterone-sterilized rats.[137] The assumption seems justified that an important component of estrogen action depends on both the *sensitivity of the organ affected and its capacity for trapping the circulating estrogens*. The studies undertaken by Szego and his group[84, 193, 194, 206] have demonstrated that injected estrogens provoke the liberation of histamine in the uterus and have attributed an important part of the overall estrogen effect to the intermediary role of histamine release. Cecil and his colleagues[34, 35] have similarly demonstrated an estrogen induced increase of vascular permeability, which could similarly be related to action of histamine. This view is shared by Ferrando and Nalbandov,[68] by Leonard[128] and by Martin.[142] Consequently, at least within the uterus, histamine seems to play an important part as an intermediary of estrogenic activity.

In the rat,[108] the content of sulfhydryl groups has been similarly shown to be directly proportional to the degree of sensitivity displayed by the tissues to estrogens. Finally, Sjoberg[187] has attached great importance to his finding that the uterine norepinephrine content in rats increased with estrogen treatment.

2.4. BIOLOGICAL ASSAY AND CHEMICAL DETERMINATION

The methods for the determination of estrogens in urine, blood and tissues will be described in Chapter 24. Most of these are of two types (1) *bioassay procedures*, and (2) *methods of direct chemical determination*. To these must be added the indirect methods of estrogen estimation which are based on the study of the response they elicit from their human targets.

2.4.1. BIOASSAY OF ESTROGENS

The bioassay procedures are based on: (1) the Allen-Doisy mouse or rat test, in which vaginal exfoliation or estrus is evaluated; (2) the test of uterine growth, which has the advantage of a logarithmically proportional relationship between the injected amount of estrogen and the incremental weight of the uterus; (3) the nipple test, which determines the increase in size of the nipples of rats or mice; (4) the tests of local intravaginal application,[117] which are the most sensitive of these tests.

2.4.2. METHODS OF CHEMICAL DETERMINATION

Enormous advances have been made in the field of chemical determination of estrogenic compounds in the last 30 years. A great number of methods are available which, for the sake of convenience, can be divided into: (1) Determination of the total of estrogens or Kober-positive steroids, by means of spectrophotometric measurement of Kober's test. (2) Fluorimetric procedures, based on the fluorescent properties of estrogens when reacting with various reagents. (3) Chromatographic procedures of extraction and separation of the different fractions, of which Brown's method[28] is currently the most commonly used procedure. For details, see Chapter 24, in which these methods are described.

2.4.3. UNITS OF ESTROGENS

The facts that by now the estrogens have all been isolated in a chemically pure state and that their structures and molecular weights are well known have resulted in a change in the method of expressing values. Estrogen values are now expressed either in micrograms or in milligrams, rather than in mouse units, rat units, etc. The levels of the hormones in body fluids are given in micrograms, whereas therapeutic products may be expressed in milligrams.

Artificial estrogens possess a somewhat different biologic activity which, in general, is considered to be greater than that of the naturally occurring estrogens. Stilbestrol and hexestrol are approximately 30 to 60 per cent more active. In this respect, there exist great disparities, which are based mainly on the mode of administration of a given hormone and on the wide range of sensitivity to different estrogens observed among experimental animals, on the one hand, and man, on the other.

Some authors, notably Kauffman and Perin, have studied the activity of the different estrogens in woman, establishing the concept of a "woman unit," comparable to existing rat units and mouse units. There is no consensus as to the magnitude of these units. This depends basically on the vehicle and mode of administration, which will be enlarged upon in a later discussion. The dosage which is necessary to regenerate the endometrium ranges from 15 mg (in the case of allenolic acid), to 30 mg (for injectable estradiol benzoate), to 150 mg (for estradiol tablets), or 200 mg (for hexestrol or doisynolic acid), all taken by the same route. It may be said, accordingly, that a woman unit in injectable form is 30 mg, whereas a woman unit with peroral administration may be as high as 150 or 200 mg.

2.5. FORMATION, METABOLISM AND EXCRETION

Estrogens are hormonal substances of widespread occurrence in nature. They are elaborated not only in the mammalian organism but also in lower animals, plants and bacteria, in which they function as growth hormones. They may even be found in carboniferous deposits. In the mammals, estrogens are biosynthesized in the ovaries, adrenals, testes and placenta. The next section will deal with the origin and formation of these compounds, as well as with their metabolism and catabolism and the forms in which they are excreted.

2.5.1. FORMATION

Estrogens are elaborated not only by the ovary but, as we have already mentioned, by the testis, adrenal and placenta. Considerable progress has been made of late in our knowledge of the enzymatic and biochemical mechanisms of their formation. Adrenal and placental elaboration of estrogen will be studied in Chapters 9 and 19. Here we shall limit ourselves to estrogen synthesis by the ovary.

The prevailing view (see Diczfalusy and Lauritzen[46]) has been that estrogens are synthesized from a cholesterol precursor, or—by direct synthesis—from squalene as the starting material, these being the first intermediary products of the steroid series. This has not been proved, since some androgens, progesterone and occasionally even some corticoids have been observed to act as precursors of estrogens, which would thus seem to place the estrogens as end products in the biosynthesis of the entire long series of steroids.

Dorfman and his group[51, 52] had demonstrated that the estrogens of the placenta were being elaborated in the presence of androstenedione. That served as the starting point for the studies of Ryan and colleagues,[176–179] who used ovarian perfusions or incubated fresh ovarian tissue with labeled steroids. Using isotope-labeled cholesterol in their experiments, they witnessed the biosynthesis of pregnenolone, dehydroepiandrostenedione and estradiol. Progesterone is formed directly from pregnenolone following the pathway shown in Figure 2–13.

The human ovary is capable of synthesizing estrogens in vitro not only in the presence of cholesterol,[177] but also in the presence of acetate alone,[94, 176] in the presence of progesterone,[75] as well as when incubated in the presence of pregnenolone.[5, 90, 178] Paradoxically, incubation with testosterone[90, 170, 183] likewise results in the formation of estrogens. All these possible synthetic pathways are taken into account in the diagram of Figure 2–13, which allows for satisfactory explanation of the conver-

Estrogens

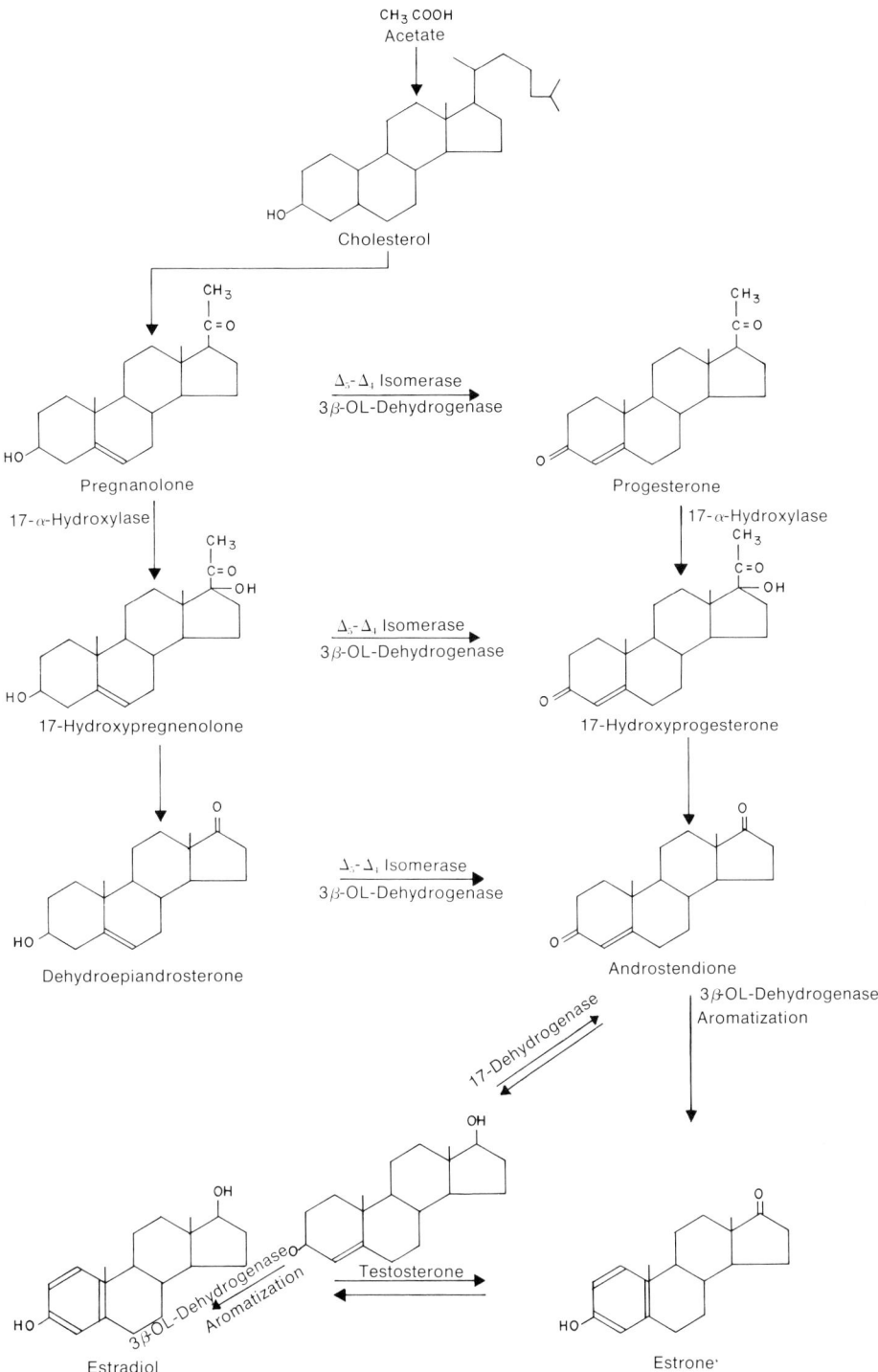

Figure 2–13. Possible metabolic pathways for ovarian estrogen biogenesis. (From Smith and Ryan: *Amer. J. Obstet. Gynec.*, 84:141, 1962.)

TABLE 2-1. Estrogen Content of Ovarian Tissue, of Ovarian Venous Blood and of Peripheral Blood, as Reported by Various Authors

SOURCE	CONCENTRATION (MCG/100 G)	AUTHOR
Entire ovary	35–57	Mahesh and Greenblatt[138]
Follicle	12–188	Smith and Ryan[189]
Corpus luteum	34–289	Zander et al.[221]
Ovarian stroma	12.1	Cedard[36]
Ovarian venous blood	9.1	Kecskes et al.[118]
Peripheral blood	1.5–5.5	Longchampt[132]
Urine	2–6	Botella-Llusiá (unpublished)

sions. It has been demonstrated that, if LH is added to a preparation of human ovary which is being incubated in the presence of any of these substances, the rate of estrogen biosynthesis is increased.[135, 170] A similar phenomenon occurs with FSH.[126] The isolation of the specific enzymes of estrogen synthesis (3β-ol-dehydrogenase and aromatizing enzymes) has been achieved in the ovaries of both rodents[67] and woman.[69, 126]

Until recently, the notion was prevalent that these estrogenic substances were being elaborated by the interstitial ovarian tissue.[105, 106, 173, 186, 213, 216] A look at Table 2-1, which sums up the concentrations reported for these compounds in different structural elements of the ovary as well as in both the venous ovarian and peripheral blood, seems to indicate clearly that the major producers are the follicle and the corpus luteum. Ryan and his co-workers,[178, 179] as well as Forleo and Collins,[75] Lisse[130] and Oakey and Stitch,[153] have incubated ovarian tissue in the presence of acetate and observed the largest amounts of synthesized estrogens in the granulosa cells and the corpus luteum.

2.5.2. CONVERSION AND INACTIVATION

If estrogens are injected into the body of normal females, as was done by Heard and Hoffmann,[98] only a very small amount will be recovered from the urine. A large part of the injected estrogens have been rapidly destroyed by the body. The organ mainly responsible for the destruction of estrogens is the liver.

The part played by the liver in the metabolism of estrogens has been the object of numerous studies, recently again resumed by Pearlman and colleagues[158] and by Jensen and Jacobson.[107] Incubation of estradiol with sliced or homogenized liver, or with free extracts from hepatic parenchymal cells, results in reduction of biologic activity of the incubated estrogen (Heller and associates[100] and Segaloff et al.[185]). Conversely, different clinical or experimentally produced lesions of the liver were noted to be associated with exaggerated biologic activity of estrogens of either endogenous or exogenous origin.

Goldzieher and Fariss[82] have demonstrated that those estrogens which are elaborated by ovarian transplants to the drainage area of the portal vein are biologically inactive. This was subsequently confirmed by other authors.[94, 107]

Evans and his colleagues[63] have studied the metabolism of hepatic steroids by means of hepatic vein catheterization. The experiment, done on nine patients with normal liver function tests, provided proof that if large amounts of estrogens were injected intravenously, their concentration in the suprahepatic vein was significantly lower than in the peripheral veins.[31] This would seem to substantiate the accepted notion that venous blood is being deprived of most of its estrogen concentration on its passage through the liver.

For the first time, in man, this experiment provided an unquestionable procedure for the demonstration of hepatic estrogenolysis. Marks and Hecker[141] have demonstrated that microsomes of hepatic cells contained NADPH and that tritiated estrogens were trapped by the cells in proportion to their content of NADPH, which would seem to suggest specific participation in the processes of estrogen transformation.

The biochemical mechanism of this conversion has been known since it was first described by Pearlman and his associates.[158] An estrinase converts alpha-estradiol to estrone and to estriol. Progesterone activates this conversion.[162] Estrone and estriol may be further converted to bile acids,[51, 52] but a considerable amount of estrogen is eliminated intact in the bile.[46, 47, 98] Diczfalusy[48] has produced evidence to the effect that more than 60 per cent of radioactive estrogens given to a woman are eliminated via feces, not in the urine.

2.5.3. REACTIVATION

The estradiol-estrone conversion reaction in the liver is reversible, so that under certain conditions, as was shown by Ryan,[177] the liver is capable of achieving resynthesis of estradiol. Considering the fact that the latter substance is more potent than estrone, the liver could possibly *reactivate* estrogenic influence. Such reconversion of estrogens has, in effect, already been demonstrated in the uterus, principally on the endometrium, by Pearlman and co-workers[158] and by Pincus,[162] and has been confirmed by others.[123, 204] The endometrium is thought to reactivate estrone by forming estradiol. Recently, the existence of an extrahepatic circulation of estrogens has been strongly supported.[97, 124] Presumably, estrogens eliminated in the bile would reenter the circulation in the bowel and eventually again reach the liver, where, depending on the necessities of the moment, they could be either inactivated or reactivated. In view of this, the circulation of estrogens through the body must be considered as touching on the following main points: in the ovary they are formed, in the liver they are destroyed or occasionally reactivated, and in the endometrium, too, they may be either destroyed or reactivated alternatively. Thus, the blood levels of estrogens, especially of those circulating in their active form, *depend not only on ovarian biosynthesis but also on the reciprocal functional interaction of the endometrium and the liver.* This is a very important concept, which will be emphasized henceforth.

2.5.4. BETA-GLUCURONIDASE

Estrogenic activity in the tissues is linked with the formation of an estrogenic complex with glucuronic acid.[100] The conjugation of estrogens in this form is brought about by an enzyme, glucuronidase, the importance of which was revealed by Fishman in 1944. In order to act upon the tissues of the genital tract, particularly the uterus, estrogens are first conjugated with glucuronic acid by the action of beta-glucuronidase which is present mainly in the liver,[26–38] kidney[47] and uterus.[169] The glucuronidase content of the uterus reflects the capacity of the latter for reacting to estrogenic stimuli.[162, 212] Castration causes the glucuronidase of the uterus, though not that of the liver or kidney, to disappear, so that the uterus of a castrated animal responds poorly to estrogenic activity because estrogens cannot be conjugated at the tissue level of the uterus itself.[170] Aside from that, they can nevertheless act in the active conjugated form, provided that the pathway of elaboration by the kidney or liver is available.[215] The action estrogens exert upon the reproductive organs results in increased glucuronidase production. This would explain the phenomenon by which estrogens are reactivated in contact with uterine tissues.

2.5.5. ESTRINASE

EXTRAOVARIAN BIOSYNTHESIS OF ESTROGENS. It is apparent that, in the absence of ovaries, estrogens can be formed by the adrenal cortex or by the placenta (see Chapters 9 and 19). However, Goldzieher and Fariss[82] report the case of a woman who eliminated 72 mcg of estradiol in 24 hours following castration and adrenalectomy. This speaks in favor of estrogen synthesis in sites other than those discussed, the exact conditions under which this can be accomplished being presently unknown.

2.5.6. CIRCULATION AND EXCRETION OF ESTROGENS

Estrogens are found above all in the ovarian follicles, both graafian and those still in process of maturation (Table 2–1). Contrary to earlier belief, based on the initial investigations, the concentration of the hormones in the follicular fluid is relatively low. Follicular hormone is also found in the rest of the ovary, including the corpus luteum.

In the blood, follicular hormone is present mainly in the serum. The serum levels of the hormone undergo cyclic variations.

However, the quantities involved are so infinitesimal that their measurement is extremely difficult.[203] Larger amounts are present in the urine, in which concentrations range from 35 to 288 mcg per 24 hours.[80] Bioassay methods are unable to differentiate estrone, estradiol and estriol from one another, which can be done by means of chemical procedures, particularly with chromatographic fractionation (method of Brown; see Chapter 23). It can thus be shown that the amounts of estradiol excreted in the urine are insignificant compared with those of other hormones. Estrone predominates during pregnancy, which, as has already been pointed out, is the result of the action that progesterone exerts upon estrone.

Very high concentrations of estrogens are found in the urine of pregnancy, as well as in the placenta. We have already indicated how estrone can be obtained by extraction from the adrenal cortex, testis and male urine, as well as from plants and other organisms.

For several years it has been postulated that, like most of the active steroids, estrogens circulated in the blood in a bound form with a *carrier protein*.[10, 175] Recent work has confirmed the existence of this carrier protein,[109, 145] and Baulieu and his group[12] have shown that estrogens can be quantitated by isolating and measuring the saturation of the carrier protein.

2.5.7. THE TRUE FOLLICULAR HORMONE

It would appear that the genuine form in which the natural estrogens are secreted is that of estradiol; they are found in the form of estradiol in the ovary, and are also carried in this form in the bloodstream. Estrone and estriol are considered as catabolites, even though they are catabolites endowed with biologic activity of their own.

2.6. PHARMACOLOGY

Section 2.5 dealt with the determination of estrogen values and with the definition of estrogen units. Therapeutic use and toxicity of the estrogens will now be summarized.

2.6.1. THERAPEUTIC PREPARATIONS

As indicated in Section 2.2, estrogens are divided into the naturally occurring forms, or estrogen hormones, and artificial forms, or estrogen drugs. From among the former, estradiol and its esters have found the most widespread applications in therapy. The main esters are estradiol benzoate and estradiol propionate. Of the artificial estrogens, the most widely used products are diethylstilbestrol, either free or in form of the dipropionic ester, hexestrol, ethinylestradiol (an artificial estrogen which in spite of its phenanthrene nucleus does not occur in nature), and the derivatives of allenolic and doisynolic acid.

Esterification of the different estrogenic substances is aimed at prolonging the duration of their effects; unesterified estradiol has a short-lived effect, whereas estradiol benzoate has a prolonged effect, and estradiol propionate has an even longer-lasting effect.

2.6.2. ROUTES OF ADMINISTRATION

The route by which estrogens are administered is of great importance. The principal and most common routes in use are the following:

ORAL USE. It has been observed that peroral administration of estrogens is relatively ineffectual.[20, 44] This happens because when estrogens are absorbed through the gut, they enter the portal circulation and are destroyed in the liver,[159, 161] as has already been noted. The capacity of the liver for destroying estrogens varies considerably from one particular type of estrogen to another, being greater for estradiol than for estrone and, in general, much greater for the naturally occurring estrogens than for the synthetic products, which are inactivated to a lesser degree.[184] In order to avoid hepatic destruction of orally administered natural estrogens, a *perlingual* form of administration has been devised. It facilitates the absorption of estrogens by the oral mucosa, particularly the mucosa of the tongue. Estrogens thus gain direct access to the general circulation while by-passing the portal vein. Perlingual absorption can be twofold: in the form of drops to be deposited in the mouth without swallowing, or in the form of buccal tablets, which are kept in the mouth long enough to melt away. While peroral use, with deglutition and intestinal absorption, is the common mode of administration for the synthetic estrogens, during the past 15 years two orally active synthetic estrogens, *Ethinylestradiol* and *Mestranol*, have largely displaced the older derivates of the stilbene series. It seems relevant to mention here the subsequent introduction of *Quinestrol*, which is excreted without being degraded[199] and, as a result of its high degree of solubility in adipose tissue,[3, 144] exerts a protracted effect which makes its actions comparable to those of long-acting "depot" substances.

PARENTERAL ADMINISTRATION. The most effective mode of administration of estrogens is parenterally. Estrogens are commonly injected *intramuscularly* and, although unesterified preparations may be used, it is customary to employ one of the esters that have been mentioned. Oil is usually an adequate vehicle, most commonly sesame oil. *Intravenous* injections are to be limited to cases in which the aim is to produce a "shock" effect, particularly for the induction of labor or for the effects necessary to precipitate menstruation. An interesting development is the injection of *suspensions of crystals*, which has acquired increasing therapeutic application. This is the mode of choice for administering preparations with slow rates of absorption. Suspensions of crystals in an aqueous medium allow the hormone to remain in crystalline form. This is similar to the implantation of tablets, to be discussed presently, except that absorption proceeds at a faster rate because of the small size of the crystals. Because most of the crystal suspensions are painful they are usually given with a small dose of novocaine. Another form of administration, as *emulsions*, has the advantage of causing less pain at the site of injection. Aqueous emulsions of water-insoluble steroids have the advantage of slow reabsorption and of prolonged duration of effects, similar to a retarded injection.[88]

LONG ACTING ESTROGEN PREPARATIONS. The use of tablet inserts for the purpose of achieving estrogen effects of prolonged duration has by now been completely abandoned. A prolonged estrogenic effect, sustained indiscriminately over a period of many months, lacks practical usefulness and is fraught with danger.

Nevertheless, some *long-acting esters of estradiol* have found a wide field of application. Junkmann and Witzel[113] used two of these esters, which were introduced into clinical practice by Boschann.[19] These are valerate and undecylate of estradiol, esters of valeric and undecylic acid, with five and 11 carbon atoms, respectively. An injection of 10 mg of estradiol valerate maintains estrogenic activity in a normal adult woman for two weeks, while the same amount of undecylate is effected for four to five weeks. For reference to the practical application of these drugs, see Chapter 27.

OTHER MODES OF ADMINISTRATION. Topical use of *lotions* has been advised for the breast, vulva and some skin conditions. Estrogens are absorbed through the skin in the same manner as the majority of the steroid hormones. The physician, however, should be alerted against the injudicious use of estrogen-based cosmetic creams which are presently so abundant on the market. Following the use of such creams, effects of chronic estrogen intoxication have been observed.

Another form of administration consists of *vaginal inserts*. Transmucosal absorption of estrogens from the vagina or cervix has also been observed and has been applied for the treatment of vaginal conditions such as leukorrhea and vaginitis, as well as for some trophic alterations of the cervix. Finally, though it has been tested in the form of suppositories, rectal administration does not seem to be practical and offers no advantage over the peroral route.

2.6.3. ANTIESTROGENS

Certain compounds possess antiestrogenic activity. In this regard, the effects of MER-25[147] have been known for some time. It has been later shown that a parent compound of the latter, Clomiphene (see Chapter 28), also possessed antiestrogenic activity and that perhaps the mode of action involved was of that type.[220] Several synthetic compounds (CN-55, 945-27 and CL-868) produce the same effect. The mode of action involved could be shown to consist in blocking estradiol uptake at the uterine receptor level.[33, 57, 220]

2.6.4. TOXIC EFFECTS

High dosages of estrogens, or *continuous, prolonged administration*, may cause *estro-*

gen intoxication. Estrogen induced intoxication may be of two types: acute and chronic. *Acute intoxication* is of a nonspecific nature and results from the action of these compounds upon the liver. The passage through the liver of an excessive dose of estrogens produces malaise, vomiting, liver tenderness and, occasionally, parenchymal cell necrosis. Other acute toxic effects are edema, premenstrual tension, headaches and aching pains in the uterus and breast.

Chronic intoxication is produced by the ingestion of smaller dosages, whose administration is sustained for long periods of time. These effects are more specific and lead to what has been called *iatrogenic hyperestrogenism*. The condition will be dealt with under the discussion of the syndromes of hyperestrogenism. It will become apparent how an imprudent and, above all, a sustained administration of estrogenic preparations, whether instituted by the physician or, as is often the case, without medical consultation, can produce uterine hemorrhage, induration and cystification of the breasts and may even, it is believed, provoke the growth of a latent malignancy. The carcinogenic effects and associated therapeutic dangers of estrogen therapy will be more fully discussed later in this book (see Chapter 46). We must point out, however, that these dangers are never so pronounced as to constitute a contraindication for a judiciously instituted therapy.

Individual susceptibility to estrogen intoxication, whether acute or chronic, varies greatly from one type of preparation to another, as well as from one individual to another. The most toxic effects upon the liver are produced by the synthetic estrogens; the natural estrogens are much less toxic. Individual susceptibility depends above all on the capacity of the liver for destroying the estrogenic compounds in question. Persons suffering from hepatic insufficiency are much more susceptible to estrogenic intoxication. Since the natural estrogens are destroyed by the liver more readily than are artificial ones, it is obvious why the latter are associated with greater toxicity. *In summary, the extent to which the body may become victim of intoxication from an estrogenic compound can be said to depend on the capacity of the liver for destroying that compound.*

REFERENCES

1. Adlercreutz, H.: *Acta Endocrinol.*, 42(Suppl. 72), 1962.
2. Aizawa, Y., and Mueller, G. C.: *J. Biol. Chem.*, 236:381, 1961.
3. Ansari, A. H.: *Fertil. Steril.*, 20:414, 1969.
4. Apelgot, S., et al.: *Ann. d'Endocr.*, 18:849, 1957.
5. Axelrod, L. R., and Goldzieher, J. W.: *J. Clin. Endocr. Metab.*, 22:431, 1962.
6. Bacon, R. L., and Kirkman, H.: *Endocrinology*, 57:255, 1955.
7. Balze, F. A., et al.: *Fertil. Steril.*, 5:421, 1954.
8. Banik, U. K., and Pincus, G.: *Proc. Soc. Exper. Biol. Med.*, 116:1032, 1964.
9. Baum, G. J., and Meyer, R. K.: *Endocrinology*, 58:338, 1956.
10. Barlow, J. J., and Logan, C. M.: *Steroids*, 7:309, 1966.
11. Basabe, J. C., Chieri, R. A., and Foglia, V. G.: *Proc. Soc. Exper. Biol. Med.*, 130:1159, 1969.
12. Baulieu, E. E., Raynaud J., and Milgrom, E.: "Measurement of Steroid Binding Proteins," in *Karolinska Symposia on Research Methods in Reproductive Endocrinology*, 2:104, 1970.
13. Beyer, A. L., and Potts, G. O.: *Endocrinology*, 70:611, 1962.
14. Bitman, J., Cecil, H. C., Menc, M. L., and Wrenn, R. T.: *Endocrinology*, 76:63, 1965.
15. Bitman, J., and Cecil, H. C.: *Arch. Biochem.*, 118:424, 1967.
16. Bo, W. J., Odor, D. L., and Rothrock, M. L.: *Anat. Rec.*, 121:163, 1969.
17. Bo, W. J.: *Amer. J. Obst. Gynec.*, 107:524, 1970.
18. Bogdanove, E. M.: *Endocrinology*, 79:1011, 1966.
19. Boschann, H. W.: *Geburtsh. u. Frauenhk.*, 15:1070, 1955.
20. Botella, J.: *Arch. Gynäk.*, 183:71, 1953.
21. Botella, J., and Nogales, F.: *Arch. Gynäk.*, 189:273, 1957.
22. Botella, J., et al.: *Amer. J. Obstet Gynec.*, 101:665, 1968.
23. Bradbury, J. T.: *Endocrinology*, 68:115, 1961.
24. Brecher, P. I., and Wotiz, H. H.: *Steroids*, 9:431, 1967.
25. Brecher, P. I., Wotiz, H. S., Vigersky, R., and Wotiz, H. H.: *Steroids*, 10:465, 1967.
26. Brooks, S. C., Horn, L., and Horwitz, J. P.: *Biochem. Biophys. Acta*, 104:250, 1965.
27. Brown, W. E., Bradbury, J. T., and Junck, E. C.: *Amer. J. Obstet Gynec.*, 65:733, 1953.
28. Brown, J. E.: *Biochem. J.*, 60:185, 1955.
29. Bullbrook, R. D., et al.: In *Endocrine Aspects of Breast Cancer*, ed. A. R. Currie. Edinburgh, E. S. Livingstone, 1958.
30. Bullogh, W. S.: *Ciba Colloquia on Endocrinology*, 6:278, 1953.
31. Butt, W. R.: *Hormone Chemistry*. London, Van Nostrand & Co., Ltd., 1967.
32. Callantine, M. R., Humphrey, R. R., and Nesset, B. L.: *Endocrinology*, 79:455, 1966.
33. Callantine, M. R., Clemens, L. E., and Shih, Y. H.: *Proc. Soc. Exper. Biol. Med.*, 128:382, 1968.
34. Cecil, H. C., Hanum, J. A., and Bitman, J.: *Amer. J. Physiol.*, 211:1099, 1966.
35. Cecil, H. C., Bitman, J., Hanum, J. A., and Trezise, L: *J. Endocr.*, 37:393, 1967.

36. Cedard, L.: *Les Oestrogenes Naturels.* Paris, Masson et Cie, 1966.
37. Chang, M. C.: *Endocrinology,* 84:356, 1969.
38. Chatterjee, A.: *Endokrinologie,* 50:1, 1966.
39. Claringbold, P. J.: *J. Biol. Sc.,* 81:396, 1955.
40. Clark, J. H., and Gorski, J.: *Science,* 169:76, 1970.
41. Csapo, A., and Corner, G. W.: *Endocrinology,* 51:378, 1952.
42. Csapo, A.: *Rec. Progr. Horm. Res.,* 12:405, 1956.
43. David, M. A., and Kovacs, K. I.: *Pathol. Biol. (Paris),* 15:182, 1967.
44. Davis, M. E.: *J. Clin. Endocr. Metab.,* 13:1551, 1953.
45. Desclin, L., et al.: *Endocrinology,* 70:429, 1962.
46. Diczfalusy, E., and Lauritzen, C.: *Oestrogene beim Menschen.* Berlin, Springer, 1961.
47. Diczfalusy, E., Katz, J., and Levitz, M.: *Steroids,* 6:855, 1965.
48. Diczfalusy, E.: *Acta Gin.,* 16:7, 1965.
49. Dickmann, Z.: *J. Endocr.,* 37:455, 1967.
50. Docke, F., and Dorner, G.: *J. Endocr.,* 33:491, 1965.
51. Dorfman, R.: *Ciba Colloquia on Endocrinology,* 12:62, 1958.
52. Dorfman, R. I., and Kincl, F. A.: *Acta Endocrinol.,* 52:619, 1966.
53. Dowling, J. T., et al.: *J. Clin Endocr. Metab.,* 16:1941, 1956.
54. Dukes, P. P., and Goldwasser, E.: *Endocrinology,* 69:21, 1961.
55. Eckstein, B., and Villee, C. A.: *Endocrinology,* 78:409, 1966.
56. Edgren, R. A., Elton, R. L., and Calhoun, D. W.: *J. Reprod. Fertil.,* 2:98, 1961.
57. Edgren, R. A., Jones, R. C., De Peterson, A. L., and Gillen, A. L.: *Acta Endocrinol. (Suppl.),* 54:115, 1967.
58. Eisenfeld, A. J., and Axelrod, J.: *J. Pharmac. Exper. Therap.,* 150:469, 1965.
59. Eisenfeld, A. J., and Axelrod, J.: *Endocrinology,* 79:38, 1966.
60. Engbring, N. H., and Engstrom, W. W.: *J. Clin. Endocr. Metab.,* 19:782, 1959.
61. Eskin, B. A., and Bogdanove, E. M.: *Endocrinology,* 59:688, 1956.
62. Eskin, B. A., Pratman, M. B., and Petit, M. D.: *Endocrinology,* 69:195, 1961.
63. Evans, J. M., et al.: *J. Clin. Endocr. Metab.,* 12:495, 1952.
64. Everett, J.: *J. Endocr.,* 24:491, 1962.
65. Fainstat, T. H.: *Endocrinology,* 71:878, 1962.
66. Feldman, J. D., and Danowsky, T. S.: *Endocrinology,* 59:463, 1956.
67. Ferguson, M. M.: *J. Endocr.,* 32:365, 1965.
68. Ferrando, G., and Nalbandov, A. V.: *Endocrinology,* 83:933, 1968.
69. Fienberg, R., and Cohen, R. B.: *Amer. J. Obstet. Gynec.,* 92:958, 1965.
70. Fisher, D. A., and Oddie, T. H.: *J. Clin. Endocr. Metab.,* 23:811, 1963.
71. Fishman, J., Hellman, L., Zumoff, B., and Gallagher, T. F.: *J. Clin. Endocr. Metab.,* 27:367, 1967.
72. Folley, S. J.: *Brit. Med. Bull.,* 11:145, 1955.
73. Fonzo, D., Mims, R., and Nelson, D. H.: *Endocrinology,* 81:29, 1967.
74. Forleo, R., and Ingrassia, E.: *Riv. Ost. Gin.,* 18:597, 1963.
75. Forleo, R., and Collins, W. P.: *Acta Endocr.,* 46:625, 1964.
76. Frantz, A. G., and Rabkin, M. T.: *J. Clin. Endocr. Metab.,* 25:1470, 1965.
77. Frieden, E. H., and Baes, F.: *Endocrinology,* 60:270, 1957.
78. Gallagher, T. F., et al.: *J. Biol. Chem.,* 233:1093, 1958.
79. Genet. P., et al.: *Ann. d'Endocr.,* 23:693, 1962.
80. Goering, R. W., Matsuda, S., and Herrmann, R. L.: *Amer. J. Obstet Gynec.,* 92:441, 1965.
81. Goldberg, B., Seegar-Jones, G. E., and Turner, D. A.: *Amer. J. Obstet. Gynec.,* 85:349, 1963.
82. Goldzieher, J. W., and Fariss, B.: *Acta Endocrinol.,* 54:452, 1967.
83. Gorski, J., Noteboom, E. D., and Nicolette, J. A.: *J. Cell. Comp. Physiol.,* 66:91, 1965.
84. Gorski, J., Notides, A., Toft, D., and Smith, D. E.: *Clin. Obstet. Gynec.,* 10:17, 1967.
85. Gottfried, H., Dorfman, R. I., and Wall, P. E.: *Nature,* 215:409, 1967.
86. Govaerts, J. M., et al.: *Endocrinology,* 59:636, 1956.
87. Greenblatt, R. B., MacDonough, P. G., and Mahesh, V. B.: *J. Clin. Endocr. Metab.,* 26:1185, 1966.
88. Greenwald, G. S.: *J. Endocr.,* 33:13, 25, 1965.
89. Greiss, F. C., and Anderson, S. G.: *Amer. J. Obstet. Gynec.,* 107:829, 1970.
90. Griffiths, K., Grant, J. K., and Symington, T.: *J. Endocr.* 30:247, 1964.
91. Grosvenor, G. E.: *Endocrinology,* 70:763, 1962.
92. Hagerman, D. D.: *Endocrinology,* 76:553, 1965.
93. Hagino, N., and Goldzieher, J. W.: *Endocrinology,* 86:29, 1970.
94. Hammerstein, J., Rice, B. F., and Savard, K.: *J. Clin. Endocr. Metab.,* 24:597, 1964.
95. Harper, M. K. J.: *Endocrinology,* 77:115, 1965.
96. Harper, M. K. J.: *J. Endocr.,* 31:217, 1965.
97. Harrington, F. E.: *Endocrinology,* 77:635, 1965.
98. Heard, R. D. H., et al.: *Rec. Progr. Horm. Res.,* 12:45, 1956.
99. Heim, L. M., and Timiras, P. S.: *Endocrinology,* 72:598, 1963.
100. Heller, J. H., et al.: *Endocrinology,* 61:235, 1957.
101. Herbener, G. H., and Atkinson, W. B.: *Proc. Soc. Exper. Biol. Med.,* 106:348, 1961.
102. Hisaw, F. L.: *Endocrinology,* 64:276, 1959.
103. Hoffmann, F.: *Geburtsh. u. Frauenhk.,* 20:1153, 1960.
104. Hoffman, F.: *Geburtsh. u. Frauenhk.,* 21:554, 1961.
105. Howard, E.: *Endocrinology,* 72:19, 1963.
106. Huang, W. Y., and Pearlman, W. H.: *J. Biol. Chem.,* 238:1038, 1963.
107. Jensen, E. V., and Jacobson, H. I.: *Rec. Progr. Horm. Res.,* 18:387, 1962.
108. Jensen, E. V., et al.: *Science,* 158:385, 1967.
109. Jensen, E. V., Suzuki, T., and Numata, M.: *Steroids,* 13:417, 1969.
110. Jepson, J. H., and Loewenstein, L.: *Endocrinology,* 80:430, 1967.
111. Jonsson, C. E., and Terenius, L.: *Acta Endocr.,* 50:289, 1965.
112. Jung, H.: *Klin. Wschr.,* 39:1169, 1961.
113. Junkmann, C., and Witzel, H.: *Erg. Vit. Horm. Forschung,* 9:227, 1958.
114. Kahwanago, I., Le Roy, W., and Herrman, W.: *Endocrinology,* 86:1319, 1970.
115. Kao, C. Y., and Gam, R. S.: *Amer. J. Physiol.,* 201:714, 1961.

116. Kato, J., and Villee, C. A.: *Endocrinology*, 80:1133, 1967.
117. Katzman, P. A.: *Endocrinology*, 76:131, 1965.
118. Kecskes, L., Mutschler, F., Than, E., and Farkas, I.: *Acta Endocrinol.*, 39:483, 1962.
119. Keever, J. E., and Greenwald, G. S.: *Acta Endocrinol.*, 56:244, 1967.
120. Ketchel, M., and Pincus, G.: *Proc. Soc. Exper. Biol. Med.*, 115:419, 1964.
121. Keyes, P. L., and Nalbanov, A. V.: *Endocrinology*, 80:938, 1967.
122. Kincl, F. A., Folch-Pi, A., Maqueo, M., Herrera-Lasso, L., Oriol, A., and Dorfman, R. I.: *Acta Endocr.*, 49:193, 1965.
123. Klebanoff, S. J.: *Endocrinology*, 76:301, 1965.
124. Klopper, A. I., and Dennis, K. J.: *Brit. Med. J.*, 2:115, 1962.
125. Kohler, P. O., and Malley, B. W.: *Endocrinology*, 81:1422, 1967.
126. Kumari, L., and Goldzieher, J. W.: *Acta Endocrinol.*, 52:455, 1966.
127. Laberge, J. L., and Rock, J.: *Fertil. Steril.*, 13:448, 1962.
128. Leonard, S. L.: *Endocrinology*, 72:865, 1962.
129. Lewis, U. J., Cheever, E. V., and Laan, W. P. van den.: *Endocrinology*, 76:362, 1965.
130. Lisse, K.: *Endokrinologie*, 53:78, 1968.
131. Liu, F. T. X.: *Amer. J. Physiol.*, 198:1255, 1960.
132. Longchampt, J. E.: In *Les fonctions endocriniennes de l'ovaire*, ed. M. F. Jayle. Paris, Gauthier-Villars, 1967.
133. Lungkvist, H. I.: *Acta Endocrinol.*, 56:391, 1967.
134. Mac Cann, S. M., and Taleisnik, S.: *Endocrinology*, 69:909, 1961.
135. Mac Donald, G. J., Armstrong, D. T., and Greep, R. O.: *Endocrinology*, 79:289, 1966.
136. Mac Gaughey, R. W., and Daniel, J. C.: *J. Reprod. Fertil.*, 11:325, 1966.
137. Mac Guire, J. L., and Kisk, R. D.: *Nature*, 221:1068, 1969.
138. Mahesh, V. B., and Greenblatt, R. B.: *Rec. Progr. Horm. Res.*, 20:341, 1964.
139. Man, E. B., Reid, W. A., Hellegers, A. E., and Jones, W. S.: *Amer. J. Obstet. Gynec.*, 103:338, 1969.
140. Manning, J. P., Tornaben, J. A., and Schwartz, E.: *Amer. J. Obstet. Gynec.*, 105:412, 1969.
141. Marks, F., and Hecker, E.: *Hoppe-Seylers Ztschr. f. Physiol. Chem.*, 349:523, 1968.
142. Martin, L.: *J. Endocr.*, 23:329, 1962.
143. Martin-Pinto, R., Lerner, U., Pontelli, H., and Robow, W.: *Compt. rend. Soc. Biol.* (Paris), 162:228, 1968.
144. Meli, A., Steinetz, B. G., and Giannina, T.: *Proc. Soc. Exper. Biol. Med.*, 127:1042, 1968.
145. Mercier-Bodard, C., Alafsen, A., and Baulieu, E. E.: *Karolinska Symposia on Research Methods in Reproductive Endocrinology*, 2:204, 1970.
146. Merrill, R. C.: *Physiol. Rev.*, 33:593, 1958.
147. Meyerson, B. J., and Lindstrom, L.: *Acta Endocrinol.*, 59:41, 1968.
148. Mirand, E. A., and Gordon, A. S.: *Endocrinology*, 78:325, 1966.
149. Mitchell, J. A., and Jochim, J. M.: *Endocrinology*, 83:691, 1968.
150. Mobbs, B. G.: *J. Endocr.*, 41:69, 1968.
151. Moricard, R.: *Ann. d'Endocrin.*, 19:943, 1958.
152. Noall, M. W., and Allen, W. M.: *J. Biol. Chem.*, 236:2087, 1961.
153. Oakey, R. E., and Stitch, S. R.: *Acta Endocrinol.*, 58:407, 1968.
154. Palka, Y. S., Ramirez, V. D., and Sawyer, C. H.: *Endocrinology*, 78:487, 1966.
155. Papanicolaou, G. N.: *Acta Cytologica*, 1:70, 1957.
156. Payne, R. W., and Runser, R. H.: *Endocrinology*, 62:313, 1958.
157. Payne, R. W., and Runser, R. H.: *Endocrinology*, 63:383, 1959.
158. Pearlman, W. H., et al.: *J. Biol. Chem.*, 208:234, 1954.
159. Peckman, B., Ladinsky, J., and Kiekhofen, W.: *Amer. J. Obstet. Gynec.*, 87:710, 1963.
160. Pereira-Luz, N., Marques, M., Ayub, A. C., and Correa, P. R.: *Amer. J. Obstet Gynec.*, 105:525, 1969.
161. Peterson, R. E., et al.: *J. Clin. Endocr. Metab.*, 20:495, 1960.
162. Pincus, G.: In *The Hormones*, ed. G. Pincus and K. V. Thimann, Vol. III. New York, Academic Press, 1955.
163. Pincus, G., and Erickson, A. E.: *Endocrinology*, 71:24, 1962.
164. Pollard, I., and Martin, L.: *J. Endocr.*, 38:71, 1967.
165. Psychoyos, A., Alberga, A., and Baulieu, E.: *Compt. rend. Acad. Sc.* (Paris), 266:1407 1968.
166. Pucoa, A., and Bresciani, F.: *Nature*, 218:967, 1968.
167. Puck, A.: *Geburtsh. u. Frauenhk.*, 18:998, 1958.
168. Ramirez, D., and Sawyer, C. H.: *Endocrinology*, 76:1158, 1965.
169. Ranney, R. E.: *Endocrinology*, 65:594, 1959.
170. Rice, B. F., Hammerstein, J., and Savard, K.: *J. Clin. Endocr. Metab.*, 24:606, 1964.
171. Roberts, J. S., and Share, L.: *Endocrinology*, 84:1076, 1969.
172. Rogers, A. W., Thomas, G. H., and Yates, K. M.: *Exp. Cell. Res.*, 40:688, 1965.
173. Romanoff, E. B., and Pincus, G.: *Endocrinology*, 71:753, 1962.
174. Rotchild, I.: *Acta Endocrinol.*, 49:120, 1965.
175. Rosenbaum, W., Christy, N. P., and Kelly, W. G.: *J. Clin. Endocr. Metab.*, 26:1339, 1966.
176. Ryan, K. J., and Smith, O. W.: *J. Biol. Chem.*, 236:705, 1961.
177. Ryan, K. J.: *Acta Endocrinol.*, 44:81, 1963.
178. Ryan, K. J., and Short, R. V.: *Endocrinology*, 76:108, 1965.
179. Ryan, K. J., and Petro, Z.: *J. Clin. Endocr. Metab.*, 26:46, 1966.
180. Saldarino, R. J., and Yochim, J. M.: *Endocrinology*, 80:453, 1967.
181. Sander, S.: *Acta Pathol. Microbiol. Scand.*, 73:29, 1968.
182. Sander, S.: *Acta Endocrinol.*, 58:49, 1968.
183. Schriefers, H., and Schmidet, E.: *Hoppe-Seylers Ztschr. f. Physiol. Chem.*, 349:1085, 1968.
184. Scott, D. B. M., and Paroshey, A. M.: *Biochem. J.*, 82:266, 1962.
185. Segaloff, A., et al.: *J. Biol. Chem.*, 173:431, 1947.
186. Short, R. V.: *J. Endocr.*, 24:59, 1962.
187. Sjoberg, N. O.: *Acta Endocrinol.*, 57:405, 1968.
188. Smith, O. W.: *Endocrinology*, 67:698, 1960.
189. Smith, O. W., and Ryan, K. J.: *Amer. J. Obstet. Gynec.*, 84:141, 1962.
190. Smith, Q. T., and Allison, D. J.: *Endocrinology*, 79:486, 1966.

191. Sol, J. R. del.: *Acta Ginecologica*, 3:337, 1952.
192. Song, C. S., Rifkind, A. B., Gilette, P. N., and Kappas, A.: *Amer. J. Obstet. Gynec.*, 105:813, 1969.
193. Spaziani, E., and Szego, C.: *Endocrinology*, 64:713, 1959.
194. Spaziani, E.: *Endocrinology*, 72:18, 1963.
195. Spaziani, E., and Suddick, R. P.: *Endocrinology*, 81:205, 1967.
196. Spratto, G. R., and Miller, J. W.: *J. Pharmacol. Exper. Therap.*, 161:1, 1968.
197. Stander, S., and Atramadal, A.: *Acta Endocrinol.*, 58:235, 1968.
198. Steinberg, M., Tolksdorf, S., and Gordon, A. S.: *Endocrinology*, 81:340, 1967.
199. Steinetz, B. G., Meli, A., Giannini, T., and Beach, V. L.: *Proc. Soc. Exper. Biol. Med.*, 124:1283, 1967.
200. Stone, G. M.: *Acta Endocrinol.*, 47:433, 1964.
201. Stone, G. M., and Bagget, B.: *Steroids*, 6:277, 1965.
202. Stone, G. M., and Martin, L.: *Steroids*, 5:791, 1965.
203. Svendsen, R., and Sorensen, B.: *Acta Endocrinol.*, 47:245, 1964.
204. Sweat, M. L., Bryson, M. J., and Young, R. B.: *Endocrinology*, 81:167, 1967.
205. Swelhaim, T.: *Acta Endocrinol.*, 49:231, 1965.
206. Szego, C., and Sloan, S. H.: *Gen. Comp. Endocr.*, 1:295, 1961.
207. Tchernichin, A. V.: *Steroids*, 10:661, 1967.
208. Terenius, L.: *Acta Endocrinol.*, 57:669, 1968.
209. Terragno, N., Gutierrez, D. A., and Botella, J.: *Acta Gin.*, 17:177, 1966.
210. Terragno, N.: Thesis, University of Madrid, 1966.
211. Twoombly, G. H., and Lewitz, M.: *Amer. J. Obstet. Gynec.*, 80:889, 1960.
212. Villee, C. A.: *Ann. N.Y. Acad. Sc.*, 75:524, 1959.
213. Vinson, G. P., Norymbersky, J. K., and Chester-Jones, I.: *J. Endocr.*, 25:557, 1963.
214. Waelbroeck, E.: *Ann. d'Endocr.*, 28:236, 1967.
215. Walrabe, V. B. R., and Turner, C. W.: *Proc. Soc. Exper. Biol. Med.*, 107:471, 1961.
216. Wiest, W. G., et al.: *Endocrinology*, 73:588, 1963.
217. Williams, H. E., and Provine, H. T.: *Endocrinology*, 78:786, 1966.
218. Witschi, E.: *Ann. N.Y. Acad. Sci.*, 75:415, 1959.
219. Wrenn, T. R., Bitmann, J., and Wood, J. R.: *Endocrinology*, 82:62, 1968.
220. Wyss, R. H., Karsznia, R., Henrichs, L. R. W., and Herrmann, W. L.: *J. Clin. Endocr.*, 28:1824, 1968.
221. Zander, J., et al.: *Acta Obstet. Gynec. Scand.*, 38:724, 1959.
222. Zarrow, M. X., and Neher, G. M.: *J. Clin. Endocr. Metab.*, 15:203, 1955.

Chapter 3
PROGESTOGENS

3.1. DEFINITION, NOMENCLATURE, HISTORY

3.1.1. DEFINITION

Progestogens, whose synonyms are *gestagens*, *progestins* or *progesteroids*, are compounds capable of provoking the *progravid* or *progestational* reaction, that is, *the preparatory process for the nidation of the ovum* in the uterine mucosa. Just as with estrogens, the biologic concept here has been left badly wanting for a chemical formulization, since under a common heading are grouped a series of compounds that in chemical terms are very difficult to categorize. In attempting to provide a chemical definition, this group of compounds might be said to consist of 3, 20 diketone derivatives of pregnane (a hydrocarbon of 21 carbon atoms) (Fig. 3–1). However, even such a definition must be but a partial one, considering the fact that there are many progestogens that, close as they may come to it, do not conform to the structural composition we have just indicated.

3.1.2. NOMENCLATURE

The natural hormone that is produced by the ovarian corpus luteum in mammals, and in some birds and reptiles,[3, 7, 84] is *progesterone* (Fig. 3–1, II), accordingly also called *luteal hormone* or *corpus luteum hormone*. Because of its action, it has also been called *progestin*. Similarly to estrogens, the number of known naturally occurring active progestogens is small, but the clinical industry has synthesized a large variety of progestogens (of which 16 formulas are shown here) that are not represented in

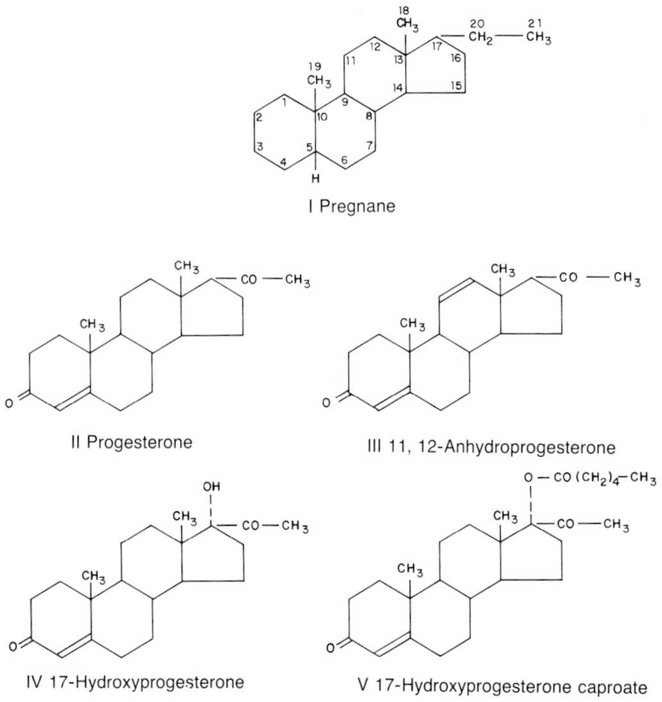

Figure 3–1. Natural and synthetic progestogens.

nature. These are endowed with, if not equal, at least similar activity to that of the *naturally occurring progestogens*. These are called *artificial progestogens* or *progestational drugs*.

3.1.3. HISTORY

Fraenkel was first to suspect the endocrine function of the corpus luteum. Resection of the ovaries of pregnant rabbits, containing corpora lutea, provoked abortion in the animals of his experiments. From this he deduced that the endocrine function of that organ was concerned with the nidation and ultimate development of the embryo. The endocrine significance of the corpus luteum was later assumed, and in part confirmed, by other authors, but no fundamental work was done until 1928, when the investigations of Corner and Allen led to the extraction of an active substance from the corpus luteum of the sow, which not only had the property of preventing abortion in ovariectomized rodents, but which also evoked morphologic endometrial changes similar to those occurring spontaneously in pseudocyesis of those animals. For these reasons, the gestation-promoting hormone was named *progestin* by the discoverers.

These same authors, as well as Clauberg in 1930, noticed that, of all the rodents, rabbits were most sensitive to corpus luteum hormone activity. These investigators devised biologic tests for the demonstration and evaluation of corpus luteum extracts, based on the progravid or progestational reaction of the rabbit uterus, thus establishing the *rabbit unit*.

In 1934, working simultaneously but independently, Butenandt, Westphal and Hohlweg, and Fels, Slotta and Ruschg in Germany, and Wintersteiner and Allen in the United States, obtained a preparation of crystallized luteal hormone whose chemical structure they were able to demonstrate. It is, as we shall see later, a steroid derived from cyclopentanophenanthrene, and chemically speaking a close relative of estrogens as well as of androgens and adrenal cortical hormones. The following year, Butenandt successfully obtained this hormone by means of partial synthesis from cholesterol as the starting material. From 1938 onwards, synthetic progesterone obtained on the basis of Butenandt's patent, or another, similar one, has been commercially available.

In 1938, Ruzicka, Inhoffen and Hohlweg simultaneously synthesized a new preparation: anhydroxyprogesterone, or pregneninolone, which became the second progestogen to be added to the progestogen series. In 1948, Tschopp and Wettstein achieved the synthesis of 11-dehydroprogesterone, a compound that is three times as active as progesterone, and subsequently Tullner and Hertz, in 1953,[158] and Djerassi et al.,[40] in 1954, synthesized the norderivatives of testosterone, whose potent progestational action was meant to revolutionize therapy.

3.2. CHEMISTRY

The hormone extracted from the corpus luteum, and crystallized by Butenandt in 1934, was progesterone (Fig. 3-1, II). It is a steroid derived from cyclopentanophenanthrene, whose three six-membered rings are saturated, with the exception of a double bond between carbons 4 and 5. The cyclopentanophenanthrene has a ketone group at carbon 3 and a ketone chain of two carbon atoms attached to carbon 17. Carbons 6 and 13 have each a methyl group, and finally, the side-chain, which contains carbons 20 and 21, has a ketone group on carbon 20. Progesterone is thus derived from a hydrocarbon of 21 carbon atoms, called *pregnane* (Fig. 3-1, I). This hydrocarbon is of great interest since it also constitutes the precursor skeleton of the adrenal cortical hormones, all of which are pregnane steroids.

Junkmann[80] showed that whereas 17-hydroxyprogesterone (Fig. 3-1, IV) had very little progestational activity its caproic ester (Fig. 3-1, V) possessed not only strong luteoid properties but in addition had a lengthened duration of effects which could be utilized as the basis for the so-called "depot" (pellet implantation) therapy.

In recent years, an enormous number of synthetic progestogens has been developed which are only remotely related to progesterone. Figure 3-2 outlines the principal changes which *potentiate progestational activity* when introduced into the molecular structure of the original hormone. The first change, which incidentally is the oldest and best known, is the substitution by an ethinyl group of

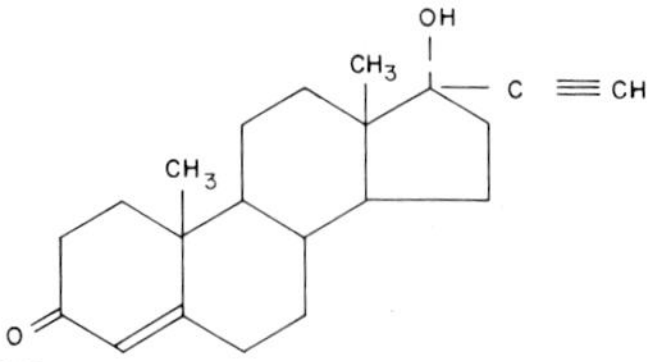

VI Pregneninolone (17-ethinyltestosterone)

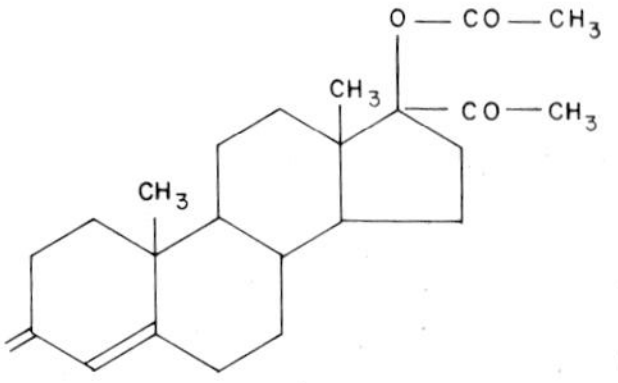

VII Hydroxyprogesterone acetate

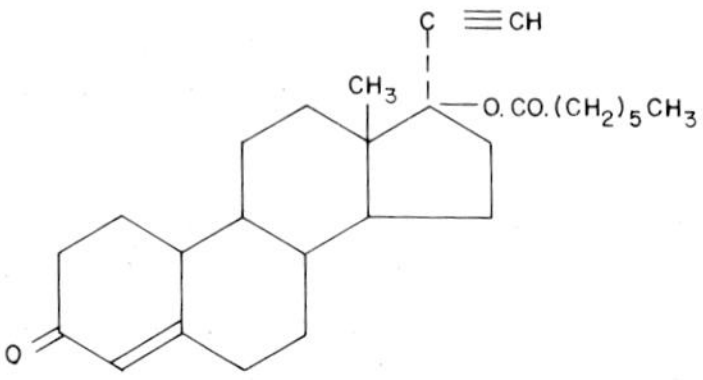

VIII 17-Ethinyl-19-nortestosterone enanthate (norpregneninolone enanthate)

Figure 3-2. Natural and synthetic progestogens (continued).

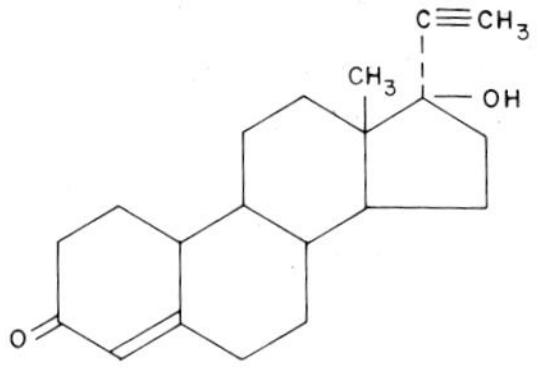

IX Norpregneninolone (17-ethinyl-nortestosterone, or Compound I of Pincus)

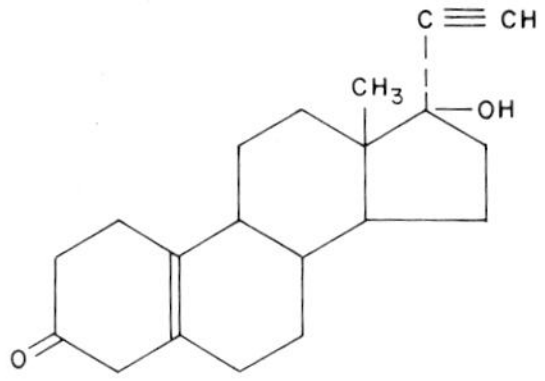

X 17α-Ethinyl-5(10)-estren-17β-3-ol-one (norethynodrel, or Compound II of Pincus)

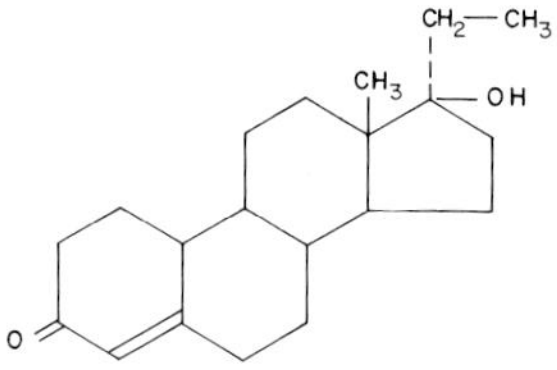

XI 17α-Ethyl-testosterone (Compound III of Pincus)

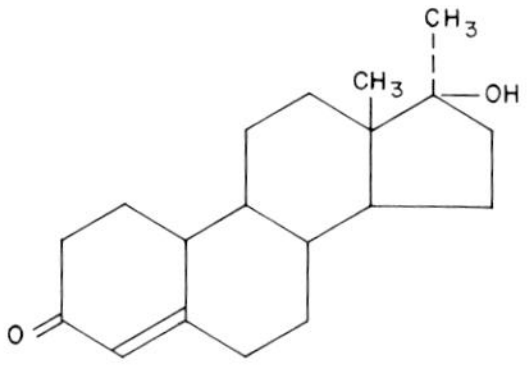

XII 17α-Methyl-19-nortestosterone (Compound IV of Pincus)

Figure 3-3. Natural and synthetic progestogens (continued)

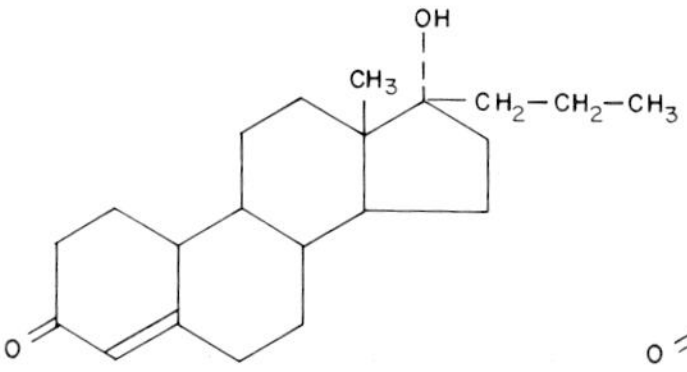

XIII Nortestosterone propionate

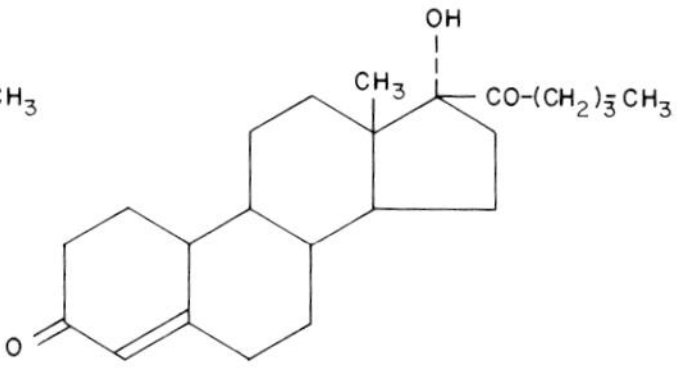

XIV Nortestosterone valerianate

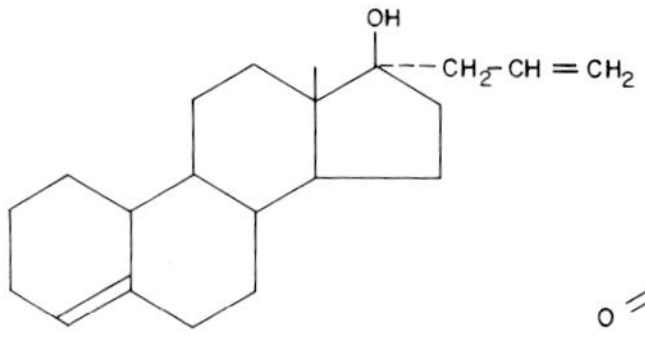

XV Allylestrenol

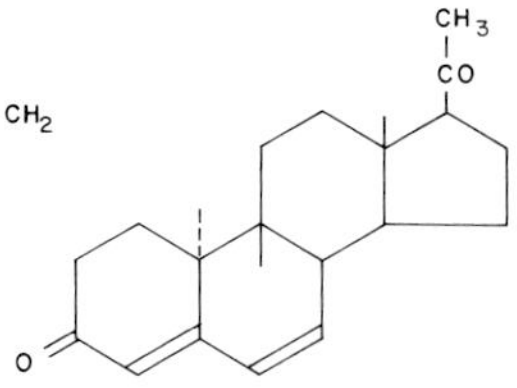

XVI Δ6-Dehydro-*retro*-progesterone

Progestogens

both the ketone and methyl group at carbons 20 and 21. This gives pregneninolone, or ethinyl-testosterone (Fig. 3–2, VI), synthesized by Inhoffen and Hohlweg in 1938.

In 1953, Tullner and Hertz[158] (and in 1954, Djerassi and his colleagues[40]) discovered that the suppression of 19-methylation, a process known as norderivation, resulted in a considerable increase of progestational potency (norpregneninolone, Fig. 3–2, IX). An isomer of this compound is ethynodrel (Fig. 3–2, X), which was synthesized by the same authors, and which was used by Pincus[120] to initiate his studies on hormonal inhibition of ovulation (see Chapter 47). The third type of modification of the progesterone molecule was proposed by Elton and Edgren[46] in 1958, and was based on the observation that esterification of the hydroxyl group at carbon 17 brought about a remarkable enhancement of progestational potency. Visser and Overbeeck[165] have synthesized another compound, allylestrenol (Fig. 3–3, XV), whose uniqueness centers on the elimination of the ketone group at carbon 3. Lynestrenol, which is a 1,3 deoxynorpregneninolone (Fig. 3–3, XII), has, in addition to its progestational action, an anovulatory effect. Another important modification reinforcing progestational activity is achieved by methylation of carbon 6 (6-methyl-17-acetoxyprogesterone, or Provera), introduced by Greenblatt[59] (Fig. 3-4, XVII). On the other hand, halogenation of carbon 6 gives rise to Chlormadinone, which has been tested by Dominguez and his colleagues[41] and by Rubio.[134] As was demonstrated by David[36] and Greenblatt and Rose,[60] esterification of the 6-methyl derivatives with acetic acid, giving C-17 acetates of these compounds, obtains the greatest intensity of progesta-

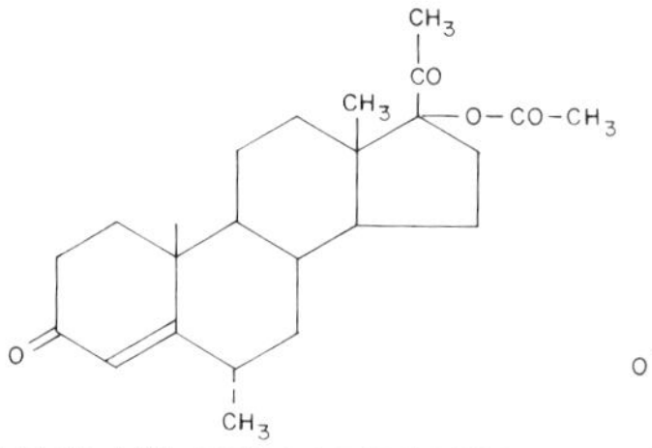

Figure 3–4. Natural and synthetic progestogens (continued).

XVII 6-Methyl-17-acetoxyprogesterone (Provera)

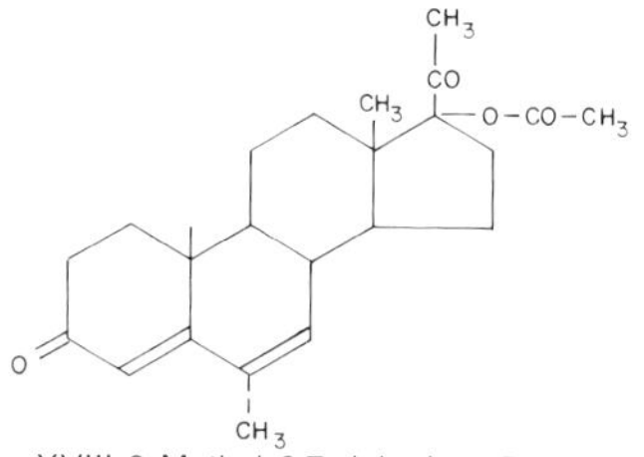

XVIII 6-Methyl-6,7-dehydro-17-acetoxyprogesterone (Megestrol acetate)

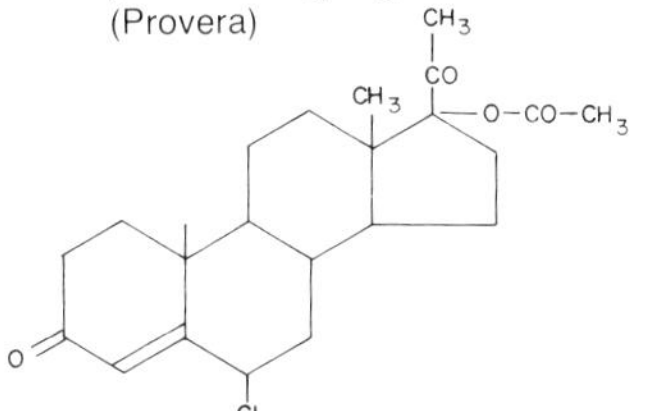

XIX 6-Chloro-17-acetoxyprogesterone

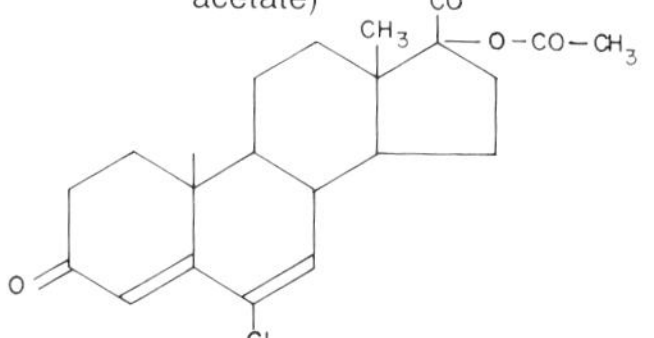

XX 6-Chloro-6,7-dehydro-17-acetoxyprogesterone (Chlormadinone)

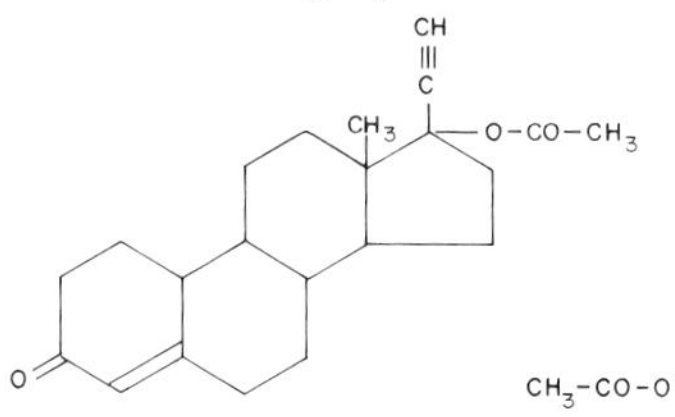

XXI Norethisterone acetate (Norlutate)

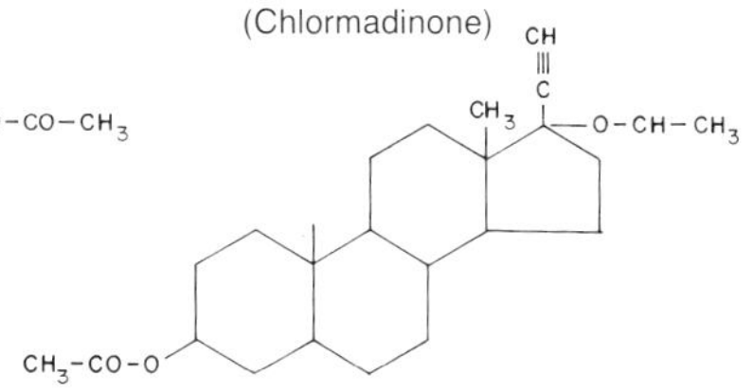

XXII Ethynodiol diacetate

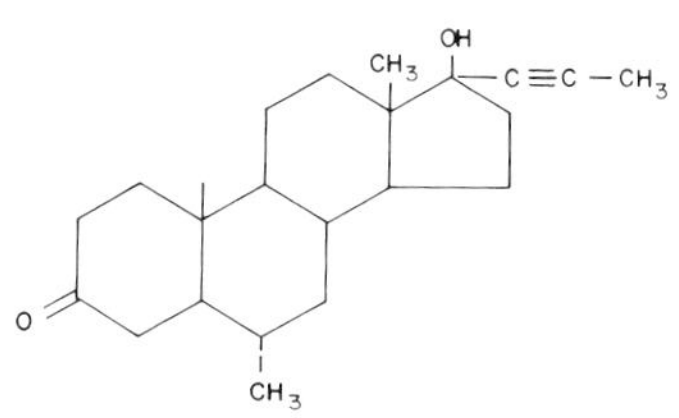

XXIII 6,21-Dimethylethisterone (Dimethisterone)

tional action. It is impossible to give a complete overview of all synthetic progestogens that are presently available commercially. Still to be mentioned, in concluding, are the derivatives of retroprogesterone (Fig. 3-3, XVI), tested by Tillinger and Diczfalusy[157] and by Backer[6] (see Fig. 3-4, XX). In Chapter 47, a final study of the chemistry of these compounds will be made.

3.3. PHYSIOLOGIC ACTION

The actions of progestogens may be described in a similar way to those of estrogens and because of the influence both hormones exert on the female sexual processes, their study from a physiologic standpoint will have to proceed by continuously drawing parallels between estrogens and progestogens.

3.3.1. EFFECTS ON THE OVARY

That progesterone inhibits ovulation in the rat has been known for some time. Studies undertaken by Smith and Bradbury[146] seem to prove that the mechanism of inhibition is mediated by the hypothalamus. The anovulatory effect by a central mechanism, notably of the synthetic compounds, is analyzed in the final paragraphs of this chapter (Section 3.7), as well as in Chapter 47. However, it seems pertinent here not to omit the fact that a direct effect on the ovary currently is suspected to inhibit the growth and rupture of the follicles, as would seem to be proved in the rat by the recent investigations of Zarrow and Hurblut.[175]

3.3.2. EFFECTS ON THE FALLOPIAN TUBES

For a long time we have entertained the likelihood of a nutritional function played by the Fallopian tubes under the influence of the corpus luteum. The ultramicroscopic studies of Stegner[152] seem to confirm this. Harper and his colleagues[66, 67, 68] have shown that ovular transport is very sluggish in the tubes of rabbits and rats treated with different progestogens, which lately has been confirmed on mice[25, 26] and on sows.[39]

We have besides been able to demonstrate the same effects in the human tubes (Terragno et al.;[62, 156] Iglesias et al.[79]). It has been noted that in the human species synthetic progestogens do not affect the rhythm of tubal contractility, but do diminish the amplitude of the contractions. Thus, it would appear that, just as they do in rodents, progestogens produce a certain degree of tubal paralysis in woman.

3.3.3. EFFECTS ON THE ENDOMETRIUM

Most important of all actions of progestogens are the effects they have on the endometrium. These are known as the *progestational reaction* and define the physiology of these compounds. *Thus, while estrogens are defined by their effects upon the vagina, progestogens are rather characterized by their effects upon the endometrium.* The progestational effects upon the uterus vary among different animal species: in the rat, the progestational reaction is characterized by scanty epithelial but pronounced stromal changes (Hooker and Forbes[76]). In the mouse, a similar phenomenon occurs. The stroma becomes loose, its nuclei proliferate and multiply, the interstitial substance absorbs water, and the uterus becomes canalized, presenting a dilated cavity. In the guinea pig, these changes assume even more conspicuous features. The mucosa not only proliferates through an expansion of its stroma and an increase in tissue fluid but also through the glands' acquiring a greater functional complexity and more extensive branching.[84] However, these endometrial changes are most marked in the rabbit. As a result of the action of progestogens, the endometrium of the rabbit is transformed, its glands proliferating to such a degree as to assume a lacework or corkscrew pattern, a reaction which is fundamental for the biologic evaluation and standardization of progestogens. An interesting feature of the progestational effect in the rabbit uterus is that, in order to come to full fruition, it must be exerted upon a previously proliferated mucosa. Consequently, direct injections of progesterone into an infantile or juvenile animal will not produce such a reaction. This may only be observed in adult animals,

Progestogens

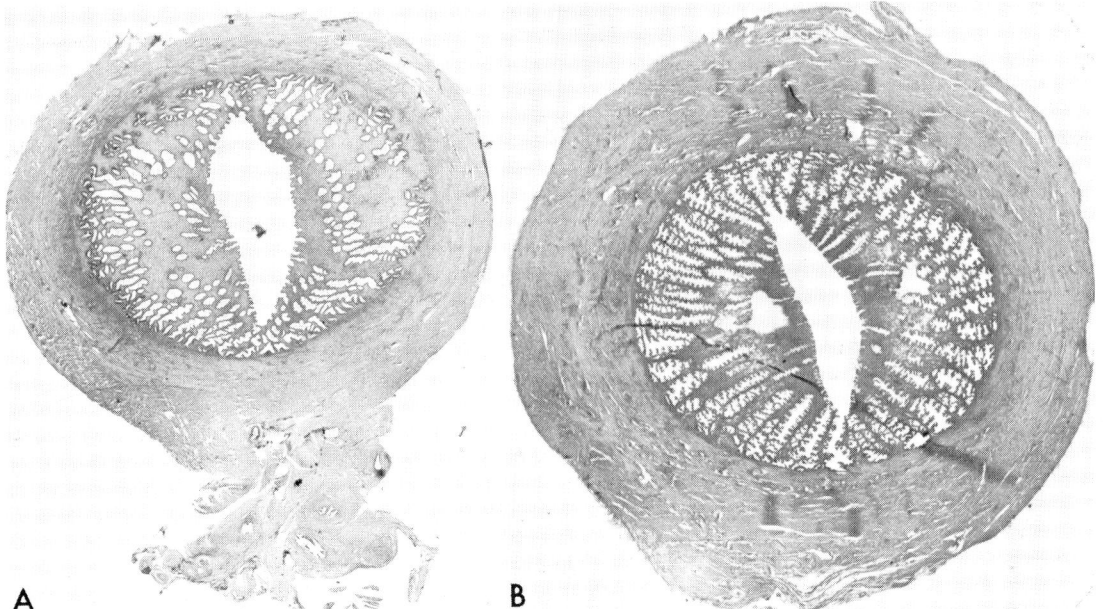

Figure 3-5. Effect of progesterone on endometrium of castrated monkey. *A*, Castrated female *Macaca mulatta*, previously treated with 0.8 mg per kg body weight of estradiol valerianate; proliferative phase (compare with Figure 2-5). *B*, Similar monkey, one week after receiving injection of hydroxyprogesterone caproate (8 mg per kg). Notice well developed secretory phase with characteristic "corkscrew" pattern of endometrial glands.

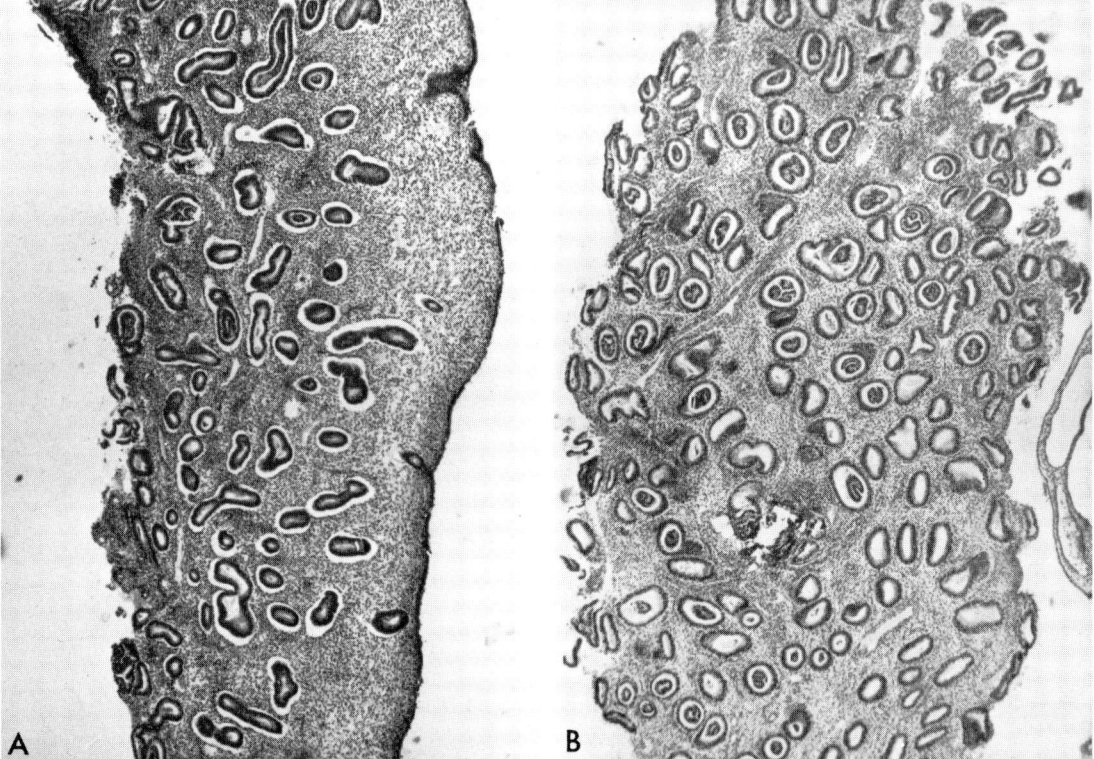

Figure 3-6. Effect of progesterone on endometrium of castrated woman. *A*, Endometrium of castrated woman who, 15 days after surgical castration, received injection of estradiol valerianate (0.8 mg per kg body weight). *B*, Same woman, following a dose of 8 mg per kg of hydroxyprogesterone caproate. First biopsy was taken 14 days after injection of estrogen, the second eight days after injection of progestogen.

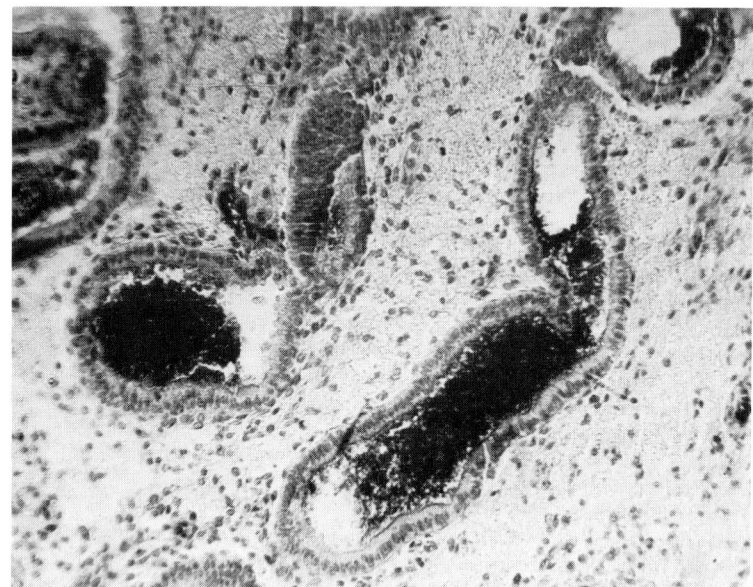

Figure 3-7. Alkaline phosphatase, stained by Gomori method, in secretory endometrium, third week of cycle. Total epithelial depletion is apparent, phosphatase positive material accumulating within lumen. This phenomenon is typical of progesterone activity during third week of cycle.

or in those castrated or juvenile animals which were previously injected with estrogens. In other words, *estrogenic priming in the form of endometrial proliferation is a prerequisite for the full effects of progesterone to be felt.* This is a general rule, which not only applies to the rabbit, but also to the human species.

In woman, progesterone produces the *secretory* phase of the endometrium. The characteristic features of this phase are the following: (1) glandular dilatation; (2) decreased height of gland epithelium, with parabasal arrangement of nuclei (Fig. 3-6); (3) festooned configuration of the glandular basement membrane, with formation of infolding connective tissue spurs; (4) great development of vascular supply, with distinct outlining of the spiral arterioles (Fig. 3-7) (this last reaction was brought to light by Moricard and by Cremades and Botella[29] only recently); (5) the appearance of glycogen in the endometrial glandular epithelium, which first localizes in the subnuclear basal portion of the cells but, in the course of major and sustained progesterone activity, becomes displaced towards the lumen-oriented pole of the cells and is eventually secreted (Fig. 3-8),[16] and (6) changes in alkaline phosphatase distribution, demonstrated by Cremades, Sanchez-Rivera and Botella,[30] which consist of deposits of the enzyme in the vascular endothelium and the depletion of phosphatase from the gland epithelium associated with its accumulation in the lumen (Fig. 3-9).

Pincus and his co-workers[112] have demonstrated that one of the very important actions of progesterone upon the endometrium is to produce in it a measurable increase of *carbonic anhydrase* activity. The phenomenon is alleged to be sufficiently specific to warrant its utilization for the bioassay of the hormone.

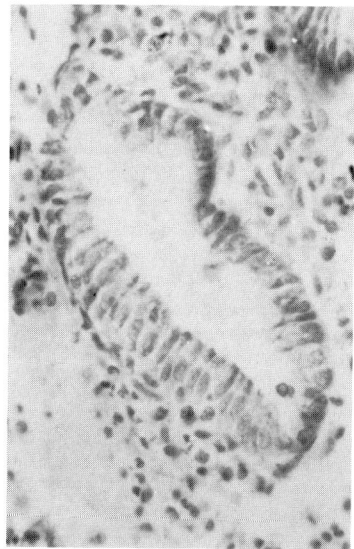

Figure 3-8. Endometrium under the effect of progesterone. Abundant glycogen within gland epithelium. Hotchkiss-MacManus reaction, with glycogen staining cherry-red.

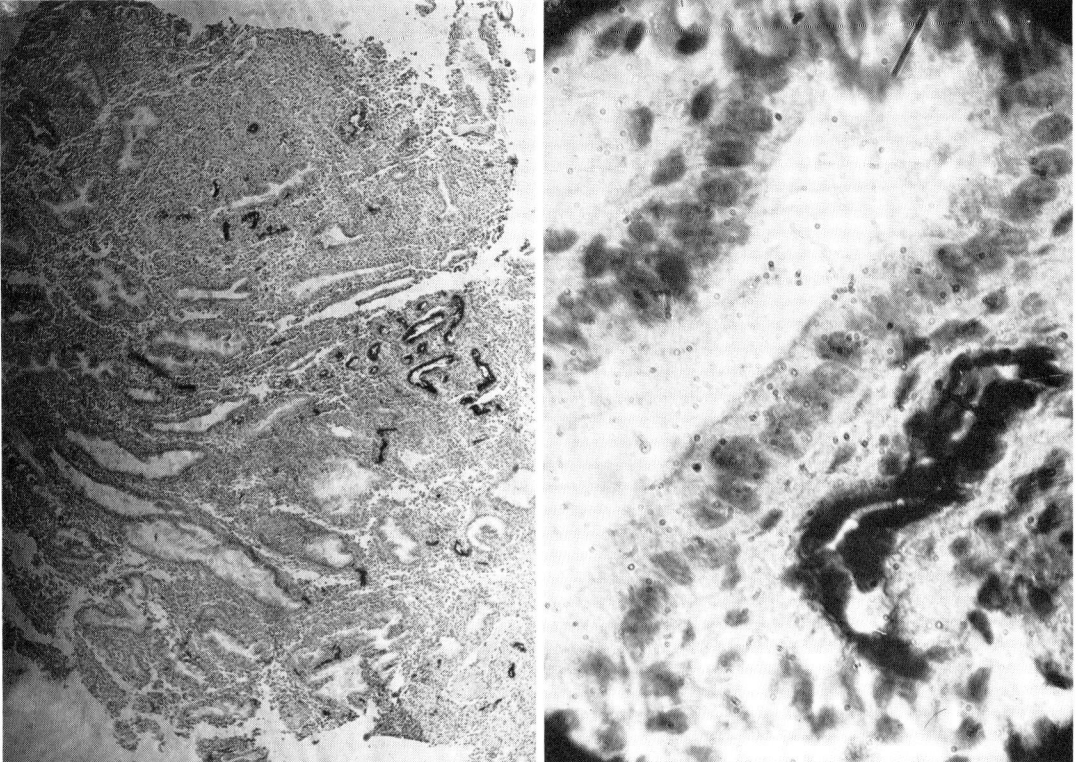

Figure 3–9. Endometrial spiral arterioles during secretory phase. Gomori stain for alkaline phosphatase. Vascular endothelium, rich in alkaline phosphatase, gives strong characteristic staining reaction, in sharp contrast against background of secretory endometrium.

3.3.4. EFFECTS ON THE MYOMETRIUM

Progesterone also exerts an action on the myometrium, as was first demonstrated by Robson and Knaus. It consists in paralyzing the spontaneous contractions of the uterus and takes place in both rodents and man. Of late, such action of progesterone on spontaneous uterine activity was also demonstrated on isolated strips of the sow uterus (Csapo[32,33]) and the uterus of woman (Sandberg and Slaunwhite[140]).

In Chapter 2, it was already mentioned that Csapo and Pinto-Dantas[34] had studied the effects of both estrogens and progesterone on the intra and extracellular sodium and potassium contents of the uterine muscle. Estrogens tend to raise the intracellular concentration of potassium while, at the same time, lowering the sodium moiety within the cell. It was possible to confirm such a mechanism of action in the last few years.[34,88]

Progesterone acts in the opposite way and thus decreases cell membrane potential.

Csapo suggested that this mode of action was not only operative at the level of the myometrial cell but was also representative of the specific activity of estrogens and progesterone in general.

Identical results concerning the action of progesterone on the myometrium were obtained from studies realized on isolated human uterine muscle.[20,24,90] Bo and his colleagues[12] have studied the ultrastructural changes occurring in the myometrium under the effect of progesterone activity. Greiss and Anderson[61] have observed increased vascularization of the uterine muscle, and Mitchell and Jochim[111] noted a rise in uterine oxygen tension under the influence of progesterone. Also, by injecting this hormone into the ewe, Hindson and his co-workers[75] have been able to delay the onset of labor.

3.3.5. EFFECTS ON THE UTERINE CERVIX

Progestogens have a strong blocking effect on the secretion of cervical mucus.

This is one of the most important mechanisms of their contraceptive action, a fact we have been able to demonstrate in our recent work.[29, 30] In cooperation with Nogales,[17] we have also found evidence that the neutral mucopolysaccharide content of the cervical glands is diminished by the action of progesterone.

3.3.6. EFFECTS ON THE ENDOMETRIAL MUCOSA IN NIDATION OF THE OVUM

Progesterone produces and favors those changes which are necessary to make nidation of the ovum possible. These changes consist in the formation of a decidua (Chapter 19), an activity of progesterone that has been demonstrated by a great many authors. Elevated levels of progesterone in rodents are capable of inducing a pseudotumoral growth of the endometrium, with the production of a deciduoma.[53, 54]

Recent studies[24, 120, 162] provide evidence that although progesterone activity is indispensable for the implantation of the blastocyst in the uterine mucosa, a certain degree of estrogen-progesterone equilibrium is also necessary. When using synthetic progestogens, we have been able to observe the loss of nidation-promoting properties of the endometrium.[31, 139]

In the mechanism of nidation, a most important intermediary function is being discharged by the activity of *carbonic anhydrase*, which has been studied by Pincus and his colleagues.[11, 112, 118] This enzyme, deposited as a result of specific progesterone activity, effects endometrial alkalinization and endometrial tissue autolysis in the presence of the egg nearing implantation.

3.3.7. EFFECTS ON THE VAGINA

The appearance of characteristically folded basophilic cells in human vaginal cytology during the luteal phase of the cycle has been well documented (Fig. 3–10).[169] Changes consisting in the *mucification* of the superficial layers of the vaginal epithelium have been observed in the rat and are particularly conspicuous in the guinea pig[24] under the effect of progesterone. A similar phenomenon had not been thought to occur in the human species, but Botella and Nogales[17] were able to confirm it by histochemical means.

Thus, the folding and basophilia of the cells, which are characteristic of vaginal smears of the second half of the cycle and of pregnancy, appear to result from a progesterone-induced accumulation of neutral mucopolysaccharides in the most superficial, shedding, layers of the mucosa.

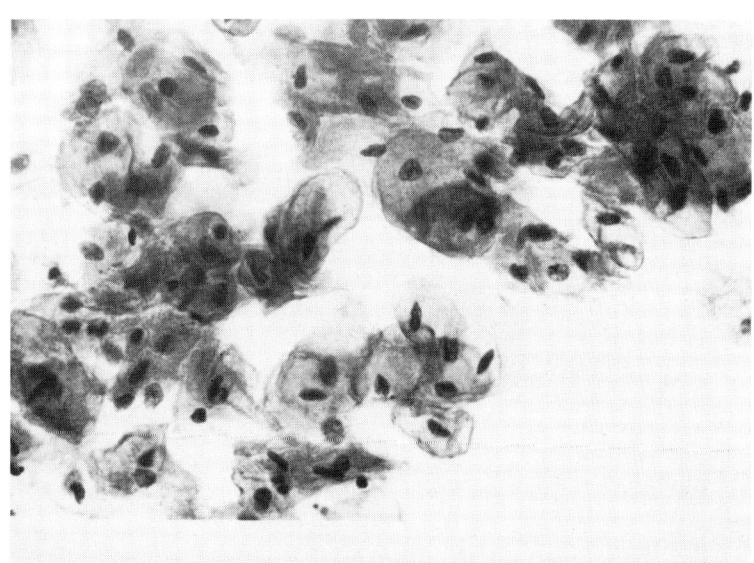

Figure 3–10. Vaginal smear from castrated woman, receiving 0.8 mg per kg estradiol valerianate 15 days after castration, followed by 8 mg per kg hydroxyprogesterone caproate 48 hours later (Compare with Figure 2–11.) Vaginal smear was taken seven days after second injection. Notice folded cells in clumps or clusters, characteristic of progestational activity. Nuclear pyknosis is no longer evident.

3.3.8. EFFECTS ON THE GLANDS OF INTERNAL SECRETION

Pituitary and hypothalamus. Sawyer and Everett[142] have demonstrated that progesterone stimulates FSH release on part of the pituitary. The release mechanism is triggered by the hypothalamus in a manner which makes the authors believe that the point of attack of the hormone is at the sexual centers of the tuber cinereum. In contrast, the hormone affects LH release conversely, by blocking it.[65, 114, 133] According to Caligaris and co-workers,[21] the dosage capable of producing an FSH "feedback" effect in woman is 2 mg, while on the other hand, our group,[139, 139a] as well as Keever and Greenwald,[85] have failed to find any effect by progesterone or its analogues on FSH release in woman.

The principal ovulation-inhibiting effect of the contraceptive drugs corresponds not to progestogens but to estrogens (see Chapter 2, Section 2.3.5, and Chapter 47). Nonetheless, a certain depressive effect is unquestionably exerted on the sexual nucleus of the hypothalamus. In recent studies with Cremades, Sanchez-Rivera and Merlo,[30, 139] we found also that some of the pure synthetic products of progestogens have a potent anovulatory action by way of the hypothalamus. Because a similar mechanism is operative with corticoids in relation to ACTH and to other hormones, it may be said in general that the addition of one hormone *determines the suppression of the release mechanism of its corresponding trophic hormone, thus bringing into play a process of hormonal equilibration or compensation* (rebound mechanism). It should be mentioned furthermore that Roberts and Share[128] have found that progesterone acts on the hypothalamus of the ewe by diminishing *oxytocin* secretion.

Thyroid. Many years ago, this author postulated an inhibitory effect of progesterone on the thyroid gland. Direct evidence of such action has ultimately been obtained.[18, 52a]

Adrenals. Progesterone produces an increase in thickness of the adrenal, particularly of the zona fasciculata.[15] All C-21 steroids are known to be linked by a common metabolism, and it might be difficult to conceive progesterone biosynthesis as occurring in any tissue without concomitant elaboration of corticoids. This is particularly true about the adrenal cortex and the placenta.[70] Therefore, progesterone is a normal component of adrenal tissue, from which it can be extracted (see Chapter 9). Progestogens moreover have an *antialdosterone effect*, blocking the activity of that hormone[43] and lowering tissue sodium retention.[105]

3.3.9. OTHER EFFECTS

Effects on the breast. Progesterone activity exerts a very important and manifest effect on the breast. In small quantities progesterone produces acinar proliferation. In higher dosages, it may provoke the onset of acinar secretion.[19] This secretion is never genuine milk—which, as we shall see later, requires a specific stimulus—but is a kind of trial-run secretion: *colostrum*. An abrupt drop from previously elevated levels of both estrogens and progesterone, such as is observed at time of delivery, may precipitate genuine secretion, which is the subject of more detailed discussion in Chapter 22.

Metabolic effects. *This hormone, as well as all other steroid hormones with a saturated ring structure (androgens and corticoids), exerts an anabolic action.* In this respect, the three hormones differ from estrogens which, on the contrary, exert a *catabolic action.*

The anabolic action of progesterone and its derivatives was recently brought to light by the studies of Landau and his colleagues.[91] Progesterone also influences lipid metabolism, by decreasing lipemia and ketonemia, and by increasing the excretion of water and sodium in the urine.[105]

As disclosed by recent studies, the anabolic action of progesterone affects very particularly the metabolism of proteins. The hormone behaves as an *anabolic steroid*,[91] although to a lesser extent than do certain androgens. This action is particularly important in regard to *the uterus*[2] *and the liver*.[50, 87, 148]

Thermogenic effect. Modern knowledge has sufficiently well established the fact that progesterone raises *basal body temperature*, an action which accounts for the increase of basal temperature during the second half of the cycle. Landau and Lughibil[91] believe that this effect is the result of stimulation of the thermoregulatory centers of the hypothalamus.

Such action cannot be ascribed to thyroid stimulation, since we believe that progesterone has been shown to have an inhibitory effect on the thyroid (see Section 3.3.8). Furthermore, Rotschild[133] has shown that in thyroprival animals, the temperature elevation reappears after injection of progesterone. The studies of Wrenn and his colleagues,[172] and of Freeman and co-workers,[55] performed on different animals, have provided proof that the thermogenic action is not dependent on the administration of estrogens or of other hormones but is a primitive and specific effect of progesterone upon the hypothalamic thermoregulatory center.

Effects on the maintenance of life in corticoprival animals. We have been able to demonstrate that the action of progesterone can be life-saving in adrenalectomized animals.[15] This action can be demonstrated not only in animals but also in the human species. In Chapter 9, the experiences which led to the establishment of this principle are discussed in detail. The idea which has gained widest acceptance is that progesterone can easily be converted to corticoids. The basic pregnane nucleus, common to all of these compounds, must be kept in mind.

Miscellaneous effects of estrogens and progesterone. In-tandem actions of estrogens-progestogens. It has long been known that the progestational changes of the uterus cannot be produced in a castrated animal, or in one lacking endogenous estrogen secretion, without pretreatment with estrogens.[73, 167] The necessity of sensitizing the animal uterus with estrogens for a meaningful bioassay of progesterone has been universally accepted. Estrogen-priming has been found equally essential in order that a whole series of progesterone effects will take place as an adequate functional response. Thus, neither the effects on the animal endometrium, nor those actions which operate upon the human endometrium, upon myometrial growth[162] and upon the growth of the breasts,[158, 159] can occur, even under the best of circumstances, unless their target organs have previously been prepared by the actions of the estrogen group of hormones. As for the stimulus necessary to precipitate menstruation or lactation, the hormone withdrawal required for either phenomenon to occur is likewise an event which neither of the isolated hormones per se is capable of accomplishing (see Chapter 12). *Progesterone, therefore, may be viewed as the continuator of estrogenic activity. Notwithstanding the antagonistic actions of the two hormones, there also exists a phenomenon of mutual continuity and integration of their effects.*

Estrogen-progestogen antagonism. Inhibition of progestational activity by estrogens and vice versa has likewise been observed by many workers.[45] Progesterone given simultaneously with estrogens reduces the proliferative effect of the latter on the endometrium.[87, 91] The anti-estrogenic effects of progesterone were lately summarized by Rudel and his colleagues.[135]

It was pointed out in Chapter 2 (see Section 2.3.8) that *not all estrogens act in a fashion equally antagonistic with regard to progesterone.* Estradiol preconditions the endometrium for the action of progesterone but, in the presence of progesterone, neutralizes its effects, whereas the action of *estriol* is synergistic with progesterone activity.

Progestogens are also known to accelerate the rate of estrogenolysis[80, 81] by speeding up the estradiol-estrone-estriol conversion process. While estrogens are known to enhance libido, progesterone has the reverse effect. This phenomenon is particularly evident in female monkeys.[71, 109]

Anesthetic action. Progesterone has a moderate anesthetic action[108]; according to Cross and Silver,[31a] this is of centrogenous origin. All synthetic progesteroids also exert a more or less defined anesthetic action,[108] and some in addition produce a hypnotic effect on the hypothalamus.[63]

Antirheumatic action. Considering the fact that progestogens are C-21 steroids with similarities to corticoids, as was pointed out previously, it is not surprising that some of them should have been shown, by Davidson and Koets,[38] to possess moderate antirheumatic action.

3.4. BIOLOGICAL ASSAY AND CHEMICAL DETERMINATION

Progesterone can be determined by either chemical or biologic means. Unlike the case with estrogens, in which biologic estimation is simple and chemical determination much more difficult, *with proges-*

togens, chemical determination is easier to perform than bioassay.

3.4.1. BIOASSAY

Except for pharmacologic purposes, the bioassay procedures of early days have fallen into disuse. Still of some practical value are the micromethods of Hooker and Forbes and that of Miyake and Pincus.

In Hooker and Forbes's[76] procedure (Fig. 3-11) progestational activity is determined by means of injecting the uterine horn of the mouse. Following ligation of the horn at two points, an infinitesimal volume of the test substance is injected between the two ligatures. As little as one tenth of a microgram of progesterone, according to the opinion of some authors, provokes the characteristic reaction in the endometrium. This consists of nuclear proliferation of the endometrial stroma associated with typical changes (Fig. 3-12). The method allows detection of minute quantities of progesterone and has been found suitable for demonstrating the presence of progesterone circulating in the blood. An improved modification of this method has recently been introduced by Leroy and his colleagues.[94]

In 1959, Pincus and his group[112] reported that progesterone quite specifically increased the content of *carbonic anhydrase* in the uteri of rats, guinea pigs and rabbits. The test, which is based on injecting progestogens into the animals and subsequently determining the uterine content of the enzyme, is claimed by the authors to be the most sensitive biologic test for the estimation of progestogens available (see Chapter 24).

3.4.2. CHEMICAL METHODS OF DETERMINATION

Until recently, there were no chemical methods available that would allow detection of progesterone in the blood. Therefore, indirect methods, which made use of procedures measuring the *urinary excretion of pregnanediol*, were necessary. Pregnanediol is a catabolite which is eliminated in the urine in considerable quantities—up to 12 mg per day of each cycle and as much as 50 mg during pregnancy near term. These quantities are large enough to permit their determination with a sufficient degree of accuracy. A detailed description of the procedure for the determination of urinary pregnanediol can be found in Chapter 24. A good review of techniques for pregnanediol has also been published by Bongiovanni and co-workers.[13]

Thanks to the recent work of Zander and his group, two complicated but precise chromatographic methods for the determination of plasma[173] and tissue[174] progesterone levels have been developed. Currently, the two techniques are credited with the measurement of minimal amounts of progesterone not merely in the blood but also in some tissues, such as the corpus luteum, the adrenals and the placenta.[137, 141, 174]

3.5. FORMATION, METABOLISM AND EXCRETION

3.5.1. SITES OF BIOGENESIS

Progesterone is elaborated in the *ovary*, in the *adrenals* and in the *placenta*. In the testis, it is possibly also formed as an intermediary stage in androgen synthesis.[102]

OVARY. It is generally admitted that the principal sites of biogenesis are the *granulosa-lutein cells* of the corpus luteum in both the progestational cycle and during gestation.[69, 70]

The progesterone concentration in the ovarian venous blood of the sow was found to be proportional to the degree of ovarian luteinization.[107] Identical results were also

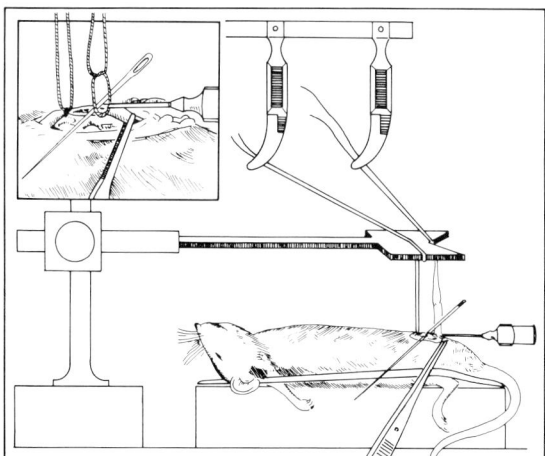

Figure 3–11. Method of Hooker and Forbes for bioassay of progesterone. (From Hooker and Forbes.[76])

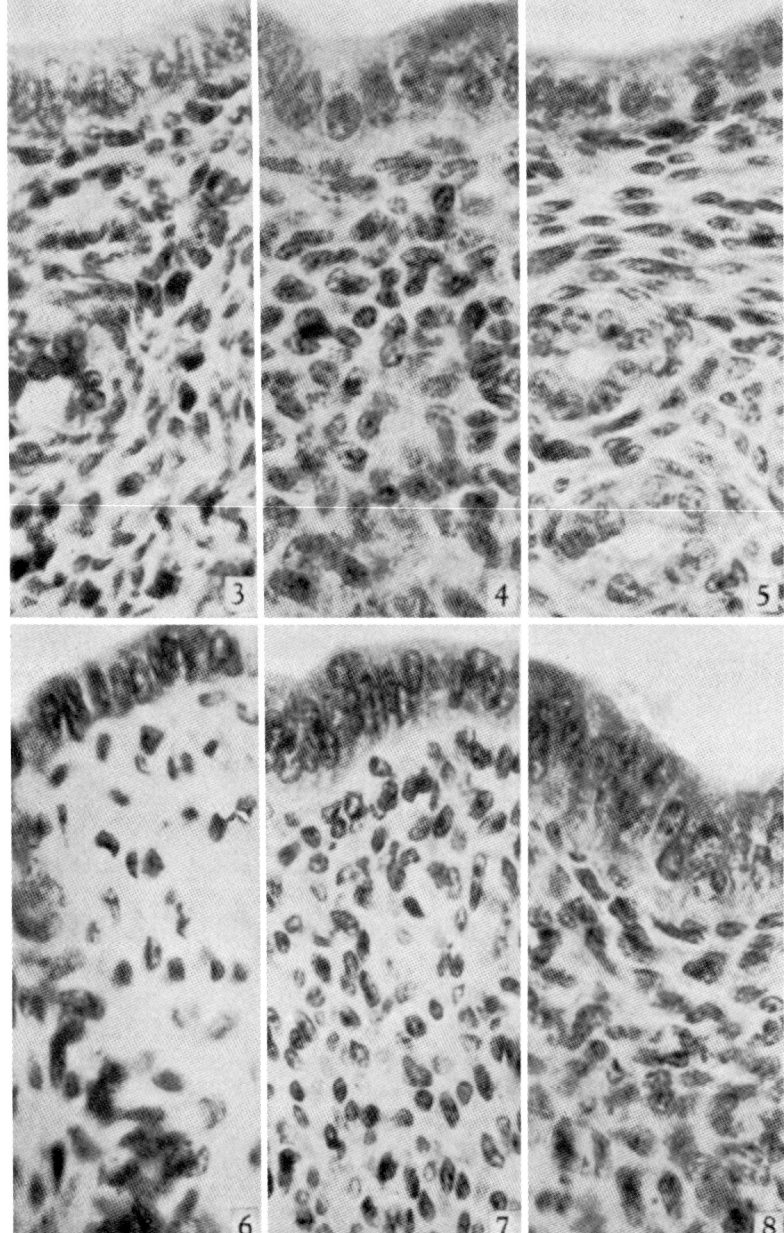

Figure 3-12. Histology of stromal cellular changes in rat endometrium with positive reaction to progesterone (4). Compare with no treatment (3), injection of sesame oil (5), deoxycorticosterone acetate (6), testosterone (7), and estradiol (8). (From Hooker and Forbes.[76])

obtained from the human ovary.[22] Perfusions of cow ovary[9] give greater yields of progesterone, if associated with injections of LH or prolactin. By incubating in vitro slices of ovary or of ovarian zones, Lisse[98] and Maire and his colleagues[104] have been able to observe progesterone synthesis to be principally bound to the theca and granulosa-lutein cells.

However, Forbes[53] and Zander,[173] with the use of their micromethods, have been able to detect a *preovulatory progesterone level* in the blood. Similar results have been reported by Van Der Molen and Groen[161] with the application of a gas-liquid chromatographic procedure. Already, more than 15 years ago, Kaufmann and Zander[82] had observed a preovulatory appearance of glycogen in the endometrium, a fact which we, in cooperation with Nogales, have been able to confirm on many occasions. The assumption would seem justified that progesterone may be elaborated in minimal quantities in the wall of the follicle, in the ovarian stroma and in the adrenal cortex.

PLACENTA. The placenta was one of the earliest recognized sources of progesterone production. Placental progesterone biosynthesis is so precocious that we were able to witness the normal continuation of pregnancy in a woman whose two ovaries had been removed on the twenty-seventh day of the cycle in which conception had taken place. It could later be established that, prior to its implantation in the uterus, the blastocyst of the rabbit was already elaborating small amounts of progesterone.[78, 95] The mechanism of placental progestogen synthesis has been studied by Smith and Ryan[145] and by Warren and Salhanick.[166] The results of these studies will be amplified in Chapter 19.

ADRENALS. The biogenesis of progesterone in the adrenals is related to its function as a precursor (see Chapter 9) in the biosynthesis of the mineralocorticoids and glucocorticoids, which, similarly to progesterone, are all closely related steroids with 21 carbon atoms (C-21 steroids). Our work of many years ago[15] had already envisaged adrenal progestogen synthesis, which by now has definitely been established. *Both adrenal and ovarian steroid biogenesis are two partial aspects of a common metabolism.* This metabolic kinship welds a close link between all steroid hormones—estrogens, progestogens, androgens and corticoids—*but very especially all steroids of 21 carbon atoms*, i.e., progestogens and corticoids.

3.5.2. BIOGENESIS OF PROGESTERONE

Experiments on ovaries perfused with radioactive substances,[69, 70] investigations of in vitro incubation of hormones,[113, 154] and an impressive array of microchemical and histochemical studies[137, 145, 146, 174] have demonstrated that progesterone is synthesized in life either from cholesterol as the starting material, or by direct synthesis through polymerization of groups of methyl acetate, giving the hydrocarbon *squalene*, which is capable of closing into an unsaturated ring structure of the estrane type. The intermediary metabolite which gives rise to progesterone is *pregnenolone*. There are three *fundamental enzymes* in progesterone synthesis: (1) *20α-hydroxydehydrogenase*, the agent of the principal, although not the only, change conducive to the conversion of cholesterol to pregnanolone, whose action was brought to light by Hechter and Pincus[70] and by Bongiovanni and colleagues[13] and was subsequently confirmed by many other workers.[10, 14, 42, 43, 69] (2) *Δ5,Δ4 isomerase*, which is responsible for the transfer of the double bond from one ring to another. (3) *3β-ol-dehydrogenase*, which converts pregnenolone (alcohol-ketone) to progesterone (diketone), thus conferring progestogenic action on the compound.

Current utilization of C-14 labeled hormones has not only brought about a number of new developments,[77, 113, 138, 144, 154, 164] but has also made it possible to isolate these enzymes, especially the first and third, from the ovary. Wiest and associates[171] and Savard and co-workers[141] succeeded in isolating 20α-hydroxydehydrogenase, and Goldberg and colleagues[58] in 1963, also obtained 3β-ol-dehydrogenase, detected and located earlier histochemically by Fuhrmann[56] *in the corpus luteum*, to the exclusion of any other ovarian tissues.

The incubation of corpus luteum tissue cultures in the presence of C-14 labeled cholesterol yields larger amounts of progesterone, if LH is added[27, 64]; however, more up-to-date reports[28, 29] claim better yields of the hormone from incubation performed in the presence of C-14 labeled acetate, instead of cholesterol. It would thus appear that acetate is a more fundamental building stone of progesterone biogenesis. Rice and Segaloff used C-14 labeled acetate in cultures of rat ovaries and reported predominant progesterone and no estrogen formation in the presence of LH.[126] The same authors[125] have demonstrated that the corpus luteum which, as a result of endogenous gonadotropin stimulation, arises in ovarian transplants to the spleen of rats does not utilize cholesterol but only acetate for its elaboration of progesterone. Consequently, the way seems to have been opened to accepting the idea that acetate, rather than cholesterol, is the starting material for the physiologic mechanism of progesterone biosynthesis in the human corpus luteum.

3.5.3. ULTIMATE CONVERSIONS OF PROGESTERONE

Contrary to earlier belief, estrogens and androgens are elaborated at the expense of progesterone, not the other way around. Therefore, progesterone is the "precursor" of the other two hormones. Figure 3–13 outlines these conversions diagrammatically. Armstrong and his group,[4,5] have

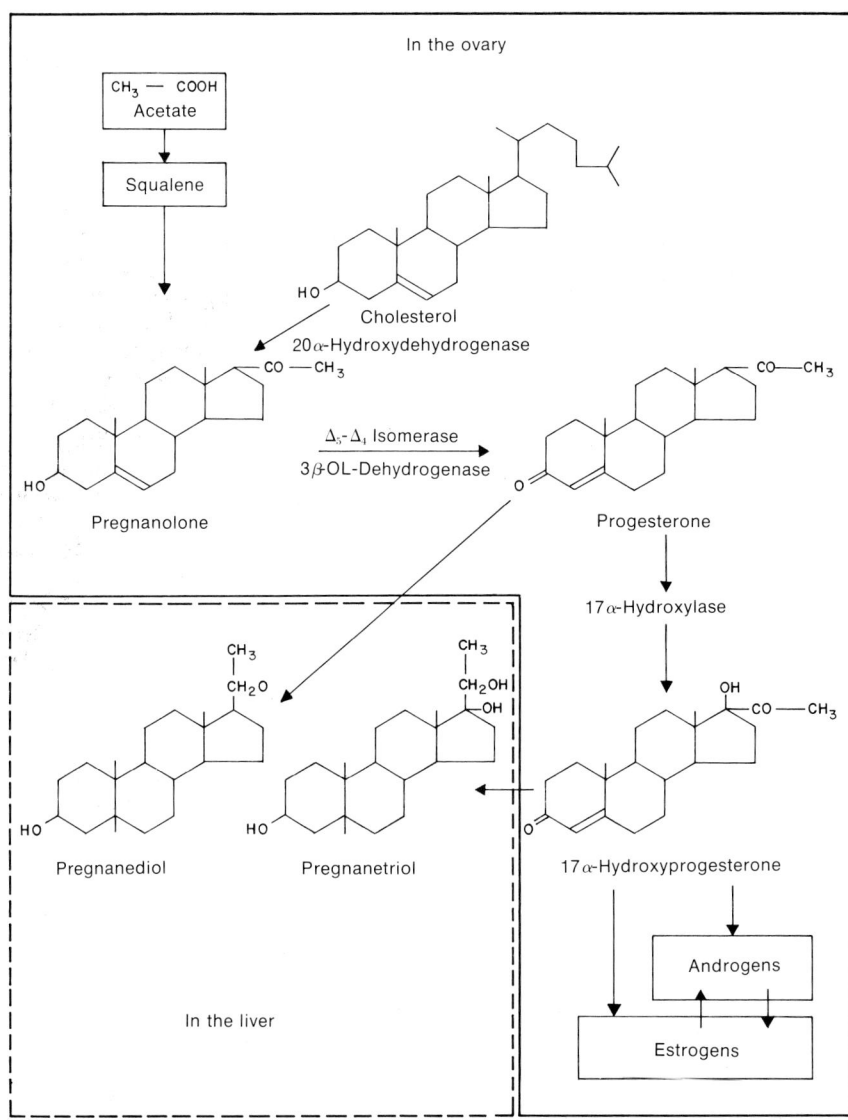

Figure 3–13. General outline of progesterone metabolism: ovarian biogenesis, conversion to androgens and estrogens, and degradation by liver.

related those processes of conversion to the actions of gonadotropins. While corticoids are probably also elaborated in the ovaries of some animal species, this is not the case in the human ovary. In woman, bilateral adrenalectomy outside pregnancy and without glucocorticoid treatment leads to death. We have been able to demonstrate that this does not occur in the rat (see Chapter 9). Vinson[164] furnishes an explanation for the discrepancy by ascertaining that the corpus luteum of both rat and mouse ovaries produces, in addition, cortisol.

3.5.4. CATABOLITES OF PROGESTERONE

The degradation of progesterone to the end product of pregnanediol, a saturated 3,20 double alcohol of pregnane, has already been indicated. The intermediary stages leading to pregnanediol, according to Dorfman,[42] are represented in Figure 3–13. According to both Dorfman and Heard and his colleagues,[69] the first step of the conversion process is a pregnene-3,20-dione resulting from simple hydrogenation of ring A of progesterone. By means of the action of a 3-hydroxylase, which is similar to the one mediating the formation of androgens at the expense of progesterone, the conversion proceeds to 3α-hydroxypregnane-20-one, and eventually, by hydroxylation of carbon 20, to pregnanediol. Hydrogenation of carbon 5 creates a stereoisomeric situation which, according to whether the hydrogen is oriented out of the plane of the ring or not, gives rise respectively to allo-pregnane-3,20-dione or to 3β-hydroxy-allo-pregnane-20-one, which in turn gives allopregnanediol. Moreover, the importance of pregnanetriol, derived from hydroxyprogesterone by the same biochemical mechanism, was lately recognized.[81, 167, 174] Keller and Houser[86] and Martin and his colleagues[106] consider pregnanetriol to be a breakdown product of the adrenocortical metabolite hydroxyprogesterone, and its excessive excretion, therefore, as indicative of adrenal cortical hyperplasia. However, there is no doubt that, as demonstrated by us and ultimately corroborated by others,[122] some corticosteroids (mainly deoxycorticosterone) are excreted in the form of pregnanediol also.

3.5.5. CIRCULATION DURING THE CYCLE

Modern techniques for blood level determinations have allowed the charting of progesterone levels along the entire cycle of both female monkeys[115] and women.[116, 127, 136, 160] The first half of the human cycle (between days one and 10) shows levels of 0.1 mcg per 100 cc of blood, i.e., next to zero levels. From days 11 to 15 of the cycle, levels of 1.60 mcg[160] have been recorded; then between days 16 and 20 a slight drop to 1.25 mcg occurs; and, finally, the level decreases to 0.44 mcg for the rest of the cycle after day 20.

These figures agree with what was previously said (Section 3.5.1) concerning the progesteronemic peak during the few days preceding ovulation. The origin of preovulatory progesterone levels is unknown.[1, 44] Curves charted on monkeys are similar, though much more elevated;[115] levels usually found between days 15 and 18 of the cycle are in the range of 3 to 4 mcg per 100 cc.

3.5.6. TRANSPORT

It has already been pointed out above (see Section 2.5.6) that steroids are transported linked to a *specific binding protein*. This is equally true of progesterone.[110, 149] Rosenthal and his colleagues,[132] as well as Westphal,[168] believe that, because it is a C-21 steroid which at the molecular level is quite similar to corticoids, progesterone may be transported by the specific binding protein of *cortisol*, particularly during pregnancy. This binding protein currently is known as *transcortin*.

3.5.7. DISINTEGRATION AND ELIMINATION

According to an already classic concept,[37, 54, 69, 70, 123, 167, 173] the liver is the site of most pregnanediol and pregnanetriol production. Because progesterone is practically equimolecular with pregnanediol, it was accepted that theoretically 1 mg of the excreted urinary diol corresponded to 1 mg of metabolized hormone. Unfortunately, that theory has been in need of a critical reappraisal, since it was demonstrated that, on the one hand, part of progesterone was

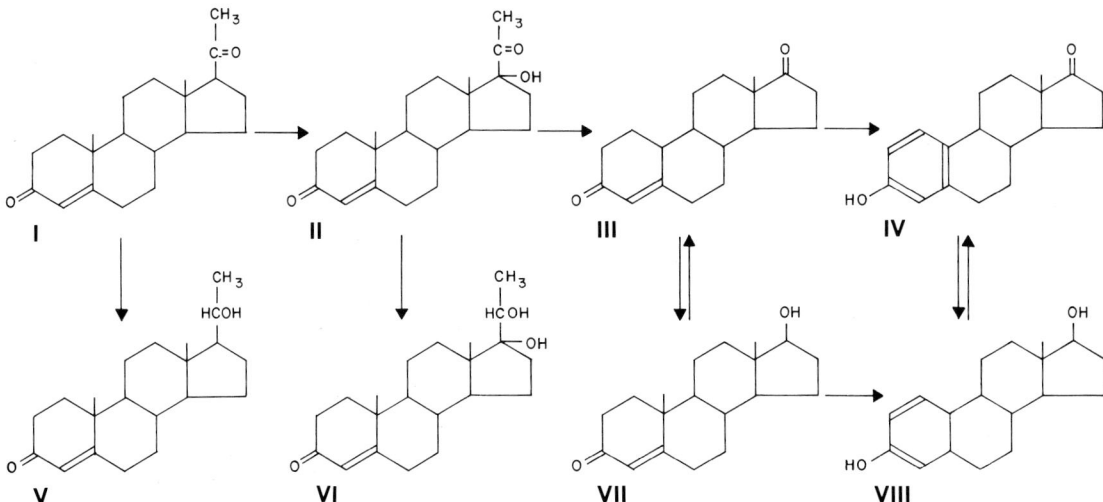

Figure 3-14. Probable metabolic pathway involved in progesterone conversion by ovarian tissue. I, Progesterone; II, 17α-hydroxyprogesterone; III, 4-androstene-3,17-dione; IV, estrone; V, 20α-hydroxy-4-pregnene-3-one; VI, 17α-dihydroxy-4-pregnene-3-one; VII, testosterone; VIII, estradiol. Note that conversion of higher forms to lower ones merely requires hydrogenation (mediated by 17- or 20-hydroxylase). (From Warren and Salhanick, *J. Clin. Endocr. Metab.*, 21:1227, 1961.)

being destroyed in the liver without degradation to pregnanediol[54, 123] and, on the other, a considerable fraction was excreted directly in the bile.[24, 155] Vermeulen and his colleagues[163] studied the fate of C-14 labeled progesterone and the manner of its elimination and found that 40 per cent was eliminated in the urine as pregnanetriol or pregnanediolone, 20 per cent was eliminated in the bile, whereas only 40 per cent of the metabolized total would wind up in the urine in the direct pregnanediol form. Consequently, if 7 mg is an estimate (Keller and Hauser[87]) of the maximal amount excreted per 24 hours of the luteal phase of the cycle, it seems reasonable to assume that the total amount produced by the cycle's corpus luteum during the same time is much more likely in the neighborhood of 20 mg.

The fact that progesterone is fat soluble[37] facilitates its storage and retention in the tissues of very obese women.

The formation and circulation of progesterone during normal pregnancy are dealt with in Chapter 19.

In Figure 3-14 an attempt has been made at representing diagrammatically progesterone metabolism: Food intake provides the liver with sufficient amounts of cholesterol, poured out into the circulation and utilized by the placenta and the adrenal cortex, where conversion to a progesterone precursor (pregnenolone) takes place. Progesterone is elaborated at the expense of this precursor and probably also in a direct manner in the ovary. The corticoids, which are intimately related to progesterone biogenetically and metabolically, are present with progesterone in the circulation.

Finally, its principal—though not only—catabolite, pregnanediol, is formed in the liver and eliminated by the kidney.

3.6. PHARMACOLOGY

3.6.1. UNITS OF PROGESTOGENS

As a result of the chemically pure and crystallized state in which progestogens are available, the necessity for using biologic units has been done away with and dosages are weighed in milligrams. *One international unit is the equivalent of one milligram of α-progesterone.* The international unit for norpregneninolone, (norethisterone), which is six times as active, is one sixth of a milligram of that compound. The 6-methylated or 6-halogenated derivatives are still more potent and, depending on the case, one international unit may be represented by as little as one tenth to one twentieth of a milligram of these compounds.

3.6.2. MODES OF ADMINISTRATION

Classically, progesterone was always used parenterally, since active oral preparations were unknown. The first active oral preparation to be used was pregneninolone, which was introduced by Hohlweg and Inhoffen in 1942. After that, the already long list of synthetic estrogens began to be matched by the supply of an equally ample range or orally active progestogens.

Injectable forms are now usually employed with long-acting preparations, such as *α-progesterone caproate*, which is used most commonly.

All synthetic norderivatives (norpregneninolone, etc.), as well as acetylated derivatives, are active when administered orally. They may be given by mouth without the risk of being inactivated by the liver. In this respect, they are similar to the synthetic estrogens, which can also be administered by the same route and in the same form.

For further reference to the therapeutic application of progesterone, see Chapter 28 (Section 28.5.1), as well as the work by Kistner.[89]

3.6.3. DOSAGE

The question of progesterone dosage has aroused considerable controversy. The original investigations of Kauffmann quoted the amount of 60 mg of progesterone as the effective dosage for the entire cycle of a woman. That was the so-called transformation dose, which the proliferative or hyperplastic endometrium was estimated to require in order to be converted to the secretory type. Further studies on endometrial biopsies from intact uteri of castrated women by Kauffmann and Zander[82] and by Ferin[52] showed that, in order to obtain a perfect secretory phase with typical glandular changes and epithelial secretion of glycogen, a dose of at least 200 mg per cycle was necessary. By necessity, several of the older precepts of progesterone therapy have been revised following realization that the dosages administered originally could not be effective. Therefore, the classical injectables, marketed in ampules of 10 mg, of which at least 20 would be needed for a period of slightly over one week's duration, were substituted by the so called "depot" preparations, each single injection of which contained as much as 125 to 250 mg of the drug. Thereby, effective and sustained activity can be assured.

3.6.4. TOXIC EFFECTS

While estrogens are notorious for their important toxic effects, no untoward toxicity has so far been described with the use of progesterone. A few workers have alluded to virilizing effects from large doses of progesterone, but such reactions have apparently not been confirmed conclusively. It is true that luteinization of ovarian tumors may be associated with virilization (see Chapter 33); however, this does not result from progestogen overproduction by the tumor cells but is probably the result of a pathologically altered progestogen metabolism leading to elevated androgen levels.

The question has similarly been raised as to whether progesterone given in large doses could inactivate ACTH secretion and therefore produce a secondary adrenocortical insufficiency. Though such an assumption seems plausible on theoretical grounds, proof to substantiate it has not been forthcoming (Barter et al.[8]).

3.6.5. ANTIGESTAGENS: ERGOCORNINE

Ergocornine, an alkaloid derived from ergot, blocks luteinization and acts as an antigestagen. Whereas, contrary to what has been held until recently, Lindner and co-workers[96] reject the assumption that this alkaloid acts by inhibiting 3β-ol-dehydrogenase, Zeilmaker[176] believes that its action is central, since it prevents the formation of the gravidic corpus luteum in the rat.

3.7. SPECIAL PROPERTIES OF SYNTHETIC PROGESTOGENS

Artificial progestogens have some properties in common with progesterone but differ from it in others. These shall now be analyzed in sequence.

3.7.1. ACTIONS SHARED WITH PROGESTERONE

PROGESTATIONAL ACTIVITY IN THE ANIMAL. All the synthetic drugs show intense progestational activity in laboratory rodents; nevertheless, certain differences in activity can be discerned; thus Zarrow and his colleagues reported that norderivatives were very effective in the Clauberg test and acted strongly on the oviducts of hens, but were ineffective in the Hooker and Forbes assay, for which natural progesterone and its caproate ester were found to possess maximum activity.

PROGESTATIONAL ACTIVITY IN WOMAN. Greenblatt and Rose[60] noted progestational changes in endometrial biopsies of ethinyltestosterone treated women. Ferin[52] studied the same drug, as well as methyl-nortestosterone, in the endometria of castrated women in order to determine the effective oral dosage, which was found to be about 150 to 300 mg per cycle, i.e., one tenth of the corresponding dose for pregneninolone. Kayser[83] indicates a daily dose of 15 mg over a period of 10 to 14 days as necessary to produce an adequate secretory phase, which is in keeping with earlier data. Shah and his co-workers[143] have studied the effects of the norderivatives on the glycogen and alkaline phosphatase contents and, finally, Pincus[120] described the effects of these compounds on the endometrial activity of carbonic anhydrase which, in the light of our present knowledge, is one of the finest tests available for the estimation of progestational activity.

THERMOGENIC EFFECTS. The thermogenic effects have been studied by Lauritzen.[92] Even though of the same nature as those produced by natural progesterone, they are more pronounced with synthetic norderivatives.

VAGINAL CYTOLOGY. Typically progestational cytologic changes, identical to those induced by progesterone, have been observed by Greenblatt and Rose,[60] Kayser,[83] and Wied and Davis.[170] The latter two have also reported inhibitory effects on cervical mucus crystallization.

PREGNANCY-PROTECTING ACTIONS. Although there are serious doubts concerning the effectiveness of progestin medication aimed at preventing abortion, lately good results were reported with peroral treatment of threatened abortion by means of synthetic 19-nor steroids.

3.7.2. ACTIONS DIFFERING FROM THOSE OF PROGESTERONE

OVULATION INHIBITION. In 1931, Haberlandt had already described the antiovulatory activity of the corpus luteum hormone, which was confirmed by Robson with pure progesterone three years later. In 1942, we listed the antiovulatory activity of progesterone, along with its physiologic actions which we believed to have been firmly established. The fact is, however, that the antiovulatory activity of progesterone is so weak as to be effective only with very high doses in animals, and never in the human species.

Since 1954, powerful ovulation- and estrus-inhibitory activity of the norderivatives, first in rats, then in rabbits, has been observed by Pincus and colleagues.[120] Rock and co-workers[129] found that the most potent antiovulatory activity was displayed by both norpregneninolone and norethynodrel, which was even more intense if small amounts of estrogens were added to these compounds. This became the basis for the recent large-scale application of oral contraceptives.[14, 44, 57, 100, 147]

The most commonly invoked mechanism by which progestogens are thought to exert this action is by blocking the production of LHRF (luteinizing hormone releasing factor) at the level of the hypothalamus.[74, 101, 138, 151]

Ovulation-inhibitory effects could be confirmed on direct examination of both animal[38] and human ovaries.[30] The effects do not appear to result from direct action upon the ovary, but to be mediated exclusively by the hypothalamus.[150] However, as was pointed out in Chapter 47, it has been fully demonstrated[97, 139] that estrogens have a more potent inhibitory effect on gonadotropin release than do progestogens, although the two are known to potentiate each other reciprocally whenever used in combination.

EFFECTS ON THE IMPLANTATION AND SURVIVAL OF THE EGG. Starup[151] and Tullner and Hertz[158] both found that, whereas the number of eggs implanting at one time in the rabbit was dependent on the amount of progesterone available, the 19-nor steroids lacked any implantation-promoting power. We have already commented on their scanty effectiveness in the Hooker-Forbes test.[53, 54] The differences in

Progestogens

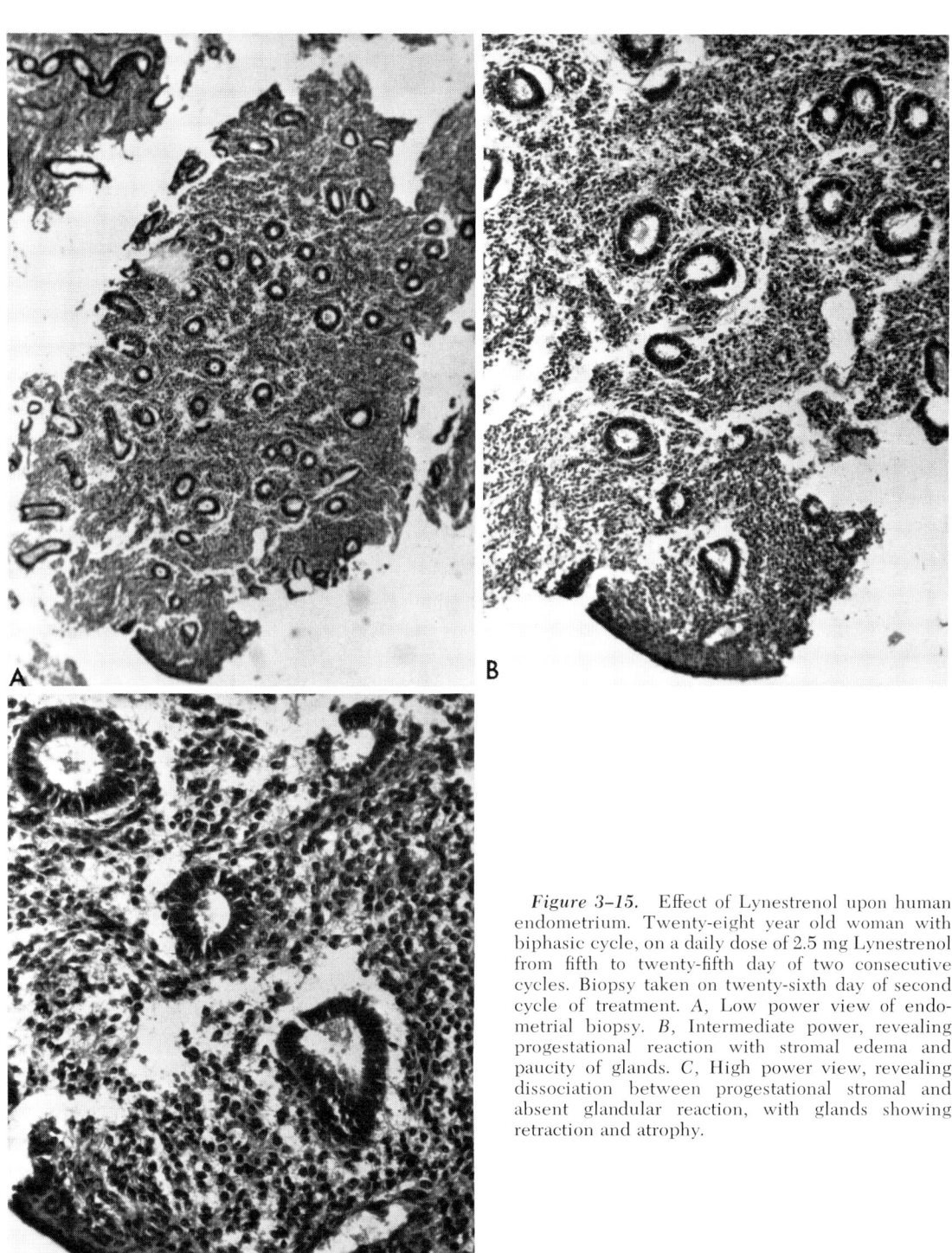

Figure 3-15. Effect of Lynestrenol upon human endometrium. Twenty-eight year old woman with biphasic cycle, on a daily dose of 2.5 mg Lynestrenol from fifth to twenty-fifth day of two consecutive cycles. Biopsy taken on twenty-sixth day of second cycle of treatment. *A,* Low power view of endometrial biopsy. *B,* Intermediate power, revealing progestational reaction with stromal edema and paucity of glands. *C,* High power view, revealing dissociation between progestational stromal and absent glandular reaction, with glands showing retraction and atrophy.

their histochemical effects on the endometrium likewise favor the conclusion that, in default of their overall progestational activity, the norderivatives are not entirely effective as regards improvement of the nutritional environment in the progravid endometrium (Fig. 3–15).

As already stated (see Section 3.3.6), implantation can be successfully performed only in the presence of a definite estrogen-progesterone balance. Should this balance be tipped in favor of either progestogen[35, 150] or estrogen[35, 37] by the addition of either hormone, implantation will fail to take place, owing to the appearance of pathologic endometrial changes, which have also already been outlined.

ESTROGENIC AND ANDROGENIC ACTIONS. Norethynodrel and Lynestrenol are both weakly estrogenic.[57, 129]

Most derivatives of nortestosterone exhibit androgenic activity.[40, 119, 165] Suchowsky and Junkmann[153] have devised a rat test for the determination of androgenic potency of commercial preparations. On the other hand, synthetic progestins derived from testosterone, such as Chlormadinone,[23, 119] lack androgenic potency completely.

As a final note of interest, we mention the finding that some of the synthetic progestogens inhibit spermatogenesis in the rabbit.[48]

MISCELLANEOUS EFFECTS ON THE ENDOMETRIUM. Because of their mild estrogenic activity, 19-nor steroids act even on previously nonproliferated endometria.[162] Roland and co-workers[130, 131] similarly have found that effects on the human endometrium are histologically rather different from those of progesterone. Effects on the glands are less pronounced, while the stroma responds by marked proliferation, with concomitant pseudodecidualization.

THROMBOEMBOLISM. A serious drawback, mainly of norethynodrel, appears to be the definite tendency to produce thromboembolic disease, which in the view of some English clinicians[103, 117, 121] is considerable and which has contributed to discrediting of norethynodrel in England. Although Rock and colleagues[129] have investigated a large series of norethynodrel treated cases, without reporting any negative effects—results which have been confirmed in a modern large series by Rice-Wray and his colleagues[124]—is one of the reasons why currently new preparations based on other progestogens than norethynodrel are being introduced.

FORM OF ELIMINATION. With the exception of the adrenogenital syndrome, progesterone is known to be excreted almost entirely in the form of pregnanediol, to which compound it corresponds in a nearly milligram per milligram fashion. On the other hand, 17-hydroxyprogesterone caproate has not been known to be excreted in the diol form.[42, 80] The same holds true for the nor-derivatives[93, 172] which, in turn, increase urinary excretion of 11-oxysteroids.[24, 51, 73] Their mode of excretion suggests that these compounds are devoid of physiologic activity and, therefore, do not partake in endogenous progesterone metabolism.

Experimental work performed with radioactive nor-steroids[3, 72] points to a difference in metabolism with regard to natural progestogens and demonstrates that they metabolize very much like testosterone, which certainly explains their androgenic fetal effects.

In summary, 19-nortestosterone derivatives have powerful progestational, weak estrogenic and variable androgenic activity. By mouth, these preparations are completely effective as drugs with progestational activity and can be used orally in small dosages to achieve therapeutic luteoid effects. Their actions, not identical with those of natural progesterone, are variable, but most important is their ovulation-inhibitory activity, which forms the basis for their current popular favor.

REFERENCES

1. Abrahamson, D.: *Ann. N.Y. Acad. Sci.*, 71:759, 1958.
2. Alberts, H. J., Bedford, J. M., and Chang, M. C.: *Amer. J. Physiol.*, 201:554, 1961.
3. Arai, K., Golab, T., Layne, D. S., and Pincus, G.: *Endocrinology*, 71:639, 1962.
4. Armstrong, D. T.: *Endocrinology*, 72:909, 1963.
5. Armstrong, D. T., Kilpatrick, R., and Greep, R. O.: *Endocrinology*, 73:165, 1963.
6. Backer, M. H.: *Obstet. Gynec.*, 19:725, 1962.
7. Barry, M. C., et al.: *Endocrinology*, 50:587, 1952.
8. Barter, F. C., et al.: *J. Clin. Invest.*, 30:327, 1951.
9. Bartosik, D., Romanoff, E. B., Watson, D. J., and Scricco, E.: *Endocrinology*, 81:186, 1967.
10. Bernerd, I., and Odano, M.: *Ann. d'Endocr.*, 21:513, 1960.
11. Bialy, G., and Brown, D. W. C.: *Endocrinology*, 72:662, 1963.
12. Bo, W. J., Odor, D. L., and Rothrock, M. L.: *Anat. Rec.*, 121:163, 1969.

13. Bongiovanni, A. M., et al.: *J. Clin. Endocr. Metab.*, 14:409, 1954.
14. Borushek, S., et al.: *Internat. J. Fertil*, 8:605, 1963.
15. Botella, J.: *Arch. Gynak.*, 183:73, 1953.
16. Botella, J.: *Actas Soc. Esp. Est. Esterilidad*, 6:56, 1958.
17. Botella, J., and Nogales, F.: *Acta Gin.*, 6:281, 1955.
18. Brown-Grant, K.: *J. Physiol.*, 190:101, 1967.
19. Bryans, F. E.: *Endocrinology*, 48:733, 1951.
20. Brydgeman, M., and Eliasson, R.: *J. Reprod. Fertil.*, 7:47, 1964.
21. Caligaris, L., Astrada, J. J., and Taleisnik, S.: *Acta Endocrinol.*, 59:177, 1968.
22. Cardeilhac, P. T., Morisette, M. C., and Calle, J. D.: *Proc. Soc. Exper. Biol. Med.*, 123:343, 1966.
23. Chambon, Y., Touret, J. L., and Depagne, A.: *Ann. d'Endocr.*, 28:333, 1967.
24. Chang, E., Slaunwhite, R., and Sanberg, A. A.: *J. Clin. Endocr. Metab.*, 20:1568, 1960.
25. Chang, M. C.: *Endocrinology*, 81:1251, 1967.
26. Chang, M. C.: *Endocrinology*, 84:356, 1969.
27. Channing, C. P., and Villee, C. A.: *Biochim. Biophys. Acta* 127:1, 1966.
28. Cook, B., Kaltenbach, C. C., Norton, H. W., and Nalbandov, A. V.: *Endocrinology*, 81:573, 1967.
29. Cremades, J., and Botella, J.: *Acta Gin.*, 17:29, 1966.
30. Cremades, J., Sanchez-Rivera, G., and Botella, J.: *Acta Gin.*, 17:167, 1966.
31. Cremades, J., and Botella, J.: *Acta Gin.*, 17:827, 1966.
31a. Cross, B. A., and Silver, I. A.: *J. Endocr.*, 31:251, 1965.
32. Csapo, A.: *Rec. Progr. Horm. Res.*, 12:405, 1956.
33. Csapo, A.: *Ann. N.Y. Acad. Sci.*, 75:790, 1959.
34. Csapo, A., and Pinto-Dantas, C. A.: *Proc. Nat. Acad. Sci.*, 54:1069, 1966.
35. Daniel, J. C., and Cowman, M. L.: *J. Endocr.*, 35:155, 1966.
36. David, A., et al.: *J. Reprod. Fertil.*, 5:331, 1963.
37. Davis, M. E., Plotz, H. J., Lupu, C. I., and Ejarque, P. M.: *Fertil. Steril.*, 11:19, 1960.
38. Davidson, R. J., and Koets, P.: *Arch. Int. Med.*, 85:365, 1950.
39. Day, B. N., and Polge, C.: *J. Reprod. Fertil.*, 17:227, 1968.
40. Djerassi, C., et al.: *J. Amer. Chem. Soc.*, 76:4092, 1954.
41. Dominguez, H., Simonovitz, F., and Greenblatt, R. B.: *Amer. J. Obstet. Gynec.*, 84:1478, 1962.
42. Dorfman, R. I.: In *The Hormones*, ed. G. Pincus and K. V. Thimann. New York, Academic Press, 1955.
43. Drucker, W. D., et al.: *J. Clin. Endocr. Metab.*, 23:1247, 1963.
44. Duncan, G. W., Lister, S. C., and Clark, J. J.: *Internat. J. Fertil.*, 8:859, 1963.
45. Edgren, R. A., Jones, R. C., Peterson, A. L. and Gillen, A. L.: *Acta Endocrinol. (Suppl.)*, 54:115, 1967.
46. Elton, R. L., and Edgren, R. A.: *Endocrinology*, 63:465, 1958.
47. Engstrom, W. W., and Munson, P. L.: *J. Clin. Endocr. Metab.*, 11:427, 1951.
48. Ericson, R. J., Dutt, R. H., and Archdeacon, J. W.: *Nature*, 204:261, 1964.
49. Eskin, B. A., Dratman, M. B., and Pettit, M.D.: *Endocrinology*, 69:195, 1961.
50. Fahim, M. S., and Hall, D. G.: *Amer. J. Obstet. Gynec.*, 106:183, 1970.
51. Feldman, E. B., and Carter, A. C.: *J. Clin. Endocr. Metab.*, 20:482, 1960.
52. Ferin, J.: *Geburtsh. u. Frauenhk.*, 17:10, 1967.
52a. Fisher, R. H., and MacColgan, S. P.: *J. Clin. Endocr. Metab.*, 13:1043, 1953.
53. Forbes, T. R.: *Endocrinology*, 53:79, 1953.
54. Forbes, T. R., Coulombre, A. J., and Coulombre, J.: *Endocrinology*, 68:859, 1961.
55. Freeman, M. E., Crissman, J. K., Louw, G. N., Butcher, R. L., and Inskeep, E. K.: *Endocrinology*, 86:717, 1970.
56. Fuhrmann, K.: *Arch. Gynäk.*, 197:383, 1962.
57. Garcia, C. R., Pincus, G., and Rock, J.: *Amer. J. Obstet. Gynec.*, 75:82, 1958.
58. Goldberg, B., Seegar-Jones, G. E., and Turner, D. A.: *Amer. J. Obstet. Gynec.*, 86:349, 1963.
59. Greenblatt, R. B.: *Ann. N.Y. Acad. Sci.*, 71:710, 1958.
60. Greenblatt, R. B., and Rose, D. F.: *Obstet. Gynec.*, 19:730, 1962.
61. Greiss, F. C., and Anderson, S. G.: *Amer. J. Obstet. Gynec.*, 107:829, 1970.
62. Gutierrez, D. A., Terragno, N., Cremades-Marco, J., Sanchez-Rivera, G., and Botella, J.: *Acta Gin.*, 18:1, 1967.
63. Gyermek, L., Genther, G., and Fleming, N.: *Internat. J. Neuropharmacol.*, 6:191, 1967.
64. Hall, P. F., and Koritz, S. B.: *Biochemistry*, 4:1037, 1965.
65. Haller, J.: *Geburtsh. u. Frauenhk.*, 22:211, 1962.
66. Harper, M. K. J.: *Endocrinology*, 77:114, 1965.
67. Harper, M. K. J.: *J. Endocr.*, 31:217, 1965.
68. Harper, M. K. J.: *Endocrinology*, 78:568, 1966.
69. Heard, R. D., et al.: *Rec. Progr. Horm. Res.*, 12:45, 1956.
70. Hechter, O., and Pincus, G.: *Physiol. Rev.*, 34:459, 1954.
71. Herbert, J., and Trimble, T. R.: *Nature*, 216:165, 1967.
72. Herrmann, U.: *Gynaecologia*, 155:187, 1962.
73. Hertz, R., and Tullner, W.: *Endocrinology*, 54:288, 1954.
74. Hilliard, J., Croxatto, H. B., Hayward, J. N., and Sawyer, C. H.: *Endocrinology*, 79:411, 1966.
75. Hindson, J. C., Schofield, B. M., and Ward, W. R.: *J. Endocr.*, 43:207, 1969.
76. Hooker, C. W., and Forbes, T. R.: *Endocrinology*, 41:158, 1947.
77. Huang, W. Y., and Pearlman, W. H.: *J. Biol. Chem.*, 238:1038, 1963.
78. Huff, R. L., and Eik-Nes, K. B.: *J. Reprod. Fertil.*, 11:57, 1966.
79. Iglesias, E., Clavero, J. A., Sanchez-Rivera, G., Cremades, J., and Botella, J.: *Acta Gin.*, 20:921, 1969.
80. Junkmann, C.: *Rec. Progr. Horm. Res.*, 13:389, 1957.
81. Junkmann, C., and Witzel, H.: *Ztschr. Vit. Horm. Forsch.*, 9:97, 1958.
82. Kaufmann, C., and Zander, J.: *Klin. Wschr.*, 34:7, 1956.
83. Kayser, R.: *Geburtsh. u. Frauenhk.*, 17:24, 1957.
84. Kao, C. Y., and Gams, R. S.: *Amer. J. Physiol.*, 201:714, 1961.
85. Keever, J. E., and Greenwald, G. S.: *Acta Endocrinol.*, 56:244, 1967.

86. Keller, M., and Hauser, A.: *Gynaecologia*, 149: 337, 1960.
87. Kessler, W. B., and Borman, A.: *Ann. N.Y. Acad. Sci.*, 71:500, 1958.
88. Kumar, D., Wagatsuma, T., Sullivan, W. J., Jr., and Barnes, A. C.: *Amer. J. Obstet. Gynec.*, 90:1355, 1964.
89. Kistner, R. W.: *The Use of Progestins in Obstetrics and Gynecology*. Chicago, Year Book Medical Publishers, 1969.
90. Kuriyama, H.: *J. Physiol.*, 159:26, 1961.
91. Landau, R. L., and Lughibil, K.: *J. Clin. Endocr. Metab.*, 21:1345, 1961.
92. Lauritzen, C.: *Geburtsh u. Frauenhk.*, 17:807, 1957.
93. Lerner, L. J., et al.: *Endocrinology*, 71:449, 1962.
94. Leroy, F., Manavian, D., and Hubinot, P. O.: *J. Endocrinol.*, 39:227, 1967.
95. Lichton, L. J.: *Endocrinology*, 76:1068, 1965.
96. Lindner, H. R., Lunenfeld, B., and Shelesnyak, M. C.: *Acta Endocrinol.*, 56:35, 1967.
97. Lisk, R. D.: *Acta Endocrinol.*, 48:209, 1965.
98. Lisse, K.: *Endokrinologie*, 53:78, 1968.
99. Little, B., and Lincoln, E.: *Endocrinology*, 74:1, 1964.
100. Livingstone, N. B.: *Internat. J. Fertil.*, 8:699, 1963.
101. Loraine, J. A., et al.: *Acta Endocrinol.*, 50:15, 1965.
102. Lynn, W. S., and Brown, R.: *J. Biol. Chem.*, 232: 1015, 1958.
103. MacIntyre, N., Phillips, M. J., and Voigt, J. C.: *Brit. Med. J.*, 2:1029, 1962.
104. Maire, W. J., Rice, B. F., and Savard, K.: *J. Clin. Endocr.*, 28:1249, 1968.
105. March, L., and Fosatti, P.: *Ann. d'Endocr.*, 23: 203, 1962.
106. Martin, M. M., Reddy, W. J., and Thorn, G. W.: *J. Clin. Endocr. Metab.*, 21:293, 1961.
107. Masuda, H., Anderson, L. L., Henricks, D. M., and Mellampy, R. M.: *Endocrinology*, 80: 240, 1967.
108. Meyerson, B. G.: *Endocrinology*, 81:369, 1967.
109. Michael, R. P., Saayman, G. S., and Zumpe, D.: *J. Endocrinol.*, 39:309, 1967.
110. Milgrom, E., and Baulieu, E. E.: *Endocrinology*, 87:276, 1970.
111. Mitchell, J. A., and Jochim, J. M.: *Endocrinology*, 83:691, 1968.
112. Miyake, T., and Pincus, G.: *Endocrinology*, 65:64, 1959.
113. Mykhail, G., Zander, J., and Allen, W. M.: *J. Clin. Endocr. Metab.*, 23:1267, 1963.
114. Nallar, R., Antunes-Rodriquez, J., and MacCann, S. M.: *Endocrinology*, 79:907, 1966.
115. Neill, J. D., Johansson, E. D. B., and Knobil, E.: *Endocrinology*, 81:1161, 1967.
116. Neill, J. D., Johansson, E. D. B., Datta, J. K., and Knobil, E.: *J. Clin. Endocr. Metab.*, 27:1167, 1967.
117. Nour-Eldin, F.: *Brit. Med. J.*, 1:1476, 1963.
118. Ogawa, Y., and Pincus, G.: *Endocrinology*, 68: 681, 1961; 70:358, 1962.
119. Peck, C. K., and LoPiccolo, J.: *Endocrinology*, 78:965, 1966.
120. Pincus, G.: *Endocrinology*, 65:819, 1959.
121. Quick, A. J.: *Brit. Med. J.*, 1:1604, 1963.
122. Ralph, C. L., and Fraps, R. M.: *Endocrinology*, 65:819, 1959.
123. Roa, L. G. S., and Taylor, W.: *Biochem. J.*, 96: 172, 1965.
124. Rice-Wray, E., Arandra-Rosell, A., Maqueo, M., and Goldzieher, J. W.: *Amer. J. Obstet. Gynec.*, 87:429, 1963.
125. Rice, B. F., and Segaloff, A.: *Acta Endocrinol.*, 51:131, 1966.
126. Rice, B. F., and Segaloff, A.: *Steroids*, 7:367, 1966.
127. Riondel, A., Tait, J. F., Tait, S. A. S., Gut, M., and Little, B.: *Endocrinology*, 52:229, 1965.
128. Roberts, J. S., and Share, L.: *Endocrinology*, 84:1076, 1969.
129. Rock, J., Garcia, C. R., and Pincus, G.: *Amer. J. Obstet. Gynec.*, 79:758, 1960.
130. Roland, M., and Ober, W. B.: *Internat. J. Fertil.*, 8:619, 1963.
131. Roland, M.: *Progestogen Therapy*. Springfield, Ill., Charles C Thomas, 1965.
132. Rosenthal, H. E., Slaunwhite, W. R., and Sandberg, A. A.: *J. Clin. Endocrinol.*, 29:352, 1969.
133. Rotschild, I.: *Endocrinology*, 70:303, 1962.
134. Rubio, B.: *Fertil. Steril.*, 14:254, 1963.
135. Rudel, H. W., Lebherz, T., Maqueo, M., Martinez-Manautou, J., and Bessler, S.: *J. Reprod. Fertil.*, 13:199, 1967.
136. Runnebaum, B., and Zander, J.: *Acta Endocrinol.*, 55:91, 1967.
137. Ryan, K. J., and Smith, O. W.: *J. Biol. Chem.*, 236:2207, 1961.
138. Ryan, K. J., Goss, D. A., and Reid, D. E.: *Amer. J. Obstet. Gynec.*, 94:515, 1966.
139. Sanchez-Rivera, G., Merlo, J. G., and Botella, J.: *Acta Gin.*, 18:193, 1967.
139a. Sanchez-Rivera, G., Cremades, J., and Botella, J.: *Acta Gin.*, 17:83, 1966.
140. Sandberg, A. A., and Slaunwhite, W. R.: *J. Clin. Endocr. Metab.*, 18:253, 1958.
141. Savard, K., Marsh, J., and Howell, D. S.: *Endocrinology*, 73:554, 1963.
142. Sawyer, C. H., and Everett, J. W.: *Endocrinology*, 65:644, 1959.
143. Shah, P. B., et al.: *Ann. N.Y. Acad. Sci.*, 71:817, 1958.
144. Short, R. V.: *J. Endocr.*, 24:59, 1962.
145. Smith, O. W., and Ryan, K. J.: *Endocrinology*, 69:970, 1961.
146. Smith, B. D., and Bradbury, J. T.: *Endocrinology*, 78:297, 1966.
147. Sobrero, A.: *Internat. J. Fertil.*, 8:721, 1963.
148. Song, C. S., Rifkind, A. B., Gilette, P. N., and Dappas, A.: *Amer. J. Obstet. Gynec.*, 105: 813, 1969.
149. Souza, M. L. A. de, Williamson, H. O., Moody, L. O., and Diczfalusy, E.: In *Karolinska Symposia, Vol. II*. Stockholm, 1970.
150. Starup, J., and Oosterggard, E.: *Acta Endocrinol.*, 52:292, 1966.
151. Starup, J.: *Acta Endocrinol.*, 51:469, 1962.
152. Stegner, H. E.: *Arch. Gynäk.*, 197:351, 1962.
153. Suchowsky, G. K., and Junkmann, K.: *Endocrinology*, 68:341, 1961.
154. Tamaoki, B. I., and Pincus, G.: *Endocrinology*, 69:527, 1961.
155. Taylor, W., and Scratcherd, T.: *Biochem. J.*, 81:938, 1961.
156. Terragno, N., Gutierrez, D. A., and Botella, J.: *Acta Gin.*, 17:177, 1966.
157. Tillinger, K. G., and Diczfalusy, E.: *Acta Endocrinol.*, 35:197, 1960.
158. Tullner, W. W., and Hertz, R.: *Endocrinology*, 52:259, 1953.

159. Tyler, E. T., and Olson, H. J.: *Ann. N.Y. Acad. Sci.*, 71:704, 1958.
160. Van Der Molen, H., et al.: *J. Clin. Endocr. Metab.*, 25:170, 1965.
161. Van Der Molen, H. J., and Groen, D.: *J. Clin. Endocr. Metab.*, 25:1625, 1965.
162. Velardo, J. T.: *Ann. N.Y. Acad. Sci.*, 71:452, 1958.
163. Vermeulen, A., Slaunwhite, W. I., and Sandberg, A. A.: *J. Clin. Endocr. Metab.*, 21:1354, 1961.
164. Vinson, G. P., Norymbersky, J. K., and Chester-Jones, I.: *J. Endocrinol.*, 25:557, 1963.
165. Visser, J. De, and Overbeeck, G. A.: *Ann. d'Endocr.*, 17:268, 1956.
166. Warren, R. P., and Salhanick, H. A.: *J. Clin. Endocr. Metab.*, 21:1227, 1961.
167. Westphal, U., Kaufmann, C., and Zander, J.: *Arch. Gynäk.*, 179:247, 1941.
168. Westphal, U.: *Hoppe-Seylers Ztschr. f. Physiol. Chem.*, 346:243, 1966.
169. Wied, G. L., del Sol, R., and Dargan, A.: *Amer. J. Obstet. Gynec.*, 75:98, 1958.
170. Wied, J., and Davis, G. L.: *Internat. J. Fertil.*, 8:601, 1967.
171. Wiest, W. G., et al.: *Endocrinology*, 73:588, 1963.
172. Wrenn, T. R., et al.: *Endocrinology*, 65:317, 1959.
173. Zander, J.: *Geburtsh. u. Frauenhk.*, 17:876, 1957.
174. Zander, J.: *Klin. Wschr.*, 33:697, 1955.
175. Zarrow, M. X., and Hurblut, E. C.: *Endocrinology*, 80:735, 1967.
176. Zeilmaker, G. H.: *Acta Endocrinol.*, 59:442, 1968.

Chapter 4
ANDROGENS IN THE FEMALE BODY

Even under normal physiologic conditions, the ovary produces androgens along with estrogens and progestogens.

4.1. DEFINITION, NOMENCLATURE, HISTORY

4.1.1. DEFINITION

The term *androgens* is applied to those steroid compounds which have masculinizing activity—viz., stimulating the development of the male genital tract. Although both progesterone and the corticosteroids display inherent low-grade androgenic activity, these are not classified as androgens. By definition, androgens comprise testosterone, androsterone and a series of derivatives of this group. Most, though not all, 17-ketosteroids are also androgenic. Moreover, androgenic activity does not appear to be inherent to any compounds other than those possessing a steroid group. Therefore, unlike estrogens, which can be divided into estrogen hormones and estrogen drugs according to structural differences, all androgens are of a steroid hormonal character.

4.1.2. NOMENCLATURE

Androgens are derived from *androstane* (Fig. 4–1), a hydrocarbon with 19 carbon atoms. The specific testicular hormone is *testosterone*, or Δ4-androsterone-17β-ol-3-one(17β-hydroxy-Δ4-androstene-3-one), whose biosynthesis by the normal ovary or adrenal cortex is at best doubtful. It seems more likely that the androgenic substances of those two glands, i.e., those exerting androgenic activity in the normal female, belong to a vast group of testosterone catabolites which, because of the presence of a ketone group on carbon 17, are referred to as *17-ketosteroids*. Estrone is also a 17-ketosteroid (see Fig. 2–2), but it is called an *acid* ketosteroid because it is obtained

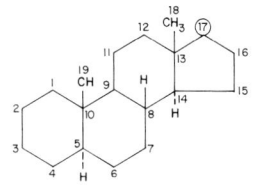
Androsterone

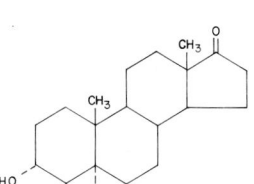
Dehydroepiandrosterone

Figure 4–1. The chemical structure of androgens. Androstane (etio-allocholane), testosterone, androsterone (etio-allocholanolone), dehydroepiandrosterone (dehydro-iso-androsterone).

from urine via acid hydrolysis. The androgens are *neutral* ketosteroids because they are obtained through neutral hydrolysis.

The principal 17-ketosteroids are *androsterone* (old name, etio-allocholanolone), mainly a product of ovarian secretion, and *dehydroepiandrosterone* (old common names, dehydroisoandrosterone, transdehydroandrosterone and dehydroandrosterone), which in turn is produced in greatest amounts by the adrenal cortex.

All of the 17-ketosteroids are more or less androgenic, though invariably to a lesser degree than testosterone. They correspond to the concept of "androgens" in a biologic sense.

4.1.3. HISTORY

The consequences of castration in males of both animals (castrated bulls, horses, fowl, etc., for domestic purposes) and man (eunuchs) have been known since time immemorial. In 1889, Brown-Sequard performed his famous and imaginative experiments which enabled him to arrive at the correct conclusion, though, as many are now convinced, he may have done so by inference rather than through an act of true observation. Nevertheless, the virilizing effects of testicular extracts, although much about them was still unknown, became a topic of discussion. The first instance of serious work on the problems of remasculinization was done in 1913 by Steinach who, by means of testicular implantation, succeeded in remasculinizing castrate male rabbits and virilizing female rabbits. The development of the concept of androgens resulted from the studies of Laqueur who, in 1927, devised the capon's comb test enabling him for the first time to estimate quantitatively the androgenic effects of testicular extracts. His co-workers successfully demonstrated the presence of a masculinizing hormone in the urine of males and, shortly thereafter, also in that of females. The latter finding was surprising and had to be demonstrated beyond any doubt before the concept of demonstrable quantities of androgens in the female urine could be convincingly established.

In 1931, Butenandt isolated from the male urine a chemically pure compound with androgenic activity which he named androsterone and, a few years later, another which he designated as dehydroisoandrosterone. In 1935, Butenandt and Ruzicka achieved the synthesis of androsterone from cholesterol. In the same year, Laqueur and David isolated a substance from a bull's testis which was much more active than androsterone and which they called testosterone. This was later shown to be the prime male hormone and the progenitor of all other androgens, which were found to be mere catabolites or intermediary metabolites of testosterone.

In 1935, Butenandt was able to establish the structural formula of testosterone. The following year, several investigators successfully synthesized testosterone and showed that its derivatives, such as methyltestosterone and testosterone propionate, were most suitable for therapeutic purposes. To date, the hormone has been used predominantly in its ester forms. In 1936, Reichstein discovered the adrenocortical androgen adrenosterone and, in the following years, Kendall, Wintersteiner and Talbot isolated several additional adrenocortical androgens. All were found to possess a ketone group on carbon 17 and were thus designated by the generic term 17-ketosteroids. In 1938, Zimmermann[104] developed a procedure for the chemical determination of 17-ketosteroids, which was as significant for the study of androgens as pregnanediol determination was for the study of progesterone metabolism.

4.2. CHEMISTRY

All androgens have the steroid cyclopentanophenanthrene nucleus. The parent hydrocarbon from which they are all theoretically derived is androstane (Fig. 4–1) which, except for the saturation of the first and second six-membered rings, has the same structural skeleton as the natural estrogens (see Chapter 2). It differs from the parent hydrocarbon of the corticoids and progesterone, pregnane, only by the absence of carbons 20 and 21.

The hormone originally isolated from the testis is testosterone, an androstene-17-ol-3-one. The most important compound among the urinary 17-ketosteroids, which are largely end-products of testosterone degradation, is androsterone (Fig. 4–1). This is an androstane-3-ol-17-one, resulting from the transposition of the ketone and hydroxyl groups and the complete saturation of the ring structure of testosterone. Dehydrogenation of androsterone, with formation of a double bond between carbons 5 and 6, gives dehydroepiandrosterone, which can be derived from cholesterol. Cholesterol, in turn, was the starting material from which Butenandt and Ruzicka achieved the synthesis of testosterone simultaneously in 1935. This fact would indicate that, rather than being a degradation product, dehydroepiandrosterone is a *precursor* in the biogenesis of the testicular hormone. It has also been isolated from urine of both males and females. Also from urine have been isolated several α and β *stereoisomers* related to androsterone. The alpha (*trans*) and beta (*cis*) designations refer to the spatial configurations of groups attached to the steroid nucleus. Some of these are etiocholanolone (stereoisomer of androsterone), 11-ketoandrosterone and 11-ketoetiocholanolone, as well as 11β-hydroxyandrosterone and 11β-hydroxyetiocholanolone.

Another compound found in the urine is Δ3,5-androstadiene-17-one (Fig. 4-2). Adrenosterone is found in the adrenal cortex. These two compounds have weak androgenic activity. A third weakly androgenic compound, 11-ketoandrosterone, which is present in large amounts in urine of both males and females, was also isolated from the adrenal cortex by Reichstein. The synthetic methylated product of testosterone, methyltestosterone (Fig. 4-2), is effective when administered orally.

Apart from variations in potency, certain minor qualitative differences in the mode of action of different androgens have been reported (Neuweiler and Richter).[66]

4.3. ACTIVITY IN THE MALE

Androgenicity in the male is reviewed here only cursorily, since the true interest of this book with regard to androgenic effects is focused on the female body. Suffice it to say that androgens act on the male genital tract principally by eliciting proliferation of the seminal vesicles and of the prostate (Fig. 4-3), although they also act on the epididymis and on the ejaculatory ducts in a more discrete way. The androgens also exert a manifest effect on secondary male sex characteristics in both animals and man. In the male fowl, they stimulate comb growth and, if injected into the capon, they induce regrowth of the comb to normal size. In the human male, they likewise influence the development of genitalia, the descent of testes into the scrotum during the final period of embryonal life, the development of the penis, the male form of hair distribution and other somatic and psychic characteristics pertaining to the male. Androgens not only exert direct morphogenetic and masculinizing effects but also have a series of general actions on the endocrine glands and on metabolism. To some extent, these actions are similar to those of progestogens and corticosteroids; all three classes of hormones have anabolic activity and stimulate those endocrine glands which are anabolically oriented (Botella[11]).

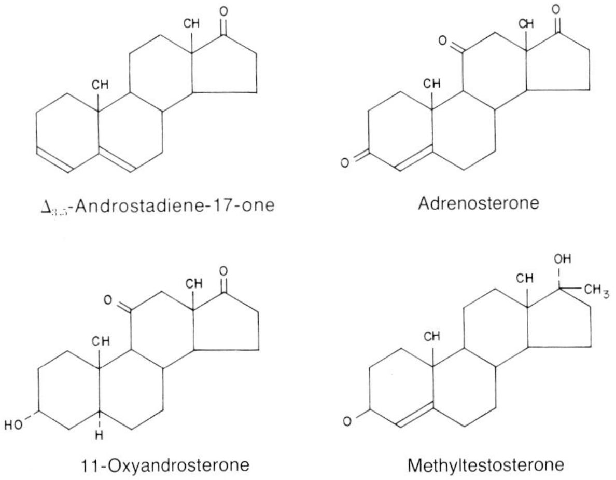

Figure 4-2. Δ3,5-Androstadiene-17-one, andrenosterone, 11-oxyandrosterone, methyltestosterone.

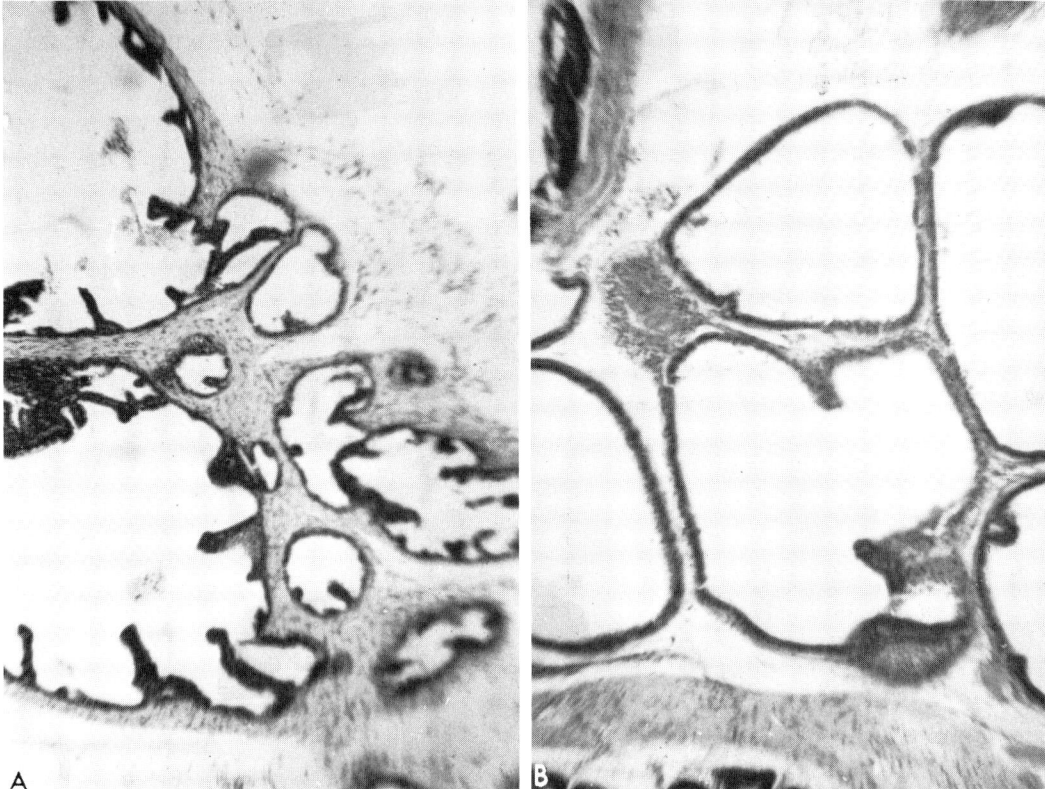

Figure 4–3. Bioassay of testosterone, using mouse seminal vesicle (test of Loewe and Voss). *A*, Before injection; *B*, after injection of testosterone. Note how seminal vesicles undergo marked dilatation.

4.4. ACTIVITY IN THE FEMALE BODY

Androgenicity in the female can be divided into two types: (1) *antifeminizing activity,* i.e., the type antagonizing the actions of estrogens, and (2) *pseudoprogestational activity,* i.e., resembling the actions of the progesterone group.

4.4.1. EFFECTS ON THE OVARY

The ovaries of immature animals are stimulated by androgens. As pointed out by MacKinney and Payne,[61] these effects are mediated by the pituitary and are the result of stimulation of gonadotropin secretion. Contradictory effects are observed in adult animals and in adult women. The administration of small amounts of hormone seems to produce a stimulatory effect on ovarian development, which is thought to result from a compensatory mechanism whereby the female gonad counters the extraneous influence of a hormone possessing antagonistic action.[46] On the other hand, large doses of androgens inhibit the ovary.[57] This seems to be due to the fact that large amounts of androgens exert an inhibitory effect on the pituitary and inactivate gonadotropin secretion. It is a general biologic phenomenon that the injection of a given hormone inhibits pituitary release of that particular trophic hormone which is specifically concerned with the physiologic secretion of the injected hormone. Accordingly, administration of a sex hormone inactivates the corresponding gonadotropin activity. Henry and co-workers[41] and Arnold and Richter[2] reported increased estrogenuria following androgen therapy. Engstrom and Munson[27] and Botella and colleagues[11, 13] found elevated urinary pregnanediol levels after injections of testosterone. These effects, which might be thought to contradict the preceding postulate and to be attributable to ovarian *stimulation,* are in fact the result of internal conversions of androgens, estrogens and, in some instances, progestogens. Androgens injected into infantile or prepubertal animals produce anovulatory ovarian cycles, owing to hypothalamic injury.[7, 31, 33, 44] Later in this chapter (Section 4.4.8), we shall emphasize this important effect.

4.4.2. EFFECTS ON THE UTERUS

ENDOMETRIUM. The effects of androgens on endometria of experimental animals are paradoxical; if they are injected into castrated animals, mild proliferative effects are apparent,[30] whereas in noncastrate adult females, the effects are much more dramatic. Various workers[8, 17, 22, 84] have been able to demonstrate unquestionable progestational effects by testosterone on rabbit, rat and guinea pig endometria. The progestational effects of testosterone are thought to be identical to those of progesterone, although the former is only about one twentieth as potent as the latter. Parkes and Zuckermann have been able to induce the growth of deciduomas with testosterone injections. Testosterone would thus appear to have weak progestogenic activity in experimental animals.

Effects on human endometria are more debatable. Although original clinical observations seemed to attribute the inhibitory effects on endometrial growth to estrogens, current thinking does not consider the favorable effects that testosterone has on functional uterine bleeding as resulting from production of endometrial atrophy but rather stemming from stimulation of secretory changes. Consequently, androgens may exert effects similar to those of progesterone.[8, 98]

EFFECTS OF THE MYOMETRIUM. Testosterone diminishes uterine vascularization[41, 56] and depresses uterine contractility, probably as a result of nonspecific activity.[2, 66] Pseudoprogestational effects had been described in earlier works.[12, 13]

4.4.3. EFFECTS ON THE VAGINA

Vaginal changes in rats have been described by Korenchewsky and Dennison as being of the progesteroid type, with concomitant appearance of superficial mucification. Similar findings in vaginas of guinea pigs were reported by Lipschutz.[57] Pundel[74] and Wied[97] have described a type of vaginal cell that is characteristic of the androgenic effect in the woman, which they call the *androgenic cell*. It resembles the cells produced during the corpus luteum phase, a fact that also supports the hypothesis of inherent pseudoprogestational activity of androgens.

4.4.4. EFFECTS ON THE VULVA

Effects on the vulva are of an altogether different nature. Unlike the purportedly progesteroid effects, weak as they may be, of androgens on the previously discussed organs of the female genital tract, androgenic effects on the vulva are frankly inhibitory of secondary female sexual characteristics. Androgens cause atrophy of the labia majora and minora and in turn stimulate the growth of both prepuce and clitoris.[51, 71, 72] Thus, for the first time, we are confronted with an instance in which stimulation of heterologous sex characteristics in the female takes place under the direct influence of androgenic activity.

4.4.5. EFFECTS ON THE SOMATIC FEATURES OF FEMININITY

Even though androgens at low levels fail to influence the bodily appearance of women,[63-68] *virilization* is the rule with sustained administration of high doses. Virilization is reflected not only by the enlargement of the clitoris and its acquisition of a peniform shape (Fig. 4-4), but also by a changed pattern of hair distribution resulting in the appearance of a male type of pilification of the upper lip and growth of a beard (Fig. 4-5). It is not unusual to observe the appearance of whiskers and beard in women treated with very large doses of androgens, such as in treatment of breast cancer (Fig. 4-5). The voice tends to become deep and coarse, and psychic function may be altered in a masculine, or at least pseudomasculine, direction. Later we shall dwell upon the extent to which sexual instincts may undergo modification under the influence of the male sex hormone, a possibility which at present is thought to be highly unlikely. In those

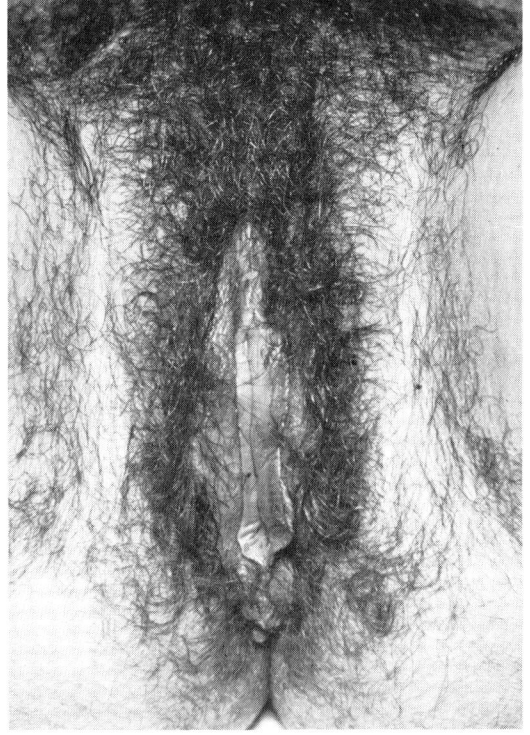

Figure 4-4. Hypertrophy of clitoris and perineal hyperpiliation in woman on long-term androgen therapy.

induces an entirely male pattern of behavior (Hart[38]).

4.4.7. EFFECTS ON EMBRYONAL MALE GENITAL TRACT RESTS

In adult females, sexual differentiation has been achieved to such a degree as to insure the complete development of the female sex organs and genital tract, with atrophy of heterologous characters, i.e., the remnants of the wolffian duct. During fetal life, however, those remnants, though already atrophied, are still highly responsive and can be stimulated to physiologic proliferation by androgens. Therefore, in those cases in which androgens are produced in abundance during embryonal development (such as the already mentioned adrenogenital syndrome), full development of the wolffian duct organs may ensue. The presence of the residual wolffian organs gives rise to what is referred to as *female pseudohermaphroditism*, to be discussed in more detail later (Chapter 37).

cases in which the body is flooded with loading dosages of androgens — viz., in cases with certain virilizing ovarian tumors and, above all, with adrenocortical adenomas exerting gonadal effects (see *Adrenogenital syndrome*, Chapter 33) — what can be seen is the development of marked hirsutism, penis-like clitoris, piliation of the abdominal linea alba and of the thighs, and growth of facial hair. Such is the clinical picture of so-called *virilism* which is present only in pathologic conditions.

4.4.6. EFFECTS ON THE FEMININE PSYCHE AND ON LIBIDO

Earlier, we questioned whether female sexual behavior can be influenced in a heterosexual sense by injections of testosterone. As a matter of fact, one of the applications of testosterone in recent times stems from its known value in the treatment of female *sexual frigidity*.

In female rats, testosterone injection

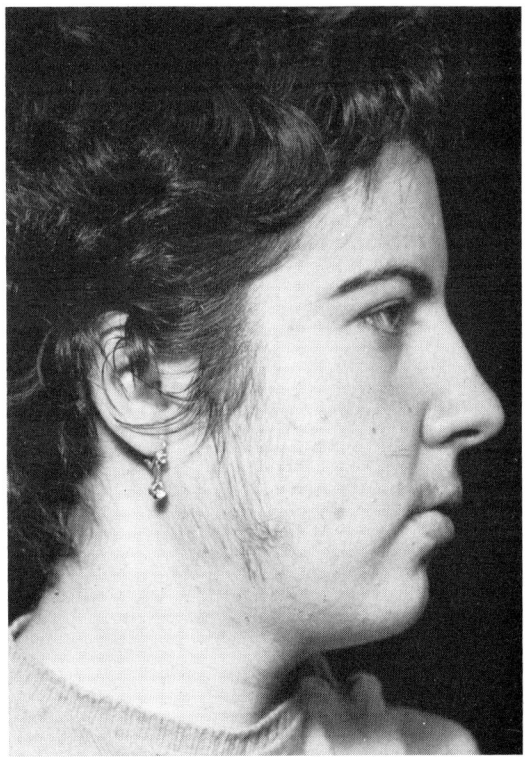

Figure 4-5. Facial hyperpiliation in woman on long-term androgen therapy.

4.4.8. EFFECTS OF ANDROGENS ON THE PREPUBERTAL FEMALE

Barraclough[7] found that if newborn rats were treated with a single dose of androgen, the animals would remain permanently sterile, even though no further androgens were given for the rest of their lives. This type of sterility is the result of production of a permanent anovulatory cycle. Sexual behavior in these animals similarly may suffer to the point of disorganization and even prevention of mating.[50] Zeilmaker[103] has shown that testosterone acts by paralyzing permanently the hypothalamic release mechanism of LH (see Chapter 8). Campbell[16] tested the effects of neonatal injections of different hormones on the hypothalamus of the rat. It would appear that injury to the sexual center can also be caused by certain progestogens and even estrogens, but to a lesser degree and with less specificity. These effects have been confirmed in mice,[93, 94] rats,[31, 37, 44, 80] guinea pigs[33] and presumably also in man.[51] The animals show loss of hypothalamic "secretory rhythm" and tend to behave like males. The sexual instinct, as we have stated, is affected by this loss of rhythm. It is believed that testicular predominance in a male fetus during gestation determines the noncyclic character of the hypophysial-hypothalamic axis (see Chapter 20). Fels and his colleagues[28] have noted, in rats treated with androgens at the moment of birth, that intrasplenic implants of ovarian tissue do not undergo luteinization, which would seem to indicate an inability of the hypothalamus to react to the lack of circulating estrogens. It is quite possible that some forms of human sterility resulting from anovulatory cycles originate in the same manner (see Chapter 41).

4.4.9. OTHER EFFECTS

EFFECTS ON THE GLANDS OF INTERNAL SECRETION. Like estrogens and progestogens, androgens also influence the glands of internal secretion. The gland in the forefront among those affected is the *pituitary*. As stated previously,[8] androgens stimulate the pituitary at low doses, whereas in large amounts they inhibit the pituitary.[9, 34] In large part, the beneficial effects androgens have in the climacterium, and in some cases of tumors of the genital organs, result from this pituitary-inhibiting activity.[59, 96]

The *adrenal cortex* likewise is affected by androgens in a definite way. Injections of small doses are stimulatory,[11, 76] and there is no doubt that stimulation is due to the intermediary function of the pituitary gland. Injection of androgens at higher dosages produces atrophy of the adrenal zona reticularis.[8, 9] Castration in rats and mice is followed by adrenocortical hyperplasia, which is brought about mainly by the overriding development of the so-called interstitial, or intermediate, *X zone* (see Chapter 9). This zone can be caused to disappear by injections of testosterone. For a long time, the inhibitory effects of testosterone were thought to be a direct action on the adrenal cortex, but present understanding, gained from hypophysectomized animals, in which these effects fail to appear, unquestionably accepts androgenic suppression of the pituitary as the mechanism involved.

Various effects of androgenic activity on the *thyroid gland* have been described, but most authors agree that the anabolic properties of androgens are opposed to those of the thyroid hormone and, therefore, are definitely beneficial in the management of hyperthyroidism.

The reported antidiabetic effect of testosterone, presumably based on stimulation of the islets of Langerhans, was shown also to be due to inhibition of pituitary secretion—in this case, of diabetogenic hormone. Androgens are therefore of value in postmenopausal diabetes (see Chapter 39), which is known to be a type of diabetes with a predominantly hypophysial component.

EFFECTS ON THE BREAST. The action exerted by androgens on the breast is partly stimulatory and partly inhibitory (see Chapter 22). However, it is pertinent to remember that some effects may not be due so much to a direct action of testosterone as to products of alterations and conversions in the body.[41, 53, 56]

EFFECTS OF METABOLISM. The metabolic actions of androgens are very interesting. They consist fundamentally in bringing about an increase of anabolic processes by elevating hepatic glycogen content,[76] by diminishing ketogenesis,[68] by promoting protein anabolism and by influencing water and electrolyte metabolism much as do the mineralocorticoids. Small amounts of androgens tend to normalize disturbances of the ionic equilibrium, but large doses may produce water and sodium retention and even edema.[34, 76]

EFFECTS ON THE EMBRYO. Androgens stimulate the development of the wolffian structures. Jost found that androgens elaborated in the embryonal testis play a decisive part in the ultimate development of the male sex. Bjorn and Gardner[9] have noted the presence of certain developmental anomalies in embryos exposed to excessive androgenic levels. The fetal body seems to be the seat of active androgen metabolism of its own, independent of the mother's androgen levels. Injections into pregnant rats of *cyproterone*, an anti-androgen to be discussed later (Section 4.7.5), inhibit the formation of testicular androgens in male embryos. This leads to disturbances in the embryonal development of male organs, resulting in experimental pseudohermaphroditism (Hohlweg[43]).

4.5. ASSAY

As with the other sex hormones, the methods of androgen assay are based on either *biologic procedures* (bioassay) or *chemical procedures.*

Bioassay procedures were the first to be employed, but have been relegated to a secondary position today. They are still of use, however, for purposes of physiologic experimentation or estimation. Chemical procedures detect only androgens with a ketone group on carbon 17 (17-ketosteroids), which, on the whole, does not yield a true index of androgenic function, owing to the fact that some 17-ketosteroids have very weak or no androgenic activity at all, whereas other potent androgens—viz., testosterone—actually are not 17-ketosteroids. Although chemical methods for the determination of androgens are rapidly replacing the bioassay procedures altogether, as is the case with estrogens, bioassay is still, for the time being, largely irreplaceable.

4.5.1. BIOASSAY

The principal procedures for the biologic assay of androgenic activity are the *test of capon's comb growth* and the *seminal vesicle growth assay.* The former test, introduced by Funk in 1930, consists in injecting a capon with the purified test substance. Comb atrophy is a known sequela of castration in the male fowl, but the comb can be restored to its normal size by injections of androgens. With this in mind, capons are injected with the androgen and the resulting incremental comb growth, if any, is measured planimetrically by means of either a millimeter scale or a photograph at a set scale, from which the surface of incremental growth can be calculated in square centimeters. Callow[15] reported that the increase in comb surface is logarithmically proportional to the amount of injected hormone.

The rat seminal vesicle method has been developed by Loewe and Voss. If a male rat is castrated, its seminal vesicles atrophy and persist in a rudimentary state. After injecting an androgen containing preparation into such an animal, the seminal vesicles respond by increasing in weight. Concomitant growth of the *ventral prostate* may also be observed, but this is less expressive. Although seminal vesicle growth may be observable grossly, it is best determined by measuring weight gain. The increase in weight of the vesicles is also logarithmically proportional to the amount of injected hormone.

4.5.2. CHEMICAL DETERMINATION

Chemical estimation of androgenic activity is done by determination of 17-ketosteroid levels. Several methods have been devised for that purpose, particularly by Zimmermann,[104] by Dobriner[23] and Kase and colleagues.[49] The three methods are based on the same principle, the colorimetric reaction of 17-ketosteroids with *meta-dinitrobenzene* after neutral hydrolysis; the red color so produced has a maximum spectral absorption in the 520 millimicron band. This colorimetric procedure can be combined with several modifications of chromatographic adsorption methods, so that as many as eight different fractions of 17-ketosteroids can be separated and determined, by various techniques, from a single urine sample (see Chapter 24). Since large amounts of sample are necessary for the extraction and concentration steps, 17-ketosteroid determinations are mainly carried out on urine. This by itself is a drawback, but it is of minor importance compared to the fact that these compounds do not constitute a direct index of androgen metabolism. A large number of urinary 17-ketosteroids, as will be seen later, not only have no androgenic activity at all, but do not even reflect androgen formation in the body. For this reason, increasing importance is being attached to urinary[25, 36] and plasma[79] *testosterone* determinations, which reflect more faithfully the androgenicity in the body. In addition, Lederer and Bataille[55] have devised a "dynamic test," which is based on determination of urinary testosterone after administration of a loading dose of 5000 IU chorionic gonadotropin.

4.6. FORMATION, METABOLISM, EXCRETION

4.6.1. ANDROPOIESIS

Androgens are elaborated by *three different endocrine glands:* (1) *the testis,* (2) *the adrenal cortex,* and (3) *the ovary.* Biogenesis in the last of the three, for a long time thought to occur only in abnormal cases, has been convincingly demonstrated to occur *in the normal ovary,* too, thanks to the recent works of Mahesh and Greenblatt,[62] Savard and colleagues,[84] Seemann and Saracino[89] and Zander.[102] Thus, while in the male 60 per cent of androgens originate in the testis and 40 per cent in the adrenal, in the female about 60 per cent of androgens are formed by the adrenal cortex and, without doubt, at least 40 per cent are elaborated by the female gonad.

TESTIS. The *Leydig cells* in the *interstitial tissue* of the testes are the principal sites of androgen biogenesis. The hormone produced, *testosterone,* is the most potent androgen of all. Knapstein and co-workers[52] have demonstrated de novo synthesis of testicular testosterone starting from acetate. As a result of research done in the last few years,[62, 85, 86, 102] there is general agreement on the existence of two main metabolic pathways for testosterone synthesis, as outlined in Table 4–1 (see also Fig. 4–6). One pathway proceeds by way of progesterone, and the other by way of dehydroepiandrosterone.

TABLE 4–1. The Two Pathways of Androgenesis*

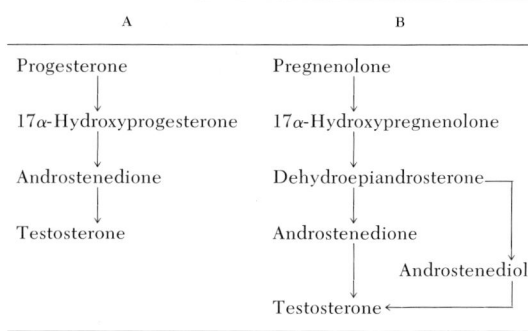

*From Butt: Hormone Chemistry. London, Van Nostrand, 1967.

There is a widely held view that most of the 17-ketosteroids appearing in the urine are of testicular origin and that, therefore, most of the metabolized androgens must likewise be derived from the gonads. This view is erroneous. It can be shown that castrated animals and men both continue eliminating 17-ketosteroids in the urine at a rate only 30 per cent below that of noncastrated animals or men.[24] The finding that testicular ablation accounts for only about one third of the urinary 17-ketosteroids would seemingly indicate the secondary role played by testicular androgen synthesis.[39, 100] However, this figure, which is obtained by estimating the neutral urinary 17-ketosteroids by the Zimmermann or similar methods, offers a misleading estimate of the androgenic potency of the hormones of both the testis and the adrenal cortex. Indeed, while the urinary 17-ketosteroid concentrations in the castrate male drop by 30 to 40 per cent, the decrease in androgenic potency is much greater.[10] Recent studies of the different types of excreted 17-ketosteroids (Fig. 4–7) by means of *chromatographic fractionation*[10, 24, 41, 60, 64] reveal that castration and adrenalectomy alike cause disappearance of *certain types* of steroids, which in each case may be considered as characteristic of either testicular or adrenal secretion. Thus, *androsterone* predominates among the testicular catabolites, whereas *dehydroepiandrosterone* must be considered as an indicator of adrenocortical activity. Adrenocortical catabolites are invariably *less androgenic* than are testicular catabolites.

In attempting to pinpoint the site of testicular testosterone biogenesis

Androgens in the Female Body 71

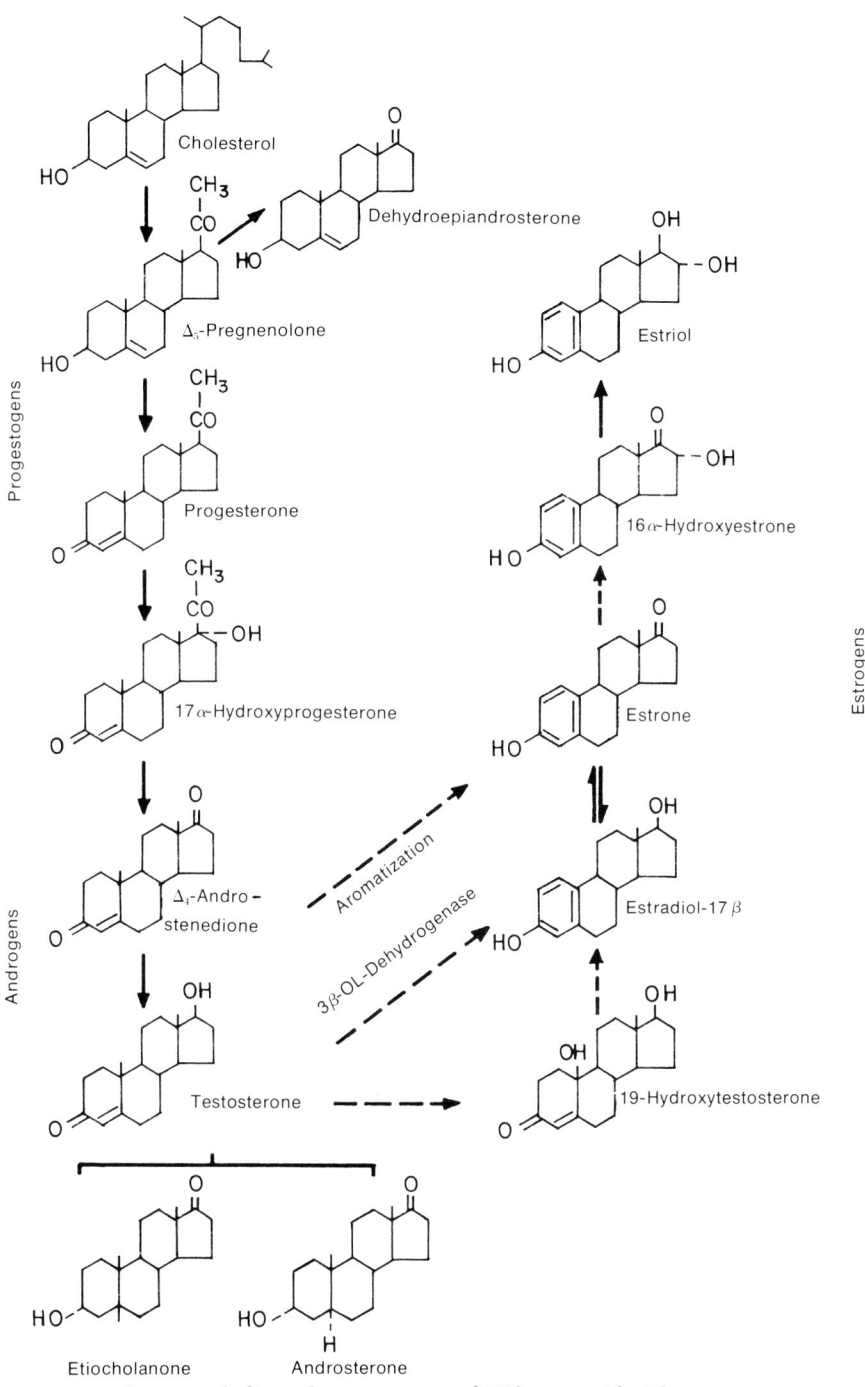

Figure 4-6. Intermediary metabolism of testosterone and 17-ketosteroids. The conversion sequence testosterone → androstenedione → androstanedione → androsterone is characteristic of the gonads. The conversion sequence etiocholanedione → etiocholanolone, and that taking place via dehydroepiandrosterone, is typical of the adrenal cortex. (After Dorfman: In *The Hormones*, Vol. III, ed. G. Pincus and K. V. Thiman. New York, Academic Press, 1955.)

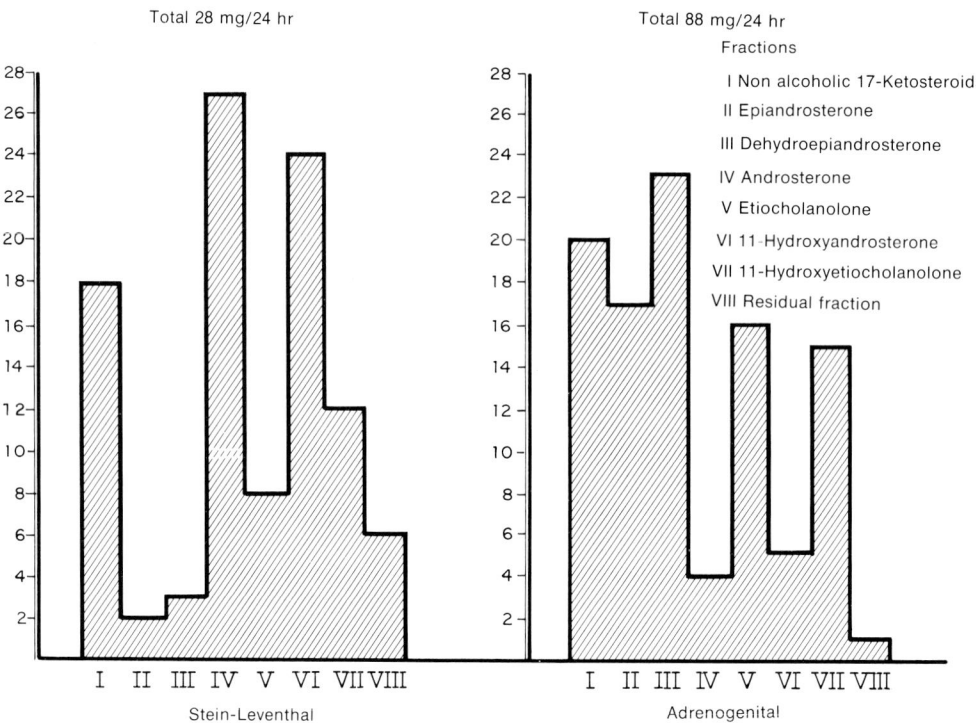

Figure 4–7. Chromatographic separation of urinary 17-ketosteroids in a case of ovarian virilism (Stein-Leventhal syndrome) and in a case of adrenal virilism (adrenogenital syndrome). Note preponderance of androsterone fraction in first case and that of epiandrosterone in the second.

precisely, recent research conducted by Baillie and Griffiths[6] and by Davies and co-workers[20] showed the presence of the enzyme 3β-ol-dehydrogenase in the Leydig cells. This enzyme is necessary for the formation of androgens (see Fig. 4–9). High temperatures partially inhibit its action,[35] which explains why there is a lowered testosterone output in ectopic testes. Investigations by Christensen and Mason[18] have also demonstrated that Leydig cells can utilize C-14 labeled progesterone to produce radioactive testosterone.

ADRENAL CORTEX. The fact we have dedicated an entire chapter (Chapter 9) to adrenocortical endocrine activity enables us to confine the present discussion to a summary presentation. The 17-ketosteroids so far have been considered as a product of specific adrenocortical activity, and the determination of their urinary excretion has been viewed as a measure of adrenocortical function. These notions, as will be pointed out, have been based on an erroneous premise. Adrenocortical androgens are formed whenever progestogens (i.e., C-21 steroids in general) have not been completely metabolized to cortisol (see Chapter 9). Thus, accumulation of 17-ketosteroids of adrenocortical origin must be considered as reflecting *enzymatic failure* in the conversion of cholesterol via pregnenolone to progesterone and then to corticoids. However, excessive hypophysial activity, mediated by ACTH or by LH, is capable of converting cholesterol to pregnenolone in amounts surpassing the needs of corticogenesis.[3, 11, 47, 101] This would lead to a surplus of unutilized 17-ketosteroid substances.

Apart from the previously mentioned dehydroepiandrosterone, the other remaining androgenic catabolites of the adrenal cortex are etiocholane-3,17-dione, with two ketone groups; etiocholanolone, an isomer of androsterone but of lesser androgenic potency; and the alcoholic derivative of dehydroepiandrosterone, androstenediol, which has both estrogenic and androgenic activity, and serves as a link with adrenal estrogen metabolism and can be utilized for therapeutic purposes (see Fig. 4–6).

OVARY. *Even under normal conditions,*

the ovary is a specific androgen producer. Considering the androgen-over-estrogen priorities in steroid biogenesis, it may be added that *without prior androgen synthesis, elaboration of estrogens would not be possible*. Ovarian androgenesis is not just an attribute of the Stein-Leventhal syndrome and of arrhenoblastomas but occurs as a normal physiologic process in the ovary.

A long time ago, Ponse[73] showed that, in rodents, LH activity stimulated the ovarian interstitial tissue to elaborate androgens, which produced virilization. A similar finding in woman was reported by Plate.[70, 71] Johnson[45] also observed virilization in both intact and castrated rats in parabiosis, which lends support to the earlier hypotheses. Culiner and Shippel[19] demonstrated that androgens induce thecal cell hyperplasia in the human ovary. Guinea pig ovaries that were incubated with pregnenolone and hydroxypregnenolone and stimulated by chorionic gonadotropin were shown to produce testosterone.[105] Similar effects have been observed in ovaries of rabbits[32] as well as those of women.[86] The site of major ovarian androgen synthesis is thought to be the *hilar region*,[26, 77] but important androgenesis has also been demonstrated in the *corpus luteum*.[32] The part played by gonadotropin hyperactivity (involving either LH or CG) seems to have been confirmed by the finding that, in rats, ovarian transplants to the spleen acquired an increased androgen-secreting capacity[73] (Fig. 4–8).

Each of the various kinds of ovarian tissues (theca, granulosa, interstitial stroma, etc.) possesses an enzyme system of its own, which, insofar as steroidogenesis is concerned, is complementary to each to the others. As a result, ovarian androgen synthesis cannot be stated to be linked to any particular type of tissue (Lisse[58]). Nevertheless, investigations by Oakey and Stitch,[69] as well as those by Schrieffers and Schmidt,[88] seem to indicate that an *incomplete* form of *estrogen synthesis* may occur in atretic follicles and in fibrothecal masses, but this is arrested at a step immediately prior to the formation of estrogens; that is, androgens are formed. In the opinion of these authors, this may explain why fibroatretic ovaries display a predominantly androgenic character.

It is probable that apart from the *ovaries* and *adrenal cortices* there are other, hitherto unknown, tissues capable of producing androgens, as one must assume from experiments with castrated or adrenalectomized animals, in whose urine androgens continue to be found.[95, 96]

MECHANISM OF ANDROPOIESIS. Inves-

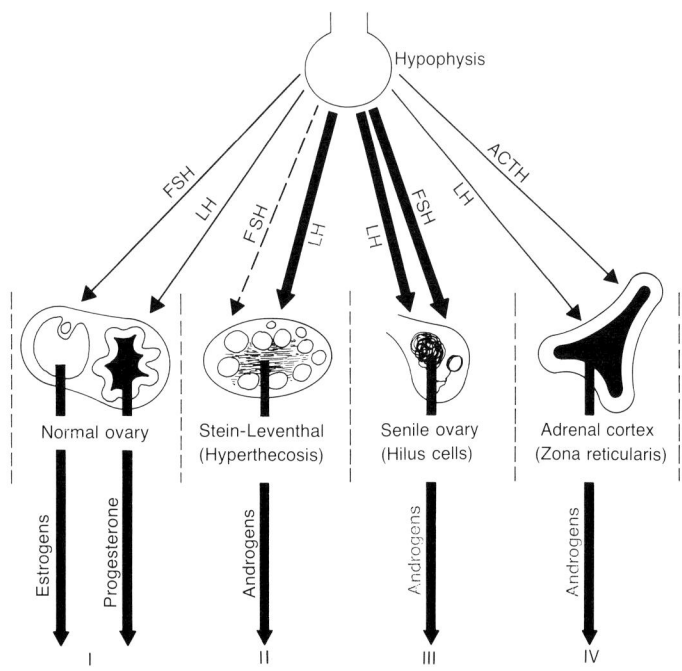

Figure 4–8. Diagram of conditions that may be associated with androgen production in the female. I, Normal ovary. Luteinizing hormone (LH) acts on ovary containing mature follicles, eliciting ovulation and luteinization. II, Stein-Leventhal syndrome. FSH deficiency and lack of normal maturation. Pathologic increase in LH in immature ovary produces hyperthecosis and abnormally elevated androgen production. III, Same effect occurring in postmenopausal ovary. There is an increase in both FSH and LH activity, but the former has no target organ to act upon, and consequently maturation does not occur. LH acts on hilus cells, the resulting hyperplasia of the latter leading to virilization. Sometimes LH also provokes cortical stromal hyperplasia. IV, LH and ACTH, acting independently or synergistically, increase androgen production.

tigations carried out during the last few years have elucidated the *mechanism of ovarian androgen biogenesis.* Zander[101] has isolated androstenedione from normal ovarian tissue, a finding also confirmed by others.[62, 91] It has been possible to isolate dehydroepiandrosterone, considered as a compound of adrenocortical origin, from normal ovaries, although it is present in much larger amounts in polycystic ovaries and in those associated with the Stein-Leventhal syndrome (see Chapter 29). Finally, Simmer and Voss,[91] as well as Mahesh and Greenblatt,[62] have found testosterone in some, though not in all, ovaries. Dehydroepiandrosterone occurs not only in the free form but also in the conjugated form. Although a cyclic secretion of androgens is postulated by Junkmann,[47] this has, in Zander's view,[102] not yet been demonstrated conclusively. If the presence of androgens does not constitute absolute proof of ovarian secretion, the finding of considerable amounts of androgens in the ovarian vein of normal ovaries[64, 89, 90] is nevertheless important evidence in favor of ovarian androgen formation. Savard and his colleagues,[85, 86] on the other hand, have been able to demonstrate the conversion of progesterone to testosterone in homogenates of testicular tissue, and Axelrod and Goldzieher,[3] Lanthier and Sandor,[53, 54, 83] as well as Zander, using radioactive substances, have been able to show that this conversion takes place in both homogenates and slices of normal human ovary. Zander condensed these ideas in the diagram shown in Figure 4–9.

As illustrated in Figure 4–9, under normal conditions androgens are indispensable building blocks in the biogenesis of estrogens. This is a most important concept since it places androgens, originally viewed as extraneous to the female body, into the category of fundamental components of the most characteristic hormonal metabolism of that sex. What is likewise corroborated by these observations is that progesterone, as we stated in the two preceding chapters, is an estrogen precursor, not the other way around. Progesterone is an extremely unstable hormone, which seemingly cannot be stabilized except in the presence of the corpus luteum. Hence, it may be pertinent

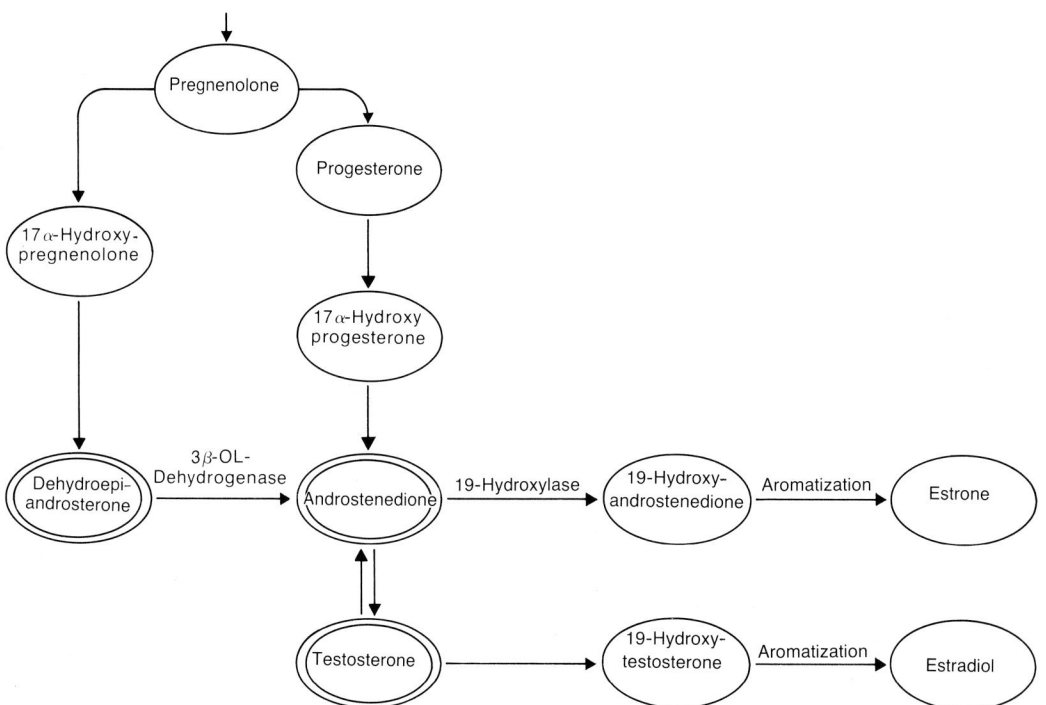

Figure 4–9. Outline of androgen biogenesis in the ovary. Note roles played by 3β-ol-dehydrogenase, by 19-hydroxylase and by aromatizing enzymes. Inactivation of the first two determines development of the Stein-Leventhal syndrome (discussed in Chapter 29). (From Zander: *Rev. Franç. Endocr. Clin. Nutr. Metab.,* 4:410, 1963.)

to assume that progesterone is continuously being produced by the ovary, the adrenal cortex and the testis, but it can be stabilized and made to persist only in the presence of granulosa-lutein cells.

The diagram also encompasses three groups of enzymes that are indispensable for steroidogenesis. These enzymes were studied in Chapter 2 (Section 2.5.1). They are 3β-ol-dehydrogenase, the histochemical demonstration of which was achieved by Ryan and Smith, 19-hydroxylase, and the aromatizing enzymes. Chapter 29 deals with the Stein-Leventhal syndrome and other ovarian androgenic states caused by enzyme deficiencies, principally of 3β-ol-dehydrogenase and of 19-hydroxylase, that block estrogen biogenesis and, by a rebound phenomenon, increase production of androgens.

4.6.2. METABOLISM OF ANDROGENS

Like androgen synthesis, androgen metabolism in the female must be discussed as a distinct process that differs from androgen metabolism in the male.

IN THE MALE. Androgen biosynthesis starts from cholesterol. Concurrent investigations by Barry and colleagues[8] and by Heard and colleagues,[40] using injections of radioactive (C-14 labeled) cholesterol, provide evidence of radioactivity in androgens recovered from tissue and urine. Zaffaroni and his co-workers,[100] perfusing adrenals with cholesterol, observed that androgens, principally dehydroepiandrosterone, were formed from cholesterol. This compound, therefore seems to be a precursor in testicular testosterone biosynthesis. This hypothesis seems more conclusive if one remembers that years ago Ruzicka had successfully synthesized testosterone from cholesterol in the laboratory. Thus, it would appear that dehydroepiandrosterone and probably some other 17-ketosteroids of adrenocortical origin are first-step intermediary metabolites arising from cholesterol that can, in turn, be further utilized for the biogenesis of testosterone. Androsterone, on the other hand, seems to be the most frequently found degradation product of testosterone, the circumstantial evidence for which lies in the fact that testosterone injections are invariably followed by maximal urinary androsterone excretion in both male and female (Fig. 4–10).

Consequently, testosterone metabolism in the male can be summarized briefly by saying that cholesterol is converted to androgenic precursors, mainly dehydroepiandrosterone, in the adrenal cortex and these precursor substances are then synthesized into testosterone in the testis. Finally, testosterone disintegrates, giving androsterone. Testosterone disintegration, with the resulting freeing of androsterone, takes place principally in the liver, as was demonstrated by various authors, including Grayhanck and Scott,[34] on hepatectomized experimental animals, in which such testosterone disintegration could not take place. *The cycle of androgen metabolism in the male can thus be conceived as proceeding from the adrenal cortex to the testis and from the testis to the liver.* This, of course, is merely a simplified outline, but it is indicative of the principal metabolic pathways taken by androgens in the male.

IN THE FEMALE. The sources of ovarian androgens and their mechanisms of conversion to estrogens have already been indicated.

The concept of *biotransformation of estrogens to androgens*, which until recently was unaccepted, has been established by Heard and colleagues.[39, 40] who injected C-14 labeled estrogens into pregnant mares. This same transformation was found to take place in the human placenta by Baggett and his co-workers[4, 5] in 1959. The relationship of androgen-progestogen interconversion has been studied by Samuels.[82] Furthermore, a relationship between 17-hydroxycorticosteroids and androgens has been envisaged by Dorfman and Shippel,[24] as well as by Brown and Migeon.[14] The boundaries determining specificity of these different hormones are therefore ill-defined. Androgens are present in nearly all pathways of steroid metabolism in both the male and the female.

Much as in the case with estrogens, androgens also have their characteristic and specific receptors at the tissue level. It is currently admitted that the syndrome of testicular feminization is caused by a congenital lack of such male receptors (see Chapter 3, Section 3.6.5.). Using tritiated testosterone, Roy and Laumas[81] observed specific uptake of the substance by the hypothalamus of female rats.

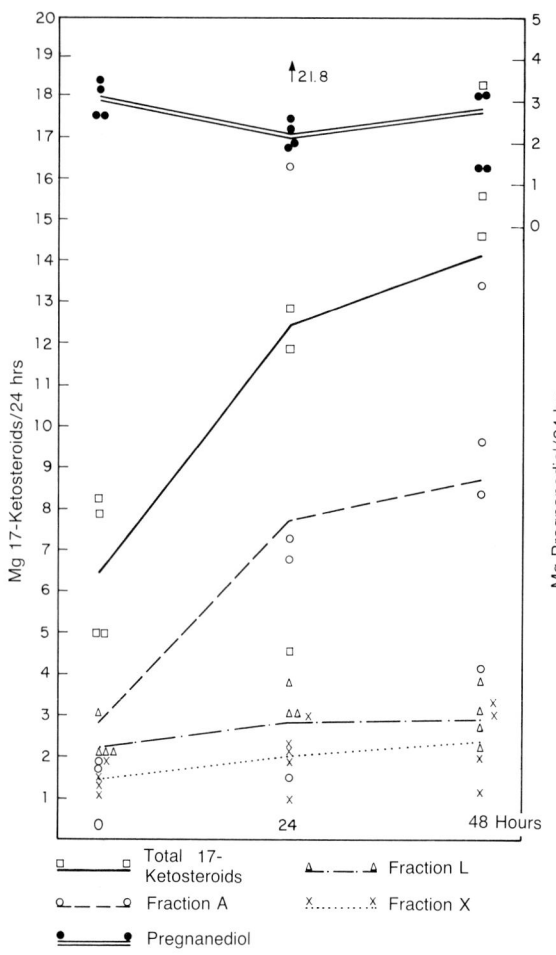

Figure 4-10. Excretion of neutral 17-ketosteroids after a loading dose of 100 mg of testosterone is given to a woman in the second half of the menstrual cycle. Most of the injected testosterone is recovered from urine in fraction A, containing androsterone. Fraction L, representing dehydroepiandrosterone and allopregnanolone, and fraction X, containing 11-oxyandrosterone, are hardly modified at all, or are so to a much lesser extent after overdose. (From Botella, Tornero and Fernández-Sánchez: *Riv. Ost. Gin.*, 9:217, 1955.)

4.6.3. ANDROGEN TRANSPORT

Like the other steroids, testosterone is bound to a specific protein which determines its transport (Southren et al.[92]).

4.6.4. EXCRETION

In our own investigations,[12, 13] we have attempted to study androgenic activity in the female by examining 17-ketosteroid excretion after a loading dose of testosterone. We found that a great deal of the injected testosterone could be recovered from the urine in the form of 17-ketosteroids and that concomitant injections of testosterone propionate were paralleled by an increase in the same urinary compounds. Part of the injected androgens were destroyed in the female body without ever appearing in the urine, this amount being constant in all cases, regardless of the injected dose. We therefore postulated a *quota of endogenous absorption* of androgens by the female body. This form of endogenous absorption varies over the course of the menstrual cycle and also with regard to age. So, during the follicular phase of the cycle, endogenous absorption in young females is scanty and reaches very large amounts during the luteal phase of the cycle. Absorption is low in postmenopausal women (Fig. 4-11). This observation, also confirmed by Engstrom and Munson,[27] seems to indicate a larger quota of endogenous absorption for the second half of the cycle or, in other words, *greater utilization of androgens during the corpus luteal phase.* We also noted that testosterone injections were followed by increased urinary pregnanediol excretions during the second half of the cycle, whereas there was no increase in diol excretion during the first half of the cycle, or in castrated and menopausal women (Figs. 4-12 and 4-13). From re-

Androgens in the Female Body

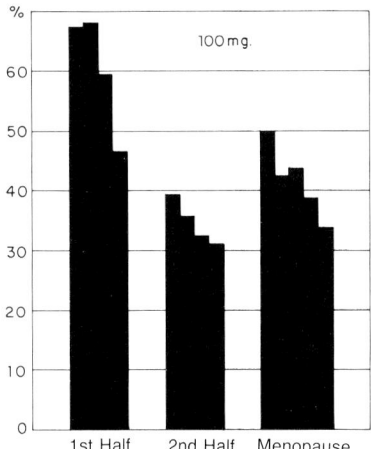

Figure 4-11. Urinary androgen recovery values in a group of normal women during first and second halves of the menstrual cycle and in a group of postmenopausal women. Endogenous androgen absorption reaches a peak during luteal phase in normal woman. (From Botella and Tornero: *Riv. Ost. Gin.*, 9:1955.)

viewing the balance sheet, we draw the conclusion that the endogenous absorption quota for androgens closely matches the amount by which excretion of pregnanediol has increased and, hence, we infer that *androgens are converted to pregnanediol during the luteal phase of the cycle.*

Because such conversion does not take place in either pregnancy or the first half of the cycle, or in castration or the menopause, we assume that the corpus luteum avails itself of injected androgens in order to convert them to compounds of the progestational series.

The aforementioned experimental observations fully coincide with the diagrammatic representation of ovarian androgen biogenesis, as outlined in Figure 4-9. Indeed, it is conceivable that injected testosterone prevents conversion of progesterone to 17α-hydroxyprogesterone and to androstenedione, whereby progesterone remains

Figure 4-12. Comparative experiment in normal woman during second half of menstrual cycle and in menopausal woman. Following testosterone injection, the normal woman excretes less androgens and more pregnanediol than the postmenopausal woman. These graphs suggest that the quota of endogenous androgen absorption is excreted in totality, or nearly so, in equimolecular quantities and in the form of pregnanediol. (From Gómez-Maestro and Botella-Llusiá: *Arch. Med. Exper.*, 18:1953.)

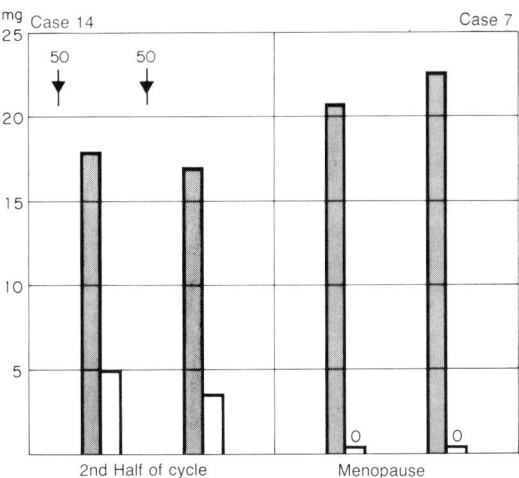

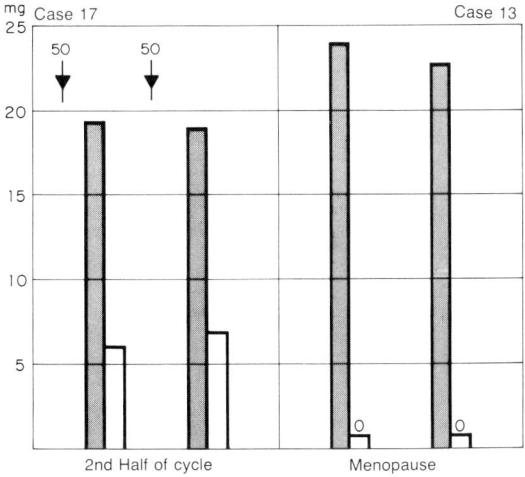

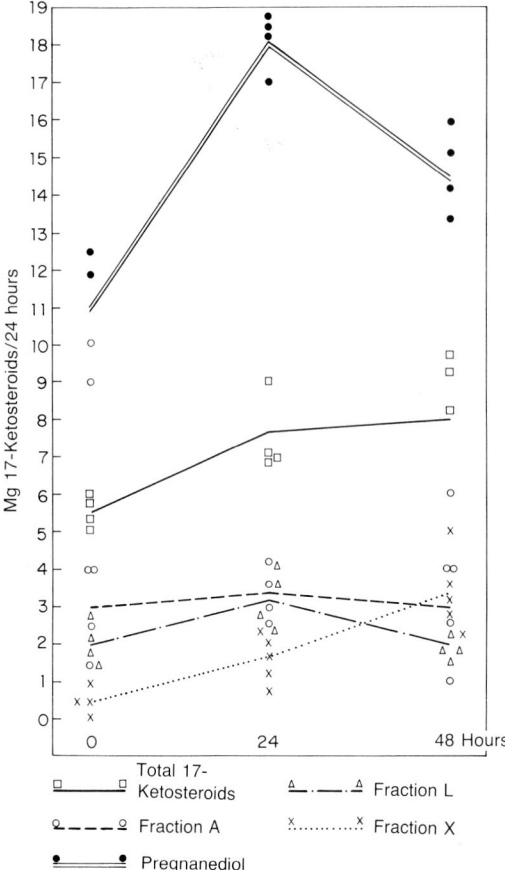

Figure 4-13. Compare with Figure 4-10. Comparison reveals that androgen injections during the second half of the menstrual cycle in women provoke elevated excretion of pregnanediol and 17-ketosteroids composing fraction X. The latter consist mainly of 11-oxyandrosterone and a group of related compounds derived directly from the adrenocortical metabolic pathway. For this reason, the injected testosterone is presumed to be converted to pregnanediol in the adrenal cortex at the same time that it is converted to fraction X. (From Botella, Tornero and Fernández-Sánchez: *Riv. Ost. Gin.,* 9:217, 1955.)

unmetabolized. Maintenance of progesterone in a stable state could only be achieved in the presence of the corpus luteum, from which it follows that only in the presence of a functional corpus luteum can androgen utilization by the ovary take place without excessive urinary androgen excretion. An increase in tolerance to androgens in active functional ovaries was reported by MacDonald and his colleagues[60] in 1963, and by Kase and co-workers,[48] as well as by Diamond and Young,[21] all in the same year. These more recent investigations support our own previous empirical observations.

4.7. PHARMACOLOGY

4.7.1. ANDROGEN UNITS

The use of biologic units, such as the capon unit and the rat unit, has fallen into disuse. A *capon unit* is the amount of hormone necessary to induce 100 per cent of comb growth in the capon under specified conditions, the description of which is beyond the scope of this book. The *rat unit* and the *mouse unit* correspond to amounts of hormone required to double the size of seminal vesicles in castrated male rats and mice, respectively, under specified experimental conditions. Values currently are expressed in terms of crystallized hormone; one capon unit, which is equivalent to one *international unit,* is one tenth of a milligram of androsterone. The international unit originally was defined as that quantity of crystallized hormone which contained one capon unit. *Testosterone has five times the potency of androsterone;* consequently, one international unit expressed in terms of testosterone is equivalent to 0.02 mg of testosterone propionate.

A rat unit is approximately half a capon unit, that is, 0.05 mg of crystallized androsterone or 0.01 mg of testosterone propionate.

4.7.2. USES AND MODE OF ADMINISTRATION

The most common mode of administration is by *intramuscular injection.* The preparation most commonly employed is *testosterone propionate* solution of sesame oil. Multiple-dose vials contain 10, 25 or 50 mg each, and the usual dosage is 25 mg. Intravenous injection is rarely used. Injections of *emulsions* or *suspensions* find special application in cases in which continuous androgenic therapy is desirable, such as in dysfunctional uterine bleeding, in certain menopausal disorders and, above all, in carcinomas. Aqueous suspensions of crystals, as well as emulsions, are prepared in dosages ranging from 50 to 250 mg.

Also currently in vogue are *topical applications of androgens.* It has been observed that absorption of these compounds by the skin (*percutaneous absorption*) is particularly effective, so that androgens can be applied in the form of lotions or solutions in oil by simple rubbing on the skin.

Oral forms of administration have the disadvantage of rapid degradation by the liver, so that *perlingual administration* in the form of linguets is preferable.

Finally, *implantation* of tablets or pellets, of 100, 200 or 250 mg, allows long-term therapy, as with other steroid hormone treatments.

4.7.3. DOSAGES

Dosages for androgens range from 10 to 250 mg. A dose of 10 mg is given either by injection or in the form of lozenges. These low dosages are applied in the treatment of functional disturbances mainly in young women apprehensive of the appearance of signs of virilization. The dosages to be employed for adult women are considerably higher, particularly for the treatment of tumors. In these cases, daily injections of 25 mg may be used, or the drug may be implanted in the form of pellets, emulsions or microcrystals, which permit administration of up to 200 or 250 mg at one time for continuous absorption extending over a period of up to one month, usually at a daily absorption rate oscillating between 5 and 25 mg. This mode of administration—by means of continuous slow absorption of not excessively high dosages (5 to 15 mg a day)—seems to be the one of choice. Higher daily absorption rates in women may lead to *virilization*. As can be inferred from our previously mentioned experience, the limit of the endogenous absorption quota for those androgens that are produced in the female body is in the neighborhood of 15 mg, so that, *as long as this limit is not exceeded, we feel confident that the female body can handle the total amount of androgens and effectively clear them from the circulation, making virilization impossible*. This seems to be one of the practical aspects of our investigations.

For the treatment of cystic glandular hyperplasia, leiomyomata, endometriosis or functional uterine bleeding, great care is required to estimate the dosages that should be given *for each cycle*. We believe that the dosage per cycle should never be in excess of 150 mg, taking into account that the total amount should be administered during the second half of the intermenstruum. For such cases, we therefore advocate the administration of 150 mg over a period of two weeks—in other words, 15 mg daily from day 15 to day 25 of the intermenstrual interval.

4.7.4. TOXICITY

While androgens are nearly free of toxic effects, their *abuse* may be conducive to conspicuous disorders in the female, which may even entail *amenorrhea*. Contrary to established beliefs, this type of amenorrhea is not due to the estrogen-antagonizing effects of androgens but to the *blocking action exerted on the pituitary*. However, the most frequently observed disturbance is *virilization*. This is a drawback of androgenic therapy of which the practicing physician must be aware, since women are particularly prone to complain about hypertrichosis of the face or legs. At any rate, unpleasant effects on the female are likely to be subjectively exaggerated, particularly through autosuggestion, when the physiologic effects of a preparation about to be injected are known beforehand. According to Swanson and Van der Werff,[93] androgens have lethal effects on embryos.

4.7.5. ANTI-ANDROGENS, CYPROTERONE

Substances attaching themselves to androgenic receptors in the manner outlined previously (see Section 4.6.2) compete with testosterone and thus prevent the latter's action at the tissue level. The synthetic progestogen *Cyproterone*, and particularly its acetate, have been found to possess highly effective anti-androgenic activity. That such activity is of local nature is shown by the fact that if this preparation is applied to rat seminal vesicle, it produces in situ inhibition of testosterone activity (Wollman[99]). Neumann[65] and Schneider and his colleagues[87] also defend this type of action. However, Hoffman and Breuer[42] observed a direct inhibitory effect by cyproterone on the testicular and adrenal biogenesis of C-19 steroids. Forsberg and Jacobson[29] reported that the administration of this substance to pregnant rats produces male pseudohermaphroditism (see Section 4.4.9).

4.8. SIGNIFICANCE OF ANDROGENS IN THE FEMALE BODY

For many years, androgens were believed to be a *pathologic element* in the woman, or perhaps an *ancestral vestige* left over from the bisexual embryonal stage and, therefore, a sort of *"error of nature."*

Nature rarely makes this type of sweeping error, and in the light of modern knowledge, androgens are accepted as basic and inseparable elements of the female physiologic makeup:

(1) *They are precursors of estrogens*, so that a metabolism of estrogens cannot be conceived without prior synthesis of androgens.

(2) They are engaged in regulating estrogenic activity and partake in a mechanism of *steroid homeostasis*.[57]

(3) They carry out certain *physiologic functions in the female body*, such as control of axillary and pubic hair growth and the maintenance of libido.

REFERENCES

1. Alloiteau, J. J., and Acker, G.: *Compt. Rend. Acad. Sci.*, 250:1566, 1960.
2. Arnold, M., and Richter, R. H. H.: *Gynaecologia*, 156:2, 1963.
3. Axelrod, L. R., and Goldzieher, J. W.: *J. Clin. Endocr. Metab.*, 22:431, 1962.
4. Baggett, B., Engel, L. L., Savard, K., and Dorfman, R. I.: *Jour. Biol. Chem.*, 221:931, 1956.
5. Baggett, B., et al.: *Endocrinology*, 64:600, 1959.
6. Baillie, A. H., and Griffiths, K.: *J. Endocr.*, 31:207, 1965.
7. Barraclough, C. A.: *Endocrinology*, 68:62, 1961.
8. Barry, M. C., et al.: *Endocrinology*, 50:587, 1952.
9. Bjorn, J. C., and Gardner, W. E. W.: *Endocrinology*, 59:48, 1956.
10. Bongiovanni, A., et al.: *J. Clin. Endocr. Metab.*, 14:409, 1954.
11. Botella, J.: *Arch. Gynäk.*, 183:73, 1953.
12. Botella, J.: *Acta Gin.*, 2:221, 1951.
13. Botella, J., et al.: *Riv. Ost. Gin (Firenze)*, 10:57, 1955.
14. Brown, C. H., and Migeon, C. A.: *J. Clin. Endocr. Metab.*, 16:1227, 1956.
15. Callow, R. K.: *Ciba Colloquia on Endocrinology*, 2:271, 1952.
16. Campbell, H. J.: *J. Physiol.*, 181:568, 1965.
17. Chang, E., Mittelman, A., and Dao, T. L.: *J. Biol. Chem.*, 238:913, 1963.
18. Christensen, A. K., and Mason, N. R.: *Endocrinology*, 76:646, 1965.
19. Culiner, A., and Shippel, L.: *J. Obst. Gynec. Brit. Emp.*, 56:439, 1949.
20. Davies, J., Davenport, R. G., Norris, J. L., and Rennie, P. I. C.: *Endocrinology*, 78:667, 1966.
21. Diamond, M. C., and Young, W. C.: *Endocrinology*, 72:429, 1963.
22. Dingemanse, E.: *Ciba Colloquia on Endocrinology*, 2:251, 1952.
23. Dobriner, K.: *Ciba Colloquia on Endocrinology*, 2:170, 1952.
24. Dorfman, R. I., and Shippel, R. A.: *The Androgens*. New York, J. Wiley & Sons, Inc., 1956.
25. Drosdowsky, M. A., Dessypris, A., Nivan, Nl. Lm., Dorfman, R. I., and Gual, C.: *Acta Endocrinol.*, 49:553, 1965.
26. Duboff, G. S., Behrman, S. J., Saraiya, H., and Catchick, J.: *Fertil. Steril.*, 15:661, 1964.
27. Engstrom, W. W., and Munson, P. L.: *J. Clin. Endocr. Metab.*, 11:427, 1951.
28. Fels, E., Moguilewsky, J. A., and Fibertun, C.: *Acta Physiol. Lat. Amer.*, 18:132, 1968.
29. Forsberg, J. G., and Jacobson, D.: *J. Endocr.*, 44:461, 1961.
30. Friedman, I. S., et al.: *J. Clin. Endocr. Metab.*, 15:1281, 1955.
31. Gorski, R., and Wagner, J. W.: *Endocrinology*, 76:226, 1965.
32. Gospodarovicz, D.: *Biochim. Biophys. Acta*, 100:618, 1965.
33. Goy, R. W., Bridson, W. E., and Young, W. C.: *J. Comp. Physiol.*, 57:116, 1964.
34. Grayhanck, J. T., and Scott, W. W.: *Endocrinology*, 48:453, 1951.
35. Hall, P. F.: *Endocrinology*, 76:396, 1965.
36. Harper, M. K. J.: *Endocrinology*, 80:1152, 1967.
37. Harris, G. W., and Levine, S.: *J. Physiol.*, 181:379, 1965.
38. Hart, B. L.: *Science*, 155:1283, 1967.
39. Heard, R. D. H., and O'Donnell, V. J.: *Endocrinology*, 54:209, 1954.
40. Heard, R. D. H., et al.: *Endocrinology*, 57:200, 1955.
41. Henry, R., Thevenet, M., Lumbroso, P., and Netter, A.: *Ann. d'Endocr.*, 21:556, 1960.
42. Hoffman, W., and Breuer, H.: *Acta Endocrinol.*, 57:623, 1968.
43. Hohlweg, W.: *Wien. Clin. Wschr.*, 80:445, 1968.
44. Jacobson, D., and Norgren, A.: *Acta Endocrinol.*, 49:453, 1965.
45. Johnson, D. C.: *Endocrinology*, 62:340, 1958.
46. Junkmann, C.: *Arztl. Wschr.*, 9:289, 1954.
47. Junkmann, C.: *Verhandl. Dtsch. Ges. Inn. Sekr.*, 11:321, 1957.
48. Kase, N., Forchielli, E., and Dorfman, R. I.: *Acta Endocrinol.*, 37:19, 1961.
49. Kase, N., Sohval, J., and Soffer, L. J.: *Acta Endocrinol.*, 44:8, 1963.
50. Kennedy, G. C.: *J. Physiol.*, 172:393, 1964.
51. Kincl, F. A., and Maqueo, M.: *Endocrinology*, 77:859, 1965.
52. Knapstein, P., Wendlberger, F., and Menzel, P.: *Steroids*, 12:191, 1968.
53. Lanthier, A., and Sandor, T.: *Metabolism*, 9:861, 1960.
54. Lanthier, A., and Sandor, T.: *Acta Endocrinol.*, 39:145, 1962.
55. Lederer, J., and Bataille, J. P.: *Ann. d'Endocr.*, 28:111, 1967.
56. Leon, N., Neves-Castro, M., and Dorfman, R. I.: *Acta Endocrinol.*, 39:411, 1962.
57. Lipschutz, A.: *Steroid Hormones and Tumors*. Baltimore, William & Wilkins, 1950.

58. Lisse, K.: *Endokrinologie*, 53:78, 1968.
59. Lloyd, C. W., and Fredricks, J.: *J. Clin. Endocr.*, 11:724, 1951.
60. MacDonald, P. C., Van de Viele, R. L., and Liberman, S.: *Amer. J. Physiol.*, 86:1, 1963.
61. MacKinney, G. R., and Payne, H. G.: *Proc. Soc. Exper. Biol. Med.*, 108:273, 1951.
62. Mahesh, V. B., and Greenblatt, R. B.: *Nature*, 191:888, 1961.
63. Marchesoni, M.: *Riv. Ost. Gin. (Firenze)*, 9:301, 1954.
64. Mikhail, G., Zander, J., and Allen, W. M.: *J. Clin. Endocr. Metab.*, 23:1967, 1963.
65. Neumann, F.: "*Res. in Reprod.*" edited by R. G. Edwards (Cambridge): 2:3, 1970.
66. Neuweiler, W., and Richter, R. H. H.: *Gynaecologia*, 152:133, 1961.
67. Noall, M. W., Alexander, F., and Allen, W. M.: *Biochim. Biophys. Acta*, 59:520, 1962.
68. Nokes, J. M., et al.: *Amer. J. Obstet. Gynec.*, 78:722, 1959.
69. Oakey, R. E., and Stitch, S. R.: *Acta Endocrinol.*, 50:407, 1968.
70. Plate, W. P.: *Gynaecologia*, 132:329, 1951.
71. Plate, W. P.: *Acta Endocrinol.*, 8:17, 1951.
72. Plate, W. P.: *Acta Endocrinol.*, 11:119, 1952.
73. Ponse, K.: *Ann. d'Endocrinol.*, 16:89, 1955.
74. Pundel, J. P.: *Acta Cytologica*, 1:82, 1957.
75. Reifenstein, E. C., et al.: *J. Amer. Geriatric. Soc.*, 2:293, 1954.
76. Remonchamps, F. L., and Guyssbrecht, P. F.: *Ann. d'Endocrinol.*, 15:229, 1951.
77. Rice, B. F., and Savard, K.: *J. Clin. Endocr. Metab.*, 26:593, 1966.
78. Rice, B. F., and Segaloff, A.: *Endocrinology*, 68:261, 1966.
79. Rivarola, M. A., Forest, M. G., and Migeon, C. J.: *J. Clin. Endocr. Metab.*, 28:34, 1968.
80. Rosner, J., Pomeau-Dellile, G., Tramezzani, J. H., and Cardinali, D.: *Compt. Rend. Acad. Sc., Paris*, 261:1113, 1965.
81. Roy, S. K., and Laumas, K. R.: *Acta Endocrinol.*, 51:629, 1964.
82. Samuels, L. T.: *Ciba Colloquia on Endocrinology*, 7:176, 1953.
83. Sandor, T., and Lanthier, A.: *Rev. Canad. Biol.*, 19:445, 1960.
84. Savard, K., Dorfman, R. I., Gaggett, B., and Engel, L. L.: *J. Clin. Endocr. Metab.*, 16:1269, 1956.
85. Savard, K., Besch, P. K., Restivo, S., and Goldzieher, J. W.: *Fed. Proceed.*, 17:1, 1958.
86. Savard, K., Gut, M., Dorfman, R. I., Gabrilove, J. L., and Soffer, L. J.: *J. Clin. Endocr. Metab.*, 21:165, 1961.
87. Schneider, H. P., Staemmler, H. J., Sachs, L., and Schwarze, M.: *Arch. Gynäk.*, 206:64, 1968.
88. Schrieffers, H., and Schmidt, E.: *Hoppe-Seylers Ztschr. f. Physiol. Chem.*, 349:1085, 1968.
89. Seeman, A., and Saracino, R. T.: *Acta Endocrinol.*, 37:31, 1961.
90. Seeman, A., Saracino, R. T., and Guerin, P.: *Acta Endocrinol.*, 41:259, 1962.
91. Simmer, H., and Voss, H. E.: *Klin. Wschr.*, 38:819, 1960.
92. Southren, A. L., Gordon, G. G., Tachimoto, S., Pinzon, G., Lane, D. R., and Stypulkowsky, W.: *J. Clin. Endocr.*, 27:686, 1967.
93. Swanson, H. E., and Van der Werff, J. J.: *Acta Endocr.*, 50:379, 1965.
94. Van Rees, G. P., and Gans, E.: *Acta Endocr.*, 52:471, 1966.
95. Wakabayashi, K., and Tamaoki, B. I.: *Endocrinology*, 80:409, 1967.
96. Warren, R. P., and Aronson, L. R.: *Endocrinology*, 58:293, 1956.
97. Wied, G. L.: *Acta Cytologica*, 1:75, 1957.
98. Wied, G. L., Sol, R. del, and Dargan, A.: *Amer. J. Obstet. Gynec.*, 75:289, 1958.
99. Wollman, A. L., and Hamilton, J. B.: *Endocrinology*, 82:868, 1968.
100. Zaffaroni, A., et al.: *J. Amer. Chem. Soc.*, 73:130, 1951.
101. Zander, J., Wiest, W. G., and Ober, K. G.: *Arch. Gynäk.*, 196:481, 1962.
102. Zander, J.: *Rev. Franç. Endocr. Clin. Nutr. Metab.*, 4:410, 1963.
103. Zeilmaker, G. H.: *Acta Endocr.*, 46:571, 1964.
104. Zimmermann, W.: *Chemische Bestimmungsmethoden von Steroidhormonen*. Berlin, Springer Verlag, 1955.
105. Zogbi, F., Begue, J. A., and Jayle, M. F.: *Compt. Rend. Soc. Biol., Paris*, 160:586, 1966.

Chapter 5
NONSTEROID OVARIAN HORMONES — RELAXIN (UTERORELAXING FACTOR)

5.1. THE FOURTH OVARIAN HORMONE

As our knowledge increased, the concept of the two ovarian hormones, estradiol and progesterone, as the only endocrine components of the female gonad had to be abandoned. Secretion of androgens has already been seen to occur in the normal ovary even under normal physiologic conditions (Chapter 4). This chapter deals with a further hormone, or rather group of hormones, which, although ignored for a long time, has regained recognition, thanks to the investigations of the last 15 years.

In 1926, when Hisaw[24] initiated his hormone studies on ovarian extracts, the properties of the corpus luteum hormone were unknown. Working on sow ovaries, he was able to obtain two different luteinic extracts: a hydrosoluble one, which caught attention because it relaxed the symphysis in guinea pigs and other rodents, and an alcohol-soluble extract, which was active mainly on the uterus, in which it elicited a certain degree of growth. While working on this second active principle in the course of the same year, Corner and Allen were rewarded with their brilliant discoveries, which were to culminate in the biochemical synthesis of pure progesterone eight years later. The importance of the alcohol-soluble principle entirely overshadowed and obscured the search for its sister, hydrosoluble fraction, so that, were it not for the tenacity of Hisaw and co-workers, nothing might have been heard for many years about the *fourth ovarian hormone*.

Rediscovery of the forgotten substance, leading to its understanding after a lapse of 30 years of obscurity, is a personal triumph of the tenacity and steadfastness of scientific commitment of one man, F. L. Hisaw.

5.2. HISTORY

Hisaw and co-workers[24, 25] discovered an active hydrosoluble principle in the sow ovary that, when injected into guinea pigs, rats or rabbits, relaxed the pubic ligaments, *which, unlike in primates, in these animals is a fundamental requirement for the realization of parturition.* The physiologic character of this substance was demonstrated by the finding that it was present in the blood of rodents during the period of gestation.

Fevold and Hisaw[15] succeeded in isolating that substance with a certain degree of purification in 1930. However, that event took place at a time when the existence of relaxin was coming under strong attack, mainly because symphysis-relaxing effects were believed to result from in-tandem actions of estrogens and progesterone. Indeed, as admitted by Hisaw[25] himself, estrogens and the corpus luteum hormone, too, have similar symphysis-loosening activity, even though to much smaller degrees and with much longer time intervals necessary to produce effects. Marois[43] reexamined the problem more recently. Estrogens would relax the symphysis in guinea pigs following treatment over a period of 10 days. If injected in combination with progesterone, clear-cut relaxation could be achieved in 36 to 38 hours, but an effect of the same magnitude could be achieved in 2 to 3 hours with injections of a relaxin preparation. On the other hand, the amount of priming by estrogen that was necessary for relaxin to produce a response was one fiftieth to one hundredth of the priming needed for progesterone. Although these arguments undoubtedly seem to favor relaxin specificity, it must be admitted that the actions of this hormone are hard to distinguish from those of other steroid hormones, to the extent of becoming unquestioningly identifiable. As a matter of fact, for many years we had had serious doubts concerning the existence of relaxin.

In 1930, Fevold[15] established the "guinea pig unit," which was defined as the minimal amount of active substance capable of provoking relaxation of the symphysis in 60 per cent of the animals within 12 hours after injection. This rather inaccurate method of bioassay nevertheless served to demonstrate the presence of the substance in the blood of pregnant animals[33] and, in 1934, Pommerenke,[45] on finding the symphysis-relaxing factor in the blood of a pregnant woman, proposed a pregnancy test based on the application of the assay to guinea pigs.

Since 1946, improved methods of bioassay have been developed (to be discussed later), which enabled Hisaw and Zarrow[25] to make estimations of values as high as 10,000 GPU per sow ovary and, at the other extreme, of amounts as small as 2 to 2.5 GPU per milliliter of serum, or 0.5 to 2.5 GPU per gram of placental weight. Finally, in 1958, Frieden[16] succeeded in isolating the active compound in a highly purified form, establishing its protein nature and showing that it was a polypeptide.

In a later study, Frieden and his group[19] were able to determine the exact composition of this polypeptide as follows:

Asparagine-alanine-arginine-(cystine)$_2$-glutathione-glycine-histidine-lysine-serine-tryptophane-valine-(leucine)$_2$.

5.3. PHYSIOLOGIC ACTIONS IN ANIMALS

These are roughly the following: (a) relaxation of symphysis pubis, (b) relaxation of uterine musculature, with paralyzing effect on contractility, (c) cervical softening and dilatation, and (d) increase in uterine weight and glycogen and water content.

5.3.1. RELAXATION OF SYMPHYSIS PUBIS

This was the first effect to be discovered.[15, 24, 25, 42, 45] It is observed, above all, in guinea pigs, but also in rats, mice and rabbits.[43] The symphysis-relaxing action has already been mentioned as forming the basis for the still used bioassay method, since of all actions of relaxin, this is the most specific and potent one. Kroc and Steinetz[35] have developed a method for its determination and exact measurement (Fig. 5–1).

Progesterone potentiates this relaxation.[22] Through its local effect on cartilage, *somatotropic hormone*[55, 56] also acts in a synergistic way. Schmidt and Leonard[52] have demonstrated that it produces an increase in mucopolysaccharide content of the symphysial ligaments, while Rudzik and Miller[50] believe such action to be mediated by local liberation of histamine.

Manning and colleagues[41] report increased phosphatase activity in epiphysial cartilage.

Relaxation of the symphysis, in the same sense of the word, does not occur in primates; however, other actions principally *on the uterus*, are observed.

5.3.2. RELAXATION OF UTERINE MUSCULATURE WITH PARALYZING EFFECT ON CONTRACTILITY

Krantz and co-workers,[34] Frieden,[16] Felton and colleagues[14] and other workers found that, while hydrosoluble ovarian extracts had no effect on the symphysis, they exerted instead a paralyzing effect on uterine muscle fibers. This phenomenon is reported to occur in rodents also.[6]

This action results in rapid and, of course, reversible effects; it does not depend on added progesterone activity and is capable

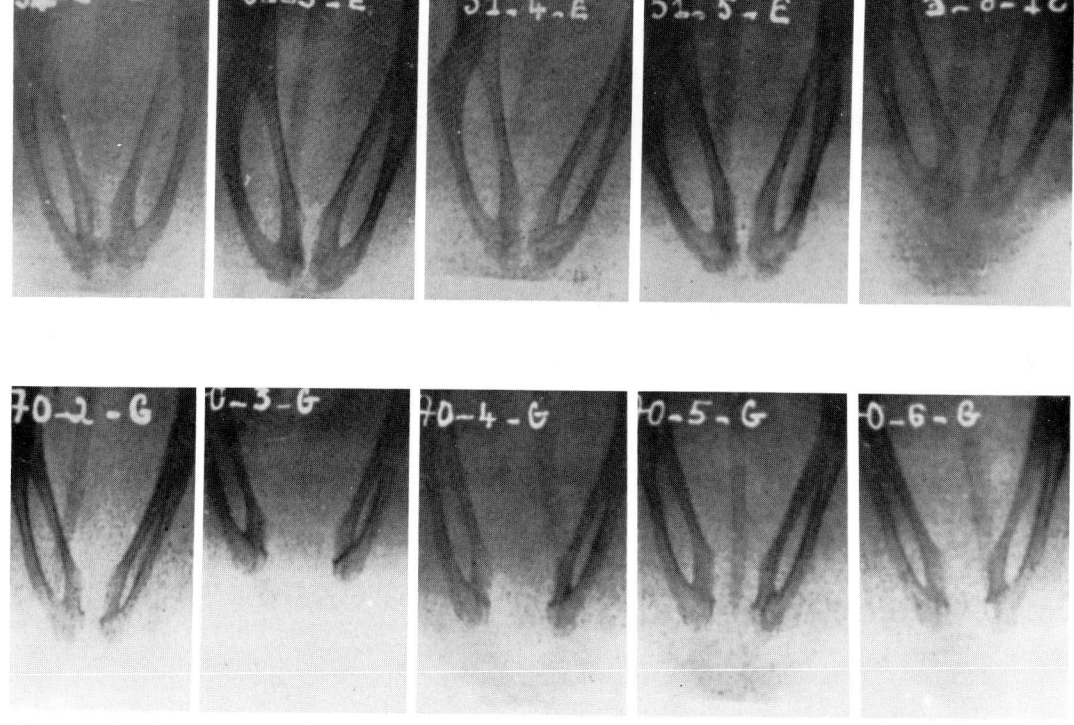

Figure 5–1. Separation of pubic symphysis in spayed guinea pig after pretreatment with 1 mg estradiol and with 2 GPU of purified hydrosoluble extract of sow ovary. A, Control animal; B, experimental animal. (From Fevold et al.[15])

of producing complete, though temporal, uterine paralysis (Fig. 5–2).

5.3.3. CERVICAL SOFTENING AND DILATATION

In cows, in which symphysial-relaxing effects are hardly noticeable, Graham and Dracy[21] noted considerable softening of the uterine cervix, allowing easy dilatation. Steinetz and co-workers[54, 55] have demonstrated that this action is more or less a general one and is operative in mice, rats, sows and women alike (see below). McGaughey and his colleagues[39] have shown that relaxation is brought about by increased water content of the cervical tissue and by "depolymerization" of the connective tissue ground substance. Admittedly, the process of cervical softening is essentially one of fluidification of cervical mucopolysaccharide constituents of the ground substance.[8, 67] This fluidification is brought about by a process of polysaccharide depolymerization which is identical in nature with that occurring in the symphysis.[35, 64, 59] *Relaxin would appear to be a substance whose basic action consists in causing disintegration of glycoproteins.*

5.3.4. INCREASE IN WEIGHT OF UTERUS AND IN ITS WATER AND GLYCOGEN CONTENT

Cervical dilatation has just been described as resulting in part from active *hydration* of cervical tissue components. An increase in uterine water content has been reported by Zarrow and his co-workers[63, 68] and subsequently by many other authors.[29, 35, 39, 54] Increased water content produces edema and, consequently, an increase in size of the organ.[6, 33, 43, 59] Velardo has demonstrated that both estrogens and progestogens are agents promoting uterine growth by a mechanism of increased interstitial water imbibition, but, in comparison, the effects of relaxin are

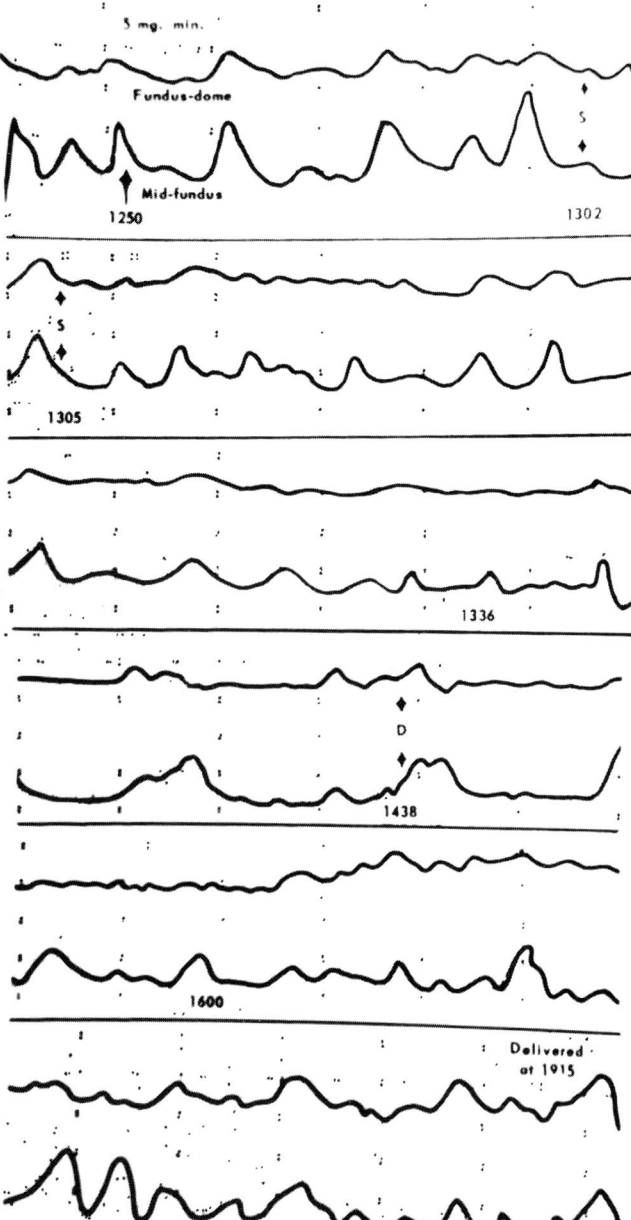

Figure 5-2. Effect of relaxin (Releasin), in an intravenous drip at 5 mg/min., on woman during stage of cervical dilatation. Note uterorelaxing and paralyzing effect, with restoration of contractile activity upon discontinuing drip. (From Eichner et al.[13])

both more rapid and more intense, as well as of longer duration.

Finally, Steinetz and Beach[55] reported increased uterine glycogen content in both gravid and nongravid rats. Such effects later could not be confirmed by Zarrow and Brennan,[66] who, however, found that in this respect relaxin *potentiated* the actions of progestogens. Thus, it is doubtful whether this effect results from relaxin activity or from, perhaps, a summation effect by persisting progesterone contaminants.

Relaxin also acts upon the *endometrium*. Hisaw and Hisaw[26] observed increased capillary permeability and vasodilation in monkey endometria. Ballenberg, Dawson and Hisaw[9] also found vasodilation, as well as secretory effects of the progestational type. Finally, Hall and Salimi-Khaligh[23] have observed that in the hamster relaxin provoked increased activity of glycogen-synthesizing enzymes, phosphorylases as well as uridine phosphorylase.

5.3.5. SYNERGISM WITH BOTH ESTROGENS AND PROGESTERONE

It has already been stated that some of the actions of relaxin could be obtained by the combined activity of injected estrogens and progesterone, although such actions are of a considerably lower degree of intensity. This, indeed, is the issue that raises most of the doubts concerning the very existence of this hormone. In order to be effective, relaxin is also known to require pretreatment of the animal with estrogens.[15, 42, 45] In gravid animals, this occurs naturally, but in order to obtain relaxinic effects in castrated animals, these must previously be injected with estrogens. In this respect, relaxin and progesterone have a property in common. However, even more noteworthy is the fact that relaxin potentiates progesterone activity. Zarrow and Brennan,[66] and Hall and his colleagues[22] have all reported typical progestational effects on rabbit endometria with as little as 0.1 mg progesterone—that is, one tenth of the otherwise minimal necessary dosage—if injections are combined with 400 to 600 GPU relaxin (Fig. 5–3). Potentiating effects on progesterone activity are similarly noted with regard to uterine motility[14, 16, 34] and to uterine content of both water and glycogen.[67] Zarrow and his co-workers[65, 66] discount any effect of relaxin on the uterine content of glycogen and believe that what relaxin really does is merely to spotlight those actions of progesterone which ineffectively small dosages would otherwise not make apparent.

Relaxin is found in great concentration in corpora lutea of rabbits[68] and also seems to have some luteinizing effects.[30]

5.3.6. ONE, TWO OR SEVERAL SUBSTANCES?

So far, relaxin preparations have been made from more or less purified hydrosoluble extracts either of corpus luteum alone or of entire sow ovaries. Thus, different preparations might be expected to have somewhat different actions. Fevold and Hisaw[15] had shown that crude extracts possess uterine relaxing activity, but they found that, with increasing purification of these extracts, there was gradual loss of

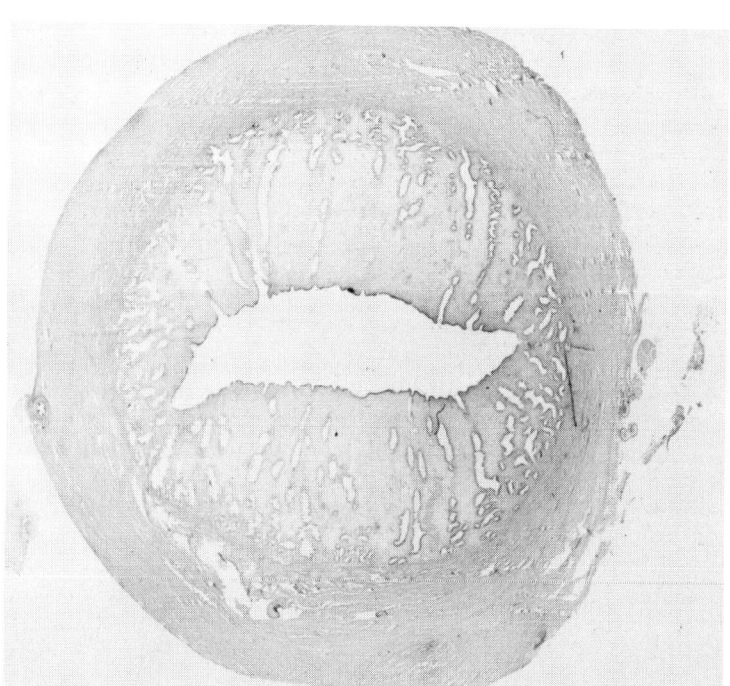

Figure 5–3. Mild degree of progestational reaction obtained in castrated *Macaca mulatta* by injection of 0.8 mg/kg estradiol valerianate plus 2000 I.U. relaxin (Releasin).

activity. Depending on the method of extraction, at least two distinct preparations have been isolated: (1) relaxin, which exerts a definite action on the guinea pig symphysis, and (2) uterus relaxing-factor (URF).[16, 17] The existence of a third factor is entertained by some. This factor is assumed to have progestational activity, to be responsible for the increase in uterine water and glycogen content and to act as a synergizer of progestogens,[35] all of which so far are merely speculative suppositions.

5.4. CLINICAL ACTIONS

Except for the symphysis-relaxing action, all other actions of relaxin described for animals can also be found in man. Clinical actions are therefore those of URF rather than those of relaxin. The following effects may be described: (1) effects on uterine motility, (2) cervical dilatation effects, and (3) uterine sedative and pain-relieving effects.

5.4.1. EFFECTS ON UTERINE MOTILITY

The effects exerted on uterine motility in the human species have been studied by Kelly[32] and by Posse and Kelly[46] by means of internal and external tocography. As do high dosages of progesterone, purified preparations of relaxin diminish spontaneous contractile activity of both nongravid and gravid uteri. Eichner and his colleagues[12, 13] have studied the effects of the hormone by means of intrapartum electrohysterography, reporting temporary inhibition with cessation of electric activity in both body and fundus. However, McGaughey and co-workers,[39] after studying the problem in vitro, expressed skepticism about those effects. In general, there is some agreement[8–10] that the paralyzing effect on contractility merely reflects progesterone activation by relaxin, which is in keeping with what was said in the preceding paragraphs.

5.4.2. CERVIX-DILATING EFFECTS

This action appears to be more generally admitted, since it is of a more obvious character. Following the finding of cervical dilatation in cows[21] and sows,[69] Birnberg and Abitbol tentatively advocated application of relaxin to achieve cervical dilatation in women at labor.[4] Their own attempts met with success, and several reports claiming accelerated dilatation have since appeared in the literature.[13, 49, 57, 58, 59] A special extract with cervix-dilating activity has been introduced for clinical application under the trade name of "Cervilaxin." Under its influence, the uterine cervix becomes soft and patulous, allowing dilatation with ease. The combination of Cervilaxin-oxytocin reportedly shortens the dilatation stage[4, 5, 49, 58] and may be employed to induce labor.[3, 57] Relaxin would thus seem to have the same actions in the human species that it has in animals.

5.4.3. UTERINE SEDATIVE AND PAIN-RELIEVING EFFECTS

It has been possible to demonstrate sedative actions on the uterus similar to those exerted by progesterone. The successful application of relaxin for this purpose has been reported in the treatment of abortion and premature labor.[1, 37, 40] Relaxin has also been applied to nongravid uteri in combatting dysmenorrhea.[2, 31, 36, 47]

Rezek[48] believes the sedative effects result from some active principal other than relaxin, so that in crude sow ovary extracts, the presence of at least three different substances would have to be admitted: (1) the first responsible for the symphysial relaxation in rodents, (2) the second, having cervix-relaxing effects in sows, cows and women, and (3) a third, with uterine sedative, anti-abortive and, perhaps, motility-inhibiting effects. It is obvious that presently available data on the specificity of these actions are still shrouded by considerable controversy. Most discrepancies stem from the fact that none of the hitherto used extracts has been completely pure, nor were their exact compositions known.

5.4.4. PROGESTATIONAL TYPE OF ACTIVITY

Relaxin activity has already been mentioned in this chapter as contributing to the maintenance of gestation in animals (Wada and Turner[60]). In some species, a secretory type of response *in the breast* has also been elicited.[60, 61] On the other hand, Slate and Mengert[53] have found no effect on lactation.

5.5. CHEMICAL COMPOSITION

Present knowledge with regard to the chemical composition of relaxin and its related substances is still incomplete. In 1953, Sawyer, Frieden and Martin[16, 44, 51] became aware of the fact that total water-soluble sow ovary extracts contained at least two different substances, one producing symphysial relaxation, the other softening of the cervix. When purified, these substances turned out to be relatively simple proteins, displaying the properties of a blend of polypeptides.[27] Frieden found that they possessed weak antigenic properties and provoked the formation of antihormones,[18, 19] a fact providing proof of their protein character.

An attempt to separate the active principles involved has been made by Frieden and his colleagues,[19, 20] using a special "countercurrent" distribution procedure with trichloracetic acid and butanol solutions (Fig. 5-4). By employing multiple purification stages, the method yielded fairly pure preparations consisting of a homogeneous protein the composition of which, however, could not yet be determined. Similar extractive procedures have been used by manufacturers presently marketing such extracts, but for the same reason, the actions of no two products can

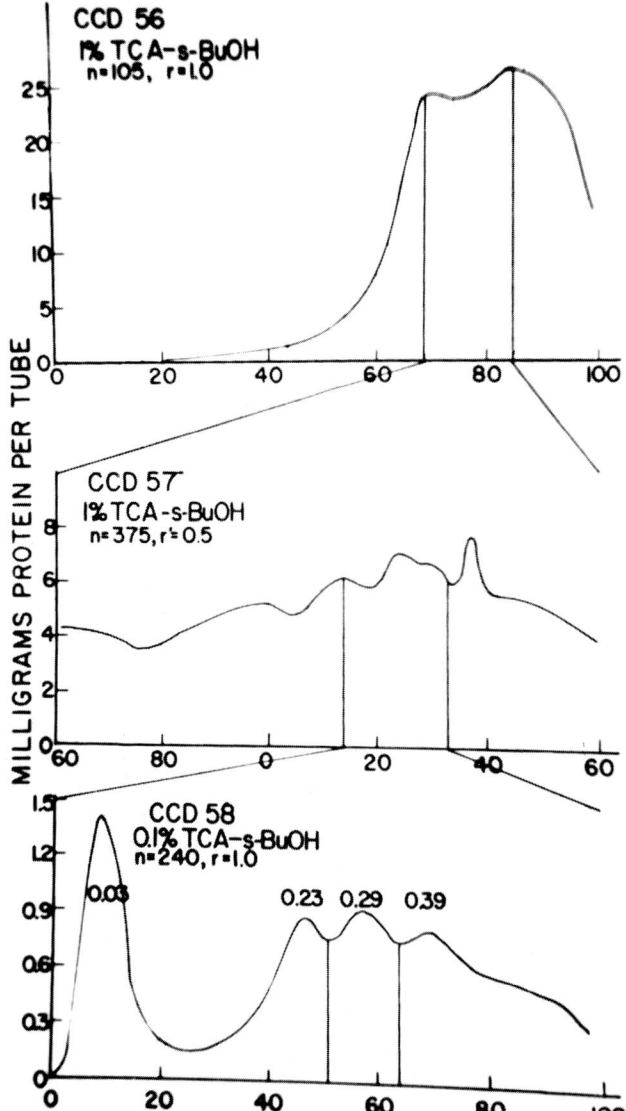

Figure 5-4. Purification of relaxin by a procedure of "countercurrent" distribution between solutions of trichloracetic acid and butanol. A protein with a global polypeptide structure, having most of the net relaxin activity, becomes deposited between 61 and 87. Successive purification of this extract, with repeat distributions, in which the relative concentrations of TCA and butanol are varied, yields a homogeneous protein with 75 per cent of the initial activity. The concentrations of two solvents are indicated in the diagram. (From Frieden and Hisaw.[17])

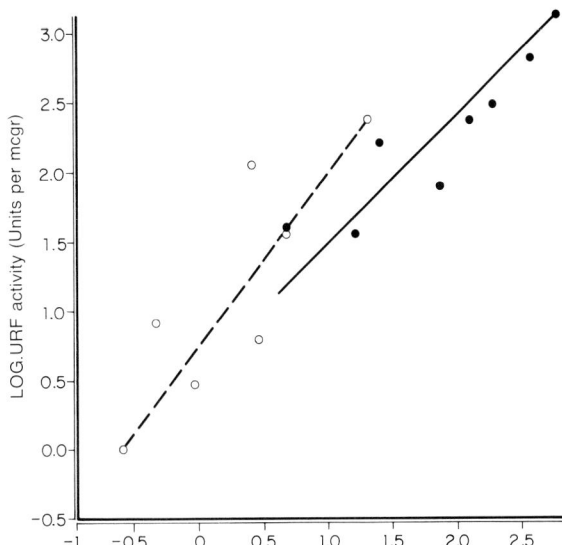

Figure 5-5. Diagram showing relationship between uterus-relaxing and symphysis-relaxing activities of two water-soluble preparations, one extracted from a nonpregnant sow, and the other from a pregnant sow ovary. The difference in distribution of the two properties suggests that the actions involved belong to two different active substances. (From Frieden.[18])

be exactly superimposed, and their basic actions on the symphysis and the uterine cervix are consequently of variable potency with each of these preparations. The higher the degree of purification, the more the dissociation of activity becomes apparent, so that one gains the clear impression of dealing with two different active principles (Fig. 5-5).

Chromatographic studies by Frieden, Noall and Alonso[20] seem to bear out the duality of the two substances, which might be called *relaxin* and *URF*, respectively, but their dual nature will not be proved definitely until the chemical structural differences involved can be defined.

The third substance still remains veiled in obscurity; it is known by the commercial name "Lutrexin" and is endowed with progesterone-potentiating and uterus-sedating actions which have already been mentioned. Rezek[47, 48] first postulated the existence of this third active principle, and Frieden[18] claims to have isolated it by means of the countercurrent distribution technique.

The recent isolation by Frieden and colleagues[19] of a specific polypeptide with relaxin activity has also been mentioned.

Asparagine-alanine-arginine-(cystine)$_2$-glutathione-glycine-histidine-lysine-serine-tryptophane-valine-(leucine)$_2$.

The different factors isolable with the countercurrent distribution procedure are currently presumed to be "analogues," having certain variations in side-chains.

As a protein hormone (or group of hormones), relaxin has *antigenic capacity*. Cohen and Steinetz[7] were able to obtain a specific antiserum in rabbits which was tested immunologically by MacClintock and Zarrow,[38] and by Struck.[59]

5.6. ESTIMATION AND UNITS OF MEASUREMENT

To date, only one type of hormonal activity has been standardized, which is that pertinent to symphysial relaxation. The original bioassay method consisted in spaying 10 virgin guinea pigs, pretreating each with 10 RU of estrogen and then injecting them with the test extract. This assay required 10 animals for each estimation. One *guinea pig unit* (GPU) is the minimal amount of hormone necessary to produce 1 cm of symphysial separation in at least six of the 10 animals. The degree of symphysial separation in the original procedure was measured by manual palpation.

Recently, Kroc and his colleagues[35] improved the method for measuring symphysial separation and proposed also new procedures based on cervical dilatation, uterine water content, increase in weight of uteri and uterine glycogen content. Since the latter actions are not specific for either relaxin or URF, and could be brought about by the actions of progesterone and estrogens, or estrogens alone, they proved to be of no practical value. And, since none of these other actions can invariably be gauged alongside the symphysis-relaxing effects, for the time being there is actually no sure and effective method of bioassay available. Despite the tediousness, inaccuracies and deficiencies with regard to direct measurement of the clinically all-important cervical dilating potency of a preparation, for lack of a better method the symphysial relaxation method in the guinea pig will have to remain the standard procedure for the time being.

5.7. ORIGIN, CIRCULATION, AND ELIMINATION

In the sow, the principal source of relaxin is the *ovary*, from which up to 10,000 GPU per gram of fresh tissue can be extracted. The *placenta* in the sow is another source, with a yield of 2.5 GPU per gram of organ weight.[25] In both mice and rabbits, placentas and ovaries likewise contain measurable amounts of the hormone.[63, 64]

While high hormone *blood levels* during pregnancy were reported, in blood of non-pregnant females no detectable amounts were found.[42, 64, 65] Blood values, of which as little as 0.2 GPU per ml of serum can be determined, rise progressively in the course of gestation, only to disappear precipitously immediately after delivery. Zarrow and Brennan[66] demonstrate a positive urinary elimination curve paralleling that of blood levels during pregnancy.

In the *human species*, Pommerenke,[45] and later Zarrow and colleagues,[64] found blood values of 2 to 5 GPU during pregnancy. In pregnant women, the placenta appears to be the primary source of relaxin, with values obtained ranging from 0.5 to 2.5 GPU per gram of fresh tissue. However, it is not certain these figures reflect the rate of hormone formation. It is pertinent to remember that demonstrable placental values for progesterone, which has been known to be formed at high rates in the placenta, are negligible (see Chapter 3).

Until the chemical composition of the substances involved can be established, and until specific and accurate methods for their determination are available, our meager knowledge of the formation, circulation and elimination of the hormone can hardly be expected to show any significant gains.

5.8. CLINICAL USES

The properties of relaxin have found ample application in clinical work with women. Before entering the subject of indications and obtained results, we shall list briefly some of the commercially available preparations.

5.8.1. COMMERCIAL PREPARATIONS

The three main commercial preparations available are all aqueous (i.e. water-soluble) extracts from sow ovaries: Releasin (Warner-Chilcott); Cervilaxin (The National Drug, Inc.); and Lutrexin (Hynson, Wescott & Dunning, Inc.). These three are dispensed in the form of injectables for parenteral intramuscular or intravenous use, and are also available in the form of tablets. The latter are barely effective since, owing to their polypeptide nature, they are attacked by pepsin and trypsin alike. Injectables contain 10, 50 or 100 mg of hormone per milliliter. One milligram of purified protein is equivalent to 150 GPU, standardized by biologic means. Recommended total dosages are 40 to 120 mg, to be divided into several doses. The total dosage thus administered amounts to 18,000 GPU. Such dosages are well tolerated and can be given even intravenously without harmful effects.

Probably because all three preparations are extracted and purified by different methods, each shows different activity and happens to correspond to one of the previously analyzed factors. Thus, Releasin is predominantly composed of the symphysis-relaxing factor, Cervilaxin of the cervix-dilating factor, and Lutrexin of the corpus luteum synergizing (and uterus-sedating) factor. The question of whether these are three different substances, or three different actions exerted by one hormone, has not been solved.

5.8.2. INDICATIONS

The principal indications for administering relaxin are: (1) dysmenorrhea, (2) prevention of abortion or premature labor, (3) uterine sedation during labor, (4) induction of labor, and (5) shortening of the stage of dilatation. The first three effects result from action of the hormone on the uterine muscle fibers; the last two result from the practical application of its effects on the cervix.

DYSMENORRHEA. In the first trial applications, Lutrexin was used and was soon recognized not to be the symphysis-relaxing factor but rather an associated uterus-sedating factor.[31, 47] More recently, purified preparations of relaxin (Releasin) provided relief from dysmenorrhea in 91 per cent of the cases.[1] Effective dosages are 20 mg (3000 GPU) intramuscularly.[2, 31, 36, 47] Satisfactory results have also been reported with the use of tablets; however, from what is known of their absorption, it seems certain that beneficial effects are, more likely than not, psychotherapeutic in nature.[28]

PREVENTION OF ABORTION AND OF PREMATURE LABOR. The uterine sedating effects of this hormone have also been found useful in the symptomatic treatment of abortion and, above all, of premature labor.[1, 37, 40, 62] According to Rezek,[48] the active substance involved would seem to be not relaxin, but the factor known as "Lutrexin," or at any rate, the factor predominating in the commercial product of that name. Effectiveness decreases with advancing pregnancy, and the preparations seem to lack any effect at all from the thirty-fourth week onward.[8, 11, 13] Tocographic tracings taken by Kelly and Posse[32a] seem to confirm these effects.

UTERINE SEDATION DURING LABOR. Some authors have tried relaxin as a uterine sedative during labor.[13] Tocographic tracings, however, would appear to confirm the previously stated fact that uterine relaxing activity is negligible from the thirty-fourth week onward. It is possible that favorable effects observed by some[37, 48] were due to potentiation of progesterone activity.

INDUCTION OF LABOR. In the human species, cervical softening and "depolymerization" are the most prominent effects produced by relaxin. Successful clinical use has therefore been achieved mainly when the preparations are used for that purpose. Several authors have used relaxin to obtain cervical softening, or "ripening," in cases requiring induction of labor by means of a continuous IV drip of oxytocin.[3, 5, 57] The absence of cervical softening is known to be the major cause of failure to induce labor by this means. Eichner and his co-workers find its application particularly useful whenever the precipitation of premature labor is necessary, in which case the artificially induced cervical ripening is of crucial importance. Stone and his colleagues[58] deliberately selected a number of poor candidates for elective induction—such as those with immature, firm, posterior cervices—but who were ideally suited for the study of relaxin effects. Each patient received 40 mg in the evening and a dose of 120 mg the following morning. Among the control group, who were given pitocin drip alone, labor was induced in 23 per cent of the patients, whereas the relaxin (Releasin) group achieved success in 72 per cent of the cases.

ACCELERATION OF DILATATION STAGE. In cases of prolonged labor or cervical rigidity, relaxin has been used to accelerate cervical dilatation, either alone,[25, 46] or in association with a running drip (in the latter case for the conduction of labor). Reports concerning results are favorable; however, the hormone does not appear so effective if administered while the fetal membranes are intact or while the cervix is insufficiently dilated.[10] Birnberg and Abitbol[4, 5] believe that the compound has no action on cervices with less than 3 cm dilatation or with incomplete effacement, for which reason they advocate association with a drip even in those cases in which the only effect sought is shortening of the dilatation stage. In this sense, it is also used by Stone and his colleagues[58], Eichner and co-workers[12] and Israel and Groeber.[28] Israel and Groeber had conducted experiments on 47 primiparous women with cervical rigidity and the results they reported were not encouraging. In general, after the initial period of enthusiasm, in later years there seems to have arisen considerable skepticism.[8, 20, 28] It must, of course, be taken into consideration how difficult it is to evaluate the cervix-dilating effects of any given drug, how often an underlying mechanical dystocia of presentation or rotation is misdiagnosed as cervical dystocia, and, finally, how association with drips really makes it barely possible to decide which of the components, oxytocin or relaxin, is at work in accelerating labor. For all these reasons, we still seem to be in the testing stage; only additional experimental data and, above all, more purified preparations will be required to arrive at a definite conclusion.

5.9. CRITICAL EVALUATION OF RELAXIN

At present, it can no longer be said that relaxin might be a product of imagination, as was done in the first edition of this book. Both its individuality and specificity have been demonstrated beyond doubt. However, there are still many dark corners left.

Considering the lack of any definite knowledge about its chemical structure, close as we may have come to solving it—and keeping in mind the facts that the only source of the preparations, pregnant sow ovaries, is limited, and further that what is isolated appears to be a blend of polypeptides rather than a single compound—it is only natural that much about the hormonal activity involved should remain unknown.

First of all, it should be pointed out that more than one substance seems to be involved. The distinctness between a symphysis-relaxing polypeptide and a cervix-softening polypeptide seems to have been borne out by the latest works of Frieden. If, apart from symphysial and cervical activity, the other features of relaxin activity are analyzed, it can be seen that all properties (uterine sedation, uterine weight increase, glycogen content increase, etc.) are also characteristic of progesterone activity. And, since it was further proved that relaxin potentiates progesterone activity, as was demonstrated in the rabbit endometrium by Zarrow and Brennan,[66] these effects cannot be assumed to be due to direct relaxin activity *but rather to some water-soluble progestogen activator contained within the corpus luteum*. Such a substance predominates in the preparation Lutrexin. In our view, a potential major field of therapeutic interest may be opened if it can be established that there is, after all, such a progestogen activator, whether it is relaxin or not, since such a substance would enjoy great application in gynecologic hormone therapy.

The symphysis-relaxing substance—that is, *relaxin* proper—is to a certain degree separable from the cervical or uterine relaxing factor (URF). However, both substances act by a similar mechanism, based on *depolymerization of mucopolysaccharides*, involving those of cartilage (sulfomucopolysaccharides) in relaxin, and those of cervical collagen (neutral mucopolysaccharides) in URF. Relaxin action could therefore be defined as glycoprotein-disintegrating and depolymerizing. If so confirmed, these substances should be of great potential importance in the treatment of rheumatoid arthritis or other chronic inflammatory disease, perhaps even in cirrhosis of the liver. Regardless of whether the progestational effect results from activity of a relaxinic complex alone or from the action of an active principle admixed to the water-soluble extracts, there is no doubt that "crude" relaxin may be defined *as a hormone which:* (1) *causes polysaccharide lysis, and* (2) *potentiates the corpus luteum hormone.*

REFERENCES

1. Abrahamson, D., and Reid, D. E.: *J. Clin. Endocr.*, 15:206, 1955.
2. Abrahamson, D., and Reid, D. E.: *Obstet. Gynec.*, 12:123, 1958.
3. Babcock, R. J., and Peterson, J. H.: *Amer. J. Obstet. Gynec.*, 78:33, 1959.
4. Birnberg, C. H., and Abitbol, M. M.: *Obstet. Gynec.*, 10:366, 1957.
5. Birnberg, C. H., and Abitbol, M. M.: *Ann. N.Y. Acad. Sci.*, 75:1016, 1959.
6. Brennan, D. M., and Zarrow, M. X.: *Endocrinology*, 64:907, 1959.
7. Cohen, H., and Steinetz, B. G.: *Proc. Soc. Exper. Biol. Med.*, 122:268, 1966.
8. Cullen, B. M., and Harkness, R. D.: *J. Physiol.*, 152:419, 1960.
9. Ballenberg, G., et al.: *Amer. J. Anat.*, 119:61, 1966.
10. Decker, W. H., et al.: *Obstet. Gynec.*, 12:37, 1958.
11. Decker, W. H.: *Ann. N.Y. Acad. Sci.*, 75:991, 1959.
12. Eichner, E., et al.: *Amer. J. Obstet. Gynec.*, 71:1035, 1956.
13. Eichner, E., et al.: *Ann. N.Y. Acad. Sci.*, 75:1023, 1959.
14. Felton, L. C., Frieden, E. H., and Briant, H. H.: *J. Pharmacol. Exper. Therap.*, 107:160, 1953.
15. Fevold, H. L., and Hisaw, F. L.: *Proc. Soc. Exper. Biol. Med.*, 27:604, 1930.
16. Frieden, E. H.: *Endocrinology*, 62:41, 1958.
17. Frieden, E. H., and Hisaw, F. L.: *Rec. Progr. Horm. Res.*, 8:333, 1953.
18. Frieden, E. H.: *Ann. N.Y. Acad. Sci.*, 75:931, 1959.
19. Frieden, E. H., Stone, N. R., and Layman, N. W.: *Science*, 130:338, 1959.
20. Frieden, H. G., Noall, M., and Alonso de Florida, F.: *J. Biol. Chem.*, 222:611, 1956.
21. Graham, E. F., and Dracy, A. E.: *J. Dairy Sci.*, 36:772, 1953.
22. Hall, E., Hoare, M., and Turner, C. B.: *J. Endocr.*, 25:271, 1962.
23. Hall, K., and Salimi-Khaligh, H.: *J. Endocr.*, 40:453, 1968.
24. Hisaw, F. L.: *Proc. Soc. Exper. Biol. Med.*, 23:661, 1926.
25. Hisaw, F. L., and Zarrow, M. X.: *Proc. Soc. Exper. Biol. Med.*, 69:395, 1948.
26. Hisaw, F. L., and Hisaw, F. L., Jr.: *Endocrinology*, 81:375, 1967.
27. Horn, E. H., and Barandes, M.: *Endocrinology*, 69:1102, 1961.
28. Israel, S. L., and Groeber, W. R.: *Obstet. Gynec.*, 15:2, 1960.
29. Jablonsky, W. J. A., and Velardo, J. T.: *Endocrinology*, 61:674, 1957.
30. Jagiello, G.: *J. Reprod. Fertil.*, 13:175, 1967.
31. Jones, G. S.: *Amer. J. Obstet. Gynec.*, 67:628, 1954.
32. Kelly, J. V.: *Ann. N.Y. Acad. Sci.*, 75:998, 1959.
32a. Kelley, J. V., and Posse, N.: *Obstet. Gynec.*, 8:531, 1956.

33. Kliman, B., and Greep, R. O.: *J. Clin. Endocr.*, 15:487, 1955.
34. Krantz, J. C., Bryant, H. H., and Carr, C. J.: *Surg. Gynec. Obstet.*, 90:372, 1950.
35. Kroc, R. L., Steinetz, B. G., and Beach, V. L.: *Ann. N.Y. Acad. Sci.*, 75:942, 1959.
36. Kupperman, H. S., Rosenberg, D., and Cutler, A.: *Ann. N.Y. Acad. Sci.*, 75:1003, 1959.
37. McCarthy, J. H., Erwing, H. H., and Laufe, L. E.: *Amer. J. Obstet. Gynec.*, 74:134, 1957.
38. McClintock, J. A., and Zarrow, M. X.: *J. Endocr.*, 36:369, 1966.
39. McGaughey, H. S., Corey, E. L., and Thornton, W. N.: *J. Endocr.*, 75:23, 1958.
40. Majewsky, J. T., and Jennings, T.: *Obstet. Gynec.*, 9:322, 1957.
41. Manning, J. P., Steinetz, B. G., Butler, M. C., and Priester, S.: *J. Endocr.*, 33:501, 1965.
42. Marder, S. N., and Money, W. L.: *Endocrinology*, 34:115, 1944.
43. Marois, M.: *Ann. d'Endocrinol.*, 19:265, 1958.
44. Martin, G. J., and Schoenbach, U.: *Ann. N.Y. Acad. Sci.*, 75:923, 1959.
45. Pommerenke, W. T.: *Amer. J. Obstet. Gynec.*, 27:708, 1934.
46. Posse, N., and Kelly, J. V.: *Surg. Gynec. Obstet.*, 103:687, 1956.
47. Rezek, G. H.: *Amer. J. Obstet. Gynec.*, 66:396, 1953.
48. Rezek, G. H.: *Ann. N.Y. Acad. Sci.*, 75:995, 1959.
49. Rothman, W. G., Bentley, E. D., and Floyd, W. S.: *Amer. J. Obstet. Gynec.*, 78:38, 1959.
50. Rudzik, A. D., and Miller, J. W.: *J. Pharmacol. Exper. Therap.*, 138:82, 1962.
51. Sawyer, W. H., Frieden, E. H., and Martin, A. C.: *Amer. J. Physiol.*, 172:547, 1953.
52. Schmidt, J. E., and Leonard, S. L.: *Endocrinology*, 67:663, 1960.
53. Slate, W. G., and Mengert, W. F.: *Obstet. Gynec.*, 15:409, 1960.
54. Steinetz, B. G., et al.: *Endocrinology*, 61:287, 1957.
55. Steinetz, B. G., and Beach, W. L.: *Endocrinology*, 72:771, 1963.
56. Steinetz, B. G., Manning, J. P., Butler, M. C., and Beach, V.: *Endocrinology*, 76:876, 1965.
57. Stone, M. L., Sedlis, A., and Zuckerman, M.: *Amer. J. Obstet. Gynec.*, 76:545, 1958.
58. Stone, M. L., et al.: *Ann. N.Y. Acad. Sci.*, 75:1011, 1959.
59. Struck, H.: *Vitamin Horm. u. Fermentforsch.*, 14:370, 1967.
60. WADA, H., and Turner, C. W.: *Proc. Soc. Exper. Biol. Med.*, 102:568, 1959.
61. Wada, H., and Turner, C. W.: *Proc. Soc. Exper. Biol. Med.*, 113:631, 1963.
62. Yochim, J., and Zarrow, M. X.: *Fertil. Steril.*, 12:263, 1961.
63. Zarrow, M. X.: *Proc. Soc. Exper. Biol. Med.*, 66:488, 1947.
64. Zarrow, M. X., Holmstrom, E. G., and Salhanick, H. A.: *J. Clin. Endocr.*, 15:22, 1955.
65. Zarrow, M. X., et al.: *Amer. J. Obstet. Gynec.*, 72:260, 1956.
66. Zarrow, M. X., and Brennan, D. M.: *Ann. N.Y. Acad. Sci.*, 75:981, 1959.
67. Zarrow, M. X., and Yochim, J.: *Endocrinology*, 69:292, 1961.
68. Zarrow, M. X., and O'Connor, W. B.: *Proc. Soc. Exper. Biol. Med.*, 121:612, 1966.

Part Two
EXTRAGONADAL FACTORS GOVERNING SEXUALITY

Gonadal function is governed by a double hormonal and neural regulatory mechanism. Although all the glands of internal secretion influence ovarian activity, it is mainly *the pituitary, the adrenal cortex and the thyroid* that are most intimately related to the female gonad. The nervous system, whose relationship to sexual processes had initially been acknowledged, only to be firmly denied subsequently, is at present known to intervene through a series of "neuroendocrine" reflexes of decisive importance in reproductive function. In the final analysis, it is the vitamins which, as biocatalysts, regulate biosynthesis of the sex hormones and their effects on target organs. This, in essence, is the subject dealt with in the next series of chapters.

Chapter 6
ADENOHYPOPHYSIS

6.1. HISTORY OF PITUITARY PHYSIOLOGY

6.1.1. ANTERIOR LOBE

Although the possibility of an endocrine function of the pituitary was entertained as early as the past century, it was not until 1921 that a definite endocrine function could be attributed to the *anterior lobe of the pituitary* as a result of the works of Evans and Long. These investigators were able to demonstrate that hypophysectomy in dogs was followed by arrest in growth of the long bones, whereas injections of pituitary extracts restored that growth. Hence, the inference of the existence of an anterior lobe *growth hormone* was made for the first time.

In 1922, the same workers made the observation that if pituitary extracts were injected into bitches, they produced certain changes in their ovaries; however, they did not attach much importance to this finding. The credit for postulating the existence of a principle capable of stimulating the ovaries went to Aschheim and Zondek, as well as to Smith, who made the discovery of a *gonadotropic hormone* in the anterior lobe of the pituitary simultaneously but independently in 1926. Shortly thereafter, in 1928, Stricker and Grueter found that hypophysectomy entailed loss of lactogenesis and, in 1931, Riddle isolated the hormone responsible for the stimulation of milk production, which was named *prolactin* or galactotropic hormone. The clinical investigations of Cushing, in 1932, and later those of Jores, Selye, Collip and Thompson, revealed the effects of pituitary function on the adrenal cortex, leading to the discovery of a corticotropic principle, or *adrenocorticotropic hormone*, whose ultimate importance in physiology would prove to be of the first order.

Aron, in 1929, and Jansen and Loeser, in 1933, first demonstrated the existence of a thyroid stimulating principle, or *thyrotropic hormone*; thus, in addition to gonadotropic and corticotropic hormone, thyrotropic hormone is currently known to be one of those unquestionable pituitary principles acting on the glands of internal secretion. In 1931, Houssay obtained a pituitary agent that caused elevation of blood sugar levels and hepatic deglycogenization, which was named *diabetogenic hormone*.

The period between 1937 and 1942 was marked by a great amount of work and effort aimed at isolating and purifying the anterior pituitary lobe principles; outstanding in this field were Evans and co-workers, and Fevold and his group. As a result of their patient and meticulous investigations, largely in the domain of biochemistry, it became evident that many of the presumed pituitary "principles" were based on invalid premises. Thus, no active principle responsible for the alleged pancreatotropic, parathyrotropic, medullotropic and thymotropic activities could be demonstrated. Instead, however, *what could be demonstrated was the fact that adrenocorticotropic hormone, thyrotropic hormone, the growth hormone and the galactotropic hormone were all well defined entities and, finally, that what heretofore had been considered a single gonadotropic hormone actually turned out to be, as previously had been postulated by Zondek, two different hormones, one stimulating the ovarian follicle and promoting testicular spermatogenesis, and the other stimulating the ovarian interstitium, promoting the growth of corpora lutea and also stimulating the interstitial cells of the testis.* The anti-insular or diabetogenic hormone, whose individuality has now likewise been established, has, however, been found to share multiple properties with the growth-promoting hormone, so that the assumption that it represents the same substance seems to be justified. Current knowledge would therefore admit as certainties the existence of the following hormones of the anterior lobe of the pituitary:

(a) Somatotropic or growth hormone (STH) (Evans, 1921).

(b) Follicle-stimulating hormone (FSH) (Zondek and Smith, 1926).

(c) Luteinizing and interstitial cell stimulating gonadotropic hormone (LH, ICSH) (Zondek and Smith, 1926).

(d) Galactotropic hormone or prolactin (Riddle et al., 1931).

(e) Diabetogenic hormone (probably identical to somatotropic hormone) (Houssay, 1931).

(f) Adrenocorticotropic hormone (ACTH) (Cushing, 1932).

(g) Thyrotropic hormone (TSH) (Aron, 1929).

It is pertinent here to mention the investigations of Pencharz and Long (1932), and those of Selye, Collip and Thompson (1933), who were first to perform serial hypophysectomies in experimental animals. Through their work, by testing the effects of extracts on hypophysioprival animals, they contributed in a decisive manner to the elucidation of many problems of pituitary physiology.

In recent years, fundamental progress was made in the field of *chemistry* of these hormones. Thanks, above all, to techniques allowing the *separation of proteins* by means of various gels, mainly Sephadex and similar preparations, it was possible to characterize six different hormones, each with a proved individuality. In addition, a large portion of the protein content in their molecules could be elucidated. For instance, the exact composition of ACTH is known, and even the chemical synthesis of some of its analogues has been accomplished. Moreover, progress in immunochemistry has facilitated the hormonal characterization of the six pituitary principles. It must not be forgotten that by virtue of the development of immunofluorescent techniques, the origin of each active pituitary principle and the identification of each type of cell composing this gland have been almost completely elucidated.

6.2. HYPOTHALAMUS AND PITUITARY

The most important advance in pituitary physiology in the last 20 years has been the understanding gained about the exact nature of pituitary-thalamic interrelationships. Both the anterior lobe (pars distalis, adenohypophysis) and the posterior lobe (pars intermedia and neurohypophysis) originally were believed to be secretory organs that received neural impulses from nerve fibers originating in hypothalamic centers which, accordingly, were thought to be the centers regulating pituitary hormonal activity.

However, in 1912, Achucarro,[1] had already called attention to the meager secretory character of the neurohypophysial cells, while at the same time emphasizing the paucity of nerve fibers in the pars distalis. Bargmann[6] and Harris[48] pointed out that the neurohypophysis was not actually an endocrine gland; the secretion of oxytocin, vasopressin and antidiuretic hormone, traditionally attributed to that gland, derived instead from the supraoptic and paraventricular nuclei of the hypothalamus, consequently representing *neurosecretion*. The part played by the pars intermedia would therefore be that of a mere "staging area."

The question of what controls the pars distalis is a problem of different nature. The fact that its vascular system is part of a single unit that also supplies the hypothalamus had already in 1933 been described by Popa and Fielding under the name of "porta-diencephalic system." Even though the existence of nerve fibers in the anterior lobe had been postulated by some authors, the idea that the agents capable of causing the cells of the adenohypophysis to secrete were *chemical mediators* soon gained ascendancy (Greer and Erwin,[44] Harris and Jacobson[47]). The regulation of gonadotropin secretion soon afterward was demonstrated to be carried out by such chemical mediators. Similarly, Harris and Jacobson[47] were able to produce evidence that secretion of both thyrotropic and corticotropic hormone was controlled by the actions of similar or identical substances.

The problem of whether neural influence is operative in gonadotropin secretion will be studied in subsequent chapters. It should be mentioned here, however, that the substances mediating such influence belong to the group of *polypeptide hormones*, such as vasopressin, oxytocin, serotonin, and many other recently discovered analogues.[82]

However, it should be made clear that these messenger substances are not exciters of anterior lobe secretion but simply provoke the *displacement from within the cells* of hormonal substances that have been produced and stored at a slow endogenous rhythm. This phenomenon of liberation, or *release*, is the essence of the action the hypothalamus exerts on the anterior lobe.

In 1963, by means of electron microscopy, Theret and Tamboise[124] found that the nerve endings in the anterior lobe themselves liberated the chemical mediators and that consequently there was no need for them to be transported by the blood-stream (see Chapter 8). This seems to be a property inherent in all substances produced by the hypothalamus so that, in addition to the chemical messengers that the anterior lobe receives via the blood flow of the hypophysioportal system, it also receives chemotransmitters from the axon cylinders, similarly to what could be seen occurring in the posterior lobe. The only difference lies in the fact that in the posterior lobe they gain direct access to the blood-stream, whereas in the anterior lobe they act upon the secretory cells.

In anterior lobe cell cultures or in pituitary transplants,[125] in which the action by hypothalamic releasing factors is bypassed, all pituitary hormones with the exception of prolactin cease to be secreted. It would therefore appear that secretion of ACTH, STH, TSH and the two gonadotropins is determined by the releasing stimulus of hypothalamic chemical mediators. Conversely, lack of hypothalamic action determines the liberation of prolactin which, in turn, is inhibited in the presence of a specific factor that is also derived from the hypothalamus. That means that secretion of all hormones proceeds in a direction opposite to that of prolactin.

The anterior lobe can thus be compared to a loaded gun that is fired under the triggering effect of hypothalamic action.

A more complete study of these interactions will be made in Chapter 8; for the time being, it will suffice here to summarize several general notions concerning the hypothalamic-pituitary interrelationships:

1. *The pituitary and hypothalamus constitute an inseparable functional unit. Pituitary hormone function is entirely under either the direct or the mediated neural control of the hypothalamus.*

2. *The paraventricular and supraoptic nuclei of the hypothalamus are endocrine organs secreting the so-called posterior lobe hormones. The posterior lobe is a mere inactive extension, a kind of excretory duct, of these nuclei.*

3. *The so-called retrohypophysial incretions are therefore neurohormones.*

4. *The anterior lobe hormones are all trophic hormones, that is to say, hormones affecting hormones, designed to stimulate other glands of internal secretion. They in turn obey hypothalamic stimuli mediated by substances likewise of hormonal character. They partake in an endocrine chain reaction that is always set into motion by the nervous system.*

5. *The hypothalamic nuclei are subordinated to higher centers, which accounts for the known fact that psychic phenomena act on the pituitary and, through it, on the rest of the endocrine system.*

6.3. ADENOHYPOPHYSIAL HORMONES

Since the neurohypophysis is not an endocrine organ but a mere extension of the hypothalamus, it will not be dealt with here. This chapter will be confined to the study of the adenohypophysis. Not so long ago, it was enough to observe the effects of a pituitary extract on a given effector in order to discover in them the actions of what was believed to be a new and independent principle. More than 20 active adenohypophysial principles were at one time or another described as distinct entities by means of similar procedures. Those old theories are currently outdated. Both the discovery of immunologic properties of the pituitary hormones and the perfected methods using gels to separate them have allowed the *purification and specific identification* of only six hormones: (1) growth hormone or somatotropic hormone (STH); (2) follicular maturation stimulating hormone (FSH); (3) luteinization stimulating hormone (LH); (4) lacteal secretion stimulating hormone (Prolactin); (5) adrenocorticotropic hormone (ACTH), and (6) thyrotropic hormone (TSH). Melanotropic hormone, which at one time was thought to be the seventh independent principle, is presently considered identical at least as far as the human species is concerned, to ACTH.

The present chapter will deal with all adenohypophysial hormones with the exception of FSH and LH which, owing to their importance in regulating sexual phenomena, deserve to be discussed in a chapter apart. Thus, Chapter 7 will be dedicated to the gonadotropins and Chapter 8 to the hypothalamus.

6.4. MORPHOLOGY OF ADENOHYPOPHYSIS

6.4.1. EMBRYOLOGY

The pituitary develops from two different anlagen. One of these is an invagination formed by an ectodermal pouch that is situated at the level of the pharyngeal membrane (Fig. 6–1). Rathke's pouch is first seen in 3 mm embryos and becomes clearly visible in 8 to 10 mm embryos. This invagination is oriented in a dorsal direction and comes to join another, similar glove-like invagination growing in an opposite direc-

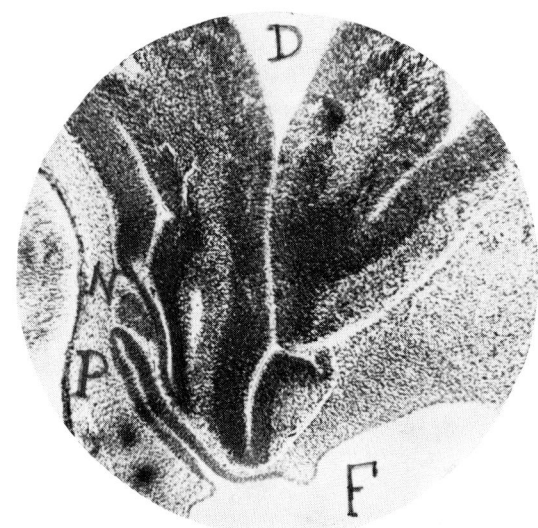

Figure 6–2. High power detail of Figure 6–1. D, Lateral ventricle with outline of eyebud. N, Median ventricle and neurohypophysis; P, adenohypophysis; F, pharynx.

tion from the highest point of the neural tube (Fig. 6–2). The invagination of ectodermal origin, that has arisen from Rathke's pouch, will give rise to the adenohypophysis (P), whereas the invagination originating in the neural tube will form the neurohypophysis (N), the latter being a prolongation of the third ventricle (see Fig. 6–2.) As shown in the figure, the junction of the two gland buds can be seen quite well in 9 mm embryos, which have 22 to 24 somites.

The pituitary does not attain a definite structure until the third or fourth month of intrauterine life. The pharyngeal recess gives rise to the anterior lobe. The intermediate lobe differentiates from this recess, and the recess of the third ventricle gives rise to the posterior lobe, which is to retain its neural structure for the rest of its existence. It will be shown later how the different embryonal origins of the pituitary lobes determine different physiologic significance.

6.4.2. ANATOMY

The pituitary is joined to the floor of the third ventricle by a slender stalk, *the pituitary stalk,* which is part of the tuber cinereum. The pituitary constitutes a kind of club-shaped enlargement with a greatest

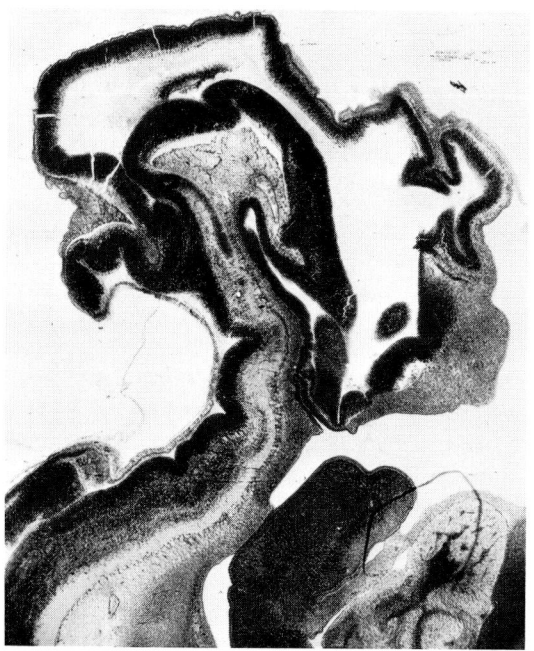

Figure 6–1. Five week human embryo in sagittal section. Anterior portion of cephalic extremity showing pharynx. Rathke's pouch and formation of pituitary bud.

TABLE 6-1. Divisions and Subdivisions of the Pituitary Gland

PRINCIPAL DIVISIONS	SUBDIVISIONS
Adenohypophysis ... Lobus glandularis	1. Pars distalis ⎫ 2. Pars tuberalis ⎬ Anterior lobe 3. Pars intermedia ....⎭ ⎫ ⎬ Posterior lobe
Neurohypophysis .. ⎧ Lobus nervosus ⎨ (neural lobe) ⎪ Infundibulum ⎩ (neural stalk)	1. Processus infunduli .. ⎭ 1. Pediculus infundibularis (stem) 2. Bulbus infundibularis (bulb) 3. Labrum infundibularis or median eminence of the tuber cinereum

diameter of 1.2 to 1.5 cm. It is lodged in the sella turcica or pituitary fossa of the sphenoid bone, which affords enclosure and protection. Its superior aspect is covered by the diaphragma sellae of the dura mater which is punctured only by the pituitary stalk. As has already been pointed out, the pituitary is divided into the anterior, intermediate and posterior lobes. The *intermediate lobe* attains unusual development in certain animals, such as fishes, batrachia and amphibians; in mammals, it is much less differentiated and in man (above all in the adult), it remains of very small size. The *posterior lobe* or *neurohypophysis* is connected directly to the floor of the brain, of which it is but an uninterrupted extension, by nervous tissue. The division into an anterior lobe (pars anterior or pars glandularis), a middle lobe (pars intermedia), and a posterior lobe (pars nervosa), is not a perfectly satisfactory one to the anatomists, who provide a more complete classification along lines indicated in Table 6-1.

A vestige of Rathke's pouch may sometimes persist buried in the posterior pharynx, constituting the so-called *pharyngeal hypophysis*, which in the normal individual is of little consequence except for the possibility of giving rise to neoplasia.

6.4.3. HISTOLOGY OF ADENOHYPOPHYSIS

The anterior lobe, or adenohypophysis, is made up of epithelial columns that are supported by a connective tissue reticulum and are surrounded by numerous sinusoids, whose walls are rich in reticuloendothelial elements. The structure of the hypophysial vasculature is very significant and will be studied in more detail in Section 6.4.5. The overall architecture of the organ is distinctly that of an endocrine gland. However, most noteworthy about the adenohypophysis is not its histology but its cytology.

6.4.4. CYTOLOGY OF ADENOHYPOPHYSIS

The various cell types described in the anterior lobe have been the object of intensive studies, particularly by the physiologists seeking to locate a distinct cell type from which each of the hormones is secreted. This goal has been only partially achieved. It may be stated that the methods used to determine the different cell types are basically four: (1) *histologic*, (2) *histochemical*, (3) *ultramicroscopic* and (4) *immunofluorescent*.

HISTOLOGIC METHODS. Time-honored, conventional methods, using routine hematoxylin-eosin stains, allow identification of three cell types: (a) Acidophilic or eosinophilic cells staining red with eosin, (b) basophilic cells staining bluish with hematoxylin, and (c) chromophobe cells that contain no specific stainable granules in their cytoplasm and therefore are not stained. It is generally admitted that hormonal secretion takes place only in the acidophilic and basophilic cells.

HISTOCHEMICAL METHODS. Important progress in pituitary cytology resulted from the introduction of the periodic acid-Schiff reaction (PAS) as a staining procedure by Hotchkiss and MacManus. This method was applied by Purves and Griesbach,[104] by Bargman[6] and by Pearse.[100] It allows identification of those hormones which contain a protein linked to a carbohydrate moiety, that is, a mucopolysaccharide; thus, thyrotropin and the two gonadotropins could be located in basophils (Pearse,[100] Purves and Griesbach[105]).

PAS positive cells received the generic name of *mucoid cells* and have been subdivided into different varieties. In some animals, e.g., the rat, as many as five different varieties of such cells (alpha, beta, gamma, delta and epsilon) could be recognized (Herlant,[55] Herlant and Pasteels[56]).

Ultimately, the employment of performic acid and alsian blue in conjunction with the PAS method (Adams and Swettenham[3]) makes the recognition of two cell types possible: one, designated R, containing neutral mucopolysaccharides, and staining red, and the other, designated S, containing acid mucopolysaccharides, and staining blue. The S cell type is rich in the sulphur-containing amino acid cystine, and can be divided, in turn, into two subtypes, S-1 and S-2. Maracek and Arendarcik[88] estimated the concentrations of FSH and LH in animal pituitaries and found that the intensity of PAS staining was proportional to the concentration of the latter two hormones, producing evidence of a PAS-gonadotropic cell relationship. *Cortisone* therapy enriches the FSH content of the anterior lobe, and the PAS positivity of that tissue increases equally.[68] However, not all PAS positive cells in the adenohypophysis are similar or have identical functions as pointed out by Conklin,[16] who distinguishes five varieties of cells giving a positive PAS reaction.

Acidophils consist of a single cell type, which is rich in tyrosine. They seem to be the source of growth hormone and prolactin secretion, both hormones having a high tyrosine content (Glenner and Lillie[38]). In man, cells secreting growth hormone cannot be distinguished from those secreting prolactin, but Barnes[7] was able to find a distinction in the rat.

ULTRAMICROSCOPIC METHODS. Electron microscopic studies undertaken by Barnes[7] and, more recently, by Vogt and Kopp,[128] and by Wilde and his colleagues,[134] also confirmed the previously recognized five varieties of cell types (Fig. 6-3) and laid the groundwork for the intracellular detection of the origin of each adenohypophysial hormone. Recently, Rambourg and Racadot,[108] as well as Siperstein and Miller,[118] have further characterized the ultramicroscopic properties of these six pituitary cell types. In Table 6-2, a tentative listing of the cell of origin of each hormone is presented. It must be said, however, that this outline is far from being definite and

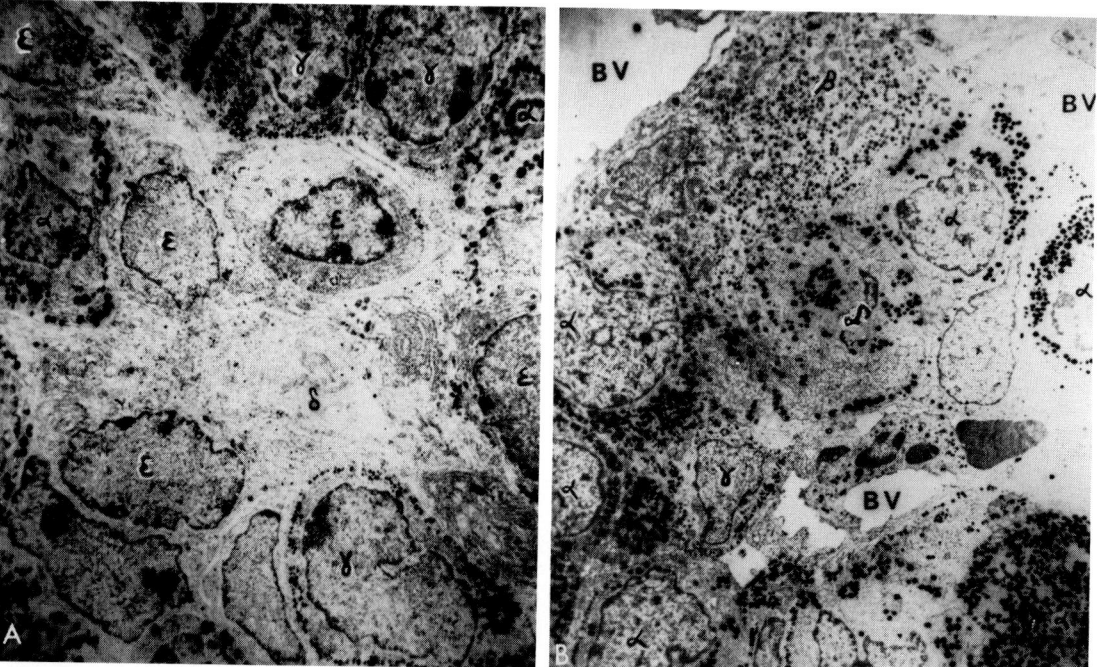

Figure 6-3. Electron micrograph of mouse pituitary. *A*, Alpha, gamma, delta and epsilon cells (3000×). *B*, Alpha, beta and gamma cells (1800×). (From Barnes, B. G.: *Endocrinology*, 71:619, 1962.)

TABLE 6-2. Functional Cytology of the Adenohypophysis*

HORMONE	KNOWN ORIGIN (CELL TYPE)	POSSIBLE ORIGIN (CELL TYPE)	ELECTRON MICROSCOPIC CORRELATION
Growth	α	$\alpha 1$	α
Prolactin	α	$\alpha 2$	ϵ
Follicle stimulating	Mucoid	S_1	β
Luteinizing	Mucoid	R1	γ
Thyrotropic	S_2	S_2	S
Adrenocorticotropic	R	R2	δ

*According to Friesen and Estwood: *New Eng. J. Med.*, 272:1218, 1965.

that investigations are still being carried on in search for the exact cellular origin of each hormone.[23, 30, 119, 134]

FLUORESCENT ANTIBODY TECHNIQUES. In 1950, Coons and Kaplan devised a technique which lends itself particularly well to the detection of cellular origin of proteic hormones behaving as antigens, which utilizes their specific fluorescein-labeled antibodies. This technique yielded specially good results in research on the adenohypophysis and enabled various authors[28, 45, 65, 80] to establish a new classification of the origin of the different pituitary hormones. By marking prolactin and somatotropin with fluorescent antibodies, it has recently been possible to trace the two hormones to acidophilic cells.[54, 119] Nayak and his colleagues[94] distinguish two subtypes of acidophilic cells, carminophilic cells containing growth hormone and orangeophilic cells containing prolactin.

Furthermore, using similar fluorescent techniques, Kracht and colleagues[72] have succeeded in locating the origin of the gonadotropins and of ACTH, and their results are essentially in agreement with the scheme already outlined. This scheme is summarized in Table 6-2.

Obviously, there still seem to be considerable discrepancies among the histochemical, immunologic and electron microscopic findings.

6.4.5. PITUITARY BLOOD SUPPLY

The blood supply to the anterior lobe differs substantially from that to the posterior lobe. In 1933, the investigators Popa and Fielding discovered in the anterior lobe the *porta-diencephalic system* which they believed conducted the blood flow in a pituitary-hypothalamic direction but which Spanner[121] subsequently demonstrated as proceeding from the hypothalamus to the pars distalis, thus really being the vector of those chemical mediators which were mentioned in Section 6.4.4. Greer and Erwin's investigations[44] showed that a similar portal system was present in quite a large number of animal species, of which they described 80 instances, ranging from cyclostomata to man. This portal system is richly endowed with vasomotor reflexes, and its blood flow is controlled by the hypothalamic centers. The diencephalic-portal system forms a *primary plexus* at the level of the median eminence of the tuber cinereum; its vessels empty into a common trunk that passes down the stalk to the pars distalis and there gives off new branches for a *secondary plexus*, which forms the venous sinuses surrounding the adenohypophysial cells (Fig. 6-4).

The venous blood coming from the sinusoids and conveying the products of anterior lobe secretion is collected by the cavernous sinus, which drains all pituitary venous channels. This vascular arrangement allows the following functional possibilities: (1) Direct passage, in the manner of a short circuit, of arterial blood through the pituitary in the resting stage, with scanty irrigation of the gland; (2) flow of venous blood from the diencephalon down the portal system, this flow in turn being regulated by a *portal sphincter*; (3) flow of arterial blood through the capillaries and pituitary sinusoids.[19] That is to say, the pituitary may receive blood predominantly from either the diencephalic portal system or the systemic arterial circulation. Whether

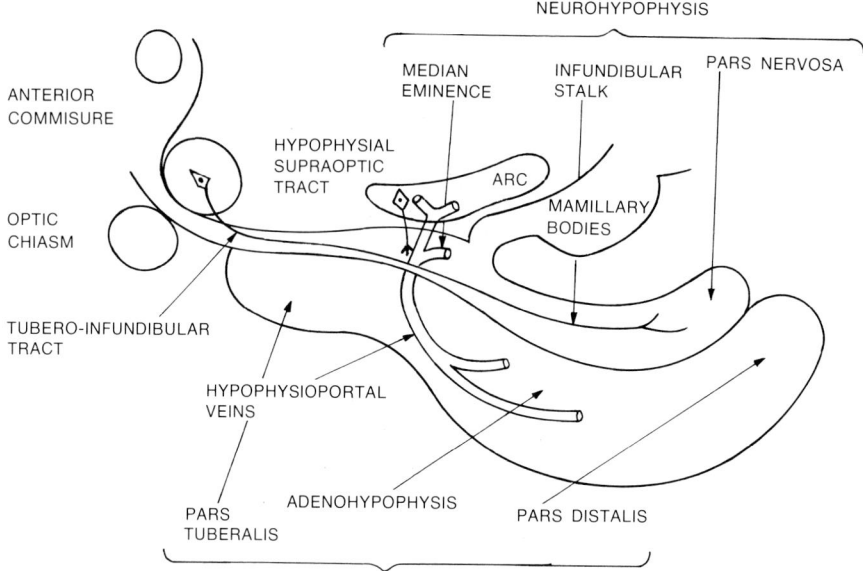

Figure 6-4. Diagram of anatomy of tuberohypophysial region in human adult.

or not it receives most of its blood from either of these vascular trunks depends on the functional state of the vascular musculature which is able to regulate the passage of the blood (Greep[43]). Porter and his colleagues[103] have been able to measure the blood flow of the portal system and to determine its neuroendocrine regulation in relation to the functional demands of the floor of the third ventricle.

6.4.6. INNERVATION

The innervation of the pituitary gland has been well documented through the investigations of Achucarro[1] and those of Ranson, of Camus and of Roussy. The recent investigations of Harris[49] and of Bargmann[6] showed that most of the pituitary innervation extends to the posterior lobe, which is extremely rich in nerve endings. According to the same authors, the anterior lobe is devoid of nerve fibers. This seems to be a revolutionary claim rebutting the traditionally accepted observations of Ranson and Spaatz, both of whom had described nerve endings in the anterior lobe. Nevertheless, more recently, Ribas-Mujal performed very meticulous research using Castro's modification of the Gross method and was able to demonstrate the existence of nerve endings in the anterior lobe of the pituitary (see Chapter 8).

Mention has already been made of the electron microscopic findings by Theret and Tamboise[124] confirming these nerve endings and the part they play in the in situ release of mediator substances.

6.4.7. INTERRELATIONSHIPS OF PITUITARY AND TELENCEPHALON BY WAY OF THE HYPOTHALAMUS

This is one aspect of pituitary physiology that until recently had been poorly understood, but which is of major interest.

The center of this interrelationship is the hypophysiothalamic system. Many psychic and sensorial impulses are currently known to be capable of modifying certain endocrine functions and these actions are believed to be produced as a result of hypothalamic control of pituitary function (Fig. 6-5). For this reason, the pathways along which impulses from the cerebral cortex reach the hypothalamus, and hence the pituitary, are of utmost importance.

Particularly conclusive in this respect is the work done by Gloor[39] in the field of neurophysiology. From his studies, it would appear that the hypothalamic centers that are related to pituitary function receive their afferent fibers from the "oldest" structures of the cortex: the hippocampus, the pyriform lobe, the cingulate gyrus, the

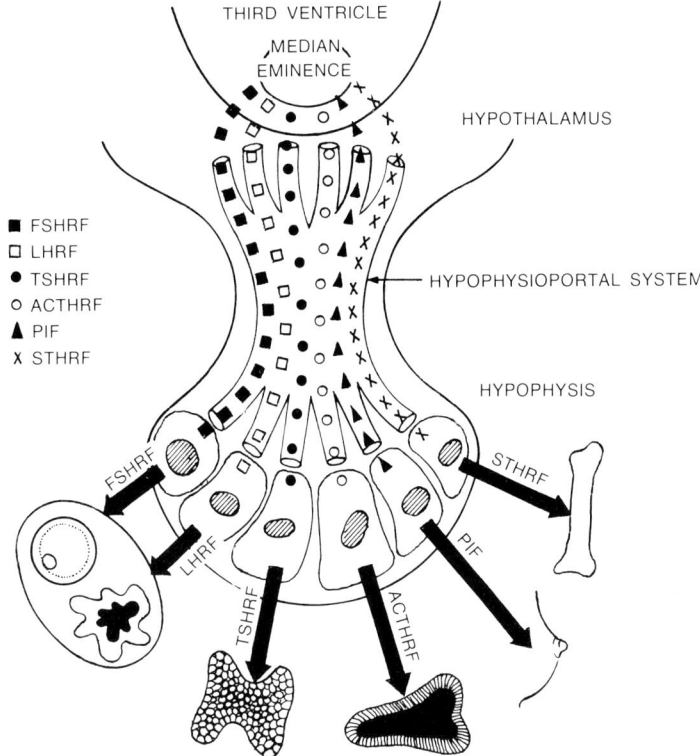

Figure 6–5. Diagram of functional relationship between hypothalamus and pituitary by means of hypophysioportal system.

anterior insula and the amygdaloid nucleus. These structures constitute what today is termed the *limbic system.*

The limbic system then controls indirectly the near totality of endocrine functions of the body by means of hypothalamic chemical mediators.

6.5. PHYSIOLOGY OF ADENOHYPOPHYSIS

6.5.1. HISTOPHYSIOLOGY

The relationship between pituitary structure and pituitary function has been the subject of many studies and of abundant speculation. The mere fact that, in addition to so complicated a glandular structure, there also exists an equally abundant and intricate vascular system allows us to assume that the mechanism of pituitary hormone secretion is a very complex one. At the same time, a close relationship to the adjacent hypothalamus and the number of the secreted hormones add to the complexity of the question.

Experiments in which the pituitary stalk was transected resulted in cessation of pituitary function.[29, 47, 131] Smith[120] subsequently proved that pituitary transplants failed to empty their products of hormonal secretion into the bloodstream but that from their macerated tissues, nevertheless, could be extracted a hormonal produce that was within normal limits; this goes to prove the earlier statement that the action of the pituitary stalk—or rather of the substances passing through it either along the axon cylinders or down the hypophysioportal system—is *not a secretory but a releasing effect.* Pituitary tissue culture studies conducted by Thompson and co-workers[125] also demonstrated that isolated pituitary tissue is capable of performing normal endocrine activity. This subject has already been broached (Section 6.2) and will be discussed more extensively in Chapter 8.

Earlier (Section 6.4.4), the relationship between cytology and hormonal biosynthesis had already been indicated. It might be added, here, that Racadot and Herlant,[107] who studied the pituitary gland in lactating animals, observed an increase in the proportion of acidophils. Leznoff and colleagues[79, 80] used a very elegant method for the detection of hormones by means of fluorescent antibody techniques, which enabled him to determine the site of somatotropin formation in the acidophils. Brown and co-workers,[9, 10] on the other hand, subjected experimental animals to stress situations with a view to determining which cell types responded by becoming hyperplastic, assuming that those would have to be the ACTH producers. This method has also been employed by Herlant and Pasteels,[56] with similar results.

Herlant and Decourt[57] have studied a clinical case of Cushing's syndrome, in which was found a chromophobe cell hyperplasia associated with the predominance of finely granular intracellular elements, or microsomes.

Pituitary cytology has been studied along similar lines in acromegaly[56] and in Basedow's (Graves') disease.[71]

Other lines of approach have resorted to histochemical and ultramicroscopic means; thanks to both, and to the works of Purves and Griesbach, we now seem to have learned a great deal about the sites of formation of LH, TSH and ACTH, as well as that of the growth hormone. Sites of FSH and prolactin formation are still being debated.

6.5.2. PITUITARY VARIATIONS RELATED TO SEX

The male pituitary is invariably smaller than that of the female.[3, 6, 28, 56] The female pituitary undergoes cyclic variations not only in function (see Chapter 12), *but also in its cytology.* Periodic changes affecting both basophils and acidophils have been known for a long time, ever since they were described by Campbell and Wolfe and by Severinghaus. More recently, Purves and Griesbach[104, 105] reported cyclic changes in those cells which stain positively in the PAS reaction. In the view of these authors, these changes were thought to reflect the morphologic variations in the differing rates of secretion of ovary stimulating hormones that determine the cyclic events in the female. Lisk[84] was able to measure the LH content of the pituitary parenchyma and noted that it likewise was subject to cyclic fluctuations.

Castration in both animal and human females, as well as *menopause* in the latter, causes the appearance of the so-called *castration cells*,[36, 37, 107] which, in Purves' opinion, are hypertrophied gonadotrophs, reflecting FSH hypersecretion in ovariprival females. In some animals, notably the rat, puberty is associated with temporary hypertrophy of the adenohypophysis.[90]

Finally, *pregnancy* is associated with the appearance of *pregnancy cells*, described by Erdheim and Stumme as far back as 1910, which are merely transformed acidophilic alpha cells and which are probably responsible for the increased production of somatotropin in the pregnant woman,[55, 56] even though in the light of the recent findings by Yen and co-workers,[138] increased somatotropin production in pregnancy may be questionable.

In the pseudogravid rat, cervical stimulation results in hypophysial changes that are similar to those of pregnancy, which might lead one to believe that the pituitary changes of pregnancy are induced by a neurohormonal reflex originating in the genitalia.

Finally, the *effects exerted upon the pituitary by estrogens* must also be considered. Estrogens have been shown to stimulate pituitary function by increasing somatotropin secretion.[35, 42] Similarly, an increase in RNA and DNA contents has been observed following estrogen administration.[62] Oxygen consumption likewise is reported to be elevated.[62] Independent of the effects that estrogens may have upon the hypothalamic sexual centers and, indirectly, upon the pituitary, a direct stimulatory effect exerted by this group of steroids upon the overall secretory activity of the adenohypophysis seems to be a well established fact.[73, 78, 129]

The male pituitary secretes the same hormones as the female pituitary, with the sole exception of lacking the cyclic character and the pregnancy changes of the latter.

6.5.3. PHYSIOLOGY OF PITUITARY HORMONES, WITH THE EXCEPTION OF GONADOTROPINS AND PROLACTIN

Here we shall study in a summary fashion the actions and properties of those hormones which are not directly implicated in the regulation of sexual function. A subsequent chapter has been reserved for a more detailed study of the gonadotropic and galactotropic hormones, both of which have a specific and obvious sex-related activity (Fig. 6–5).

SOMATOTROPIC HORMONE. Somatotropic hormone, also known as growth hormone, is secreted by the acidophils (eosinophilic cells) and has the chemical structure of a protein, which was recently isolated in its crystallized form by Li.[81, 82] It is known to stimulate longitudinal growth of the long bones in young animals and in young persons, provided that chondrogenesis in the epiphysial growth plate remains active. Once ossification has been completed in adults, it can no longer effect bone growth in length but it can cause certain parts of the body to jut out, as occurs with hands, feet, chin or nose in *acromegaly*.

Bioassay is performed on rats by measuring radioactive sulphur (^{32}S) deposition in the distal cartilages of the long bones. Its origin, as already pointed out (Section 6.4.4), has been proved beyond doubt to be in the acidophils of the subtype alpha.[45, 79, 89] This could also be confirmed with eosinophilic adenomas of the alpha cell type, which are well known to be associated with acromegaly.[139] Apart from its stimulative effect on growth, the hormone also has a lactogenic effect, as will be shown in Chapter 22. However, in adult animals and in the adult woman, its most important effects are exerted on the metabolism of proteins, by contributing to protein synthesis (Korner[70]), and on the metabolism of carbohydrates, by virtue of its well known diabetogenic effects.[17, 21, 24]

Even so, somatotropic hormone is not without practical interest in the field of gynecology.

The traditional view, postulating increased somatotropin activity during pregnancy, presently is undergoing revision.[5, 126, 138] It would now seem more likely that elevated diabetogenic activity of pregnancy is the result of placental lactogen (see Chapter 18). Although somatotropic hormone is not believed to cross the placental barrier,[75] a teratogenic effect has nevertheless been described in rats[12] following injection of somatotropin. This, of course, is an effect that could possibly be induced indirectly by the fetus rather than by the passage of injected hormone.[138] The physiopathologic significance of somatotropin and placental lactogen will be re-examined in greater detail in our discussion of diabetes of pregnancy (see Chapter 45).

Earlier, somatotropin was believed to be the *"hormone of infancy,"* which ceased being secreted at puberty. The investigations of Gershberg[36] and those of Wright[136] have provided evidence to the contrary. Hormone values secreted in adulthood are comparable to those found in children. What actually happens is that there is a *different response of the target organs* and, in the presence of somatotropin, the long bones no longer grow. At puberty, somatotropin is converted to diabetogenic hormone.

THYROTROPIC HORMONE. The investigations of Aron[4] established the existence of a thyroid stimulating pituitary principle. This active principle has been found to produce characteristic and significant stimulatory changes in the histologic appearance of the thyroid, such as reabsorption of colloid and increased mitotic activity, with proliferation and stratification of the epithelium.[11] In animals injected with the hormone, thyroid stimulation leads indirectly to the elevation of the basal metabolic rate, to the depletion of hepatic glycogen, to the appearance of ketonuria and to increased resistance to acetonitrile.[4] Since all of the latter reactions are absent in thyroprival animals, there is no doubt that stimulation of these functions takes place indirectly by means of the thyroid gland.

Estimation of thyrotropin activity by bioassay currently is achieved by procedures measuring radioactive iodine (^{131}I) uptake by the thyroid of a hypophysectomized animal treated with thyrotropin. It has already been indicated that thyrotropin seems to be elaborated by basophils of the subtype S-2.[100, 101]

The effects of thyrotropin activity have been revised by Keating and co-workers.[64] During the last few years, its exophthalmos-producing effects have been much emphasized. Morris[91] has insisted that there are no two distinct substances involved, but that both the thyrotropic and exophthalmogenic effects are produced by one and the same purified compound. It should be pointed out that there seem to be two thyrotropic substances: one, whose actions are acute, and which corresponds to what is termed TSH, and the other, possessing a prolonged action, called LATS (long-acting thyroid stimulator), which was described and isolated by Adams.[2, 3]

Thyrotropic hormone plays an important role in pregnancy, as will be seen later (Chapter 20). This author has demonstrated elevated TSH values during pregnancy, which are important because they account for both the hyperfunctioning thyroid of pregnancy and some other gestational manifestations (Chapters 20 and 41). The hormone is likewise an important factor in shaping fetal thyroid function. By crossing over into the placental circulation, TSH is capable of stimulating the fetal thyroid and, under certain circumstances (Chapter 20), of initiating the metabolic functions of the embryo.

Greer and Erwin,[44] and later Yamada,[137] found the regulatory centers for thyroid function and TSH secretion to be located in the anterior hypothalamus.

ADRENOCORTICOTROPIC HORMONE. Adrenocorticotropic hormone of the anterior lobe of the pituitary has been demonstrated by Anselmino and Hoffmann and by Jores. From the anterior lobe of the pituitary, these authors extracted a principle capable of stimulating the adrenal cortex of the mouse. Selye, Collip and Thompson found atrophy of the adrenal cortex in hypophysectomized animals. This hormone, which is also known by the synonyms of corticotropin and ACTH, stimulates adrenal cortical function, producing mainly an increase in thickness of the zona fasciculata and increasing cortical hormonal production, particularly that of the glucocorticoids: cortisone, dehydrocortisone, etc. It influences the output of mineralocorticoids to a lesser degree, elevating them slightly notwithstanding, and it produces increased 17-ketosteroid excretion, also to a lesser degree than with glucocorticoids. It is doubtful whether increased 17-ketosteroid excretion reflects stimulation of metabolic or sexual cortical function (see Chapter 9). By virtue of its adrenal cortical stimulatory action, adrenocorticotropic hormone exerts very important effects on carbohydrate metabolism by increasing glycemia and by mobilizing carbohydrate deposits towards the liver. It also produces alterations in electrolyte levels by elevating serum chloride and by promoting tissue sodium retention. On injection, other noticeable effects produced are *eosinopenia* and *lymphocytosis,* decrease in fatigability and stimulation of metabolic rate of muscle, as well as increased rate of phosphorylation and enhanced resistance to stress and to infection. However, none of these effects result from a direct action by ACTH, since they can be suppressed by adrenalectomy, which is proof that they are mediated by the adrenal cortex.

The recent investigations of Kline[69] and Sandberg and co-workers[114] demonstrated that ACTH promoted synthesis of acetyl groups and their polymerization via squalene, with eventual conversion to cholesterol or to C-21 steroids (see Chapters 2 and 3). This action would seem to explain why, in castrated and adrenalectomized women, ACTH injections nevertheless produce increased levels of estrogen, undoubtedly as a result of synthesis of these compounds starting from simple chains in organs other than the gonad or the adrenal cortex.

Certain centers, as yet poorly characterized, which are believed to regulate body defenses and response to stress, recently were found to stimulate ACTH secretion. Guillemin[46] succeeded in provoking increased secretion of 11-oxysteroids by stimulating different areas of the hypothalamus, and Van Wick and his colleagues[127] reported the absence of a stress response after transection of the pituitary stalk. The same effect can allegedly be obtained with reserpine or chlorpromazine which, by virtue of their gangliopegic action, inhibit the centers of the tuber cinereum (Kitay et al.,[67] Sewy et al.[116])

Hypothalamic control of ACTH secretion has been confirmed by a great many workers.[13, 86, 95, 132] Aspects concerning that subject will be dealt with in greater detail in Chapter 8. Sayers' method[115] for the determination of ascorbic acid depletion in the adrenal cortex has already become the classic bioassay for corticotropin. As indicated previously, the principal action of corticotropin consists in stimulating adrenocortical steroidogenesis, which has been demonstrated in vitro.[113] Extracortical actions of ACTH are mainly those activating the phosphorylases[52] and those affecting lipid metabolism.

Regarding the cell type in which it originates, immunofluorescence[17, 80] and histochemical[101] studies seem to be in accord in that ACTH is elaborated by mucoid cells of subtype R (see Section 6.4.4).

In recent years, discussion has arisen as to whether melanogenic hormone and

Adenohypophysis

ACTH are one or two substances. In mammals, at least, there would seem to be only one substance.[27, 117] This hormone plays a significant part in sexual processes. Insofar as the rat is concerned, at least, ACTH secretion apparently is enhanced by estogens.[33] ACTH was also shown to exert a discrete effect on the ovary, causing in it increased steroidogenesis.

The hormone is excreted in the urine in larger amounts during pregnancy than at other times and is found in even greater quantities in certain pathologic conditions of pregnancy, such as, for instance, the toxemias of pregnancy (see Chapter 40).

FOLLICLE-STIMULATING HORMONE (FSH). As was stated previously, this substance shall be studied in Chapter 7.

LUTEINIZING HORMONE (LH). This hormone likewise will be studied in Chapter 7.

PROLACTIN (LTH). Although prolactin will be discussed in more detail in Chapters 7 and 22, a few facts concerning it must be mentioned here. Prolactin was discovered by Riddle and co-workers in 1932. As Rao and colleagues[112] have found, it is the only hormone that the adenohypophysis keeps elaborating after its neurovascular connections are severed. It seems to originate in the acidophilic cells,[7, 8] even though it is admitted that a special kind of acidophil, called epsilon cells,[28, 58] are the true prolactin producers, and that these have been observed to proliferate in pituitary explants.

Prolactin also possesses gonadotropic activity (see Chapter 7) and is responsible for the maintenance of the corpus luteum, by preventing its regression. Hence, it is called "luteotropin" or LTH.

6.5.4. WHAT IS MEANT BY "PITUITARY HORMONES"?

Melanogenic hormone has by now been identified with ACTH. Similarly, diabetogenic hormone has been found to be identical to somatotropin. Consequently, only the following hormones are to be regarded as true pituitary hormones:

(1) Somatotropin or growth hormone (STH)
(2) Thyrotropin or thyroid-stimulating hormone (TSH)
(3) ACTH
(4) Follicle-stimulating hormone (FSH)
(5) Luteinizing hormone (LH)
(6) Prolactin (LTH)

6.6. CHEMISTRY OF ANTERIOR LOBE HORMONES

Knowledge of the chemical composition of the pituitary hormones has been lagging considerably compared to our knowledge of the chemistry of other hormones. The reason for this is the protein nature and high molecular weight of these substances. In most instances, it has been impossible to achieve crystallization of the pituitary hormones, and, except for rough approximations, their constitutional formulas can not otherwise be derived. The isolation of one of these hormones in its pure state indeed constitutes the first proof of its unquestionable individuality.[26, 61]

6.6.1. SOMATOTROPIC HORMONE

In 1955, Li[81] obtained a preparation of growth hormone in pure form from an alkaline extract of bull pituitary. Electrophoretic studies have shown the homogeneity of that product. Li and Papkoff[82] have dedicated their efforts to elucidating the chemical structure of that compound.

Growth hormone was found to be a protein with a molecular weight of 4400, which is practically insoluble in water and can be destroyed by either pepsin or trypsin. It is heat coagulable at 70° C.

Its composition and structure were revealed by Hays and Steelman[51] in 1955, and by Li and Papkoff[82] in 1956. These authors availed themselves of microbiologic procedures, mainly by using strains of lactobacilli that are capable of fermenting the hormone. With this original technique and by means of colorimetric determination of the amino acid content, they were able to establish the proportions in which the different components of the hormone were represented. Furthermore, Lewis and co-workers[78] established the amino acid makeup of that basic polypeptide whose definite structure was eventually brought to light by Ellis[25] in 1961. It is made up of two biologically active proteins. One of them is composed of alanine, phenylalanine and free terminal NH_2 groups. The other contains alanine and methionine, and links up with the amino groups of the former. This results in formation of a large ellipsoidal molecule, whose dissymmetry constant is 1.31 and whose ratio of long axis to broad axis is 6 to 1.[97]

It should be mentioned, finally, that electrophoresis made possible the complete separation of prolactin and growth hormone, hitherto always mutually contaminated. Thus, we are only a step or two away from being able to obtain a pure preparation with known formula.

6.6.2. FOLLICLE-STIMULATING HORMONE (FSH)

It has been possible to obtain FSH in a state of purity. Isolation of the hormone in the pure state was achieved by Steelman and colleagues[122] in 1958. From the work of that author, it would appear to be a glycoprotein with a high sugar content, but without galactose. Its carbon content is reported to be 44.95 per cent, that of hydrogen 6.67 per cent and that of nitrogen 15.10 per cent. It is said to contain 4.3 per cent tyrosine, 0.6 per cent tryptophan, 13 per cent hexoses and 0.6 per cent hexosamine. At variance with other pituitary hormones, it is characterized by the absence of precipitation with ammonium sulfate. Electrophoretic analysis demonstrated a glycoprotein component that could be isolated, revealing the existence of mannose as one of its constituents. Its molecular weight, calculated by MacShan and Meyer,[87] is in the neighborhood of 200,000. However, the latest findings by Li[82, 83] would appear to contradict those figures.

6.6.3. LUTEINIZING HORMONE (LH)

The clinical properties of this hormone are very similar to those of FSH. It was isolated by Raben[106] in 1957. It also seems to be a glycoprotein with an elevated hexosamine and tyrosine content. Its molecular weight is estimated to be approximately 40,000. These data were confirmed by Wilhelmi[135] in 1961. By means of gel filtration using Sephadex 50 and g-100 (soluble filtration), Papkoff and co-workers[98, 99] have isolated ovine LH, which has a molecular weight of only 15,000. Currently, the various proteins making up the different specific gonadotropins are thought to differ greatly from each other chemically.

Earlier data concerning FSH and LH were nearly all obtained from the study of hormones of nonhuman origin, mainly those of sheep.[63] Isolation of human gonadotropins from pituitaries (HPG) of cadavers or from menopausal urine (HMG)[22] allowed the establishment of the fact that the molecular weights of both HPG and HMG amount to approximately 30,000.[96]

Human LH is present in variable amounts in pituitary extracts (see Chapter 7) and has been found to contain sialic acid, hexoses (galactose and mannose), glucosamine, galactosamine, proline, serine, threonine, glutamic acid, lysine, alanine, aspartic acid and valine.[63]

6.6.4. PROLACTIN

Li[83] and Wilhelmi[135] were able to obtain chemically pure prolactin and established its percentage composition as: carbon, 50.72 per cent; hydrogen, 6.66 per cent; nitrogen, 15.86 per cent; sulfur, 1.79 per cent. In the view of most workers, there is no phosphorus in the molecule. The sulfur contained in prolactin seems to pertain to the SH groups, mainly those of cysteine, that enter into the constitution of its molecule. The cysteine content amounts to 3 per cent of the total composition. According to Li, the methionine content is 4.31 per cent.

Moreover, the hormone would appear to contain 5 per cent tyrosine and 1.3 per cent tryptophan. There would also seem to be 12.3 per cent glutamic acid and 8.37 per cent arginine.

Recently, Ferguson[32] and Reisfeld[111] obtained highly purified extracts from gels of prolactin. The amino acid composition of these extracts could be determined and was found to contain a large amount of threonine and alanine.[15] The modern studies of Dixon[20] succeeded in establishing part of the structural formula of prolactin.

6.6.5. ACTH

Just as the other pituitary hormones, ACTH is a protein, which is made up of 46.3 per cent carbon, 5.89 per cent hydrogen, 16.65 per cent nitrogen and 2.3 per cent sulfur.

It contains neither phosphorus nor cysteine and, in contrast to the other hormones, contains no carbohydrates, and is not a glycoprotein. According to Li's work in 1959, the following amino acids would seem to be represented: tryptophan, 1 per cent; tyrosine, 4.5 per cent; methionine, 1.93 per cent; and cystine 7.19 per cent. According to more recent investigations, the NH content of purified hormone is 4.70 per cent, that is, frankly on the acid side. Its molecular weight was estimated by Sayers[115] to be approximately 20,000.

The addition of formaldehyde, which is known to block function of the primary amines, depresses ACTH's adrenocortical stimulatory activity, so that the amino acids that are found in ACTH are believed to be implicated directly in the mechanism of action of the hormone. Tyrosine is of fundamental importance for its activity, since the destruction of tyrosine radicals by iodine entails a considerable loss of ACTH activity. This led Li to the conclusion that the presence of both free amine and tyrosine groups is indispensable for the hormone to exert its activity.

A decisive advance in the understanding of the structure of ACTH was made by Lee and colleagues,[76] who isolated and crystallized the pure hormone and determined its amino acid composition.

In 1963, Currie and Davis[18] found that ACTH is a polypeptide composed of 39 amino acids and, the following year Hofmann established its constitutional formula, which is shown in Figure 6-6.

This, then, is the first adenohypophysial hormone whose structure has been fully characterized and which is already available commercially in synthetic form.

6.6.6. THYROTROPIC HORMONE

Thyrotropic hormone has been obtained in a highly purified form by Steelman and colleagues[122] and by Elrick and co-workers.[26] This preparation contains a high proportion of both acidic and basic amino acids, and these are linked to a smaller amount of carbohydrates yet to be identified. The compound contains no free amine groups and is readily dialyzable, which allows for calculation of its molecular weight, provided that it is less than 10,000. Thyrotropic hormone is therefore a compound of a smaller molecular size than the gonadotropins. In spite of this, it seems to lack the facility to penetrate the placental barrier.[14, 102]

The fact that several amino acids in TSH

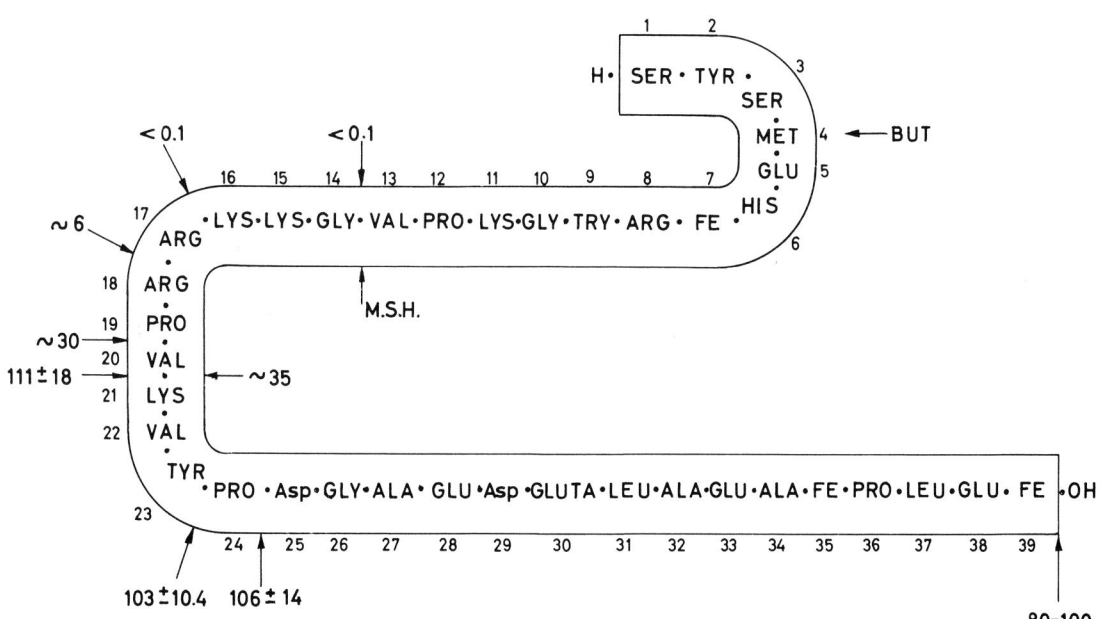

Figure 6-6. Expanded formula of sequences of ACTH. (From Currie and Davies: *Acta Endocr.*, 42:69, 1963.)

are coupled with a prosthetic carbohydrate group, along with the physical properties of this compound, made Steelman and colleagues[53, 122] assume that it is, like the other gonadotropins, a glycoprotein.

6.7. IMMUNOLOGIC PROPERTIES OF ANTERIOR LOBE HORMONES

As we have just seen, all anterior lobe hormones are proteins. It has been many years now since Zondek[140] demonstrated that gonadotropins provoked the formation of antibodies or *antigonadotropins*. These antibodies are not formed against gonadotropins of the same species, but against those of other species, a fact which allows an animal to be immunized with human gonadotropin and a woman to be immunized with gonadotropins of animal origin. These properties are shared by the other pituitary hormones and have been used as the basis for the development of *immunobiologic methods* for the determination of such compounds.

Two possibilities regarding the practical application of our new knowledge derived from these investigations are apparent: the first, the devising of methods of hormone assay that are more sensitive and more accurate than those currently in use, and, the second, the use of *immunochemical methods* that may contribute towards the elucidation of the chemical structures involved. The results of recent studies in this field concerning each of the pituitary hormones is briefly summarized here:

6.7.1. SOMATOTROPIN

Immunologic methods for the determination of somatotropin were proposed by Keele and Webster[66] in 1961, and by Read and colleagues,[109] Dominguez and Pearson[21] and Franchimont and Salon[33] in 1962. In 1963, Laron and Assa[74] employed this method to separate purified preparations of prolactin and somatotropin. Moudgal and Li[92, 93] had earlier (1961) used such methods to complete their extensive studies on the chemical composition of STH. In 1962, moreover, Hayashida[51] had reported that pure crystallized somatotropin is, immunologically speaking, composed of five different components, a fact which has complicated considerably the problem of the definite structure of this hormone, which earlier work had given every reason to believe had been definitely solved.

6.7.2. PROLACTIN

Levy and Sampliner[77] in 1961, and Hayashida[50] in 1962, were able to develop a procedure for the estimation of prolactin based on hemagglutination inhibition. These studies were further pursued by Irie and Barrett[59] in 1962.

6.7.3. THYROTROPIN AND ACTH

These hormones are among the least studied immunologically. MacGarray was able to isolate an antibody to human ACTH, whereas Werner,[130] in 1962, obtained another with analogous properties with regard to thyrotropin. Attempts have been made to evaluate both hormones by means of immunologic methods.

6.7.4. GONADOTROPINS

Chapter 24 shall treat in more detail the importance of immunologic reactions for the demonstration of chorionic gonadotropin, as well as for diagnostic pregnancy tests. Discussion is limited here to the technical aspects of pituitary gonadotropin determination. The problem concerning FSH was studied by Lunenfeld[85] in 1961, and by Wide and Gemzell[133] in 1962.

Luteinizing hormone has been studied more extensively, and exact methods for its determination were developed by Wide and Gemzell[133] in 1962, as well as by Goss and Taymor[40] in the same year. In 1964, Goss and Lewis[41] achieved the separation and immunologic characterization of luteinizing gonadotropin of both the pituitary and placenta.

Though hardly begun, this chapter in the search for greater knowledge holds high promise for the future. In the next few months or years, understanding of pituitary physiology is certain to receive far-reaching contributions from these studies, which, at the same time that they permit purification of the hormones involved, allow the characterization of their chemical structure and their determination in minimal concentrations in blood, body fluids and tissues.

REFERENCES

1. Achucarro, N.: *Trab. Lab. Invest. Biol.*, 11:187, 1911.
2. Adams, D. D.: *J. Clin. Endocr. Metab.*, 18:699, 1959.
3. Adams, C. W. H., and Swettenham, R. V.: *J. Path. Bact.*, 75:95, 1958.
4. Aron, M.: *Ann. d'Endocr.*, 12:994, 1951.
5. Assenmacher, I., Tixier-Vidal, A., and Astier, H.: *Ann. d'Endocr.*, 26:1, 1965.
6. Bargmann, W.: *Das Zwischenhirn-Hypophysensystem.* Berlin, Springer Verlag, 1954.
7. Barnes, B. G.: *Endocrinology*, 71:618, 1962.
8. Barnett, R. J., Roth, W. D., and Salzer, J.: *Endocrinology*, 69:1047, 1961.
9. Brown, J. H., Lavella, F. S., and Ulvedal, F.: *Endocrinology*, 66:1, 1960.
10. Brown, J. H., and Ulvedal, F. S.: *Endocrinology*, 66:175, 1960.
11. Campbell, J., et al.: *Endocrinology*, 46:273, 1950.
12. Carpent, G., and Desclin, L.: *Acta Endocr.*, 55:10, 1967.
13. Chauvet, J., and Acher, R.: *Ann. d'Endocr.*, 20:111, 1957.
14. Carsten, M. E., and Pierce, J. G.: *J. Biol. Chem.*, 238:1724, 1963.
15. Cole, R. D., Geschwind, I. I., and Li, C. H.: *J. Biol. Chem.*, 224:399, 1957.
16. Conklin, J. L.: *Anat. Rec.*, 160:59, 1968.
17. Cruickshank, B., and Currie, A. R.: *Immunology*, 1:13, 1958.
18. Currie, A. R., and Davies, B. M. A.: *Acta Endocr.*, 42:69, 1963.
19. David, M. A., Csernay, L., Laszlo, F. A., and Kovacs, K.: *Endocrinology*, 77:183, 1965.
20. Dixon, J. S., and Li, C. H.: *Metabolism*, 13:1093, 1964.
21. Dominguez, J. M., and Pearson, O. H.: *J. Clin. Endocr. Metab.*, 22:865, 1962.
22. Donini, P., Puzzuoli, D., D'Alessio, I., Lunenfeld, B., Eskohl, A., and Parlow, A. F.: *Acta Endocr.*, 52:169, 1966.
23. Dubois, P., and Giroud, C.: *Compt. Rend. Soc. Biol., Paris*, 158:21202, 1965.
24. Elert, R.: *Arch. Gynäk.*, 183:229, 1953.
25. Ellis, S.: *Endocrinology*, 69:554, 1961.
26. Elrick, H., et al.: *J. Clin. Endocr. Metab.*, 23:694, 1963.
27. Engel, F. L.: *Vitamins Hormones*, 19:189, 1961.
28. Emmart, E. W., Bates, R. W., and Turner, W. A.: *J. Histochem. Cytochem.*, 13:182, 1965.
29. Everett, N. B.: *Endocrinology*, 58:786, 1956.
30. Ezrin, C., et al.: *J. Clin. Endocr. Metab.*, 18:917, 1958.
31. Fawcett, C. P., Reed, M., Charlton, H. M., and Harris, G. W.: *Biochem. J.*, 106:229, 1968.
32. Ferguson, K. A., and Wallace, A. L. C.: *Rec. Progr. Horm. Res.*, 19:1, 1963.
33. Fonzo, D., Mims, R., and Nelson, D. H.: *Endocrinology*, 71:29, 1967.
34. Franchimont, P., and Salon, J.: *Ann. d'Endocr.*, 23:556, 1962.
35. Frantz, A. G., and Rabkin, M. T.: *J. Clin. Endocr. Metab.*, 25:1470, 1965.
36. Gershberg, H.: *Endocrinology*, 61:160, 1957.
37. Girod, C.: *Compt. Rend. Soc. Biol., Paris*, 156:845, 1963.
38. Glenner, G. C., and Lillie, R. D.: *J. Histochem. Cytochem.*, 7:416, 1959.
39. Gloor, P.: *Hypothalamic-Hypophysial Interrelationships*, ed. Fields, Guillemin and Corton, Springfield, Ill., Charles C Thomas, 1956.
40. Goss, D. A., and Taymor, M. L.: *Endocrinology*, 71:321, 1962.
41. Gross, D. A., and Lewis, J.: *Endocrinology*, 74:83, 1964.
42. Greenblatt, R. B., McDonough, P. G., and Mahesh, V. B.: *J. Clin. Endocr. Metab.*, 26:1185, 1966.
43. Greep, R. O.: "Physiology of Anterior Hypophysis," In Young, W. C.: *Sex and Internal Secretions*, 3rd ed., Baltimore, Williams & Wilkins, 1961.
44. Greer, M. H., and Erwin, M. L.: *Endocrinology*, 58:665, 1956.
45. Grumbach, M. M.: *Ciba Colloquia on Endocrinology*, 14:373, 1962.
46. Guillemin, R.: *Ann. Rev. Physiol.*, 29:313, 1967.
47. Harris, G. W., and Jacobson, D.: *Proc. Roy Soc., London (Ser. B.)*, 139:263, 1953.
48. Harris, G. W.: *Arch. Gynäk.*, 183:35, 1953.
49. Harris, J. I., et al.: *J. Biol. Chem.*, 209:133, 1959.
50. Hayashida, T.: *Ciba Colloquia on Endocrinology*, 14:338, 1962.
51. Hayashida, T., and Grunbaum, B. W.: *Endocrinology*, 71:734, 1962.
52. Haynes, R. C., Sutherland, E. W., and Rall, T. W.: *Rec. Progr. Horm. Res.*, 16:121, 1960.
53. Hays, E. E., and Steelman, S. L.: In *The Hormones*, ed. G. Pincus and K. V. Thimann, Vol. III. New York, Academic Press, 1955.
54. Herbert, D. C., and Hayashida, T.: *Science*, 169:378, 1970.
55. Herlant, M.: *Compt. Rend. Acad. Sci.*, 248:1033, 1959.
56. Herlant, M., and Pasteels, J. L.: *Compt. Rend. Acad. Sci.*, 249:2625, 1960.
57. Herlant, M., and Decourt, J.: *Ann. d'Endocr.*, 24:497, 1963.
58. Hymer, W. C., MacShan, W. H., and Christiansen, R. R. G.: *Endocrinology*, 69:81, 1961.
59. Irie, M., and Barrett, R. J.: *Endocrinology*, 71:277, 1962.
60. Jarrett, R. J.: *Endocrinology*, 76:434, 1965.
61. Jones, A. E., Fisher, J. N., Lewis, U. J., and Valderlaan, W. P.: *Endocrinology*, 76:578, 1965.
62. Kar, A. B., et al.: *Steroids*, 5:519, 1965.
63. Kathan, R. H., Reichert, L. E., and Ryan, R. J.: *Endocrinology*, 81:45, 1967.
64. Keating, F. R., et al.: *Endocrinology*, 36:137, 1945.
65. Kofler, D., and Fogel, M.: *Proc. Soc. Exper. Biol. Med.*, 115:1080, 1964.
66. Keele, D. K., and Webster, J.: *Proc. Soc. Exper. Biol. Med.*, 106:168, 1961.
67. Kitay, J. I., et al.: *Endocrinology*, 65:548, 1959.
68. Klastersky, J., and Herlant, M.: *Ann. d'Endocrinol.*, 28:127, 1967.
69. Kline, I. T.: *Endocrinology*, 63:335, 1958.
70. Korner, A.: *Biochem. J.*, 92:449, 1964.
71. Korspassy, B.: *Ann. d'Endocr.*, 22:417, 1961.
72. Kracht, J., Hachmeister, U., Breustedt, H. J., and Zimmermann, H. D.: *Excerpta Med. Sect. III*, 22:67, 1968.
73. Lajos, L., et al.: *Gynaecologia*, 156:234, 1964.

74. Laron, Z., and Åssa, S.: *Nature*, 197:299, 1963.
75. Laron, Z., Mannheimer, S., and Guttmann, S. S.: *Experientia*, 22:831, 1967.
76. Lee, T. H., Lerner, A. B., and Janusch, V. B.: *J. Biol. Chem.*, 236:2970, 1961.
77. Levy, R. P., and Sampliner, J.: *Proc. Soc. Exper. Biol. Med.*, 106:214, 1961.
78. Lewis, U. J., Cheever, E. V., and Van der Laan, W. P.: *Endocrinology*, 76:732, 1965.
79. Leznoff, A.: *Proc. Soc. Exper. Biol. Med.*, 104:232, 1960.
80. Leznoff, A., et al.: *J. Clin. Invest.*, 41:1720, 1962.
81. Li, L. H.: *Acta Endocr.*, 10:255, 1952.
82. Li, C. H., and Papkoff, H.: *Science*, 124:1293, 1956.
83. Li, C. H.: *Ciba Colloquia on Endocrinology*, 14:20, 1962.
84. Lisk, R. D.: *Neuroendocrinology*, 3:18, 1968.
85. Lunenfeld, B.: *Acta Gynecologica*, 18:629, 1967.
86. MacCann, S. M.: *Endocrinology*, 60:644, 1957.
87. MacShan, W. H., and Meyer, R. K.: *Endocrinology*, 50:294, 1952.
88. Maracek, I., and Arendarcik, J.: *Endocr. Exper. (Bratislava)*, 2:225, 1968.
89. Meneghelli, V., and Scapinelli, R.: *Acta Anatomica*, 51:198, 1962.
90. Morehead, J. R., and Morgan, C. F.: *Fertil. Steril.*, 18:530, 1967.
91. Morris, C. J.: *Proc. Roy. Soc. Med.*, 55:540, 1962.
92. Moudgal, N. R., and Li, C. H.: *Endocrinology*, 68:704, 1961.
93. Moudgal, N. R., and Li, C. H.: *Nature*, 191:192, 1961.
94. Nayak, R., MacGarry, E. E., and Beck, J. C.: *Endocrinology*, 83:731, 1968.
95. Nichols, B., and Guillemin, R.: *Endocrinology*, 64:914, 1959.
96. Odell, W. D., Swann, R. W., and Nydlick, M.: *J. Clin. Endocr. Metab.*, 24:1266, 1964.
97. Papkoff, H., and Li, C. H.: *Metabolism*, 13:1082, 1964.
98. Papkoff, H., and Anantha-Samy, T. S.: *Biochem. Biophys. Acta*, 147:175, 1967.
99. Papkoff, H., Mahlaman, L. J., and Li, C. H.: *Biochemistry*, 6:3797, 1967.
100. Pearse, A. G. E.: *Histochemistry*, 2nd ed., London, Churchill Ltd., 1960.
101. Pearse, A. G. E., and Van Noorden, S.: *Canad. Med. Ass. J.*, 88:462, 1963.
102. Pierce, J. G., et al.: *Ann. N.Y. Acad. Sci.*, 86:613, 1960.
103. Porter, J. C., Hynes, M. F. M., Smith, K. R., Repass, R. L., and Smith, A. J. K.: *Endocrinology*, 80:503, 1967.
104. Purves, H. D., and Griesbach, W. E.: *Endocrinology*, 56:374, 1955.
105. Purves, H. D., and Griesbach, W. E.: *Ciba Colloquia on Endocrinology*, 10:51, 1957.
106. Raben, M. S.: *Science*, 125:883, 1957.
107. Racadot, J., and Herlant, M.: *Ann. d'Endocr.*, 21:828, 1960.
108. Rambourg, A., and Racadot, J.: *Compt. Rend. Acad. Sci., Paris*, 266:153, 1968.
109. Read, C. H., et al.: *Ciba Colloquia on Endocrinology*, 14:45, 1962.
110. Reisfeld, R. A., et al.: *Endocrinology*, 71:559, 1962.
111. Reisfeld, R. A., et al.: *J. Biol. Chem.*, 239:1777, 1964.
112. Rao, P. M., Robertson, M. C., and Winnick, M.: *Endocrinology*, 80:1111, 1967.
113. Saffran, M., and Schally, A. V.: *Endocrinology*, 56:523, 1955.
114. Sandberg, H., et al.: *J. Clin. Endocr. Metab.*, 18:1268, 1958.
115. Sayers, M. A., Sayers, G., and Woodbury, L. A.: *Endocrinology*, 42:379, 1948.
116. Sewy, R. W., et al.: *Endocrinology*, 61:45, 1957.
117. Shimizu, N., et al.: *J. Clin. Endocr. Metab.*, 25:984, 1964.
118. Siperstein, E. R., and Miller, K. J.: *Endocrinology*, 86:45, 1970.
119. Siperstein, E. R., and Allison, V. F.: *Endocrinology*, 76:70, 1965.
120. Smith, P. E.: *Endocrinology*, 68:131, 1961.
121. Spanner, R.: *Klin. Wschr.*, 721:1, 1952.
122. Steelman, S. L., Segaloff, M. G., and Mays, G. M.: *Arch. Biochem.*, 78:262, 1953.
123. Stokes, H., and Boda, J. M.: *Endocrinology*, 83:1362, 1968.
124. Theret, C., and Tamboise, E.: *Ann. d'Endocr.*, 24:241, 1963.
125. Thompson, K. W., et al.: *Proc. Soc. Exper. Biol. Med.*, 102:403, 1959.
126. Van Rees, G. P., and Rott, C. A. de: *Acta Endocr.*, 49:370, 1965.
127. Van Wyck, J. J., et al.: *J. Clin. Endocr. Metab.*, 20:157, 1960.
128. Vogt, A., and Kopp, R.: *Nature*, 202:1350, 1964.
129. Waelbroeck, E.: *Ann. d'Endocr.*, 28:236, 1967.
130. Werner, S. C.: *Ciba Colloquia on Endocrinology*, 14:225, 1962.
131. Westman, A. L.: *Arch. Gynäk.*, 183:131, 1953.
132. Wied, D., Buman, P. R., and Smelik, P. G.: *Endocrinology*, 62:605, 1958.
133. Wide, I., and Gemzell, C. A.: *Ciba Colloquia on Endocrinology*, 14:296, 1962.
134. Wilde, C. E., Orr, H. A., and Bagshave, K. D.: *Nature*, 205:191, 1965.
135. Wilhelmi, A. E.: *Canad. J. Biochem.*, 39:659, 1961.
136. Wright, J. E., et al.: *Amer. J. Med. Sci.*, 38:449, 1965.
137. Yamada, T.: *Endocrinology*, 65:216, 1959.
138. Yen, S. C., Pearson, O. H., and Stratman, S.: *J. Clin. Endocr. Metab.*, 25:655, 1965.
139. Young, D. G., Bahn, R. C., and Randall, R. V.: *J. Clin. Endocr. Metab.*, 25:249, 1965.
140. Zondek, B.: *Ann. Ost. Gin.*, 81:29, 1959.

Chapter 7
GONADOTROPIC HORMONES

Chapter 6 dealt with the pituitary in general terms. *The study of the actions exerted by the pituitary on sex has been deliberately omitted.* Pituitary influence on the sexual sphere is mediated by three hormones: (1) *follicle-stimulating hormone* (FSH), which stimulates gametogenesis in both the male and the female; (2) *luteinizing hormone* (LH, ICSH), which promotes formation of the corpus luteum and stimulates the testicular interstitium, and (3) *luteotropin* (LTH), which maintains corpus luteum activity and is identical to *prolactin*, known to stimulate mammary secretion.

7.1. PHYSIOLOGIC ACTION

Gonadotropins are hormones that act by stimulating the gonads, both the ovaries and the testes. We have been able to demonstrate that gonadotropins also stimulate that portion of the adrenal cortex which is concerned with sexual processes (see Chapter 9). But for this sole instance of extragonadal activity, however, all other gonadotropin actions are exerted *upon the gonads.*

7.1.1. EFFECT OF PITUITARY EXTRACTS UPON THE OVARY

The first discoveries to be made in this field, by Zondek and Aschheim and by Smith and Engle, demonstrated that when pituitary extract was injected into a female rat or young mouse, the following modifications took place: (1) follicular maturation; (2) ovulation, followed by formation of a corpus luteum, and (3) proliferation of the theca and of the interstitial tissue (Fig. 7–1).

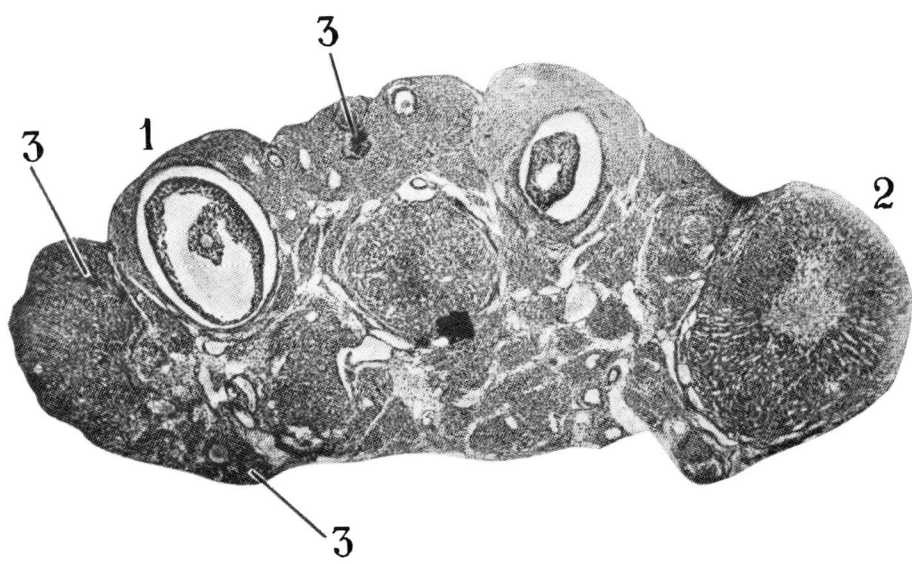

Figure 7–1. Ovary of immature young rat weighing 20 gm, which was injected with a mixture of gonadotropins, showing three characteristic reactions described by Zondek: (1) follicular maturation; (2) corpora hemorrhagica, and (3) corpora lutea.

Of these, in fact, only the first and third are specific reactions, since the second results from the combined effects of the other two.

From the work of Zondek and Smith, the first effect (follicular maturation) has been attributed to a specific follicle-stimulating hormone (FSH), also called gonadotropin A, or, since it stimulates development of gametes in both ovary and testis, gametokinetic gonadotropin.

The second hormone stimulates the formation of the corpus luteum, hence the term luteinizing hormone (LH), or gonadotropin B. Corpus luteum formation is the result of joint FSH and LH activity. When acting alone LH produces a stimulatory effect on both the ovarian and testicular interstitium, hence it is also termed ICSH (*interstitial cell stimulating hormone*).

This duality of gonadotropic principles has not been accepted without reservation. As pointed out in the preceding chapter, the chemical structure of neither hormone has been perfectly defined, which so far has constituted the main obstacle to their characterization as two compounds of distinct composition existing independently of each other. For the same reason, Albert and his colleagues[3,4] postulated the existence of just one hormone, admitting the possibility that the two distinct effects might be the result of action of different side chains on the same molecule.[4] Nevertheless, chemically as well as electrophoretically and above all immunologically, it seems clear that we are dealing with *two different hormones*. Since 1963, highly purified extracts of LH have been obtained.[135, 136] The effects of the two hormones on the ovary are to be studied as they occur, first in animals, then in woman.

ACTION OF FSH AND LH ON THE ANIMAL OVARY. The effects of the two gonadotropins on the animal ovary were already studied by Zondek and Aschheim and by Smith and Engle 40 years ago. While recent work with mice,[138, 161] rats,[1, 36, 81] rabbits,[146] sows[43, 71] and cows[8] supports these classical descriptions, it has moreover brought to light the biochemical mechanism of action. FSH produces increased glycogen[73] and nucleic acid[36] content in rat ovaries as well as enhanced enzyme activity by 3β-ol-dehydrogenase.[146] FSH also increases oxygen consumption of the isolated rat ovary.[72] LH, on the other hand, seems to be a decisive factor in the process of cholesterol-pregnenolone conversion and in addition activates the same enzyme system (3β-ol-dehydrogenase).[40, 107, 146] The present tendency, however, is to attribute the acetate-squalene-pregnenolone-progesterone conversion process to LH[7, 43, 79, 80, 94] and to exclude any mechanism of biosynthesis involving utilization of cholesterol as the starting point. Nevertheless, Herbst[78] observed that LH raised cholesterol concentrations in rat ovaries, which would appear to contradict the foregoing conclusions. The study of LH-induced corpora lutea in rat ovaries has shown that there is increased oxygen consumption,[1] characteristic ascorbic acid depletion,[127] greater glycogen deposition and enhanced phosphorylase activity,[161] as well as accumulation of adenosine triphosphate (ATP).[112] Hypophysectomy abolishes all of these biochemical modifications.[87, 88, 92] Under the influence of LH, the corpus luteum produces not only progesterone but also estrogens,[103] yet if such an ovary is transplanted to the spleen,[137, 138] progesterone alone, without estrogen, is produced.

These changes can be well followed in ovarian transplants to the anterior chamber of the eye.[10, 30, 113] Moreover, Pavic[128] and Blandau[21] have noted in vitro stimulation of granulosa cells by FSH.

Finally, it must be mentioned that as a result of LH activity the ovarian interstitial tissue also elaborates both estrogens and progesterone, as shown by Hilliard and co-workers[81] in in vitro experiments. While the preceding data have so far been confined predominantly to ovarian effects in rodents, Bennett[15] has also studied extensively the effects of FSH and LH on monkey ovaries. Channing[39] has cultured monkey granulosa cells in vitro, noting that they likewise underwent luteinization under the influence of LH activity.

FSH AND LH EFFECTS ON THE HUMAN OVARY. Until recently, gonadotropins in use were of animal origin (equine gonadotropins). In man, they were associated with the production of antigonadotropins, and their action on the human ovary was therefore uncertain. Gemzell and colleagues[65-67] initiated the extraction of gonadotropins from pituitaries of cadavers and subsequently, Donini and his co-workers[52] likewise obtained gonadotropins of human pituitary origin from postmenopausal urine. The effects produced by these extracts correspond to those of a mixture of FSH and LH in which the former predominates.

Gonadotropic Hormones

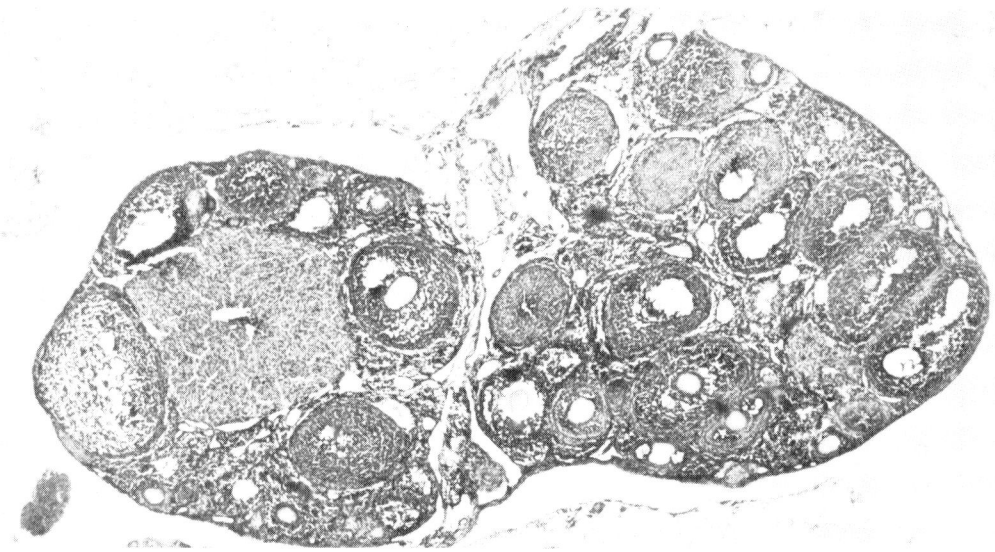

Figure 7–2. Ovary of immature mouse injected with LH, revealing numerous atretic follicles and a corpus luteum.

Their in vitro action upon the ovary is roughly comparable to effects described previously.[86] The importance of these preparations in clinical therapy shall be apparent later (see also Chapter 6, Section 6.5 and Chapter 41, Section 41.1.1). Gonadotropin activity, particularly that of FSH, is not concerned only with follicular maturation and corpus luteum formation; Moricard[120] has in addition demonstrated an effect on the maturation of the oocyte.

OVULATION INDUCING EFFECT OF GONADOTROPINS. The mechanism of ovulation will be studied in Chapter 12. It is mediated by combined FSH and LH activity. Without the associated (i.e., follicle-stimulating) effect of the first, LH stimulates only the interstitial tissue[114] (Fig. 7–2), whereas FSH by itself is incapable of provoking follicular rupture in either animals[11, 12, 15] or woman.[67] The question of in what proportions the two hormones must act in order to trigger ovulation has in recent years been a matter of extensive debate.[17, 19, 52, 104] It will be the subject of a more detailed study in Chapter 12 (see also Fig. 7–3).

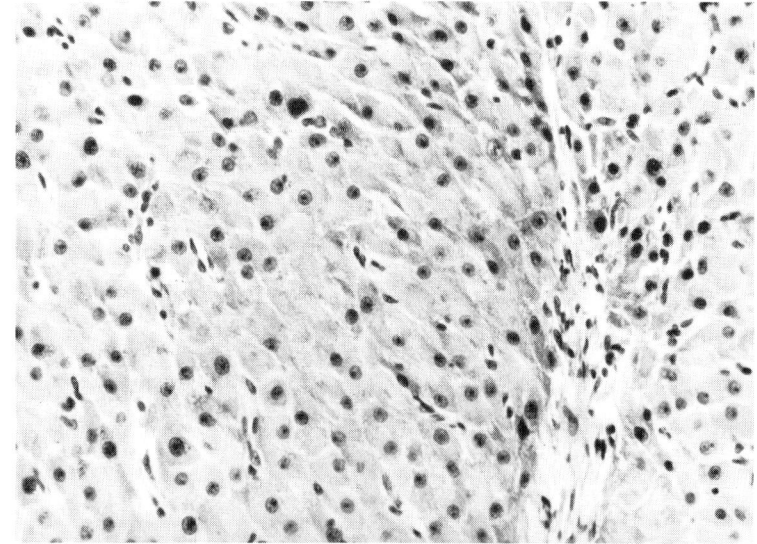

Figure 7–3. Ovary of woman suffering from anovulatory cycle, infertility and amenorrhea, treated during one cycle with 10,000 IU of Pergonal (gonadotropin extracted from menopausal urine), plus 15,000 IU of Primogonyl (gonadotropin extracted from pregnancy urine). Treatment resulted in ovulation, followed by formation of corpus luteum. Biopsy was performed on the twenty-sixth day of the cycle.

7.1.2. ACTION OF PITUITARY EXTRACTS UPON THE TESTIS

The two active principles involved also exert different effects upon the testis. The response evoked by follicle-stimulating hormone is one of spermatogenesis,[23, 109] (Fig. 7-4), whereas luteinizing hormone produces growth of the Leydig cells in testicular interstitial tissue. Using FSH and LH tagged with fluorescent isothiocyanate, Mancini and co-workers[110] observed that FSH did appear preferentially in the seminiferous tubules, while LH would localize in the interstitial Leydig cells. It follows that follicle-stimulating hormone undoubtedly promotes growth of the gamete-producing apparatus, which prompted some authors to designate it as *gametokinetic gonadotropin*. Similarly, luteinizing hormone stimulates the interstitial tissue of the testis and has therefore also been designated as *interstitial cell stimulation hormone* (ICSH).

ACTION IN MALE ANIMALS. Recent work on dogs[83] and rats[171] has clarified the effects of testicular perfusion with C-14 labeled cholesterol and with gonadotropins. In addition to testosterone, the presence of progesterone and estrogens in the testicular vein could also be determined. The maximal output of the male hormone has been obtained with LH, a finding lending support to the assertion that the main source of testosterone production is the interstitial tissue, which is specifically stimulated by LH (in this case, referred to as ICSH).

EFFECTS OF GONADOTROPINS ON THE HUMAN TESTIS. In males suffering from various forms of oligospermia and oligoasthenospermia,[24, 104] spermatogenesis has been successfully restored by injections of gonadotropins of human origin (Fig. 7-5). MacLeod and his co-workers,[105] as well as Gemzell,[67] reported successful restitution of spermatogenesis in two males, both of whom had become azoospermic following hypophysectomy for an intracranial neoplasm. Mancini[108] examined 44 male patients by means of testicular biopsy. Half of these had been hypophysectomized. The atrophic seminiferous tubules of the testis were observed to regenerate after injection of human gonadotropin from menopausal urine (HMG). The remaining 22 cases were children with primitive hypogonadism, but similar results were obtained. Although there is still considerable debate going on with regard to this issue, Steinberger and Duckett[163] have shown that FSH produced an increase in the number of motile spermatozoa in the human ejaculate.

This author[25] has besides been able to demonstrate that the rate of spermatozoal progression was heightened as a result of combined HMG and HCG treatment. As a matter of fact, it was not apparent whether this was due to a direct effect on sperma-

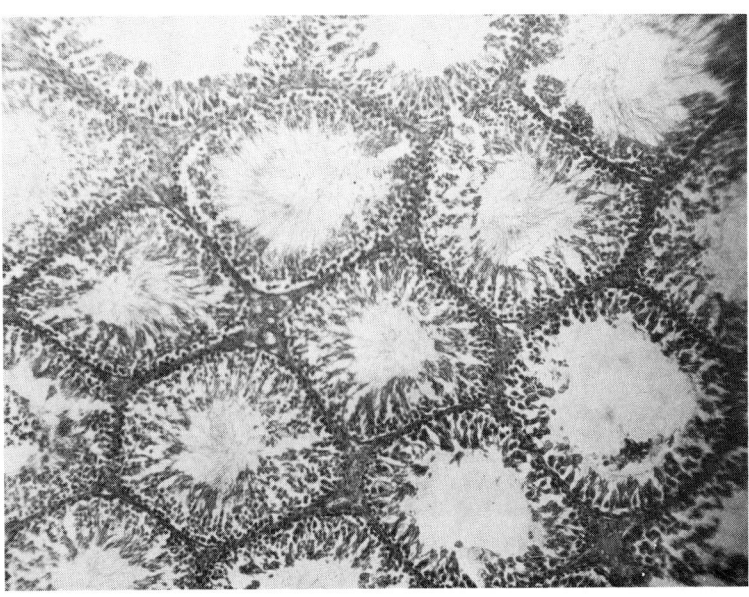

Figure 7-4. Testis of immature mouse treated with 20 IU pregnant mare serum (Anteron). Note extensive spermatogenesis.

Gonadotropic Hormones

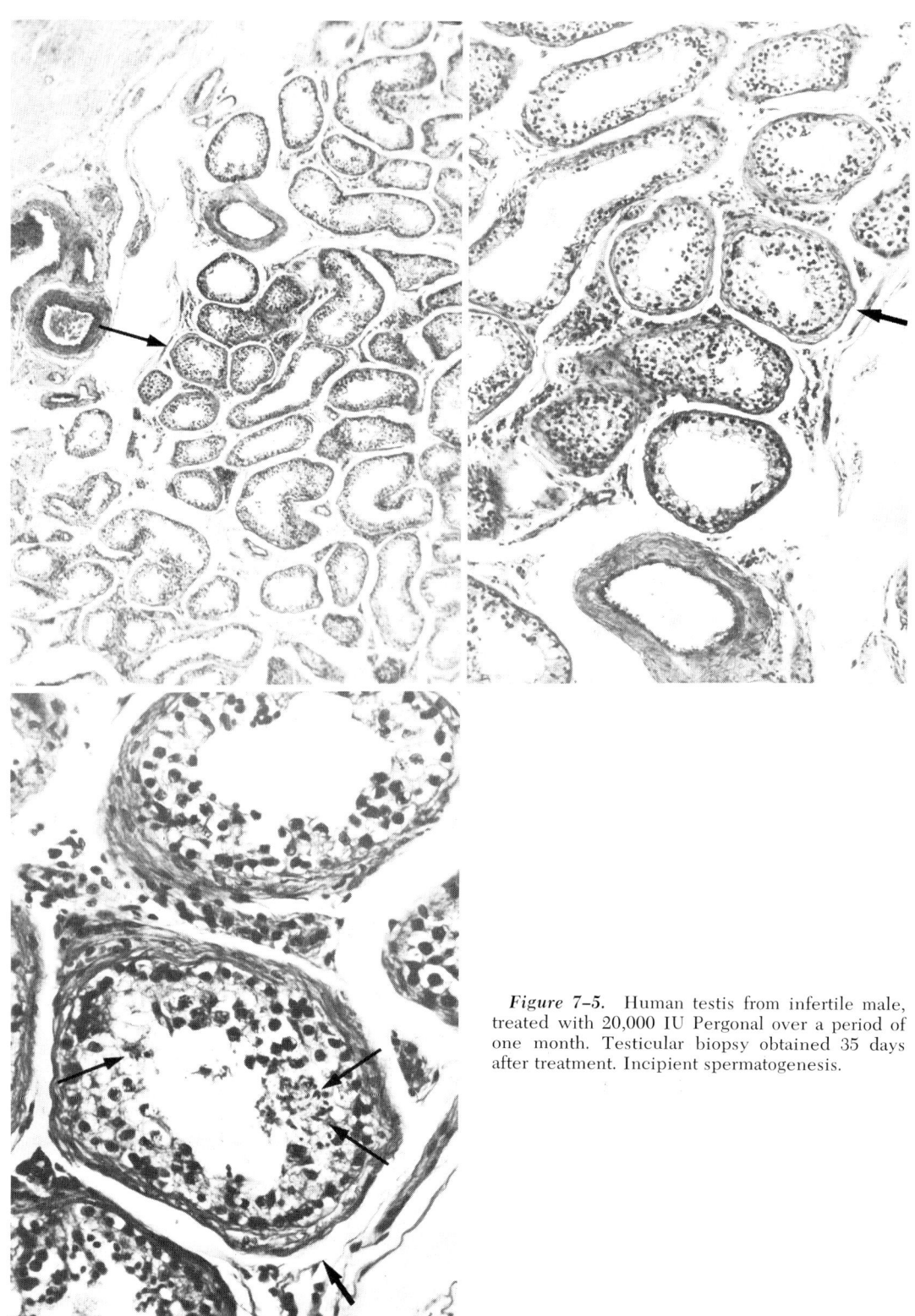

Figure 7-5. Human testis from infertile male, treated with 20,000 IU Pergonal over a period of one month. Testicular biopsy obtained 35 days after treatment. Incipient spermatogenesis.

togenesis or whether, as a result of increased testosterone secretion by the testicular interstitium, this was brought about by biochemically more favorable conditions in the seminal plasma.

7.1.3. EFFECT OF GONADOTROPINS ON HYPOPHYSECTOMIZED ANIMALS

Meyer and MacShan[114] have shown that regression of oocytes occurred after hypophysectomy and that their demise could be averted with injections of FSH.

If used in the pure state, *luteinizing hormone* (LH) has no effect on the ovaries of hypophysectomized animals.[122, 177] This has been reported to hold true not only in rats but also in ewes,[87, 88] monkeys[92] and women. Hence, strictly speaking, LH is the luteinizing hormone only if its action is primed by FSH. Whenever LH is injected into an animal or woman with an intact hypophysis the small amount of endogenous FSH present is sufficient to produce the required preparatory effect. In the absence of the pituitary gland, and without adding the necessary amount of exogenous FSH, LH only stimulates the interstitial tissue and does not induce the formation of corpora lutea. This is the reason why some authors, as mentioned previously, prefer the term ICSH (interstitial cell stimulating hormone).

7.1.4. EFFECTS OF GONADOTROPINS OF PREGNANCY

It should be mentioned in the first place that Bedford and Shalkowsky[14] have shown that gonadotropins impair spermatic capacitation in the uterus and have an adverse effect on implantation, which would seem to denote a direct antiuterine effect.

In the placentas of both woman and the mare, gonadotropic hormones are elaborated that have properties similar, although not quite identical, to those of gonadotropins elaborated by the pituitary.[177] In the urine of pregnancy, as well as in placental extracts, the occurrence of gonadotropins with properties similar to those of LH has long been known. Luteinizing hormone produces ovarian luteinization when acting upon mature follicles (Fig. 7–1) but has no effect on the ovaries of hypophysectomized animals.

The gonadotropin of pregnant mare's serum[3, 21] possesses properties that are different from those of human chorionic gonadotropin (Fig. 7–4). Its action is similar to that of FSH; that is to say, it produces follicular maturation but has little or no luteinizing activity.[4, 33, 78]

7.1.5. NOMENCLATURE OF GONADOTROPINS

Follicle stimulating hormone, or FSH, has a maturing effect on ovarian follicles and on testicular spermatogenesis. The chemical composition of this gonadotropin is different in each species. Recent immunologic studies have shown FSH to be distinctive of each animal species, for which reason FSH should be qualified by origin (human, porcine, bovine, etc.).

Luteinizing hormone or LH, has a luteinizing effect on mature ovarian follicles, no effect on ovaries in resting stage and an interstitium-exciting effect in testis. In the same manner as referred to in the preceding paragraph, LH, too, is endowed with animal specificity and should be identified by the animal from which it is derived.

Human chorionic gonadotropin (HCG) is identical with pituitary gonadotropin B or LH, but in addition it exerts a hyperemia-inducing effect on ovaries, which LH lacks. HCG produces luteinization of ovaries with mature follicles (Fig. 7–6), has no effect on ovaries in resting stage and stimulates the Leydig cells of the testis.

Equine chorionic gonadotropin (PMS or pregnant mare serum) is produced by the mare's placenta, but it is not eliminated in the urine. This hormone is identical to pituitary gonadotropin A (FSH) and has a follicle-stimulating effect on the ovary and a gametokinetic effect on the testis.

Human pituitary gonadotropin (HPG), obtained by Gemzell and colleagues[65] from pituitaries of human cadavers, contains FSH and LH, with the former predominating.

Human menopausal gonadotropin (HMG), isolated by Donini and colleagues[52] has a composition similar to HPG.

Gonadotropic Hormones

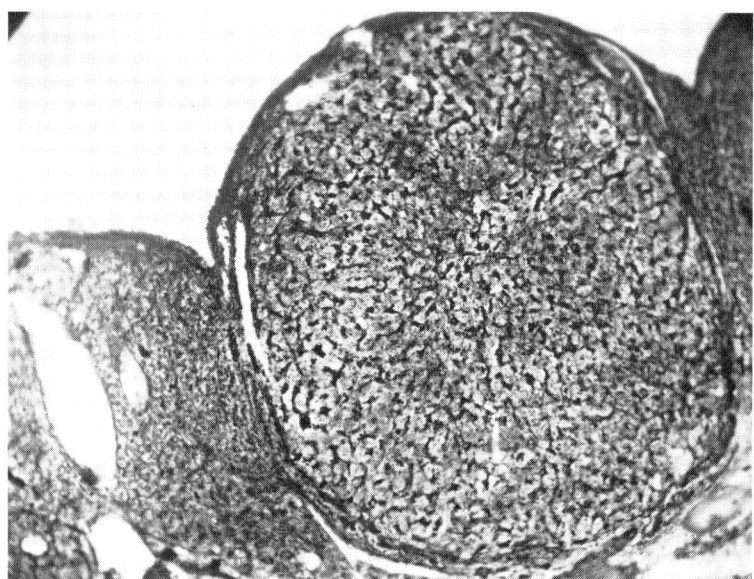

Figure 7-6. Effect of chorionic gonadotropin on ovary pretreated with FSH. Formation of perfect corpus luteum.

7.1.6. EFFECT OF GONADOTROPINS ON OVULATION

For a number of years now, ovulation has been known to be induced by the combined actions of FSH and LH. It is generally admitted that, for ovulation to be triggered, different species of animals require different proportions of the hormones, usually with predominance of FSH.

Studies conducted on laboratory rodents by Sawyer and his colleagues[11, 12, 58, 59, 122] have considerably clarified the mechanism involved. The present consensus is that ovulation can be induced only in mature

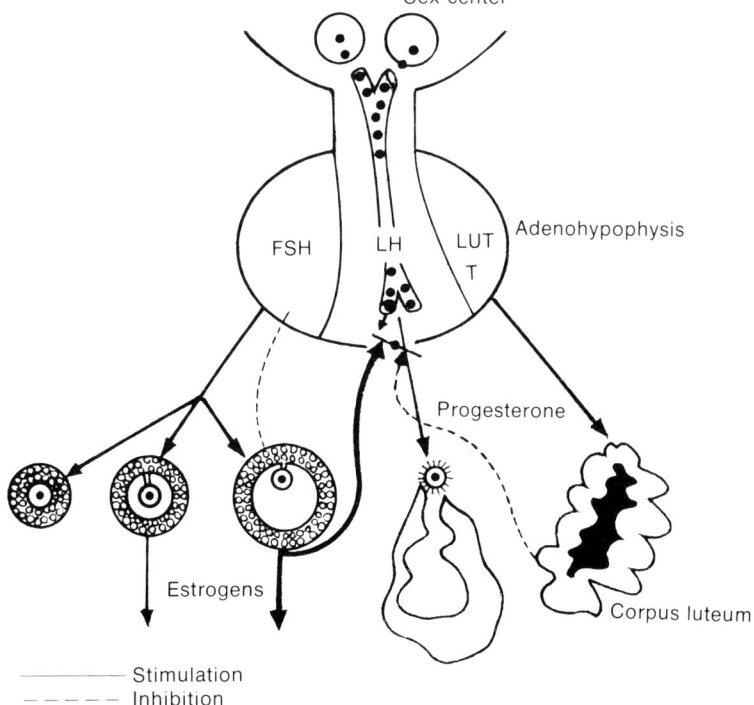

Figure 7-7. Diagram of LH release mechanism and ovulation. FSH stimulates follicular maturation and estrogen production; estrogens increase LH secretion and decrease FSH secretion by the pituitary. Estrogens contribute to LH release (diagrammed as valve that opens in response to estrogenic hormonal stimuli). Chemical mediators, conveyed by the pituitary portal strengthening the hormonal mechanism of LH release. By acting on a mature follicle, LH elicits ovulation. The ruptured follicle becomes luteinized by ulterior LH activity. Progesterone tends to close that valve. Prolactin or luteotrophic factor (LUT T) maintains corpus luteum.

follicles. Follicular maturation requires FSH activity. After the FSH has brought the follicle to a point near rupture, a discharge of LH precipitates ovulation. According to Lamond and Emmens,[97] the ovulation-inducing effect can be produced only by *pituitary* luteinizing hormone (LH) and not by other gonadotropins, such as are obtained from pregnant women or pregnant mares. Similarly, Ladman and Runner[96] found that ovarian susceptibility to this action by LH varied a great deal according to the age of the animal or person.

Pituitary LH secretion, intended to trigger ovulation, is not an instantaneous process. LH is secreted gradually and progressively over the entire first half of the cycle as a result of estrogen activity.[59, 60] At the moment immediately preceding ovulation, high estrogen levels force the opening of the hormonal "gateway," resulting in the sudden liberation or release of LH and the precipitation of ovulation (Fig. 7-7).

As shall be shown later (Chapter 8), the phenomenon of release is governed by an important central nervous system control mechanism. For this reason, ovulation is only partially a hormonal phenomenon. The realization of this fact constitutes a considerable advance in the field of endocrinology of the past few years in that it delineates more exactly the role played by the hypothalamus and by the neurohormones in the production of LH release and ovulation.

7.1.7. LUTEOTROPIC EFFECT

In 1941, Evans and co-workers demonstrated that conjoint injection of FSH and LH into hypophysectomized animals produced only transient ovarian luteinization. In addition, the corpora lutea thus formed would fail to persist for several days unless a separate principle, extracted from the anterior lobe of the pituitary, was injected. By inference, the existence of two luteinizing hormones had to be entertained: *one, which is necessary for the formation of the corpus luteum (that is, a luteinizing hormone in the proper sense of the word), and the other, which is indispensable for the formed corpus luteum to remain viable (that is, a luteotropic hormone)*. Subsequent investigations proved that the corpus luteum of pregnancy could not come to fruition without the associated activity of this second hormone. Experimental induction of deciduomas in rats and rabbits can only be achieved by means of the associated activity of luteotropic hormone.[106, 114, 177]

Administration of LH alone is incapable of maintaining the corpus luteum in the rat[144, 159] and in the rabbit.[164] Greenwald and colleagues[70] found that for that to be achieved, the action by another factor, which they called the "luteotropic factor," was necessary. This factor was later to be identified as prolactin.

The mission to be accomplished by the gonadotropins can be summed up as follows:

(1) FSH: Stimulation of follicular development.

(2) LH: When acting upon follicles previously subjected to FSH activity, induction of ovulation and initiation of corpus luteum formation.

(3) Prolactin or luteotropic factor (LTH): Maintenance of formed corpora lutea.

7.1.8. FEEDBACK EFFECT

What is understood by the term *feedback effect* or *rebound phenomenon* (see Chapter 8, Section 8.4), is the regulating effect exerted by the sex hormones on the hypothalamic median eminence. The same effect, though to a lesser extent, is also exerted by the gonadotropins.[44, 45, 150] Excessive activity by either gonadotropin seems to act on the hypothalamus by inhibiting the production of the corresponding releasing factor (see Chapter 8).

7.2. SECRETION, METABOLISM AND EXCRETION OF GONADOTROPINS

Gonadotropins are secreted by the pituitary and by the chorion. Little is known about their endogenous metabolism in spite of the fact that their excretion in the urine and the conditions influencing their secretion and elimination are perfectly well known.

7.2.1. SECRETION

PITUITARY CYCLE. Both FSH and LH are secreted by the pituitaries of both sexes *without quantitative differences.* However, unlike in the male, *secretion by the female pituitary is cyclic.* The occurrence of cyclic changes in pituitary cytology has been described by Hellbaum and co-workers.[76] The acid phosphatase reaction, thought to represent an index of secretory pituitary cell activity, has been found by Sobel[156] to follow an up-and-down pattern. Similarly, the gonadotropin content of pituitary tissue, studied by Schwartz and Bartosik[154] in the rat and by Santolucito and colleagues[151] in the ewe, has been found to fluctuate. Electron microscopic studies[169] agree with the assessment of periodic variations paralleling estrus in female animals and the menstrual cycle in women.

Finally, the pituitary gonadotropin content[48, 93] undergoes cyclic oscillations in the female but not in the male. The latter phenomenon, however, may be more apparent than real. As a matter of fact, even secretion in the female may be less of a cyclic phenomenon than previously was assumed. Nikitovitch and Everett[122] recently demonstrated that LH secretion by pituitaries of female animals takes place continuously but what imparts the appearance of cyclicity to blood levels is the manner in which LH is released. In other words, periodicity in the female pituitary lies not in *secretion* but in *discharge* of its hormones into the blood. The pituitary cycle, then, is not determined by the manner of secretion but by the manner of release. That this phenomenon is in large part of neural origin has been shown by means of pituitary transplants, in which both FSH and LH secretion have been found to be acyclic and constant (Everett[58] and Smith[155]).

Consequently, the hormonal difference between man and woman does not lie in the pituitary gland; secretion by that gland is equal in both sexes. *The difference lies in the mechanism of hypothalamic control, which is cyclic in the female and constant in the male.*

Thus, *it is the hypothalamus which imposes a cyclic rhythm on female life. The ovary merely responds to the pituitary and the latter, in turn, responds to the gray nuclei at the base of the brain, which is where such cyclicity originates.*

SECRETORY CELLS. Until recently, there was considerable controversy regarding the type of pituitary cells that give rise to the different hormones. At least in part, this problem has now been solved. The discovery of the structure of LH, revealing the presence of sialic acid,[69, 132] as well as the exact characterization of FSH, showing its content of amino acids and of glucosamine,[162] have greatly facilitated the histochemical or immunofluorescent localization[48, 93] of the site or origin of the two gonadotropins (see Chapter 6, page 110).

7.2.2. FACTORS INFLUENCING GONADOTROPIN SECRETION

Pituitary gonadotropin secretion is influenced by the following factors: (1) the hypothalamus and, by way of it, the central nervous system; (2) the ovarian hormones; (3) other hormones; (4) substances acting as antigonadotropins.

HYPOTHALAMUS AND GONADOTROPINS. The influence of the hypothalamus and of its nuclei upon gonadotropin secretion is considerable.[50, 58] Its main function, as stated earlier, is to control the release of gonadotropins by means of *chemical mediators* or *neurohormones.*

The hypothalamic control of the pituitary (see Chapter 8) preferably is defined as of humoral rather than neural variety, since there are only very few nerve endings among the cells of the anterior lobe and no systematized hypothalamo-adenohypophysial bundles have been found. Instead, a "porta-diencephalic" system (see page 103) conveys all products of these nuclei to the pituitary.

Chapter 8 enlarges in greater detail on the mechanism through which the hypothalamus controls pituitary gonadotropin release. Anesthesia with Nembutal or with other gangioplegic agents provokes paralysis of gonadotropic function.[11, 12, 58, 59] Reserpine is specially effective in this respect.[12, 59, 122] There are two hypothalamic substances that regulate the liberation of gonadotropins: one, acting on FSH (FSH releasing factor or FSHRF), and the other, acting to release LH (LH releasing factor or LHRF). Both of these shall be studied in greater detail in Chapter 8.

ESTROGENS AND PITUITARY. Estrogen action on the process of gonadotropin production is twofold: (a) direct action on the pituitary and (b) indirect action, via the sexual nucleus of the hypothalamus.

(a) *Direct action on the pituitary.* This has already been discussed in Chapter 2.

There is evidence that gonadotropin synthesis is enhanced under the influence of estrogens[144]; as a result of estrogenic activity, there is an increase in the secretory granules of gonadotropin producing cells.[169]

(b) *Action on the hypothalamus.* This second action is even more important.[51, 134] At dosages of less than 10 mcg estrogens concentrate in the medial hypothalamus (see Chapter 2) and induce formation of LHRF. At higher dosages—as a rule above 100 mcg—they block LHRF and are anovulatory. The latter fact serves as the basis for the so-called "sequential" contraceptive therapy, which will be considered in Chapter 47.

ACTION OF OTHER HORMONES ON PITUITARY GONADOTROPIN SECRETION. Thyroid hormone produces increased FSH secretion whereas, in contrast, thyroidectomy entails lack of gonadotropin secretion, causing arrest of follicular maturation (Janes[85]). Soffer and Fogel[158] have shown that *cortisone* enhances the rate of pituitary FSH production while slowing down the formation of gonadotropin B. Under stress conditions, increased production of LH can be observed in conjunction with increased ACTH output. The latter fact has been invoked as proof that stress-producing substances, regardless of whether they may be specific agents or hormonal compounds of the epinephrine type, are involved in exciting not only the hypophysio-adrenal but also the hypophysio-ovarian axis.[157]

EFFECT OF LIGHT ON GONADOTROPIN SECRETION. The classic observations by Bisonette and by Benoit (see Chapter 12) had already demonstrated the effects of *illumination* on animal estrus. The influence of environmental illumination is a determining factor in gonadotropin secretion in the rat[99] and also in woman.[98] The pituitary gonadotropin content is elevated in animals that have been subjected to intense illumination.[111]

7.2.3. METABOLISM OF GONADOTROPINS

No reliable data are available as to the possible precursor substances of the pituitary hormones. Considering the chemical composition of gonadotropins, such precursors must undoubtedly comprise amino acids and sugars, particularly glucosamine.[172] There is no evidence to suggest that gonadotropins are destroyed by the liver in the same manner as are estrogens and other steroids. Instead, the peculiarities of the renal excretion of gonadotropins are well known. Investigations by Lunenfeld and colleagues[101] have shown that, contrary to common earlier assumptions, only about 6 per cent of an injected dose of gonadotropin is eliminated via the kidney, which leaves an amount of up to 94 per cent to be accounted for by the rest of the body. This phenomenon of endogenous destruction of a hormone is not without interest. Two main factors intervene in the destruction of gonadotropins: first, utilization by target organs, and second, the presence of *antigonadotropic substances.*

The first of the two factors, that is, utilization of the gonadotropins and their degradation in the process of acting, was shown to be related to the volume of the target organ, which thus determines both the blood level and rate of urinary excretion of these hormones.[176] Hence, the absence of an ovary produces a pathologic elevation of urinary FSH,[34, 95] regardless of whether absence of an ovary is the result of castration or of agenesis, as may be the case in Turner's syndrome. It is a proved fact that the lack of a target organ leads to increased gonadotropin excretion. In concrete terms, this means that in the absence of an organ to be acted upon, the hormone is wasted. Conversely, if there is a target organ to act upon, the amount of hormone utilized has been found to be proportional to the volume of tissue acted upon.

The second factor, destruction of the hormones by the action of antigonadotropic substances, will be discussed later in this chapter.

7.2.4. CIRCULATION AND EXCRETION OF GONADOTROPINS

Gonadotropins are found in the blood and in the urine. The study of the circulation and elimination of chorionic gonadotropins will be dealt with in Chapter 19, so that the present discussion can be confined exclusively to pituitary gonadotropins. As pointed out previously, follicle-stimulating hormone (FSH) is found primarily in the blood and urine of individuals without gonadal

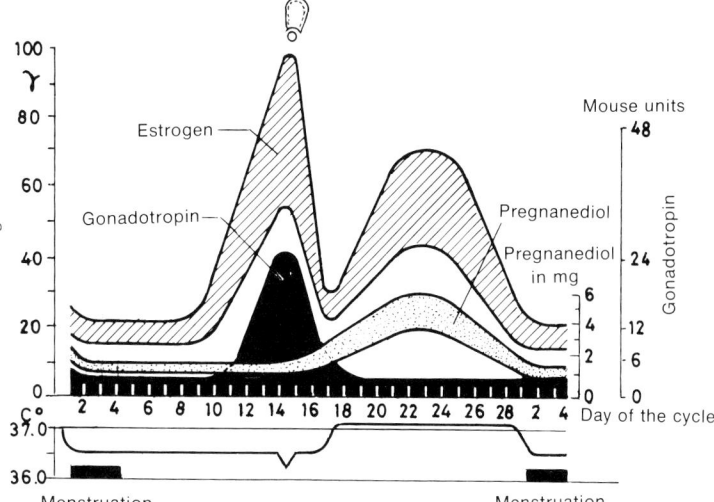

Figure 7-8. Diagram of urinary excretion of sex hormones throughout the cycle. (From Hammerstein: Arch. Gynäk., 196:504, 1961.)

function. Belonging to this category are postmenopausal women, surgically castrated women and cases of primary ovarian insufficiency, such as occurs in ovarian aplasia or hypoplasia.[100] In all these cases, a considerable amount of follicle-stimulating hormone is eliminated in the urine. FSH levels are also elevated during the first half of the menstrual cycle,[98, 166] particularly immediately prior to ovulation, and have been found to be similarly elevated in certain cases of pituitary pathology. The hormone occurs in the urine in relatively large quantities, ranging from 50 to 250 IU in the urine of castrated women, and from 10 to 50 IU during the first half of the menstrual cycle (Fig. 7-8).

7.2.5. CYCLIC FLUCTUATIONS IN GONADOTROPIN PLASMA LEVELS

Using modern, ultrasensitive, radioimmunologic methods, various authors have investigated the plasma levels of FSH and LH separately. There is general agreement that cyclic variations do not occur in male plasma.[124, 125, 173]

In contrast, the variations noted by different workers with plasma of women are of great interest. There is no doubt that LH levels, which are low throughout the cycle, spike to a "preovulatory peak." Already, in 1961, Brown and co-workers[29] showed the existence of a preovulatory peak by means of bioassay procedures. This was subsequently confirmed with radioimmunoassay techniques by Fukushima and colleagues[63] in 1964. Recently, the occurrence of an LH peak has been demonstrated in women,[37, 116, 167, 168, 170] as well as in female monkeys.[90] As a result, this point seems to have been established beyond any doubt (Fig. 7-9). On the other hand, there is no agreement regarding the behavior of FSH. As a result of their studies with biologic methods, Perloff and Steinberger[129] had already, in 1965, hinted at the impossibility of establishing a set pattern for FSH elimination during the cycle. Later studies with radioimmunoassay procedures, undertaken by various authors, failed to produce any consensus on the matter. Thus, Vorys and his group gave a curve in which, as shown in Figure 7-9, there seems to be an FSH peak around the time of menstruation, a progressive downhill deflection until ovulation and a repeated upswing before the following menstruation. A similar curve, apparently the reverse of the LH curve, has been obtained by Cargille and co-workers[37] and by Taymor and co-workers.[167, 168] Conversely, Midgley and Jaffe[116] described a radically different situation in which, as shown in Figure 7-10, there is an FSH peak coincident with a maximal LH peak. It should be mentioned, finally, that neither Thomas and Ferin[170] nor Rosemberg and his colleagues[146] have found any appreciable variations of FSH levels in the course of the cycle, which led them to believe that they were dealing with a rather flat curve.

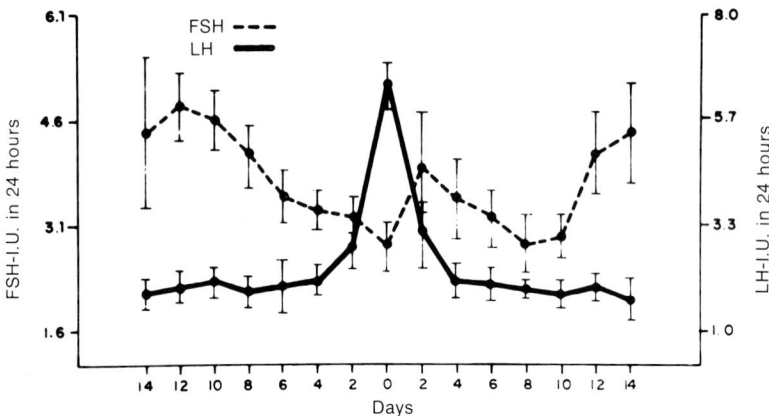

Figure 7-9. Fluctuations of FSH and LH in the course of the human cycle. (From Fukushima, Stevens, Gant and Vorys: *J. Clin. Endocr.*, 24:205, 1964.)

Faiman and Ryan[61] demonstrated the existence of a day-to-night circadian rhythm in plasma LH concentrations. Eleftheriou and colleagues[55] observed comparable variations in response to stimulating the amygdaloid nucleus. As a final note of interest, Conway and co-workers[42] have demonstrated cyclic variations in gonadotropin levels in the efferent venous blood of the pituitary.

7.3. NATURAL AND ARTIFICIAL ANTIGONADOTROPINS

Antigonadotropic substances are antibodies which are formed in response to the antigenic capacity of gonadotropins. In addition, there are also some drugs that display antigonadotropic activity.

7.3.1. ANTIBODIES TO GONADOTROPINS

Because of their protein as well as mucopolysaccharide nature, gonadotropins possess strong *antigenic properties*. These properties are not *individual* but *species* specific. This means that human gonadotropins are antigenic in animals, and those of animal origin — e.g., the mare — produce antihormones when used therapeutically in humans. A good review of the problem has been written by Oostergaard.[126]

In recent years, knowledge of such properties has been used for the isolation and characterization of these compounds, as well as for their detection and immunologic estimation (see Section 7.4).

Knobil and Josimovitch[91] made the interesting observation that the more remote two species are, the greater is the difference in composition of their gonadotropins and, therefore, the greater is the mutual antigenicity of their gonadotropins.

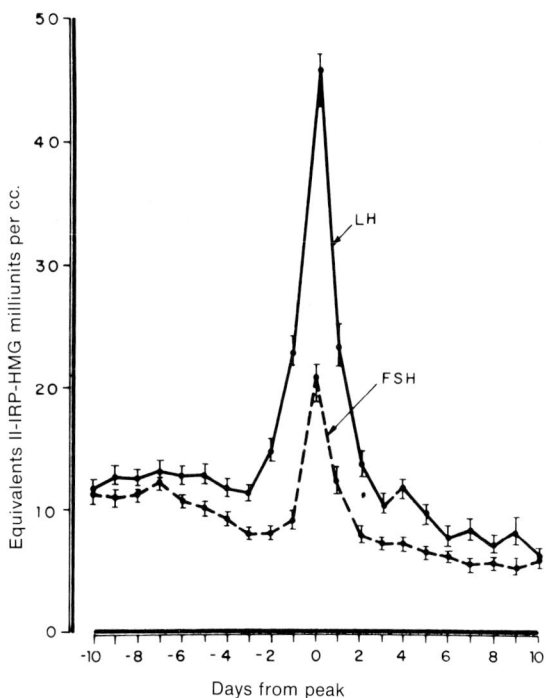

Figure 7-10. Fluctuations of FSH and LH in the course of the cycle. (From Midgley and Jaffe: *J. Clin. Endocr.*, 28:1699, 1968.)

Research on the subject of antigonadotropins has made significant progress in recent years. Tamada and co-workers[165] have succeeded in isolating and purifying human anti-FSH and anti-LH antigonadotropins. A method for their estimation has been devised by Diczfalusy and his group.[141] Similarly, an anti-FSH substance has been recovered from the urine of female monkeys,[146] which was found to be inactive against human gonadotropins. In the same way, the absence of cross-reactions between women and monkeys, as well as between rodents and women, could be demonstrated by other authors.[68, 121]

Antigonadotropins play an important role in senility according to Soffer and his colleagues,[157, 158] who reported that, with advancing age, the presence of urinary antigonadotropins[49, 74] increased and so did the antigonadotropic potency of the serum.[57, 118] Keele and his associates[89] found that FSH and LH injections produced specific antibodies in rabbits, which made it possible for Brody and Carlstrom[28] to devise a method for the detection and characterization of FSH, and enabled Hayashida and Contropoulos[41, 75] to achieve the immunologic differentiation of FSH and LH.

The specificity of the two antigonadotropins, anti-FSH and anti-LH, has been questioned by Franchimont and van Cauwenberghe[62] and by Lunenfeld and associates.[101] However, later work by Gemzell's group,[66, 67] who in our view have most thoroughly studied the question, leads one to believe that if the preparations used to immunize animals are *pure*, the antibodies obtained are equally pure and are absolutely specific.

The practical results of the discovery of antigonadotropins are:

(1) Proof of two distinct gonadotropins (FSH and LH) existing in fact and not as a result of two side chains on the same molecule (see Section 7.2).

(2) The feasibility of detecting and estimating these two compounds by means of immunoassay, instead of bioassay, technique (see Section 7.4).

(3) An explanation for some paradoxical reactions observed with gonadotropin injections in animals and in women (see Bourdel and Li[26]).

(4) The ineffectiveness of therapy based on animal gonadotropins (such as pregnant mare serum).

7.3.2. ANTIGONADOTROPIC DRUGS

The compound known by the name of MER 25 is not only an antisteroid but also a potent inhibitor of gonadotropic activity. It mainly inhibits LH activity (Cutler and his associates[47]).

From the plant *Lithospermum ruderale* and, in smaller amounts, from the common pea (*Pisum sativum*), an active principle called *lithospermine* has been extracted. According to the studies by Ringler and Kliman,[139] it inhibits gonadotropin secretion, which has more recently been confirmed by Brennemann and colleagues.[27] The latter authors also found that it inhibited the formation of *oxytocin*, a discovery of great clinical and potentially therapeutic significance. At the same time, it would seem to be of considerable theoretical interest since one might assume that lithospermine acts on the hypothalamic centers by suppressing the production of neurohormones of the polypeptide type, that is, the chemical mediators that are known to stimulate the formation of gonadotropins. Its action would thus seem to be of the "indirect" type.

7.4. BIOASSAY, IMMUNOASSAY AND RADIOIMMUNOASSAY OF GONADOTROPINS

The first immunologically oriented investigations were undertaken by Gemzell and his group in 1960.[66] Soon thereafter it was shown that the immunoassay could be perfected and converted into a radioimmunoassay by using labeled gonadotropins in the competitive test. This subject is discussed in more detail in Chapter 24.

7.4.1. BIOASSAY OF CHORIONIC GONADOTROPIN (HCG)

The different gonadotropins are determined by various bioassay procedures. The first ones to be developed were adequate for the demonstration of urinary chorionic gonadotropin and have since been employed for many years in the *biologic pregnancy test*. These methods will be described in detail in Chapter 24 and are outlined here only briefly.

The Aschheim-Zondek reaction for the demonstration of chorionic gonadotropins is based on detecting the effects of the latter on follicular maturation, formation of hemorrhagic follicles and ovarian luteinization in infantile mice.

The Friedman test is also an assay for chorionic gonadotropin based on the formation of hemorrhagic follicles and corpora lutea in juvenile rabbits.

The Hogben test determines the deposition of eggs by the female South African toad *Xenopus laevis*.

The *reactions in batrachian males*, of either frogs or toads (*Rana esculenta, Rana pipiens, Bufo bufo* and *Bufo arenarum*) constitute a fourth test.

The preceding reactions currently have all been superseded by Wide and Gemzell's immunologic reaction[66] and its modifications[102] (see Chapter 24).

7.4.2. BIOASSAY OF FSH

The hormones of the pituitary cannot be estimated with these tests which, at best, may serve to detect chorionic gonadotropin, provided that the latter is present in sufficient quantities. The following methods for the determination of FSH have been proposed:

Method of Levin and Tyndale, which consists in measuring the increment in weight of the infantile mouse uterus. It is based on an indirect effect reflecting follicular maturation. FSH acts on the infantile mouse ovary (in the resting stage, in which it is producing no estrogens) and induces sudden maturation of some or all of its follicles, thus leading to production of estrogens which in turn act on the uterus, increasing the weight of the latter.

Induction of estrus in immature mice, according to the methods of Zondek, Loeser and others. This is also based on an indirect effect. Estrogens secreted by the ovary, brought to maturation by FSH pretreatment, act upon the vagina and provoke estrus which otherwise would not occur in immature mice.

The Evans test, based on the appearance of follicular maturation in hypophysectomized animals after they are injected with FSH. This is a direct test and is the most precise of all currently known methods.

Immunologic methods. Crooke and Cunningham,[46] as well as Iserski, Lunenfeld and Shelesnyak,[84] introduced two similar methods for the immunologic estimation of FSH. Their results are excellent and have only been surpassed by radioimmunologic techniques.

Radioimmunologic techniques[60, 117] have made it possible to assay FSH with greater precision. During the past years, a number of techniques have been introduced to improve on the radioimmunoassay of FSH.[5, 119, 133, 152] Nevertheless, as late as 1968, a man of such unquestionable authority on the subject as Albert,[2] still defended the bioassay for FSH as superior to radioimmunologic techniques.

7.4.3. BIOASSAY OF LH

The following procedures have been devised for the determination of LH:

Determination of *weight increment of the anterior lobe of the prostate*, according to Van Dyke and Greep.

Determination of *weight increment of seminal vesicles*, according to Fevold (Figs. 7–11 and 7–12). As with the preceding one, this procedure is an indirect method and is similar to those used for the determination of FSH. As mentioned previously in discussing the action of FSH on indirect

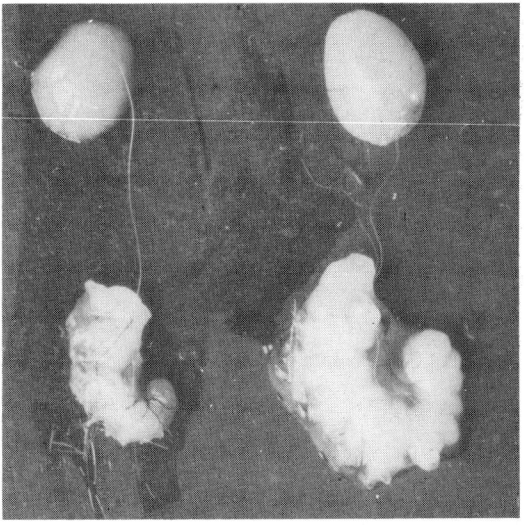

Figure 7–11. Effect of LH on rat seminal vesicle and testis. Left, seminal vesicle and testis of immature male rat. Right, following injection with LH. Testis increases in size as a result of interstitial cell proliferation and seminal vesicle grows noticeably under the influence of androgens elaborated by LH-stimulated testis.

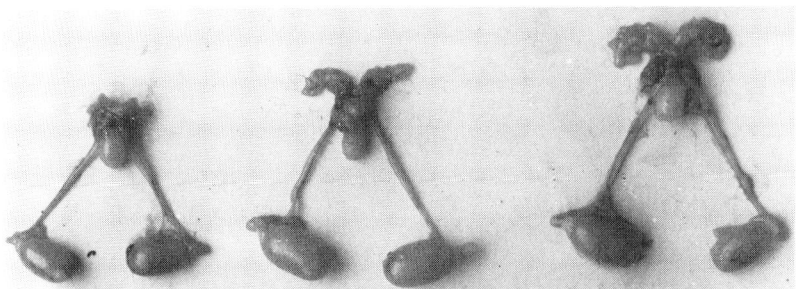

Figure 7–12. Comparison of FSH and LH effects upon genital tract of immature male rat. From left to right: Control animal, animal injected with FSH, animal injected with LH. Note lack of increase in size of testes as well as absence of longitudinal growth of vas deferens and absence of growth of either prostate or seminal vesicles following FSH injection. On the other hand, injection of LH produces proliferation of testicular interstitium, increase in size of the testes, increased production of androgens and, consequently, overall development of target organs.

effectors, FSH exerts a greater effect in females by virtue of the fact that the production of estrogens, which produce the increase in weight of the female genital organs, depends precisely on FSH activity. In the male, on the other hand, the increase in weight of the prostate and seminal vesicles, that is, the indirect gonadotropin effectors, is brought about by the activity of androgenic hormone and, since the latter is secreted by the interstitium, its production is primarily dependent on the level of LH (or ICSH) activity. *Consequently, in the bioassay procedures for gonadotropin A, the criterion used is the increase in weight of the female tract organs, whereas in the bioassay of gonadotropin B, what is measured is the increase in weight of the male organs.* This, however, does not mean that gonadotropin A is to be considered as primarily feminizing or gonadotropin B as primarily masculinizing, since both hormones affect both sexes.

Another procedure for the estimation of LH, based on restitution of the testicular interstitial tissue in hypophysectomized rats, was also devised by Evans and is similar to his method for the determination of FSH.

According to Jansen and Loeser, LH can also be determined by means of inducing the *formation of corpora lutea in infantile animals* that have been previously injected with FSH.

Currently, a very popular procedure devised by Farris for the quantitative determination of LH is one that assays the degree of *ovarian hyperemia.* This method was subsequently modified by a number of authors. Two to four hours after gonadotropin B is injected into an animal an acute congestion of the ovary takes place, which the authors claim to be entirely specific.

All the foregoing procedures have the drawback of not being fully specific for LH since many of the same effects, though to a lesser extent, can be produced by the action of FSH. A procedure worked out by Parlow[127] that is highly specific is based on the phenomenon of *ascorbic acid depletion.* This method has received favorable comment from other workers.[22, 117, 149, 153]

Brody and Carlstrom[28] were first in attempting a *hemagglutination* technique, similar to that of Wide and Gemzell, for the determination of chorionic gonadotropin. The main difficulty encountered apparently consisted in obtaining a specific antibody, which seems to have been finally achieved by several investigators.[56, 57, 160] Lately, Rizkallah and co-workers[140] published an improved method of immunoassay. The most accurate methods, however, resort to radioimmunologic techniques in which a labeled antigen competes for antibody fixation with the test antigen.[9, 115, 123] These techniques are dealt with in greater detail in Chapter 24.

Just as with FSH, the most accurate and specific methods for the determination of LH are based on *radioimmunological techniques.* The more recent ones to be listed among the latter are those of Albert and colleagues,[5] Ryan[147] and Saxena and co-workers.[152] This subject is equally covered in detail in Chapter 24.

7.4.4. EFFECTS OF FSH AND LH ON BATRACHIA

Batrachia (see Chapter 24) are most suitable animals for the detection of urinary gonadotropins in pregnancy and are used for pregnancy tests. However, a point of major interest is a peculiar side effect these gonadotropins have on the testes of male batrachia. FSH, which normally stimulates spermatogenesis, in this respect has no noticeable effect, whereas LH, as well as chorionic gonadotropin, elicits spermiation. The mechanism of the latter effect has been brought to light by the work of Houssay's associates[82] and that of our own group.[23] Just as it does in mammals, FSH accelerates spermatogenesis in batrachia but the newly formed spermatozoa remain attached to the Sertoli cells and are not expelled from the testis. As a result of LH action, the spermatozoa are freed from their attachment to the germinal epithelium by lysis of the Sertoli cells. The resulting *release of sperm* is known by the name of *spermiation*. Lysis of the Sertoli cells is associated with highly interesting alterations of their intracellular mucopolysaccharides. These compounds are depolymerized, setting free sugars (probably fructose) that provide the sperm with nutrition during migration. Hence, besides the known interstitial cell stimulating effect of LH on the testis, in batrachia an additional effect must be taken into consideration: *spermiation* (see Fig. 7–13).

7.4.5. UNITS OF GONADOTROPINS

Attempts at expressing values in mouse units or *rat units* (Armstrong and Greep[6]) have been abandoned in favor of the establishment of international standards for measurement of gonadotropic potency of a given preparation. These can be applied equally well for bioassay, immunoassay or radioimmunoassay. The only type of comparison they do not lend themselves to is a ponderal comparison, because the gonadotropic potency per unit of weight for each preparation is different.

Robyn[142] has compared equivalent values as applied to international standards, as follows:

Table 7–1 shows the equivalencies between the first and second international reference preparations (IRP) of gonadotropins extracted from human menopausal urine.

TABLE 7–1

1.0 of LH activity equivalent to 2 mg of first IRP (WHO 1964)*
1.0 of FSH activity equivalent to 7 mg of first IRP (WHO 1964)†

---

*Based on weight increment of ventral prostate in male rat.
†Based on weight increment of ovaries in immature female rat.

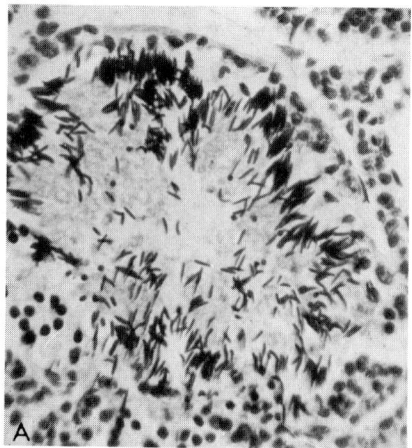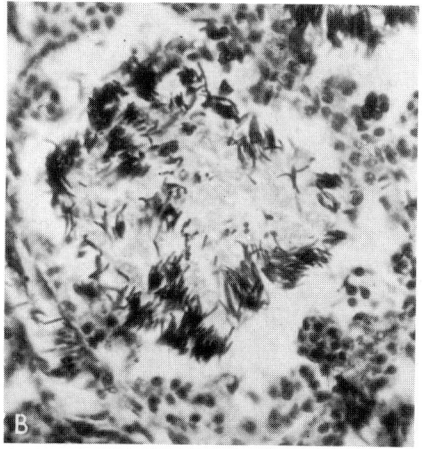

Figure 7–13. Effect of human chorionic gonadotropin upon the testis of male *Rana esculenta*. A, Prior to injection. B, After injection of 1000 IU of HCG. The resulting reaction is not one of spermatogenesis but one of spermiation, which is characterized by "release" of mature spermatozoa, detached from the walls of the tubules through lysis of Sertoli cells. (From Botella et al.: *Studies of Fertility*, 8:58, 1956. Blackwell, Oxford, England.)

Table 7-2 shows equivalencies, estimated by bioassay, between the second international standard of human chorionic gonadotropin (HCG) and the second reference preparation of gonadotropin from human menopausal urine (HMG).

TABLE 7-2

1.0 IU HCG equivalent to 6.25 IU of LH activity*
1.0 IU HCG equivalent to 3.00 IU of LH activity†

*From Cargille et al.,[37] based on weight increment of seminal vesicles in male rat
†From Robyn et al.,[141] based on test of ventral prostate in male rat.

Table 7-3 shows equivalencies, estimated by bioassay, between the second international reference preparation of HMG and the standards of ovine FSH and LH of the National Institutes of Health (NIH-FSH and NIH-LH).

TABLE 7-3

1.0 mg NIH-LH equivalent to 1500 IU LH*
1.0 mg NIH-LH equivalent to 66.6 IU LH†
1.0 mg NIH-FSH equivalent to 22.7 IU FSH‡
1.0 mg NIH-FSH equivalent to 26.3 IU FSH§
1.0 mg NIH-FSH equivalent to 27.7 IU FSH**

*From Reichert and Parlow,[135] based on ascorbic acid depletion in rat ovary.
†From Rosemberg et al.,[145] based on weight increment of ventral prostate in male rat.
‡From Reichert and Parlow,[135] based on weight increment of immature rat ovaries, according to Steelman and Poohley.
§From Diczfalusy et al., based on weight increment of immature rat ovaries, according to Steelman and Poohley.
**From Robyn et al.,[141] based on weight increment of immature rat ovaries, according to Steelman and Poohley.

7.5. THERAPEUTIC APPLICATIONS OF GONADOTROPINS

Hormone therapy by means of pituitary extracts has not yet been fully developed, owing to the low concentrations in which such extracts are obtained from animal pituitaries. Only those manufacturers that can avail themselves of the services of large slaughterhouses could aspire to obtain total pituitary extracts with a gonadotropin concentration high enough to be suitable for therapeutic application. Preparations that are rich in gonadotropins can be obtained by extracting concentrated urine of pregnancy, but such preparations have only a limited therapeutic value because chorionic gonadotropin exerts a scanty stimulatory effect on the human ovary.

In Table 7-4, a synopsis of the principal commercial preparations of gonadotropins is listed.

During the last few years, great progress has been achieved through the introduction of preparations of *human pituitaries* obtained from cadavers. The idea, originally proposed by Gemzell and co-workers,[65-67] has now been adopted by other investigators, principally by Bettendorf and associates.[18-20]

However, this is an enormously costly procedure. To carry out his treatment, Bettendorf needed extracts from no less than 3000 pituitary glands. For this reason, Benz and co-workers,[16] Donini and associates[52] and Kovacic and Loraine[95] have come up with the ingenious procedure whereby pituitary gonadotropins are extracted from the urine of postmenopausal women who are known to excrete it in increased amounts (see Chapter 17). Although Bettendorf[20] voices his reservations about the efficacy of preparations obtained in such a manner, we as well as a number of other authors have had satisfactory results with them.[24, 53, 101, 108]

This type of therapy has now reached widespread usage, especially in the treatment of female infertility[66, 67] and male sterility,[24, 108] and shall be further enlarged upon in Chapter 41 (Section 41.11.14).

7.6. LACTOTROPIC HORMONE OR PROLACTIN

7.6.1. DEFINITION, NOMENCLATURE, HISTORY

The term *prolactin* or *lactotropic hormone* refers to a pituitary anterior lobe hormone that stimulates milk secretion by acting on the acini of the mammary gland. Milk is a specific product of acinar secretion. The hormone involved has also been called *lactotropin, galactotropic hormone, galactogenic hormone* or LTH. Its individuality has been fully demonstrated and the hormone has been identified with the so-called *luteotropic factor*, or *factor of corpus luteum persistence*.

TABLE 7-4. Commercial Preparations with Gonadotropin Effect

NAME OF PRODUCT AND MANUFACTURER	MODE OF ADMINISTRATION
(1) Preparations of whole pituitary	
Pituitary gland (Parke, Davis & Co.)	Injectables of 0.065 gm (65 mg)
(2) Total pituitary extracts containing FSH	
Antephysan (G. Richter)	Tablets and vials equivalent to 1 gm of fresh gland
Anterior pituitary extract (Parke, Davis & Co.)	Vials
Hypophysen vorderlappen (Dr. Georg Henning)	Vials containing 0.5 gm of fresh gland
Pituitary anterior extract (Eli Lilly & Co.)	Vials with 1.2 gm of fresh gland
Pituitary anterior lobe extract (Armour)	Tablets of 0.13 gm and vials of 0.01 gm
Praephyson (Promonta)	Tablets and vials of 25 rat units
Preloban (Hoechst)	Pellets containing 5 maturing units and vials in dry powder containing 25 maturing units
(3) Purified preparations of gonadotropins of anterior lobe of pituitary	
Praehormon (Promonta)	Vials containing 100 rat units of dry extract
(4) Preparation of gonadotropins of pregnant mare serum	
Anteron (Schering)	Vials containing 500, 1000 and 5000 I.U. of dry extract
Gestil (Organon)	Vials containing 200 and 400 I.U. of dry extract
Antex (Leo)	Vials containing 300 and 1000 I.U. of dry extract
(5) Preparations of human urinary chorionic gonadotropins	
Antuitrin S. (Parke, Davis & Co.)	Injectables of 100 and 500 I.U. per cc
A.P.L. (Ayerst)	Injectables in vials containing 500 and 1000 I.U. per cc
Pregnyl (Organon)	Vials containing 100, 500, 1500 and 5000 I.U. of dry extract
Physex (Leo)	Vials containing 500 and 1500 I.U. of dry extract
Prolan (Bayer)	Vials containing 100, 500 and 2000 I.U. of dry extract
Primogonyl (Schering)	Vials containing 300, 1000 and 5000 I.U. of dry extract
(6) Postmenopausal human urinary FSH	
Humegon (Organon Oss)	Vials containing 500 and 1000 I.U. for intramuscular injection
Pergonal (Serono)	

The idea that milk secretion is under pituitary control is an old one and is derived from the discoveries of Stricker and Grueter who, in 1928, demonstrated that pituitary extracts produced increased secretion of milk in female rabbits. In 1933, Riddle, Bates and Dikshorn made the observation that the gland in the pigeon's crop (the function of which in the nutrition of the offspring is identical to that of the mammary gland) is stimulated by way of the anterior lobe of the pituitary gland. As a result of this observation, they devised the so-called "pigeon test" for the bioassay of prolactin in pituitary extracts. The following year, they were able to demonstrate the existence of a pituitary hormone possessing a complete biologic individuality, which was capable of provoking the growth of the gland of the avian crop as well as mammary gland development and secretion in mammals.

In 1933, Selye, Collip and Thompson found that loss of lactation resulting from hypophysectomy in female rats could be restored by injections of pituitary extracts. In 1935, Riddle and Bates successfully obtained a relatively pure preparation of prolactin by means of an isoelectric precipitation technique and, the following year, Lyons obtained an even purer preparation. Finally, employing a procedure similar to that used to extract insulin from the pancreas, White and co-workers, in 1937, achieved the isolation of crystallized prolactin. This hormone thus became the first pituitary hormone to be obtained in pure form. This made it possible to establish an international unit for it, equivalent to a tenth of a milligram of the pure crystallized preparation. In 1942, Lyons and collaborators determined the molecular weight of prolactin to be 32,000.

7.6.2. CHEMISTRY OF PROLACTIN

Despite the large number of active preparations isolated in the past years, purified[80] and crystallized[177] hormone preparations have been obtained only by means of starch gel electrophoresis. According to Butt,[35] ovine prolactin, so far the most purified and best known preparation, has an isoelectric point (pH) of 5.74, a sedimentation coefficient of 2.17, a diffusion constant of 8.62×10^{-7} and a molecular weight of 23,400. Its potency corresponds to 30 IU per milligram of product. By sequential analysis of this purified product, 18 different amino acids are obtained in ratios that could not be fully determined. It is a terminal C polypeptide, the sequence of which has of late been characterized with certainty as follows:

$$H_2N\text{-Thr-Pro-Val-Thr-Pro-} \atop \overline{CyS\text{-Tyr-Leu-Asp}(NH_2)\text{-CyS-COOH}}$$

7.6.3. PHYSIOLOGY

Prolactin produces secretion of milk. However, it does not produce that effect unless the mammary gland has previously been acted upon by estrogens or by the corpus luteum hormone. The large quantities of both of the latter hormones that are elaborated during pregnancy prepare the breast for secretion to be initiated by the pituitary release of prolactin during the puerperium. It is presently held that the combined actions of estrogens and progesterone during pregnancy provoke pituitary secretion of considerable amounts of prolactin but, at the same time, they block that hormone within the pituitary cells so that its release can take place only after the activity of the ovarian hormones has stopped.[31] In that way estrogens and progesterone act as stimulators of pituitary prolactin secretion while at the same time blocking prolactin release.

As to the release mechanism involved, prolactin behaves inversely with regard to all other adenohypophysial hormones. While a hypothalamic factor is known to be responsible for *inhibiting* prolactin release, no factor is known to be responsible for stimulating its release. The inhibiting factor, which has been isolated and characterized, has been designated PIF (*prolactin inhibiting factor*) (see Chapter 8). For that reason, anesthesia, destruction or inhibition of the medial neurogenic nucleus of the hypothalamus produces, besides amenorrhea (through loss of releasing factors for FSH and LH), galactorrhea (through inhibition of PIF). That is the basis of the Chiari-Frommel syndrome, which will be studied later (see Chapter 31, Section 31.4.4).

It has already been mentioned that LH possesses luteinizing, but not luteotrophic,[144, 151] activity; in contrast, prolactin activity is aimed at the maintenance of the corpus luteum. (An example is the rat, whose ovary remains luteinized during the entire period of lactation; see Chapter 22.) If cow ovaries are perfused with prolactin their progesterone output is 10 times greater than when they are perfused with LH.[13] Bryans[31] found elevated progesteronemia after prolactin injection, and Greenwald and his colleagues[70] noted that, unless hamsters were also injected with prolactin, FSH and LH alone failed to bring about formation of secretory corpora lutea. Judging from available evidence, this hormone should be considered as a *third gonadotropin*.

Prolactin is elaborated by the gamma cells of the pituitary.[131] The hypertrophy these cells experience in association with active prolactin formation gives them a characteristic appearance during pregnancy, resulting in what Erdheim and Stumme had designated *pregnancy cells*.

Apart from its previously mentioned effect on the breast, prolactin has also been shown to exert a decisive effect on the maintenance of the corpus luteum, which earned for it the name *luteotrophic hormone*. Luteotrophic hormone or LTH was first described by Evans in 1939, and its existence was subsequently confirmed by Albert and his colleagues[34] and by Cashida and associates.[38, 164] The complete identity of the two hormones was established more recently so that there is no longer any doubt that prolactin is the same compound that is responsible for prolonging the life of the corpus luteum.[143, 174] In this respect, it behaves as an additional gonadotropic factor. While gonadotropin A "primes" the follicle for ovulation and eventual luteinization and gonadotropin B initiates the very process of luteinization, prolactin is the only hormone capable of impressing persistent activity upon the corpus luteum.[130] As pointed out in Chapter 11, chorionic gonadotropin also possesses luteotrophic activity, while pituitary gonadotropin B (LH) completely lacks such activity; therefore, the periodic action of prolactin during the second half of the interphase is indispensable for the ovary to maintain corpus luteum activity over the span of 1 to 10 days of its physiologic duration (see Chapter 12).

7.6.4. ESTIMATION

Prolactin determinations can be performed by means of bioassay, immunoassay and radioimmunoassay.

BIOASSAY OF PROLACTIN. There are two classic tests, that of the pigeon crop, which was introduced by Riddle and co-workers and popularized by Gati and co-workers[64] in 1969, and that of MacShan and Meyer,[106] which is based on the study of the histologic changes occurring in the gland of the crop. Finally, Wolthuis and de Jongh[175] in 1963 based a bioassay procedure on the luteotrophic action of prolactin on the corpus luteum of rodents.

IMMUNOASSAY. Hayashida[75] described an immunologic method for the determination of prolactin. It is based on the application of a double diffusion technique in agar using as antigen serum of immunized female rabbits.

RADIOIMMUNOASSAY. The preceding techniques are being rapidly replaced by the much more accurate radioimmunoassay procedures, recently championed mainly by Bryant and Greenwood,[32] who employed them for the estimation of ovine, caprine and bovine plasma prolactin values.

7.6.5. THERAPEUTIC APPLICATION

Prolactin has been used therapeutically for two purposes: (1) to stimulate the formation of a corpus luteum, and (2) to stimulate lactation.

Table 7-5 lists the principal commercial preparations of prolactin.

The only disadvantage about the use of prolactin preparations is that injections are painful and may cause local tissue irritation.

7.7. SYNOPSIS OF PITUITARY HORMONES

The preceding two chapters have dealt with the hormones of the pituitary. Notwithstanding the fact that only three of these—FSH, LH and prolactin—act upon the gonads, *the majority of the pituitary hormones are more or less directly involved in the phenomena of sexual life.* Thus, the stimulus of growth hormone is indispensable for embryonal development; similarly, thyrotropic hypersecretion during pregnancy fulfills a physiologic function; so does diabetogenic hormone, the participation of which in some pathologic conditions of woman is very important; and lastly, ACTH plays a most important role in controlling adrenal cortical function, especially during pregnancy. Of the posterior lobe hormones, oxytocin is also very intimately implicated in reproductive processes and, similarly, the vasopressor and antidiuretic hormones exert unquestionable effects on certain pathologic conditions of pregnancy.

The most important aspect of pituitary physiology is regulating the correlation of endocrine and metabolic functions. *The anterior pituitary may be viewed as the site at which neural stimuli are converted to hormonal reactions, whereas the posterior pituitary gives rise to chemical mediators, destined to carry the influence of the nervous system beyond the reach of nerve*

TABLE 7-5

NAME OF PRODUCT AND MANUFACTURER	MODE OF ADMINISTRATION
Prolactin (Armour)	Injectables containing 100 IU per cc
Prolactin (Ayerst Mac-Kenna)	Injectables containing 100 IU per cc
Prolactin (Schering Bloomfield)	Vials containing 100 IU in dry powder

endings. This is why the study of pituitary physiology or physiopathology no longer allows that gland to be separated from the nearby hypothalamus with which it constitutes the *hypophysiohypothalamic unit.*

As is made clear in the following chapter, this hypothalamic-pituitary center constitutes the crossroads at which relational life and vegetative life interact. Consequently, the pituitary is the gland that impresses rhythmicity upon the inner microcosmos of the body. Sexual life and its rhythm depends on the rhythm of the pituitary gland. While the pituitary of woman displays a monthly cyclic rhythm, that of the male *differs from the female pituitary only by the absence of that cycle.* Insofar as reproductive processes are concerned, man is a *stable* organism, whereas woman is an eminently *mutable* organism. Stability in one sex, just as mutability in the other, depends fundamentally on hypothalamic control.

REFERENCES

1. Ahren, K. E. B., Hamberger, A. C., and Hamberger, L. A.: *Endocrinology,* 77:332, 1965.
2. Albert, A.: *J. Clin. Endocr.,* 28:1683, 1968.
3. Albert, A., and Derner, I.: *J. Clin. Endocr. Metab.,* 20:1059, 1960.
4. Albert, A., and Kobi, J.: *J. Clin. Endocr. Metab.,* 21:1, 1961.
5. Albert, A., Rosemberg, E., Ross, G. T., Paulsen, C. A., and Ryan, R. J.: *J. Clin. Endocr.,* 28:1214, 1968.
6. Armstrong, D. T., and Greep, R. O.: *Endocrinology,* 70:701, 1962.
7. Armstrong, D. T., O'Brien, J., and Greep, R. O.: *Endocrinology,* 75:488, 1964.
8. Armstrong, D. T., and Black, D. L.: *Endocrinology,* 78:937, 1966.
9. Bagshave, K. D., Wilde, C. E., and Orr, A. A.: *Lancet,* 1:1118, 1966.
10. Balboni, G. C.: *Arch. Ital. Anat. Embriol.,* 65:115, 1960.
11. Barraclough, C., and Sawyer, C. H.: *Endocrinology,* 61:341, 1957.
12. Barraclough, C., and Sawyer, C. H.: *Endocrinology,* 65:503, 1959.
13. Bartosik, D., Romanoff, E. B., Watson, D. J., and Scricco, E.: *Endocrinology,* 81:186, 1967.
14. Bedford, J. M., and Shalkowsky, R.: *J. Reprod. Fertil.,* 13:361, 1967.
15. Bennett, P.: *J. Reprod. Fertil.,* 13:357, 1967.
16. Benz, F., et al.: *J. Endocr.,* 19:158, 1959.
17. Bergers, A. C., and Hao-Li, C.: *Endocrinology,* 66:255, 1960.
18. Bettendorf, G., Apostolakis, M., and Voigt, K. D.: *Acta Endocr.,* 41:1, 1962.
19. Bettendorf, G., Boetticher, U., Le Coultre, C., and Maas, H.: *Klin. Wschr.,* 41:398, 1963.
20. Bettendorf, G.: *Internat. J. Fertil.,* 8:799, 1963.
21. Blandau, R. J., and Rumeri, R.: *Fertil. Steril.,* 13:335, 1963.
22. Bogdanove, E. M., and Gay, V. L.: *Endocrinology,* 81:1104, 1967.
23. Botella, J., Plaza, F., and Del Sol, R.: *Studies on Fertility* (Oxford), 8:58, 1956.
24. Botella, J.: *Actas Soc. Esp. Esteril.,* 11, 1957.
25. Botella, J.: *Acta Gin.,* 19:59, 1968.
26. Bourdel, G., and Li, C. H.: *Acta Endocr.,* 42:473, 1963.
27. Brennemann, W. R., et al.: *Endocrinology,* 67:583, 1960.
28. Brody, S., and Carlstrom, G.: *J. Clin. Endocr. Metab.,* 22:564, 1962.
29. Brown, P. S., et al.: *J. Endocr.,* 18:191, 1961.
30. Browning, H. C., and Larke, G. A.: *Proc. Soc. Exper. Biol. Med.,* 118:913, 1965.
31. Bryans, F. E.: *Endocrinology,* 48:733, 1951.
32. Bryant, G. D., and Greenwood, F. C.: *Biochem. J.,* 109:831, 1968.
33. Burt, A. S., and Velardo, J. T.: *J. Clin. Endocr. Metab.,* 14:979, 1954.
34. Butt, W. R.: The Chemistry of the Gonadotropins. Springfield, Ill., Charles C Thomas, 1967.
35. Butt, W. R.: Hormone Chemistry. London, Van Nostrand, 1969.
36. Callantyne, M. R., Humphrey, R. R., and Lee, S. L.: *Endocrinology,* 76:332, 1965.
37. Cargille, C. M., Ross, G. T., and Yoshimi, T.: *J. Clin. Endocr.,* 29:12, 1968.
38. Cashida, L. E., et al.: *Endocrinology,* 51:148, 1952.
39. Channing, C. P.: *Endocrinology,* 87:49, 1970.
40. Channing, C. P., and Villee, C. A.: *Biochim. Biophys. Acta,* 127:1, 1966.
41. Contopoulos, A. N., and Hayashida, T.: *J. Endocr.,* 25:451, 1963.
42. Conway, L. W., Schalch, D. S., Utiger, R. D., and Reichlin, S.: *J. Clin. Endocr.,* 29:446, 1969.
43. Cook, B., Kaltenbach, C. C., Norton, H. W., and Nalbandov, A. V.: *Endocrinology,* 81:573, 1967.
44. Corbin, A., and Daniels, E. L.: *Experientia,* 24:1260, 1968.
45. Corbin, A., Daniels, E. L., and Milmore, J. E.: *Endocrinology,* 86:735, 1970.
46. Crooke, A. C., and Cunningham, F. J.: *Biochem. J.,* 81:596, 1961.
47. Cutler, A., et al.: *Endocrinology,* 69:473, 1961.
48. David, M. A., Fraschini, F., and Martini, L.: *Compt. Rend. Acad. Sci.,* 261:2249, 1965.
49. Davis, J. C., Hyde, T. A., and Hipkin, L. J.: *J. Clin. Endocr. Metab.,* 26:1123, 1966.
50. Desclin, L.: *Ann. d'Endocr.,* 13:137, 1952.
51. Döcke, F., and Dörner, G.: *J. Endocr.,* 33:491, 1965.
52. Donini, P., Puzzoli, D., and d'Alessio, I.: *Actas Soc. Esp. Esteril.,* 11:17, 1967.
53. Dörner, G., Zabel, R., and Stahl, F.: *Klin. Wschr.,* 39:1196, 1961.
54. Eckstein, B., and Landsberg, R.: *Acta Endocr.,* 42:480, 1963.
55. Eleftheriou, B. E., Desjardins, C., and Zolovic, A. J.: *J. Reprod. Fertil.,* 21:249, 1970.
56. Ely, C. A., and Chen, B. L.: *Endocrinology,* 79:362, 1966.
57. Ely, C. A., and Chen, B. L.: *Endocrinology,* 81:1033, 1967.

58. Everett, J. W.: *Endocrinology*, 58:786, 1956.
59. Everett, J. W., and Sawyer, C. H.: *Endocrinology*, 47:198, 1950.
60. Faiman, C., and Ryan, R. J.: *J. Clin. Endocr. Metab.*, 27:444, 1967.
61. Faiman, C., and Ryan, R. J.: *Nature*, 215:857, 1967.
62. Franchimont, P., and Van Cauwenberghe, H.: *Ann. d'Endocr.*, 23:247, 1962.
63. Fukushima, M., Stevens, V. C., Gantt, C. L., and Vorys, N.: *J. Clin. Endocr.*, 24:265, 1964.
64. Gati, I., Odszpod, J., and Preisz, J.: *Acta Physiol. Acad. Sci. Hung. (Budapest)*, 32:115, 1967.
65. Gemzell, C. A., Diczfalusy, E., and Tillinger, K. G.: *Acta Obstet. Gynec. Scand.*, 38:465, 1959.
66. Gemzell, C. A.: *Ciba Colloquia on Endocrinology*, 13:191, 1960.
67. Gemzell, C. A.: *Actas Soc. Esp. Esteril.*, 11:7, 1967.
68. Glass, R. H., and Mroueh, A.: *Amer. J. Obstet. Gynec.*, 97:1082, 1967.
69. Got, R., and Bourrillon, R.: *Nature*, 189:234, 1961.
70. Greenwald, G. S., Keever, J. E., and Grady, K. L.: *Endocrinology*, 80:851, 1967.
71. Hall, P. F., and Koritz, S. B.: *Biochemistry*, 4:1037, 1965.
72. Hamberger, L. L. A.: *Acta Physiol. Scand.*, 74:410, 1968.
73. Hamberger, L. A., and Ahren, K. E. B.: *Endocrinology*, 81:93, 1967.
74. Hahn, H. B., and Albert, A.: *J. Clin. Endocr. Metab.*, 25:409, 1965.
75. Hayashida, T.: *J. Endocr.*, 26:75, 1963.
76. Hellbaum, A. A., et al.: *Endocrinology*, 68:144, 1961.
77. Henry, R.: Etude génerale sur les dosages des gonadotropines, in *Les gonadotropines en gynécologie*. Paris, Masson et Cie., 1962.
78. Herbst, A. L.: *Endocrinology*, 81:54, 1967.
79. Helling, H. R., and Savard, K.: *J. Biol. Chem.*, 240:1957, 1965.
80. Helling, H. R., and Savard, K.: *Biochemistry*, 5:2944, 1966.
81. Hilliard, J., Penardi, R., and Sawyer, C. H.: *Endocrinology*, 80:901, 1967.
82. Houssay, B. A.: *Acta Fisiol. Latinoamer.*, 4:2, 1954.
83. Ibayashi, H., et al.: *Endocrinology*, 76:347, 1965.
84. Iserski, C., Lunenfeld, B., and Shelesnyak, M. C.: *J. Clin. Endocr. Metab.*, 23:54, 1963.
85. Janes, R. G.: *Endocrinology*, 54:464, 1954.
86. Kaiser, J.: *Acta Endocr.*, 47:676, 1964.
87. Kaltenbach, C. C., Graber, J. W., Niswender, G. D., and Nalbandov, A. V.: *Endocrinology*, 82:753, 1968.
88. Kaltenbach, C. C., Graber, J. W., Niswender, G. D., and Nalbandov, A. V.: *Endocrinology*, 82:818, 1968.
89. Keele, D. K., et al.: *J. Clin. Endocr. Metab.*, 22:287, 1962.
90. Kirton, K. T., Niswender, G. D., Midgley, A. R., Jaffe, R. B., and Forbes, A. B.: *J. Clin. Endocr.*, 30:105, 1970.
91. Knobil, E., and Josimovitch, J. B.: *Endocrinology*, 69:139, 1961.
92. Knobil, E., Neill, J. D., and Johansson, E. D. B.: *Endocrinology*, 82:410, 1968.
93. Kofler, D., and Fogel, M.: *Proc. Soc. Exper. Biol. Med.*, 115:1080, 1964.
94. Koritz, S. B., and Hall, P. F.: *Biochemistry*, 4:2470, 1965.
95. Kovacic, N., and Loraine, J. A.: *Endocrinology*, 68:356, 1961.
96. Ladman, A. J., and Runner, M. N.: *Endocrinology*, 65:581, 1959.
97. Lamond, D. R., and Emmens, C. W.: *J. Endocr.*, 18:251, 1959.
98. Lawton, I. E., and Schwartz, N. B.: *Endocrinology*, 76:276, 1965.
99. Lawton, I. E., and Schwartz, N. B.: *Endocrinology*, 81:497, 1967.
100. Louchart, J., Trouffert, J., and Decourt, J.: *Acta Endocr.*, 49:293, 1965.
101. Lunenfeld, B., Iserski, C., and Shelesnyak, M. C.: *J. Clin. Endocr. Metab.*, 22:555, 1962.
102. Lunnen, J. E., and Foote, W. C.: *Endocrinology*, 81:61, 1967.
103. MacDonald, G. J., Armstrong, D. T., and Greep, R. O.: *Endocrinology*, 79:289, 1966.
104. MacLeod, J., Pazianos, A., and Ray, B. S.: *Lancet*, 1:1196, 1964.
105. MacLeod, J., Pazianos, A., and Ray, B. S.: *Fertil. Steril.*, 17:7, 1966.
106. MacShan, W. H., and Meyer, R. K.: *Endocrinology*, 50:294, 1952.
107. Major, P. W., Armstrong, D. T., and Greep, R. O.: *Endocrinology*, 81:19, 1967.
108. Mancini, R. E.: *Actas Soc. Esp. Esteril.*, 11:65, 1967.
109. Mancini, R. E.: *Testiculo Humano*. Buenos Aires, Ed. Panamericana, 1968.
110. Mancini, R. E., Castro, A., and Seiguer, A. C.: *J. Histochem. Cytochem.*, 15:516, 1967.
111. Marik, D. K., Matsuyama, E., and Lloyd, C. W.: *Endocrinology*, 77:529, 1965.
112. Marsh, J., Butcher, R. W., Savard, K., and Sutherland, E. W.: *J. Biol. Chem.*, 241:22, 1966.
113. Meyer, C. J.: *Gynaecologia*, 151:143, 1961.
114. Meyer, R. K., and MacShan, W. H.: In *Menstruation and its Disorders*, ed. E. T. Engle. Springfield, Ill., Charles C Thomas, 1950.
115. Midgley, A. R.: *Endocrinology*, 79:10, 1966.
116. Midgley, A. R., and Jaffe, R. B.: *J. Clin. Endocr.*, 28:1699, 1968.
117. Mills, J. M., and Schwartz, M. B.: *Endocrinology*, 69:844, 1961.
118. Mori, K. F.: *Endocrinology*, 81:1241, 1967.
119. Mori, K. F.: *J. Endocr.*, 42:55, 1968.
120. Moricard, R.: *Rev. Franç. Gynec. Obstet.*, 63:643, 1968.
121. Neill, J. D., Peckham, W. D., and Knobil, E.: *Nature*, 213:1014, 1967.
122. Nikitovitch, M., and Everett, J. W.: *Endocrinology*, 82:523, 1968.
123. Odell, W. D., Ross, G. T., and Rayford, P. L.: *Metabolism*, 15:287, 1966.
124. Odell, W. D., Ross, G. T., and Rayford, P. L.: *J. Clin. Invest.*, 46:248, 1967.
125. Orr, A. H., Ward, A. P., and Bagshave, K. D.: *J. Reprod. Fertil.*, 21:307, 1970.
126. Oostergaard, E.: Les antihormones dues aux gonadotropines, in *Les gonadotropines en gynécologie*. Paris, Masson et Cie., 1962.
127. Parlow, A. F., and Reichert, L. E.: *Endocrinology*, 72:955, 1963.

128. Pavic, D.: *J. Endocrinol.*, 26:531, 1963.
129. Perloff, W. H., and Steinberger, E.: *Acta Gin.*, 16:455, 1965.
130. Quilligan, E. J., and Rotchild, I.: *Endocrinology*, 67:48, 1960.
131. Racadot, J., and Herlant, M.: *Ann. d'Endocr.*, 21:828, 1960.
132. Rafelson, M. E., Clauser, H., and Legault, J.: *J. Biochem. Biophys. Acta*, 47:406, 1961.
133. Raiti, S., and Blizzard, R. M.: *J. Clin. Endocr.*, 28:1719, 1968.
134. Ramirez, D., and Sawyer, C. H.: *Endocrinology*, 76:1158, 1965.
135. Reichert, L. E., and Parlow, A. F.: *Endocrinology*, 73:224, 1963.
136. Reichert, L. E.: *Endocrinology*, 80:319, 1967.
137. Rice, B. F., and Segaloff, A.: *Acta Endocr.*, 51:131, 1966.
138. Rice, B. F., and Segaloff, A.: *Endocrinology*, 68:261, 1966.
139. Ringler, I., and Kliman, A.: *Endocrinology*, 63:135, 1958.
140. Rizkallah, T.: Taymor, M. L., Park, M., and Batt, R.: *J. Clin. Endocr. Metab.*, 25:943, 1965.
141. Robyn, C., Diczfalusy, E., and Finney, D. J.: *Acta Endocr.*, 58:593, 1968.
142. Robyn, C.: Unités biologiques et immunologiques des gonadotropines, in *L'ovulation*, ed. R. Moricard and J. Ferin. Paris, Masson et Cie., 1969.
143. Rotchild, I.: *Endocrinology*, 67:9, 54, 1960.
144. Rotchild, I.: *Acta Endocr.*, 49:107, 120, 1965.
145. Rosemberg, E., Joshi, S. R., and Nwe, T.: *J. Clin. Endocr.*, 28:1419, 1968.
146. Rubin, B. L., Hilliard, J., Hayward, J. N., and Deane, H. W.: *Steroids*, 5(Suppl. 1):121, 1965.
147. Ryan, R. J.: *J. Clin. Endocr.*, 28:866, 1968.
148. Sairam, M. R., Mahdwa-Raj, H., and Moudgal, N. R.: *J. Endocr.*, 40:165, 1968.
149. Sakiz, E., and Guillemin, R.: *Endocrinology*, 72:813, 1963.
150. Samli, M. H., and Geschwind, I. I.: *Endocrinology*, 81:835, 1967.
151. Santolucito, J. A., Clegg, M. T., and Cole, H. H.: *Endocrinology*, 66:273, 1960.
152. Saxena, B. B., Demura, H., Gandy, H. M., and Peterson, R. E.: *J. Clin. Endocr.*, 28:519, 1968.
153. Schmidt-Elmendorff, H., and Loraine, J. A.: *J. Endocr.*, 23:413, 1962.
154. Schwartz, N. B., and Bartosik, D.: *Endocrinology*, 71:756, 1962.
155. Smith, P. E.: *Endocrinology*, 68:131, 1961.
156. Sobel, P. E.: *Endocrinology*, 69:1108, 1961.
157. Soffer, L. J., Salvaneschi, J., and Futterweit, W.: *J. Clin. Endocr. Metab.*, 22:532, 1962.
158. Soffer, L. J., and Fogel, M.: *J. Clin. Endocr. Metab.*, 23:870, 1963.
159. Spies, H. G., Conn, L. L., and Gier, H. T.: *Endocrinology*, 78:67, 1966.
160. Spies, H. G., and Quadri, S. K.: *Endocrinology*, 80:1127, 1967.
161. Stansfield, D. A., and Robinson, J. W.: *Endocrinology*, 76:390, 1965.
162. Steelman, S. L., Segaloff, A., and Andersen, R. N.: *Fed. Proceed.*, 18:330, 1959.
163. Steinberger, E., and Duckett, G. E.: *J. Reprod. Fertil.*, Suppl. 2:75, 1967.
164. Stormshak, F., and Casida, L. E.: *Endocrinology*, 77:337, 1965.
165. Tamada, T., Soper, M., and Taymor, M. L.: *J. Clin. Endocr.*, 27:379, 1967.
166. Taymor, M. L., Goss, D. A., and Tamada, T.: *Fertil. Steril.*, 17:613, 1966.
167. Taymor, M. L., Aono, T., and Phatplace, C.: *Acta Endocr.*, 59:298, 1968.
168. Taymor, M. L., Liberman, B., and Rikzallah, T. H.: *Fertil. Steril.*, 20:267, 1969.
169. Theret, C., and Tambois, E.: *Ann. d'Endocr.*, 24:421, 1963.
170. Thomas, K., and Ferin, J.: Les gonadotropines plasmatiques ou sériques au cours du cycle menstrual; leur evaluation radioimmunologique, in *L'ovulation*, ed. R. Moricard and J. Ferin. Paris, Masson et Cie., 1969.
171. Wakabayashi, K., and Tamaoki, B. I.: *Endocrinology*, 80:409, 1967.
172. Ward, D. N., Walborg, E. F., and Adams-Mayne, A.: *Biochim. Biophys. Acta*, 50:224, 1961.
173. Wilde, C. E., Orr, A. H., and Bagshave, K. D.: *J. Endocr.*, 37:23, 1967.
174. Wilhelmi, A. E.: *Canad. J. Biochem.*, 39:659, 1963.
175. Wolthuis, O. L., and DeJongh, S. E.: *Acta Endocr.*, 43:271, 1963.
176. Yen, S. S. C., Llerena, O., Little, B., and Pearson, O. H.: *J. Clin. Endocr.*, 28:1763, 1968.
177. Zarrow, M. X., and Quinn, D. L.: *J. Endocr.*, 26:181, 1963.

Chapter 8
NERVOUS SYSTEM AND ENDOCRINE GLANDS

8.1. NEW CONCEPT IN ENDOCRINE PHYSIOLOGY

The most important advance in endocrinology over the past 10 years has been the demonstration of the fact that the *vegetative nervous system and the endocrine glands function as a single unit.*

It may be well to review the stages modern thinking had to pass through in order to arrive at this realization: (1) first it was learned that nearly all endocrine glands were controlled by the pituitary; (2) it became apparent that the pituitary was intimately related to the nervous system and that secretion took place on command from the hypothalamus, with which the pituitary acted in concert; (3) it was realized that some nervous centers, particularly those at the level of the hypothalamic region, elaborated "neurohormones" capable of regulating pituitary secretion and of acting on other distant organs through a new modality of reflexes, i.e., "neurohormonal reflexes," in which both the afferent pathway and central elaboration were neural but the efferent pathway of the reflex arc was humoral. As a result, the assertion by Harris[80] that *the endocrine glands were effectors of the nervous system* was recognized to be correct. And (4), it was found that, conversely, the nervous system, especially the hypothalamus, was influenced by, and modified its reactions in response to, hormonal activity, which is the basis of what is currently known as "feedback" effect.[165] Consequently, in addition to the science of *neuroendocrinology,* there exists the science of *endocrinoneurology,* representative of the latter being the works by Bleuler and those by Meng.

Having studied the pituitary as well as the gonadotropic hormones produced by the latter, it shall now be necessary to examine the relationship between the pituitary and the hypothalamus and the *control exerted by the nervous system over sexual function.*

8.2. INNERVATION OF FEMALE GENITAL TRACT

The autonomous nerve supply to the female genital apparatus is complex and important. Recent investigations by Mitchell,[123] Reynolds[149] and Jabonero[90] have greatly contributed to its systematization. Doyle[51] outlined the afferent neurovegetative fibers as composed of two main components: an adrenergic component comprising sympathetic fibers and a cholinergic component represented by parasympathetic fibers. The fibers of the adrenergic system originate in the sympathetic lumbar chain and link up with each other over the anterior aspect of the sacrum, forming the so-called "presacral plexus." Another important afferent sympathetic plexus is the utero-ovarian plexus, a satellite of the utero-ovarian artery and a homologue of the spermatic plexus in the male (Fig. 8–1).

The afferent parasympathetic fibers form a common trunk mainly in the pelvic nerve which, proceeding from the pelvic ganglion, reaches the uterus by way of the utero-sacral ligament. Those three systems constitute a network of nerve fibers that run along the entire uterine margin from the cervix to the point of emergence of the Fallopian tube and, from there, to the mesosalpinx and mesoovary, and as far as the most lateral portions of the broad ligament. A thickening of the lowermost seg-

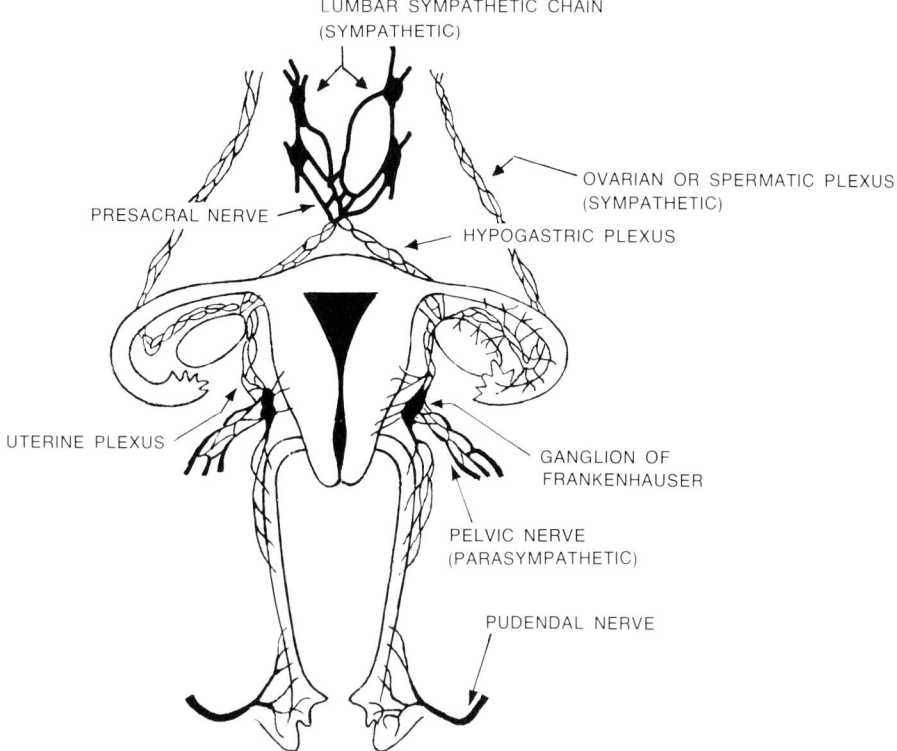

Figure 8–1. Diagram of autonomous innervation of genital tract.

ment of that plexus, inconsistently present, is known as *Frankenhäuser ganglion*.

Thus, what could be termed the *lateral müllerian autonomous plexus*, because it flanks all müllerian organs from the vagina to the abdominal extremity of the Fallopian tube, has a double sympathetic-parasympathetic structure. This system gives off branches that innervate the ovary, Fallopian tube, corpus uteri and the vagina.

8.2.1. OVARY

The nerve supply to the ovary has been studied by Hansel,[78] by Reynolds[149] and recently by Tcheng.[181] This innervation is twofold: a *parenchymal nerve supply*, and a *vascular nerve supply*. The parenchymal nerve supply is particularly important with regard to the corpus luteum, in whose formation and maintenance neurogenic stimuli are believed to play a fundamental role. The perivascular nerve supply serves a system of spiral arterioles (see Chapter 12) which were discovered and described in laboratory animals as well as in man by Reynolds.[148] Its terminal network, essentially of a vasomotor character, is implicated in the phenomenon of vasospasm responsible, as shall be pointed out later, in triggering ovulation. Therefore, a direct anatomic-functional relationship is apparent between the neurovegetative system on the one hand and ovulation and the maintenance of the corpus luteum on the other. The first of these functions is disengaged by the perivascular system, the second by the parenchymal system.

8.2.2. FALLOPIAN TUBE

In recent years, the nerve supply to the Fallopian tube has been studied by Decio[40] and by Garcia-Hernández. Analogous in function to the small bowel, this organ is similarly provided with an autonomous nervous system, and with ganglion cells in the muscle coat which are responsible for the pseudoperistaltic movements of the tube. The investigations by Rodríguez-Galindo, conducted in our laboratory, reveal that the autonomous nervous system is fundamental for the preservation of tubal motility.

8.2.3. UTERUS

We are indebted to Jabonero[90] for a complete systematization of the autonomous nerve supply to the uterus. This author found a nerve plexus in the wall of the human uterus, formed by a network of protoplasmic fibers in which interstitial cells make up the neural pole of a plexiform synapsis of remote control performance, while the other pole consists of the effector cells. In the strict sense of the word, this cannot be ascribed to the individual intervention by either these cells or the uterine walls, but rather to a global influence of the neural syncytium by means of a chemical mediator, thought to be discharged in the interstitial spaces and to act on the nonneural elements of the wall as a whole. These neural elements extend only to the musculature and to the basal layer of the endometrium.

A highly interesting question concerning the nerve supply to the uterus is whether there are any nerve fibers in the endometrium. This problem has been examined by Krantz.[104] Apparently, well outlined nerve fibers can be observed in the basal layer and around the vascular anastomoses occurring in that zone. As to the functional layer and the surroundings of the spiral arterioles, State and Hirsch in 1941 failed to recognize any kind of nerve endings. Nevertheless, it cannot be ruled out that syncytial neural elements, such as have been described by Jabonero in the endometrium, could reach the uppermost layers of the endometrium and serve as vectors of those chemical mediators which produce premenstrual vasospasm.[78] There is evidence that this may be the case under both physiologic and clinical conditions in those numerous instances in which menstruation can be precipitated by means of physostigmine or other cholinergic drugs of that group.

8.2.4. UTERINE CERVIX

According to the investigations by Suranyi,[175] the uterine cervix contains very important baroreceptor nerve endings which are responsible for the occurrence of neurohormonal reflexes whenever the cervix is induced to dilate (reflexes of Harris and Ferguson; see Section 6.8.2). The implications are that the nervous system of the female genital apparatus is involved directly in at least the following actions: (1) ovulation; (2) maintenance of the corpus luteum; (3) uterine contractility; (4) menstruation; (5) cervical dilatation, and (6) tubal motility.

8.3. THE RELEASING FACTORS OF THE HYPOTHALAMUS

As far back as 1942, we already stated the following: "For all, or at least most of all, the functions the pituitary is capable of controlling, there is a specific diencephalic center. The existence of a sexual center in the tuber cinereum can be considered as certain. That center must control pituitary secretion, since the pituitary stops secreting gonadotropins whenever the pituitary stalk is transected. Those diencephalic centers seem to control, in one way or another, the motor functions of the pituitary."

We have since come a long way in our understanding of the relationship that exists between the hypothalamus and the nearby pituitary. Though, at one time, there was no explanation for such a relationship other than *neural contact*, it has now long been known that *chemical mediators of neurohormonal nature* do provide an effective link between the gray nuclei of the base of the brain and the secretory cells of the anterior lobe by means of the hypophysioportal system (see Fig. 8-10).

During the past 10 years, enormous progress has been made concerning the nature, physiologic properties, as well as the isolation and purification of these substances. Although their chemical composition is not yet entirely known, indications are that we are dealing with polypeptides of relatively simple structure.

8.3.1. GENERALITIES

Critchlow[32] found that ovulation could be produced in rats by stimulating the hypothalamus electrically. The stereotaxic localization of the sexual center (Fig. 8-3) has been achieved by Everett,[57] by Lisk[112] and by Gorski.[66] Similar studies to localize that center in batrachia have been undertaken by Dierick.[44]

The various hypothalamic centers excite not only gonadotropic activity but other types of pituitary activity. They have been shown to stimulate thyroid function,[81] ad-

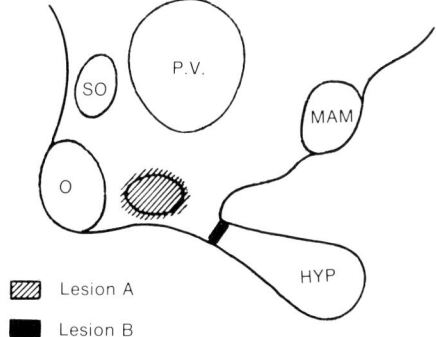

Figure 8–2. Effect of injury to hypothalamic area on sexual function in the ewe. Lesion A produces sexual frigidity, but neither ovarian maturation nor the cycle is interrupted. Lesion B causes arrest of the cycle but does not alter sex attraction. SO, Supraoptic nucleus; P.V., paraventricular nucleus; O, optic chiasm; MAM, mamillary body; HYP, hypophysis. (From Clegg and Ganong: *Endocrinology*, 67:179, 1960.)

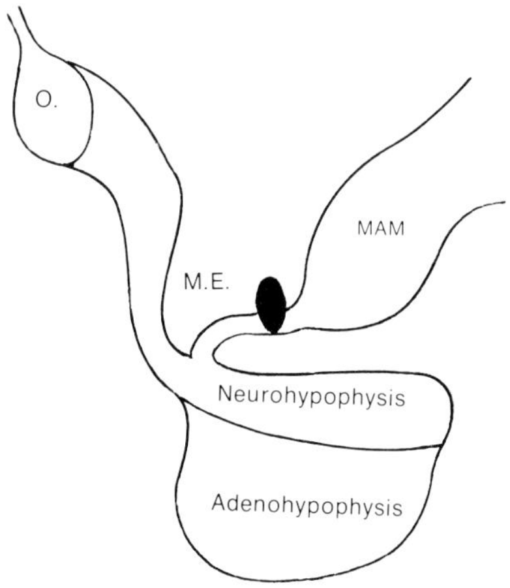

Figure 8–3. Location of sexual center in the median eminence of the rat. M.E., Median eminence; MAM, mamillary body; O, optic chiasm. (From Sawyer et al.: *Endocrinology*, 73:342, 1963.)

renal cortical function,[141] growth hormone activity,[162] and in some animals, the secretion of melanogenic hormone.[94] In addition, electrical stimulation of those centers has been shown to inhibit the secretion of prolactin.[120] Consequently, adenohypophysial function in its entirety would appear to be regulated by the centers of this region (Figs. 8–4 and 8–5).

The realization that, contrary to earlier belief, the regulatory mechanism involved is of humoral, and not neural, nature has evolved only recently. While stimulation of the hypothalamic median eminence produces ovulation in rats,[57] ovulation fails to occur if the pituitary stalk has previously been severed. It has also been shown that pituitary transplants to the kidney lose all secretory activity except for prolactin. However, if the same pituitary tissue is retransplanted to the hypothalamus,[41, 52, 133] it retrieves its capacity for secreting all of the principles. Apart from that, Moghilewsky and his colleagues[124] have found that, as far as the entire region of the median eminence of the rat hypothalamus is concerned, *oxygen consumption* is *cyclic* in the female but it is not so in the male. This

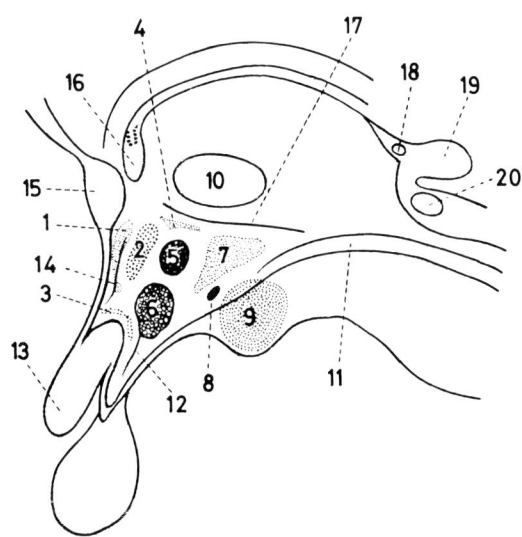

Figure 8–4. Diagram of the basal gray nuclei and their relationship to the pituitary. 1, Supraoptic nucleus; 2, paraventricular nucleus; 3, lower portion of supraoptic nucleus; 4, dorsal hypothalamic area; 5, dorsomedial hypothalamic nucleus; 6, ventromedial hypothalamic nucleus; 7, posterior hypothalamic nucleus; 8, premamillary nucleus; 9, mamillary nucleus; 10, intermediate mass; 11, limiting sulcus; 12, lateral infundibular sulcus; 13, optic chiasm; 14, anterior intracerebral sulcus; 15, anterior commissure; 16, interventricular foramen; 17, ventral diencephalic sulcus; 18, habenular commissure; 19, epiphysis; 20, posterior commissure.

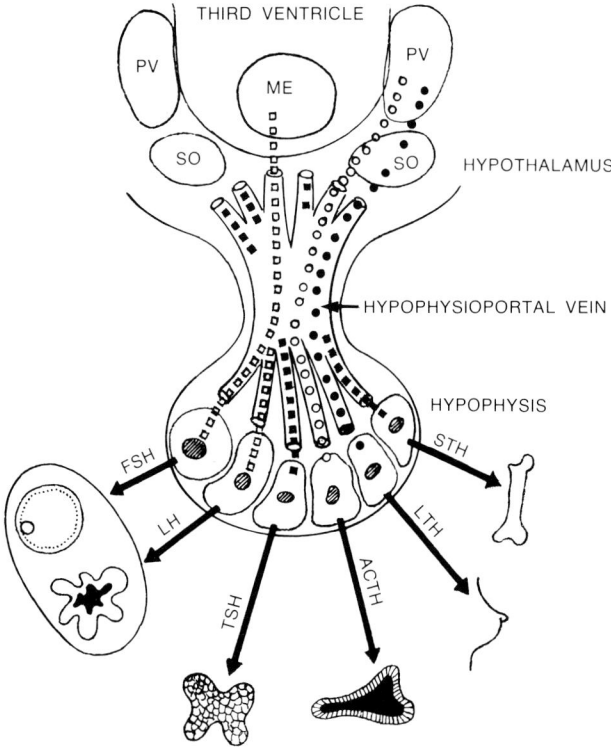

Figure 8–5. Diagram of hypothalamic action on the adenohypophysis by means of chemical mediators. ME, Median eminence; PV, paraventricular nucleus; SO, supraoptic nucleus.

raises the question of a possible hypothalamic cycle, existing alongside that observed in the pituitary (see page 123) and that seen in the genital organs (see Chapter 13).

An excellent recent review of the whole question of hypothalamic influence on adenohypophysial function has been made by Schally and Arimura.[165]

In the same way, if extracts from the hypothalamic median eminence are locally injected into a pituitary with a previously transected stalk, restitution of lost pituitary function ensues.[114, 163] Intracarotid injections of hypothalamic extracts are capable of eliciting discharges of different pituitary principles.[133] None of these phenomena would be possible if the connections in-

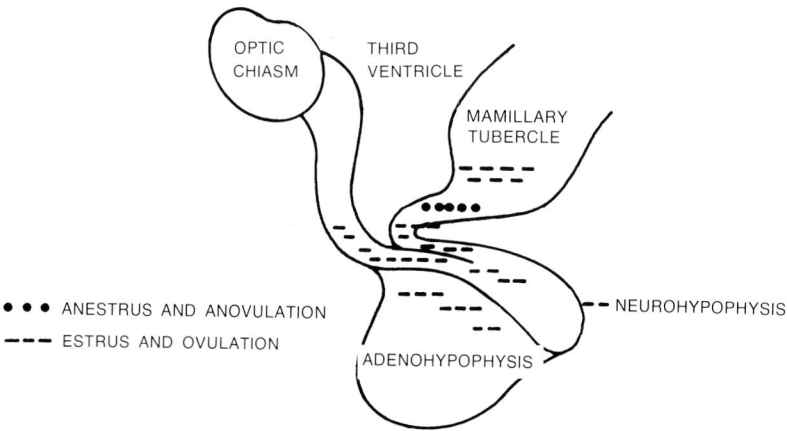

Figure 8–6. Results of stereotaxic stimulation of the hypophysiothalamic region in the rat. (From Harris, Reed and Fawcett: *Brit. Med. Bull.*, 22:266, 1966.)

volved were neural; to account for the transmission of the stimuli to the adenohypophysis, it is necessary to admit the existence of a blood-borne humoral substance, in this case conveyed by the hypophysioportal system.

It has additionally been shown[57, 109, 115] that injection of hypothalamic extracts resulted in decreased presence of active pituitary principles. Such an effect by hypothalamic extracts would therefore not seem to be consistent with biocatalytic action on pituitary hormone synthesis but rather with action involving *"release"* of pituitary hormones.

Hence, the term *"releasing factors"* has been given to the agents under consideration. In the abbreviated form, they are designated with the capital letters RF.

Currently, at least five different hypothalamic principles of this type are presumed to exist:

LHRF or releasing factor for luteinizing hormone.

FSHRF or releasing factor for follicle-stimulating hormone.

CRF or releasing factor for corticotropin.

TRF or releasing factor for thyrotropin.

GHRF or releasing factor for growth hormone.

Also isolated in some animals was MRF, or releasing factor for melanocyte-stimulating hormone.

There seems to be no special releasing factor for prolactin, but there does exist an inhibiting factor (PIF or factor inhibiting prolactin secretion) which also originates in the hypothalamic centers.

In a recent publication, Ratner and associates[145] considered the following tests as necessary for the demonstration of the existence of a specific factor:

(1) Destruction of a given area of the hypothalamus must produce a change in the secretion of a particular hormone.

(2) The factor in question must be extracted from the hypothalamus.

(3) The factor must modify the secretion of the tropin in question. In that case, the ideal animal test would be one in which a hypothalamic lesion, e.g., section of the pituitary stalk, interrupts neural control of the pituitary.

(4) The factor must be effective when applied directly to the pituitary in vivo, for instance, by means of microinjection of the test substance into the gland.

(5) The factor must be effective when applied directly to pituitary tissue in vitro.

(6) The factor must be detectable in the blood of the hypophysioportal system.

(7) In order to demonstrate that the factor plays a true physiologic role in controlling a given pituitary hormone, it is necessary to prove that factor blood levels are altered in those conditions that affect secretion of the hormone involved. For example, FSHRF in castration, etc.

8.3.2. LHRF (LUTEINIZING HORMONE RELEASING FACTOR)

This factor was first discovered and has been studied in most detail. In 1961, MacCann and Taleisnik[113] became aware of the fact that when extracts from the median eminence were injected into rats, the LH blood levels of the injected rats would rise, which has subsequently been confirmed by Gay and his colleagues.[64] The concentration of the latter principle has been found to be elevated in the blood of the hypophysioportal system.[60, 98] It was later shown that injection of such extracts produced ovulation in the same animal.[134] The injection of hypothalamic extract into the pituitary stalk also caused increased LH production.[129, 130] Highly suggestive in this respect are the observations by Ramirez and Sawyer[143] who reported that at the time of ovulation, with rising LH concentrations in the blood and urine, the adenohypophysial content of the same hormone decreased and the hypothalamic content of LHRF was equally minimal. That observation was later confirmed by Chowers and MacCann.[30] Intrapituitary injection of that extract,[25, 52] as well as addition of such extract to pituitary tissue cultured in vitro,[155] caused increased LH production.

It was further possible to demonstrate that coitus in rats provoked a reflex discharge of that principle and that illumination had a favorable effect on LHRF production.[79] If the suprachiasmatic neurogenic connections were severed,[1] the production of LHRF was interrupted.

This factor plays a role not only in males but also in females. Yamashita[197] has shown that the release of ICSH is controlled by an analogous substance originating in the median eminence of the tuber cinereum.

Electron microscopic studies by Knowles and Bern,[101] as well as by Ishii,[89] have revealed the presence of neurosecretory granules within the cells of the median eminence in rats. Those granules are most abundant in conjunction with estrus and decrease in number after the onset of ovulation. It should be kept in mind that, as a result of interrupting the connections between the suprachiasmatic region and the median eminence of the hypothalamus, ovulation in female rats is blocked, which justifies the assumption that the median eminence of the hypothalamus is subject to neural stimuli originating in other parts of the brain. This substance has been conclusively shown to be distinct from FSHRF (follicle-stimulating hormone releasing factor), which is discussed subsequently. The methods used to achieve purifications of this type shall be indicated when discussing the chemistry of these compounds.

The purified product contains neither FSHRF[31] nor PIF (prolactin inhibiting factor), as demonstrated by Arimura and colleagues.[3] Finally, it should be pointed out that MacCann and his group[116] have been unable to reproduce any of the effects of LHRF either with oxytocin, vasopressin or serotonin, or with any other compounds of this group. However, modern studies[99, 107, 177, 198] have shown that *pentothal*, *chlorpromazine* and *reserpine* all inhibit the sexual center and block secretion of LHRF.

8.3.3. FSHRF (FOLLICLE-STIMULATING HORMONE RELEASING FACTOR)

Though customarily FSH is considered before luteinizing gonadotropin because of the fact that its action precedes that of LH in time, this order has been inverted here because of the later discovery of FSHRF. Indeed, a great many authors believed[56, 57, 88, 129, 143] that a single factor released both gonadotropins. However, recent investigations by Schally and associates[163] produced evidence of two distinct factors which by chromatography on Sephadex-25 give two separate and independent bands.

A special characteristic of FSHRF is that of being inactivated by both Puromycin and Actinomycin.[193]

Upon injection, the compound isolated in a pure state[154, 164] has been shown to cause the depletion of pituitary FSH but not that of LH.[88, 106] Recent studies concerning purification of that factor demonstrate that it is a polypeptide with an approximate molecular weight of 2000.[43, 163] Therefore, it would seem to differ from LHRF whose molecular weight is lesser (approximately 1400). Experimental work with the purified compound has demonstrated effects on both females and males, by indirectly producing follicular maturation in the former and by eliciting spermatogenesis in the latter.[162, 163]

It would also seem that in terms of responding to local injection of steroids into the hypothalamus, this substance behaves in a different way since, while estrogens produce release of LHRF, progestogens are responsible for releasing FSHRF.

In recent years, the possible mode of action of these substances has been under scrutiny. Classically,[36] they were thought to act by virtue of altering membrane permeability of the cells of the adenohypophysis, enabling the corresponding gonadotropin to escape across the membrane. However, more recent studies by Justisz and associates[92, 93] and by Taymor[180] seem to support the concept that they act not only as releasing agents of the cell-confined gonadotropins of the adenohypophysis but also as biocatalysts necessary for the synthesis of the same hormones.

As yet, there is no consensus on the subject. While Schally's group claims to have encountered gonadotropin depletion of the pituitary following injection of the releasing factors, French scholars,[72, 92, 93] on the other hand, believe that synthesis of the glycoprotein moiety of gonadotropins is thereby enhanced.

8.3.4. PIF (PROLACTIN-INHIBITING FACTOR)

It has been a well known fact[32, 56, 57, 161] for some time that destruction of the median eminence of the hypothalamus by different pathologic processes gives rise to a syndrome characterized by amenorrhea, galactorrhea and lack of ovulation, which has been known by the name of Chiari-Frommel syndrome or, in one given case, by the name of "syndrome of Argonz and del Castillo." Conversely, stimulation of the median eminence produces enhanced ovarian activity,[112] but also inhibition of mammary secretion.[134] It has already been pointed out that, in transplants of pituitary tissue to sites outside its natural localization—for example, the kidney[59, 61, 133, 134, 135]—the gland ceases to elaborate all of the hormonotropic principles with the exception of prolactin. All this would seem to suggest that pituitary function, insofar as prolactin secretion is concerned, is diametrically opposed to that of the other hormones, and that what the median eminence secretes is not a prolactin-releasing factor but, quite the contrary, a *prolactin-inhibiting factor.*

As shown by Sinha and Meites,[172] hypothalamic extracts excite ovarian activity at the same time that they inhibit mammary activity. In contrast, ideas prevailing until recently[32, 56, 163] postulated that one and the same compound both stimulated the release of gonadotropin and inhibited the release of prolactin. At any rate, recent studies do not seem to support this view.

First of all, pituitary cells cultured in vitro[179] secrete no gonadotropic hormone other than prolactin. However, addition to the culture media of purified hypothalamic extracts induces production of the remaining gonadotropins[4] without inhibiting the continued elaboration of prolactin. The inavailability of sufficiently purified extracts in earlier experiments[159] to allow differentiation of prolactin-inhibiting effects from gonadotropin-stimulating effects. However, this has become possible recently.[4, 41, 183]

Attention must be called to the fact that both suckling of the nipple and administration of reserpine are capable of blocking the inhibitory effect on prolactin activity, by depressing the release of PIF,[120, 122] without affecting the rate of gonadotropin production. In the same way, if estrogens are introduced into the median eminence,[194] or into the amygdaloid nucleus,[183] a stimulatory effect on gonadotropin function is produced without altering the rate of prolactin secretion.

Finally, it must be emphasized that the role of the prolactin-inhibiting factor in birds is quite different.[103, 130] Those animals produce a factor that stimulates prolactin release and, indirectly, enhances the secretory activity of the gland of the crop. Though exerting a similarly positive action, that factor is distinct from the gonadotropin-releasing factor.

Therefore, the property of the pituitary to produce prolactin when free from inhibitory influences, and to cease releasing prolactin whenever in direct contact with hypothalamus-derived chemical mediators, is an *exclusive characteristic of the mammalian pituitary.*

Though it is equally well governed by the hypothalamus, prolactin is the only pituitary hormone that is not stimulated but is on the contrary inhibited by the hypothalamus.

8.3.5. TRF (THYROTROPIN RELEASING FACTOR)

A centrogenic regulatory mechanism of thyroid function, as exemplified by the term "hypothalamic hyperthyroidism," has long been suspected. Harris,[81] in 1959, and Blanquet[17] in 1961, found that electric stimulation of the hypothalamus in experimental animals produced hyperplasia of the thyroid gland. In 1962, Shizume and Matsuda demonstrated increased trapping of ^{131}I by the thyroid glands of rats after the animals' hypothalami had been electrically stimulated. Greer and Erwin[69] showed that propylthiouracil had no effect on the thyroid of those animals in which the hypothalamus had previously been destroyed.

Evidence that the releasing factor involved was essentially identical with previously studied factors was obtained by Guillemin's group.[71, 72] In fact, pituitary transplants to the kidney lacked any thyrotropic activity, but if reimplanted into the region of the hypothalamus, such activity was reestablished.[41, 52, 130, 132, 133] Averill and his colleagues[6, 7] demonstrated the presence in the hypophysioportal system of a factor that stimulated thyrotropin secretion.

By means of a test performed on mice, Redding and associates[146, 147] proved that factor to be different from vasopressin, serotonin, norepinephrine and oxytocin.

Purification of this factor has been achieved by both Schally's group[162] and Guillemin's group.[21] Four micrograms of bovine or porcine hypothalamic extract are sufficient to release TSH in rat pituitaries. It is not certain whether this active extract is a polypeptide, as has so far been believed, since it is not affected by either pepsin or trypsin.[21, 72]

Nevertheless, there is no doubt that we are dealing with one more factor playing a most important role in controlling adenohypophysial function.

8.3.6. CRF (CORTICOTROPIN RELEASING FACTOR)

It has been generally assumed[73, 136] that corticotropin release was mediated by vasopressin. However, up-to-date studies indicate that although vasopressin indirectly favors this release,[73] *it is not an active ACTH releasing agent.*

Laszlo and Wied[108] observed that after sectioning the pituitary stalk, the pituitary-adrenal axis tests (Thorn test, etc.) became negative. Similarly, according to Halasz and co-workers,[76] stimulation of the medial basal hypothalamus led to a discharge of ACTH. The stimulative response normally elicited by various compounds, such as epinephrine, serotonin, vasopressin, or simply stress agents, is absent if the median eminence has been injured (Porter and co-workers[141]). Arimura and his associates[4] developed a bioassay procedure for the demonstration of CRF (corticotropin releasing factor) and have been able to demonstrate that CRF secretion is inhibited by dexamethasone, chlorpromazine or morphine. Of all hypothalamic factors, this is perhaps the one that is most actively stimulated by various neurohormones. What has long been suspected has been confirmed by Chambers and co-workers,[28] viz., that vasopressin acts on the median eminence by eliciting a discharge of CRF. This reaction, however, is absent if the median center of the hypothalamus is destroyed.

Thus, not only the gonadotropins and thyrotropin but also ACTH is controlled by the median eminence of the hypothalamus by means of a releasing factor whose chemical structure appears to be simple but is not yet fully known.

8.3.7. GHRF (GROWTH HORMONE RELEASING FACTOR)

Until relatively recently, growth hormone was not thought to be controlled by any releasing factor. In general, all adenohypophysial hormones are subject to a rapid rhythm of secretion, and this determines the necessity for their prompt release and for their short-lived action. Growth hormone is admittedly the only hormone to be endowed with a less rapid mode of action and has therefore not been suspected to be involved in "rapid neurohormonal reflexes." There is no doubt that growth hormone, or STH as it is also called, intervenes in regulating carbohydrate metabolism, a poorly studied and poorly known subject, in which the need for an "acute" neural regulatory mechanism most certainly must be envisioned.

Demonstration of the releasing principles for growth hormone has required above all the development, in this case by Krulich and MacCann[105] and by Müller and Pecile,[126] of bioassay methods similar to the ones applicable to other releasing factors.

A substance has been obtained from the hypothalamus of sows, cows and ewes which, when properly purified and injected into the carotid artery of a rat, produces depletion of ACTH (Müller and co-workers[127, 128]). Similarly, when bovine hypothalamic extract is added to cultures of pituitary tissue or is injected into the pituitary locally,[162] it produces release of STH, a fact upon which the corresponding test, using the distal cartilage, etc., is based. It was also possible to demonstrate that resected rat pituitaries, grafted beneath the renal capsule,[96, 127, 164] no longer stimulated growth of the long bones but, in turn, would again do so if they were removed from that location and reimplanted into the region of the hypothalamus. In keeping with the previously stated postulates, this seems to be sufficient evidence to accept the existence of a releasing factor for growth hormone, GHRF, which, as will be seen later, has already been isolated and purified.

A most interesting feature about this factor is the finding that the hypothalamus of experimental animals is highly sensitive to hypoglycemia to which it reacts by discharging this factor.[96, 127] *This means that the hypothalamus partakes in regulating glycemia by means of discharges of the releasing factor for the hyperglycemia inducing hormone.* The classic experiment described by Claude Bernard, in which puncture of the hypothalamus produced diabetes in a rabbit, probably resulted from stimulation of the median eminence of the hypothalamus, apparently the site the eminent French physiologist had stimulated with his famous "puncture."

It should be further stressed that drugs causing norepinephrine depletion, such as reserpine and the like, also produces release of this factor.[128] When injected into the vicinity of the median hypothalamic center, epinephrine and norepinephrine both provoke a discharge of GHRF and, as a result, hyperglycemia. Is this possibly one of the mechanisms of action on glycemia by epinephrine?

8.3.8. MSHRF (MELANOCYTE-STIMULATING HORMONE RELEASING FACTOR)

Schally and his group,[94, 162] as well as Taleisnik and Tomats,[176] have detected the presence of a factor in animals, causing release of melanocyte-stimulating hormone. In the human species and in higher mammals, this principle is apparently devoid of action and its presence in the human hypothalamus has not been demonstrated. However, it has been found to be present in some animals, e.g., the bull and the hog, that would seem to have no active melanogenic function.

8.3.9. CHEMISTRY OF RELEASING FACTORS

At present there is no doubt that the previously mentioned releasing factors can be separated from oxytocin and vasopressin and that they have a distinct individuality. MacCann and Ramirez[114] have undertaken the exhaustive task of extracting active principles from the median eminence, from the preoptic, supraoptic and paraventricular nuclei and from other hypothalamic centers. They concluded that only extracts from the median eminence possessed releasing activity; in comparison, the supraoptic and paraventricular nuclei, known to produce vasopressin and oxytocin, have been found by them to be functionally inert in that respect. MacCann and his group[115, 116] have been able to show that thioglycolate, which inactivates both vasopressin and oxytocin, does not affect the activity of either TRF or CRF.

Dhariwal[43] has isolated various active principles from bovine hypothalamic extracts. The method used was chromatography with Sephadex G-25, giving distinct distribution bands for FSHRF and LHRF, as well as for TRF, CRF and GHRF.

The studies of the above authors suggest that we are dealing with a group of possible polypeptide compounds, the molecular weight of which oscillates between 1400 and 2000, which would indicate that they are relatively simple compounds. However, in view of the finding that they are resistant to pepsin or trypsin digestion and that some of them are devoid of sulfur, there may be some doubt as to whether they indeed are polypeptides. This question is still open to debate. Though the chemical composition of these factors is as yet unknown, it is to be hoped that, at the present advanced stage of research into their biochemistry, the next few months or years will reveal the definite chemical structure of these important compounds.

Work so far has been focused mainly on the separation and purification of the releasing factors for FSH and for LH, and on that of PIF. Currently, it can be stated that these objectives have been fully accomplished for each of the three factors by four different groups of investigators: one in Paris (Guillemin[72]), one in Texas (MacCann and Dhariwal[116]), another in Oxford (Fawcett and colleagues[58]), and a fourth in New Orleans (Schally and co-workers[162–164]).

The approximate structural formula of LHRF was first suggested by the New Orleans group. Guided by that formula, Schally[158] recently synthesized LHRF and obtained a synthetic product of exactly the same composition, revealing identical releasing properties as those of purified extracts of the median eminence. The experimental efforts aimed at cracking the complete formula of LHRF have thus been completed.

Recently, Butt[21] has also indicated the formula of CRF. Here too it can be clearly seen that we are dealing with polypeptides, composed of chains of amino acids linked up in a manner similar to oxytocin (discussed later), vasopressin, serotonin and other neurohormones.

8.4. RELATIONSHIP OF HYPOTHALAMUS TO THE REST OF THE BRAIN

The hypothalamic center is unquestionably a regulatory organ of utmost importance, since it purveys adenohypophysial function as a whole. Regarding sexual function, which has been the question by far the best studied, there is no doubt whatsoever that the hypothalamus is the center of control in both the female and the male, particularly of the cycle in the former. The female sexual cycle, which is a phenomenon of "internal rhythm of the body," must necessarily be controlled by a neural organ and not by an endocrine one. In this respect, it is of interest to consider the connecting pathways linking this center to the cerebral cortex and particularly to the limbic system.

According to numerous reports,[2, 37, 77] transection of the neural connections to the median eminence results in suspension of cycling in rats. Similarly, neurogenic isolation of the median eminence is followed by the disappearance of pseudocyesis.[27] Of special importance are the connections of the sexual center with the limbic system, primarily the *amygdaloid nucleus*, destruction of which causes loss of LHRF in mice[53] and rats,[54] whereas conversely, stimulation of which produces increased plasma LH concentrations in rats.[186]

8.5. EFFECT OF STEROIDS ON THE MEDIAN EMINENCE

However, one aspect of major interest to be visualized only recently is the fact that the hypothalamus itself is in turn the "chemoreceptor" of a series of humoral alterations that precipitate its own activity and, consequently, its very action as a regulator. This has been illustrated in a preceding chapter in connection with the matter of hypothalamic control of hypoglycemia; it is therefore not surprising that the variable hormone levels occurring in the female in the course of the cycle should determine fluctuations in median eminence function, and that the variable, albeit noncyclic, testosterone levels in the male could be the determinant of sexual activity.

Indisputable evidence is accumulating that estrogens, androgens, as well as progestogens, exert definite effects on this center.

8.5.1. ESTROGENS

Some years ago, Westman[195] was able to demonstrate that labeled estrogens were trapped by the hypothalamus. More recently, this finding was confirmed by Kato and Villee.[95] If microcrystals of estrogens are stereotaxically implanted in the median eminence or any other part of the hypothalamus or anterior pituitary, the resulting effects that are observed differ according to the site of implantation. Implantation in the anterior pituitary produces increased secretion of both gonadotropins; in the nonsexual portion of the hypothalamus, estrogens produce no effect; whereas implantation in the median eminence produces release of LHRF and inhibits the synthesis of FSHRF.[137] The studies by Palka and Sawyer[136, 157] have shown that the only estrogen-sensitive site in the anterior hypothalamus is the premamillary zone, right in the median eminence. Chowers[30] and Doecke[46] reported that local injection of microquantities of estrogens in this zone caused local depletion of LHRF but, conversely, increased the amounts of the latter substance in the blood of the porta-pituitary vein, which can be construed as evidence that estrogens provide the stimulus necessary for the release of LH, just as has been suspected on the basis of indirect tests, the above experiments being the first instance in which objective evidence to this effect has become available (Fig. 8–7).

Nallar and MacCann[129] have shown that the plasma LHRF content, the determination of which has recently become possible, is considerably elevated in hypophysectomized animals. A compensatory phenomenon, due to absent pituitary function, is undoubtedly involved. However, if such a hypophysectomized animal is injected with estrogens, secretion and appearance in the peripheral blood of LHRF ceases immediately, which seems to underscore the fact that once the ultimate objective, that is, maintenance of steroid homeostasis and estrogen balance, is achieved, the hypothalamus suspends its function. Similar phenomena have also been described by Piacsek and Meites.[138, 139]

Estrogens probably also act on other areas of the cerebrum than the median eminence, which are neurally interconnected with it, though at some distance from the latter. Thus, the preoptic region, known to be linked by nerve fibers to the median eminence, is just as sensitive to local injection of estrogens, the response being the same as that obtained with local estrogen injection into the hypothalamic sexual center (Lincoln and Cross[110]). The same is true if estrogens are implanted in the *amygdaloid nucleus* (Tindall and colleagues[183]). This of course means that, in addition to the sexual nucleus itself, the

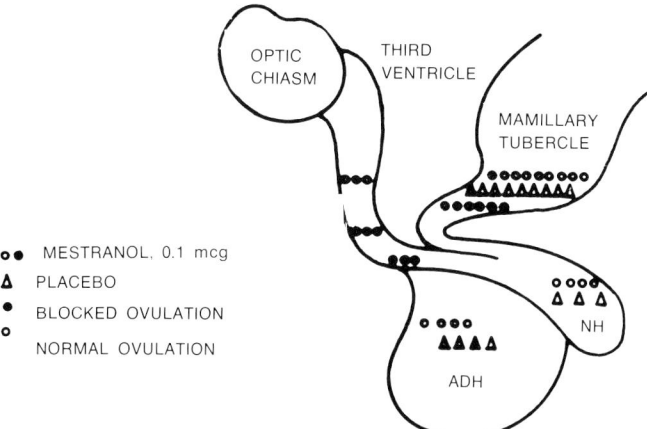

Figure 8–7. Effects of implantation of estrogen microcrystals (Mestranol) into the hypothalamico-pituitary region in female rat. (Based on data from Starup: *Acta Endocr.*, 51:469, 1966.)

higher centers that regulate the activity of the sexual nucleus are equally susceptible to changes in estrogen levels.

It has recently been asserted (Ratner and colleagues[145]; Motta and co-workers[125]) that the sexual centers are specially sensitive to estrogens during certain periods of life. One of these is the prepuberal age, another the puerperium. It must be kept in mind that, immediately after parturition, estrogens may exert quite dangerous and irreversible effects on the sexual center of the hypothalamus.

The "feedback" effect on the median eminence by estrogens is biphasic: Goldzieher and associates[74] have shown that whereas such small dosages of estrogens as are encountered under physiologic conditions during the cycle in both women and female rodents produce the release of LH, synthetic estrogens (Ethinylestradiol or Mestranol) in dosages exceeding 100 mcg a day inhibit LHRF and suppress ovulation in women, as will be pointed out in detail in the final part of this book (see Section 47.3.1, Table 47–1). Moreover, it should be noted that, independently of this unquestionable effect on the hypothalamus, estrogens also have a *direct effect* on the pituitary.[97, 168]

8.5.2. PROGESTOGENS

Sawyer and Kawakami[157] have been able to inhibit LHRF secretion in the median eminence by means of locally implanting microcrystals of progesterone. Radford and co-workers[142] believe that secretion of LHRF is equally dependent on either increased estrogen activity or the reduced inhibitory action by progesterone. On the contrary, Caligaris and colleagues[24] have found that progesterone as well as synthetic progestogens enhance the production of FSHRF in rats. However, our own observations on humans, and more recently those of Keever and Greenwald,[100] seem to indicate that progesterone has no effect on FSH release in the human species (this will be discussed later).

8.5.3. ANDROGENS

The effects of androgens on the hypothalamus have been brought to light by recent studies.[45, 118, 138, 192] Small dosages apparently produce stimulatory effects while, just as with the other steroids, large dosages are inhibitory. This phenomenon is of special importance in weanling rats and, in general, in young females. Wagner and associates[192] have found that neonatal treatment with microcrystals of androgens implanted in the hypothalamus *sterilizes the rats*, a finding also confirmed by Matsuyama and co-workers.[118] According to Doecke and Koloczek,[45] such sterilization is not due to suppression of sexual function of the median eminence but simply to the fact that *testosterone interrupts the alternate rhythm between LHRF and FSHRF, whereby the cycle disappears and the animal is rendered anovulatory.* A similar pathogenetic mechanism is possibly also involved in certain types of human sterility (Greenblatt, Botella) that are due to a moderate increase of androgenic activity, and, in the former author's view, this is also the pathogenesis of the anovulatory cycle in the Stein-Leventhal syndrome (see Chapter 29). As a final note of interest, it should be mentioned that if androgenized juvenile rats are injected with the anti-androgenic agent *cyproterone* (Section 4.7.5), the inhibitory hypothalamic effect does not take place.[2a]

8.6. GENERAL SIGNIFICANCE OF THE NEUROHORMONES OF THE MEDIAN EMINENCE

Thus, after having for many years believed that the organ controlling endocrine economy is the pituitary, we are now learning that the driver's seat actually belongs to the hypothalamus. It has been known for several decades that the posterior pituitary, or neurohypophysis, is really not a secretory organ but an organ responsible for channeling the neurohormones into the peripheral circulation. Thanks to the eventual isolation of the releasing factors, it has now become evident that the adenohypophysis, or anterior pituitary, is in fact but an obedient instrument manipulated by that crucial center, the median eminence of the tuber cinereum, which seems to regulate not only sexual activity but all phenomena of stress, thyroid function, glycogenolysis and lactation.

In the course of the past few years, special importance has been attached to the *role played by the hypothalamus in initiating puberty.* Indeed, puberty would seem to be determined by setting off the cyclic release of the gonadotropins of the anterior pituitary. The capacity of the adenohypophysis for secreting these compounds would seem to have been established in advance, and it behooves the hypothalamus, as the regulator of the rhythmic phenomena of the economy, to determine the precise time for the onset of puberty. The studies of Elwers and Critchlow,[55] and those of Ramirez and Sawyer,[143] reveal the fundamental part played by the sexual center of the hypothalamus in setting off puberty in rats. There is no doubt that the same phenomenon that has been reported by these investigators to occur in rodents also occurs in the human species, in which the occurrence of both pure neurogenic precocious puberty, without any endocrine alteration, and retarded puberty, determined by neuropathic phenomena, are only too well known.

8.6.1. EFFECT OF LIGHT ON THE PITUITARY

In the same way, a number of effects that sensory organs seem to exert on sexual life may be explained as resulting from a similar mechanism. For instance, the effect of light on animal estrus, described by Benoit and Bisonette more than 30 years ago, has now been found—as reported by Lincoln and Cross[110] and by Piacsek and Meites[138,139,140]—to be due to stimulation of the median eminence by *light* via the optic tracts of association.

Conversely, Donovan,[50] Singh and Greenwald[171] and Hoffmann,[87] among others, have shown that prolonged darkness produced equally prolonged anestrus in rats and mice. Aside from this, Relkin[148] reported the appearance of precocious puberty as a consequence of constant illumination of the litter, and Negro-Vilar and colleagues[131] found continuous elevation of FSHRF values under such conditions. It therefore seems certain that the release of gonadotropins by light is carried out by way of *optic-hypothalamic connections.*

Work by Grosvenor and Mena[70] revealed the fact that visual stimuli may affect secretion of milk. The inhibitory factor for milk secretion (PIF) can be stimulated not only by visual but also by auditory and olfactory stimuli. Those observations have been corroborated by Minagouchi and Meites.[122]

8.6.2. EFFECT OF CATECHOLAMINES ON THE HYPOTHALAMIC SEXUAL CENTER

An interesting development of the last years, which offers further proof of the functional interrelationships between the autonomous nervous system and sexual function, is the finding that catecholamines have an effect on the hypothalamic sex centers. Donoso and colleagues[48,49] came up with evidence that castration in rats resulted in increased hypothalamic norepi-

Nervous System and Endocrine Glands

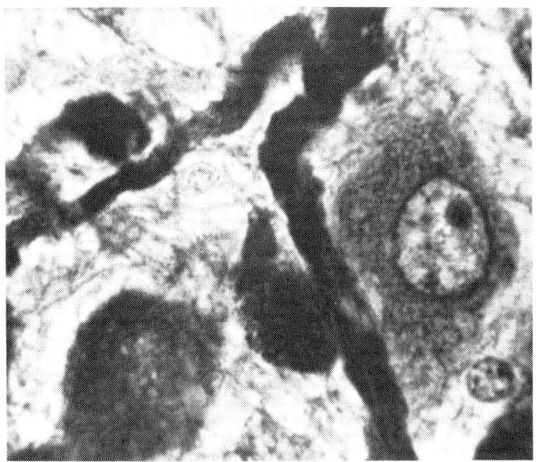

Figure 8-8. Neuron in the supraoptic nucleus of a dog, with scanty secretion. Adjacent to it is the process of another neuron completely filled with secretion. (From Bargmann.[10])

nephrine concentrations, while Stefano and Donoso[174] and Sandler[156] found that the hypothalamic norepinephrine content varied in accordance with the different stages of the cycle. Norepinephrine inhibits LHRF (Lippmann and colleagues[111]) as well as PIF (Birge and co-workers[15]). In dosages stimulating LH release, estrogens reduce hypothalamic catecholamine concentrations (Deutsch[42]), a finding that correlates well with the preceding data. Lending support to the above findings are also the observations by Kamberi[99] and Schneider,[167] both colleagues of MacCann's, that *dopamine* enhances the release of both FSH and LH.

It has been established that catecholamines inhibit LHRF and PIF production by the median eminence, which has led to speculation (Halasz and Gorski[77]) that the mode of action whereby the epiphysis as well as other zones of the cerebrum inhibit puberty may be mediated by the inhibitory action of norepinephrine or other substances of this group.

8.7. OXYTOCIN AND VASOPRESSIN

8.7.1. SITE OF ORIGIN OF THE SO-CALLED RETROHYPOPHYSIAL HORMONES

Our ideas concerning oxytocin and the other hormones of the "posterior lobe of the pituitary" have undergone profound modifications during the last years. The fundamental investigations by Bargmann,[10] Harris[80, 81] and Hild[85, 86] produced evidence that these substances did not originate in the neurohypophysis, as had hitherto been presumed, but were simply transferred there from nerve endings into the vascular tree. The presumptive retrohypophysial hormones are thought to be secreted within the cytoplasm of the neurons of the hypothalamic centers: the *supraoptic nucleus* and the *paraventricular nucleus*. From there they are believed to be conveyed along axon cylinders down to where, at the

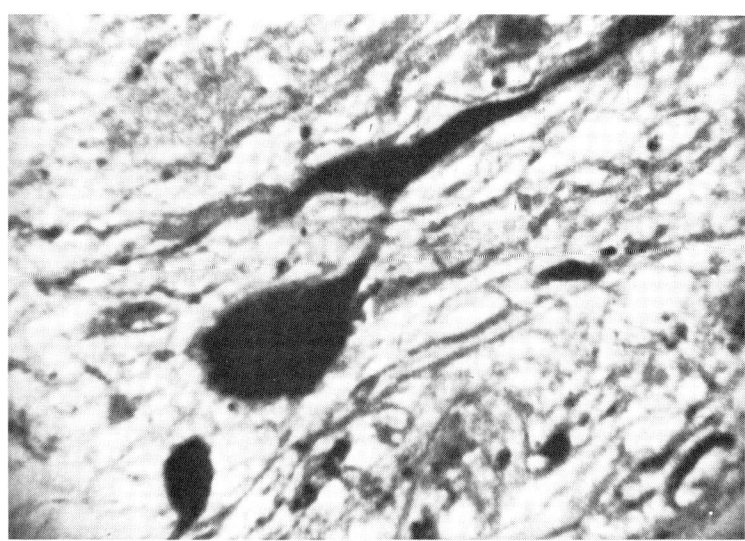

Figure 8-9. Secretion-laden cell processes in the posterior lobe of the dog pituitary. (From Bargmann.[10])

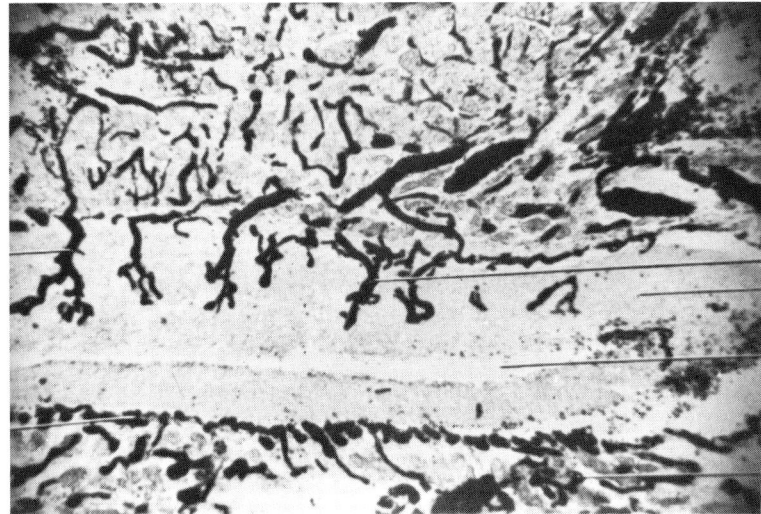

Figure 8-10. Hypophysioportal system, exposed by injection of infundibular region in rat. (From Bargmann.[10])

level of the posterior lobe of the pituitary, they gain entry into the bloodstream (Figs. 8-11 and 8-12).

This is what constitutes neurosecretion in the true sense of the word; and the cells of the gray nuclei at the floor of the third ventricle are true neurosecretory cells, by Scharrer's standards,[166] so that the floor of that ventricle may be conceived of as an *organ of internal secretion*. From now on, oxytocin and vasopressin will be referred to as neurohormones.

The neurohormones possess properties that are somewhat different from those of ordinary hormones. Their secretion can only be induced by neural impulses. Such impulses are propagated more or less directly from the periphery by means of complex pathways of association in which the neurohormones can be considered as the centripetal limb of a reflex arc whose afferent limb is neurovegetative. *They are therefore the executorial agents of a neurohormonal reflex.*

While certain endocrine secretions of a different type act in slowly fluctuating waves of secretion, the action of the neurohormones is based on a rapid discharge.

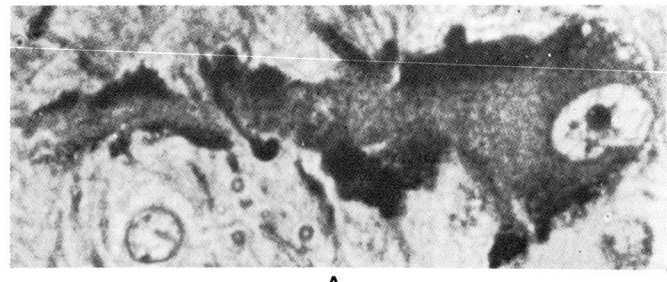

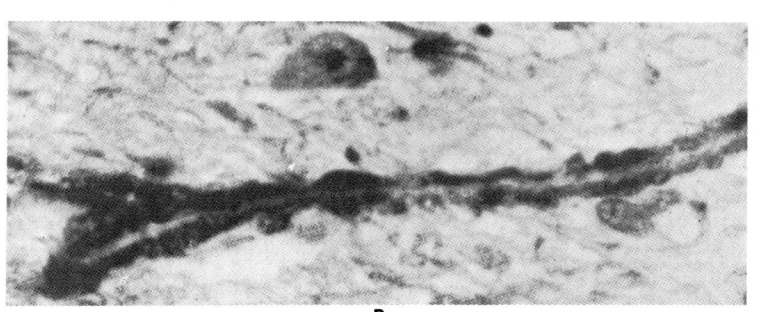

Figure 8-11. A, Secretion-containing neuron in supraoptic nucleus of dog. B, Process of same neuron within tract of pituitary stalk. (From Bargmann: *Arch. Gynäk.*, 183:14, 1953.)

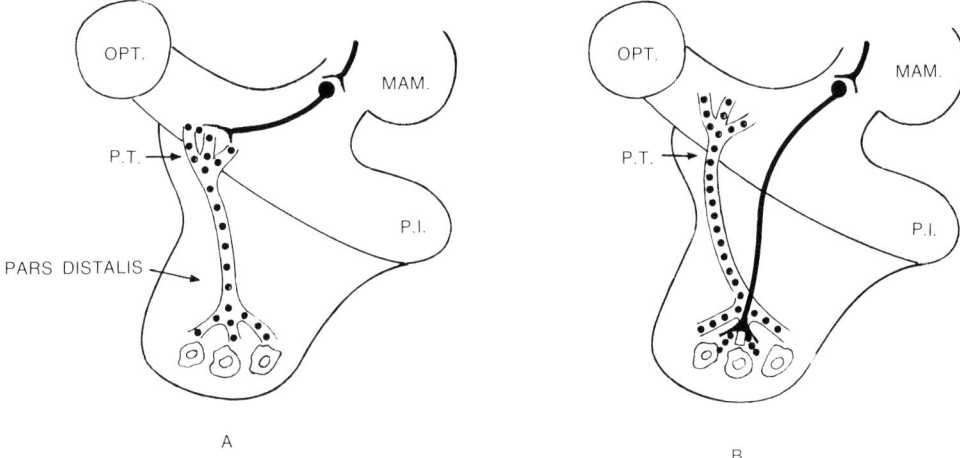

Figure 8–12. Diagram depicting humoral excitation by means of chemical mediators of the cells in the anterior lobe of the pituitary. *A*, Chemical excitation of anterior lobe cells by means of mediators transported by the hypophysioportal system. *B*, Apart from humoral excitation mediated by the portal system, direct excitation may also take place by means of substances released by nerve endings. OPT., optic chiasm; MAM., mamillary body; P.T., pars tuberalis; P.I., pars intermedia.

Much like the *peripheral neurohormones*, norepinephrine and acetylcholine, the central neurohormones react in a rapid, almost instantaneous manner to neural impulses, their effects likewise ceasing almost immediately. Rydén and Sjöholm[153] have measured the "half-life" of oxytocin, which is but a few minutes. Consequently, the *effect* of these substances is *extremely short-lived.* The blood, specifically during gestation, has been found to contain *oxytocinase*,[26, 91, 169] an enzyme that inactivates oxytocin. A specific *vasopressinase*[11, 83, 84] has also been discovered. After being rapidly released under the impulse of neural stimuli, the corresponding hormone exerts its action for a short period of time only to be subsequently inactivated by its specific blood enzyme. Thus, the acute character of these hormonal effects has become evident. It is no wonder that in the past, with the exception of Hawker and Robertson[83, 84] who were able to measure infinitesimal amounts of oxytocin (see Chapter 21), most investigators failed to detect any oxytocin in the blood under these circumstances.

Bargmann[10] has been able to pinpoint the

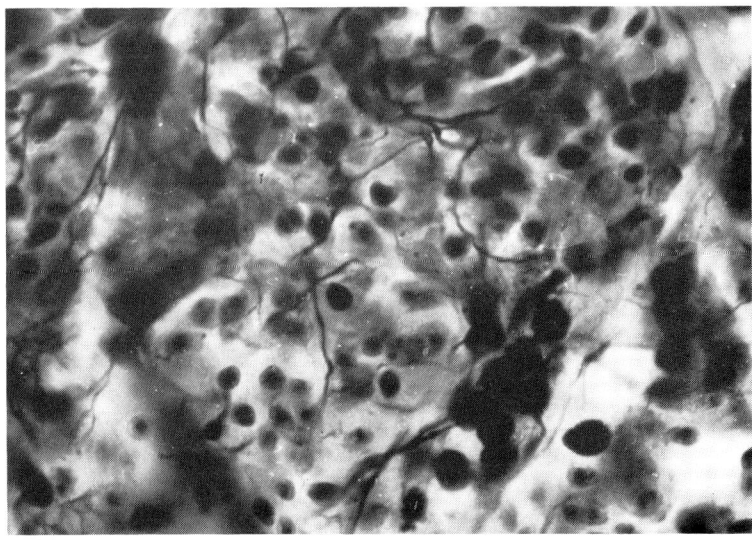

Figure 8–13. Innervation of intermediate lobe of bull pituitary, stained by Bielchowsky-Gross method. (From Ribas-Mujal.[150])

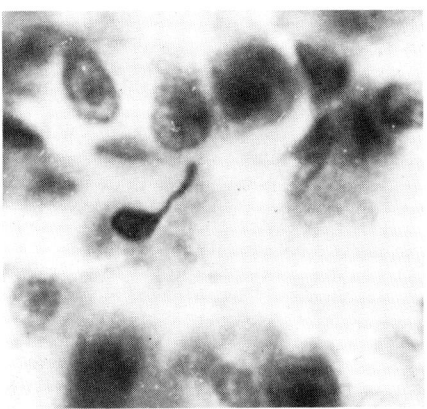

Figure 8–14. Nerve endings in intermediate lobe of bull pituitary, stained by Bielchowsky-Gross method. (From Ribas-Mujal.[150])

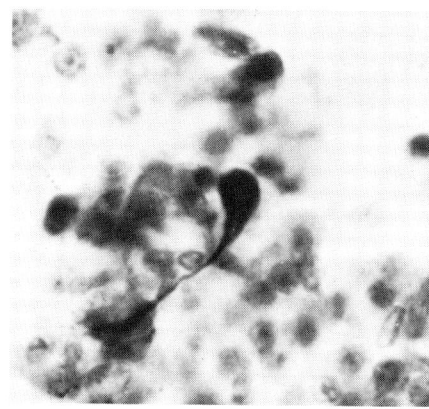

Figure 8–15. Nerve endings in intermediate lobe of bull pituitary, stained by Bielchowsky-Gross method. (From Ribas-Mujal.[150])

intracellular location of these neurosecretions by means of Gomori's *hematoxylin-phloxin* stain (see Fig. 8–11). The secretions are not delivered into the porta-diencephalic system, as is the case with the chemical mediators acting on the anterior pituitary lobe, but progress along the axon-cylinders of the neurons, as shown in these illustrations.

Following injection of tritiated (H-3 labeled) oxytocin, the latter localizes mainly in the liver and kidney (Sjöholm and Rydén[173]), which is in keeping with its previously mentioned rapid inactivation and clearance.

It seems pertinent to point out that, in Gerschenfeld's view,[65] most of the chemical mediators to the adenohypophysis are likewise not conveyed by the portal system but are propagated along the course of the nerve fibers and set free in situ. An important argument in support of this theory has been advanced by the research of Ribas-Mujal,[150] who found abundant nerve endings in the adenohypophysis (see Figs. 8–13 to 8–16).

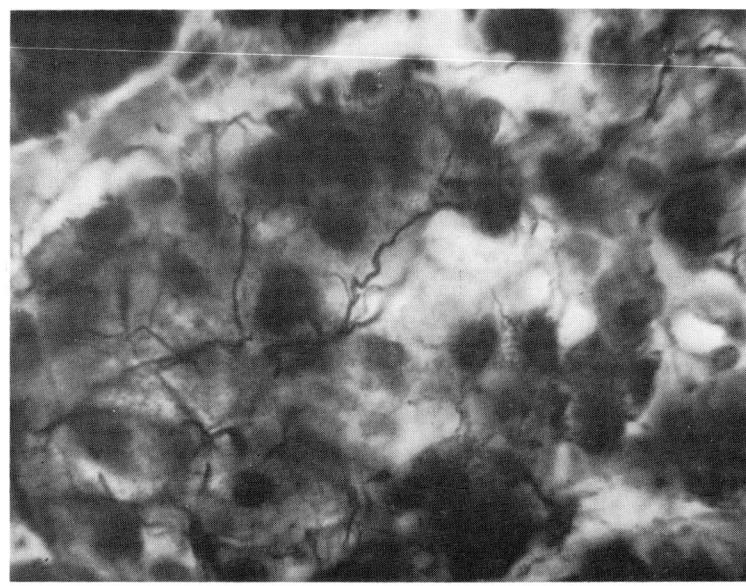

Figure 8–16. Innervation of intermediate lobe of mule pituitary, stained by Bielchowsky-Gross method. (Courtesy of Ribas-Mujal.[150])

8.7.2. PHYSIOPATHOLOGY OF NEUROHORMONAL REFLEXES

Hild and Zetler[85] have called attention to the fact that, as a result of withholding water from dogs, the dogs revealed hypersecretion of antidiuretic hormone. Verney[187] postulated that secretion of antidiuretic hormone was elicited by a reflex mechanism initiated by the *glomus carotideum*, in which osmoreceptor nerve endings were in this way responsible for regulating water balance. Evidence of such osmoreceptors has been brought to light by Baratz.[9] Since the organ of the carotid is at the same time a center controlling arterial pressure, it may be justified to assume that a similar reflex is operative in a parallel fashion insofar as vasopressin is concerned.

As for oxytocin, its secretion by reflex impulses has currently been well documented. One such reflex originating in the nipple has been demonstrated by Harris,[80] Folley,[62] Cross[33, 34] and lately by Debackere and co-workers.[39] In breast-feeding, the human newborn or animal sucklings excite the nerve endings of the nipple and create an impulse which, through a reflex arc passing through the sympathetic ganglia and the spinal cord, reaches the supraoptic and paraventricular nuclei and there induces secretion of oxytocin hormone, contributing to the contracture of the smooth muscle fibers of the nipple and those of the lactiferous ducts and facilitating the outflow of milk. However, hypothalamic secretion of oxytocin is not only induced in a reflex fashion from the nipple but probably also *from the uterine cervix*. Suranyi and colleagues[175] found evidence of baroreceptor endings in the cervix, while Cross[33] was able to produce increased intramammary pressure in rats (owing to increased oxytocin release) by stimulating the uterine cervix. For this reason, it is now generally admitted that stimulation of either the nipple or the uterine cervix, or both, leads to stimulation of the supraoptic and paraventricular nuclei and to increased output of oxytocin hormone.[80, 170]

Van Denmark and Hays[185] have observed that, in cows following coitus, spermatozoa appeared in the upper passages of the genital apparatus much more rapidly than could be explained on the basis of simple active progression of sperm. A similar phenomenon has been noted in women by our colleagues Ateca and Puras.[5] At present, such a phenomenon is thought to be due to "active suction" of spermatozoa by the uterus and is also believed to be a neurohormonal reflex that is triggered by coitus (probably, by vaginal distention) and leads to oxytocin release.

Nevertheless, because Hawker and Robertson[83] also detected oxytocin in the semen, the latter phenomenon could be accounted for without the need for invoking a reflex mechanism.

Furthermore, the coital reflex has been found to occur in a number of animals, such as the rabbit (Green and Harris[68]), the ewe (Hawker et al.[84]), and even the camel (Adamson et al.[1]).

Electric stimulation of the uterine cervix produces a discharge of oxytocin (Tindall et al.[178]), and mechanical distention of the vagina of lactating ewes elevates oxytocinemia (Roberts and Share[151]).

In the same way as described for the cow, coitus provokes secretion of oxytocin in all these animals, stimulating uterine contractions and facilitating the ascending transport of sperm.

Consequently, oxytocin must be viewed in a new light: not as a substance that, in view of its invariably elevated blood level before term and during labor, determines any sustained effect, but rather as a humoral component of a mixed reflex arc, designed to exert, as do other neurohormones, a *very rapid, transient effect of a regulatory character*. In order to fully understand the clinical effect of oxytocin and why this hormone must *never be administered in a manner leading to cumulative high levels* (to be discussed later), it is of great importance to bear this fact in mind.

As a final note of interest, it may be pointed out that nicotine enhances the rate of oxytocin release.[22]

8.7.3. ROLE OF OXYTOCIN IN INDUCING AND MAINTAINING UTERINE CONTRACTIONS

The idea that labor is precipitated by progressive accumulation of oxytocin in the blood near term is erroneous. Hawker and Robertson,[83] who achieved the detection of oxytocin in blood, failed to find any pre- or intrapartum elevations that would correlate with the onset of obstetric activity.

For many years, it has been suspected that the most important factor initiating labor was *increased sensitivity of the uterine fibers to various excitants*. Studies by Csapo[35] concerning the mechanism of action by estrogens and progesterone on the myometrial ionic content totally bear out this long-standing suspicion. What takes place is not increased action by excitants but increased excitability of the uterine muscle (see Chapter 21).

That this is actually so has been shown by a number of recent observations, mainly with regard to such changes in vaginal cytology as are interpreted to indicate impending labor.

In recent studies,[117, 151, 191] it has been possible to show that while *estrogens increase the response in the Ferguson-Harris reflex*, progesterone reduces it.[152]

However, it is to be emphasized later that oxytocin alone does not seem to be the only agent responsible for initiating labor. This can be inferred from experimental observations that hypophysectomy,[144] section of the pituitary stalk[195] and destruction of the hypothalamic region[67, 68] do not interfere with labor, and from clinical observations that human diabetes insipidus is compatible with a normal onset of labor, even though the subsequent course of labor itself is usually marked by secondary hypodynamia.[135]

Therefore, possibly other substances acting on the uterine smooth muscle fiber—and which have unquestionably been proved to be present in increased amounts in the blood and tissue fluids of pregnant women near term—may be admitted to substitute for oxytocin, and it may even be postulated that these, rather than oxytocin, are the initial labor-inducing oxytocic agents. The substances referred to are *acetylcholine*,[132] *histamine*[23, 40] and, possibly, *serotonin*.[196]

A detectable increase of oxytocin blood values can be observed during labor only after the beginning of cervical dilatation.[82, 83, 84] This would lead one to assume that active release by the hypothalamic gray nuclei of this hormone really only takes place during labor as a result of a reflex originating in the uterine cervix as the latter is being dilated or compressed by the fetal head or by the presenting fetal part. There are a number of clinical findings that indicate that dilatation and compression of the cervix causes more vigorous contractions (for further details, refer to bibliography of the article by Suranyi and coworkers[175]). *It may thus be asserted that the real function of oxytocin is not that of initiating labor but that of maintaining the contractions once these have started. The latter function is thought to be realized by virtue of a neuroendocrine reflex arc that is activated by cervical dilatation.*

8.7.4. EFFECT OF OXYTOCIN ON MILK EJECTION

Another important action by oxytocin, to be studied more comprehensively later (Chapter 22), is exerted on the muscular elements of the breast, determining the *suckling reflex* and ejection of milk. Through stimulating the nerve endings in the nipple, the breast-feeding baby excites the supraoptic and paraventricular nuclei whereby a discharge of oxytocin takes place and the lactiferous ducts in the breast contract (Fig. 8–17).

This reflex has been well studied by Harris[80] and subsequently by Caldeyro-Barcia's group.[22, 23] Based on this effect, Mendez-Bauer,[120a] as well as Tindall and Yokoyama,[182] have developed some of the finest bioassay methods for oxytocin currently known.

Hence, the reflex of oxytocin discharge is a double one or, as it were, a *crossed reflex* (Fig. 8–17), which can be excited either at the level of the uterine cervix or at the level of the nipple, the action in turn being exerted either at the level of the breast or at the level of the uterus. For practical purposes, this means that there may be noticeable uterine contractions during breast-feeding (Fig. 8–18) and, conversely, that the uterine contractions during labor are associated with increased intramammary pressure (Fig. 8–19).

8.7.5. CHEMISTRY OF OXYTOCIN

Ever since 1941, when it was isolated in a pure state, oxytocin has been known to be a polypeptide containing in its molecule sulfur[13, 18] in addition to nitrogen. In 1953, Tuppy[184] and Du Vigneaud[188, 189] both simultaneously and independently determined the exact formula of this polypeptide as:

L-cysteinyl-L-tyrosyl-L-isoleucyl-
L-glutaminyl-L-asparaginyl-L-cysteinyl-L-
prolyl-L-leucyl-glycinamide.

Nervous System and Endocrine Glands

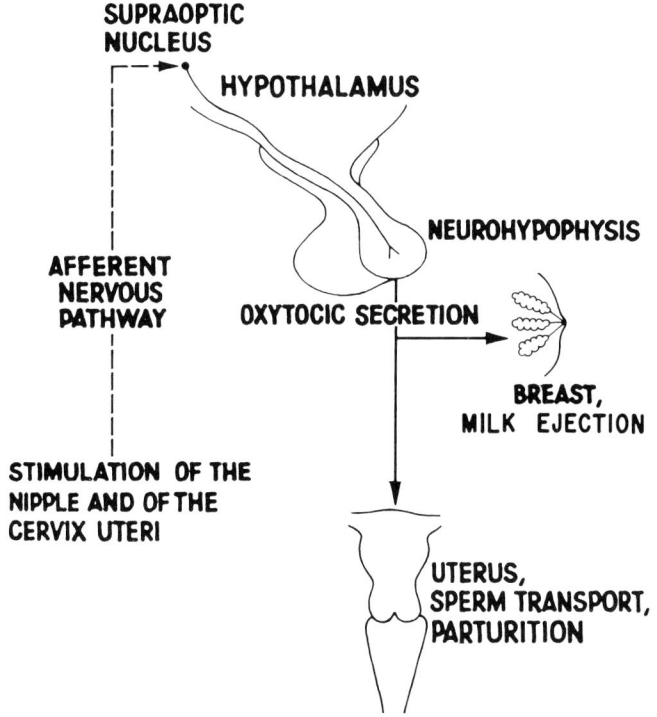

Figure 8-17. Diagram of neuroendocrine correlations of the posterior lobe.

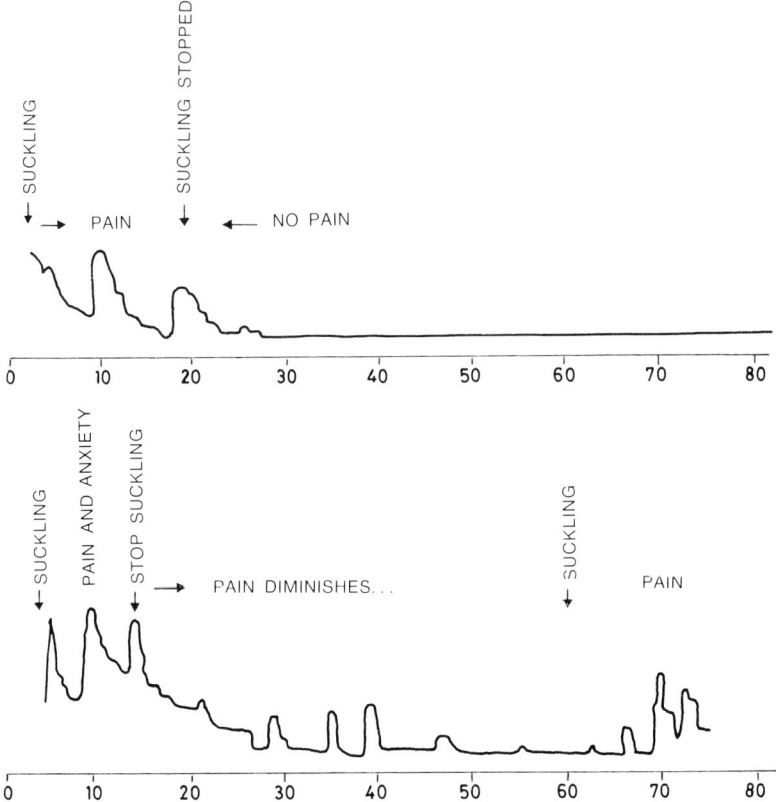

Figure 8-18. Uterine contractions registered by external tocography during suckling of nipple. They are induced by the reflex of oxytocin release. (From Dominguez and Pereira: *Acta Gin.*, 10:405, 1959.)

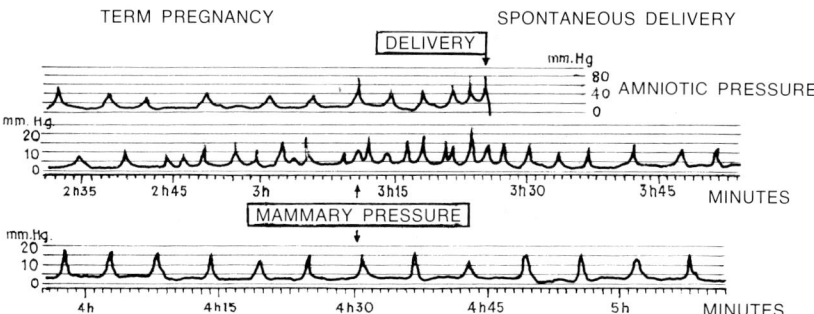

Figure 8–19. Increase of intramammary pressure, registered by means of introducing catheter with micromanometer through nipple, during labor. Notice how uterine contractions, produced by discharges of oxytocin, are accompanied by increased intramammary pressure as a result of contraction of the smooth muscle fibers in that organ. (From Sica-Blanco et al.: *Arch. Gin. Obst. (Montevideo)*, 17:63, 1959.)

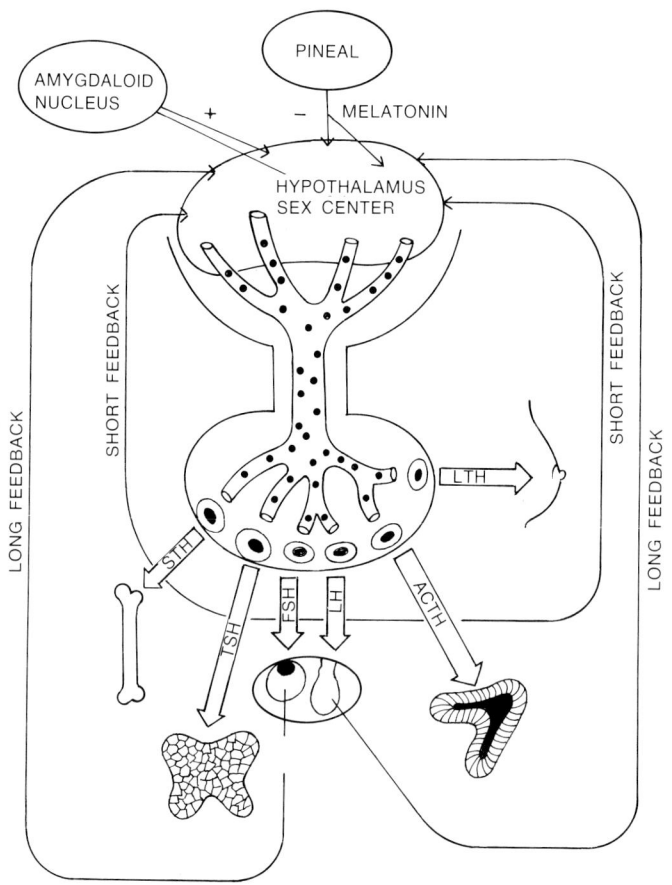

Figure 8–20. Diagram of endocrine correlations of the anterior lobe, illustrating stimulative action by amygdaloid nucleus on hypothalamic sex center and reciprocally inhibitory action of pineal, mediated by melatonin. Diagram also shows long feedback mechanism from gonads to hypothalamic sex center, as well as short feedback effect by gonadotropins on hypothalamic sex center.

Nervous System and Endocrine Glands

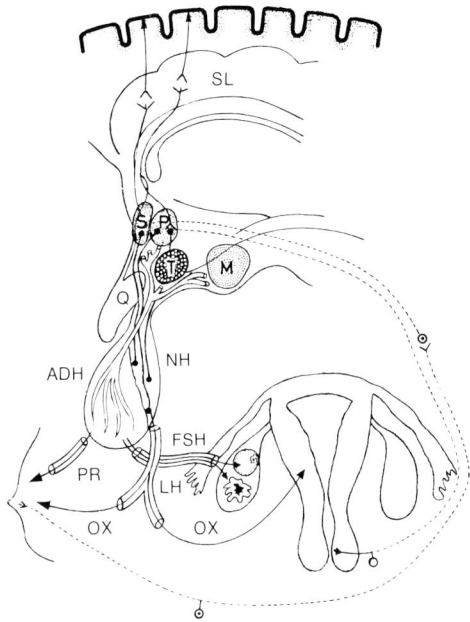

Figure 8-21. Relationships of the hypothalamic sex center with the limbic system. Note that, by means of its connections with the hypothalamic nuclei, the limbic system controls the function of the latter, and, by means of the portal diencephalic system, also represented here, controls secretion by the anterior lobe. Also represented in the figure are the cervico-hypothalamic and the mammary-hypothalamic reflexes (reflexes of Ferguson-Harris). ADH, Adenohypophysis; NH, neurohypophysis; PR, prolactin; OX, oxytocin; M, mamillary body; O, optic chiasm; S, supraoptic nucleus; P, paraventricular nucleus; T, nucleus of tuber cinereum; SL, limbic system.

That is to say, oxytocin is a polypeptide composed of the following amino acids, all of which are levorotatory: cysteine, tyrosine, isoleucine, glutamic and aspartic acid, proline, leucine and glycinamide. They are linked into a ring structure in the following fashion:

```
           Tyrosine————————Isoleucine
Cysteine                      |
   |       Asparagine————————Glutamine
   |           |                |
Proline——Leucine———————————Glycinamide
```

the expanded formula of which is:

$$\begin{array}{c}
\text{C}_6\text{H}_4\text{OH} \quad \text{C}_2\text{H}_5 \\
\text{NH}_2 \;\; \text{O} \quad \text{CH}_2 \;\; \text{O} \quad \text{CH—CH}_3 \\
\text{CH}_2\text{—CH—C—NH—CH—C—NH—CH} \\
\text{S} \quad\quad\quad\quad\quad\quad\quad\quad\quad\quad \text{C=O} \\
\text{S} \quad\quad\quad \text{O} \quad\quad\quad\quad\quad \text{NH} \\
\text{CH}_2\text{—CH—NH—C—CH—NH—C—CH} \\
\text{C=O} \quad\quad \text{CH}_2 \quad\quad \text{CH}_2 \\
\text{CH}_2\text{—N} \quad\quad \text{CONH}_2 \quad \text{CH}_2 \\
\text{CH—C=O} \quad\quad\quad\quad \text{CONH}_2 \\
\text{CH}_2\text{—CH}_2 \quad \text{NH} \;\; \text{O} \\
(\text{CH}_3)_2\text{·CH—CH}_2\text{—CH—C—NH—CH}_2\text{—CONH}_2
\end{array}$$

Du Vigneaud and colleagues[188,189] have confirmed this structure after synthesizing the hormone in 1954. One year later, Boissonnas and his co-workers[18] developed a second method for synthesis, which has been applied for industrial purposes by Sandoz of Basel, the resulting preparation having been marketed under the name of Syntocinon. Synthetic oxytocin has exactly the same biologic properties as the naturally occurring product[13,14,18,135] and can be applied under the same indications and in similar dosages. In addition, Berde,[14] in 1957, obtained four synthetic analogues of oxytocin with comparable pharmacologic action.

8.7.6. ACTIONS BY PURE OXYTOCIN

When pure, both natural and synthetic forms of oxytocin are devoid of such side effects as were commonly associated with earlier total retrohypophysial extracts as a result of contamination with vasopressin. The action of the synthetic hormone, as compared to that of an international standard of purified oxytocin, has been studied in animals by Berde and Cerletti,[13] and in women by Francis and Winifred,[63] Bainbridge and co-workers[8] and Nixon.[135] The synthetic product offers one obvious advantage over the natural hormone in that it never contains admixtures of other hormones.[18]

The effect of the hormone on the breast is of great interest. It has already been pointed out that oxytocin increases the rate of milk ejection, an effect of potential utilization by the veterinarian[33, 34] or the clinician[102, 135] to facilitate milking or breastfeeding, respectively. The experimental effect of oxytocin on the breast of the rabbit has been studied by Berde and Cerletti[13]; however, recent work by Benson and co-workers[12] seems to reveal a new and interesting finding, namely, that oxytocin stimulates prolactin secretion by the adenohypophysis, which, if valid, would indicate that *the effect of oxytocic hormone on the maintenance of lactation is a double one.*

8.7.7. VASOPRESSIN

Already, in 1930, vasopressin was described by Kamm as the hormone responsible for stimulating the vascular wall and producing hypertension. It was isolated and identified by Heller in 1941. In contrast, it has not been possible to identify a separate antidiuretic hormone, called *adiuretin*, which had once been believed to be intimately related to vasopressin.

The formula of vasopressin is that of a polypeptide, similar to oxytocin.

A neurohormonal reflex for the regulation of arterial pressure has also been described. It has already been mentioned that the uterine cervix contains baroreceptors for the transmission of neural stimuli to the hypothalamus. Such baroreceptors are currently well known to monitor *arterial pressure* and are located in the glomus carotideum.[9] Any lowering of arterial pressure automatically excites the supraoptic and paraventricular nuclei, resulting in a discharge of vasopressin. The phenomenon under discussion has been explored by Bargmann[10] who observed increased amounts of Gomori-positive substances in the mentioned nuclei as well as in the pituitary stalk of dogs with experimentally induced hypotension.

The function of the *osmoreceptor nerve endings*, which are distributed in different parts of the vascular tree, particularly in the glomus carotideum,[9, 11] is to make sure that any reduction in the level of blood water content is promptly followed by inhibition of diuresis. This has been clearly demonstrated in thirsty dogs by Hild and Zetler.[85]

Without entering into in-depth discussion of the important functions exercised by vasopressin in renal and circulatory physiology, it is evident that this hormone is equally associated with rapid neurohormonal reflexes of a regulatory nature. In addition to a specific enzyme for oxytocin, the blood contains a specific enzyme for vasopressin, *vasopressinase*.[11, 82] Thus, the mission of the hypothalamic-neurohypophysial system may be summed up as follows: The real endocrine gland is located in the supraoptic and paraventricular nuclei of the hypothalamus. There, the neurohormones that regulate uterine contractions, arterial pressure and diuresis are secreted and released in brief, rapid discharges in response to afferent neural impulses. The regulatory neurohormonal reflex arc is thereby closed. In other words, *the hypothalamic-neurohypophysial system is a vital exchange center of neurohormonal reflexes of a regulatory nature.*

8.7.8. ANALOGUES OF OXYTOCIN AND OTHER NEUROHORMONES

There are a series of polypeptides, all originating in the hypothalamic nuclei, which act as chemical emissaries and constitute the family of *polypeptide hormones*. Because oxytocin is the best known and is considered representative of this group, the remaining hormones are designated by the generic name of "oxytocin analogues."

Knowledge concerning these analogues is still in its infancy. Some of them do not occur naturally but can be produced by simple synthesis, possessing nevertheless useful pharmacologic effects. For example, *octapressin* has been used as a vasoconstrictor in surgery (Botella[19]).

Antidiuretic hormone, the individuality of which had been in doubt, has been identified by Mayer[119] as arginine-vasopressin. At present, a great deal of work is in progress to establish the composition and individuality of these emissary agents mediating the release of anterior pituitary hormones but, at this stage, few concrete data seem to be available.

Some of the analogues are preparations possessing greater potency than the naturally occurring substances in pure form. For instance, *desamino-oxytocin*[29, 189, 190] is twice as potent, and *vallyl-oxytocin*[12] is five times as potent, as natural oxytocin.

Lastly, an *arginine vasotocin-like* substance has been found in the pineal gland by Milcu and his colleagues,[121] raising the possibility that pineal physiology may after all be based on secretion of this type (see Chapter 10).

8.8. CONCLUSION

It has now become apparent that many biologic actions which for many years have been believed to be subject to a hormonal mechanism of control are actually under the control of the nervous system. In contrast, some phenomena that have passed for classic examples of neurogenic activity can now be explained on the basis of a hormonal mechanism. *This really proves but one thing: that there are no separate theories, one neural and another hormonal, to account for the phenomena of sexual life, just as there are none to explain any other problem in physiology.*

Chapter 1 mentioned the fact that each individual's life could be viewed as composed of a sexual sphere, a vegetative sphere and a relational sphere. These three spheres, though independent of each other, are interrelated through the hypophysiothalamic system which, therefore, is the great coordinator of all physiologic correlations. *The process of coordination involved is at the same time both neural and hormonal; the hormones regulate the activity of the centers and the latter, in turn, stimulate the secretion of the former. The neuroendocrine and endocrinoneural reflexes are thus the agents of sexual control.*

REFERENCES

1. Adamson, K., et al.: *Endocrinology*, 58:272, 1956.
2. Antunes-Rodrigues, J., and MacCann, S. M.: *Endocrinology*, 81:666, 1967.
2a. Aray, Y., and Gorski, R. A.: *Proc. Soc. Exper. Biol. Med.*, 127:590, 1968.
3. Arimura, A., et al.: *Endocrinology*, 80:972, 1967.
4. Arimura, A., et al.: *Endocrinology*, 81:235, 1967.
5. Ateca, M., and Puras, A.: *Rev. Franç. Gynec. Obstet.*, 52:365, 1967.
6. Averill, R. L. V., Salaman, D. F., and Curtis, W. W.: *Nature*, 211:144, 1966.
7. Averill, R. L. V., and Kennedy, T. H.: *Endocrinology*, 81:112, 1967.
8. Bainbridge, W. N., et al.: *Brit. Med. J.*, 1:1133, 1956.
9. Baratz, D., Doig, A., and Adatto, J. J.: *J. Clin. Invest.*, 39:1359, 1960.
10. Bargmann, W.: *Das Zwischenhirn-Hypophysensystem.* Berlin, J. Springer, 1954.
11. Barnes, A. C., and Sawyer, J. B.: *Amer. J. Obstet. Gynec.*, 79:1053, 1960.
12. Benson, G. K., Folley, S. J., and Tindall, J.: *J. Endocr.*, 20:106, 1960.
13. Berde, B., and Cerletti, A.: *Gynaecologia*, 144:257, 1957.
14. Berde, B.: *Recent Progress in Oxytocin Research.* Springfield, Ill., Charles C Thomas, 1959.
15. Birge, C. A., Jacobs, L. S., Hammer, C. T., and Daughaday, W. H.: *Endocrinology*, 86:120, 1970.
16. Bisonette, T. H.: *Amer. J. Anat.*, 45:289, 1930.
17. Blanquet, P.: *J. Med. Bordeaux*, 8:979, 1961.
18. Boissonas, A. A., et al.: *Helv. Chim. Acta*, 38:149, 1955.
19. Botella, J.: *Arch. Fac. Med. Madrid*, 2:165, 1962.
20. Botella, J., Merlo, J. G., and Sanchez De Rivera, G.: *Amer. J. Obstet. Gynec.*, 101:665, 1968.
21. Burgus, R., Sakiz, E., Ward, D. N., and Guillemin, R.: *Compt. Rend. Acad. Sci. (Paris)*, 262:2643, 1966.
21a. Butt, W. R.: *Hormone Chemistry.* London, Van Nostrand, 1969.
22. Caldeyro-Barcia, R., and Poseiro, J. J.: *Ann. N.Y. Acad. Sci.*, 75:813, 1959.
23. Caldeyro-Barcia, R., and Poseiro, J. J.: *Symposium sobre Oxitocina.* Montevideo, Editorial Caldeyro-Barcia, 1960.
24. Caligaris, L., Astrada, J. J., and Taleisnik, S.: *Acta Endocr.*, 59:177, 1968.
25. Campbell, H. J., and Gallardo, E.: *J. Physiol.*, 186:689, 1966.
26. Carballo, M., and Mendez-Bauer, C.: *II Congreso Uruguayo de Ginecologia*, 1957.
27. Carrer, H. F., and Taleisnik, S.: *Endocrinology*, 86:231, 1970.
28. Chambers, W. F., et al.: *Gerontologia*, 12:65, 1966.
29. Chan, W. Y., O'Connell, M., and Pomeroy, S. R.: *Endocrinology*, 72:279, 1963.
30. Chowers, I., and MacCann, S. M.: *Endocrinology*, 76:700, 1965.
31. Crighton, D. B., Schneider, H. P. G., and MacCann, S. M.: *J. Endocr.*, 44:305, 1969.
32. Critchlow, B. V.: *Anat. Rec.*, 127:283, 1957.
33. Cross, B. A.: *Brit. Med. Bull.*, 11:151, 1951.
34. Cross, B. A., and Harris, G. W.: *J. Endocr.*, 8:148, 1952.
35. Csapo, A.: *Rec. Progr. Horm. Res.*, 12:402, 1956.
36. David, M. A., Fraschini, A., and Martini, L.: *Compt. Rend. Acad. Sci. (Paris)*, 261:2249, 1965.
37. Davidson, J. M., and Zondek, B.: *Endocrinology*, 80:365, 1967.
38. Davis, M. E.: *Rec. Progr. Horm. Res.*, 16:135, 1960.
39. Debackere, M., Peeters, G., and Tuyttens, N.: *J. Endocr.*, 22:321, 1961.

40. Decio, R.: *Riv. Ost. Gin. (Firenze)*, 12:234, 1957.
41. Desclin, L., and Flament-Durand, J.: *Z. Zellforsch.*, 69:274, 1966.
42. Deutsch, S. F.: *Psychosomatics*, 9:127, 1968.
43. Dhariwal, A. D. S., Nallar, R., Batt, M., and MacCann, S. M.: *Endocrinology*, 76:291, 1965.
44. Diereck, K.: *Naturwiss.*, 56:279, 1966.
45. Doecke, F., and Koloczek, G.: *Endokrinologie*, 50:225, 1966.
46. Doecke, F., and Doerner, G.: *Endocr. Exper. (Bratislava)*, 1:65, 1967.
47. Donnet, V., et al.: *Compt. Rend. Soc. Biol. (Paris)*, 156:1123, 1962.
48. Donoso, A. O., and Stefano, F. J. E.: *Experientia*, 23:665, 1967.
49. Donoso, A. O., Stefano, F. J. E., Biscardi, A. M., and Ciker, J.: *Amer. J. Physiol.*, 212:737, 1967.
50. Donovan, B. T.: *J. Endocrinol.*, 39:105, 1967.
51. Doyle, J. B.: *Fertil. Steril.*, 5:105, 1954.
52. Ducommun, S., and Guillemin, R.: *Proc. Soc. Exper. Biol. Med.*, 122:1251, 1966.
53. Eleftheriou, B. E., Zolovic, A. J., and Norman, R. L.: *J. Endocr.*, 38:469, 1967.
54. Eleftheriou, B. E., Desjardins, C., and Zolovic, A. J.: *J. Reprod. Fertil.*, 21:249, 1970.
55. Elwers, M. B. S., and Critchlow, B. V.: *Amer. J. Physiol.*, 211:1103, 1966.
56. Everett, J. W.: Preoptic Region of the Brain and its Relation with Ovulation, in *Control of Ovulation*, ed. C. A. Villee. New York, Pergamon Press, 1961.
57. Everett, J. W.: *Physiol. Revs.*, 44:373, 1964.
58. Fawcett, C. P., Reed, M., Charlton, H. M., and Harris, G. W.: *Biochem. J.*, 106:229, 1968.
59. Feyel-Cabanes, T.: *Ann. d'Endocr.*, 21:217, 1960.
60. Fink, G.: *Nature*, 215:159, 1967.
61. Fiske, V. N., and Greep, R. O.: *Endocrinology*, 64:175, 1959.
62. Folley, S. J.: *Brit. Med. Bull.*, 11:145, 1955.
63. Francis, H. H., and Winifred, J. A.: *Brit. Med. J.*, 1:1136, 1956.
64. Gay, V. L., Niswender, G. D., and Midgley, A. R.: *Endocrinology*, 86:1305, 1970.
65. Gerschenfeld, H. M., Tramezzani, J. H., and De Robertis, E.: *Endocrinology*, 66:471, 1960.
66. Gorski, R. A.: *Anat. Rec.*, 157:63, 1967.
67. Green, J. D.: *Amer. J. Anat.*, 88:225, 1951.
68. Green, J. D., and Harris, G. W.: *J. Anat.*, 80:247, 1946.
69. Greer, M. A., and Erwin, H. L.: *Endocrinology*, 58:665, 1956.
70. Grosvenor, C. E., and Mena, F.: *Endocrinology*, 80:840, 1967.
71. Guillemin, R., et al.: *Compt. Rend. Acad. Sci. (Paris)*, 262:2278, 1966.
72. Guillemin, R.: *Ann. Rev. Physiol.*, 29:313, 1967.
73. Gwinup, G., et al.: *J. Clin. Endocr. Metab.*, 27:927, 1967.
74. Hagino, N., and Goldzieher, J. W.: *Endocrinology*, 86:29, 1970.
75. Halasz, B., and Gorski, R. A.: *Endocrinology*, 80:608, 1967.
76. Halasz, B., Vernikos-Danellis, J., and Gorski, R. A.: *Endocrinology*, 81:921, 1967.
77. Halasz, B., and Gorski, R. A.: *Endocrinology*, 80:608, 1967.
78. Hansel, W.: *Internat. J. Fertil.*, 6:241, 1961.
79. Harrington, F. E., Eggert, R. G., and Wilbur, R. D.: *Endocrinology*, 81:877, 1967.
80. Harris, G. W.: *Arch. Gynäk.*, 183:35, 1953.
81. Harris, G. W.: *Brit. Med. Bull.*, 22:195, 1966.
82. Hawker, R. W.: *J. Endocr.*, 14:400, 1957.
83. Hawker, R. W., and Robertson, P. A.: *J. Clin. Endocr. Metab.*, 17:448, 1957.
84. Hawker, R. W., et al.: *Endocrinology*, 69:391, 1961.
85. Hild, W., and Zetler, G.: *Arch. Exper. Path.*, 213:139, 1951.
86. Hild, W.: In *Hypothalamic-Hypophyseal Interrelationships*, ed. R. Guillemin and S. Fields. Springfield, Ill., Charles C Thomas, 1956.
87. Hoffmann, J. C.: *Neuroendocrinology*, 2:1, 1967.
88. Igarashi, M., and MacCann, S. M.: *Endocrinology*, 74:446, 1964.
89. Ishii, S.: *Endocrinology*, 86:207, 1970.
90. Jabonero, V.: *Acta Anatomica* (Basel), 18:295, 1953.
91. Jung, H., and Klock, F. K.: *Gynaecologia*, 167:28, 1969.
92. Justisz, M., et al.: *Compt. Rend. Acad. Sci. (Paris)*, 248:3, 1963.
93. Justisz, M., Berault, A., Novella, M. A., and Chapeville, F.: *Compt. Rend. Acad. Sci. (Paris)*, 263:664, 1966.
94. Kastin, A. J., and Schally, A. V.: *Endocrinology*, 79:1018, 1966.
95. Kato, J., and Villee, C. A.: *Endocrinology*, 80:567, 1967.
96. Katz, S. H., Dhariwal, A. P. S., and MacCann, S. M.: *Endocrinology*, 81:333, 1967.
97. Kahwanago, I., Le Roy, W., and Herrmann, W.: *Endocrinology*, 86:1319, 1970.
98. Kamberi, I. A., Mical, R. S., and Porter, J. C.: *Science*, 166:388, 1969.
99. Kamberi, I. A., Schneider, H. P. G., and MacCann, S. M.: *Endocrinology*, 86:278, 1970.
100. Keever, J. E., and Greenwald, G. S.: *Acta Endocr.*, 56:244, 1967.
101. Knowles, F., and Bern, A.: *Nature*, 210:271, 1966.
102. Konzett, H., Berde, B., and Cerletti, A.: *Schw. Med. Wschr.*, 86:226, 1956.
103. Kraft, C. L., and Meites, J.: *Endocrinology*, 76:1169, 1965.
104. Krantz, K. E.: *Ann. N.Y. Acad. Sci.*, 75:770, 1959.
105. Krulich, L., and MacCann, S. M.: *Proc. Soc. Exper. Biol. Med.*, 122:668, 1966.
106. Kuroshime, A., et al.: *Endocrinology*, 78:1105, 1966.
107. Labsetwar, A. P.: *Endocrinology*, 81:357, 1967.
108. Laszlon, F. A., and De Wied, D.: *Endocrinology*, 79:547, 1966.
109. Lincoln, D. W.: *J. Endocr.*, 37:177, 1967.
110. Lincoln, D. W., and Cross, B. A.: *J. Endocr.*, 37:191, 1967.
111. Lippmann, W., Leonardi, R., Bali, J., and Coppola, J. A.: *J. Pharmacol. Exper. Therap.*, 156:258, 1967.
112. Lisk, R. R.: *J. Exper. Zool.*, 161:129, 1966.
113. MacCann, S. M., and Taleisnik, S.: *Endocrinology*, 68:1023, 1961.
114. MacCann, S. M., and Ramirez, V. D.: *Rec. Progr. Horm. Res.*, 20:131, 1964.
115. MacCann, S. M., Antunes-Rodrigues, J., and Dhariwal, A. D. S.: *Proceed. XXIII Internat. Congr. Physiol. Sci.*, p. 292, 1965.
116. MacCann, S. M., and Dhariwal, A. D. S.: "Hypo-

thalamic Releasing Factors," in *Neuroendocrinology*, ed. L. Martini and W. F. Ganong. New York, Academic Press, 1966.
117. Martin-Pinto, R., Lerner, U., Ponetlli, H., and Rabow, W.: *Compt. Rend. Soc. Biol. (Paris)*, 162:228, 1968.
118. Matsuyama, E., Weisz, J., and Lloyd, C. W.: *Endocrinology*, 79:261, 1966.
119. Mayer, F. S.: *Acta Endocr.*, 35:568, 1960.
120. Meites, J., and Nicoll, C. S.: *Ann. Rev. Physiol.*, 28:57, 1966.
120a. Mendez-Bauer, C., Cabot, H. M., and Caldeyro-Barcia, R.: *Science*, 132:299, 1960.
121. Milcu, S. M., et al.: *Endocrinology*, 72:563, 1962.
122. Minagouchi, H., and Meites, J.: *Endocrinology*, 80:603, 1967.
123. Mitchell, G. A. G.: *Anatomy of the Autonomous Nervous System*. Edinburgh, E. & S. Livingstone, 1963.
124. Moghilewsky, J. A., Libertun, C., Schiaffini, O., and Schwarzfarb, B.: *Neuroendocrinology*, 3:193, 1968.
125. Motta, M., Fraschini, G., Guillani, G., and Martini, L.: *Endocrinology*, 83:1101, 1968.
126. Müller, E. E., and Pecile, A.: *Endocrinology*, 79:448, 1966.
127. Müller, E. E., Saito, T., Arimura, A., and Schally, A. V.: *Endocrinology*, 80:77, 1967.
128. Müller, E. E., Savano, J., Arimura, A., and Schally, A. V.: *Endocrinology*, 80:431, 1967.
129. Nallar, R., and MacCann, S. M.: *Endocrinology*, 76:272, 1965.
130. Nallar, R., Grosvenor, C. E., and MacCann, S. M.: *Endocrinology*, 76:883, 1965.
131. Negro-Vilar, A., Dickerman, E., and Meites, J.: *Proc. Soc. Exper. Biol. Med.*, 127:751, 1968.
132. Nickerson, H. K., et al.: *Amer. J. Obstet. Gynec.*, 67:1028, 1964.
133. Nikitowitsch-Wiener, M. B.: *Endocrinology*, 70:350, 1962.
134. Nikitowitsch-Wiener, M. B., and Everett, J. W.: *Endocrinology*, 63:917, 1958.
135. Nixon, W. C. W.: *Triangulo "Sandoz,"* 3:329, 1958.
136. Palka, Y. S., and Sawyer, C. H.: *J. Physiol.*, 185:251, 1966.
137. Palka, Y. S., Ramirez, V. D., and Sawyer, C. H.: *Endocrinology*, 78:487, 1966.
138. Piacsek, B. E., and Meites, J.: *Endocrinology*, 79:487, 1966.
139. Piacsek, B. E., and Meites, J.: *Endocrinology*, 81:535, 1967.
140. Piacsek, B. E., and Meites, J.: *Neuroendocrinology*, 2:129, 1967.
141. Porter, J. C., Dhariwal, A. D. S., and MacCann, S. M.: *Endocrinology*, 80:679, 1967.
142. Radford, H. M., Wheatley, L. S., and Wallace, A. L. C.: *J. Endocr.*, 44:135, 1969.
143. Ramirez, V. D., and Sawyer, C. H.: *Endocrinology*, 72:282, 1965.
144. Ranson, S.: *Ergeb. Physiol.*, 41:56, 1939.
145. Ratner, A., Dhariwal, A. D. S., and MacCann, S. M.: *Clin. Obstet. Gynec.*, 10:106, 1967.
146. Redding, T. W., Bowers, C. Y., and Schally, A. V.: *Endocrinology*, 79:229, 1966.
147. Redding, T. W., and Schally, A. V.: *Endocrinology*, 81:918, 1967.
148. Relkin, R.: *Endocrinology*, 82:865, 1968.
149. Reynolds, S. R. M.: *Physiology of the Uterus*. New York, Hoeber, 1949.
150. Ribas-Mujal, D.: *Ztschr. f. Zellforsch.*, 48:356, 1958.
151. Roberts, J. S., and Share, L.: *Endocrinology*, 83:272, 1968.
152. Roberts, J. S., and Share, L.: *Endocrinology*, 84:1076, 1969.
153. Rydén, G., and Sjöholm, I.: *Acta Obstet. Gynec. Scand.*, 48:Suppl. 3, 1969.
154. Saito, T., et al.: *Endocrinology*, 80:313, 1967.
155. Samli, M. I., and Geschwind, I. I.: *Endocrinology*, 81:835, 1967.
156. Sandler, R.: *Endocrinology*, 83:1383, 1968.
157. Sawyer, C. H., and Kawakami, M.: "Interreactions Between Central Nervous System and Hormones Influencing Ovulation," in *Control of Ovulation*, ed. C. A. Villee. New York, Pergamon Press, 1961.
158. Schally, A. V.: *Acta Gin. (Madrid)*, 21:709, 1970.
159. Schally, A. V., Meites, J., Bowers, C. Y., and Ratner, A.: *Proc. Soc. Exper. Biol. Med.*, 117:252, 1964.
160. Schally, A. V., and Kastin, A. J.: *Endocrinology*, 79:768, 1966.
161. Schally, A. V., et al.: *Endocrinology*, 79:1087, 1966.
162. Schally, A. V., et al.: *J. Clin. Endocr. Metab.*, 27:755, 1967.
163. Schally, A. V., Bowers, C. Y., White, W. F., and Cohen, A. I.: *Endocrinology*, 81:77, 1967.
164. Schally, A. V., Bowers, C. Y., White, W. F., Arimura, A., Sito, T., and Savano, S.: *Endocrinology*, 81:882, 1967.
165. Schally, A. V., Arimura, A., and Bowers, C. Y.: *Rec. Progr. Horm. Res.*, 24:497, 1968.
166. Scharrer, E., and Leveque, T. F.: *Endocrinology*, 52:436, 1953.
167. Schneider, H. P. G., and MacCann, S. M.: *Endocrinology*, 87:249, 1970.
168. Schneider, H. P. G., and MacCann, S. M.: *Endocrinology*, 87:330, 1970.
169. Semm, K.: *Arch. Gynäk.*, 199:265, 1963.
170. Sica-Blanco, I., et al.: *Arch. Gin. Obstet. Montevideo*, 17:63, 1959.
171. Singh, K. B., and Greenwald, G.: *J. Endocr.*, 38:389, 1967.
172. Sinha, D. H., and Meites, J.: *Endocrinology*, 80:131, 1967.
173. Sjöholm, J., and Rydén, G.: *Acta Endocr.*, 61:432, 1969.
174. Stefano, F. J. E., and Donoso, A. O.: *Endocrinology*, 81:1405, 1967.
175. Suranyi, S., Kovacs, T., and Molnar, G.: *Ztschr. f. Geb. u. Gyn.*, 144:268, 1955.
176. Taleisnik, S., and Tomats, M. E.: *Endocrinology*, 81:819, 1967.
177. Tejasen, T., and Everett, J. W.: *Endocrinology*, 81:1387, 1967.
178. Tindall, J. S., Knaggas, G. S., and Turvey, A.: *J. Endocr.*, 40:205, 1968.
179. Tiwalker, P. K., Ratner, A., and Meites, J.: *Amer. J. Physiol.*, 205:213, 1963.
180. Taymor, M. L.: *Clin. Obstet. Gynec.*, 10:670, 1967.
181. Tcheng, K. T.: *Compt. Rend. Soc. Biol. (Paris)*, 151:1838, 1958.
182. Tindall, J. S., and Yokohama, A.: *Endocrinology*, 71:196, 1962.
183. Tindall, J. S., Knaggs, G. S., and Turvey, A.: *J. Endocr.*, 37:279, 1967.
184. Tuppy, H., and Du Vigneaud, V.: *Biochim. Biophys. Acta*, 11:449, 1953.

185. Van Denmark, N. L., and Hays, R. L.: *Fertil. Steril.*, 5:131, 1954.
186. Velasco, M. E., and Taleisnik, S.: *Endocrinology*, 84:132, 1969.
187. Verney, E. B.: *Proc. Roy. Soc., London, (Ser. B.)*, 135:27, 1947.
188. Vigneaud, V. du, et al.: *J. Biol. Chem.*, 205:949, 1953.
189. Vigneaud, V. du, et al.: *J. Biol. Chem.*, 235:64, 1960.
190. Vigneaud, V. du, and Chang, W. Y.: *Endocrinology*, 71:977, 1962.
191. Vorherr, H., Kleeman, C. R., and Lehmen, E.: *Endocrinology*, 81:711, 1967.
192. Wagner, J. W., Erwin, W., and Critchlow, V.: *Endocrinology*, 79:1135, 1966.
193. Watanabe, S., Dhariwal, A. D. S., and MacCann, S. M.: *Endocrinology*, 82:674, 1968.
194. Welsch, C. W., Sar, M., Clemens, J. A., and Meites, J.: *Proc. Soc. Exper. Biol. Med.*, 129:817, 1968.
195. Westman, A.: "Neurohormonale Steuerung des Hypophysen-Zwischenhirnsystems und Ihre Störungen," in *Biologie und Pathologie des Weibes*, 2nd ed. Vol. I, ed. L. Seitz and I. Amreich. Vienna, Urban and Schwarzenberg, 1957.
196. Yamada, T.: *Endocrinology*, 65:216, 1959.
197. Yamashita, K.: *J. Endocr.*, 35:401, 1966.
198. Zeilmaker, G. H., and Moll, J.: *Acta Endocr.*, 55:378, 1967.

Chapter 9
ADRENALS AND SEXUAL FUNCTION

9.1. INTRODUCTION

That a relationship exists between the adrenal cortex and sexual function has been known for more than a century and a half. Already, in 1800, Haller had realized that certain anomalies of genital development were associated with congenital alterations of the adrenal cortex, implying a causal relationship between the two. In 1803 and 1804, respectively, Cooke and Bevern, as well as Roemhil, described the first known instances of the congenital adrenogenital syndrome, calling attention to the existing hyperplasia or tumor of the adrenal cortex in these cases. In the following years Tilesius and Meckel established the foundations for the adrenocortical theory of certain genital anomalies. Meckel went even further and postulated that the adrenal cortex determined the development of sex. This theory was far ahead of its time and, despite its extraordinary clairvoyance, was, understandably perhaps, doomed to fall into oblivion.

Of course, no one at that time could have predicted that the relationship between the adrenals and the gonads would one day prove to be much more intimate than suspected. Not only is there a physiologic and anatomic relationship between the two glands but, what is more important, the adrenals and the gonads are related to each other *embryologically*, since both are derived from a common anlage. Moreover, experiments of the past few years have revealed that steroid hormone metabolism is not exclusively dependent on the gonads and the interrenal system but is established by a metabolic chain some stages of which take place in the adrenal glands while others take place in the ovary or testis, respectively.

Accordingly, the relationship between the adrenal cortex and the ovary has to be examined from the following viewpoints: (1) embryological; (2) chemical; (3) physiological, and (4) pathological and clinical. The next sections deal with these criteria.

9.2. EMBRYOLOGY

The gonad and the adrenal cortex have much in common in terms of embryonal development. It must not be forgotten that both organs are derived from the coelomic crest, which is located away from the midline on both sides of the posterior wall of the primitive peritoneal cavity. The development of the adrenal cortex is discernible at an even earlier stage than that of the gonad. The coelomic crest appears as early as the fourth week of embryonal life and turns into the anlage of the *interrenal system*.

The rise of a separate gonadal bud somewhat below the previously formed crest, representing the sexual portion of the mesonephros (see Chapter 15, Section 15.1.1.), cannot be observed until the end of the fifth week. Either the wolffian body or the interrenal system by itself in embryos ranges over a greater number of somites than would correspond to the eventually formed respective glands, and the caudal pole of the interrenal bud therefore extends beyond the superior pole of the wolffian body. However, owing to progressive shrinkage of these two embryonal buds in the course of their development, the adult gonad is eventually located at the level of the terminal sacral segments, whereas the interrenal system rests against the diaphragm at the level of the last dorsal vertebra.

It is of interest to note that not only does the interrenal system appear earlier and

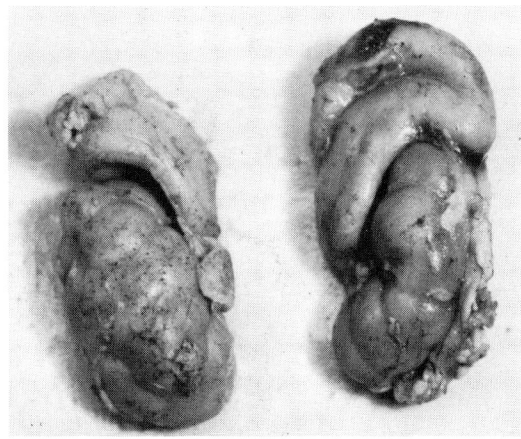

Figure 9-1. Kidneys and adrenals of a five-month female fetus. Notice large size of adrenals compared to kidneys.

develop more precociously than the gonad, but *the adrenal cortex moreover shows signs of much greater activity than the gonad during the entire embryonal era.* Beginning with approximately the third month of intrauterine life, and up to the fifth or sixth months, the adrenal cortex is one of the most voluminous intraabdominal organs (Fig. 9-1). If such bulky adrenals of a five-month fetus are examined histologically, the most striking finding is that they are not made up of the three classical zones of the adult adrenal, i.e., zona glomerulosa, zona fasciculata and zona reticularis. Instead, the embryonal adrenal is composed of tissue that is similar in appearance to that of the last of the three zones, and comprises the full thickness of the organ.

This tissue has histologic and chemical features that are identical to those of the zona reticularis (Fig. 9-2). This phenomenon is not confined to man and to the primates but can also be observed in rodents, particularly the mouse, the embryo

Figure 9-2. Histologic preparation of adrenal cortex of 14-week fetus. Structural features are identical with those of the zona reticularis. There is no trace of either glomerular or fascicular zone.

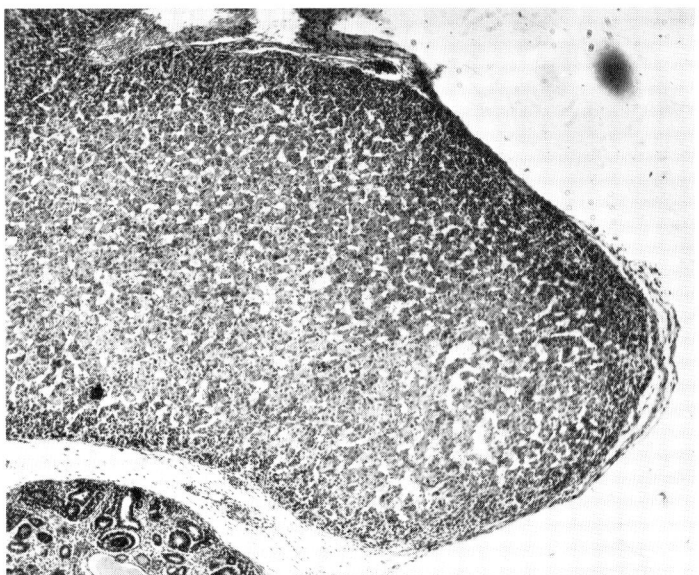

Figure 9-3. Histologic preparation of adrenal of fetal mouse at term, revealing the same fundamental structure as that of human fetal adrenal.

of which has an adrenal structure quite similar to that of man (Fig. 9-3).

Elsewhere, this author[19] advanced the theory that, because it consisted only of reticularis-like tissue, *the fetal adrenal was an organ embryologically and functionally distinct from the adult adrenal cortex which, in comparison, consisted mainly of the glomerular and fascicular zones.*

That such hyperplastic fetal adrenals were the site of active steroidogenesis could be shown in different animals. Thus, Roos[89] in rats, and Bloch and Benirschke[11] in armadillos, found that fetal adrenals elaborated corticoids, estrogens as well as progesterone. Active steroidogenesis in the human species has been shown to occur from the third month onwards by Cavallero and his colleagues.[28] Bengtsson and his associates[5] observed that injections of C-14 labeled cholesterol produced great concentrations of radioactivity in the adrenals of six-month fetuses. Further supportive evidence was reported by Villee and Loring,[103] who studied fetal adrenals in vitro. These and similar data would seem to bear out the morphologic finding of fetal adrenal hyperactivity by biochemical means.

At about the sixth month, another type of tissue begins to be formed alongside the precociously developed reticular zone and is clearly distinguishable from the latter (Figs. 9-4 and 9-5) by virtue of the fact that *it arises from an inwardly growing subcapsular blastema,* as opposed to the reticular zone, which arises from *an out-*

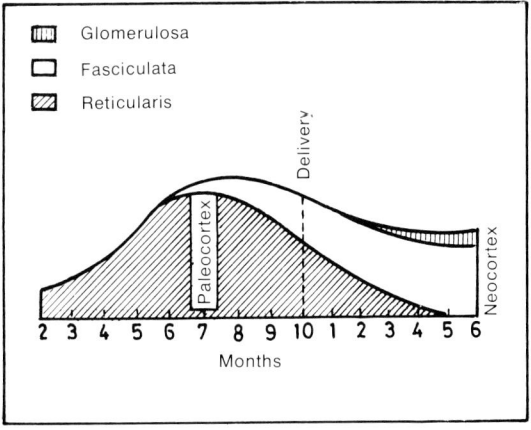

Figure 9-4. Diagram of development of primitive cortex (paleocortex) and definitive cortex (neocortex). (From Botella: *Arch. Gynäk.*, 183:75, 1953.)

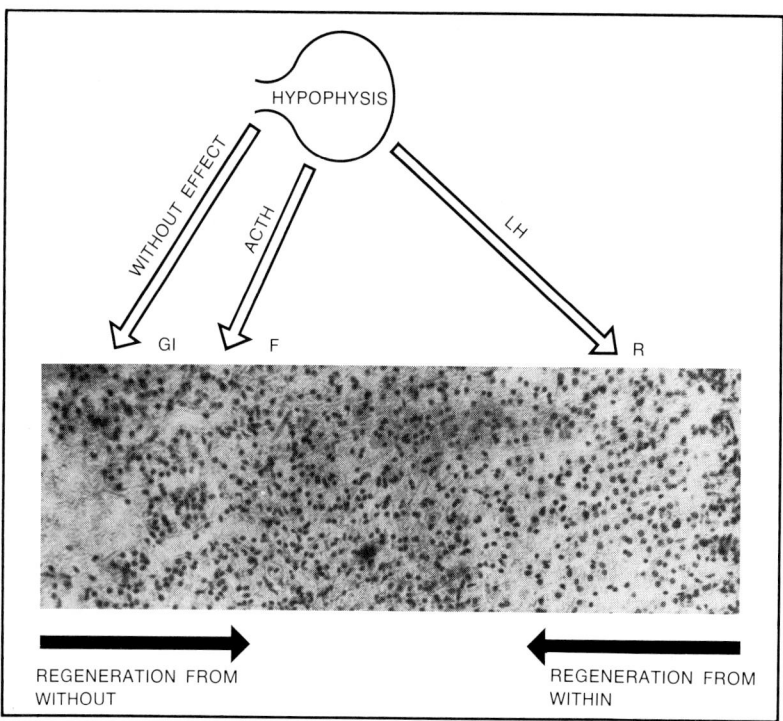

Figure 9-5. Diagram of regeneration in adult adrenal at the expense of subcapsular blastema (neocortex) and juxtamedullary blastema (paleocortex), with indication in each instance of the trophic hormone that stimulates the corresponding zone. (From Botella: in E. Romero: *Hipófisis*. Barcelona, Editorial Científico-Médica, 1954, p. 195.)

wardly growing *juxtamedullary blastema.* Cortical regeneration proceeds in the same manner throughout the rest of an individual's life, starting from these two different foci which, one may be led to assume, belong in fact to different stocks of tissue. In the female, this process of regeneration is always more intensive than it is in the male.[65]

This author has therefore proposed that a distinction be made between the *primitive cortex,* or *paleocortex,* and the *definitive cortex,* or *neocortex.*[19] Their respective characteristics are represented in Table 9-1.

A similar systematization can also be seen in Figure 9-3. *In the course of this study, it should become apparent that these two embryologic units also behave as two functionally independent units.*

Our theory was subsequently shown to be correct.[9, 10, 34, 45, 70, 85]

The term *postnatal degeneration*[6, 7, 30, 49] refers to the phenomenon of adrenal regression which, though apparent as early as the seventh month, becomes much more pronounced after birth (Fig. 9-4). Postnatal degeneration or atrophy occurs as a consequence of the disappearance of the paleocortex, which has almost completely disappeared by the time a child reaches the age of six months.

In mice and in wild rodents,[34, 35] postnatal atrophy is even more striking.

Inclusions of interrenal tissue in the vicinity of, or within, the gonads had been demonstrated long ago by Marchand. These were called *accessory adrenals,* since their embryologic origin could obviously be attributed to the close proximity of the two embryonal buds. Since this discovery, we

TABLE 9-1.

PALEOCORTEX	NEOCORTEX
Zona reticularis	Zona glomerulosa and fasciculata
Juxtamedullary origin and regeneration	Subcapsular origin and regeneration
Transitional zone	Definitive zone
Synthesis of C-19 steroids	Synthesis of C-21 steroids
Sex hormones	Corticoids

have become accustomed to finding inclusions of adrenal tissue in the gonads.

It has been this author's repeated contention that the adrenal cortex should be viewed as a "third gonad," in view of the now universally accepted fact that the cortex elaborates sex hormones.

9.3. POSTNATAL DEVELOPMENT AND REGENERATION

The *definitive cortex*, or *neocortex*, develops after birth and persists for the rest of life. Its function is to produce corticoids, the hormones indispensable for metabolism and the maintenance of life. The *primitive cortex*, or *paleocortex*, of utmost importance in the fetus, after birth persists in a state of atrophy and only during later life may show fleeting episodes of activity. It experiences a first transient phase of development at *puberty* (see Chapter 16). The question of whether the paleocortex again increases in thickness during *pregnancy* is still a matter of debate. It may be said that, at least in some women, it does. However, there is no doubt that the zona reticularis regains considerable importance during the *climacterium*, or during an *artificially induced climacterium*, resulting from castration in both man and animals. Thus, it may be stated that, *with the exception of transient episodes of development, the paleocortex disappears between birth and the menopause*.

The paleocortex does not reach its greatest degree of development in normal individuals. It may appear surprisingly well developed in pathologic states. Hyperplasia of this tissue is responsible for the syndrome known by the name of *adrenogenital syndrome* (Chapter 32).

The special features of this tissue with regard to its histologic and histochemical properties are to be reviewed in a later section. For the time being, it seems of interest to point out that both histologic observations of the regenerative process and experimental data of adrenal cortex regeneration in animals[7] indicate that, *while the glomerular and fascicular zones regenerate at the expense of the subcapsular blastema—that is, in a centripetal way, from without inward—the paleocortex does so from the juxtamedullary blastema,* *that is, growing in a centrifugal way, from within outward* (Fig. 9–5). This diverse mode of regeneration by itself would seem to be enough evidence to assume that the tissues involved are of different origins and have different functions. However, what is more, the two types of tissue also behave in totally distinct manners insofar as function, histologic texture and response to pituitary hormones are concerned. *In conclusion, present knowledge concerning the development and the vicissitudes of life of the adrenal cortex would appear to indicate that the latter consists of two different entities. These two different entities are subsequently shown to play equally different roles in the physiology of sex.*

9.4. EFFECT OF SEX HORMONES ON THE CORTEX

Castration produces profound changes in the structure of the adrenal cortex.[6, 13, 33, 34, 66] As a result, both ovarian and testicular hormones have been assumed to modify adrenal function. The problem can be examined from the following three angles: (1) castration; (2) structural changes in the cortex under the effect of sex hormones; and (3) variations in corticoid blood levels under the effect of the same hormones.

9.4.1. CHANGES IN THE ADRENAL CORTEX RESULTING FROM CASTRATION

As indicated previously, the adrenal cortex undergoes hypertrophy following castration.[6, 13, 33, 34, 64] Houssay and his co-workers,[56] and more recently Altman and co-workers,[1] found a high incidence of adrenal adenomas in castrated rats and mice. Nandi and colleagues[79] reported that steroidogenesis was accelerated in castrated mice (for further details, see Section 9.9.2).

9.4.2. STRUCTURAL CHANGES IN THE CORTEX UNDER THE EFFECT OF SEX HORMONES

In the course of our earlier investigations,[13] estrogen injections were found to produce thickening of the cortex, with predominance of the zona reticularis, whereas progestogens produced predominant thickening of the zona fasciculata (Fig. 9–6). Similar patterns of cortical thickening were subsequently reported by various investigators.[6, 7, 32, 33, 35, 85, 87, 98] Thus, both progesterone and estrogens seem to produce an increase in cortical thickness and function. In contrast, testosterone[65, 66] reduces the thickness of the adrenal gland.

9.4.3. EFFECT OF SEX HORMONES ON CORTICOID BLOOD LEVELS

Estrogen injections provoke an increase in the level of circulating corticoids.[68, 77, 105] It has also been shown that progestogens produce increased aldosterone synthesis.[68, 72] The latter action by progestogens, however, is associated with the antagonistic influence of progesterone on aldosterone activity at the tissue level, as already mentioned in Chapter 3 (Section 3.8.3).

Two possible explanations have been suggested for the action by the ovarian hormones on corticoid blood levels. Sandberg and his colleagues[94, 95] believe that the action involved is one affecting transport, since estrogens increase *transcortin* values. On the other hand, Kitay[66] offers a much more simple explanation: both estrogens and progesterone are known to induce pituitary secretion of ACTH.

9.5. HORMONE METABOLISM OF THE ADRENAL CORTEX

The presence of at least the following steroids in the cortex has been demonstrated:

1. *Specific adrenocortical hormones* (corticoids):
    a. *mineralocorticoids* (deoxycorticosterone, aldosterone)
    b. *glucocorticoids* (corticosterone, dehydrocorticosterone, cortisone, cortisol)
2. *Sex hormones:*
    a. *androgens* (17-ketosteroids, more than 20 having been isolated)
    b. *estrogens* (primarily estrone)
    c. *progestogens* (progesterone and a series of intermediary products of progesterone and corticoids) (Fig. 9–7)

9.5.1. DEMONSTRATION OF SEX HORMONES IN THE ADRENAL CORTEX

Already early classical investigations (see summaries in Botella,[13] Courrier et al.,[30] Dorfman[38]) had led to the demonstration of estrogens, progesterone and androgens in adrenocortical tissue. By means of extractive chemical methods, several workers (Baulieu et al.[3]; Dorfman[37, 38]; Hechter and Pincus[53]; Oertel and Eik-Nes[80]; Peron[83] and Welicky and Engel[106]) more recently achieved the isolation of the active principles estrone, progesterone and androsterone, as well as that of a large number of

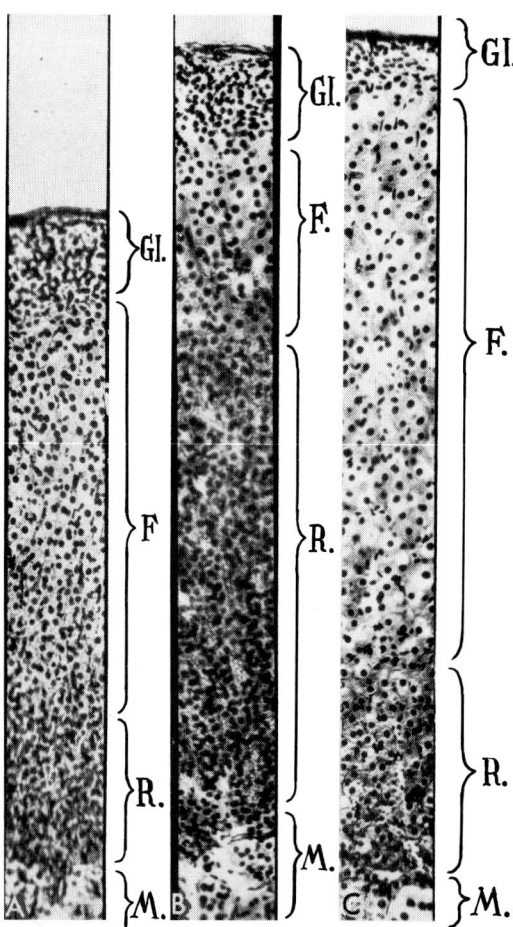

Figure 9–6. Effect of ovarian hormones on adrenal cortex of rat. A, Control. B, Injected with estrogens. C, Injected with progesterone. (From Botella: *Suprarrenales y Función sexual*. Madrid, Morata, 1946.)

Adrenals and Sexual Function

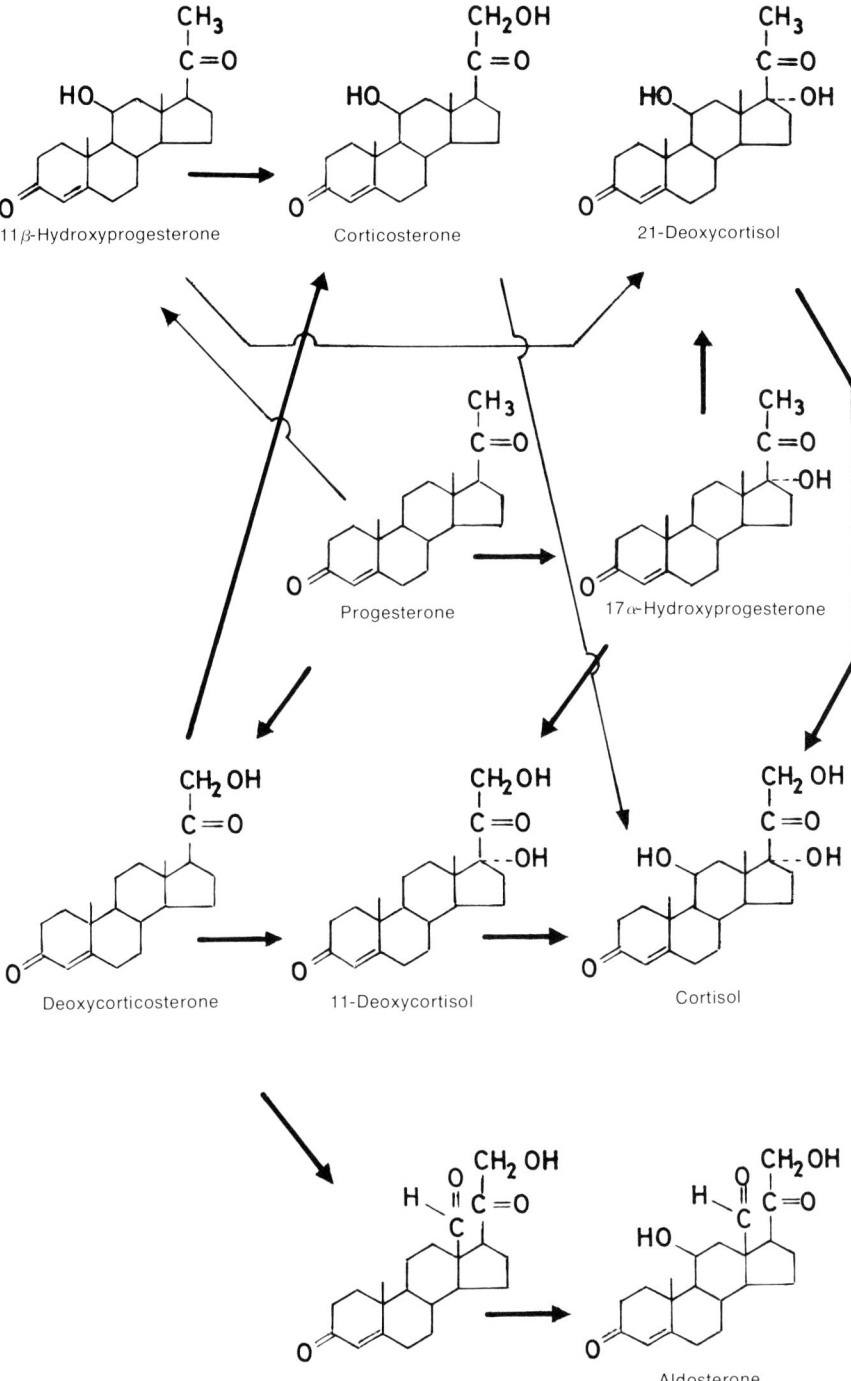

Figure 9-7. Diagram of biogenesis of adrenocortical C-21 steroids, according to Dorfman (somewhat modified). Progesterone, represented as the central product, is formed from cholesterol by way of pregnanolone. Progesterone undergoes 17-hydroxylation and is converted to 17-hydroxyprogesterone which, by means of 21-hydroxylation, is converted to 11-deoxycortisol, and the latter, in turn, by means of 11-hydroxylation, gives the basic glucocorticoid, cortisol. At the same time, through 21-hydroxylation, progesterone is converted to deoxycorticosterone and the latter, after undergoing 11-hydroxylation and 18-oxidation, to aldosterone. As can be seen, three specific hydroxylases (11-, 17- and 21-) and one oxydase (18-) are the basic enzymes of the entire corticoid steroidogenesis.

intermediary catabolites, some (not all) of which are listed in Table 9-2.

Observations of particular interest have been made on extracts of adrenal tumor tissue by Dorfman[37] and by Symington and his colleagues,[99] and similarly, on normal adrenals removed in cases of breast cancer, by Lombardo and colleagues[58, 74] and by Berliner and associates.[8]

Camacho and Migeon[24] have isolated testosterone, a most uncommon finding, from hypertrophic adrenals. Goldzieher and Fariss[47] have been able to obtain estrogens from the adrenals of surgically castrated women. According to both Vecsei and co-workers[101] and Pierson,[84] adrenocortical tumors are capable of metabolizing large quantities of progesterone. Those are but a few isolated instances, gleaned from an enormous amount of recent literature, of reports dealing with the presence of practically every single sex steroid in either normal or pathologically altered adrenal tissue.

While studying adrenal steroidogenesis in vivo, Desphande and his colleagues[36] discovered the presence of sex steroids in the adrenal vein from which they could all be obtained. For corticoid synthesis, the adrenal utilizes primarily progesterone.[110] Kazekas and Kokai[64] have isolated large amounts of estrogens from progesterone-perfused adrenals of rats.

9.5.2. URINARY EXCRETION OF STEROIDS IN CASTRATED ANIMALS AND WOMEN

The question of elevated urinary steroid elimination in the syndromes of adrenocortical hyperfunction is to be discussed in Chapter 33. This aspect is therefore not insisted upon here although it represents further evidence of adrenal biogenesis of sex hormones. We shall nevertheless briefly point out a fact that is of utmost importance in clinical gynecology: *the continued urinary elimination of sex steroids after castration.* Currently, this is a perfectly well known fact which has been analyzed by numerous investigators.[20, 21, 26]

TABLE 9-2. Steroids Isolated by Perfusion of Adrenals

SUBSTRATE	PRODUCT	AUTHOR
	6β-HYDROXYLATION:	
Progesterone	6β-hydroxyprogesterone	Levy et al.: *J. Biol. Chem.*, 203:433, 1953
Androstenedione	6β-androstenedione	Meyer et al.: *J. Biol. Chem.*, 203:463, 1953
	11β-HYDROXYLATION:	
11-Deoxycorticosterone	Corticosterone	Hechter et al.: *Rec. Progr. Horm. Res.*, 6: 215, 1951
11-Deoxycortisol	Cortisol	Ungar et al.: *J. Biol. Chem.*, 207:375, 1954
Progesterone	11β-hydroxyprogesterone	Levy et al. (loc. cit.)
Progesterone	Corticosterone	Hechter et al. (loc. cit.)
17α-Hydroxyprogesterone	Cortisol	Levy et al.: *J. Biol. Chem.*, 208:156, 1955
Epiandrosterone	11β-hydroxyandrosterone	Meyer et al. (loc. cit.)
Testosterone	11β-hydroxytestosterone	Meyer et al. (loc. cit.)
Progesterone	11-deoxycortisol	Levy et al. (loc. cit.)
Progesterone	17α-hydroxyprogesterone	Hechter et al. (loc. cit.)
Progesterone	Cortisol	Ungar et al. (loc. cit.)
3β-Hydroxypregnen-20-one	Cortisol	Hechter et al. (loc. cit.)
	21-HYDROXYLATION:	
Progesterone	11-deoxycortisol	Hechter et al. (loc. cit.)
	Corticosterone	Ungar et al. (loc. cit.)
	Cortisol	Dorfman: *Ciba Coll.*, VI:134, 1954
17α-Hydroxyprogesterone	Cortisol	Dorfman (loc. cit.)
	16α-HYDROXYLATION:	
Progesterone	16α-R-progesterone	Weliky et al.: *J. Biol. Chem.*, 238:1302, 1963
Progesterone	11-ketoprogesterone	Oertel et al.: *Endocrinology*, 70:39, 1962
	18α-HYDROXYLATION:	
Progesterone	18α-hydroxyprogesterone	Peron: *Endocrinology*, 70:386, 1962

It should be added that data obtained by us on the urine of surgically castrated women[21, 33] make the extragonadal (adrenocortical) origin of those sex hormones abundantly clear.

9.5.3. METABOLISM OF CORTICAL C-21 STEROIDS

The term C-21 steroids is used to designate steroids of 21 carbon atoms, i.e., derivatives of *pregnane* (Fig. 3–1), which, in addition to all natural progestogens, comprise corticoids of both the mineralo- and glucocorticoid variety (see Fig. 9–7).

The chemical similarities between progestogens and corticoids have been brought to light through investigations concerning the biosynthesis of corticoids, which revealed *progesterone to be an intermediary metabolite between cholesterol and corticoids.*

This is a new and very interesting concept in endocrinologic biochemistry, that has been developed principally by Hechter's group.[53] As a result, progesterone no longer figures as just one more adrenocortical sex hormone that is specific of the "adrenal sexual zone," or "third gonad," but actually is a *pivotal component of the metabolic chain that leads to the synthesis of corticoids.*

Figure 9–7 reproduces the metabolic relationships of those compounds, while Figure 9–13 shows their enzymatic correlation.

The enzyme *21-hydroxylase* deserves special mention. By attaching a hydroxyl group to 17-hydroxyprogesterone, it converts the latter to 11-deoxycorticosterone. Bongiovanni and his associates[12] have shown that disruption of this enzymatic process results in failure to form glucocorticoids at the expense of progesterone and is the underlying cause of the *adrenogenital syndrome* (see Chapter 33).

9.5.4. BIOSYNTHESIS OF ADRENOCORTICAL STEROIDS

The studies of Hechter and Pincus[53] and those of Heard,[52] in which human adrenals were perfused with radioactive materials (C-14 labeled steroids), have produced a wealth of data concerning corticoid biosynthesis. In recent years, a large amount of research[3, 26, 40, 80, 82, 106] has been devoted to exploring almost every step of the intermediary steroid metabolism in the adrenal cortex.

It has become apparent that the adrenal gland serves as a central staging area for the intermediary metabolism of all cyclopentanophenanthrene derivatives. Figure 9–7 illustrates the fact that the cardinal role in all those metabolic processes is played by progesterone. By definition, C-21 steroids (see Chapter 3, Section 3.2) are pregnane-derived steroids, that is, compounds with 21 carbon atoms. Pregnanolone and progesterone are the two basic compounds from which all other corticoids of the C-21 steroid variety are derived. Accordingly, progesterone may also be classified as a corticoid, since it originates specifically in the adrenal cortex and is essential for the biogenesis of the remaining adrenocortical hormones.

A series of data, obtained by means of perfusion studies with radioactive steroids, has been hypothetically constructed in Figure 9–13. Progesterone synthesis utilizes cholesterol, which is first converted to pregnanolone. 3β-ol-dehydrogenase, known to be present as well in the ovary (see Chapter 2, Section 2.5.1, and Chapter 3, Section 3.5.2), converts pregnanolone to progesterone. Through the intervention of 21-hydroxylase, a specific adrenal enzyme that is not found in the ovary, progesterone is transformed into deoxycorticosterone. At the same time, 17-hydroxylation of progesterone (a process also operative in the ovary) gives hydroxyprogesterone, which serves as an intermediate stage for the synthesis of cortisol. An essential step in the synthesis of cortisol, as well as that of aldosterone, is 11-hydroxylation. Thus, apart from 21-hydroxylase, 11-hydroxylase is another highly specific adrenal enzyme. Aldosterone biosynthesis further requires the presence of 18-oxidase, which seems to be a specific enzyme of the zona glomerulosa. The different enzymes are by no means spread throughout the cortex in a diffuse manner but have a specific distribution within the different zones.

9.5.5. URINARY EXCRETION OF ADRENOCORTICAL STEROIDS

The hormones originating in the adrenal cortex are corticoids (gluco- and mineralocorticoids, estrogens, progesteroids and androgens. Among these, androgens and corticoids are the most genuine representatives of adrenocortical excretion.[37, 38, 82] While urinary corticoids represent the surplus from a completed cycle of synthesis urinary 17-ketosteroids reflect interruption of that cycle (see Fig. 9–13). Therefore, urinary 17-ketosteroid values are elevated in those conditions in which there is faulty cortisol synthesis owing to 21-hydroxylase deficiency.[12] It follows that urinary 17-ketosteroids cannot be regarded as a true index of adrenocortical function. *The genuine representatives of adrenal function are the corticoids, whereas 17-ketosteroids reflect the fact that adrenal function is disturbed.*

Two inactive catabolites of adrenal origin deserve to be mentioned here: *pregnanediol*, a catabolite of progesterone, including progesterone of ovarian origin, and *pregnanetriol*, which is a specific catabolite of 17-hydroxyprogesterone. As a typical adrenal metabolite, pregnanetriol reflects adrenal, not ovarian, progestational activity (Finkelstein and Goldberg[43]).

9.6. THE SEXUAL ZONE OF THE ADRENAL CORTEX

Based on the embryologic and histologic background of the two tissue stocks of the adrenal cortex, and in the presence of convincing evidence that sex hormone synthesis in fact takes place in the cortex, it seems logical to attribute such synthesis to either tissue in question. Hence the concept of a *sexual zone of the adrenal cortex*, a concept that rests on a series of physiologic tests. The sexual cortex corresponds to a zone, earlier described by us as primitive cortex, or paleocortex, solely because of its precocious embryonal origin, which in the strict physiologic sense of the word does not really have the character of an adrenal cortex but rather that of an *accessory gonad*, intervening in processes of sexual function only during phases of eclipse or failure of the true gonad. It can thus be conceived as a kind of *vicarious sex gland* that appears to function: (1) *during embryonal life*, the gonad still being immature; (2) *during puberty*, the gonad not having matured fast enough to meet the body's demands for sex hormones; (3) *during pregnancy*, or at least during some phases of it, in order to strengthen the chorio-ovarian endocrine system; (4) *during the climacterium or menopause*, in order to avert absolute and total lack of sex hormones and the resulting serious consequences for genital trophism and endocrine balance, and (5) *in some pathologic states*, without serving any compensatory purpose, as a simple primary abnormal event.

Various authors have described definite morphologic structures, differentiated within the adrenal cortex, as responsible for sexual activity. For instance, Grollmann[51] has described what he calls the *androgenic fetal zone*, which corresponds to our *paleocortex*. According to Grollmann, this zone develops during the embryonal period and its mission is to secrete androgens in order to counteract the flood of estrogens of female origin and to allow the development of the wolffian organs, that is, the male genital tract. (For further data concerning the androgenic zone and the mechanism of action involved, see Chapter 15). Let us add, however, that in Grollmann's view, the androgenic fetal zone secretes androgens exclusively and therefore develops only in males, so as to create the necessary conditions for the development of male characteristics.

In 1928, Deanesly and Howard[57] described the presence in rats of a well differentiated zone, lying between the medulla and the cortex, which they denominated "X zone." Judging by their original account, their X zone could be inferred to have features similar to those of Grollmann's androgenic zone or to those of what we call the paleocortex in man. In agreement with these findings, we were able to demonstrate[16] that the X zone under consideration gave the specific reactions of the sexual zone. However, in later years, Benua and Howard[6] questioned the sexual nature of that zone, and presently there is still no consensus as to whether or not the X zone should be regarded as identical to the sexual zone. It is our opinion that the X zone of small rodents is unquestionably the equivalent of the sexual zone in man.

In the golden hamster, the existence of a rich sexual zone has also been demonstrated.[49, 61] This animal's zone is particularly reactive and its reactions are quite similar to those described by us in the

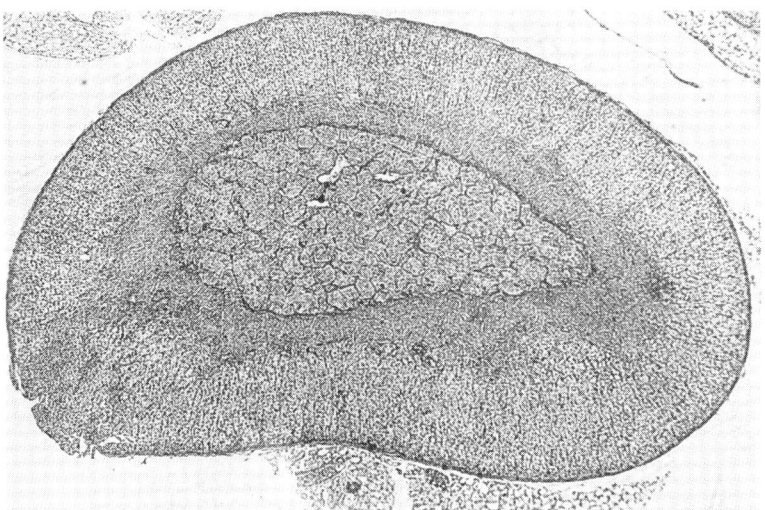

Figure 9–8. X zone in adrenal of spayed mouse. Notice good differentiation of intermediate zone between cortex and medulla. Unlike the case in the human species, the X zone of the mouse can be distinguished from the zona reticularis.

human adrenal, including the intense postcastration reaction. In addition, its histochemical features match perfectly those of the human sexual zone.

In 1938, while studying adrenals of the adrenogenital syndrome that had been removed by the surgeon Broster, the English histologist Vines came up with a specific staining reaction with Ponceau fuchsin in which the granulations of the sex hormone-bearing adrenal zone stained red. He further found that such staining was most prominent in the zona reticularis and was invariably associated with sexual activity of pathologic adrenals. We have verified the occurrence of such fuchsinophilic staining not only in adrenals of the adrenogenital syndrome (see Chapter 32) but also in the paleocortex (the so-called androgenic zone) of the fetus (Fig. 9–10) and the X zone of castrated mice as well (Fig. 9–8); this seems to denote a close relationship between the fuchsinophilic human sexual zone, which we call paleocortex, and the X zone of animals. Ashbel and Seligman later developed a staining procedure with Nile blue with which they claim to have achieved specific staining of the carbonyl groups of 17-ketosteroids. Although the specificity of this reaction, just as that of Vines' reaction, is open to question, the fact is that Ashbel and Seligman's method stains exclusively both the androgenic fetal zone and the postmenopausal human adrenal while at the same time, according to Benua and Howard,[6] failing to stain the X zone of

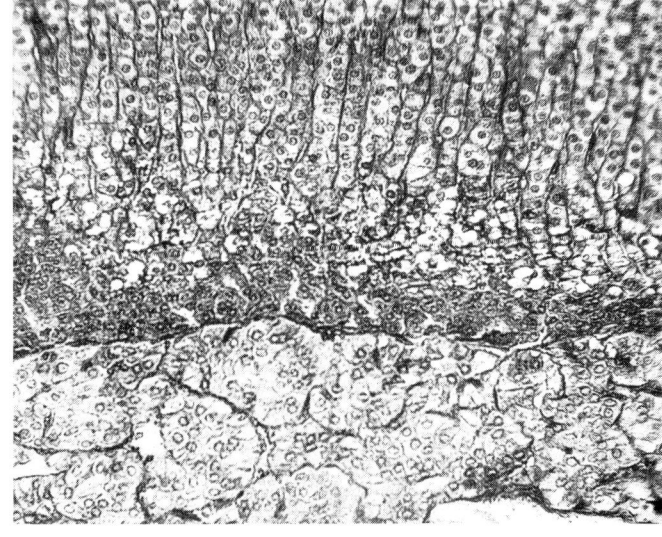

Figure 9–9. Area from Figure 9–8 at a higher magnification. Difference between reticular zone and X zone is distinguishable.

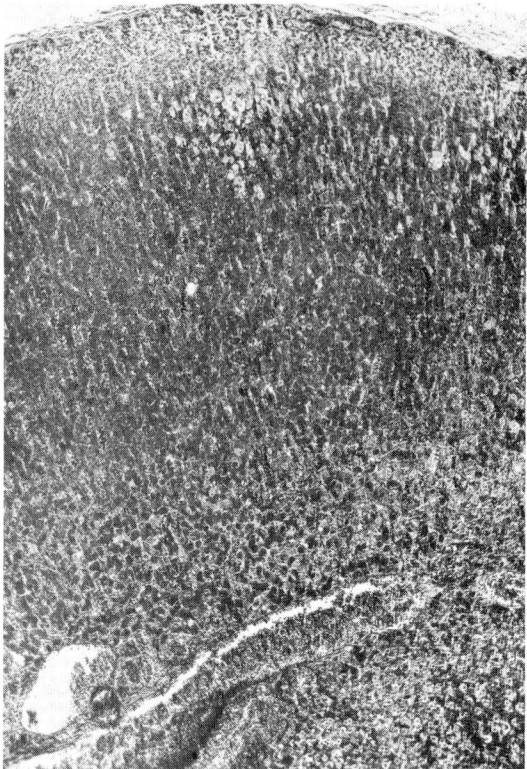

Figure 9-10. Adrenal of seven-month female fetus. Marked development of sexual zone seen with strongly positive Ponceau fuchsin stain (fuchsinophilic zone in photomicrograph appears black).

castrated mice. Apart from that, the presumptive "sexual zone" reveals other characteristic features, such as the presence of birefringent lipoids[7] and sudanophobia, compared to the other layers of the cortex, which are sudanophilic.

The same characteristics of the sexual zone or X zone that are found in laboratory rodents and in the human species are also present in wild rodents (Delost[35]). Studies by Jones[63] have shown that the cortical metabolism of X zone slices consists in preferably synthesizing testosterone at the expense of progesterone, which seems to corroborate our earlier hypothesis.

Lastly, let us call attention to the very interesting work of Houssay's group[56] concerning the occurrence of spontaneous tumors in castrated rats. In certain strains of rats, castration produces adrenal hyperplasia to a much greater extent than it does in women. The mechanism involved is believed to consist in a compensatory effort on part of the pituitary, resulting in a high rate of gonadotropin secretion. In some strains, on the other hand, this may lead to the induction of truly neoplastic growths. While hyperplastic reactions are estrogenic, tumoral growths are strongly androgenic and are associated with virilization.

There is no doubt in our mind that the zone we are referring to is distinctive enough to have a special place assigned to it in what is commonly known as the adrenal cortex, and deserves the name of *sexual adrenal* or *sexual zone of the adrenal cortex*, whereas the rest of the cortex may be qualified as the *metabolic adrenal* or *metabolic zone of the adrenal cortex*.

9.7. EFFECT OF PITUITARY ON THE ADRENAL CORTEX

9.7.1. ACTH AND THE ADRENAL CORTEX

The action exerted by the pituitary on the adrenal cortex by means of adrenocorticotropic hormone, or ACTH, is well known. The intimate mechanism of ACTH action, as it appears in the light of modern ideas, has been outlined in one of the preceding paragraphs.

The fact that ACTH enhances sex steroid synthesis by the cortex is generally less well known. Caldwell and colleagues[23] have observed increased enzyme activity of 3β-ol-dehydrogenase within mitochondria of adrenal tissue under the influence of corticotropin. Estrogen synthesis in perfused adrenals has been found to be stimulated by ACTH.[44,60] While androgen[93] and progesterone[88] biogenesis is similarly increased in castrated animals and humans, ACTH administration is known to increase the rate of urinary 17-ketosteroid excretion. Thus, it is obvious that, under the specific stimulus of ACTH, the adrenal cortex produces not only corticoids but also sex steroids.

9.7.2. LH AND THE ADRENAL CORTEX

Regrettably, few investigators have cared to analyze the *effect of gonadotropins on the adrenal cortex*. Yet, it is clear that if the gonadotropins are biocatalysts of estrogen, androgen and progestogen synthesis, and provided that these three groups of hormones are physiologically present in the adrenal cortex, then the latter three hormones might be expected as well to exert some kind of effect on the adrenal cortex.

In 1950, our group, in cooperation with Cano,[16-19] investigated this question and believe the following facts to have been established: first, that chorionic gonadotropin (LH) markedly increased the thickness of the zona reticularis in experimental animals; second, that there was a widening of the fuchsinophilic zone, with enhancement of granularity; and, third, that the uterus and vagina of castrated females, or the vesicles and prostate of castrated males, increased in weight under the influence of this gonadotropic hormone (Fig. 9-11). *We concluded that, under gonadotropic influence, the adrenal cortex of a castrated animal in each case secreted the sex hormone of the corresponding sex. Thus, the sexual zone of the adrenal cortex functions endocrinologically as a true gonad, not merely on account of its embryologic and physiologic properties but, also because it is subject to the same pituitary control and susceptible to the same gonadotropic hormone that stimulates the gonads.*

Modern studies have established the stimulatory effect of LH on the adrenal cortex in rats,[4, 22, 25, 27, 48, 59] monkeys[55, 100] and, thanks mainly to the work of Jones,[63] Farnsworth,[41] Lanman,[70] Plate,[86] Rosenfeld[92] and our own group, also in women.

According to recent observations on dogs by Cushman,[31] LH does not seem to affect the rate of 17-ketosteroid excretion. On the other hand, Lantos and co-workers[71] hold the view that, although hydroxylation of C-21 steroids is a specific ACTH effect on the adrenal cortex, LH activity may be involved in adrenal steroid synthesis at some earlier phase.

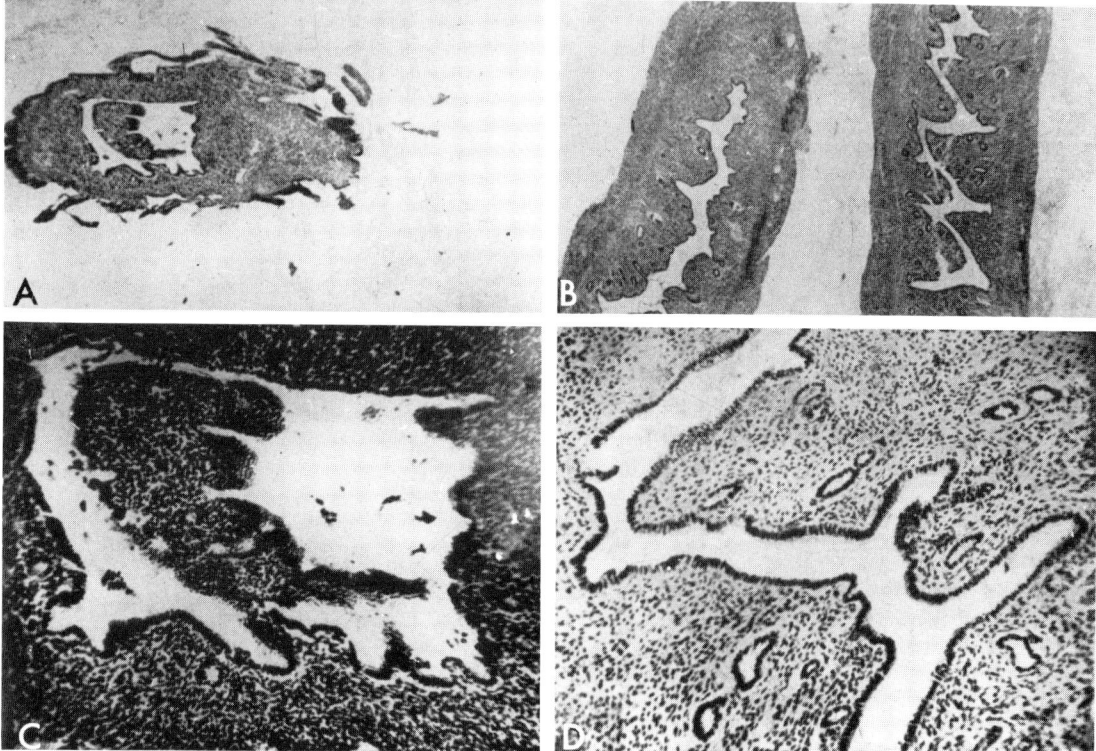

Figure 9-11. Indirect effect, mediated by adrenal cortex, of chorionic gonadotropin on uterus of castrated albino mouse. *A,* Castrated mouse with atrophy of uterus. *B,* Same, at higher magnification. *C,* Castrated animal, treated with 1000 I.U. of chorionic gonadotropin. Note hyperplasia and regeneration of uterus. *D,* Higher magnification of C. Experimental conditions were similar to those in Figure 9-11. (From Botella and Cano: *Arch. Med. Exper.,* 13:81, 1950.)

9.7.3. STH AND THE ADRENAL CORTEX

Division of the adrenal cortex into three zones: *glomerulosa, fasciculata* and *reticularis*, is classical. The studies by Greep and Deane,[49] and those by Giroud and his colleagues,[46] have confirmed the zonal distribution of gluco- and mineralocorticoids. Accordingly, glucocorticoids originate in the *zona fasciculata*, whereas mineralocorticoids are believed to be elaborated in the *zona glomerulosa*. With the exception of progesterone—the synthesis of which is linked with glucocorticoid synthesis (discussed previously), and which therefore presumably takes place in the zona fasciculata—the sex hormones are thought to be a product of the zona reticularis.

While LH appears to be the appropriate exciting agent for the reticular zone and for the biogenesis of sex hormones, ACTH stimulates the zona fasciculata as well as glucocorticoid synthesis. The question as to which is the appropriate exciting agent for mineralocorticoid synthesis by the glomerular zone remains unanswered. Until recently it had been suspected that the latter zone might not be subject to pituitary control.

Investigations by Giroud's group,[46] by Farrel,[42] by Hilton and colleagues[54] and by Jenkins[62] would seem to indicate that aldosterone secretion is under hypothalamic control.

On the other hand, the idea put forth several years ago that STH provided the stimulation for aldosterone biosynthesis seems to have received no confirmation[75, 102] and remains a moot point in adrenal physiology.

In summary, ACTH may be concluded to be the most general and most common stimulant of each adrenocortical zone; LH exerts mainly a stimulatory effect on sexual steroidogenesis; and vasopressin seemingly plays a specific role in the biosynthesis of aldosterone. Thus, the question of specific hormonal stimulation for the three zones by three different hormones seems to have been settled.

9.8 PLACE OF THE "SEXUAL ZONE" IN THE ENDOCRINE SYSTEM

The sexual zone functions as an accessory sexual gland. It is stimulated by a trophic

TABLE 9–3

ZONE	HORMONE SECRETED	SPECIFIC STIMULANT
Glomerulosa	Mineralocorticoids	Vasopressin?
Fasciculata	Glucocorticoids	ACTH
Reticularis	Sex hormones	LH

hormone of interstitial nature which is the same as that which stimulates the gonads. Its place in the endocrine system is assigned to a function of a compensatory nature. Through the action of gonadotropin A, the pituitary can be said to excite testicular gametogenesis and the development of the ovarian follicular apparatus. Through the action of gonadotropin B, it excites the ovarian stroma and corpus luteum on the one hand, and the testicular stroma on the other. At the same time, it stimulates the development of the adrenocortical sexual zone. Finally, by means of ACTH, the pituitary stimulates the zona fasciculata of the cortex, promoting the production of glucocorticoids.

In the absence of either the male or the female gonads, the adrenal cortex is thus capable of assuming the task of compensating, if but in part, for any existing deficit. During those periods of life in which the demand for sex hormones is particularly strong, owing to a nonfunctioning gonad in either sex, the sexual zone of the adrenal cortex enters into action.

It is a well known fact that *castration* in both males and females stimulates pituitary gonadotropin production (see Chapter 18). Consequently, the functional inactivation of either testes or ovaries immediately brings about gonadotrophic hyperactivity and results in activation of the compensatory capacity of the adrenal cortex by the respective gonadotropic hormone.

During *intrauterine life*, adrenal sexual zone function is probably upheld by the action of maternal gonadotropins, reaching the fetal circulation through the placenta. Although the question of whether chorionic gonadotropin is capable of penetrating the placental barrier is still unsettled, it can be assumed that small quantities of the hormone, undoubtedly smaller than those reaching the maternal blood, can reach the fetal circulation.

The sexual cortex can then be admitted to hold the position of a vicarious gland which, geared as it is into the system of pituitary regulation, serves as a ballast or equilibrator in cases of gonadal insufficiency. A mechanism devised by nature, it provides for the maintenance of what has elsewhere been referred to as *steroid homeostasis*. What must be foremost in mind regarding the regulation of steroid homeostasis are first, that the sex hormone that is lacking must be substituted (estrogens in females and androgens in males), and second, that the adrenal probably intervenes in balancing steroid homeostasis by means of the heterosexual hormone, e.g., in females, by elaborating the androgens that under physiologic conditions circulate in the female blood (the physiologic and equilibrating function of this phenomenon has been outlined in Chapter 4).

9.9. OTHER SEXUAL ASPECTS OF ADRENAL PHYSIOLOGY

9.9.1. UNITY OR PLURALITY OF ADRENAL FUNCTION

What has already been said concerning the biogenesis of adrenal steroids illustrates the fact that all of these are linked in a common metabolic chain. This unquestionable fact reflects the *unitarian* character of adrenocortical function. Rather than resulting from the union of three different glands, as suggested earlier, the adrenal cortex is seen as a single tissue, possessing the overall capacity for elaborating a variety of hormonal catabolites, linked into a single cycle but endowed with divergent actions that have a bearing on sex, carbohydrate metabolism and water and mineral metabolism.

On the other hand, however, it is clear that each of the three zones responds to a specific pituitary excitant, that each may enter phases of activity or rest on its own and, finally, that each is capable of displaying its own pathologic syndromes, which moreover are characterized by precise histopathologic substrates.

Two theories, one "unitarian" and the other "pluralistic," have thus evolved. Modern studies, however, have made it possible to account for the phenomena of plurality without giving up the accepted fact of a single and common metabolic cycle.

Van Dorp and Deane[39] and Deane[33] have confirmed our own[19] and Rotter's[91] findings that regeneration of the reticularis and that of other zones is dependent on distinct blastemas. In reptiles and in prototheria (*Ornithorhynchus*), in which the reticularis (paleocortex) and the fasciculata (neocortex) are two distinct organs, Wright and Chester-Jones[108] and Prunty[87] have also confirmed the existence of the same duality.

However, a most important argument is based on evidence that the different types of basic enzyme activity involved in adrenocortical steroidogenesis (11- and 21-hydroxylases, 3β-ol-dehydrogenase and 18-oxidase) (Fig. 9–12) can be *localized in different cortical zones, each zone thereby assuming different functions.*

Specific enzyme localization in *slices* of different cortical layers had already been achieved by Giroud's group[46, 97] and again more recently by Williams and his colleagues in 1962, by Griffiths and co-workers[50] and by Vinson and Chester-Jones[104] in 1963, and by Baille and co-workers[2] and by Klein and Giroud[67] in 1966.

Metopirone, known to specifically inhibit 11- and 21-hydroxylase, acts only on the fasciculata and not on the remaining zones, nor does it act on *slices* taken separately from either remaining zone.[29, 76]

These ideas are reproduced in Figure 9–13. Each cortical zone is clearly shown to be an *independent entity within the framework of a harmonious and common metabolism*. In addition, each of them obeys a specific higher command and functions in a totally characteristic and individual way in response to hypothalamic and pituitary activity.

Another feature characteristic of adrenal zoning is the fact that the reticularis constitutes a "preparatory" zone for the biogenesis of sexual steroids. Among the latter, progesterone is a precursor of corticoids, and both androgens and estrogens are catabolites of progesterone metabolism whenever the progesterone-corticoid conversion step is blocked. *Secretion of sexual steroids by the adrenal cortex therefore reflects failure of the gland to complete its work (adrenal hypofunction).*

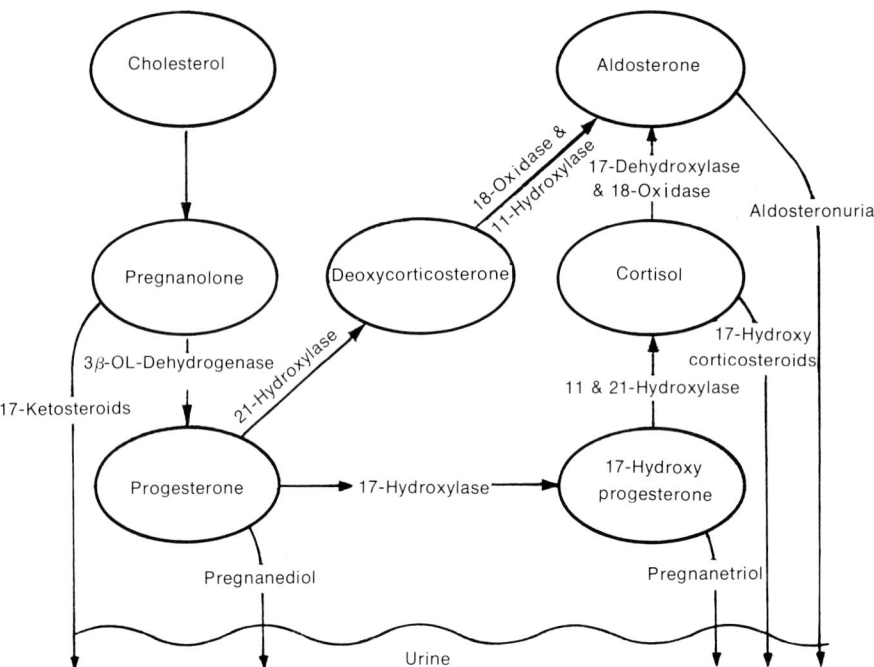

Figure 9-12. Simplified diagram of enzyme interactions in C-21 steroidogenesis. (Synopsis of data reported by Hechter, Pincus, Heard and Dorfman).

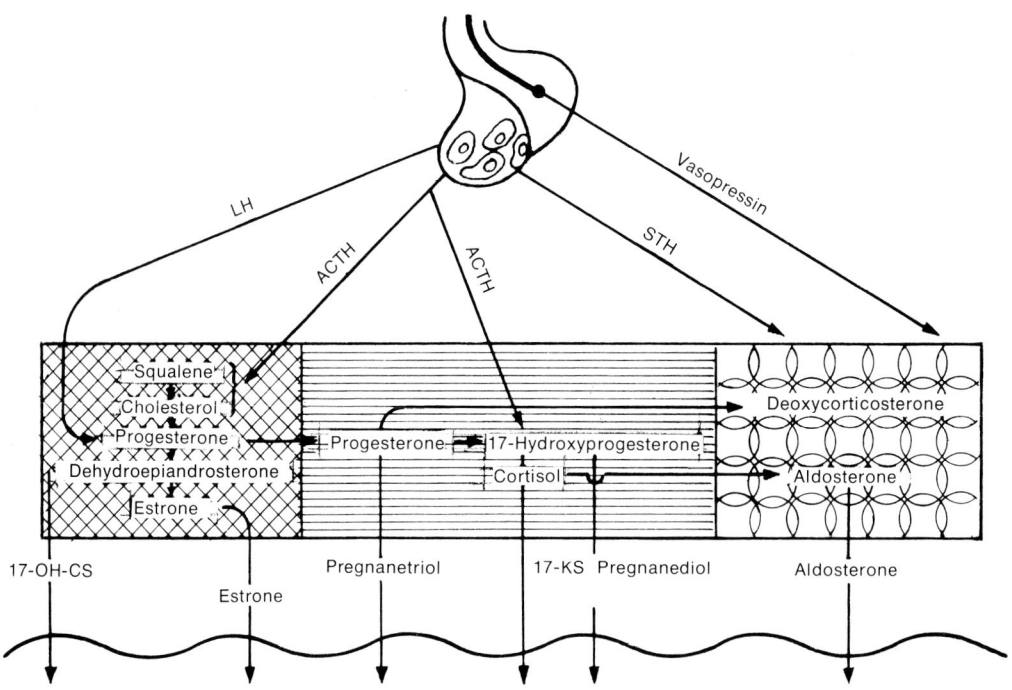

Figure 9-13. Diagram designed to interpret our hypothesis concerning the hormonal cycle of C-21 steroidogenesis and other adrenal steroids, including the interzonal overlap of the cycle. The most simple steroids are synthesized in the reticularis. Starting from squalene and from cholesterol, the product obtained is progesterone, which seems to be the basic steroid. Dehydroepiandrosterone and related 17-ketosteroids, as well as estrone, are progesterone catabolites in this zone. The specific catalyst for the conversion of cholesterol to sex hormones is thought to be LH, which, just as it does in the testis and ovary, possesses the capacity for stimulating sexual steroidogenesis quite characteristically. Of all the steroids of the reticular zone, only progesterone is believed to spill over into the zona fasciculata, where it can be converted to cortisol by virtue of the biocatalytic activity of ACTH. As to the glomerulosa, it seems likely that aldosterone is elaborated in it starting from DOCA, derived from progesterone as well as directly from cortisol derivatives. In this still little known conversion, STH and vasopressin might be the necessary biocatalysts. It is probable that ACTH, as shown in the figure, acts on the reticularis by stimulating steroid synthesis from squalene as the starting point.

9.9.2. THE THIRD GONAD

The pathology of the adrenal sexual zone (dealt with in Chapter 33) similarly corroborates the concept of a zone made up of gonadal interstitial tissue. To recapitulate, the following statements can presently be made: *Within the framework of the interrenal system, two genetically distinct formations must be distinguished. One, the cortex, commonly known to elaborate corticoids and to regulate metabolism, appears in human embryos relatively late, around the seventh month of intrauterine life; this is called by us the "neocortex." The other, an embryologically older formation, which constitutes the sex hormone-secreting cortex that in the human species begins to atrophy at seven months, is completely atrophied after birth; for this zone we propose the term "paleocortex."* Those two formations are regenerated by two different blastemas (the subcapsular blastema in the first case, and the juxtamedullary blastema in the second) and also have different hormone synthesizing functions in that the "neocortex" secretes corticoids whereas the "paleocortex" produces sex hormones. They respond to different specific excitants and, in the course of life, behave in divergent, if not counteracting, ways. Their tissues possess different tinctorial properties, the first staining with sudan but not with fuchsin, the second staining in the opposite way. Finally, as is pointed out in Chapter 33, the endocrine syndromes determined by either cortical insufficiency or cortical hyperfunction—that is, Addison's or Cushing's disease, respectively—are quite different from the diseases or pathologic syndromes caused by either hyper- or hypofunction of the sexual zone (the adrenogenital syndrome and congenital adrenocortical insufficiency). As a result, syndromes combining hyperfunctional states of one zone, with hypofunction of the other zone, or vice versa, e.g., Addison's disease associated with adrenogenital syndrome, may also occur. The functional divergence between the two glands has been indicated in Table 9–4, which summarizes our point of view on the subject.

Because of the marked differences just indicated, because of the occasional direct intervention of the sexual cortex in the regulation of reproductive phenomena and, above all, because of the supplementary gonadal nature and gonad-like embryologic origin of a portion of the adrenal cortex, we have been led to regard that portion of the cortex as a *functional unit that is independent of the metabolic cortex, thereby distinguishing two different glands in the interrenal system:* the sexual cortex and the metabolic cortex. In view of the distinctive properties of the former, we have proposed the designation "third gonad" for the sexual zone.

9.9.3. SEXUAL ACTIONS BY CORTICOIDS

In preceding sections, the adrenocortical sexual zone is discussed as a compensatory system of gonadal secretion, intermittent in function, but possessing features of an independent endocrine gland. However, it must not be forgotten that the

TABLE 9–5

ZONE: ENZYME:	RETICULARIS 3β-OL-DEHYDROGENASE	FASCICULATA 11- AND 21-HYDROXYLASE	GLOMERULOSA 18-OXIDASE
STEROIDS PRODUCED:	Squalene Cholesterol Pregnanolone Progesterone Dehydroepiandrosterone ↓ Estrone	Deoxycorticosterone Corticosterone ↓ Cortisol	Aldosterone

TABLE 9–4

SEXUAL CORTEX	METABOLIC CORTEX
	(a) *Embryology*
Precocious origin from primordium adjacent to that of gonad (paleocortex)	Late origin from subcapsular blastema (neocortex)
	(b) *Variations in course of life*
Temporary cortex, postnatal involution	Permanent cortex; no involution
	(c) *Hormones*
17-Ketosteroids Estrone	Progesterone Cortisol Aldosterone
	(d) *Histologic features*
Fuchsinophilia Sudanophobia	Fuchsinophobia Sudanophilia
	(e) *Specific excitant*
Gonadotropin (LH)	Corticotropin (ACTH); vasopressin.
	(f) *Pathologic hyperfunction*
Adrenogenital syndrome	Cushing's disease; aldosteronism.
	(g) *Pathologic hypofunction*
Congenital adrenocortical insufficiency	Addison's disease

cortical hormones proper—strictly speaking the corticoids—are compounds that are metabolically related to the sex hormones in a most intimate fashion, particularly as regards the products of the corpus luteum series.

SEXUAL ACTION BY CORTICOIDS. Various workers[16, 30, 109] have injected animals, especially rats and rabbits, with deoxycorticosterone acetate. In conveniently prepared uteri of rabbits, they were able to induce progestational reactions analogous to those provoked by the corpus luteum hormone. The only differences noted concerned intensity of effect, deoxycorticosterone producing effects five to 10 times less pronounced than those obtained with progesterone under identical conditions. In women, the problem has been studied by Neumann and by ourselves.[15, 19] In our studies, induction of a progestational phase in women was achieved with 250 mg deoxycorticosterone acetate. Injections of half a gram of that compound elicited detectable deposits of glycogen. The progestational effect of deoxycorticosterone is exerted not only at the endometrial level but is also reflected in vaginal smears, as reported by Montalvo[78] (Fig. 9-14), further, in the dynamics of the myometrium,[85] and even in pregnancy maintenance in castrated rodents.[30]

Deoxycorticosterone also exerts an effect on the male sex organs. We have been able to detect growth of the seminal vesicles in castrated rats following injection of 100 mg of that substance. Similar results have been observed by other authors, proving that corticoids exert a virilizing action in both experimental animals and man.

Although deoxycorticosterone would appear to have quite marked sexual actions, such is not the case with cortisone. The latter has been found to have a paralyzing effect on the endometrium and, in both animals and humans,[25] causes decreased 17-ketosteroid excretion[73] as well as regression of male characteristics. Hence, it is of interest to note that deoxycorticosterone possesses weak progestational and mild androgenic activity which, on the other hand, is not shared by the compounds of the 11-oxysteroid series. The reason for this remains obscure.

CORTICOID ACTION BY SEX HORMONES. Sex hormones appear to play a certain role in the maintenance of corticoprival animals, as noted by us in 1941 in a series of experiments on castrated rats.[13, 14, 19] Adrenalectomized female rats showed a very low rate of mortality. At first, this was thought to result from the presence of possible accessory adrenal tissue, as suggested by other investigators. However, it soon became apparent that even in the complete absence of any other interrenal tissue, laboratory rats were able to live and even gain weight for many months (Fig. 9-15). Later experiments showed that adrenalectomized male rats died rapidly if subjected to bilateral orchidectomy (Fig. 9-16). Unilateral orchidectomy was not enough to kill the animals, but after the removal of the contralateral testis, death ensued, with a picture of acute adrenal insufficiency. The inference we drew from these experiments was that the presence of one testis was sufficient to compensate for the absence of the adrenal glands in these animals. Mortality rates were much higher when the experiments were repeated on females. Anatomic examination of those female rats that had died following adrenalectomy disclosed that their ovaries were devoid of corpora lutea, whereas those rats whose ovaries contained corpora lutea were able to survive bilateral resection of the adrenals under the same conditions that had been used for the experiments on males (Fig. 9-17). We could not fail but to conclude that testicular hormone as well as corpus luteum hormone were capable of maintaining life in animals that had been deprived of their adrenal cortex. Estrogens, by contrast, failed to exert that effect.

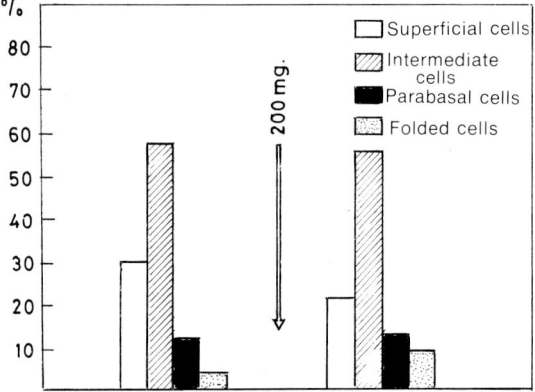

Figure 9-14. Progestational effect on vaginal smear by administration of 200 mg DOCA. Observe increased number of folded cells with luteal features. (From Montalvo-Ruiz: Arch. Med. Exper., 16:371, 1953.)

Adrenals and Sexual Function

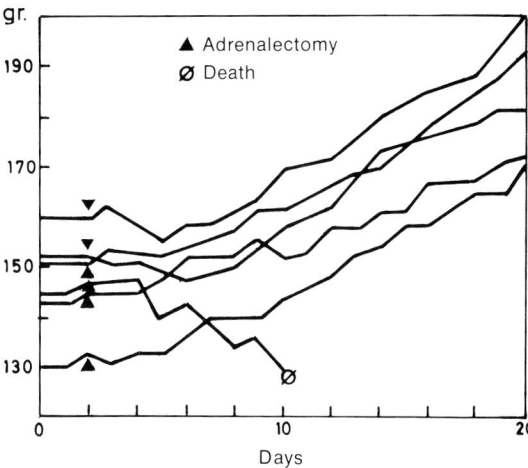

Figure 9-15. Slight lethal effect of adrenalectomy in adult male rat. Survival is possible owing to active testis. (From Botella: *Rev. Clin. Esp.*, 1:4, 1941.)

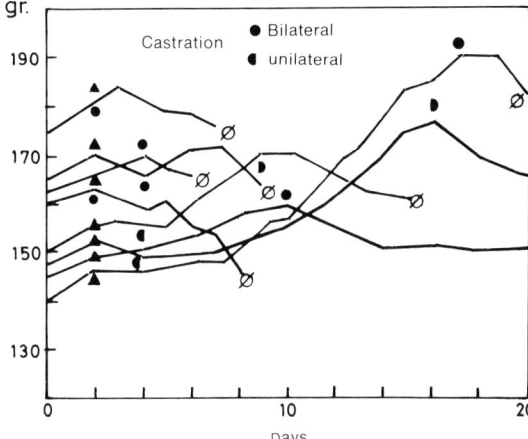

Figure 9-16. Experiment similar to the one in Figure 9-16. However, after adrenalectomy, animals are also castrated. Notice how castration leads to death of animals. Those with unilateral castration survive for as long as the other gonad is not removed.

Figure 9-17. Six adrenalectomized female rats, each treated with chorionic gonadotropin (each arrow indicates 50 mouse units). Among these, four survive. All four had corpora lutea in ovary, formed under the influence of the injected gonadotropin. Of the two that died, one showed atrophic ovaries, the other ovaries with corpora hemorrhagica but without corpora lutea. This is evidence in support of the hypothesis that presence of a corpus luteum averts death in corticoprival animals.

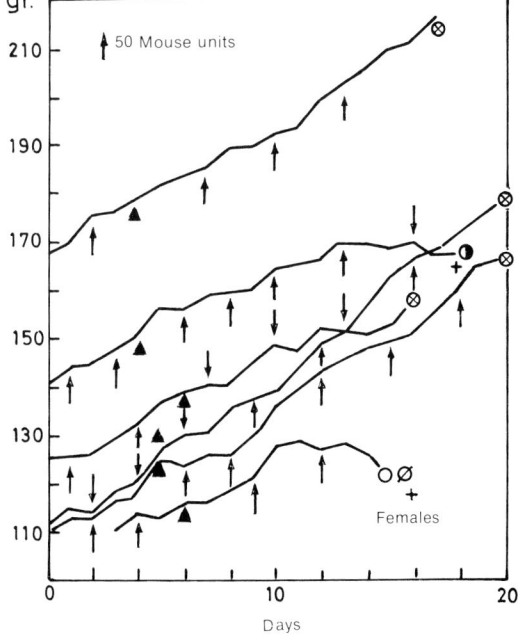

Later studies conducted for the same purpose on animals undergoing both castration and adrenalectomy simultaneously showed that such animals could be kept alive with injections of either progesterone or testosterone (Figs. 9–18 and 9–19). Subsequent experimental work by other authors has fully confirmed those findings. In his clinical experience with patients, Marañón has demonstrated a noticeable improvement in individuals suffering from Addison's disease after injections of testosterone or elevated dosages of progesterone.

The conclusion that we feel justified to draw is that both progesterone and testosterone exert an unquestionable corticoid action. This action is not unexpected in the light of our earlier discussions in Chapters 3 and 4, in which we reported that androgens and progesterone both possessed metabolic activity of anabolizing nature, especially with regard to carbohydrate metabolism, which, if not identical, is quite similar to the type of effect exerted by corticoids.

Analogous results were obtained by Seliger and his colleagues[96] in 1966, who worked with adrenalectomized squirrels. However, they ascribed that effect to corticoidogenic activity by proliferations of clear cells in the ovarian hilum.

For whatever reason, it is a fact that the capacity of certain animal species for survival following bilateral adrenalectomy is assured by the presence of the gonad.

THE HORMONAL TRIANGLE. Our present study may be completed by recalling

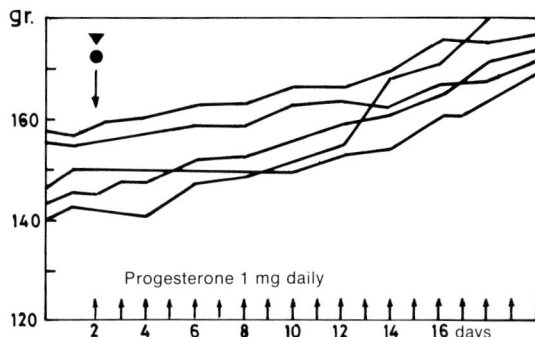

Figure 9–19. Experiment identical to that of Figure 9–18, but using progesterone. Corpus luteum hormone similarly prevents animals from dying.

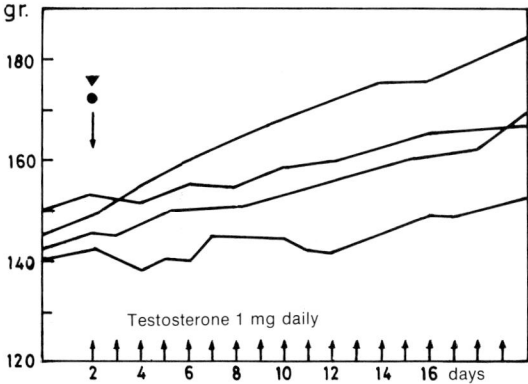

Figure 9–18. Castrated and adrenalectomized animals kept alive by administration of testosterone. (From Botella: *Suprarrenales y Función Sexual.* Madrid, Morata, 1946.)

that, as stated in Chapter 3, progesterone possesses weak androgenic activity. We were able to show, as others did, that androgens were substances having weak progestational effects. Our recent studies, mentioned in Chapter 4, revealed that testosterone injections in women were followed by elevated urinary pregnanediol excretion, probably due to a progesterone-like effect. Each of these groups of hormones possesses specific activity: metabolic in corticoids, androgenic in androgens and progestational in progestogens. At the same time, however, each of these groups may exert paraspecific effects, duplicating, though to a lesser degree of intensity and efficiency, the effects of the other two: progesterone having androgenic and at the same time corticogenic effects, corticoids having progestational and at the same time androgenic effects, and, lastly, testosterone having corticogenic and progestational effects. A system of mutual endocrine compensation is thus established, the reason for which lies certainly in the profound structural similarities shared by all three groups of hormones.

In summary, it may be said that the classical description of the adrenal gland encompasses but one aspect of the gland's overall activity. The common concept of the adrenal as the regulator of mineral and carbohydrate metabolism, the physiology of muscle and the fight against "stress" and infectious agents, covers only part of the total physiology of that gland. Aside from the metabolic adrenal, there exists a sexual adrenal or "third gonad," whose mission is to provide a system for the substitution and compensation of the gonadal hormones. In terms of hormone secretion, the sexual adrenal is a "third gonad" whose participation has to be counted upon in all schemes of neuroendocrine control of sexual function.

However, the relationship between the adrenal cortex and sex is not limited to this aspect, important as it may be: in addition, by virtue of being closely related to the gonadal hormones, the adrenal hormones are linked into a common metabolism with the latter, with reciprocal conversions between them having been convincingly demonstrated. Therefore, not only is adrenal cortical intervention in sex hormone synthesis possible, but it must also be admitted that the hormones of the gonads and those of the cortex substitute each other in their functions under given circumstances, normal as well as pathologic.

REFERENCES

1. Altman, N. H., Street, C. S., and Terney, J. Y.: *Amer. J. Veter. Res.*, 30:583, 1969.
2. Baille, A. H., Calman, K. C., Ferguson, M. N., and Hart, D.: *J. Endocr.*, 34:1, 1966.
3. Baulieu, E. E., Wallace, E., and Liebermann, I.: *J. Biol. Chem.*, 238:1316, 1963.
4. Bayer, J. M., Breuer, H., and Nocke, W.: *Klin. Wschr.*, 38:1143, 1960.
5. Bengtsson, G., Wiquist, N., Ullberg, S., and Diczfalusy, E.: *Acta Endocr.*, 46:544, 1964.
6. Benua, R. S., and Howard, E.: *Bull. Johns Hopkins Hosp.*, 86:200, 1950.
7. Bergner, G. H., and Deane, H. W.: *Endocrinology*, 43:240, 1948.
8. Berliner, M. L., Berliner, D. L., and Dougherty, T. F.: *J. Clin. Endocr.*, 18:109, 1958.
9. Bloch, E., Benirschke, K., and Hertig, A. T.: *Endocrinology*, 58:958, 1956.
10. Bloch, E., and Benirschke, K.: *Endocrinology*, 60:789, 1957.
11. Bloch, E., and Benirschke, K.: *Endocrinology*, 76:43, 1965.
12. Bongiovanni, M., Elberlein, W. R., and Cara, J.: *J. Clin. Endocr.*, 14:409, 1954.
13. Botella, J.: *Suprarrenales y Función Sexual, la Tercera Gonada*. Madrid, Morata, 1946.
14. Botella, J.: *Rev. Clin. Esp.*, 1:4, 1941.
15. Botella, J.: *Zbl. Gynäk.*, 66:287, 1942.
16. Botella, J., and Cano, A.: *Gynaecologia*, 124:466, 1947.
17. Botella, J., and Cano, A.: *Arch. Med. Exper.*, 13:65, 75, 81, 1950.
18. Botella, J.: *Gynaecologia*, 133:80, 1952.
19. Botella, J.: *Arch. Gynäk.*, 183:74, 1953.
20. Botella, J., Gómez-Maestro, D. V., and Santos Ruiz, A.: *Arch. Med. Exper.*, 15:79, 1952.
21. Botella, J., Santos-Ruiz, A., and Gómez-Maestro, D. V.: *Arch. Med. Exper.*, 16:51, 1953.
22. Bühner, P., Rindt, W., and Oertel, G. W.: *Endokrinologie*, 51:303, 1967.
23. Caldwell, B. V., Peron, F. G., and MacCarthy, J. L.: *Biochemistry*, 7:788, 1968.
24. Camacho, A. M., and Migeon, C. J.: *J. Clin. Endocr. Metab.*, 26:893, 1966.
25. Cañadell, J. M., and Rodríguez-Soriano, J. A.: *Rev. Esp. Fisiol.*, 7:281, 1951.
26. Carcatzolulis, S.: *Presse Medicale*, 53:2437, 1961.
27. Cattaneo, P., and Hecht-Lucari, G.: *Bol. Soc. Ital. Biol. Sper.*, 28:383, 1952.
28. Cavallero, C., Magrino, U., Dellepiane, M., and Cizelj, T.: *Ann. d'Endocr.*, 26:409, 1965.
29. Chart, H., et al.: *Experientia*, 14:151, 1958.
30. Courrier, R., Baclesse, M., and Marois, M.: *J. de Physiol.*, 45:327, 1953.
31. Cushman, P.: *Amer. J. Obstet. Gynec.*, 107:519, 1970.
32. David, M. A., and Kovacs, K. I.: *Pathol. Biol. (Paris)*, 15:182, 1967.
33. Deane, H. W.: *Handbuch der experimentellen Pharmakologie*, Vol. XIV, 1. Berlin, Springer, 1962.
34. Delost, P.: *Les Corrélations Genito-Surrénaliennes*. Paris, Masson et Cie, 1956.
35. Delost, P.: *J. de Physiol.*, 47:164, 1965.
36. Desphande, N., Jensen, V., Bulbrok, R., and Douss, T. W.: *Steroids*, 9:939, 1967.
37. Dorfman, R. I.: *Ciba Colloquia on Endocrinology*, 8:112, 1955.
38. Dorfman, R. I.: In *The Hormones*, ed. G. Pincus and K. V. Thimann, Vol. III. New York, Academic Press, 1955.
39. Dorp, A. W. Van and Deane, H. W.: *Anat. Rec.*, 107:265, 1950.
40. Dyrenfurth, I., Beck, J. C., and Venning, E. H.: *J. Clin. Endocr.*, 20:751, 1960.
41. Farnsworth, W. E.: *J. Clin. Endocr.*, 16:947, 1956.
42. Farrel, G. L.: *Endocrinology*, 65:29, 1959.
43. Finkelstein, M., and Goldberg, S.: *J. Clin. Endocr.*, 17:1063, 1957.
44. Gemzell, C. A.: *Acta Endocr.*, 11:221, 1952.
45. George, A. M., Arey, J. B., and Bongiovanni, M.: *J. Clin. Endocr.*, 16:1281, 1956.
46. Giroud, C. J. P., et al.: In *Aldosterone*, ed. A. F. Müller and C. M. O'Connor. London, Churchill, 1958.
47. Goldzieher, J. W., and Fariss, B.: *Acta Endocr.*, 54:452, 1967.
48. Gonzalo-Sanz, L.: *Rev. Med. Est. Gen. (Navarra, Pamplona)*, 1:219, 1957.
49. Greep, R. O., and Deane, H. W.: *Endocrinology*, 40:417, 1949.
50. Griffiths, J. K., Grant, J. G., and Symington, T.: *J. Clin. Endocr.*, 23:776, 1963.
51. Grollman, A.: *The Adrenals*. Baltimore, Williams & Wilkins, 1936.
52. Heard, R. D. H.: *Rec. Progr. Horm. Res.*, 12:45, 1956.
53. Hechter, O., and Pincus, G.: *Physiol. Revs.*, 34:459, 1955.
54. Hilton, J. G., et al.: *Endocrinology*, 67:299, 1960.
55. Hopper, B. R., and Tullner, W. W.: *Endocrinology*, 82:876, 1968.
56. Houssay, B. A., et al.: *Rev. Soc. Arg. Biol.*, 29:170, 1953.
57. Howard, E., and Benua, R. S.: *J. Anat.*, 42:157, 1950.
58. Hudson, P. H., and Lombardo, M. E.: *Proc. Soc. Exper. Biol. Med.*, 95:311, 1957.

59. Incerti-Bonini, L. D., and Pagani, C.: *Biológica Latina*, 5:428, 1952.
60. Jarrett, R. J.: *Endocrinology*, 76:434, 1965.
61. Jayle, M. F.: *Ann. d'Endocr.*, 12:404, 1951.
62. Jenkins, J. S.: Biochemical Aspects of the Adrenal Cortex. London, Arnold Ltd., 1968.
63. Jones, I. C.: *The Adrenal Cortex*. Cambridge, Cambridge University Press, 1957.
64. Kazekas, A. G., and Kokai, K.: *Steroids*, 9:177, 1967.
65. Kitay, J. I.: *Endocrinology*, 68:818, 1961, and 73:253, 1963.
66. Kitay, J. I.: *Acta Endocr.*, 43:601, 1963.
67. Klein, G. P., and Giroud, C. J. P.: *Canad. J. Biochem.*, 44:1005, 1966.
68. Laidlaw, J. C., Ruse, J. L., and Gornal, A. G.: *J. Clin. Endocr.*, 22:161, 1962.
69. Landing, B. H.: *Ciba Colloquia on Endocrinology*, 8:52, 1955.
70. Lanman, J. T.: *Endocrinology*, 61:684, 1957.
71. Lantos, C. P., Birmingham, M. K., and Traitkov, H.: *Acta Physiol. Lat. Amer.*, 17:42, 1967.
72. Layne, D. S., Meyer, C. J., Vaishwanar, P. S., and Pincus, G.: *J. Clin. Endocr.*, 22:107, 1962.
73. Lewis, A. W., et al.: *J. Clin. Endocr.*, 10:703, 1950.
74. Lombardo, M. E., et al.: *J. Clin. Endocr.*, 16:1283, 1956.
75. Lucis, O. J., and Venning, E. H.: *Canad. J. Biochem.*, 38:1069, 1960.
76. Migliavacca, A., and Bompiani, A.: *Ann. d' Endocr.*, 23:95, 1962.
77. Mills, I. H., et al.: *J. Clin. Endocr.*, 20:515, 1960.
78. Montalvo, L.: *Arch. Med. Exper.*, 16:371, 1955.
79. Nandi, J., Bern, H. A., Biglieri, E. G., and Pieprzyk, J. K.: *Endocrinology*, 80:576, 1967.
80. Oertel, G. W., and Eik-Nes, K. B.: *Endocrinology*, 70:39, 1962.
81. Okinara, S., et al.: *Endocrinology*, 67:319, 1960.
82. Pasqualini, J. R., and Jayle, M. F.: *Biochem. J.*, 81:147, 1961.
83. Peron, F. G.: *Endocrinology*, 70:386, 1962.
84. Pierson, R. W.: *Endocrinology*, 81:693, 1967.
85. Planel, H.: *Arch. d'Anat. d'Histol. d'Embryol.*, 41:117, 1958.
86. Plate, W. P.: *Acta Endocr.*, 8:17, 1951, and 11:119, 1952.
87. Prunty, F. T. G.: *Brit. Med. J.*, 2:615, 673, 1956.
88. Resko, J. A.: *Science*, 163:70, 1969.
89. Roos, T. B.: *Endocrinology*, 81:716, 1967.
90. Rosner, J., Charreau, E., Houssay, A. B., and Epper, C.: *Endocrinology*, 79:681, 1956.
91. Rotter, W.: *Virchows. Arch.*, 316:590, 1949.
92. Rosenfeld, G.: *Endocrinology*, 56:649, 1955.
93. Roy, S., and Mahesh, V. B.: *Endocrinology*, 74:187, 1964.
94. Sandberg, H., et al.: *J. Clin. Endocr.*, 18:1268, 1958.
95. Sandberg, H., and Slaunwhite, W. R.: *J. Clin. Invest.*, 38:1290, 1960.
96. Seliger, W. G., Blair, A. J., and Mossman, H. W.: *Amer. J. Anat.*, 118:615, 1966.
97. Stachenko, J., and Giroud, C. J. P.: *Endocrinology*, 64:730, 743, 1959.
98. Suchowsky, G.: *Acta Endocr.*, 27:225, 1958.
99. Symington, T., et al.: *Ciba Colloquia on Endocrinology*, 12:102, 1958.
100. Tullner, W. W.: *Endocrinology*, 79:745, 1966.
101. Vecsei, P., et al.: *Acta Endocr.*, 53:24, 1966.
102. Venning, E. H., and Lucis, O. J.: *Endocrinology*, 70:486, 1962.
103. Villee, C. A., and Loring, J. M.: *J. Clin. Endocr. Metab.*, 25:307, 1965.
104. Vinson, G. P., and Chester-Jones, I.: *J. Endocr.*, 26:407, 1963.
105. Wallace, E. Z., and Carter, A. C.: *J. Clin. Invest.*, 39:601, 1960.
106. Weliky, I., and Engel, L. L.: *J. Biol. Chem.*, 238:1302, 1963.
107. Williams, H. E., Johnson, P. I., and Field, J. B.: *Endocrinology*, 71:293, 1962.
108. Wright, A., and Chester-Jones, I.: *J. Endocr.*, 15:83, 1957.
109. Yoffey, J. M.: *Ciba Colloquia on Endocrinology*, 8:18, 1955.
110. Youdaev, N. A., and Droujinina, K. V.: *Europ. J. Steroids*, 2:93, 1967.

Chapter 10
INFLUENCE OF OTHER ENDOCRINE GLANDS ON SEX

Although the pituitary and the adrenals are the principal glands of internal secretion that are related to sexual activity, the remaining components of the incretory system are, at times, quite intimately related to sexual function. For instance, while its activity is closely linked with the process of ovarian maturation, the *thyroid* gland in turn depends on direct or indirect stimuli from the ovary to discharge its own function. The *pancreas* influences sexual life mainly through the reproductive cycle, while the *parathyroids* are inextricably implicated in regulating certain female vegetative processes. Finally, the *pineal* and the *thymus* have an antagonistic and retardatory action on sexual maturity, the intimate mechanism of which remains to date unknown.

10.1. THYROID GLAND AND SEXUAL FUNCTION

A good many years ago, the thyroid was usually featured as possessing feminizing activity, whereas to the adrenal was ascribed a tendency to produce virilization (Marañón[85]). These early notions have now been discarded. Nonetheless, it is true that over the past years the adrenal gland has been shown to have the potential for producing either feminizing or masculinizing tendencies (see Chapter 9), whereas the thyroid may be said to profoundly affect the development of the female gonad, without altogether lacking influence on the maturation process of the male gonad.

10.1.1. THE NORMAL THYROID

The average weight of a normal thyroid is about 25 gm; however, the variations among the population at large, and even in the same individual, may cover a wide range. Significantly, the weight of the female thyroid varies greatly. *In general*, as had been observed many years ago by Seitz and Engelhorn, *the thyroid of females is larger than that of males.* The thyroid of children and adolescents, too, is proportionately larger than that of adults or older individuals.

The blood supply to the thyroid gland is of great importance. It had been asserted that the total circulating blood volume (3.8 to 4 liters in a woman of average build) could pass through the gland once every hour, or, during pregnancy, even once every 40 minutes. Obviously, this by itself would seem to suggest some significance of the gland in the reproductive physiology of woman.

During pregnancy, the thyroid increases in weight and is much more compact in consistency than it usually is. The follicles are reduced in caliber and the colloid is in part reabsorbed (see Chapter 20, Section 20.1.3).

In recent years, a second hormone, called *thyrocalcitonin*, has been discovered in the thyroid gland. This is a polypeptide which lowers plasma calcium levels and is an antagonist of parathyroid hormone (Kracht et al.[77]). The manifestations of osteoporosis associated with various states of sexual function are to a considerable extent attributable to changes in thyrocalcitonin secretion.[73, 77, 94, 110, 140]

Let us briefly review some of the modern tests of thyroid function most commonly referred to in this book:
PBI: Protein Bound Iodine
BEI: Butanol Extractable Iodine
TBG: Thyroxin Binding Globulin

TBPA: Thyroxin Binding Prealbumin

The radioactive iodine (^{131}I) uptake test is done in association with a scintiscan of the thyroid gland.

10.1.2. THYROID CHANGES RELATED TO SEXUAL FUNCTION

Through careful studies, Peterson and his colleagues[104] in 1952 confirmed the validity of the ancient idea that the female thyroid is not only larger than that of the male, but it is also of greater structural complexity, invariably showing signs of greater functional activity. During puberty, during the course of the sexual cycle and during pregnancy, as well as after castration and menopause, very important changes take place in the makeup of the female thyroid. These can be either anatomic or functional, or both.

PUBERTY. Various authors[36, 51, 144] have observed thyroid enlargement during puberty. Marañón, who in particular stressed that phenomenon, believed that it was not always indicative of hyperfunction but was sometimes of a purely degenerative nature. Nevertheless, thyroid hyperfunction would seem to be a necessary prerequisite for normal pubertal development, considering that both cretins and patients with myxedema show retarded puberty and, occasionally, essential amenorrhea.[37] In his studies on the clinical aspects of the pubertal thyroid, Lerman[81] calls attention to the fact that thyroid hyperfunction occurs not only during puberty but also during the prepubertal period and is implicated in the phenomena of growth and morphogenesis of adolescence. In lower animals, there is an antagonism between thyroid and pituitary action on growth and metamorphosis. The early investigations by Gudernatsch on tadpoles revealed that, while pituitary growth hormone produced growth in size but inhibited metamorphosis, thyroxin, conversely, provoked precocious metamorphosis but inhibited growth. No similar antagonism between growth and sexual development is readily apparent in the human species, in which thyroid hormone is admitted to stimulate both growth and sexual maturation. *Prepubertal and pubertal thyroid hyperfunction is therefore believed to be aimed not only at stimulating sexual maturation but probably also at contributing toward the somatic development of the individual.*

Russell[121] has stressed the occurrence of *elevated PBI values at puberty.* Standard PBI determinations are at present among the most useful tests for the diagnosis of thyroid hyperfunctional states and, on the basis of elevated pubertal levels, would seem to bear out the existence of *pubertal thyroid hyperfunction.*

THE CYCLE. The early literature makes ample reference to changes observed in the thyroid during the different phases of the sexual cycle. *Premenstrual hyperthyroidism* has been described, mainly on the basis of clinical evidence, such as increased basal metabolic rates. At the time of estrus, all thyroid function tests in the ewe show values above normal (Robertson and Falconer[117]). Thyrotropin secretion in rats has been found to follow a cyclic pattern (Bocabella and Alger[13]). Nonetheless, it is important to remember that estrogens, too, tend to exert a hyperdynamic action that may raise the rate of metabolic turnover and that the period we are referring to corresponds precisely to the presence of increased amounts of estrogens in females. On the other hand, evidence of neurovegetative lability in a woman may also raise the question of *false hyperthyroidism.* However, it is a fact that, despite modern techniques, no demonstrable variations in thyroid function could be shown to occur in the course of the menstrual cycle. Thus, Russell[121] Singh and Bennett,[126] Czerniak and Italson[26] and Engstrom and Marquardt,[37] all of whom had studied PBI and ^{131}I uptake on human as well as animal thyroids, have never been able to detect any variations that would correlate with the reproductive cycle. It can therefore be concluded that *the thyroid is not subject to cyclic changes, as was assumed in the past.*

PREGNANCY. During pregnancy, the thyroid gland undergoes highly significant changes,[29, 34, 123] which are discussed in detail in Chapter 20.

The relationship between the fetal and maternal thyroid has recently been reexamined by means of modern exploratory techniques of thyroid function.[10, 18, 27, 28, 38, 46, 96] For the time being, suffice it to say that the thyroid seems to have a decisive influence on the course of pregnancy and on fetal morphogenesis.

CASTRATION AND MENOPAUSE. There is nearly unanimous agreement that menopause may induce hyperthryoidism, described as "climacteric hyperthyroidism" by Marañón.[85] The degree of the resulting hyperfunction may vary considerably from case to case and depends above all on constitutional factors. Grumbrecht and Loeser[51] ascribe it to increased thyrotropin activity during the climacterium. Increased activity of that adenohypophysial hormone apparently goes hand in hand with increased activity of other pituitary factors (FSH, etc.).

In contrast, castration seems to reduce thyroid function. Numerous authors have reported thyroid hypofunction in animals after castration.[32, 43, 65] As for man, Beckers and Vischer[9] and Stoddard and his colleagues[130] likewise found low PBI and triiodothyronine blood levels and reduced radioactive iodine uptake values in surgically castrated women. At first sight, the discrepancy between menopause and castration may seem paradoxical if one overlooks the fact that the two conditions are far from being identical (see Chapter 17). According to our current ideas concerning the climacteric, menopause is followed, at least quite frequently, by a state of hyperestrinism. Except for some cases of adrenal overcompensation, estrogen levels in castrated individuals, on the contrary, are diminished. In recent years, estrogens have been regarded unanimously as thyroid stimulators. Far from being an obscure, paradoxical phenomenon, the difference between thyroid function at menopause and after castration may be viewed as further evidence that an ovarian-thyroid interrelationship does exist.

10.1.3. EFFECT OF THYROID HORMONE ON THE OVARY

There is no question that thyroid hormone has an effect, and an important one at that, on the ovary. That the ovary is stimulated by thyroxin can be substantiated by the following: (1) the effect of thyroidectomy on ovarian function; (2) the effect of thyroid extracts on ovarian structure and function; (3) the effect of thyrosuppressive drugs on ovarian function; and (4) the effect of experimentally induced hyperthyroidism on ovarian function.

EFFECT OF THYROIDECTOMY ON OVARIAN FUNCTION. Ross and his colleagues[119] and Thorsöe[135] found that thyroidectomy in rats arrested the maturation process of the ovarian follicles, resulting in death and atresia of ovules. Chu and co-workers[23] and Fredrikson and Ryden[45] also noted that the follicles of thyroidectomized rabbits failed to mature, and in addition thyroprival animals required much greater amounts of gonadotropic hormone to produce luteinization than did normal animals (Fig. 10–1).

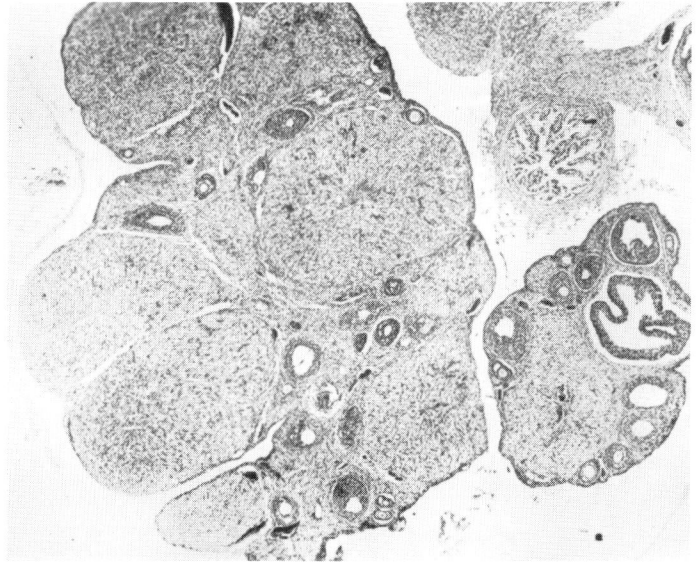

Figure 10–1. Ovary of thyroidectomized rat injected with urine of pregnancy. Corpora lutea are being formed as expected; however, no evidence of follicular maturation can be observed.

Lederer and Meyer[79] and Williams and his co-workers[141] both admitted that thyroid function was necessary for corpora lutea to be formed in a normal fashion. Parriot[101] reported lower indices of fertility in partially thyroidectomized rats.

EFFECT OF THYROID HORMONE ON THE OVARY. Even though thyroidectomy seems to have a clear-cut and uniform effect on the female gonad, the corresponding effect of thyroid hormone itself does not appear to be quite as unequivocal. Thus, Chu and Yu[22] showed that administration of dried thyroid extracts to rats produced a decrease in the number of ovarian follicles. However, other workers, such as Fishman and co-workers,[39] Kotz and Herrman,[76] Wilson and co-workers[143] and Young and colleagues,[154] reported that the rate at which follicles were being formed increased in thyroxine-treated animals, and so did the total weight of their ovaries.

Knobil and co-workers[74] discovered that dried thyroid extracts had to be supplemented with FSH and LH in order to produce ovulation in hypophysectomized monkeys. Milcou[89] showed that there was increased radioactive phosphorus uptake by the ovaries of thyroxine-treated animals.

Thyroxine also enhances the effect of gonadotropins on the testis.[136] Conversion of estradiol to estriol and hydroxyestrone in woman is believed to depend on the level of circulating thyroid hormone.[40] Finally, the relationships between thyroid function and fertility[59] and breast development[8] are generally well known, and are discussed in Chapters 22 and 41.

EFFECT OF THYROSUPPRESSIVE DRUGS ON THE OVARY. The present use of compounds with strong antithyroid actions, capable of completely blocking thyroid function, has made it desirable to test the effect on the ovary of such substances as *thiouracil*. Recent investigations on rats by Folley,[43] on rabbits by Krohn[78] and on humans by Williams and co-workers[142] have shown that thiouracil causes ovarian atrophy, with arrest of follicular maturation. At toxic levels, it produces polymicrocystic ovaries in ewes (Nesbitt et al.[99]). This has given rise to speculation that Stein-Leventhal's syndrome might, after all, result from diminished thyroid function.

Thyroidectomy, or treatment with thyrosuppressive drugs, blocks the implantation of blastocysts in rats (Holland et al.[60]).

Conversely, blastocyst implantation as well as fertility are regained in thyroidectomized rats following thyroid hormone administration (Holland et al.[61]). *While fully agreeing with earlier findings that thyroidectomy is followed by ovarian paralysis, the results of the above investigations illustrate the fact that one of the physiologic functions of the thyroid gland is to stimulate the ovary.*

EFFECT OF EXPERIMENTALLY INDUCED HYPERTHYROIDISM ON THE OVARY. Various authors (Korenchewsky and his colleagues,[75] Janes and Bradbury[64]) have studied the effect of experimentally induced hyperthyroidism on the ovary. For that purpose, they employed injections of thyrotropic hormone. While some of their experimental animals showed disappearance of estrus, others, on the contrary, showed an increase in the frequency of estrus. Despite this, ovarian function in all cases examined appeared to reflect a stimulatory effect, whereas the variable effect on estrus appeared to be of an indirect nature and secondary to the altered rhythm of maturation.

To summarize these observations, thyroid hormone can be said to stimulate follicular maturation, provided that there is no interference from other endocrine interactions. Its effect on ovulation and the corpus luteum—admittedly somewhat debatable on the latter—is currently recognized. Thus, the thyroid must be regarded as an important accessory gland of sexual function, as had already been postulated by Marañón.

10.1.4. EFFECT OF THYROID ON THE FEMALE GENITAL TRACT

Numerous clinical observations can be construed as contributory evidence that the thyroid acts on the female genital tract. For instance, the frequent occurrence of amenorrhea or oligomenorrhea in hypothyroidism,[69, 76, 90] and the fact that instances of copious menstrual flow or true metrorrhagia are often associated with hyperthyroidism,[75, 104] would also seem to indicate a relationship between the clinical condition of the thyroid gland and estrogen levels in woman. Goldsmith and his colleagues[50] studied menstrual patterns in women suffering from thyroid disorders and came to contradictory conclusions. Nonetheless, Lederer and Meyer,[79] as well as Hoar and his co-workers,[56] have come up with evidence that the menstrual cycle, interrupted following thyroidectomy, can be reestablished normally by injections of thyroxine. In experimental animals, injections of thyroid hormone have similarly produced growth in size and weight of the uterus,[97] increased development of the vaginal mucosa and increased frequency and desquamation during estrus.[76, 116]

10.1.5. EFFECT OF THYROXINE ON THE BREAST

The effect of thyroxine on the breast is of great significance and is dealt with in Chapter 21. In passing, however, attention is called here to the frequency with which gynecomastia is observed in hyperthyroidism, as was shown by, among others, Marañón[85] and Berson and Schreiber.[11] Under experimental conditions, injections of thyroid hormone produce mammary hyperfunction. It has been suggested that the presence of thyroxine activity is necessary for the production of milk (Becker et al.,[8] Folley[43]).

10.1.6. EFFECT OF THYROXINE ON THE MALE GENITAL TRACT

That there is a relationship between the thyroid and testicular function has been convincingly demonstrated. Hotchkiss had already indicated the high incidence of defectively formed spermatozoa in hypothyroid males. Our own experimental and clinical observations have led us to similar conclusions. Only too frequently, men with a low basal metabolism and a tendency to obesity, apart from other signs of hypothyroidism, are found to have below normal sperm counts and are particularly prone to reveal hypomotility of spermatozoa. The studies by Young and co-workers[154] on experimental animals showed that thyroid hormone enhanced spermatogenesis. Giarola and Ballerio[48] encountered higher sperm counts with increased motility of cells after thyroxine administration in infertile males. In our experience, thyroid therapy also increases the *speed of spermatozoal progression* (Fig. 10-2). This

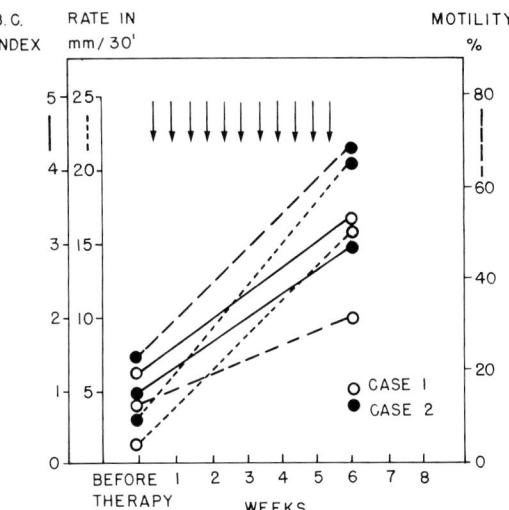

Figure 10-2. Effect of daily administration of thyroid tablets (Leo No. 4) for eight weeks to two hypofertile males. Effect on kinetics of spermatozoa. Note the increased percentage of motile forms, increased rate of linear progression and increased B.C. index. The B.C. index is the index of male fertility, according to Botella and Casares (see Botella-Llusiá and Ruiz-Velasco: *Internat. J. Fertil.*, 5:301, 1960). The rate of spermatic progression is measured by the method of Botella-Llusiá: *Internat. J. Fertil.*, 1:115, 1956.

observation is significant since it establishes a parallel with the stimulatory action of thyroxine on the ovarian follicular development. By demonstrating that spermatogenesis, too, is favorably influenced by thyroxine, the latter can be reliably classified as a *gametokinetic hormone, stimulating the development of gametes and the gametogenic organs in both male and female.*

10.1.7. EFFECT OF OVARY ON THE THYROID

According to a number of earlier investigators, both ovarian and placental extracts would seem to have a stimulatory effect on the thyroid gland.[124] In 1936, we conducted our own studies[16] on the subject by injecting ovarian hormones into rats that had previously been on a thyroid resting diet to keep their thyroids in a basal functional state. Under those experimental conditions, we were able to ascertain that estrogens had a strong stimulatory effect on the thyroid epithelium and induced the reabsorption of colloid (Fig. 10-3). In comparison,

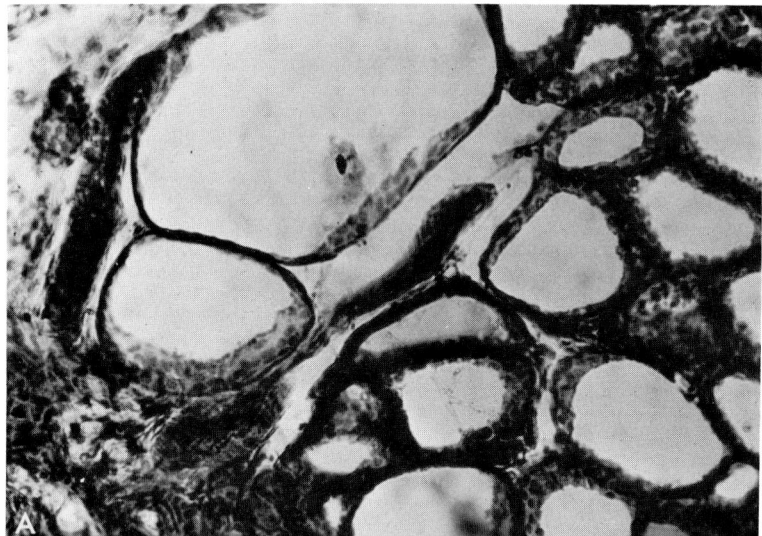
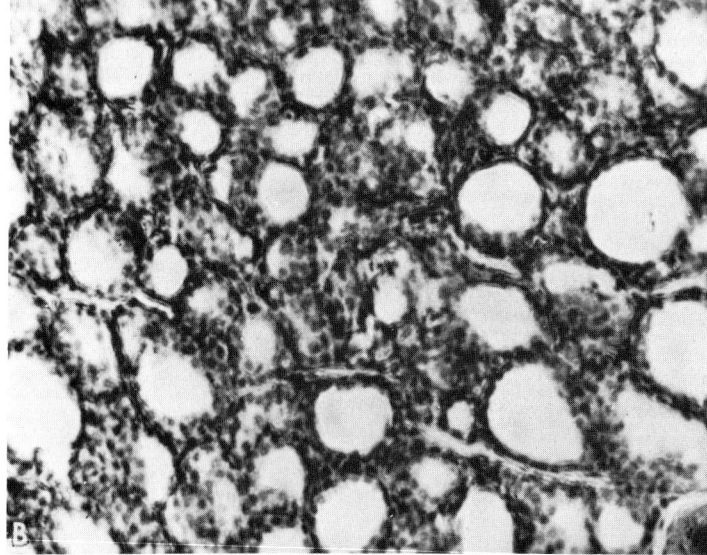

Figure 10–3. A, Thyroid of rat kept on thyroid resting diet. Large follicles lined by single layer of flattened epithelial cells indicate functional resting stage of gland. (According to Oehme and Paal.) B, Thyroid of rat, similar to preceding one, injected with estradiol benzoate (1 mg daily for 10 days). Histologically, the thyroid reveals proliferation and multistratification of epithelium, colloid reabsorption and small follicles, features indicative of a highly active state. (From Botella, Amilibia and Mendizábal: *Klin. Wschr.*, 2:1001, 1936.)

progesterone seemed to have an inhibitory action on the thyroid, if it produced any effect at all. Grumbrecht and Loeser[51] later investigated the effect of estradiol on the thyroid epithelium of rats and rabbits, using a technique similar to ours. Results comparable to ours were also obtained by Emge and Laqueur[35] and by Chu and Yu.[22] As a result of these studies, there would seem to be sufficient *evidence that estrogens exert a thyrotropic effect*, recognizable by the resulting proliferation of the epithelium of the thyroid follicles.

More recent research by Engbring, Engstrom and Marquardt[36, 37] has shown that the amount of precipitable serum iodine is an index of circulating thyroxine and that elevated values are indicative of increased thyroid function. Estrogen treatment produces a rise in that iodinemic fraction. Similarly, Russell[121] found increased PBI values after estrogen injections, and Dowling and his colleagues,[33a] in addition to confirming the same observations, reported increased TBP (thyroxine-binding protein) levels. The TBG (thyroxine-binding globulin) fraction is also increased as a result of estrogen activity.[84, 108] Very interesting studies using radioiodine (^{131}I) have been carried out by Money and co-workers,[90] by Becker and his colleagues[8] and by Czerniak and Italson.[26] Radioactive iodine uptake by the thyroid seems to be a dependable index of thyroid function. Thyrotropic hormone is known to enhance selective trapping of this isotope by the thyroid. According to Czerniak and Italson,[26] *estrogens increase radioiodine uptake by the thyroid gland.* Testosterone produces identical results, whereas progesterone, as shown by Brown-Grant,[17] reduces ^{131}I uptake much in the same way ACTH and cortisone does, the latter two being well known for their antagonistic action on thyroid function. *In conclusion, thyroid function is stimulated by estrogens in the female and by testicular hormone in the male, whereas it is depressed by progesterone, cortisone and ACTH alike.*

10.1.8. THYROID AND GONADOTROPINS

Increased gonadotropin levels in hypothyroid animals appear to be of a reactive nature and are aimed at stimulating an ovary that is less responsive, as suggested by Evans and Simpson in 1930, and shown by Cohen[25] in 1945 and by Reforzo-Membrives[111] in 1958. Because similar conditions of pituitary function are known to develop in rats after castration, it is believed that the pituitary response must be compensatory in nature. While studying the pituitaries of thyroid-fed animals histologically, Severinghaus and co-workers in 1934 observed that the number of basophils, as well as the amount of granulation within acidophils, increased. In 1939, Severinghaus reviewed the literature dealing with the effect of hyperthyroidism on the pituitary and reproductive physiology. Meyer and his colleagues,[87] among others, interpreted this type of pituitary reaction as proof of a thyroxine-mediated response to compensate for ovarian atrophy. Judging from our own experience, we believe quite the opposite, that is, that thyroprival animals have to cope with deficient ovarian follicular maturation and thus are liable to develop anestrus and sterility. As a result, we infer that thyroid hormone is necessary for a normal ovarian response to gonadotropins. This has recently been confirmed by Knobil and his colleagues[74] and by Timonen and Hirvonen.[137]

Some comment must also be made here concerning the nature of ovarian stimulation by thyroid hormone. In the opinion of Vaes,[138] thyroxine enhances the ovarian response to gonadotropin A. We have already pointed out that follicular maturation is affected by thyroidectomy, whereas luteinization is not. As a result, it can be concluded that thyroxine acts by heightening follicular sensitivity to the action of FSH. The hypothalamus, too, is modified by thyroidectomy, as was recently shown by Talanti.[132] Hypophysioprival animals show no response either to thyroidectomy or to injections of thyroid hormone. *It may therefore be stated that thyroid hormone acts on the ovary in synergy with FSH activity.*

10.1.9. SYNOPSIS OF THYROID-OVARIAN INTERACTIONS

The pathology affecting the relationship between thyroid function and reproduction will be discussed extensively in the clinical part of this book. It has been known for a long time that hypothyroid women are sterile, abort with ease, frequently have longer phases of amenorrhea or other menstrual disturbances, generally show diminished libido and, in terms of femininity, show diminished somatic as well as psychic development. It has equally been emphasized that marked fluctuations in thyroid function may occur during puberty, during the different phases of the menstrual cycle, or after menopause; it has been learned that castration, too, can produce profound changes in thyroid function. Even though, as was stated earlier, there is no real consensus as to the specific mechanism involved in these phenomena, the circumstances surrounding them are all well known.

The fact that thyroidectomy is followed by alterations in ovarian function is unquestionable. And it is also true that the effect of thyroid hormone on the female gonad is in the first place a trophic one, permitting the stimulatory action by gonadotropin A to be exerted at the target level and to maintain the physiologic development of both the follicle and the ovum contained in the follicle. *Because thyroid hormone has been observed to stimulate gametogenesis in the male as well, it may be qualified as a gametokinetic hormone, that is to say, a hormone capable of stimulating the development of the gametes* of either sex, and of safeguarding the life and maturation of those gametes. With this in mind, it may be further said that *thyroxine is necessary, in the broadest sense of the word, for the development of the germinal plasma, the latter protective action starting with the ovule and sperm, extending to the fertilized ovum, and terminating with the somewhat more mature embryo.* Conceivably, lack of thyroid hormone may thus be responsible for failure of the reproductive mechanism as a result of what may be instances of most precocious "death" of ova or spermatozoa still within their respective gametogenic carriers, or as a result of the death of male fertilizing elements shortly after ejaculation (oligoasthenospermia of hypothyroidism), or else, owing to premature death of the ovum after expulsion from the ovary. Unfortunately, no research whatsoever has been devoted to the question of oocyte maturation and chromatin reduction processes as regards hypothyroidism, despite clear indications that thyroid function is intimately involved in the phenomena of germ cell maturation. Even after fertilization, thyroid hormone may still be necessary for the young germinal elements to develop normally. Thus, Courrier has shown that blastocysts of thyroidectomized animals tend to perish without achieving implantation, which results in considerable early embryonal mortality.

For the future, thyroxine must be counted upon as one more hormone serving the needs of the reproductive process, with special protective action on the germinal plasma.

10.2. PANCREAS AND SEXUAL FUNCTION

A possible relationship between the pancreas and the gonads has long been entertained (see recent reviews by De Meyer[88] and by Quinto and colleagues[109]). *However, the contradictory nature of experimental data concerning the subject must be emphasized.* Castillo and Calatroni[19] have been unable to recognize any changes in the onset of sexual maturity and appearance of sexual development among various young rodents that had been treated with insulin. On the other hand, Herlant[54] reported an increased pituitary content of gonadotropic hormone in rats treated with insulin. It was his opinion that insulin enhanced gonadotropin (LH) secretion by the anterior pituitary and that sustained activity of that hormone, by luteinizing the ovary, inhibited ovarian function, thereby preventing the formation of new follicles, and maintaining the animals in a state of anestrus and sterility. However, it seems pertinent to point out that investigations of that type yield isolated data that have not been sufficiently substantiated and therefore must be admitted with discretion.

Remote and indirect as they may be, *the actions exerted by the ovarian hormones on the pancreas* are nevertheless real. The effect of castration on the pancreas has been studied by Hoffmann and Reiter[58] who found evidence of islet cell proliferation. The average diameter of the islets was found to increase by 80 per cent in animals following castration. As a result of their observations, these authors concluded that the gonads acted on the pancreas by inhibiting the development of the insular apparatus. Cavallero[20] encountered insular hypertrophy after treatment with synthetic progestogens. This question has been raised repeatedly in connection with modern observations that oral contraceptives were associated with a diabetogenic effect (see Chapter 47, Section 47.8.8). Basabe and his colleagues[6] reported that estrogens increased the degree of insulinemia. On the other hand, Spellacy and co-workers[129] maintain that, while estrogenic activity indeed causes elevation of insulin levels, the same effect is produced by both natural and synthetic progestogens to a much greater extent.

The relationships between the gonads and carbohydrate metabolism are manifold and significant. In cooperation with Amilibia and Mendizábal,[16] we studied the effect of estrogens and progesterone on blood sugar levels in rabbits and found that while estrogens produced hyperglycemia, progesterone had the opposite effect, causing hypoglycemia. We observed similar effects in estrogen treated rats, which revealed reduced glycogen storage in the liver and concomitant elevation of ketonuria and glycemia, whereas progesterone increased hepatic glycogenesis and reduced ketogenesis and glycemia in the same animals. Aside from this, rats treated with estrogens for long periods of time devel-

Influence of Other Endocrine Glands on Sex

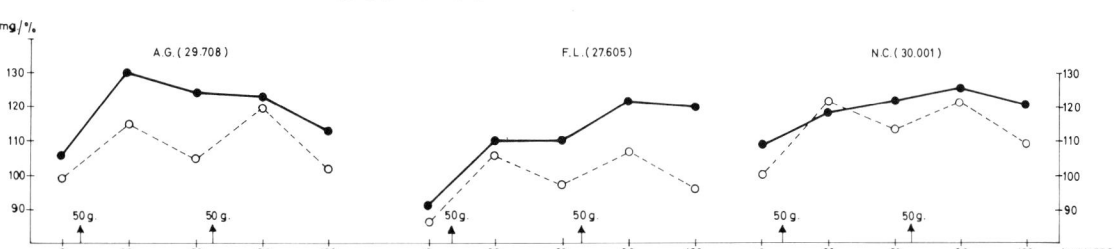

Figure 10-4. Two-dose glucose tolerance curve, Exton-Rose type, in three patients on birth control therapy for a period of six months. The contraceptive used contained 0.5 mg Norgestrol and 0.05 mg Ethinylestradiol per tablet, and was given in the conventional mode of administration, from fifth through twenty-fifth day of the cycle, inclusive. In each of the three cases, some elevation of the tolerance curve, though still within normal limits, was observed. (Dundov and Botella-Llusiá: unpublished data.)

oped the symptomatology of experimental diabetes with chronic glycosuria and ketonuria. In view of these results, we reached the conclusion that estrogens had a hyperglycemia inducing effect, while progesterone produced hypoglycemia. These conclusions were subsequently confirmed by various investigators. Though apparently attributable to gonadal action on the pancreas, we believe that these effects are due to *extrainsular* causes. The hyperglycemia-inducing effect of estrogens becomes apparent in an indirect way through the application of oral contraceptive steroids (see Chapter 44) which causes, among other things, lowered glucose tolerance[38, 42, 69] (see Figs. 10-4 and 10-5).

The findings concerning the effect of castration on glycemia are contradictory. While some seem to deny that castration produces hyperglycemia,[65] others have shown that castrated animals have diminished tolerance to glucose,[131] and still others emphasize the primary role of menopause in predisposing to and initiating diabetes. In fact, postmenopausal women

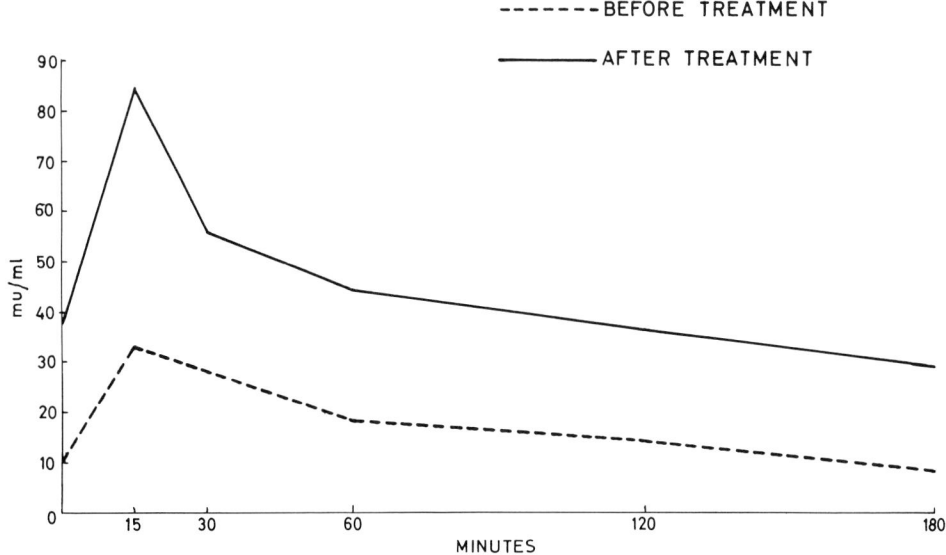

Figure 10-5. Insulinemia following intravenous glucose tolerance test (0.5 g per kg). Radioimmunologic determination of plasma insulin levels by method of Hales and Randle. The dashed line represents a 28-year-old woman before treatment with oral contraceptives. The solid line represents results obtained on same patient after six months' uninterrupted "combined" therapy, each tablet containing 150 mcg Mestranol and 2500 mcg Lynestrenol (Lyndiol-2'5, Organon). Mode of administering contraceptive consisted of one tablet daily between fifth and twenty-fifth day of the cycle, inclusive. (Dundov and Botella-Llusiá: unpublished data.)

quite frequently are seen to develop the symptoms of diabetes for the first time in their lives. This is certainly due to the same type of pituitary reaction that is seen in castration and in the climacterium, as has been indicated previously (Chapter 6), and as will be covered again in Chapter 36. Indeed, the existence of reactive climacteric hyperpituitarism is now admitted. This results in production of a contrainsular hormone, a diabetogenic factor. However, other than the just-mentioned relationship, which actually indicates an indirect gonadal effect on carbohydrate metabolism by way of the pituitary, there really is no biochemical or experimental evidence to uphold the view that sex hormones act on the pancreas. It is obvious, therefore, that while insulin seems to exert a certain remote and mild action on sexual function, the gonadal hormones, conversely, have no effect on the pancreas. The effect of gonadal hormones on carbohydrate metabolism and diabetes is of extrainsular origin.

In conclusion, the reciprocal interactions between the gonads and the pancreas can be stated as being much less pronounced than those between the gonads and the thyroid gland. Thus, whereas the thyroid, in conjunction with the adrenals and the pituitary, is part of the accessory endocrine system of sex, the pancreas, on the other hand, has no specific relationships with the gonads—other than relationships of the general type that interrelate all endocrine glands to each other—and there is no direct gonado-insular interaction to speak of.

10.3. PARATHYROID GLANDS AND SEXUAL FUNCTION

Recently, Littledike and Hawker[83] succeeded in purifying an active extract of hog parathyroids. It has a molecular weight of 9622 and is a diamino-12-peptide, with the following sequence:

(Methionine-Threonine-Proline-Histidine-Arginine-Glycine-Alanine-Valine-Asparagine-Lysine-Leucine-Glutamine-Phenylalanine)—$CONH_2$.

This hormone is closely linked to changes in calcium mobilization and calcium metabolism that are observed in relation to ovarian function. As with the pancreas, the parathyroid glands undergo important changes during pregnancy (see Chapter 20).

Some of the observed sexual effects on *calcemia* are of interest. Holtz and Rossmann studied the influence of sex hormones on the levels of calcemia and noted that estrogens lowered serum calcium values. The same effects were observed in both normal and parathyroprival animals, though differing in that the hypocalcemia-inducing effect in the latter occurred more promptly and was more pronounced. It is of interest to note that while estrogens reduce serum calcium levels, progestogens do not. Whether this effect of estrogens is a direct one or is mediated by the parathyroid glands is not yet known. Charles and Hogben,[21] as well as Pfeiffer and Gardner,[105] studied the same problem in birds, in which an unusually marked calcium-depressing effect by estrogens may be related to requirements for the building of a calcareous egg shell. These authors reached the conclusion that the effect under consideration was mediated by the parathyroid glands under the influence of pituitary "parathyrotropic hormone" stimulation. Apart from the estrogen-induced depression of serum calcium, they also reported significant histologic structural changes in avian parathyroids. Zwarenstein likewise believes that parathyroid glands are stimulated by estrogens indirectly by way of the pituitary.

A further physiologic consideration favoring the existence of a relationship between sex hormones and parathyroid function is the facility with which tetany seems to occur in pregnancy. According to Parriot and colleagues[101] parathyroidectomy during pregnancy rapidly leads to death, whereas nonpregnant control animals survive five times as long. Aceto and his colleagues[1] observed compensatory hypertrophy of fetal parathyroids in response to the extirpation of the maternal glands (see Chapter 19). The hypocalcemia that is observed in the newborn[139] persists for the first week of postnatal life.

Pathologic mobilization of calcium in osteoporosis, such as develops in castrated animals and climacteric women,[85, 119] is well known. Similarly, Polin and Sturke[107] have found hypercalcemia in spayed hens. Thyrocalcitonin also seems to play an important role in climacteric osteoporosis.[110, 140]

Although the relationship between the parathyroid glands and sexual function is a very remote one, an effect by estrogens on calcium metabolism that is antagonistic to parathyroid function can be admitted. Accordingly, parathormone is thought to raise serum calcium levels, whereas estrogens are believed to lower them. It cannot at present be ascertained whether or not those effects result from opposite and antagonistic actions exerted at the level of the target organs, those of estrogens favoring calcium uptake (e.g., by the egg shell), and those of parathormone mobilizing calcium. The fact that estrogens should play as important a role as they do in enhancing phosphatase activity in many organs and tissues (see Chapters 2 and 3) would seem to be an argument in favor of their direct action on calcium metabolism.

10.4. EFFECT OF THYMUS ON SEXUAL FUNCTION

Early anatomic investigations had disclosed the fact that thymic involution takes place about the time of puberty. Since, by increasing and accelerating the rate of thymic involution, pregnancy must have a particularly depressing effect on the thymus, it may be surmised that castration, on the contrary, would inhibit thymic involution. Unquestionably, as was shown by Lenhart[80] in a variety of laboratory animals, the arrest of thymic growth can be prevented and thymic involution can be averted at will by means of castration. The classical studies by Tandler and Gross had long ago confirmed the same fact in man: castration—above all, if performed on young individuals—averts thymic involution. According to Cohen,[25] curves obtained by plotting thymic growth and involution of both castrated and normal rats prior to puberty are of the same height but differ in showing a delayed downward slope in castration, with eventual involution occurring in both groups. That is to say, castration *delays* thymic involution but does not prevent it.

The opposite situation, that is, *the onset of precocious puberty* as a result of thymectomy, is a well known fact, suggesting an antagonistic relationship between the thymus and the gonads (Chapter 34). Pereira-Luz and co-workers[103] demonstrated that administration of *estradiol valerianate* induced accelerated atrophy of the thymus in spayed immature female rats.

Early researchers stressed the antagonism between the pituitary and the thymus. Thus, Evans stated that pituitary extracts accelerated thymic involution. More recently, Bearn[7] showed that both the adrenal and the pituitary inhibited thymic growth. Fetuses of hypophysectomized and adrenalectomized rabbits show exaggerated thymic enlargement at birth. Administration of gonadotropins or corticoids prevents such thymic hypertrophy from developing.

This is probably the etiology of the giant thymus found in *anencephalic fetuses*. Because of lack of pituitary development, the adrenals remain stunted and the thymus undergoes hypertrophy.

It has also been observed recently (Kincl et al.[67]) that thymic extracts block the action of testosterone on the rat hypothalamus, preventing the development of so-called "androgenic sterility."

Gonadal function and thymic function are then antagonistic. This antagonism is difficult to prove by any direct action of thymic extracts on the gonads. For the time being, thymic extracts are nonspecific and no generic thymic hormone has to date been isolated. In contrast, the effect of sex hormones on the thymus is clearly antagonistic. The same holds true for the effect of thymectomy, which has been proved to induce precocious puberty not only in the laboratory but also in clinical experience (see Chapter 34).

In summary, it may be asserted, first that thymic function and gonadal function are antagonistic to each other in both sexes. Second, by the time the thymus is at its functional peak, the gonads are barely in their infancy. Third, by the time the gonads have matured, the thymus begins to undergo involution. Fourth, by eliminating gonadal function a priori, *castration in young animals extends the vital capacity of the thymus for longer periods of time, and fifth, the destruction, inactivation or removal of the thymus results in much more precocious and rapid development of the gonads.* It is also necessary to point out that destruction of the thymus does not produce gonadal hyperfunction but simply advances in time the rhythm of sexual maturation. Whether these effects are direct, resulting from a hormone-to-hormone antagonism, or whether they are merely apparent, owing possibly to an intermediary pituitary control mechanism, may be revealed only by further research. In comparison to both those glands that stimulate sexual function (pituitary, adrenals and thyroid) and those glands that do not, such as the pancreas and the parathyroids, *the thymus must be classified as a gland acting in opposition to the gonads.*

10.5. PINEAL GLAND AND SEXUAL FUNCTION

Until recently, knowledge concerning the physiology of the pineal was indeed quite meager. It has been known, for instance, that pineal tumors (see Chapters 34 and 37) may cause *precocious puberty* (Heubner[55]), but there was no agreement as to how this is brought about. Though early investigations by Achúcarro and Sacristán[2] seemed to ascribe to the pineal a secretory function, the fact remained that no true pineal "hormone" has been isolated in the course of 30 years of painstaking research. Recently (1963), Milcou and his colleagues[89] isolated a polypeptide, seemingly an arginine-vasopressin complex, from the pineal glands of animals. Also, Rodríguez-Pérez, at the Instituto Cajal de Madrid, found electron microscopic evidence that pineal cells and their processes contained holocrine granules (Figs. 10–6, 10–7, and 10–8), not unlike those described in the cells of the supraoptic and paraventricular nuclei. This would appear to suggest that pineal secretion, *rather than being endocrine in nature, is actually neuroendocrine*, a concept already proposed on the basis of histochemical studies by Dempsey and Wislocky[145] a number of years ago.

10.5.1. EXTRAGENITAL EFFECTS OF THE PINEAL

Original studies in comparative anatomy (see Achúcarro and Sacristán[2]) seemed to suggest that the pineal was an analogue of the *dorsal eye* of some lower vertebrates. This ancient concept has gained new ascendancy since Roth and his associates[120] demonstrated that the pineal of birds controlled adaptation of sexual behavior to light. Fiske and his co-workers[41, 42] observed atrophy of the pineal gland in rats that had been subjected to continuous intense illumination for long periods of time. *Hence the pineal gland would seem to be, at least in certain animals, a neuroendocrine organ serving the needs of physiologic adaptation to environmental illumination.*

Another type of extragenital activity,

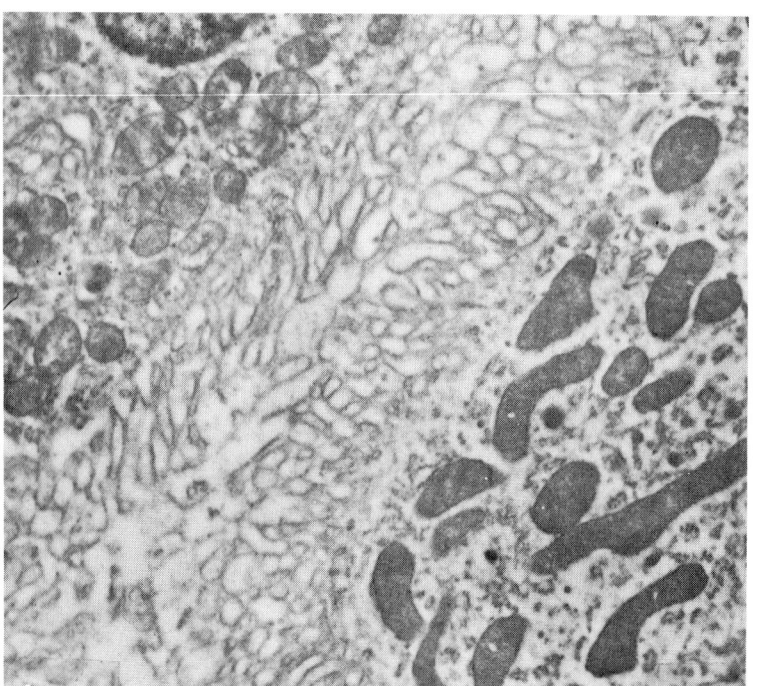

Figure 10–6. Stalk of pineal gland of a cat (26,000×), showing gland-like cavity. (From Rodríguez-Pérez: *Investigaciones Inéditas.* Madrid, Instituto Cajal, 1964.)

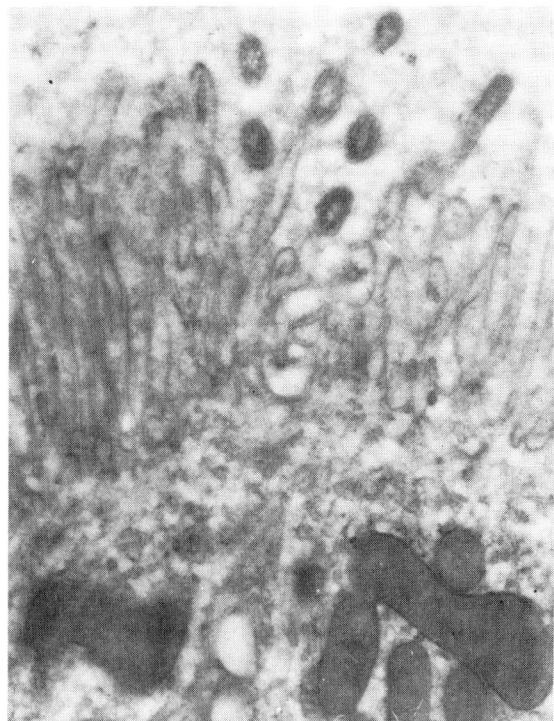

Figure 10-7. Stalk of pineal gland of cat (60,000×). Note ciliary appendages and apparent holocrine secretion. (From Rodríguez-Pérez: *Investigaciones Inéditas*. Madrid, Instituto Cajal, 1964.)

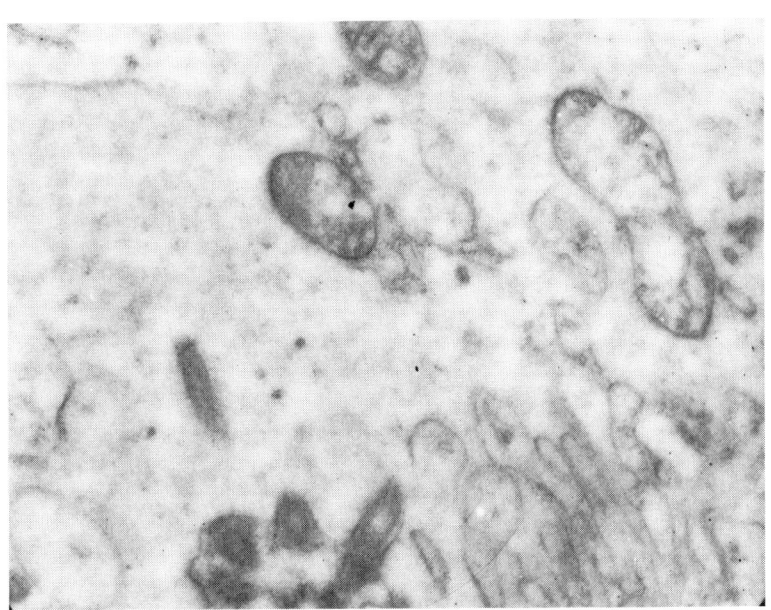

Figure 10-8. Stalk of pineal of cat (110,000×). Phenomena of apparent holocrine secretion. (From Rodríguez-Pérez: *Investigaciones Inéditas*. Madrid, Instituto Cajal, 1964.)

which at present seems to be highly significant and, perhaps, the best known function of the pineal, is the *role played by the pineal in regulating natremia*. Hungerford and Panagiotis[62] made the observation that pinealectomized animals lost the capacity for regulating serum sodium levels, even though the levels of the remaining electrolytes showed no deviation from normal. Romani and associates[118] relate the pineal to sodium retention which, they believe, is implemented *by means of aldosterone*. This assumption seems to harmonize well with the previously mentioned discovery by Milcou and co-workers[89] that the pineal elaborates an arginine-vasopressin complex in response to aldosterone activity. *Thus, it seems plausible to regard the pineal as a neurosecretory center related to the regulation of sodium metabolism.*

10.5.2. THE PINEAL AND THE OPTIC SYSTEM

Whereas in keeping with the classical concept that the pineal is a homologue of the "dorsal eye" of some vertebrates, the pineal of batrachia and reptiles is directly stimulated by luminous impulses (Wurtman[151]), the mammalian pineal, on the other hand, is "blind" and is unable to respond to direct optic stimuli. However, by way of intermediary connections with the inferior accessory optic tract, the mammalian pineal, too, is capable of being influenced by light, if but in an indirect fashion.[113, 148, 159]

The pineal is not really an endocrine gland but functions as a "neuroendocrine transducer," in the terminology of Wurtman.[151] That is to say, it serves as a kind of device through which neural stimuli are converted to hormonal stimuli.

10.5.3. SEXUAL EFFECTS OF THE PINEAL

The existence of a close relationship between the pineal and certain reproductive functions in mammals has been acknowledged.[30, 71, 72] In female rodents, pinealectomy results in early development of vaginal patency, precocious puberty, ovarian hypertrophy and an increase in cornified cells in vaginal smears.[72, 125] In males, it similarly produces testicular hypertrophy and increased size of the prostate.[63, 68, 93, 146] These effects of pinealectomy can be reversed through the administration of pineal extracts.[47, 87, 89] Bovine pineal extracts depress gonadal size in rats.[70] *Castration* causes increased neurosecretory activity of the pineal, as suggested by the electron microscopic observations of Bostelmann.[15] On the other hand, pinealectomy in young animals is associated with increased pituitary secretory activity.[12, 24] An earlier hypothesis that antigonadotropins might originate in the pineal has not been borne out by recent studies.[122] The pineal has further disclosed a rich enzyme content[100, 133, 134] very similar, but not identical to the enzyme composition of the hypothalamic region.[133] This suggests that a polypeptide of a specific nature may be elaborated at this locus.[66, 102]

10.5.4. PINEAL INCRETION: MELATONIN

A specific neurosecretory product called melatonin[47, 152, 153] or 5-methoxy-N-acetyltryptamine[82, 93] (see Fig. 10–9), has been isolated from the pineal gland. It has been postulated that this might be *the pineal hormone* in view of the fact that the pineal is the only structure in the body of higher mammals that contains the specific enzyme hydroxyindole-O-methyl transferase (HIOMT), which is fundamental for the biosynthesis of melatonin. This hypothesis is supported by a variety of studies revealing that both pineal weight[23, 44] and HIOMT activity decrease considerably under certain experimental conditions, such as exposure to light, which, in contrast, provokes a

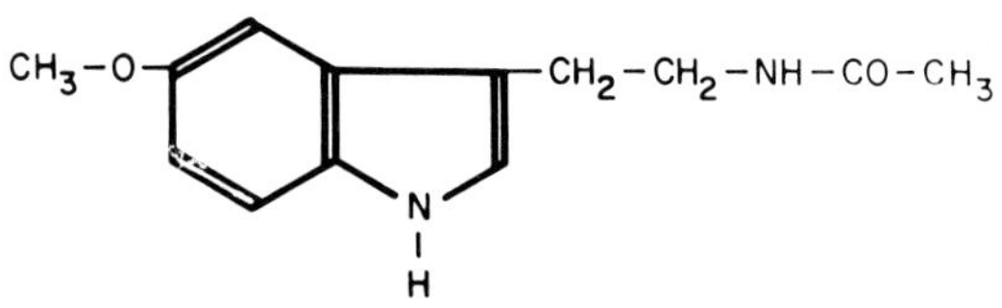

MELATONIN
(5-METHOXY-N-ACETYLTRYPTAMINE)

Figure 10–9. Melatonin.

Influence of Other Endocrine Glands on Sex

marked increase in gonadal activity of rodents (see Chapter 8).

Parenteral administration of melatonin has been found to prevent some, though not all, of the effects of pinealectomy. Melatonin reduces ovarian weight,[3, 23] delays the onset of puberty in immature rats[152, 153] and diminishes estrous activity in the same animals.[48, 145] It equally reduces the weight of the prostate and seminal vesicles in males.[31, 68, 86, 93]

The foregoing data suggest strongly that this substance may be the specific secretion of the pineal gland. Lately, melatonin has been shown to inhibit FSH[31] and LH secretion at the level of the anterior lobe, probably by means of an antirelease mechanism, acting in an opposite, though exactly parallel, direction as regards LHRF.[44]

10.5.5. BIOSYNTHESIS OF MELATONIN

Melatonin synthesis has been well clarified by the writings of Wurtman and Axelrod and their colleagues.[4, 147, 151] This neurohormone is derived from tryptophan which, when oxidized to 5-hydroxytryptophan, can be converted to the melatonin precursor *serotonin*. Most of serotonin is destroyed or metabolized by monoamine oxidase (MAO), an enzyme present in the pineal in high concentration.[100, 128] However, a small fraction of serotonin is acetylated to N-acetylserotonin, which is converted to melatonin by the action of the previously mentioned enzyme, hydroxyindole-O-methyl transferase (HIOMT), according to the scheme shown at the bottom of the page.*

The pineal gland also reveals changes in relation to sexual function and the menstrual cycle.[41, 42, 89] The early neurologic studies by the Spanish school, above all those of Achúcarro and Sacristán,[2] had brought to light the presence of important neural pathways of association between the pineal and the pituitary. Moszkowska[91] contends that the purpose of these pathways is to inhibit the pituitary. However, currently any antagonism that might be involved is thought to be *humoral* in nature and probably results from anti-LH-releasing activity of melatonin.

10.5.6. THE PINEAL AND ENVIRONMENTAL LIGHTING

As indicated previously, the pineal of lower vertebrates is directly related to the optic system, whereas the mammalian pineal has lost its direct connections with the second cranial nerve. In spite of this, other connections are maintained with the *indirect tracts of association*. Pineal activity is endowed with distinct *circadian rhythmicity*.[5] It is well known that constant

---

*Melatonin synthesis, according to Wurtman.[151]

Tryptophan → 5-Hydroxytryptophan → MAO ← Serotonin → N-Acetylserotonin → HIOMT → Melatonin

exposure to light induces ovarian changes as well as estrous activity in a great variety of animals.[33, 98, 106, 127, 155] This reaction does not develop in previously blinded[112, 155] or pinealectomized[92, 117] animals. Light-induced precocious puberty is inhibited by pinealectomy[52, 53] or by severing all neural connections to the pineal.[57, 150]

The pineals of animals "blinded" by such procedures reveal abundant secretory granules.[14, 114] In the final analysis, all indications are that *the pineal is a neuroendocrine organ, a "transducer" in Wurtman's sense of the word, secreting a serotonin-related compound called melatonin, which is a neurosecretory hormone inhibiting FSH and LH release in the median eminence and consequently possessing indirect antigonadotropic activity. Its activity appears to depend directly (in lower vertebrates) or indirectly (in mammals) on the second cranial nerve, through which the pineal assumes the role of mediating cyclic sexual activity in response to environmental lighting.*

REFERENCES

1. Aceto, T., Batt, R. E., Bruck, E., Schulz, R. B., and Pérez, R.: *J. Clin. Endocr. Metab.*, 26:487, 1966.
2. Achúcarro, N., and Sacristán, J. M.: *Trab. Lab. Invest. Biol.*, 10, 1912.
3. Adams, W. C., Wan, L., and Sohler, A.: *J. Endocr.*, 31:295, 1965.
4. Axelrod, J., and Weissbach, H.: *J. Biol. Chem.*, 236:21, 1961.
5. Axelrod, J., Wurtman, R. J., and Snyder, S. H.: *J. Biol. Chem.*, 240:949, 1965.
6. Basabe, J. C., Chieri, R. A., and Foglia, V. G.: *Proc. Soc. Exper. Biol. Med.*, 130:1159, 1969.
7. Bearn, J. G.: *Endocrinology*, 80:979, 1967.
8. Becker, K. L., Winnacker, J. L., Mathews, M. J., and Higgins, G. A.: *J. Clin. Endocr. Metab.*, 28:277, 1968.
9. Beckers, C., and Vischer, M. De: *Ann. d'Endocrinol.*, 18:1, 1957.
10. Beierwaltes, W. H.: *Endocrinology*, 80:545, 1967.
11. Berson, S. A., and Schreiber, S. S.: *J. Clin. Endocr. Metab.*, 13:1126, 1953.
12. Bindoni, M., and Raffaele, R.: *J. Endocrinol.*, 41:451, 1968.
13. Bocabella, A. V., and Alger, E. A.: *Endocrinology*, 81:121, 1967.
14. Bostelmann, W.: *Endokrinologie*, 53:365, 1968.
15. Bostelmann, W.: *Endokrinologie*, 54:56, 1969.
16. Botella, J., Amilibia, E., and Mendizábal, M. M.: *Arch. Gynäk.*, 160:532, 1936.
17. Brown-Grant, K.: *J. Physiol.*, 190:110, 1967.
18. Burrow, G. N.: *J. Clin. Endocr. Metab.*, 25:403, 1965.
19. Castillo, E. B., and Calatroni, C. C.: *Compt. Rend. Soc. Biol.*, 102:455, 1929.
20. Cavallero, H.: *Die Endokrine Regulation des Kohlehydratstoffwechsels*. Berlin, Springer Verlag, 1961.
21. Charles, E., and Hogben, L.: *Quart. J. Exper. Physiol.*, 23:243, 1933.
22. Chu, J. P., and Yu, S. S.: *J. Clin. Endocr.*, 4:116, 1944.
23. Chu, E. W., Wurtman, R. J., and Axelrod, J.: *Endocrinology*, 75:238, 1964.
24. Clementi, F., De Virgilis, G., and Mess, B.: *J. Endocrinol.*, 44:241, 1969.
25. Cohen, R.: *Amer. J. Anat.*, 56:143, 1945.
26. Czerniak, P., and Italson, I.: *Internat. J. Fertil.*, 5:163, 1960.
27. D'Angelo, S. A.: *Proc. Soc. Exper. Biol. Med.*, 121:555, 1966.
28. D'Angelo, S. A.: *Endocrinology*, 81:132, 1967.
29. David, M., Dikstein, S., and Sulman, F. G.: *Proc. Soc. Exper. Biol. Med.*, 121:873, 1966.
30. Davis, L., and Martin, J.: *Arch. Neurol.*, 23:34, 1940.
31. Debeljuk, L., Feder, V. M., and Paolucci, O. A.: *J. Reprod. Fertil.*, 21:363, 1970.
32. Delost, P., and Delost, H.: *Compt. Rend. Acad. Sci.*, 245:208, 1957.
33. Donovan, B. T.: *J. Endocrinol.*, 39:105, 1967.
33a. Dowling, J. T., Freinkel, N., and Ingbar, S. H.: *J. Clin. Endocr. Metab.*, 16:1491, 1956.
34. Dworkin, H. J., Jacquez, J. A., and Beierwaltes, W. H.: *J. Clin. Endocr. Metab.*, 26:1329, 1966.
35. Emge, L. A., and Laqueur, G. L.: *Endocrinology*, 29:96, 1941.
36. Engbring, N. N., and Engstrom, W. W.: *J. Clin. Endocr. Metab.*, 19:783, 1959.
37. Engstrom, W. W., and Marquardt, B.: *J. Clin. Endocr. Metab.*, 14:215, 1954.
38. Fioretti, P., and Carretti, N.: *Riv. Ital. Ginec.*, 50:170, 1966.
39. Fishman, J., Hellman, L., Zumoff, B., and Gallagher, T. F.: *J. Clin. Endocr. Metab.*, 22:389, 1962.
40. Fishman, J., Hellman, L., Zumoff, B., and Gallagher, T. F.: *J. Clin. Endocr. Metab.*, 27:367, 1967.
41. Fiske, V. M., Bryant, G. K., and Putnan, J.: *Endocrinology*, 66:489, 1960.
42. Fiske, V. M., Pond, J., and Putnan, J.: *Endocrinology*, 71:130, 1962.
43. Folley, S. J.: *J. Physiol.*, 93:401, 1938.
44. Fraschini, F., Meis, B., and Martini, L.: *Endocrinology*, 82:919, 1968.
45. Fredrikson, H., and Ryden, H.: *Acta Physiol. Scand.*, 14:136, 1947.
46. Geloso, J. P.: *Ann. d'Endocrinol.*, 28, Suppl. 1, 1967.
47. Giarman, N. J., and Day, M.: *Biochem. Pharmacol.*, 1:235, 1959.
48. Giarola, A., and Ballerio, K.: *Ann. Ost. Gin.*, 75:179, 1959.
49. Gittes, R. F., and Chu, E. W.: *Endocrinology*, 77:1061, 1965.
50. Goldsmith, R. E., Sturgis, S. H., Lerman, L., and Stanbury, J. B.: *J. Clin. Endocr. Metab.*, 12:486, 1952.
51. Grumbrecht, P., and Loeser, A.: *Arch. Gynäk.*, 167:199, 1936.
52. Herbert, J.: *J. Endocrinol.*, 41:20, 1968.

53. Herbert, J.: *J. Endocrinol.*, 43:625, 1969.
54. Herlant, M.: *Compt. Rend. Soc. Biol. (Paris)*, 129:157, 1938.
55. Heubner, R.: In *The Pineal Gland*, ed. J. I. Kitay and M. D. Altschule. Cambridge, Mass., Harvard University Press, 1954.
56. Hoar, R. M., Goy, R. W., and Young, W. C.: *Endocrinology*, 60:337, 1957.
57. Hoffmann, J. C.: *Neuroendocrinology*, 2:1, 1967.
58. Hoffman, R. A., and Reiter, R. J.: *Science*, 148:1609, 1965.
59. Hohlwag, W., Dörner, G., Schumann, B., and Spode, E.: *Endokrinologie*, 47:179, 1964.
60. Holland, J. P., Dorsey, J. M., Harris, N. N., and Johnson, F. L.: *J. Reprod. Fertil.*, 14:81, 1967.
61. Holland, P., Calhoun, F. J., Farris, F. J., and Walton, N. W.: *Acta Endocrinol.*, 59:335, 1968.
62. Hungerford, G. F., and Panagiotis, N. M.: *Endocrinology*, 71:936, 1962.
63. Ifft, J.: *Endocrinology*, 71:181, 1962.
64. Janes, R. G., and Bradbury, J. T.: *Proc. Soc. Exper. Biol. Med.*, 97:187, 1952.
65. Jores, A.: In *Biologie und Pathologie des Weibes*, ed. L. Seitz and A. I. Amreich. Berlin, Urban & Schwarzenberg, 1953.
66. Jouan, P., Garreu, A., and Samperez, S.: *Ann. d'Endocrinol.*, 26:535, 1965.
67. Kincl, F. A., Oriol, A., Folch, P. A., and Maqueo, M.: *Proc. Soc. Exper. Biol. Med.*, 120:252, 1965.
68. Kincl, F. A., and Benagiano, C.: *Acta Endocrinol.*, 54:189, 1967.
69. Kitay, J. I.: *Endocrinology*, 54:114, 1954.
70. Kitay, J. I., and Altschule, M. D.: *The Pineal Gland.* Cambridge, Mass., Harvard University Press, 1954.
71. Kitay, J. I.: *J. Clin. Endocr. Metab.*, 14:623, 1954.
72. Kitay, J. I., and Altschule, M. D.: *Endocrinology*, 55:782, 1955.
73. Klein, D. C., Morii, H., and Talmage, R.: *Proc. Soc. Exper. Biol. Med.*, 124:627, 1967.
74. Knobil, E., Kostyo, J. L., and Greep, R. O.: *Endocrinology*, 65:487, 1959.
75. Korenchewsky, W., Hall, H., and Clapham, B.: *Brit. Med. J.*, 1:235, 1943.
76. Kotz, H. L., and Herrman, W.: *Fertil. Steril.*, 12:96, 1961.
77. Kracht, J., Hachmeister, U., and Kruse, H.: *Münch. Med. Wschr.*, 110:203, 1968.
78. Krohn, J.: *J. Endocrinol.*, 7:307, 1947.
79. Lederer, J., and Meyer, R.: *Ann. d'Endocrinol.*, 18:570, 1957.
80. Lenhart, G.: *Erg. Inn. Med.*, 50:1, 1956.
81. Lerman, J.: "The Thyroid in Gynecology," in *Progress in Gynecology*, ed. S. H. Sturgis and J. V. Meigs. New York, Grune & Stratton, 1950.
82. Lerner, A. B., Case, J. D., and Takahashi, Y.: *J. Biol. Chem.*, 235:1992, 1960.
83. Littledike, E. T., and Hawker, C. D.: *Endocrinology*, 81:262, 1967.
84. Man, E. B., Reid, W. A., and Hellegers, A. E.: *Amer. J. Obstet. Gynec.*, 103:338, 1969.
85. Marañón, G.: *El Climaterio de la Mujer y del Hombre.* Madrid, Espasa Calpe, 1936.
86. Martini, L., Fraschini, F., and Motta, M.: *Rec. Progr. Horm. Res.*, 24:439, 1968.
87. Meyer, C. J., et al.: *Endocrinology*, 68:795, 1961.
88. Meyer, R. De: *Etude experimental de la glucoregulation gravidique.* Paris, Masson et Cie., 1961.
89. Milcou, M., Pavel, S., and Neascu, C.: *Endocrinology*, 72:563, 1963.
90. Money, W. L.: *J. Clin. Endocrinol.*, 10:285, 1950.
91. Moszkowska, A.: *Ann. d'Endocrinol.*, 19:69, 1958.
92. Moszkowska, A., and Scemamma, A.: *Compt. Rend. Soc. Biol. (Paris)*, 162:636, 1968.
93. Motta, M., Fraschini, F., and Martini, L.: *Proc. Soc. Exper. Biol. Med.*, 126:431, 1967.
94. Motta, M., Fraschini, F., and Martini, L.: *Proc. Soc. Exper. Biol. Med.*, 126:461, 1967.
95. Munson, P. L., Hirsch, P. H., and Brewer, H. B.: *Rec. Progr. Horm. Res.*, 24:589, 1968.
96. Nataf, B. M., Rivera, E. M., and Chaikoff, I. L.: *Endocrinology*, 76:35, 1965.
97. Nathanson, I. R.: *Proc. Soc. Exper. Biol. Med.*, 43:737, 1940.
98. Negro-Vilar, A., Dieckermen, E., and Meites, J.: *Proc. Soc. Exper. Biol. Med.*, 127:751, 1968.
99. Nesbitt, R. E. L., Abdul-Karim, R. W., Prior, J. T., Shelley, T. F., and Rourke, J. E.: *Fertil. Steril.*, 18:739, 1967.
100. Otani, T., Gyorkey, F., and Farrell, G.: *J. Clin. Endocr. Metab.*, 28:349, 1968.
101. Parriot, M. W., Johnston, M. E., and Durbin, P. W.: *Endocrinology*, 67:467, 1960.
102. Pavel, S.: *Endocrinology*, 77:812, 1965.
103. Pereira-Luz, N., Marques, M., Ayub, A. C., and Correa, P. R.: *Amer. J. Obstet. Gynec.*, 105:525, 1969.
104. Peterson, R. R., et al.: *Endocrinology*, 51:504, 1953.
105. Pfeiffer, C. A., and Gardner, M. W.: *Endocrinology*, 23:485, 1938.
106. Piasceck, B. E., and Meites, J.: *Neuroendocrinology*, 2:129, 1967.
107. Polin, D., and Sturke, P. D.: *Endocrinology*, 63:177, 1959.
108. Portioli, I., Avanzini, L., Merialdi, A., and Rochi, F.: *Monit. Ost. Gin. Endocr. Metab.* 39:589, 1968.
109. Quinto, P., Bottiglioni, F., and Orlandi, C.: *Metabolismo Glicidico e Stato Puerperale.* Bologna, Ed. Capelli, 1964.
110. Raisz, L. G., and Niemann, I.: *Nature*, 214:486, 1967.
111. Reforzo-Membrives, J.: *Compt. Rend. Soc. Biol.*, 127:695, 1958.
112. Reiter, R. J.: *Neuroendocrinology*, 2:138, 1967.
113. Reiter, R. J.: *Fertil. Steril.*, 19:1009, 1968.
114. Relkin, R.: *Endocrinology*, 82:865, 1968.
115. Relkin, R.: *Endocrinology*, 82:1249, 1968.
116. Rio-Hortega, P. del: *Cytol. Cell. Pathol. Nerv. System*, 2:635, 1932.
117. Robertson, H. A., and Falconer, I. L.: *J. Endocrinol.*, 22:133, 1961.
118. Romani, J. D., Keller, A., and Piotti, L. E.: *Ann. d'Endocrinol.*, 21:612, 1960.
119. Ross, G. T., et al.: *J. Clin. Endocr. Metab.*, 18:492, 1958.
120. Roth, W. D., Wurtman, R. J., and Altschule, M. J.: *Endocrinology*, 71:888, 1962.
121. Russell, K. P.: *Obstet. Gynec. Surv.*, 9:157, 1954.
122. Schneider, H. P., Staemmler, H. J., Sachs, L., and Glockner, C.: *Arch. Gynäk.*, 206:72, 1968.
123. Schulz, M. A., Forsander, J. B., Chez, R. A., and Hutchinson, D. L.: *Pediatrics*, 35:743, 1965.

124. Siegert, F.: In *Biologie und Pathologie des Weibes*, ed. L. Seitz and A. I. Amreich, Vol. I. Vienna, Urban & Schwarzenberg, 1953.
125. Simonnet, H., Thiebolt, L., and Melik, T.: *Ann. d'Endocrinol.*, 12:202, 1951.
126. Singh, B. O., and Bennett, R. L.: *Amer. J. Obstet. Gynec.*, 71:839, 1956.
127. Singh, K. B., and Greenwald, G.: *J. Endocrinol.*, 38:389, 1967.
128. Singh, K. B., Narang, G. D., and Turner, C. W.: *J. Endocrinol.*, 43:489, 1969.
129. Spellacy, W. N., Buhi, W. C., Spellacy, C. E., Moses, L. E., and Goldzieher, J. W.: *Amer. J. Obstet. Gynec.*, 106:173, 1970.
130. Stoddard, F. J., et al.: *J. Clin. Endocr. Metab.*, 17:561, 1957.
131. Stora, C.: *Ann. d'Endocrinol.*, 22:305, 1961.
132. Talanti, S.: *Acta Physiol. Scand.*, 70:80, 1967.
133. Thieblot, L., Bastide, P., Blaise, S., Boyer, J., and Dastugue, G.: *Ann. d'Endocrinol.*, 26:313, 1965.
134. Thieblot, L., et al.: *Ann. d'Endocrinol.*, 27:1, 1966.
135. Thorsöe, H.: *Acta Endocrinol.*, 41:441, 1962.
136. Tienhoven, A. Van, Simkin, D., Weke, J., and Barr, G. R.: *Endocrinology*, 76:194, 1965.
137. Timonen, S., and Hirvonen, E.: *Geburtsh. Frauenhk.*, 22:948, 1962.
138. Vaes, G.: *Ann. d'Endocrinol.*, 21:955, 1960.
139. Wagner, G., Transbol, I., and Melchior, J. C.: *Acta Endocrinol.*, 47:549, 1964.
140. Wase, A. W., Solewsky, J., Rockes, E., and Seidenberg, J.: *Nature*, 214, 388, 1967.
141. Williams, C., Phelps, D., and Burch, I. C.: *Endocrinology*, 29:373, 1941.
142. Williams, R. H., Weinglass, A. R., Russell, G. W., and Peters, J.: *Endocrinology*, 34:31, 1944.
143. Wilson, E. D., Chai, L. K., and Roscoe, B.: *J. Endocrinol.*, 24:431, 1962.
144. Wilson, E. D., Runner, M. N., and Zarrow, M. X.: *J. Reprod. Fertil.*, 5:233, 1963.
145. Wislocky, G. B., and Dempsey, E. W.: *Endocrinology*, 42:56, 1948.
146. Wurtman, R. J., Altschule, M. D., and Holmgren, U.: *Amer. J. Physiol.*, 197:108, 1959.
147. Wurtman, R. J., Axelrod, J., and Phillips, L. S.: *Science*, 142:1071, 1963.
148. Wurtman, R. J., and Axelrod, J.: *Science*, 143:1329, 1964.
149. Wurtman, R. J., and Axelrod, J.: *Sci. Amer.*, 213:50, 1965.
150. Wurtman, R. J., and Axelrod, J.: *Arch. Neurol.*, 18:208, 1968.
151. Wurtman, R. J.: *Amer. J. Obstet. Gynec.*, 104:320, 1969.
152. Wurtman, R. J., Axelrod, J., and Chu, E. W.: *Science*, 141:277, 1963.
153. Wurtman, R. J., Axelrod, J., Snyder, S. H., and Chu, E. W.: *Endocrinology*, 76:798, 1965.
154. Young, W. C., et al.: *Endocrinology*, 51:12, 1952.
155. Zacharias, L., and Wurtman, R. J.: *Science*, 144:1154, 1964.

Chapter 11
VITAMINS AND SEXUAL FUNCTION

Although, strictly speaking the exclusive theme of this book is endocrinology, the influence of vitamins on the reproductive organs is so closely related to that of hormones that the solution of many problems encountered in this field requires an understanding of the physiology of vitamins. The therapeutic handling of many female endocrine disorders, too, often resorts to the use of vitamins, if but as auxiliary remedies. For these reasons, a general review of the significance of this group of compounds in the processes of reproduction seems to be in order.

11.1. GENERALITIES

By vitamins we understand organic substances that, contained in food, are ingested in minute amounts and are indispensable for nutrition and development. This classical definition, formulated by Ammon and Dirscherl,[2] exludes, because of their inorganic nature, certain salts or mineral elements, such as iodine and calcium, which may be just as indispensable for nutrition and development. This definition might equally be expanded by adding that *vitamins are substances that are also necessary for the reproductive process.* Lack of adequate vitamin intake in animals suspends estrous activity and causes sterility (Moe et al.[59]); furthermore, as has been shown by Warkany[90] and Watteville and his colleagues,[91] faulty vitamin intake by pregnant mothers may give rise to various developmental alterations and even congenital anomalies in the fetus.

The distinction between vitamins and hormones seems to be simple in terms of the preceding definition, since vitamins are not synthesized by the body whereas hormones are, and are so, moreover, by organs specifically designed for that purpose—the glands of internal secretion. Nevertheless, easy as it may seem, this distinction is far from being clear-cut. Thus, for instance, the fact that thyroxine synthesis requires ingestion of iodine obviously is not in keeping with the provision that hormones should be totally and exclusively synthesized from endogenous products, and may not in the least be dependent on dietary constituents. On the other hand, some vitamins have long been known to be synthesized within the body—e.g., *vitamin D*, which is produced from ergosterol in the skin as a result of the action of ultraviolet light. This means that the body utilizes sterols or analogous compounds as *provitamins* for almost the entire process of vitamin D synthesis. In Chapters 3 and 4, we have indicated how adrenal perfusion studies have revealed partial synthesis of progesterone, corticoids and, probably, androgens from cholesterol as the starting point. *In this respect, vitamin D$_2$ and some of the sexual steroids would seem to have a similar origin.* When we apply only these criteria, therefore, a distinction between vitamins and hormones may prove difficult. This point might further be exemplified by citing hepatic conversion of carotene to vitamin A and the finding, reported by several workers,[21, 24, 68] that both the adrenal cortex and the ovary are capable of synthesizing ascorbic acid. For these reasons, *a topographic definition would be more meaningful and preferable to a chemical definition of vitamins.* Under such a definition, most, though not all, vitamins would thus be formed outside the organism and most of them, too, would therefore have to be ingested with food, but *what above all* defines them as distinct from the hormones is the fact that there is no specific organ to elaborate them, that is, no counterpart of an endocrine gland. Vitamins differ from hormones on another count in that *neither their elaboration nor their mode of action is regulated by the nervous system.* Finally, the actions exerted by hormones are of much greater specificity than those of vitamins, a secondary but nevertheless important distinction; as an example, vitamins as biocatalysts participate in a variety of metabolic processes going on simultaneously in quite different effector organs.

The distinction between an "enzyme" and a "vitamin" may be even more difficult. Most of the roles of vitamins are enzymatic actions in which the vitamins are biocatalysts, acting by virtue of being present in minimal quantities. However, by definition, an enzyme is an intrinsic biocatalyst, one that is bound to the cells in which the substrate is to be transformed. Because vitamins are of exogenous origin they can be defined as *exogenous biocatalysts.* For the sake of a working hypothesis, biocatalysts may therefore be divided as follows:

Biocatalysts
- Exogenous
  - Biocatalysts exogenous to the cell, elaborated by a specific organ and secreted under the influence of the nervous system (*hormones*).
  - Biocatalysts exogenous to the organism, ingested with food, without any specific organ for their production and independent of the nervous system (*vitamins*).
- Endogenous
  - Endogenous biocatalysts, elaborated in the cells in whose cytoplasm they exert their activity (*enzymes*).

11.2. MODE OF ACTION OF VITAMINS

Originally, the mode of action of vitamins was assessed on the basis of the effects caused by their deficiency. By studying animals under controlled conditions of food intake in which certain nutritive elements were withheld alternately, any resulting pathologic disturbances could be correlated with the absence of specific purified principles. If added to the diet, such purified principles had to be capable of reverting those pathologic disturbances (that is, the manifestations of deficiency). Vitamins were thus defined as antirachitic, antixerophthalmic, etc. Such *negative definitions* were of course not conducive to a full understanding of the true nature of these biocatalysts, because most of the time the deficiencies involved were complex phenomena. In addition, it was impossible to separate the primary disturbances from possible secondary manifestations with any degree of certainty.

11.2.1. VITAMINS AS BIOCATALYSTS

Until vitamins were finally synthesized or obtained in a pure state there was no way of determining their mode of action other than by purely *pharmacologic* studies. The effect of *pure vitamins* thus became the object of studies on experimental animals similar to those carried out with *pure hormones.* Instead of removing the original gland, a prerequisite for appreciating exactly the effect of a given hormone, vitamin research resorted to withholding the vitaminic factor in question from the diet. It was thus learned that vitamins were not nutrient substances. Although their deficiency apparently gives rise to disturbances similar to those which might be caused by lack of a given mineral or chemical substance, the last 30 years of research have made it abundantly clear that they are active substances, biocatalysts, which affect cellular metabolism and regulate chemical processes. It has also been learned that vitamins are basic elements in the biosynthesis of enzymes, since the latter were shown by Euler[21] to be actually made up of two parts: one, a protein carrier of a high molecular weight, called *apoenzyme,* which is inactive so long as it does not join the other group. The latter is smaller in size, and serves as a prosthetic group to the protein carrier; it is called a *coenzyme* or active group. The enzyme is not formed unless these two groups are joined together. Some vitamins, particularly the phosphoric esters, are coenzymes; such is the case with all or nearly all vitamins of the B group. For instance, phosphorylized vitamin B_1 is *cocarboxylase,* and vitamin B_2 in similar phosphoric union is *Warburg's yellow respiratory enzyme.*

11.2.2. VITAMINS AND METABOLISM

The actions of vitamins unfold at the *metabolic level*. Vitamins regulate respiratory processes of tissues, are active in carbohydrate catabolism and influence the synthesis or degradation of certain amino acids. Such processes as intestinal absorption of neutral fats and regulation of calcium and phosphorus metabolism are equally affected by certain vitamins. Those other vitamins that have no known metabolic actions but are believed to exert distant effects on some systems (bone marrow, etc.) most likely are endowed with some actions of the intermediary metabolic type.

11.2.3. VITAMINS AND REPRODUCTION

As for the effect of vitamins on reproductive processes, it must be remembered that reproduction is a special form of growth (Chapter 1). Like growth, sexual physiology in its entirety is governed by the actions of vitamins. By and large, vitamins are promotors of growth. Even though classically the effects of some vitamins on development were believed to have a stimulatory specificity, currently their growth-promoting action is known to result from generally favorable effects on metabolism. Many of the growth-promoting factors in lower animals are vitaminic in nature. For instance, some protozoal species have been found to possess substances of the *crocin* type, closely related to vitamin A, which not only stimulate development but also activate reproduction of clones, in this case again a form of growth. An essential growth-promoting element in vertebrates, vitamin A functions as a sexual substance in simpler forms of animal life. Moewus has drawn a parallel between the effects of crocin and those of estrogens (see Chapter 14). While estrogens act as growth-promoting substances in certain protozoa, exerting a stimulatory effect on cellular metabolism comparable to that exerted by vitamins in higher animals, crocin acts on reproduction in protozoa in a way similar to estrogens in higher animals. The crocin-estrogen inversion of effects becomes more apparent as one ascends the animal scale, a striking example of how similar the actions of vitamins may be to those of sex hormones under certain circumstances.

In higher animals, various vitamins clearly are implicated in gonadal development and biogenesis of some of the sex hormones. Vitamin C seems to be necessary for the synthesis of certain steroids of the pregnane group, such as mineralocorticoids and progesterone. This effect is undoubtedly due to metabolic redox activity, for which ascorbic acid is perfectly adapted. So far as the mammalian reproductive cycle during pregnancy as well as during lactation is concerned, the significance of vitamins is extraordinary. In addition to acting as metabolic regulators in the mother, they influence the development and nutrition of the fetus. Although suppression of some vitamins in animal research has produced fetal deficiency states associated with developmental alterations, deficiencies encountered in human clinical experience do not seem to reach sufficient severity to completely drain the fetal circulation of vitamins and to give rise to fetal avitaminosis. Nonetheless, vitamin deficiencies of the gestational period do affect the eventual nutritional state of the newborn during lactation. Consequently, the reproductive process in general may be profoundly affected or modified by these nutritional factors.

11.3. VITAMINS AND HORMONES

The preceding paragraphs seem to us indispensable for understanding the effects of vitamins on the endocrine system. The purpose of this chapter is not to enter into a detailed study of all possible relationships existing between vitamins and sexual function but rather to clarify the relationship between *vitamins and the sex hormones*. This relationship is closer than might be suspected, since the ranges of vitamin and hormone activity cannot be exactly demarcated. There is evidence that in the rat vitamin C is elaborated by an endogenous process of adrenocortical synthesis so that, at least in this species, ascorbic acid might have to be considered a hormone rather than a vitamin.

The relationship between hormones and vitamins may then be explored under these aspects: (1) chemical relationship between hormones and vitamins, and (2) similarities in synthesis.

11.3.1. CHEMICAL RELATIONSHIP BETWEEN HORMONES AND VITAMINS

In our view, some of the most interesting instances of chemical relationship between hormones and vitamins are those existing between *steroids and vitamin D*, between *thyroxine and vitamin A*, between *epinephrine and vitamin C*, and between *insulin and vitamin B*. Vitamin D has the same structural ring as the sex hormones (estrogens, androgens, progesterone) and the cortical hormones (mineralo- and glucocorticoids). The possibility of conversion of vitamin D to androgenic compounds has been inferred by some researchers on the basis of weak virilizing activity of some of the vitamins mentioned. As indicated previously, this entire group of compounds can be regarded as having a common origin in stigmasterol and cholesterol.

Eufinger and Gottlieb[20] reported that carotene and thyroxine tended to maintain a reciprocal equilibrium by counteracting each other's activity. Abelin found that the same antagonism obtained in vitro—viz., that the two substances mutually inactivated each other. The antagonism under consideration would therefore seem to be chemical in nature, only in this case the chemical relationship would be the opposite of the preceding example. Aside from this, Abderhalden and Schroeder have shown that oxidation of epinephrine is inhibited by ascorbic acid, the action of epinephrine thereby being potentiated. Similarly, vitamin C is involved in oxidative conversion of progesterone to deoxycorticosterone and vice versa.

As a result of the work of Euler[21] and Högberg, it is now admitted that insulin contains aneurin in its molecule, this vitamin thus having turned out to be a component of a hormonal molecule.

11.3.2. SIMILARITIES BETWEEN VITAMIN AND HORMONE SYNTHESIS

Some vitamins, such as vitamins A and D, are thought to be elaborated in the body at the expense of certain simpler compounds, or *provitamins*. This raises the question of whether, in the strict sense of the word, vitamins A and D might not be thought of as hormones rather than vitamins. Similarly, while vitamin C behaves as a true vitamin in the guinea pig as well as in the human species—that is, it must be *entirely acquired from outside*—rats can be maintained on vitamin C deficient diets for entire generations without ever becoming afflicted with scurvy. At present, it is known that rats as well as the human fetus are capable of synthesizing ascorbic acid in the adrenal cortex. This may give rise to a hormonal concept concerning these vitaminic substances. The fact that some vitamins display these features only in certain animals can best be exemplified among the vitamins of the B complex. Thus, factors B_3 and B_5, which, in conjunction with vitamin B_1, are indispensable for growth as far as the pigeon is concerned, are instead dispensable in the human species, a fact lending support to the idea that, since there exist no fundamental differences between animal and human metabolism as regards the most elementary chemical reactions, *the human species undoubtedly must be forming those otherwise unobtainable substances within their own bodies.*

11.4. VITAMIN A AND SEXUAL FUNCTION

Vitamin A is a liposoluble vitamin. Its deficiency in experimental animals causes xerophthalmia and arrest of growth associated with multiple epithelial alterations. It is therefore a growth-promoting factor and a protector of epithelial structures. This compound is a polyenic alcohol, with the following composition:

$$\text{CH}_3\ \text{CH}_3$$
$$\begin{array}{c}\diagup\\\diagdown\end{array}\!\!\!-\text{CH}=\text{CH}-\underset{\underset{\text{CH}_3}{|}}{\text{C}}=\text{CH}-\text{CH}=\text{CH}-\underset{\underset{\text{CH}_3}{|}}{\text{C}}=\text{CH}-\text{CH}_2\text{OH}$$
$$-\text{CH}_3$$

Vitamin A usually is not ingested preformed as such except in relatively small quantities. Most of the vitamin to be utilized is derived from the conversion of a provitamin, *carotene*, present in abundance in certain roots and vegetables, such as carrots, beets, and so forth. The carotene-vitamin conversion takes place in the liver under the influence of a specific enzyme: *carotenase*. Both vitamin A and carotene are present in the circulating blood and can be estimated by chemical photometric procedures. Estimated daily consumption in man ranges from a minimal 1 mg to an optimal 5 mg of carotene, in the presence of a normally functioning liver. Vitamin A consumption consequently depends on the condition of the liver so that, provided liver function is adequate, an individual may do well with practically no ingestion of preformed vitamin. As is the case with all other liposoluble vitamins, the intestinal capacity for their absorption depends on the *dietary content of fats*.

11.4.1. EFFECT OF VITAMIN A ON THE OVARY

Because of its role in protecting epithelia, this vitamin is *necessary for the development of the ovarian follicle*. Lack of it provokes degenerative changes in the follicle and causes arrest of ovarian maturation (Fig. 11–1). Consequently, avitaminosis A results in suspension of the menstrual cycle and, at the same time, causes decreased estrogen synthesis (Gaethgens[24]).

MacCarthy and Cerecedo[50] observed that vitamin A deficiency in rats produced anovulation. Lutwak-Mann[48] also found absence of follicular maturation, and Highnett[37] moreover described anestrus and sterility in rats and mice kept on a diet free of vitamin A and carotene.

11.4.2. EFFECT OF VITAMIN A ON THE TESTIS

Avitaminosis A produces quite noticeable effects, primarily by diminishing spermatogenesis, and vitamin A can be inferred to be a gametokinetic agent, necessary for the development of germ cells as well as the gametogenic apparatus (Fig. 11–2).

Hence, its effect on the testis is quite evident, as has been recently confirmed by various investigators. In the male rat,[47] the ram,[17] the mating bull[11, 19] and in man,[15] vitamin A deficiency leads to oligospermia or azoospermia and eventual sterility.

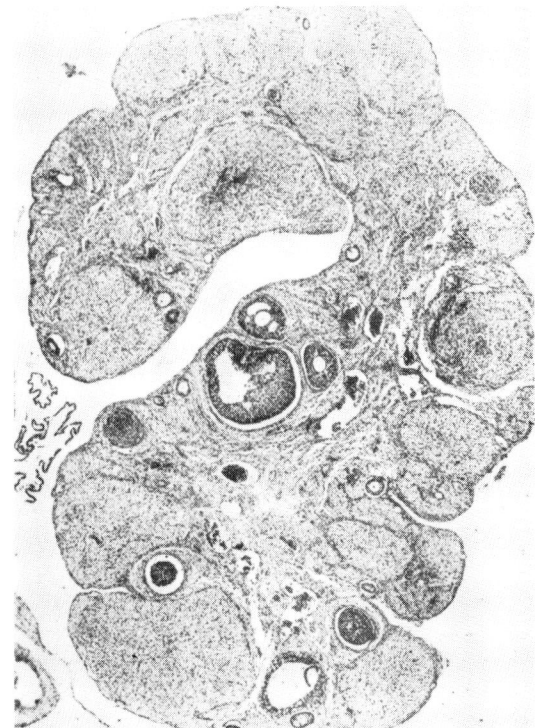

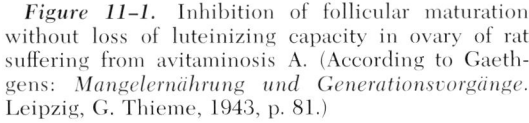

Figure 11–1. Inhibition of follicular maturation without loss of luteinizing capacity in ovary of rat suffering from avitaminosis A. (According to Gaethgens: *Mangelernährung und Generationsvorgänge*. Leipzig, G. Thieme, 1943, p. 81.)

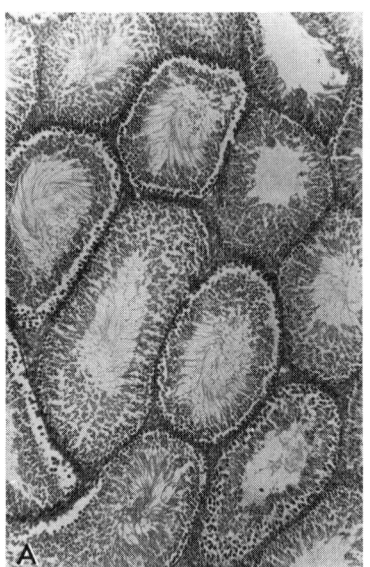 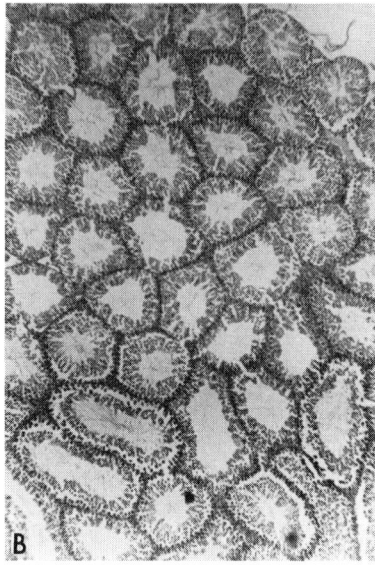

Figure 11–2. Effect of vitamin A deficient diet on rat testis. A, Control animal. B, Animal suffering from avitaminosis A. Notice atrophy of seminiferous tubules and absence of spermatogenesis.

11.4.3. EFFECT OF VITAMIN A ON THE UTERUS AND VAGINA

Vitamin A deficiency causes lack of mucosal development. In some cases, amenorrhea has been found to respond favorably to vitamin A treatment.[10] Vitamin A deficiency has a remarkable effect *on the vagina*. The consequence is development of colpokeratosis, first described by Hohlweg and Dohrn in 1930, and recently studied by Laurence and Sobel.[43] The occurrence of colpokeratosis in rodents has given rise to the erroneous assumption that avitaminosis A was responsible for inducing permanent estrus. On the contrary, vitamin A is capable of regenerating the atrophic vaginal epithelium in deficient animals, as shown by Murray.[61]

11.4.4. VITAMIN A AND PREGNANCY

Vitamin A is of considerable importance to the mother. Gaethgens[25] has shown that during pregnancy, even in well-fed women, vitamin A blood levels decreased, whereas carotenemia increased. Because the corresponding conversion process takes place in the liver, it is admitted that functional insufficiency of the latter may be associated with inadequate carotene-vitamin A conversion in pregnancy. Gaethgens[24] also found that the placenta was similarly capable of converting carotene to vitamin A. As a result, in the absence of adequate dietary vitamin A and fat intake, pregnant women are prone to develop the symptoms of vitamin deficiency (Botella and Hernández-Araña[10]). It would thus appear that during pregnancy the site of carotene-vitamin conversion is displaced from the liver to the placenta (Fig. 11–3). Recently, Laurence and Sobel[43] found that considerable fluctuations in vitamin A blood concentrations occurred in the course of the menstrual cycle, with peak values coinciding with the time of ovulation. The interpretation the authors offered for the phenomenon was that provitamin was being actively converted to vitamin as a result of *maximal carotenase activity under the effect of estrogens.* It might be speculated that the greater metabolic turnover of estrogens in the liver during certain phases of the cycle might be associated with greater hormone concentrations in the hepatic cells and that the resulting estrogenic activity might be responsible for the higher rate of vitamin production. During pregnancy, the greater concentration of estrogens in the placenta and the metabolic utilization of these hormones by this organ, rather than by the liver, suggest that the site of carotenase activity may be transferred to the placenta.

Thus, a close relationship seems to exist between estrogen concentrations of parenchymal cells and their capacity to convert provitamin to vitamin, as a result of which a certain degree of synergism can be assumed to exist between estrogen and vitamin A activity.

The sexual effect of vitamin A may be summed up by stating that, *whereas vitamin A is necessary for the development of the follicle and, consequently, for estrogen synthesis, estrogens in turn seem to advance the process of carotene-to-vitamin conversion and thereby promote production of the latter vitamin within the body.* In the same way, the protective effect exerted by vitamins on the seminiferous tubules of the testis brings on increased estrogen synthesis even in male animals, and, what is more, synergism exists between the actions of estrogens and those of vitamin A in males as well. As a result, *vitamin A is a vitamin possessing feminizing activity.*

11.4.5. EFFECT OF VITAMIN A ON FETAL DEVELOPMENT

Studies by Warkany and his co-workers,[89, 90] Wilson and Barch,[92] Watteville and colleagues[91] and Laschet and Weise[42] appear to have revealed an *important role played by vitamin A in the development of the embryo.* In rats maintained on vitamin A-free diets from 13 days prior to mating up to the time of littering, there was evidence that the litter had been only slightly affected by embryonal alterations. If, however, vitamin A deficient dieting was started one month prior to mating, the systematic appearance in the offspring of anophthalmia, microphthalmia and such other malformations as congenital absence of limbs, agenesis of portions of the endoderm, as well as similar anomalies, was the rule. This indicates that only in cases with pronounced degree of maternal avitaminosis is there a sufficient loss of vitamin to affect embryonal development. The circumstances surrounding maintenance of vitamin A levels during pregnancy, as well as the capacity of the placenta to convert provitamin to vitamin, account for the fact that maternal deficiency with diets containing carotene but no vitamin A may assume serious proportions; on the other hand, as soon as provitamin is converted by the placenta it is assimilated and fixed in situ by both the placenta and the fetal organism, thereby alleviating the fetal deficiency state while leaving maternal deficiency unaffected. *It follows that, by virtue of the displacement of carotenase activity toward the placenta, a selective system of fetal protection is established,* which vividly illustrates the validity of Hammond's[34] general law concerning the priorities of ovular nutrition.

Vitamin A deficiency also decisively affects the weight and resistance of the offspring. The litter from mothers that had been deprived of vitamin A prior to pregnancy were found to show less resistance, to have less vitality and to be underweight.

It should be further stressed that prolonged conditions of avitaminosis in animals of either sex, preceding the date of conception by more than two months, produce sterility—in the male because of absent spermatogenesis, and in the female because of anovulation.

11.4.6. HYPERVITAMINOSIS A

That excessive amounts of vitamin A may be toxic has long been known. Hypervitaminosis A produces some significant sexual effects. Laschet and co-workers[41] reported that daily administration of 60,000 I.U. to female rats caused sterility. With somewhat larger dosages, of the order of 250,000 I.U., Maddock and his colleagues[52] succeeded in inducing testicular degeneration in males of the same species. Randaz-

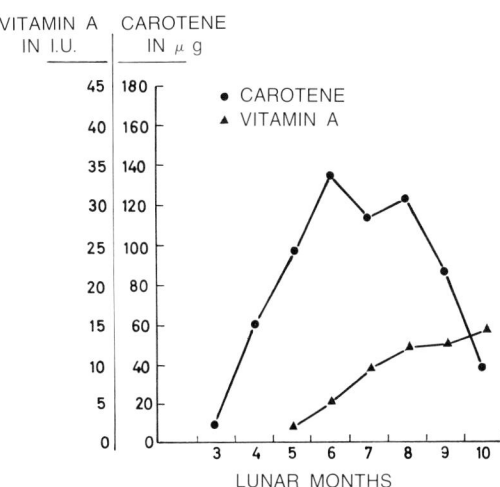

Figure 11–3. Placental storage of vitamin A. (From Gaethgens: *Der Vitaminhaushalt in der Schwangerschaft.* Dresden, Th. Steinkopff, 1937.)

zo[72] claimed that hypervitaminosis A depressed estrogen synthesis in the human species.

11.5. THE VITAMIN B COMPLEX

11.5.1. VITAMIN B₁ (ANEURIN, THIAMINE)

Vitamin B₁ belongs to the group of hydrosoluble vitamins. Deficiency of this factor in man is the cause of beriberi, with a clinical picture in which polyneuritis predominates. Currently, however, polyneuritis is suspected of being in part the result of associated deficiencies of other group B factors. The manifestations of experimentally induced beriberi polyneuritis can also be duplicated in animal research, particularly in domestic fowl and pigeons. This vitamin, the main source of which is the husk of the rice grain, has the following formula:

$$H_3C-\underset{N-C-NH_2}{\overset{N=CH}{C}}\quad C-CH_2-\underset{HC}{\overset{Cl}{N}}\underset{S}{\diagdown}\overset{C-CH_3}{\underset{C-CH_2-CH_2OH}{\|}}$$

Although vitamin B₁ is stored by parenchymal cells in smaller amounts than other vitamins, it is nevertheless widely distributed throughout the body, owing to the fact that thiamine diphosphate is *cocarboxylase*, an enzyme that is intimately associated with phosphorylation processes of carbohydrate metabolism.

Vitamin B₁ may be estimated either by biologic methods (using mainly pigeons, chickens or rodents) or by chemical methods (based on diazo coupling to give *diazo reactions*, or else on its conversion to a *thiochrome*), and subsequent spectrophotometric measurement. Thiamine is amply represented in the vegetable kingdom and its synthesis is linked mainly to green plants. Some microbes and lower protists are capable of partial thiamine synthesis from thiazole, but this is not possible in higher animals. Thiamine is absorbed by the gut in simple form and is subject to phosphorylation by different parenchymal cells, mainly those of the bowel wall, the kidney and the liver. Since thiamine contains a sulfur atom in its molecule, its metabolism can be studied by utilizing radioactive sulfur. Using a similar approach, Borsook and his associates[8] were able to demonstrate the existence of an endogenous absorption quota for thiamine, which varied in relation to different physiologic and pathologic conditions.

THIAMINE AND REPRODUCTION. The existence of a *relationship between vitamin B₁ and reproduction* is unquestionable, although many aspects of it are still poorly understood. The occurrence of amenorrhea and gonadal atrophy have been convincingly proved to be part of the clinical picture of beriberi. Similarly, Sánchez-Rodríguez and Morros-Sardá[74] were able to show that atrophy of the genital apparatus in pigeons with beriberi could be prevented by estrogen administration. These findings permit the assumption of an existing synergism between the respective activities of follicular hormone and thiamine, based on the premise that B₁ avitaminosis suppresses estrogen secretion by the avian ovary, resulting in adverse effects on the genital tract which could therefore be avoided through the administration of estrogens. Coward and his associates[14] reported finding follicular atrophy with loss of cyclic activity in guinea pigs affected by B₁ avitaminosis. Gaethgens[25] observed multiple ovarian atresias (Fig. 11-4) associated with atrophy of the uterus and vaginal epithelium (Fig. 11-5) in animals kept in a state of avitaminosis, as a result of which the animals developed anestrus. According to Pfaltz and Severinghaus,[70] the capacity of such animals for conceiving is diminished. Even though gestation may be achieved, an infrequent occurrence in vitamin B₁ deficient animals, abortion or reabsorption of the fetus almost invariably follows. The testes are particularly affected and undergo atrophy, attaining barely half the size of normal testes. This effect on the testes is especially conspicuous *in man*. Lutwak-Mann[48] reported that clinical B₁ hypovitaminosis in man was associated with a marked drop in 17-ketosteroid excretion, and Mann[53] made the observation that Leydig cell activity was significantly reduced. Rather than being the result of direct action on the gametes, these effects appear to be endocrine in nature, since affected individuals do not develop azoospermia in spite of lowered endocrine testicular activity. A small amount of yeast or vitamin

Figure 11-4. Effect of vitamin B₁ deficient diet on the rat ovary. Note ovarian atresia with absent follicular maturation and many atretic corpora lutea. (From Gaethgens: *Der Vitaminhaushalt in der Schwangerschaft.* Dresden, Th. Steinkopff, 1937.)

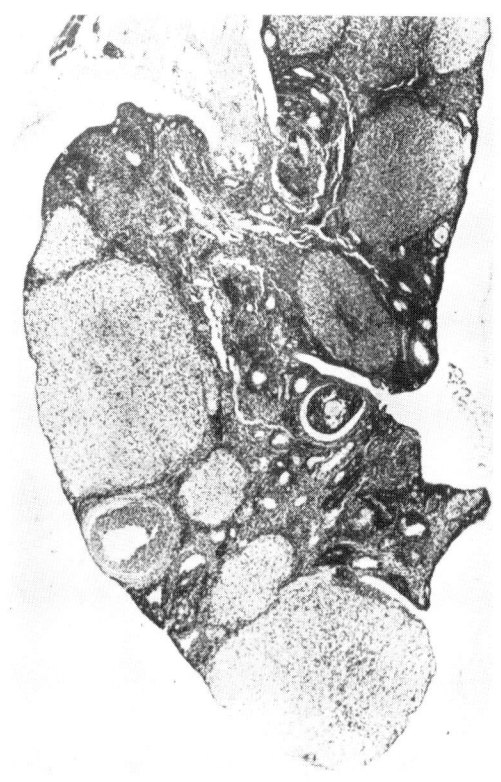

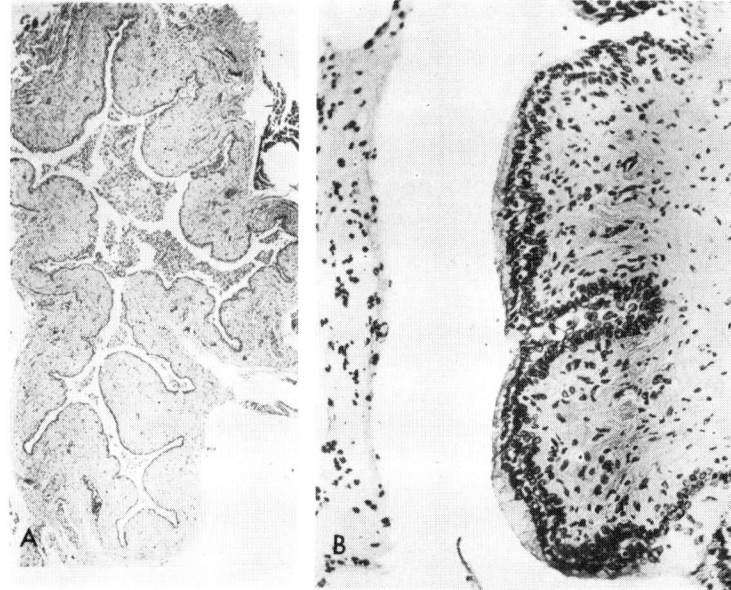

Figure 11-5. Effect of vitamin B₁ deficiency on the rat vagina. Note the vaginal epithelial atrophy. (From Gaethgens: *Der Vitaminhaushalt in der Schwangerschaft.* Dresden, Th. Steinkopff, 1937.)

is sufficient to protect the sexual organs from the effects of vitamin B_1 deficiency. The fact that vitamin B_1 deficiency merely slows down rather than totally inhibits gonadal activity has been shown by Siddall,[77] who was able to restore sexual function in animals with experimental B_1 avitaminosis by treating them with gonadotropins.

The effect of vitamin B_1 deficiency on *uterine motility* has also been described. Spontaneous uterine contractions have been observed to decrease in animals with experimental avitaminosis, so that vitamin administration is at present assumed to stimulate uterine contractions. This effect is probably related to the role played by thiamine in carbohydrate metabolism.

THIAMINE AND PREGNANCY. Vitamin B_1 requirements during pregnancy are markedly increased, owing to the active role of vitamin B_1 in carbohydrate metabolism and to enhanced glycogenolysis, which causes accumulation of tricarbons and increases the demand for cocarboxylase to degrade them.[32, 44] Daily thiamine requirements are doubled or trebled as a result. Gaethgens[24] finds that thiamine blood concentrations in the fetus are invariably higher than those in the mother, assigning to the placenta an active role in elevating thiamine concentrations in the fetal circulation (Fig. 11–6). Fetal organs, particularly the liver, kidneys, adrenals and bowel, have been shown to be rich in thiamine. As revealed by the work of Hildebrandt[38] and Staehler,[80] gestational vitamin B_1 deficiency is of great clinical importance. *A deficit in thiamine body saturation has been detected in approximately 17 per cent of normal pregnancies, in about 40 per cent of pregnancies presenting with vomiting and in about 62 per cent of normal lactating women, whereas B_1 hypovitaminosis was present in 100 per cent of pregnancies complicated by toxemia.* Hypovitaminosis of vitamin B_1 in pregnancy is responsible for the appearance of *polyneuritis of pregnancy*, an important clinical syndrome, the description of which is beyond the scope of this book. However, it is pertinent to point out that some *cardiac disturbances* of pregnancy also have the same etiology. In general, milk contains but scant amounts of vitamin B_1, cow's milk even less so than human milk.

11.5.2 OTHER VITAMINS OF THE B COMPLEX

The remaining vitamins of group B comprise a very heterogeneous assortment of compounds which, although originally extracted from identical sources, have currently been demonstrated to be independent and diversified. The following elements are included:

Vitamin B_2 (lactoflavin, riboflavin).

Vitamin B_3, known to promote growth in pigeons.

Vitamin B_4, known to promote growth in rats.

Vitamin B_5, possessing growth-promoting properties in both pigeons and rats. (These three substances are distinct, though difficult to separate from each other.)

Vitamin B_6 (adermine, pyridoxine).

Pantothenic acid.

Nicotinic acid, and

A vast group of hematogenic factors, the most important of which are *folic acid* (vitamin B_{11}) and *cobalamin* (vitamin B_{12}). Little is known about the relationship of most of these vitamins to sexual function. In recent years, important relationships have been demonstrated to exist between riboflavin, pyridoxine and pantothenic acid and reproduction, especially as regards the capacity of these vitamins to *protect embryonal development. Their deficiency may cause abortion or congenital malformations.*

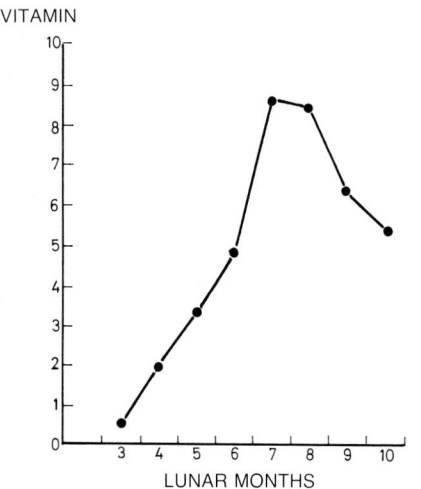

Figure 11–6. Placental storage of vitamin B_1. (From Gaethgens: *Der Aneurinhaushalt in der Schwangerschaft.* Leipzig, G. Thieme, 1939.)

RIBOFLAVIN. Coward and his colleagues[14] reported that riboflavin deficiency in rats caused suspension of estrous activity. However, the most significant effect associated with riboflavin deficiency is a *teratogenic effect.*

Warkany[88] produced congenital anomalies in fetuses of rodents maintained on deficiency diets for the entire B complex. However, more selective investigations, using thiamine, riboflavin, niacin, pyridoxine and pantothenic acid, all in crystalline form, have shown the inability of these compounds to completely prevent the development of malformations. Nevertheless, *riboflavin* is an element necessary for the prevention of teratogenic effects. Malformations resulting from riboflavin deficiency develop at a very early stage of embryonal life. Precursors of bone are affected before the onset of ossification. Thus, riboflavin apparently influences the formation of the bony skeleton at a very early phase. In rats, the effects of deficiency become apparent before the thirteenth day of gestation. Riboflavin administration after that date no longer contributes toward the protection of the newborn from congenital malformations. These important and decisive findings by Warkany have been confirmed by other investigators (Giroud and Boisselot,[27, 28] Leinbach,[45] Noback and Kupperman,[65] Piccioni and Bologna,[71] and Pfaltz and Severinghaus[70]). The occurrence of such malformations is of extraordinary importance since it suggests that certain alterations in the development of human skeletal morphology, as well as the presence of voluminous congenital anomalies, may result from riboflavin deficiency at the beginning of pregnancy. Watteville and his colleagues[91] later also reiterated that these congenital alterations were due to vitamin B_2 deficiency and emphasized the fact that the congenital malformations involved were of the classical type, such as exencephaly, microphthalmia and others, which also occurred in man. In order to interpret the possible etiologic role of riboflavin in the development of these malformations, it would therefore be of interest to assess the conditions of riboflavin metabolism in relation to the internal secretions.

Verzar[87] has identified riboflavin phosphate with Warburg's respiratory yellow enzyme, and showed that this substance

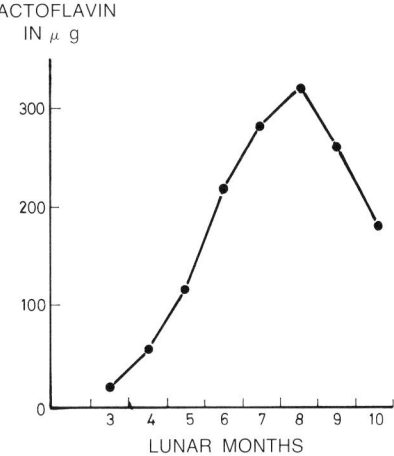

Figure 11-7. Placental storage of vitamin B_2 (lactoflavin). (From Neuweiler: *Ergeb. Ber. Vit. u. Horm. Forsch.*, 8:1, 1943.)

was capable of preventing the appearance of acute adrenal insufficiency in adrenalectomized animals. Subsequent studies revealed that vitamin B_2 consumption was increased in all those cases in which unusually heavy demands were imposed on adrenocortical function owing to, among other things, stress, Addison's disease and serious infections. In pregnancy, in which relative adrenal insufficiency is almost always the rule (see Chapter 10), an associated increase in riboflavin consumption has by now been conclusively demonstrated. Research by Neuweiler[64] revealed that *riboflavin was stored in the placenta* (Fig. 11-7). This suggests that the maternal body tends to protect the fetus from vitamin B_2 deficiency. Results of studies on the possible existence of riboflavin avitaminosis in pregnancy and, conceivably, of related effects on the human embryo have so far been quite unsatisfactory. Nevertheless, there is evidence that riboflavin consumption in pregnancy is elevated, apparently owing to the presence of relative adrenal insufficiency, and in view of available evidence relating riboflavin deficiency to serious congenital anomalies in animals, there is every reason to believe that any type of disturbances jeopardizing the supply of this substance to the egg is liable to play an equally significant role in the pathogenesis of abortion, particularly with regard to the development of teratologic fetuses in the human species.

PYRIDOXINE. Studies by Nelson and

Evans and their colleagues[22, 62, 63] seem to attach extraordinary importance to the role played by pyridoxine deficiency in the course of reproductive processes. Rats kept on diets devoid of this vitaminic principle show atrophy of corpora lutea, apparently as a result of absent gonadotropic stimuli and, at the same time, lack of progesterone synthesis.

In rats, pyridoxine (vitamin B$_6$) deficiency produces disturbances in the reproductive apparatus and suspension of estrous activity which, according to Lyons[49] and to Pfaltz and Severinghaus,[70] are due to deficient biogenesis of ovarian hormones, viz., estrogens and progesterone. Gestational pyridoxine deficiency leads to abortion (Lyons[49]). Nelson, Lyons and Evans[62, 63] have subsequently demonstrated that gonadotropin administration was capable of averting abortion in rats. Moreover, they found that the effects of pyridoxine deficiency were actually intermediary pituitary effects.[63] Pyridoxine is necessary for the action of gonadotropins on the ovary of hypophysectomized animals to be effective (Wooten et al.[93]). In the absence of pyridoxine, pituitary follicle-stimulating and luteinizing activity is impaired. Therefore, it may currently be admitted that pyridoxine is an element that is indispensable for the biosynthesis of pituitary gonadotropins and that the effects of pyridoxine deficiency on the reproductive apparatus are mediated by pituitary activity. Sawyer[83] has demonstrated that pyridoxine deficiency in woman may cause sterility.

It seems possible therefore that pyridoxine may be implicated in gonadotropin B (LH) biogenesis as well as in normal corpus luteum metabolism. Pyridoxine deficiency in pregnant rats was found to produce abortion. Nelson and colleagues[63] did not believe that these abortions were attributable to congenital malformations resulting in fetal expulsion but rather that they were due to *failure of the corpus luteum to be formed*. Since the corpus luteum is not indispensable for human gestation (see Chapter 19), *it does not seem likely that pyridoxine deficiency in the female might cause abortion unless the vitamin is in some way related to placental hormone synthesis* (a problem which, to our knowledge, has so far not been investigated). Watteville and associates[91] have studied the deficiency effects in rats in relation to the appearance of congenital anomalies. Pyridoxine deficiency was found to be associated with congenital malformations less frequently than is riboflavin deficiency; nonetheless, such anomalies as *syndactyly, clubfoot* and *exencephaly* have been described. This means that even though pyridoxine deficiency is of far less concern in the possible development of congenital anomalies, it nevertheless exerts some influence on the development of the conceptus, by acting instead as a synergizer of corpus luteum activity.

PANTOTHENIC ACID. Seemingly, pantothenic acid deficiency may also cause congenital malformations. Warkany[90] has noted the occurrence of hydrocephalus in pantothenic acid deficient hogs and, similarly, O'Dell and co-workers,[66] Pfaltz and Severinghaus,[70] and Giroud and Boisselot[28] observed ocular congenital defects attributable to pantothenic acid deficiency. As with riboflavin, little is known about the mode of action involved. At any rate, the specificity of action of this compound has been questioned by some investigators who believe that pantothenic acid deficiency may be associated with riboflavin deficiency, the latter causing the congenital malformations, which is a view also advocated by Watteville and his colleagues.[91] Ullrey and associates[85] reported that pantothenic acid deficient sows developed ovarian atrophy.

FOLATES. Folic acid, or vitamin B$_{11}$, was the original name given to a vitaminoid substance that was extracted from spinach leaves in 1941. However, pteroylmonoglutamic acid, which was isolated in pure form from the above extract and used for clinical therapeutic purposes, was not found to produce the true action of the vitamin in the body. Instead, the action of this substance is due to a series of derivatives, designated generically as "folates." Giroud[27] and Nelson and his colleagues,[63] who were able to produce folate deficiency in pregnant rats, also noted the presence of malformations in the offspring. Rats can grow and reproduce while on a folate free diet so long as this substance is being formed by the intestinal flora. In order to induce a deficiency state, rats were fed a vitamin free diet with concurrent administration of succinylsulfathiazole. When such a regimen was strictly observed, reabsorption of embryos would occur, or, on about the tenth day of gestation, the rats would abort malformed fetuses.

Until recently, it was not known whether folate deficiency could give rise to any similar complications in *human gestation.* The discovery by Hibbard and colleagues[35, 36] that large amounts of *formiminoglutamic acid (FIGLU)* were excreted in the urine of pregnant women whenever there was associated folate deficiency resulted in a simple test for folate deficiency based on the assay of urinary FIGLU. Aside from causing *megaloblastic anemia,* lack of folates in woman has thus been found to also cause *abortion,*[36, 54] *abruptio placentae*[35, 56] and even *fetal deformities and death.*[35, 36, 54, 56] Because all of the above conditions are usually associated with elevated urinary FIGLU values, the routine determination of FIGLU excretion has become an important tool of modern obstetrics.

OTHER FACTORS. Chamberlain and Nelson[13] pointed out that *niacin* deficiency in rats also produces malformations.

It is clear that lack of any of these various components of the B complex must have some repercussions not only on pregnancy but also on the physiology of the ovary, testis and other parts of both the male and the female genital tract. The reason why only congenital malformations have so far been described may be because these defects are quite conspicuous, whereas possible alterations at the histologic level may be overlooked. The observation that animals maintained in a state of deficiency of all these principles long enough become sterile may be construed as evidence that, while *acute* deficiencies may produce malformations in the offspring, *chronic* varieties of deficiency may affect the progenitors' reproductive system as well. We are here confronted with an unexplored, or nearly unexplored, area of sexual physiology.

11.5.3. INFLUENCE OF B COMPLEX ON HEPATIC ESTROGENOLYSIS

Biskind[4, 5] has shown that dietary vitamin B complex deficiency produces *experimental hyperestrinism* in rats because the liver loses its capacity for detoxifying estrogens. By the same token, Segaloff[75] found that vitamin B deficient rats exhibited increased responsiveness to estrogens. If yeast extracts were added to the diet, this sensitivity to estrogens disappeared.

Singer and his co-workers[78] showed that the above phenomenon was due to the fact that deficiencies of thiamine, riboflavin, pyridoxine and pantothenic acid, alone or in combination, resulted in impairment of hepatic degradation of estrogens.

These ideas are supported by the observation that deficiency in man of any of these principles may be associated with hemorrhages (György and Goldblatt[33]). Finally, Ayre[3] postulates that B avitaminosis predisposes to uterine cancer by virtue of the fact that it tends to be associated with hyperestrinism.

11.6. VITAMIN C (ASCORBIC ACID)

Vitamin C, deficiency of which causes scurvy, once the scourge of whale hunters and polar explorers, is perhaps the most widely distributed and best known vitamin. This is not only because of the significance of the symptoms caused by its deficiency in the human species, but more importantly because its relatively simple chemical structure made possible first the isolation and characterization of the vitamin, and then its synthesis by Szent-György. The composition of *ascorbic acid* is as shown:

$$CH_2OH-CHOH-CH-COH=COH-C=O$$
$$|\underline{\qquad\qquad O \qquad\qquad}|$$

Vitamin C is a carbohydrate present in abundance in all kinds of fruits and plants, particularly oranges, lemons, tomatoes and peppers. It can be estimated relatively easily, thanks to its reducing properties, which can be determined with methylene blue, sodium thiosulfite or dichlorophenolindophenol. Ascorbic acid, or hexuronic acid, is widely distributed in nature. While the higher animals (for instance, man) are incapable of synthesizing it, many lower animals, including some mammals (e.g., rats), are able to synthesize ascorbic acid as an intermediary product of their carbohydrate metabolism. By and large, most of ascorbic acid synthesis takes place in the adrenal cortex, which is why a *semihormonal* character has been ascribed to ascorbic acid by many. Some authors have contended that *embryonic tissue is capable of ascorbic acid synthesis* and claim to have shown this in the human fetus. Because of its reducing capacity, ascorbic acid falls into a special category, that of a *regulator of the body's redox reactions* and, consequently, serves as a biocatalyst of many chemical processes requiring the intervention of oxidase. Vitamin C is readily stored in the body, primarily in the liver, then in the adrenal cortex or, during pregnancy, in the placenta, all of which have a high vitamin C content. Thus, vitamin C is an important factor in the intermediary metabolism of cortical steroids and of some of the sex hormones. The previously mentioned chemical procedures make its estimation fairly simple, so that most data concerning its urinary excretion, circulating blood levels, as well as metabolism in general, are currently well known. This has also facilitated better understanding of the important role played by vitamin C in reproduction and of its metabolic relations.

11.6.1 VITAMIN C AND THE OVARY

Various authors (Giroud,[27] Parlow and Reichert[68]) have encountered elevated ascorbic acid concentrations in the ovary. Of all ovarian structures, the one containing this compound in largest amounts is the corpus luteum (Biskind,[5] Fujita and Ebihara,[23] Miller and Everett[57]). Ascorbic acid concentrations in the latter may exceed values of 100 mg per cent, second only to those of the adrenal cortex and equaling those found in the pituitary. Our own quantitative determinations of corpus luteum ascorbic acid content (Fig. 11-8) revealed that it was related to that gland's functional activity and presented regular oscillations in the course of the menstrual cycle. Histochemical studies (Giroud[27] and Tonutti and Plate[84]) have revealed that some ascorbic acid is also located in the theca interna and granulosa of the follicle, though to a lesser degree. At present, the most specific test for measuring corpus luteum stimulation by LH is based on *ascorbic acid depletion*, a method introduced by Parlow.[68] This test is modeled on an identical phenomenon, that of adrenal ascorbic acid depletion in response to ACTH stimulation, for which Sayers had devised a specific reaction many years ago. As with the adrenal and the pituitary, the ascorbic acid in the ovary was found by Fujita and Ebihara[23] to be present largely in its reduced form. Histochemically, ascorbic acid in the corpus luteum cells and other ovarian cells was pinpointed in the Golgi apparatus, a localization of profound functional significance, indicating a relationship to secretory activity. The fact that vitamin C is stored in the adrenal cortex, whose hormone synthesis is chemically quite similar to that of the corpus

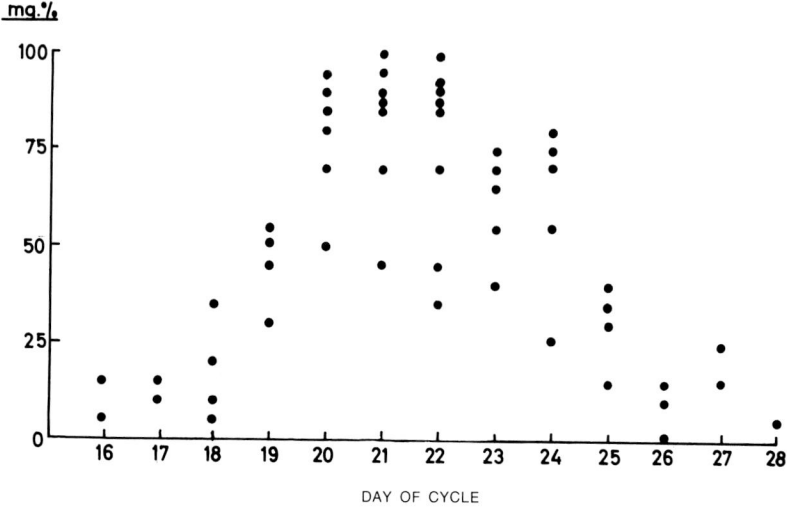

Figure 11-8. Corpus luteum storage of vitamin C, as determined by the biochemical method of Martini and Bonsignore on extracts from fresh corpora lutea removed by laparotomy. (Botella-Llusiá: unpublished data.)

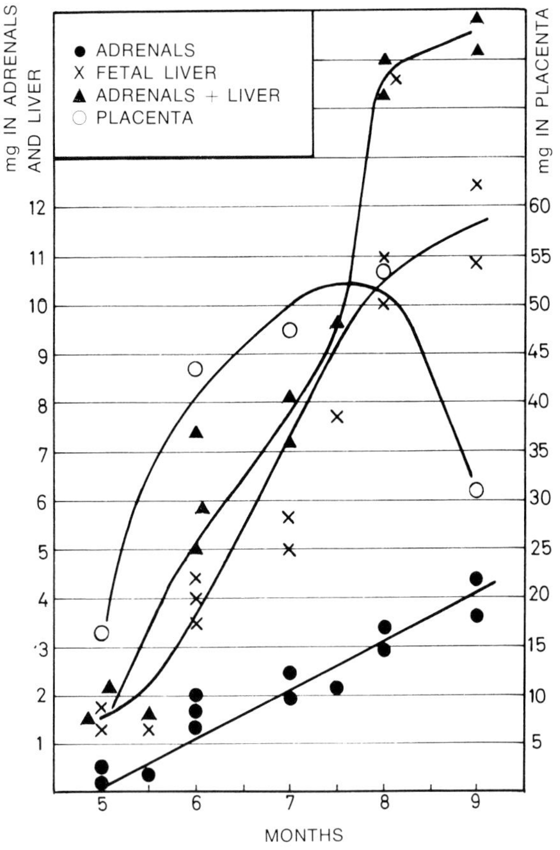

Figure 11-9. Balance of fetal ascorbic acid. Note that the total present in the fetal body corresponds to the amount transferred from the placenta, which refutes the assumption of active storage by the fetus. (From Botella: *Rev. Esp. Farmac.*, 1:350, 1940.)

luteum, and the proved fact that this vitamin is essential for cortical function bring up the *possibility that ascorbic acid may be a fundamental element in the biosynthesis of pregnane-derived hormones.*

The testicular vitamin C content is more exiguous, although equally important. Investigations by Giroud and Boisselot[27, 28] have shown that compound to be present in testicular tissue in about the same concentrations as are found in ovaries devoid of corpora lutea.

11.6.2. ASCORBEMIA, ASCORBURIA AND SEXUAL FUNCTION

Biskind[5] reported that peak vitamin C excretion coincided with the corpus luteum phase. Similar cyclic fluctuations in ascorbemia were recorded by Neuweiler.[64] While postmenopausal women revealed lowered blood ascorbic acid levels, pregnant women showed markedly elevated levels, according to Neuweiler. All indications are that there is a very close relationship between gonadal activity and corpus luteum ascorbic acid metabolism.

11.6.3. PREGNANCY

Ascorbic acid plays a role of extraordinary importance in pregnancy.[9, 10]

As shown by us, and confirmed by a number of investigators,[28, 64, 84] the placenta stores ascorbic acid. During pregnancy, ascorbic acid progressively accumulates, reaching a maximum at term. Blood levels and urinary excretion values experience a similar progressive rise during pregnancy. Not infrequently, placental storing may drain this vitamin from the maternal body and a relative maternal deficiency may coexist along with an abundance of the vitamin in the placenta and in the fetal body.

Fetal storage of ascorbic acid, particularly by the adrenal cortex and the liver, acquires considerable importance near term. From our studies on vitamin balance (Fig. 11-9), in which the amount of ascorbic acid in the adrenal cortex during the last month of pregnancy was found to be directly proportional to the amount by which placental content in ascorbic acid had decreased, we arrived at the conclusion that ascorbic acid is not synthesized, but merely stored, by the fetus.[9]

The net amount of ascorbic acid deposited in the placenta is considerable, as shown in Fig. 11-9. Placental concentrations, expressed in milligrams per cent, are higher than those of most other organs and body fluids, although they are not as high as those of the large adrenal deposits. However, since the weight of the placenta is many times that of the adrenal cortex, the net amount stored in the placenta is greater than that of the fetal adrenal and nearly as great as that of the adult adrenal.

Vitamin C was shown by Neuweiler[64] to be also present in high concentrations in the lactating breast, which suggests that it is essential for, or at least plays an important role in, the secretion of milk.

11.6.4. VITAMIN C AND THE ADRENAL

Although the amount of outstanding work published on the subject cannot be reviewed here in its entirety, we must content ourselves with pointing out that in the light of present-day knowledge, adrenocortical vitamin C storage not only constitutes an important reservoir for the body *but in fact reflects the functional state of the adrenal cortex*. Cortical vitamin C content is depleted under conditions of stress and in absolute or relative adrenocortical insufficiency. Ever since the time of Sayer's discovery, it has been known that the most specific test for the assay of ACTH effect on the adrenal cortex is the test of ascorbic acid depletion, currently used in the bioassay for corticotropin. In an analogous fashion, ovarian ascorbic acid depletion serves as the most specific test for LH activity. This means that, as a result of specific endocrine stimulation, ascorbic acid disappears precisely from the two endocrine glands that are known to contain it in highest concentrations. Ascorbic acid would therefore appear to be utilized by those glands for the synthesis of hormones, in this instance C-21 steroids specifically.

Employing C-14 labeled cholesterol, Peric-Godia and colleagues[69] were able to demonstrate the essential role played by vitamin C in adrenal corticoid synthesis.

11.6.5. SIGNIFICANCE OF VITAMIN C IN GENITAL HORMONOPOIESIS

Vitamin C is currently held to be directly implicated in the synthesis of both corticoids and progesteroids. To support this view, we quote the following experimental and clinical data:

1. Ascorbic acid avitaminosis in experimental animals causes lack of corpus luteum formation and symptoms of adrenal insufficiency.

2. In addition to serious disturbances of adrenocortical origin, clinical scurvy equally leads to suspension of menstruation, as well as to sterility or frequent abortion.

3. Vitamin C is stored specifically in those organs which, like the adrenal, produce corticoids or, like the corpus luteum, the placenta and the adrenal cortex, produce progesterone.

4. The amount of vitamin C stored in the placenta forms a curve that parallels that of progesterone synthesized by the placenta.

5. Vitamin C deposits in the fetal adrenal are not apparent before the seventh month of pregnancy—that is, *not until the gland has started secreting corticoids*. Both androgen and estrogen syntheses by the adrenal cortex during the first months of gestation, when there are still no ascorbic acid deposits, have been demonstrated to occur.

6. Our own investigations have convinced us that the reciprocal effects by the adrenal cortex and the corpus luteum failed to be operative in vitamin C deficient animals. In this respect, we have been able to demonstrate that rats could still be maintained alive indefinitely after bilateral adrenalectomy provided either that their ovaries contained corpora lutea or that they were treated with progesterone (see Chapter 9, Figs. 9-16, 9-17 and 9-20). Conversely, we have been able to show that deoxycorticosterone injections in experimental animals provoked a progestational uterine phase, with progestational-like changes in the vagina (Chapter 9, Fig. 9-15).

These effects of mutual substitution, discussed previously, have been ascribed to interconversion of one hormone into the other rather than to existing similarities between them. Animals maintained on vitamin C deficient diets for more than one month failed to survive adrenalectomy. Obviously, despite the presence of corpora lutea, rats with experimentally induced scurvy lost their capacity to withstand bilateral adrenalectomy. Injections of LH or progesterone into control animals failed to produce any signs of improvement, which seems to indicate that, in the absence of ascorbic acid, progesterone cannot be converted to corticoids, and thus cannot prevent death in adrenoprival animals. Another group of control animals treated with ascorbic acid were able to survive the effect of adrenalectomy even without progesterone administration.

The significance of these findings seems to deserve some further comment concerning the *existence of a fundamental difference between the human species and certain animal species with regard to their respective capacity for endogenous vitamin C synthesis.* Because vitamin C is not synthesized within the human body, women depend entirely on dietary supply in order to maintain the necessary requirements for this biocatalyst. In contrast, the reproductive capacity of the rat, which is capable of synthesizing this substance, is hardly affected by dietary vitamin C intake; however, if this source of vitamin C production in the rat (the adrenal) is removed, *the biocatalyzing action by vitamin C is completely lost. Even though the exact biochemical mechanism involved is not known, it seems plausible to assume that vitamin C acts as a biocatalyzer of C-21 steroid synthesis and that it therefore intervenes in a decisive manner in progesterone and corticoid biogenesis.*

11.6.6. EFFECT OF ASCORBIC ACID DEFICIENCY ON PREGNANCY

Both clinical and experimentally induced vitamin C deficiencies have been found to be important factors in the etiology of abortion. The mechanism of action involved in producing abortion is self-explanatory, on the basis of the foregoing discussion. By completely blocking progesterone synthesis, not only in the ovary (which in the human species would be of little consequence) but also in the placenta and the adrenal, vitamin C deficiency leads to complete failure of the entire hormonal system responsible for protecting gestation. By depressing adrenal function during pregnancy, vitamin C deficiency may equally well play an important role in the genesis of some pathologic conditions of pregnancy, particularly that of hyperemesis gravidarum (see Chapter 44). This accounts for the beneficial effects obtained with vitamin C administration in preventing abortion as well as in handling intractable vomiting. Vitamin C deficiency seems to have no adverse effect on the progeny in terms of congenital deformities, as none have been observed either in experimental animals or in man.

11.6.7. EFFECT OF VITAMIN C DEFICIENCY ON MENSTRUATION

Menstrual anomalies may appear as a result of scurvy. At present, however, subclinical vitamin C deficits are believed to play an equally significant role in the pathogenesis of some endocrine ovarian alterations, particularly *functional bleeding*, as a result of faulty corpus luteum formation. In this respect, two important facts deserve mention: (1) *In the Northern hemisphere*, functional bleeding is more likely to be observed on a *seasonal basis in relation to dietary vitamin C deficits.* (2) Vitamin C has a *favorable therapeutic effect* on certain forms of metropathia haemorrhagica.

11.7. VITAMIN D

Known for a long time for its antirachitic activity, vitamin D is a steroid which from a chemical standpoint shows a highly interesting similarity to sex hormones. Thanks to studies by Windaus, its chemical composition has been characterized following its crystallization. In pure form, it is called vitamin D_2, to distinguish it from the previously isolated vitamin D_1, which is a mixture of vitamin D_2 and lumisterol. Vitamin D_3 can be obtained synthetically by means of irradiating dehydrocholesterol. A detailed study of the biochemical peculiarities of this vitamin would seem to us superfluous at this point. We shall confine ourselves to outlining the structural formulas involved:

[Structural formula of Vitamin D₂]

[Structural formula of Vitamin D₃]

These formulas reveal the striking similarity between this vitamin and the phenanthrene-derived steroids, as well as its resemblance to cholesterol. As we have indicated in the corresponding chapters (Chapters 3, 4 and 9), cholesterol is utilized by the adrenal, by the corpus luteum and by the testis as the *starting material for the synthesis of saturated steroids,* viz., androgens, corticoids and progestogens. Vitamin D, which can be formed in the body by a semisynthetic procedure utilizing the effect of ultraviolet light on ergosterol, has a marked similarity to the above group of steroids, a similarity even extending into certain physiopathologic phenomena.

11.7.1. EFFECT OF VITAMIN D ON THE GENITAL TRACT

Because only minor gonadal alterations have been observed in vitamin D deficiency, there is a dearth of clinical and experimental work published on the subject. The effects on the testis seem to be of much greater relevance than those on the ovary. While testicular alterations in rachitic animals have been described by Demole,[16] ovarian alterations in the same type of animals, described by Guggisberg,[32] seem to occur much less frequently and less consistently. According to Guggisberg follicular development is lacking. However, these observations are not free from objections, considering the possibility that the type of avitaminosis involved in these studies might not have been of the pure variety and might have included associated effects from vitamin A deficiency. Investigations by Sánchez-Rodríguez would seem to indicate that vitamin D in toxic dosages may be associated with a virilizing effect. The latter could result from conversion of excessive vitamin D to compounds of the androgenic series. That this may be so is supported by the finding of elevated urinary 17-ketosteroid values following the administration of a vitamin D overdose. A certain functional synergism might therefore be postulated to exist between vitamin D and androgens, in which case lack of vitamin D would lead to testicular hypofunction, whereas excess would induce overproduction of androgens. Similarly, roosters treated with high dosages of calciferol develop exaggerated growth of the comb. Even though sexual alterations in females suffering from rickets have been described, with the implication of possible relationships among vitamin D, osteomalacia and ovarian function, data presently available on the subject are highly contradictory and shall not be examined further here. It seems highly probable that most of the diverse effects recorded were the result of multiple deficiencies of nonspecific factors.

11.7.2. SIGNIFICANCE OF VITAMIN D IN PREGNANCY

According to Guggisberg[32] and Neuweiler,[64] vitamin D is stored in the placenta (Fig. 11–10). Placental storage, as well as increased daily needs and utilization of calciferol in pregnancy, indicates a fetus-oriented anabolism of this compound. Hence, pregnant women in general, and particularly those in northern countries, are highly sensitive to vitamin D deficiency, so that from the standpoint of clinical management and prophylaxis, vitamin D administration is of extraordinary importance. However, the most interesting aspect of vitamin D deficiency is related to the occurrence of congenital anomalies. In this regard, the studies done by Warkany[88] are significant. By maintaining pregnant rats in a state of D avitaminosis, Warkany found that the litter of those rats in which avitaminosis was of recent onset showed lack of ossification of long bones, primarily the

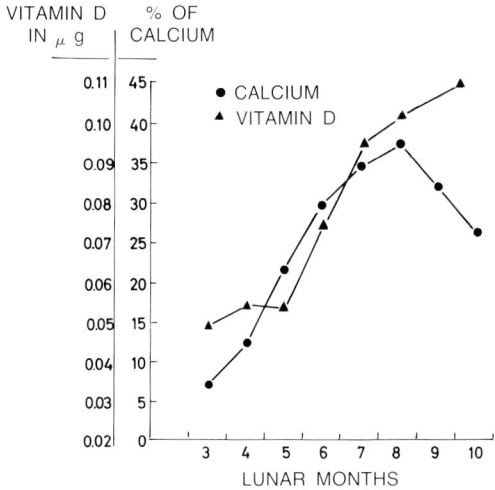

Figure 11-10. Placental storage of vitamin D₂. Calcium content is expressed in milligrams per 100 grams of fresh tissue. (From Neuweiler: *Ergeb. Ber. Vit. u. Horm. Forsch.*, 8:1, 1943.)

ulna, radius, tibia and fibula. If, however, vitamin deficiencies were of longer standing, they resulted in *congenital malformations*, with lack of development of long bones. Vitamin D therefore seems to play an important role in the genesis of certain congenital malformations. Nevertheless, it is true that while similar malformations may be observed quite clearly in experimental animals, the degree of nutritional deficiencies in humans hardly ever reaches such extremes in the mother as to affect the offspring. Also of interest is the finding that large amounts of vitamin D are present in milk, both of woman and animals (cow, etc.). The antirachitic properties of vitamin supplemented milk are well known. Nonetheless, the milk of those women who have been on low vitamin D diets during pregnancy may completely lack this ingredient, owing to the fact that the reserves of this principle have been exhausted in favor of placental deposition, and consequently their breast-fed babies may develop rickets. Although signs of avitaminosis D in human pregnancy are seldom noted, these signs, if present, may appear as delayed manifestations, such as rickets of early infancy.

11.8. VITAMIN E

Of all vitamins, vitamin E has the most bearing on the reproductive processes. As early as 1922, Evans and Bishop showed that a dietary factor, present in the oil of seeds and therefore liposoluble, was necessary for the normal development of pregnancy in rats. Sure,[82] in 1924, called this substance vitamin E. Its existence was confirmed in 1926 by Evans and Burr, who devised a method for the bioassay of vitamin E. Lack of this vitamin in the pregnant female manifests itself through abortion—which occurs more early the more pronounced the degree of avitaminosis—and through the appearance of sterility and absent spermatogenesis in the male. Thus, while necessary for the maintenance of pregnancy in the female, this substance seems to be necessary for gametogenesis in the male. Although the occurrence of avitaminosis E in rats and other animals has been demonstrated, *it has not been possible to demonstrate the clinical existence of E avitaminosis in the human species*. This is why the effect of therapeutic vitamin E applications seems to be what at one time we chose to call *pharmacologic action* of vitamins. The chemical composition of vitamin E has been brought to light by Karrer and consists of three distinct substances: α, β and γ tocopherol, all three having a hexagonal (anthracene) double ring and differing from each other only in the structure of their lateral chains. Vitamin E is widely distributed in nature, and is so abundantly present in the human diet that any dietary situation leading to deficiency is extremely unlikely. Probably the only possibility of such a deficiency would appear with an inability to *utilize* the vitamin.

11.8.1. EFFECT OF VITAMIN E ON THE FEMALE SEX

Apart from the previously mentioned effect (abortion), vitamin E deficiency would appear to have a definite effect on the ovary. Thus, several authors (Euler,[21] Staehler and Hopp[81]) reported that rats suffering from E avitaminosis were unable to form corpora lutea. In female bitterlings, Duyvenné De Witt[18] found that tocopherol had an effect similar to that of progesterone. Progestational effects by tocopherol in rodents have been described by various authors.[37, 80, 81] However, these result from a stimulatory effect of tocopherol on the corpus luteum rather than from any progesterone-like action by the vitamin. Evidence to this effect has been provided by the experiments of Guggisberg,[32] who used gonadotropin injections to compensate for vitamin E induced absence of corpora lutea. Müller[60] views the effects of vitamin E on the ovary as of the same type as those produced by the hormone from pregnant women's urine. The theory developed by Verzar[87] postulates that vitamin E is a *protohormone* of the anterior pituitary hormones. This theory is supported by the fact that the manifestations of E avitaminosis in rats are very similar to those of experimental hypophysectomy. However, other workers, such as Müller[60] and Rowlands,[73] have been unable to find any pituitary alterations in vitamin E deficient animals. Bomskov and Kaulla,[7] among others, therefore repudiate the possibility of any specific effect on the ovary by vitamin E.

11.8.2. EFFECT OF VITAMIN E ON THE TESTIS

Vitamin E exerts a readily apparent, early and pronounced effect on the testis. Blaxter and Brown[6] and Linder[47] have shown that under experimental conditions vitamin E stimulates the development of the germinal epithelium. Vitamin E deficiency causes rapid atrophy of that epithelium and brings about sterility in the male (Vecchietti[86]).

The nature of the effect exerted by vitamin E on the testis would therefore appear to be different from that exerted on the ovary. In the latter, vitamin E acts as a luteinizing, *interstitium-exciting* agent, whereas in the male gonad it acts as a *gametokinetic* substance.

Since the human species does not seem to be affected by E avitaminosis, it has not been possible to determine to what extent tocopherol might be responsible for oligospermia and infertility in the male. Nevertheless, vitamin E therapy has in fact been found to be of value in effectively correcting asthenospermia (Giarola and Ballerio[26]).

11.8.3. EFFECT OF VITAMIN E ON PREGNANCY

The notion that vitamin E is an indispensable factor for the maintenance of pregnancy is based on the fact that increasing vitamin E deficiency in experimental animals, particularly in rats, as had been shown by the early investigations of Evans and Burr, produces abortions of commensurately progressive precocity. In this connection, the observations by Shute[76] are also of interest. Bees were noted to feed their queens a special diet containing vitamin E, but whenever the workers were deficient, the queens failed to develop their reproductive capacity. Shute moreover also believed that lack of tocopherol could be an etiologic factor in human abortion and advocated the use of tocopherol in cases of threatened abortion or in habitual abortion. A great deal of therapeutic information concerning the use of vitamin E in the treatment of abortion has so far been published. However, the results of both endocrine and vitamin prophylaxis of abortion have been reexamined recently, and, on the basis of claimed therapeutic results, they do not seem to warrant any conclusions concerning the etiology of abortion.

Lately, the fact that vitamin E can be used effectively in the treatment of toxemia of pregnancy has been greatly stressed (Mastboom and Sikkel[55] and Ingelman-Sunberg[39]).

11.8.4. PLACENTAL STORAGE OF VITAMIN E

Evans and co-workers[22] and Neuweiler,[64] among others, have showed that the placenta also selectively stores vitamin E. Since the ultimate purpose of such storage undoubtedly is that of supplying the fetus with tocopherol, it constitutes one more piece of evidence of how important this vitamin is for the evolution of gestation.

Vitamin E has been shown to pass through the placenta, and its presence in the fetal circulation has been demonstrated by Gounelle and his associates.[30]

It is of interest to point out that E hypovitaminosis is associated with the production of *congenital anomalies* in rats. The investigations of Vecchietti[86] have revealed that rats maintained on tocopherol deficient diets for relatively short periods of time would mate and conceive in a normal manner but that the fetuses would suffer premature death or reabsorption. Many such fetuses are actually *abortive eggs* in which death results from pathologic or teratoid development of the embryo. Warkany,[90] too, holds that vitamin E deficiency leads to the production of embryonic developmental anomalies.

11.8.5. MODE OF ACTION OF TOCOPHEROL

It is true that little is known at present concerning the mechanism of action involved. According to the previously mentioned hypothesis of Verzar,[87] this compound is required for the elaboration of pituitary hormones. Favoring this view is the fact that the pituitary has an unusually high tocopherol content. This compound, however, differs fundamentally from the proteic structure of anterior lobe hormones and does not appear to be either related to, or implicated in, the metabolism of those mucoproteins that normally make up the substrate of the "trophic" adenohypophysial hormones. On the other hand, the fact that normal pituitaries have been found in animals suffering from complete vitamin E deficiency would seem to speak against such a hypothesis. Other investigators would instead assume that vitamin E exerts a stimulatory effect on the growth of embryonal tissues and promotes the growth of germinal organs, including that of the ovary and testis. The latter concept would seem to explain the embryonal and testicular effects; however, it would fail to account for the luteinizing effect of vitamin E.

Research done by Griesbach and coworkers[31] revealed that vitamin E deficiency in animals was associated with disappearance of gonadotropic cells in the pituitary, as well as with loss of PAS positive glycoprotein substances contained within those cells. This would seem to be a decisive argument in favor of Verzar's theory.

Another question that must be raised here is whether there are two distinct vitamin E complexes. Since the exact chemical structure of tocopherol is known, it may seem impossible to uphold such a view. What seems certain, however, is the fact that vitamin E exerts actions of two types: (1) *A luteinizing action on the ovary, similar to that of LH*, and (2) *a growth-promoting action on germinal elements, testicular as well as embryonal.* As a result of some recent investigations, moreover, vitamin E has been asserted to activate synthesis of the corpus luteum hormone directly rather than by way of the pituitary.

Several other vitamins, such as vitamins K, H, P, and the presumptive vitamin T, are much less directly involved in reproductive processes and shall not be studied here.

11.9. GLOBAL DEFICIENCY

Up to this point, we have examined the occurrence of specific vitamin deficiencies and related effects on reproduction. However, it must be acknowledged that specific and selective deficiency states occur quite seldom. Much more common in human clinical experience are global deficiency states involving various dietary principles at the same time. Such deficiency states (customarily associated with "underdeveloped" countries, but which have also been observed in hyperdeveloped countries as a result of war inflicted calamities) do have a profound effect on the endocrinosexual system. Smith[79] reported that 50 per cent of the women in Rotterdam were infertile from malnutrition during the years of occupation. Adams[1] noted that a poor diet caused anovulation in rabbits. Glass and Lazarus[29] obtained cures in some cases of human infertility merely by improving the diet, whereas Carroll and Noble[12] emphasized the value of foods rich in amino acids in safeguarding fecundity.

Global protein deficiency causes arrest of estrous activity[46] and suspends the endocrine function of the placenta in rats.[40] Similarly, low protein diets in mice abolish the ovarian response to exogenous gonadotropins.[46]

Leathem[44] likewise indicates that lysine, tryptophan and several other amino acids are essential for reproduction which, without them, fails.

Fat free diets, in the view of Panos,[67] result in lack of ovarian and testicular secretion, whereas MacClure[51] and Millen[58] point out the harmful effect on the fertility of laboratory animals caused by deficiency of nutrient principles.

REFERENCES

1. Adams, C. E.: *Ciba Colloquium on Mammalian Germ Cells.* London, Churchill, 1953.
2. Ammon, R., and Dirscherl, W.: *Fermente, Hormone, Vitamine,* 3rd ed. Stuttgart, G. Thieme, 1960.
3. Ayre, E. J.: *Amer. J. Obstet. Gynec.,* 54:363, 1947.
4. Biskind, M. S., and Biskind, G. R.: *Science,* 94:462, 1941.
5. Biskind, M. S.: *Vitamins Hormones,* 4:147, 1946.
6. Blaxter, K. L., and Brown, F.: *Nutr. Abstr. Rev.,* 22:1, 1952.
7. Bomskov, C., and Kaulla, H. von: *Klin. Wschr.,* 20:334, 1941.
8. Borsook, W. J., Hachter, L., and Yost, G. H.: *J. Appl. Physiol.,* 12:325, 1941.
9. Botella, J.: *Rev. Esp. Farmacol.,* 1:527, 584, 1940.
10. Botella, J., and Hernández-Araña, F.: *Sem. Med. Esp.,* 5:242, 439, 1942.
11. Bratton, R. W., et al.: *J. Dairy Sci.,* 31:779, 1948.
12. Carroll, K. K., and Noble, R. L.: *Canad. J. Biochem. Physiol.,* 35:1093, 1957.
13. Chamberlain, J. G., and Nelson, M. M.: *Proc. Soc. Exper. Biol. Med.,* 112:836, 1963.
14. Coward, K. H., Morgan, B. G. E., and Waller, L.: *J. Physiol.,* 100:423, 1942.
15. Da Rugna, D.: *Schw. Med. Wschr.,* 88:563, 1958.
16. Demole, W.: *Ztsch. f. Vit. Forsch.,* 8:338, 1939.
17. Dutt, B.: *Brit. Vet. J.,* 115:236, 1959.
18. Duyvenné De Witt, P.: *Klin. Wschr.,* 20:1171, 1941.
19. Erb, R., et al.: *J. Dairy Sci.,* 30:687, 1947.
20. Eufinger, H., and Gottlieb, R.: *Klin. Wschr.,* 12:1397, 1933.
21. Euler, H. Von: *Ergeb. Physiol.,* 34:360, 1933.
22. Evans, H. M., Scott, W. I., and Bishop, R. M.: *J.A.M.A.,* 81:889, 1933.
23. Fujita, I., and Ebihara, H.: *Biochem. Z.,* 290:201, 1937.
24. Gaethgens, G.: *Arch. Gynäk.,* 171:417, 1941.
25. Gaethgens, G.: *Mangelernährung und Generationsvorgänge im Weiblichen Organismus.* Leipzig, G. Thieme, 1943.
26. Giarola, A., and Ballerio, C.: *Ann. Ost. Gin.,* 5:179, 1959.
27. Giroud, A.: *Ann. d'Endocr.,* 12:733, 1951.
28. Giroud, A., and Boisselot, J.: *Compt. Rend. Soc. Biol.,* 145:526, 1951.
29. Glass, S. J., and Lazarus, M. L.: *J.A.M.A.,* 154:908, 1954.
30. Gounelle, H., et al.: *Gynec. Obstet.,* 54:334, 1953.
31. Griesbach, W. E., Bell, M. E., and Livingstone, M.: *Endocrinology,* 60:729, 1957.
32. Guggisberg, H.:: "Die Vitamine und Ihre Beziehungen zur Fortpflanzung," in *Biologie und Pathologie des Weibes,* Vol. II. Vienna, Urban & Schwarzenberg, 1951.
33. György, P., and Goldblatt, H.: *Z. Exper. Med.,* 75:355, 1942.
34. Hammond, J.: *Proc. Nutr. Soc.,* 2:8, 1944.
35. Hibbard, B. M., Hibbard, E. D., and Jeffcoate, T. N. A.: *Acta Obstet. Gynec. Scand.,* 44:375, 1965.
36. Hibbard, B. M., and Hibbard, E. D.: *Brit. Med. Bull.,* 24:10, 1968.
37. Highnett, S. L.: *Proc. Nutr. Soc.,* 19:8, 1960.
38. Hildebrandt, W.: *Arch. Gynäk.,* 170:540, 1940.
39. Ingelman-Sunberg, H.: *Gynaecologia,* 134:391, 1952.
40. Kinzey, W. G.: *Endocrinology,* 82:266, 1968.
41. Laschet, U., et al.: *Internat. Ztschr. Vit. Forsch.,* 30:77, 1959.
42. Laschet, U., and Weise, W.: *Internat. J. Fertil.,* 5:317, 1960.
43. Laurence, P. A., and Sobel, A. E.: *J. Clin. Endocr.,* 13:1192, 1953.
44. Leathem, J. H.: *Rec. Progr. Horm. Res.,* 14:141, 1958.
45. Leinbach, D. G.: *Rev. Internat. Vit.,* 21:222, 1949.
46. Lerner, L. J., and Turkheimer, A. R.: *Endocrinology,* 76:359, 1965.
47. Linder, E.: *Ztschr. Vit. Forsch.,* 29:33, 1958.
48. Lutwak-Mann, C.: *Vitamins Hormones,* 16:35, 1958.
49. Lyons, W. R.: *Proc. Soc. Exper. Biol. Med.,* 54:65, 1953.
50. MacCarthy, P. T., and Cerecedo, L. R.: *J. Nutr.,* 46:361, 1952.
51. MacClure, T. J.: *J. Physiol.,* 147:221, 1959.
52. Maddock, C. L., et al.: *Arch. Pathol.,* 56:333, 1953.
53. Mann, T.: *Proc. Nutr. Soc.,* 19:15, 1960.
54. Martin, R. H., Harper, T. A., and Kelso, W.: *Lancet,* 1:670, 1965.
55. Mastboom, J. L., and Sikkel, A.: *Gynaecologia,* 134:391, 1952.
56. Menon, M. K. K., Sengupta, M., and Ramaswamy, N.: *J. Obstet. Gynec. Brit. Comm.,* 73:49, 1966.
57. Miller, D. C., and Everett, J. W.: *Endocrinology,* 42:421, 1948.
58. Millen, J. W.: *The Nutritional Basis of Reproduction.* Springfield, Ill., Charles C Thomas, 1962.
59. Moe, P. G., Caughey, J. E., and Dutz, W. E.: *Amer. J. Clin. Nutr.,* 20:1179, 1967.
60. Müller, C.: *Arch. Gynäk.,* 169:482, 1939.
61. Murray, T. K.: *Proc. Soc. Exper. Biol. Med.,* 111:609, 1962.
62. Nelson, M. M., and Evans, H. M.: *J. Nutr.,* 43:281, 1951.
63. Nelson, M. M., Lyons, W. R., and Evans, H. M.: *Endocrinology,* 52:585, 1953.
64. Neuweiler, W.: *Ergeb. Vit. Horm. Forsch.,* 8:1, 1943.
65. Noback, C. R., and Kupperman, H. S.: *Proc. Soc. Exper. Biol. Med.,* 57:183, 1944.
66. O'Dell, W. G., et al.: *Proc. Soc. Exper. Biol. Med.,* 76:349, 1951.
67. Panos, T. C., et al.: *J. Nutr.,* 68:509, 1959.
68. Parlow, A. F., and Reichert, L. E.: *Endocrinology,* 72:955, 1963.
69. Peric-Godia, L., Eik-Nes, K., and Jones, R. S.: *Endocrinology,* 66:48, 1960.
70. Pfaltz, H., and Severinghaus, E. L.: *Amer. J. Obstet. Gynec.,* 72:265, 1956.
71. Piccioni, V., and Bologna, U.: *Clin. Ost. Gin.,* 54:994, 1947.
72. Randazzo, G.: *Arch. Ost. Gin.,* 61:291, 1956.
73. Rowlands, C. I.: *J. Physiol.,* 86:323, 1936.
74. Sánchez-Rodríguez, J., and Morros-Sardá, J.: *Ztschr. Vit. Forsch.,* 6:193, 1937.
75. Segaloff, A., and Segaloff, I.: *Endocrinology,* 34:346, 1944.
76. Shute, E.: *Amer. J. Obstet. Gynec.,* 35:429, 1938.
77. Siddall, P. C.: *Amer. J. Obstet. Gynec.,* 35:662, 1938.

78. Singher, H. O., et al.: *J. Biol. Chem.*, 154:79, 1944.
79. Smith, C. A.: *Amer. J. Obstet. Gynec.*, 53:599, 1947.
80. Staehler, E.: *Ztschr. Vit. Forsch.*, 10:26, 1940.
81. Staehler, E., and Hopp, W.: *Klin. Wschr.*, 21:58, 1942.
82. Sure, B.: *J. Nutr.*, 13:513, 1937.
83. Sawyer, G. I. M.: *Brit. J. Nutr.*, 3:100, 1949.
84. Tonutti, W., and Plate, W. P.: *Arch. Gynäk.*, 164:36, 1937.
85. Ullrey, D. E., et al.: *J. Nutr.*, 57:401, 1955.
86. Vecchietti, G.: "Vitamina E nella Ginecologia," *Atti del Terzo congresso Internazionale della Vitamina E, Venezia, 1955*, Verona, Ed. Valdonega, 1956.
87. Verzar, E.: *Ztschr. Vit. Forsch.*, 1:116, 1942.
88. Warkany, J.: *Amer. J. Dis. Child.*, 66:511, 1943.
89. Warkany, J., Monroe, B. B., and Sutherland, B. S.: *Amer. J. Dis. Child.*, 102:249, 1961.
90. Warkany, J.: *Maternal Nutrition During Pregnancy and its Relationship to Reproductive Failure*, Actas del Congreso Internacional de Obst. y Ginec., Geneva, 1954. Geneva, Libraire P. Georg, 1955.
91. Watteville, H., De Jürgens, R., and Pfaltz, H.: *Schw. Med. Wschr.*, 84:30, 1954.
92. Wilson, J. G., and Barch, S.: *Proc. Soc. Exper. Biol. Med.*, 72:687, 1949.
93. Wooten, E., et al.: *Endocrinology*, 56:59, 1955; 63:860, 1958.

Part Three
THE SEXUAL CYCLE

In Parts One and Two, we have studied the internal secretions of the ovary, as well as the hormonal, neural and vitaminic factors that govern the biosynthesis of ovarian hormones. These are the basic elements of sexual physiology. In Part Three, we shall describe how these elements are linked up with each other within the reproductive mechanism.

Sexual life, as was indicated in Chapter 1, cannot be lived in a self-contained enclosure; for, in order for the individual to accomplish the most important act, that of fertilization, it cannot do without a mate and, therefore, without the external environment. Preparation for fertilization then depends on environmental elements and, since these must be kept up with as they arise, a continuous cyclic activity has to be instituted. Our present concern will be the study of this cycle. Having studied sexual endocrinology "at rest," we shall now analyze it "in motion."

Chapter 12

ESTABLISHMENT OF THE SEXUAL CYCLE: THE OVARIAN CYCLE

The preceding chapters dealt with the elements of female endocrinology: the gonadal hormones, their physiology, and the presence or absence of humoral influences in controlling gonadal function. Having studied the hormones involved in their "static" condition, it is now fitting to examine their dynamics throughout the different phases of the sexual cycle of woman.

12.1. ESTABLISHMENT OF THE SEXUAL CYCLE

Vertebrates produce three kinds of eggs (Chapter 1): *aquatic eggs*, which derive nutrition from the surrounding environment; *cleidoic eggs*, which contain a nutritional reserve provided by the mother, and *placental eggs,* in which the embryo is fed at the expense of substances obtained by diffusion from the maternal body. These reflect the fact that, as one advances along the animal scale, one is bound to find increasingly better developed systems of embryonal nutrition. At the same time, however, higher development entails greater complexity and greater measures of independence of embryonal development from impositions by the environment.

Significantly, any greater measure of independence from the cosmos is achieved at the expense of having to create a correspondingly more complex reproductive system. In lower animals, there is but one physiologic circle: the sphere of vegetative life, in which are implicated both reproduction and external relations. In higher animals, more advanced vegetative development on the one hand and reproductive complexity on the other lead to greater independence of the three spheres of vegetative life, relational life and reproductive life.

12.1.1. SEXUAL LIFE, VEGETATIVE LIFE AND RELATIONAL LIFE

In those animals which lay aquatic eggs, the preparatory process for reproduction is minimal. On the other hand, any animal requiring extensive preparation for reproduction, such as birds and to some extent mammals, is *not fertile at all times but only at a point in life when preparedness for reproduction has reached a certain degree of maturity*. However, upon reaching that degree of maturity in the female, the whole preparatory effort would be necessarily wasted unless it can be salvaged from outside by the fertilizing male impulse. Only if the fertilizing element can be made to *coincide in space and time* with the element to be fertilized, under conditions of necessary preparedness for fertilization, can the latter event be accomplished and gestation ensue. The new being, which is to depend entirely on the gestating body for its nutrition, therefore requires that *the mother's vegetative sphere be adapted to its needs*. Thus, the sphere of *relational life* and that of *sexual life* have to be synchronized to permit fertilization to take place. To an equal degree, *vegetative life* and *sexual life* in turn must also be correlated in order to make gestation after fertilization possible.

These three spheres—sexual, vegetative and relational—must then be accurately geared so as to allow harmonious interactions for the purpose of perpetuating the species. The foregoing chapters described the existence of a system, specifically the hypophysiothalamic system, that serves as the link between the external environment and reproductive life, between the environment and vegetative life and between the latter and reproduction. *In essence, then, the sexual cycle is nothing else but the means of correlating these three spheres once they are duly coordinated in space and time by the action of the hypophysiothalamic system.*

12.1.2. THE PHENOMENON OF ESTRUS

Two conditions must be fulfilled in mammals for the realization of fertilization: (1) *that the gametes of both sexes meet at a given place and time*, and (2) *that, once formed, the egg be provided with a proper site for nidation*. These requirements presuppose the double coincidence of a mature ovum being encountered by a mature sperm at a precise moment and in a propitious nidatory terrain. In other words, for reproduction to succeed, two things are necessary:

1. That the expulsion of the gametes in both sexes coincide with copulation (within the limits of the animal's own "timetable").
2. That ovulation be associated with the preparation of an adequate implantation site in the uterus of the female.

In birds, only the first of the two prerequisites must be met. For fertilization to take place, copulation must coincide with the expulsion of the ovum, or else fertilization does not occur if the male meets the female and she has no ova available. Coincidence of ovulation with fertilization requires coordination of the physiology of the female with that of the male, but such coordination can only be provided by nature, that is, through the intervention of relational life. Nature solves the problem of this coordination by means of the phenomenon called *estrus*. At a given time in sexual life, the gonad of either sex can be aroused into activity, which then induces the gametes to start maturing and concurrently stimulates gonadal endocrine function. While the sexual cells are being readied for their mutual union, the hormones produced by the ovary as well as the hormones produced by the testis provide for mutual sexual attraction and, in addition, facilitate the preparation of the soil necessary for fertilization and eventual implantation in the female. That is to say, ovarian function is excited both as regards gametokinetic and endocrine activity, as a result of which the female possesses an ovum ready for fertilization and also has been "saturated" with estrogenic hormone, causing the genital apparatus to react in a specific way in preparation for fertilization as well as for attracting the male. However, in order to be attracted to the female at that propitious moment, the male must simultaneously be subjected to the same external stimulus that affects the female. By a design of nature, sexual arousal, or estrus, occurs simultaneously in both animals.

12.1.3. INFLUENCE OF HYPOTHALAMUS ON ESTRUS

The external influence causing estrus in wild animals is naturally exerted by way of the nervous system. This phenomenon can best be studied in birds. Benoit and co-workers,[11] Bisonnette,[13] Lamond and Braden,[79] and Lehrman and associates[80] have all shown that environmental illumination triggered estrous activity in birds and in certain wild rodents. Delost[33] found that wild animals lose their responsiveness to light after becoming domesticated. Fiske and Lamond,[49] as well as Lamond and Braden,[79] have demonstrated that light acts by producing release of neurosecretory substances which in turn excite the anterior lobe of the pituitary.

The role of light in regulating hypothalamic function was analyzed in Chapter 8. The effects involved have been shown to be mediated by the pineal,[45, 150] as indicated in Chapter 10 (Section 10.5.2). McCormack and Bennin[89] made the observation that while exposure to light induced ovulation in adult rats, it caused a delay in the appearance of ovulation in immature animals. Human blindness at birth is known to be associated with precocious puberty. In rats, these reactions are blocked by pinealectomy.[150] It is probable that estrogens increase the sensitivity of the hypothalamic nuclei to light. According to Tejasen and Everett,[133] the vector of sensory impulses initiating estrous activity is the *preoptico-tuberal pathway* (see Chapter 10, Section 10.5.2).

Other external influences may similarly modify or provoke estrus. Grindeland and Folk[57] have noted that low temperatures suspended estrus in hamsters, whereas Folman and Drori[46] were able to induce estrous activity in rats by means of certain odors.

It is therefore evident that in wild animals, in which environmental exigencies impose a seasonal pattern on estrous activity, such factors as changes in light, environmental temperature and sensory, particularly olfactory, stimuli must excite the sexual centers of the hypothalamus through the sensory organs in order to produce estrus.

That estrous activity is indeed regulated by the nervous system can be inferred from the following items:

1. The relationship that exists between the sensory organs and the sexual cycle (light, temperature, odors).

2. The well known fact that in some animals, e.g., the rabbit,[129] ovulation in the female is induced by mere coming into contact with the male.

3. The finding that ovulation and estrus can be produced by means of experimental vaginal stimulation in some rodents (Sawyer et al.,[119] Sturkie and Freedman[127]).

4. The demonstration of a *sexual center* in the median eminence of the tuber cinereum (see Chapter 8), stimulation of which provokes estrus.[30, 73, 79]

5. The finding of characteristic *electroencephalographic changes* at the time of estrus.[3, 73]

6. The fact that estrous activity in rats, rabbits and sheep can be blocked by means of pentothal,[44, 59, 108] chlorpromazine[61, 112] or reserpine.

The neuroendocrine physiology of sexual secretion has already been explained in Chapter 8. The sexual center of the median eminence of the tuber cinereum *also controls ovulation* through discharges of gonadotropins. In the well known experiment of Westman,[146] ovulation in the female rabbit induced by coitus or simply the male presence, is suspended by means of sectioning the pituitary stalk. Similar results have been obtained by Kawakami and Sawyer[73] by destroying the premamillary zone of the floor of the third ventricle. Interestingly, MacArthur and co-workers[87] produced ovulation in a variety of animals by *locally injecting* estrogens into this zone, which suggests that the mechanism of ovulation release, thought to result from a cumulative rise in estrogen blood levels toward the end of the follicular phase, is mediated by stimulation of this center.

12.1.4. ESTRUS AND RELATIONAL LIFE

It can be concluded that estrus, of all the types of sexual activity, is most closely related to relational life. Not only is estrus initiated by sensory stimuli, such as light or perception of male odors, but the relationship between the hypothalamic sexual centers and the limbic system (see Chapter 9) also makes it possible for *estrus to be entirely controlled by emotions.* Thus, estrus in wild animals may be induced by hypothalamic stimulation of the following type:

1. Emotions, either instinctive or conscious in nature, in the presence of members of the opposite sex.

2. General corporal stimuli, physical in nature, resulting from seasonal changes, such as light or heat.

3. In females, stimulation through being in contact with, being pursued by, or involved in a struggle with, the male — in other words, through intensification of the level of activity related to the "sexual struggle." Estrus in turn exerts an influence on relational life, by provoking greater psychic activity and enhanced neuromuscular excitability.[75]

A diagrammatic representation of the neurohormonal correlations determining the appearance of estrus is shown for the entire mammalian scale in Figure 12.1.

12.1.5. ESTRUS IN RODENTS

Essentially the same mechanism as that already outlined is responsible for estrus in laboratory animals. As a matter of fact, most of our experimental data have been obtained from just these animals. However, as a result of comparative studies of the passage of certain species of rodents from

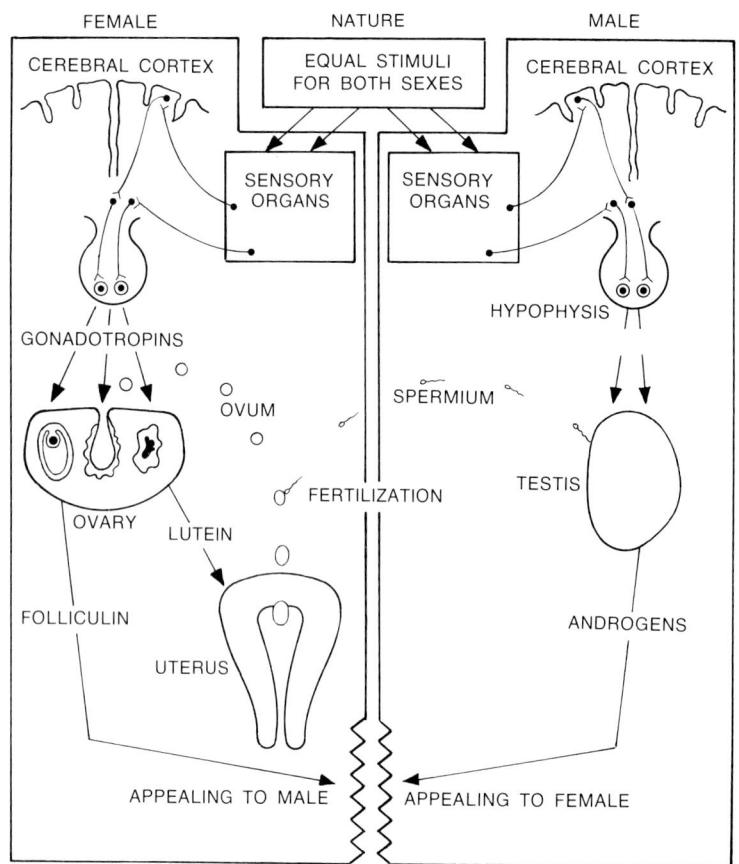

Figure 12-1. Scheme of the phenomenon of estrus in the female and in the male.

the wild state to captivity, some investigators, among them Delost,[33] describe a progressive loss of external influences on sexual life in the domesticated group. *Domestication, then, means a greater measure of independence for both sexual and relational life and, at the same time, greater autonomy of the endocrine system, as well as less intervention by the nervous system into the reproductive cycle.*

The phenomenon of estrus in the rat and in the mouse has been extensively studied by numerous investigators[143, 155] (Fig. 12-2). The phenomenon is almost identical in both species and in addition is quite similar in the guinea pig. In contrast, the *female rabbit* differs significantly. Ovulation in rabbits does not occur spontaneously and therefore there is no spontaneous estrus. Because estrus only appears on physical contact with the male,[129] the female rabbit closely resembles wild animals insofar as initiation of estrous activity is concerned. In the presence of the male, the female rabbit takes exactly 9 hours to ovulate,[50] which is about the same time it takes the sperm to reach the tube. A similar situation exists in *Microtus agrestis*.[18] Westman[146] and Jacobson and Norgren,[68] as well as a number of other investigators (see Harris[62]), showed that ovulation could be blocked by sectioning the pituitary stalk, a clear indication that we are dealing with a neurohormonal reflex phenomenon mediated by hypothalamic-pituitary pathways. This means that ovulation, estrous activity and the entire process of setting up the conditions necessary for fertilization are all initiated by the female rabbit's sensory perception of and sexual "struggle" with the male. A diagrammatic explanation of this phenomenon is given in Figure 12-1. It is of interest to note that ovulation in the rabbit and ovulation in either the mouse or rat exemplify two opposite types of ovulatory reactions occurring in mammals. Whereas in either rats or mice this process is spontaneous and therefore cannot be provoked by external stimuli involving the nervous system, the reaction in rabbits seems to be primarily dependent on neurogenic activity, so much so that it obeys external stimuli rapidly and automatically. Various investigators (Brinkley and Nalbandov,[20] Duncan et al.,[39] Harper[60] and Sawyer et al.[119]) have found that estrogen injections into female rabbits fail to produce release of luteinizing gonadotropin (LH) (see Chapter 8). On the other hand, Everett[44] and Velardo[142] have verified previous findings that rats respond to estrogens with a characteristic release of gonadotropic hormone. *This means that whereas pituitary gonadotropin production in animals with neurogenic ovulation, such as rabbits, is barely, if at all, subject to hormonal regulation, gonadotropin production in animals with spontaneous rhythmic ovulation, which is stimulated preferably by estrogenic activity, depends on the rhythm of ovarian-hypothalamic-pituitary interactions.*

12.2. THE SEXUAL CYCLE IN PRIMATES AND IN WOMAN

Just as in rats, ovulation in these mammals appears spontaneously, *but with a rhythm that rodents do not possess.* This rhythmic event occurs at four week intervals, at which time *ovulation invariably takes place* in the sexually mature female. Ovulation, periodically repeated in the ovary, is also constantly being stimulated at stated intervals with secretion of sex hormones, the latter inducing regular changes in the genital tract, and indeed the entire body, of female primates and woman, which recur each month with similar characteristics, in a cyclic manner. Such factors as seasonal changes, environmental circumstances, neurogenic stimuli or pathologic alterations may, though only superficially, modify this menstrual rhythm, as nature tends to compensate for such influences by maintaining regulation of the four-week cycle as completely as possible. The most important event of this cycle—ovulation, which is the *primum movens* of all the rest—takes place in the ovary. However, the most conspicuous happening of the entire cycle is the monthly shedding of the uterine mucosa, called *menstruation*. Menstruation is known to occur only in primates. Periodic pseudomenstrual bleeding has been observed during estrus in some animals, e.g., the bitch, the cat and the cow, but such hemorrhage is not menstruation, as will be explained in Chapter 13. *Menstruation is a phenomenon that is exclusive of the order of primates and that results from failure of the endometrium, which has undergone a preparatory process for a special type of ovular nidation, to achieve its goal.*

12.2.1. INTERNAL "RHYTHM" IN THE CYCLE OF PRIMATES

An interesting feature about the sexual cycle in primates is its fixed, built-in periodicity of four weeks. Not imposed by external influences, this periodicity is endogenous, a phenomenon of *internal "timing."*

Van Waagenen and Simpson[141] noted that

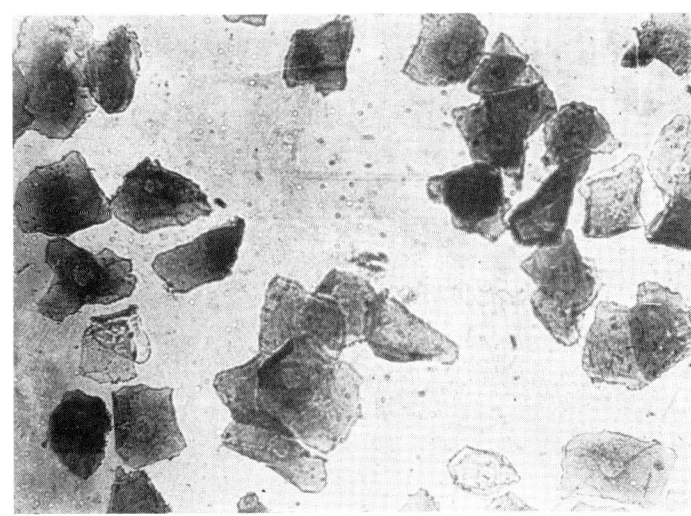

Figure 12-2. Vaginal smear from rat, showing typical desquamation of estrus.

certain species of monkeys tended to have short cycles (e.g., 6.5 days in *Macaca mulatta*), while Collett and associates[26] recently found that the internal rhythm in the human species was subject to alterations after the age of 30, and that women maintained the precision of their internal rhythm unaltered only during the third decade of their lives.

Another interesting phenomenon concerning the cycle in primates in general is the occurrence of *anovulatory cycles. Such cycles*, in which an ovarian follicle matures to the point of rupture but fails to rupture and no corpus luteum is formed, were described by Hartman (in the monkey) and Novak (in woman). The presence of an anovulatory cycle, or *anovular menorrhea*, is physiologic in woman only at puberty and at menopause; however, it is an important cause of *sterility* (Chapter 41). On the other hand, anovular menorrhea in monkeys is physiologic during the summer months.[95, 141, 152]

12.2.2. DIFFERENCES BETWEEN THE MALE AND FEMALE CYCLE

Although in recent years a certain degree of cyclicity in testicular function has been described,[46, 154] there is no male sexual cycle, in the proper sense of the word, in either man or lower animals. The male hypothalamus does not discharge the releasing factors LHRF and FSHRF in a cyclic fashion, as is the case in the female. It has been discovered over the past few years that the *rhythmic pattern of secretion* in both the hypothalamus and the pituitary of female weanling rats or mice *was lost as a result of androgen injections.*[24, 54, 63, 68, 128, 153] Greenblatt postulates that the anovulatory cycle in woman has a similar etiology, owing to abnormal androgen production by the ovary under certain circumstances (see *Stein-Leventhal syndrome*, Chapter 29).

12.2.3. EXOGENOUS INFLUENCES ON THE CYCLE OF PRIMATES

The very nature of the internal rhythm of the cycle in primates suggested that, unlike the case with other animals in the wild, it was not subject to exogenous influences. Even though Van Waagenen and Simpson[141] and Schrank and Koch[120] have shown that ovulation in monkeys and women, respectively, was not induced by coitus, it must be remembered that Stieve[125] had demonstrated that, if coitus could not, at least such other factors as emotion, fear, anxiety, and so forth, could provoke alterations or disappearance of the cycle. The many clinical aspects concerning influences of the nervous system on the female cycle are discussed in Chapter 34.

The following sections are concerned with the cycle in woman, starting with the study of the ovarian cycle.

12.3. THE OVARIAN CYCLE

The ovary is a small gland of ovoid shape, lodged in the pelvis minor, whose average greatest dimensions are 3 to 5 × 2 to 3 × 1 to 1.5 cm. It reaches its greatest size at puberty and during the first years of sexual maturity, decreasing little by little afterwards. The fetal ovary is characterized by proliferation of *oogonia* (phase of multiplication or oogenesis, according to Boveri) until the end of intrauterine life. Beginning with birth, this process of multiplication ends, so that the number of germ cells contained in both ovaries, making up a woman's germinal pool, no longer can increase. The number of follicles, is estimated at between 300,000 (Schroeder) and 450,000 (Watzka[145]). After birth, oogonia are transformed into primary oocytes and begin their process of maturation by entering and remaining in the *diplotene* stage, further evolution being blocked throughout infancy until puberty or until that moment in a woman's life when follicular growth is set into motion (Ohno and Smith[105]).

The ovarian cortical zone of a newborn female contains an impressive number of oocytes (Fig. 12–3), surrounded by a layer of flattened cells (the future granulosa layer). Follicles containing an oocyte in a state of arrested development are referred to as *primordial follicles* or *primordia* (Watzka[145]). Such follicles remain at a resting stage for long periods of time—involving years—after which they begin, one by one, to develop further. Once begun, this developmental process of the follicle goes ahead at a steady pace. One follicle is thus "set in motion" in each cycle

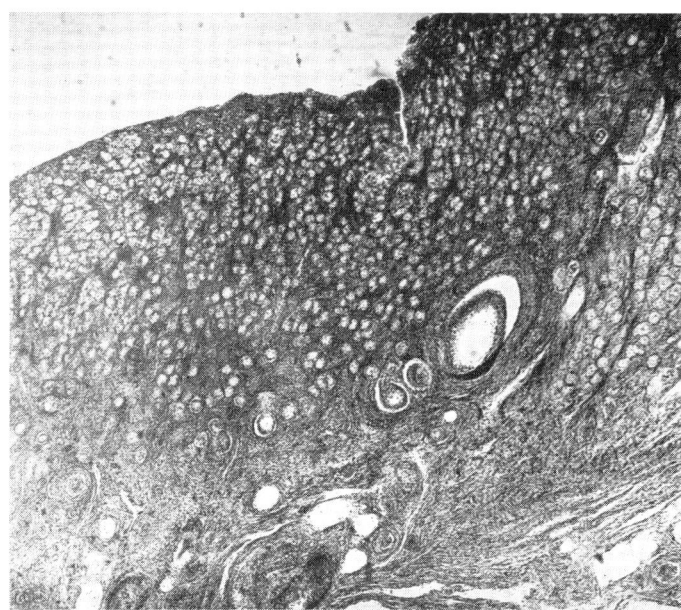

Figure 12-3. Section of the ovary of a young girl, revealing an enormous number of primordial follicles.

and, by maturing, these follicles eventually give rise to a *complete* ovarian unit.

Koppen,[77] Zuckermann[155] and MacKay and colleagues[91] found that the old idea, according to which follicles no longer were formed after birth, was erroneous. Neoformation of oogonia, even though only to a moderate extent, goes on in the human ovary throughout life. However, with advancing age, the proliferative capacity of oogonia wanes. Behrman and Duboff[9] have shown that, in addition to the absence of germ cell multiplication, the senescent ovary is characterized by modifications in the gland's carbohydrate metabolism.

12.3.1. HISTOLOGIC FEATURES

The first event to occur in the developing *primary* follicle is prompt differentiation of its single epithelial layer into two layers. One of these retains its concentric arrangement of flattened cells, with simultaneous accentuation of its mesenchymal features, giving rise to the *theca*. The innermost portion, in contact with the ovum, differentiates into a thin layer of cuboidal cells, with prominent nuclei but little cytoplasm, not exceeding 5 to 6 microns in diameter. The latter is known as the *granulosa layer (membrana granulosa)*. The resulting structure, made up of the germ cell encircled by the granulosa theca, receives the name of *secondary ovarian follicle*. From this stage on, the ovarian follicle begins to grow in size, and is referred to as a *growing follicle* (Fig. 12-4). Follicular growth is associated with growth of the oocyte (growth phase of Boveri). The growing germ cell surrounds itself by a hyaline membrane, consisting of a mucoid substance (*zona pellucida* or *oolemma*). By a process of vacuolization and fusion of some of the granulosa cells, follicular growth creates a central cavity, small initially but eventually becoming bigger and bigger, until there is complete separation of the centrally placed ovum, surrounded only by a peninsula-like aggregate of granulosa cells (*cumulus oophorus*), from the remainder of the granulosa layer, which at this stage is adherent to the wall of the follicle and is made up of five to six rows of cuboidal cells (Figs. 12-5 and 12-6). Outside this granulosa membrane, in the meantime, the theca differentiates into an internal layer, which acquires a rich vascular supply (*theca interna* or *vascular theca*), and an external layer, which undergoes fibrosis in order to protect the follicle from external pressure (*theca externa* or *fibrous theca*). The follicular cavity is filled with a clear transparent fluid, containing estrogenic hormone in high concentration, which receives the name of *liquor folliculi*.

The position of the follicle in relation to

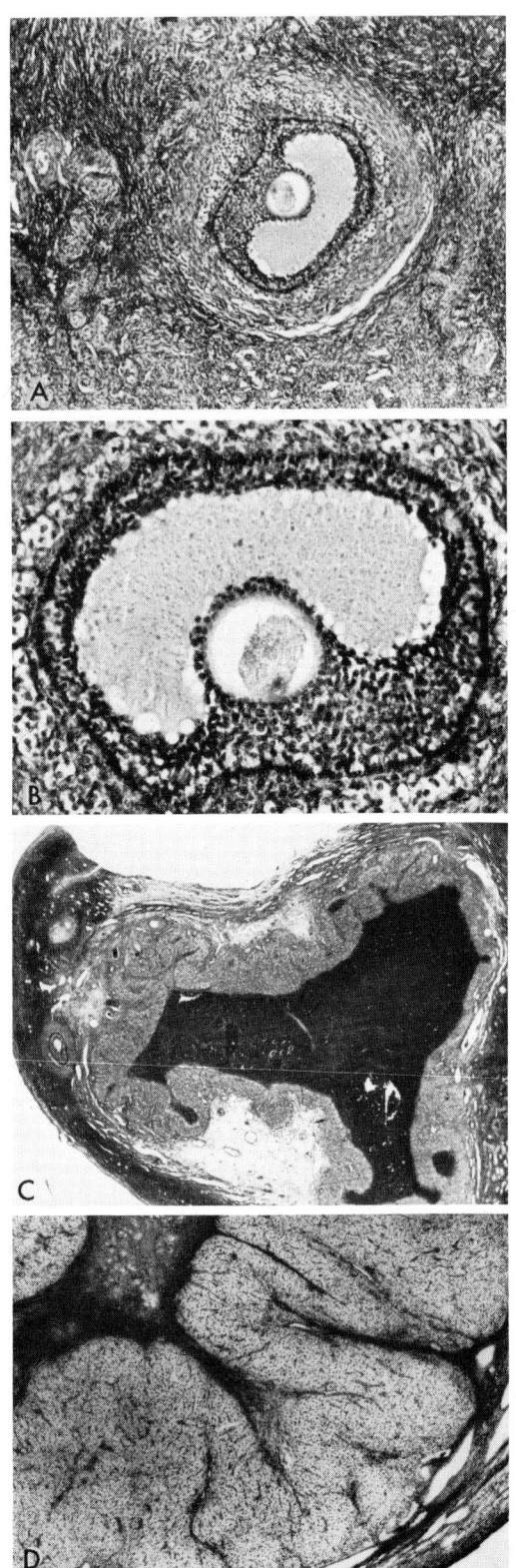

Figure 12–4. The ovarian cycle in woman. *A*, Maturing follicle in the ovary of a 28-year-old woman at low magnification (100×). *B*, Same, at higher magnification (300×). The secretory theca interna, composed of large, clear cells, is clearly discernible from the surrounding fibrous theca externa. The cumulus oophorus contains the ovum with apparently shrunken cytoplasm due to processing artifacts. *C*, Corpus luteum in ovary of 29-year-old woman (4×), shown at higher magnification (100×) in *D*.

Figure 12-5. Follicular maturation in *Macaca mulatta* ovary. A, Under low magnification (50×), numerous follicles in various stages of maturation are seen in the ovarian cortex. B, Higher power (100×) reveals maturing follicle containing well preserved oocyte with distinctly outlined nucleus. The granulosa layer is well developed and the theca well differentiated. C, High power view of cortical zone, showing follicle in early phase of maturation, in which oocyte exhibits distinct nucleus, nucleolus and membrana pellucida.

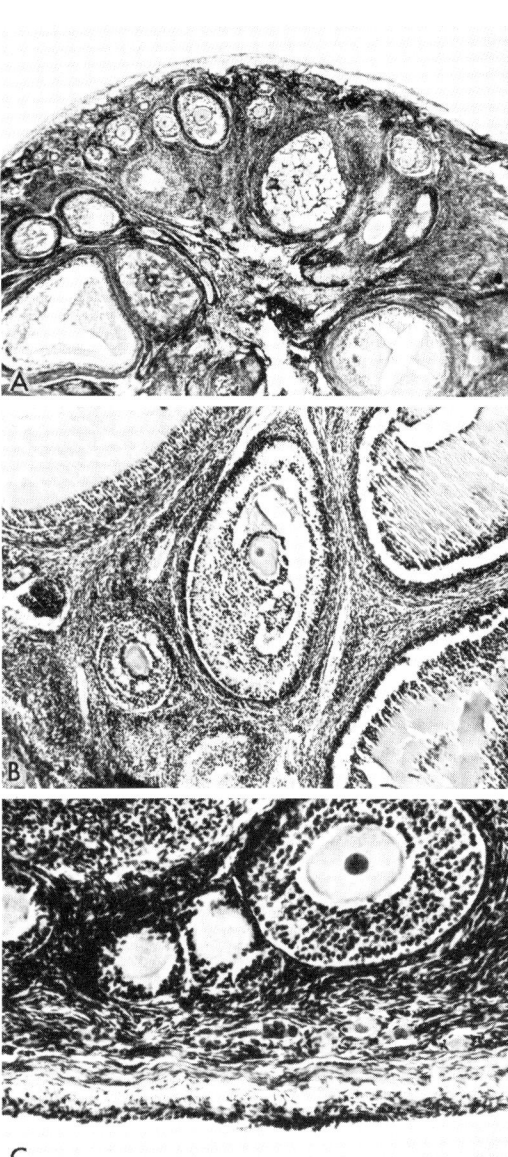

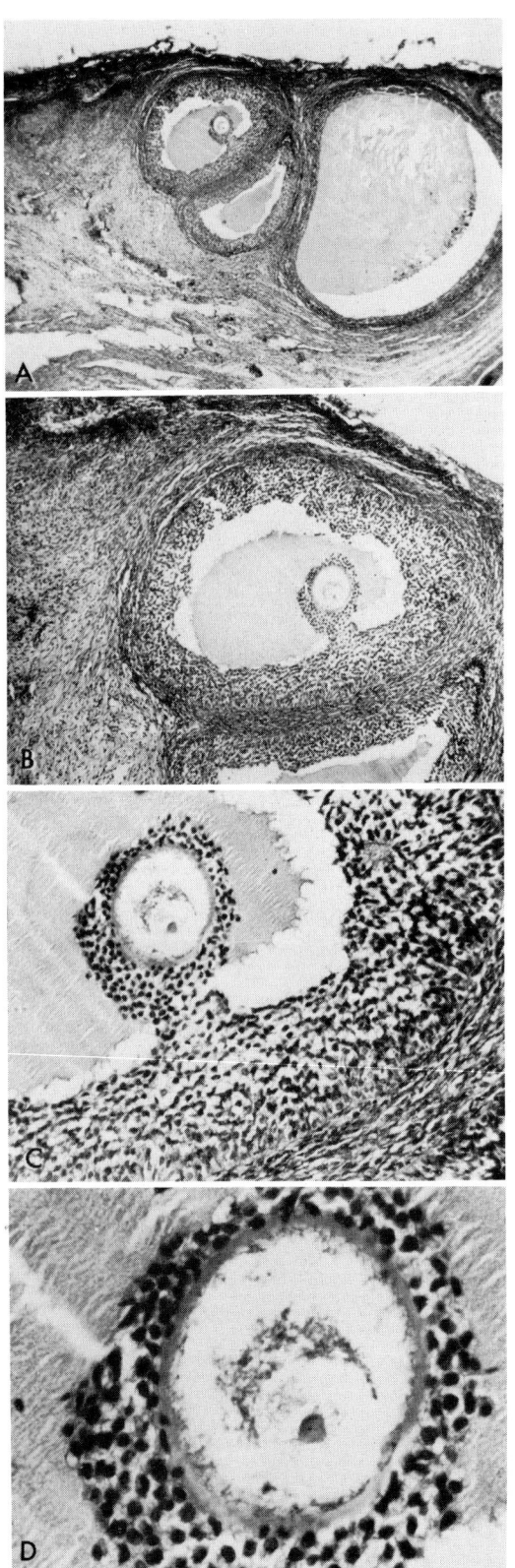

Figure 12-6. Maturing follicle in ewe ovary, seen in a series of increasing magnifications: *A*, 100×; *B*, 200×; *C*, 300×; *D* 900×. Note details of cytoplasm, nucleus, and nucleolus of ovum, cumulus oophorus, and granulosa layer, as well as theca interna and theca externa.

the ovarian surface varies in the course of follicular development. At first, the follicle grows toward the medulla, that is, centripetally; after reaching a diameter of about 4 mm, however, it can no longer expand in the direction of the ovarian center and encounters less resistance in growing toward the periphery, where it eventually bulges out over the ovarian surface. As the follicle opens its way toward the free surface, the internal theca forms a cellular wedge that, by inserting itself between the overlying mesenchymal elements of the ovarian stroma, facilitates the outward displacement of the follicle (Fig. 12-15). This wedge, first described by Strassmann,[126] certainly plays a significant role in the mechanism of follicular rupture and ovulation. By the time a follicle is about to rupture, it is known as a *mature, tertiary* or *graafian follicle* (in honor of its discoverer, Regnerius de Graaf). The graafian follicle consists of the same elements that have been described previously: the two theca layers, the granulosa layer, and the follicular cavity with the cumulus oophorus and the ovum. The cumulus oophorus is continuous with the membrana granulosa by means of a small isthmus, which imparts the appearance of a peninsula to that part of the follicle comprising the cumulus and the ovum (Fig. 12-6).

Ovulation occurs on the fourteenth day of the intermenstruum, in keeping with the long known observations of Schroeder and Meyer, although slight physiologic variations may be observed in this regard, depending on the internal *rhythm*. As a result of ovulation, the internal pressure of the follicle drops suddenly, owing to the egress of follicular fluid and the ovum. Consequently, the wall of the follicle folds up as it retracts, causing shrinkage and wrinkling of the granulosa, while the concomitant sudden drop of intracavitary pressure leads to abundant hemorrhage in the theca interna. This gives rise to a *hemorrhagic follicle,* displaying a folded contour, formed on the inside by the granulosa and on the outside by the theca, the latter assuming a wavy configuration that is punctuated by occasional penetrating spurs of tissue. The stoma of the ruptured follicle is occluded by a fibrinous plug and subsequently the hemorrhagic follicle turns into a *corpus luteum* (Figs. 12-4,C, and 12-8). After extrusion of the ovum, both the granulosa and theca cell components in the wall of the collapsed and flaccid follicle begin to proliferate. Contrary to earlier belief, the first signs of proliferation in the corpus luteum are seen in the theca interna, with the appearance of large polyhedral cells containing abundant lipid. These are the so-called *theca lutein cells* (Fig. 12-4,B). The theca lutein cells actually begin to appear prior to follicular rupture,[98] which accounts for the fact that the presence of progesterone in the circulating blood of woman can be demonstrated before ovulation. Immediately following proliferation of theca lutein cells, there is also vigorous proliferation of the cells of the granulosa layer. Because of poor vascularization of the granulosa, the latter cells contain less lipid material than the theca lutein cells. There is no evidence that the granulosa layer experiences any increase in vascularity during this first phase of corpus luteum formation (Rennels[109]).

This first proliferative stage, during which the corpus luteum is organized by means of a luteinic reaction, involving first the theca, then the granulosa, is followed by a second stage: that of *vascularization*. Three to four days after rupture, numerous capillaries sprout from the theca interna and begin growing into the granulosa. This process is associated with growth in size of the granulosa cells, which assume a polyhedral shape; soon outstripping in growth the theca cells, these cells become an element of utmost importance for the corpus luteum, which does not, until this time, acquire its characteristic luteal appearance. By the eighth day after ovulation, the corpus luteum displays its maximal activity and has entered the phase of maturity. The granulosa layer has reached its greatest thickness and is bright yellow in color. The dentate and festooned appearance of this yellow zone at this time is more prominent than ever because of lack of space. The initially important theca lutein cells begin to decay. Dubreuil[38] is correct in pointing out that the corpus luteum owes its name to a pigment that, rather than reflecting the true function of this tiny incretory gland, is really degenerative in nature. He proposes the name of *corpus progestativum* for the corpus luteum of the cycle, and that of *corpus gestativum* for the corpus luteum of pregnancy.

In most of the mammals, including the human species, evolution of the corpus progestativum into the corpus gestativum

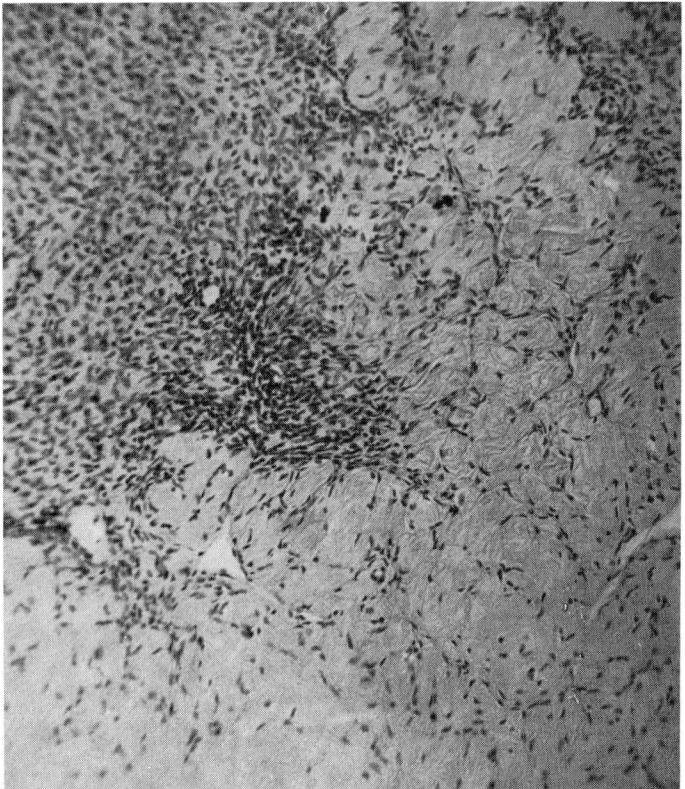

Figure 12-7. Detail of a corpus albicans.

is accomplished without any transition, merely taking place because fertilization itself has taken place; however, in some species, such as the badger, the bison and the marten, in which nidation occurs in a stepwise and deferred manner, transformation of a simple transient corpus luteum into a definitive corpus luteum of pregnancy is progressive and passes through several stages.[15]

Green and co-workers[56] have been able to discern ultrastructural differences between the progestational and the gestational corpus luteum. Though most mammals reveal no essential light microscopic differences in this regard, there appear to be significant differential features present at the ultrastructural level.

If gestation fails to take place, the *corpus luteum regresses* (Williams[148]). According to studies by Corner,[28, 29] the process of corpus luteum decay sets in between the eighth and the tenth day after ovulation. The granulosa lutein cells become vacuolated and degenerate. Their nuclei undergo pyknosis and chromatolysis and their cytoplasm reveals hyaline degeneration.

The thecal cells persist but acquire more and more a connective tissue appearance; the thecal septa are gradually invaded by fibroblasts, and a dense scar tissue is formed around the outline of what vaguely resembles the folded structures of granulosa lutein cells. The result is a *corpus albicans* (Fig. 12-7), whose remnants of variable size will persist in the ovarian hilus indefinitely, although Joel and Foraker[70] have shown that most corpora albicantia disappear without leaving a trace.

In some animals, as well as in the human species, the *ovarian interstitial tissue*, too, undergoes cyclic histologic changes.[58, 98, 111] These changes are believed to be related to the *secretion of androgens* by the ovarian interstitium, this process too possessing to some extent features of cyclicity.[55]

12.3.2. HISTOCHEMICAL MODIFICATIONS IN THE OVARIAN CYCLE

A great deal of histochemical investigations concerning the sexual cycle have recently been carried out on both the uterus and the ovary. Most of the work has been concerned with the study of lipids, phosphatase activity, presence of carbonylic groups, succinic dehydrogenase activity and the types of enzymes implicated in hormone synthesis.

FLUORESCENCE, BIREFRINGENCE AND SUDANOPHILIA. The ovarian lipid content was studied by MacKay and colleagues[91] in 1961 by means of a combination of these three methods. Their studies revealed a close correlation between the presence of detectable lipids and endocrine activity. The lipid content of the corpus luteum has been the object of a great deal of study.[7, 32, 95] The highest concentrations have been observed between the twenty-second and twenty-sixth day of the cycle. The decadent corpus luteum loses its lipid content.

CARBONYLIC GROUPS. Ashbel and Seligman[4] have devised a diazo reaction capable of revealing the carbonylic groups of steroids in tissues. Both authors, as well as Barker,[7] have shown that the corpus luteum, particularly the granulosa lutein cells, and to a lesser degree the theca lutein cells, gives a positive reaction.

PHOSPHATASES. *Glycerophosphatases* play a special role in corpus luteum function. Dempsey and his colleagues[35] have found that alkaline glycerophosphatase activity was proportional to the degree of development of the gland, while Corner[29] suggested that the appearance of that enzyme in the ovary was the result of a specific effect of LH activity. Stafford and colleagues,[23] Lobel and co-workers[83] and MacKay and co-workers[91] have also studied acid glycerophosphatase activity in relation to alkaline glycerophosphatase and arrived at the conclusion that the alkaline counterpart was characteristic of a young corpus luteum in development, whereas acid phosphatase activity was exclusively present in mature corpora that were undergoing regression. *Aminopeptidase* activity[82] appears to run parallel to acid glycerophosphatase and is most pronounced in the corpus gestativum.

Studies concerning *adenosine triphosphatase* activity have been conducted by Meyer and his co-workers.[95] Such activity is localized principally in the corpus luteum and can be considered as an index of that gland's activity.

Our own observations show alkaline phosphatase activity present in the theca interna and above all in perivascular locations within the corpus luteum in the stage of vascularization (Figs. 12–8 and 12–9). However, a finding that we consider of great interest is the presence of phosphatase activity in corpora atretica which is much more pronounced than that of normal follicles, and nearly as marked as that of corpora lutea. This observation, it is felt, may strengthen the argument that these structures fulfill an active secretory function.

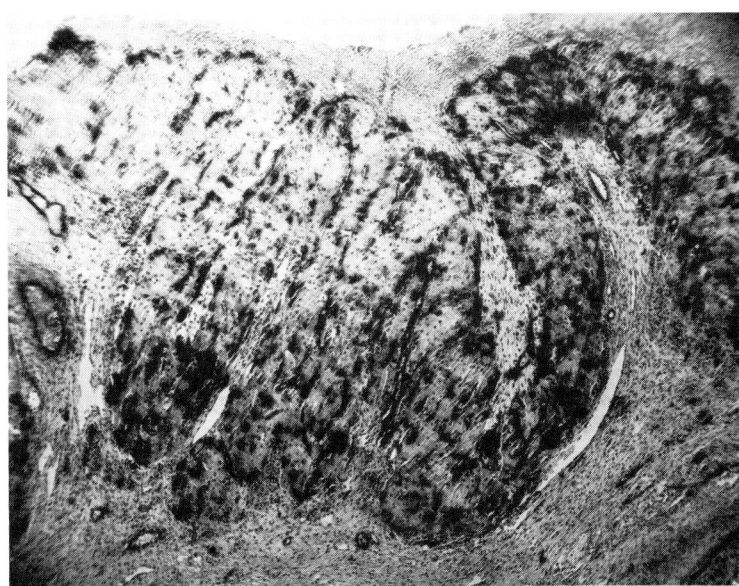

Figure 12–8. Human corpus luteum, showing alkaline phosphatase reaction. Notice perivascular distribution of alkaline phosphatase.

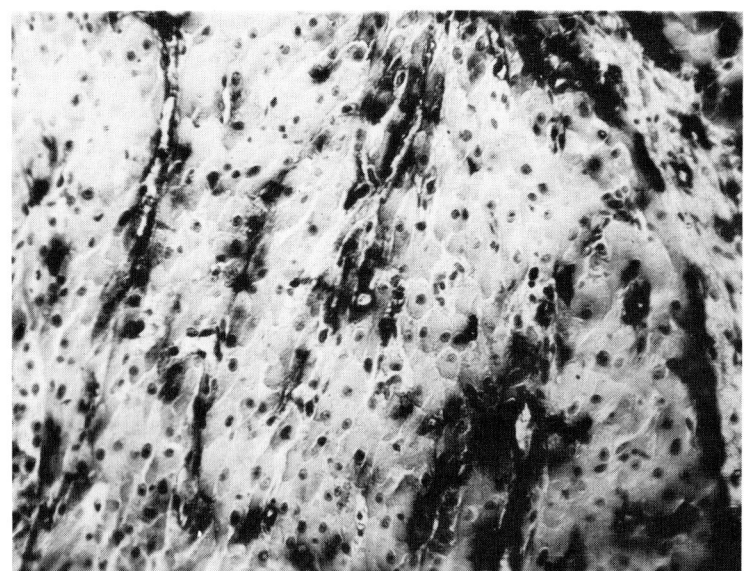

Figure 12-9. Detail of Figure 12-8, at higher magnification.

SUCCINIC DEHYDROGENASE. Meyer and his associates[95] attach special importance to the high concentrations of succinic dehydrogenase found by them in the corpus luteum, where, they believe, the enzyme exercises a highly specific type of activity aimed at partaking in progesterone biosynthesis in a yet unknown manner.

3β-OL-DEHYDROGENASE. The significance of 3 β-ol-dehydrogenase for progestogen synthesis has been explained in Chapter 3 (see Section 3.5.2). The presence of this catalyst in the corpus luteum has been demonstrated by the histochemical studies of Taylor[132] and subsequently confirmed by Ryan and Smith,[116] Deane and colleagues[32] and Brandau and colleagues.[17] The last group of investigators found that dehydrogenase activity was present in both the follicular and luteal theca, as well as in the granulosa lutein cells, but not in the ovarian structures.

12.3.3. CYCLIC EVOLUTION OF THE FEMALE GAMETE

The oocyte constitutes a cellular element in the ovary completely distinct from all other ovarian structures. It must be remembered that, while the ovary arises through differentiation of the retrocoelomic mesenchyme (see Chapter 15), the oocyte is derived from gonocytes and, therefore, is part of the *germinal route* which, being clearly separated from the soma, belongs to that abstraction which we have come to call "the germ." In the adult ovary, Seitz pointed out, there exists an antagonism between the ovarian mesenchyme and the germ cells. The latter are encircled by the membrana granulosa in what appears to be a protective screen erected in defense of the germ against the cells of the soma. Destruction of the granulosa layer has been shown to entail immediate destruction of the ovum by the surrounding ovarian mesenchyme. The ovary has a rich autonomous innervation whose nerve fibers were shown by Reynolds[110] not to penetrate beyond the theca-granulosa interface, possibly indicating that, by not receiving the same inervation and blood supply, both the granulosa and the ovum are meant to be independent stocks of tissue. The electron microscopic studies by Stegner and Wartenberg[124] have brought to light the fact that the demarcation between the granulosa and the oocyte is not as neat as it was originally believed to be. Tiny cytoplasmic processes from the cells of the "corona radiata" penetrate the pellucida and appear to convey secretions or possibly nutrients into the interior of the germ cell (Fig. 12–10).

It has been suggested that the role of evocator, played by the gonocyte in the embryonal ovary, has been retained by the oogonium and by the oocyte for the rest of life. In the past, German investigators often referred to the principle of *ovular primacy,* which holds that the follicle develops only on behalf of the oocyte. If the latter does not develop, follicular growth does not proceed and the follicle undergoes atresia (Moricard and Gothie[98]). By removing oocytes from follicles of rabbit ovaries through puncture and aspiration, El Fouly and his colleagues[41] showed that follicular maturation was arrested and that such follicles failed to undergo luteinization. The ovary of a newborn, as indicated previously, contains approximately 300,000 primordial follicles, of which only as few as one thousandth, that is, about 300, achieve maturity in the course of life. The vast majority of primordial follicles are subject to atresia at some point or another of their development. Atresia is thought to result from the demise of the germ cell, since as soon as death of the ovum occurs, follicular development is arrested. In mice, Edwards[40] found that the nuclear chromatin of oocytes underwent degenerative changes as soon as the follicles containing them were arrested in their development and started showing signs of atresia. Since atresia is nothing else but premature involution of the theca, and since the same thecal changes are known to occur in both follicular atresia and corpus luteum formation, we can generalize by saying that *the death or loss of an oocyte may be considered to bring about a phenomenon of proliferation and secretory activity on part of the thecal tissue.* Thus, follicular function is essentially conditioned by growth of the ovum. *Loss of the ovum determines loss of follicular growth, and, as a result, the follicle undergoes atresia or luteinization.*

12.3.4. OVULAR DEATH RATE IN THE COURSE OF THE CYCLE

Austin[5] called attention to the fact that the chromosomes of oocytes in female rabbits experienced steady deterioration with increasing age. It must be remembered that the passage from the oogonium to the oocyte and the beginning of the dictyotene stage in the human female is still accomplished in the embryonal stage. In some women an interval of many years must go by before one of those oocytes can complete its maturation process and gets a chance to

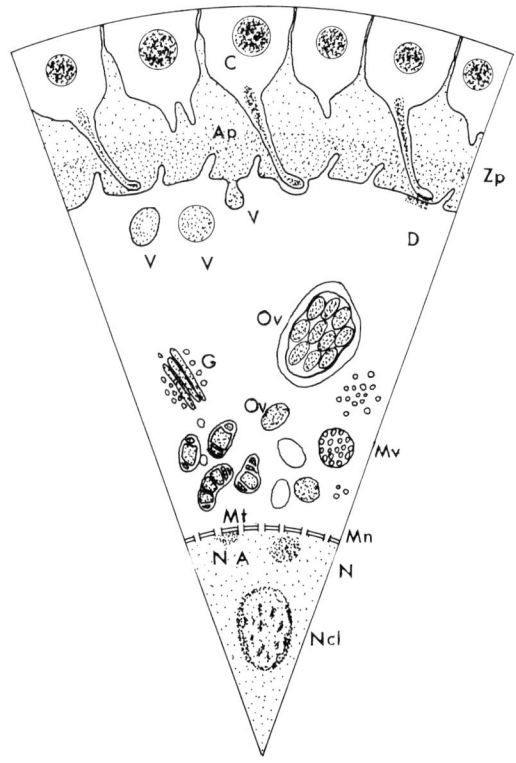

Figure 12–10. Diagrammatic representation of a segment of human ovum. *C*, Granulosa cells; *Zp*, zona pellucida, crossed by protoplasmic processes of granulosa cells (*Ap*) which, as can be seen, are nutritional elements of the oocyte cytoplasm. The cellular membrane is almost nonexistent, but in it certain structures connecting it to the corona radiata, or desmosomes (*D*), are conspicuous. Oval bodies (*Ov*) are seem in the cytoplasm, either in aggregates or scattered singly, as well as a Golgi apparatus (*G*), mitochondria (*Mt*) in various stages of development, and so-called "multivesicular" bodies (*Mv*). The nuclear membrane (*Mn*) is perforated and the nuclear chromatin substance (*N*), is of low density. The nucleolus (*Ncl*) and paranucleoli (*NA*), can also be seen. (From Stegner and Wartenberg: *Arch. Gynäk.,* 196:23, 1961.)

be fertilized. It is therefore not surprising that women in the older age groups should show a higher incidence of abortion from chromosomal aberrations[121] as well as a higher incidence of hydatidiform mole and of babies with Down's syndrome. *Delayed ovulation* in rats was shown by Butcher and his colleagues[21, 22] to result in chromosomal anomalies. McGaughey and Chang[90] found the same result in mice.

12.4. REGULATION OF THE OVARIAN CYCLE

As an adjunct to Chapter 7, in which we discussed pituitary control over the cyclic activity of the ovary and the effects of gonadotropic hormones on ovarian function, the following sections are intended to give a global overview of the facts that provoke the cyclic effect of the pituitary on the ovary, the reciprocal interactions between the two, and the role played by the hypothalamus in controlling this entire complex.

12.4.1. THE ROLE OF GONADOTROPINS IN THE REGULATION OF THE MENSTRUAL CYCLE

As was pointed out in Chapters 6 and 7, the female pituitary differs from the male pituitary in that it presents a monthly, cyclic pattern of activity. This *monthly pituitary cycle* in the female can be demonstrated by cytologic studies of the pituitary.

Until recently, it was not known what the actual rhythm of FSH and LH secretion during the cycle was. Thanks to accurate bioassay methods (method of Parlow, etc.) and, above all, to radioimmunologic procedures, it has been possible to establish the approximate rhythm of secretion, or release, of both gonadotropins of the cycle, as well as to demonstrate the effect they exert on the ovary. The studies of Loraine and Bell and their colleagues[10, 84] first established the presence of an *LH peak* at the midpoint on the cycle, but they failed to detect any definite pattern of FSH excretion. Such a *preovulatory peak* of LH release was later confirmed by Becker and Albert[8] and by Anderson and MacShan.[2] Rosemberg and Keller[75, 113] observed that FSH levels were elevated between the seventh and eighth days of the cycle, and again between the thirteenth and fourteenth days. However, more accurate observations have recently been achieved by means of *radioimmunoassay* techniques. There is general agreement that luteinizing hormone levels (see Chapter 7, Section 7) indeed appear to remain low throughout the entire cycle except for an elevation occurring about the thirteenth or fourteenth day, called the *preovulatory peak*.[25, 52, 76, 97, 103, 106, 134, 137, 147] In contrast, there is still little consensus regarding follicle-stimulating hormone (FSH). As indicated previously (Chapter 7, Section 7), the most widely held view is that the curve of FSH activity follows the reverse pattern, showing a maximal upswing during the menstrual phase and a downswing at the time of ovulation.[25, 52, 114, 134] However, significantly different curves for FSH have also been suggested.[97, 135, 137, 147] At this time, therefore, a cyclic pattern of FSH elimination seems far from established. The problem is further complicated by the known fact that FSH release by the pituitary follows a *circadian pattern*.[27, 47] Heald and his associates[64] found that variations in the adenohypophysial content of LH followed a similar pattern.

The respective curves of FSH and LH activity explain the development of the ovarian cycle. During the first half, high levels of the former induce follicular maturation, whereas the preovulatory *peak* of LH, *acting on a ripened follicle*, initiates ovulation and ultimate formation of the corpus luteum.

It is still a moot point whether in addition there is a cycle of *luteotropic hormone* secretion (LTH). Stafford[123] believes that a discharge of luteotropin is necessary for the corpus luteum to remain active over the period of 10 to 12 days that its secretory activity persists normally. However, it has been shown in bitches that hypophysectomy immediately following ovulation does not interfere with the normal duration of the corpus luteum.[20, 125]

12.4.2. THE ROLE OF THE OVARY IN GONADOTROPIC REGULATION, THE FEEDBACK MECHANISM

The median eminence is a receptor of steroid stimuli (Chapter 8, Section 8.5).

In adequate dosages, estrogens stimulate production of LHRF, whereas progestogens have the opposite effect.[88] Thus, while adequate levels of FSH activity induce follicular maturation and, consequently, the production of estrogens, the latter in turn provoke the release of the counteracting hormone and in this way the opposite phase is established in the ovary. Alternatively, once the corpus luteum has achieved its functional capacity, it provides the necessary stimulus for the pituitary to release once more FSH, thus leading to renewed maturation of other follicles that in the next cycle are to take the place of the decaying corpus luteum. Although attempts have been made to explain the chronologic regulation of the 28 day cycle as a *rebound phenomenon* subject to the physicochemical law of mass action, it is evident that the constant and fixed rhythm at which these reactions occur *cannot be based exclusively on hormonal interrelationships.* Undoubtedly, the existence of a *neural factor* must be invoked in order to explain what impresses an alternating rhythm on these pituitary-ovarian interactions (see Fig. 12–16).

12.4.3. ROLE OF HYPOTHALAMUS IN REGULATING THE OVARIAN CYCLE

That the sexual cycle in rodents is controlled by the hypothalamus has been known ever since publication of the pioneering experiments of Everett and his group.[44, 45, 93] In Chapter 8, we made it clear that the rhythm of pituitary secretion depends on the action of "releasing factors," which are derived from the median eminence, on the sexual center of the "tuber cinereum." Elaboration of FSHRF and LHRF is conditioned by ovarian steroid activity, viz., activity of estrogens and progestogens. Thus, the *hormonal rebound* mechanism seems to have been conclusively established. In any case, *the alternating endocrine rhythm under consideration is recognized as being determined by an inherent property of the hypothalamus* whose role as pacemaker of the internal rhythm of the body (nocturnal rhythm, rhythm of metabolism, etc.) is readily apparent.

The part played by the nervous system in the sexual cycle is particularly evident in the human species, in which emotional factors are known to affect ovarian function as well as menstruation. Many years ago, Stieve[125] had demonstrated the influence of emotion on *ovarian* activity. The influence of emotional factors on *menstrual* alterations is discussed in clinical terms in Chapter 32.

12.5. OVULATION

The phenomenon of ovulation merits special consideration in this chapter. Here we shall study the normal process in detail, but the clinical diagnostic problems concerning ovulation will be dealt with in Chapter 23 and following chapters.

12.5.1. DESCRIPTION OF OVULATION

The phenomenon of ovulation has been studied by a great many investigators in rats, rabbits and, less frequently, women.[143] According to Schroeder, as well as, more recently, Strassmann,[126] Corner[28] and Blandau,[14] ovulation in rats is preceded by progressive displacement of the follicle toward the ovarian surface. A wedge of theca interna is driven between the elements of the albuginea until this layer is effaced at the point of direct contact with the theca and granulosa and separated from the free surface merely by a thin layer of germinal epithelium. At this point, a small herniation of the granulosa develops through this surface and, shortly thereafter, the follicle ruptures and the follicular fluid is ejected. It has been possible to visualize this physiologic phenomenon directly. As early as 1928, Walton and Hammond were able to contemplate the occurrence of ovulation in a rabbit through a plastic window placed in the animal's abdomen. In 1934, availing himself of the same method, Smith studied ovulation in rabbits and rats. Reynolds[110] also happened to observe ovulation in the course of laparotomies performed on experimental animals. In several instances, it has been possible to visualize the process of ovulation even in the human species by means of culdoscopy. Interestingly, in some women the incidence of ovulation can be felt by virtue of the so-called "ovulation pain," which in some patients may be so selective that ovulation can be recognized in each cycle to occur either in one ovary or the other.

12.5.2. CAUSES OF OVULATION

Ovulation results from the combined actions of several factors—endocrine, vascular, nervous and enzymatic.

ENDOCRINE FACTORS. Maturation of the follicle is at present known to be an effect of FSH activity, whereas *ovulation is due to the action of LH*.[12, 85, 144] Buxton and Herrmann,[23] as well as Velardo,[142] have seen ovulation in the rat occur solely under the effect of chorionic gonadotropin while, on the contrary, the hormone of follicular maturation in this case was found to be incapable of inducing ovulation. Ovulation in rats can be produced by the injection of LH, either alone[130] or in equal parts with FSH,[86] these animals reacting readily to LH, as shown by Bettendorf[12] and by Saunders.[118] Johannison and his group[71] have shown that chorionic gonadotropin does not produce ovulation in the human species and that results are equivocal when gonadotropin of pregnant mare serum is used. Better results are obtained with injections of purified extracts of human pituitaries.[12, 71] Such extracts, containing predominantly, though not exclusively, FSH, are effective by themselves in provoking ovulation; however, their effects are strengthened by the addition of chorionic gonadotropin which, when given alone, is totally ineffective.

While FSH alone can induce ovulation in the cow,[92] the presence of LH is necessary to produce ovulation in the monkey.[87, 141] LH activity is similarly indispensable for the induction of ovulation in rabbits.[19, 60]

At present, the most commonly held view[23, 71, 143, 144] is that, just as in monkeys and rabbits, LH is the *decisive ovulation-inducing factor* in woman, provided its action is exerted on completely mature follicles, that is, follicles previously acted upon by FSH. Johanisson and his colleagues[71] have found that the period of time that must be let elapse between the injection of FSH and that of LH for this purpose is 96 hours.

VASCULAR MECHANISM OF OVULATION. In 1947, a system of spiral arteries, very similar to that found in the endometrium and unquestionably playing a role in ovulation, was described by Reynolds[110] in the rabbit ovary. In 1948, the presence of such spiral vessels was also demonstrated in the human ovary.[34] Reynolds had shown that the spiral vessels in the rabbit ovary responded in a characteristic way to chorionic gonadotropin activity, which caused them to proliferate. The vascular reaction to chorionic gonadotropin in the rabbit is equivalent to that seen in rats in the so-called *ovarian hyperemia test*. Various authors (Kupperman et al.,[78] Fried and Rakoff,[51] and Albert and Berkson[1]) have verified the fact that LH produces a characteristic hyperemic reaction in the rat ovary. This is the same type of hyperemic reaction that in a previous section was described as immediately preceding ovulation. LH can therefore be assumed to produce hyperemia of the ripened follicle and to contribute to the development of Reynolds' spiral arteries, which trigger ovulation. It will be pointed out in Chapter 13 that menstruation is due to a very similar mechanism. It is possible that certain neurogenic factors, such as chemical mediators exerting a direct vascular effect on vasomotor nerve endings, are at play in producing hyperemia by controlling the function of the spiral vessels. This would certainly explain the neurogenic mechanism of ovulation, which is discussed in the following section.

Ovarian vascularization is less pronounced in older animals, in which ovulation is proportionately more difficult (Zarrow and Wilson[152]).

Thorsoe[138] and Blandau[14] believe that ovulation is precipitated by an abrupt rise in intrafollicular pressure owing to sudden depolymerization of mucopolysaccharides within the follicular cavity. Thyroid hormone presumably speeds up the rate of that depolymerization and is thus believed to be a factor indirectly implicated in ovulation.

NEUROGENIC FACTORS IN OVULATION. In some animals, such as the rabbit (Section 12.1.5), the fact that the nervous system intervenes in ovulation is quite apparent; however, considering what we have so far learned about the role of the median eminence (see Chapter 8, Section 8.5), neural regulation of ovulation is clearly evident in all species. A complete review of the subject may be found in a recent report by Harris.[62]

Meyerson and Sawyer[96] have brought to light the action exerted by *monoamines* on LHRF and on ovulation. Experiments on this subject have been performed by Nikitovitsch,[102] who was able to produce ovulation in rats by means of locally injecting pituitary transplants with hypothalamic extracts. These experimental findings turned out to be the missing link that closed what had for many years been a hypothetical circuit, now proved to actually exist.

While ovulation in some animals, such as rats, is regulated primarily by endocrine processes, it is invariably also influenced by neural factors. In other animals, such as rabbits, ovulation occurs by virtue of a pure neuroendocrine reflex. However, the situation in woman is an intermediate one in that the endocrine chain of events terminating in ovulation is set off by an all-important reflex that originates in the target organs, is transmitted by the spinal cord and is elaborated in the hypothalamus, specifically in the median eminence.

PSYCHIC FACTORS IN OVULATION. In view of the profound influence wielded by the central nervous system on the course of ovulation, it is only natural to assume that ovulation must also be subject to psychogenic causes. In rodents, a series of behavioral factors are known to affect ovulation.[37, 94] Botella and Sanchez-Garrido[117] found that, as a result of captivity, female monkeys developed anovulatory cycles. Psychoanalytic considerations in human ovulation have been described by Nesbitt and co-workers.[101]

ENZYMATIC FACTORS IN OVULATION. As early as 1916, Schochet voiced the opinion that rupture of the ovarian follicle was caused by digestion of the follicle wall. The presence of a proteolytic enzyme in sow follicles was later demonstrated by Held. Moricard and Gothie[98] believed that the activity of this proteolytic enzyme was stimulated by gonadotropins. However, most of these ideas were based on mere speculation. Ultrastructural studies of the ovarian follicle seem to suggest the involvement of enzyme activity in follicular rupture (Espey[43]). Espey and Lipner[42] reported the finding of a *collagenolytic enzyme* that produced ovulation. By injecting small amounts of bacterial collagenase into the antrum of large follicles, they achieved follicular rupture that was indistinguishable from genuine ovulation.

12.6. THE OVARIAN HORMONAL CYCLE

The preceding sections dealt with the ovarian cycle and the underlying hormonal and neural causes. After having gained some understanding of these aspects, we may now proceed to considering again the consequences of the ovarian cycle. In terms of genetics, the immediate consequence of the ovarian cycle is the *expulsion of the ovum*. In terms of endocrinology, the immediate consequence is the creation of a cycle of hormone secretion involving alternate predominance of estrogens and progesterone.

12.6.1. CYCLIC SECRETION OF ESTROGENS

Most of the early data concerning periodic estrogen production were based on *urinary values*. Reliable information on plasma values have been a relatively recent acquisition.

ESTROGENURIA DURING THE CYCLE. The first determinations of urinary estrogens known to have been achieved with a certain degree of accuracy were those reported by D'Amour[31] in 1940, and by Jayle[69] in 1945. We owe it mainly to the work of Diczfalusy and Lauritzen,[36] as well as Loraine and Bell,[84] that precise data concerning urinary excretion of total and fractionated estrogens are now available. Recent studies by Goering's group,[53] and by Svendsen and Sörensen,[131] confirm these earlier results as essentially correct.

The curve of estrogenuria shows an upswing during the first half of the cycle, experiencing afterwards a slight dip at the time of ovulation. It keeps rising during the luteal phase and descends ultimately and definitively in the premenstrual period. This double humped estrogen excretion curve is the result of superposition of two partial estrogen curves, the first produced by follicular activity, the second by corpus luteum activity, the latter also constituting an important source of hormone, as has already been pointed out (Chapter 2).

PLASMA ESTROGEN LEVELS DURING THE CYCLE. Plasma estrogen values during the cycle have been studied by means of biologic procedures (Markee and Everett[93]), and by biochemical methods (Diczfalusy and Lauritzen,[36] Oertel and Kaiser,[104] and Baird and Guevara[6]).

The plasma curves run parallel to the urinary curve, showing a rise during the first half of the cycle, a drop at the time of ovulation and a second rise during the luteal phase.

Soliman and Nasr[122] have been able to demonstrate increased estrogenuria during estrous activity in rats.

These recent observations, performed with reliable and objective methods on sufficient numbers of cases, fully confirm early assumptions regarding the shape of the hormonal curve during the cycle as well as the role of estrogens in initiating menstruation (see Chapter 13).

12.6.2. PROGESTERONE

Progesterone is not known to be eliminated in the urine other than in the form of a catabolite, pregnanediol. Pregnanedioluria and progesteronemia of the cycle will therefore be studied separately.

PREGNANEDIOLURIA DURING THE CYCLE. Modern studies compiling a great number of pregnanediol determinations during the ovarian cycle may be found in publications by Jayle[69] and in more recent works by Leventhal and his colleagues.[81] Tornero, at our laboratory, has performed a large number of determinations on isolated cases which may be integrated into Figure 12–11. Both this figure and Figure 12–13, taken from Brown, show that pregnanediol values are practically zero during the first half of the cycle, are positive only during the progestational phase and decrease at the time of ovulation. It must be recalled, however, that some investigators (Taymor[133] and Hilliard et al.[65]) described the presence of a *preovulatory elevation of pregnanediol values* corresponding to a *parallel elevation of progesteronemia.*

The first attempts at discerning any existing pattern of fluctuation in progesteronemia levels had already been made by the methods developed by Hooker and Forbes (see Chapter 3). Later, thanks mainly to the work done by Zander and co-workers,[115, 151] it was possible to study progesterone concentrations by means of microchemical methods. An initial tentative curve was drawn up by Riondel and his associates[111] and later by Van der Molen and his co-workers,[139, 140] as well as by Hobzova and Novak.[66] The latter two in-

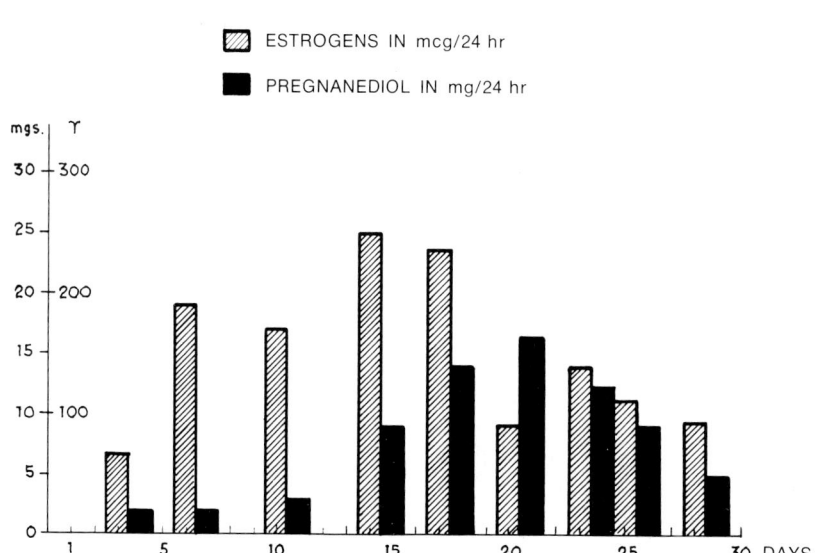

Figure 12–11. Elimination of total estrogens and pregnanediol in the course of normal cycle. (From Tornero.)

Establishment of the Sexual Cycle: the Ovarian Cycle 251

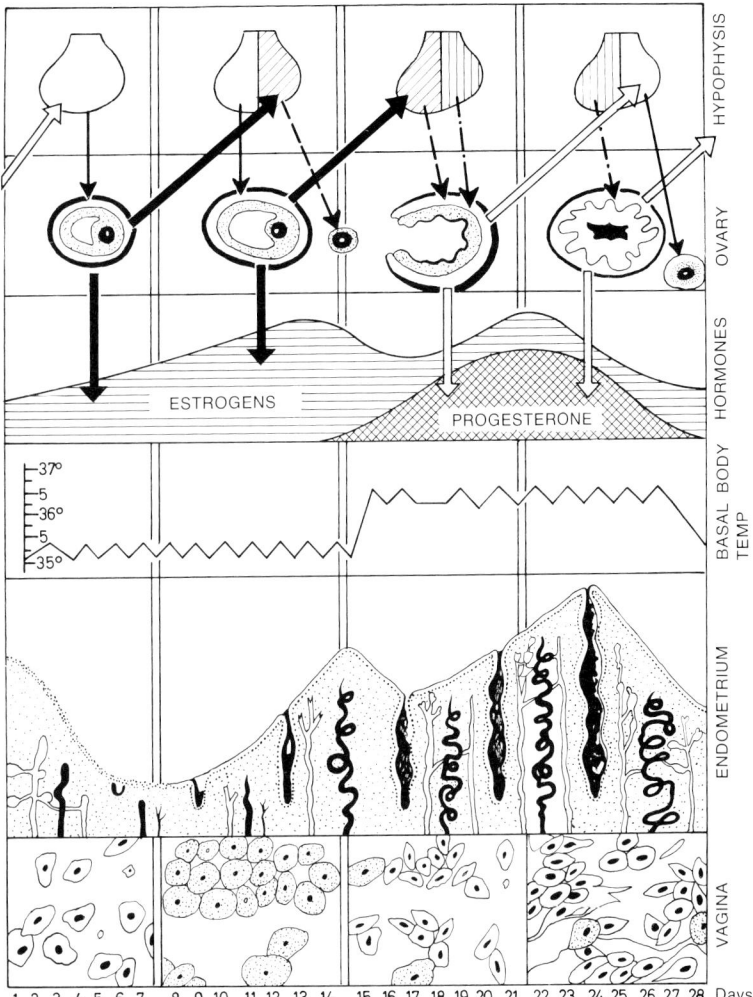

Figure 12-12. Diagram of menstrual cycle.

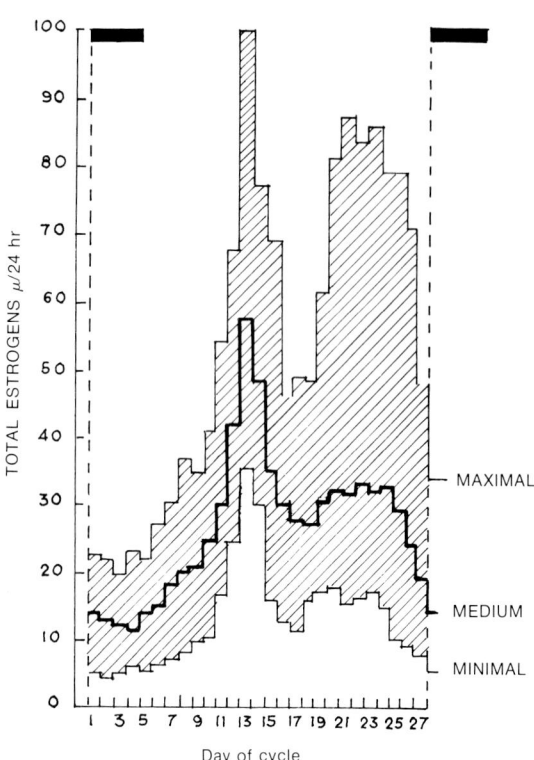

Figure 12-13. Fluctuations in total estrogen levels in the course of the cycle, as revealed by daily determinations among a group of 16 women with normal cycles. (From Brown, Keller, and Mathew: *J. Obstet. Gynec. Brit. Emp.*, 66:177, 1959.)

Figure 12-14. Excretion of total gonadotropins, pregnanediol, estriol, estrone and estradiol in the course of cycle in normal woman. (From Brown, Klopper, and Loraine: *J. Endocr.*, 17:401, 1958.)

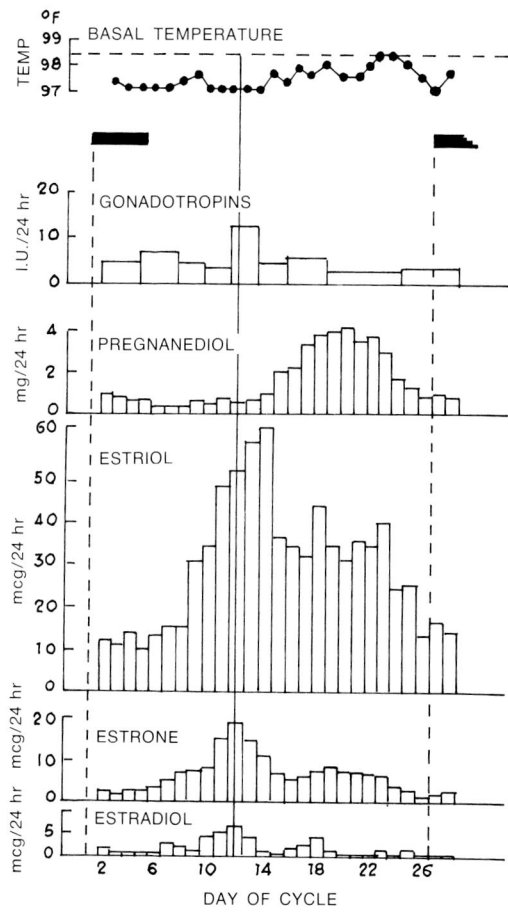

Establishment of the Sexual Cycle: the Ovarian Cycle   253

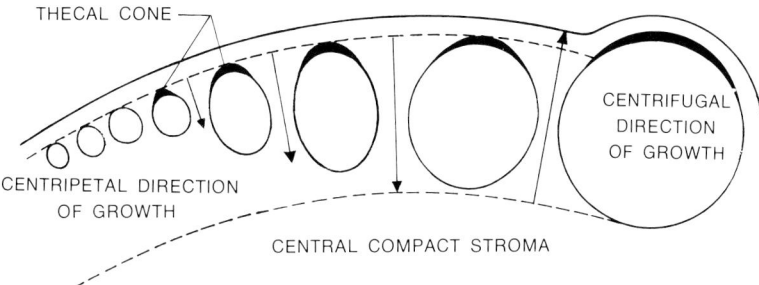

Figure 12-15. Diagram of follicular growth. Initial growth results in centripetal displacement. Once its size reaches central fibrous stroma, follicle can no longer grow inwards and begins growing in a centrifugal direction, with resulting bulge over surface. The "thecal cone," described in the human species by Strassmann, is the result of centripetal growth. (From Botella-Llusiá et al.; *Fertilidad y Esterilidad Humanas,* 2nd ed. Barcelona, Editorial Científico-Médica, 1971.)

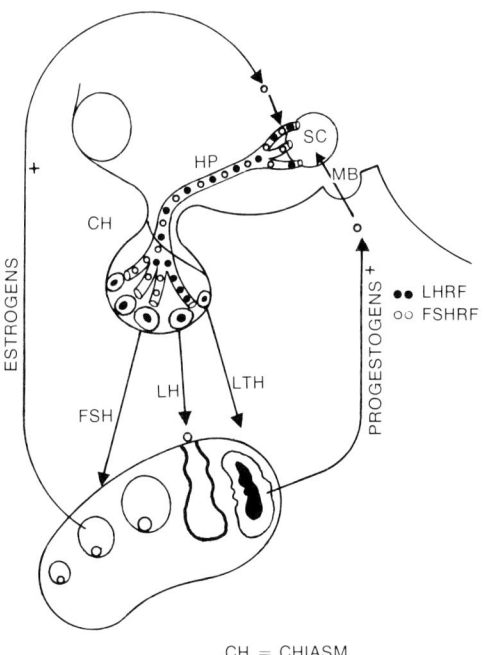

Figure 12-16. Diagram of "feedback" mechanism involved in human ovulation.

CH = CHIASM
HP = HYPOPHYSIOPORTAL VEIN
SC = SEX CENTER
MB = MAMMILLARY BODY

vestigators found that normal values ranged from less than 0.1 mcg between the first and tenth days of the cycle, to 1.60 mcg between the eleventh and fifteenth days, 1.25 mcg between the sixteenth and twentieth days, and 0.44 mcg from the twentieth day onwards. This curve is of interest because, as we pointed out previously, it actually indicates progesterone production *prior to ovulation, probably by the mature follicle.* Progesterone production by mature cow follicles has been recorded by Lisse and Schürenkämper.[82] Recently, Neill and colleagues[99, 100] reconstructed the progesteronemia curve for woman and for the female monkey. It closely resembles that obtained by Van der Molen and reveals a similar preovulatory peak, which has given rise to much speculation. Rising preovulatory progesteronemia values have lately also been confirmed by Neill and his colleagues[99] and by Hopper and Tullner[67] in female monkeys, and by Kazama and Hansel[74] in cows.

The existence of variations in estrogen and progesterone levels during the ovarian cycle is no longer a matter of speculation but is based on dependable data concerning the manner in which these two hormones and their catabolites are excreted and, what is more important, the manner in which their blood levels are modified.

12.7. SYNOPSIS OF THE OVARIAN CYCLE AND ITS EFFECTS

The ovarian cycle and its relationships with the pituitary and the target organs are summarized in Figure 12-12. This figure also reproduces estrogen and progesterone secretion curves as computed on the basis of current research, and indicates changes in basal body temperature, in endometrial morphology and in vaginal cytology.

In summing up this chapter, it must be emphasized that the sexual cycle in the human species is autoregulated at a constant and fixed internal rhythm, which is independent of outside influences to a much greater extent than is that of lower animals.

It is apparent that, as a species becomes increasingly domesticated and gains a greater measure of independence from the environment, it creates its own reproductive microcosmos, in contradistinction to the wild animal, which lives engulfed in the macrocosmos.

The relatively constant manner in which ovarian hormone secretion influences the hypothalamus and the hypothalamus in turn influences the adenohypophysis, the regularity throughout the cycle with which the pituitary releases its gonadotropins in a rhythmic fashion and, finally, the manner in which this concerted teamwork influences the sexual target organs constitute one of the most admirable and precise mechanisms of reproductive physiology.

REFERENCES

1. Albert, A., and Berkson, S.: *J. Clin. Endocr.,* 11:805, 1951.
2. Anderson, R. R., and MacShan, W. H.: *Endocrinology,* 78:976, 1966.
3. Aron, G., Asch, C., Asch, L.: *Gynec. Obstet.,* 62:53, 1953.
4. Ashbel, R., and Seligman, A. M.: *Endocrinology,* 44:565, 1949.
5. Austin, C. R.: *Nature,* 213:1018, 1967.
6. Baird, D. T., and Guevara, A.: *J. Clin. Endocr.,* 29:149, 1969.
7. Barker, W. L.: *Endocrinology,* 48:772, 1951.
8. Becker, K. L., and Albert, A.: *J. Clin. Endocr. Metab.,* 25:962, 1965.
9. Behrman, S. J., and Duboff, G. S.: *Fertil. Steril.,* 11:210, 1960.
10. Bell, E. T., Mukerjee, S., Loraine, J. A., and Lunn, S. F.: *Acta Endocr.,* 51:578, 1966.
11. Benoit, J., Assenmacher, I., and Berard, E.: Action de l'eclairement prolongé sur l'evolution testiculaire du canard de Peking," in *Le Sexe.* Paris, Masson et Cie., 1960.
12. Bettendorf, G.: *Arch. Gynäk.,* 202:132, 1965.
13. Bisonette, T. H.: *Quart. Rev. Biol.,* 11:271, 1936.
14. Blandau, R. J.: *Clin. Obstet. Gynec.,* 10:347, 1967.
15. Bonnin-Laffargue, M., and Canivenc, R.: *Ann. d'Endocr.,* 23:164, 1962.
16. Borell, U., and Westman, A.: *Acta Endocr.,* 3:111, 1949.
17. Brandau, H., Remlinger, K., and Luh, W.: *Acta Endocr.,* 56:433, 1967.
18. Breed, W. G., and Clarke, J. R.: *J. Reprod. Fertil.,* 22:173, 1970.
19. Brinkley, H. J., and Nalbandov, A. V.: *Endocrinology,* 73:515, 1963.
20. Brinkley, H. J., Norton, H. W., and Nalbandov, A. V.: *Endocrinology,* 74:914, 1964.
21. Butcher, R. L., and Fugo, N. W.: *Fertil. Steril.,* 18:297, 1967.
22. Butcher, R. L., Blue, J. D., and Fugo, N. W.: *Fertil. Steril.,* 20:223, 1969.
23. Buxton, C. L., and Herrmann, W.: *Amer. J. Obstet. Gynec.,* 81:585, 1961.
24. Campell, H. J.: *J. Physiol.,* 181:368, 1965.

25. Cargille, C. M., and Ross, G. T.: *J. Clin. Endocr.*, 29:12, 1969.
26. Collett, M. E., Wertenberger, M. E., and Fisk, V. M.: *Fertil. Steril.*, 5:437, 1954.
27. Conway, L. W., Schalch, D. S., Utiger, R. D., and Reichlin, S.: *J. Clin. Endocr.*, 29:446, 1969.
28. Corner, G. W.: *Contrib. Embryol.*, 31:117, 1947.
29. Corner, G. W.: In *Menstruation and its Disorders*, ed. E. T. Engle. Springfield, Ill., Charles C Thomas, 1950.
30. Critchlow, W.: *Endocrinology*, 63:596, 1958.
31. D'Amour, G.: *Amer. J. Obstet. Gynec.*, 40:598, 1940.
32. Deane, H. W., Lobil, B. L., and Rommey, S. L.: *Amer. J. Obstet. Gynec.*, 83:281, 1962.
33. Delost, P.: *Arch. d'Anat. Microsc.*, 45:11, 1956.
34. Delson, B., Lubin, S., and Reynolds, S. R. M.: *Endocrinology*, 42:124, 1948.
35. Dempsey, E. W., Greep, R. O., and Deane, H. W.: *Endocrinology*, 44:88, 1949.
36. Diczfalusy, E., and Lauritzen, C.: *Oestrogene beim Menschen*. Berlin, Springer, 1961.
37. Doerner, G., Doecke, F., and Mustafa, S.: *J. Reprod. Fertil.*, 17:583, 1968.
38. Dubreuil, G.: *Ann. d'Endocr.*, 23:1, 1962.
39. Duncan, G. W., et al.: *Endocrinology*, 68:199, 1961.
40. Edwards, R. G.: *Nature*, 196:446, 1962.
41. El Fouly, M. A., Cook, B., Nekola, M., and Nalbandov, A. V.: *Endocrinology*, 87:288, 1970.
42. Espey, L. L., and Lipner, H.: *Amer. J. Physiol.*, 208:208, 1965.
43. Espey, L. L.: *Endocrinology*, 81:267, 1967.
44. Everett, J. W.: *Endocrinology*, 80:145, 1967.
45. Everett, J. W., and Tejasen, T.: *Endocrinology*, 80:790, 1967.
46. Exley, D., and Corker, S. C.: *J. Endocr.*, 35:83, 1966.
47. Fayman, C., and Ryan, R. J.: *Nature*, 215:857, 1967.
48. Folman, Y., and Drori, D.: *J. Reprod. Fertil.*, 11:43, 1966.
49. Fiske, R. I., and Lamond, D. R.: *Endocrinology*, 64:175, 1959.
50. Fox, R. R.: *Proc. Soc. Exper. Biol. Med.*, 128:639, 1968.
51. Fried, P. H., and Rakoff, A. E.: *J. Clin. Endocr. Metab.*, 10:423, 1950.
52. Fukushima, M., Stevens, V. C., Gant, C. L., and Vorys, N.: *J. Clin. Endocr. Metab.*, 24:205, 1964.
53. Goering, R. W., et al.: *Amer. J. Obstet. Gynec.*, 92:441, 1965.
54. Gorski, R., and Wagner, W. J.: *Endocrinology*, 76:226, 1965.
55. Gospodarovicz, D.: *Biochim. Biophys. Acta*, 100:618, 1965.
56. Green, J. A., Garcilaso, J. A., and Maqueo, M.: *Amer. J. Obstet. Gynec.*, 99:855, 1967.
57. Grindeland, R. E., and Folk, G. E.: *J. Reprod. Fertil.*, 4:11, 1962.
58. Guraya, S. S., and Greenwald, G. S.: *Amer. J. Anat.*, 114:495, 1964.
59. Hagino, N., Ramaley, J. A., and Gorski, R. A.: *Endocrinology*, 79:451, 1966.
60. Harper, M. J. K.: *J. Endocr.*, 26:307, 1963.
61. Harrington, F. E., Eggert, R. E., Wilbur, R. D., and Linkenhaimer, W. H.: *Endocrinology*, 79:1130, 1966.
62. Harris, G. W.: *Amer. J. Obstet. Gynec.*, 105:659, 1970.
63. Harris, G. W., and Levine, S.: *J. Physiol.*, 181:379, 1965.
64. Heald, P. J., Furnival, B. E., and Rookledge, K. A.: *J. Endocr.*, 37:73, 1967.
65. Hilliard, J., et al.: *Endocrinology*, 72:79, 1963.
66. Hobzova, J., and Novak, M.: *Endokrinologie*, 52:366, 1967.
67. Hopper, B., and Tullner, W. W.: *Endocrinology*, 85:1225, 1970.
68. Jacobson, D., and Norgren, A.: *Acta Endocr.*, 49:453, 1965.
69. Jayle, M. F.: *L'ovaire et ses fonctions*. Paris, Gauthier Villars, 1966.
70. Joel, R. V., and Foraker, A. G.: *Amer. J. Obstet. Gynec.*, 80:314, 1960.
71. Johanisson, E., Gemzell, C. A., and Diczfalusy, E.: *J. Clin. Endocr. Metab.*, 21:1068, 1961.
72. Kaufmann, C., Westphal, U., and Zander, J.: *Arch. Gynäk.*, 179:357, 1951.
73. Kawakami, M., and Sawyer, C. H.: *Endocrinology*, 65:631, 1959.
74. Kazama, N., and Hansel, W.: *Endocrinology*, 86:1252, 1970.
75. Keller, P. J., and Rosemberg, E.: *J. Clin. Endocr.*, 25:1050, 1965.
76. Kirton, K. T., Niswender, G. G., Midgley, A. R., Jaffe, R. B., and Forbes, A. D.: *J. Clin. Endocr.*, 30:105, 1970.
77. Koppen, K.: *Zbl. Gynäk.*, 78:915, 1950.
78. Kupperman, H. S., MacShan, W. H., and Meyer, R. K.: *Endocrinology*, 43:275, 1948.
79. Lamond, D. R., and Braden, A. W. H.: *Endocrinology*, 64:921, 1961.
80. Lehrman, P. S., Brody, P. N., and Wortis, R. P.: *Endocrinology*, 68:507, 1961.
81. Leventhal, J. M., Roman, F. F., and Wotiz, H. H.: *Boston Med. Quart.*, 11:46, 1960.
82. Lisse, K., and Schürenkämper, P.: *Acta Endocr.*, 50:429, 1965.
83. Lobel, N. L., Rosenbaum, R. M., and Deane, H. W.: *Endocrinology*, 68:232, 1961.
84. Loraine, J. A., and Bell, E. T.: *Lancet*, 1:1340, 1963.
85. Loraine, J. A., and Bell, E. T.: *J. Obstet. Gynec. Brit. Comm.*, 75:71, 1968.
86. Lostroh, A. J., and Johnson, R. E.: *Endocrinology*, 79:991, 1966.
87. MacArthur, J. W., et al.: *J. Clin. Endocr. Metab.*, 18:1186, 1958.
88. MacCann, S. M., et al.: *Amer. J. Physiol.*, 202:601, 1963.
89. MacCormack, C. E., and Bennin, B.: *Endocrinology*, 86:611, 1970.
90. MacGaughey, R. W., and Chang, M. C.: *J. Exper. Zool.*, 170:937, 1969.
91. MacKay, D. G., Pinkerton, J. H., and Hertig, A. T.: *Obstet. Gynec.*, 18:13, 1961.
92. Marden, W. G. R.: *Endocrinology*, 50:546, 1951.
93. Markee, J. E., and Everett, J. W.: *Rec. Progr. Horm. Res.*, 7:139, 1952.
94. Matsumoto, S., Igarashi, M., and Nagaoka, Y.: *Internat. J. Fertil.*, 13:15, 1968.
95. Meyer, R. K., MacShan, W. H., and Erway, W. F.: *Endocrinology*, 37:431, 1945.
96. Meyerson, B. J., and Sawyer, C. H.: *Endocrinology*, 83:170, 1968.
97. Midgley, A. R., and Jaffe, R. B.: *J. Clin. Endocr.*, 28:1699, 1968.

98. Moricard, R., and Gothie, S.: *Ciba Colloquium on Mammalian Germ Cells.* London, Churchill, 1953.
99. Neill, J. D., Johansson, E. D. B., and Knobil, E.: *Endocrinology,* 81:1161, 1967.
100. Neill, J. D., Johansson, E. D. B., Datta, J. K., and Knobil, E.: *J. Clin. Endocr. Metab.,* 27:1167, 1967.
101. Nesbitt, R. E. L., Holander, M., Fisher, S., and Sosofsky, H. J.: *Fertil. Steril.,* 19:778, 1968.
102. Nikitovitsch, M. B.: *Endocrinology,* 70:351, 1962.
103. Odell, W. D., Ross, G. T., and Rayford, P. L.: *J. Clin. Invest.,* 46:248, 1967.
104. Oertel, G. W., and Kaiser, E.: *Klin. Wschr.,* 39:492, 1961.
105. Ohno, S., and Smith, J. B.: *Cytogenetics,* 3:324, 1964.
106. Orr, A. H., Ward, A. P., and Bagshave, K. D.: *J. Reprod. Fertil.,* 21:307, 1970.
107. Pinkerton, J. H. M., et al.: *Obstet. Gynec.,* 18:152, 1961.
108. Radford, H. M.: *J. Endocr.,* 34:135, 1966.
109. Rennels, E. G.: *Endocrinology,* 79:373, 1966.
110. Reynolds, S. R. M.: *Rec. Progr. Horm. Res.,* 5:186, 1950.
111. Riondel, A., et al.: *Endocrinology,* 25:229, 1965.
112. Robertson, H. A., and Rakha, A. M.: *J. Endocr.,* 32:383, 1965.
113. Rosemberg, E., and Keller, P. J.: *J. Clin. Endocr. Metab.,* 25:1262, 1965.
114. Rosemberg, E., Joshi, S. R., and Nwe, T. T.: *J. Clin. Endocr.,* 28:1419, 1968.
115. Runnebaum, B., and Zander, J.: *Acta Endocr.,* 55:91, 1967.
116. Ryan, H. J., and Smith, O. W.: *Acta Endocr.,* 44:81, 1963.
117. Sanchez-Garrido, F., Nogales, F., and Botella, J.: *Acta Gin.,* 21, 1970.
118. Saunders, F. J.: *Endocrinology,* 40:1, 1947.
119. Sawyer, C. H., Everett, J. W., and Markee, J. E.: *Endocrinology,* 44:218, 234, 1949.
120. Schrank, P., and Koch, K. H.: *Ztschr. Geb. Gyn.,* 130:200, 1948.
121. Singh, R. P., and Carr, D. H.: *Obstet. Gynec.,* 29:806, 1967.
122. Soliman, F. A., and Nasr, H.: *Nature,* 194:154, 1962.
124. Stafford, R. O., et al.: *Endocrinology,* 41:45, 1947.
124. Stegner, H. E., and Wartenberg, H.: *Arch. Gynäk.,* 196:23, 1961.
125. Stieve, H.: *Arch. Gynäk.,* 183:178, 1953.
126. Strassmann, E. O.: *Internat. J. Fertil.,* 6:135, 1961.
127. Sturkie, P. D., and Freedman, S. L.: *J. Reprod. Fertil.,* 4:81, 1962.
128. Swanson, H. E., and Van der Werff, J. J.: *Acta Endocr.,* 47:37, 1964.
129. Staples, R. E.: *J. Reprod. Fertil.,* 13:429, 1967.
130. Sugawara, S., and Takeuchi, S.: *Endocrinology,* 86:965, 1970.
131. Svendsen, R., and Sörensen, B.: *Acta Endocr.,* 47:245, 1964.
132. Taylor, E. B.: *Acta Endocr.,* 136:361, 1961.
133. Taymor, M. L.: *J. Clin. Endocr. Metab.,* 21:976, 1961.
134. Taymor, M. L., Aono, T., and Pheteplace, C.: *Acta Endocr.,* 59:298, 1968.
135. Taymor, M. L., Lieberman, B., and Rikzallah, T. H.: *Fertil. Steril.,* 20:267, 1969.
136. Tejasen, T., and Everett, J. W.: *Endocrinology,* 81:1387, 1967.
137. Thomas, K., and Ferin, J.: In *L'ovulation,* ed. R. Moricard and J. Ferin. Paris, Masson et Cie., 1969.
138. Thorsoe, H.: *Acta Endocr.,* 41:441, 1963.
139. Van der Molen, H., et al.: *J. Clin. Endocr. Metab.,* 25:170, 1965.
140. Van der Molen, H., and Groen, D.: *J. Clin. Endocr. Metab.,* 25:1625, 1965.
141. Van Waagenen, G., and Simpson, M. E.: *Endocrinology,* 61:316, 1957.
142. Velardo, J. T.: *Science,* 137:357, 1960.
143. Villee, C. A.: *Control of Ovulation.* New York, Pergamon Press, 1961.
144. Wallach, E. W.: *Clin. Obstet. Gynec.,* 10:361, 1967.
145. Watzka, M.: "Ovarium," in Von Moellendorf, *Handbuch der Mikroskopischen Anatomie,* Vol. VII. Munich, J. F. Bergmann, 1957.
146. Westman, A.: *Arch. Gynäk.,* 183:131, 1953.
147. Wilde, C. E., Orr, A. H., and Bagshave, K. D.: *J. Endocr.,* 37:23, 1967.
148. Williams, P. C.: In *Ciba Colloquia on Ageing,* Vol. II. London, Churchill, 1956.
149. Woolever, C. A.: *Amer. J. Obstet. Gynec.,* 85:981, 1963.
150. Wurtman, R. J., et al.: *Endocrinology,* 81:509, 1967.
151. Zander, J.: *Arch. Gynäk.,* 196:481, 1962.
152. Zarrow, M. X., and Wilson, E. D.: *Endocrinology,* 69:851, 1961.
153. Zellmaker, G. H.: *Acta Endocr.,* 46:571, 1964.
154. Zogbi, F., Begue, J. A., and Jayle, M. F.: *Compt. Rend. Soc. Biol. (Paris),* 160:586, 1966.
155. Zuckermann, S.: *The Ovary,* Vol. I. London, Churchill, 1961.

Chapter 13
SEXUAL CYCLE IN TARGET ORGANS

The ovarian cycle determines the alternate secretion of the two female sex hormones: estrogen and progesterone. The manner in which these two incretory substances are elaborated in the course of the cycle was analyzed in Chapter 12. By exercising control over the physiology of the genital tract and affecting quite distant organs and tracts, these two hormones determine the occurrence of cyclic changes in the entire female body. The physiology of woman as a whole may be said to be affected in one way or another by the monthly alternation of ovarian hormone activity.

This chapter deals with the cycle as it involves the Fallopian tube, the uterus, the uterine cervix and the vagina. In addition, we shall analyze the changes produced in the breast and in the endocrine glands, concluding with a discussion of such systemic cyclic phenomena as are observed to take place in metabolism and basal body temperature.

13.1. TUBAL CYCLE

Estrogenic hormonal activity produces a *proliferative phase* in the tubal mucosa, resulting in increased height of epithelial cells and some pseudostratification, the tubal epithelium assuming a picket fence appearance. In contrast, progesterone produces a *secretory phase* in the same epithelium, resulting in considerably diminished epithelial height, with nuclei aligned in a row and with appearance of goblet cells, whose secretion can be observed in the lumen. This tubal cycle has been described at our clinic by Cortés-Ruiz.[34] These cyclic tubal changes take place in order to provide nutrition for the egg or the ovum on its passage through the organ. Consequently, the embryo passes through a *tubotrophic phase of nutrition* (Botella[18]). Recently, Stegner[109] studied the tubal cycle with the electron microscope and indeed verified the existence of an initial proliferative phase, followed by a short period in midcycle during which *secretory changes* are quite apparent. The tubal musculature in addition experiences *cyclic movements*, which have been studied by De la Fuente[48] at our clinic. Spontaneous motility in this organ is minimal during the postmenstrual phase but gradually increases until reaching a maximum on the fifteenth day of the cycle, after which it again decreases little by little until the time of menstruation (Fig. 13-1).

The *rate of ovitransportation* has also

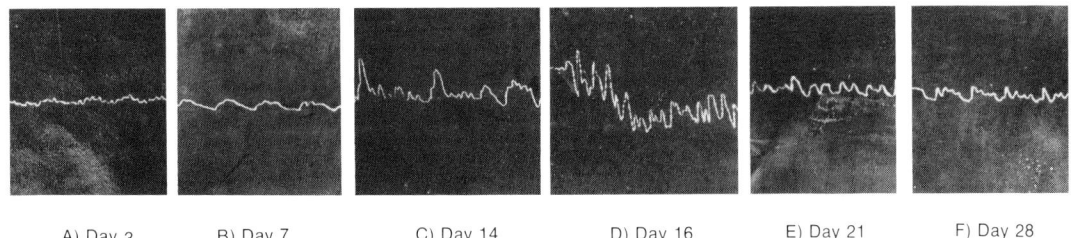

A) Day 3   B) Day 7   C) Day 14   D) Day 16   E) Day 21   F) Day 28

Figure 13-1. Tubal cycle: motility of "in vitro" isolated human tube in the course of the cycle. (From La Fuente and Botella: *Acta Gyn. Endocr.*, 2:62, 1949.)

been estimated by various authors.[35, 100] Estrogens speed up the rate at which the ovum is transported (Chapter 2), whereas progestogens slow it down (Chapter 3). Thus, the tube has its own cycle, apparent mainly in terms of tubal *motility*.

13.2. UTERINE CYCLE

Within the context of female endocrinologic processes, the uterine cycle is of utmost importance. Although the major onus of cyclic transformations is borne by the endometrium, the myometrium and the uterine cervix also partake in the monthly changes. We shall therefore study successively: (1) the endometrial cycle; (2) menstruation; and (3) the myometrial cycle.

13.2.1. ENDOMETRIAL CYCLE

The first histologic studies on menstruation appeared over a hundred years ago (Kiwisch, 1855). In 1865, Pflüger for the first time established a relationship between menstruation and ovulation but failed to appreciate any typical characteristic oscillations in the cycle. First to describe the existence of a cycle in the uterine mucosa were Kundrat and Engelman in 1873. However, their work has by now been almost completely forgotten. The discovery of the uterine cycle has been attributed to Hitschmann and Adler, although their work, significant as it was, was of a much later date than that of Kundrat and Engelman. A complete description of the endometrial cycle may be found in the writings of Schröder and Meyer, published simultaneously and independently in 1913. Their descriptions are classical and still serve as a model.

The uterine mucosa is divided into two parts: a basal layer and a functional layer (Fig. 13-2). While the basal layer remains unaltered, the functional layer undergoes cyclic changes and is shed at the time of menstruation. On the first day after the end of the monthly bleeding, the endometrium consists only of a thin basal layer (Fig. 13-3,A), not yet lined with surface epithelium and presenting a raw surface. In the following days, both the stromal and glandular components of the mucosa start to grow rapidly at the expense of the tubular glands of the zona basalis. Already, by the seventh day of the cycle, a functional zone, proliferating toward the surface, is clearly distinguishable from the basal zone. This phase is known as the *proliferative phase*. During the first week of the cycle, the functional layer consists of a dense and abundant stroma traversed by scanty epithelial tubules exhibiting a nearly rectilinear course (Fig. 13-3,B). Starting from the seventh day onwards, during the second week of the cycle, the functional layer becomes thicker and thicker, so that the glands contained in it undergo an eight- to

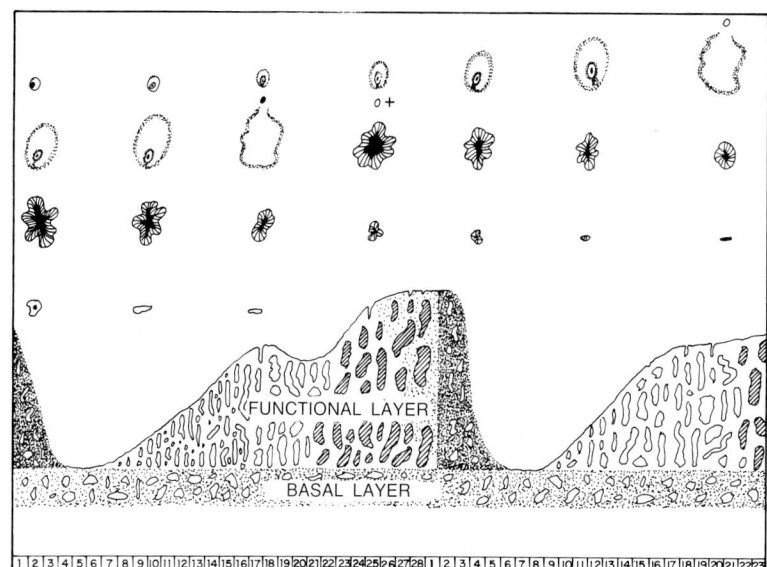

Figure 13-2. Schröder's classical scheme of the cycle. (From Botella: *Endocrinologia de la Mujer*, 1st ed. Madrid, Aquado, 1942.)

Sexual Cycle in Target Organs

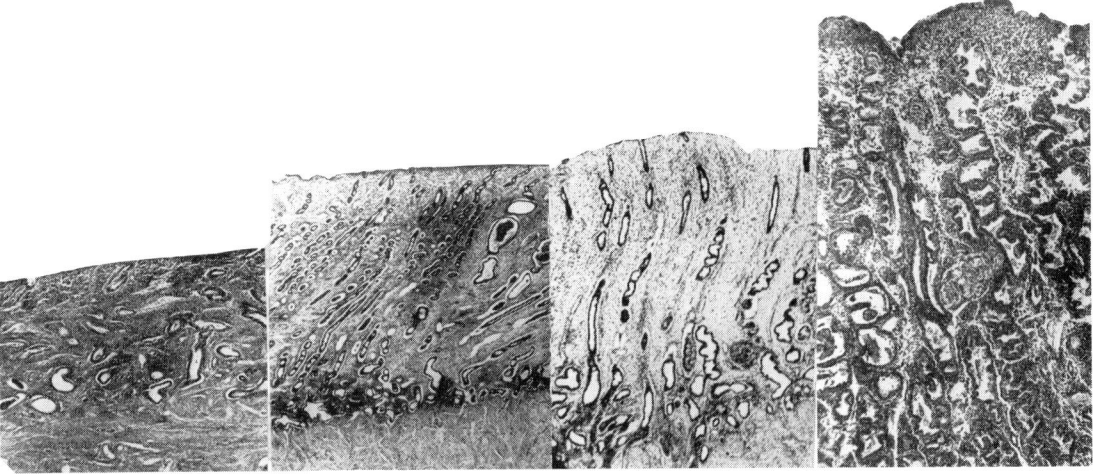

Figure 13-3. Histologic features of human endometrium in the course of the cycle (30×). A, Immediately postmenstrual; B, on the twelfth day of the cycle; C, on the sixteenth day of the cycle; D, on the twenty-sixth day of the cycle.

ten-fold increase in length. Even though the stroma is growing as well, its rate of expansion lags behind the rate of glandular growth, which obliges the glands to double up and to assume a zig-zag configuration (Fig. 13-4). As the moment of ovulation is reached, estrogenic activity ceases, or rather, ceases to be exerted independently and starts to be associated with progesterone activity. Here the proliferative phase comes to an end and the glands subsequently grow in length very little, if at all. Under the effect of progesterone activity from now onwards, the endometrial glands start to secrete, the epithelium experiencing very interesting changes that consist in dilatation and development of a characteristic acinar pattern between the fourteenth and twenty-first days, that is, during the third week of the cycle (Fig. 13-3,C). The *secretory phase* is thus fully established. During the fourth week of the cycle, which

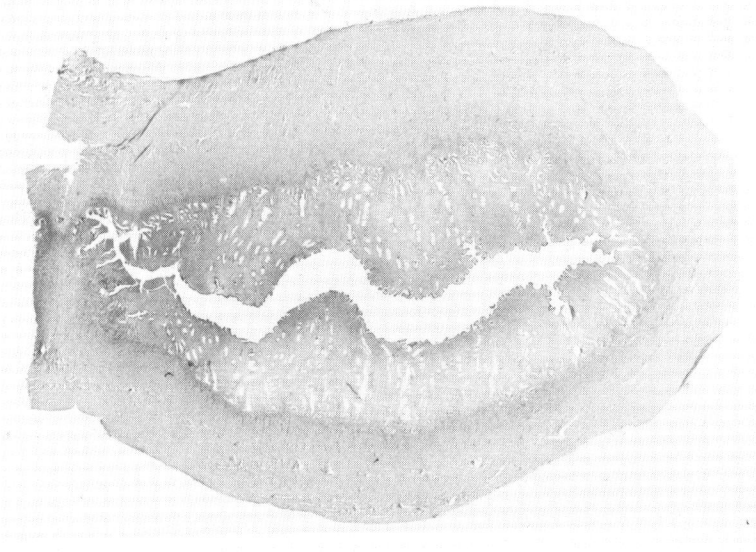

Figure 13-4. Cross section of human uterus on the twelfth day of the cycle, revealing proliferative phase at low magnification.

in a four-week cycle is between the twenty-first and twenty-sixth days, the secretory phase is at its strongest and stromal edema, as well as marked glandular dilatation with abundant products of secretion, is most pronounced (Fig. 13-3,D). Starting with the twenty-sixth day of the cycle, interstitial hemorrhages appear in the stroma and occasional areas of necrosis may begin to develop in the functional layer. This marks the onset of what is known as the *premenstrual phase*, which ends two to three days later with the complete shedding of the mucosa, whereby the endometrium is once more reduced to the starting point, that is, stripped to the basal layer.

This basal layer does not undergo any structural changes at any time during the cycle. Its histologic texture remains constant, as though it were made up of a stock of reserve cells from which the other layers periodically arise, evolve and then are shed. Every 28 days, the endometrium reenacts the same changes.

Among the various investigators who recently studied the structural changes of the endometrial glands are Moricard,[77] Hertig and Rock,[59] and Brewer and Jones,[24] as well as Philippe and his colleagues,[89] and Dallenbach-Hellweg.[38] These investigators paid special attention to the *histologic appearance* of the endometrium in relation to the different days of the cycle. During the first week, the epithelial tubules have a very narrow lumen and consist of a tall epithelium with nuclear pseudostratification. The stroma in this phase is dense and is composed of fusiform or oval connective tissue cells with scanty intervening ground substance and therefore in close proximity to each other. Although there is considerable widening of the gland lumen during the second week of the cycle, the epithelium retains the same characteristics. A finding of interest at this stage is the presence in it of mitotic figures. The stroma is less compact than in the first week. The epithelial changes are most interesting during the third week of the cycle. Mitotic figures are absent and so is pseudostratification of nuclei, which instead are lined up in a single row in the midportion of the cells. Finally, the stroma at this stage becomes looser and looser and shows a moderate degree of edema.

Highly typical glandular changes occur during the fourth week of the cycle. The epithelium becomes even more flattened, nuclei are closer to the basal pole of the cell and the cytoplasm of the luminal pole is seen disintegrating into the gland lumen. Glands are filled with abundant secretion and their contour is so tortuous that the stroma penetrates between their convolutions in the form of what Moricard[77] has termed *connective tissue spurs* (Fig. 13-3,D). A markedly edematous stroma reveals many venous lakes and foci of spotty hemorrhage.

In recent years, most interesting studies have been made concerning the ultrastructure of the endometrium. Clyman[32] and

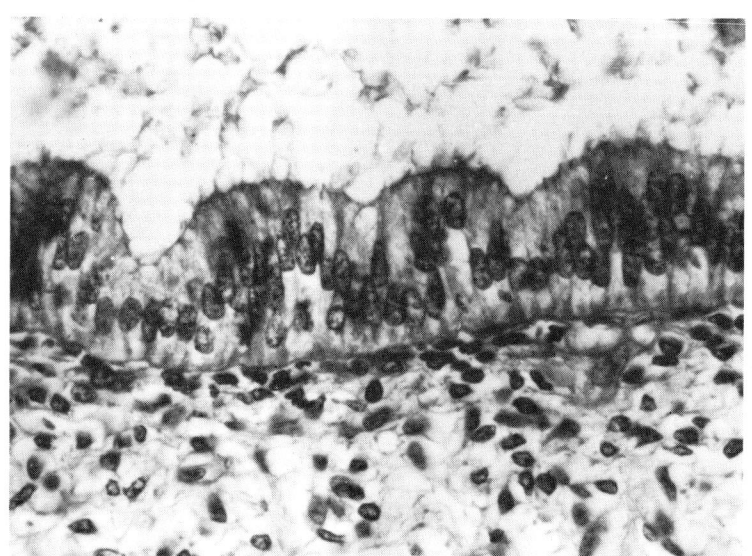

Figure 13-5. High power view of late proliferative phase in a castrated monkey (*Macaca mulatta*), injected with 0.8 mg of estrogen per kg of body weight. Note the tall epithelium with pseudostratification.

Sexual Cycle in Target Organs 261

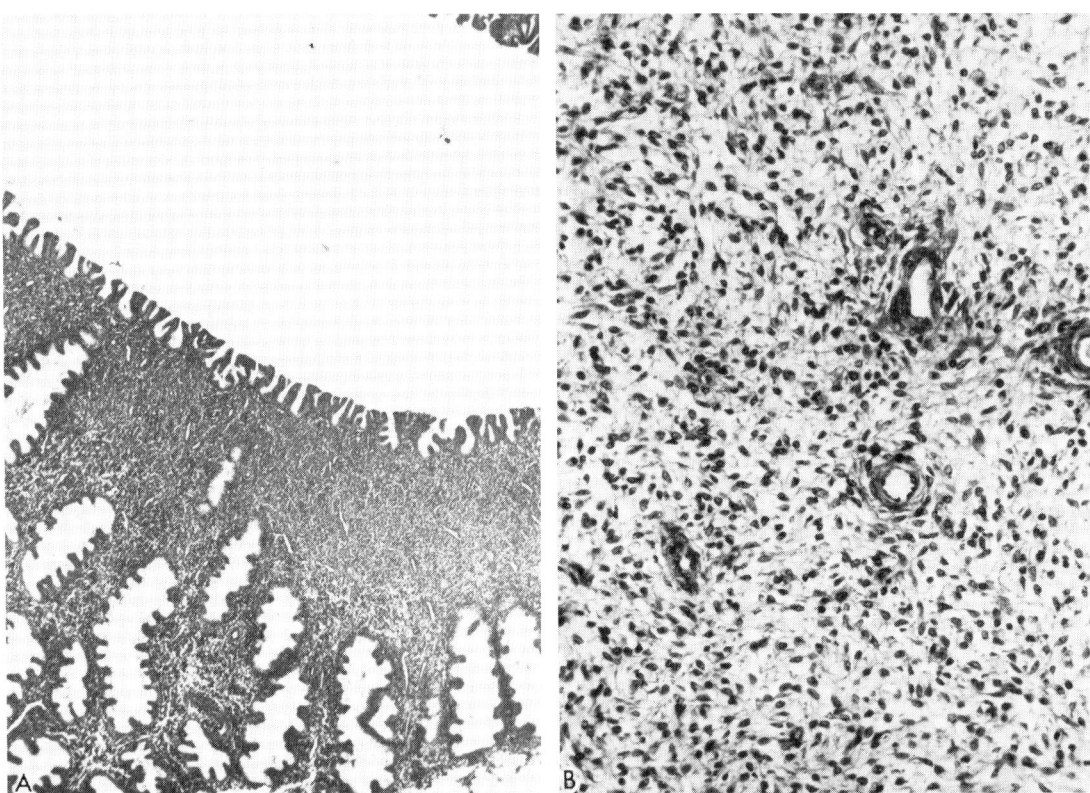

Figure 13-6. Secretory phase in castrated monkey (*Macaca mulatta*), obtained by means of consecutive injections of 0.8 mg/kg estradiol valerianate and 8 mg/kg hydroxyprogesterone caproate. *A*, Gland detail at intermediate power. *B*, Stromal detail at higher power, revealing spiral vessels.

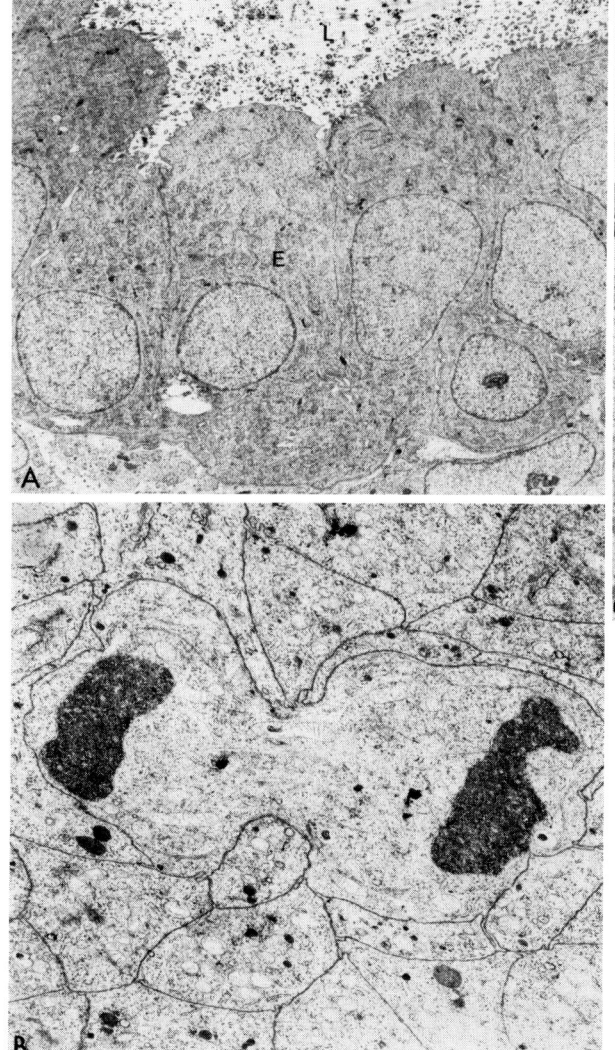
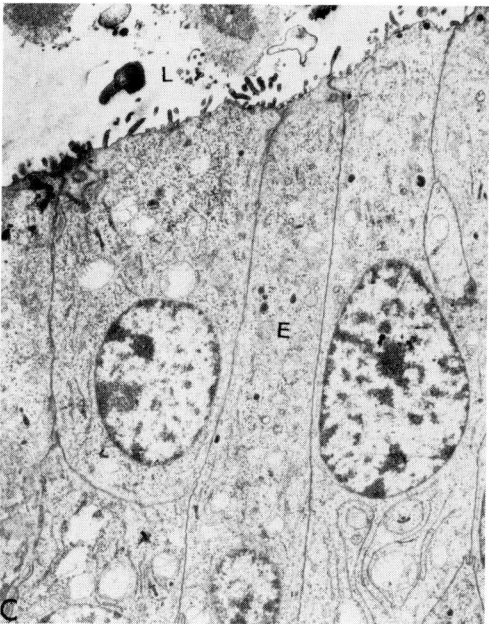

Figure 13–7. Ultrastructural features of the human endometrial cycle. *A*, Early proliferative phase (12,000×). *B*, Mitosis in anaphase in epithelial cell near end of proliferative phase (16,000×). *C*, Early secretory phase, with numerous microvilli on luminal surface, nucleus displaced toward lumen and scattered glycogen granules in cytoplasm (15,000×). E, Epithelium; L, gland lumen.

Gompel[52] have described cyclic changes in the gland epithelium and in the villous processes of the epithelial surfaces, as well as other peculiarities of endometrial fine structure.

Wynn and Wooley,[118] Cavazos and co-workers,[29] and Bickers and Krone[13] all subsequently repeated and amplified those studies on women. In addition, an interesting study on the ultrastructure of the endometrial cycle has been conducted by Cardell and co-workers,[28] using castrated female monkeys treated with known dosages of sex hormones.

Complementary enzymologic studies on the ultrastructural level have been published by Banon and his associates,[7] Bryson and Sweat[26] and Warren and co-workers.[117] Rather than entering into descriptive details concerning those findings, we refer the reader to the expressive illustrations in figure 13–7, which were obtained at our laboratory.

13.2.2. VASCULAR CYCLE OF THE ENDOMETRIUM

For many years this type of histologic change was believed to be the only change occurring in the endometrium during the menstrual cycle. By transplanting homografts of endometrial tissue into the anterior chamber of the eye in monkeys, Markee[72] was able to observe how the grafts "took" and by means of a corneal microscope succeeded in studying the vascular changes taking place in the grafted pieces of tissue. Even though the phenomena observed under these conditions cannot be likened entirely to those occurring in human menstruation, Markee was nevertheless able to recognize vascular endometrial changes induced by endocrine activity. Bartelmez,[8,9] and subsequently Daron,[39] carried such studies a step farther by analyzing the anatomic disposition of the vessels in question on the basis of intravascular injections of monkey endometria and, later, Brewer and Jones,[24,25] Okkels[85] and Kayser[63] performed similar studies on the vascular system in woman.

First, let us consider the general disposition of the uterine vessels. The main arterial network in this organ is derived from the branches of the uterine arteries and consists of the so-called *arcuate arteries* (Fig. 13–8), which run through the myometrium parallel with the serosal surface and give off, at right angles, the so-called *external radial arteries* reaching out to the peritoneal surface, and the *internal radial arteries*, directed toward the basalis of the endometrium. The internal radial arteries are provided with a powerful muscular coat and, since they are surrounded by smooth muscle in their course through the submucosal layers of the myometrium, contractions of the myometrium may cause ischemia of the entire mucosa, as shown by Faulkner[44] and Prill and Gotz.[92] On entering the basal layer of the endometrium, these arteries become the *basal arteries* (Fig. 13–8), which give rise to a rich network of branches and anastomoses in this portion of the endometrium. Because none of the arteries described to this point are affected by the sex hormones, they are not subject to cyclic changes. However, on penetrating into the functional layer, the basal arterioles become terminal arterioles which no longer anastomose and which, owing to their spiral trajectory, are known as *spiral arteries*. The latter undergo cyclic changes.

The tortuosity and spiral course of the spiral arteries is minimal at the beginning of the proliferative phase but reaches its utmost at the end of the secretory phase. By proliferating during the proliferative phase and continuing to grow during the secretory phase, when they reach their greatest degree of development, the spiral arterioles in terms of growth closely follow the evolutions of the endometrium. Regarding the histology of the endometrial glands, a distinction must be drawn between the proliferative phase and the secretory phase:

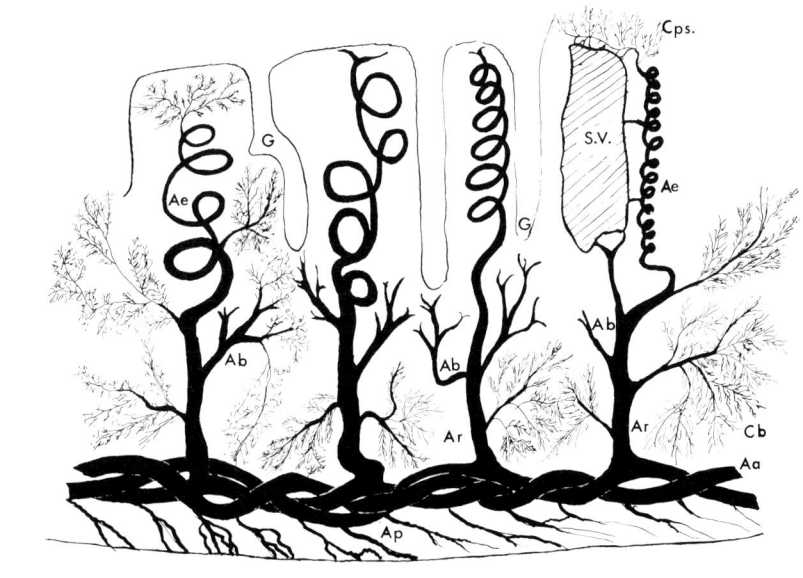

Figure 13–8. Scheme of uterine vascular supply: *Aa*, Arcuate arteries; *Ar*, radial arteries; *Ab*, basal arteries (anastomosing); *Ae*, spiral arteries (terminal); *Cps*, capillaries; *SV*, venous sinuses; *G*, glands; *Ap*, parietal arteries; *Cb*, basal capillaries.

as far as the vascular apparatus is concerned, the *proliferative phase is continuous from the beginning to the end of the cycle*. This proliferative phase is stimulated first by the action of estrogens and then continues to be stimulated by the combined action of estrogens and progesterone.

It is of interest to point out that Zweifach and Shorr[122] have brought to light the presence of numerous *precapillary sphincters* in the spiral arteries. Several Danish workers (Schlegel,[105] Dalgaard[37] and Okkels[85]) have shown that the spiral arterioles present a great many *arteriovenous anastomoses* connecting them with the venous sinuses that develop in large numbers in the endometrium during the secretory phase. These arteriovenous anastomoses are thought to be implicated in the mechanism of menstruation. The capillaries in the endometrium are disposed in the form of a subepithelial network running parallel to the epithelial basement membrane. This capillary network is particularly dense around the glands and, above all, below the surface epithelium of the decidua compacta. It originates by fine dichotomization and branching of arteries and arterioles; however, instead of eventually joining a system of larger and larger capillary veins, it opens abruptly into the large venous vessels, which are disposed in the form of true venous sinuses (Reynolds and colleagues[94, 95]).

Obviously, these vascular changes lead to associated variations in the intrauterine pO_2. The intrauterine oxygen tension in rats has been measured by Mitchell and Jochim,[76] who found that it varied in the course of the estrous cycle.

13.2.3. RELATIONSHIPS BETWEEN STROMA, GLANDS AND VESSELS

Elsewhere,[16] we have already called attention to the fact that the rate at which the individual components of the endometrium—the stroma, the glands and the vessels—develop is not uniform. In general, it may be asserted that growth of the stroma proceeds at a rate of linear progression, that of the glands at a rate of geometric progression and that of the vessels at a rate of cubic progression. This means that because the glands grow during the cycle at a faster rate than the stroma, they are compelled to double up for lack of space and, since the spiral arteries grow at an even faster rate than either the glands or the stroma, they achieve maximal tortuosity (Fig. 13-9).

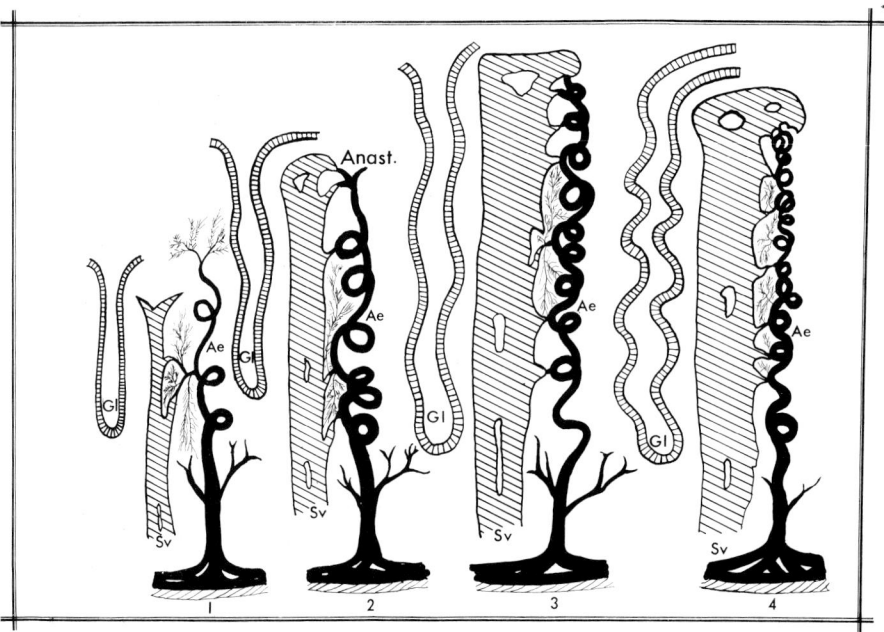

Figure 13-9. Reciprocal disposition of glands, stroma, arteries and venous sinuses over the four week span of the cycle. Gl, Glands; Sv, venous sinuses; Ae, spiral arteries; Anast., anastomosis.

13.2.4. HISTOCHEMICAL CHANGES DURING THE ENDOMETRIAL CYCLE

In recent years, extraordinary importance has been attached to endometrial histochemistry as a means of elucidating the biochemical changes that take place in the endometrium in order to facilitate implantation and nutrition of the egg. As a result of these studies, the presence of the following main substances in the endometrium has been shown to be cyclic in nature: (1) glycogen; (2) ascorbic acid; (3) alkaline glycerophosphatase; (4) β-glucuronidase; (5) nucleic acids; and (6) mucopolysaccharides.

GLYCOGEN. Moricard,[77] Hughes and colleagues,[58] Noyes,[83] and Botella and Nogales[20] have repeatedly emphasized the importance of the presence of glycogen in the endometrium. The observations of the foregoing workers have subsequently been completed and confirmed by numerous studies.[22, 30, 46, 58, 66, 110]

Glycogen is a characteristic element of the progestational phase and therefore denotes progesterone effect. Zander and Ober[120] have detected its presence in the endometria of castrated women as early as two hours following the injection of progesterone. A number of years ago, we showed that also corticosterone increased endometrial glycogen deposition and, more recently, Vaes[114] found that the same was true about cortisone. Paradoxically, endometrial glycogen deposition takes place independently of the action of insulin.[111]

Since progesterone appears in the bloodstream shortly before ovulation (see Chapter 12), glycogen too actually begins to be stored within the cells of the endometrial glands before ovulation. It afterwards accumulates in the basal pole of the cells until about the twentieth day of the cycle. The glycogen is then found to migrate toward the luminal pole of the cells prior to being secreted. Little by little, this polysaccharide is extruded into the gland lumen during the fourth week of the cycle and will have completely disappeared from the cells by the time of menstruation. If fertilization is achieved, the glycogen persists in the epithelium and is also deposited in the stroma, where its presence may be considered as histochemical evidence of early pregnancy. Quantitative glycogen

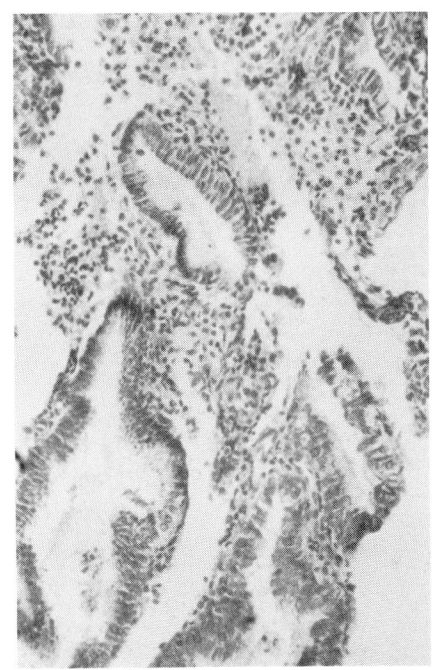

Figure 13–10. Endometrial glycogen on the twenty-third day of the cycle. Some glycogen can still be found in the subnuclear location, with the rest in the luminal portion of the cell. (Periodic acid-Schiff stain.)

determinations will be discussed later in this chapter.

ASCORBIC ACID. Vitamin C, or ascorbic acid, has also been found in the endometrium by various investigators.[11, 115] Like glycogen, it is absent during the proliferative phase but appears during the secretory phase as an integral constitutent of the nutritional secretion which, under the influence of the corpus luteum, is intended to prepare the mucosa for the reception of the egg.

PHOSPHATASES. Using his original histochemical method for phosphatase, Gomori was first to demonstrate the presence of alkaline glycerophosphatase (AGP) in the endometrium, a finding that was later confirmed by Atkinson and Engle.[4] This enzyme has since been demonstrated by numerous authors, among them Dempsey and Wislocky.[116] We have conducted our own studies on the cyclic activity of endometrial phosphatase.[18, 19]

Our results are summarized in Figure 13–11. During the *first week* of the cycle, phosphatase activity is apparent within the cytoplasm as well as in the nuclei of the

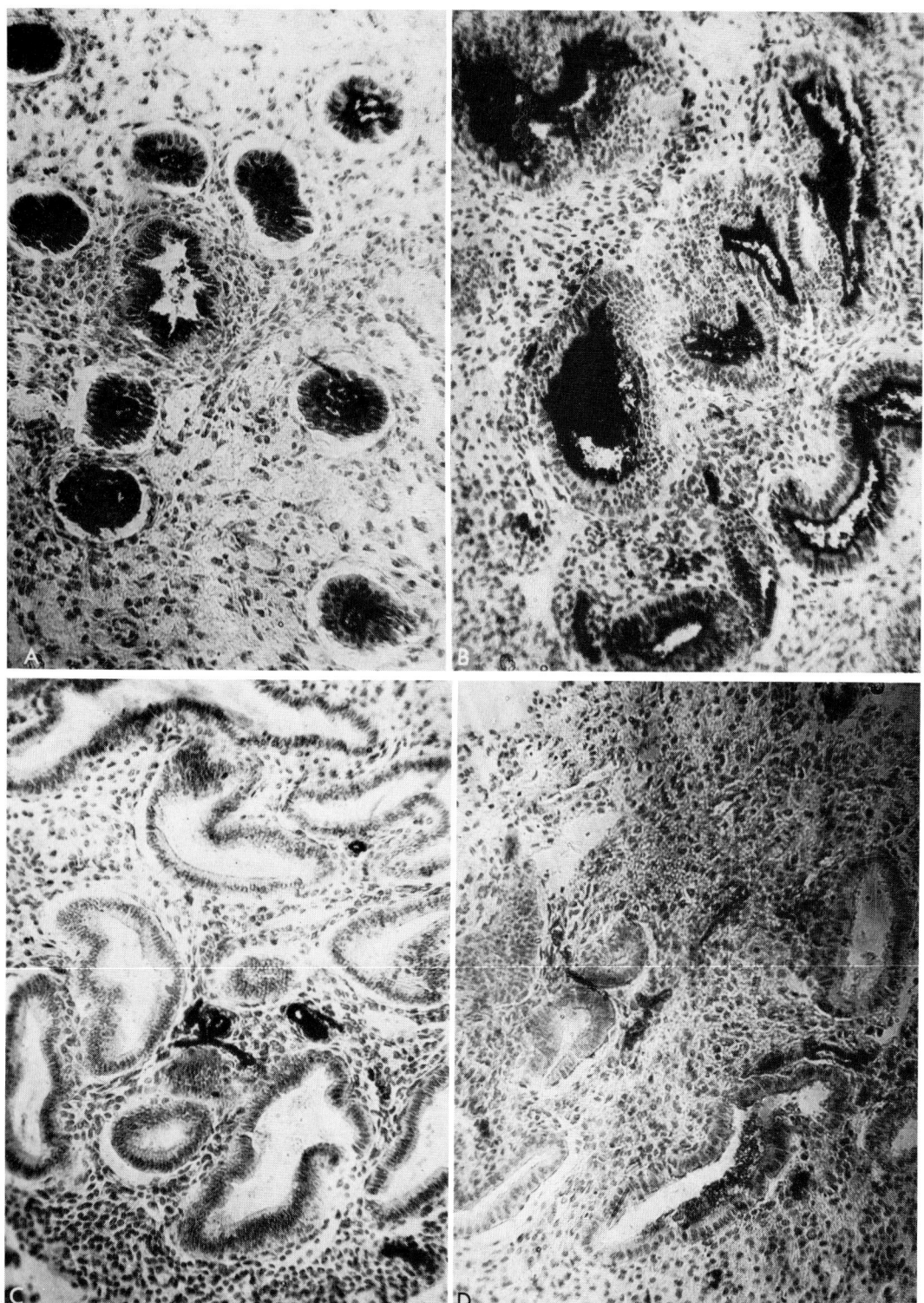

Figure 13–11. Gomori reaction for alkaline glycerophosphatase (AGP) in endometrium during the cycle. *A*, First week of cycle. Nondilated glands lack AGP activity in lumen, and there is tall columnar epithelium with a high rate of AGP activity. *B*, Beginning of third week. There are low columnar epithelium with scanty AGP activity and dilated glands with AGP positive content. *C*, Fourth week of cycle. Total absence of AGP activity from both epithelium and lumen. Vessels are well outlined. *D*, End of fourth week (intramenstrual). Both glands and vessels are AGP negative and appear collapsed (4505×). (From Botella and Nogales: *Arch. Med. Exper.* 18:33, 1955.)

cells of glands. During the *second week* of the cycle, enzyme activity has a similar distribution, but some spillage into the lumen can be observed. Most active outpouring into the lumen occurs during the *third week*, and is associated with an interesting phenomenon: the epithelium ceases to exhibit any enzyme activity, denoting complete passage of the enzyme into the secretion. During the *fourth week* of the cycle, the glands are totally devoid of any AGP activity, both in the lumen and in the secretory products contained in it, and Gomori's reaction is positive only in the vascular endothelium which, on account of the degree of development attained by the arterial vessels, produces a well defined and distinct image. A similar vasvular localization of enzyme activity has also been demonstrated in the cow endometrium by Moss and co-workers.[78] In addition, on the basis of estimating alkaline phosphatase activity by a biochemical procedure, Fuenzalida[49] concluded that a cycle similar to that established by us did exist.

Acid glycerophosphatase has been investigated by us[20] and subsequently by Foraker and Marino[46] and by Boutselis and his colleagues.[22] The observed variations in activity are also cyclic in nature, though less typical than those of alkaline phosphatase.

Apart from histochemical studies, phosphatase activity in the human endometrium during its cycle has also been studied by means of quantitative determinations (Gautray et al.[51]), with results that are essentially in agreement with morphologic observations.

On the other hand, the role played by both alkaline and acid phosphatase in implantation has been brought to light by Manning and co-workers.[71]

In addition, Hughes and his colleagues,[59] as well as Foraker and Marino,[46] have studied glucose-6-phosphatase and phosphorylase, the two enzymes that are directly implicated in glycogen synthesis. The endometrium contains both in high concentrations. Epinephrine has been found to modify phosphorylase concentration,[59] a fact which is undoubtedly related to the mechanism of glycogen deposition.

β-GLUCURONIDASE. In Chapter 2, we emphasize the important role of β-glucuronidase as an activator of estrogenic activity in the uterus. Boutselis and his colleagues,[22] Fishman[45] and Prahlad[91] investigated the question of endometrial β-glucuronidase activity in the course of the cycle and were able to show a peak in the enzyme's activity during the proliferative phase.

NUCLEIC ACIDS. Several workers (Atkinson et al.,[5] Bremer et al.[23]) have reported the presence of histochemically demonstrable DNA in the course of the endometrial cycle. A characteristically increased DNA content is present in epithelia undergoing mitotic activity and, consequently, is found during the proliferative phase but not during the secretory phase. As already indicated, during the second week of the endometrial cycle, numerous mitotic figures appear in the endometrial glandular epithelium. The finding of deoxyribonucleic acid is coincident with this period of mitotic activity and is not unexpected.

MUCOPOLYSACCHARIDES. A method combining the PAS stain with the Alcian blue stain enabled Runge and his associates[103] to detect the presence of both *acid and neutral mucopolysaccharides* in tissue sections. With this method, Merlo[75] at our clinic was able to characterize the occurrence of polysaccharides in relation to cycle (Fig. 13–12). Acid mucopolysaccharides abound in the stroma during the proliferative phase and in the glands during the secretory phase; on the other hand, neutral polysaccharides appear in the stroma during the secretory phase. Boutselis and colleagues[22] and Strauss,[110] by histochemical means, and Loewi and Consden,[68] by means of electrophoretic procedures, recently confirmed the results of Merlo's work.

CARBONIC ANHYDRASE. Pincus and his group[90] have discovered that the finest assay for the estimation of progesterone activity in the rodent uterus is to determine the presence of *carbonic anhydrase*. On the basis of later studies on human endometria, they reported that this enzyme clearly was predominant during the progestational phase.

SUMMARY. Figure 13–12 represents a synthesis of the cyclic events involving glycogen, AGP and acid and neutral mucopolysaccharides according to observations made at our own laboratory. The graph has been obtained by integrating the many observations made by Nogales, Merlo and Botella.[18, 75, 80] In summary, *the proliferative phase* may be said to be *characterized*

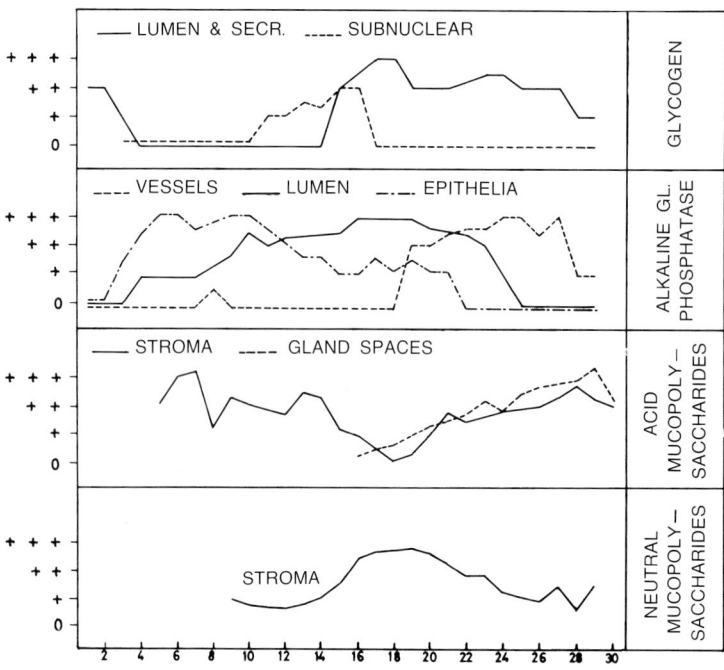

Figure 13-12. Diagram integrating various histochemical reactions in endometrium as they occur during the cycle. (Based on integrated data from Botella, Nogales and Merlo.)

by: (1) *absence of intraglandular glycogen;* (2) *abundant AGP activity in the gland epithelium;* (3) *abundance of stromal mucopolysaccharides,* and (4) *a rich nuclear DNA content.* The secretory phase is characterized by: (1) *the appearance of glycogen first in the basal pole, then in the luminal pole of the gland cells, as well as in the secretion;* (2) *the appearance of AGP first in the gland lumen and then in the vascular endothelium;* (3) *the gradual accumulation of acid mucopolysaccharides in the gland lumen and of neutral mucopolysaccharides in the stroma,* and (4) *nuclear DNA depletion.*

In order to establish the functional diagnosis of the endometrium, the exact evaluation of these conditions is of utmost importance.

13.2.5. BIOCHEMICAL CHANGES IN THE ENDOMETRIUM IN THE COURSE OF THE CYCLE

During the past few years, great advances have been made in the study of the endometrium, not only concerning histochemistry but particularly *quantitative biochemistry.* At present, the detailed mechanism involved in the action of sex hormones on the uterine tissues is in the process of being elucidated. However, it is not the purpose of this work to go into details, which belong instead to the study of biochemistry. We shall confine ourselves to simply listing those cyclic biochemical and enzymatic changes that have been observed to occur in the endometrium.

WATER AND MINERAL CONCENTRATION. Johnson[62] recently described the changes occurring in human endometrial water, sodium, chloride and potassium concentrations. Prior to ovulation, there is a slight increase of water content, which falls after ovulation, only to rise again conspicuously during the fourth week of the cycle. While potassium and chlorides predominate during the proliferative phase, a large amount of potassium is found in the stroma during the secretory phase.

GLYCOGEN. As was already indicated, glycogen can be demonstrated in great detail by histochemical means. In their recent studies with the anthrone method, Payne and Latour[88] achieved quantitative measurements of endometrial glycogen for the different phases of the cycle. A sudden increase is noted from the fourteenth day onwards, reaching a maximum between the seventeenth and eighteenth days, followed by a decrease until the twenty-first day and afterwards a slight rise again until the end of the cycle. The first of the two peaks corresponds chronologically to the early secretory phase, when glycogen deposition is evident in subnuclear location while the second represents the late secretory phase, when glycogen appears both in the stroma and within the products of gland secretion.

LIPIDS. Changes in cholesterol content during the cycle have been indicated by Leathem,[65] Everett[43] and Frieden and Bates.[47] In the stroma, cholesterol characteristically increases during the secretory phase.

NITROGEN. In this regard, investigations of particular interest have been undertaken by Leathem[65] and by Frieden and Bates.[47] The endometrial glycine content increases progressively and reaches a high level during the secretory phase. These changes, as well as the changes observed in the cholesterol content, are probably related to the processes taking place in preparation for the nutrition of the embryo.

ASCORBIC ACID. The use of histochemical methods for the demonstration of ascorbic acid has already been mentioned. This compound has been studied by Leathem, who reported finding increased amounts during the secretory phase.

CATECHOLAMINES. Wurtman and his associates[119] found a great increase of these compounds in the rat endometrium during estrous activity. Catecholamines are believed to play an important role in the implantation of the egg.

ENZYME ACTIVITY. While the greatest number of substrate deposits seems to be found during the secretory phase, enzyme activity is most pronounced during the proliferative phase. This is accounted for by active endometrial growth during this phase, associated with the necessary preparations for the anabolic reactions of the secretory phase. Rosa and Velardo[101] have studied the system of oxidative enzymes (DPN-diaphorase and TPN-diaphorase, as well as succinic dehydrogenase). Villee[115] and Bever[12] have investigated the enzyme system of the intermediary carbohydrate metabolism (LDH, glucose-6-phosphodehydrogenase, isocitric dehydrogenase and transdehydrogenase). Probably estrogens act on the endometrium by means of activating transdehydrogenase. Beta-glucuronidase, the phosphatases and carbonic anhydrase have been discussed in the preceding section.

All this wealth in enzymes and nutritional substrates points to one thing: the endometrium is getting ready for the implantation and the extraordinary nutritional demands of the embryo.

LUTEOLYTIC ACTIVITY. The role played by the endometrium in the disappearance of the corpus luteum involves a humoral "rebound" mechanism that regulates the duration of the secretory phase.[69]

ESTROGEN RECEPTORS IN THE ENDOMETRIUM. Gorski and his associates[53] have demonstrated the presence of specific receptors for estrogens in the uterus. This question has already been discussed in Chapter 2 (see Section 2.3.9).

Although small in extension and volume, the endometrium is one of the richest and most important nutrient parenchymas of the body. It gives rise to the maternal placenta on which, along with the fetal placenta, everything depends once gestation has become a fact.

13.3. MENSTRUATION AND ITS MECHANISM

Let us now analyze the phenomena associated with menstruation and their causes. Attention must be drawn to the fact that menstruation, defined as hemorrhage accompanied by the shedding of the endometrial mucosa, is known to occur only in the primates, that is, woman and female monkeys and apes. In lower animals, other types of bleeding occur, but none is an example of true menstruation. Such, for instance, is the periodic bleeding seen in bitches or that produced in female rabbits by injecting massive doses of estrogenic hormone. Because the latter types of bleeding are neither associated with the shedding of the mucosa nor preceded by such vascular changes as are characteristic of menstruation, they must be considered as instances of possibly traumatic uterine bleeding rather than menstrual bleeding.

13.3.1. DEFINITION OF MENSTRUATION

What is understood by menstruation is *the type of periodic hemorrhage occurring in females of primates in conjunction with the shedding of an endometrium that ex-*

hibits the features of the secretory phase.[16] This definition is intended to exclude any other type of hemorrhage, such as, for example, bleeding by diapedesis, in which there is no detachment of the uterine mucosa. It was the view of Meyer that menstruation resulted from failure of the ovum to be fertilized. According to this view, the secretory transformation of the mucosa takes place only to provide a site for gestation. When gestation fails, the mucosa is expelled with hemorrhage. In modern times, objections to this concept have been raised by Novak and a number of his followers. In their view, the term menstruation can be applied to *any kind of periodic hemorrhage, provided it is associated with the shedding of the mucosa.* Hartman found that during the summer months female monkeys experienced periodic shedding of the mucosa with the same characteristics as normal menstruation except for the *absence of previous transformation of the mucosa into a secretory type.* Later, Novak, Rock, Bartlett, and Matson, as well as Abarbanel and Leathem,[1] showed that the shedding of a proliferative, instead of a secretory, type of mucosa also commonly occurred with some regularity in women. This is what is known as *anovulatory menstruation,* monophasic menstruation, or *anovulomenorrhea.* This phenomenon will be discussed in detail in Chapter 16. Should anovulomenorrhea be considered as menstruation? In an earlier statement,[18] we favored an affirmative answer. Therefore, we consider any periodic hemorrhage that is accompanied by mucosal shedding, *whatever the functional condition of the involved mucosa may be,* as consistent with menstruation. In the already mentioned monograph, we explained the reasons for admitting this concept, which here would be too lengthy to restate. The reader is therefore referred to the original. Kayser[63] found that menstruation in American monkeys occurred without the presence of vascular changes. This would seem to indicate that vascular changes too may not be absolutely necessary in defining menstruation. To be able to call an instance of uterine hemorrhage menstruation, Markee[72] insistently emphasized, the endometrium must not only be shed but, as has been pointed out here earlier, shedding must be preceded by those vascular changes which are characteristic of menstruation, and which will be analyzed later. Nevertheless, the fact that menstruation without associated vascular changes does occur in some animals, such as American monkeys, suggests that they are not essential either for the induction or for the definition of menstruation.

13.3.2 ENDOCRINE CAUSES OF MENSTRUATION

The concept of Schröder and Meyer that menstruation is controlled by the ovarian hormones has been universally accepted. In the following sections, we shall analyze the hormonal processes involved in the determination of the uterine cycle and in the initiation of menstrual bleeding.

The classic doctrine held that the onset of menses coincided with the beginning of corpus luteum regression, which began as soon as the corpus luteum-derived hormonal stimulus, responsible for those changes, ceased to act. According to this concept, then, menstruation was a *negative phenomenon* resulting from the abolition of something set up for a definite purpose that could no longer be served. It was also a negative phenomenon in that it was believed to be due to decreased levels of one of the circulating hormones (progesterone).

These classic ideas have been modified during the past 20 years. Allen discovered that a few days after an adult female monkey was castrated, it developed a regular pattern of menstrual bleeding. Such menses appeared regardless of whether there were corpora lutea in its ovaries or not. Later, Robertson and his co-workers showed that if, following castration, such monkeys were injected with estrogens they failed to develop menstruation and that, conversely, whenever estrogen administration was discontinued, even after therapy extended over several months, they developed menstruation. These experiments, which were later repeated by Van Waagenen and Aberle, brought home the fact that what produced menstruation in these monkeys was not the decline of corpus luteum activity but *an abrupt fall in the level of circulating estrogens.* It could be shown by Bedoya at our clinic that castrated women treated with estrogens similarly developed menstruation after a short period of latency of 2 to 3 days' duration. Such menstruation in castrated women could be deferred indefinitely with sustained estrogen injections but would reappear as soon as estrogens were allowed to disappear from the circulation. Zuckerman[121] subsequently conducted an extensive series of experiments which clarified the various aspects of this phenomenon. In order for menstruation to occur, it is not only necessary that there be a sudden drop in the blood level of estrogens but moreover that that drop be of sufficient magnitude to descend below a certain level or below the hormonal threshold. Unless this threshold is exceeded, menstruation does not appear. The threshold level has been estimated to be approximately 100 I.U. of estrogen per 1000 ml of blood, but it varies among the different species of primates. If a drop takes place in an equally sudden manner but without passing below the menstrual threshold, menstruation does not occur (Fig. 13-13). Similarly, no menstruation appears if such drop takes place in a slow and gradual manner, even though subliminal levels are reached. As is graphically shown in Figure 13-13, the occurrence of menstruation is therefore conditioned by a sudden drop in the level of circulating estrogens down to values below 100 I.U. per 1000 ml, and is further conditioned by the rapidity with which such drop occurs. The drop must not be gradual, nor must it allow maintenance of an estrogen level above the threshold level.

Progesterone injections into castrated monkeys or women do not cause menstruation if the treatment is suddenly discontinued. If, however, a woman has been previously treated with estrogens, and estrogen administration is suddenly stopped and replaced by progesterone administration, a phenomenon described by Corner[33] as *delayed* or *deferred menstruation* occurs. Progesterone therefore does not seem to play any role in the initiation of menstrua-

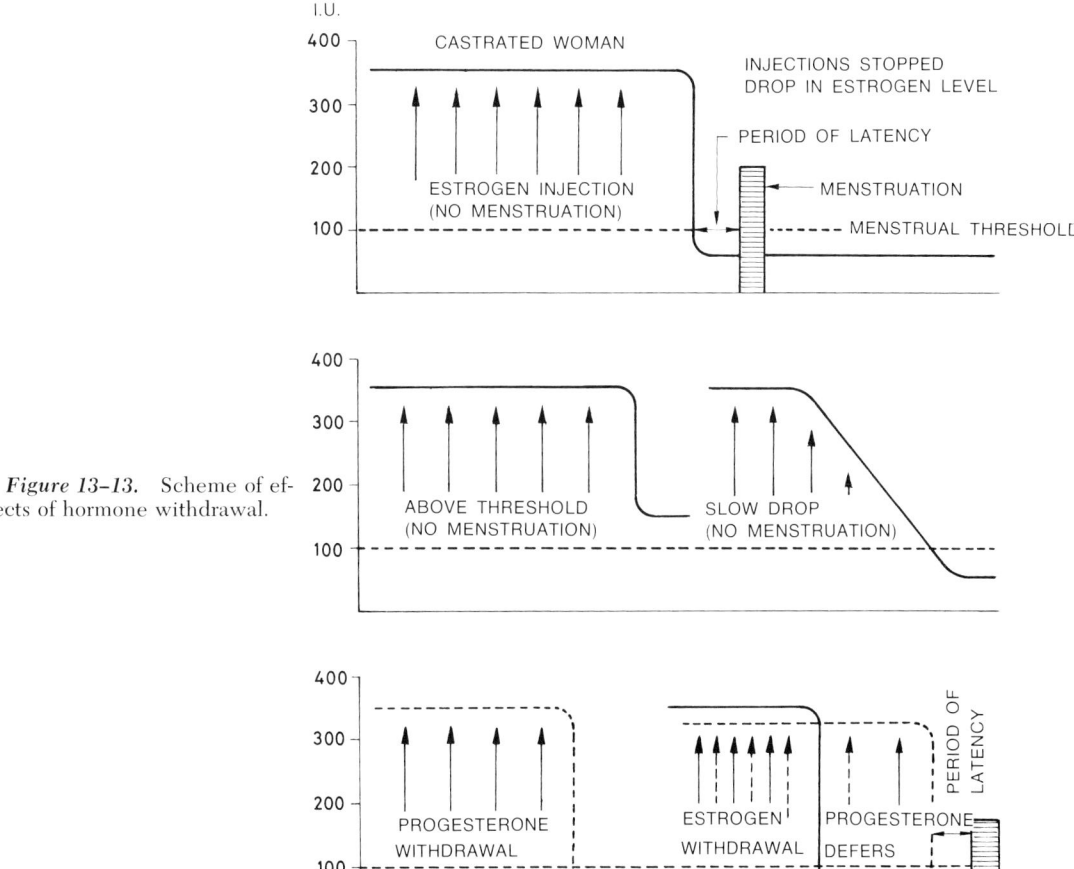

Figure 13-13. Scheme of effects of hormone withdrawal.

tion; it does however seem capable of deferring or delaying the appearance of the type of menstruation that is provoked by estrogen withdrawal.

How then is menstruation brought about in the light of the cyclic ovarian hormonal changes that were analyzed in Chapter 12? It has been pointed out that estrogen levels during the first half of the cycle rise gradually in a manner commensurate with follicular maturation. At the time of follicular rupture, there is a transient decrease in estrogen levels, followed again by a rise caused by estrogenic activity of the corpus luteum (Fig. 13–14). During this phase of the cycle, the second upswing of the estrogen curve goes hand in hand with an approximately parallel upswing in the progesterone curve. Although a dip occurs consistently between the first (follicular) and the second (corpus luteum-induced) upswings in the estrogen curve, the rate of hormone withdrawal involved in the process is never so pronounced as to reach menstrual subthreshold levels, and therefore menstruation does not take place. The ovulatory, or intermenstrual, bleeding observed in some women can probably be accounted for by an exceedingly deep dip between the two peaks of the estrogen curve. In the premenstrual phase, toward the end of the cycle, a parallel drop occurs in both estrogen and progesterone levels, so that the onset of menstruation can be attributed to estrogen withdrawal alone, without the need to invoke progesterone participation in the menstruation-triggering mechanism. When such early writers as Halban, in 1914, and Prat, in 1927, noticed that the resection of the corpus luteum resulted in development of menstruation, they, among others, committed an error in interpretation by assuming that the onset of menstruation was precipitated by lack of progesterone; *actually, the reverse was true—corpus luteum resection results in lack of estrogens.* Another question that must be raised is why decreased estrogen production by the regressing corpus luteum is not taken over by a new maturing follicle. Studies on perfused ovaries by Dorfmann[40] showed that the cyclic ups and downs of ovarian estrogen production are much less pronounced than one might expect from the morphologic changes taking place in the ovary, and are much less than we had been led to believe on the basis of classical notions. Rather than off-and-on estrogen synthesis, the ovary maintains a *wave-like pattern of estrogen production.* Under these circumstances, it is hard to understand how this can give rise to a drop in estrogen levels sufficiently abrupt to create hormonal deprivation leading to menstruation. We shall reiterate the fact that menstruation may fail to develop even in the presence of an ovarian cycle because estrogen levels do not fall with sufficient abruptness (see Chapter 16). Consequently, it may be suspected that a *chemical cycle in estrogen metabolism* could in addition cause estrogens not only

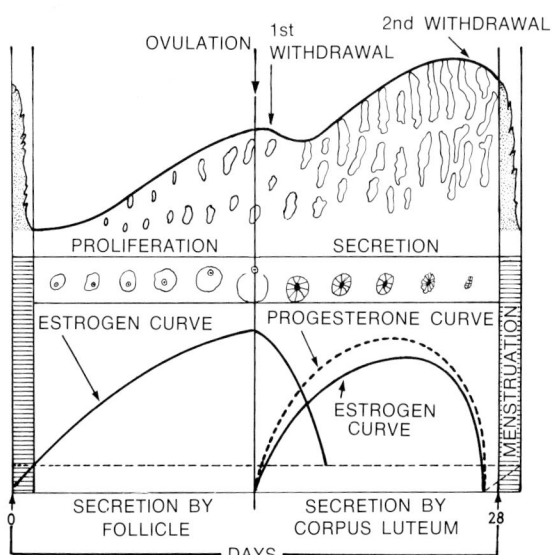

Figure 13–14. Effect of ovarian hormone activity on the course of the endometrial cycle and on the precipitation of menstruation.

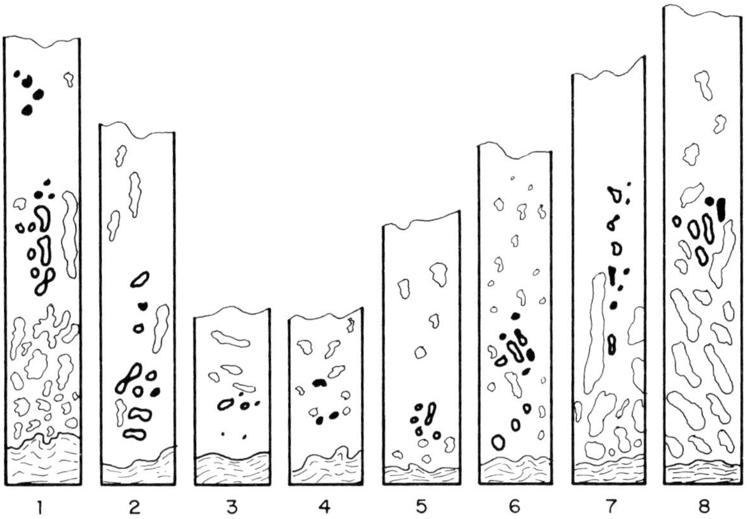

Figure 13-15. Sketch of endometrial vascular disposition during the cycle. 1, Premenstrual; 2, menstrual; 3 and 4, early proliferation; 5, late proliferation; 6, ovulation; 7, early secretion; 8, late secretion.

to be elaborated in smaller amounts but also *to be destroyed at a much faster rate* during the premenstrual phase. In this connection, the work done by Smith and Smith[108] is of interest because it provides evidence to the effect that progesterone activates degradation of estrogens, their conversion to estrone and estriol and their elimination by the kidneys. In their studies concerning the process of hepatic degradation of estrogens, already discussed in Chapter 2, Schiller and Pincus believe to have detected the existence of a certain rhythm in this degradation. From these findings, one might infer that owing to progesterone activity or, perhaps, to other as yet poorly understood influences, estrogens are in some way or other degraded much more rapidly during the premenstrual phase, which therefore leads to an abrupt lack of estrogens. Therefore, it is apparent that the mere fact that ovarian estrogen production occurs in an ebb-and-flow fashion does not by itself cause hormonal deprivation in a sufficiently abrupt manner to induce menstruation; probably other factors, such as rapid catabolization of the hormone in the premenstrual phase, are involved in bringing about the necessary abrupt fall in estrogen levels.

13.3.3. VASCULAR CAUSES INVOLVED IN MENSTRUATION

For many years, the interpretation of menstrual phenomena has been based mainly on endocrinologic studies. The study of the mucosa during the cycle was believed to be of utmost importance, and menstruation was seen at best as a negative phenomenon of desquamation. During the last 15 years, however, the concept of menstruation as a *positive phenomenon* has been gaining acceptance. Far from being useless, necrotic tissue, the mucosa is not shed in a passive way but is actively expelled, and its elimination is facilitated by a series of events which we shall analyze subsequently. The studies of Bartelmez,[8, 9] Daron[39] and Markee[72] have revealed the important function carried out by the endometrial vascular tree in the course of the menstrual cycle. The spiral vessels have been observed to grow in structural complexity throughout the proliferative phase and to develop even more during the progestational phase. Using endometrial homografts on the anterior chamber of the eye of female monkeys, Markee has been able to observe through the corneal microscope that menstruation was preceded by intense spasmodic constriction of the endometrial vessels. This type of vasoconstriction produces endometrial ischemia, which is thought to lead ultimately to hemorrhage, initiating menstruation. In 1948, we enunciated a hypothesis concerning the manner in which the vascular phenomena leading to menstruation are brought about (see Fig. 13-16).

As pointed out previously, the thickness of the endometrial stroma depends in great measure on the existing stromal water con-

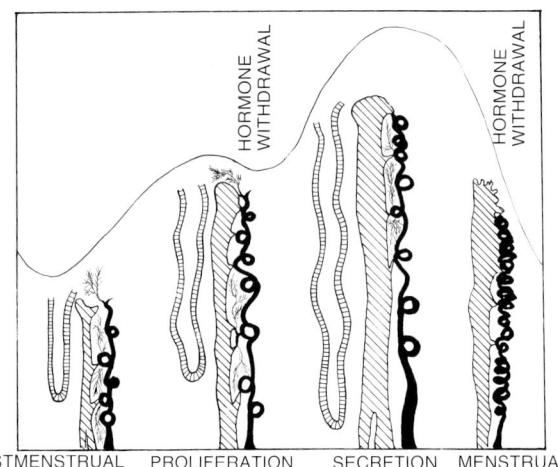

Figure 13–16. Variations in thickness of endometrial mucosa throughout the cycle, in relation to disposition of glands and vasculature.

tent and consequently it depends directly on the level of estrogenic activity. Contrary to earlier belief, the endometrium continues to experience a considerable increase in thickness during the progestational phase, reaching a maximal thickness between the twenty-fourth and twenty-sixth day of the cycle. Therefore, the ensuing estrogen deprivation causes sudden endometrial dehydration and, as a consequence, reduction in thickness. The resulting shrinkage of the stroma causes both glands and vessels to become more tortuous than ever (see Fig. 13–9). At the same time, certain humoral factors, which we shall discuss later, produce constriction of the spiral vessels; this constriction, together with the spring-like retraction of these vessels, gives rise to sudden ischemia of the entire capillary bed of the endometrium. It is well known today that any organ at its full functional activity is irrigated by its capillary network, whereas any collapse of functional activity determines closure of the precapillary sphincters of Zweifach and Shorr[122] and causes the blood flow to be withdrawn from the capillary territory, diverting it through an alternate route. This is exactly what takes place in the premenstrual endometrium where, owing to the vasospasm and specifically the spasm of the precapillary sphincters, the blood is rechanneled toward other routes. In most other organs, under these circumstances, the blood would be passed from the arterial to the venous system through a connecting artery ("meta-artery"). However, in the endometrium, where such arteries either do not exist or lack functional significance, this function is performed by a highly developed system of arteriovenous anastomoses (Fig. 13–17). Because the capillary bed is no longer accessible, the blood is forced into the venous system through such anastomoses (Fig. 13–18) and, as a result, the venous lakes, which are so well developed in the endometrium, are subjected to excessive pressure by the passage of arterial blood and, as shown in Figure 13–18, burst and initiate the hemorrhage. The more edematous and necrotic the stroma, the greater the ease with which extravasation spreads and produces a hematoma between the basal and the functional layers, causing detachment of the functional layer and giving rise to the menstrual flow.

13.3.4. HUMORAL FACTORS INVOLVED IN VASOSPASM

Up to this point, it may have seemed clear that estrogen deprivation and endometrial retraction explain in part the appearance of the menses as well as the associated vascular phenomena. At the same time, however, the question arises as to whether vasospasm, especially that involving the precapillary sphincters, may not after all be the result of active factors or *positive phenomena*. In general terms, vasospasm may possibly be induced by either *humoral* or *neural* agents. Among the first, three main groups of substances capable of producing vasospasm must be

Sexual Cycle in Target Organs

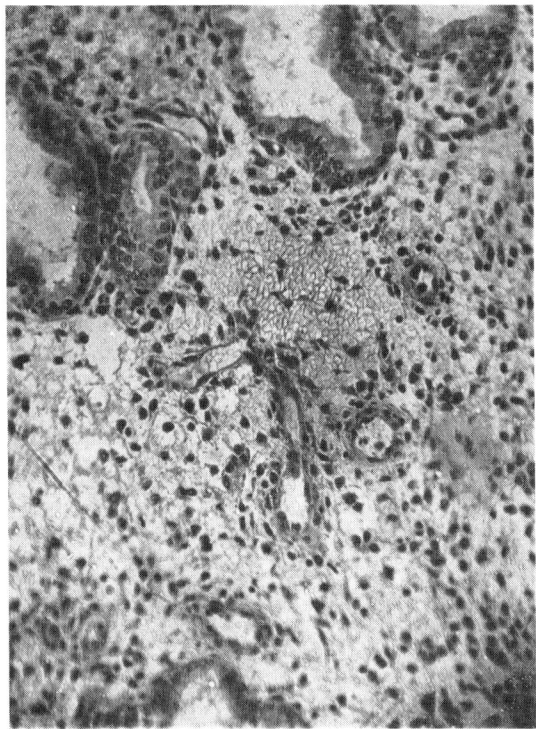

Figure 13-17. Arteriovenous anastomoses in premenstrual endometrium.

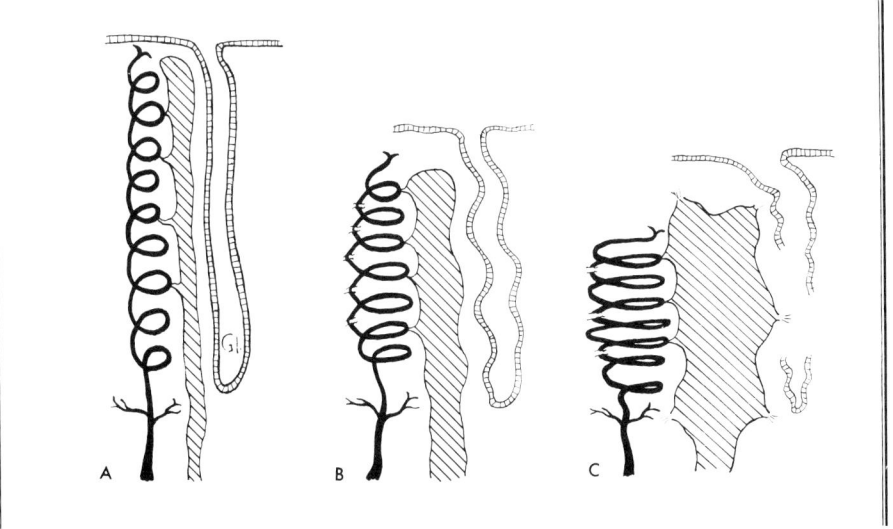

Figure 13-18. Diagram of vascular etiology of menstruation. See text for details.

considered: (1) hormones, in the strict sense of the word; (2) incretions, or tissue hormones, and (3) toxins.

HORMONAL FACTORS. Although playing a predominantly negative role, estrogens may possibly induce vasospasm in an indirect way. We have already called attention to the fact (Chapter 2) that estrogens are active dilators of the endometrial vasculature. Cessation of vasodilative action may produce the opposite effect. Based on capillaroscopy of the nail bed, various workers have been able to show that the onset of menstruation is associated with discernible vasoconstriction. On the other hand, the investigations of Okkels and Engle,[85] and those of Traut and Kuder,[112] would seem to indicate that progesterone may similarly play a significant role in these reactions, and that progesterone withdrawal may involve removal of an important stimulus that keeps precapillary sphincters patent and dilated. In general, it may be asserted that the high degree of development and function reached by the endometrium in the secretory phase is comparable to the highest degree of hyperfunction of active parenchymal tissues. Just as the blood flow through the capillary territory of the latter disappears as soon as their functional activity is inhibited, so also, when active endometrial function—which is maintained by the actions of estrogens and progesterone or, preferably, the two hormones in combination—disappears, a state of general functional collapse of the endometrial tissue ensues. In the final analysis, it is this which is responsible for the associated vascular changes. Seen from this viewpoint, the role played by ovarian hormones, if not an active one, is nevertheless an important negative one in that it produces the type of vasospasm that results from cessation of hormonal stimuli.

PHARMACOLOGIC FACTORS. Reynolds[94, 95] calls attention to the fact that the vasoconstrictive effect under consideration is not a continuous but a rhythmic one, of the same type described by Markee[72] in the anterior chamber of the eye, which means that it must result from some compound that is endowed with a rapid mode of action but which, at the same time, is subject to rapid degradation. The substance involved may be assumed to be a compound possessing neuromimetic activity, so that the finding of catecholamines in the endometrium[119] acquires added significance. Reynolds,[94] moreover, has been able to show that the vascular effect involved was of the *acetylcholine variety*. Soskin and his colleagues, among various investigators, suspected that certain menstrual abnormalities resulted from the abnormal release in the uterus of similar cholinergic substances and, in addition, corroborated the menstruation-inducing effect of *physostigmine*.

Over the past years, the role of *histamine* in regulating vascular tissue processes has been greatly emphasized (see Chapter 2). For the time being, little is known concerning the possibility that histamine may be involved in triggering menstruation; nevertheless, its action, particularly in regard to certain instances of hemorrhage by diapedesis, may be admitted.

TOXIC FACTORS INVOLVED IN MENSTRUATION. In 1938, Smith and Smith[108] discovered in the endometrium a toxic substance which they likened to the *menotoxins* of the early investigators. The substance is an estrone derivative and has vasoconstrictive properties. It has been found to be bound to a carrier protein and can be isolated from the blood in a bound form with fraction 3 of Kohn. Smith and Smith later showed that menstrual uterine extracts, when injected into experimental animals, caused generalized constriction of capillaries. The toxic substance in question is known to possess fibrinolytic properties and probably plays an important role in a series of pathologic conditions that we shall analyze later (Chapter 16). By injecting this substance into the anterior chamber of the eye of a female monkey to which he had previously transplanted endometrial tissue, Markee[72] was able to ascertain a vasostimulant effect of this substance on the endometrial vessels. Based on this observation, Smith and Smith postulated that the substance involved was the menotoxin, capable of inducing both vasospasm and menstrual hemorrhage.

13.3.5. NEURAL FACTORS INVOLVED IN ANGIOSPASM

Having realized the importance of the part played by the vasculature in the production of menstruation, it is easy to understand that the phenomenon of menstruation is subject to modification by certain neural impulses. It is common knowledge that, as a result of a frightening experience or a nervous reaction, a woman's menstrual pattern may be altered, menses being either suppressed or advanced in time. Interesting in this respect are the investigations of Van Waagenen, who provoked the appearance of pseudomenstrual hemorrhage, with concomitant paralysis of ovarian maturation, in monkeys by transecting the spinal cord. This same author later demonstrated that uterine denervation was followed by amenorrhea in monkeys. This, however, correlates poorly with the fact that Markee recorded the occurrence of normal menstrual phenomena in endometrial transplants in the anterior chamber of the eye. It may nevertheless be concluded that, even though denervated and explanted endometrial tissue may be perfectly capable of carrying on its cyclic activity, the in situ endometrium, that is, one that preserves its innervation intact, is subject to neural influences that determine the appearance of menstruation. The influence of the nervous system on the regulation of sexual phenomena was discussed in Chapter 8. In Chapter 32, we shall study the significance of these phenomena which, though not decisive, may nevertheless play an ancillary role in the appearance of pathologic alterations of menstruation.

13.3.6. MECHANISM OF ENDOMETRIAL SHEDDING AND REGENERATION

The classic descriptions of endometrial desquamation, as formulated by Meyer and Schröder, has in recent times undergone profound modifications. In 1957, Bartelmez[9] pointed out that extensive stretches of the endometrium may not be shed but may involute without detaching. More recently, MacLennan and Rydell[70] were able to demonstrate that the endometrium was shed only over limited areas of the surface of the uterine cavity.

Recent investigations of our own group (Nogales, Martinez and Parache), working on whole transected uteri (Fig. 13-19), have yielded evidence of a mechanism that differs from the classical concept of endometrial shedding and regeneration. From the study of the available material, it is evident that the shedding process, while affecting the entire endometrial surface, does not extend deep enough to involve the basalis which, in the opinion of the authors, is at any rate hard to demarcate clearly. On the contrary, a significant portion of the "functional" layer is retained, and, in their view, it is at the expense of the latter that the process of endometrial regeneration is initiated. The regenerative process becomes apparent as early as 35 hours after the onset of menstruation, that is, *at a time when the shedding process is still in progress*, since it usually goes on for a period of 48 to 56 hours.

Regeneration starts *selectively* from the *necks* or surface openings of gland stumps. The latter reveal *increased cellular proliferation, as compared to the remaining portions of the glands.* The cells become cylindrical, pale and eosinophilic, tall and vacuolated, with oval or slightly irregular nuclei that are located basally and contain a finely granular chromatin meshwork.

Epithelia in normal stages of regeneration reveal no mitoses or direct divisions.

Frank regeneration appears and becomes quite manifest in about 50 hours. By this time, cellular proliferation has extended beyond the gland stumps and has started to *reepithelialize the denuded surface*, "climbing," so to speak, over any obstacles in its way, whether these be torn-off tissue particles or collections of clotted blood. The cellularity of the new epithelium is even greater than the foci of glandular cellularity from which regrowth has originated.

The glands underneath the regenerating epithelium, even though apparently collapsed, retain their secretory features, so much so that in a number of instances we have even been able to demonstrate the presence of scanty and irregularly distributed *glycogen* in both the gland epithelium and the lumen.

Regeneration is *nearly completed* by the fourth day (96 hours). The type of regeneration described by Schröder's followers, consisting of, first, detachment of the compacta and then dissolution of the spongiosa (Behrens), have not been recognized in our studies. Instead, our findings revealed that significant portions of the functional layer above the *basalis had not been shed*, appearing somewhat retracted and depleted, but present *in amounts that varied from case to case*.

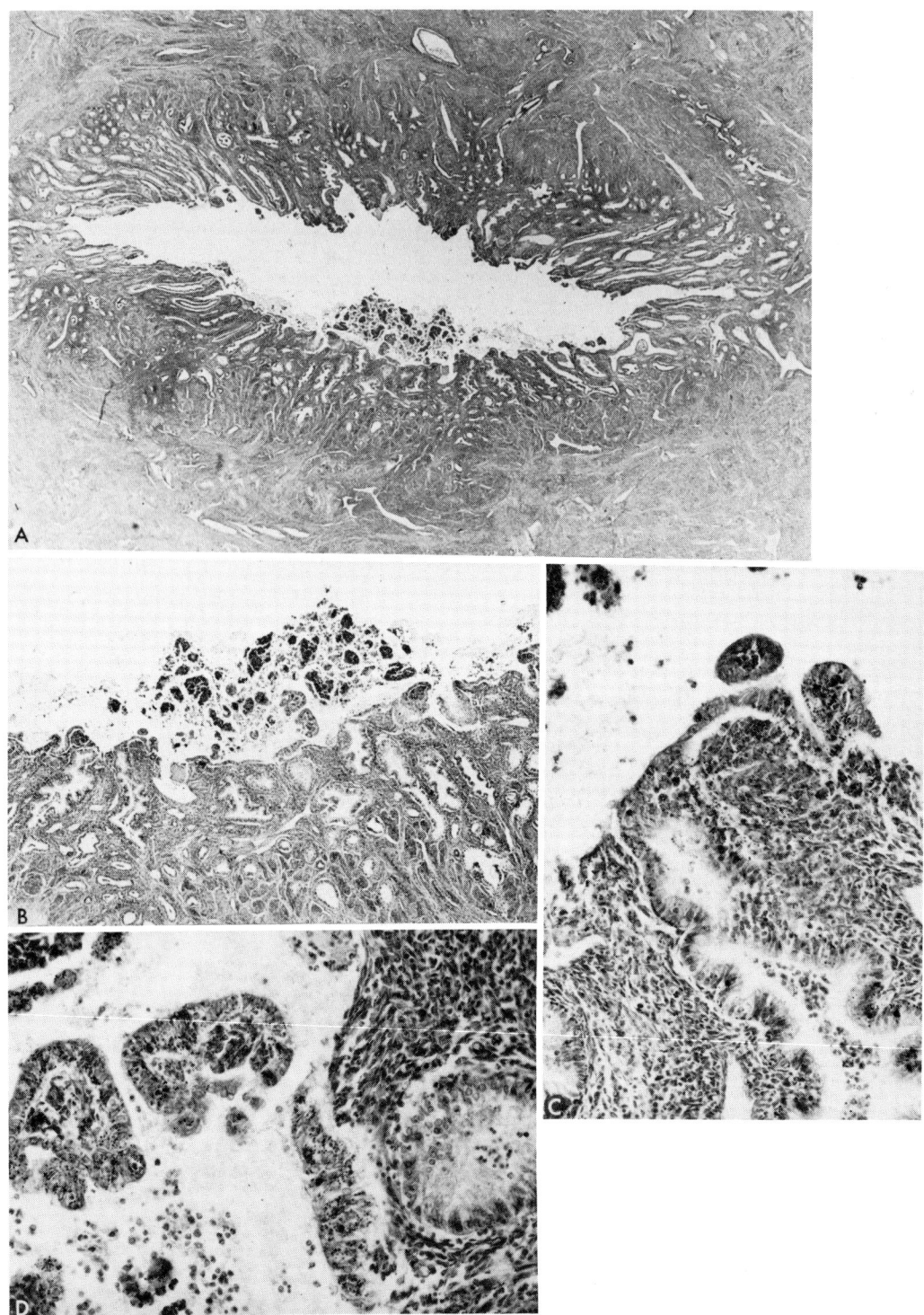

Figure 13-19. A, Cross section of uterus on fifth day of the cycle, at low magnification. Process of endometrial regeneration is seen to be well advanced; most of the surface epithelium, except for some angles, has been re-epithelialized. B, Detail of preceding section, revealing newly formed epithelium covering all aspects of the uneven mucosal surface. C, Detail of epithelial regeneration: Two regenerative papillary columns, cross sectioned, with syncytial epithelial mass beneath. D, High power view of gland openings, spared by the shedding process, beginning active proliferation, with noticeable increase in the number of cells. Proliferating cell masses are comparable to "lava" spreading over volcanic soil. (From Nogales, Martinez, and Parache. *Gynäk. Rundsch.*, 7:292, 1969.)

On the other hand, the classical criteria for what constitutes the basalis layer should be revised.

In our view, the basal portion of a gland extending into the functional zone cannot be separated from the rest of the same gland, because the entire gland is a whole, that is, a morphologic and functional unit with fundamental structure and biologic properties, notwithstanding the fact that some portion of that gland may have adapted itself to less favorable conditions, rendering its nutrition more difficult. In the basal layer, the stroma is *denser*, its fibers *thicker* and its vascular supply *less developed* than that of the functional layer in which the connective tissue is *looser*, made up of finer reticulin fibers and apparently *better vascularized*. It may be argued that under special circumstances the basalis gives rise to endometrial regeneration, as may be the case postpartum, following instances of deep curettage or in continuous metrorrhagia. This is not unexpected, considering the fact that every gland constitutes an anatomic and functional entity, with all its parts possessing *identical* biologic properties. Apart from the secretory morphology, we have been able to show the presence of *glycogen synthesis* in the so-called basalis layer by histochemical means. What actually happens is that regeneration starting from the basal layer is more laborious, slower and difficult, because the ovarian hormones that facilitate regeneration diffuse more readily in the loose stroma of the better vascularized functional layer.

Although we have been unable to identify the manner in which the cells of the regenerating epithelium multiply from examining surgical specimens, nevertheless, in material from prolonged metrorrhagia and from uterine curetting, we have recognized instances of atypical epithelial regeneration in the form of highly cellular masses exhibiting numerous *direct amitotic divisions*, which we have been able to photograph.

In contrast, we have noted numerous mitotic divisions within the epithelium of the glands in the retained portions of the functional layer after the latter was already covered by a regenerated surface epithelium. Such divisions occurred between the third and fourth days of the cycle, and during the following days were also noted within glands of the secretory type, which in some instances revealed the presence of intracytoplasmic glycogen while division was in progress.

From the foregoing observations, we conclude that the surface epithelium regenerates by means of *direct division*, whereas the gland epithelium does so by means of *mitotic division*.

Bartelmez[9] and Rockenschaub[97,98] believe that the mechanism of regeneration at the expense of the endometrium of the preceding cycle, as well as nondesquamative menstruation, are quite common in the human species, though by no means constant.

13.3.7. MENSTRUATION AS A PASSIVE EVENT

Let us consider the significance of endometrial shedding in primates. Such nonprimate animals as the rat and the rabbit, whose reproductive efficacy is incomparably higher than that of woman, have no menstruation. Obviously, this can only mean that the endometrial build-up necessary for the implantation of the egg can be effectively dismantled without any associated menstrual bleeding.

Participation of active vascular phenomena in the menstrual process is tantamount to indicating that nature disposes of a device for the highly effective elimination of an endometrium in secretory transformation. In an earlier publication,[17] we questioned the significance of menstruation as a positive phenomenon that is exclusive of the primates. In the first place, we pointed out that no other type of endometrium had so complex a vascular organization as the endometrium of woman or, for that matter, that of monkeys. This is a result of the fact that primates have a hemochorial placenta (see Chapter 19), differing from that of lower animals in that hemochorial nutrition, in which the chorionic villi must be bathed in the maternal venous lakes, requires a great deal of decidual vascular preparation. Seen in this context, the endometrial vascular system lays the groundwork for a hemochorial type of nutrition. In such animals as the sow, in which nutrition is derived at the expense of endometrial gland secretion in an epitheliochorial placenta (see Chapter 19), the most important nutritional factor is the endometrial *glands*. On the other hand, in the placenta of the ewe, in which nutritional requirements are met by the chorionic villi through a process of imbibition in the endometrial stromal lacunae, the most important element is the endometrial *stroma*. In the placenta of the primates, in which nutrition is accomplished by virtue of the chorionic villi being bathed in maternal blood, the most important element is the endometrial *vascular tree*. Table 13-1 summarizes these differences.

TABLE 13-1

TYPE OF PLACENTA	TYPE OF NUTRITION	PREDOMINANT ELEMENT IN ENDOMETRIUM
Epitheliochorial	Glandulotrophic (at expense of gland secretion)	Glands
Syndesmochorial	Syndesmotrophic (at expense of fluid in interstitial connective tissue)	Stroma
Hemochorial	Hemotrophic (at expense of maternal blood)	Vessels

13.3.8. MENSTRUATION AS AN ACTIVE EVENT

Conceived as a mere process of dismantling a no longer useful vascular apparatus, menstruation can be viewed only as a negative phenomenon. However, we have indicated that it also offers some positive aspects. In the light of investigations by Hertig and Rock,[57] the incidence of implantation in the endometrial mucosa of pathologic embryos is extraordinarily high (see Chapter 38). Most of such abortive or pathologic eggs, however, are eliminated with the next menstrual shedding. In a hypothesis we have voiced elsewhere,[17, 18] we have equated menstruation to an act of rejection by the body, undertaken to dispose of any abnormal eggs or any faultily implanted eggs. Only normal and well implanted eggs, having developed normal trophoblastic function, are believed able to withstand the onslaught of the next menstruation and, therefore, to survive and initiate pregnancy. *Thus, it is our belief that menstruation is a process of active endometrial desquamation, designed to eliminate any pathologic conceptus undeserving of continued gestation.* Menstruation also fulfills another important function. Periodic endometrial shedding and regrowth enhances the functional efficacy of the endometrium manifold in that, by "sporting" a new endometrium in each cycle, it constitutes a very important factor in prevention of inflammatory processes that may affect this type of tissue. The pathology of the endometrium, particularly as regards inflammation, would be undoubtedly significantly greater were it not for this periodic monthly shedding. The fact that endometrial neoplasia appears predominantly years after cessation of menses may also argue in favor of a prophylactic role of endometrial shedding in the prevention of uterine neoplasia. Thus, the menstrual shedding of the endometrium, far from representing merely passive elimination of a no longer useful mucosa, is an active phenomenon, carefully regulated by nature for the twofold purpose: (1) *to eliminate defective conceptions, and* (2) *to maintain a continuously fresh and newly formed mucosa, ready for possible implantation.*

These concepts of menstruation were offered by us in 1951.[18] In 1959, Rock and his associates[96] published similar ideas and conclusions.

13.4. MYOMETRIAL CYCLE

The contractile properties of the myometrium similarly undergo cyclic modifications. As early as 1929, Knaus demonstrated that the isolated rabbit uterus in the follicular phase exhibited more intense contractions than in the secretory uterus. By inflating a human uterus with a balloon in 1933, the same author was able to demonstrate that spontaneous uterine contractions during the first half of the cycle were more intense than during the second half of the cycle. A method based on these studies (known as the "Knaus test") has been used in clinical work to calculate the date of ovulation. After reviewing the literature on the subject, Reynolds[94] concluded that the follicular phase of the human and monkey menstrual cycles was characterized by hypermotility of the uterine body which ceased during the luteal phase, giving way to a period of rest. Reynolds and associates[95] reached identical conclusions after conducting comparative experimental studies on female animals and women. Thus, uterine muscle motility is cyclic, gradually increasing during the proliferative phase, reaching a peak at ovulation, and slowly decreasing according to some authors, or remaining elevated, according to others, until the time of the following menstruation. Del Sol, at our clinic, obtained recordings on strips of isolated human uterus (Fig. 13-20) revealing elevated motility between the tenth and fifteenth days of the cycle, with complete loss of motility occurring during the secretory phase. Recently, confirmation of such a *dynamic cycle* has been provided by Liu and Chai[67] and Chang and his colleagues.[31]

It may therefore be asserted that the uterine musculature contracts with greater intensity during the first and second weeks of the cycle and reaches peak contractility at the time of ovulation. Aside from this, Palmer and Ayala[86] have investigated the motility of the uterine isthmus as it can be appreciated in hysterosalpingographies, arriving at the conclusion that the isthmus and the body behave in diametrically opposed ways. Thus, it became apparent that while contractions in the body gain in strength, the isthmus is relaxed during the follicular phase, and that, conversely, the body is relaxed whereas the isthmus experiences contractions and spasms during the secretory phase. These findings are of interest because, in addition to throwing light on some of the mechanisms involved in sterility caused by cervical factors, they seem to explain the part played by progesterone in maintaining gestation by preventing cervical dilatation and may elucidate the mechanisms involved in certain types of dysmenorrhea.

13.5. THE CERVICAL CYCLE

The uterine cervix has been shown by extensive studies to play a role of extraordinary importance in fertilization and to participate actively in the reproductive process. It would therefore be only natural to expect that, like the other components of the genital tract, the cervix, too, undergoes a cyclic process of preparation for reproduction. Such a cycle has in fact been known for some time to exist and to be reflected by the amount and properties of products of cervical secretion, the *cervical mucus*. Until very recently, however, no conclusive histologic evidence had been available as to comparable changes taking place in the cervical mucosa.

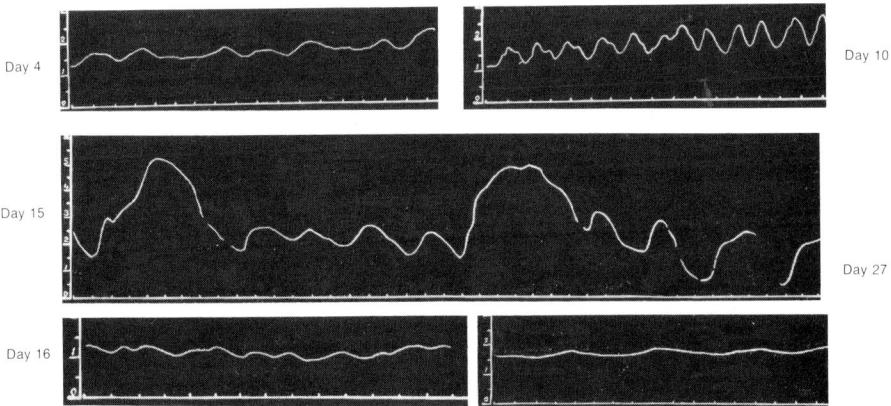

Figure 13-20. Changes in spontaneous motility of strips of human uterus, isolated in vitro during various days of the cycle. Notice the maximal motility during the proliferative phase, with a peak around the fifteenth day. (From Del Sol: *Acta Gin.*, 2:257, 1951).

13.5.1. CYCLE OF CERVICAL SECRETION

It is commonly known that cervical secretion is increasingly abundant up to the fourteenth day of the cycle, gradually decreasing afterwards. As the cycle progresses, cervical mucus, as shown by, among others, Bergman and Lund,[11] increases not only in quantity but also in fluidity. One of the properties related to the degree of fluidity is *stringiness*, the capacity of the mucus to string out, also called *Spinnbarkeit* (Fig. 13-21). This permits cervical mucus to be pulled into threads which, at the time of ovulation, may measure up to 12 cm or more in length. Another property of cervical mucus, discovered by Rydberg[104] and subsequently studied by Campos da Paz[27] as well as by de la Fuente[48] in Spain, is its ability to crystallize, owing to the presence in mucus of dissolved crystalloid substances. Crystallization takes place in the form of fern leaves, pertaining to the tetragonal system (Fig. 13-22), and becomes increasingly more pronounced as the cycle advances, reaching a maximum at the time of ovulation. After ovulation, the ability of the mucus to crystallize decreases gradually during the progestational phase and is totally lost by the fourth week of the menstrual cycle.

The property of crystallization of cervical mucus displays hormonally induced cyclic variations and is related to a hormonal determinism so intimately that Urdan and Kurzon[113] recently suggested that it might serve as a clinical index for determining the moment of ovulation as well as the level of estrogenic activity.

Such other properties of cervical mucus as its osmolality, studied by Bergman and Lund,[11] undergo similar cyclic modifications, and the same has been observed concerning the chemical composition of mucus, and its content of lipids, phosphorus, mucopolysaccharides, galactose, etc.

One further parameter exhibiting cyclic features is the *sodium chloride content* of cervical mucus. The latter increases after menstruation and reaches maximal concentrations at the time of ovulation, as had been shown by the studies of Joel many years ago. MacSweeney and Sbarra have devised a simple method using a paper indicator, called estrus indicator or "Estrindex," which is bleached upon contact with NaCl. Aside from permitting the demonstration of an additional type of cyclic activity of cervical secretion, this indicator is accurate enough to determine the moment of ovulation (see Chapter 24).

As a result, it may be asserted that cervical mucus reveals cyclic variations in all its properties, which reach a high point at the time of ovulation and diminish afterwards. Thus, from the time of menstruation to the time of ovulation—that is, during the estrogenic phase—its fluidity, quantity, capacity for crystallization and stringiness show ascending curves. At the same time, the rate of carbohydrate release as well as the richness in content of hydrolyzed mucin may be observed to

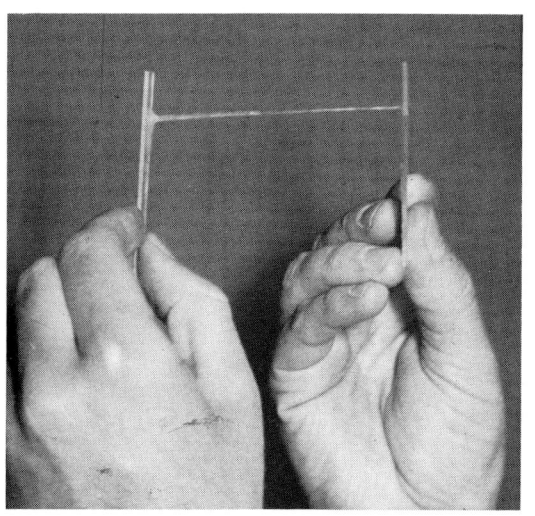

Figure 13-21. Stringiness ("Spinnbarkeit") of cervical mucus.

Sexual Cycle in Target Organs

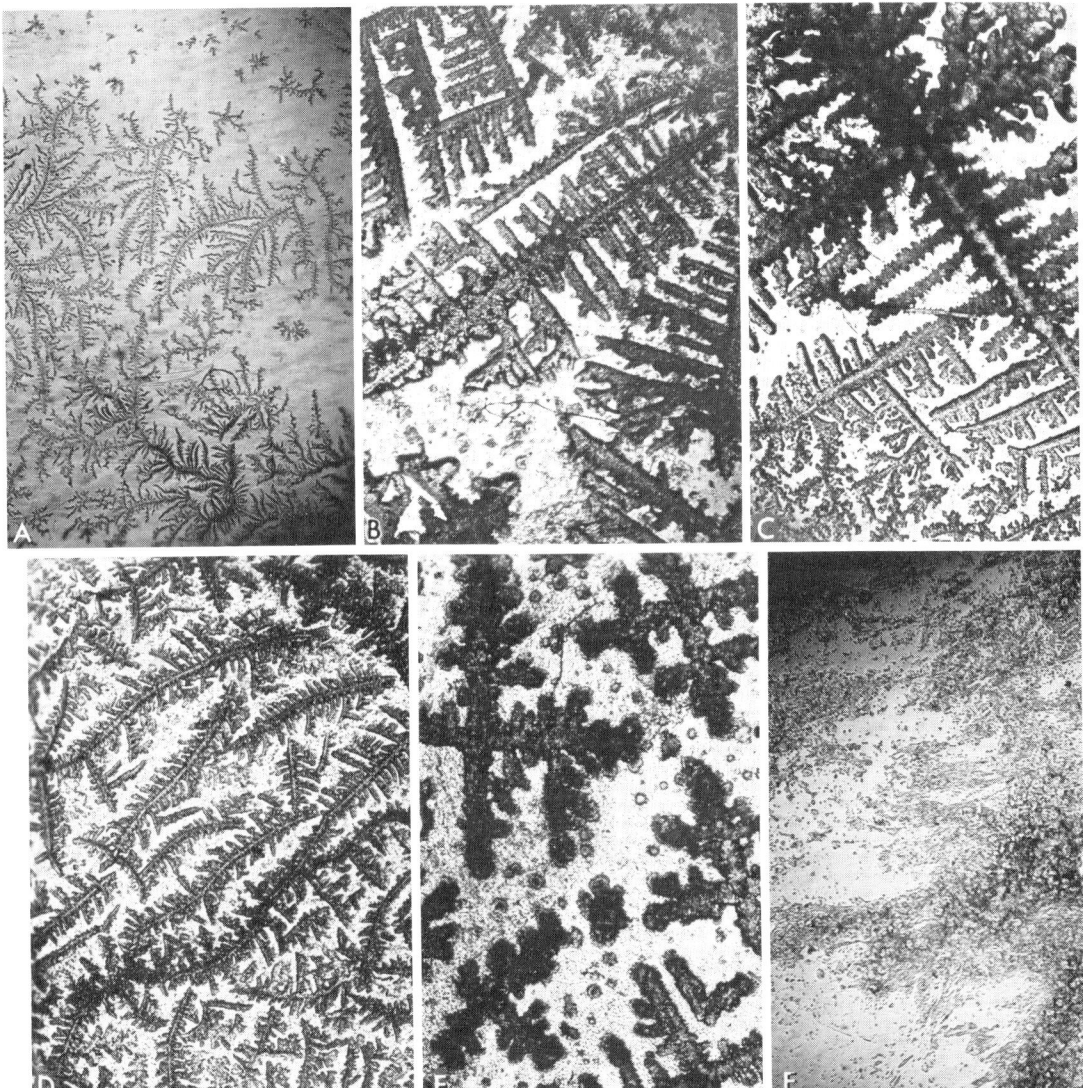

Figure 13-22. Crystallization of cervical mucus on the basis of the cycle. *A*, Fifth day of cycle with scanty crystallization in fine tufts. *B*, Tenth day, with marked crystallization in large tufts. *C*, Fourteenth day of cycle, showing maximal crystallization. *D*, Seventeenth day, with crystallization beginning to recede. *E*, Twentieth day, showing crystallization in scattered foci. *F*, Twenty-sixth day with absence of crystallization.

rise commensurately. All these changes, designed to facilitate spermatic penetration, begin to decline slowly from the moment of ovulation until the onset of the following menstruation. Consequently, the existence of a *cycle in cervical secretion* is a proved fact, its characteristics justifying the assumption that it is aimed at facilitating fertilization. It is perhaps relevant to point out here that *nasal mucus* likewise crystallizes in a cyclic manner similar to cervical mucus (Henderson[56]), and so does saliva (Andreoli and Della Porta[3]).

What is the ultimate purpose of this cycle of cervical mucus and what are its hormonal causes? The works of Noyes[83] and those of Botella and Gomez-Ruiz[21] revealed beyond any doubt that *the highest rates of spermatic penetration occur during the days of the midcycle, that is, when fluidity, crystallization and hexose content are all at their highest levels.*

Regarding the question of *hormonal determinism* of the cycle, it must be remembered that all these progressive changes affecting cervical mucus are subject to estrogenic stimulation. This has recently been demonstrated by several authors.[48, 78, 112] However, the question of whether progesterone partakes in any of these effects remains to be solved, in view of the fact that such properties of the cervical mucus are not maintained during the second half of the cycle, while estrogen levels continue to be elevated.

13.5.2. THE CYCLE IN THE ENDOCERVICAL MUCOSA

It would only be natural to expect that the presence of a cycle, evident in the product of secretion, should also be detectable in the corresponding secretory organs. However, simple histologic techniques have so far failed to demonstrate such a cycle in the cervical mucosa. Nevertheless, using improved techniques, such a cycle has been brought to light by means of: (1) histochemistry; (2) radioactive scanning techniques; and (3) the electron microscope.

HISTOCHEMISTRY. Nogales and Botella[80, 81] detected cyclic variations in reduction of methylene blue and in the content of neutral mucopolysaccharides and alkaline glycerophosphatase in endocervical glands. The reduction of methylene blue is a dependable test of great interest, since the fertilizing capacity of spermatozoa has been shown by de la Cruz and Puras,[35] at our laboratory, to depend on the ability of the medium to reduce methylene blue. Later, Scott and Parksley[107] demonstrated the existence of a cycle in the content of sulfhydryl groups, and Smith and Smith[108] found that the content of PAS positive material in the collagenous ground substance of the cervix also varied in a cyclic manner.

RADIOACTIVE SCANNING METHODS. At Moricard's laboratory, Rodríguez-Galindo[99] found that ^{35}S uptake increased around the midcycle.

ELECTRON MICROSCOPE. Nilson and Westman[79] have obtained beautiful electron micrographs which leave no doubt as to the existence of a proliferative and a secretory phase in the cervical glands, in which the high point of the secretory phase corresponds to the time of ovulation.

Consequently, there exists a cervical cycle which parallels the cycle of the remaining components of the genital tract but, unlike the endometrial cycle, does not present a proliferative phase and a secretory phase but, instead, is characterized by progressive secretory activity during the first half of the intermenstruum, reaching a peak at ovulation and decreasing afterwards. The purpose of these changes is to facilitate fertilization.

13.5.3. THE CYCLE OF THE CERVICAL AND ISTHMIC MUSCULATURE

Besides the cyclic changes occurring in the endometrium, Chapter 12 had dealt with those occurring in the uterine muscle. In addition to the changes taking place in the cervical mucosa, this chapter will describe in addition the changes occurring in the musculature of both the cervix and the isthmic sphincter.

Palmer and Ayala[86] have studied the behavior of the isthmic sphincter over the course of the cycle. They employed a radiographic method using manometric hysterosalpingography. If lipiodol is injected into the uterine cavity and the pressure of injection is recorded kymographically, it may be observed that, on removing the cannula, the uterine cavity empties rapidly during the follicular phase, whereas the contrast medium is retained if the experiment is performed during the progestational phase. Pressure readings at the same time may reveal high pressure during injection which drops rapidly on removing the cannula in procedures done during the proliferative phase, whereas during the progestational phase injection pressures are low and, in contrast, fail to descend after the cannula is removed. This is a clear indication that the uterine cervix is hypotonic and the uterine body hypertonic in the first half of the cycle, whereas during the second half, the opposite is true: the isthmic sphincter is closed while the uterine cavity is relaxed. From this we can infer that *the progestational phase is characterized by closure of the isthmic sphincter, whose cyclic behavior is the reverse of that of the body.*

13.6. THE VAGINAL CYCLE

The typical cyclic changes that occur in the vagina of rodents are well known and have served as the basis for experimental research on estrogens. The recognition of a vaginal cycle in the human species posed greater difficulties, but such a cycle has now been demonstrated to occur beyond any shadow of doubt. In 1927, Dierks described cyclic vaginal alterations that were thought to be related to the ovarian cycle. He distinguished the following three vaginal layers: the basal, the intermediate and the superficial, or functional, zone. In his descriptions, the two upper zones were thought to be desquamated during menstruation and to be progressively regenerated during the following cycle. Later, Zondek and Friedman failed to verify the occurrence of such histologic changes in the vaginal mucosa. In 1936, the problem was approached in a new way by Papanicolaou. Just as it is more difficult to recognize any modifications in the cervical mucosa than it is in the products of cervical secretion, it is more difficult to appreciate any possible cyclic changes in the wall of the vagina *than it is among the products of vaginal exfoliation*. This realization led Papanicolaou, and later Murray, to typify the different varieties of cells appearing in the vaginal exudate and, by counting them proportionately, they came to the conclusion that cytologically the vagina in fact revealed characteristic cyclic changes. One of the first studies concerning this question was pioneered by this author in cooperation with Asín, in 1941.

13.6.1. CELL TYPES FOUND IN THE EXUDATE

The study of vaginal cytology has been considerably simplified by Papanicolaou who, by introducing a special staining method, was able to characterize the various cell types that appear at different intervals of the cycle.[87] Having devoted Chapter 25 to a detailed study of vaginal cytology, we shall confine ourselves here to merely listing the three fundamental cell types that must be distinguished: (1) Large polyhedral cells with abundant, predominantly basophilic staining cytoplasm and a small nucleus, which are characteristic of the first week of the cycle. (2) Cells resembling the basophilic cells but for an even smaller, pyknotic nucleus and *eosinophilic* cytoplasm, which are characteristic of the pronounced estrogen effect at the close of the second week of the cycle. (3) Cells similar to the preceding types but whose cytoplasm is folded around the margins, assuming a navicular rather than polyhedral shape. These *folded* or navicular cells are characteristic of the secretory phase (Fig. 13–23). The moiety of eosinophilic cells receive the name of "eosinophilic" or "acidophilic" index, while that of the cells with pyknotic nuclei is designated "karyopyknotic" index. Both indices usually correlate with and are characteristic of the follicular phase. On the other hand, the "index of folded cells" and the index of clumped cells are consistent with the secretory phase. As shall be seen later (see Chapter 25), the study of the different types and subtypes of cells and their careful categorization allows us to follow up not only normal cycles but also to diagnose, on the basis of vaginal cytology, the presence of pathologic cycles.

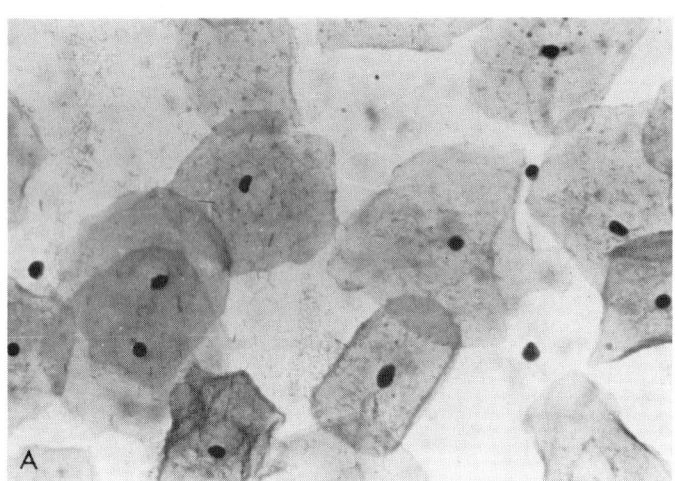
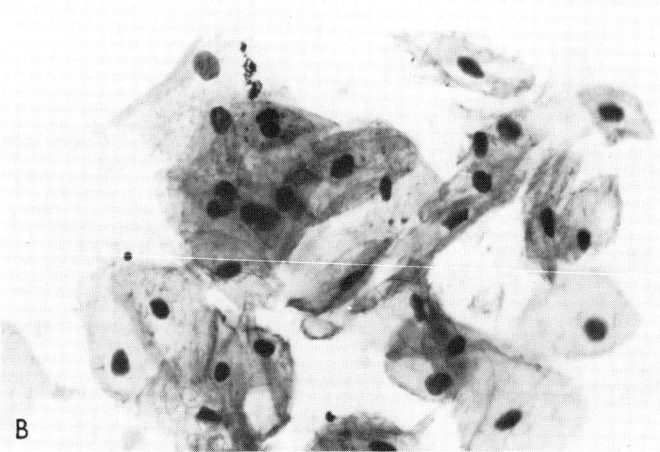

Figure 13–23. A, Typical appearance of exudate during follicular phase of cycle; karyopyknotic cells with acidophilic cytoplasm (staining pink). B, Typical appearance of exudate during luteal phase of cycle: folded cells, predominantly basophilic cytoplasm (staining blue) (500×). Papanicolaou stain.

13.6.2. RELATION OF GLYCOGEN TO THE VAGINAL CYCLE

The occurrence of glycogen in the epithelial wall of the vagina is a well known fact. Rakoff and his associates[93] established the relationship between vaginal epithelial glycogen deposits and estrogens, which was later confirmed by various authors. For many years since, it had been an article of faith to consider increased glycogenization of vaginal cytology as indicative of similarly increased estrogenic influence on the vagina.

This belief, however, has lately been challenged by contradictory findings. Montalvo, at our clinic, made the observation that glycogen appeared in the vagina of newborns after the fifth day of life, by which time a situation of marked estrogen deprivation had already developed. Similarly, Ayre and Ayre[6] in 1949 showed that estrogen injections did not provoke any demonstrable increase in vaginal glycogen whereas, in contrast, estrogen deprivation did. Again, Ayre has shown more recently that glycogen does not appear in vaginal smears of women suffering from hyperestrinism. In cooperation with Nogales,[18, 80, 81] we have been able to verify this in our histochemical studies of the vaginal wall. Glycogen is deposited mainly in the intermediate layer and only very scantily in the superficial cornified layer of the vagina. Though some PAS positive material may occasionally be detected in the superficial layer, it has been shown to be a mucopolysaccharide rather than glycogen. It appears as a result of a progesterone-induced effect and consequently occurs during the second half of the cycle, representing the equivalent, in woman, to the superficial mucification in the guinea pig. As a rule, in neither the proliferative phase nor the secretory phase does glycogen appear in the superficial layer, but it is found only in the deeper layers.

Whenever, as a result of severe hormonal deprivation, the deep vaginal layers are desquamated, glycogen can be found in them, which is not the case when there are high estrogen levels. This explains the phenomenon described by Montalvo.

Other investigators[61, 73, 106] subsequently were able to confirm the fact that highly estrogenic and karyopyknotic smears contain no glycogen. Smears with abundant intermediate cells, on the other hand, usually show the presence of glycogen. The eosinophilic cells in the Papanicolaou stain do not contain glycogen. A detailed synthesis of our ideas on the subject is presented in Table 13-2.

TABLE 13-2. The Vaginal Cycle

FOLLICULAR PHASE	OVULATION	LUTEAL PHASE
I. *In histologic sections:* Thick intermediate zone; Abundant glycogen; Thin "functional" zone	Same as in follicular phase	Thin intermediate zone; Scanty glycogen; Thick functional zone with abundant mucin
II. *In smears:* Karyopyknotic cells; Intermediate cells with glycogen; No folded cells	Abundant mucus and leukocytes originating in cervix	Karyopyknotic cells; No glycogenized cells; Numerous folded cells containing mucus

13.6.3. CYCLIC CYTOLOGIC CHANGES IN OTHER ORGANS

Cyclic changes in cell structure and pattern of exfoliation are not confined to the vagina but are seen in *buccal* smears, in cells of the *urinary sediment* (Galli-Mainini et al.[50]), as well as in gastric cytology (Henderson[56]), all occurring in relation to the female sexual cycle. Exfoliated cells in the male, as might be expected, do not reflect any cyclic variations.

13.7. THE CYCLE IN THE BREAST AND IN ENDOCRINE GLANDS

The organs we have so far studied all depend directly on the sex hormones and are involved in the complex mechanism of the sexual cycle. The cyclic events occurring in the Fallopian tubes, in the uterus and its diverse components, and in the vagina are all processes that are necessary for the realization of fertilization and nidation. The glands to be examined here, even though directly influenced by the ovarian hormones, partake in the process of fertilization only in a remote way and therefore do not reveal equally clear-cut cyclic changes, albeit such changes are unquestionable.

13.7.1. MAMMARY CYCLE

An ovarian hormone-dependent mammary cycle also exists and parallels the cycle in the rest of the genital apparatus. This will be studied in Chapter 22.

13.7.2. PITUITARY CYCLE

The existence of a pituitary cycle, exclusive to the female and not known to occur in the male, has already been discussed (Chapter 6). *Much more functional than morphologic* in nature, this cycle is apparent above all in the degree of FSH and LH release in response to impulses reaching the pituitary by means of chemical mediators from the hypothalamus. Modern studies deny the existence of a cytologic pituitary cycle, as it had been described by Campbell, Wolfe and Severinghaus. D'Amour[36] and Ecker[41] were unable to find any evidence of consistent cytologic changes, but found that the hormonal content was variable.

13.7.3. THYROID CYCLE

The question of variations in thyroid function as related to sexual life has been discussed at length in Chapter 10. A cyclic type of hyperfunction seems to have been recognized in the rat.[14] One of the most dependable modern methods for the evaluation of thyroid function is based on the determination of protein-bound iodine (PBI). Using this method, Heineman and his colleagues[55] and Russell[102] *failed to find any significant variations* that would indicate premenstrual thyroid hyperfunction.

13.7.4. ADRENAL CYCLE

Early investigations (see Chapter 9) referred to certain cyclic features in adrenal morphology, recurring, particularly in rodents, in association with estrous activity, at which time the gland was observed to be thickened.

There is a complete lack of precise morphologic studies concerning the human adrenal, mainly owing to the difficulties involved in obtaining study material from young women. Indirect changes suggesting a functional cycle have already been touched upon in Chapter 9 (see Section 9.4). More recently, Engstrom and Munson[42] found that the rate of androgen metabolism differed between the first and the second halves of the cycle, which they attributed to an adrenocortical cycle. In Chapter 4, we questioned these data. As a result, while the occurrence of cyclic events in the pituitary and in the thyroid appears to be relatively clear, *so far we possess no concrete data that would allow us to assert the existence of a monthly cycle in the adrenal cortex.*

13.7.5. CHANGES OCCURRING IN OTHER GLANDS OF INTERNAL SECRETION

It seems possible that *pancreatic function* undergoes cyclic changes. The hyperglycemic effect of estrogens, described by us (see Chapters 2 and 10), indicates a probable relationship between follicular hormone and the pancreas, and the possibility that the latter gland may experience correlative cyclic changes.

Insofar as *parathyroid function* is concerned, there seems to be no relationship between the parathyroid and ovarian function. Calcemia levels and calcium absorption rates remain unaltered during the cycle. The same is true concerning the remaining glands of internal secretion—the pineal and the thymus—neither having been shown to be affected by the cycle.

13.8. SYSTEMIC CHANGES DURING THE CYCLE

Were we now to analyze organ by organ in search for changes related to the female cycle, the list would indeed be interminable. Nevertheless, certain concrete aspects of the cycle are of interest not only from the physiologic standpoint but also from the standpoint of the clinician, and are briefly reviewed here.

13.8.1. CYCLIC CHANGES IN BODY TEMPERATURE

Of all systemically observed changes, those affecting the basal temperature curve are most significant. Benedek and Rubenstein[10] described the presence of *relative hyperthermia* in the premenstrual phase, followed by a rapid fall in temperature during the course of menstruation, and continued low temperatures during the follicular phase of the cycle. These observations were later amplified by a great many investigators. The cyclic vicissitudes of basal body temperature show great individual variations, as well as marked variations from cycle to cycle in the same woman. However, speaking in general terms, it may be stated that basal temperatures tend to be low immediately after menstruation and during the first and second weeks of the cycle. An abrupt fall at the time of ovulation has been described by some but has not been confirmed by all. Nonetheless, one of the observations that can be made consistently is that a rapid, ladder-like elevation of temperature occurs at the beginning of the secretory phase, just after ovulation, and there is a subsequent persistent elevation of up to 1°C above that of the follicular phase during the entire secretory phase. Menstruation is followed by a drop in basal temperature of 0.5°C to 1°C, occasionally even more (Fig. 13–24). Individual variations are highly significant because they provide a relatively simple and exact guide for estimating the pattern of a woman's cycle, thereby serving as a substantial corollary for the functional study of a female patient, for the diagnosis and treatment of sterility and for the control of endocrine therapy. Modern studies by Masters and Magallón seem to have borne out the fact that the hyperthermia of the progestational phase definitely results from the action of luteal hormone, since the same happens in castrated women treated with progesterone, and since elevations of basal body temperature can also be observed in early pregnancy and in women undergoing progesterone therapy (see Chapter 3). This by no means invalidates the previously mentioned possibility that there exists a relationship between this thermal elevation and thyroid function, which, if true, would necessarily imply a stimulatory effect of progesterone on thyroid function. Based on results of our own studies (see Chapter 9), it seems unlikely that a stimulative progesterone effect on the thyroid exists. Thus, the whole issue remains unsettled. What is unquestionable is the fact that, during the second half of the cycle, women have a tendency to experience a rise in

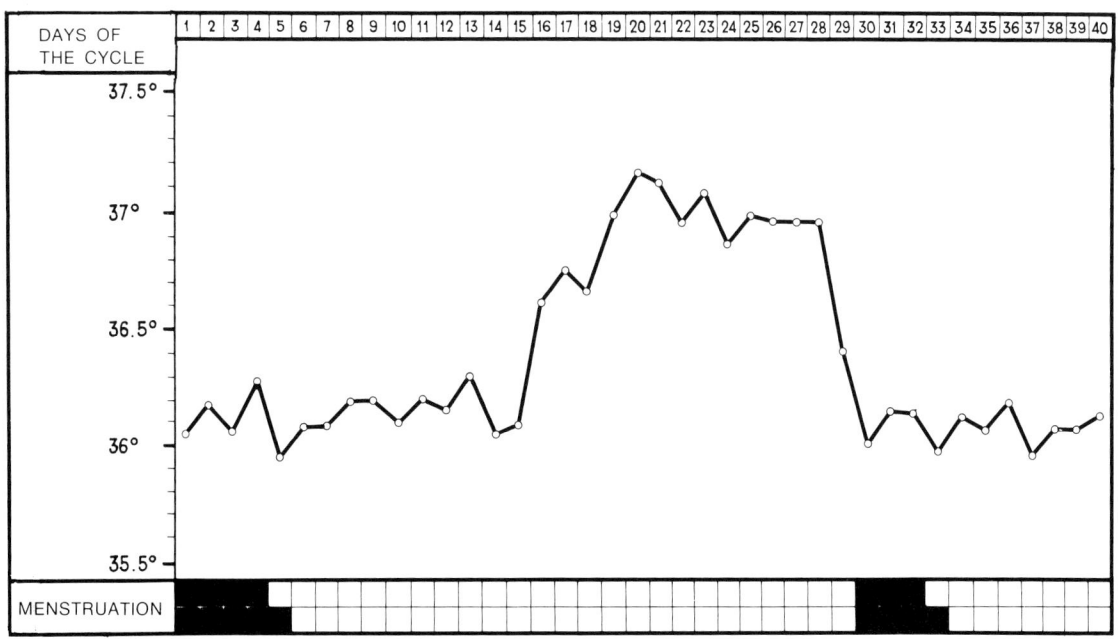

Figure 13–24. Graph of typical basal body temperature in biphasic cycle.

basal body temperature owing to the action of the corpus luteum.

13.8.2. METABOLIC CHANGES

Changes in the basal metabolic rate in relation to the cycle, and in conjunction with a premenstrual elevation of metabolism, have been referred to by many authors. The presence of cyclic changes in carbohydrate metabolism have also been brought to light; these have been reviewed by us extensively in an earlier publication.[15] Of no lesser interest are modifications observed to affect the water and mineral metabolism. A tendency toward water and sodium retention on part of the tissues has been noted to occur in the premenstrual phase. Water retention has been shown by various authors to be an estrogen-induced effect that can be incremented or potentiated by the action of progesterone. It is beyond the scope of this book to digress into those changes which may be found in protein metabolism, acid-base equilibrium and other partial aspects of metabolism in general, all of which indicate that the female body is profoundly influenced by the sexual cycle in all its organs and systems. The influence of sexual life may be even more profound and overwhelming in lower animals, in which the metabolic changes of the estrous cycle may be of such magnitude that, for example, in some species of mice estrus may be associated with a 100 per cent increase of catabolism.

13.8.3. HEMATOLOGIC CHANGES

A decrease in circulating erythrocytes associated with leukocytosis in peripheral blood has been reported (Duckles and Elvejhem) to occur in the immediately premenstrual phase. Leverton estimated menstrual iron loss at an average of 18 mg for each day of the period. Since such large amounts of iron often are not available in the diet, unusually copious menses may become an important factor in the pathogenesis of sideropenia. However, it must be admitted that, in normal women, the effect of the menstrual loss of iron is of no consequence. Blood coagulability decreases during menstruation, while capillary fragility increases, a circumstance which accounts for the greater tendency to develop peripheral hemorrhages, which we shall study in greater detail in Chapter 16.

13.8.4. ALLERGIC AND IMMUNOLOGIC CHANGES DURING THE CYCLE

A great deal of the clinical data available indicate that the response to allergic or immunologic phenomena undergoes modifications in relation to the cycle. Allergic women often experience an aggravation of their symptoms just prior to the onset of menstruation. Similarly, tuberculous females have been noted to run higher temperatures during the days of menstruation. In the view of Pastor, bronchial asthma usually also reveals a relationship to the menstrual cycle insofar as the timing of flare-ups is concerned. It seems plausible to assume that similar effects result from estrogen-induced exacerbation of allergic reactions. Using guinea pigs for experimental estrogen injections, Schäfer has found evidence that one of the experimental estrogen effects is that of enhancing allergic phenomena.

In addition, an interesting finding about the menstrual cycle is related to immune response. Ross and Pfeizer found that titers of protective antibodies, developed against a special type of pneumococcus, revealed fluctuations in the course of the cycle, which reached their highest levels immediately before and after menstruation. Hudson and co-workers similarly have observed that the function of the reticuloendothelial system is influenced by estrogens and that estrogen injections stimulate antibody production. Hansen and Raymond[54] also find that estrogens enhance the defensive reaction of the female body against different antigens injected by intravenous route. All these findings would seem to indicate that allergic and immune responses are exalted during the premenstrual phase, and that this occurs by virtue of a stimulative effect exerted by estrogens on the reticuloendothelial system.

13.8.5. PSYCHOSEXUAL CHANGES

More than 20 years ago, Benedek and Rubinstein[10] devoted an entire book to the description of the psychologic changes encountered in the normal and pathologic cycles. Two later monographs[64, 74] were largely concerned with the same problem. Recently, a well documented work by Abramson and Torghele[2] has been published. The foregoing studies all agree on the occurrence of important psychic changes during the premenstrual phase, which undoubtedly are responsible for the fact that many instances of psychopathy are triggered off during the days of the menses. This topic, which is extremely absorbing, covers a wide range, going far beyond the scope of this book.

13.9. SUMMARY OF CYCLIC EVENTS IN THE FEMALE BODY

As far as participation in the cycle is concerned, three categories of organs must be distinguished in the female body: In the first place, the ovary presents an autochthonous cycle, and its secretion is the prime mover of all other monthly phenomena. In the second place, the organs derived from the müllerian duct, designed for direct participation in the reproductive process, are directly and primordially influenced by the ovarian hormones and present a most conspicuous cycle, above all at the level of the endometrial mucosa. *In the third place, various other organs,* such as the breast, the glands of internal secretion and, in general, all those elements concerned with the regulation of the autonomous system, similarly show cyclic modalities of responses which perhaps are more evident in some organs than in others but, which nevertheless, are real. These determine a fluctuating type of response in metabolism, in body temperature, in frame of mind – in a word, in all aspects of both vegetative and relational life. In Chapter 1, we emphasized the fact that sexual life, vegetative life and relational life are intimately interrelated and that woman's monthly cycle of reproduction indicates how very close these relationships are.

Concerning the way different organs respond to cyclic phenomena, two distinct types of response may be encountered. Some organs, for instance, the endometrium and the muscular coat of the uterus, respond to both estrogens and progesterone. The response involved is specific and char-acteristic for each hormone. Such organs thus have a *biphasic cycle,* in which we are able to distinguish a *follicular* and a *luteal phase.* But there are other organs that respond exclusively to estrogens in a manner which causes their response to be equally cyclic in nature, presenting a peak that correlates with peak estrogen levels, and not being affected in the least by the action of progesterone. Instances of this type of response are seen mainly in the cervix and in the vagina. Finally, some factors, such as basal body temperature, do not seem to respond to estrogens but instead respond exclusively to progesterone. *This means that, depending on whether a given effect responds to either or both hormones, the cycle in the corresponding organ is either monophasic or biphasic.* Whatever the case, a large number of organs of the body are affected by woman's monthly cycle.

REFERENCES

1. Abarbanel, A. R., and Leathem, C.: *Amer. J. Obstet. Gynec.,* 50:562, 1945.
2. Abramson, M., and Torghele, J. R.: *Amer. J. Obstet. Gynec.,* 81:223, 1961.
3. Andreoli, C., and Della Porta, M.: *J. Clin. Endocr.,* 17:13, 1957.
4. Atkinson, W. B., and Engle, E. T.: *Endocrinology,* 40:327, 1947.
5. Atkinson, W. B., et al.: *Cancer,* 3:132, 1949.
6. Ayre, E. J., and Ayre, W. B.: *J. Clin. Endocr.,* 11:103, 1951.
7. Banon, P., Brandes, D., and Frost, J. R.: *Acta Cytol.,* 6:416, 1964.
8. Bartelmez, G. W.: *Physiol. Revs.,* 17:28, 1937.
9. Bartelmez, G. W.: *Amer. J. Obstet. Gynec.,* 74:931, 1957.
10. Benedek, T., and Rubenstein, B. B.: *El Ciclo Sexual Femenino* (Spanish ed.). Buenos Aires, El Ateneo, 1942.
11. Bergman, P., and Lund, G. G.: *Acta Obstet. Gynec. Scand.,* 30:267, 1951.
12. Bever, A. T.: *Ann. N.Y. Acad. Sci.,* 75:373, 1959.
13. Bickers, K., and Krone, H. A.: *Beitr. Path. Anat.,* 136:180, 1967.
14. Bocabella, A. V., and Alger, E. A.: *Endocrinology,* 81:121, 1967.
15. Botella, J., et al.: *Arch. Gynäk.,* 159:435, 1935.
16. Botella, J.: *Fisiología de la Menstruación.* Lisbon, II Congreso Hispano-Português de Ginecología, 1948.
17. Botella, J.: *Para qué sirve la Menstruación.* Barcelona, Actas del III Congreso Hispano-Português de Ginecología, 1950.
18. Botella, J.: *Rev. Franç. Gynec. Obstet.,* 46:197, 1951.
19. Botella, J., and Nogales, F.: *Acta Gin.,* 6:281, 1955.

20. Botella, J., and Nogales, F.: *Actas Soc. Esp. Esterilidad*, 3:5, 1955.
21. Botella, J., and Gómez-Ruiz, J.: *Acta Gin.*, 10:439, 1959.
22. Boutselis, J. G., et al.: *Obst. & Gynec.*, 21:423, 1963.
23. Bremer, E., et al.: *Arch. Gyn.*, 181:96, 1951.
24. Brewer, J. I., and Jones, H. O.: *Amer. J. Obstet. Gynec.*, 38:389, 1939.
25. Brewer, J. I., and Jones, H. O.: *Amer. J. Obstet. Gynec.*, 54:561, 1948.
26. Bryson, M. J., and Sweat, M. L.: *Endocrinology*, 81:729, 1967.
27. Campos Da Paz, A.: *Fertil. Steril.*, 4:137, 1953.
28. Cardell, R. R., Hisaw, F. L., and Dawson, S. B.: *Amer. J. Anat.*, 124:307, 1969.
29. Cavazos, F., Green, J. A., Hall, D. G., and Lucas, F. V.: *Amer. J. Obstet. Gynec.*, 99:833, 1967.
30. Cecil, H. C., Bittman, J., Connoly, M. R., and Wrenn, T. R.: *J. Endocr.*, 21:69, 1962.
31. Chang, W. Y., O'Connell, M., and Pomeroy, S. R.: *Endocrinology*, 72:279, 1963.
32. Clyman, M. J.: *Internat. J. Fertil.*, 10:359, 1965.
33. Corner, G. W.: *Contrib. Embryol.*, 31:117, 1945.
34. Cortés-Ruiz, J.: *Thesis, University of Madrid*, 1951.
35. Cruz, J. de la, and Puras, A.: *Actas Soc. Esp. Esterilidad*, 3:70, 1955.
36. D'Amour, F. E.: *Amer. J. Obstet. Gynec.*, 40:598, 1970.
37. Dalgaard, J. B.: *Acta Obstet. Gynec. Scand.* 26:342, 1947.
38. Dallenbach-Hellweg, G.: *Das Endometrium*. Berlin, J. Springer, 1969.
39. Daron, G. H.: *Amer. J. Anat.*, 58:439, 1946.
40. Dorfman, R. I.: *Endocrinology*, 36:347, 1945.
41. Ecker, A. D.: *J. Clin. Endocr.*, 1:442, 1941.
42. Engstrom, W. W., and Munson, P. L.: *J. Clin. Endocr.*, 11:427, 1951.
43. Everett, J.: *J. Endocr.*, 24:491, 1962.
44. Faulkner, R. L.: *Amer. J. Obstet. Gynec.*, 49:1, 1951.
45. Fishman, W. H.: *J. Biol. Chem.*, 169:7, 1947.
46. Foraker, A. G., and Marino, G. A.: *Obstet. Gynec.*, 17:311, 1961.
47. Frieden, E. H., and Bates, F.: *Endocrinology*, 60:270, 1957.
48. Fuente, F. de la: *Actas Soc. Esp. Esterilidad*, 3:70, 1955.
49. Fuenzalida, F.: *Endocrinology*, 45:321, 1949.
50. Galli-Mainini, C., Castillo, E. del and Argonz, J.: *J. Clin. Endocr.*, 8:76, 1948.
51. Gautray, J. P., Couderc, P., Colomb, M. C., Sibut, H., and Maurenl, C.: *Amer. J. Obstet. Gynec.*, 104:818, 1969.
52. Gompel, C.: *Amer. J. Obstet. Gynec.*, 84:1000, 1962.
53. Gorski, J., Toft, D., and Shymala, G.: *Rec. Progr. Horm. Res.*, 24:45, 1968.
54. Hansen, O. C., and Raymond, R.: *J. Clin. Endocr.*, 3:81, 1943.
55. Heineman, M., et al.: *J. Clin. Invest.*, 27:91, 1948.
56. Henderson, I. D.: *J. Clin. Endocr.*, 16:905, 1956.
57. Hertig, A. T., and Rick, J.: In *Menstruation and its Disorders*, ed. E. T. Engle. Springfield, Ill., Charles C Thomas, 1950.
58. Hughes, E. C., Ness, A. W., and Lloyd, C. W.: *Amer. J. Obstet. Gynec.*, 59:1291, 1950.
59. Hughes, E. C., Jacobs, R. D., Rubulis, B. S., and Husney, R. M.: *Amer. J. Obstet. Gynec.*, 85:594, 1963.
60. Jaeger, J., and Dallenbach-Hellweg, G.: *Gynaecologia*, 168:117, 1969.
61. James, V. H. T.: *J. Endocr.*, 22:195, 1961.
62. Johnson, T. H.: *Amer. J. Obstet. Gynec.*, 75:240, 1958.
63. Kayser, I. H.: *Endocrinology*, 43:127, 1948.
64. Kroger, W. S.: *Psychosomatic Obstetrics, Gynecology and Endocrinology*. Springfield, Ill., Charles C Thomas, 1962.
65. Leathem, J. H.: *Ann. N.Y. Acad. Sci.*, 75:463, 1959.
66. Leonard, S. L.: *Endocrinology*, 71:803, 1962.
67. Liu, F. T., and Chai, C. K.: *Proc. Soc. Exper. Biol. Med.*, 106:521, 1961.
68. Loewi, G., and Consden, R.: *Nature*, 195:148, 1962.
69. Lukaszewska, J. H., and Hansel, W.: *Endocrinology*, 86:261, 1970.
70. MacLennan, C. E., and Rydell, A. H.: *Obstet. Gynec.*, 26:605, 1965.
71. Manning, J. P., Steinetz, B. G., Giannina, T., and Meli, A.: *Proc. Soc. Exper. Biol. Med.*, 125:508, 1967.
72. Markee, J. E.: *Contrib. Embryol.*, 24:223, 1940.
73. Martin, L., Cox, R. I., and Emmens, C. W.: *J. Endocr.*, 22:129, 1961.
74. Meng, H.: *Psyche und Hormon*. Bern, H. Huber, 1960.
75. Merlo, J. G.: *Acta Gin.*, 11:450, 1960.
76. Mitchell, J. A., and Jochim, J. M.: *Endocrinology*, 83:701, 1968.
77. Moricard, R.: In *Colloques sur la Fonction Lutéale*, Vol. I. Paris, Masson et Cie., 1954.
78. Moss, S., et al.: *Endocrinology*, 55:261, 1954.
79. Nilson, O., and Westman, A.: *Acta Obstet. Gynec. Scand.*, 40:223, 1961.
80. Nogales, F., and Botella, J.: *Acta Gin.*, 9:1, 1958.
81. Nogales, F., and Botella, J.: *Arch. Gynäk.*, 189:273, 1957.
82. Nogales, F., Martinez, H., and Parache, J.: *Gynäk. Rundschau* (Basel), 7:292, 1969.
83. Noyes, R. W.: *J. Endocr.*, 18:165, 1959.
84. Ogawa, Y., and Pincus, G.: *Endocrinology*, 67:551, 1960.
85. Okkels, H.: In *Menstruation and its Disorders*. Springfield, Charles C Thomas, 1950.
86. Palmer, R., and Ayala, G.: *Actas Soc. Esp. Esterilidad*, 3:271, 1955.
87. Papanicolaou, G. N., Traut, H. F., and Marchetti, G.: *The Epithelia of Woman's Reproductive Tract*. New York, The Commonwealth Foundation, 1948.
88. Payne, H. W., and Latour, J. P. A.: *J. Clin. Endocr.*, 15:1106, 1955.
89. Philippe, E., Ritter, J., Reneard, R., and Gander, R.: *Rev. Franç. Gynec. Obstet.*, 60:405, 1965.
90. Pincus, G., et al.: *Ann. N.Y. Acad. Sci.*, 71:677, 1958.
91. Prahlad, K. V.: *Acta Endocr.*, 31:407, 1962.
92. Prill, H. J., and Gotz, F.: *Amer. J. Obstet. Gynec.*, 82:103, 1961.
93. Rakoff, A. E., et al.: *Amer. J. Obstet. Gynec.*, 47:467, 1944.
94. Reynolds, S. R. M.: *Physiology of the Uterus*. New York, Hoeber, 1949.
95. Reynolds, S. R. M., Harris, J. S., and Kayser, I. H.: *The Measurement of Uterine Forces*

96. Rock, J., Garcia, C. R., and Menkin, M. F.: *Ann. N.Y. Acad. Sci.*, 75:831, 1959.
 97. Rockenschaub, A.: *Gynaecologia*, 149:179, 1960.
 98. Rockenschaub, A.: *Ztschr. Geb. Gynäk.*, 155:105, 1960.
 99. Rodríguez-Galindo, M.: *Rev. Franç. Gynec.*, 55:583, 1960.
100. Rorie, D. K., and Newton, J.: *Fertil. Steril.*, 16:27, 1965.
101. Rosa, C. G., and Velardo, J. T.: *Ann. N.Y. Acad. Sci.*, 75:491, 1959.
102. Russell, K. J.: *Obstet. Gynec. Surv.*, 9:157, 1954.
103. Runge, H., et al.: *Deutsch. Med. Wschr.*, 81:351, 1957.
104. Rydberg, E.: *Acta Obstet. Gynec. Scand.*, 28:172, 1948.
105. Schlegel, J. V.: *Acta Anat.* 1:1285, 1945.
106. Schramm, B.: In *Colloques sur la fonction lutéale*, Vol. I. Paris, Masson et Cie., 1954.
107. Scott, D. B. M., and Parksley, A. M.: *Biochem. J.*, 83:266, 1962.
108. Smith, G. V., and Smith, O. W.: *J. Clin. Endocr.*, 6:475, 1946.
109. Stegner, H. E.: *Arch. Gynäk.*, 197:351, 1962.
110. Strauss, G.: *Arch. Gynäk.*, 197:524, 1962.
111. Swigart, R. H., Wagner, C. H., Herbener, G. H., and Atkinson, W. B.: *Endocrinology*, 70:600, 1962.
112. Traut, H. F., and Kuder, A.: *Amer. J. Obstet. Gynec.*, 61:145, 1945.
113. Urdan, B. E., and Kurzon, A. M.: *Obstet. Gynec.*, 5:3, 15, 1955.
114. Vaes, G.: *Acta Endocr.*, 39:513, 1962.
115. Villee, C. A.: *Ann. N.Y. Acad. Sci.*, 75:524, 1959.
116. Wislocky, G. B., et al.: In *Menstruation and its Disorders*. Springfield, Ill., 1950.
117. Warren, J. C., Chathun, S. L., Greenwald, G. S., and Barker, K. L.: *Endocrinology*, 80:714, 1967.
118. Wynn, R. M., and Wooley, R. S.: *Fertil. Steril.*, 18:721, 1967.
119. Wurtman, R. J., Chu, E. W., and Axelrod, J.: *Nature*, 198:547, 1963.
120. Zander, J., and Ober, G. K.: *Arch. Gynäk.*, 196:481, 1962.
121. Zuckerman, S.: *The Ovary*. London, Churchill, 1962.
122. Zweifach, B. W., and Shorr, E.: In *Menstruation and its Disorders*. Springfield, Ill., Charles C Thomas, 1950.

Part Four
THE EVOLUTION OF SEX

In the first three parts of this book, dealing with the subjects of sex hormones, control of gonadal function and the reproductive cycle, we have presented an outline of what we believe to be a sufficiently approximate scheme of female sexual life "in space." These same concepts now remain to be developed "in time." The analysis of how sex is generated and how it evolves in the course of life shall constitute the main topic of the following chapters.

Chapter 14

ORIGIN OF SEX: GENETIC SEX

by PROF. J. A. CLAVERO-NÚÑEZ
*Department of Gynecology,
Medical Faculty of the
University of Madrid*

14.1. REPRODUCTION: THE GAMETES

The purpose of sexual reproduction has already been explained (see Chapter 1, Section 1.0.0). Essentially, sex is aimed at achieving genetic variation by virtue of pairing two cells, the sexual cells, each derived from different progeny and each bearing a distinct genetic message. In order to maintain the number of chromosomes constant and to preserve the genetic code, the sexual cells to be conjugated must contain half the number of chromosomes of the species. The number of chromosomes in a cell is expressed by the letter N, and a cell bearing a single set of chromosomes is known as *a haplont, with a haploid number of chromosomes*. The union of two haplonts (each with N chromosomes) gives rise to a *diplont* (2N chromosomes), and a pair of diplonts, in turn, generate a *tetraploid* cell (4N). Were there no *reduction division* (known as meiosis), which transforms the diploid number into the haploid number, the pairing of two 2N cells would result in tetraploid (4N) cells, and the number of chromosomes would thus increase geometrically in each successive generation, giving rise to mutation of the species. Meiosis is therefore necessary for the conservation of species immutability on the animal scale *through a type of division designed to preserve the characteristic diploid number of chromosomes by means of producing haploid cells, namely the gametes, the union of which restores the* 2N *number of chromosomes typical of the species.*

Sexual reproduction, then, may be defined as an exchange of genes through pairing of chromosomes, followed by meiotic division, which yields the gametes.

In the case of *isogamous* beings, there is no morphologic differentiation into sexes, such differentiation emerging only as a later feature of reproduction. Nevertheless, a relative biochemical sexual distinction is apparent even here in that an isogamete may be spoken of as either male or female,[40, 50] depending on the nature of its would-be mate. This stage has been carried a step further among bacteria. In *Escherichia coli*,[52, 119] the organism on which most research has been done, fertilization is accomplished by the passage of the only existing chromosome from one cell (the male) to another (the female), a subsequent reduction division completing the cycle of reproduction. This simple process involves a type of "functional differentiation" that brings us closer to morphologic differences between the sexes and is itself, of course, a form of "sexual differentiation."

14.2. SEXUAL DIFFERENTIATION

Even though lower unicellular organisms, as we have seen, have no true sexual differentiation, but rather a form of "relative differentiation," the presence of dimorphism throughout the rest of the biologic scale is quite evident, *provided that it is understood that such duality may affect either both gametes and somatic morphology (phenotype) or only the gametes (in the case of hermaphroditism). We shall therefore be concerned with two types of sexual differentiation: gametic differentiation, and phenotypic, or somatic, differentiation, the two not necessarily coexisting in a given biologic species, as they do in hermaphrodites, under physiologic conditions.*

By definition, all heterogamous beings undergo sexual differentiation (at least, insofar as their gametes are concerned); in addition, in some species there exist male organs side by side with female organs in the same individual (hermaphrodites), which must be interpreted as the next step in phylogeny toward complete separation of the sexes, that is, *higher differentiation*. We shall then discuss two types of heterogamous individuals: those in which no phenotypic sexual separation takes place, viz., hermaphrodites, and those presenting complete sexual differentiation.

14.3. HERMAPHRODITISM

Having already defined hermaphroditism, we shall now briefly describe the existing gradations among hermaphrodites, which range up to true sexual dimorphism.

Generally speaking, "true hermaphrodite" frequently evokes in one's mind the image of a worm, since it is well known that in the annelid *Sagitta*, a worm studied by Witschi,[116] the germ cells located in the midsegment develop into ovules, whereas those remaining in the tail of the worm give rise to sperm. Similarly, the germ cells of *Helix pomatia*[101] may differentiate either way, depending on their location, and the same occurs in *Valvea crestata*, a mollusk studied by Furrow,[29] in which the same bisexual gland contains ovules in the cortex and seminal cells in the medulla.

It follows that the germ cells of this type of animals have the potential for bivalent development, evolving, according to where they are located, either into sperm or into ovules through the action of different inductors present in the internal environment. Significantly, those germ cells of *Valvea crestata* which are surrounded by several nutritional cells (in the cortex of the gland) give rise to ovules, whereas those which are clustered around a single nutritional cell evolve into spermia. While, on the one hand, nutrition would seem to play an essential role in sexual differentiation, on the other hand, the already mentioned disposition of cells is strikingly similar to that adopted by the germ cells of vertebrates, with the ovum lying in the granulosa and the spermatocytes developing around a single Sertoli cell.

Representative of the second group of hermaphrodites are *Ophryotrocha puerilis* (a sea worm) and some other annelids, such as isopods and mollusks, in which sexual dimorphism *evolves with advancing age*, so that while younger individuals are male, they change into female as they grow older. Hartmann[40] asserts that even tiny particles of *Ophryotrocha* are able to develop into full males by virtue of the regenerative process that is peculiar to these annelids. The occurrence of age-linked sexual duality in the same individual presupposes a potential of the male cells to transform into female cells depending either on the aging process itself or on the presence of a rudimentary female gland which, at a given time in the animal's life, is able to reach full development while the male gonad undergoes atrophy. In either case, the unquestionable fact is that these animals are hermaphrodites since, however transiently, they possess both female and male gonads at the same time.

Finally, a third group of hermaphrodites has features overlapping with true sexual dimorphism. As an example, we cite *Bonellia viridis*, a worm studied by Baltzer[2,3] and Herbst,[43] in which sexual dimorphism is determined by certain substances secreted by the mother's tube which cause those larvae in contact with the mother to become male individuals, while causing those larvae that remain unattached to become female individuals. In this instance, sexual dimorphism of both somatic and gametic variety is achieved by the action of the external environment, that is, substances of hormonal nature and of maternal origin. Yet, it is evident that these are nevertheless a variety of hermaphroditism, even though borderline, because their eggs are sexless and because sex in their larvae is induced by special *mediators*, a clear indication that they possess a common organ, or undifferentiated gonad (ovotestis), which has the potential to develop in either direction.

This, as we pointed out earlier, is the common denominator for all hermaphrodites.

Even though the gametes of hermaphrodites may undergo sexual differentiation, it is evident that, by themselves, they are unable to establish either genotypic or phenotypic dimorphism. Only by virtue of certain internal or external conditions, such dimorphism may later eventually be established.

Seen from this point of view, what differentiates hermaphroditism from true sexual dimorphism is the fact that the gametes of hermaphrodites, even if morphologically distinct, are not inherently endowed with sex-determining faculties, as are animals higher on the biologic scale, but require internal (lower hermaphrodites) or extrinsic (higher hermaphrodites) stimuli for their gonads to be differentiated, which thus gives rise to false sexual dimorphism, as in the case of Bonellia.

14.4. TRUE SEXUAL DIMORPHISM

The stimulus, or genetic principle, *per se* capable of determining sex emerged on the biologic scale in the course of evolution. According to Witschi's calculations,[117] it was during the Jurassic period, 150 million years ago, that mammalian genes underwent mutation, possibly imposed by the influence of the phenotype on the genotype, whereby the already morphologically distinct male and female gametes became also genetically distinct.

The imposed mutation possibly involved a simple translocation of some genes, that is, the acquisition on the part of one chromosome of some genes pertaining to the opposite gamete, instead of equitably sharing the genes, as occurred in hermaphrodites. *From then on, the resulting genetic difference gave rise to a new development in sexual evolution, that is, to true and complete dimorphism of animals higher on the biologic scale.*

This was an unprecedented event. As a result, there were two types of gametes carrying complementary genetic material, giving rise to equally different chromosomal constitutions. What is more, these gametes were capable by themselves of producing different sexes, each endowed with a distinct genotype, a distinct soma and gonads specific to the particular sex involved.

True sexual dimorphism can only be admitted to occur in animals fulfilling the following two conditions: (1) presence of gametes with different chromosomal constitution for each sex, and (2) presence of specific gonads for each sex.

14.5. GAMETOGENESIS IN EACH SEX

For the sake of clarity, let us recall Boveri's scheme of gametogenesis, as modified by modern knowledge. This is illustrated in Figure 14–1, for the development of both the oocyte (oogenesis) and the spermatocyte (spermatogenesis). Gonadal differentiation, as will be described in a subsequent chapter (Chapter 15, Section 15.1.1), is accomplished by migratory cells, known as gonocytes, which are endowed with ameboid motility. Originating in the primitive gut, these cells migrate through the mesentery until they reach the genital primordium or "Anlage." There, they are transformed into either oogonia (the future oocytes) or spermatogonia, depending on their genetic constitution—XX or XY—respectively.

In the embryonal and fetal ovary, oogonia undergo proliferation and rapid multiplication. However, after the sixth or seventh month of intrauterine life, this proliferative process ceases and (generally speaking) there is no further increase in the number of oogonia. In comparison, spermatogonia keep proliferating and multiplying throughout a man's life, well into advanced age. Thus, while *oogenesis* in the female is a process of *limited duration*, *spermatogenesis* in the male may be considered a *continuous* process.

After the seventh month of intrauterine life, oogonia remain in a "fixed" state. At this stage, they begin to undergo their first maturation division, during which each oogonium engenders a primary oocyte. Böving[11] has shown that the process of chromosomal reduction (that is, a 50 per cent decrease in the number of chromosomes) already starts in primary oocytes, although the latter are still diplonts and although genuine meiosis does not occur until they become secondary oocytes. Since

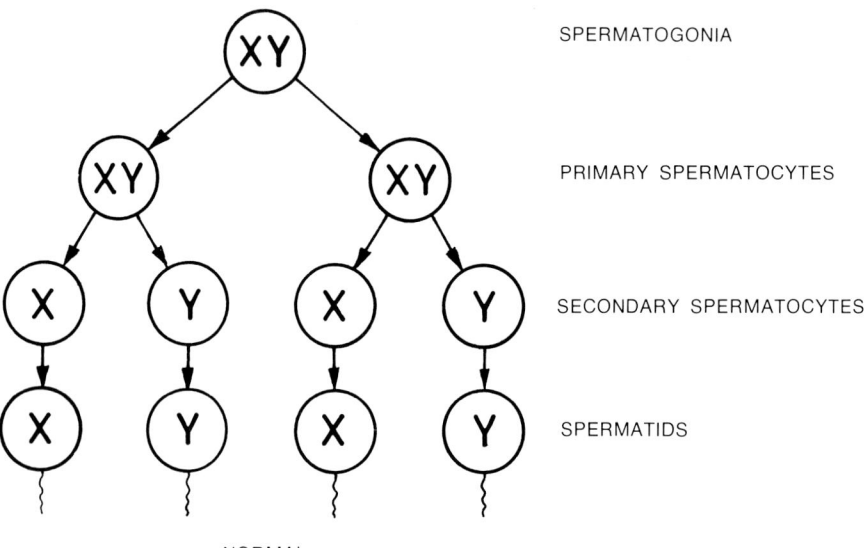

Figure 14-1. Spermatogenesis in man, resulting in formation of spermatids, or mature male gametes, from spermatogonia (immature gametes).

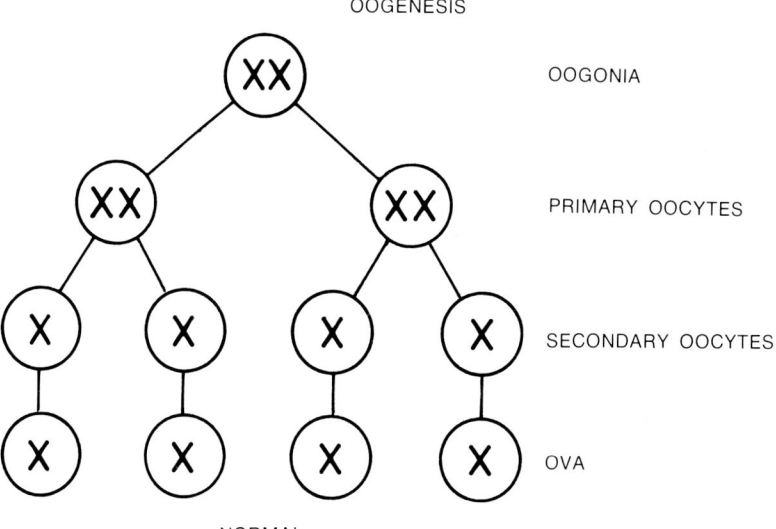

Figure 14-2. Formation of ova from oogonia. To stress the similarity to spermatogenesis, the polar bodies, which have no germinal function, have been omitted.

this point in the development of the primary oocyte, as well as the beginning of the dictyotene stage, is reached during the seventh month of intrauterine life, it is quite obvious that the time interval elapsing between the occurrence of the first phases of meiosis and completion of meiosis must be of many years' duration, from 13 to 14 years for the first ovulation, up to 45 years or more for the last one. In the meantime, the oocyte rests in the ovary in a state of hibernation, during which the process of chromosomal reduction is arrested.

The same cannot be said about the spermatocyte. The entire process of multiplication, meiosis and differentiation, from the moment a spermatogonium first undergoes division until maturation of the spermatozoon is completed, has been shown to take 32 days in studies with tritiated thymidine conducted by Clermont.[17] As a result, the mature spermatozoon is a recently formed cell, as compared with the mature oocyte, or, using Böving's terminology, the *ootid*, which is a cell whose maturation has been delayed and arrested for a long time.

14.6. THE CHROMOSOMES

The idea of possible chromosomal differences between nuclei, allowing one to distinguish a male from a female in all their cells, both the autosome and the gametes, was first entertained by Henking[42] in 1891 when, in the course of a study on spermatogenesis in the bug *Pyrhocoris apterus*, he observed the presence in a dividing nucleus of a peculiar chromatinic element. However, he failed to recognize its significance and mistook it for a nucleolus.

In 1899, McClung identified this element as an "accessory chromosome" and, in 1902, proposed an unusually bold hypothesis for that time, namely, that the element in question was somehow involved in determining sex.[59] Although this hypothesis was greeted with mixed reactions of surprise and alarm, following intensive studies, particularly by Wilson and Stevens, this theory eventually became fully accepted and, at the same time, recognized to be applicable to all animals. As a result, chromosomes have been divided into two categories: one, called *autosomes*, responsible for somatic growth and development, the other, *heterochromosomes or gonosomes*, responsible for the origin of sex.

In 1912, von Winiwarter[115] developed a new technique for the visualization of mitoses in the cells of the testis and introduced the term *diploid* (2N). He believed, mistakenly, that there were two kinds of spermatozoa, one with a single heterochromosome (XO), the other with two X chromosomes, each carrying a total of 23 or 24 chromosomes, respectively. Ovules were believed to invariably possess two X chromosomes. The fusion of an XO gamete with an XX ovum was thought to give rise to a male with 47 chromosomes, whereas the union of an XX spermium with an XX ovum produced a female with 48 chromosomes, four of which presumably were heterochromosomes.

In 1921, Painter[73] found that the number of chromosomes was identical in both sexes, noting that only one of the two heterochromosomes was different: the Y chromosome of the male. Aside from this, however, Painter was undecided as to whether the total number of chromosomes was 46 or 48. Interestingly, still later (in 1923)[74] he decided that the correct figure was 48, which was to remain the accepted number until 1956, at which time the true number was definitely established as 46, as a result of the convincing studies of fetal lung cells in abortuses by Tjio and Levan.[110] In the same year, Ford and Hamerton[24] confirmed the fact that the spermatogonia of the male had 23 chromosomes, of which one was unequivocally a Y chromosome.

Thanks to technical innovations, introduced mainly by Makino and Mishimura[60] in 1952 (hypotonic solutions, producing swelling of cells in mitosis and causing breakup of the spindle at metaphase, with release and separation of individual chromosomes), it was possible to establish that the number and shape of chromosomes, with the exception of one of the heterochromosomes (XX in females, XY in males), was constant for a given species. This gave impetus to exhaustive clinical research and new technical developments. The feasibility of obtaining excellent leukocyte cultures from a simple venipuncture has contributed enormously to progress in this branch of science, which is termed *cytogenetics*. In the process, new light has been shed on the pathogenesis of countless alterations of sex, soma and psyche, which shall be studied extensively later (see Chapter 35).

We shall now consider the role of chromosomes in determining sex.

14.7. DETERMINATION OF SEX

The anlage of the gonad does not take shape until after the arrival in it of certain migratory cells, called *gonocytes* by Fischer, which are derived from the coelomic epithelium and the underlying mesenchyme (see Chapter 15). These cells constitute the "germinal route," composed of an ensemble of cells thought to have a twofold mission: (1) to determine the sex of an individual and to induce development of that sex, and (2) to produce the gonia, or gametes, which transmit hereditary characteristics.

14.7.1. THE GERMINAL ROUTE

Politzer,[78] in 1933, was first to describe a germinal route (Keimbahn), no mention of which is made in the classic works of Stieve,[104] Simkins,[96] or Swezy and Evans.[106] Recent studies seem to confirm its existence in man (Everett,[21,22] Gillman[32] and Witschi[118]). Germ cells can first be recognized in the yolk sac of 2.8 mm embryos (in Streeter's Horizon XI, which usually appears 24 days from the time of ovulation and comprises embryos of 13 to 20 somites). From here they migrate through the caudal part of the primitive gut and reach the undifferentiated gonad at Horizon XV (31.5 days after ovulation, which corresponds to 7.5 mm embryos) (Witschi[119]). Blandau found that migration of such germ cells in the mouse was made possible by their capacity for ameboid motion. The extraordinary importance all this has for the development of the gonads is apparent from the experiment of Everett.[21,22] If the sexual zone of a mouse is transplanted to the kidney before it reveals any primitive cells, the sex cords do not develop, whereas, in the presence of primitive sexual cells in the transplanted tissue, typical ovaries or testes are formed in the animals with the transplants. A similar observation made in birds by Dantschakoff[19] and by Grünwald[39] some time ago revealed that gonadal differentiation failed to take place if migration of these primitive cells was blocked.

Under normal conditions, the germ cells are obviously capable of determining and developing sex by virtue of their genetic chromosomal differentiation, which gives rise to true sexual dimorphism, as distinct from hermaphroditism. Although a very early stage in the life of vertebrates may be spoken of as a stage of gonadal undifferentiation, the ultimate destiny of the gonad is irrevocably sealed from the very moment of fertilization, since the genes involved in the fusion of the spermium and the ovum inherently carry the appropriate stimulus for the origin of sex.

14.7.2. SPERMATIC DIMORPHISM

Unlike the case with higher hermaphrodites, we are witnessing the complete emancipation of sexual determination and development from the influence of the external or internal environment. Hereditary in nature, this emancipation is transmitted through the germinal route.

In fact, some of the spermatozoa carry 22 autosomes plus one X chromosome, while others carry the same number of autosomes plus one Y chromosome. This unequal apportionment, bestowing "sexual personality" on spermatozoa, takes place during the conversion of spermatogonia (diplonts) to spermatids (haplonts).

In the scheme proposed by Boveri (Fig. 14–1), genetic dimorphism among spermatids is already apparent. By comparing this with Figure 14–2, which illustrates oogenesis, it becomes evident that ovules invariably possess one X chromosome, whereas spermatozoa have either one X chromosome or one Y chromosome.

Shettles,[90–94] and Fariñas and Botella[23] observed the fact that spermatozoa have a dual morphology: some have small and rounded heads (very numerous), and some have large, elongated heads (less numerous). The first seemed to be Y chromosome carriers, the second X chromosome carriers (Figs. 14–3 and 14–4).

Oogonia, on the other hand, give ovules with only one X chromosome although, as will be seen later, there seems to be a fundamental biochemical difference be-

Origin of Sex: Genetic Sex

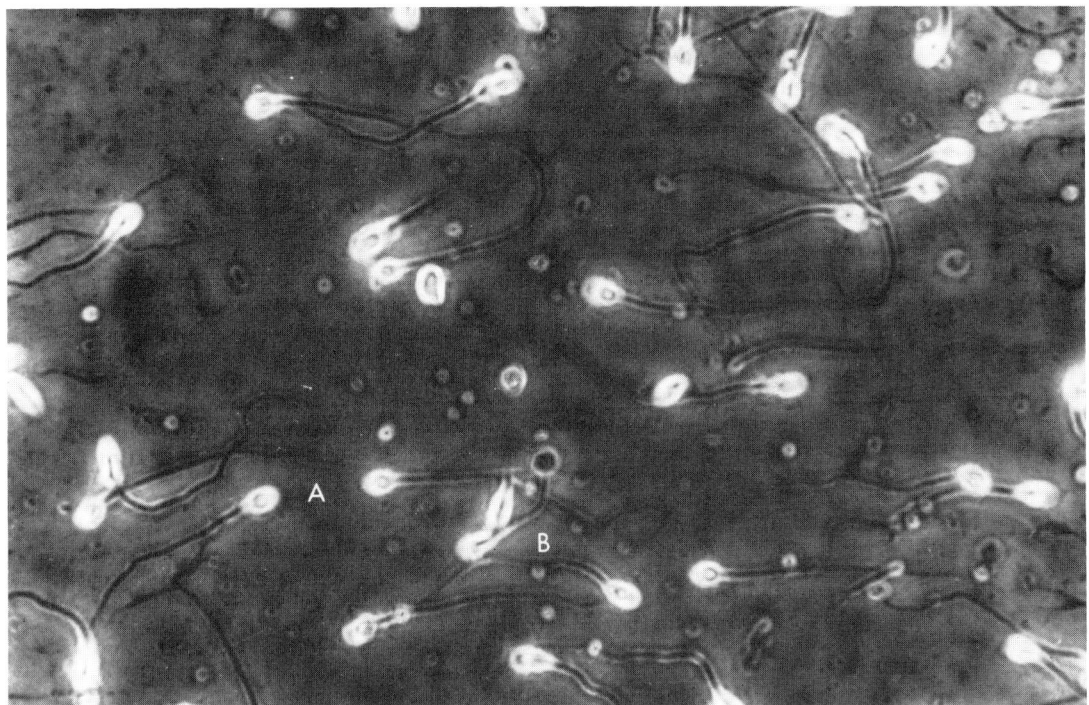

Figure 14-3. Dried, thin film preparation of normal human sperm, viewed by means of phase contrast microscope (480×). Two types of spermatozoa are distinctly noted—one with an elongated head, and the other, which is smaller in size, with a round head.

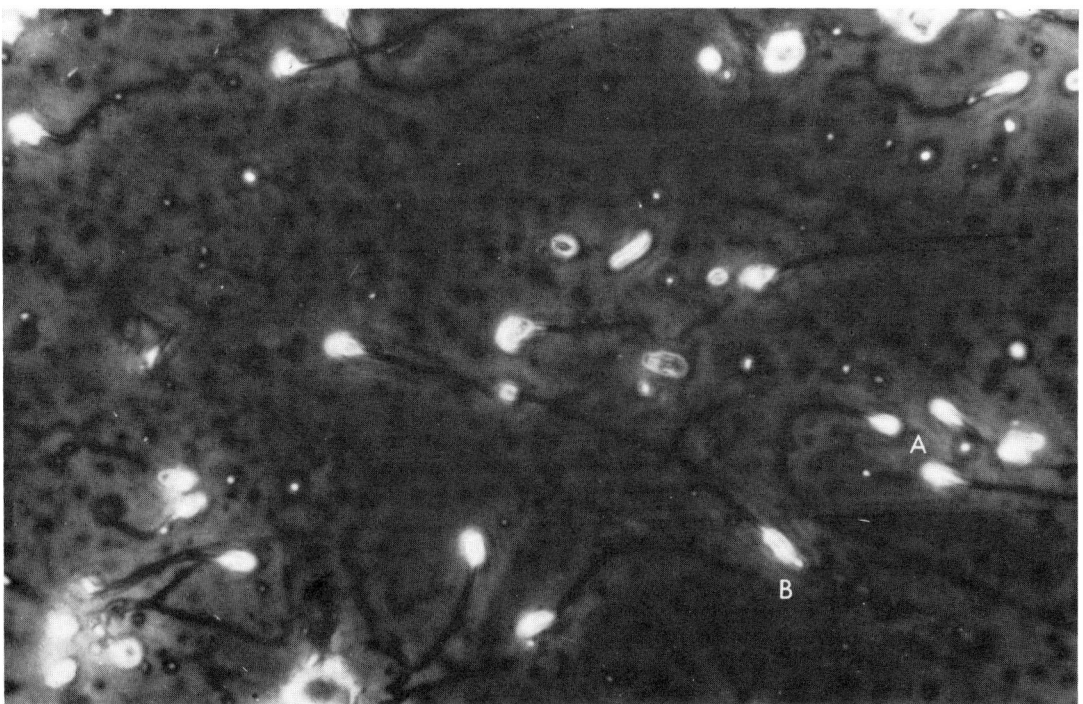

Figure 14-4. Dried, thin film of normal human sperm (phase contrast, 480×). Spermatozoa A have a round, small head. Spermatozoa B have an elongated, large head.

tween the two components of the bivalent XX. Boveri's scheme raised even more questions concerning oogenesis than concerning spermatogenesis. In the first place, Boveri, along with most classical proponents, subscribed to the belief that the first division occurred by means of meiosis and not mitosis. Accordingly, an oogonium in the ovary was thought to proceed only halfway through meiosis (the diplotene stage) only to "hibernate" during a subsequent resting period, as we have indicated above. Blandau[7] has shown that the process of meiosis is not completed until the primary oocyte divides, leaving behind the secondary oocyte and the first polar body.

Böving[11] has introduced the notion that the first division is by mitosis and not by meiosis. Furthermore, he rejects the term ovule as unrealistic. In his opinion, an oocyte II (a fertilizable female gamete) does not give off a polar body II unless fertilized, in which case both the polar body and the ootid actually result from meiotic division. Aware of the arguments involved, we have retained a somewhat modified scheme, which most clearly illustrates the fact that chromosomal distribution in oogenesis is apparently even. The fusion of an X spermatozoon with an X ovum is thought to produce a normal female (44 + XX), whereas the fusion of a Y spermatozoon with an X ovum gives a normal male (44 + XY).

14.7.3. THE ACTIVE X CHROMOSOME

Overzier[71, 72] enunciated the theory that, in monogametic sex (female), a single X chromosome is specific of femininity, being transmitted specifically to daughters, whereas the other X chromosome (nonspecific) is transmitted to sons. In this way, the pairing up of an "active" maternal X chromosome with a male Y chromosome would be impossible, as would also that of an "inactive" female X with a similar male X chromosome.

Studies on tritiated thymidine labeled chromosomes by Giannelli,[31] among others, seem to indicate that indeed only one X chromosome is active, and that this one is actually the chromosome present within the chromatin mass or the Barr body, which has also been referred to as the "hot" chromosome (Turpin and Lejeune[114]) (see Fig. 14–6).

14.7.4. SEXUAL DIFFERENTIATION AMONG DIFFERENT SPECIES

The question of whether heterochromosomes partake in determining sex had long been a matter of debate. It has already been mentioned that von Winiwarter[115] explained the process of sexual determination in the human species without the participation of a male-specific Y chromosome. In 1923, while studying *Drosophila melanogaster* (a fly in which the Y chromosome is not necessary for the formation of a male), Bridges[12] formulated his famous laws concerning the need for balance between the number of autosomes and that of X heterochromosomes in order to produce either male or female individuals. Ponse,[79] in 1949, and Hartmann,[41] in 1953, were convinced that sexual determination was linked to a factor of realization located in the X chromosome. If there was only one X chromosome, the male type predominated; if there were two, there was female predominance.

This type of determination can be observed in the hemipterous insect *Protenor belfragii*, in which only one X heterochromosome is present in the male and two in the female. Wilson draws a distinction between this type and that observed in the insect *Lygaeus bicrucis*, in which the male has a bivalent XY and the female an XX.

The way sexual differentiation takes place in the *Lygaeus* model is believed to be as follows: autosomes carry a number of male genes and female genes in an equilibrium which is unbalanced by the presence of the pairs XY or XX. Because the Y chromosome predominates over the X chromosome, a male develops whenever the former is present and, vice versa, its absence always results in a female. It was actually Goldschmidt who, in 1917, advanced the theory of dominance of the Y over the X chromosome in the sense that the presence of a Y chromosome induces the development of a male.

In 1942, Westergard observed that in plants with an XX (female) and XY (male) genotype, XXXY individuals were male. The same effect was observed by Kanaka, in 1953, in *Bombyx mori* (males, ZZ; females, ZW) in which a ZZW constitution produced females, and by Ford, in 1961, in butterflies. These experiments proved the existence of a "strong" chromosome in digametic sex. The observation that men with the Klinefelter's syndrome may have an XXY, XXYY, XXXY, XXXXY or XXXYY constitution (see Chapter 35) proves the existence of Y chromosome dominance in the human species also, though to a lesser extent, since such individuals are far from being normal.

Based on the foregoing considerations, the gametes of the human species can be concluded to have a distinct constitution, possessing the inherent faculty of determining and developing sex. Their fusion gives a diploid zygote which, although it is morphologically a hermaphrodite in the earliest stage, eventually evolves into the sex irrevocably determined by its chromosomes, without need for any other external or internal stimuli.

14.7.5. CHARACTERIZATION OF X AND Y CHROMOSOMES

The feasibility of identifying the "hot" X chromosome by means of tritiated thymidine labeling (Giannelli[31]) has already been referred to. It should be added that, as recently as 1970, Pearson and co-workers,[77] as well as George,[30] have demonstrated selective Y chromosome staining with quinacrine chlorhydrate or quinacrine mustard, facilitating, among other things, detection of the double Y chromosome (the so-called chromosome of aggressivity) in buccal smears.

14.7.6. EXPERIMENTALLY INDUCED DETERMINATION OF SEX

In 1949, Bengtson[8] maintained that, on the basis of statistical data, coitus between the eleventh and fifteenth days of the cycle was likely to result in a higher ratio of males than coitus between the fifteenth and twentieth days, which was associated with a greater proportion of females. Shettles[94] attempted to explain this by prostulating that because Y chromosome-carrying spermatozoa, identifiable in cytologic preparations by their smaller heads, were characterized by a higher rate of motility, they exhausted their available energy pool faster, thereby shortening the duration of their motile life. In contrast, the slower moving spermatozoa with large heads, presumptive X chromosome carriers, were believed to enjoy a longer span of active life. Though supported by O'Ferrall and his associates[67] and recommended by Shettles himself as the method for choosing the desired sex by timing coitus, this hypothesis could not be confirmed by subsequent experimental studies on artificial fertilization (Lindahl[56] and Kleegman[47]). While reaffirming the statistical data of Bengtsson as basically correct, Cederqvist and Fuchs[16] have similarly been unable to come up with a satisfactory explanation.

Notwithstanding the fact that all kinds of similar attempts in humans so far have been based on more or less hypothetical grounds, artificial insemination in animals has actually solved the problem of achieving the desired sex, thanks to various procedures which allow X spermia to be separated from Y spermia. For this purpose, for instance, Lindahl[56] used a countercurrent centrifugation procedure. Lewin[55] and Gordon[34] employed electrophoresis. Other experiments, using various modifications of countercurrent distribution techniques, have also been tested by, among others, Schilling[86] and Sevinç,[89] while Rotschild[83] employed a selective hemagglutination procedure.

By and large, while separation of the two kinds of spermatozoa, Y carriers from X carriers, no longer poses any unsurmountable problem, induction of the desired sex can for the time being not be achieved by ordinary means, other than artificial insemination.

14.8. DIAGNOSIS OF SEX: CHROMATINIC SEX AND CHROMOSOMAL SEX

Findings such as those summarized in preceding sections have obliged clinicians to search for adequate diagnostic means that would elucidate the problem of intersexuality. Tangible results in advancing the understanding of sexual genetics have been achieved in practice with the introduction of so-called "karyotype" or "chromosome maps," which shall be studied in the following section.

14.8.1. THE SEX CHROMATIN

Some progress in this respect was made as early as 1949 by Barr and Bertram,[4] who described what later was to prove a discovery of exceptional significance. While studying the nuclei of the hypoglossal nerve of a female cat, they became aware of a small accumulation of chromatin, in the form of a hump, present in about 40 per cent of the nuclei. They designated it "nucleolar appendage," or "satellite." Similar satellites were almost never observed in nuclei of male cells. Subsequent investigations on tissue from other parts of the nervous system of the same and other laboratory animals showed that the nuclear appendage, or satellite, appeared also in Betz cells, in Purkinje cells and, quite prominently, in cells of the sympathetic ganglia, but that this was invariably the case in nuclei of female cells but not in those of male cells.

In 1950, Barr and his associates[5] discovered the presence of similar nucleolar appendages in human cells. Later, Graham and Barr,[36, 37] Moore and Barr,[64] as well as Takahashi,[107] found that the occurrence of such bodies extended to nearly all mammals (rabbits, rats, mice, macaques, and various types of domestic animals).

Of even greater significance was the finding that sex chromatin could be demonstrated in all human tissues, especially skin, adrenal cortex, liver and mucosas (see Figs. 14–5 and 14–6). Studies in this field were pioneered mainly by Prince and his colleagues[80] and by Lang and Hansel.[51]

However, perhaps the greatest practical advances in the diagnosis of sex have been made possible through the development of readily available and easily studied cytologic preparations of vaginal smears, buccal smears, amniotic fluid and thin smears of peripheral blood.

ORAL MUCOSA. Marberger and his associates,[61] as well as Moore and Barr,[65] described a simple technique that yielded excellent results, which subsequently received prompt endorsement from Greenblatt and co-workers.[38]

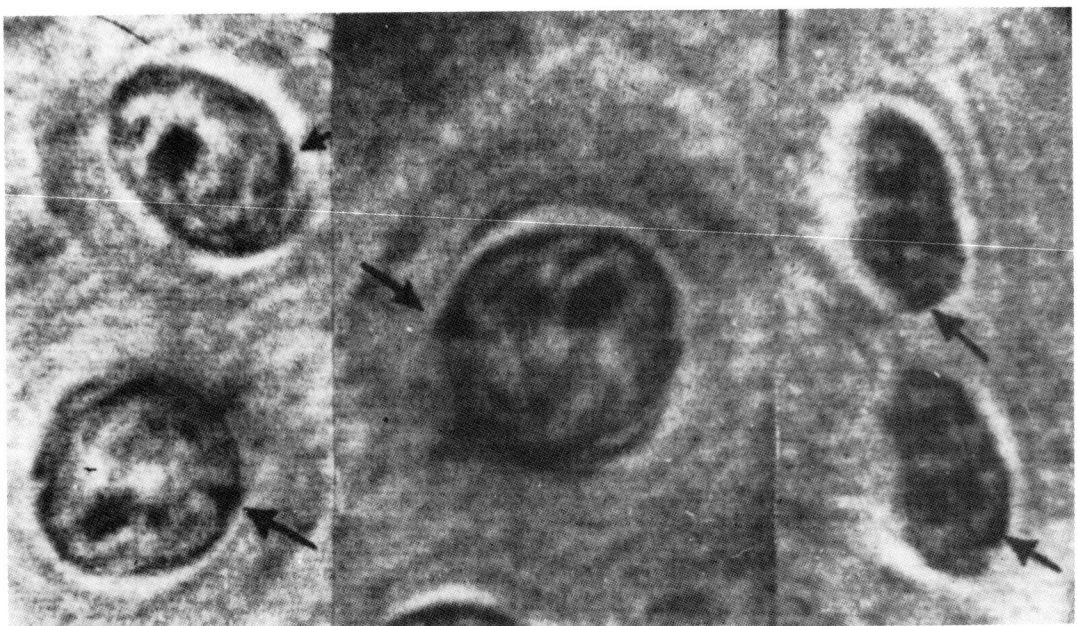

Figure 14–5. Sex chromatin in the form of a wedge-shaped chromatin mass beneath the nuclear membrane of a malpighian cell of the skin. This case, which is Barr body positive, is discussed in a different context in Chapter 36 (case of true hermaphroditism). (From Botella et al.: *Acta Gin.*, 12:139, 1961.)

Figure 14–6. Sex chromatin in exfoliated cells: *A*, buccal smear; *B, C, D*, vaginal smears.

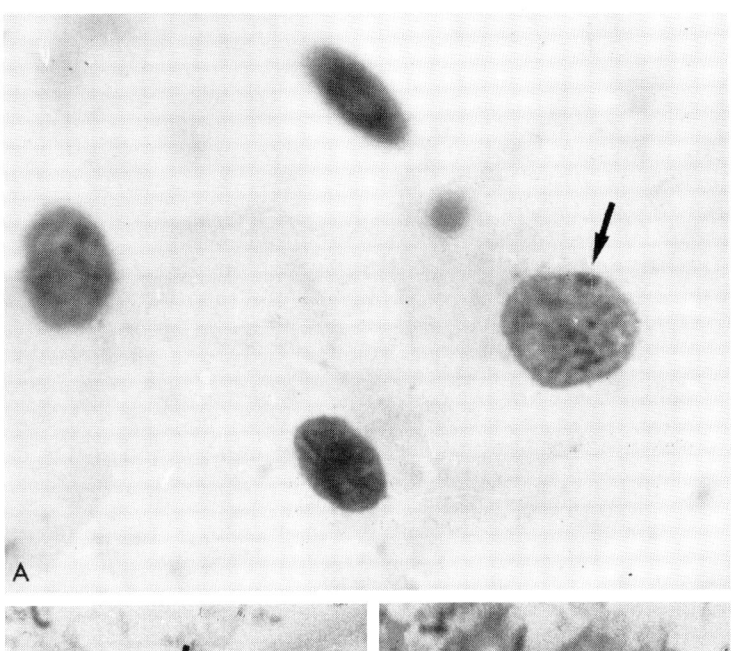
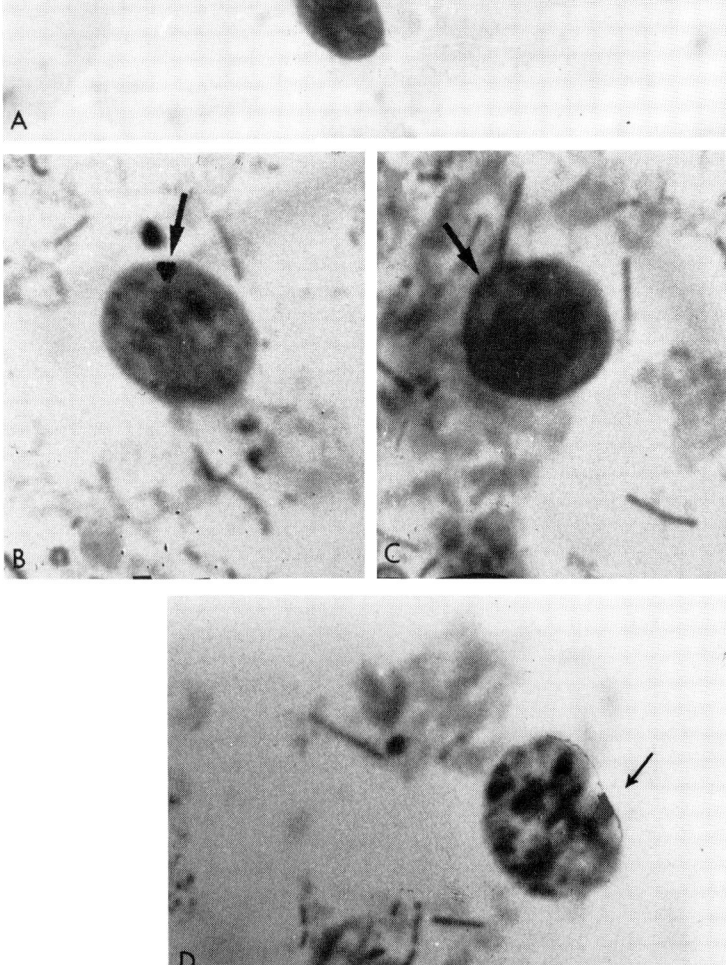

VAGINAL MUCOSA. Carpenter and his colleagues[14, 15] reported that a higher percentage of Barr bodies could be visualized in cells of ordinary vaginal smears than in buccal smears that were prepared by the same technique.

AMNIOTIC FLUID. The sex of the fetus can be detected by studying exfoliated fetal cells, obtained by centrifugation of amniotic fluid, with a margin of error that is less than 10 per cent, according to various investigators (Sachs et al.,[84] Shettles,[95] James,[46] Dewhurst,[20] Sohvall et al.[99] and Montalvo[63]).

BLOOD SMEARS. One to two per cent of polymorphonuclear leukocytes from females were described by Davidson and Robertson-Smith to have a nuclear appendage in the form of a drumstick; this appendage was practically never observed in males (less than one in 500). This gave rise to a new method for the determination of sex, which was popularized by Danon,[18] and Rakoff[105] and Briggs and Kuppermann.[13] However, results with this method have not been found to be as reliable as those obtained with other methods we have described, and results may differ in the same individual. Drumsticks do not seem to respresent the same entity that makes up the Barr chromatin (Fig. 14-7).

In cytologic preparations, the Barr body appears as a triangular or discoid mass, ranging in size from 0.3 to 1.1 microns, resting directly against the nuclear membrane. The consistency with which it can be visualized depends on the type of tissue and staining technique employed, as well as the thickness of the smear. Sachs and Danon[85] reported that the best results were obtained by studying prickle cells of the skin by means of the Feulgen reaction (95 per cent).

CHARACTERISTICS OF THE SEX CHROMATIN. The appearance of sex chromatin in the embryo is coincident with the blastocyst stage (Barr,[6] Austin and Amoroso,[1] Glenister,[33] Park[75] and Klinger[48]) and, although much has been said about its immutability throughout life, Taylor,[108] Gordon and Dewhurst,[35] as well as Smith and colleagues,[98] have observed that the percentage of Barr bodies increases ap-

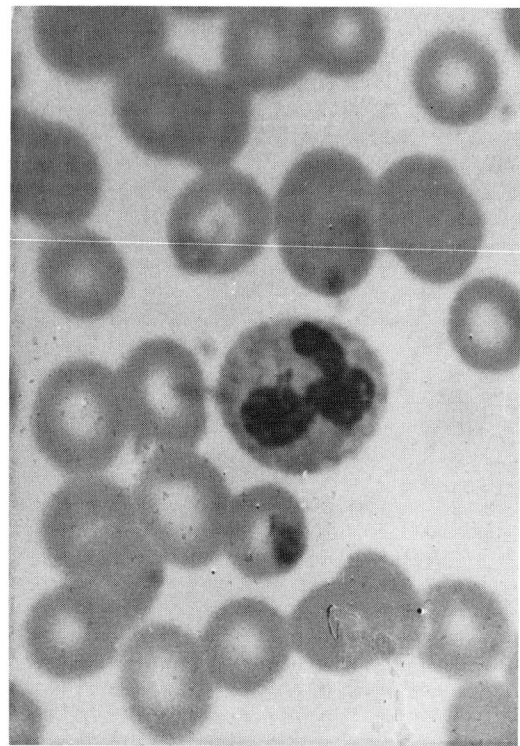

Figure 14-7. Double "drumstick" in neutrophil of female.

proximately 48 hours after birth. Should the fetus die prior to that time, a rapid increase in the number of Barr bodies is also noted, which Taylor[109] attributes to the hormonal effect of the maternal environment, since the opposite reaction may also be observed in the presence of certain substances. For instance, hydrocortisone and ACTH are capable of reducing the number of observable sex chromosomes, though only in a transient way.

Antibiotic therapy is alleged to cause reduction in the size of the chromatin mass, without affecting its incidence (Sohvall and Bruce Casselman[100]), which may give rise to discrepant results following such therapy.

SIGNIFICANCE OF THE SEX CHROMATIN. The sex chromatin is generally accepted to be of chromosomal origin. The material of chromosomal derivation it contains displays the characteristic property of heteropyknosis. However, neither a nonchromosomal origin, as postulated by Tobias,[112, 113] nor an autosomal or nonheterochromosomal origin (Segal and Nelson[87]), can be ruled out entirely. Nevertheless, the works of Reitalu,[81, 82] Klinger,[48, 49] Serr and colleagues[88] and Fraccaro and Lindsten,[26] based on studies of the transformation of chromosomes into chromatin, seem to have established a chromosomal origin.

Graham and Barr[36] had assumed that the nuclear sex chromatin contained the heteropyknotic portions of both X chromosomes. This hypothesis had several vulnerable points, among them the assumption that the crossing over of X chromosomes occurred in nuclei at interphase.

Stewart[102] and, almost simultaneously, Ohno and his colleagues,[68, 69] reached the conclusion that the sex chromatin was formed from a single X chromosome. Regarding the question of whether that heterochromosome was pyknotic in its entirety, Stewart[103] added that only its long arms were pyknotic, the short (or eupyknotic) arms presumably comprising the following loci: blood group Xg (Mann et al.[60a]), hemophilia, color blindness, muscular dystrophy and glucose-6-phosphate dehydrogenase deficiency. Ohno and Makino,[69] McLean,[58] Turpin and Lejeune[114] and Simpson and Christakos[97] similarly believe that only a portion of the chromosome is incorporated into the nuclear sex chromatin.

More recently, however, the arguments advanced by Miles,[62] and particularly the studies of Giannelli,[31] which have already been mentioned, seem to confirm the fact that only one of the X chromosomes of the bivalent sexual complex is heteropyknotic, and is so in its entirety.

The entire mass of the Barr body, then, would appear to be made up of a single X chromosome, derived from the mother, which is the chromosome of "femininity." The paternal X is believed to be euchromatic and, hence, invisible at interphase.

14.9. THE NORMAL KARYOTYPE

While the sex of a species can be recognized by examining nuclei at rest or interphase, as a result of the incidence of Barr bodies (apparently each representing a single X chromosome), the individual chromosomes of the nuclear spindle can be sorted out and readily identified by studying nuclei in the reproductive phase. This is of great practical significance because, in addition to the autosomes, *it enables us to visualize the sexual chromosomes with all clarity.*

Prior to 1956, it was hard to come by microscopic preparations of sufficient quality to allow determination of the number of chromosomes in an unequivocal manner. Since then, the number of chromosomes in the human species has been established at 46, with 44 autosomes and two heterochromosomes, or sex chromosomes. Thus, the female sex is monogametic (XX), whereas the male sex is di- or heterogametic (XY). It has been suggested that, at least at the biochemical or genetic level, the female, too, may be heterogametic in view of the fact that only one of her X chromosomes, the one that is transmitted to daughters, seems to be sex-specific, while the other is more or less inert and is the one that is transmitted to male offspring.

Two developments, more than anything else, have contributed toward achieving clear visualization of chromosomes: first, the introduction of hypotonic solutions which, by penetrating into the nucleoplasm, cause the nucleus to burst, thus setting free the chromosomes (Makino and Mishimura[60]), and, second, the application of antimitotic or cytostatic agents (colchicine) by Ford and Hamerton[24] to prevent chromatids from splitting into two—in other words, to cause arrest of mitoses at metaphase, the

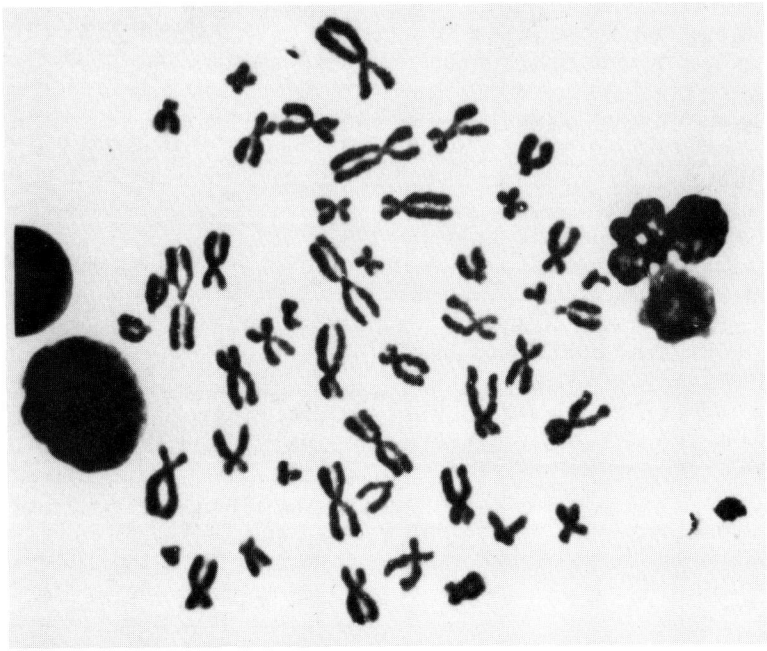

Figure 14-8. Metaphase chromosomes in normal woman obtained from culture of peripheral blood, from which chromosomes are separated (see text).

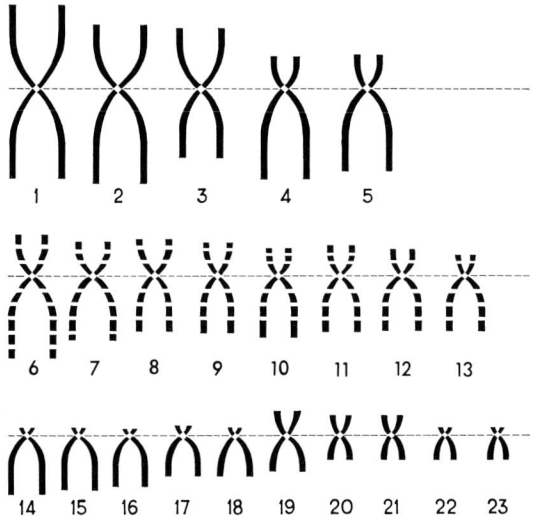

Figure 14-9. Classification of chromosomal pairs of normal woman, according to Denver system.

stage of choice for the study of chromosomes (Fig. 14-8).

To obtain adequate chromosomal spreads for karyotyping, three basic procedures are utilized:

(1) Bone marrow cultures, (2) tissue cultures, and (3) leukocyte cultures.

14.9.1. BONE MARROW CULTURES

Ford and co-workers,[25] as well as Fraccaro and his group,[27] advocate the use of fresh bone marrow cells obtained by means of sternal puncture. Because of abundant mitotic activity in the normal bone marrow, only a short period of incubation is necessary to obtain a sufficient number of cells at metaphase. This procedure is still much in use and is, by and large, the simplest if not the most perfect method currently available.

14.9.2. TISSUE CULTURES

Tissue cultures are much more complex and cumbersome to perform but have the added advantage of permitting isolation of aberrant cell lines that cannot be detected in marrow or blood cultures (see Chapter 35). Many quite different methods have been employed: some investigators (Tjio and Puck,[111] Ingenito et al.,[45] Fraccaro et al.[27]) culture small pieces of skin. Lejeune and his colleagues[53, 54] and others, on the other hand, use particles of fascia lata. In any kind of tissue culture, whatever the tissue involved, it is important to achieve growth of fibroblasts, which requires rather long periods of incubation, during which it is necessary to perform several successive passages, preceded by trypsinization.

14.9.3. LEUKOCYTE CULTURES

The ease with which excellent preparations of cultured mononuclear leukocytes can be obtained with a simple venous puncture constitutes the most important advance in recent years in the technical field of human cytogenetics. Cultures grown for only three days are sufficient to yield a rich harvest of excellent mitoses. Currently, the technique used universally is one introduced by Moorhead and co-workers[66] as a modification of earlier techniques developed by Osgood and Brooke[70] and by Hungerford and co-workers.[44]

14.9.4. THE DENVER SYSTEM

The wealth of new findings reported since 1956 as a result of improved methodology called for a universally acceptable nomenclature for chromosomes. At the Denver, Colorado, meeting of an international group of geneticists, a new classification system was introduced which took into consideration the size of the two chromatids and the position of the centromere (Fig. 14-9.)[10, 11] Chromosomes were divided into long, medium and short, and subdivided into metacentric, submetacentric and acrocentric, according to whether the centromere was in the midportion of the chromosome or more or less displaced toward one of its ends (Fig. 14-10). In the human species, there is actually no perfectly metacentric chromosome (except for the pathologic "isochromosomes" — see Chapter 34 — described by Fraccaro and his colleagues[28] and Lindsen[57]), although some pairs are so designated for practical purposes to distinguish them from more obviously submetacentric pairs. It was agreed that pairs should be numbered from 1 to 22 in descending order of length, while setting the sex chromosomes into a group apart. A set of chromosomes arranged in this order is called a *karyotype,* the term *idiogram* remaining reserved for the diagrammatic representation of the cells of an individual.

Patau and his associates[76] prefer to classify chromosomes into seven groups (designated with the letters A to G) according to size since, in practice, it is often impossible to differentiate correlative pairs. Nonetheless, the Denver system has been accorded worldwide acceptance by all geneticists and will be used in this book.

In addition to the karyotypes of a normal man (Fig. 14-11) and normal woman (Fig. 14-8), we conclude this chapter with a table (Table 14-1) summarizing the characteristics of chromosomes according to the Denver system.

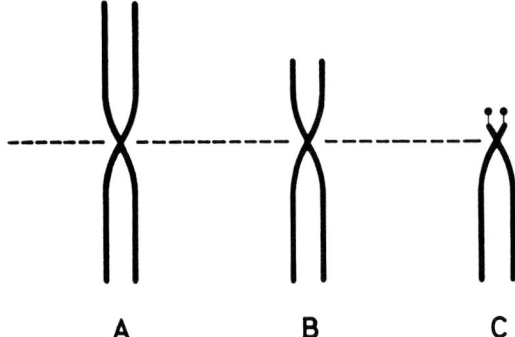

Figure 14-10. Schematic representation of different human chromosomes. *A*, Metacentric chromosome, with centromere equidistant from both extremes. *B*, Submetacentric chromosome, with centromere displaced towards one of the extremes. This point thus delimits the "long arms" and the "short arms." *C*, Acrocentric chromosome, with subterminal centromere. The short arms practically disappear; however, certain prolongations ("satellites"), which are not always visible, consistently occur in their rudiments.

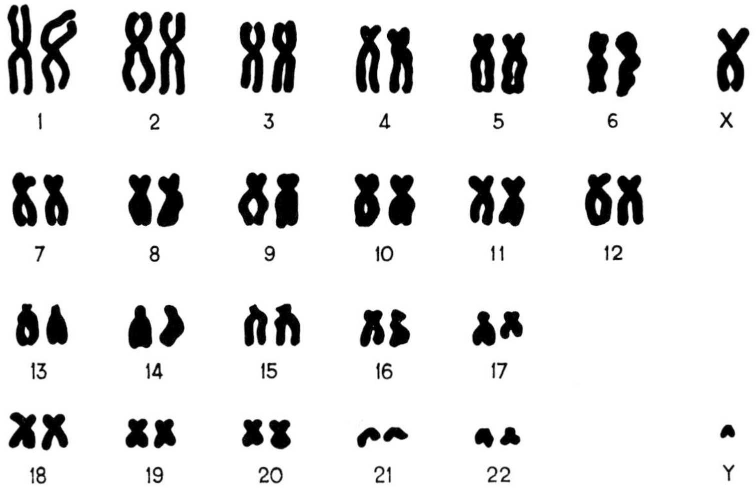

Figure 14-11. Normal male karyotype.

TABLE 14-1. Order of Arrangement of Chromosomes in the Denver System

	METACENTRIC			SUBMETACENTRIC			ACROCENTRIC		
Pairs	Large	Medium	Small	Large	Medium	Small	Large	Medium	Small
1–5	1st	–	3rd	2nd	4th	5th	–	–	–
6–12	6th–7th	8th	11th	9th	10th	12th	–	–	–
13–20	16th	19th	20th	17th	–	18th	13th	14th	15th
21–22	–	–	–	–	–	–	21st	–	22nd

REFERENCES

1. Austin, C. R., and Amoroso, E. C.: *Exper. Cell Res.*, 13:419, 1957.
2. Baltzer, F.: *Verh. Deutsch. Zool. Ges.*, 273, 1928.
3. Baltzer, F.: *Rev. Suisse Biol.*, 40:243, 1933.
4. Barr, M. L., and Bertram, E. G.: *Nature*, 163:676, 1949.
5. Barr, M. L., Bertram, E. G., and Linsay, H. A.: *Anat. Rec.*, 107:283, 1950.
6. Barr, M. L.: *Second International Conference on Congenital Malformations*, New York, July 14–19, 1963.
7. Blandau, R. J.: *Clinical Obstet. Gynec.*, 10:347, 1967.
8. Bengtsson, L. P.: *Gynec. Obstet.*, 48:474, 1949.
9. Bök, J. A., et al.: *Lancet*, 1:1063, 1960.
10. Bök, J. A., et al.: *J.A.M.A.*, 174:159, 1960.
11. Böving: *Preimplantation Stages of Pregnancy*, CIBA Symposium, 1965.
12. Bridges, C. B.: *Jour. Exp. Zool.*, 15:587, 1923.
13. Briggs, D. K., and Kuppermann, H. S.: *J. Clin. Endocr.*, 16:1163, 1956.
14. Carpenter, B. J.: *Bull. Soc. Roy. Belg. Obst. Gyn.*, 20:21, 1956.
15. Carpenter, B. J., Stolte, L. A. M., and Visschers, G. P.: *J. Clin. Endocr.*, 16:155, 1956.
16. Cederqvist, L. L., and Fuchs, F.: *Clin. Obstet. Gynec.*, 13:159, 1970.
17. Clermont, Y.: In *The Human Testis*, ed. E. Rosemberg and C. H. Paulsen. New York, Plenum Press, 1970.
18. Danon, M.: *Schw. Med. Wschr.*, 87:294, 1957.
19. Dantschakoff, V.: *I. Zschr. Zellforsch.*, 14:323, 1932.
20. Dewhurst, S. J.: *Lancet*, 1:471, 1956.
21. Everett, N. B.: *J. Exp. Zool.*, 92:49, 1943.
22. Everett, N. B.: *Biol. Rev., Cambridge Philos. Soc.*, 20:45, 1945.
23. Fariñas, M., and Botella-Llusiá, J.: *Acta Ginec.*, 8:281, 1962.
24. Ford, C. E., and Hamerton, J. L.: *Nature*, 178:1020, 1956.
25. Ford, C. E., Jacobs, A., and Lajdha, L. G.: *Nature*, 181:1565, 1958.
26. Fraccaro, M., and Lindsten, J.: *Exp. Cell Res.*, 17:536, 1959.
27. Fraccaro, M., Kaijser, K., and Lindsten, J.: *Ann. Hum. Genet.*, 24:45, 1960.
28. Fraccaro, M., et al.: *Lancet*, 2:1144, 1960.
29. Furrow, C. L.: *Zschr. Zellforsch.*, 22:282, 1935.
30. George, K. P.: *Nature*, 226:80, 1970.
31. Giannelli, F.: *Lancet*, 1:863, 1963.
32. Gillmann, J.: *Contrib. Embryol. Carnegie Inst. Wash.*, 32:81, 1948.
33. Glenister: *Nature*, 177:1135, 1956.
34. Gordon, M. J.: *Proc. Nat. Acad. Sci.*, 43:913, 1957.
35. Gordon, R. R., and Dewhurst, C. J.: *Lancet*, 2:872, 1962.
36. Graham, M. A., and Barr, M. L.: *Anat. Rec.*, 112:709, 1952.
37. Graham, M. A., and Barr, M. L.: *Arch. Anat. Micros. (Paris)*, 48:111, 1954.
38. Greenblatt, R. B., de la Costa, O. A., Vazquez, E., and Mullins, O. F.: *J.A.M.A.*, 161:683, 1956.
39. Grünwald, P.: *Roux Arch.*, 136:389, 1937.
40. Hartmann, M.: *Die Sexualität*. Stuttgart, Gustav Fischer, 1956.
41. Hartmann, M.: *Allgemeine Biologie*. Stuttgart, Gustav Fischer, 1953.
42. Henking, H.: *Z. Wiss. Zool.*, 51:685, 1891.
43. Herbst, C.: *Roux Arch. Entwicklungsmechanik Org.*, 139:282, 1939.
44. Hungerford, D. A., Donelly, A. J., Nowell, P. C., and Beck, S.: *Amer. J. Hum. Genet.*, 11:215, 1959.
45. Ingenito, E. F., Craig, J. M., Labesse, J., Gautier, M., and Rutstein, D.: *Arch. Path.*, 65:365, 1958.
46. James, F.: *Lancet*, 1:202, 1956.
47. Kleegman, S.: In *Advances in Sex Research*, ed. H. G. Beigel. New York, Hoeber, 1963.
48. Klinger, H. P.: *Acta Anat. (Basel)*, 30:371, 1957.
49. Klinger, H. P.: *Exp. Cell Res.*, 14:207, 1958.
50. Kniep: *Die Sexualität der Niederen Pflanzen*. Jena, Gustav Fischer, 1928.
51. Lang, D. R., and Hansel, W.: *J. Dairy Sci.*, 42:1330, 1959.
52. Lederberg, J.: *Harvey Lectures Ser.*, 52:69, 1959.
53. Lejeune, J., Gautier, M., and Turpin, R.: *Compt. Rend. Acad. Sci. (Paris)*, 248:602, 1959.
54. Lejeune, J., and Turpin, R.: *Les chromosomes humains*. Paris, Gauthier-Villars, 1965.
55. Lewin, S.: *Brit. Veter. Journ.*, 112:549, 1956.
56. Lindahl, P. E.: *Acta Agricol. Scand.*, 8:226, 1968.
57. Lindsen, J.: *Lancet*, 2:1228, 1961.
58. McLean, N.: *Lancet*, 2:1154, 1962.
59. McClung, C. E.: *Biol. Bull.*, 3:43, 1902.
60. Makino, S., and Mishimura, I.: *Stain Technol.*, 27:1, 1952.
60a. Mann, J., Cahan, A., Gelb, A. G., Fisher, N., Hamper, J., Tippett, B., Sanger, R., and Race, R. R.: *Lancet*, 1:8, 1962.
61. Marberger, E., Boccabella, R. A., and Nelson, W. U.: *Proc. Soc. Exp. Biol. Med.*, 89:488, 1955.
62. Miles, C. C.: *Lancet*, 2:660, 1962.
63. Montalvo, L.: *Actas del 1-er Congreso Mundial de Citologia*. Vienna, 1961.
64. Moore, K. L., and Barr, M. L.: *J. Comp. Neurol.*, 98:213, 1953.
65. Moore, K. L., and Barr, M. L.: *Lancet*, 2:57, 1955.
66. Moorhead, T. S., Nowell, T. C., Mellmann, W. J., Batipps, D. M., and Hungerford, D. A.: *Exp. Cell Res.*, 20:613, 1960.
67. O'Ferrall, G. J. M., Meacham, T. N., and Foreman, W. E.: *J. Reprod. Fertil.*, 16:243, 1968.
68. Ohno, S., and Hauschka, C. S.: *Cancer Res.*, 20:451, 1960.
69. Ohno, S., and Makino, S.: *Lancet*, 2:78, 1961.
70. Osgood, E. E., and Brooke, J. H.: *Blood*, 10:1010, 1955.
71. Overzier, C.: *La Intersexualidad*. Barcelona, Editorial Científico-Médica, 1963.
72. Overzier, C.: *Acta Ginec.*, 1:57, 1962.
73. Painter, T. S.: *Science*, 53:503, 1921.
74. Painter, T. S.: *J. Exper. Zool.*, 37:291, 1923.
75. Park: *J. Anat.*, 91:369, 1959.
76. Patau, K., Smith, E., Therman, E., Inhorn, S. L., and Wagner, H. P.: *Lancet* 1:790, 1960.
77. Pearson, P. L., Bobrow, M., and Vosa, G. G.: *Nature*, 226:78, 1970.
78. Politzer, G.: *Zschr. Anat.*, 100:334, 1933.

79. Ponse, K.: *La différentiation du sexe et l'intersexualité chez les vertebrés. Facteurs héréditaires et hormones.* Lausanne, Rouge Cie., 1949.
80. Prince, R. H., Graham, M. A., and Barr, M. L.: *Anat. Rec.*, 122:153, 1955.
81. Reitalu, J.: *Acta Genet. Med. Gemellol.*, 6:393, 1957.
82. Reitalu, J.: *Hereditas*, 44:488, 1958.
83. Rotschild, V.: *Brit. Med. J.*, 2:743, 1962.
84. Sachs, L., Serr, J. A., and Danon, H.: *Science*, 123:548, 1956.
85. Sachs, L., and Danon, H.: *Genetica*, 28:201, 1956.
86. Schilling, E.: *J. Repro. Fertil.*, 11:469, 1966.
87. Segal, S. J., and Nelson, W. O.: *J. Clin. Endocr.*, 17:676, 1957.
88. Serr, J. A., Ferguson-Smith, M. A., Lennox, B., and Paul, J.: *Nature*, 182:124, 1958.
89. Sevinc, A.: *J. Reprod. Fertil.*, 16:7, 1968.
90. Shettles, L. B.: *Nature*, 186:648, 1960.
91. Shettles, L. B.: *Nature*, 187:524, 1960.
92. Shettles, L. B.: *Obstet. Gynec.*, 16:10, 1960.
93. Shettles, L. B.: *Fertil. Steril.*, 12:20, 1961.
94. Shettles, L. B.: *Fertil. Steril.*, 12:502, 1960.
95. Shettles, L. B.: *Amer. J. Obstet. Gynec.*, 71:834, 1956.
96. Simkins, C. S.: *Amer. J. Anat.*, 41:249, 1928.
97. Simpson, J. L., and Christakos, A. C.: *Obstet. Survey*, 24:580, 1969.
98. Smith, D. W., Marden, P. M., McDonald, M. S., and Speckhard, M.: *Pediatrics*, 30:707, 1962.
99. Sohvall, A. R., Gaines, J. A., Strauss, L.: *Ann. N.Y. Acad. Sci.*, 75:905, 1959.
100. Sohvall, A. R., and Bruce Casselman, W. G.: *Lancet*, 2:1386, 1961.
101. Stern, C.: *Triangulo Sandoz*, 5:131, 1960.
102. Stewart, J. S.: *Lancet*, 1:825, 1960.
103. Stewart, J. S.: *Lancet*, 2:1269, 1962.
104. Stieve, H.: *Zschr. Mikrosk. Anat. Forsch.* (Leipzig), 10:225, 1927.
105. Sun, C. C. Y., and Rakoff, A. E.: *J. Clin. Endocr.*, 16:55, 1956.
106. Swezy, O., and Evans, H. M.: *J. Morph.*, 49:543, 1930.
107. Takahashi, M.: *Zool. Mag.*, 61:26, 1952.
108. Taylor, A.: *Lancet*, 2:1059, 1962.
109. Taylor, A.: *Lancet*, 1:912, 1963.
110. Tjio, J. H., and Levan, A.: *Hereditas*, 42:1, 1956.
111. Tjio, J. H., and Puck, T. T.: *J. Exp. Med.*, 108:259, 1958.
112. Tobias, P. V.: *S. Afr. J. Med. Sci.*, 19:57, 1954.
113. Tobias, P. V.: *Lect. Univ. Johannesburg*, 27:7, 1958.
114. Turpin, R., and Lejeune, J.: *Les chromosomes humains.* Paris, Gauthier-Villars, 1965.
115. Winiwarter, H. von: *Arch. Biol.*, 27:91, 1912.
116. Witschi, E.: In *La Intersexualidad*, by C. Overzier. Barcelona, Editorial Científico-Médica, 1963.
117. Witschi, E.: *Science*, 130:274, 1960.
118. Witschi, E.: *Contrib. Embryol. Carnegie Inst. Wash.*, 32:67, 1948.
119. Wollmann, E. L., Jacob, F., and Hayes, W.: *Cold Spring Harbor Symp. Quant. Biol.*, 21:141, 1956.

Chapter 15

DEVELOPMENT, EMBRYOGENESIS AND EMBRYOMECHANICS OF SEX

The study of sexual development is essential for a full understanding of female endocrinology. The processes involved must be studied at two different levels: the *morphologic level* and the *functional level*. In terms of morphology, a great deal of data concerning sexual development have been known for many years. These were the objects of study of classical embryology and will be reviewed here only cursorily, the reader being referred to textbooks of embryology for further information. On the other hand, the study of *embryomechanics*, that is, the functional phenomena conditioning morphogenesis of sex, is at present an issue of great novelty and interest, and must be discussed here not only because it is essential for the understanding of endocrine physiology but also — and more importantly — because hormones play an important role in the embryomechanics of sex.

Matter and energy, which may be said to be expressed in biologic terms as *form and function*, are actually one and the same thing. For many years, morphologic changes, that is to say, changes affecting matter, have been described without attempting to go beyond what meets the eye, that is, without due consideration for the nature of the underlying energy changes and biochemical process involved. The purpose of *chemical embryology*[13, 63] is to correlate changes in morphology with the biochemical reactions that cause and condition them. The present chapter has accordingly been divided into two parts: one dealing with morphologic embryology and the other with chemical embryology.

15.1. EMBRYOLOGIC DEVELOPMENT OF THE GENITAL TRACT

In view of the numerous and accurate classic descriptions of the embryology of the genital tract,[1, 30, 33] any detailed analysis of the subject here would be redundant; what follows is a mere condensed summary.

15.1.1. DEVELOPMENT OF THE GONAD

The genital apparatus is derived from the embryo's intermediate layer, the mesoderm, on the posterior aspect of the coelomic cavity. The genital eminence, a protuberant region medial to the wolffian body, emerges on both sides of the coelomic cavity and originally extends from the cranial to the caudal end of the embryo, although its length subsequently decreases owing to atrophy of its extremes. The cells composing the genital eminence are already differentiated during the earliest stages of embryonic development, so that by the time an embryo is 5 weeks old, the genital crest is fully formed. This crest consists of a ridge that runs medially parallel to the fold of the urinary portion of the wolffian body. Currently, the genital eminence is held to develop in response to stimuli originating in certain cells, which have migrated to this region at an earlier stage of development and which are believed to act as inductors of the development of this structure. These cells must undoubtedly begin to differentiate before

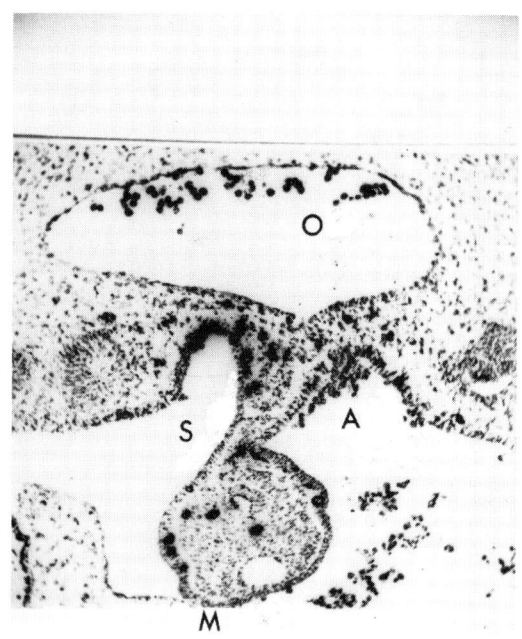

Figure 15-1. Cross section of coelomic cavity of 32 day old, 5 mm human embryo, stained for alkaline glycerophosphatase. Black staining gonocytes are seen migrating from the gut through the mesentery to the region of the gonadal anlage. M, Terminal gut; S, mesentery; O, dorsal aorta; A, anlage of gonad. (From Hertig: *Contributions to Embryology*. Baltimore, Carnegie Institution, 1958.)

the initial stages of segmentation; they can later be spotted in the posterior wall of the primitive gut, from where, by virtue of ameboid motility, they travel through the mesentery and eventually reach their final destination, remaining lodged in the genital crest. These migrating or motile cells are known as *gonocytes* and, in the view of some authors (Mintz[55]), give rise directly to the sexual cells (Figs. 15-1, 15-2 and 15-3). Direct visualization of ameboid movements by rat gonocytes was recently reported by Blandau and co-workers.[7] Brachet[13] does not believe that these cells are precursors of the germ cells, viz., ova and spermatozoa, but that they are meant merely to induce development of the genital eminence and to disappear afterwards. He therefore calls them *primary gonocytes*, to distinguish them from the *secondary gonocytes*, a second generation of sexual cells, which are to remain incorporated in the gonad and

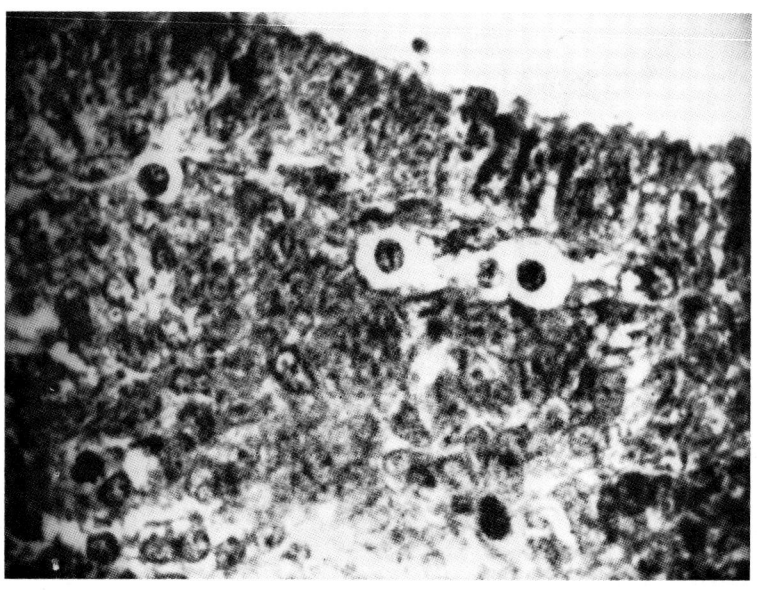

Figure 15-2. Longitudinal section of primitive mesentery of a 31-day-old, 4 mm embryo. The coelomic epithelium is seen above and, below, in the form of clear cells, gonocytes may be seen in the process of migration. (From Boyd and Hamilton, in *Modern Trends in Obstetrics and Gynecology*. London, Butterworth, 1955.)

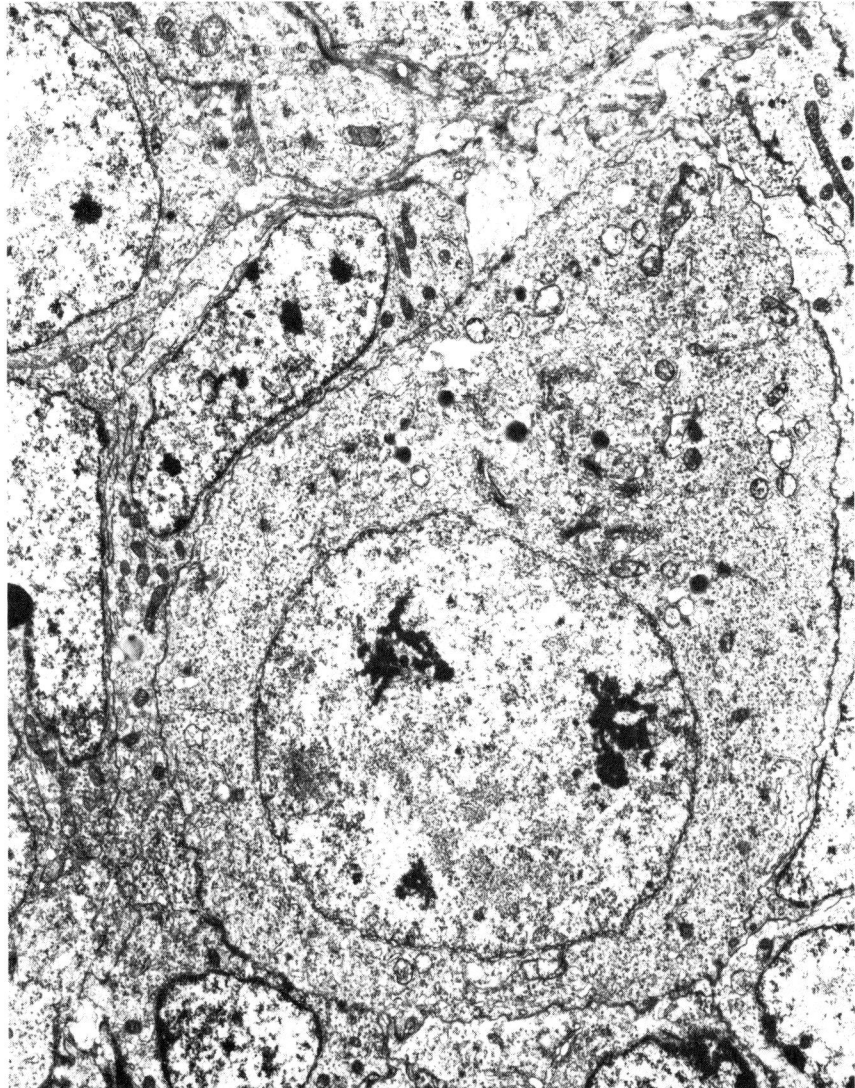

Figure 15-3. Gonocyte of chick embryo after seven days of incubation (10,350×). (Courtesy of Dr. R. Gonzalez-Santander, Department of Embryology, Faculty of Medicine of Madrid.)

are to induce the appearance of either oogonia, or spermatogonia.

At any rate, a considerable amount of modern opinion tends to consider gonocytes as representing the germinal route and to believe that either these cells by themselves or other cells derived from them give rise, in a primary or secondary way, to the germ cells. According to Brachet[13] and Needham,[63] the two generations of gonocytes are postulated to be involved in gonadal organogenesis in quite different ways. *The first generation of gonocytes presumably induces development of the gonad and degenerates before the individual attains sexual maturity, while the second generation is involved in unfolding the functional activity of the gonad.* In light of present day knowledge, the production of some teratomas and perhaps even development of some anomalies of the interrenal system may be thought to result from a pathologic process of induction on the part of primary gonocytes. Gonocytes do not only invade the gonadal anlage; Capurow[16] has demonstrated that tissue transplants to the retrocoelomic area are also invaded and are converted to aberrant gonads.

The inductive action exerted on the genital crest by gonocytes can be divided into three successive stages. The first stage marks the appearance of the *primary bilateral anlagen*, in the posterior region of the trunk as an anterolateral thickening of the mesoblast in both its splanchnic and its somatic layers. Very early, this primary mesodermal thickening becomes independent of the scleromyotome, of the nephrotome and of the lateral plate, as a result of the emergence of three different planes of segmentation. The mesoderm is thereby divided into three portions: (1) the scleromyotome; (2) the nephrotome; and (3) the *genital eminence* proper, which eventually gives rise to the gonad.

The second stage, that of the *primary unpaired anlage*, is of little consequence for the question under consideration, but the third stage is of great interest because during it the so-called *secondary bilateral (or definitive) anlagen* are formed, which contribute to the development of the gonads in a decisive manner (Figs. 15–6 and 15–7). Some investigators assume that the cells arising through an active process of proliferation in the genital eminence on the arrival of the gonocytes become the germinal epithelium of the sexual gland, whereas others believe that the only proliferation taking place is that of mesenchymal cells, and that development of the germinal epithelium represents a reaction of the coelomic epithelium to growth of the genital crest. Brachet[13] believes that during this stage, the primary gonocytes degenerate and merge with the surrounding coelomic system, thereby setting up a primitive genital system that is bound to disappear in higher animals.

Let us now consider the question of *organogenesis of the genital crest.* The crest is located medial to the wolffian body, beyond which it extends at both the cranial and caudal poles. Its bulk increases not only as a result of growth provoked by the arrival of the gonocytes but also because of considerable hyperplasia of its cellular components. Little by little, it separates from the wolffian body until the two formations are connected only by a mesenchymal bridge, which constitutes the genital mesentery. The wolffian body similarly is connected to the posterior wall by means of an analogous fold, which is the wolffian mesentery. Into the lower and upper ends

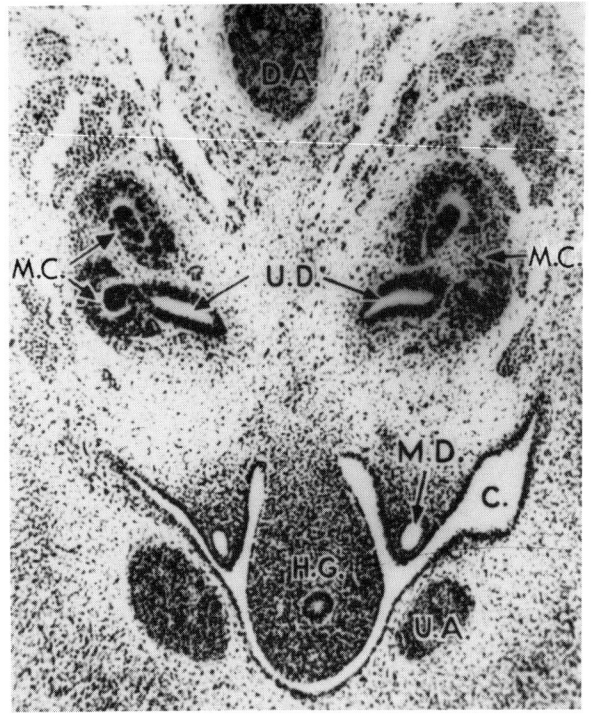

Figure 15–4. Cross section of a human embryo, measuring 13 mm from crown to rump, at the level of the transverse intestine. *M.C.,* metanephros; *U.D.,* ureteral diverticulum; *H.G.,* hindgut; *C.,* primitive peritoneum or coelom; *M.D.,* mesonephric duct (wolffian duct); *D.A.,* dorsal aorta; *U.A.,* umbilical artery. (From Harrison: *Textbook of Human Embryology.* Oxford, England, Blackwell, 1959.)

Figure 15-5. Section of the urinary and genital portions of a still undifferentiated wolffian body in a 12.5 mm human embryo. *G,* Undifferentiated gonadal crest; *T,* mesonephric tubes; *D,* mesonephric duct (wolffian duct). (From Giroud: In *La fonction spermatogenique du testicule.* Paris, Masson et Cie, 1958.)

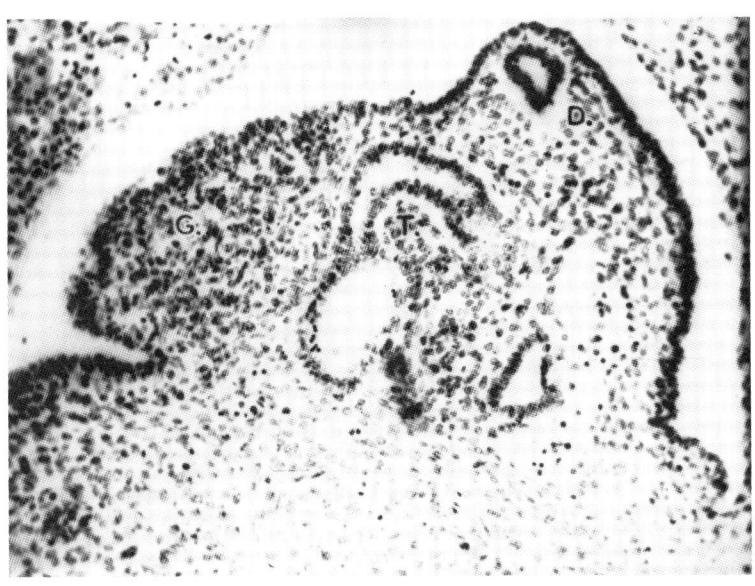

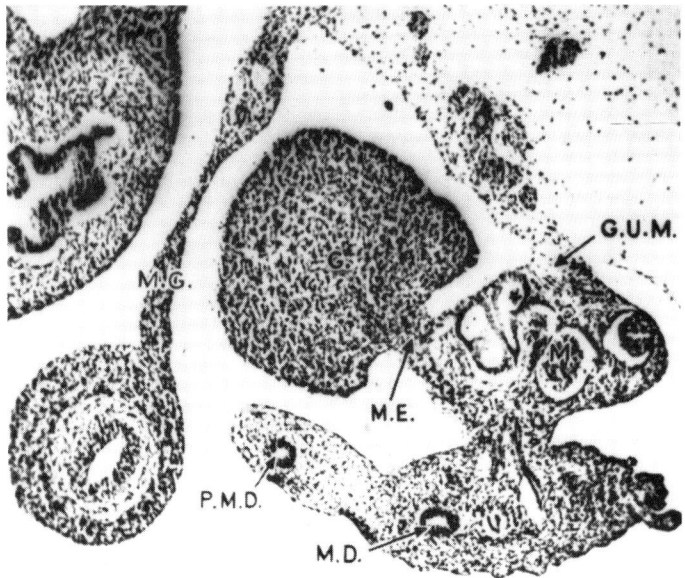

Figure 15-6. Cross section of posterior wall of coelomic cavity in a 28.5 mm human embryo. The gonad has already separated from the wolffian body, and in embryos of this age, ovaries and testes are microscopically distinguishable. Such distinction is, incidentally, not apparent in this section, owing to the level at which it is cut. *G.U.M.,* genitourinary mesentery; *M.E.,* gonadal mesentery; *G,* gonad; *P.M.D.,* paramesonephric duct (müllerian duct); *M.D.,* mesonephric duct (wolffian duct); *M.G.,* mesentery, with gut visible at one extreme. (From Harrison: Textbook of Human Embryology. Oxford, England, Blackwell, 1959.)

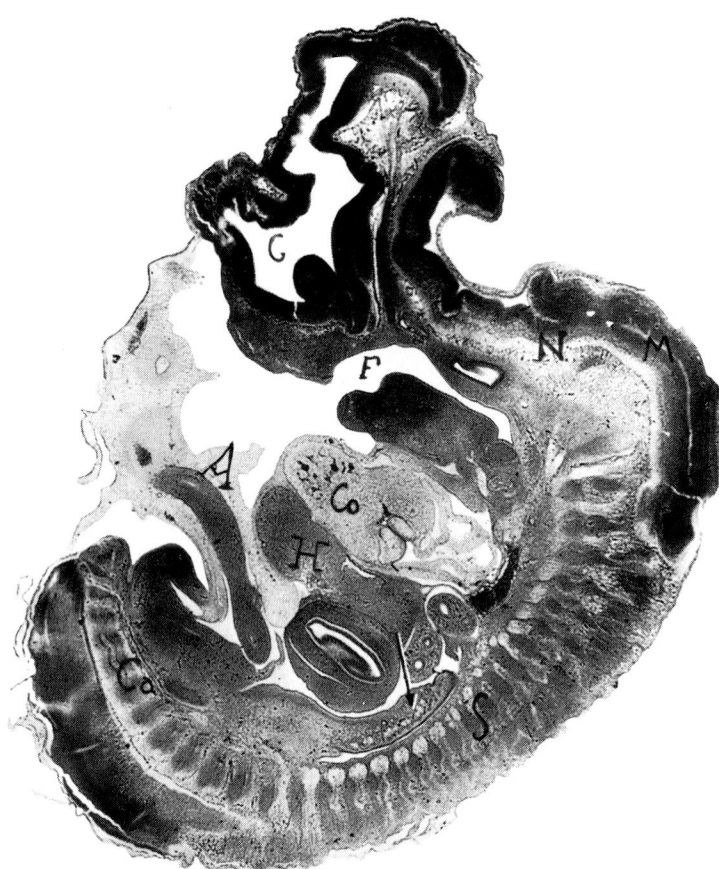

Figure 15-7. Five week old human embryo. Development of wolffian body (arrow). *C*, Head; *F*, pharynx; *N*, notochord; *M*, spinal cord; *A*, allantoic stalk; *Co*, heart; *H*, liver; *Ca*, caudal end; *S*, spine.

of the genital mesentery insert two ligaments, a superior one connecting to the subdiaphragmatic area, and an inferior one, extending to the pelvic region. These two ligaments are of importance in the eventual topographic evolution of both the ovary and the testis. Before either the ovary or the testis becomes organized, the genital eminence passes through an undifferentiated stage. It is possible that, rather than being truly undifferentiated, the sex in this stage has already been latently established within the anlage, although our present-day analytic methods, especially the microscope, are unable to reveal this. Nevertheless, we are now certain that, at least insofar as amphibia and lower animals are concerned, the gonad's differentiation into either sex can be manipulated at will during this stage of development. This is to say, at this stage the gonad in lower animals is *truly undifferentiated*.

The manner in which an ovary or a testis develops from this undifferentiated anlage has been explained by Felix.[23] According to his views, proliferation of the cortical portion and regression of the medullary portion of the undifferentiated gonad gives rise to an ovary, whereas proliferation of the medullary portion and regression of the cortex gives rise to a testis.

OVARY. The proliferative process in the superficial or germinal epithelium of the ovary starts in the dorsal portion of the genital anlage, proximal to the fold joining the latter to the wolffian body. The resulting cellular buds in this area are to become the future *medullary cords* of the ovary. The existence of these cords is short-lived, since a subsequent new proliferative process starts in the superficial germinal epithelium, giving rise to the *cortical,* or secondary, *cords.* The latter develop from without inward, rather than from within outward, and from this point on begin producing the structures of the primordial ovarian follicles (Fig. 15-8). Within the thickness of the secondary cords, there now appear some clear, large cells, which are the *primordial ovules.* Their significance is comparable to that of *oogonia.* It is still debatable whether, as we have mentioned earlier, these oogonia are to be considered as direct descendants of gonocytes, or whether they are an outgrowth of a secondary kind of proliferation. The theory of Pflüger, postulating a coelomic epithelial origin for the gonia, appears to have been abandoned. We would prefer to believe that the oogonia evolve in the same area from differentiated mesenchymal cells under the impact of arriving gonocytes. Although the question has not been settled definitely, we shall adhere to this hypothesis. The course of peripheral ovarian development apparent in later life indeed suggests, as was pointed out by Gillman,[25] that the evolutionary processes of three elements play a fundamental role. The three elements in question are: (1) the components of the *germinal route,* the gonocyte or descendant of the gonocyte, which is the future source of ovules; (2) derivatives of the *coelom,* descended from the secondary ovarian cords, which are the future source of the follicular envelope and the granulosa layer; (3) the *mesenchyme,* converted into a true endocrine gland of the gonad, in which embryologic induction determines the specificity of the hormone to be produced, as will be described later in this chapter.

Until recently, the fetal ovary was thought to maintain its germ cells in a phase of multiplication, that is, to contain nothing but oogonia (see Fig. 14-2). Baker and Franchi,[4] as well as Blandau,[8] have found evidence that oocytes in the dictyotene stage are already present in human embryos over 17 cm long, consequently corresponding to the sixth month of intrauterine life. Prior to this time—that is, in embryos younger than six months—oogonia grow, divide and display ameboid motility. During the remaining four months of gestation, however, the number of germ cells becomes stationary and all germ cells are converted to oocytes.

TESTIS. In the testis, no comparable penetration of primary or secondary cords into the germinal epithelium has been recognized. The testicular cords appear to be the product of mesenchymal cell differentiation, although some authors still consider the possibility that they might originate from proliferating gonocytes. These cords, evolved at the expense of mesenchymal elements, give rise to an anastomosing reticular system known as the *testicular blastema* (Fig. 15-9). From it, the seminiferous tubules and the anlage of the *rete testis* are derived. For a long time, the rete testis had been assumed to arise from the wolffian duct but it is now known to result likewise from differentiation of the primitive blastema. Lack of space prevents us from going into further detail in reviewing this subject.

In summary, it may be stated that both gonads, the ovary as well as the testis, arise on the posterior aspect of the coelom from anlagen derived from, and in intimate contact with, the wolffian body. Growth of the genital anlage is initiated by the arrival of a special kind of migratory cell, the gonocytes, originating in the primitive gut and possibly representing what is known as the germinal route. Either directly, or through a second generation of cells, gonocytes are continuous in lineage with oogonia and spermatogonia, thereby establishing the continuity of the cells assigned for reproduction. The gonads of either sex develop within retrocoelomic mesenchymal tissue which, under the influence of inductive sexual differentiation, acquire the ability to be converted into an *endocrine sexual*

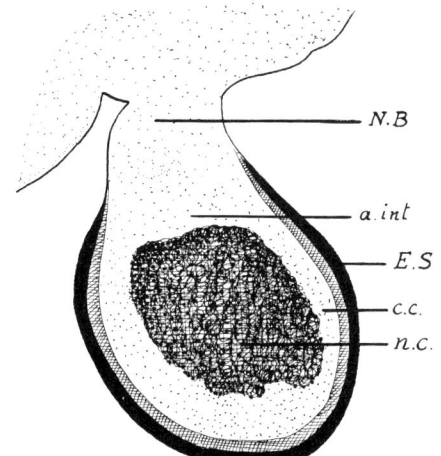

Figure 15-8. Undifferentiated gonad evolving into ovary through proliferation of superficial blastema. (From Felix.)

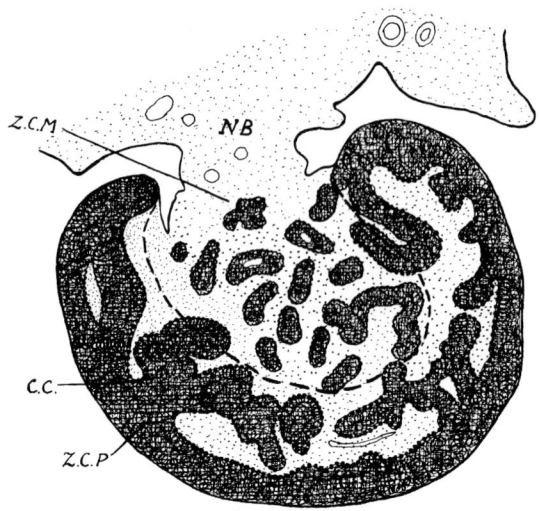

Figure 15-9. Gonad evolving into testis through proliferation of deep blastema. (From Felix.)

gland. Finally, it should be reiterated that while the ovary develops from the most superficial portion of the gonadal anlage, the development of a testis results from proliferation of the medullary zone.

15.1.2. DEVELOPMENT OF THE FEMALE GENITAL TRACT; THE MÜLLERIAN DUCT

The wolffian ducts, or excretory ducts of the mesonephros, can already be distinguished in 11 mm embryos. At this stage, a second series of genital ducts becomes apparent next to the cephalic extremity of the mesonephros, which little by little begins to extend caudad, assuming a lateral disposition alongside the wolffian duct. These are the müllerian ducts which at this stage, according to Koff,[44] begin to converge downwards and medially, the two contralateral ducts eventually merging and reaching the urogenital sinus at the tubercle of Müller. At about 8 weeks (25 mm stage), the embryo has two sets of genital ducts. If the primary gonad is a testis the wolffian duct remains, in the words of Jost,[40] "fixed" and gives rise to the vasa deferentia and to the seminal vesicles, while the müllerian duct is inhibited and regresses, persisting in the adult male only as the prostatic utricle. If, on the other hand, the gonad is an ovary, the wolffian duct undergoes atrophy and the müllerian duct prevails, its fused portion giving rise to the uterus and to the superior segment of the vagina, and its free portions becoming the Fallopian tubes.

In the female sex, the genital tract is known to be formed from the *müllerian duct*. At its upper end, the müllerian canal opens into the coelomic cavity above the level of the upper pole of the wolffian duct and laterally into the gonadal anlage, that is, on the outward side of the latter. At its lower end, its downward trajectory is at first lateral to the wolffian duct until *it crosses the latter and finally courses along the medial side of the latter.* For a considerable length of time, the müllerian duct is a simple cord-like structure, rather than a true tube, despite the fact that it initially takes shape as a groove that invaginates, so that it must not be thought of as having a lumen right from the start. *The acquisition of the lumen is a secondary phenomenon, a minor detail which is nevertheless of great importance in understanding the structure of the genital apparatus and the etiology of its anomalies.* However, by the seventeenth week of embryonic development, a lumen has developed throughout its length and is lined with a simple cylindrical epithelium. Distally, the müllerian duct converges on, and fuses with, the duct of the opposite side and then opens into the urogenital sinus. At the site of confluence of the two fused müllerian ducts, a prominent area, called *tubercle of Müller,* is formed.

In approaching the midline, the müllerian

duct crosses the wolffian duct. At about the same point, it also crosses the inferior ligament of the gonad, which is formed by a fold with a thickened mesentery. The point at which the duct crosses *Hunter's ligament* is an important landmark in the later evolution of the müllerian duct. The portion of the latter superior and lateral to Hunter's ligament persists throughout life without fusion as a paired organ, in symmetry with its contralateral counterpart. This organ is the *tubal canal* from which the Fallopian tube develops at a later stage. Below the point at which it crosses Hunter's ligament, the müllerian duct fuses with that of the other side, forming a common duct, the *uterovaginal duct*, which gives rise successively to the uterus and to the vagina. While the wall of the upper portion of the müllerian duct shows a relatively mild increase in thickness, the wall of the lower portion becomes significantly thicker, gaining increasingly in sturdiness, and its epithelium undergoes important transformations. *The upper half of the uterovaginal canal gives rise to the uterus*, whose epithelium, although remaining atrophic to the very time of birth, is already structurally reminiscent of the basal layer in the adult woman. In its lowermost portion, the müllerian duct is invaded secondarily by a process of epidermidization at the expense of cells lining the urogenital sinus, that is, by squamous polystratified epithelium. Meyer[52] had shown that, notwithstanding the fact that the vagina is originally a tubal structure of müllerian derivation, its epithelium is histologically derived from the cloacal epithelium and is closely related to the epithelia that line the vulvar vestibulum and the urinary bladder.

It is hoped that the foregoing details, though only a summary, will nevertheless facilitate the understanding of many aspects of female physiology and pathology.

15.1.3. DEVELOPMENT OF THE WOLFFIAN DUCT

The wolffian duct is the excretory duct of the mesonephros, or the *mesonephric duct*. While the mesonephros itself undergoes atrophy, its duct persists and, in the male, gives rise to the excretory channels of the testis: the coni epididymidis, the epididymis, the vas deferens and the ejaculatory canal. Though the embryology of these structures in the male is not indicated here, it will be pertinent to analyze which elements in the female are derived from the wolffian duct (Fig. 15–11). The upper segment of the wolffian duct persists at the level of the ovarian end of the Fallopian tube, constituting the pedunculated hydatid (appendix epididymis), which is analogous to a similar formation in the testis (appendix testis). In the paragenital region, remnants of the wolffian duct persist as a mesonephric tubule on each side and, in the broad ligament, as the epoophoron, or

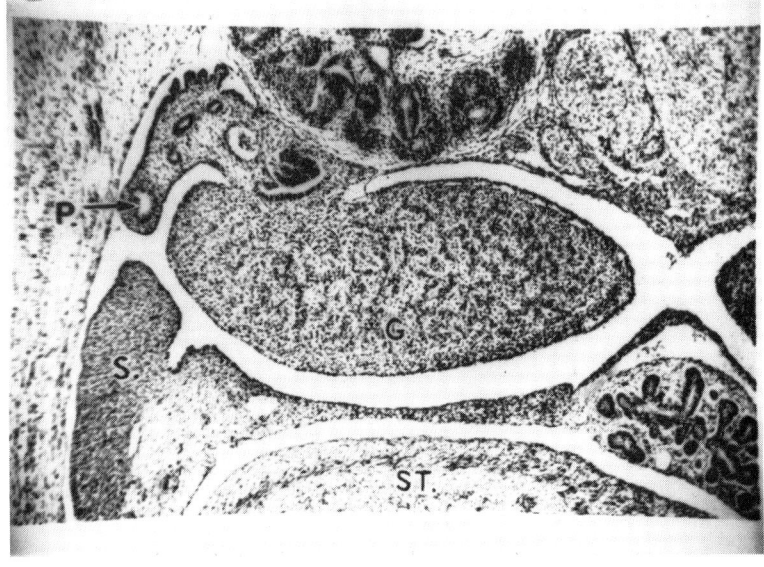

Figure 15–10. Histologic section of recently differentiated testis in a 20 mm male embryo. G, Gonad with well developed rete testis; S, spleen; ST, stomach; P, müllerian duct. (From Giroud: in *La fonction spermatogenique du testicule.* Paris, Masson et Cie., 1958.)

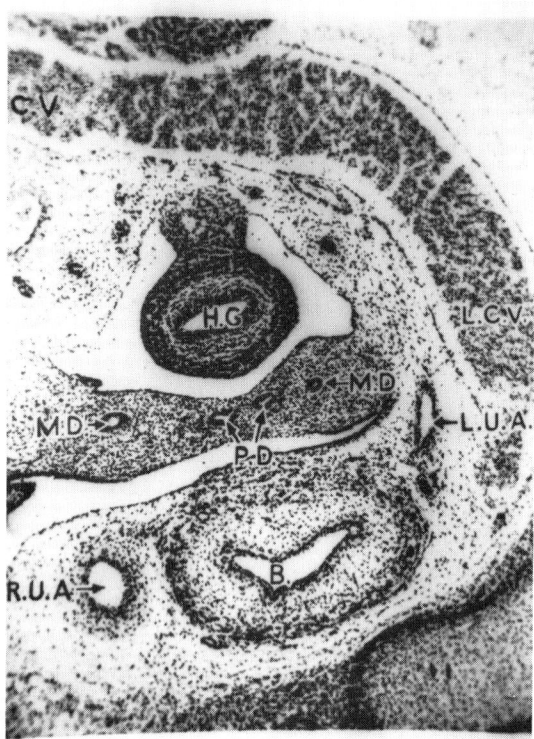

Figure 15–11. Cross section of 28 mm human embryo through caudal portion of trunk. M.D., Wolffian duct; P.D., müllerian duct; H.G., hindgut; B, bladder. Both the wolffian and the müllerian ducts are located in a transverse septum called *urogenital septum*. (From Harrison: *Textbook of Human Embryology.* Oxford, England, Blackwell, 1959.)

organ of Rosenmüller, consisting of mesonephric tubules with a segment of wolffian duct. The mesonephric tubules join a common trunk running parallel with the Fallopian tube, which is called the epoophoron duct.

Vestigial wolffian structures are scattered all along the genital tract, including the paravaginal region down to the vulva, where they constitute Gartner's duct, the pathology of which is also of interest.

The embryologic evolution of the external genitalia, which are derived from the *urogenital sinus* and from the *cloaca*, is beyond the scope of this book.

15.2. EMBRYOMECHANICS OF SEX AND OF SEXUAL DETERMINATION

The term "sexual determination" refers to a series of phenomena aimed at defining the nature of sex. This subject has been studied in Chapter 14. *As distinct from this, by "sexual differentiation" we mean the morphogenetic development of sex as a result of the tendencies established by sexual determination.* For many years, we have subscribed to the belief that sexual determination was strictly a chromosome-linked phenomenon and was irrevocably determined at the moment of fertilization. This classic idea, though essentially correct, will be shown to be subject to many exceptions.

15.2.1. GOLDSCHMIDT'S THEORY AND PROTOPLASMIC INHERITANCE OF SEX

It must be pointed out that, precise as the data in Chapter 14 may seem to be, they have nevertheless drawn serious criticism. One of the first to start questioning the rigid concept of chromosomal determination of sex was Goldschmidt.[27] This author postulated that all animals are originally hermaphrodites and that all initially produce both male and female substances in approximately equal ratios, but that at a certain point in development, called the *turning point*, either a male or a female influence breaks the balance and becomes predominant. Goldschmidt and his followers assume that the influences involved can be divided into three different types: (1) *chromosomal determination*, (2) *secondary, or embryonic determination*, and (3) *tertiary, or terminal determination*. Goldschmidt admits the validity of the chromosomal type of influence, though with some reservations. In the second type, sex is determined by substances secreted during the embryonal era, which are capable of influencing the process of gonadal differentiation by altering the primitive disposition of heredity, that is, by modifying or ammending the genetic makeup. The tertiary types of influence are no longer believed to modify the actual nature of the gonads, but to affect the development of both the genital apparatus and somatic morphology. As will be pointed out later in this chapter, such tertiary influences have later been likened to *sex hormones*.

Goldschmidt performed his investigations on the butterfly, *Lymanthria dispar*, which is widely distributed throughout most of the world. When a European butterfly was cross-mated with a butterfly of Japanese origin, some individuals among the offspring were intermediate between females and males, and were designated by the author as *gynandromorphous*, that is, intersexual. Goldschmidt made the observation that, in the biologic sense of the word, the Japanese breed was stronger than the European breeds and that whenever cross-mating of butterflies of a male of Japanese race with a female of European race was accomplished, the offspring invariably consisted of either all males or intersexual females. Conversely, whenever a European male, presumably a weaker breed, was mated with a Japanese female, a strong breed, the resulting second generation of butterflies consisted predominantly of females, and many among the minority group of males were intersexual males. Considering that cross-mating between strong and weak races resulted in imposing the sex of the stronger mate on the offspring, this must happen, Goldschmidt concluded, because in the process some substance was being transmitted to the weaker race that was capable of influencing the direction of gonadal development. These secondary type substances could not be fully characterized by Goldschmidt but have later been identified with considerable accuracy, so that today the secondary effects described by Goldschmidt are no longer questioned. However, his theory also raises the important question of extrachromosomal transmission of hereditary characters. If one analyzes the genetically possible combinations resulting from crosses of *Lymanthria*, as they were described by Goldschmidt, it becomes apparent that the type of sexual determination involved is *protandry*, that is, the number of heterochromosomes in the male is always even (for example, MM), while that in the female is odd (M). The determinative potency of the chromosomes is influenced by substances of the humoral type, to be discussed later, which are responsible for the fact that heterochromosome-linked male or female tendencies are either strong, if the race is strong, or weak, if the race is weak. However, Goldschmidt has equally well demonstrated that in the female the chondriome of the ovule is the carrier of sexual hereditary tendencies, whereas the male sperm, which is devoid of protoplasm, lacks hereditary protoplasmic tendencies. As a result, cross-breeding between a strong male and a weak female leads to the production of two types of genetic combinations: in one, there is a strong X chromosome (M), derived from the father, and a weak X chromosome (m), derived from the mother, both linked to a feminizing tendency F, imbued in the protoplasm of the egg, which originates exclusively in the mother. In this case a male animal MmF develops because the sum of the two heterochromosomes outweighs the cytoplasmic tendency. But, in the other possible combination, a female will be produced, which has one heterochromosome from the father; she will inherit no female sex chromosome from the mother but will, instead, inherit the mother's protoplasmic F. However, because we are dealing with a weak race in which cytoplasmic heredity is minimized, the result will be a female intersex (MF).

Concerning the possible genetic combinations resulting from a reverse cross-mating, this is, one between a weak European male and a strong Japanese female, no noteworthy change is observed in the first generation, but beginning with the second generation it may be noted how the dominant tendencies, particularly those inherited from the mother, prevail over the chromosomal tendencies (M) inherited from the father and cause the production of predominantly female and intersex offspring. The determinative force of the sex chromosomes may be enhanced or diminished during the earliest stages of embryonic development, first by substances secreted in the embryo and then by substances inherited through the protoplasm of the ovule.

The existence of *protoplasmic transmission of sexual heredity* (by and large, a protoplasmic type of transmission is also involved in carcinogenic tendencies) is of interest because it explains the predominant and progressively feminizing tendency observed in *Lymanthria*. Because of its chromatinic formula, this animal is a protandric animal, that is, one that evolves toward feminization. On the other hand, in those species that are noted for protogyny, this cytoplasmic tendency simply serves to strengthen the basic sex. *Therefore, it is more difficult to obtain instances of intersex in protogynic species because, unlike* in protandric species, their female inheritance, inherent in their ovular protoplasm, favors the basic sex, as compared with protandric species in which it opposes the basic sex. This probably explains why *Lymanthria*, together with the other insects of the same group, as well as some birds, reptiles and some species of frogs, are all animals of choice when it comes to obtaining instances of intersex.

15.2.2. THE CHEMICAL BASIS FOR THE DETERMINATION OF SEX

The nucleus is far from being a simple conglomeration of chromosomes; on the contrary, it is the director of cellular nutrition. The chromosomes are the morphologic expression of a substrate of chemical entities whose biocatalytic mission lies in morphogenesis. Chromosomes must be conceived of as comprising a set of chemical substances acting in a manner comparable to that of a *biocatalyst*. Consequently, sexual determination cannot be accepted as linked exclusively to heterochromosomes. Investigations by Bridges have revealed that *what really matters in sexual embryogeny is not the heterochromosomes* but the state of balance established between the latter and the ordinary chromosomes (autosomes) (see Chapter 14, Section 14.6). In the light of Goldschmidt's hypothesis, protoplasmic intervention was shown to modify chromosomal balance and to influence sexual determination. Finally, humoral factors in embryonal development are also able, as we have stated previously, to modify the balance of sexual determination. It is therefore fitting to speak, along with Hartmann,[31] about *genotypic and phenotypic sexual determination*, that is, one type of sexual determination motivated by genes, and another type conditioned by the external environment. Lubs and Ruddle[50] have reported that 1.5 per cent of all newborns had chromosomal anomalies, but only one fourth of these (0.36 per cent) revealed alterations of phenotype. Obviously, in a large number of instances, chromosomal alterations do not affect embryogeny. Recent research has produced a series of examples in which phenotypic sexual determination is quite clear.

IN INVERTEBRATES. The most typical example is that of *Bonellia viridis*. Details concerning sexual determination in this species were worked out by Moewus and Kuhn.[56, 57]

Bonellia viridis is a sea-worm. The female measures 7 to 8 cm in length but has a reproductive tube measuring about 1 mm in length. The male hardly reaches 2 mm in length and is a parasite living within the gut of the female. The fate of the swimming larvae, hatched from fertilized eggs, differs depending on whether they attach themselves to the mother or to some inert object. Baltzer[5] discovered that when *larvae attached themselves to the mother's tube, they developed into males, whereas, when separated from the mother, the larvae developed into females.* Herbst[32] ascribed this effect to the masculinizing nature of a chemical substance secreted by the mother's tube. Further investigations by Nowinski[65] have led to the extraction of a hormonoid type of substance, soluble in acetone, capable of masculinizing *Bonellia* larvae. Rather than affecting the sex characteristics, the masculinizing effect is exerted on the genetic makeup of the larvae itself, so that *Bonellia* larvae treated with this substance are converted to genetic males. This is the first known instance in which genetic transformation of sex has been induced by means of a chemical type of action.

Another example has been provided through the investigations of Moewus and Kuhn[57] on a unicellular alga, *Chlamydomona eugametos*. This organism can reproduce either by simple division (asexual or agamic mode) or by conjugation of gametes. Whenever cultured on agar, it multiplies only asexually, but if the cells are introduced into a rich nutritional medium and, in addition, are illuminated, flagella appear and a type of isogamic reproduction takes place. This has been inferred to result from some light-activated substance, capable of provoking sexual reproduction in the above type of alga. The substance referred to has been proven by Moewus and Kuhn's investigations to be crocine, which is an ester of crocetine and of the carbohydrate gentiobiose. Moewus[48, 56] observed that if an extract of female gametes is added to sexually undifferentiated cells, all cells become female, whereas, inversely, addition of male gamete extract converts the cells to males. Substances with this kind of effect have been denominated *termones*. Kuhn and his colleagues[48] called *gynetermones* those substances which converted undifferentiated cells to females, and *androtermones* those producing males. The chemical composition of androtermones has been identified as that of *saffronal*, an odorific derivative of saffron, whereas gynetermones have been reported to be identical with *picrocine*, the bitter principle of saffron. In brief, both *Bonellia* and *Chlamydomonas* have been found to contain substances (those of the latter analyzed in a chemically pure state), that are capable of modifying the chromosomal machinery of sexual determination. *In other words, these sexual biocatalysts can alter the nuclear chromosomal formula by acting on the sex chromosomes which they modify.* There is little doubt that sexual determination in invertebrates is not invariably a genetic process and that *phenotypic sex, or chemically induced sex, may occur in addition to genotypically determined sex.*

IN VERTEBRATES. The process of sexual determination in vertebrates is more difficult to study than it is in lower animals. That sex in vertebrates is determined genetically is a matter of common knowledge. In relatively modern times, Waddington[85] reviewed the question of sexual determination in higher animals as a whole. As was pointed out in our earlier descriptive summary of embryology, the question of male versus female development depends on the type of mesenchymal cells proliferating in the gonadal primordium. The arrival of endoderm-derived germ cells, the gonocytes, gives rise to two types of mesodermal development in the anlage of the gonad: the *cortex*, with feminizing potentiality, and the *medulla*, with masculinizing potentiality. The question of which of these two regions is to unfold depends wholly on the animal's genetic constitution. While the eventual development of a müllerian duct in the female, and a wolffian duct in the male, depends in part on such masculinizing or feminizing potentialities, it is also the consequence of an *endocrine orientation*. Thus, the primitive fact to be determined—and, by what is so far known, determined in a genetic manner—is development of either the male or the female gonad. Nevertheless, investigations by Witschi[90] on amphibians reveal that *the autochthonous tendency of the gonadal anlage to develop the genetic sex may be conditional.* That investigator placed in parabiosis amphibian larvae of opposite sex, maintaining them in that state until they reached sexual maturity. In toads, the resulting effects were negligible, apparently because the active substances involved are poorly diffusible. However, in frogs, the presence of a gonadal medulla possessing masculinizing potency suppressed ovarian development. Apparently, any substance with similar activity is not transported by the circulation but rather by direct diffusion, as there was evidence in these experiments that the influence of the agent was greater or lesser, depending on the reciprocal positions in which the larvae were implanted. In cooperation with Mintz and Foote, Witschi also succeeded in producing sexual inversion in frog larvae by means of testosterone[54] (Fig. 15–12). The inhibitory influence exerted by the gonad was found to be even greater in newts, in which the active substance is more diffusible. Depending on the species, one or the other gonad predominates. For instance, in frogs, the male sex predominates over the female sex, as a result of which there is a tendency toward masculinization, whereas in toads and newts, the opposite is true: the female sex is predominant and there is a tendency toward feminization. *In short, diffusible substances, secreted by the gonads of Batrachia and Amphibia, are able to inhibit the development of the gland of the opposite sex.* Depending on the species, the presence in the immediate environment of an ovary may prevail over a testis and transform the latter into another ovary, or vice versa, the testis may dominate the ovary and induce conversion of the latter to a testis. *The contest between the sexes unfolds in such a way that it faithfully reflects the contest between the cortex and medulla, which are present in both gonads.*

Witschi[92] has demonstrated that elevated temperatures favor the development of the medulla at the expense of the cortex in the Batrachia and Amphibia. The active gonadal substances have been called *cortexine* (feminizing) and *medullarine* (masculinizing). These substances were subsequently shown, by Witschi and his colleagues,[91,92] not to be exclusive to amphibians but also to occur in higher animals, and to most

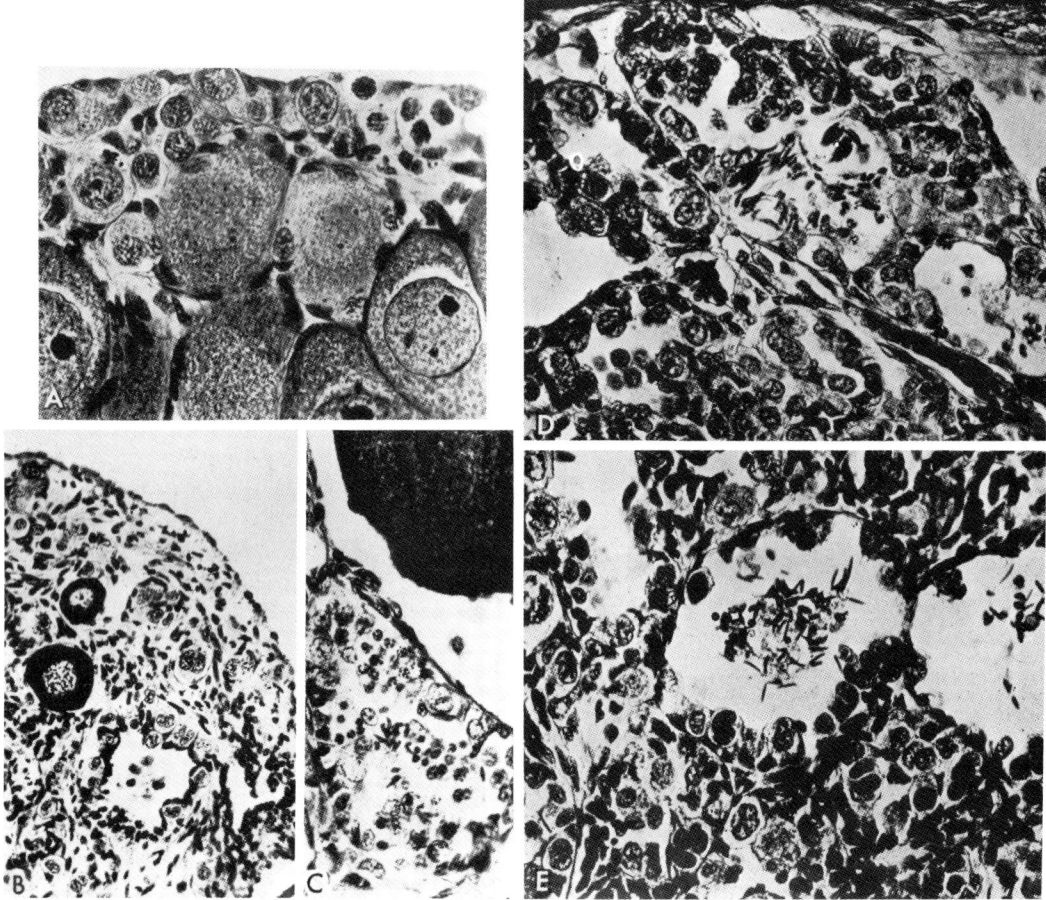

Figure 15–12. Action of testosterone on sexual inversion of larvae of *Rana clamitans*. A, Ovary of larva sacrificed in May, showing seasonal proliferation of oocytes. B, Ovary converted to testis by injection of 1.1 mg testosterone dipropionate administered over a period of 151 days. The gonocytes have migrated deeper into the medullary cords, away from the cortex. C, Complete inversion of gonad by August, after having received a total dose of 8.5 mg testosterone in 280 days. Note tubule containing spermatids and several spermia. Part of a degenerating egg can still be noted (right top). D, Another field from the gonad of same animal, revealing well formed spermia. E, Control male, sacrificed at the same time as preceding metamorphosed female and showing similar stage of sexual development as in D. (From Mintz, Foote and Witschi.[54])

likely be *protein-bound complexes of estradiol and testosterone, respectively.* Experimental gonadal induction by means of either androgens or estrogens was later clearly demonstrated in frogs,[48] amphibians[24] and elasmobranchial fishes.[16] Although sex hormones do not invariably produce the same effect, salamander tadpoles treated with estrogens have been observed to undergo feminization, whereas androgen-treated frog tadpoles have been reported to reveal musculinization (Needham[63]).

Successful research on birds along similar lines has been undertaken by three groups of investigators: Dantschakova and co-workers,[21] Wolff and colleagues[93] and Willier's group.[88, 89] The methods employed by these investigators consisted of injecting male or female hormones into eggs of chickens or other birds. The hormonally induced effects were found to be quite variable, depending on the type of animal studied. Complete feminization of genetic males was achieved by Dantschakova and Massavicius with injections of estrone in a oily vehicle into the allantoic cavity on the fourth day of incubation.

However, if testosterone propionate was introduced in the same way, the embryos died. To some extent, the mechanism involved in the lethal effect seems to result from *precocious transformation of the mesonephros into epididymis*, causing failure of the intermediary renal system with consequent development of fatal edema. Conversely, Dantschakova was able to produce complete masculinization in a mammalian (guinea pig) embryo by introducing testosterone propionate, in a single drop of oily solution, into the amniotic cavity at a very early stage of gestation. Korenchewsky[46] obtained similar results with injections of male hormone into pregnant animals. Subsequently, the same phenomenon was observed to occur accidentally in humans; injections of androgens or norprogesteroids in pregnant women produce fetal virilization (see Chapter 39). As a matter of fact, what we are witnessing here is but an experimentally induced imitation of an otherwise naturally occurring phenomenon, which has been well known ever since it was described by Lillie in 1916 — the occurrence of freemartins. A phenomenon of parabiosis occurs in calf twins, whose fetal membranes have a common third circulation, that is similar to that occurring in human parasitic or papyraceous fetuses. Under such conditions, the female parabiont shows marked deviation in a male direction, producing an intersex animal with well developed testes and wolffian ducts. Jainudeen and Hafez[37] have obtained freemartins by injecting pregnant cows with androgens. Hughes demonstrated that the same phenomenon could be produced in the sow. It may safely be assumed that a similar development occurs in human parasitic fetuses, which fails to produce manifestations because of the lethal nature of its effects on parabiosis. Whether we are dealing in this case with a premature masculine transformation of the wolffian body, with death of the fetus owing to *mesonephric insufficiency*, remains to be elucidated. However, according to modern ideas, *such transformations can only be achieved if they occur in the direction of the basic sex* (see preceding section). This means that, *in protogynic animals, such as mammals, the deviation occurs in the direction of the male sex*, as exemplified by freemartins, while *in protandric animals, such as birds, the transformation takes place in a female direction*, as has been shown in Dantschakova's investigations. It remains to be seen why transformations in the opposite direction do not occur; probably it is because an individual cannot acquire an additional X chromosome but, on the other hand, it can indeed lose one. On the other hand, Dantschakova assumed that the lethal nature of the masculinizing influence in birds, and the feminizing influence in mammals, results from associated urinary anomalies.

There is no doubt that *inversion of gonadal sex does occur. If the gonad is admitted to be determined genetically, this must be possible only through inversion of the genetic machinery of sexual determination.*

Interestingly, the prevailing trend over the past few years has been to supplant the theory of direct gonocyte-induced action by that of *chemically-induced (evocator-induced) action*. Evocators have been demonstrated in mollusks by Streiff.[82] Hoffenberg and Jackson[34] have been able to locate the effect of evocator activity in the gonad of various vertebrates, which was confirmed by Witschi and his colleagues[92] in the course of the same year. Substances of the evocator type in the newt have been long known to be conveyed by the mesonephric duct, so that destruction of the latter results in gonadal dysgenesis (Houillon[35]). Seemingly, the same phenomena may have been observed in the human species in view of the findings, reported by Carpenter and Potter,[17] that gonadal agenesis is frequently associated with the absence of mesonephric rests.

15.2.3. SUMMARY

Let us review briefly the current concept of sexual determination. *Sexual determination means the establishment of an individual's sexual nature.* Since, fundamentally, this is based on the nature of his or her gonad, sexual determination may be considered equivalent to the *establishment of the gonad*. In morphologic terms, sexual determination is characterized by the development of the *cortical zone in the female* and the *medullary zone in the male*. This kind of gonadal polarity is essentially similar in all animal species. In theory, sex is predetermined from the very moment of fertilization. The chromosomal formula resulting from the conjugation of female and male pronuclei establishes the sexual character of all somatic cells and, as a result, also the direction in which the gonad of a newly created individual will tend to evolve in its development. Theoretically speaking, between the moment of fertilization and the time the gonad has reached development, there elapses an interval during which, *though it is not demonstrable, sex in a sense has already been determined.* Our inability to recognize the embryo's sex during this interval stems from the inadequacy of our analytic methods. While most of the already mentioned events may occur in accordance with classical theory, a number of recent developments would lead us to believe that, *during the phase of gonadal undifferentiation, genetic sexual determination can be modified by humoral factors. If this is true, then embryonic undifferentiation at this stage is not merely an apparent entity, covering up the reality of predetermination, but is in fact a state of real undifferentiation, in which humoral factors can modify the definitive sex.*

In lower animals, such humoral factors have been brought to light in a convincing way. They probably also exist in higher animals and perhaps even in man. Substances that affect gonadal determination have been designated respectively as *medullarine* and *cortexine*. These are believed to possess a sexual activity and to be closely related to the specific sex hormones, that is, testosterone and estrogen. Obviously, *there are two modalities of sexual determination: a genotypic one and a phenotypic one.* Both types are operative in a phase of embryonal life interposed between fertilization and sexual gland development of either male or female nature. Genetic determination establishes the basic tendency of one particular sex, but humoral factors can modify that tendency, giving rise to a gonad of the sex opposite to the primitively established one. In lower organisms, such as *Bonellia* as well as the *Chlamydomonas*, substances capable of determining phenotypic sex apparently are able to affect the entire somatic cell population by rendering them male or female, respectively. However, in vertebrates, the process is confined to the gonads, the cells of the soma retaining the sexual formula that corresponds to them by virtue of the genetically established sex. Expressed in a different way, this means that *the genetic female of higher animals*, for instance, *is characterized by a female pattern of chromosomes despite the possible presence of a testis rather than an ovary.* Our long-standing belief that sex is defined by the male or female nature of the gonad notwithstanding, it is obvious that *what actually defines sex is the number of chromosomes present in the nucleus.* Thus, when faced with discrepancies between number of nuclear chromosomes and nature of the gonad, we must admit the fact that *phenotypic inversion of the determined sex does occur, and accept the sex indicated by the individual's nuclear chromatin formula as the individual's genetic sex.* This concept is of utmost importance because, as we shall see in Chapter 35, in discussing the subject of hermaphroditism, what really defines an individual's sex is not the sexual gland but the immanent genetic nature of all cells of the body as a whole.

15.3. SEXUAL DIFFERENTIATION

Sexual differentiation denotes establishment of gonadal sex. *By sexual differentiation, we mean development of the genital apparatus in the direction of the corresponding sign of the gonad.* This definition, which is the classic one, must nevertheless be modified in view of what has already been stated. According to the revised concept, *sexual determination is chromosomal determination reflected in somatic cells; the gonad is a product of differentiation, achieved by means of a series of factors that cooperate with genetic factors in male or female development.*

15.3.1. SUBSTANCES STIMULATING MÜLLERIAN DUCT DEVELOPMENT

A number of observations permit us to assume that *müllerian duct development takes place owing to stimulation by ovarian hormones.* Estrogens injected into the amniotic cavity of birds or mammals arrest the development of the wolffian duct and stimulate that of the müllerian ducts. In cultures of chicken oviduct, Kohler and Malley[45] found that estrogens elicited differentiation of fibroblasts. By the same token, experimental feminization following parabiosis, such as can be produced in amphibians,[53, 90] seems to indicate that the feminizing substance is estrogenic hormone. The effects of estrogens become clearly manifest when studied in the opposite sex. Even in male embryos, both systems of ducts, male and female, can be stimulated. Estrogens produce no visible alterations in the female sex because their action coincides with the genetically determined direction of differentiation of the müllerian duct. In contrast, in embryos of the male sex, they stimulate the development of structures that otherwise would undergo atrophy. Laccassagne[49] reported that estradiol benzoate, injected into male baby rabbits, induced müllerian duct development, in spite of the fact that these were newborn animals; moreover, after several months, uteri developed giving rise to pseudohermaphroditism in these animals. Similar experiments were performed by Burrows[15] on newborn mice in which subcutaneous implants of estrogen crystals would lead to sexual inversion. Price and Pannabecker[73] cultured embryonic tissue from both wolffian and müllerian ducts in vitro, and recorded specific stimulative effects by androgens and estrogens, respectively. Similar results were obtained by means of stilbestrol administration to rats and mice. With injections of estradiol into female opossums Burns[14] achieved comparable results. The persistence of müllerian structures in male birds hatched from eggs into which estrogens had been injected was reported by Willier and his co-workers,[87] who introduced either estrone or estradiol into the yolk sac of chicken eggs during the second day of incubation. Analogous research has been carried out by Forbes on the opossum, and by Green and colleagues,[28] as well as by Raynaud,[78] on pregnant rats and mice. It is of interest to point out that regression of wolffian ducts was not observed in any of the foregoing experiments, whereas development of müllerian ducts was invariably found to be enhanced, which favors the conclusion that *estrogens act on the male embryo by provoking development of dormant female rests rather than causing atrophy or inhibition of elements of the genital apparatus pertaining to the male sex.*

15.3.2. EFFECTS OF ANDROGENS

Investigations have also been undertaken on the effects of androgens on the wolffian system of the embryo. Androgenic hormone likewise has been observed to affect the development of the wolffian ducts of female embryos significantly. Steinach studied the effects of testicular transplants in spayed female guinea pigs, noting that the wolffian ducts persisted. Afterwards, Minoura and Greenwood repeated these experiments, arriving at the same conclusion. Wolff,[94] who injected chick embryos with androgens from the third day of incubation onwards, observed that female embryos revealed markedly developed wolffian ducts and, in fact, became pseudohermaphrodites. In similar experiments, as already mentioned, Raynaud[77] injected pregnant rats with 5 to 10 mg testosterone propionate daily. Sometimes this treatment resulted in abortions; however, in those animals that did not abort, embryos of the female sex had well developed wolffian ducts. These findings were confirmed in guinea pigs by Dantschakova,[21] and in birds' eggs by Willier.[89] Significant in this respect were the findings from similar experiments with androgen injections reported by Greene and co-workers.[28] In pregnant rats, they found the appearance of female progeny with persistent wolffian ducts and with epididymis, vasa deferentia, seminal vesicles and prostate. Coexisting with those organs were normal oviducts, uteri and superior portions of the vagina. As far as the external genitalia were concerned, the presence of a penis was observed. This again seems to provide evidence to the effect that wolffian duct development is furthered by androgens in the same way as that of müllerian ducts is by estrogens. However, here, too, one would have to infer that androgens exert no inhibitory effects on the müllerian ducts. What is even more interesting in the case of androgens is the observation of Witschi and Fugo[91] that androgen injections may occasionally cause growth in size not only of the wolffian organs but *also that of the oviduct.* This seems to be in keeping with clinical observations that adult women receiving androgen therapy in some cases reveal stimulatory effects on uterine growth.

Based on the foregoing arguments, *androgens may be concluded to be specific stimulators of male tract development not only in adult life but during embryonic life as well.* Estrogens seem to carry out an analogous function with regard to the female tract. A natural phenomenon, which in human clinical experience substantiates this assertion, can be found in the *adrenogenital syndrome* (described in Chapter 32). The latter exemplifies a disturbance in embryonal development whereby, as a result of a pathologic alteration in adrenocortical development, the body is flooded with androgens of the corticoid variety. In girls, these androgens produce the appearance of a peniform clitoris and the development of male structures of wolffian origin. The ovaries in those cases are perfectly well developed and present no anomalies. Less commonly, the syndrome appears in males and is of the opposite type, that is, the adrenals elaborate excessive amounts of estrogenic substances. In these cases, the cloaca develops a female character, resulting in a penis with hypospadias, and sometimes a rudimentary vagina as well as a rudimentary uterus. The testicles are usually well formed and well developed in these cases, only the genital tract being affected by feminization.

15.3.3. AUTONOMY OF DIFFERENTIATION OF THE DUCTS OF WOLFF AND DUCTS OF MÜLLER

Pincus and Hopkins[69] failed to produce sexual inversion very early in the course of a regimen of large doses of synthetic estrogens. In recent publications, Witschi and his colleagues[91, 92] admitted the pronephric origin of the müllerian duct, postulating that induction of the latter occurred solely by virtue of its pronephric nature and without any participation by steroid hormones. In their view, *what initiates the development of the future female genital tract are nonsteroid autonomous evocators.* Only after having attained a certain degree of development does the genital tract begin to respond to estrogenic stimuli. Similar views were advocated by Jost[40, 41] with regard to the male genital tract.

15.3.4. ORIGIN OF SEXUAL INCRETIONS DURING EMBRYONIC LIFE

The embryogeny of the genital apparatus would certainly appear clear if both the testis and ovary of the embryonic phase were mature glands whose functional conditions were comparable to those of adult glands, and if each were able to secrete sufficient quantities of their specific hormones, since such a situation would explain what stimulates the development of the respective genital tracts. However, during embryonal life, the ovary, at least, seems to lack sufficient incretory capacity to discharge that function. On the other hand, both the placenta and the adrenal cortex intervene in a decisive manner in the production of sex steroids. The organs producing the sex steroids and determining the development of the corresponding genital tracts during embryonal life are: (1) the placenta, (2) the adrenal cortex, and (3) the fetal testis.

EFFECT OF PLACENTAL INTERNAL SECRETION. The placenta secretes abundant estrogens (Chapter 19) throughout gestation. These estrogens are highly diffusible, so that elevated estrogen concentrations are found in the fetal body during pregnancy (Phoenix and co-workers[68]). A number of investigators (Jost,[42, 43] Rosa,[80] Zuckermann and Van Waagenen[95]) believe that the estrogens inundating the body during pregnancy initiate a feminizing trend in sexual development. Thus müllerian duct development is presumably a simple consequence of the genital tract being, so to say, "dragged in" passively. On the contrary, the development of male structures from the wolffian duct would require the action of some secretion with a male effect to oppose environmental feminizing influences.

Whatever the case may be, it is important to realize that fetuses are exposed to elevated levels of feminizing hormones, regardless of sex and conditions under which they undergo differentiation.

EFFECT OF ADRENAL STEROIDS. The adrenal, as already pointed out in Chapter 9, and as we shall again stress (Chapter 20), is a very important organ during the first months of embryonic life. Secretion of steroids, androgens as well as estrogens, by the fetal adrenal has been demonstrated by numerous investigators (Grollman,[29] Jayle,[38] Tonutti and Fetzer,[84] Price[72] and Botella[11]). Our own studies (Cano and Botella[9, 10]) have demonstrated the ambisexual nature of the fetal cortex, so that the adrenal may be admitted to be equally capable of secreting estrogens and androgens. Excessive adrenal development preceding weight increase of the gonads during embryonic life, the occurrence of pseudohermaphroditism in congenital adrenal hyperplasia (adrenogenital syndrome, see Chapter 33), as well as the appearance of disturbances of sexual differentiation in anencephalic fetuses with adrenal aplasia (Botella[12]), are all instances favoring the assumption that the sex hormone of the interrenal system is of utmost significance during embryonic life.

FETAL TESTIS. Jost[39] and Moore[59] succeeded in castrating rodent embryos. Testicular ablation in those animals seems to entail the transformation of genetic males into females. Since signs of interstitial activity in the fetal testis can be detected as early as the initial stages of embryonal life, the testis must undoubtedly be taken into consideration as an important testosterone supplier in male embryos.

Bengtsson and his colleagues[6] have demonstrated that injections of C-14 labeled cholesterol into human fetuses between the age of six and seven months resulted in considerable concentration of radioactivity in the testis, which seems to indicate an active role of the testis in steroid hormone synthesis. Cavallero and co-workers[18] have similarly demonstrated steroidogenic enzyme activity in the human fetal testis. Rice and his colleagues[79] incubated a testicle of a 21 cm fetus with C-14 labeled acetate and found large amounts of androsterone, androstenedione and progesterone in the culture fluid. Goldman and his co-workers[26] have shown the presence of 3β-hydroxysteroido-dehydrogenase in the testicular primordium of two month old fetuses. Likewise, 3β-ol-dehydrogenase, known to be the most specific enzyme of testicular and ovarian steroidogenesis, has been identified in the fetal testis of rats[81] and man.[3]

FETAL OVARY. Even though the fetal ovary may be admitted to display less endocrine activity than the fetal testis (see Chapter 20), the presence of active steroid hormone synthesis has also been demonstrated in both avian[83, 86] and human[6, 26] embryos. Evidently, results of modern biochemical and enzymological experiments concur in ascribing steroid-synthesizing capacity to the testis and, to a lesser degree, the ovary, at a very early stage of fetal life.

15.3.5. EFFECTS OF EMBRYONIC CASTRATION ON SEXUAL DIFFERENTIATION

The bihormonal theory of sexual differentiation, as just presented here, has been borne out by experiments involving removal of embryonal gonads. Because this is an extremely difficult operation to perform, on birds as well as mammals, relatively little research has so far been done with this approach. Fortunately, the special conditions offered by the opossum, in which the baby in the pouch, even though already born, is at a stage of differentiation analogous to that of an embryo, have helped shed considerable light on this problem. Moore and his colleagues[59, 60, 62] castrated such animals on the twentieth day of development. At this age, the testis and the ovary are both still attached to the medial aspect of the mesonephros and both the male and female ducts on both sides are simple, undifferentiated tubes. The male prostate, which serves as an indicator of androgenic activity, appears on the sixteenth day as a tiny cellular anlage. Even after the testis is removed on the twentieth day of development, prostatic growth is observed to continue unchecked, and ultimate prostatic development is comparable to that of noncastrated animals. In later experiments, the same authors observed that castration of male embryos similarly failed to produce atrophy or lack of development of Cowper's glands. In contrast, female structures derived from the müllerian ducts were noted to undergo a similar degree of atrophy in castrated as in intact male embryos.[34]

Female embryos, ovariectomized at the same stage of development, similarly failed to show any developmental impairment of the müllerian organs. The uterus was exactly the same size as that of nongonadectomized females. Nor did ovariectomized animals subsequently reveal any persistence of wolffian ducts. In conclusion, these experiments may be said to have demonstrated that the embryonal gonads have absolutely no effect on the development of the genital tract either in the male or in the female. Jost[40, 41] performed identical studies on rabbit embryos. By means of an admirably delicate intervention, he was able to extract the embryos from the mother's uterus, to gonadectomize them, and to replace them in the uterus, which he afterwards sutured. Thus, in some cases, uninterrupted gestation was achieved.

In a second series of experiments, Jost[42] performed hypophysectomies on rabbit embryos. In female embryos, hypophysectomy was found to have no effect whatsoever on sexual development, while in male embryos, on the contrary, hypophysectomy caused atrophy of the testis and subsequent development of an intersex animal of female appearance. Those results enabled Jost to locate the missing link in his hypothesis, admitting not only that the testis exerted an influence on wolffian duct development but that testicular activity of the embryonic era was under pituitary control.

15.3.6. PRODUCTS OF EXTRACTION FROM THE EMBRYONAL GONAD

Other investigators turned their attention to the study of active substances in embryonal gonads. Womak and Koch extracted fetal bovine testes shortly before term and found that such extracts behaved as androgens in the capon's comb test. However, they were unable to extract any free substances and speculated that perhaps the embryonal bovine testis secreted small amounts of testicular hormone without releasing it. Atsumi[2] conducted similar studies on calf fetuses in conjunction with bioassay procedures in rats and mice, and was able to demonstrate the presence of both estrogenic and androgenic substances. However, Moore[61] was unable to confirm those results and expressed skepticism concerning any possible gonadal hormone activity in these animals. As far as the human species is concerned, the ovarian function in term fetuses was studied by Phillipp[67] histologically. The histologic features observed in these ovaries were judged to be suggestive of some hormonal activity. Some follicles were still in the process of maturation, while others exhibited proliferation of the granulosa and theca. Montalvo and Shocker[58] at our Clinic similarly noted that the genital organs of term fetuses usually reveal evidence of some cell proliferation consistent with estrogenic effect. As a result, one might assume that during the last hours of embryonic life, because of gonadotropin-induced stimuli, both the testis and the ovary may be stirred into a transient phase of activity. This may be the reason for the so-called *genital crisis,* a phenomenon of sexual hyperactivity at time of birth. At any rate, at this stage of embryonic life, both male and female genital organs are well developed. However, there is no evidence of similar gonadal activity during the first months of gestation, which is precisely the time during which the wolffian and müllerian ducts develop in the human species. *Whether male or female, the gonad may then be assumed to secrete no active substance capable of stimulating the development of the müllerian and wolffian ducts. To explain the development of these ducts, we may have to invoke the hypothesis of adrenal activity or that of combined placental-adrenal activity.*

15.3.7. EFFECTS OF PARABIOSIS AND TRANSPLANTATION OF THE GONAD

The results obtained by means of parabiosis and transplantation of the gonad, particularly in nonmammalian vertebrates, are interesting enough to deserve some comment. The parabiotic union between amphibians in the larval stage can be achieved by a relatively simple technique, which makes it possible to maintain two individuals, joined heterosexually, in a state of embryonal development and to study the resulting interactions between them. This type of research has been carried out by Witschi and his colleagues,[92] Burns,[14] Humphrey[36] and Ponse.[70, 71] Larvae grown in parabiotic union are observed to develop gonadal deviations. Gonadal inversion of sex takes place in a way similar to what is known to happen in freemartins. Depending on the species, the tendency to inversion may be linked to either sex. In the frog, for instance, the testis predominates over the ovary, inducing transformation of the latter into an ovotestis. Thus, parabiotic union between a male larva and a female larva results in development of a testis in the male and that of an ovotestis in the female. The opposite effect is observed in toads and newts. In these latter species, parabiosis between male and female larvae allows the female to develop ovaries normally but causes the male to develop ovotestes. The magnitude of this effect has been found to be proportional to the distance between the gonads of the two parabionts. Thus, the resulting effect is mild if parabionts are implanted tail first, but is most pronounced if the animals are implanted in such a way that their gonadal anlagen are adjacent. This, as well as the fact that the degree of diffusibility of the feminizing or masculinizing substance (whichever the case may be) varies according to the species, raises the question of whether the observed interactions of parabiosis, rather than being the result of sex hormones, may be due instead to nonhormonal components of the *local inductor* type, secreted by the gonads and probably identical to *medullarine* and *cortexine*, which were mentioned previously. In those animals in which gonadal function is physiologically undifferentiated, phenotypic determination of sex seems to play a much more important role than it does in higher animals, particularly mammals.

The studies by Davis and Potter[22] on human embryos, in which intraembryonal injections of large amounts of estrogens and androgens were used, revealed that sex hormones failed to exert any noticeable effects on human sexual determination. In no case was it possible to achieve inversion of gonadal sex by means of injecting the opposite hormone. Despite the fact that such inversion effects as are seen in experiments with parabiosis seem to result from the actions of cortexine and medullarine, rather than sex hormones, the latter, too, in effect, have been quite convincingly shown to be able to produce inversion of the gonad in amphibian larvae. Padoa[66] has injected estrogens into toad larvae noticing transformation of the testis into an ovotestis. The opposite effect, obtained in frogs by Mintz and his colleagues,[54] has already been described (Fig. 15–12). These results were later confirmed by Gallien,[24] Puckett[74] and Witschi.[90] Although the inversion effect on the sexual glands of Batrachia is produced in a physiologic way by substances of the inductor type, whose mode of action in parabiosis is known, experimental estrogen administration may be inferred to be capable of producing effects similar to those of cortexine. Kornfeld and Nalbandov[47] later carried out similar investigations by injecting hormones into the eggs of birds during development and arrived at similar conclusions. It thus seems evident that, while sex hormone activity is apparently not involved during the embryonic stage, sex hormones injected artificially produce an extraphysiologic effect which is of the same sign and direction as the effect produced by inductors. In other words, *when injected in large quantities, sex hormones may act as inductors, despite the fact that the physiologic inductors secreted by the gonads during the embryonic era are believed to be cortexine and medullarine.*

Another conclusion to be drawn from the foregoing observations is the fact that, while sex hormones are able to modify the development of a female or male genital tract in mammals, they are unable to produce inversion of gonadal sex in mammals, though they can do so in lower vertebrates. Consequently, *in higher vertebrates, particularly mammals, the role of hormones in endocrine development is limited to acting as biocatalysts in the development of both the wolffian and müllerian ducts, whereas, in lower animals, such as birds, amphibians, etc., the sex hormones—or in their stead the inductors—fulfill a much more fundamental function in that they are involved in the evolution of undifferentiated sexual glands into either ovaries or testes. As one ascends on the animal scale, genetic determination of sex may be asserted to rest on increasingly firm grounds while, in equal measure, sex becomes decreasingly less susceptible to being modified by humoral factors.* If gonadal development in lower animals is allowed to proceed in the absence of humoral influences, gonadal sex undergoes no modifications, and the gonads develop in accordance with their genetic sex. Evidence to this effect has been provided by Wolff and Haffen,[94] who cultured gonads of chick embryos in vitro, observing that they developed in accordance with their genetic sex.

15.4. SYNOPSIS OF SEXUAL DIFFERENTIATION AND EMBRYOMECHANICS OF SEX

In conclusion, the following three issues, which are considered essential, must be discussed: (1) hormonal theories of sexual differentiation; (2) influence of genetic sex and target organ response in sexual differentiation; and (3) basic sex and evolution of sexuality.

15.4.1. THEORIES OF SEXUAL DIFFERENTIATION

As indicated previously, the placenta, the fetal adrenal and the fetal testis all intervene in sexual differentiation by virtue of being the principal producers of steroids. Since their actions are sometimes directly opposed to each other, the reciprocal equilibrium among them is believed to play an influential role in the development of the wolffian and müllerian ducts. However, it must be pointed out that, as shown by Witschi and his colleagues,[91, 92] hormonal influence is *confined to accelerating growth of the wolffian and müllerian primordia already in existence and can by no means create a new primordium where there had been none before*. The action of steroids may thus be defined as *sexokinetic* but not *sexogenic*.

To explain this phenomenon three fundamental theories have been proposed:

GROLLMAN'S THEORY. Grollman[29] theorized that placental estrogen secretion during embryonic life drove the embryo inevitably along the road of feminization, but that androgen secretion on the part of the male adrenal could efficiently oppose and even overcome this feminizing influence. Accordingly, male embryos were postulated to have an adrenal *androgenic fetal zone*, absence of which in female embryos was responsible for the development of the müllerian duct. Consequently, *femininity resulted from the absence of an androgenic zone*. A scheme of Grollman's theory is shown in Figure 15-13.

JOST'S THEORY. Based on his own research, Jost postulated that the androgenic influence Grollman thought was necessary to oppose the feminizing effect of placental estrogens did not originate in the adrenal but in the testis, whose activity during embryonic life was considerable when compared to that of the underdeveloped ovary. Jost's theory represents an important contribution toward explaining the genesis of Turner's syndrome (Chapters 27 and 35)

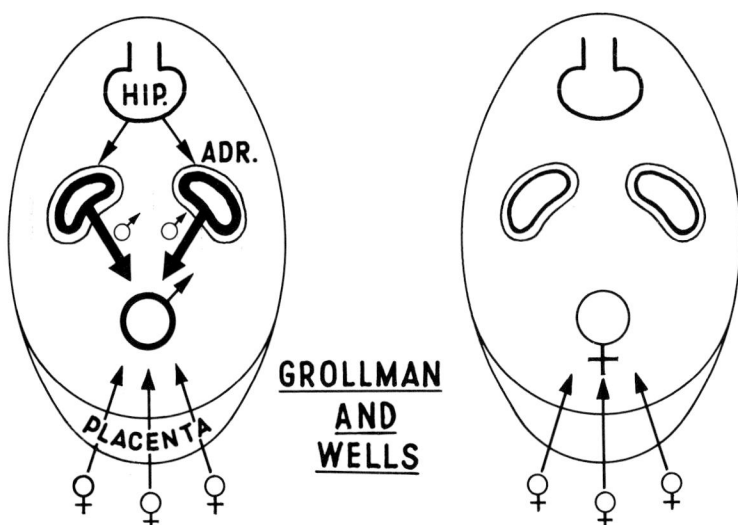

Figure 15-13. Diagram representing sexual differentiation as proposed by Grollman and Wells. The fetus is subjected to the continuous feminizing influence of placental estrogens. In the absence of any counterbalancing action by androgens, all embryos, including those with male genetic sex, would differentiate into females. The androgenic stimulus necessary for the development of males is provided by the adrenocortical sexual zone, or "androgenic fetal zone," which secretes androgens. HIP., hypophysis.

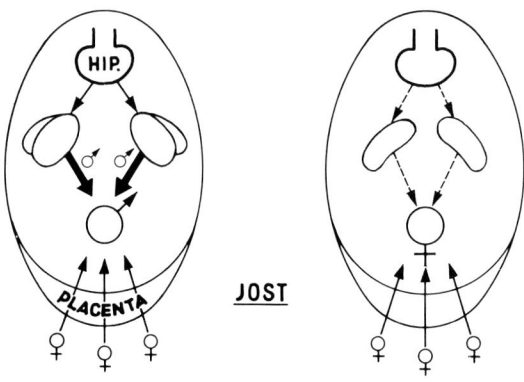

Figure 15–14. Schematic representation of sexual differentiation according to Jost. The mechanism is identical to that proposed in Figure 15–14, except for the assumption that androgens originate in the fetal testis, from where they are secreted under the influence of pituitary stimulation. HIP., hypophysis.

and has been reproduced graphically in Figure 15–14.

OUR OWN THEORY. It has been our belief that the two preceding theories are open to criticism. A number of investigators have shown (see Chapter 19) that there was no clear predominance of estrogens in urine of pregnancy until well beyond the fourth month of gestation, by which time the genital tract is undoubtedly well developed. During the critical months when the wolffian and müllerian ducts develop in their respective physiologic direction, there is a state of androgen-estrogen balance in the urine and blood of pregnant women and, we presume, also in the fetal circulation. On the other hand, as already pointed out, the fetal adrenal has been shown[10] to display histophysiologic features of active secretion in the male as well as in the female. We therefore assume that, even though the testis is able to exert a masculinizing influence and the placenta a feminizing influence, the two influences are in a stalemate up to the fifth month of gestation. At that time, adrenal secretion, exerting a feminizing effect in the female and a masculinizing effect in the male, for the first time acquires a decisive influence. Our hypothesis has been reproduced in the diagram of Figure 15–15.

The question of why the adrenal should secrete androgens in some cases and estrogens in others remains unsolved. However, this is also true in adults with the adrenogenital syndrome; some show frank virilization, whereas others reveal complete feminization, in the absence of any known reason for adrenal hyperplasia to manifest itself in either direction. We speculate that, since gonadal incretory activity during the embryonal period is induced by evocators organizing the gonadal mesenchyme as a secretory organ, influences of the same type could in a similar way reach the interrenal anlage, close as the latter is to that of the gonad, and cause similar changes in the latter's mesenchyme. However, this remains no more than theory.

Nevertheless, we believe that the adrenal cortex plays a primordial role in the sexual development of the genital organs.

15.4.2. INFLUENCE OF GENETIC SEX AND TARGET ORGAN RESPONSE IN SEXUAL DIFFERENTIATION

It must not be forgotten that the *sex chromosomes confer a sexual character on every cell in the body.* As a result of the presence of a distinctive number of chromosomes, sexuality is immanent in all cells. Thus, in addition to the nature of the hormonal stimulus, *the mode of response on*

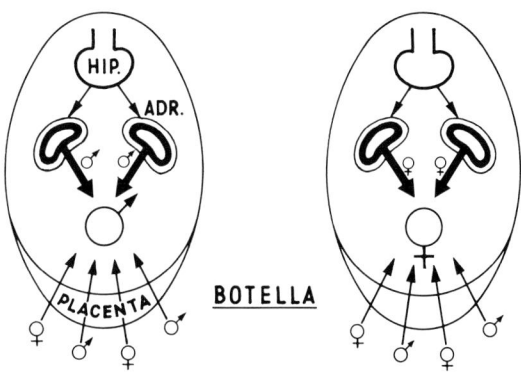

Figure 15–15. Diagram representing sexual differentiation according to our own ideas. During the period between the fourth and sixth weeks, while the genital tract develops, placental estrogen production is low and maternal estrogenemia is adequately counterbalanced by high androgen levels. The impulse delivered by way of the placenta is therefore bisexual. What makes differentiation in terms of sex possible is the fetal adrenal, which is able to secrete either estrogens or androgens, facilitating the development of female or male sex, respectively. HIP., hypophysis.

part of the organism undergoing differentiation must be taken into account. By and large, genetic males are believed to have a special tendency to respond to male hormones, whereas genetic females have a special capacity for responding to estrogens. Clark and Gorski[20] have reported the presence of an estrogen binding protein, or "estrogen receptor," in the uterus of female rat fetuses. It has been found to reach a peak on the tenth day of intrauterine life and to decrease gradually afterwards, presumably indicating a high degree of sensitivity of the müllerian duct to estrogens. Seen in this context, although the response of a given target organ is subject to hormonal stimulation, the type of response is not, since it is invariably oriented in a genetically determined direction. *As far as sexual differentiation is concerned, hormones are mere factors of realization of genetically preestablished phenomena.* It must not be overlooked that this refers to both physiologic and pathologic phenomena.

15.4.3. BASIC SEX AND EVOLUTION OF SEXUALITY

In a preceding section, we referred to *basic sex* as that sex which, in a given species, has an even number of X chromosomes. It is also referred to as monogametic sex as distinct from digametic sex, in which the sex chromosomes are asymmetrical or unpaired. The basic, monogametic sex of both mammals and frogs is female. On the other hand, in reptiles, newts and toads, the basic sex is male. As a rule, it is easier to lose an X chromosome than to acquire one, which is why evolution invariably moves from basic sex to heterogametic sex. In the human species, such evolution of sex only takes place in rare pathologic states (Chapter 35), whereas in reptiles, amphibians and birds, it is a habitual phenomenon, giving rise to so-called "Pflüger hermaphrodites." Because sexual evolution always proceeds, as pointed out above, from the basic sex to the other, *all animals with a female basic sex are invariably protogynic, whereas those with a male basic sex are always protandric.* Many years ago, Marañón[51] had expressed the belief that femininity is an intermediate stage in the evolution of a male individual to manhood, which represented his *"theory of evolution of sexuality."* This assertion of his, based on purely clinical and constitutional observations of external appearances and hormonally induced conditions, such as tertiary sex characters (see Chapter 18), may have a deeper significance than it might appear. Although there is no undifferentiated gonad in the human species, capable, as in Amphibia, of transforming or inverting its nature in response to hormonal stimuli, and although genetic sex in man is established on comparatively much more solid grounds, we have nevertheless become aware of a few rare pathologic cases in which such gonadal transformation had actually occurred, and, in each case, it occurred in a female-to-male direction.

REFERENCES

1. Arey, L. B.: *Developmental Anatomy*, 6th ed. Philadephia, W. B. Saunders Co., 1956.
2. Atsumi, C. R.: *J. Clin. Endocr.*, 10:942, 1950.
3. Baillie, A. H., Ferguson, M. M., and Hart, D. M. K.: *J. Clin. Endocr. Metab.*, 26:738, 1966.
4. Baker, G., and Franchi, L. L.: *Chromosome*, 22:258, 1967.
5. Baltzer, F.: *Arch. Exper. Zellforsch.*, 22:276, 1939.
6. Bengtsson, G., Ullberg, S., Wiqvist, N., and Diczfalusy, E.: *Acta Endocr.*, 46:544, 1964.
7. Blandau, R. J., White, B. J., and Rumery, R. E.: *Fertil. Steril.*, 14:482, 1963.
8. Blandau, R. J.: *Amer. J. Obstet. Gynec.*, 104:311, 1969.
9. Botella, J., and Cano, A.: *Arch. Med. Exper.*, 13:81, 1950.
10. Botella, J., and Cano, A.: *Gynaecologia*, 124:166, 1947.
11. Botella, J.: *Arch. Gynäk.*, 183:73, 1953.
12. Botella, J.: *Arch. Esp. Morfol.*, 2:145, 1942.
13. Brachet, J.: *Embryologie Chimique*. Paris, Masson et Cie., 1947.
14. Burns, R. K.: *Cold Spring Harbor Symp. Quant. Biol.*, 9:125, 1942.
15. Burrows, H.: *The Biological Action of the Sex Hormones*. Cambridge, Cambridge University Press, 1945.
16. Capurow, A.: *Compt. Rend. Acad. Sci. (Paris)*, 256:4736, 1963.
17. Carpentier, P. J., and Potter, E. L.: *Amer. J. Obstet. Gynec.*, 78:235, 1959.
18. Cavallero, C., Magrini, U., Dellepiane, M., and Cizelj, T.: *Ann. d'Endocr.*, 26:409, 1965.
19. Chieffi, G.: In *Le sexe*. Paris, Masson et Cie. 1960.
20. Clark, J. H., and Gorski, J.: *Science*, 169:76, 1970.
21. Dantschakova, V.: In *La differentiation sexuelle chez les vertebrés*. Paris, Masson et Cie., 1951.
22. Davis, M. E., and Potter, E. L.: *Endocrinology*, 42:370, 1948.
23. Felix, W.: In *Handbuch der Entwicklungsgesch-*

ichte. Ed. Keibel and Mall, Vol. II. Berlin, Springer, 1910.
24. Gallien, L.: In *Le sexe*. Paris, Masson et Cie., 1960.
25. Gillman, J.: *Contrib. Embryol.*, 32:200, 1948.
26. Goldman, A. S., Yakovac, W. C., and Bongiovanni, A. M.: *J. Clin. Endocr. Metab.*, 26:14, 1966.
27. Goldschmidt, R.: *Physiological Genetics*. New York, McGraw-Hill, 1938.
28. Greene, R. R., Burrill, M. W., and Ivy, A. C.: *Proc. Soc. Exper. Biol. Med.*, 43:32, 1940.
29. Grollman, A.: *The Adrenals*. Baltimore, William & Wilkins Co., 1936.
30. Harrison, R. G.: *Textbook of Human Embryology*. Oxford, Blackwell, 1959.
31. Hartmann, M.: *Naturwiss.*, 19:8, 1931.
32. Herbst, C.: *Naturwiss.*, 20:375, 1932.
33. Higuchi, I.: Arch. Gynäk., 249:144, 1932.
34. Hoffenberg, R., and Jackson, W. P. V.: *J. Clin. Endocr.*, 17:454, 1957.
35. Houillon, C.: *Compt. Rend. Acad. Sci.*, 236:1079, 1953.
36. Humphrey, R. R.: *Cold Spring Harbor Symp. Quant. Biol.*, 9:81, 1942.
37. Jainudeen, M. R., and Hafez, E. S. E.: *J. Reprod. Fertil.*, 10:281, 1965.
38. Jayle, M. F.: *Ann. d'Endocrinol.*, 12:404, 1951.
39. Jost, A.: *Arch. d'Anat. Micro. Morphol. Exper.*, 36:151, 242, 147, 1947.
40. Jost, A.: In *La differentiation sexuelle chez les vertebrés*. Paris, Masson et Cie., 1951.
41. Jost, A.: *Rec. Progr. Horm. Res.*, 7:3739, 1953.
42. Jost, A.: In *Probleme der Fetalen Endokrinologie*, ed. by H. Nowakowsky. Berlin, Springer, 1956.
43. Jost, A.: In *Le sexe*. Paris, Masson et Cie., 1960.
44. Koff, A. K.: *Contrib. Embryol.*, 24:50, 1933.
45. Kohler, P. O., and Malley, B. W.: *Endocrinology*, 81:1422, 1967.
46. Korenchewsky, V.: *Ergeb. Vit. Horm. Forsch.*, 2:418, 1938.
47. Kornfeld, W., and Malbandov, A. W.: *Endocrinology*, 55:751, 1951.
48. Kuhn, R., Moewus, F., and Wendt, G.: *Ber. Deutsch. Chem. Ges.*, 72:1702, 1939.
49. Laccassagne, A.: *Compt. Rend. Soc. Biol.*, 116:95, 1934.
50. Lubs, A. N., and Ruddle, F. H.: *Science*, 169:495, 1970.
51. Marañón, G.: *La evolución de la sexualidad y los estados intersexuales*. Madrid, Morata Ed., 1927.
52. Meyer, R.: Arch. Gynäk., 169:322, 1939; 170:85, 1940.
53. Mintz, B.: *Anat. Rec.*, 89:538, 1944.
54. Mintz, B., Foote, C. L., and Witschi, E.: *Endocrinology*, 37:286, 1945.
55. Mintz, B.: In *Le sexe*. Paris, Masson et Cie., 1960.
56. Moewus, F.: *Naturwiss.*, 27:97, 1939.
57. Moewus, F., and Kuhn, R.: *Ber. Deutsch. Chem. Ges.*, 73:547, 1940.
58. Montalvo, L., and Slocker, C.: *Acta Gin.*, 2:187, 1951.
59. Moore, C. R.: *Amer. J. Anat.*, 76:1, 1945.
60. Moore, C. R.: *Embryogenic Sex Hormones and Sexual Differentiation*. Springfield, Ill., Charles C Thomas, 1947.
61. Moore, C. R.: *J. Clin. Endocr.*, 10:942, 1950.
62. Moore, K. L., et al.: *Surg. Gynec. Obstet.*, 96:641, 1953.
63. Needham, J.: *Biochemistry and Morphogenesis*. Cambridge, Cambridge University Press, 1950.
64. Nowakowsky, H.: *Probleme der foetalen Endokrinologie*. Berlin, Springer, 1956.
65. Nowinsky, N. N.: *Biochem. J.*, 33:978, 1939.
66. Padoa, F.: In *La differentiation sexuelle chez les vertebrés*. Paris, Masson et Cie., 1951.
67. Phillipp, E.: Arch. Gynäk., 166:185, 1938.
68. Phoenix, C. H., et al.: *Endocrinology*, 65:369, 1959.
69. Pincus, G., and Hopkins, T. F.: *Endocrinology*, 62:41, 1958.
70. Ponse, K.: *La differentiation du sexe et la sexualité chez les invertebrés*. Lausanne, Rouge et Cie., 1949.
71. Ponse, K.: In *La differentiation sexuelle chez les vertebrés*. Paris, Masson et Cie., 1951.
72. Price, D.: In *Gestation*, ed. C. A. Villee. New York, The Josiah Macy Foundation, 1957.
73. Price, D., and Pannabecker, R.: In *Le sexe*. Paris, Masson et Cie., 1960.
74. Puckett, W. O.: *J. Exper. Zool.*, 84:39, 1940.
75. Raynaud, A.: *Compt. Rend. Soc. Biol.*, 129:289, 528, 632, 637, 1938.
76. Raynaud, A.: In *La differentiation sexuelle chez les vertebrés*. Paris, Masson et Cie., 1951.
77. Raynaud, A., and Frillen, M.: *Ann. d'Endocrinol.*, 11:32, 1960.
78. Raynaud, A.: In *Le sexe*. Paris, Masson et Cie., 1960.
79. Rice, B. F., Johansson, C. A., and Sternberg, W. H.: *Steroids*, 7:79, 1966.
80. Rosa, P.: *Endocrinologie sexuelle du Foetus feminin*. Paris, Masson et Cie., 1955.
81. Schlegel, R. J., Farias, E., Russo, N. C., Moore, J. C., and Gardner, L. I.: *Endocrinology*, 81:565, 1967.
82. Streiff, W.: *Ann. d'Endocrinol.*, 28:461, 1967.
83. Taber, E., Knight, J. S., Ayers, C., and Fishburne, J. L., Jr.: *J. Gen. Comp.*, 4:343, 1964.
84. Tonutti, E., and Fetzer, S.: In *Probleme der Foetalen Endokrinologie*. Berlin, Springer, 1956.
85. Waddington, C. H.: *An Introduction to Modern Genetics*. London, Allen & Unwin, 1939.
86. Weniger, J. P.: *Compt. Rend. Soc. Biol. Paris*, 158:175, 1964.
87. Willier, B. H., Gallagher, T. F., and Koch, F. C.: *J. Biol. Chem.*, 109:371, 1935.
88. Willier, B. H., Gallagher, T. F., and Koch, F. C.: *Anat. Rec.*, 61:50, 1935.
89. Willier, B. H.: In *La differentiation sexuelle chez les vertebrés*, Paris, Masson et Cie., 1951.
90. Witschi, E.: In *Gestation*. New York, The Josiah Macy Foundation, 1957.
91. Witschi, E.: *Ann. N.Y. Acad. Sci.*, 75:412, 1959.
92. Witschi, E., Nelson, W. O., and Segal, J. T.: *J. Clin. Endocr.*, 17:737, 1957.
93. Wolff, E., and Giglinger, A.: *Compt. Rend. Soc. Biol.*, 120:909, 1312, 1935.
94. Wolff, E.: In *La differentiation sexuelle chez les vertebrés*. Paris, Masson et Cie., 1951.
95. Zuckermann, S., and van Waagenen, G.: *J. Anat.*, 69:497, 1935.

Chapter 16

PUBERTY

16.1. GENERALITIES

Puberty marks the beginning of woman's active sexual life. The word *active* is stressed here as distinct from *latent*, since latent sexual life begins at the very moment of fertilization.

16.1.1. DEFINITION

Puberty is difficult to define. From the etymological point of view, the Latin word *pubere* meaning "to become grown over with hair," puberty denotes the phase during which sexual hair growth becomes first apparent. A fuller and more accurate definition had been rendered by Marañòn, who stated that puberty was a "pluriglandular crisis affecting the entire body and marking the beginning of sexual life." The foregoing definition might be completed by adding that puberty is *that period of time in life during which tertiary sex characters begin to develop. By and large, puberty may be said to be the phase in life during which active sexuality begins, marked by the development of somatic or tertiary sex characters and by the development of a pluriglandular endocrine crisis that is designed to set up a new endocrine balance. Female cyclic activity, hallmarking the phase of sexual maturity, has its onset at the time of puberty.*

It is important to realize that puberty is not a calendar date but a period of several years, during which there is an overlap between, on the one hand, imperceptible continuation of childhood and, on the other, gradually advancing maturity. A definite age for puberty can therefore not be set, nor can limits be set for its beginning and end. Nevertheless, a concrete date that must be singled out is that of the beginning of menstruation, or *menarche*. However, a girl who has reached menarche is far from being sexually developed. What must mark the end of puberty, therefore, is the time at which a woman reaches complete maturity, the so-called phase of *nubility*. For the sake of convenience, puberty may be subdivided into three phases. The first, the *prepubertal phase*, or prodromal pubertal phase, begins approximately at the age of 10 and ends at menarche, which on the average occurs at about 13 years of age. After that comes the *pubertal phase*, in the proper sense of the word, lasting from menarche to about the age of 16, when a woman apparently reaches full development. In general, however, functional maturation of the genital apparatus at this age has not been completed, which means that the woman has not actually reached nubility. Between the age of 16 and 18, a woman achieves full maturity. This is the *postpubertal phase*, which terminates in nubility.

16.1.2. AGE OF PUBERTY

Because of ill-defined limits, it is practically impossible to give any exact dates for any of the different phases of puberty. Menarche is a definite event and the date of its occurrence can be recorded, but the age at which menarche may occur is highly variable. Precise statistical data concerning the age of menarche have been published by Skerlj,[85] Hoseman[42] and Schreibner,[79] based on compilations of worldwide statistics comprising thousands of cases (Table 16-1).

As can be inferred from these statistics, the age of menarche is quite variable. It is also apparent that latitude is a significant factor, a fact well known since antiquity.

TABLE 16-1. Age at Menarche

AUTHOR	COUNTRY	NO. OF CASES	AVERAGE AGE
Engelman	United States	19,405	13 years 9 months
Rosi Doria	Italy	31,659	14 years 3 months
Yamasaki	Japan		14 years 10 months
Doktor	Hungary	9600	15 years 4 months
Schafer	Germany	11,550	15 years 7 months
Grusdeff	Russia	10,000	15 years 9 months
Rodserwitch	Northern Russia	12,000	16 years 5 months
Botella	Spain	10,000	13 years 3 months
Marañón	Spain		13 years 6 months

Table 16-2, taken from Engelman and Leicester, illustrates the point.

Within Spain alone, there are noticeable regional differences in the age of menarche. In Andalucia, for instance, menarche frequently occurs at 12 or even 11, whereas in Galicia and along the Cantabrian coastline, menarche is commonly observed at 15.

Nevertheless, there seems to be no exact correlation between geographical latitude, climate and menarche. Possibly, *racial factors*, way of life and certain geologic influences (composition of water) may also modify the age of menarche.

As regards the age limits of the other phases of puberty, there is even less agreement. Marañón considered the age of 11 to 12 as the beginning of prepubertal changes, and the age of 13, marked by the onset of pubic hair growth, as the beginning of puberty proper. Between 13 and 14, menarche occurred, and between 15 and 18 was the postpubertal phase, the latter terminating in woman's complete development and nubility.

16.1.3. CHRONOLOGY OF PUBERTY

The preceding attempt at setting a date for puberty obliges us to discuss the question of the existing chronologic order or periodic succession of different events in puberty. Thus, Marañón gave the chronologic sequence of pubertal events in both the female and the male, which is shown in Table 16-3.

In the female as well as in the male, puberty is noted to begin, as a rule with growth in stature, of the sexually undifferentiated type, which is associated with many still equivocal morphologic aspects. Males still tend to show markedly feminoid features (see Chapter 17), while females, perhaps owing to frame of mind rather than physical configuration, tend to look like tomboys. This period of growth often may be associated with eunuchoid features, predominant development of extremities, particularly arms and legs, a small trunk and quite exaggerated cubitus valgus. In the female, this phase usually occurs earlier than in the male, that is, girls usually "stretch out" earlier than boys (between ages 10 and 12, as compared to ages 12 and 13 in boys).

Before growth in stature is completed, at approximately 11 years of age, there is usually a marked increase in female mammary and pelvic development. In males, too, this phase of breast development may become apparent as a transient turgescence of the nipple. The female sexual hair begins to develop at about the age of 12 to 13, first the pubic hair then the axillary hair. Pubic hair in the male appears somewhat later. Coincident with secondary hair growth in the female, menarche makes its appearance, as indicated previously, between the ages of 13 and 14. At 15, a female's pubic hair is ostensibly, if not completely, grown and her breasts are well, if not fully, developed. Aside from this, psychologic changes, marking the transition

TABLE 16-2.

COUNTRY	AGE AT MENARCHE
Arctic zone	16 years and 6 months
Holland and Denmark	15 years and 5 months
North America	13 years and 9 months
Spain	13 years and 3 months
Tropical zone of America	12 years and 6 months
Equatorial belt	12 years and 3 months

TABLE 16-3. Chronologic Sequence of Events in Puberty

AGE	FEMALE	AGE	MALE
10–12	Critical phase in statural growth, with still equivocal morphology	12–13	Critical phase in statural growth, with still equivocal morphology
11–12	Initial development of breast and pelvis	13–14	Initial pubic hair growth, juvenile type
12–13	Initial pubic hair growth, juvenile type	14–15	Intensification of thoracic and muscular development
13–14	Initial axillary hair growth	14–15	Initial axillary hair growth
13–14	Menarche	14–16	Increase in size of genital organs
15–18	Acquisition of definitive female shape and psyche	16–18	Beginning of frank facial hair growth
		19–22	Completion of virile shape and psyche

to adulthood, become apparent. The morphologic evolution of woman is thus completed at 18, or at the latest, at 19.

In our experience, these stages of development in the male are reached somewhat later. Axillary hair does not develop until after 14, although between the ages of 13 and 14 boys grow more robust and stronger, as regards both thoracic development and growth of body musculature as a whole. At 15, males have well grown axillary and pubic hair although their facial hair develops last, usually not growing fully until after the age of 20. The male's psychological development is attained also at a later age.

From the foregoing brief outline, puberty (and particularly female puberty) can be inferred to encompass four major changes. The first is *prepubertal growth;* the second is characterized by *growth of sexual hair;* the third change is *menarche;* and in the fourth, *the female acquires her definite feminine body shape,* her hair develops fully and she matures psychologically. It may also be said that during the last stage the maturation process of the female sexual apparatus is completed for reproduction, usually after no less than four years from the onset of the menses. Thus, we must distinguish a first *prepubertal* phase, a second *pubertal* phase and a third *postpubertal* phase. The first comprises the statural growth phase and initial sexual hair development. The second coincides with maximal sexual hair development and terminates in full development of breasts and female curves, with menarche occurring in between. The third covers the interval between the establishment of complete external female morphology and that of sexual maturity, including fertility.

16.1.4. PUBERTY AND NUBILITY

In accordance with the preceding definition, puberty means, in addition to the appearance of menarche, development of female morphology, as regards both somatic female morphology and local morphology of the genital apparatus. On the average, female puberty is all but over at 15 or, at the latest, 16. However, as we have just pointed out, a puberal female has not yet reached the degree of sexual maturity necessary to be fertilized and to be able to achieve pregnancy. Instead, there is a more or less extended period of time, lasting up to five years from the time of menarche, before complete morphological and functional maturity is reached in woman. The time at which she reaches that degree of maturity that allows her to become a mother is called *nubility.* It is a well known fact, particularly recorded by ethnologists (see Ploss and Bartels[66]), that in those countries in which women marry quite young, such as for instance India, Indochina or some native black communities in Africa, it may take a woman several years before she develops her first pregnancy. Thus, it is not unusual for girls in those countries to marry at the age of 12 or 13 and to practice regular marital sex without begetting children until four or five years later. (From this we can infer that there is a *physiologic period of pubertal infertility* which lasts from the onset of puberty until nubility.)

Anatomic studies on monkeys by Hartman[36] revealed a similar period of physiologic pubertal infertility. This phenomenon was thought to stem from the fact that both menstruation and maturation of ovarian follicles in these animals begin at the same time and that follicles must undergo maturation for some time before being able to rupture, so that no corpora lutea were formed in the meantime. Consequently, the period of physiologic infertility between puberty and nubility results from absence of ovulation. In modern times, Ashley-Montagu[2] have studied the statistics of physiologic pubertal infertility on a large number of women from many countries, noting that such infertility disappears with nubility. *In summary, although menarche marks the onset of the menstrual cycle, that cycle is sterile, anovulatory. As a rule, several years have to go by before the puberal woman develops ovulatory cycles and is able to become pregnant.* Nubility marks the time at which the genital apparatus, having reached a maximal degree of functional development, becomes fully capable of discharging its reproductive function.

16.2. CLINICAL ASPECTS OF PUBERTY

A brief clinical description of the puberal process has already been made. Here we shall deal with the changes taking place in the female body during puberty, dividing these into three major groups: (1) Local changes involving the genital apparatus, (2) systemic changes, and (3) psychological changes.

16.2.1. LOCAL CHANGES IN THE GENITAL APPARATUS

The evolution of the female genital apparatus in the course of puberty is of utmost interest. We shall study successively: (1) the prepuberal genital apparatus, (2) ovarian changes at the onset of puberty, (3) tubal and uterine changes, (4) vaginal changes, (5) external genital organs and breast, and (6) the mechanism involved in the first menstruation.

THE PREPUBERAL GENITAL APPARATUS. The ovary of the newborn contains an enormous number of oogonia, which represent, so to speak, the woman's lifelong stock of germ cells. These oogonia, as well as the primordial follicles in which they are enclosed, remain in a stationary phase throughout infancy and childhood. There is hardly any difference between the ovary of a girl (Figs. 16–1 and 16–2) and that of a fetus. In spite of this, the belief that the ovary does not "get going" until after the age of 13, in conjunction with the ostensible phenomena of puberty, is erroneous. On the contrary, reliable observations from autopsies, as well as modern endocrinologic studies, have shown a certain degree of latent ovarian activity before the age of 10, beginning at about 8 or 9 years of age. Cordier and his colleagues,[15] and subsequently Dubreuil and Rivière,[17] have found that the ovaries in girls older than nine years revealed evidence of incipient follicular maturation. At the same time, there was evidence that the uterus and the Fal-

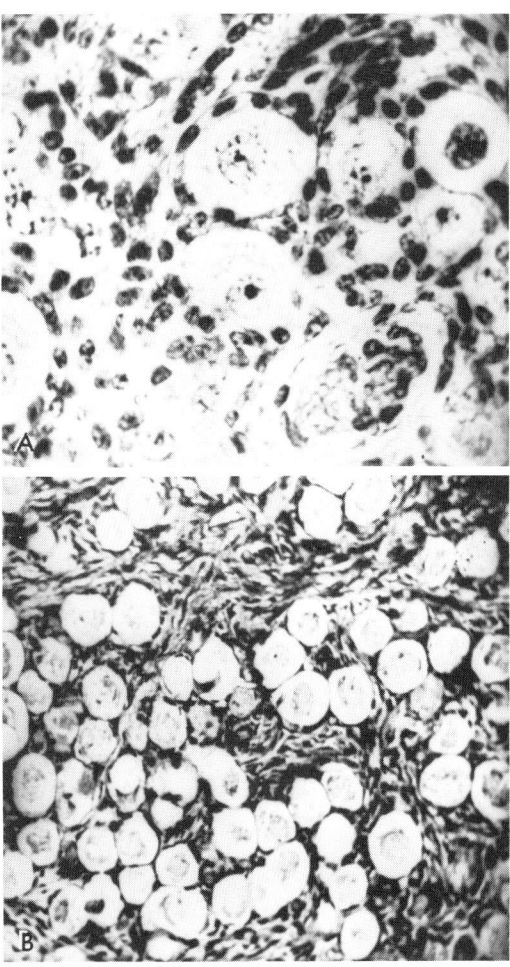

Figure 16–1. A, Section of ovary of a five and a half month female fetus, showing oogonia and differentiated mesenchymal cells (500×). B, Section of ovary from newborn female infant. Note vast number of oogonia (120×).

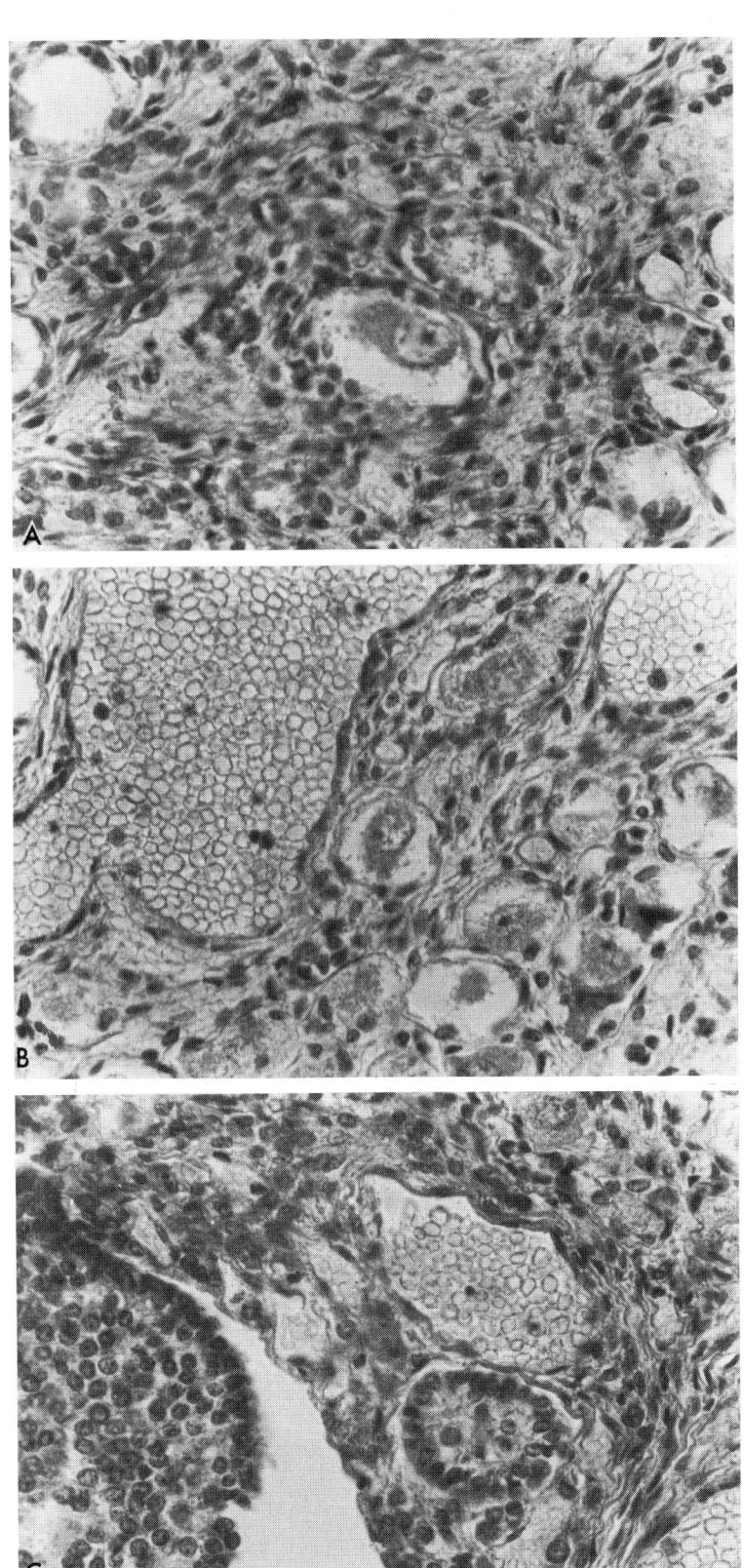

Figure 16-2. Ovarian histology in a five-year-old girl. *A*, Cortical zone of ovary, revealing presence of primordial follicles, one with conspicuous oogonium. Other follicles show incipient development of granulosa, with disappearance of oogonia (premature atresia). *B*, Abundance of oogonia in ovarian midzone, in vicinity of large dilated vessel. *C*, Proliferation of germ cells together with pseudogranulosa elements and absence of oogonia in hilar region of ovary, adjacent to cortical zone.

lopian tubes were similarly undergoing development. As shown by Jayle,[43] urinary estrogen excretion during this phase of life is first minimally, then unequivocally, increased. Nathanson and co-workers[62] demonstrated that the increase in urinary estrogens already occurred between the ages of 10 and 11 — in general, two to three years before the appearance of the first signs of puberty. Similarly, Koch[49] found that urinary androgens (as determined by bioassay) in males began rising from the age of 11 onwards, and Talbot and his colleagues[90] reported an increase in urinary 17-ketosteroids in 10 to 11 year old girls, from levels of 1.2 mg per 24 hours to 3.7 mg per 24 hours. Thus, gonadal activity, and possibly adrenal activity, would seem to be considerably enhanced before the onset of puberty. By means of estimating estrogenic activity in the vagina, these results have been confirmed by Pundel,[67] who observed that the complete absence of karyopyknotic cells, characteristic of the infantile vagina, gradually gave way to the appearance of partly cornified and karyopyknotic cells beginning with the age of 9 or 10, although complete transformation of the vagina, indicative of full ovarian secretion, was not observed until the age of 15. As a result, it must be concluded that the ovary experiences a slow awakening even before puberty and that, contrary to common belief, the transition from infancy to sexual maturity is not abrupt but rather slow, commensurate with a gradually swelling tide of ovarian hormonal function. For practical purposes, however, the human ovary is inactive until puberty. On the other hand, in some animals — for instance the giraffe (Amoroso,[1] Kellas and co-workers[46]) — the fetal ovary displays marked activity, with mature follicles and corpora lutea, which regresses in infancy. This may be viewed as an instance of true "fetal puberty" which is followed by postnatal ovarian regression, in a way similar in origin to postnatal regression of the adrenal cortex.

ONSET OF PUBERTY: THE OVARY. With the beginning of puberty, the ovaries increase in volume, particularly between the ages of 12 and 15. The process of ovarian maturation starts with the simultaneous growth of several follicles. For this reason, the ovary of a prepuberal girl acquires the gross appearance of a polymicrocystic ovary (Fig. 16–4). For a period of time, the maturing follicles compete in growth and seem to hold each other back from attaining full maturation until one of them gains the "upper hand" and soon thereafter is converted to a mature graafian follicle, ready to rupture. Because menarche has been shown not to occur during the phase of progressive follicular growth, the first menstruation is often delayed in girls with polymicrocystic ovaries, whose follicles are about 1 cm in diameter.[50, 59, 63, 95] *The*

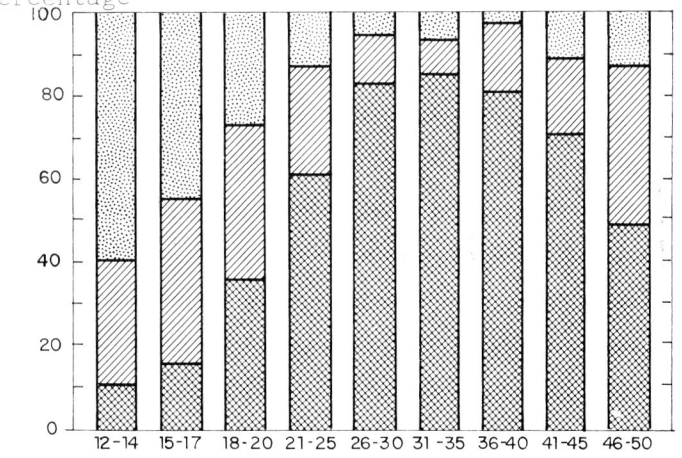

Figure 16–3. Diagram showing incidence of anovulatory, hypoluteal and normal cycles among different age groups, based on basal body temperature curves for 3264 cycles among 481 women. (From U.N. World Health Organization: *Biology of Birth Control by Periodic Continence*, Geneva, 1967.)

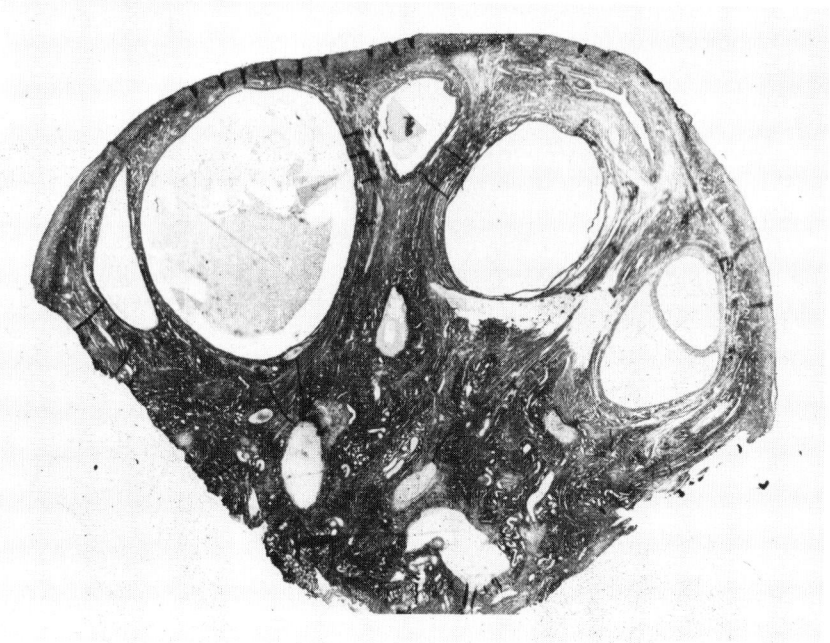

Figure 16-4. Juvenile type of polymicrocystic ovary in a girl, age 18.

onset of menarche is concurrent with the first signs of follicular atresia or regression. This can be explained by what is known about the mechanism of menstruation (Chapter 13). The menstrual flow has been shown to result from *hormonal deprivation*, either involving only estrogens, in which case menstruation is anovulatory, or involving both estrogens and progesterone, in which case there is normal menstruation. Ovarian follicular regression is therefore a necessary requirement for menstruation to occur. No corpora lutea can be observed in ovaries of impuberal girls. During the pubertal phase, only mature follicles but no corpora lutea were found to be present in the ovaries of humans by Breipohl,[12] Mickulicz-Radecky and Kausch,[58] Effkeman[18] and Eckstein,[19] and those of females of *Pithecus rhesus* monkeys (Hartman[36]). The follicles described by the foregoing investigators were functionally normal in appearance, with both granulosa and theca layers apparently fully developed. The oocytes they contained were apparently normal morphologically, although some writers[59] expressed doubts concerning their ability to develop fully. In short, the pubescent ovary develops a follicular thecal apparatus but is not yet capable of developing the corresponding luteal apparatus. Ovulation and well developed corpora lutea first occur only during the phase of nubility. Quoting Fluhmann,[26] *the pubertal female is "physiologically sterile."*

One of the essential features of the pubertal ovary is *dysrhythmia*, causing follicular maturation and atresia to go on in a manner that is at times sporadic, at times tumultuous, rather than at regular, evenly spaced monthly intervals. This is why, as shall be pointed out again, the first menses are often quite irregular.

FALLOPIAN TUBES AND UTERUS. The Fallopian tubes undergo a process of growth and development similar and parallel to that of the ovaries. At puberty, the tubes begin to show contractile properties they had heretofore lacked. The uterus undergoes a marked increase in bulk. According to data supplied by Tisserand,[92] the uterus of a 10 year old girl weighs approximately 28 gm, whereas at the age of 13, the average weight of the uterus is 50 gm. Thus, its weight has nearly doubled in three years. Anatomic studies[35, 88] have shown that the uterine lining at this stage also proliferates and is transformed into a mucosa quite similar to that of the adult uterus.

Puberty

The studies concerning the question of hormonal influences in uterine growth have been resumed over the past years (Hisaw et al.,[40] Velardo,[93] Lerner et al.[52]). The principal growth-promoting agent seems to be estradiol, but other steroid compounds, such as progesterone, corticosterone and related compounds in this group, are essential in supplementing the effects of estrogens on uterine development. This explains why the uterus of animals and humans alike at puberty grows only slightly during the first phase (estrogenic phase) but develops at a much faster pace once the estrogens derived from net ovarian maturation start acting in unison with progesterone and corticoids. Consequently, normal ponderal development of the uterus, and probably that of the Fallopian tubes and vagina as well, depends not only on ovarian estrogen synthesis *but on ovarian luteinization and on adrenocortical maturation.*

This is important because ovarian estrogen synthesis, as mentioned previously, starts at a very early stage of prepubertal development without inducing active, frank development of the uterus.

VAGINAL CHANGES. The morphologic changes involving the internal genitalia at puberty are poorly known, owing to the paucity of surgical and autopsy material available from this age group. In comparison, the accessibility of the vagina has made a thorough study of the puberal changes in this organ possible. The vagina of girls has been studied by Hamblen,[35] Rakoff and colleagues,[69] Pundel[67] and Shorr[81] from cytologic and histologic points of view. Histologically, the impuberal vagina is characterized by a markedly flattened epithelium, composed exclusively of a basal cell layer and a thin discontinuous layer of intermediate cells. At puberty, the basal layer proliferates conspicuously and assumes a papillary configuration owing to the development of a thick intermediate layer and, especially, to the appearance of a superficial layer, separated from the intermediate layer by a transitional layer, or zone of Dierks. These new developments are also reflected by changes in vaginal exfoliative cytology. In the prepuberal phase, the predominant cells in the microscopic field are intermediate and basal cells, as well as leukocytes, whereas after the onset of puberty there appear numerous karyopyknotic and acidophilic cells, reflecting an ever increasing estrogen effect. Consequently, there is a parallel between vaginal epithelial proliferation, as evident in vaginal cytology, and the degree of ovarian maturation.

EXTERNAL GENITALIA AND BREAST. In infancy, as well as during the prepuberal phase, the vulva faces forward and is denuded. As a result of the remarkable changes occurring with puberty, the *vulva* becomes covered and, instead of facing forward, faces downward. The labia majora

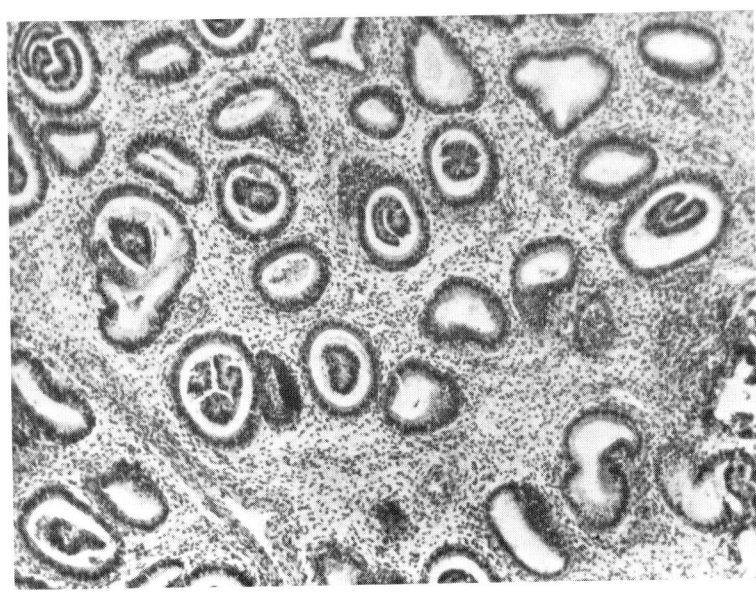

Figure 16–5. Proliferative endometrium obtained by biopsy on the twenty-sixth day of the cycle (same case as in Figure 16–4).

and minora develop and close the introitus. At the same time, the clitoris and the erectile system develops and so do the Bartholin glands. Finally, the mons pubis as well as the external aspect of the labia majora become covered with hair.

The *breasts* develop almost completely, although histologically such development takes place predominantly *in the lactiferous ducts*. There is scanty participation of mammary acini, which are unable to secrete colostrum. Thus, the histology of the puberal breast is the expression of the breast's responding exclusively to estrogenic stimuli, to the exclusion of luteinic stimuli.

MECHANISM OF MENARCHE. Menstrual bleeding occurs at about the age of 13. Significantly, menstrual activity as a rule is not rhythmic immediately after the first bleeding episode but usually consists first of a more or less extended phase of amenorrhea, followed by a phase during which menstrual periods are discontinuous or appear in a highly haphazard manner. Thus, though the menstrual nature of the bleeding is established with the first bleeding episode, the corresponding menstrual rhythm develops little by little. The slow pace at which the menstrual rhythm is acquired results from the fact that ovarian maturation is similarly sluggish. As has been pointed out previously, the ovaries of this phase of life often reveal persistence of mature follicles for more or less protracted periods of time, or growth arrest, at a similar stage of development, of a good many follicles in what grossly appear to be polymicrocystic ovaries. This leads to occasionally quite long phases of elevated and continuous estrogen production, without any sudden drops to produce hormonal deprivation. Since menstrual bleeding is known to occur as a result of sudden hormone withdrawal, it is only natural that *lack of ovarian rhythmicity should be associated with irregularities in menstruation*.

Consequently, the so-called *anovulatory cycle* of puberty is a physiologic development (Figs. 16-2, 16-3 and 16-4). *Follicular persistence* is an equally common, if not physiological, finding in puberty. In the minds of some authors, both findings bear out the existence of a *pubertal* variety of *hyperestrinism* (see Chapter 29). Although, in our opinion, puberal hyperestrinism cannot, at least in a quantitative sense, be asserted to occur, it can nevertheless be admitted to constitute an entity insofar as rhythm alone is concerned. While under normal conditions manifestations of *hyperfolliculinism* do not occur in puberal girls, this phenomenon is particularly prone to develop in this phase of life as the underlying cause of what we shall later describe as pathologic disturbances of puberty, with special reference to so-called *juvenile metropathy* (see Chapter 37).

The mechanism involved in menstruation at puberty is that of anovulatory menstruation. Pubertal menstrual irregularities result from associated irregularities in the maturation pattern of the ovarian follicular system.

16.2.2. SYSTEMIC CHANGES AT PUBERTY

CHANGES IN STATURE. As confirmed by the statistical observations of Greulich[32] and Bayer,[5] puberal changes in stature *occur mainly during the prepubertal phase*. Growth continues during the pubertal phase, so that *prepubertal* somatic growth must be distinguished from *pubertal* somatic growth, the two having different characteristics. The first form of growth is mainly longitudinal, involving the limbs, arms and legs, whereas pubertal growth *primarily involves the trunk. While growth of the long bones of the extremities is nonspecific in character, pubertal statural growth, by increasing the size of the trunk, involves a secondary sex character*. Thus, whereas the distal end of the ulna in an 11 year old girl reaches the upper third of the thigh, in a 15 year old girl this point of the wrist barely reaches the greater trochanter. The S-B index, that is, length of lower extremity divided by length of trunk, decreases progressively between the age of 9 and 16.

MUSCULAR AND PONDERAL GROWTH. Skeletal growth is followed by *muscular growth*, which in the female is less important than in the male but, unlike the case in males, is supplemented by the development of a subcutaneous fat panniculus that is mainly responsible for changing the habitus of a girl to that of an adult woman. Histologically, the prepubertal muscle is rich in sarcoplasm but poor in fibrils.

Beginning with puberty, the fibrillary structure grows and the potency and efficiency of the muscular system undergoes significant development.

Fat becomes deposited in the subcutaneous tissue, leading to roundness in shape that is distinctive of the feminine type, which must also be considered a sex character. Deposits of adipose tissue affect certain parts of the body, mainly the hips, buttocks, abdomen and shoulders, imparting the characteristic female habitus. At the same time, skeletal development produces fundamental effects on the pelvic girdle, resulting in an increase of the bispinous and bitrochanteric diameters, so that these exceed the same diameters in males.

As a result of statural growth, muscular growth and growth of adipose tissue during puberty, the overall weight increases considerably. The weight-stature quotient rises from 1.62 at 6 years of age, to 1.90 at 9, 2.39 at 12, and 3.16 at 17 years of age. Thus, the body evidently grows not only in stature but also in transverse diameter, gaining in girth and at the same time acquiring the typical female morphology.

CHANGES IN THE SKIN AND IN THE PILAR SYSTEM. Concomitant with external sexual differentiation at puberty, a number of interesting modifications are noted to involve the integument and hair. A woman's hair grows in length, assuming a characteristic pattern of development over the scalp, where it grows at a faster rate than does the hair in the male. Over the mons pubis, it develops in a triangular fashion characteristic of woman. The distribution of early pubic hair growth is different in each sex. In the female, hair growth begins along the free borders of the labia majora and stops at the level of the upper border of the pubis, forming a horizontal line. As a result, hair growth over a girl's mons pubis assumes the shape of an isosceles triangle with a superior base. In the male, in contrast, hair growth does not stop at this point but extends along the linea alba up to the vicinity of the umbilicus, the area involved assuming a diamond shape with an acute infraumbilical vertex. The axillary hair of both male and female makes its appearance in a similar way, without showing any distinctive disposition in either sex. However, inhibition of hair growth over some regions is characteristic of femininity. Not only is there no development of hair on the upper lip, the masseteric region and the chin, but in addition even the light downy growth, usually observed over those regions in infancy, tends to disappear completely. Interesting in girls, too, is the disappearance of body hair over the limbs. Whether male or female, a child usually has a soft lanugo covering forearms and calves. At the time of puberty, this growth undergoes active development in the male to make up the future normal body hair over a man's limbs. In woman, the same regions become progressively hairless, and so do the regions of the chin and the upper lip. *Not only is there a specifically female form of hair development over some regions of the body, but there is also a specifically female lack of hair development over others.*

The female skin becomes progressively smoother and softer over most of the body. Over the breasts, the skin begins to develop its periareolar pigmentation and the characteristic appearance of the nipple of adult woman. Sebaceous gland excretion increases at the time of puberty and, finally, woman's skin becomes less dry and her hair softer than that of a child.

CHANGES IN OTHER ORGANS AND SYSTEMS. *The circulatory system* undergoes a steady process of growth, without any abrupt acceleration during puberty. This is a part of the uniform growth process begun in infancy and continuing into adult life. The pulse becomes less frequent and arterial pressure rises slightly from the prepubertal phase to the pubertal phase.

Quite interesting changes can be observed in the *respiratory tract*. The changes involving the larynx also have a specific character. These were recently studied by Greene[31] who found that the high pitch of a woman's voice is due to a less developed larynx. Apart from remaining smaller than that of the male, the female larynx has a different configuration, which allows not only emission of higher tones but also facilitates special modulation of such tones.

Although increase in thoracic capacity and pulmonary development at this stage is primarily a male trait, women also display an increase in thoracic size and in capacity of pulmonary ventilation.

Whether the *blood* undergoes any changes during female puberty has been a matter of conjecture. Serial observations have indeed shown that a minor decrease in the number of red blood cells takes place.

From a statistical viewpoint, this is a significant decrease, since the lesser number of red blood cells in females, as compared to males, persists throughout woman's life.

A tendency to *cyclic changes in body temperature* is observed beginning with the postpubertal phase. These become more noticeable at the time of nubility when typical elevations of basal body temperature occur during the second half of the cycle, which have been described in Chapter 13 (Fig. 16-6).

Changes involving the digestive tract, the liver and metabolism have also been described, but these are largely the result of nonspecific effects attributable to increased body stature.

16.2.3. PSYCHIC CHANGES OF PUBERTY

To engage in an assay of psychological changes in female puberty is beyond the scope of this book. In the female, as well as in the male, puberty is associated with the *development of intelligence, character and personality*. These three psychological parameters do not, of course, come into existence for the first time at puberty, but were already established in infancy as a result of two kinds of factors: hereditary, or atavistic, factors, and educational as well as familial factors. The psychological propensities of a child are occult but develop rapidly in the years preceding and following puberty. Since the era of Freud, this *acceleration of psychokinetics at the time of puberty* has been attributed to the influence of sexuality. Although by no means derogating whatever part sexuality may play in the development of such psychic phenomena, we believe it to be of quite secondary importance. It would seem to us that the great spurt in psychological development between the ages of 12 and 18 is the result of exogenous factors which are alien to the sexual sphere. These include the following: (1) An increase in, and progressive maturation of, intelligence, taking place in an autochthonous and constant manner; (2) an educational effort, which in our type of society is at a maximum at this stage of life; (3) the very consciousness of sexuality, whether or not associated with imagination, which is acquired through conversations with, or comments on the part of, persons of the same age. In this way, the *development of the female temperament is guided by the external environment rather than by woman's bodily changes*. It is a fairly frequent observation that *somatic sexual precociousness is seldom or never associated with, or is even*

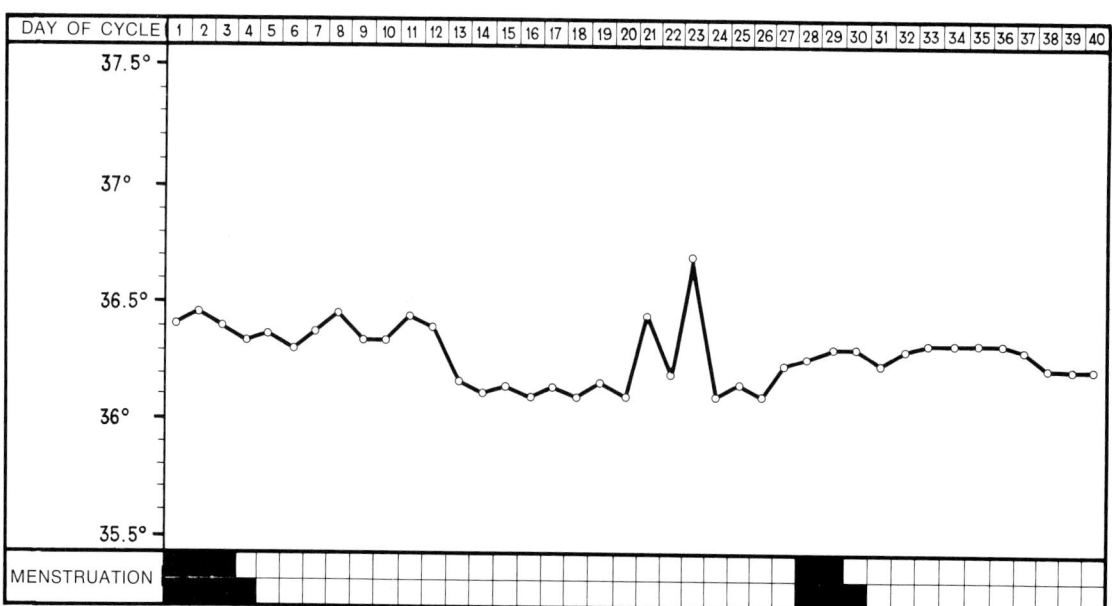

Figure 16-6. Basal body temperature curve, corresponding to case shown in Figures 16-4 and 16-5.

diametrically opposed to, psychic precociousness. Girls that are markedly retarded in terms of sexual and endocrine development are prematurely sex conscious, whereas, on the contrary, somatically and sexually well developed girls tend to remain in a state of great ignorance and indifference concerning the very process of their puberty. There is invariably an endocrine factor in such problems, since there are psychological differences between male and female. However, as we have been able to infer from our observations of intersexual states (see Chapter 36), development of both male and female psychology is linked to the type of male or female oriented education an individual receives rather than to the nature of the gonad involved. *We therefore insist that the psychological features described as characteristic of femininity at puberty are, to a minor degree, endocrine, but in a large measure are exogenous in nature.*

16.3. ENDOCRINOLOGY OF PUBERTY

During puberty, in addition to gonadal maturation, we observe an overall change in endocrine correlations. On the one hand, the sexual glands enter their phase of activity. On the other, the physiology of functionally related glands undergoes modifications, and, finally, such inhibitory factors as those originating in the pineal and in the thymus are abolished as a result of decisive atrophy of these two glands. We shall therefore study successively the changes occurring during puberty in the ovaries, pituitary, adrenals, thymus and pineal, and finally discussing the influence that the nervous system exerts on endocrine regulation during this phase of life.

16.3.1. OVARIAN FUNCTION DURING PUBERTY

Some of the morphologic changes taking place in the ovary before and during puberty have already been mentioned. Progressive maturation of ovarian follicles at this time results in increased hormone production. The hormone increased first is estrogen; only later does progesterone appear on the endocrine scene. In 1939, Gallagher and co-workers[29] became aware of increased urinary estrogen excretion during puberty. Daily amounts of up to 200 mcg of estrogenic hormone were found in the urine of pubescent girls. Such amounts are approximately equal to those found in adult women and are 10 to 20 times greater than those found during the prepubertal phase. Based on similar observations, Glass and Bergman[30] later gave figures of 300 mcg of hormone excreted per day during puberty. These figures, even though comprising total estrogens, are considerably elevated and support the previously made assumption concerning the occurrence of a transient form of hyperestrinism at puberty. The pubertal tendency to elevated estrogens, occasionally beyond normal limits, has also been confirmed by Nathanson and co-workers.[62] Pundel[67] similarly reported the occurrence of a very abrupt increase in the number of estrogenic cells in the Papanicolaou test, which speaks in favor of a rather sudden elevation of estrogenic activity. The vaginal karyopyknotic index of puberal girls tends to be higher than that of many adult women, which likewise may be construed as indicating the presence of hyperestrinism, however mild in degree. On the other hand, Dorfman and his colleagues[16] failed to find any evidence of estrogens having been increased above normal levels during puberty, reporting slowly and progressively rising values between the ages of 10 and 16, without exceeding the norm.

The fundamental triggering role of estrogens is proved by the fact that precocious puberty occurs with the infantile type of polymicrocystic ovaries,[87] as well as in cases with granulosa cell tumor.[64] These aspects of puberal pathology shall be covered in Chapter 38.

Pregnanediol excretion was studied by Hamblen,[35] who reported that this catabolite was absent from pubertal urine up to the age of 17 or 18. These data are in full agreement with our own observations. We never encountered folded vaginal cells, which would indicate luteal activity, until sexual maturity was well advanced. This, too, is in favor of what we have indicated previously—namely, that acquisition of corpora lutea is a late event.

Puberty then is characterized by *maturation of the follicular portion of the ovary, without maturation of the luteal portion, the latter taking place at a later date.*

Such folliculinic ovaries produce a continuous estrogen output, one that, rather than consisting in an increased amount of estrogens, results in sustained estrogenic activity. In conjunction with the absence of any periodic rhythm during the initial stages of puberty, this steady type of estrogen production often gives rise to conditions of follicular persistence with rhythmic hyperestrinism which have been mistaken for conditions of follicular hyperfunction by many authors. The ovary at puberty may thus be characterized by the presence of a state of irregular maturation, with persistence of follicles and with an anovulatory cycle and, as as a consequence, with accumulation of estrogens in time and absence of corpus luteum hormone.

16.3.2. PITUITARY

If the changes that are observed in the maturation process of the genital apparatus, such as growth of the uterus, proliferation of the vagina, development of the breasts and development of external sex characters, are to be ascribed to the beginning of ovarian estrogen synthesis, then the natural question that must be raised is why ovarian estrogen synthesis is turned on so suddenly at puberty as an active regulator of sexual processes. *The cause may be assumed to lie in the pituitary.* It has been known for many years that destruction of the pituitary in prepubertal animals was followed by failure of sexual development. In 1926, Zondek[102] injected prepubertal mice with anterior pituitary lobe extracts and observed that the animals became sexually mature. The pituitary has ever since been designated the *gland of puberty*. In the first edition of this book, we stated that by means of its somatotropic secretion, the pituitary governed growth of the soma during the entire period of infancy and that, with the arrival of puberty, pituitary secretion changed in type, because the pituitary ceased to secrete somatotropin and started secreting gonadotropin. The changed nature of pituitary secretion causes arrest of the somatic development begun at the beginning of puberty, and in turn produces progressive sexual maturation. According to Seitz,[80] the antagonism between somatic growth and sexual development, an essential characteristic of puberty, is an illustrative example of the *struggle between soma and germ cell*, witnessed in the developmental process of all species. The soma, representative of the individual, is thus seen to "oppose" the germ cell, representative of the species. Growth of the soma leads to attainment of the organism's specific shape (see Chapter 1) and, once the latter is attained, reproduction becomes necessary lest growth of living matter extend beyond the size and shape that are specific for the species. *Reproduction, we have pointed out previously, is therefore a mere extension of the growth process, and thus puberty represents the process whereby somatic growth is translated into reproductive growth, that is to say, into growth of the species.* Consequently, the *primum movens* of puberty is a change in pituitary activity.

Early investigations by Neumann and Peter,[63] and those by Katzman and Doisy,[45] had indicated that there was a relationship between gonadotropins and pubertal maturation. In recent years, Arslan and his colleagues,[3] as well as Beltermann and Stegner,[6] were able to induce precocious puberty in animals by injecting them with gonadotropins.

In the human species, too, there seems to be a relationship between adenohypophysial secretion and puberty. Thus, gonadotropin concentrations in 24 hour urine specimens of prepubertal girls were found to vary from 3 to 10 mouse units, whereas after the onset of puberty the figure rose to between 50 and 100 units. Those results were confirmed by von Haam[34] and by Catchpole and Greulich.[13] Using various bioassay procedures, Freed,[28] Kammlade and co-workers[44] and Ramirez and McCann[71] all demonstrated a considerable prepubertal increase in gonadotropin levels. These classic data have recently been amplified by radioimmunoassay studies. Kulin and co-workers[51] have shown that gonadotropin levels begin to rise slowly as much as several years before menarche. Radioimmunoassay studies on FSH were performed by Raiti and co-workers,[68] Rifkind and co-workers[76] and Yen and Vicic.[99] The last two investigators found that FSH excretion values in school-age boys and girls increased five- to tenfold with the beginning of puberty, with the recorded values exceeding adult rates of gonadotropin excretion by a significant margin. Not only were follicle-stimulating hormone values elevated but, what at the outset appeared even more striking, so were LH excretion values. Grunewald and Heugel,[33] Rifkind and co-workers[76] and Yen and associates[98] performed radioimmunoassay studies on LH, finding similarly a five- to tenfold increase in excretion values coincident with the onset of puberty. Also of great interest are the results obtained by Witschi and Riley,[96] who demonstrated that hormonal extracts from puberal girls' pituitaries showed not only increased amounts of gonadotropin secretion but also a marked increase of thyrotropin secretion, which was recently confirmed by Singh and co-workers.[84] Hence it may be concluded that, in addition to the gonads, the thyroid is also stimulated during female puberty.

16.3.3. THYROID

The role of the thyroid in puberty is a particularly interesting one. According to Marañón,[54,55] the thyroid acts as a feminizing gland, being involved in stimulating the unfolding of female puberty. As early as 1921, increased thyroid activity at puberty was suspected by Benedict and Talbot,[7] who had found that basal metabolic rates were elevated in puberal girls. Marañón[54] and Seitz,[80] as well as Eufinger,[22] called attention to the occurrence of "pubertal goiters" which, though transient, were nonetheless quite apparent in many girls. Studying iodine blood levels and basal metabolic rates before, during and after puberty, King and Hamilton[48] also arrived at the conclusion that thyroid function was enhanced during this phase of woman's sexual life. Clegett and Hathaway[14] stressed the common finding of increased caloric output, slight tachycardia and increased psychic and neuromuscular excitability in puberal girls and likewise concluded that these resulted from thyroid hyperfunction. Similarly, Fashena[23] later studied iodine blood levels during puberty and described the occurrence of puberal hyperiodinemia. More recently, following an in depth review of the pathognomonic significance of PBI (protein-bound iodine) levels during the various phases of female sexual life, Fisher[24] drew attention to the fact that increased values of this iodemic fraction during puberty reflected *pubertal hyperthyroidism.*

Regarding the significance of this kind of thyroid reaction at puberty, some authors believe that it might be a manifestation secondary to the pituitary and the ovarian reactions. As has been pointed out in Chapter 10, estrogens stimulate thyroid function, a fact which alone could account for thyroid hyperfunctional activity. We have also previously mentioned the fact that thyrotropic hormone is present in increased amounts in the pubertal pituitary, so that thyroid hyperfunction may have no physiologic significance. However, in accordance with our own recently formulated ideas, we would view the thyroid instead as playing a significant role in the development of female puberty. The thyroid may be considered as an accessary gland of sexuality, whose feminizing character had been repeatedly emphasized by Marañón. Thyroid hormone seems to be indispensable for the development of the ovarian follicular apparatus (Chapter 10), as well as for the development of corpora lutea. It would appear that follicular maturation at puberty requires not only the gonadotropic impulse to stimulate massive development of the ovarian follicular system but possibly the trophic activity of the thyroid as well. This point of view is supported by the investigations of Siegmund,[82] who found that gonadotropins alone were not enough to produce ovarian maturation in thyroidectomized animals and that it was necessary to inject a mixture of thyroid extracts and gonadotropins to obtain follicular maturation and to induce experimental puberty in laboratory rodents. Subsequently, Fränkel and his colleagues[27] have also shown beyond doubt that, in order to produce precocious puberty in experimental animals by means of gonadotropin injections, it was necessary to supplement the injections with thyroid hormone.

16.3.4. ADRENALS

At puberty, the adrenal cortex also experiences a period of growth. As mentioned earlier, our own investigations,[11] and principally those of Rotter,[77] have revealed the occurrence of postnatal atrophy of the adrenal cortex. This type of atrophy (see Chapter 9) occurs mainly at the expense of the sexual zone, which regresses and disappears. In the infant, as a result, the adrenal consists essentially of the zona glomerulosa and zona fasciculata, the two layers that are to gain predominance for the entire period of infancy. Adrenal weight increases at puberty. This has been shown by, among others, Scammon and his colleagues[78] and Benner.[8] Studies by Riddle,[75] conducted on pigeons and other birds, have shown that the beginning of sexual maturity in these species is associated with striking adrenal enlargement. These observations were confirmed in mice by Swingle and Pfiffner[89] by means of planimetric studies. Data obtained at autopsy demonstrated that the zona fasciculata and zona reticularis of human adrenals both widen at puberty.[11, 77] Thus, the adrenals of both animals and man have been shown to grow in size during puberty.

The presence of pubertal adrenal hyperfunction, suggested by the anatomic findings, appears to be substantiated by the pattern of 17-ketosteroid and 11-oxysteroid excretion. Koch[49] had demonstrated the presence of androgens in the urine of pubertal girls. As pointed out previously, female androgens are known to be derived largely from the adrenals, so that a hyperfunctional state of that gland can be taken for granted. Similarly, the observations reported by Talbot and colleagues[90, 91] seem to have demonstrated the presence of increased 17-ketosteroid excretion during the prepubertal and pubertal phases; those observations have been confirmed by Baumann and Metzger.[4] According to data supplied by Metzger, urinary 17-ketosteroid levels during female puberty may reach 11 mg per 24 hours, values which are well above those occurring during infancy or during later years of life. Visser and Degenhart[94] found that premature development of axillary and pubic hair in young girls was always associated with a sudden elevation of 17-ketosteroid excretion. Studies in young females[94] have revealed a moderate rise in 11-oxysteroid excretion values, reaching figures slightly above those found in infancy or during the later phase of sexual maturity. Consequently, these findings also seem to lend support to the idea that, during puberty, at least in a transient way, *the adrenal experiences an increase in function and structural complexity.*

In birds, pubertal adrenal hypertrophy is a factor that determines sexual maturity.[75] In the human species, the adrenal cortex seems to be responsible for the process of pubic and axillary hair growth at puberty.[11, 92, 94]

16.3.5. FACTORS INHIBITING PUBERTY

The extraordinary importance of the *pineal* and of the *thymus* as inhibitors of puberty and antagonists of sexuality has been indicated in Chapter 10. Present-day knowledge concerning the physiology of these two glands is highly unreliable and is based mainly on empirical and clinical observations (Fig. 16–7). The pathology of puberty, including the description of such conditions as precocious puberty, resulting from destructive processes involving the pineal, and delayed puberty, resulting from the persistence of the thymus, shall be discussed in Chapter 37.

PINEAL. The antagonistic action of the pineal on puberty was reported in the early literature.[20, 25, 101] A form of "pineal precocious puberty," resulting from destruction of that gland by neoplasia or other pathologic processes (Heubner[39]), shall be mentioned in Chapter 38. In Chapter 10

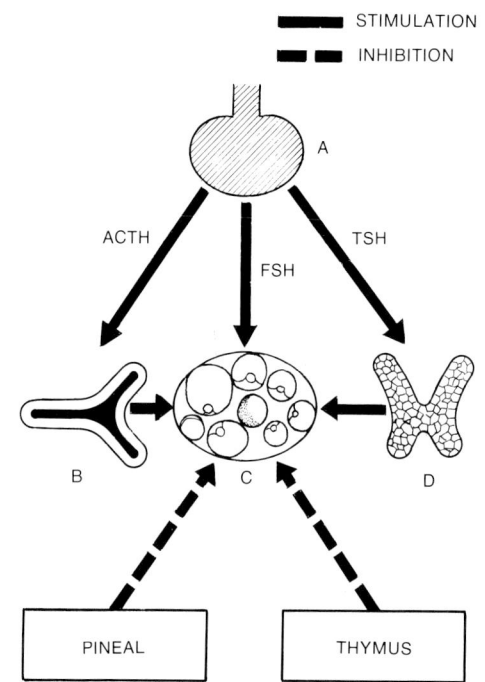

Figure 16–7. Diagram of pubertal endocrinology. *A,* Pituitary; *B,* adrenal; *C,* ovary; *D,* thyroid.

(Section 10.5.2), some new ideas were developed concerning the possible significance of the pineal incretion, *melatonin*, which is thought to act on the sex nucleus of the median eminence by blocking its function.

It is a well documented fact that pineal activity not only blocks the onset of puberty but also suppresses the hypothalamus during the prepuberal phase. The pineal is also known to be the agent which, in certain animals, determines the relationship between puberty and environmental lighting (see Section 16.3.7).

THYMUS. As a result of ancient observations, the thymus was ascribed the role of delaying sexual maturity. Persistence of the thymus does delay onset of puberty (see Chapter 38), and thymic extracts inhibit sexual maturation in experimental animals.[1] The physiology of the thymus is covered in Chapter 10.

MALNUTRITION. Another factor that inhibits puberty is *malnutrition*. It is well known that starvation in infancy and during the prepubertal phase results in human pituitary insufficiency, causing delayed sexual maturation and late onset of puberty, occasionally leading to sterility.

Kennedy and Mitra[47] studied the effects of malnutrition on sexual maturation in rats and found that rats receiving diets deficient in amino acids, niacin and biotin remained impuberal until their diet was enriched.

16.3.6. HYPOTHALAMIC INFLUENCE ON THE ONSET OF PUBERTY

Puberty is initiated by the release of adenohypophysial gonadotropins. However, it is well known today (see Chapter 8, Section 8.3) that the stimulus for the liberation of these hormones originates in the sex nuclei of the median eminence of the tuber cinereum. Neoplasms that destroy the mamillary bodies delay the onset of puberty,[21, 73] whereas electric stimulation of that zone[73] in experimental animals produces premature sexual maturation. Liu and co-workers[53] have demonstrated the presence of characteristic electroencephalographic alterations in precocious puberty. On the other hand, it is a well known fact that purely hypothalamic alterations, without associated endocrine dysfunction of any sort, can also produce precocious puberty. Administration of reserpine delays puberty in rats if the hypothalamic region is anesthetized.

It should be mentioned, finally, that Smith and Davidson,[86] as well as Motta and co-workers,[61] have shown that estrogen insertion into the median eminence of the rat provoked precocious puberty and vaginal patency.

The sexual center remains inactive before puberty owing to inhibition of other hypothalamic areas and probably of the pineal, as has been proven by Ramley and Gorski,[70] who, by severing all connections of the median eminence, have been able to induce precocious puberty in rats. *There is no reason why puberty, which marks the beginning of the sexual rhythm, may not equally be assumed to be under hypothalamic control. As regards puberty, the hypothalamus "sounds the alarm clock" for sexual awakening, serving, once more, as the timing device of bodily function.*

16.3.7. ILLUMINATION AND PUBERTY

The close relationship that exists between environmental lighting and the appearance of puberty in rodents has been found to be mediated by the pineal, as has been explained in Chapter 10 (Section 10.5.2). Wurtman and Axelrod[97] have demonstrated that luminous impulses reach the pineal through sympathetic fibers by way of the superior cervical ganglia. The pineal may be "blinded" by severing this pathway, and may thus be prevented from reacting to luminous stimuli.

Rats subjected to continuous illumination have been found to develop precocious puberty.[65, 73, 83] On the other hand, permanent darkness delays sexual awakening in these animals.[41] All the previously mentioned reactions may be abolished by extirpating the pineal.[37, 38, 74] While puberty fails to appear in blinded hamsters, removal of the pineal in such hamsters produces puberty.[60, 72] Bostelmann[9] studied the ultrastructure of pineals from animals subjected either to continuous illumination or to constant darkness, reporting absence of secretory granules in the former and abundance of such granules in the latter.

A similar phenomenon is believed to

occur in the human species, in view of the finding reported by Zacharias and Wurtman[100] that blindness since birth is associated in girls with *precocious puberty* (see Chapter 38, Section 38.3.5).

16.4. SUMMARY OF PUBERTY

First, puberty is neither a sudden event nor one occurring at a specific date in life, but rather a *slow process of transformation that continues imperceptibly from infancy and blends, also imperceptibly, into maturity*. It is a transition or evolution, if you wish, but by no means a change or a revolution. Sexual awakening does not consist in ovarian maturity alone but involves changes in all glands of internal secretion. The endocrine influences acting in puberty are represented schematically in Figure 16-7. *The ovary is stimulated and brought to maturity by the action of pituitary gonadotropic hormones*, which are the driving force behind sexual awakening, from which the pituitary justifiably deserves the name of "gland of puberty." However, gonadotropic function, in turn, is subject to hypothalamic stimulation; in close cooperation with the nervous system, the hypothalamus coordinates the task of shaping sexuality with the processes of maturation and evolution of the other functions of the body. The two pituitary gonadotropic hormones do not enter into action at the same time. FSH seems to govern exclusively the rhythm of ovarian maturation during the entire period of time extending from puberty to nubility, whereas LH activity marks the beginning of nubility and, consequently, the beginning of complete sexual maturity.

The thyroid plays an important role in the unfolding of puberty. The morphogenetic action of the thyroid is exerted on the ovary and is necessary for complete ovarian maturation. The feminizing tendency of thyroid activity is particularly apparent during puberty. *The adrenal cortex passes through a phase of transient hyperfunction at puberty*. Although the exact scope of this adrenal hyperfunctional state has not been fully determined, it is believed to play an important part in initiating the metabolism of the sex hormones, as is suggested at puberty in both males and females by the increased rate of adrenocortical hormone synthesis, that of ketosteroids as well as that of corticoids.

Both the pineal and the thymus act as inhibitors of puberty. Finally, although the role of the hypothalamus in sexual awakening is not altogether well known, there is no doubt that the influence of the hypothalamus as the coordinator of the biologic rhythm is a decisive one.

REFERENCES

1. Amoroso, E. C.: *Brit. Med. Bull.*, 11:117, 1955.
2. Ashley-Montagu, M. F.: *Human Fertil.*, 2:33, 1947.
3. Arslan, M., Wolf, R. C., Meyer, R. K., and Prasad, M. R. N.: *J. Reprod. Fertil.*, 17:119, 1968.
4. Bauman, E. J., and Metzger, N.: *Endocrinology*, 27:664, 1940.
5. Bayer, L. M.: *J. Pediat.*, 17:331, 1940.
6. Beltermann, R., and Stegner, H. E.: *Acta Endocr.*, 57:279, 1968.
7. Benedict, F. G., and Talbot, F. B.: *Carnegie Inst. of Wash.*, 302, 1921.
8. Benner, M. C.: *Amer. J. Path.*, 16:787, 1940.
9. Bostelmann, W.: *Endokrinologie*, 53:365, 1968.
10. Botella, J.: *Endocrinologia de la Mujer*, 1st ed. Madrid, Aguado, 1942.
11. Botella, J.: *Suprarrenales y Función Sexual. La tercera Gonada*. Madrid, Morata, 1946.
12. Breipohl, C.: *Zbl. Gynäk.*, 58:1998, 1935.
13. Catchpole, H. R., and Greulich, W. W.: *Amer. J. Physiol.*, 129:331, 1940.
14. Clegett, D. D., and Hathaway, M. L.: *Amer. J. Dis. Child.*, 62:967, 1941.
15. Cordier, P., Pevos, L., and Gineste, J. D.: *VIII Congr. Gynec. Langue Française*, Lille, France, May 27–30, 1939.
16. Dorfman, R. I., et al.: *Endocrinology*, 21:741, 1947.
17. Dubreuil, G., and Rivière, M.: *Ann. d'Endocr.*, 11:62, 1950.
18. Effkemann, G.: *Zbl. Gynäk.*, 63:154, 1937.
19. Eckstein, P.: *Old Age in Modern World*. Edinburgh, E. S. Livingstone, 1955.
20. Engel, P.: *Z. Exper. Med.*, 94:333, 1934.
21. Eronould, H. J., Thibaut, A., and Decamps, G.: *Ann. d'Endocr.*, 26:181, 1965.
22. Eufinger, H.: *Arch. Gynäk.*, 143:338, 1930.
23. Fashena, G. J.: *J. Clin. Invest.*, 17:179, 1938.
24. Fisher, J. J.: *Obstet. Gynec. Surv.*, 9:479, 1954.
25. Fleischmann, W., and Goldhammer, P.: *Klin. Wschr.*, 1:415, 1934.
26. Fluhmann, C. F.: *The Management of Sex Disorders*. Philadelphia, W. B. Saunders, 1956.
27. Frankel, R. K., Evans, H. M., and Simpson, J. P.: *Endocrinology*, 27:670, 1940.
28. Freed, S. C.: *J.A.M.A.*, 117:103, 1941.
29. Gallagher, T. F., et al.: *J. Clin. Invest.*, 16:695, 1937.
30. Glass, I. J., and Bergman, H. C.: *Endocrinology*, 23:625, 1938.
31. Greene, J. S.: *J.A.M.A.*, 120:1193, 1942.
32. Greulich, W. W.: *J. Pediat.*, 19:302, 1941.

33. Grunewald, C., and Heugel, M.: *Presse Med.*, 77:297, 1969.
34. Haam, G. von: *Amer. J. Clin. Path.*, 10:205, 1940.
35. Hamblen, E. C.: *Endocrinology of Women*. Springfield, Ill., Charles C Thomas, 1945.
36. Hartman, C. G.: *Contrib. Embryol.*, 134:1, 1932.
37. Herbert, J.: *J. Endocr.*, 43:625, 1969.
38. Herbert, J.: *J. Endocr.*, 41:20, 1968.
39. Heubner, R.: In *The Pineal Gland*, ed. J. I. Kitay and M. D. Altschule. Cambridge, Mass., Harvard University Press, 1954.
40. Hisaw, F. L., Velardo, J. T., and Goolsby, C. M.: *J. Clin. Endocr.*, 14:1134, 1954.
41. Hoffmann, J. C.: *Neuroendocrinology*, 2:1, 1967.
42. Hoseman, H.: *Ztschr. Geburtsh.*, 128:170, 1947.
43. Jayle, M. F.: *Conf. Congr. Jub. Gynecologie*. Paris, L'Expansion Scientifique Française, 1951.
44. Kammlade, W. G., Welch, J. A., Nalbandov, A. V., and Norton, H. W.: *J. Anim. Sci.*, 11:646, 1952.
45. Katzman, P. A., and Doisy, E. A.: *J. Biol. Chem.*, 106:125, 1934.
46. Kellas, L. M., Lenner, E. W. van and Amoroso, E. C.: *Nature*, 181:487, 1958.
47. Kennedy, G. C., and Mitra, J. M.: *J. Physiol.*, 166:408, 1963.
48. King, J. D., and Hamilton, F. E.: *West. J. Surg. Obstet. Gynec.*, 49:231, 1941.
49. Koch, F. C.: *Bull. N.Y. Acad. Med.*, 14:655, 1938.
50. Krohn, P. L.: *Schw. Med. Wschr.*, 87:417, 1957.
51. Kulin, H. E., Rifkind, A. B., Ross, G. T., and O'Dell, W. D.: *J. Clin. Endocr.*, 27:1123, 1967.
52. Lerner, J. F., Holthaus, J., and Thompson, C. R.: *Endocrinology*, 63:295, 1958.
53. Liu, N., Grumbach, M. M., Napoli, R. A., and Morishima, A.: *J. Clin. Endocr. Metab.*, 25:1296, 1965.
54. Marañon, G.: *Estudios de Fisiopatologia Sexual*. Barcelona, Marín, 1931.
55. Marañon, G.: *Med. Ibera*, 25:449, 1931.
56. Marañon, G.: *El Crecimiento y sus Trastornos*. Madrid, Espasa Calpe, 1953.
57. Marañon, G., Richet, C., and Rymer, M.: *Pathologie de l'hypophyse*. Paris, Balliere, 1948.
58. Mickulicz-Radecky, F. von and Kausch, G.: *Zbl. Gynäk.*, 59:2296, 1935.
59. Moricard, F.: *Hormonologie Sexuelle Humaine*. Paris, Masson et Cie., 1943.
60. Moszkowska, A., and Scemmama, A.: *Compt. Rend. Soc. Biol. (Paris)*, 162:636, 1968.
61. Motta, M., Fraschini, G., Giuliani, G., and Martini, L.: *Endocrinology*, 83:1101, 1968.
62. Nathanson, I. T., et al.: *Endocrinology*, 24:335, 1939.
63. Neumann, H. O., and Peter, E.: *Z. Kinderheilk.*, 52:24, 1932.
64. Niswander, K. R., and Courey, N. G.: *Obstet. Gynec.*, 26:381, 1965.
65. Piacseck, B. E., and Meites, J.: *Neuroendocrinology*, 2:129, 1967.
66. Ploss, H., and Bartels, M. P.: *Das Weib*. Berlin, Neufeld & Henius, 1927.
67. Pundel, P. P.: *Les Frottis Vaginaux et Cervicaux*. Liege, Masson & Desoer, 1950.
68. Raiti, S., Light, C., and Blizzard, R. M.: *J. Clin. Endocr.*, 29:884, 1969.
69. Rakoff, A. E., et al.: *Amer. J. Obstet. Gynec.*, 47:467, 1944.
70. Ramley, J. A., and Gorski, R. A.: *Acta Endocr.*, 56:661, 1967.
71. Ramirez, D. V., and McCann, S. M.: *Endocrinology*, 72:452, 1963.
72. Reiter, R. J.: *Neuroendocrinology*, 2:138, 1967.
73. Relkin, R.: *Endocrinology*, 82:865, 1968.
74. Relkin, R.: *Endocrinology*, 82:1249, 1968.
75. Riddle, O.: *Endocrinology*, 15:27, 1931.
76. Rifkind, A. B., Kulin, H. E., and Ross, G. T.: *J. Clin. Invest.*, 46:1925, 1967.
77. Rotter, W.: *Virchows. Arch.*, 316:190, 1949.
78. Scammon, R. E., et al.: *The Measurement of Man*. Minneapolis, Minnesota University Press, 1940.
79. Schreibner, H.: *Ztschr. Geburtsh.*, 116:37, 1937.
80. Seitz, L.: *Wachstum, Geschlecht und Fortpflanzung*. Berlin, J. Springer, 1939.
81. Shorr, E.: *J. Pediat.*, 19:327, 1941.
82. Siegmund, P.: *Arch. Gynäk.*, 142:702, 1930.
83. Singh, K. B., and Greenwald, G.: *J. Endocr.*, 38:389, 1967.
84. Singh, D. V., Narang, G. D., and Turner, C. W.: *J. Endocr.*, 43:489, 1969.
85. Skerlj, J.: *Arch. Gynäk.*, 159:12, 1935.
86. Smith, E. R., and Davidson, J. M.: *Endocrinology*, 82:100, 1968.
87. Steiner, M. M., and Hadawi, S. A.: *Amer. J. Dis. Child.*, 108:28, 1964.
88. Stieve, H.: *Der Einfluss des Nervensystems auf Bau and Tätigkeit der Weiblichen Genitale*. Stuttgart, G. Thieme, 1952.
89. Swingle, W., and Pfiffner, J. J.: *Proc. Soc. Exper. Biol. Med.*, 38:876, 1939.
90. Talbot, W. B., et al.: *New Eng. J. Med.*, 223:369, 1940.
91. Talbot, W. B., et al.: *Amer. J. Dis. Child.*, 65:364, 1943.
92. Tisserand, M.: *La Puberté Feminine*, in the *Encyclopedie Med.-Chir.*, Gynecologie, Vol. I, Fasc. 145, Paris, A. Laffont, 1939.
93. Velardo, J. T.: *Ann. N.Y. Acad. Sci.*, 75:441, 1959.
94. Visser, H. K. A., and Degenhart, H. J.: *Helv. Paed. Acta*, 21:409, 1966.
95. Wilkins, L.: *Diagnosis and Treatment of Endocrine Disorders in Childhood and Adolescence*, 2nd ed. Springfield, Ill., Charles C Thomas, 1957.
96. Witschi, E., and Riley, G. M.: *Endocrinology*, 26:565, 1940.
97. Wurtman, H. J., and Axelrod, J.: *Arch. Neurol.*, 18:208, 1968.
98. Yen, S. S. C., Vicic, W. J., and Karchner, D. V.: *J. Clin. Endocr.*, 29:382, 1969.
99. Yen, S. S. C., and Vicic, W. J.: *Amer. J. Obstet. Gynec.*, 106:134, 1970.
100. Zacharias, L., and Wurtman, H. J.: *Science*, 144:1154, 1964.
101. Zephiroff, R.: *Compt. Rend. Soc. Biol.*, 154:77, 1940.
102. Zondek, B.: *Die Hormone des Ovariums und der Hypophysenvorderlappen*. Berlin, J. Springer, 1931.

Chapter 17

THE CLIMACTERIUM

17.1. CONCEPT

Menopause is not the end of woman's sexual life; it merely means cessation of menstrual periods and therefore involves the loss of one of the symptoms, or external manifestations, of female sexual life. However, female sexual life extends beyond menopause, sometimes into far advanced age. Conversely, even the presence of menstrual periods in a woman does not mean sexual maturity is preserved, since, long before menstrual activity ceases, deficiency changes become apparent to indicate that the sexual apparatus is undergoing involution.

17.1.1. MENOPAUSE

What we call *menopause* refers to the external manifestation consisting in the *cessation of menstrual periods*. However, before a woman may be accepted as having reached menopause, a certain length of time must be allowed to elapse since the date her menstrual activity terminated, a time lapse of six months' duration currently being considered as acceptable. During this phase, a woman's menstrual periods may be suspended, only to reappear afterwards. Therefore, total suspension should not be admitted unless amenorrhea has been present for more than six months. Unless this precaution is observed, a woman may be believed to be postmenopausal when, in fact, she is not yet so in definite terms.

17.1.2. THE CLIMACTERIUM

By *climacterium*, we mean the endocrine and vegetative crisis associated with woman's decline in fertility. Climacterium and menopause are two events that are usually coincident, but which are different in nature. *While menopause is a simple external or symptomatic phenomenon, the climacterium is a fundamental and profound phenomenon, affecting the entire body and of a more or less extended period in a woman's sexual life. Menopause may thus be defined as one of the symptoms accompanying the climacterium.*

17.2. EVOLUTION

The idea that the climacterium and menopause occur at the same time needs some clarification. The climacterium generally starts *before* menopause, its phenomenology usually culminates at the time of the occurrence of menopause, and its endocrine and vegetative processes are prolonged even after menses have disappeared. As a result, menopause usually occupies a *central position in the course of the climacterium*. While most commonly true, this however is not the absolute rule, since in some cases the entire climacteric endocrine crisis may precede menopause, and still in some other instances, menstruation may cease and the disturbances of the climacterium proper may become manifest only afterwards.

Let us examine the sequence of events occurring during the climacterium, concentrating first on the local processes that involve the *genital apparatus*, and following up with a general examination of what takes place in the *glands of internal secretion* and in the rest of the body. The corresponding phenomenology must be divided into three fundamental phases: premenopausal, menopausal and postmenopausal.

17.2.1. PREMENOPAUSAL PHASE

The premenopausal phase is the period of time preceding the cessation of menses, the phase during which woman is apparently normal, though inapparent and yet undeveloped involutional processes are already under way in her.

There is a phase in puberty, discussed in Chapter 16, during which menstrual activity is present but ovulation does not occur—a period of *physiologic sterility*. In the same way, having surpassed her phase of sexual maturity, woman moves along the same itinerary, but in the opposite direction. It is a well established fact that woman seldom retains her capacity for conception after the age of 40, and that the fertility index rapidly declines after the age of 45. *The lowering of the fertility index* results from progressive disappearance of ovarian corpus luteum activity, as a result of which a physiologic anovulatory cycle[26] develops in premenopausal ovaries, in which ovarian follicles mature almost to the rupture point, but rupture does not occur and ova are not extruded, so that the follicles undergo atresia little by little. Naturally, ovarian involvement of this type is reflected in the endometrium by a persistent state of proliferation, and women in the preclimacteric phase are prone to develop the symptoms of hyperestrinism. This is the age of hemorrhagic metropathy, uterine fibroids and endometriosis. Bonfirraro and Sensi[6] have shown that only 71 per cent of women between age 40 and 47 ovulate. The incidence of ovulation drops rapidly in women over 40 (Fig. 17–2).

Although corpora lutea usually are no longer formed during the menopause, this is by no means a constant finding. Sharman[66] recently called attention to the fact that women over 50, in most cases presenting with definite amenorrhea, frequently showed evidence of secretory phase patterns in their endometria. Husslein[29] reported the finding of an active corpus luteum in an 80 year old woman. We have also encountered well developed corpora lutea in women of advanced climacteric age (Fig. 17–3). Finally, Nogales and Martinez[47] found that many instances of "hemorrhagic metropathy" of the climacteric age were nothing else than overlooked, short-lived abortions, and provided evidence to the effect that ovulation did in fact occur during that phase of life, although the corpora lutea formed were most often insufficient.

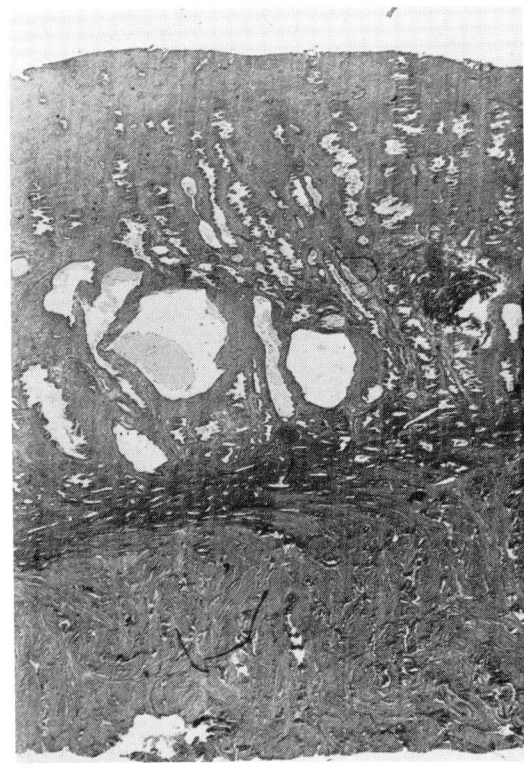

Figure 17–1. Endometrium of 52-year-old woman one year after menopause, revealing imperfect though evident secretory phase with cystic dilatation of some glands.

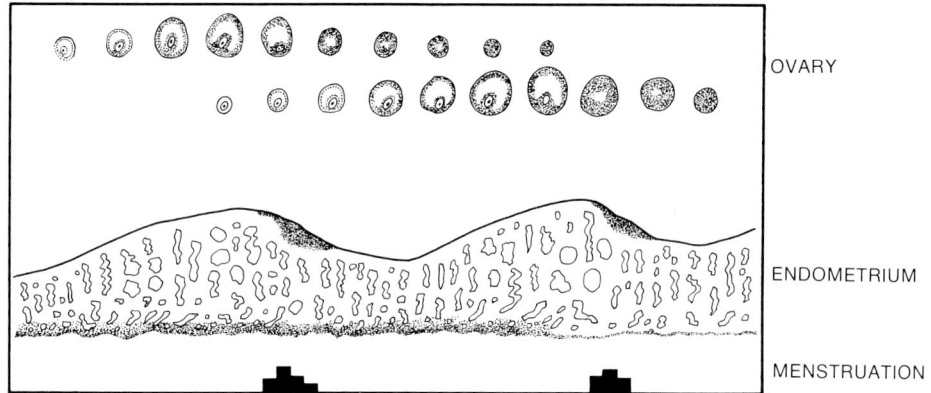

Figure 17-2. Anovulatory cycle, showing a flat menstrual curve which nevertheless is compatible with the occurrence of menstruation (pseudomenstruation).

17.2.2. MENOPAUSAL PHASE

Within a short time, the climacteric crisis sets in unmistakably; the woman begins to present with manifestations of disturbed endocrine balance that is consistent with sexual decline. These manifestations are of two types, *local and general*. All are due to decadence of and alterations in ovarian hormone production. The presence of an *altered menstrual rhythm* indicates the existence of an underlying ovarian dysfunction.

Depending on the estrogen output, *ovarian dysfunction* can be classified into essentially three types. Ovaries manifesting alterations in rhythm rather than quantity of secretion may be termed *normoestrogenic ovaries*. Hypoestrogenic ovaries are those in which rhythms may have remained unaffected but the amount of secretion has diminished. And, finally, *hyperestrogenic ovaries*—a variety much more commonly encountered than was once believed—are those in which rhythm is normal or altered, but in which estrogen output is elevated.

17.2.3. MECHANISM INVOLVED IN THE CESSATION OF PERIODIC BLEEDING

One way or another, any of the three types of ovarian alterations eventually leads to the cessation of menstrual bleeding. Although menstrual bleeding is determined by vascular phenomena that are regulated by ovarian activity and by the level of estrogen synthesis, menstruation is precipitated specifically by sudden withdrawal or deprivation of estrogens (Chapter 13). Therefore, what most often causes menstruation to be discontinued is *not an absolute quantitative decrease in estrogenic activity but*

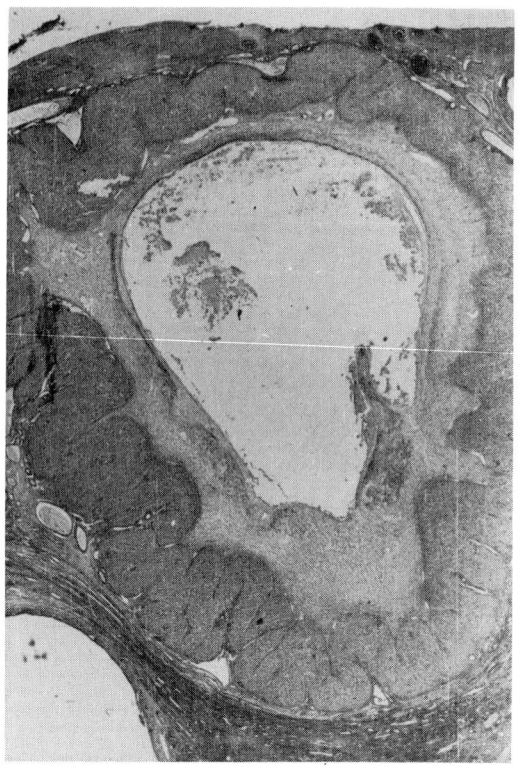

Figure 17-3. Ovary from same case as in Figure 17-1. A well developed corpus luteum is present. Compared with the endometrium, the ovary in this case is relatively better developed, which would indicate a sort of "metrosis of receptivity."

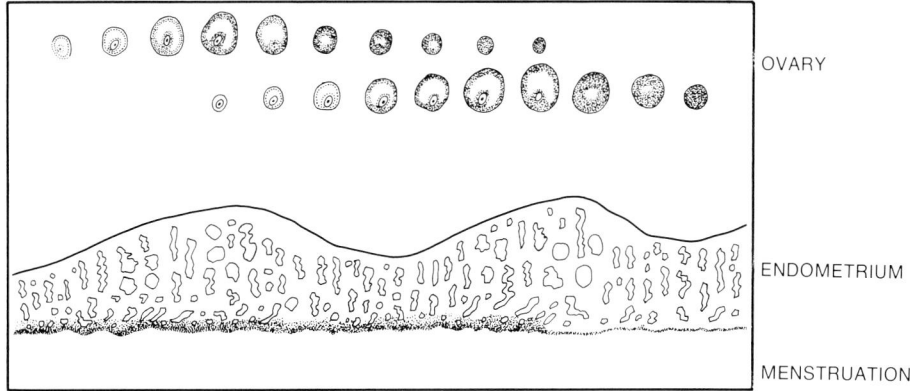

Figure 17–4. More advanced stage than that of Figure 17–3. There is disappearance of the menstrual curve and of menstruation, even though the ovary and endometrium remain morphologically unchanged.

rather the loss of alternating rhythmicity in estrogen synthesis. Menopause does not occur because the ovary suddenly stops secreting altogether but rather because, *even in the presence of above normal or, at any rate, normal hormonal levels, the necessary fluctuations to produce hormonal deprivation are missing, as a result of which menstruation fails to occur* (Figs. 17–4 and 17–5). Despite adequate estrogen synthesis, amenorrhea may develop if the level of hormone activity is continuous and sustained, that is, by a mechanism similar to that producing *hyperhormonal amenorrhea,* which shall be discussed in Chapter 28.

The foregoing mechanism differs fundamentally from the one involved in women with below normal estrogen synthesis, in whom there are neither hormone level fluctuations nor any proliferative endometrial activity to speak of. The mechanism involved in the latter is radically different from the preceding one, resembling instead the mechanism involved in amenorrhea due to hypoestrinism.

Suspension of menstruation does not necessarily mean a collapse of ovarian secretory function. Although in a number of cases, ovarian activity has in fact declined, in others the ovary remains active and active estrogen synthesis may be present in spite of absent menstruation.

Nor does cessation of menses invariably occur in an abrupt and sudden manner. It

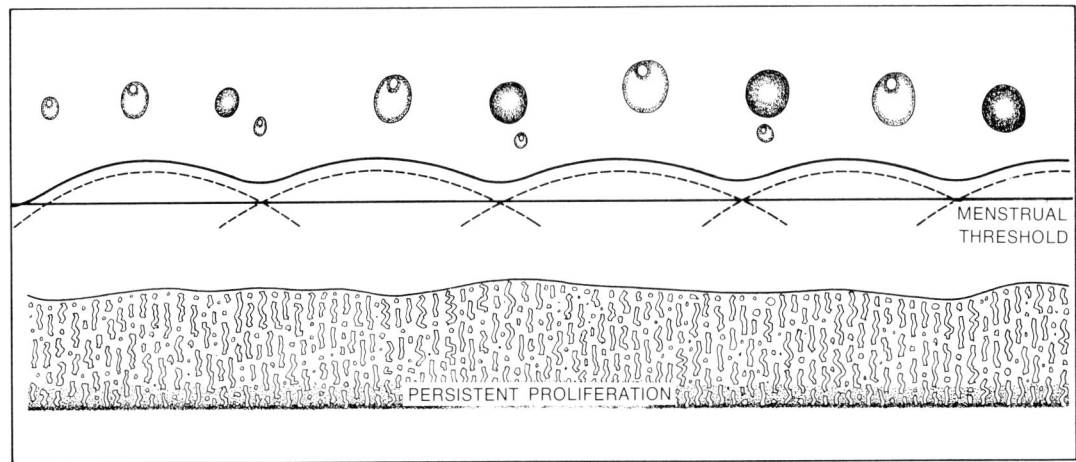

Figure 17–5. Polymicrocystic ovary, amenorrhea with sustained hyperestrinism and persistent proliferation. (From Botella-Llusiá: *Enfermedades del aparato genital femenino,* 5th ed. Barcelona, Editorial Científico-Médica, 1959.)

must not be assumed that large amounts of estrogens and sudden hormone withdrawal are involved in every cycle, and that all at once menstruation fails to occur in one particular cycle. During the phase of woman's sexual maturity, the abruptness of hormonal fluctuations may be mitigated by a deficit in corpus luteum function (corpus luteum hormone representing one of the factors that promote elimination of estrogens and contribute toward rapidly lowering estrogen levels), so that hormone withdrawal deflections may be less abrupt, although they may still be of sufficient magnitude to produce menstrual bleeding. However, little by little they become sluggish and finally "plateau." Ultimately, whether or not menstruation takes place depends on the menstrual threshold (Fig. 17-5). Of course, there is no reason why a casual drop in the hormonal curve may not occur in any of the subsequent cycles, in which case menstruation may again occur. Irregular fluctuations of that kind may or may not involve menstrual subthreshold levels, which is why the phenomenon of periodic bleeding does not terminate abruptly and why menstrual bleeding may recur.

Occasionally, perhaps less commonly, amenorrhea may also develop in association with a *flat-curved cycle*. These are otherwise normal ovulatory cycles but in which the pattern of hormone withdrawal necessary for menstruation does not occur. This type of cycle is associated with postmenopausal amenorrhea in the presence of positive pregnanediol excretion (see Table 17-1).

Anovulatory cycles in conjunction with sustained estrogenic curves may be encountered with polymicrocystic ovaries, of common occurrence at menopause. Amenorrhea in such cases has essentially the same mechanism as that described previously (Fig. 17-5).

17.2.4. POSTMENOPAUSAL PHASE

Last to appear, the *postmenopausal phase* is one in which the ovary appears to have lost all trace of activity, at least in the majority of cases. We possess no statistical data concerning the type of woman involved and the age group in which complete cessation of estrogen synthesis occurs, but approximately 70 per cent of all postmenopausal women may be estimated to be subject to a more or less gradual decrease in estrogenic activity, eventually leading to complete absence, at which stage curettage reveals only atrophy of the endometrium and no proliferation whatsoever. Nevertheless, a certain percentage of postmenopausal women reveal active proliferative endometria despite absent menses (Fig. 17-7). What is more, in these cases, studies of urinary hormone content may reveal continued estrogen elimination in large amounts, occasionally as large as those found in normal women. This means that some ovaries may still secrete appreciable amounts of hormones at this late phase and that, for all the external appearances, their sexual life has not yet terminated.

Colpocytologic examinations tend to confirm these findings. Already, in the second Spanish edition of this book, we had stated that postmenopausal smears suggested the presence of hypoestrinism only on rare occasions. Montalvo,[43] Osmond-Clarke and Murray,[49] Masukawa[42] and Stoll and Ledermair[68] all pointed out that postmenopausal women seldom revealed totally atrophic smears, exhibiting intermediate or frank estrogenic patterns much more frequently. Struthers[70] reported estrogenic smear patterns in up to 79 per cent of postmenopausal women. Wied[76] gave comparable figures of 65 per cent, and Boschann[8] of 50 per cent, of endometria

TABLE 17-1. Urinary Steroid Excretion in Postmenopausal Women

GROUP	YEARS AFTER MENOPAUSE	ESTROGENS (MCG) Average	Range	PREGNANEDIOL (MG) Average	Range	17-KETOSTEROIDS (MG) Average	Range
I	3 to 5	180	0-615	4	0-9	7.9	5-14
II	6 to 10	100	0-300	2.8	0-8	8.6	4-16
III	more than 10	70	0-200	0.9	0-2.5	8.5	4-15

revealing cytologic evidence of activity at that phase of life. Magee,[39] as well as Sedlis and co-workers,[65] noted that only 46 to 50 per cent of postmenopausal women revealed atrophic vaginal cytology, the rest revealing estrogenic or intermediate patterns. In Table 17-3, we have summarized our own observations on postmenopausal women, in a large number of whom vaginal estrogenic activity is evident many years after the cessation of menses. In addition, their vaginal epithelia continue to contain abundant glycogen.

While from a clinical standpoint, menstruation may be viewed as the yardstick of menopause, the condition of the vaginal mucosa might well be considered as an index of the climacterium. It might be added that a woman has indeed reached this stage when her vaginal mucosa begins to show signs of atrophy and altered, pathologic desquamation.

17.3. ENDOCRINOLOGY OF THE CLIMACTERIUM

17.3.1. THE OVARY

The preceding data indicate clearly that the climacteric ovary does not stop secreting but merely *loses its capacity for rhythmic estrogen synthesis.*[23] The follicles of postmenopausal ovaries have been found to cease maturing in a regular rhythmic fashion. In addition, they generally fail to achieve full maturation and remain incompletely developed, and then either undergo atresia or persist for a long time in a cystic stage without ever rupturing. Although some ovaries may lack follicles altogether, estrogen synthesis may be carried on by atretic follicles or by fibrothecal cells. As a result of dynamic tests in which the ovary is stimulated by means of gonadotropins, Poliak and co-workers[55] believe that the ovarian response is normal. However, such findings may be questionable, since they appear to contradict the rather common observation that women with high gonadotropin levels usually have small, hypoplastic ovaries. *The postmenopausal ovary then must be admitted to continue secreting hormones even though it may lose the capacity to do so in a monthly rhythmic fashion.*

The classical concept of menopause must therefore be rectified by accepting the fact that menses cease not because the sexual glands cease elaborating estrogens but rather because estrogens no longer gain the circulation in surging waves whenever the rhythm of the cycle weakens or disappears.

17.3.2. ESTROGEN EXCRETION AT MENOPAUSE

Alterations in the rhythm of ovarian secretion are generally associated with *elevated urinary estrogen excretion.* Such estrogen excretion may reach significant levels. According to Klotz and Jayle,[32] values as high as 300 mcg of Kober positive steroids (total estrogens) may be found in climacteric women. We obtained similar values in 1956[11, 12, 13] (see Tables 17-1 and 17-3). These results were subsequently confirmed by a number of investigators. Randall and co-workers[57] found increased estrogens in 50 per cent of their cases. On the other hand, MacBride[37] found that urinary estrone and estriol concentrations in young women during the "resting" phase of the cycle did not differ from those of postmenopausal women. Similarly, Buzzoni and co-workers,[17] as well as Subrizi and co-workers,[71] reported elevated values of menopausal estrogenuria.

What accounts for the apparent paradox is, in the first place, the fact that both thecal cells and fibrothecal cell masses in the ovary are no less important agents of estrogen synthesis[20, 75] than ovarian follicles themselves. In the second place, the fact that, owing to absent luteal activity—which, as was pointed out previously, usually has disappeared several years earlier—estrogen production proceeds at a steady pace. Hyperestrinism is known to result from a continuous type of action rather than from any single episode of massive hyperproduction (Botella[12]). Finally, not to be discounted is the fact that declining and frequently insufficient hepatic function, prone to occur in that phase of life, facilitates the accumulation of estrogens through *failure of estrogen degradation* (see Chapter 28).

17.3.3. INCREASED GONADOTROPIN ACTIVITY

This paradoxical behavior of the ovary may be ascribed to enhanced production of gonadotropins. Zondek[77] had demonstrated the presence of increased FSH excretion in castrated animals, a finding which later was convincingly corroborated. Modern studies[38,50] have produced evidence to the effect that castration elevates not only FSH but also LH levels, which is a finding of extraordinary importance when it comes to explaining the thecal and interstitial reaction occurring in postmenopausal ovaries of both female animals and women. The pituitaries of castrate animals as well as those of postmenopausal women have been shown histochemically[53,56] and endocrinologically[21,63] to reflect such heightened rates of gonadotropin *production*.

In menopausal women, the increased rate of urinary gonadotropin excretion is equally apparent, so much so that menopausal urine is at present utilized as the commercial source of human FSH for therapeutic purposes (see Chapters 7 and 40).

Increased FSH values have been reported by Albert and co-workers,[1,2] Paulsen and co-workers,[52] Veziris,[72] Brown,[16] Rosemberg and Engel[62] and Coble and colleagues.[19] However, recent studies have shown that FSH is not the only type of gonadotropin that is elevated, and that considerable quantities of LH are also excreted, which explains why such ovaries display predominantly excitatory interstitial reactions, whereas postmenopausal adrenals show evidence of pituitary effect (to be discussed later). The finding of LH in climacteric and postclimacteric urine was reported by Albert and Rosemberg,[2,61] Brown,[16] Kovacic and Loraine,[33] Vignes[73] and Coble and colleagues.[19] The role played by these two gonadotropins in climacteric endocrine phenomena has been illustrated in figure 17–11. Recent studies by Roos[60] and by Parlow and Hendrich[51] have revealed a markedly elevated gonadotropin concentration in climacteric pituitaries. Bostelman,[9] who studied pineals of castrated animals, found that the number of secretory granules in such pineals was reduced in relation to enhanced pituitary function.

17.4. THE POSTCLIMACTERIC AND SENILE PHASE

Undoubtedly, the question of much greater interest is whether estrogenic hormone is still being elaborated *during the later phases, when the endocrine crisis is over and woman finds herself on the threshold of old age.* Estrogenic hormone does not cease being elaborated during this phase, though it has been found to be produced in much smaller amounts than in the immediately preceding phase. The classic concept held that in postmenopausal woman estrogenic activity had been wiped out completely by the time woman entered the postclimacteric phase. Nonetheless, as shown by modern investigations and particularly by our own research, the female body continues to actively elaborate estrogens long after menopause, even though woman's reproductive life by that time appears to have been left far behind.

The presence of estrogenic activity in postclimacteric women may be demonstrated in three different ways: (1) through the presence of urinary estrogens; (2) through evidence of endometrial activity, and (3) through vaginal cytology. These will be discussed here.

17.4.1. POSTCLIMACTERIC ESTROGENIC ACTIVITY

URINARY ESTROGENS. Zondek[77] found estrogens in the urine of a woman who was 18 years beyond menopause. Modern investigations have all confirmed these results (Bret and Bardiaux,[15] Jayle et al.,[30,31] MacBride,[37] Randall et al.[57] and Carcatzoulis[18]). Our own findings have corroborated the presence of elevated urinary estrogens in women 10 or more years after menopause (Tables 17–1 and 17–2).

Analogous values, as we shall point out later, have been found in surgically castrated women, a fact that shall enable us to discuss the possible source of persistent follicular hormone production.

ENDOMETRIAL ACTIVITY IN THE POSTCLIMACTERIC PHASE. Evidence that the senile endometrium retains its capacity to proliferate in many instances has been provided by the fairly common finding of great functional reactivation, with marked hyperplasia of the endometrium (see Figs. 17–6, 17–7 and 17–8), in association with, among other conditions, granulosa cell tumors in old women. Proliferative endometrial changes in women over 50 have

The Climacterium

TABLE 17-2. Urinary Steroid Excretion (in Group of Women from Table 17-1, with Breakdown of Increased, Normal or Decreased Values)*

GROUP	ESTROGENS (MCG)			PREGNANEDIOL (MG)			17-KETOSTEROIDS (MG)		
	Decreased 0–100 mcg	Normal 100–200 mcg	Increased >200 mcg	Decreased 0–6 mg	Normal <10 mg	Increased >10 mg	Decreased 0–8 mg	Normal 8–13 mg	Increased >13 mg
I	44.6%	44.6%	10.8%	74.0%	26.0%	0%	24.5%	55.5%	20%
II	50.8	40.3	8.9	90.1	9.9	0	20.0	60.5	19.5
III	60.1	30.2	9.7	90.4	9.6	0	35.7	62.3	2.0

*Figures indicate percentage of total number of cases.

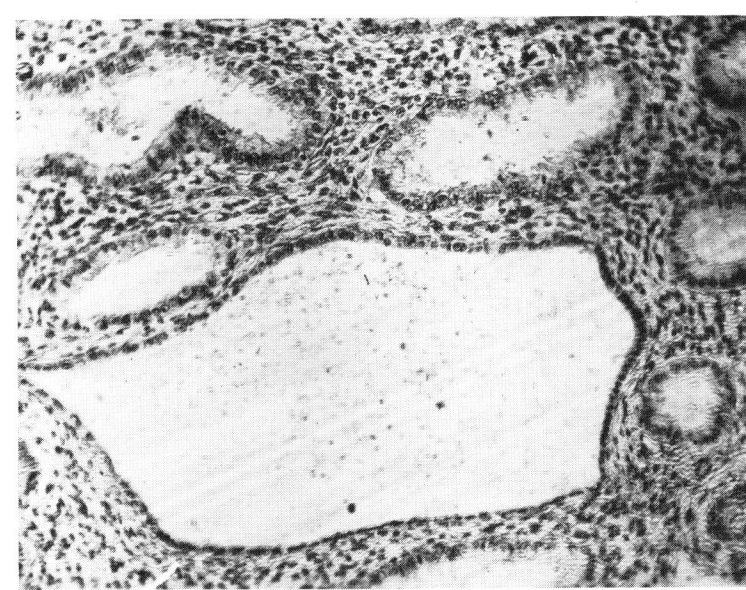

Figure 17-6. Endometrium with cystic glandular hyperplasia in a woman six months after her last menstrual period.

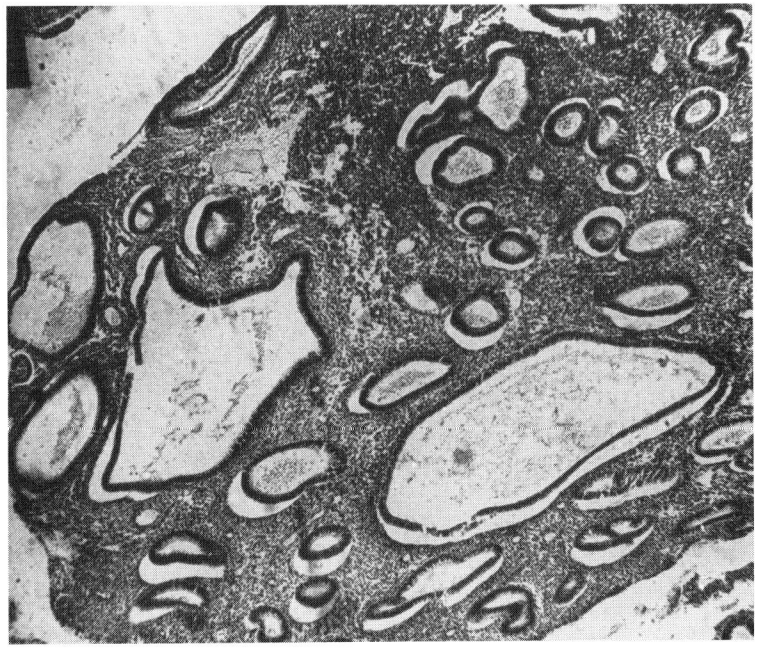

Figure 17-7. Active endometrial hyperplasia in postmenopausal woman. (From Nogales: *Arch. Med. Exper.*, 11:123, 1948).

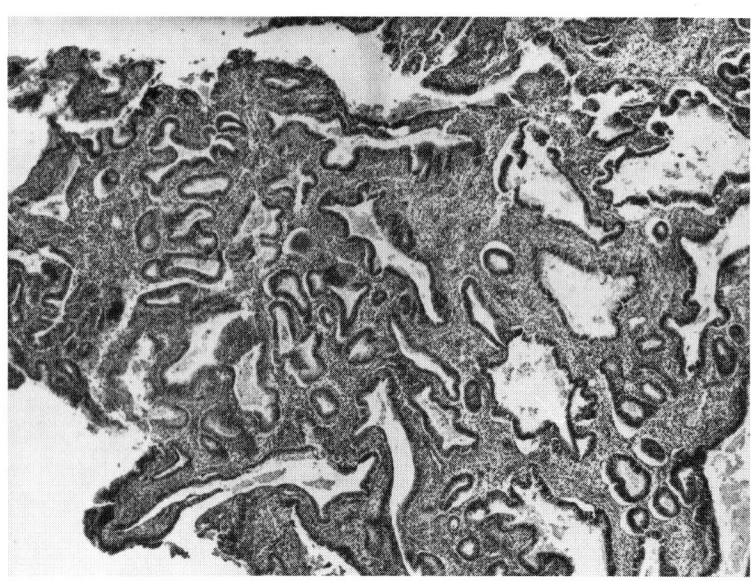

Figure 17–8. Atypical hyperplasia in a postmenopausal woman.

already been described by Novak and Richardson[48] and, more recently, by Roddick and Greene,[59] Bigelow[7] and MacBride.[37] At our clinic, Nogales[46] studied the endometria of a large series of postmenopausal women by means of microcurettage. In 30 cases (25 per cent of all cases), he found endometria of the proliferative type (Fig. 17–7), while none of his cases revealed the presence of secretory patterns.

We have studied postmenopausal endometria in 98 cases, in some of which menstrual periods had been absent for over 15 years.[13] The study material was divided into three groups: Group I, 3 to 5 years after menopause; Group II, 6 to 10 years; and Group III, 10 or more years after menopause (see Table 17–3). Even after classifying the instances of regressive hyperplasia encountered among degenerative changes, there still remains a total of 35 per cent of active endometria, and in Group III, 7 of 21 cases (33 per cent) revealed equivocal signs of endometrial activity.

Our studies showed fairly accurate correlation between urinary estrogen excretion and vaginal cytology (Fig. 17–9). On the other hand, after having examined the ovaries and endometria of a large series of postmenopausal women, Bigelow[7] maintained that ovarian histology (nearly always revealing hyperthecosis) correlated well

TABLE 17–3. Condition of Endometrium in Postmenopausal Women (Nonbleeding Endometria)*

GROUP	Atrophy and Hypoplasia	Proliferation	Secretion	Active Hyperplasia	Regressive Hyperplasia
I	15 cases	12 cases	3 cases	3 cases	3 cases
II	17 cases	8 cases	0 cases	2 cases	3 cases
III	13 cases	4 cases	1 case	2 cases	1 case
Total: 98 cases	45 (45%)	24 (24%)	4 (4%)	7 (7%)	7 (7%)

*Endometria studied histochemically by means of PAS and alkaline glycerophosphatase reaction.

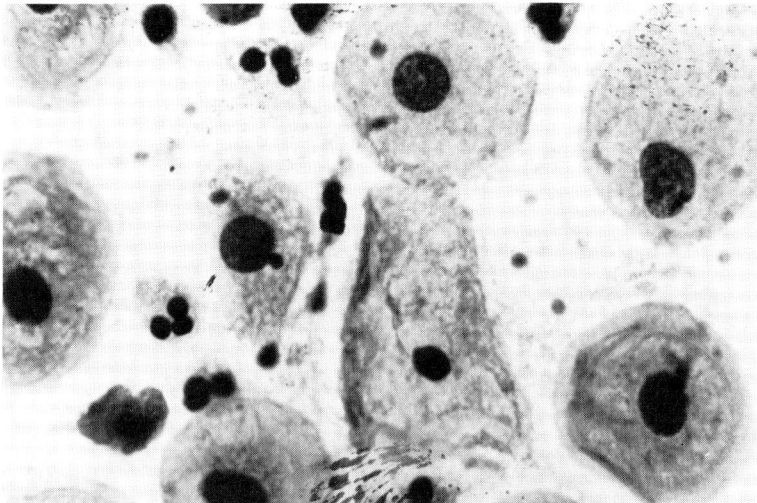

Figure 17-9. Vaginal smear illustrating atrophy in a case of syndrome of hypoestrinism in a postmenopausal woman. Parabasal cells predominate.

with the finding of endometrial proliferation.

VAGINAL ESTROGENIC EFFECT. It is of interest to note that, based on the study of vaginal cytology in postmenopausal women, Montalvo[44] reported cytologic evidence of estrogen deficiency in only 40 per cent, that is, in less than half the cases. Other authors, such as Bourg and Pundel,[14] Struthers[70] and Wied,[76] also reported the presence of estrogenic effect in smears from women three or more years after menopause. Four cases, reported by Folsome and co-workers,[26] are remarkable in that estrogenic smears were obtained from women over 80 years of age. In recent times, Masukawa,[42] Osmond-Clarke and Murray[49] and Stoll and Ledermair[68] have also described persistent karyopyknotic cytology in the old age group.

TABLE 17-4. Colpocytologic Findings in Women After Menopause. Most of the Cases Are From the Same Series as in Table 17-3.

GROUP	TYPE OF CYTOLOGY			
	Atrophic	Weakly Estrogenic	Moderately Estrogenic	Markedly Estrogenic
I	13 cases	6 cases	2 cases	0 cases
II	10 cases	5 cases	1 case	4 cases
III	18 cases	4 cases	2 cases	1 case
	11 (61%)	15 (22%)	5 (7%)	5 (7%)

Our own studies included 67 postmenopausal women classified by age into three categories (Table 17-4). As may be appreciated, the results indicate a high percentage of markedly estrogenic smears even in the far advanced postmenopausal group.

Subsequently, Montalvo[44] repeated the same type of study on a much larger number of cases; his results showed discrepancy insofar as there was an even higher percentage of estrogenic cytology. Other investigators, as already pointed out, have obtained similar results.

Interestingly, results obtained on *surgically castrated women* are roughly comparable (Boschann,[8] Ferin[25]). Ferin found atrophic smears in only 32 per cent of his cases of surgically castrated women, a really surprising finding. As a result, one might have to consider a probable *extraovarian origin*, if but in part, for postmenopausal estrogen secretion.

In summary, then, it must be said that studies of urinary hormones, endometria and, finally, vaginal cytology would all seem to indicate that estrogenic hormone continues being elaborated in some part of the body after the apparent cessation of woman's reproductive activity. In a later section, we shall determine in which site this belated type of hormone production takes place, but first let us examine the question of the other sex hormones in the climacterium.

17.4.2. DEMONSTRATION OF ANDROGENIC ACTIVITY DURING AND AFTER THE CLIMACTERIUM

Signs suggesting viriloid deviations[49] may appear in women as early as the preclimacteric phase or during the months of menopause proper. In the course of subsequent years, such trends tend to become more accentuated. The presence of androgenic activity pertaining to this phase in woman's life can be determined by the following means: (1) somatic and psychologic evidence of a tendency toward virilization; (2) biologic determination of urinary androgens, and (3) chemical determination of 17-ketosteroids. The climacteric ovary, in the view of Mattingly and Huang,[41] loses its ability to aromatize steroids, as a result of which the absence of the androstenedione-estrone and testosterone-estradiol conversion process leads to excessive production of androgenic substances.

TENDENCY TOWARD VIRILIZATION. The fact that women tend toward virilization when reaching the critical age has been well known. Marañón[40] viewed such virilization in the light of his own theory on sexual evolution. Elsewhere, we have mentioned the occurrence of a genuine variety of "climacteric virilism" and stressed its adrenocortical origin.[26] The menopausal symptomatology frequently goes beyond mere virilization of a certain degree of hirsutism and may involve typical features of masculine psychology. It is at this stage of life that women, when widowed, may unexpectedly display extraordinary firmness of character and assume the role of the father of the family, sometimes with remarkable efficiency.

While there is little doubt that development of the somatic features mentioned depends on increased male hormone activity, it is not certain whether the second group of features, involving masculine psychologic attributes, are equally hormone dependent.

URINARY ANDROGENS. Increased amounts of urinary 17-ketosteroids during the climacterium have been reported by this writer[13] (see Table 17-5).

Table 17-5 is informative insofar as it shows the pattern in which 17-ketosteroids are increased during the phase of sexual decline. This increase in 17-ketosteroids corresponds mainly to the age group between 50 and 55, that is, following menopause. These data also afford an indication of the origin of this postmenopausal hormonal hyperactivity, as we shall see later.

In summary, androgenic activity during the climacterium may be said to be enhanced, experiencing a marked upswing toward the end of that phase as well as during the immediately following postclimacteric phase. Compared to estrogenic activity which, when persistent, follows a downhill rather than a rising course, androgenic activity undergoes a genuine upswing above and beyond normal limits.

17.4.3. THE PITUITARY AND GONADOTROPINS

Increased urinary gonadotropin excretion in climacteric and postclimacteric women was generally suspected before it was actually discovered. Zondek[77] and Zuckerman[78] were first to describe the presence of considerable amounts of urinary gonadotropic hormone in such women. On the basis of the original investigations, FSH was believed to be the only hormone eliminated, but it is now known that appreciable amounts of LH are also eliminated. By means of comparative studies,[21, 62, 64] it could be established that pituitaries of postclimacteric women contained about 50 times more FSH and two to five times more LH than normal controls.

Histologically, such pituitaries are also consistent with a state of hyperactivity. Histochemical studies (Purves and Griesbach,[56] Pearse[53]) have likewise revealed an increase of so-called "gonadotropic" PAS-positive elements. Thus, there is no

TABLE 17-5. 24 Hour Urinary Excretion of Neutral 17-Ketosteroids in Castrated and Climacteric Women

CONDITION	NUMBER OF CASES	AVERAGE, IN MG
Normal women, age 30 to 40	4	5.686
Climacteric women, age 42 to 48	6	9.333
Postclimacteric women, age 54 to 70	6	4.285
Surgically castrated women	6	7.184

doubt that, *in the absence of the suppressive effect on the pituitary by normal ovarian function, the pituitary responds with a compensatory form of hyperfunction during the climacteric and postclimacteric phases, so that the resulting increased FSH, LH and possibly also ACTH activity stimulates the interstitial tissue of both the ovary and the adrenal, and thereby gives rise to compensatory production of steroids.*

17.4.4. BELATED LUTEAL ACTIVITY

In the course of our own investigations,[11, 12] we only seldom found positive pregnanedioluria in postmenopausal women; however, in this regard, special mention must be made of a case, reported by Husslein,[29] in which a well developed endometrial secretory phase was observed in a woman over 80 years old. In a few exceptional cases, we have also encountered postmenopausal endometrial secretory activity (Figs. 17–1 and 17–2). Sharman,[66] too, relates similar occurrences.

17.4.5. DEMONSTRATION OF ADRENAL HYPERACTIVITY DURING THE CLIMACTERIUM

For many years, we considered the adrenal origin of postclimacteric estrogen synthesis as certain. This assumption of ours was later questioned.[18, 45] We are presently inclined to admit that senile ovaries occasionally, though not always, produce considerable quantities of estrogens. Naturally, the very rare functional tumors of either the feminizing or masculinizing variety are exceptions to the rule. The origin of the hormones present in the urine, estrogens as well as androgens, must be attributed to some other organ. Moreover, those cases in which, following surgical castration, there is continued excretion of the same hormonal products, would lead us to strongly suspect that *sex hormones may be also derived from extraovarian sources.* In an earlier extensive publication and in several monographs[10] (see Chapter 9), we have attempted to explain the reasons for considering the adrenal as a "third gonad," capable of elaborating gonadal steroids during those periods of life in which the need for such hormones cannot be satisfied by their specific glands of origin. Accordingly, the presence of both estrogens and androgens in the urine of postmenopausal women ought to be attributed to an interrenal source of origin. In the same way, our histologic studies have enabled us to demonstrate that the so-called *sexual* zone of the adrenal cortex, which stains characteristically with Vines's fuchsin, is equally well developed in the innermost zone of the reticularis of both men and climacteric and postclimacteric women (Fig. 17–10).

Of the six cases listed in Table 17–6, the ovaries, uteri and vaginas were also examined at autopsy; four of these cases revealed signs of estrogenic activity in their uteri and vaginas; five of the six cases, however, showed totally involuted and atrophic ovaries, leaving no doubt that the estrogenic effect, which in four cases was observed to be of sufficient intensity to produce endometrial proliferation, must have been of extragonadal origin, presumably arising in the adrenal.

Perhaps the findings relative to urinary 17-ketosteroid excretion provide even more decisive information. As already pointed out, elimination of these compounds has nowadays come to be considered as an exponent of adrenal sexual activity.[58] On recalling what has been said here concerning the subject earlier, it should be perfectly plain that the estrogens and androgens occurring in the urine of climacteric individuals, as well as those occurring in surgically castrated women, are all of adrenocortical origin. The presence of adrenal hyperplasia in castrated animals, presenting primarily as a thickening of the reticularis, which is thus transformed into a kind of X zone containing abundant fuchsinophilic inclusions, has been known for a long time. It has already been mentioned that, by means of estrogen injections, the associated fuchsinophilic deposits can be caused to disappear completely.

17.4.6. GONADOTROPINS AND SEXUAL CORTEX

The relationship between LH and the sexual zone of the adrenal cortex was discussed in Chapter 9. Modern literature contains abundant reference to the finding that *interstitial cell stimulating gonado-*

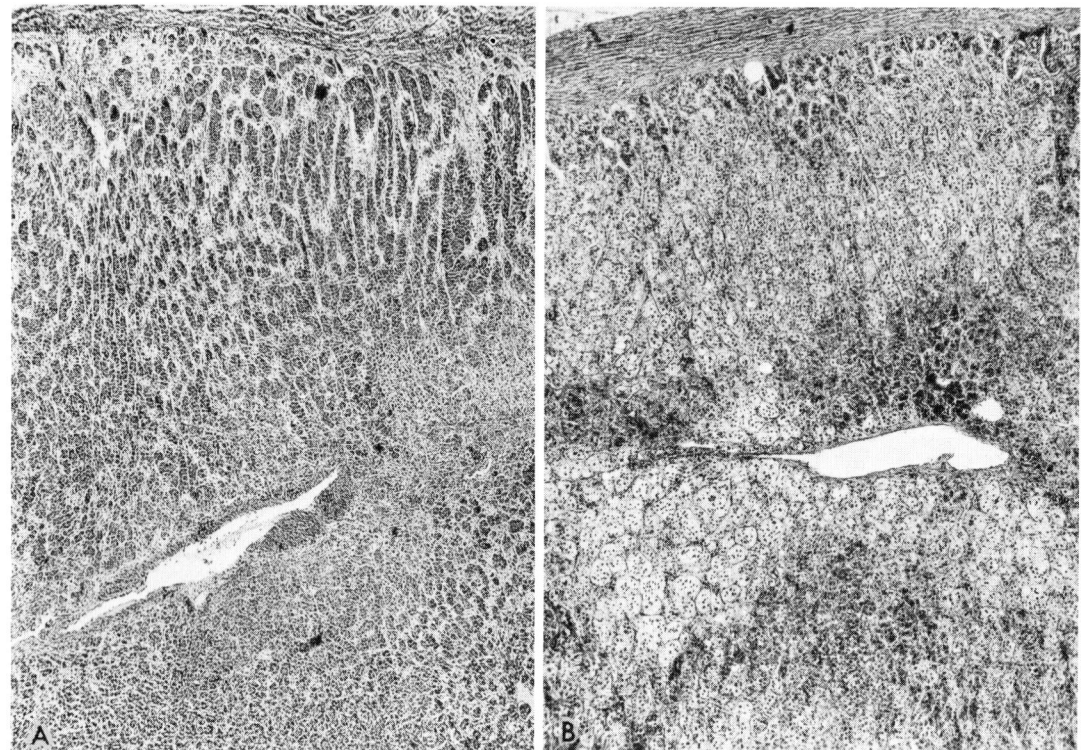

Figure 17-10. A, Adrenal cortex of 35-year-old male adult, who died accidentally; although it is well developed, the zona fasciculata lacks fuchsinophilic cells. B, Adrenal of a man aged 73, who had sclerosis of the adrenal cortex, particularly involving capsule and zona glomerulosa; fuchsinophilic cells, staining black, are present in large numbers. (From Botella and Cano: *Gynaecologia (Basel)*, 127:133, 1947.)

tropin (LH) also stimulates the adrenal interstitium, that is, the sex hormone-producing X zone.[10, 36, 58] That something of this sort occurs in castration has been brought to light by our own work,[10] as well as by the castration experiments on rats by Houssay[28] and Fekete and Little.[24] Evidence that LH activity increases during the climacterium and afterwards makes such an assumption plausible.

TABLE 17-6. Histologic Findings in the Adrenal Cortex of Climacteric and Postclimacteric Individuals

WOMEN (6 CASES)	MEN (4 CASES)
Age: 48 to 55	Age: 65 to 76
Positive fuchsinophilic reaction in five cases, negative reaction in one case	Positive fuchsinophilic reaction in all four cases

17.4.7. ARE POSTMENOPAUSAL ESTROGENS OF ADRENAL OR OF GONADAL ORIGIN?

This, of course, is a question that must be raised before completing our present discussion. If estrogens keep being eliminated in the urine after menopause, often for many more years, and their effects on the end organs, the uterus and vagina, continue to be perceived, what origin should we ascribe to these compounds?

EVIDENCE FAVORING AN ADRENAL ORIGIN. The adrenal, as we have already mentioned here, *increases in thickness in conjunction with the appearance of an "interstitial fuchsinophilic zone" that appears to be invariably associated with adrenal sex hormone synthesis.* It must be added that hypertrophy of the latter zone is known to occur in response to LH activity, under the influence of which the zone is known to produce both androgens and estrogens (Botella[10]). According to Berger,[5] ACTH also stimulates biogenesis of adrenal estrogens.

Even in the absence of gonads, such as occurs following animal or human castration, estrogens continue to be encountered in the urine (see Chapter 45). Finally, it must be said that the simultaneous elevation of both estrogens and 17-ketosteroids in the postmenopausal period seems to prove the postmenopausal adrenal origin of both.

EVIDENCE FAVORING AN OVARIAN ORIGIN. *Thecal hyperplasia* is currently known to involve active estrogen synthesis (Wall et al.,[74] Husslein,[29] Roddick and Greene,[59] Morris and Scully[45]). Thecal hyperplasia may sometimes occur in quite small ovaries that grossly appear insignificant. However, Craig[22] denies the significance of cortical stromal hyperplasia. Similarly, Morris and Scully,[45] as well as Lauber and Sulman,[34] have called attention to the possible feminizing effect of *hilar cell hyperplasia*, which to date has been believed to be exclusively associated with virilization (see Chapter 29). Of no less importance, it must be realized that *small thecomas* or *minute granulosa cell tumors* may be inadvertently overlooked in the course of exploratory examinations and even in gross postmortem specimens. Yet, these are precisely the type of tumors that may generate considerable amounts of estrogenic hormone. Further details concerning this subject may be found in Chapters 28 and 30.

Thus, there seems to be no absolute need, after all, to invoke the adrenal in explaining the genesis of these paradoxical estrogens. Mainly for these reasons, many authors have repudiated our doctrine of *the third gonad.*

EXTRAGONADAL AND EXTRACORTICAL ORIGIN OF ESTROGENS. Through his investigations, initiated at our laboratory and then continued in Italy, Lenzi[35] arrived at the surprising conclusion that, *even without adrenals and ovaries, animals are able to continue forming estrogens as long as they are under the effect of adequate pituitary stimulation.* These results were later confirmed in the human species after the introduction of combined oophorectomy and adrenalectomy for the treatment of breast cancer (Struthers,[70] Strong,[69] Gompel,[27] Brown,[16] Diczfalusy et al.[23]). Further reference to this question is made in Chapter 45. There is no doubt that, under the influence of gonadotropin and ACTH activity (see Chapter 2), sex steroid synthesis may be initiated from very simple compounds (acetate-squalene) and that, at least under certain circumstances, this type of hormone synthesis may take place in tissues other than the adrenal or the ovary.

TOWARD A NEW CONCEPT OF THE "SEXUAL MESENCHYME." Although there is no question that the adrenal elaborates estrogens at menopause and, in general, in all those moments of life marked by the imperative need to supplement failing ovarian function, it is also evident that the ovary, as well as other hitherto unknown tissues, are able to engage in estrogen synthesis in the aged woman, much in the same way they are known to partake in such synthesis—and this is a very important fact—under conditions of neoplasia. To take a one-sided view of these developments would seem to us irrational. We must not lose sight of the fact that in the embryonic era both the interrenal system and the gonads arise in closely juxtaposed embryonic primordia, both derived from a common retrocoelomic mesenchyme. Thus, the mesenchyme of the posterior wall of the primitive abdomen may be assumed to possess the potentiality for sex steroid synthesis. In all likelihood, the adrenal sexual zone, as well as the stromal and thecal structures of the ovary, are nothing else than potentially active vestiges of that mesenchyme. LH is thought to be the specific stimulator of the "sexual mesenchymal system." However, it is entirely possible that the mesenchyme, diffusely disseminated in the perirenal compartment or in the broad ligament, possesses the potentialities of the type just mentioned and, without constituting any definite organ per se, is able to respond by synthesizing estrogens whenever the normal synthetic system itself—the ovary and the adrenal—fail to do so.

This is only a hypothesis but, at the actual stage of sexual endocrinology, 20 years after having enunciated our doctrine of *the third gonad,* this generalization has become necessary.

Our ideas have been diagrammed in Figure 17-11.

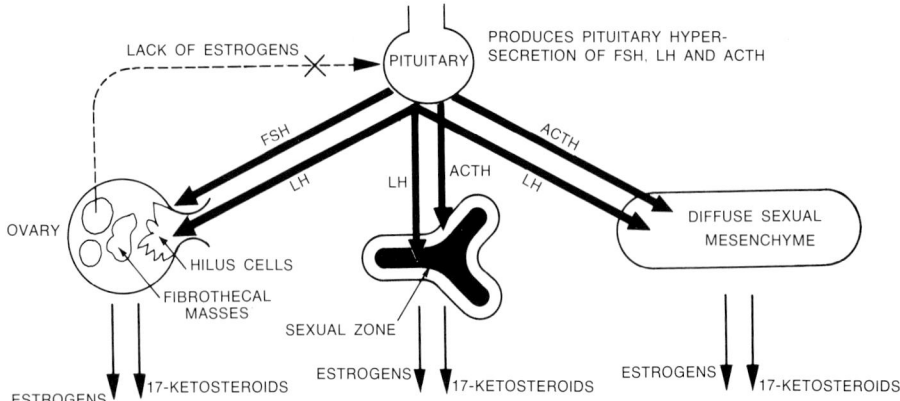

Figure 17-11. Diagrammatic outline of estrogen and androgen biogenesis by the sexual mesenchyme in the adrenal and in the ovary.

17.4.8. LIVER FUNCTION IN RELATION TO SEX HORMONES

We have already drawn attention to the frequency with which endometrial hyperplasia occurs in old age. Also to be discussed in the following paragraph is the occurrence of a genuine type of metropathy at this age (senile metropathy), which has by now been recognized as an entity in gynecologic clinical experience.[49, 50] However, in order to explain the unusual and paradoxical production of the anatomic and clinical symptomatology of hyperestrinism on the mere basis of a certain, invariably lower than normal, level of estrogenic activity, it is necessary to resort to a second contributing factor: the liver. That the liver plays an essential role in metabolizing and inactivating estrogens is common knowledge.[4, 54, 67]

Progesterone has been found to intervene in activating hepatic estrogen breakdown in a decisive manner. During the phase of woman's sexual maturity, progesterone partakes in the methodical degradation of excess estrogens in each cycle. Once cyclic activity is terminated, and with it the process of luteinization, these estrogens, their generally lower levels notwithstanding, become more dangerous because their presence is no longer opposed by the lytic effect of antagonistic hormones. By and large, hepatic parenchymal disturbances and metabolic liver insufficiency are not uncommon conditions in late life. Ayre has shown the presence of hepatic insufficiency with hypothiaminosis in elderly women suffering from the syndrome of hyperestrinism.

Accumulation of estrogens in postmenopausal women, and the pathologic consequences resulting from such cumulative effects, would thus appear to be due to *failure of estrogen breakdown* rather than *excessive estrogen synthesis.*

17.4.9. HEPATIC INSUFFICIENCY IN THE CLIMACTERIUM

Hormonal factors play an important part in hepatic insufficiency of the climacterium, causing, in turn—as we have just indicated—hyperestrinism through faulty inactivation of estrogens. Liver disturbances in women of that age group are common enough to have prompted French authors to describe a "hepato-ovarian syndrome," which shall be discussed in a later chapter (Chapter 28). It is also possible that, in association with the increasing incidence of hepatic parenchymal pathology during the climacterium, the uterine enzyme system catalyzing estrogen degradation is weakened.

17.5. CLINICAL EFFECTS OF SEXUAL SECRETION IN WOMEN AFTER THE CLIMACTERIUM

Two clinical problems, intimately related with the foregoing considerations, deserve some comment. One involves the question of senile metropathy, the other that of malignant degeneration in the uterus and breast of aged women.

17.5.1. SENILE METROPATHY

Under the name of senile or postclimacteric metropathy we classify those cases of functional metrorrhagia which have their onset at least two years after menopause. At our clinic, Nogales[46, 47] made a detailed study of such cases. For many years, only theca and granulosa tumors were thought to produce such syndromes; today, they are known to occur in the presence of atretic and afunctional ovaries. The mechanism involved has already been described. Metropathy is caused by hyperestrinism, which in turn can be attributed to adrenal estrogen synthesis coincident with deficient hepatic estrogen degradation. The loss of estrogen-inactivating capacity by the senile body is decisively aggravated by lack of progesterone activity.

17.5.2. MALIGNANT DEGENERATION OF THE UTERUS AND BREAST

In a recent publication,[12] we examined the question of postclimacteric estrogens in relation to the genesis of some hormone-dependent carcinomas, such as those of the breast and those of the endometrium. Concerning this topic, the reader is referred to Chapter 45. Although a direct relationship between estrogens and such tumors has not been established, there is nevertheless reason to believe that hyperestrogenism may facilitate the development of malignancy. The type of hyperestrinism involved is one of *rhythm* rather than *quantity*. On the other hand, such hyperestrinism has been also observed to occur in women without carcinoma with nearly the same frequency. At any rate, there is no doubt that *the frequent occurrence of elevated and continuous levels of estrogenemia in women over 50 is a factor predisposing to carcinogenesis at this phase of life.*

REFERENCES

1. Albert, A., et al.: *J. Clin. Endocr.*, 18:453, 1958.
2. Albert, A., and Rosemberg, E.: *J. Clin. Endocr.*, 19:518, 1959.
3. Albeaux-Fernet, M., et al.: *L'Année Endocrinologique*, 18:165, 1966.
4. Albeaux-Fernet, M., et al.: *Sem. Hôp. Paris*, 3:79, 1950.
5. Berger, J.: *Acta Cytol.*, 1:78, 1957.
6. Bonfirraro, G., and Sensi, G.: *Riv. Ost. Ginec. (Firenze)*, 21:668, 1966.
7. Bigelow, B.: *Obstet. Gynec.*, 11:487, 1958.
8. Boschann, H. W.: *Acta Cytol.*, 2:611, 1958.
9. Bostelmann, W.: *Endokrinologie*, 54:56, 1969.
10. Botella, J.: *Arch. Gynäk.*, 183:75, 1953.
11. Botella, J.: *Rev. Iber. Endocr.*, 4:417, 1957.
12. Botella, J.: *Proceed. 1st Internat. Cong. Exfoliative Cytology*, Vienna, 1961. Philadelphia, J. B. Lippincott, 1962.
13. Botella, J.: *Arch. Fac. Med. (Madrid)*, 3:307, 1963.
14. Bourg, R., and Pundel, J. P.: *Acta Obst. Gyn. Hisp. Lus.*, 1:62, 1961.
15. Bret, J., and Bardiaux, M.: *Rev. Franç. Gynec.*, 50:295, 1955.
16. Brown, P. S.: *J. Endocr.*, 25:427, 1963.
17. Buzzoni, P., Curiel, P., and Noci, L.: *Riv. Ost. Ginec. (Firenze)*, 23:457, 1968.
18. Carcatzoulis, S.: *Presse Med.*, 52:2375, 1961.
19. Coble, Y. D., Kohler, P., Cargille, C. M., and Ross, G. T.: *J. Clin. Invest.*, 48:359, 1969.
20. Corner, G. W.: *Contrib. Embryol.*, 45:344, 1948.
21. Cozens, D. A., and Nelson, M. M.: *Endocrinology*, 68:767, 1961.
22. Craig, J. M.: *Amer. J. Obstet. Gynec.*, 97:100, 1968.
23. Diczfalusy, E., and Lauritzen, C.: *Oestrogene beim Menschen.* Berlin, Springer, 1961.
24. Fekete, E., and Little, C.: *Cancer Res.*, 5:220, 1945.
25. Ferin, J.: *Acta Cytol.*, 1:80, 1957.
26. Folsome, C. E., Napp, E. E., and Tanz, A.: *J.A.M.A.*, 161:1447, 1956.
27. Gompel, C.: *Bull. Soc. Roy. Belg. Obstet. Gynec.*, 28:71, 1958.
28. Houssay, B. A.: *Actas del II Congreso Mundial de Obst. Ginec.*, Geneva, 1954.
29. Husslein, H.: *Zbl. Gynäk.*, 73:1649, 1951.
30. Jayle, M. F.: *Ann. d'Endocr.*, 12:933, 1951.
31. Jayle, M. F., Vallin, M., and Bret, P.: *Ann. d'Endocr.*, 10:68, 1949.
32. Klotz, H. P., and Jayle, M. F.: *Ann. d'Endocr.*, 12:931, 1951.
33. Kovacic, W., and Loraine, J. A.: *Endocrinology*, 68:356, 1960.
34. Lauber, A., and Sulman, F. G.: *J. Clin. Endocr.*, 16:1151, 1956.
35. Lenzi, E.: *Acta Gin.*, 9:23, 1958.
36. Limburg, H.: *Arch. Gynäk.*, 180:260, 1961.
37. MacBride, J.: *J. Clin. Endocr.*, 17:1440, 1957.
38. MacCann, S. M., and Taleisnik, S.: *Endocrinology*, 69:909, 1961.
39. Magee, T. P.: *Acta Cytol.*, 11:179, 1967.
40. Marañón, G.: *El Climaterio de la Mujer y del Hombre.* Madrid, Espasa-Calpe, 1937.
41. Mattingly, R. F., and Huang, W. Y.: *Amer. J. Obstet. Gynec.*, 103:679, 1969.
42. Masukawa, T.: *Obstet. Gynec.*, 16:407, 1960.
43. Montalvo, L.: *Acta Cytol.*, 4:111, 1960.
44. Montalvo, L.: *Citologia vaginal, cervical y endometrial, hormonal y maligna*, 2nd ed. Barcelona, Editorial Científico-Médica, 1967.
45. Morris, J. M. L., and Scully, R. E.: *Endocrine Pathology of the Ovary.* St. Louis, C. V. Mosby, 1958.

46. Nogales, F.: *Arch. Med. Exper.*, 11:129, 1948.
47. Nogales, F., and Martínez, H.: *Acta Gin.*, 15:427, 1964.
48. Novak, E., and Richardson, J. W.: *Amer. J. Obstet. Gynec.*, 42:564, 1941.
49. Osmond-Clarke, F., and Murray, M.: *Brit. Med. J.*, 1:307, 1958.
50. Parlow, A. F.: *Endocrinology*, 74:102, 1964.
51. Parlow, A. F., and Hendrich, C. E.: *Endocrinology*, 87:444, 1970.
52. Paulsen, C. A., et al.: *J. Clin. Endocr.*, 15:846, 1955.
53. Pearse, A. G. E.: *Histochemistry*, 2nd ed. London, Churchill, 1960.
54. Plate, W. P.: *Acta Endocr.*, 11:119, 1952.
55. Poliak, A., Seegar-Jones, G., and Goldberg, B.: *Amer. J. Obstet. Gynec.*, 101:731, 1968.
56. Purves, H. D., and Griesbach, W. E.: *Endocrinology*, 56:374, 1955.
57. Randall, C. L., et al.: *Amer. J. Obstet. Gynec.*, 74:719, 1957.
58. Reifenstein, E. C., et al.: *Amer. J. Med. Sci.*, 4:466, 1948.
59. Roddick, J. W., and Greene, R. R.: *Amer. J. Obstet. Gynec.*, 75:235, 1016, 1958.
60. Roos, P.: *Acta Endocr.*, 59:151, 1968.
61. Rosemberg, E., and Engel, J.: *J. Clin. Endocr.*, 20:1576, 1960.
62. Rosemberg, E., and Engel, J.: *J. Clin. Endocr.*, 22:377, 1962.
63. Ryan, R. J.: *J. Clin. Endocr.*, 22:300, 1962.
64. Sala, G.: *Minerva Ginec.*, 21:185, 1969.
65. Sedlis, A., Turkell, W. V., and Stone, D. F.: *Bull. N.Y. Acad. Med.*, 45:271, 1969.
66. Sharman, A.: "The Menopause," in *The Ovary*, ed. Sir Solly Zuckerman. New York, Academic Press, 1962.
67. Smith, G. van, Smith, O. W., and Schiller, S.: *Amer. J. Obstet. Gynec.*, 44:455, 1942.
68. Stoll, P., and Ledermair, O.: *Geburtsh. Frauenhk.*, 20:263, 1960.
69. Strong, J. A.: *Lancet*, 2:955, 1952.
70. Struthers, R. A.: *Brit. Med. J.*, 1:1331, 1956.
71. Subrizi, D. A., Curiel, P., and Gentili, G.: *Riv. Ost. Ginec.*, 22:484, 1967.
72. Veziris, C. D.: *Ann. d'Endocr.*, 18:120, 1957.
73. Vignes, P.: *Gynec. Obstet.*, 61:321, 1962.
74. Wall, E., Hertig, A. T., Smith, G. van, and Salmson, L. C.: *Amer. J. Obstet. Gynec.*, 56:617, 1948.
75. Wallart, E.: *Contrib. Embryol.*, 45:118, 1948.
76. Wied, G. L.: *Acta Cytol.*, 1:75, 1957.
77. Zondek, B.: *Proc. Soc. Exper. Biol. Med.*, 43:570, 1940.
78. Zuckerman, Sir Solly: *The Ovary*. New York, Academic Press, 1962.

Chapter 18
FEMALE CONSTITUTION, EVOLUTION OF SEXUALITY AND SEX CHARACTERS

18.1. INTRODUCTION

Although we have endeavored so far to present as realistic as possible an explanation of existing endocrine correlations in woman, we fear our descriptions may have adhered to too rigid a cast. Reviewing the long list of physiologic phenomena enumerated, some based on human statistical data and some on animal experimentation, the fundamental fact that woman is not a statistic or a test tube but a human being endowed with a firm *individuality,* among other intangibles, may perhaps have been overlooked. Phenomena described as physiologically normal are the expressed average of many observations. The exact age at menarche, or, for that matter, the average weight of the ovary or the average height of woman, may be given in terms of the mean value obtained on the basis of many observations; yet, it would be difficult to find any individual in whom the exact measurements of what is thus considered as normal or average are reproduced. Women may be tall or short, and their organs may weigh more or less than their peers'—in a word, all the physiologic constants are subject to variability curves. There is great risk of error in *statistical medicine* of overlooking this simple fact, which is even more important in endocrinology than it is in other branches of medicine. It must be emphasized that there is no such absolute entity as "the woman," but only "women," and that if we must resort to making abstractions of woman it is only because of our need to be methodical in the pursuit of our study.

Having examined the endocrine correlations of normal woman in general, we must now analyze female individuality as a whole, but trying to distinguish not what all women share equally but, quite on the contrary, what is specific to each woman. Seen in this context, the individuality of a person is called *constitution.*

18.2. BIOTYPOLOGICAL CLASSIFICATION OF WOMAN

There are many constitutional classifications of woman; however, none is entirely satisfactory because nearly all are based on mere external physical appearances. Some of the accepted classifications rely on dividing women into longilineal or brachylineal, asthenic or pyknic, hypoplastic or hyperplastic, hypogynic or hypergynic types. However, such definitions emphasize *morphologic* features. Although external appearances serve as our most direct mode of recognizing female constitution, they are not really the true essence of individual differences—which resides instead in more profound phenomena—but are mere external manifestations of the underlying essence.

The biologic types of woman can be classified only by taking into account woman's physiologic characteristics and her genuine mode of reacting in the face of her reproductive endocosmos. It must be kept in mind that woman, as such, has her own raison d'être in the phenomenon of reproduction. Independently of sex, each human individual possesses constitutional characteristics affecting male and female equally but, inasmuch as each individual belongs to either one or the other sex, he or she thereby must have a *sexual constitution*, that is, a sex-linked characteristic as well. Essentially, female constitution is a woman's personal way of behaving with regard to the reproductive process and all its consequences.

18.2.1. THE TWO PHASES IN FEMALE LIFE

The ovary, as we have learned, is not a single gland but a double gland of internal secretion. Two distinct hormones are elaborated in it. Whereas, as regards reproduction as a whole, these different hormones act synergistically, their actions are antagonistic to each other in many aspects of reproduction. In the first place, they are *antagonists* in time, though they equally share the role of influencing woman's sexual life, since half of each cycle falls under the endocrine influence of the follicle, and the other half under the influence of the corpus luteum. Throughout the period of sexual maturity, the same cycle repeats itself uniformly, woman reproducing successively a follicular and a luteal phase, each different from and, in a way, opposed to the other. The follicular phase signifies the time of heightened femininity, whose end is facilitating fertilization (and, incidentally, attracting the male by virtue of maintaining physical feminine attributes). Once that final purpose is accomplished and fertilization achieved, the hormone of the corpus luteum appears on the scene in order to facilitate implantation and development of the ovum. Thus, while the follicular hormone is the hormone of femininity, the luteal hormone is the hormone of maternity. Femininity and maternity, although essentially meaning the same thing, and although one is the culmination of the other, are nevertheless two quite distinct phenomena. During the first, woman might be said to be oriented toward the external cosmos, living a full relational life; during the second, woman creates her own *endocosmos* in which, and for which, she lives. The cycle, which passes from the follicular phase to the luteal phase, is the ever-present leitmotif of woman's existence, taking her in circles around her twofold theme, always consisting of these two phases, follicular and luteal.

By virtue of the endocrine relationships of the two glands under consideration, the rest of the endocrine system—the pituitary, the thyroid, the adrenals—also pass through cycles which, though attenuated, are nevertheless real. In a remote way, woman's metabolism, autonomic nervous system and mental frame reflect a parallel phasic duality. Every woman is balanced between these two tendencies, which are completely equilibrated in what in the strict sense of the word is "normal woman." During the first half of the cycle, the tendency is strictly follicular and therefore directed toward femininity; during the second half, predominantly luteal, woman is oriented toward maternity. Normal woman presents balanced ovarian phases. She does not tip their balance an iota either way; she remains infinitely harmonious in her dual role of being both woman and mother.

18.2.2. THE FOLLICULAR SYSTEM

The ovarian follicle, main estrogen producer and hence promotor of feminizing changes, is functionally linked to the other glands of internal secretion, acting with them in concert. Follicular hormone influences the pituitary by provoking increased production of certain pituitary hormones (see Chapter 2). The latter are mainly gonadotropin B (LH) and thyrotropin. In response to estrogenic stimuli, the pituitary thus produces, on the one hand, ovarian luteinization, thereby completing and synchronizing the cycle, and, on the other, a thyroid hyperfunctional tendency, the latter also directly aided by the thyrostimulatory effect of estrogens (Botella et al.[2]). Since the mission of the pituitary acidophils is to promote growth and that of the thyroid to promote active morphogenetic changes, the existing ovarian follicle-pituitary acidophil-thyroid synergism leads to a frank tendency toward longitudinal forms of development, that is, the longilineal type. As already indicated in Chapter 2, the catabolizing effects of estrogens tend to enhance metabolic function and to reduce weight. Adding to this the effect of thyroid hormone, which is known to act in the same direction, it becomes obvious that, in terms of constitution, conditions of hyperfolliculinism lead at once to leanness, elongated forms, increased metabolism and moreover predominantly adrenergic reactivity of the neurovegetative system.

Naturally, it is realized that the above formulations are much too general and schematized. However, they enable us to better understand, as pointed out by Marañón, the fundamental characteristics of what later is to be referred to as the *asthenic type*.

18.2.3. THE LUTEINIC SYSTEM

Owing to its extraordinary biochemical similarity to the adrenal cortex, the corpus luteum functions in close synergism with that gland. At the same time, luteal hormone stimulates the pituitary in its basophilic components, producing follicle-stimulating hormone and possibly also ACTH. This closes a symmetrical endocrine cycle—however, one that is opposed to the previously outlined cycle in the acidophilic pituitary and the thyroid, creating repercussions of a totally opposite effect to the former. The glands stimulated in the process, the adrenal cortex as well as the corpus luteum, possess anabolic activity, which determines a tendency toward obesity and economy of energy. At the same time, the vegetative nervous system is attuned to a cholinergic type of reactivity, so that under the predominant influence of the corpus luteum, women grow more obese, they display economy of metabolic function, their nervous system becomes more stable and calmer, and their psychology is reoriented in an endogenous direction, all features characteristic of the pregnant woman.

In women that are well balanced insofar as their cycles are concerned, these two opposite tendencies are evenly matched, from the resulting equilibrium emerging "normal woman." However, the prototype of "perfect" normal woman is extremely rare. While ideal, it is certainly not encountered every day. Usually, a woman's constitution is not so ideally balanced, and she is dominated by either one or the other endocrine component; consequently a woman usually belongs to one of two main constitutional types, as tentatively outlined below.

18.2.4. ASTHENIC HABITUS AND PYKNIC HABITUS

Both the asthenic and pyknic habits are usually described together as manifestations of external morphology. The term *asthenic* applies to individuals in whom longitudinal dimensions predominate. Such individuals are slender and tall, and their fat panniculus is scanty. Their long bones are delicate and elongated. Similarly, the trunk is narrow and long, and the costal margins form acute angles (Fig. 18–1). These individuals have a tendency to develop visceral ptosis and low blood pressure.

In contrast, the *pyknic* habitus is defined as pertaining to individuals, male as well as female, in whom transverse dimensions predominate (Fig. 18–2). Such individuals are brachylineal, short in stature, with robust and solid limbs, well developed musculature and hair, with generally higher arterial pressure and a wider xyphoid angle. However, defined on the basis of their somatic exterior as they are, these types are of little consequence for female biotypology. If encountered in women at all, *neither type occurs solely as the expression of external appearances but rather as the manifestation of two radically opposed modes of sexual constitution*. Thus, the asthenic woman is hyperfollicular and hyperthyroid, slender, feminine and high-strung, as outlined previously; on the other hand, the pyknic woman is hypercortical, obese, robust, prone to maternity, with pituitary basophilic, adrenocortical and corpus luteum predominance of her endocrine system.

As far as their physiology and pathology are concerned, these two types have highly singular characteristics. Asthenic women tend to have an exaggerated follicular phase. As a result, they are prone to develop hyperfolliculinism, with accentuation of strictly feminine features. Their skin is soft and transparent, completely devoid of hair-

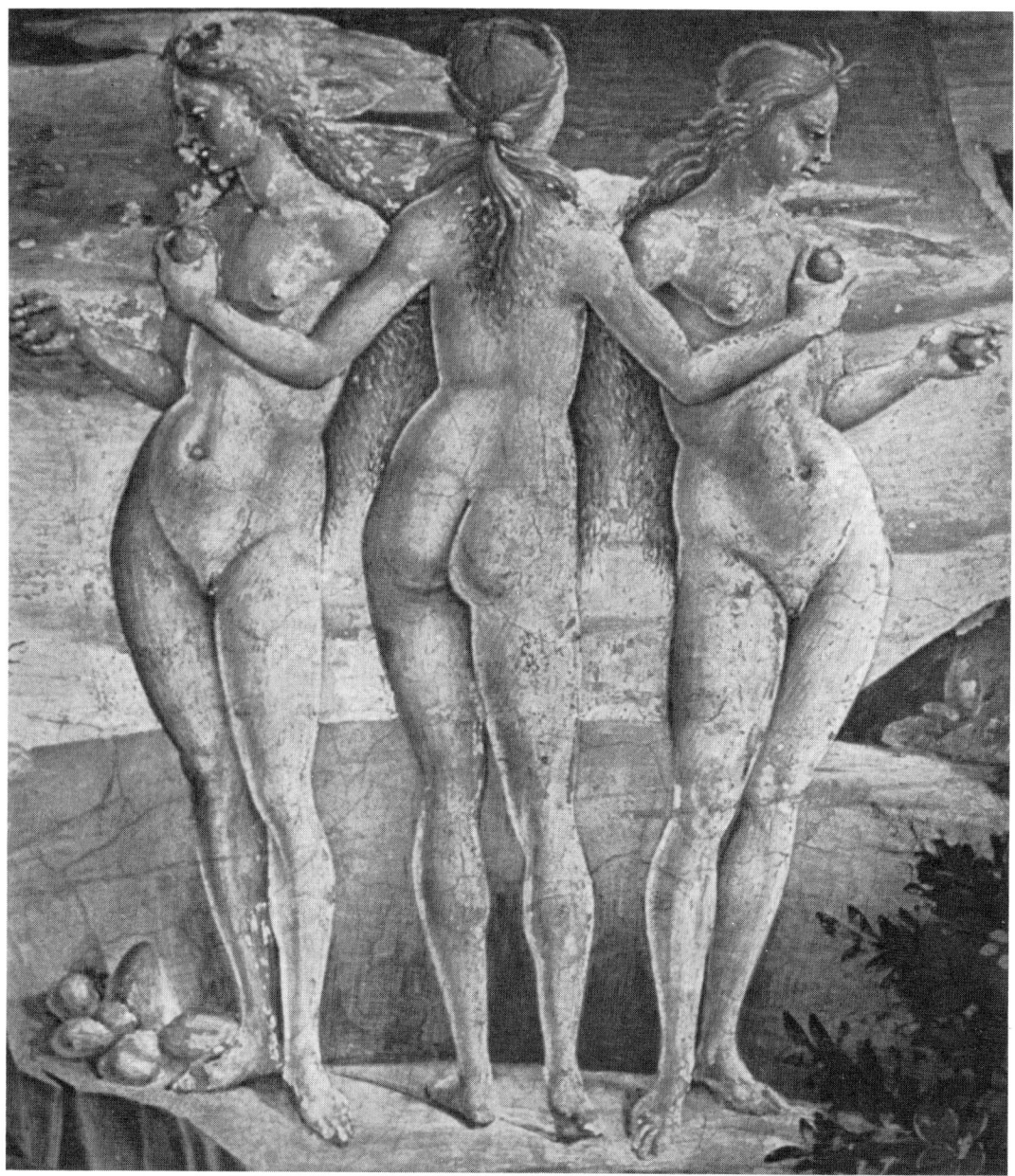

Figure 18-1. Asthenic woman in art. F. del Cossa: "The Three Graces," Schifanoia Palace, Ferrara, Italy.

Female Constitution, Evolution of Sexuality and Sex Characters

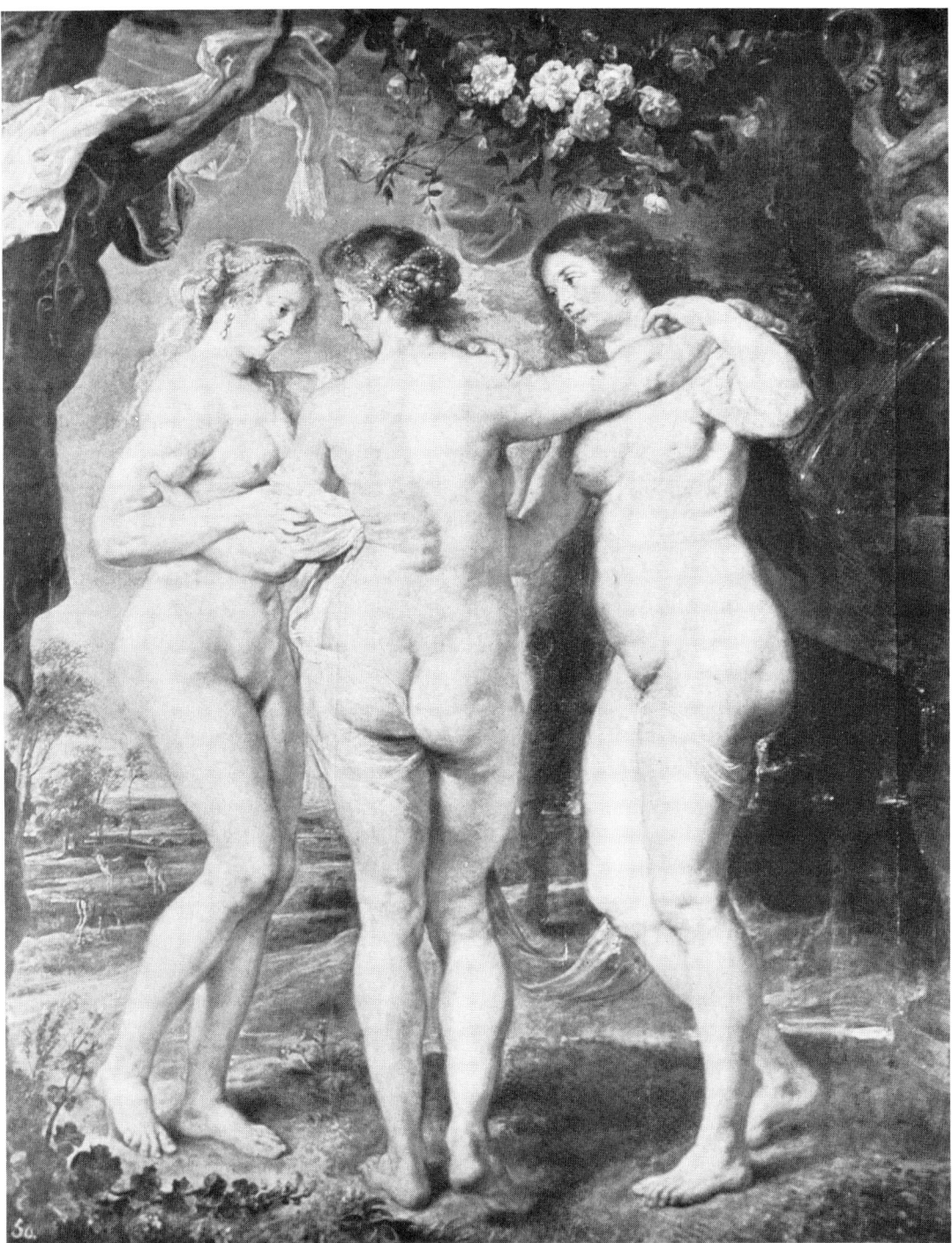

Figure 18-2. Pyknic woman in art. P. P. Rubens: "The Three Graces," Del Prado Museum, Madrid, Spain.

iness except for those areas that are normally covered with hair in women. Their shapes are graceful and elongated, and because, as we mentioned earlier, pituitary growth hormone predominates in them, they are tall women with relatively small transverse diameters and pronounced longitudinal proportions. Somatically, the asthenic type develops as a result of depressed activity on part of the system pertaining to the opposite phase, the adrenocortical system, which in this case acts "by default." This picture is due in large measure to the hyperthyroid tendency of these women and to their elevated metabolism. Asthenic women are very feminine but less fertile; they appeal to the male but lack the deep-rooted drive for motherhood and do not usually have many children. Confronted with pregnancy, labor and the puerperium, they behave as the constitutionally weaker type, predisposed to vomiting and habitual abortion. The frequent presence of a retroflexed uterus plays a contributory role in abortion. Labor in these women is usually prolonged because uterine contractions are less energetic, and also because the occurrence of narrow pelves in them is not uncommon. Finally, after delivery they are poor nursing mothers. In essence, this broadly outlined picture represents what we shall call asthenic habitus, understanding full well that, so far as we are concerned, the term does not denote any actual somatic morphologic character, as it may to most other authors, but rather a *sexual state* which expresses itself through a constellation of functional and morphologic manifestations.

The opposite biotype, that of the hyperluteinic woman, as we have indicated above, refers to the hypercortical and basophilic hyperpituitary woman. Predominance of this second kind of endocrine makeup makes for a short woman with a tendency to obesity. Her transverse diameters are wider than those of the asthenic type and her morphologic appearance is brachylineal. Adrenocortical predominance imparts to her musculature a more vigorous tonus, while pituitary predominance predisposes her to plethora and hypertension. The progestational phase is accentuated and anovulatory cycles are rare. Better developed genitalia render her more fertile and more liable to achieve pregnancy. Her less excitable, more relaxed frame of mind makes her more quiet and affable. On account of associated virilizing adrenal effects, these women tend to be slightly hypertrichous and in general less feminine than the other type. Their gestations generally have an uneventful course, their deliveries are easy and they usually nurse well.

This type has perhaps been somewhat caricatured in comparison to the preceding one. Apart from existing in the minds of physicians and biologists, the forms described for each type can also be encountered in art and in literature. In the first edition of this book,[1] we drew attention to the fact that the women depicted by Botticelli or by the early Flemish and Italian masters were predominantly of the asthenic type, whereas the women in the paintings of Rubens, Jordaens, Rembrandt and other Dutch masters represented the typical pyknic habitus (Fig. 18-2). Perhaps the most abstract and idealized prototype of woman of the Middle Ages and the initial period of the Renaissance comes closer to the asthenic type than it does in later centuries, which were marked by the prevailing pyknic ideal of the baroque period. Esthetic ideas undergo changes constantly, and so present trends in fashion have again made the first biotype, so to say, the woman of the day. In addition, literary works also describe the spiritual attributes of these two types of woman. In modern times, Maurois[11] reflected on the two contrasting characters involved in one of his best-known novels. But even the ordinary man's view of what woman should be like may range from an asthenic ideal to a pyknic ideal, a clear indication that interpretation of these values is to a great extent subjective and dependent on each person's own set of values. Thus, for instance, while Don Quijote saw in Dulcinea the quintessence of idealized womanhood, and the reader is certainly swayed to see her through the nobleman's eyes in the same light, the more realistic Sancho presented her as a refreshing robust country girl, certainly a potentially good mother of family, that is, of a pyknic habitus.

It may be agreed, however, that neither type is actually 100 per cent woman. Only a mixture containing ingredients of both types in exact proportions could give the average or standard woman.

Such a perfect example of balance

between womanhood and motherhood, between asthenic and pyknic, would be perfect woman. Let us not commit the error, though, in believing that, because it represents the model of "perfect" femininity, such woman must occur normally, in other words, in commonplace existence. The type of woman encountered in ordinary life is equally divided between more or less asthenic and more or less pyknic, because real balance between the two types is extremely difficult to achieve.

18.3. CONSTITUTIONAL FORMS OF DEVELOPMENT

We have so far considered constitution solely on the basis of the inherent balance between the follicular and the luteal phases of the cycle. Thus, we have not taken into account the fact that woman's sexuality actually develops throughout the course of her life in a continuous process of growth, reaching its peak at maturity and slowly declining until the climacterium. Accordingly, the presence of insufficiently pronounced female sex characters may be viewed as reflecting a juvenile or infantile constitutional state, whereas, in the light of the doctrine of evolution of sexuality, excessive characterization of such sex traits enables us to suspect a biotype that is deviated toward the male sex. Up to this point, we have contemplated the question in a dimension that, so to say, passes transversely from the asthenic to the pyknic type. Let us now examine woman's constitutional evolution in a chronologic order of sequence, as it takes place between childhood and senility.

It may then be realized that woman does not represent any fixed entity. She begins by being a girl and, after a variable evolution, reaches climacterium by presenting a tendency to virilization. Were we now to compare an adult woman with both a child and a man, it would be evident that, biotypologically, adult woman represents an intermediate stage between the latter two (Seitz[15]). On this basis, Marañón[9] formulated his theory of evolution of sexuality, which has been amply outlined in his works and will be later analyzed here. According to this view, *the female sex does not represent an end stage of evolution but a state intermediate between infancy and virility*. A number of endocrine characteristics, which are discussed below, rather than woman's somatic features, enable us to view female constitution in a new dimension, ranging from the infantile constitution to the viriloid or intersexual type. Just as normal woman stands halfway between the asthenic and the pyknic types, when seen in a different light, she also stands midway between the hypoplastic and intersexual types. Woman enters sexual life at puberty still with infantile features. Should the latter persist, she will retain those infantile characteristics throughout life, most probably in the form of a hypoplastic and babylike appearance. With increasing age, the feminine features grow more pronounced. However, once the phase of sexual maturity is over, the virile characters become apparent with the beginning of the climacterium, as indicated in more detail in Chapter 17. In this way, woman is always more or less intersexual in the closing years of her life, and while her feminine features are being gradually effaced, other, frankly heterologous features, those pertaining to the opposite sex, begin to predominate.

18.3.1. CHARACTERISTICS OF THE HYPOPLASTIC BIOTYPE

The features characterizing the hypoplastic type are well known. These are usually women that are short in stature, with scanty somatic development. Their short stature, however, must not be confused with dwarfism, which is a pathologic state usually stemming from a pituitary condition, though occasionally also directly related to ovarian function and to sexual life. Short as they are, hypoplastic women are never dwarfish. Their somatic development is exiguous, they are usually not obese and their bony skeleton is small, light and graceful, similar to the infantile skeleton. The external sex characters are poorly developed. Breasts are small and occasionally absent. The pubic hair is poorly developed and generally silky and thin. Axillary hair is similarly scanty and may sometimes be absent. The hair of the scalp is fine, similar to that of a child. The skin of these women is pale and soft. Their voices are high pitched and their temperaments are ingenuous and placid. As for their genitalia, the uterus is usually hypoplastic or infantile, menses are scanty and puberty frequently has a late onset. In short, at the age of 30 or even later, these women may still appear to be at puberty.

Endocrinologically speaking, these women are, as shall be seen later, protagonists of ovarian insufficiency. On rare occasions, such ovarian insufficiency may manifest itself by congenital ovarian atresia (Turner's syndrome). It is of interest to note that features already outlined are precisely most pronounced in Turner's syndrome (see Chapter 27).

18.3.2. CHARACTERISTICS OF INTERSEXUAL WOMAN

The intersexual woman, on the other hand, is well developed. Occasionally, her musculoskeletal system is comparable to that of the male. Shoulder girth may be so well developed as to exceed pelvic measurements. Female curves are equally poorly developed, while hair growth is abundant, assuming a viriloid distribution, filling the mons pubis and extending in the midline toward the umbilicus. Axillary hair is also abundant and so may be the hair over the upper and lower extremities. Not infrequently, light fuzzy growth may appear over the upper lip and chin. Nevertheless, such viriloid manifestations are very discreet and barely perceptible in the intersexual habitus. Whenever apparent in an ostensible manner, they indicate a frankly pathologic condition, discussed in a corresponding chapter (virilization). The muscular system in an intersexual woman resembles that of the male, and her fat panniculus is less abundant, giving her body a male contour. These women similarly show poorly developed female forms and their genital tracts may reveal defective development. Endocrinologically speaking, they are hypoestrogenic but, unlike hypoplastic women who in addition to being hypoestrogenic reveal scanty androgenic activity with low rates of 17-ketosteroid excretion, these women in contrast show evidence of hyperandrogenicity, excreting urinary 17-ketosteroids in excess of normal values. Psychologically, these women also show male traits of character and adapt themselves readily to male types of occupations, so that they may be encountered, among other diverse walks of life, in the liberal professions as well as in business. Women belonging to a more moderate variety of this type abound in our times, and are usually successful in sports and in what are traditionally male professions, contributing their own features of perspicacity with a resolute, jovial and masculine character. To a large extent the image of the stylized modern woman, broad-shouldered and narrow-hipped, agile and sporty, has been patterned on this type of intersexual woman. Both this and the hypoplastic biotype reveal poor adaptation to the reproductive process and usually experience difficulties at labor. Perhaps the increasing frequency with which difficult labor is encountered in primiparas is connected with the rising incidence of this biotype in modern society.

18.3.3. INTEGRATION OF THE FEMALE BIOTYPES

We have just described four fundamental biotypes. Two are oriented, so to say, transversely with regard to the theme of the sexual cycle of woman. The other two are oriented crosswise with relation to the foregoing, that is, in a plane encompassing vertically the entire length of biologic evolution of the female sex.

These four types are then *the asthenic, the pyknic, the hypoplastic and the intersexual biotypes.* By carefully examining in a step-by-step fashion the events that occur in the life of a woman, one may realize that asthenic features predominate in the first stage of her life, corresponding to the juvenile phase of her sexual life, and that little by little woman becomes pyknic, particularly as she achieves motherhood. Finally, virilization, although discreet during the climacterium, becomes a physiologic manifestation during the decline of her sexual life. Woman may consequently be viewed as an essentially changeable entity that, as a natural part of her life phases, passes through all the constitutional biotypes, evolving from the hypoplastic physiology of her pubertal period, through the asthenic type of her first years of maturity, becoming pyknic at the peak of the reproductive process and, finally, ending as an intersexual type after menopause. These four biotypes integrate female constitution as a whole. Intermediate forms between any two of the four indicated biotypes may also be found. Among these, one might mention a hypoplastic-asthenic type, a hypoplastic-intersexual type and, finally, a pyknic-viriloid or pyknic-intersexual type, although, to a variable degree, these states are usually the result of superimpositions of isolated features of one or another of the main types.

18.4. THE DOCTRINE OF "SEXUAL EVOLUTION"

18.4.1. GENERALITIES

In the first chapter of this book, we analyzed the true significance of sexual life. We have learned that sex arises as a consequence of a process of adaptation to the more complex requirements of metazoal reproduction. The emergence of sexual dimorphism, of relatively late advent on the phylogenetic scale, reflects the need for sharing the physiologic workload, as a result of which the species is divided into two kinds of individuals: one, carrier of the macrogramete, and the other, carrier of the microgametes. This kind of arrangement, whereby the sexual workload is shared by two distinct individuals, is only exceptionally seen in plants (dioicous plants) and, as a rule, exists only in higher animals. Within the realm of all living creatures, there are numerous species in which both sexes, that is, both types of gametes, are represented in one and the same individual. For instance, on the plant scale and, to a lesser extent, on the animal scale, there exists a vast group of hermaphroditic species in which the same individual is the carrier of both sexes. It would seem to us that differentiation of the species — and in this concrete case, that of the human species — into two sexes is consistent with the nature of life itself, so that our conception of the individual makes it extremely difficult to abstract these two sexes. Nevertheless, on giving due thought to the progressive degree of complexity involved in the human organism, it becomes apparent that division of the species into male and female sex is a differentiatory phenomenon of relatively late emergence.

On the other hand, in some species, such as bees and ants, individuals are divided into three, rather than just two, groups, viz., sexual individuals, male and female, respectively, and a third, asexual group of individuals, in charge of performing most of the collective work and the tasks concerned with relational life. Hence, in order to understand what we have undertaken to discuss in this paragraph, we must accept first of all the fact that sexual differentiation is a relatively late development on the animal scale and that division of a given species into male and female individuals is something relatively mundane as regards the nature of life itself in the individuals involved.

18.4.2. PREMATURE AND DELAYED SEXUAL DIFFERENTIATION

If the preceding assertions are valid with regard to phylogenetic evolution, they are certainly also valid as far as ontogeny is concerned. Sexual differentiation in all kinds of embryos occurs after a relatively long period, during which the individual has remained in an indifferent state. Even after the future sex has been determined as a result of gonadal differentiation in either male or female direction, many years are still to pass (13 or 14 years of postnatal life in the case of a woman), in addition to her entire embryonal period of development, before sexual differentiation is eventually translated into behavior, external appearance and sentiments. Therefore, the appearance of sexuality is a fairly late event even as regards the sexual development of the individual, even though bisexual somatic and functional features coexist in the sexually indifferent individual long before. Before the fifth week of intrauterine life, the gonad is undifferentiated. Until nearly halfway through the gestational period, the wolffian ducts, slightly atrophied as they may be in the female, persist next to the müllerian ducts. Conversely, the wolffian ducts of the male predominate only slightly over the müllerian ducts during the early phase of ontogenic development. Although the distinctive organs of the dominated, or rather, subjugated, sex undergo atrophy in the course of later life, they may persist in a latent form and may be discovered, at least microscopically, as vestiges of the heterologous sex, such as, for instance, are found within or in the vicinity of woman's genital tract. However, by comparison with the latent intersexualism present at the anatomic level, *the intersexualism persisting at the functional level is much more pronounced*. Thus, androgen synthesis in woman does not stop after sexual differentiation is completed, not even after the ovary has matured in puberty, but continues throughout life in amounts only slightly below those found in males, and androgens and 17-ketosteroids can be detected in the blood and urine of women. Conversely, estrogens are present in the male's testis, blood and urine. As a result, the sex hormone composition of the male cannot be accepted as different from that of the female, at the present time. At best, we may refer to female hormone predominance in the latter and to male hormone predominance in the former.

The latent presence of physiologic intersexualism comes to the surface under certain abnormal circumstances. For instance, coexistence to a greater or lesser extent of both male and female parts in the same genital tract gives rise to the phenomenon known as either hermaphroditism or pseudohermaphroditism (see Chapter 35).

Although it is of late appearance in man, sexual differentiation occurs even later in some animal species, particularly in newts and batrachia. In the latter animals, a kind of transmutation of one sex into the other takes place in parallel with larval metamorphosis and with the conformation of adult individuals. Depending on the species, some larvae with a predominant female sex may be observed later to undergo masculinization and to end their lives behaving as fertilizing males, whereas in other instances the opposite may take place (see Chapter 15). The phenomenon we are describing is known by the name of *Pflüger's hermaphroditism*. Generally, the species involved reveal a differentiated ovary on one side and an ovotestis on the other. The sex is changed by a process whereby the ovary atrophies and the ovotestis undergoes male differentiation, in which case the individual is converted into a male, or conversely, by atrophy of the testis and proliferation of the ovarian portion of the ovotestis, in which case a male is converted into a female. The occurrence of sexual evolution of this type in later life can be explained on the basis of bisexual permanence in all animals. Transformations similar to those taking place in Pflüger's hermaphrodites are not known to occur in the human species. Human hermaphroditism is invariably congenital but secondary conversions in terms of sex characters developing in either a feminizing or a virilizing direction are observed among clinic patients quite commonly. This means that the only difference between one group of species and another consists in the fact that mutability of sexual features in some species is fixed early, whereas in others it is fixed at a later stage. For instance, mammals are known to be species with *early sexual fixation*, as compared with amphibians and reptiles in which *sexual fixation occurs late*.

18.4.3. THE THEORY OF MARAÑÓN

In 1929, Marañón[9] enunciated the following theory: the female sex is an intermediate state between infancy and virility. The human species is born into the infantile state, evolves subsequently in a feminine direction and acquires masculinity only in the final stages of evolution. The male's puberal awakening of masculinity is preceded by a brief, nevertheless perfectly appreciable, period of femininity. It is during this ephebe phase when his forms are equivocal, his chin is beardless and there often is minor areolar engorgement announcing his transient feminization, pronounced in some instances, more discreet in others, but invariably present, only to readily open the way to the subsequent appearance of frank masculinity. By comparison, woman, so to say, awakens into femininity and passes from infancy to maturity without any transitional intermediate heterosexual stage, only to develop a viriloid tendency when she reaches the climacterium. Although climacteric masculinization may occasionally be quite subtle, it is undoubtedly always detectable.

According to Marañón, both sexes therefore evolve from infancy, and pass through femininity toward masculinity; masculinity is the end-stage of sexual differentiation in the human species.

This observation is within the reach of any clinician. It has been confirmed by a number of authors. Interestingly, in his book *Growth, Sex and Reproduction*, which must be ranged among the classics of reproductive science, Seitz professes the same ideas. Regrettably, he does not refer to Marañón in any way, apparently having been unaware of the latter's work. Marañón's ideas have similarly been ignored by the modern geneticists, who discovered that sexual evolution occurs on a much larger scale and much more distinctly in lower vertebrates than in the human species.

Marañón believed that evolution of sexuality actually resulted from an evolutionary tendency in the biogenesis of sex hormones, by which he meant that, since estrogens, of all hormones, were easiest to synthesize, they were formed in the body first, progestogens and androgens being derived from them later, in that order. We must confess that for many years we also subscribed to the same view concerning sexual evolution, explaining *biotypologic sexual evolution* on the basis of a *chemical sexual evolution*. However, the work of geneticists of the past few years has provided us with a more satisfactory explanation for this phenomenon, while at the same time confirming the prophetic nature of Marañón's observations.

18.5. GENETIC EXPLANATION OF THE THEORY OF SEXUAL EVOLUTION

The role of sex chromosomes in sexual determination is well known (see Chapter 14). In the human species, the female has two X chromosomes, while the male has one X and one Y chromosome. The same pattern occurs in all mammals, the male being always XY, the female XX. Man and donkey, or monkey and rat, for that matter, differ only in the number of autosomes associated with the pair of sex chromosomes: 44 autosomes in the human species and a variable number in other animal species.

During the chromosomal reduction process of gametogenesis, the male with a diploid XY constitution engenders two distinct varieties of spermia, one carrying a single X chromosome, the other a single Y chromosome. In comparison, each ovule is well known to invariably carry at least one X chromosome. The term "digametic sex" refers to the presence of two distinct modalities, or "clones," of sexual cells. The term "monogametic sex" is used when all germ cells are of a single modality. In mammals, the female is always the monogametic sex, while the male is invariably the digametic sex.

Monogametic sex may sometimes be converted into digametic sex, but not vice versa. This type of conversion occurs in lower vertebrates—for example, in fishes and in amphibians. In mammals, and above all in the human species, no such dramatic event as woman changing into man is ever possible naturally. What is possible is evolution of feminine features into virile features. The law of sexual evolution, as enunciated by Marañón, is a natural consequence of monogametism in the female and digametism in the virile sex.

18.6. EVOLUTION OF SEX IN LOWER VERTEBRATES

The uniform pattern of sex determination that occurs in all mammals (see Table 18–1) does not always occur in other vertebrates. For instance, the reverse combination occurs in birds. In these species, the sex-determining chromosomes are not the X and the Y chromosomes but two different types of chromosomes, called Z and W. Female birds have a sexual pair ZW and, consequently, are digametic, whereas male birds without exception have the ZZ combination, which makes them monogametic. Also, in some reptiles, the male snake, lizard or crocodile is ZZ, whereas the female is ZW. But even more interesting are the amphibians. Some of these have sex constitutions similar to mammals, while others resemble saurians. As in the human species, the male sex of the common frog is XY, while that of the female is XX, whereas the reverse is true in the toad: the male is ZZ, the female ZW. The South African frog *Xenopus laevis* falls into the same category and so does *Ambystoma mexicanum*, or axolotl, as well as the strange animal designated by naturalists as *Pleurodeles waltii*. The homogametic sex of batrachians and amphibians is always the male sex, with the exception of the frog, in which the homogametic sex is the female sex. Animals like these have served as ideal study models for biologists. Witschi[17] and his co-workers Foote and Mintz in the

TABLE 18-1. Mono- and Digametic Sex in Different Species

	SPECIES	MALE	FEMALE	CONVERSION	AUTHOR
Mammals	Human	XY	XX	Female-Male	
	Monkey	XY	XX	Female-Male	
	Rat	XY	XX	Female-Male	
Amphibia	Rana esculenta	XY	XX	Female-Male	Witschi (1923)[17]
	Bufo vulgaris	ZZ	ZW	Male-Female	Ponse (1925)[12,13]
	Xenopus laevis	ZZ	ZW	Male-Female	Gallien (1955)[3]
	Ambystoma mexicanum	ZZ	ZW	Male-Female	Humphrey (1945)[7]
	Pleurodeles waltii	ZZ	ZW	Male-Female	Gallien (1955)[3]
Fishes	Lebistes reticulatus	XY	XX	Female-Male	Winge (1922)[16]
	Platipoecilus maculatus	ZZ	ZW	Male-Female	Gordon (1946)[4]
Birds		ZZ	ZW	Male-Female	Gowen (1961)[5]

United States, as well as Gallien[3] in France, availed themselves of amphibians for the experimental study of sexual evolution. As a matter of fact, the embryonal period of undifferentiation is extremely short in the human species and in mammals in general, amounting to the first five or six weeks in man. In contrast, the period of embryonal undifferentiation in amphibians is much longer because sexual differentiation is not achieved until after metamorphosis at the larval stage is completed. Such animals therefore pass through a physiologic period of hermaphroditism. The latter lasts several weeks, allowing the animals to be studied under laboratory conditions, through subjecting them to different endocrine influences. In this way, it has been established that the homogametic sex can be readily diverted toward the heterogametic sex, but not vice versa. Androgens, for instance, are capable of modifying the original sex of larval frogs in the sense that in the adult period genetic female frogs turn out to be males. Significantly, the inverse phenomenon, that is, inversion of a gametic male frog by means of estrogens, cannot be achieved. The exactly opposite phenomenon occurs in toads. By treating toad larvae with estrogens, adult females can be obtained from genetic males. The validity of Marañón's theory of sexual evolution can thus be verified on these lower animals. The sex of frogs, which have the same genetic formula as the human species, evolves from female to male, but in toads, axolotls and *Pleurodeles* sexual evolution takes place in the opposite direction (Table 18-1).

This is further exemplified by Pflüger's hermaphrodites. These are undifferentiated hermaphroditic batrachians in which sexual evolution and development during the transitional phase from larvae to adult individuals are incomplete. Both these hermaphrodites and their larvae reveal the same phenomenon, namely, that virilization can be achieved in those species in which the monogametic sex is the female sex, whereas if the monogametic sex is the male sex, feminization is the rule.

18.7. PROTOGYNY AND PROTANDRY

The term *protogyny* denotes the existence of a monogametic female sex. The monogametic sex is also referred to as the *basic sex*. On the other hand, *protandry* is the presence of a basic male sex, that is, male sex with a homogametic composition of two similar sex chromosomes.

Accordingly, mammals are always protogynic, and birds and reptiles protandric, whereas some species of amphibians are protogynic (frogs) while others, such as newts and toads, are protandric.

It remains still to be seen whether the profound transformations observed in the course of amphibian sexual evolution involve any associated modifications or mutations of the pair of sex chromosomes. For the time being, this would seem to be the case; however, this is still an open question that has not been fully investigated. *Acquired chromosomal changes*, associated with sexual evolution, are currently known to occur only in worms. Baltzer has studied the sea worm *Bonellia viridis*. The male of this species is much smaller than the female which is equipped with a proboscis, or tube, to which the male attaches himself during reproduction. *Bonellia* larvae swimming at some distance from the mother's body are transformed into females and remain such for the rest of their lives. Larvae adhering to the maternal tube *are transformed into male larvae.*

All of this has been known for a long time, but what must be considered as a surprising revelation is the discovery by Humphrey and Frankhauser[8] that those larvae which, by virtue of their attachment to the maternal tube, acquire a male character do so by losing one sex chromosome. The evolution of sexuality has thus been clarified in this species not only in its morphologic but also in its chromosomal aspects.

The phenomenon therefore reflects an occurrence of general order which can be summarized by saying that masculinization of protogynic species, as well as feminization of protandric species, consists in simple atrophy or loss of one heterosexual chromosome.

18.8. MALE DOMINANCE IN MAMMALS

Predominance of the male sex in mammals can be inferred on the basis of many physiologic and pathologic data. Of utmost interest in this respect is the discovery by Jost concerning the mode of differentiation in rodents. This investigator opened the abdomen of pregnant rabbits, extracted the embryos and, after successfully castrating them, reinserted them into the abdominal cavity. The mothers' uteri were then sutured and, as a result of such almost magic surgery, the effects of embryonic castration on development and on sexual differentiation could be studied. Jost thus found that if males were castrated in the embryonal stage, they changed into females, whereas castration of females left the original sex unaltered. What at first sight might seem to contradict our previous assertions is in fact further proof of sexual evolution. It means that the genital tract of each embryo evolves toward the female sex and that only interference by embryonal testicular incretion determines that the eventual outcome be a male. This phenomenon, which owing to a fortuitous experiment of nature is also known to occur in Turner's syndrome of the human species, demonstrates once more that the basic sex of mammals is the female sex, and that the male sex is the result of evolution or differentiation. In the latter case, a male is "produced" by the androgenic effect of the fetal testis.

Much the same situation applies to the *adrenogenital syndrome*.[14] At one time believed to occur exclusively in females, its clinical picture also occurs in males. However, it is much less frequently seen in men, simply because adrenal sexual zone hyperplasia is less likely to be capable of causing feminization in the male. This is so because, as a result of the monogametic constitution of the female sex, and therefore protogynic constitution of the human species, any female-male direction in evolution is possible and indeed easy to realize, whereas evolution in the opposite direction is extremely difficult and highly improbable.

In other chapters of this book, it has already been pointed out that *sex hormones play a less important role in sex determinism than originally thought.* By acting on the end organs in their capacity as biocatalysts and morphogenetic agents, the sex hormones stimulate the development of sex characters. However, what imparts the specific response, and obliges those sex organs to develop in one direction rather than in another, is invariably the underlying genetic impulse present. This is what led us to assert earlier that sex hormones should be conceived not as nourishing agents but rather as decisive agents, necessary for the impulsion of the sex organs. *For many years we believed that the occurrence of chemical hermaphroditism in the human species might be the explanation for intersexual states. Without denying the limited role occasionally assigned to the sex hormones in producing deviations of sex, we currently concede much more importance to the role played by genetic factors in producing such alterations.* We therefore believe that *receptivity to substances endowed with feminizing and estrogenic activity steadily declines throughout life in the human species and, instead, there is increasingly greater receptivity to substances endowed with androgenic activity.*

Consequently, it is our view that, although it is remiss in achieving sexual mutation as complete in character as that achieved by lower species, or as that occurring in the course of the embryonal development of hermaphrodites, the human species nonetheless shows a definite tendency toward evolution of genetic sexuality from the female sex to the male sex.

18.9. SEX CHARACTERS

The term "sex characters" has been used frequently in the few preceding chapters. It refers to *those morphologic or functional features which are proper to the sex involved.* For instance, the male is morphologically defined by the fact that he possesses testes, a penis and other male sex organs, by his body shape and characteristic hair distribution, by his voice and by his character. On the other hand, the female is distinguished by the fact that she possesses ovaries, vagina, uterus, tubes, and developed breasts, as well as by her general body shape, hair distribution, tone of voice and feminine psychology.

Much as we may dwell on male or female features enumerated above so briefly, it is obvious that, insofar as their importance and the time of appearance of each are concerned, most of these corresponding features are in quite different categories. So, of all the characters listed, differentiation of the testis in the male, and of the ovary in the female, is first to appear during embryonic life. Only later, and depending on the degree of differentiation of the gonads, we may observe the development of either male or female internal as well as external genital organs. By the time of birth, the sexual apparatus of the newborn is composed of the gonads and a well differentiated genital tract, leaving no doubt as to the nature of the baby's sex. However, other than that, the body of a baby boy cannot be told from that of a baby girl. External or somatic undifferentiation persists throughout infancy and not until puberty does the male begin to be externally distinguishable from the female. Such female features as growth of pubic, scalp or axillary hair, tone of voice, breast development and rounded shape do not become manifest until adolescence. Much the same may be said concerning the corresponding characters of the male.

TABLE 18–2. Sex Characters

Primary:	Chromosomal (genetic sex)	Presence of XX complex in woman and XY in man
Secondary:	Gonadal (gonadal sex)	Presence of ovary in woman and testis in man
Tertiary:	Genital (morphologic sex)	Presence of vulva, vagina, uterus and tubes in woman, and penis, prostate, seminiferous ducts and accessory organs in man
Quaternary:	Corporeal (apparent sex)	Presence of female physical appearance in woman and male physical appearance in man

In the third Spanish edition of this book, we proposed dividing sex characters along lines suggested by Havelock-Ellis[6]: (1) *primary sex characters*, the gonads; (2) *secondary sex characters*, the genital tract, male or female, respectively; and (3) *tertiary sex characters*, features representative of femininity or virility, respectively. However, this apparently natural classification has been obscured by the concept of genetic sex (see Chapter 14). *If the sex of the gonad is determined by the sex chromosome, then the gonad is no longer a primary but a secondary sex character.* Sex characters would therefore have to be established and classified as in Table 18–2.

18.9.1. TIME TABLE OF SEX CHARACTER DEVELOPMENT

The *chronology of sex character development* varies greatly. Thus, the primary characters are developed most early—they could not be less so—since they are established *at the very moment of fertilization.* The secondary characters are established in conjunction with gonadal differentiation, about the *fifth week of development.* The tertiary characters are initiated shortly afterwards but are not clearly established until the tenth week of intrauterine life. Last of all, the quaternary characters do not develop until *puberty.*

18.9.2. DETERMINISM OF SEX CHARACTERS

As indicated in Chapters 14 and 15, the determinism of sex characters is variable, depending on the type of character involved. Primary characters are determined by the combinations of chance; the secondary characters are the consequence of the *inducing action of germ cells;* tertiary characters are produced by the *combined actions of evocators and fetal sex hormones;* and, finally, quaternary characters are the product of pituitary hormone activity (the gonadotropins) which, by acting on the respective gonads, provoke sexual awakening.

The sex characters are hierarchical. They are interdependent on each other in the same order we have described them in.

REFERENCES

1. Botella, J.: *Endocrinología de la Mujer*, 1st ed. Madrid, Afrodisio Aguado, 1942.
2. Botella, J., Amilibía, E., and Mendizábal, M. M.: *Klin. Wschr.*, 16:1001, 1936.
3. Gallien, L.: "Analyse des effets des hormones steroides dans la differenciation sexuelle des amphibiens," in *Le sexe*, ed. R. Courrier. Paris, Masson et Cie., 1960.
4. Gordon, R.: *Genetics*, 32:817, 1947.
5. Gowen, J. W.: "Genetic and cytologic foundations for sex," in *Sex and Internal Secretions*, ed. W. C. Young. Baltimore, The Williams & Wilkins Co., 1961.
6. Havelock-Ellis: *Man and Woman*. Boston, Houghton Mifflin, 1929.
7. Humphrey, R. R.: *Amer. J. Anat.*, 76:33, 1945.
8. Humphrey, R. R., and Frankhauser, G.: *J. Morphol.*, 98:161, 1956.
9. Marañón, G.: *La Evolución de la Sexualidad y los Estados Intersexuales*. Madrid, Morata, 1927.
10. Marañón, G.: *Ginecologia Endocrina*. Madrid, Espasa-Calpe, 1935.
11. Maurois, A.: *Climats*. Paris, Grasset Ed., 1929.
12. Ponse, K.: *Compt. Rend. Soc. Biol.*, 92:592, 1925.
13. Ponse, K.: *La différenciation du sexe et l'intersexualité chez les vertébrés*. Lausanne, F. Rouge Ed., 1949.
14. Riegel, B., Harton, W. L., and Rittinger, G. W.: *Endocrinology*, 47:311, 1950.
15. Seitz, L.: *Wachstum, Geschlecht und Fortpflanzung*. Berlin, J. Springer, 1939.
16. Winge, O.: *Compt. Rend. Trav. Lab. Carlsberg*, 17:1, 1922.
17. Witschi, E.: *Biol. Zblt.*, 43:83, 1923.

Part Five
GESTATION, LABOR AND THE PUERPERIUM FROM THE ENDOCRINE POINT OF VIEW

The menstrual cycle, usually covered in the first part of a textbook on female endocrinology, is merely intended to prepare the way for the true reproductive cycle of woman—the *gravidic cycle*. The latter begins whenever the ovum is fertilized, about halfway through the monthly cycle. The implantation of the resulting conceptus in the uterus marks the beginning of gestation. Implantation, pregnancy, labor and the puerperium are all associated with specific endocrine phenomena of utmost importance. Our study of these phenomena will conclude that part of the book which is concerned with physiology.

Chapter 19

ENDOCRINE PROTECTION OF PREGNANCY; TROPHOBLAST AND PLACENTA AS ENDOCRINE ORGANS

19.1. ADAPTATION TO VIVIPARITY

As indicated in Chapter 1, the transition from oviparity to viviparity involves very important changes as regards both the egg and the mode of embryonal nutrition. *New hormonal correlations are created by the development of a uterus, the necessity to prepare an implantation site in this organ, and the presence of the corpus luteum as the center controlling those changes.*

Viviparity is a phenomenon that is not confined to mammals but also occurs in fishes and reptiles. Especially in mammals, viviparity is associated with certain innovations relative to reproduction which, according to Amoroso,[5,6] may be summarized as follows:

1. *Reduction in the number of extruded ova.* Oviposition of hundreds or literally thousands of ova in lower animals is reduced to less than a dozen ova in mammals and to just one ovum in the human species.

2. *Highly improved mechanisms of internal fertilization.* As a result, fertilization becomes a complex physiologic process, giving rise to abundant pathology and, for the first time on the animal scale, to the problem of *sterility*.

3. *Utilization of the yolk sac or the allantois*, and structures derived from the latter (in mammals, the placenta), for absorbing the nutritional substrate and for eliminating waste products.

4. *Intracorporeal maintenance of the embryo* until the latter is sufficiently developed and, hence, the need for a new organ: *the uterus.*

5. *Emergence of endocrine correlations*, designed to maintain the egg in the uterus until term, far beyond the duration of the normal menstrual cycle—hence, the creation of the *corpus luteum* and *internal placental secretion*.

6. *Origin of lactation* as the means to feed the newborn.

The next four chapters deal with the subject of endocrine control of these phenomena.

19.2. NUTRITION PRIOR TO IMPLANTATION

It is a common misconception to believe that embryonal nutrition begins with the implantation of the blastocyst in the uterus. Westman's investigations demonstrated that castration of rabbits immediately following coitus led to the demise of the conceptus in the tubes and that this could be prevented with injections of corpus luteum extract. The presence of some nutritional substance in the tubal wall was therefore suspected.

The studies of Chang[36,37] seem to prove that a hitherto unknown substance, secreted in the tubal wall, is necessary for fertilization to be successful and for the morula to derive its nutrition while passing through the tube. Balmi[11] similarly postulates that some nutritional product, secreted by the mucosa of the oviduct, is indispensable for fertilization.

Mastroianni and his colleagues,[122a] using female albino rabbits, and Tanaka and Nakajo,[171] using hens, demonstrated the presence of a nutrient secretion in the tubal wall, the release of which was dependent on the action of progesterone.

In connection with the foregoing findings, the possible existence of a *nutritional tubal cycle* has been under investigation for many years (see Chapter 13), but results have so far been contradictory or negative, with the exception of those obtained by means of *electron microscopic techniques*, which enabled Bjorkman and Fredrickson,[19] as well as Stegner,[165] to confirm the presence of a tubal epithelial secretory process that is subject to cyclic changes.

The regulation of this "tubotrophic" nutrition, which is probably necessary for fertilization as well as maturation of the blastocyst, has been reproduced diagrammatically in Figure 19–1.

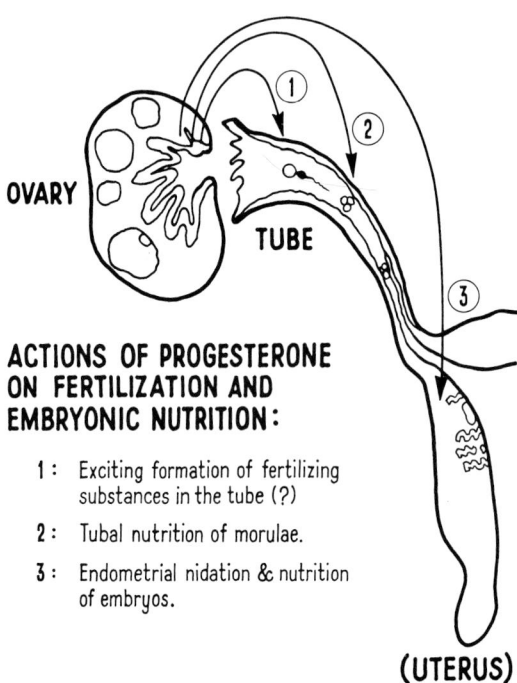

Figure 19–1. Scheme of nutrition prior to implantation. (From Botella-Llusiá: *Obstetrical Endocrinology.* Springfield, Ill., Charles C Thomas, 1961.)

19.3. ENDOCRINOLOGY OF IMPLANTATION

The process of implantation in mammals and its hormonal control have been the subject of extensive modern research.[33, 36, 116, 152, 153] Implantation takes place while the embryo is in the blastocyst stage, in woman on the seventh day (Fig. 19–2), and in the monkey on the ninth day (Wislocky[192]) after fertilization. Eckstein and his co-workers[53] investigated the question of which day implantation occurs on in different species (the sixth day in rodents, the thirteenth day in cats). Recent reviews concerning the physiology of implantation have been published by Canivenc and Meyer,[33] by Boving,[27] by Lutwak-Mann,[116] and by Shelesnyak.[152] In Chapter 2 (Section 2.3.9), the role of histamine in relation to the action of estrogens was mentioned; histamine equally plays an important part in the process of implantation.[122]

19.3.1. HORMONAL CONTROL OF IMPLANTATION

The process of implantation is mainly under the control of *progesterone*, but estrogens and *luteotrophic* hormone are also involved.

PROGESTERONE. A good many years ago, Courrier and Kehl showed that castration after coitus in various rodents blocked implantation and thereby prevented pregnancy. While repeating the same experiment in conjunction with the administration of progesterone in physiologic dosages, Mayer[124] observed that implantation did take place. However, if progesterone administration was discontinued at a certain moment, the development of the blastocysts was arrested and implantation failed. Similar experiments on hamsters by Orsini and Meyer[132] revealed that the number of blastocysts implanted was proportional to the dosage of progesterone. Fowler and Edwards[60] expressed the belief that progesterone could not act alone and had to be associated with estrogens in order to exert its action; nevertheless, Meyer and Cochrane,[125] as well as Hafez,[79] demonstrated that the simple addition of an adequate dose of progesterone alone was enough to

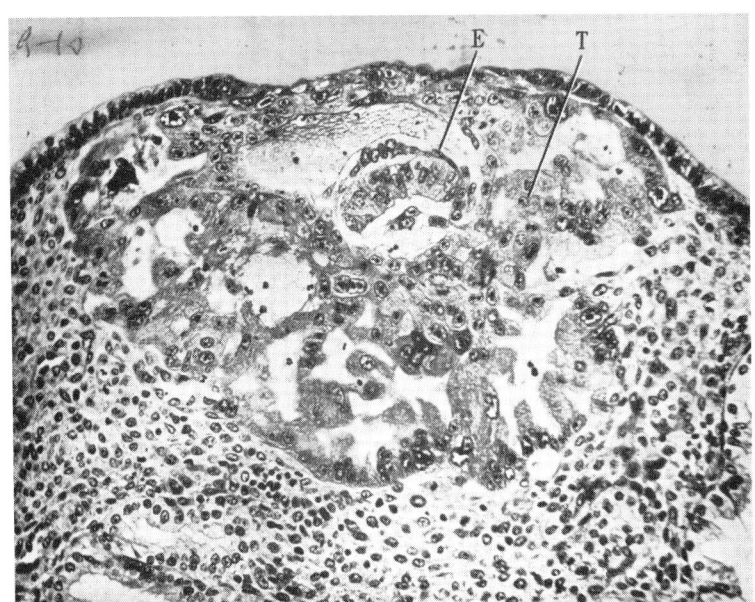

Figure 19-2. Human embryo, nine to 10 days old. *E*, Embryo; *T*, trophoblast. (From Hertig and Rock: *Contrib. Embryol. Carnegie Inst.*, 31:65, 1945.)

facilitate implantation in castrated and adrenalectomized animals.

ESTROGENS. As regards the mechanism of nidation, Fowler and Edwards,[60] Psychoyos,[139] Deanesly[43] and Smith and Biggers[159] emphasize the essential function of estrogens as *auxiliaries to progesterone*. The question has already been raised as to whether nidatory function is subject to progesterone control alone. The prevalent view today is that a certain ratio of joint progesterone-estrogen action is necessary in most species for implantation to be possible.[79, 118, 126, 153] Sugawara and Hafez[169] found that, as a result of castration, rabbits lose their capacity for implantation. The number of blastocysts implanted was shown to be greater when the animals were treated with a combination of estrogen and progesterone than when treated with progesterone alone. Estrogens are believed to cause release of histamine which, together with carbonic anhydrase,[136, 153] is thought to be essential for the alkalinization of the endometrium and for the process of implantation (see Chapter 3, Section 3.3.6).

LUTEOTROPHIC HORMONE. Berswordt-Wallrabe and Turner,[18] as well as Cochrane and his colleagues,[39] consider LTH necessary for implantation. It is not known whether the action of LTH is a direct one or whether it is mediated by a larger output of progesterone as a result of special stimulation of the corpus luteum.

MECHANICAL STIMULI. Implantation in rodents is known to be preceded by marked decidual hyperplasia, giving rise to a *deciduoma*, which must be formed in order for implantation to occur.[117, 125, 200] Masuda and co-workers[123] noted that simple mechanical irritation of the progravid sow uterus caused the progesterone level in the ovarian vein to rise. Orsini and co-workers[133] showed that local conditions created by the implantation of the trophoblast could be reproduced by means of mechanical or physical irritation of various types. De Feo[54] underscored the role of mechanical and probably *chemical* irritation caused by the egg in the production of the *decidual reaction without which implantation is impossible*.

HISTAMINE. Histamine has previously been mentioned as playing an important role in nidation, as borne out by the work of Shelesnyak's group.[122, 153] Ferrando and Nalbandov[55] found evidence that estrogens induced the mast cells to produce histamine, which is possibly related to the favorable effect of estrogens on implantation.

19.3.2. DEFERRED IMPLANTATION

The mechanism of implantation can be better understood by studying the phenomenon of deferred implantation. The occurrence of deferred implantation was discovered in deer by Harvey as far back as the middle of the seventeenth century and was scientifically described in the armadillo by Hamlett. It is observed in animals that once fertilization has been achieved and the conceptus has developed to the stage of blastocyst, rather than implanting, the blastocyst remains within the endometrial cavity in a retarded state of latency. It may live as such for several months only to resume development and to eventually implant. A kind of "ovular hibernation" is thus involved here, which stops ontogenic development for a considerable length of time. Amoroso[5, 6] has verified the occurrence of this phenomenon in the armadillo, the deer, the badger and some bats. The European badger particularly has become the object of extensive studies (Harrison and Neal,[81] Canivenc and Mayer,[33] Mayer[124]). The last mentioned author found that in the absence of progesterone implantation did not take place. On the other hand, Holkomb[89] noted that in the bison, another animal in which deferred implantation is known to occur, the period of latency is shortened by progesterone injections. Estrogens would seem to be equally involved, to the extent that a certain degree of estrogen-progesterone equilibrium, apparently in a ratio of 1/2000 (5 mcg/10 mg) is necessary for successful implantation of the blastocyst.

A similar ratio between estrogens and progesterone was reported to be most efficient in producing the necessary condition to enable the egg to implant at a certain depth in both the human and the rodent endometrium (Hertig et al.[85]).

19.3.3. ENDOMETRIAL HISTOCHEMISTRY AND IMPLANTATION

The fact that the presence of *endometrial glycogen* is important for implantation has been brought to light by several investigators (Hughes,[90] Botella,[25] Boyd[28]). Judging by the observations of MacLaren and Mitchell[120] on mouse uteri, in which only glycogen-containing zones were receptive to nidation, there is apparently a relationship between the capability of the blastocyst to implant and the presence of glycogen. In the human species, too, it has been found that lack of glycogen prevents the blastocyst from lodging in the endometrium (Botella[25]).

Significant progress in elucidating the *biochemical mechanism of implantation* has been made during the last few years. Whereas Vokaer and Leroy[185] believe that implantation occurs by "athrocytosis," American investigators attach much importance to enzyme activity in conditioning the nidation bed. Boss and Craig[22] stress the role of *succinic* and *isocitric dehydrogenases*. Prahlad[137] points out that endometrial β-glucuronidase activity is necessary to promote implantation.

Investigations by Pincus[136] have confirmed the presence of *carbonic anhydrase* in the endometrium. It is the view of various authors[27, 28, 116] that carbonic anhydrase produces endometrial alkalinization, necessary for the egg to be fixed by the endometrium. The earlier assumptions that had attributed tryptic properties to the trophoblast have thereby been disproved.

Before it is implanted, and during its first contacts with the endometrium, the blastocyst derives nourishment from endometrial gland secretion (Hertig et al.,[85] Lutwak-Mann[116]). However, this phase is short-lived in woman, usually lasting not longer than five days. In animals with deferred implantation, it may last for months, and in the sow, for instance, it is actually a physiologic state lasting for the entire duration of gestation. As shown by Grosser, the placenta of these latter animals does not implant and derives nutrition by absorbing endometrial secretion (uterine milk).

During the subsequent phase, the nascent trophoblast burrows into the endometrial stroma. There, it initially feeds by imbibition, that is, by establishing a *syndesmotrophic* type of nutrition, as we have termed it elsewhere.[25]

The endometrial glycogen content, analyzed in Chapter 13, also reflects the localization of these two types of nutrition with considerable clarity. While the glycogen within the glands is undoubtedly designed to meet the nutritional needs of the blastocyst, the glycogen in the stromal decidual cells would instead seem to be concerned with the nutrition of implanted eggs whose trophoblast is already well developed.

Hence, the distinction between glands and stroma—the two different elements involved in histiotrophic nutrition—acquires added significance. Modern investigations employing new synthetic progestogens (Pincus[136]) prove that these produce marked regressive changes in the glands. Under the resulting circumstances of stromal-glandular dissociation, the embryos fail to implant.

It is therefore important to realize that both *adequate development of endometrial glands and the presence of endometrial secretion are indispensable conditions for the implantation of the conceptus.*

The embryo, once successfully lodged in the stromal connective tissue and receiving a syndesmotrophic type of nutrition, has yet to develop its chorionic villi, and is in the "previllous" stage. The appearance of the first chorionic villi is coincident with an episode of implantation bleeding, known as the *placental sign of Hartman,* which occurs when the conceptus is 15 days old, that is, at the time of the first missed menstruation. Elsewhere (see Chapter 13), we called attention to the significance of that event. It actually marks the beginning of *hemotrophic nutrition.*

The phenomenon of implantation ends, so to speak, with the occurrence of implantation bleeding and the institution of a hemotrophic type of nutrition.

In this way, the normal boundaries of the hormone-conditioned correlations of gestation are demarcated. The trophoblastic villi will give rise to the chorion and, in due time, to the placenta, which will impose itself as the endocrine gland of pregnancy.

At the same time, and shortly before the time of the first missed menstruation, the cyclic corpus luteum (*progestational corpus luteum*) turns into a corpus luteum of pregnancy (*gestational corpus luteum*). This transformation is mediated by trophoblastic gonadotropin which henceforward is present in the blood. As a result, although the life of the embryo begins with the very moment of fertilization, *gestation, as such, is not established until after implantation.*

19.4. ESTABLISHMENT OF GRAVIDIC CORRELATIONS

The stimulus provided by the activity of chorionic hormone, which begins to be secreted by the trophoblast of nearly all animals at the moment of implantation, produces a new wave of corpus luteum secretion. In this way, the progestational corpus luteum is transformed into the corpus luteum of pregnancy.

In terms of duration, *the implantation phase* may be defined as the period of time corresponding to *the first two weeks of the embryo's life.* During it, *the function of protecting the new being is entirely discharged by the progestational corpus luteum,* by inducing the following changes:

1. Prefertilization changes in the Fallopian tubes.
2. Secretion of a tubomorphic substance by the same organ.
3. Endometrial gland secretion and nutrition of the blastula (glandulotrophic nutrition).
4. Stromal decidual reaction and appearance of syndesmotrophic nutrition.

19.4.1. PROGESTATIONAL REACTION OF HYPERPLASIA

It must be emphasized that up to the twenty-second day of the cycle the endometrium reveals the same histologic pattern regardless of whether or not fertilization has been achieved. After that date, however, a *hyperplastic progestational reaction of the endometrium* is observed[27, 28, 53, 153] whenever fertilization and subsequent implantation have taken place. This reaction alone allows the experienced observer, trained in histopathology, to suspect the presence of early pregnancy even though the embryo is not apparent (White et al.[188]). It has been debated (Foote,[57] Hertig et al.[85]) whether this hypersecretory reaction is caused by increased corpus luteum secretion in response to the incipient action of the fetal trophoblast, or whether it is the result of local mechanical irritation by the recently implanted embryo, in a manner analogous to the production of deciduomas in rodents.

19.4.2. THE GESTATIONAL CORPUS LUTEUM

The new set of gravidic correlations is established as soon as the progestational corpus luteum is converted to a gestational

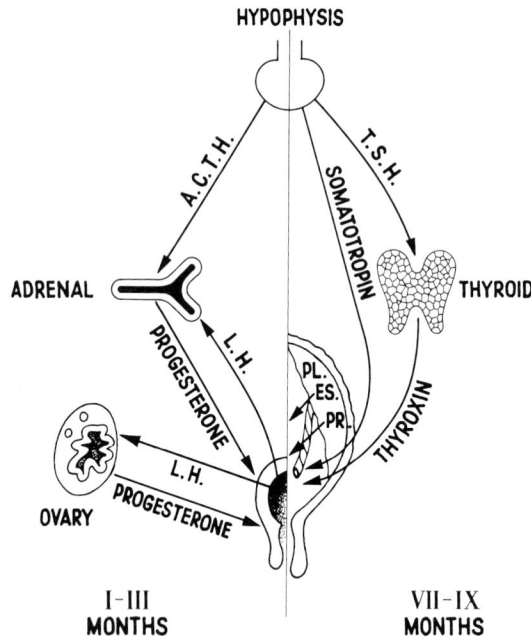

Figure 19–3. Diagram illustrating principal endocrine interrelationships of pregnancy during first and last trimesters. While progesterone is necessary for the maintenance of gestation for the entire length of pregnancy, during the first trimester it mainly comes from the gestational corpus luteum, whereas in the subsequent stages it originates in the placenta. PL., Placenta; ES., estrogens; PR., progesterone. (From Botella-Llusiá: *Obstetrical Endocrinology*. Springfield, Ill., Charles C Thomas, 1961.)

corpus luteum by the action of trophoblastic gonadotropin. The cardinal point in this change is the fact that, *from that moment onward, the pituitary surrenders control of gonadal activity to the chorion*. The corpus luteum thus formed is not equally important in all animals for the course of gestation. Studies in comparative physiology by Amoroso[6] revealed that lutectomy may be performed in women, monkeys, mares, cats, some viviparous snakes and salt water fishes from a certain stage of pregnancy on without causing abortion. On the other hand, bilateral ovariectomy was found to cause abortion[120] in rodents and in a large number of other mammals, irrespective of the phase of gestation at which it was performed. It has been shown by others, and also observed by ourselves (Fig. 19–4), that if a pregnant rodent (rat, mouse or rabbit) is castrated bilaterally and all fetuses except one or two are removed, but all placentas of the total number of implanted embryos are left behind, abortion does not follow despite ovariectomy.[6, 53] This means that the internal secretion elaborated by the placenta is not of the magnitude required to maintain the embryo by itself, but that the sum of progesterone-secreting capacity of all placentas is sufficient to maintain one or two embryos. In other words, the placenta never ceases to be a source of progesterone; what happens is that, while its progesterone output in some animals is sufficient to subsidize all needs of gestation, in others it is not.

Thus, by elaborating additional amounts of progesterone, the ovary is an indispensable auxiliary in the maintenance of gestation. Our own findings would indicate that the human trophoblast produces sufficient amounts of progesterone to be self-sufficient at a very early phase, occasionally perhaps as early as the beginning of the *villous phase*, and that even early lutectomy produces no effects. As also shown in Figure 19–5, we have collected sufficient evidence that *the adrenal, too, may aid placental function*. The trophoblast in young embryos of this early phase is already active and secretes small but sufficient amounts of gonadotropin that stimulate the formation of the corpus luteum. This amount of chorionic gonadotropin can be detected in the blood as early as the twenty-fifth day of the cycle (Albert and Berkson,[4] Bedoya et al.[14, 15]). Beginning with this moment, it determines the *persistence of the corpus luteum*, by converting the latter from a *menstrual (progestational) corpus luteum* to a *gravidic (gestational) corpus luteum*.

Once the egg is implanted, a new element is for the first time introduced in the

Endocrine Protection of Pregnancy; Trophoblast and Placenta as Endocrine Organs 399

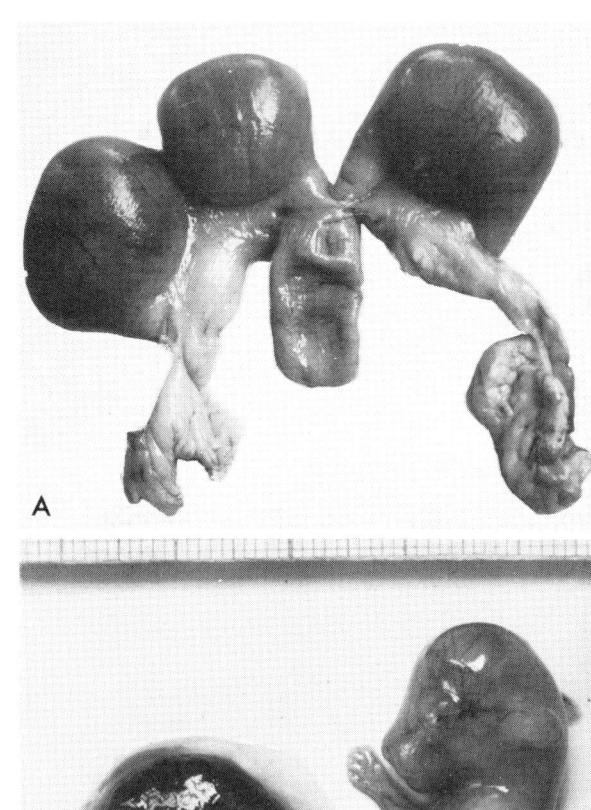

Figure 19–4. A, Unilateral castration of pregnant rabbit resulting in expulsion of two fetuses of five, while the other three remain retained. Gross appearance of removed uterus, revealing the three sacs. B, One of the expelled embryos, with its placenta.

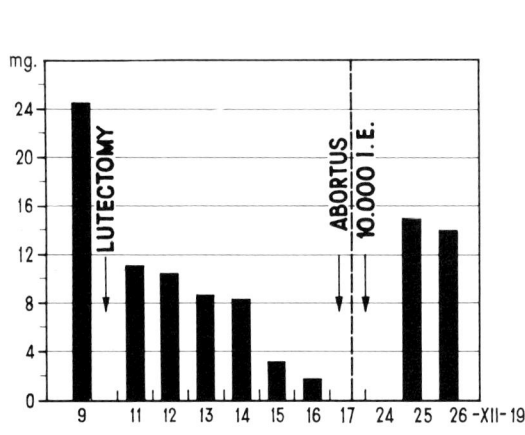

Figure 19–5. Pregnanediol excretion in a case of lutectomy followed by abortion. One week after abortion (with subsequent curettage), injection of 10,000 IU chorionic gonadotropin (CG) caused a rise in pregnanediol values. In the absence of both the placenta and the corpus luteum, excreted pregnanediol is believed to be derived from progesterone elaborated in the adrenal. (From Botella: *Arch. Gynäk.*, 183:83, 1953.)

mother's endocrine correlations, interrupting the menstrual cycle and creating a new situation, called gestation. In endocrine terms, gestation begins with implantation and with the secretion of chorionic gonadotropin, as a result of which control over hormonal correlations, formerly held by the pituitary, is henceforward taken over by the embryo.

19.5. THE PLACENTAL HORMONES

The concept of internal placental secretion has undergone a number of revisions in past years.[5, 30, 48, 192] What seems certain is that the human placenta produces two types of hormones: *human chorionic gonadotropin* (HCG) and *human placental lactogen* (HPL). Aside from this, a large variety of steroids are produced: estrogens, progestogens, androgens and corticoids, not exclusively by the placenta but also within the framework of the steroid synthesizing function of the feto-placental unit as a whole.

It is doubtful whether any of the other hormones postulated to be elaborated in the placenta are actually synthesized by that organ. These include relaxin, melanogenic hormone, somatotropin, ACTH, prolactin and thyrotropin.

Recently, while studying a rare instance of ectopic pregnancy that progressed to term, Friedman and co-workers[64] left a viable placenta intact at the insertion site within the mother's abdominal cavity. As a result, they were able to verify the fact that the retained placenta remained active and caused continued urinary excretion of large amounts of estrone, estriol, pregnanediol, HCG and HPL. In view of this, the foregoing substances may be assumed to be elaborated by the placenta independently of the presence of a live fetus.

19.5.1. CHORIONIC GONADOTROPIN (CG)

If there was any doubt initially as to whether the gonadotropins found in the urine of pregnancy were derived from the placenta or from the pituitary, there has been solid evidence, for the last 20 years,

TABLE 19-1. C-21 Steroids Isolated Chromatographically from Human Placental Extract* (See also Figure 19-16)

COMPOUND	AMOUNT (MICROGRAMS/KG)
Tetrahydrocortisone	6
Cortisol	4
Pregnanetriol-dione	20
Cortisone	90
Aldosterone	3
Dehydrocorticosterone	45
Progesterone	980

*From Salhanick, H. H.: *The Placenta and Fetal Membranes*. Baltimore, Williams and Wilkins, 1960.

proving their placental origin. Diczfalusy and Troen,[50] and Fuchs,[67] as well as this author,[25] have all argued in favor of a chorionic origin for the biosynthesis of gravidic gonadotropin, by now universally designated *(human) chorionic gonadotropin (HCG)*. Among the evidence are the following:

1. Diczfalusy[47] isolated chorionic gonadotropin from placental tissue. Its eventual purification was achieved by Adams and co-workers[1] and by Ashitaka and co-workers.[8] Midgley and co-workers[129] were able to prove definitively that HCG could be separated immunologically from LH.

2. Albert and Berkson[4] isolated it from the blood of pregnant women.

3. Gey and his colleagues[71] isolated CG from cultures of placental tissue, a finding to be later confirmed by Waltz and associates[186] and by Uher and co-workers.[178]

4. Stewart[167] similarly isolated CG from transplants of placental tissue to the anterior chamber of the eye.

5. A number of investigators performed hypophysectomies in monkeys[174] and women[111, 112, 171, 188] during pregnancy. In 1958, Little and colleagues[112] demonstrated that normal amounts of urinary CG continued to be excreted despite hypophysectomy.

6. By means of the PAS reaction, Botella and co-workers[24] and Zilliacus[201] demonstrated the characteristic presence of glycoprotein in the Langhans layer of chorionic villi, particularly in immature placentas. In view of the known glycoprotein nature of CG and the fact that the gonadotropic cells of the pituitary give a similar reaction—a reaction that is markedly enhanced by

castration—these authors feel justified in their assumption that the glycoprotein demonstrated by their studies corresponds either to the hormone itself or to a closely related substance.

7. Various authors[16, 17, 108] have isolated the same substance from the umbilical cord blood and have characterized it immunologically.

8. Finally, radioimmunologic studies[128, 191] have made identification of urinary HCG possible with a protein isolated electrophoretically from the placenta by Got and Bourrillon.[75] The identical electrophoretic properties of the two substances constitute a decisive argument in favor of their being identical.

19.5.2. PLACENTAL LACTOGEN (HPL)

The second of the placental hormones is placental lactogen, isolated in 1962 by Josimovitch and MacLaren[96] from placental extracts. Because its properties are similar to those of prolactin, with which it was confused initially, it has been designated placental lactogen. Turkington and Topper[175, 176] found that it likewise possessed somatotropic activity, promoting growth much in the same way as the somatotropic principle of the adenohypophysis (see Chapter 6, Section 6.5.3). Although lactogen is known to cross-react immunologically with the other two hormones, it has also been found to be independent of both. It may thus be considered to have an action intermediate between that of prolactin and that of somatotropin. Its purification has been achieved by several investigators.[56, 65, 177] With the use of lead perchlorate, Bollengier and Hubinot[20] lately obtained a preparation with a high degree of purity. Its estimated molecular weight of 20,000 was subsequently determined by Andrews.[7] It is a polypeptide which readily incorporates injected tritiated leucine (Friesen[66]). The site in which it is synthesized could thus be convincingly traced to the syncytial cells, bearing out what Sciarra[149] had earlier postulated on the basis of the close correlation he had observed between the degree of syncytiotrophoblastic growth and the rate of urinary HPL excretion.

PHYSIOLOGIC ACTIONS. There is agreement among most investigators[77, 98, 145, 155] that lactogen has an important diabetogenic action which is responsible for eliciting increased plasma insulin levels[76, 161] and increased plasma free fatty acid levels.[12, 77]

To a lesser degree, lactogen also possesses anabolic activity, inducing storage of nitrogen[12, 150, 161] and increased hepatic amino acid utilization as well as enhanced hepatic protein synthesis.[32] On the other hand, it differs from growth hormone in that it does not enhance radioactive sulfate uptake[87] by the epiphysis of long bones.[77, 145, 161, 176]

Like prolactin, placental lactogen exerts an important luteotrophic action, as has been shown by Grumbach and Kaplan[76] and by Sciarra.[149]

DETERMINATION OF LACTOGEN. Saxena and co-workers,[147] as well as Varma and co-workers,[181] introduced two methods for the rapid determination of lactogen, the former based on radioimmunoassay, the latter on complement microfixation.

PROGNOSTIC SIGNIFICANCE IN PREGNANCY. It has recently been recognized that lactogen determinations are of great value in the assessment of placental function (Josimovitch et al.,[97] Selenkow et al.,[151] and Singer et al.[156]) (Fig. 19–17). The relative simplicity of the above mentioned methods makes this an important future test of placental function (see Chapter 44, Section 44.5.4).

In Chapter 45 (Section 45.4.1), we shall mention some of the recent work that would indicate that placental lactogen may be implicated in the pathogenesis of gravidic prediabetes (see also Spellacy et al.[162]).

19.5.3. ESTROGENS

It is now known with certainty that the placenta—and even before that, the trophoblast—secretes estrogens. The main arguments favoring such secretion are:

1. The finding of high concentrations of free estrogens in the placental tissue (Diczfalusy[49]).

2. The fact that the fractions obtained from the placenta agree in composition and quantity with the estrogen fractions obtained from the blood[51, 138] and urine[31] of pregnant women.

3. Estrogens continue to be eliminated in the same proportions and quantities in the urine of women even after the ovaries

(Diczfalusy and Troen,[50] Diczfalusy and Borell[51]), pituitary (Little et al.[112]) or adrenals (Ryan,[143] Knowlton et al.[105]) are extirpated.

4. Animals with viable placental transplants to the anterior chamber of the eye continue to excrete estrogens even if they have previously been castrated (Stewart[167]).

5. Though Gey and colleagues[71] failed to extract estrogens from cultures of placental tissue, this result was subsequently achieved by Declerck.[44]

6. A final decisive argument comes from placental perfusion experiments conducted by Salhanick[146] and Ryan[144] in 1959 and 1960, respectively. By using C-14 labeled steroids, both were able to demonstrate estrogen and progesterone synthesis from cholesterol as the starting material. Ryan,[143, 144] and after him various other authors,[3, 141, 158] succeeded in isolating from the placenta components of the same estrogen synthetic enzyme system that is found in the ovary (see Chapter 2, page 28). It is, however, only fair to point out that not all estrogens produced by the gravid organism are of placental origin, since Cassmer[35] and Diczfalusy and Lauritzen[49] alike produced evidence that at least part of these estrogens are synthesized by the fetal organism (see Chapter 19, Section 19.7.2).

19.5.4. PROGESTERONE

Evidence of placental progestogen synthesis is based on the following facts:

1. Elimination of elevated amounts of pregnanediol in urine of pregnancy.[120] This is indirect evidence, but supported by the fact that such elevated levels are known to occur only in the presence of functioning placenta.

2. The presence of elevated blood progesterone values in pregnant women (Zander[197]), which disappear with the death or expulsion of the placenta.

3. The persistence of elevated progesteronemia and pregnandioluria after bilateral oophorectomy in pregnant women (Botella,[23] Diczfalusy and Troen,[50] Little and Rossi[111] and Loraine[114]).

4. The finding of high progesterone concentrations in the placenta, first reported by Adler, de Fremmery and Tausk in 1933, and recently confirmed by means of accurate methods by Salhanick[146] and by Zander and Münstermann.[198]

5. The previously mentioned experiments of placental perfusion which also demonstrate a high rate of progesterone biosynthesis in perfused placental tissue.[143, 144]

6. Venning and co-workers[183] have shown that women, castrated and adrenalectomized during pregnancy, continue to eliminate normal amounts of urinary pregnanediol.

7. Van de Wiele and Jailer[180] have found that the placenta contains specific enzymes that convert pregnenolone to progesterone, known to be also present in the ovarian corpus luteum (see Chapter 3, Section 3.5.2).

8. Some of the data concerning progesterone biogenesis by the placenta have been clarified by recent investigations. Jungman and Schweppe[99] reported the presence in the human placenta of all those enzymes of progestogen synthesis that are normally encountered in the ovary. Experimental studies on placental perfusion by Hellig and associates[82] revealed progesterone biogenesis at the expense of cholesterol. Aside from this, the placenta is capable of degrading progesterone to pregnanediol,[40] the latter being able to pass to the fetus where pregnanediol can be conjugated mainly as sulfate by the fetal liver (Cooke et al.[40]).

19.5.5. CORTICOIDS

The occurrence of an increased rate of urinary corticoid excretion has been fully demonstrated in pregnancy.[110, 183] Resection of both adrenals in pregnant bitches has been shown not to be followed by death because the placenta is capable of compensating for adrenal function at a very early stage. Ryan,[143, 144] in 1962, expressed the belief that corticoids in the placenta were formed only from intermediary metabolites rather than from end-products. Although this is true in the case of androgens, there is considerable evidence that the placenta produces corticoids and that the latter are utilized as products of secretion during pregnancy (see Chapter 20).

In their studies with placental perfusion, Salhanick,[146] in 1960, and Troen,[173] in 1961, both found evidence that all the corticoids, of the aldosterone as well as the cortisol series, can be synthesized in the placenta. From studies on interrupted non-term pregnancies, Pasqualini and co-workers[134] arrived at identical conclusions.

19.5.6. HORMONES NOT CONCLUSIVELY DEMONSTRATED IN THE PLACENTA

A number of hormones have been described as being elaborated by the placenta; however, their placental origin is still very much in dispute.

SOMATOTROPIN. Although Josimovitch and MacLaren[96] initially believed they isolated it from the placenta, they, as well as several others,[12, 144, 176] later identified the isolated substance as lactogen.

MELANOGENIC HORMONE AND ACTH. Shizume and Lerner[154] and Varon[182] found melanogenic hormone in placental tissue. The melanogenic factor is increased in the urine of pregnant women (discussed later) and the occurrence of "chloasma gravidarum" is well known fact. ACTH has likewise been isolated from human placenta by Cassano and Tarantino,[34] Jailer and Knowlton[92] and Lundin and Holmdahl.[115] Significantly, Smith and Hagerman[157] observed that, unless given ACTH, hypophysioprival pregnant animals died. Chorionic ACTH secretion would therefore seem to be necessary for the production of corticoids at the level of the placenta, the fetal adrenal as well as the maternal adrenal. Placental ACTH production would account for the fact that adrenalectomy is better tolerated during pregnancy. The modern trend to identify melanogenic hormone with ACTH has been commented on in Chapter 6. It is our belief that both types of gravidic secretions are one and the same substance.

THYROTROPIN. It is generally recognized that blood and urine thyrotropin levels during pregnancy are increased (see Chapter 20). Until now, there has been no evidence that thyrotropin is synthesized by the placenta. Recently, however, Hennen and associates[83] and Hershman and Starner[84] described a protein apparently elaborated in the placenta which, while possessing thyroid-stimulating properties, is distinct from thyrotropin both chemically and immunologically. At this stage, therefore, any definite conclusions seem premature.

RELAXIN. Steinetz and his colleagues[166] and Zarrow and co-workers[199, 200] encountered elevated placental relaxin concentrations in rabbits. The placental origin of the latter, however, cannot be demonstrated conclusively, since it is impossible to maintain gestation in ovariectomized rabbits. In the human species, this hormone does not seem to be isolable from chorionic tissue.

ANDROGENS. The previously mentioned experiments by Salhanick[146] and Troen[173] have led to the isolation of some 17-ketosteroids from placental perfusates. However, Diczfalusy[48] and Ryan[144] have never been able to isolate androgens from placental tissue, which seems to indicate that whatever androgens are produced in the placenta are not end products but rather intermediary products that rapidly disappear, giving rise to other hormones.

Despite isolation of testosterone and androstenedione in large amounts by Mizuno and co-workers,[130] and that of retrotestosterone by Dell'Acqua and associates,[45] from placental blood, the placenta does not seem to be a specifically androgenic organ. It must be realized that androgens are intermediary catabolites in estrogen synthesis and are, therefore, bound to be encountered, fleeting as their presence may be, in all those tissues which synthesize estrogens.

The placenta is evidently an important endocrine organ. Rather than producing any specific hormones of its own, however, it characteristically produces imitations or replicas of hormones of such other endocrine organs as the pituitary, the adrenal and the ovary.

19.6. SITE OF HORMONE SYNTHESIS IN THE PLACENTA

The site in which the placental hormones are produced has been the subject of much dispute. Three different criteria may be followed in determining the site of hormone production: (1) drawing a parallel between the degree of development reached by certain tissues and the rate of hormone excretion; (2) studying tissue cultures of chorionic cells; and (3) using histochemical methods.

Our own studies of estrogen and gonadotropin elimination in the course of pregnancy, as compared with the observed quantitative development of the Langhans layer and that of the syncytiotrophoblast, indicate that peak gonadotropin elimination is coincident with the period of maximal cytotrophoblastic development, whereas maximal estrogen excretion corresponds chronologically to maximal syncytial development. Nevertheless, electron microscopic studies have indicated that the Langhans layer persists to the end of pregnancy (Strauss[168]). From these and similar observations, it might be inferred that the site of estrogen synthesis is the syncytiotrophoblast, whereas the gonadotropins are elaborated by the Langhans layer.

The drawback of placental tissue culture techniques is the fact that tissues growing in culture media rapidly lose cytomorphologic and architectural features, so that it soon becomes impossible to tell which elements correspond to the cytotrophoblast and which to the syncytiotrophoblast.

So far, most data have been obtained by means of histochemical methods. In this respect, valuable information has been provided by the works of Wislocky and Padykula.[192, 193] From a large series of histochemical experiments, used mainly to detect glycoproteins and steroid carbonyl groups, the authors conclude that gonadotropin is synthesized in the Langhans layer, whereas steroids are the product of syncytiotrophoblastic cells and Hofbauer cells. The findings by Purves and Griesbach,[140] Zilliacus[201] and Botella and colleagues[24] concerning the correlation between PAS staining and gonadotropin values, have already been cited (Fig. 19-7). We further assume that the alkaline glycerophosphatase reaction is connected with estrogen biosynthesis.[25] Similar points of view are held by Lobel and colleagues[113] and by Bargmann.[9]

Puzzling indeed is the finding that gonadotropin production should continue till the very end of pregnancy (see Figures 19-8, 19-9 and 19-10). Deane and colleagues[42] and Weber[187] assume that this is possible because gonadotropin production is linked to cytotrophoblastic islets of the basalis, which persist till the end of pregnancy, rather than to the absorptive integument of

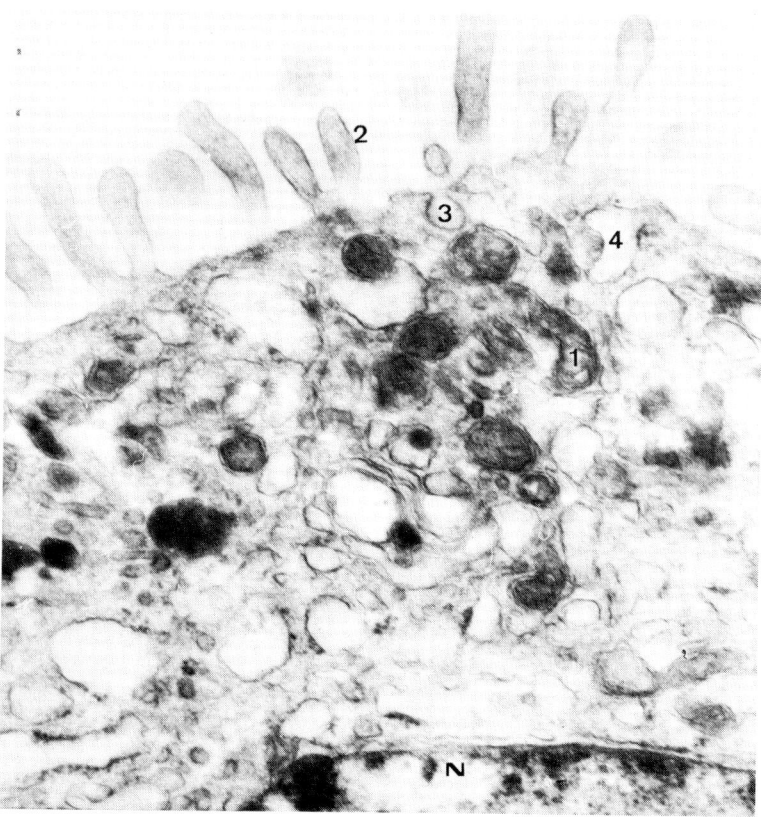

Figure 19-6. Fine structure of placental syncytium (37,200×). 1, Mitochondrion; 2, microvilli; 3, surface invagination (pinocytosis?); 4, pseudovacuole; N, nucleus.

Endocrine Protection of Pregnancy; Trophoblast and Placenta as Endocrine Organs 405

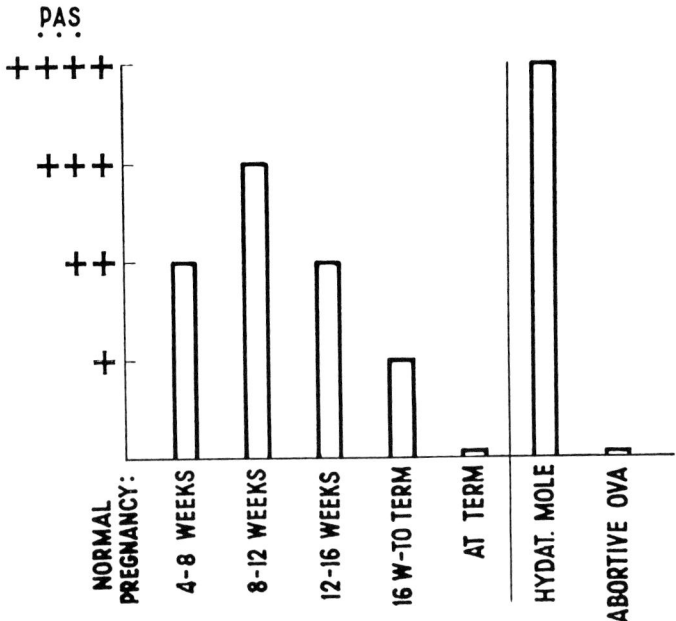

Figure 19-7. Intensity of PAS staining reaction for glycoproteins in chorion and placenta at different stages of pregnancy. Note that highest degrees of intensity of reaction correspond to peaks of urinary gonadotropin excretion. (From Botella-Llusiá: *Obstetrical Endocrinology.* Springfield, Ill., Charles C Thomas, 1961.)

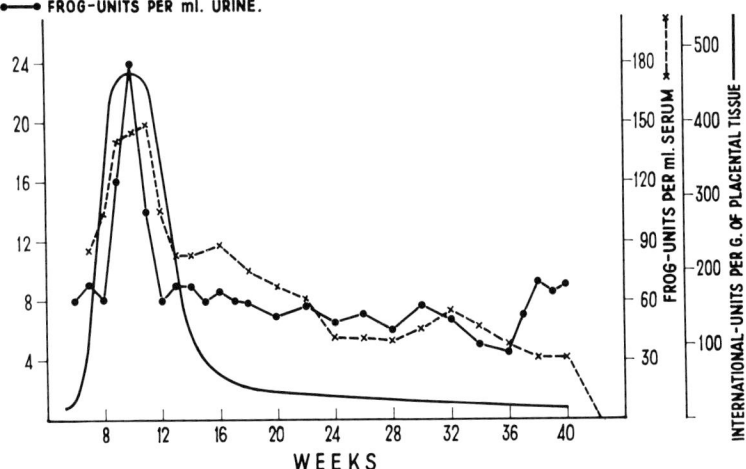

Figure 19-8. International units of chorionic gonadotropin per gram of placental tissue (from Diczfalusy), compared with esculenta units in urine and serum, based on data obtained at our laboratory. The three curves are similar.

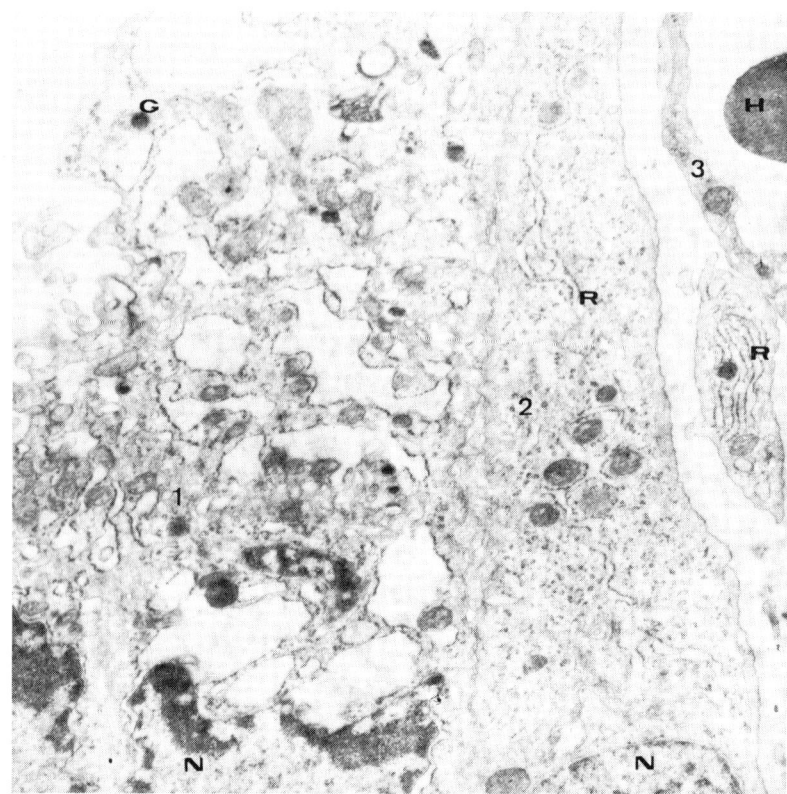

Figure 19-9. Fine structure of mature placental tissue (6300×). 1, Syncytiotrophoblast; 2 and 3, Langhans cell with endoplasmic reticulum (R) revealing evidence of active gonadotropin synthesis; N, nuclei pertaining to both Langhans and syncytial layers; H, erythrocyte in villous vascular space; G, vacuolar spaces within syncytium. Electron microscopic details shown here confirm persistence of Langhans layer to term and explain why chorionic gonadotropin secretion is similarly maintained till the final phase of gestation, as indicated in Figures 19-8 and 19-10.

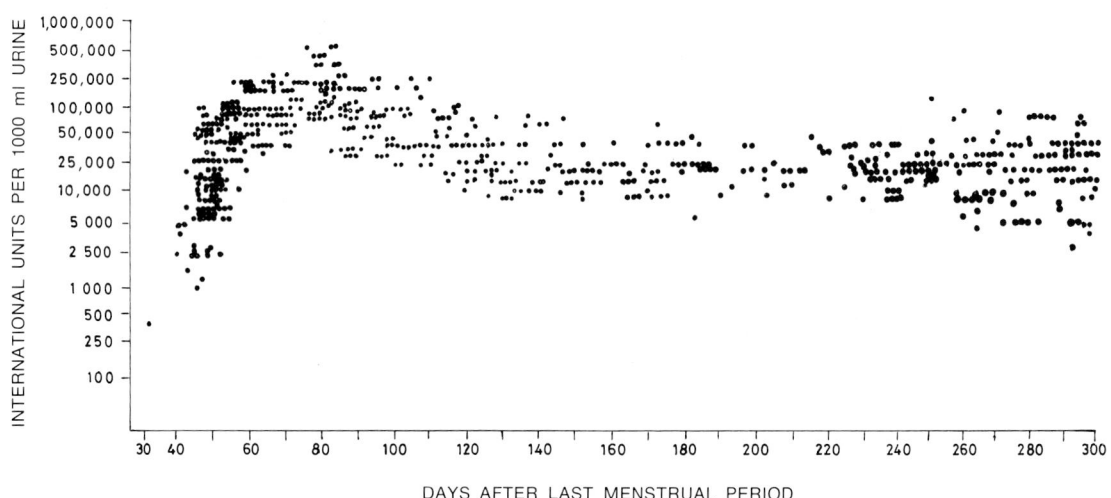

Figure 19-10. Gonadotropinuria curve during pregnancy, based on a large series of determinations by means of the hemagglutination method. (From Wide and Gemzell: *Ciba Colloquia on Endocrinology*, 14:300, 1962.)

the villi, from which the cytotrophoblast seems to disappear around the fifth or sixth month. However, as already pointed out, electron microscopic observations by Strauss[168] indicate that Langhans cells are present underneath the syncytial investment until the end of pregnancy (see Figure 19–9).

Incidentally, dietary deficiency is known to reduce the rate of endocrine secretion by the rat chorion,[101] while hypophysectomy reduces the gonadotropin content of mouse placenta, perhaps suggesting the possibility that gonadotropin is merely stored in the mouse placenta.[97] Finally, the so-called chorionic gonadotropin of the human species has recently been postulated to consist of actually two immunologically distinct substances.[80]

Additional and decisive confirmatory evidence concerning the site of placental hormone synthesis has been obtained by means of *immunofluorescent techniques*,[128, 191] which seem to pinpoint the localization of HCG to the cytotrophoblast of both young and mature placentas.

19.7. HORMONE EXCRETION DURING PREGNANCY

Placental biosynthesis of chorionic gonadotropins, estrogens, progesterone and corticoids raises considerably blood levels and rates of urinary excretion of the corresponding hormones. The wealth of information presently available in the literature on the subject is reviewed briefly below.

19.7.1. CHORIONIC GONADOTROPIN

Thanks to Zondek and Pfeiffer,[202] chorionic gonadotropin has been known to be produced in greater amounts at the beginning than toward the end of gestation, that is, to be primarily a product of the young chorion. Also, as regards its concentration per gram of placental tissue, the highest values have been recorded by Diczfalusy[48] between the eighth and sixteenth weeks (see Figure 19–8). Various authors[13, 51, 114] have investigated the question of gonadotropinuria during pregnancy, reporting peak values between the first and third months of gestation.

Maximal excretion rates, reaching up to 300,000 IU, are observed about the fifty-fifth day of pregnancy. Recently, Gemzell,[69] Brody and Carlstrom,[29] MacKean[119] and Wide and Gemzell[189] obtained similar curves using immunologic data (Fig. 19–10). It is debatable whether a second peak in gonadotropinuria occurs during the last months of gestation. Such a peak was mentioned in the original observations by Venning and colleagues,[120] and although it was subsequently denied, was described again in Gemzell's studies. We may then have to admit that gonadotropinuria increases toward the end of pregnancy.

The occurrence of pathologic forms of gonadotropin excretion and its semeiotic significance shall be dealt with extensively in our discussion of moles (Chapter 43) and abortion (Chapter 42). For the time being, suffice it to say that multiple pregnancies are associated with higher values (Neuwirth et al.[131]), and so are pregnancies of female fetuses (Brody and Carlstrom[29]). Finally, postpartum values remain positive for a week, or occasionally longer, until circulating amounts of HCG are eliminated totally by renal clearance (Insler et al.[91]).

As far as serum concentrations are concerned, these follow a parallel course.[15, 48, 50] In Figure 19–8, the superposition of three curves may be noted, the first representing placental concentrations, the second serum concentrations and the third urinary excretion. Notice that all three are parallel.

19.7.2. ESTROGENS

Estrogen synthesis and elimination curves during pregnancy are well known.[172] They are the reverse of gonadotropin curves, showing a minimum at the beginning and a maximum at the end of gestation (Fig. 19–11). Here, too, the curves representing plasma concentration and urinary concentration, as shown in the diagram, are more or less parallel (Diczfalusy and Lauritzen[49]).

Heusghem,[86] Hobkirk,[88] and Frandsen and Lundvall[62] fractionated the various estrogen compounds encountered in urines of pregnancy. The main components consist of estrone, estradiol and estriol; however, considerable amounts of α-*ketoestrone*, *methoxyestrone* and *epiestriol* also are eliminated. Special importance has been

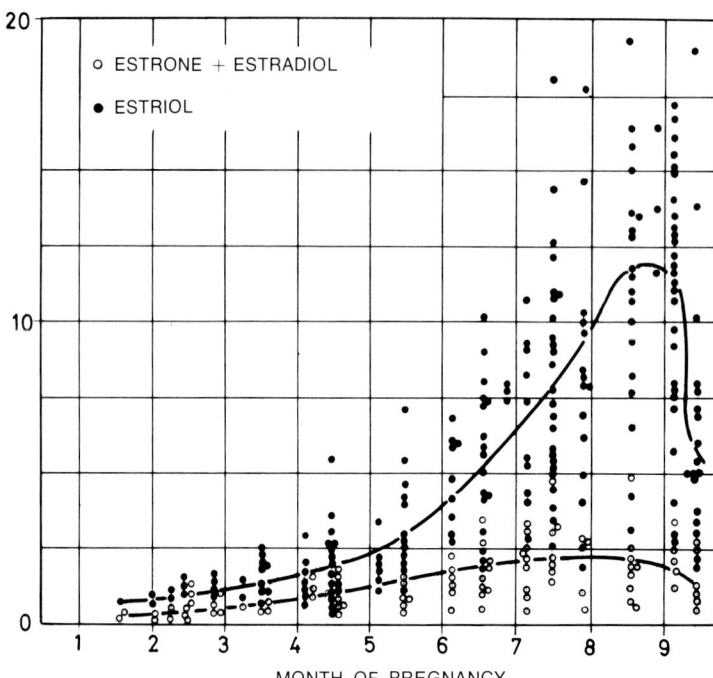

Figure 19-11. Urinary excretion of different fractions of estrogens during pregnancy. (From Heusghem.[86])

attached to the rate of estriol excretion as an index of placental maturity and, in the case of a falling rate, as an eventual sign of placental insufficiency. Cortisol is not produced by the ovary; it is a product of liver catabolism.

It is impossible to describe placental estrogen synthesis without taking into consideration the existence of the fetoplacental unit.[45, 47, 195] The placenta utilizes cholesterol and pregnenolone available in the maternal circulation to synthesize progesterone, which is converted by the fetal adrenal—and near the end of pregnancy possibly also by the fetal liver—to dehydroepiandrosterone sulfate (DHEA-SO$_4$). On its passage through the placenta, DHEA-SO$_4$ is converted to estradiol, estrone and estriol. The ability of the placenta to aromatize androgens, thereby carrying out their conversion to the foregoing estrogens, has been demonstrated by Reynolds and colleagues[141] and by Sybulsky.[170] Wu and co-workers[194] have shown that the young placenta is capable of converting tritiated DHEA to estrone, giving, however, a much greater yield in estrone if incubated in the presence of fetal liver homogenate, which seems to be a further argument in support of the active role played by the fetal liver in these processes.

19.7.3. PROGESTERONE

The curve of progesterone synthesis parallels that of estrogen synthesis but is inverted with regard to that of gonadotropin synthesis. Serum progesterone concentrations have been measured by Forbes and Hooker[58, 59] and by Zander and his associates.[198, 199] Urinary pregnanediol excretion rates are generally known to run a parallel course[25, 31, 50, 110, 138] (Fig. 19-12).

19.7.4. FETO-PLACENTAL STEROIDOGENIC UNIT

While the placental protein hormones (HCG and HPL) are synthesized strictly within the placental compartment, all steroids are linked in a common maternofetal chain of biogenesis (Younglai and Solomon[195]). Since there is now no doubt that estriol cannot be formed without previous conjugation with sulfate by the fetus, determination of estriol values offers a faithful means for assessing the gravidic condition of the fetus[68, 103, 104] (see Chapter 45). In contrast, aromatization of DHEA-SO$_4$ takes place only in the placenta,[38, 45, 121] so that estriol cannot accumulate in the amniotic fluid in the absence of normal placental activity.[127] Bolte and co-workers[21] believe that all estriol present in the term placenta is of fetal origin. Basing their ideas on the knowledge that aromatization of estriol precursors (DHEA-SO$_4$) takes place only in the placenta, and that progesterone synthesis is equally an exclusive function of placental tissue, but that these two types of steroid formation do not necessarily take place in parallel, Lamb and his associates[107] and Villee[184] postulate the existence of *two different placental compartments* so far as steroid synthesis is concerned.

19.7.5. CORTICOIDS

Urinary corticoid excretion during pregnancy has been the object of extensive research.[34, 92, 135, 183] The outline of the excretion curve has been defined by Venning and colleagues.[183] It reveals a gradually rising slope until the third month of pregnancy, a dip between the fifth and sixth months, and a second upswing with a peak about the eighth month, after which there is a downward slope during the last month of gestation.

19.8. BIOGENESIS OF PLACENTAL STEROIDS

Data obtained by means of placental perfusion[102, 109] and by enzymologic studies[93, 94, 95] have clarified the *biochemical mechanism of placental steroidogenesis.*

19.8.1. ESTROGENS

As early as 1954, Pearlman[135] used deuterium in the study of the metabolism of placental estrogens. Joel and his associates[94] incubated slices of placenta with ^{14}C and were able to follow estrogen synthesis by monitoring radioactivity. But it was above all Ryan[143, 144] who, in 1962, performed a more thorough study of estro-

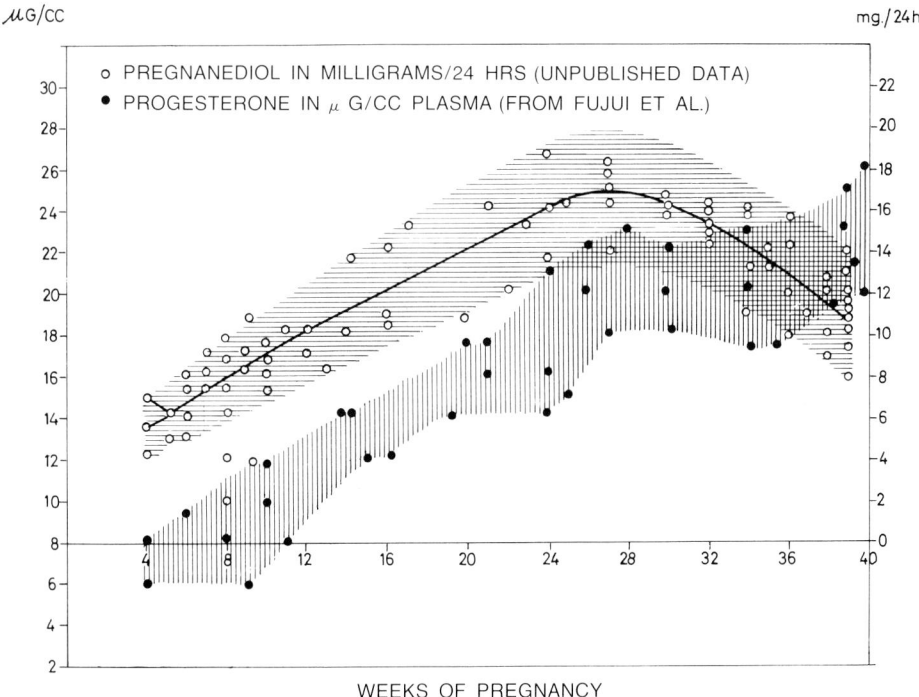

Figure 19-12. Progesterone blood levels and rates of human urinary pregnanediol excretion by month of pregnancy.

gen synthesis by chorionic tissue, the results of which were later confirmed by Baulieu.[10]

Further details pertaining to placental estrogen synthesis were brought to light by the consecutive works of Diczfalusy and his group (Goebelsmann et al.[72, 73]), Ryan[2, 143, 144] and Smith and Hagerman.[157] Although, as a rule, the placenta, like the ovary, utilizes the pregnenolone-progesterone-androgen pathway for estrogen production, considerable amounts of estrogens are produced from adrenal precursors (Frandsen,[61] Goebelsmann et al.[72, 73]). Despite the fact that estrogens may be synthesized by placental tissue incubated in vitro with testosterone,[154a] this does not seem to be the most likely conversion pathway involved, since neither testosterone nor androstenedione is ordinarily encountered in placental tissue.[78, 102] Hence, all indications are that Diczfalusy's theory is the correct one, and that placental estrogen synthesis utilizes dehydroepiandrosterone sulfate (DHEA-SO$_4$) of fetal adrenal origin as the main, if not the only, source of estrogens (see Chapter 20).

On the other hand, Koon and Looke[106] demonstrated the presence of aromatizing enzymes which, according to Wilcox and Engel,[190] are localized in the microsomes of the syncytiotrophoblast. In addition, small amounts of equilenin have been reported to be elaborated by the human placenta (Starka et al.[164]).

19.8.2. PROGESTERONE

Davis and his associates,[41] using radioactive progesterone, have studied progesterone metabolism in the placenta, which, as we have seen, is intimately intertwined with that of estrogens. A great contribution toward elucidating the question of placental progestopoiesis has been made by Zander and Münstermann.[198] Eventually, the placental biogenesis of progesterone was fully explained in a recent publication by Ryan[144] (Fig. 19–14).

Like in the ovary, progesterone is synthesized in the placenta from pregnenolone, and the latter, in turn, is synthesized from cholesterol. Likewise as in the ovary, 3β-ol-dehydrogenase is the fundamental enzyme of progestogen production (Botte et al.[26]). By means of a process of 20-hydroxylation, progesterone gives two isomeres, α- and β-hydroxypregnenolone, differing from each other only by the position of their OH group on carbon 20. Other than this, the metabolism of placental progestogen synthesis is identical to that of ovarian progestogen synthesis. Van Leusden and Villee[179] found that HCG was also involved in the process.

Failure of 3β-ol-dehydrogenase activity, as in the ovary, results in deficient progesterone synthesis, giving rise to the Stein-Leventhal syndrome as a result of excessive estrogen and androgen production; there has been some speculation over whether a similar reaction in the placental tissue, involving lack of progesterone and excess of estrogens, might not be a possible cause of abortion. Nevertheless, the fact that placental androgen synthesis has not been demonstrated either in this or in any other case would seem to indicate that the processes involved are not exactly the same as those taking place in the female gonad.

19.8.3. CORTICOIDS

Hirschmann and co-workers [7] and Troen,[173] by means of chromatographic fractionation of placental extracts, as well as later Salhanick[146] and Solomon,[163] by both perfusing placentas with radioactive cholesterol and then fractionating the steroids isolated from the efferent blood, accounted for the presence of deoxycorticosterone, 11-deoxycortisone, cortisol, aldosterone and several other derivatives (Fig. 19–15 and Table 19–1), representing almost the entire series of mineralo- and glucocorticoid regulators. These are intimately related to progesterone synthesis and somewhat indirectly to estrogen formation. This is only natural since, as was pointed out in Chapter 9 and indicated in Figure 19–15, progesterone is a pivotal link in the metabolism of all corticoids.

19.9. SUMMARY

The endocrinology of the placenta is complex, though no less so than other biologic aspects of this organ. Its role as provider of embryonal nutrition makes the placenta assume a variety of functions which, outside pregnancy, are discharged
(Text continued on page 415)

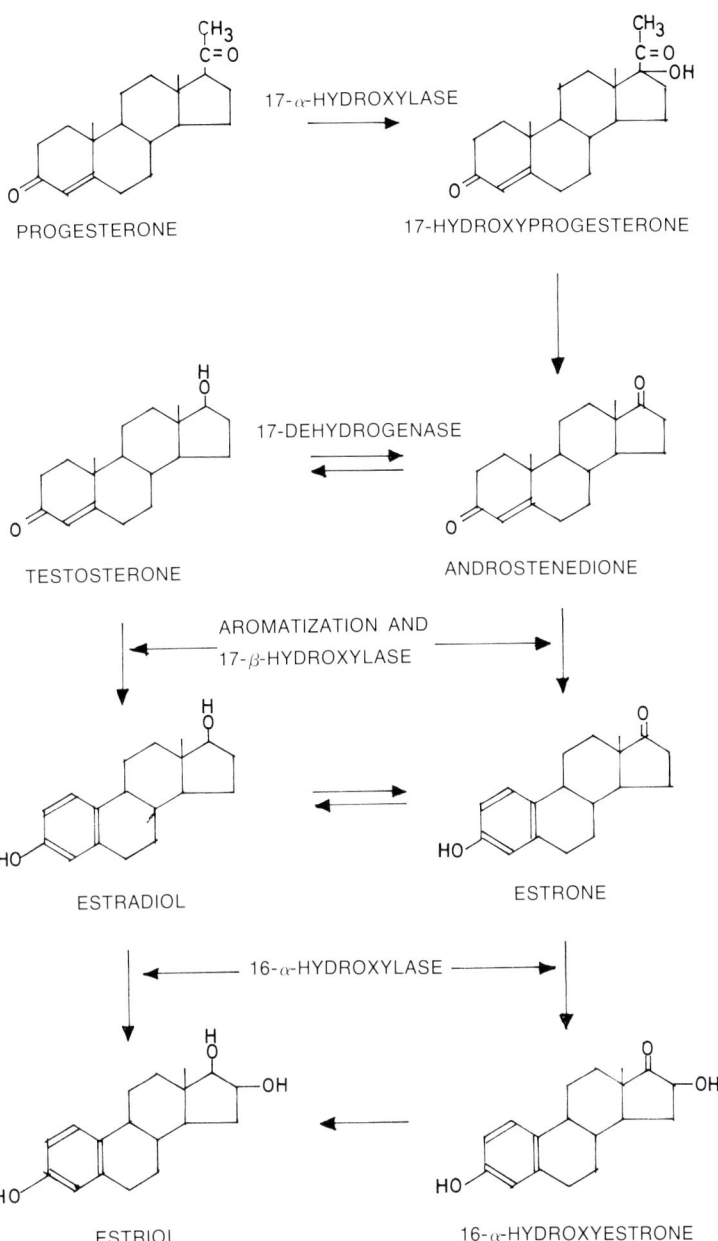

Figure 19-13. Biosynthesis of estrogens by the human placenta. See text for details. (From Ryan: *Amer. J. Obstet. Gynec.*, 84:1705, 1962.)

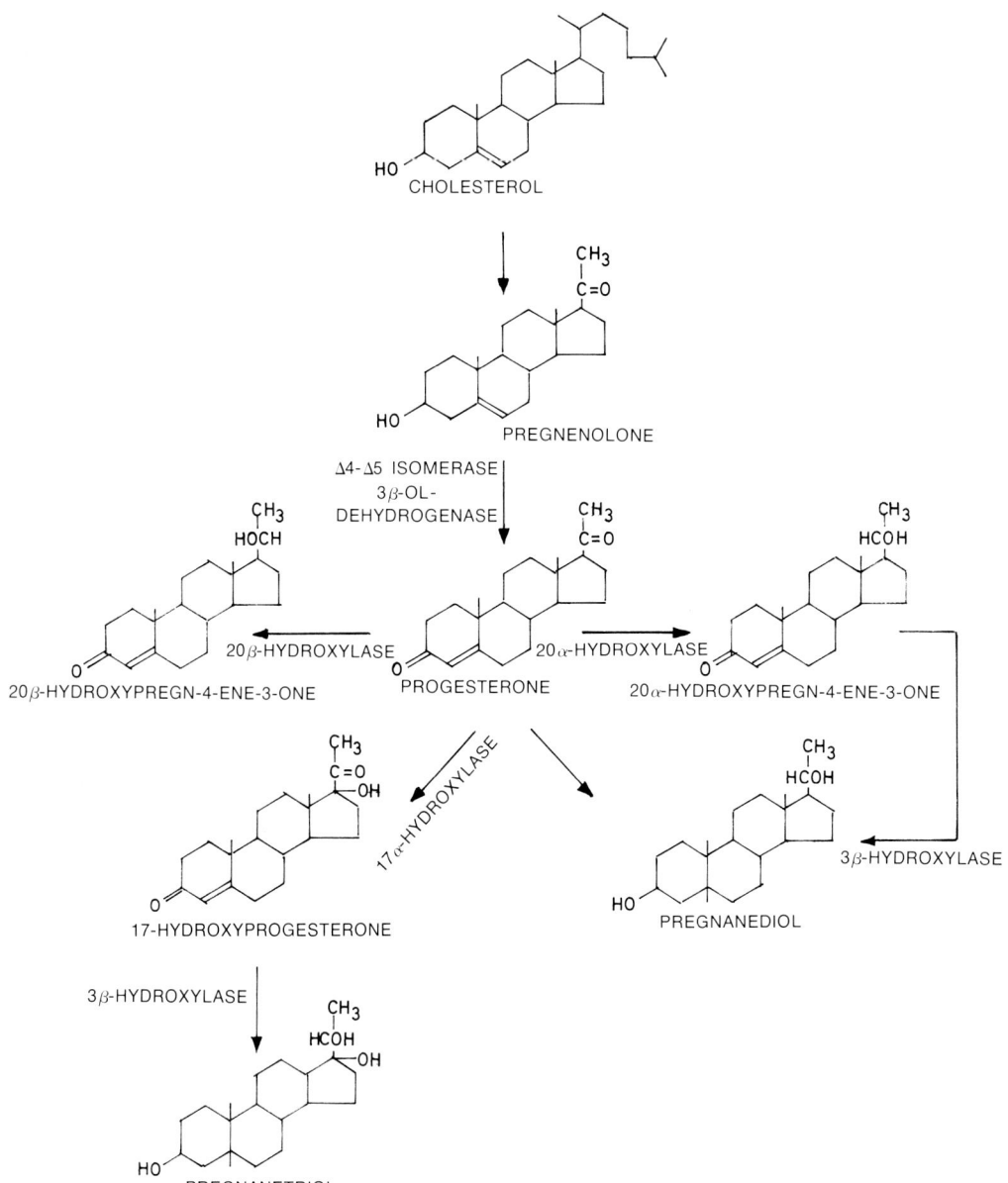

Figure 19-14. Biosynthesis of progesterone by the human placenta. See text for details. (From Ryan: *Amer. J. Obstet. Gynec.*, 84:1702, 1962.)

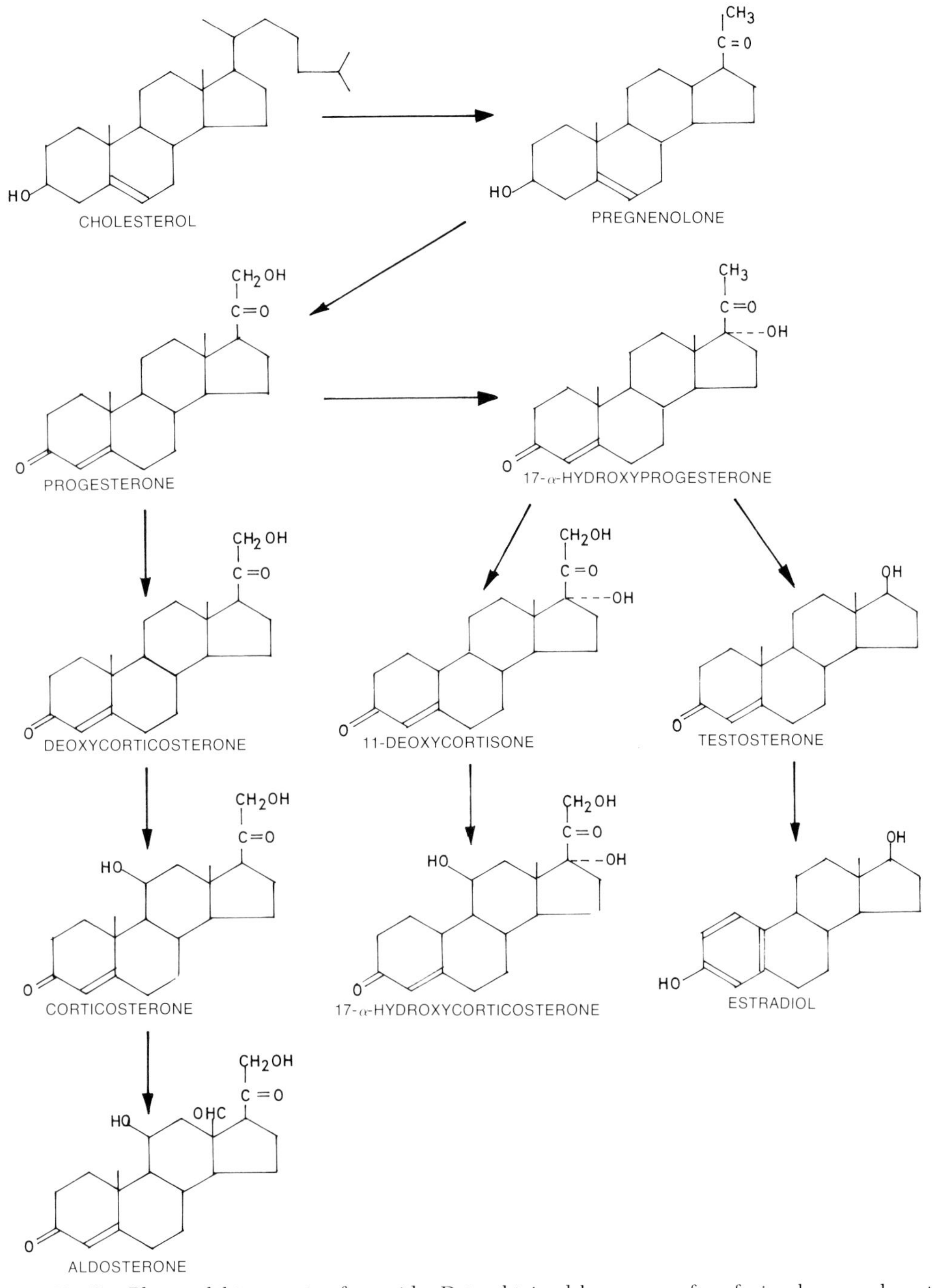

Figure 19-15. Placental biogenesis of steroids. Data obtained by means of perfusing human placenta with C-14 labeled cholesterol. (From Solomon.[163])

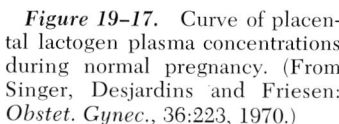

Figure 19–16. Principal corticoids isolated from placenta by Salhanick,[146] in 1960. I, Cortisol; II, tetrahydrocortisone; III, pregnenedioltrione; IV, cortisone; V, aldosterone; VI, dehydrocorticosterone. (See Table 19–1.)

Figure 19–17. Curve of placental lactogen plasma concentrations during normal pregnancy. (From Singer, Desjardins and Friesen: *Obstet. Gynec.*, 36:223, 1970.)

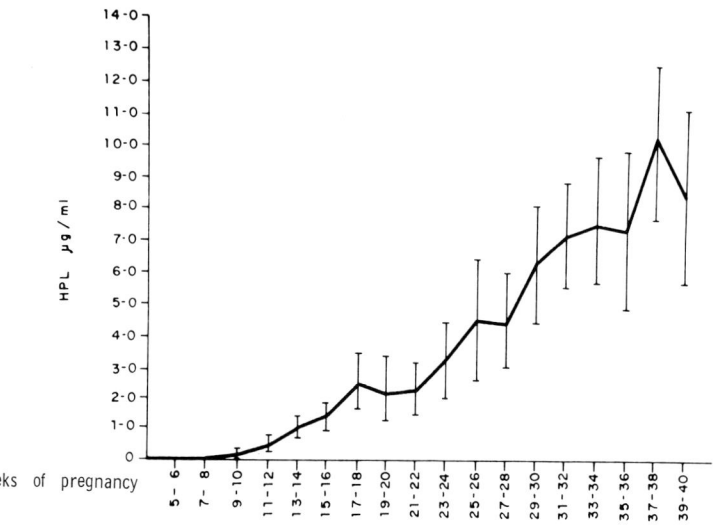

by other endocrine glands, such as the pituitary, adrenals and ovaries. *There is no single placental hormone;* the placenta produces *counterparts of other glands' hormones.* There is similarly no characteristic placental steroid synthesizing system, although *the placenta duplicates in every detail the synthesis of C-21 steroids as it occurs in the adrenal cortex.*

While the immature placenta (trophoblast and chorion) imitates the pituitary (production of CG), the mature placenta instead duplicates primarily the metabolism of the adrenal and that of the corpus luteum. On the histologic level, these two different functions are characterized by two distinct entities: *the cytotrophoblast (Langhans layer), which is the site of pituitary type secretion, and the syncytiotrophoblast, which is the site of steroid biogenesis and metabolism.*

REFERENCES

1. Adams, E. C., Chambliss, K. W., and Longman, B. E.: *J. Clin. Endocr.*, 27:509, 1967.
2. Ainsworth, L., and Ryan, K. J.: *Endocrinology*, 79:875, 1966.
3. Ainsworth, L., Daenen, M., and Ryan, K. J.: *Endocrinology*, 84:1421, 1969.
4. Albert, A., and Berkson, J.: *J. Clin. Endocr. Metab.*, 11:801, 1951.
5. Amoroso, E. C.: *Ann. N.Y. Acad. Sci.*, 75:855, 1959.
6. Amoroso, E. C.: In *The Placenta and Fetal Membranes*, ed. C. A. Villee. Baltimore, Williams & Wilkins, 1960.
7. Andrews, P.: *Biochem. J.*, 111:799, 1969.
8. Ashitaka, Y., Tokura, Y., Tane, M., Mochizuki, M., and Tojo, S.: *Endocrinology*, 87:233, 1970.
9. Bargmann, W.: *Geburtsh. u. Frauenhk.*, 17:865, 1957.
10. Baulieu, E. E., and Dray, F.: *J. Clin. Endocr. Metab.*, 23:1299, 1963.
11. Balmi, H.: *Amer. J. Obstet. Gynec.*, 76:30, 1958.
12. Beck, P., and Daughaday, W. H.: *J. Clin. Invest.*, 46:103, 1967.
13. Bedoya, J. M., and Puras, A.: *Geburtsh. u. Frauenhk.*, 10:492, 1950.
14. Bedoya, J. M., and Plaza, F.: *Geburtsh. u. Frauenhk.*, 10:507, 1950.
15. Bedoya, J. M., and Rodriguez, M.: *Acta Gin.*, 2:499, 1951.
16. Berle, P., and Schultze-Morgau, H.: *Acta Endocr.*, 58:339, 1968.
17. Berle, P.: *Acta Endocr.*, 61:369, 1969.
18. Berswordt-Wallrabe, R., and Turner, C. W.: *Proc. Soc. Exper. Biol. Med.*, 108:212, 1961.
19. Bjorkman, N., and Fredrickson, B.: *Internat. J. Fertil.*, 7:259, 1962.
20. Bollengier, F., and Hubinot, P. O.: *Compt. Rend. Acad. Sci. (Paris)*, 267:653, 1968.
21. Bolte, E., Gattereau, D., Joly, M., and Lefevre, Y.: *Acta Endocr.*, 61:307, 1969.
22. Boss, J. H., and Craig, J. M.: *Obstet. Gynec.*, 20:272, 1962.
23. Botella, J.: *Arch. Gynäk.*, 183:73, 1953.
24. Botella, J., Nogales, F., and Duran, J. M.: *Arch. Gynäk.*, 188:269, 1957.
25. Botella, J.: *Obstetrical Endocrinology.* Springfield, Ill., Charles C Thomas, 1961.
26. Botte, V., Metterazzi, G., and Chieffi, G.: *J. Endocr.*, 34:179, 1966.
27. Boving, B. G.: *Ann. N.Y. Acad. Sci.*, 75:700, 1959.
28. Boyd, J. D.: In *Implantation of Ova*, ed. P. Eckstein, M. C. Shelesnyak and E. C. Amoroso. Cambridge, Cambridge University Press, 1959.
29. Brody, S., and Carlstrom, G.: *J. Clin. Endocr. Metab.*, 25:792, 1965.
30. Brody, S.: "Protein Hormones and Hormonal Peptides from the Placenta," in *Fetus and Placenta*, ed. A. Klopper and E. Diczfalusy. Oxford, Blackwell, 1969.
31. Brown, J. B.: *Lancet*, 1:704, 1956.
32. Burt, R. L., Pegram, P. S., and Leake, N. H.: *Amer. J. Obstet. Gynec.*, 103:44, 1969.
33. Canivenc, R., and Mayer, G.: *Ann. d'Endocr.*, 16:1, 1955.
34. Cassano, F., and Tarantino, C.: *Folia Endocr.*, 7:165, 1954.
35. Cassmer, O.: *Acta Endocr.*, 45, Suppl. 1, 1959.
36. Chang, M. C.: *J. Exper. Zool.*, 128:379, 1955.
37. Chang, M. C., and Yanimagichi, R.: *J. Exper. Zool.*, 154:173, 1963.
38. Charreau, E., Jung, W., Loring, J., and Villee, C. A.: *Steroids*, 12:29, 1968.
39. Cochrane, R. L., Prasad, M. R. N., and Meyer, R. K.: *Endocrinology*, 70:228, 1962.
40. Cooke, I. D., Wiqvist, N., and Diczfalusy, E.: *Acta Endocr.*, 56:43, 1967.
41. Davis, M. E., et al.: *Fertil. Steril.*, 11:19, 1960.
42. Deane, H. W., et al.: *Endocrinology*, 70:497, 1962.
43. Deanesly, R.: *J. Reprod. Fertil.*, 5:49, 1963.
44. Declerck, P.: In *Le placenta humain*, ed. J. de Snoeck. Paris, Masson et Cie., 1958.
45. Dell'Acqua, S., Mancuso, S., Ericsson, G., and Diczfalusy, E.: *Biochim. Biophys. Acta*, 130:241, 1966.
46. Dell'Acqua, S., Mancuso, S., Wiqvist, N., Ruse, J. L., Solomon, S., and Diczfalusy, E.: *Acta Endocr.*, 55:389, 1967.
47. Diczfalusy, E.: *Acta Endocr.*, 12, Suppl. 1, 1953.
48. Diczfalusy, E.: In *Probleme der foetalen Endokrinologie*, ed. A. Nowakowsky. Berlin, Springer, 1957.
49. Diczfalusy, E., and Lauritzen, C.: *Oestrogene beim Menschen.* Berlin, Springer, 1961.
50. Diczfalusy, E., and Troen, P.: *Vitamins Hormones*, 19:229, 1961.
51. Diczfalusy, E., and Borell, U.: *J. Clin. Endocr. Metab.*, 21:1119, 1961.
52. Dutt, R. H.: *J. Anim. Sci.*, 13:469, 1964.
53. Eckstein, P., Shelesnyak, M. C., and Amoroso, E. C.: *Implantation of Ova.* Cambridge, Cambridge University Press, 1959.
54. Feo, V. J. de: *Endocrinology*, 72:305, 1963.
55. Ferrando, G., and Nalbandov, A. V.: *Endocrinology*, 83:933, 1968.

56. Florini, J. R., et al.: *Endocrinology*, 79:692, 1966.
57. Foote, R. H.: *Internat. J. Fertil.*, 3:78, 1958.
58. Forbes, T. R.: *Endocrinology*, 49:218, 1951.
59. Forbes, T. R., and Hooker, C. W.: *Endocrinology*, 61:381, 1957.
60. Fowler, R. E., and Edwards, R. D.: *J. Endocr.*, 20:1, 1960.
61. Frandsen, V. A.: *Rev. Europ. Endocr.*, 1:227, 1965.
62. Frandsen, V. A., and Lundvall, F.: *Acta Endocr.*, 53:93, 1966.
63. Frantz, A. G., Rabkin, M. T., and Friesen, H.: *J. Clin. Endocr. Metab.*, 25:1136, 1965.
64. Friedman, S., Gans, B., and Eckelring, B.: *J. Obstet. Brit. Emp.*, 76:554, 1969.
65. Friesen, H.: *Endocrinology*, 76:369, 1965.
66. Friesen, H. G.: *Endocrinology*, 83:744, 1968.
67. Fuchs, F.: *Acta Obstet. Gynec. Scand.*, 41 (Suppl. 1):7, 1962.
68. Galbraith, R. S., Low, J. A., and Boston, R. W.: *Amer. J. Obstet. Gynec.*, 106:352, 1970.
69. Gemzell, C. A.: *CIBA Colloquia on Endocrinology*, 14:296, 1962.
70. Georgakopoulos, P. A.: *Acta Endocr.*, 49:221, 1965.
71. Gey, G. O., Seegar-Jones, G., and Helman, L. M.: *Science*, 88:306, 1938.
72. Goebelsmann, U., Eriksson, G., Wiqvist, N., and Diczfalusy, E.: *Acta Endocr.*, 50:273, 1965.
73. Goebelsmann, U., et al.: *Acta Endocr.*, 52:550, 1966.
74. Goecke, C., and Timonen, S.: *Arch. Gynäk.*, 203:118, 1966.
75. Got, R., and Bourrillon, R.: *Biochim. Biophys. Acta*, 39:241, 1960.
76. Grumbach, M. M., and Kaplan, S. L.: *Trans. N.Y. Acad. Sci.*, 27:167, 1964.
77. Grumbach, M. M., Kaplan, S. L., Abrams, C. L., Bell, J. J., and Conte, F. A.: *J. Clin. Endocr. Metab.*, 26:478, 1966.
78. Gurpide, E., et al.: *J. Clin. Endocr. Metab.*, 26:1355, 1966.
79. Hafez, E. S. E.: *J. Reprod. Fertil.*, 7:241, 1964.
80. Hamashage, S., Astor, M. A., Arquilla, E. R., and Van Thiel, D. H.: *J. Clin. Endocr.*, 27:1690, 1967.
81. Harrison, R. G., and Neal, E. G.: In *Implantation of Ova*, ed. P. Eckstein, M. C. Shelesnyak, and E. C. Amoroso. Cambridge, Cambridge University Press, 1959.
82. Hellig, H., Gattereau, D., Lefebvre, Y., and Bolte, E.: *J. Clin. Endocr.*, 30:624, 1970.
83. Hennen, G., Pierce, J. G., and Freuchet, P.: *J. Clin. Endocr.*, 29:581, 1969.
84. Hershman, J. M., and Starner, W. R.: *J. Clin. Invest.*, 48:923, 1969.
85. Hertig, A. T., Rock, J., Adams, E. C., and Mulligan, W. J.: *Amer. J. Anat.*, 98:435, 1956.
86. Heusghem, C.: *Contribution à l'étude analytique et biochimique des oestrogenes naturels*. Paris, Masson et Cie., 1957.
87. Hirschmann, H., Hirschmann, F. B., and Zala, A. P.: *J. Biol. Chem.*, 236:3141, 1961.
88. Hobkirk, R., and Nilsan, L.: *J. Clin. Endocr. Metab.*, 22:134, 1962.
89. Holkomb, L. C.: *Ohio J. Sci.*, 67:24, 1967.
90. Hughes, E. C., Ness, A. W., and Lloyd, C. W.: In *Pregnancy Wastage*, ed. E. T. Engle. Springfield, Ill., Charles C Thomas, 1953.
91. Insler, V., et al.: *Monit. Ost. Gin. Endoc. Metab.*, 36:129, 1965.
92. Jailer, J. W., and Knowlton, A. I.: *J. Clin. Invest.*, 29:1430, 1950.
93. Jayle, M. F., and Crepy, O.: In *Colloques sur la fonction luteale*, Vol. II. Paris, Masson et Cie., 1954.
94. Joel, P. B., Hageman, D. D., and Villee, C. A.: *J. Biol. Chem.*, 236:3151, 1961.
95. Johnson, R. H., and Haines, W. J.: *Science*, 116:456, 1962.
96. Josimovitch, J. B., and MacLaren, J. A.: *Endocrinology*, 71:209, 1962.
97. Josimovitch, J. B., Kosor, B., Boccella, L., Mintz, D. H., and Hutchinson, D. L.: *Obstet. Gynec.*, 36:244, 1970.
98. Josimovitch, J. B., Kosor, B., and Mintz, D. H.: "Role of Placental Lactogen in Fetal-Maternal Relations," in *Fetal Autonomy*, ed. G. E. W. Woltelholme and M. O'Connor, Symposium, CIBA Foundation. London, Churchill, 1969.
99. Jungman, R. A., and Schweppe, J. S.: *J. Clin. Endocr.*, 27:1151, 1967.
100. Kazeto, S., and Hreshchyshyn, M. M.: *Amer. J. Obstet. Gynec.*, 106:1229, 1970.
101. Kinzey, W. G.: *Endocrinology*, 82:266, 1968.
102. Kirschner, M. A., Wiqvist, N., and Diczfalusy, E.: *Acta Endocr.*, 53:584, 1966.
103. Klopper, A.: "The Assessment of Placental Function in Clinical Practice," in *Fetus and Placenta*, ed. A. Klopper and E. Diczfalusy. Oxford, Blackwell, 1969.
104. Klopper, A.: *Amer. J. Obstet. Gynec.*, 107:807, 1970.
105. Knowlton, A. I., Mudge, G. H., and Jailer, J. W.: *J. Clin. Endocr. Metab.*, 9:514, 1949.
106. Koon, T. I., and Looke, K. H.: *Steroids*, 8:385, 1966.
107. Lamb, E., Mancuso, S., Dell'Acqua, S., Wiqvist, N., and Diczfalusy, E.: *Acta Endocr.*, 55:263, 1967.
108. Lauritzen, C., Lehman, W. D., and Bambas, W.: *Endokrinologie*, 52:248, 1967.
109. Levitz, M., Condom, G., and Dancis, J.: *Endocrinology*, 58:376, 1956.
110. Li, C. H., and Evans, H. M.: In *The Hormones*, ed. G. Pincus and K. V. Thiman, Vol. IV. New York, Academic Press, 1958.
111. Little, B., and Rossi, E.: *Endocrinology*, 61:111, 1957.
112. Little, B., et al.: *J. Clin. Endocr. Metab.*, 18:425, 1958.
113. Lobel, B. H., et al.: *Amer. J. Obstet. Gynec.*, 83:295, 1962.
114. Loraine, J. A.: *CIBA Colloquia on Endocrinology*, 11:19, 1957.
115. Lundin, P. M., and Holmdahl, S.: *Acta Endocr.*, 26:388, 1957.
116. Lutwak-Mann, C.: In *Implantation of Ova*, ed. P. Eckstein, M. C. Shelesnyak, and E. C. Amoroso. Cambridge, Cambridge University Press, 1959.
117. Lyons, W. R., Simpson, M. E., and Evans, H. M.: *Endocrinology*, 51:173, 1953.
118. MacDonald, G. J., Armstrong, D. T., and Greep, R. O.: *Endocrinology*, 80:172, 1966.
119. MacKean, C. M.: *Amer. J. Obstet. Gynec.*, 80:956, 1960.
120. MacLaren, A., and Mitchell, D.: In *Implantation*

of Ova, ed. P. Eckstein, M. C. Shelesnyak, and E. C. Amoroso. Cambridge, Cambridge University Press, 1959.
121. MacNaughton, M.: "Endocrinology of the Fetus," in *Fetus and Placenta*, ed. A. Klopper and E. Diczfalusy. Oxford, Blackwell, 1969.
122. Marcus, G. J., and Shelesnyak, M. C.: *Endocrinology*, 80:1028, 1967.
122a. Mastroianni, L., Beer, F., Shah, V., and Cleve, T. H.: *Endocrinology*, 68:92, 1961.
123. Masuda, H., Anderson, L. L., Hendricks, D. M., and Mellampy, R. M.: *Endocrinology*, 80:240, 1967.
124. Mayer, G.: *Ann. d'Endocr.*, 21:501, 1960.
125. Meyer, R. K., and Cochrane, R. L.: *J. Endocr.*, 24:77, 1963.
126. Meyer, R. K., and Nutting, E. F.: *J. Endocr.*, 29:243, 1966.
127. Michie, E. A., and Livingstone, J. R. B.: *Acta Endocr.*, 61:320, 1969.
128. Midgley, A. R.: *Endocrinology*, 79:10, 1966.
129. Midgley, A. R., Fong, I. F., and Jaffe, R. B.: *Nature*, 213:733, 1967.
130. Mizuno, M., Lobotsky, J., and Lloyd, C. W.: *J. Clin. Endocr.*, 28:1133, 1968.
131. Neuwirth, R. S., et al.: *Amer. J. Obstet. Gynec.*, 91:982, 1965.
132. Orsini, M. W., and Meyer, R. K.: *Proc. Soc. Exper. Biol. Med.*, 110:713, 1962.
133. Orsini, M. W., Wynn, R. M., Harris, J. A., and Bulmash, J. M.: *Amer. J. Obstet. Gynec.*, 106:14, 1970.
134. Pasqualini, J. R., Mozere, G., Wiqvist, N., and Diczfalusy, E.: *Acta Endocr.*, 60:237, 1969.
135. Pearlman, W. H.: *CIBA Colloquia on Endocrinology*, 11:233, 1957.
136. Pincus, G.: In *Gestation*, Vol. III. New York, The Josiah Macy Foundation, 1956.
137. Prahlad, K. V.: *Acta Endocr.*, 39:407, 1962.
138. Preedy, J. R. K., and Aitken, E. H.: *Lancet*, 1:191, 1957.
139. Psychoyos, J.: *Compt. Rend. Acad. Sci.*, 253:1616, 1961.
140. Purves, H. D., and Griesbach, W. E.: *Endocrinology*, 49:244, 1951.
141. Reynolds, J. W., Mancuso, S., Wiqvist, N., and Diczfalusy, E.: *Acta Endocr.*, 58:377, 1968.
142. Riggi, S. J., Boshart, C. R., Bell, P. H., and Ringler, I.: *Endocrinology*, 79:709, 1966.
143. Ryan, K. J.: *Endocrinology*, 69:613, 1961.
144. Ryan, K. J.: *Amer. J. Obstet. Gynec.*, 84:1695, 1962.
145. Saaman, N., et al.: *J. Clin. Endocr. Metab.*, 28:485, 1968.
146. Salhanick, H. A.: *Clin. Obstet. Gynec.*, 3:295, 1960.
147. Saxena, B., Refetoff, F., Emerson, K., and Selenkow, H. K.: *Amer. J. Obstet. Gynec.*, 101:874, 1968.
148. Schindler, A. E., and Herrmenn, W. L.: *Amer. J. Obstet. Gynec.*, 95:301, 1966.
149. Sciarra, J. J.: *Clin. Obstet. Gynec.*, 10:132, 1967.
150. Schulz, R. B., and Blizzard, R. M.: *J. Clin. Endocr. Metab.*, 26:291, 1966.
151. Selenkow, H. A., Saxena, B. N., Dana, C. L., and Emerson, K.: "Measurement and Pathophysiological Significance of Human Placental Lactogen," in *The Feto-Placental Unit*, ed. A. Pecile and C. Finzi. Amsterdam, Excerpta Medica Foundation, 1969.
152. Shelesnyak, M. C.: *Acta Endocr.*, 23:106, 1956.
153. Shelesnyak, M. C.: *Acta Endocr.*, 50:452, 1965.
154. Shizume, K., and Lerner, A. B.: *J. Clin. Endocr. Metab.*, 14:1491, 1954.
154a. Siitere, O. W., and Hagerman, D. D.: *J. Clin. Endocr. Metab.*, 26:751, 1966.
155. Simmer, H. H.: "Human Placental Lactogen," in *Biology of Gestation*, Vol. I, ed. N. S. Assali. New York, Academic Press, 1968.
156. Singer, W., Desjardins, P., and Friesen, H. G.: *Obstet. Gynec.*, 36:222, 1970.
157. Smith, O. W., and Hagerman, D. D.: *J. Clin. Endocr. Metab.*, 25:732, 1965.
158. Smith, E. R., and Kellie, A. E.: *Biochem. J.*, 104:83, 1967.
159. Smith, D. M., and Biggers, J. D.: *J. Endocr.*, 41:11, 1968.
160. Spellacy, W. N., Carlson, K. L., and Birk, S. A.: *Amer. J. Obstet. Gynec.*, 95:118, 1966.
161. Spellacy, W. N., Carlson, K. L., and Birk, S. A.: *Amer. J. Obstet. Gynec.*, 96:1164, 1966.
162. Spellacy, W. N., Cohen, W. D., and Carlson, K.: *Amer. J. Obstet. Gynec.*, 97:560, 1967.
163. Solomon, S.: In *The Placenta and Fetal Membranes*, ed. C. A. Villee. Baltimore, Williams & Wilkins, 1960.
164. Starka, L., Breuer, H., and Cedard, L.: *J. Endocr.*, 34:447, 1966.
165. Stegner, H. E.: *Arch. Gynäk.*, 187:351, 1962.
166. Steinetz, B. G., Beach, V. L., and Krog, R. L.: *Rec. Progr. Endocr. Reprod.*, p. 389. New York, Academic Press, 1959.
167. Stewart, H. L.: *Amer. J. Obstet. Gynec.*, 61:900, 1951.
168. Strauss, F.: "Die normale Anatomie der menschlichen Placenta," in *Handbuch der speziellen pathologischen Anatomie und Histologie*, Henke-Lubarsch. ed. E. Uehlinger. Berlin, Springer, 1967.
169. Sugawara, S., and Hafez, E. S. E.: *Anat. Rec.*, 158:281, 1967.
170. Sybulsky, S.: *Amer. J. Obstet. Gynec.*, 105:1055, 1969.
171. Tanaka, K., and Nakajo, S.: *Endocrinology*, 70:453, 1962.
172. Taylor, E. S., Heppner, H. J., and Drose, V. E.: *Amer. J. Obstet. Gynec.*, 76:983, 1958.
173. Troen, P.: *J. Clin. Endocr. Metab.*, 21:895, 1511, 1961.
174. Tullner, W. H., and Hertz, R.: *Endocrinology*, 78:1076, 1966.
175. Turkington, R. W., and Topper, Y. J.: *Endocrinology*, 79:175, 1966.
176. Turkington, R. W.: *Endocrinology*, 82:575, 1968.
177. Turtle, J. R., Beck, P., and Daughaday, W. H.: *Endocrinology*, 79:187, 1966.
178. Uher, H., Jirasek, J., and Herzman, J.: *Gynaecologia*, 161:21, 1966.
179. Van Leusden, H., and Villee, C. A.: *Acta Endocr.*, 6:31, 1965.
180. Van de Wiele, R. L., and Jailer, J. W.: *Ann. N.Y. Acad. Sci.*, 75:889, 1959.
181. Varma, S. K., et al.: *Amer. J. Obstet. Gynec.*, 107:472, 1970.
182. Varon, H. H.: *Proc. Soc. Exper. Biol. Med.*, 100:609, 1959.
183. Venning, E. H., et al.: *J. Clin. Endocr. Metab.*, 19:1486, 1959.
184. Villee, C. A.: *Amer. J. Obstet. Gynec.*, 104:406, 1969.

185. Vokaer, R., and Leroy, F.: *Amer. J. Obstet. Gynec.*, 83:141, 1962.
186. Waltz, H. K., et al.: *J. Nat. Cancer Inst.*, 14:1173, 1954.
187. Weber, J.: *Acta Obstet. Gynec. Scand.*, 40:139, 1961.
188. White, R. A., et al.: *Contrib. Embryol.*, 24:55, 1951.
189. Wide, L., and Gemzell, C. A.: *Acta Endocr.*, 35:261, 1960.
190. Wilcox, R. B., and Engel, L. L.: *Steroids*, Suppl. 2:249, 1965.
191. Wilde, C. E., Orr, A. H., and Bagshave, K. D.: *Nature*, 205:191, 1965.
192. Wislocky, C. B.: *CIBA Colloquia on Ageing*, 2:105, 1956.
193. Wislocky, C. B., and Padykula, H.: In *Sex and Internal Secretions*, Vol. II, 3rd ed. Baltimore, Williams & Wilkins, 1961.
194. Wu, C. H., Touchstone, J. C., and Flickinger, G. L.: *Amer. J. Obstet. Gynec.*, 102:862, 1968.
195. Younglai, E. V., and Solomon, S.: "Neutral Steroids in Human Pregnancy," in *Fetus and Placenta*, ed. A. Klopper and E. Diczfalusy. Oxford, Blackwell, 1969.
196. Yousem, H., Seitchnik, J., and Solomon, D.: *Obstet. Gynec.*, 28:491, 1966.
197. Zander, J.: *Arch. Gynäk.*, 198:113, 1963.
198. Zander, J., and Münstermann, A. M: *Klin. Wschr.*, 34:944, 1956.
199. Zarrow, M. X., and Neher, G. M.: *Endocrinology*, 56:1, 1955.
200. Zarrow, M. X., Holstrom, E. G., and Salhanick, H. A.: *J. Clin. Endocr. Metab.*, 15:22, 1955.
201. Zilliacus, H.: *Gynaecologia*, 135:141, 1953.
202. Zondek, B., and Pfeiffer, V.: *Acta Obstet. Gynec. Scand.*, 38:742, 1959.

Chapter 20

INCRETORY SYSTEMS OF THE MOTHER AND FETUS DURING GESTATION

In discussing the endocrinology of the placenta in Chapter 19, we stressed its importance in the physiology of pregnancy and in the maintenance of endocrine correlations. Since the evolution of a placenta means that a new organ has become part of the incretory system, the remaining glands of internal secretion undergo compensatory changes in function. As a result, woman's endocrine balance as a whole is altered by the emergence of the placenta as the incretory organ of gestation. This gives rise to a situation in which, in response to the emergence of a new and different type of endocrine function—that of the chorion, which from now on must be taken into account—the remaining glands of internal secretion also undergo noteworthy variations and changes in function. While studying successively the *maternal* and the *fetal incretory systems*, we shall not lose sight of the fact that this arbitrary division is not based on two truly independent entities but is merely adopted here for the sake of clarity. *The maternal and fetal systems together constitute a biologic unit that is governed by reciprocal relationships.*

20.1. THE MATERNAL INCRETORY SYSTEM

The changes occurring in the maternal incretory system affect all glands of internal secretion, but those most notably affected, in the order of decreasing importance, are the ovary, the pituitary, the adrenal and the thyroid. However, the adrenal medulla, the parathyroid and the pancreas also undergo significant alterations during pregnancy, which we shall analyze subsequently.

20.1.1. OVARIAN FUNCTION

During pregnancy, the ovary passes through two quite different phases. Persistence of the corpus luteum is characteristic of the first weeks of pregnancy. The *gravidic corpus luteum* lasts until the twelfth week of gestation, although it begins to be affected by regressive changes even before that time. Subsequently, the rate of corpus luteum regression is increasingly accelerated, so that, by the fifth month, the ovary is observed to contain only a degenerative corpus luteum. Follicular maturation is inhibited, probably by the combined actions of chorionic gonadotropin, estrogens and progesterone.

For the purposes of our study, we shall analyze three different aspects of the ovary of pregnancy: (1) the gravidic corpus luteum; (2) the ovary during the second half of gestation; and (3) the interstitial ovarian gland.

THE GRAVIDIC CORPUS LUTEUM. The onset of pregnancy is associated with the occurrence of evident changes in the corpus luteum. If gestation takes place, the menstrual corpus luteum, usually in full regression from the twenty-fourth day of the cycle (Corner[44]; see Chapter 12), persists, and regressive changes fail to set in. The classic idea[54, 66] has been that nidation of the egg, along with chorionic gonadotropin secretion by the incipient trophoblast, is sufficient *per se* to maintain the viability of the corpus luteum, and these are, in effect, determinant factors in corpus luteum persistence. However, since under normal conditions the corpus luteum would be expected to undergo atrophy by not later than nine days after fertilization it must be admitted that chorionic gonadotropin secretion by a nine day old conceptus is capable of maintaining the functional activity of the corpus luteum.

As mentioned in Chapter 19, the action of chorionic gonadotropin would not appear to be exactly identical with that exerted by pituitary LH. *The latter possesses luteinizing but no luteotrophic activity.* In order to last for eight or nine days, the menstrual corpus depends on the action of galactogenic hormone. Because chorionic gonadotropin of the rat possesses less luteotrophic activity than the human variety, the gravidic corpus luteum of the rat depends for its maintenance on the action of prolactin during the entire first half of gestation (Greenwald and Johnson[87]). In contrast, the activity of trophoblastic incretion alone is enough to make the corpus luteum last for three months. Obviously, then, the gravidic corpus luteum persists not just because it is stimulated by a new hormone, namely chorionic gonadotropic hormone, but also because the new gonadotropic hormone exerts a *luteotrophic rather than luteinizing action.*

Having explained the reasons for the persistence of the gravidic corpus luteum, let us now examine what characterizes such a corpus morphologically. The gravidic corpus luteum has been studied in detail by Corner[44] and by Dubreuil and Marc-Riviere.[58] According to the descriptions given by these authors, which are roughly in agreement with each other, the gravidic corpus luteum may be said to develop from the menstrual corpus luteum in its final phase, namely, the phase of vascularization. Its vascularity is markedly increased and there is discernible proliferation of lutein cells. The central hemorrhagic area remains unchanged or occasionally may even grow in size. In the latter case, gravidic corpora lutea often have a pseudocystic appearance, which may cause them to be confused with true ovarian cysts (Fig. 20-1). The histologic architecture of the gravidic corpus luteum (Fig. 20-2) is characterized by the following features: (1) proliferation of the cells of the luteinic layer, whose cytoplasm becomes increasingly lipid-laden and denser. (2) Markedly increased vascularization, as reflected clearly by a richer capillary network, stainable with the Gomori technique for phosphatase. These vessels are seen to give off numerous branches to the thecal septa and to penetrate into the luteal structure where they form an extensive lacunar network between the secretory cells, enveloping them nearly completely. (3) A pronounced *luteal reaction* in the theca. The period of time during which the corpus luteum of pregnancy is active is a relatively

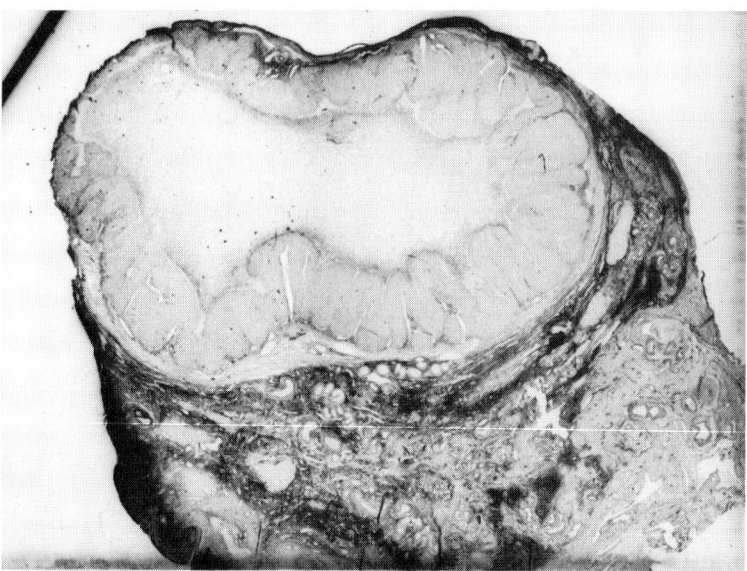

Figure 20-1. Low power view of gravidic corpus luteum (corpus luteum graviditatis), which occupies most of ovary.

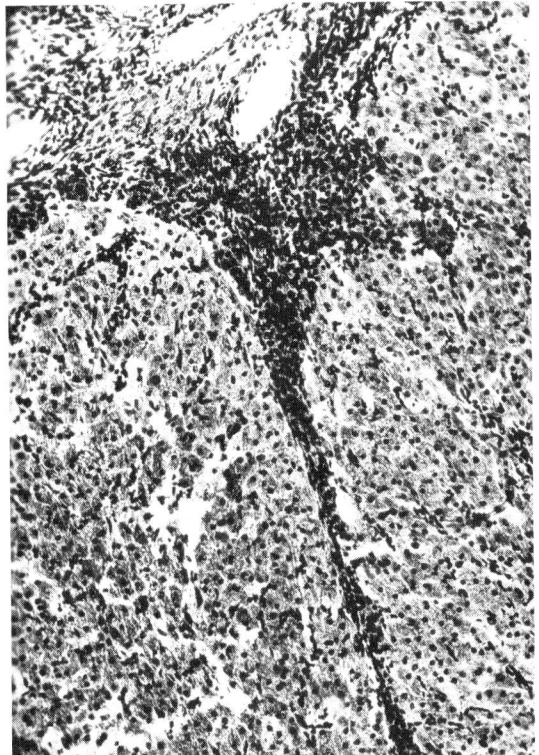

Figure 20-2. Structural detail of gravidic corpus luteum.

short one. Enzyme studies[129, 216] have revealed that its activity reaches a peak by the fourth week, after which it slackens till the tenth week. By that time, new follicles begin to grow,[84] marking the beginning of the decline of the corpus luteum of pregnancy.

Thecal luteinization is not so important in the human species as it is in rodents.[37] The gravidic corpus luteum in some of the latter animals, e.g., the rabbit and the hare, is formed as a result of exuberant theca-lutein proliferation (Fig. 20-3), which eventually involves the surrounding stroma and the ovary as a whole, converting the latter into a single diffuse corpus luteum.

Over the past years, the fine structure of the corpus luteum has been studied by Rennels,[155] Adams and Hertig,[4] and Pedersen and Larsen,[147] to mention just a few of the more important works. These studies seem to bear out the validity of the previously mentioned enzymologic data regarding evidence of declining activity after the tenth week.

Contrary to classic ideas, the amount of secretion produced by the gravidic corpus luteum is not excessive.[69] Pregnanediol excretion during the first half of pregnancy reaches values only slightly above those found during the second half of the physiologic cycle. During the progestational phase of the cycle, pregnanediol values average 10 to 12 mg per 24 hours; during the first half of pregnancy, 24 hour urinary pregnanediol values never exceed 20 mg.[86, 188] *Hence, the significance of the conspicuous histologic changes in the ovary must be related to the function of maintaining the persisting corpora lutea rather than to actual superproduction of luteal hormone.*

METABOLISM OF THE GRAVIDIC CORPUS LUTEUM. Mikhail and colleagues,[137] as well as Ryan, availed themselves of perfusion techniques for the study of gravidic corpora lutea in rabbits and women, respectively. According to their ideas, progesterone production in rabbits experiences a rise during the first half of gestation, only to fall afterwards. Obviously, in rabbits as in women, the placenta in conjunction with the ovary is necessary toward the end of pregnancy to assure the maintenance of gestation. This has also been confirmed by the studies of, among others, Csapo and Lloyd-Jacob.[45] Ryan[166] has been able to follow the intermediary metabolism of C-21 steroids by means of perfusing human ovaries, containing gravidic corpora lutea, with radioactive carbon-labeled pregnenolone and progesterone. In addition, the gravidic corpus luteum has been found to produce considerable amounts of estrogens by utilizing the following conversion route: pregnenolone → progesterone → 17-hydroxyprogesterone → androstenedione → estradiol. Essentially, its metabolism does not differ from that of the nongravidic corpus luteum.

The metabolism of the gravidic corpus luteum is basically identical to that of the menstrual corpus luteum (see Chapter 3). Hilliard and his associates[97] observed that cholesterol metabolism is quantitatively enhanced. This effect can be ascribed to greater luteotrophic activity of CG. Harbert et al.[91] and Zander and Rünnebaum[220] studied the behavior of radioactive progesterone in the maternal and fetal compartments separately, finding that progesterone was degraded at a much slower rate in the former.

THE CORPUS LUTEUM OF THE SECOND HALF OF GESTATION. After the first trimester, regressive changes in the human ovary become noticeable.[58, 80, 81, 85] According to

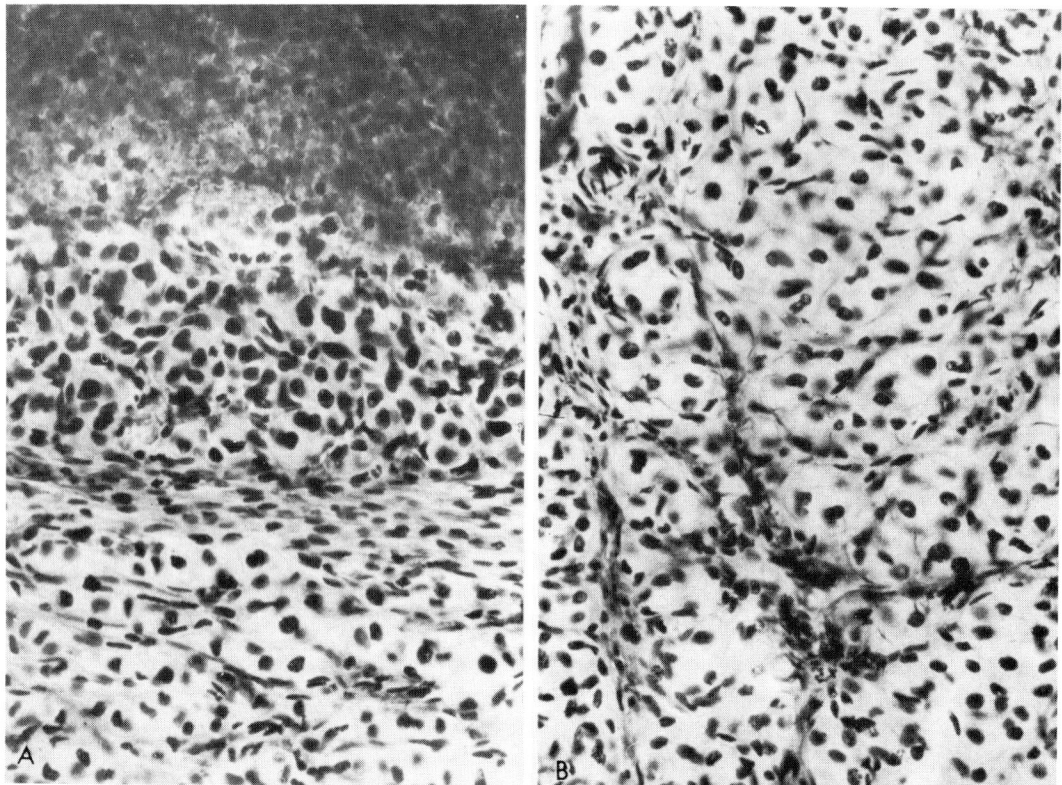

Figure 20-3. Diffuse luteinization of the ovary of a pregnant rabbit. *A*, Luteinized theca; *B*, interstitial luteinization.

investigations by Nelson and colleagues,[142] the life of the gravidic corpus luteum is actually shorter than previously believed. It reaches a functional peak about the sixth week; however, by the eighth week initial degenerative changes have already set in, which culminate during the seventeenth week, after which function all but vanishes totally.[171] In this respect, there is a radical difference between the ovary of woman and that of rodents, the latter retaining activity throughout gestation. Ovarian regression after the first trimester of gestation is characteristic of all primates, with major or minor variations according to species. Neither in woman nor in the various simian species is corpus luteum function necessary for the entire duration of gestation, but it is indispensable for the initial period of gestation. The process of follicular maturation resumes before the end of pregnancy (Fig. 20-4). Dubreuil and Marc-Riviere[58] have called attention to the fact that follicular maturation is initiated during the second trimester. Corpus luteum activity would otherwise inhibit maturation of new follicles, and unless the corpus regresses new follicles cannot grow. Lynch and co-workers[130] and Rathmacher and his associates[152] recently reported the finding of *hyperthecosis* during the first trimester of gestation and during the corpus luteum phase, occurring in parts of the ovary removed from the corpus luteum site and, as would be expected, in the contralateral ovary. They believed that elevated CG concentrations during the first phase of pregnancy were responsible for gestational hyperthecosis. *Since hyperthecosis stops the maturation process of new follicles* (see Chapter 28), *one must assume that paralysis of follicular maturation prior to the seventeenth week of pregnancy is, in the final analysis, due to predominance of CG.*

Various authors[44, 58, 207] have stressed the occurrence of *follicular atresia* as characteristic of this phase of pregnancy. In our view, atresia, as well as hyperthecosis, can be attributed to chorionic gonadotropin activity.

It is therefore evident that placental CG

secretion throughout pregnancy constitutes a permanent influence conducive to follicular atresia, which prevents complete maturation of follicles during pregnancy. *The changes that are observed in the gravidic ovary can all be imputed to the action of elevated concentrations of CG.*

THE OVARIAN INTERSTITIAL GLAND. Follicular involution resulting in atresia in the course of pregnancy stimulates development of a true interstitial gland. Many years ago, Angel and Bouin saw in such interstitial proliferation during the second half of pregnancy the emergence of a new endocrine gland, the interstitial gland, designed to insure myometrial and decidual development. In their day, the incretory function of the placenta was still unknown and there seemed to be no need to search for any other gland besides the ovary to account for the unquestionable estrogenic effect observed during pregnancy. The existence of the interstitial gland was later upheld by Seitz, Dubreuil and Marc-Riviere[58] and others.[97, 155]

There is no doubt that the "interstitial gland" secretes estrogens during pregnancy, but these do not seem to play a primordial role. The fact that gestation in ovariectomized rats and mice may be maintained with injections of progesterone, but not with estrogens (Amoroso[6]), and the fact that ovariectomy may be performed in the human species at any time during gestation without causing disappearance of estrogens from the urine, indicate that, in the absence of the interstitial gland, the placenta and the fetus together are a sufficiently powerful source of estrogen production.

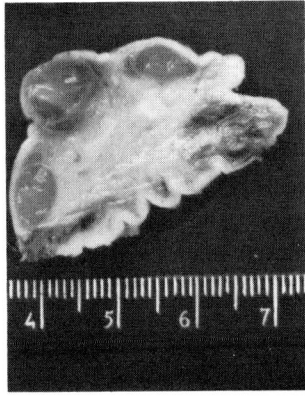

Figure 20-4. Ovary of pregnant woman near term, showing large central interstitial mass and incipient maturation of some follicles.

20.1.2. THE PITUITARY IN PREGNANCY

MORPHOLOGY. Years ago, Erdheim, Stumme and Berblinger described a certain type of *pregnancy cell*, arising from chromophobe cells through a process of transformation. Subsequent studies by Lajos and colleagues[122] and by Swanson and Ezrin[189] questioned the functional significance of these cells. The concept that the pituitary displayed hyperfunction of certain of its elements during pregnancy, which was prevalent for many years and shared by us (see previous editions of this book), seems to have lost ground during the last years, as shall be pointed out.

According to Swanson and Ezrin,[189] the gravidic pituitary is characterized by the absence of δ (delta) cells. In the opinion of Lajos and co-workers,[122] the above-mentioned pregnancy changes result simply from the action of estrogens, as indicated by their finding that the pituitaries of patients with advanced carcinomatosis, who were treated with massive dosages of estrogens, reveal identical "gravidic" changes at autopsy.

HYPOPHYSECTOMY AND GESTATION. The morphologic changes we have just described are not essential for the course of gestation. It is known, for instance, that hypophysectomy does not interrupt gestation either in rats or in rabbits.[180] Anderson and colleagues[7] have in addition shown that transection of the pituitary stalk does not cause interruption of pregnancy in the sow. In more recent times, this has also been found to be the case in Macaca monkeys (Smith,[179] Hutchinson et al.[103]). As for man, Little had extirpated the pituitary of a woman in the twenty-sixth week of pregnancy without causing interruption of gestation, the patient eventually being delivered of a live fetus. Later, Kaplan[112] removed a pituitary chromophobe adenoma during the third month of pregnancy and reported no subsequent adverse effects. However, although the women of both cases gave birth to live infants, they were unable to breast feed them and had to receive supplementary cortisone therapy (see Chapter 45).

GROWTH HORMONE. Early investigations[42, 77, 85] indicated the presence of increased somatotropic hormone activity during pregnancy. After the discovery of *placental lactogen* (see Chapter 19, Section 19.5.5), and following the introduction of specific immunologic methods for the determination of circulating STH (Gitlin et al.,[79] Kaplan and Grumbach,[113] Schalch and Reichlin[167]), it was found that growth hormone was *not increased in pregnancy and that positive bioassay results were attributable to the effects of lactogen.* A great deal of modern research,[149,180,181,216,217] based on specific radioimmunoassay techniques, has failed to reveal any evidence of increased somatotropic activity in gravid women or in gravid animals. Nevertheless, Tyson and his co-workers[195] maintain that somatotropin activity is increased in both normal and pathologic pregnancies. On the other hand, Beaton and colleagues[13] and Tuchmann-Duplessis[194] found that hypophysectomized mothers bore underweight fetuses. Similarly, in a case reported by Little (see Chapter 45), in which the pituitary was extirpated at 26 weeks of pregnancy, the weight of the live-born fetus was markedly decreased. It would therefore seem likely that STH does play some role in gestation after all, although to a lesser extent than formerly was postulated.

GONADOTROPIC HORMONES. We have long been convinced that the urinary gonadotropins excreted during pregnancy were of chorionic and not of pituitary origin (see Chapter 19). In this regard, the findings by Phillip[148] that the pituitary gonadotropin content at pregnancy is practically nil are of interest. Hypophysectomy does not interfere with pregnancy; in hypophysioprival animals, the corpus luteum persists and pregnancy proceeds in a normal way. For these reasons, it must be concluded that the gravidic pituitary *does not secrete gonadotropins.* As a matter of fact, one of the most characteristic phenomena of gestation is precisely the shift of gonadotropin-secreting function from the pituitary to the trophoblast. Nonetheless, Goss and Lewis[83] recently reported finding FSH, immunologically reacting as if it were of pituitary origin, in the urine of pregnant women; they therefore believe that, despite pituitary gonadotropin suppression, the pituitary continues producing some FSH during gestation.

In contrast, in some animals, the pituitary gonadotropin content during pregnancy is quite elevated, but the mechanism of pituitary gonadotropin release is inhibited, as has been shown by, among others, Schwarz and Talley.[173]

THYROTROPIC HORMONE. In 1940, this author showed that the serum of pregnant women contained a thyrotropic principle capable of stimulating the thyroid gland of rats (Fig. 20–5). Sethre and Wells demonstrated that thyrotropin was able to pass across the placental barrier in rodents, but not, according to Green[88] and to Knobil and Josimovitch,[119] in the human species. *Being poorly permeable to large molecules, the*

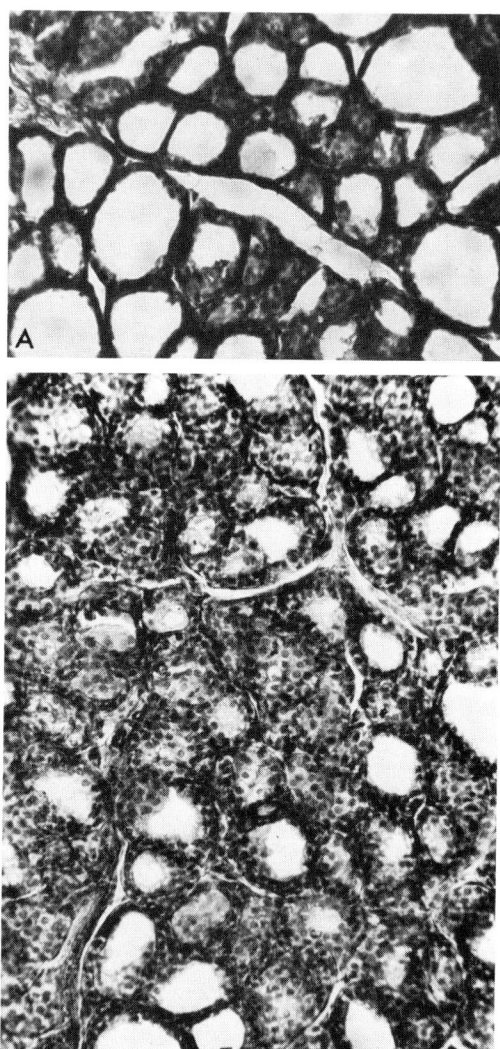

Figure 20–5. Demonstration of thyrotropic hormone in circulating blood during pregnancy. *A*, Control animal, maintained on a thyroid resting diet. Large follicles with flattened, nonproliferative epithelium. *B*, Similar animal, but treated for 10 days with 1 ml per day of pregnant mare serum. A proliferative reaction appears in the thyroid, associated with diminution of follicles, polystratification and cuboidalization of epithelium, which is indicative of functional hyperactivity. (From Botella-Llusiá: *Medicina Española*, 3: 116, 1940.)

human placenta allows almost no passage of pituitary hormones, all of which are proteins of high molecular weight.

PROLACTIN. Blood and urinary prolactin values during pregnancy are not increased. Particularly near term, however, the pituitary secretes prolactin, which is stored in chromophobe cells and is abruptly released during labor (see Chapter 22).

ACTH. As indicated in Chapter 19, adrenocorticotropin is probably not generated in the placenta. However, a certain degree of pituitary overproduction of ACTH seems likely during pregnancy if one considers the fact that pregnant women reveal increased amounts of this tropic substance in their urine (Schmidt and Hoffmann[169]) and blood (Lanman and Dinerstein[126]). This conclusion is supported by the findings of Poulton and Reece[151] who reported that the pituitaries of pregnant rats revealed a considerably increased ACTH content.

NEUROHORMONES. As indicated in Chapter 8, those hormones that in the past were attributed to the posterior lobe of the pituitary, viz., oxytocin, vasopressin and antidiuretic hormone, are actually synthesized by the supraoptic and paraventricular nuclei of the anterior hypothalamus. The functional activity of these nuclei is enhanced during pregnancy. Increased blood levels of oxytocin have been reported by Dieckmann and co-workers[54] and by Hawker,[95] and vasopressin levels would also appear to be elevated (Robinson et al.[158]). Modern immuno-endocrinologic studies have likewise revealed increased pitocinase and oxytocinase activity.[49]

A detectable immune response to the above-mentioned neurohormonal principles is indirect evidence that the latter are increased in pregnancy. Working with recently developed accurate bioassay methods for vasopressin, Robinson and co-workers[158] and Eglin and Jessiman[62] have been able to determine a *definite gravidic elevation of the vasopressin factor.*

While, contrary to earlier belief, the gestational adenohypophysis cannot be qualified as experiencing a phase of hyperfunction, the hypothalamus of pregnancy, on the other hand, is engaged in frank hyperproduction of neurohormones.

CATECHOLAMINES: SEROTONIN. The fact that catecholamine production is increased during pregnancy has been brought to light by Zuspan.[222]

Increased serotonin levels in pregnancy have been reported by Van Den Driesche,[197] Beller and Pollich[19] and Israel and his associates.[105] The physiologic significance of serotonin is open to question but seems to be related to certain abnormalities associated with toxemia of pregnancy (see Chapter 44).

20.1.3. THYROID AND PREGNANCY

The existence of *thyroid hyperfunction* in pregnancy, which had been suspected for decades, has been confirmed through a series of anatomic as well as functional data: (1) thyroid hypertrophy; (2) elevated PBI values; (3) increased levels of thyroxine binding protein (TBP); and (4) increased radioactive iodine (^{131}I) uptake by the thyroid.

THYROID HYPERTROPHY AND HYPERPLASIA. A 65 per cent increase in the volume and weight of thyroid glands in pregnant women was reported by Stander. The studies of Stoffer and colleagues[186] have corroborated the finding of *gravidic thyroid hypertrophy.* Histologically, Herold described *hyperplasia of thyroid follicles* (Fig. 20–6), a finding confirmed by Singh and Morton,[177] Stoffer and co-workers,[186] Bartolomei and Tronchetti,[10] Dowling and colleagues,[57] and Walser.[206] *From the very beginning of gestation, the thyroid grows in size and weight, it becomes hyperemic, its histologic elements undergo hyperplasia, and the colloid is reabsorbed.*

PROTEIN-BOUND IODINE. It is generally well known that the basal metabolic rate is of little value in diagnosing thyroid hyperfunction. This test is even less helpful in pregnancy because of increased metabolism. Protein-bound iodine (PBI) levels are recognized as much more informative, since they are always increased in pregnancy in a constant and regular fashion (Heineman et al.,[96] Man et al.,[132] Mowbray and Tickner,[140] Russell et al.,[165] Ferraris and Scorba,[67] Singh and Morton,[177] Stoffer et al.,[186] Benson et al.[21]). The *butyl-extractable iodine* (BEI) fraction is equally increased (Benson et al.,[21] Kerr[115] and Man et al.[134]). Similarly elevated values have been reported for other thyroid function tests, e.g., thyroxine-binding globulin (Hirschfeld and Söderberg[99]).

THYROXINE-BINDING PROTEIN (TBP). This constitutes another thyroid function

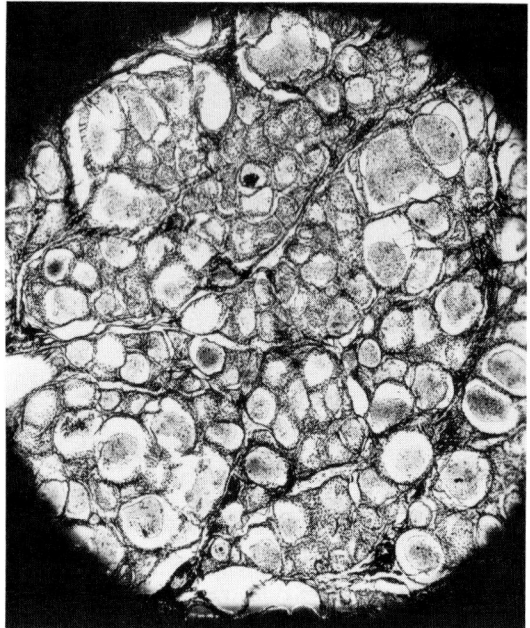

Figure 20-6. Thyroid of pregnancy, showing epithelial proliferation and partial reabsorption of colloid, which are histologic features indicative of a transient state of hyperfunctional activity.

test, considered important in recent times, which shows similarly increased values (Dowling et al.,[57] Carr et al.,[38] Dworkin et al.,[59] and Friedrich et al.[74]).

RADIOACTIVE IODINE (^{131}I) UPTAKE. This routinely employed test has also been applied to the study of thyroid function in pregnant animals (Iino and Greer,[104] Ferraris and Scorba[67]) and in pregnant women (Hodges et al.,[101] Benson et al.,[21] Dowling et al.,[57] Robertson and Falconer[157]), *showing consistently increased values.*

OTHER TESTS INDICATING THYROID HYPERFUNCTION. Plasma thyroxine levels have also been found to be elevated.[78, 176] Finally, Parker and Beierwaltes[145] have reported increased amounts of *antithyroid substances* in the blood of pregnant women, one more argument in favor of gravidic hyperfunction of the thyroid.

THE ORIGIN OF GRAVIDIC HYPERTHYROIDISM. The fact that thyrotropin activity during pregnancy increases has already been mentioned. This is probably the primary cause of the thyroid reaction. Dowling and colleagues[57] found no thyroid hyperfunction in cases with chorioepithelioma, which would seem to eliminate chorionic gonadotropin from among a number of agents possibly causing hyperfunction.

Burger[34] reported that human placental extracts exhibited slight thyrotropic activity and wondered whether chorionic tissue might not secrete small amounts of TSH (Chapter 19, Section 19.5.4) or, alternatively, whether HCG might not inherently possess weak thyrotropic activity.

"COMPENSATORY" HYPERTHYROIDISM. One might expect that Basedow's disease and other functional hyperthyroid states should be aggravated by pregnancy. In reality, just the opposite occurs, as has been stressed by Marañón. Even when thyroid function tests show unusually elevated values—for instance, a PBI of 13 to 18 mcg (normal, 5 to 8 mcg)—pregnant women display no clinical signs of hyperthyroidism (palpitations, tremor, anxiety, exophthalmos, etc.). On the contrary, they tolerate higher amounts of thyroxine than do nonpregnant women (Dowling et al.,[57] Werner[208]). In Chapter 41, we shall again emphasize the fact that hypothyroidism produces abortion and that fetal thyroxine requirements are related to morphogenetic processes. *At present, therefore, we believe that the hyperthyroidism occurring in pregnancy is compensatory in nature, aimed at meeting the increased demands for thyroid hormone of the maternal, and above all, the fetal metabolism. It must be recalled that thyroxine is a morphogenetic agent which accelerates tissue metamorphosis and is apparently also necessary for embryonal development.* Dokumow,[56] Stempak[185] and Schultz and colleagues[172] *consider hyperthyroidism of pregnancy as a compensatory phenomenon.*

20.1.4. THE PARATHYROIDS IN PREGNANCY

During pregnancy, the parathyroid glands enlarge in size, which is believed to be related to the calcium requirements of fetal growth.

Serum calcium levels decrease considerably during pregnancy (Wagner et al.[205]) although phosphorus levels remain unaffected. Pregnancy no doubt puts heavy demands on parathyroid function. Throughout pregnancy, there is a heightening of neuromuscular excitability, which in the past was ascribed to parathyroid hypofunction, or at least to relative parenchymal cell insufficiency in pregnancy.[6, 125] Increased quantities of guanidine bases are also encountered, all of the foregoing data suggesting insufficiency of the gland. However, this is not in keeping with the previously mentioned enlargement of the parathyroid glands and the presence of hyperplasia, principally of the chromophilic cell components. Van Arsdel[196] reported a case of maternal hyperparathyroidism with compensatory atrophy of the fetal parathyroids. Increased production of amine bases, leading to accumulation of *guanidine*, is known to occur in pregnancy. This presumably also imposes an additional strain on the parathyroids.

Parathyroid function during pregnancy may be defined as hyperfunction resulting from increased demands which, if unable to cover existing requirements, may occasionally result in a state of *relative insufficiency*.

20.1.5. PANCREAS IN PREGNANCY

Pregnancy is known to be associated with a tendency toward the development of diabetes. In many women, latent diabetes manifests itself for the first time during gestation (see Chapter 45). On the other hand, multiple pregnancies seem to predispose to pancreatic diabetes. This, and the relative ease with which glycosuria appears in pregnancy, has been thought to be adequate proof of *pancreatic insufficiency in pregnancy*. According to Burt and Pullian,[36] hyperlactacidemia is a sign of pancreatic insufficiency of pregnancy. Nevertheless, the occurrence of *insular hyperplasia* in pregnancy has been reported by various authors.[6, 125] Spellacy and his co-workers,[179] Trayner and associates[192] and Jiménez-Quijada (personal communication) have all reported elevated *insulinemia* in pregnancy by means of accurate radioimmunologic techniques. These findings are in agreement with our own observations[146] (Fig. 20–10), as well as with those of Beck[15] and Kalkhoff and co-workers.[111] The last-mentioned authors have observed similar conditions after the administration of both naturally occurring and synthetic progestogens, and believe that enhancement of insulinic function in pregnancy is a progesterone-induced effect. Finally, Goodner and Freinkel,[81] who studied endogenous insulin consumption by means of radioactive insulin, found that pregnancy consumption rates were twice as high as those found outside pregnancy. This would seem to explain the reason for gestational insular hyperplasia, as well as the fact that gravid women are *insulin-resistant*. Thus, *the pancreas, too, performs a compensatory function during gestation*.

20.1.6. ADRENALS AND PREGNANCY

In Chapter 19, we examined some aspects of corticoid production by the placenta. The ability of the placenta to produce corticoids by no means precludes the occurrence of *gravidic adrenocortical hyperfunction*,[67, 127] which will be discussed later.

CORTICAL HYPERTROPHY AND HYPERPLASIA. In the course of gestation, the adrenal cortex increases in size (Botella[28]) and reveals hyperplasia histologically. This proliferative process involves mainly the fascicular zone (Fig. 20–7) and is associated with an increased lipid content and with

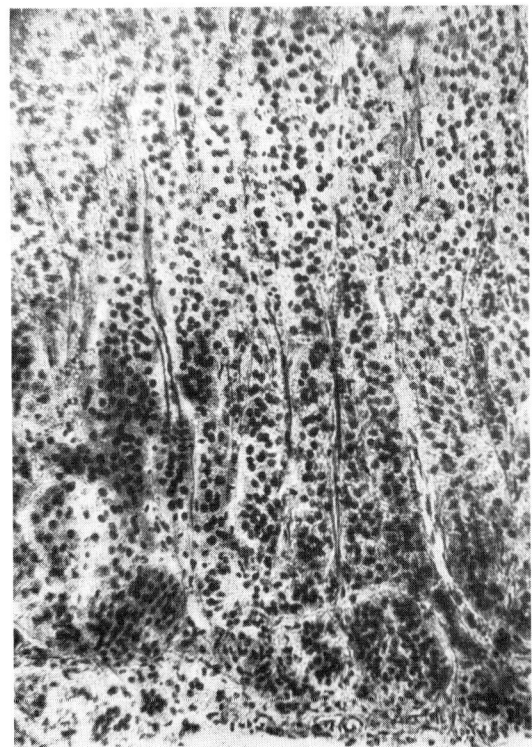

Figure 20–7. Hyperfunctional features in the adrenal cortex of pregnancy. There is pronounced proliferation in the zona fasciculata.

increased vascularization. In contrast, the reticular layer (sexual zone; see Chapter 8) is relatively decreased in thickness, so that the distinctive *fuchsinophilic reaction* otherwise shown by this zone is almost nonexistent in pregnancy.

As pointed out in Chapter 19 (see Fig. 19-3), the adrenal is an additional source of gravidic progesterone and constitutes a sort of "solder" between the luteal phase and the period of placental progestogen synthesis. However, according to our own ideas (see Chapter 9), it would be most unusual to have sex steroid synthesis in the absence of sexual zone hyperplasia. At present, it is well recognized that, of all sex steroids involved in corticoid metabolism, progesterone, a C-21 steroid, is the only one originating in the zona fasciculata. The presence of hyperplasia of the zona fasciculata, without involvement of the reticularis, would therefore be the expected pattern in pregnancy.

CORTICOIDS IN BLOODSTREAM AND URINE DURING GESTATION. *In the bloodstream*, Bayliss and co-workers,[11] Gemzell[77] and Robertson and Falconer[157] found *glucocorticoid* levels to be elevated; Kumar and associates (see Chapter 45) found elevated *mineralocorticoids*, while Bryans and Beitler,[33] Dässler[50] and Rivarola and colleagues[156] encountered increased 17-ketosteroids, although not all of these were believed to be of adrenal origin. High corticoid-binding protein (transcortin) titers in pregnancy have been demonstrated by Doe and his associates,[55] Gala and Westphal,[75] and Rosenthal and co-workers.[163]

In the urine, Porter-Silber positive chromogens in twice as high as normal amounts have been demonstrated by Dässler and Kyank,[49] Sybulsky and Venning,[190] and Cassano and associates.[39] Staemmler[183] and Williams[210] refer to positive aldosteronuria in pregnancy. Lastly, a great number of investigators,[31, 33, 39, 50, 156, 183, 184, 193] among them Rodriguez-López,[159] have reported an increase in one or another of the urinary corticoid fractions. Urinary 17-ketosteroids are also increased in pregnant women, although only part of these are of adrenal origin (Fig. 20-7).

ADRENALECTOMY AND GESTATION. Adrenalectomy is well tolerated during gestation, undoubtedly as a result of placental function. Pregnant bitches do not need any further treatment. In women, adrenalectomies performed during pregnancy have been well tolerated with simple addition of 50 to 60 mg cortisone (Davis and Plotz,[51] Laidlaw et al.,[21] and Bergman et al.[22]), or no supportive therapy at all (Estrada et al.,[66] Brownley et al.,[32] Barber et al.[9]). In all the reported cases, normal amounts of 11-oxysteroids continued to be excreted in the urine, although 17-ketosteroid values were markedly decreased.[92, 93]

TOLERANCE TO CORTISONE DURING GESTATION. Frazer and Fainstat[72] drew attention to the *occurrence of congenital anomalies in the newborn as a result of cortisone therapy in the mother*. Great caution has since been recommended in the use of corticoids in pregnant women.[61] However, reexamination of this problem by Varangot,[199] as well as statistical data obtained by Kostyo,[120] and studies on rats by Curry and Beaton,[46] would seem to indicate that cortisone therapy really involves less danger than originally assumed. Nevertheless, doses of 50 mg a day, or more, during the first trimester may expose patients to unnecessary risks. Such risks are negligible, however, if smaller dosages are used or if therapy is instituted after the first trimester.

Another danger involved in cortisone therapy has been called recently to attention by Hottinger.[102] This is the danger of causing *compensatory atrophy of the fetal adrenal, producing Addison's disease in the newborn.*

Finally, a further hazard associated with hypercorticism of pregnancy, whether endogenous or exogenous, is development of *toxemia of pregnancy*, which shall be discussed in Chapter 44.

SUMMARY: CORTICO-PLACENTAL EQUILIBRIUM IN STEROID SYNTHESIS. *Compensatory hyperfunction of the adrenal cortex indeed occurs in pregnancy. At the same time, the placenta temporarily assumes the function of the cortex. This means that gestation relies on a double system—a security system, so to speak—to meet the markedly increased demands for corticoids. This system operates in a balanced manner. Placental function and cortical function adjust to each other's needs, and both in turn to woman's needs.*

20.2. FETAL INCRETORY SYSTEM

In the beginning of embryonic life, the fetal endocrine glands are immature and un-

Incretory Systems of the Mother and Fetus During Gestation 429

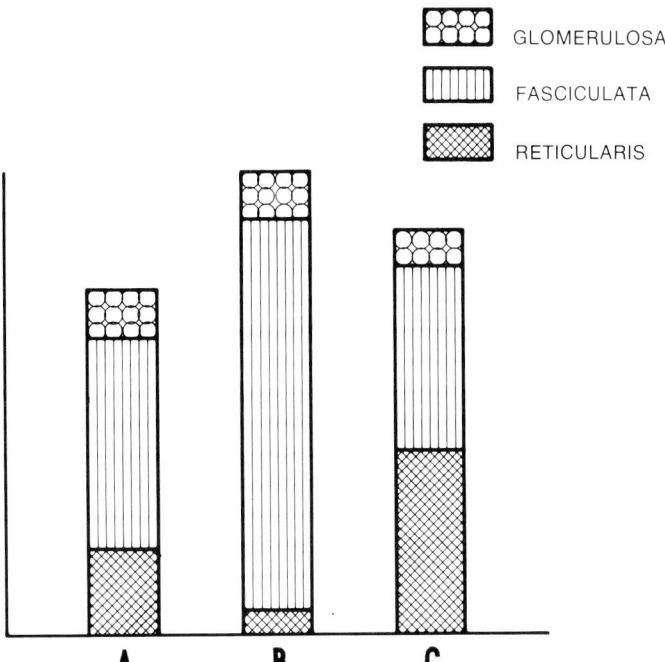

Figure 20–8. Proportional correlations of cortical zones during different phases of woman's sexual life, as revealed by planimetric measurements of adrenals at autopsy. A, Normal woman. B, Eighth month of pregnancy. C, Surgically castrated woman. (From Botella-Llusiá: *Obsterical Endocrinology.* Springfield, Ill., Charles C Thomas, 1961.)

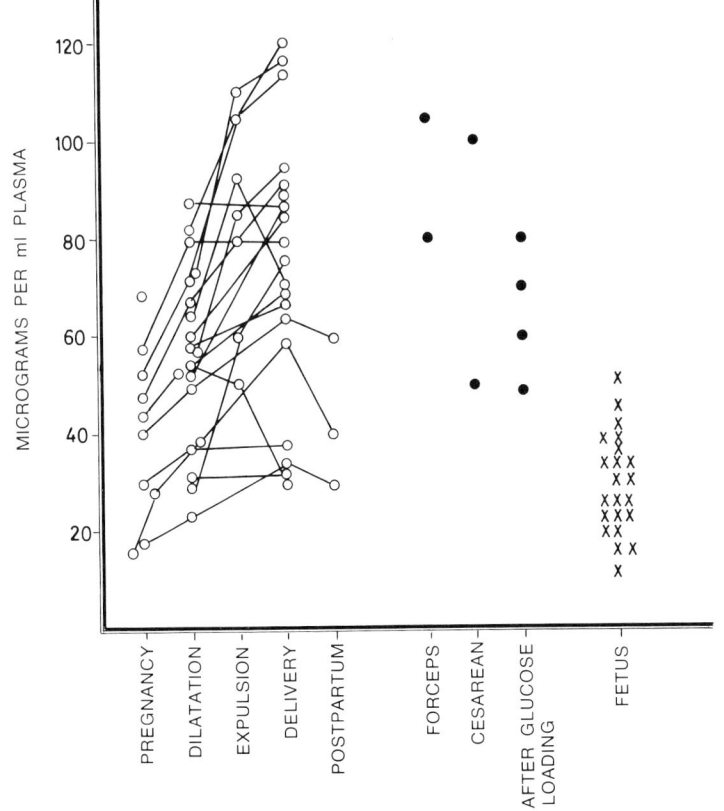

Figure 20–9. Plasma cortisol levels during pregnancy and labor and postpartum, along with fetal levels (method of Valor and Erroz). Note elevated plasma cortisol during pregnancy and labor. (From Botella-Llusiá and Clavero-Nuñez: *Fisiologia Femenina,* 9th ed. Barcelona, Editorial Científico Médica, 1971.)

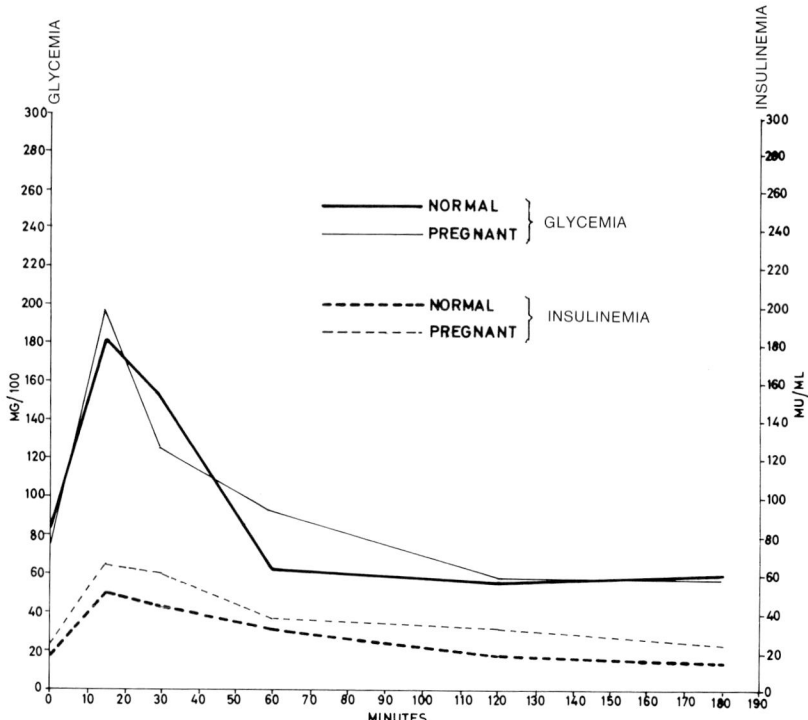

Figure 20-10. Plasma insulin levels in six pregnant women during the third trimester and six nonpregnant controls, determined by means of the technique of Hales and Randle (radioimmunoassay after giving 0.5 g/kg loading dose of intravenous glucose). A significant increase in the level of insulin reserve is noted in normal gestation. (From Botella-Llusiá et al.: *Acta Gin.*, 21:569, 1970.)

able to perform any function. But by midterm some of them start to show signs of activity, activity which may become very important before term. We owe a detailed study of fetal endocrine gland evolution to Tonutti[191] (Fig. 20-11) and to MacNaughton.[131] We shall examine successively: (1) the gonads; (2) the adrenals; (3) the thyroid; (4) the pancreas; (5) the pituitary; (6) the parathyroids; (7) the thymus; (8) the liver.

20.2.1. THE GONADS DURING FETAL LIFE

The possibility that the embryonal gonads secrete hormones has been discussed in Chapter 15. The embryonic gonads probably produce a hormonoid substance, consisting of estrogens and androgens in conjunction with a protein, possibly a globulin. This gives rise to *estroproteins* and *androproteins*, respectively, for which other workers have used the terms *cortexine* and *medullarine*.

GENERAL CONSIDERATIONS. As already mentioned in Chapter 15, the embryonal gonads display a certain degree of steroidogenic activity. There are significant differences between the behavior of the ovary and that of the testis. While the ovary appears to have scanty endocrine activity during embryonic life, the testis displays precocious activity, intervening in the process of wolffian duct differentiation (Chapter 15, page 331), as had been shown by the classic works of Jost and associates.[108, 109]

The enzyme 3β-ol-dehydrogenase serves to indicate the onset of steroidogenic activity in embryonal gonads. Baillie and colleagues[8] detected the presence of this enzyme in the genital crest of a 14 mm human fetus. The quite early appearance of this steroidogenic enzyme in the fetal testis has also been reported by Bloch and Benirschke,[25] Cavallero and co-workers,[40] Botte and Chieffi,[30] and Schlegel and co-workers.[168] The occurrence of pseudohermaphroditism was observed by Elger[64] among the males of the litter of pregnant rabbits treated with cyproterone on the tenth day of gestation, which would indicate testicular endocrine activity in rabbits as early as the tenth day of gestation. Serra and colleagues[174] have also found the fetal testis to be capable of synthesizing testosterone directly from cholesterol, without intermediate precursors, which seems to suggest a remarkable degree of steroidogenic maturity.

Ovarian endocrine maturation, on the other hand, lags far behind. Bengtsson and his co-workers[20] failed to detect any C-14 labeled cholesterol uptake by human fetal ovaries. Similarly, no estrogen synthesis was noted by Jungman and Schweppe[110] to take place in homogenates of ovary incubated in the presence of C-14 labeled acetate. Investigations aimed at detecting 3β-ol-dehydrogenase in the embryonic ovary have likewise yielded consistently negative results.[30, 168]

Bedoya and Rodríguez,[16] at our laboratory, measured fetal serum HCG concentrations. The amounts found were less than 1 IU per milliliter and, thus, a hundred times lower than those circulating in the mother's bloodstream at the same time. Consequently, because of the large size of the molecules involved, these investigators rejected the possibility of HCG passage into the fetal blood, and believed that, since it was secreted by the trophoblast, HCG reached the maternal compartment by diffusion much more readily than it entered the fetal compartment.

We believe that the selective passage of gonadotropins to the mother serves the purpose of *preserving the fetal gonad from excessive gonadotropin stimulation*. The fetal gonad, particularly the testis, is thought to be subject to stimulation by the action of the fetal pituitary itself, possibly induced, in turn, by estrogens of chorionic origin.

STRUCTURE AND FUNCTION OF FETAL OVARIES NEAR TERM. Although the fetal ovary, unlike the testis (see Chapter 15), reveals no endocrine activity at midterm, it does undergo a period of activity toward the end of gestation. Investigations undertaken by Rodríguez-Soriano,[160] and, more recently, by Merlo and Riaza at our clinic, have implied this is the case. Figure 20-12 reveals the appearance of ovaries of fetuses approaching maturity.

FETAL STEROIDOGENESIS. There are many reports bearing witness to steroid

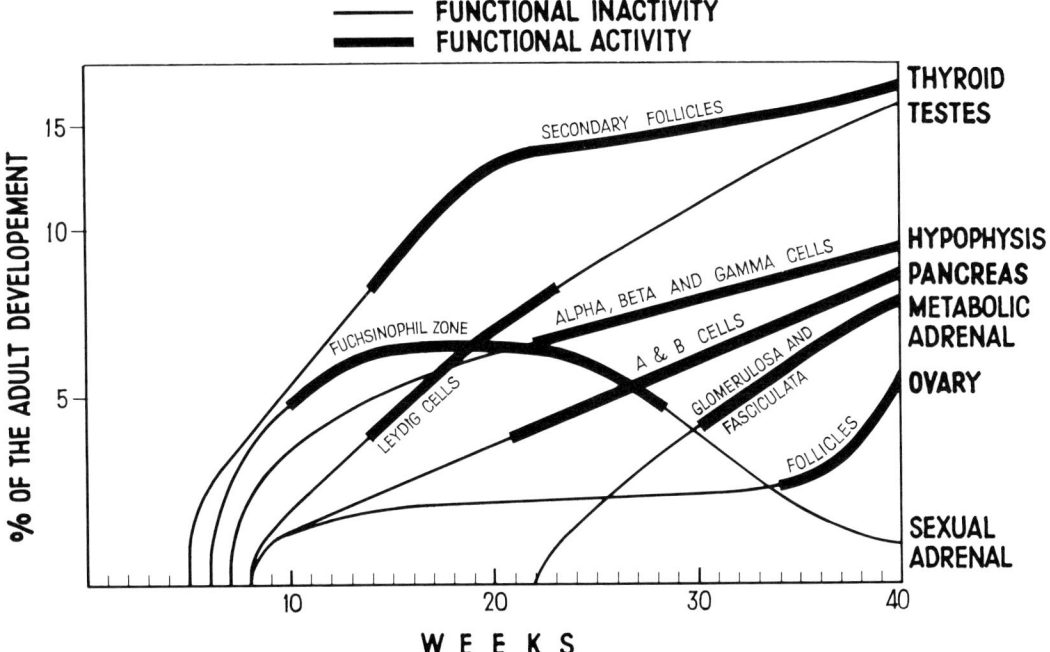

Figure 20–11. Development of fetal endocrine glands in terms of percentage of adult development. Fine lines represent phases of functional inactivity; thick lines denote presence of histologic (or other type) of evidence of functional activity. Note the presence of two kinds of transient activity, that of testis and that of sexual adrenal. The remaining glands enter into action near the end of pregnancy, in preparation for the activities of extrauterine life. (From Botella-Llusiá: *Obstetrical Endocrinology.* Springfield, Ill., Charles C Thomas, 1961.)

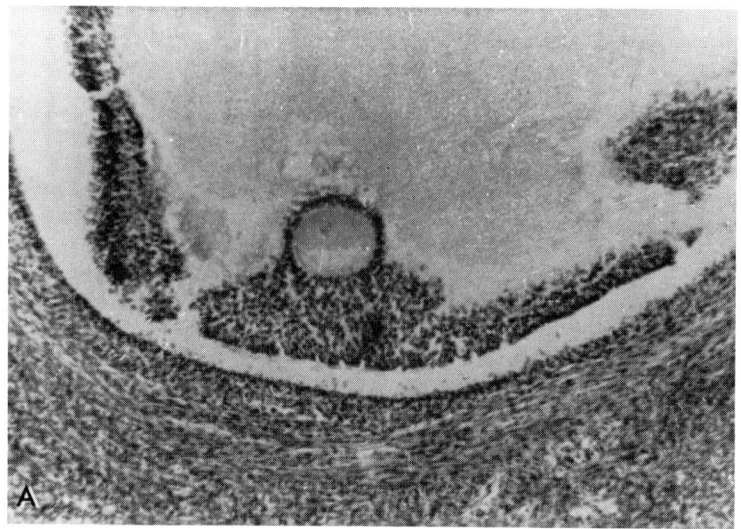
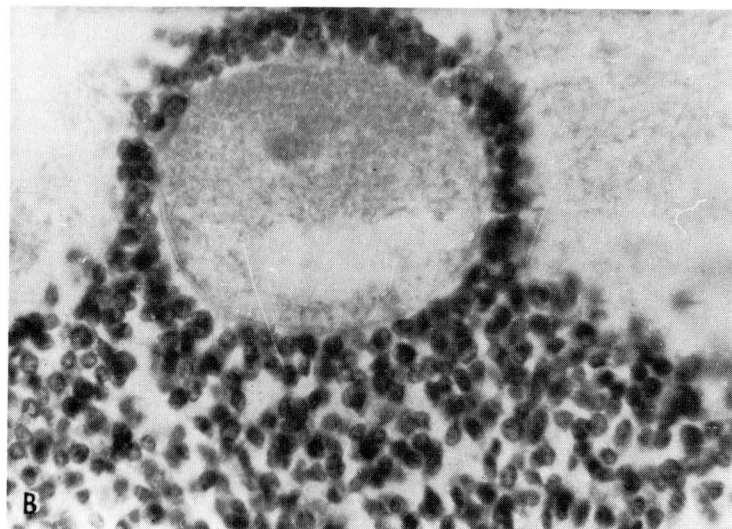

Figure 20-12. Mature follicle in fetal ovary at term. A, 100×; B, 450×.

biogenesis in the fetal body, involving estrogens,[53, 71, 135, 136] androgens[2, 108, 109, 143] and progesterone.[153, 200, 203, 219] However, fetal steroid synthesis cannot be ascribed exclusively to the fetal gonads, since it is mainly a product of the interplay between the *fetal adrenal and the placenta*, with some participation by the *liver*, as has been shown by the modern studies in Stockholm (Diczfalusy[53]). For this reason, we devote a separate section to examining this question later in this chapter.

20.2.2. THE ADRENAL DURING FETAL LIFE

Apart from the medulla, whose development and secretory activity in the fetus have been clarified by the investigations of Lewis,[128] the most important aspect concerning the embryonal adrenal is the *physiology of the adrenal cortex*. As pointed out in Chapter 9, the adrenal cortex is one of the most important organs lying within the abdominal cavity during embryonal life (Fig. 20-13). It develops and unfolds to peak performance about the fourth month of gestation.

PALEOCORTEX AND NEOCORTEX. In the course of our studies,[28] we found that the fetal cortex, which first exhibits obvious hypertrophy in four month old fetuses, has a different histologic architecture from that of the adult adrenal under physiologic conditions. It bears a much closer resemblance to the zona reticularis or to the X zone of rodents, described by a number of authors to undergo postnatal involution (see Chapter 9). A similar phenomenon occurs in the human species. Before the seventh month of gestation, the cortex consists almost exclusively of zona reticularis-like tissue, whereas the fascicular and glomerular zones begin to show some development only after the seventh or eighth month of gestation. Histogenetic studies of these zones would seem to indicate that the fasciculata and glomerulosa, on the one hand, and the reticularis, on the other, have distinct origins. While the first two arise through proliferation of the *subcapsular blastema*, the third arises from the *juxtamedullary blastema*. In our opinion, then, the fetal adrenal cortex consists of two functionally different components. The first of these, the *sexual adrenal*, is, as we shall explain subsequently, deeply involved in sexual steroid metabolism, viz., that of estrogens and androgens; the second, the *metabolic adrenal*, develops much later and is concerned with corticoid synthesis. Beginning with birth, the sexual adrenal undergoes atrophy, giving rise to what is known as *postnatal atrophy* of the gland, observed to occur also in rats and mice,[28] whereas the metabolic adrenal proliferates and will persist as the exclusive zone of infancy. Because of this, we have also used the terms *temporary zone* and *permanent zone* in referring to these entities. A similar point of view has later been espoused by Christianson and Jones[41] and by Levine.[127]

MATURATION OF THE FETAL METABOLIC ADRENAL. Prior to the twenty-sixth week of fetal life, the cortex consists exclusively of the paleocortex. Bech and co-workers[14] noted that this intermediate zone underwent involution while fetuses were still immature. After that, corticoid synthesizing activity becomes perceptible. According to Verne and Herbert,[201] there is as yet no corticoid production apparent in seven month old fetuses. From fetuses less than seven months old, Bloch and Benirschke[25] have been able to obtain only 17-ketosteroids, whereas 17-hydroxyprogesterone could be obtained only from older fetuses.

In vitro steroid synthesis has been observed to occur in slices of fetal adrenal by Lanman[124] and Villee.[202] Adrenalectomy in the mother was found to produce compensatory fetal hyperfunction (Davis and Plotz,[51] Verne and Herbert,[201] Knobil and Briggs[118]). Alexander and co-workers,[5] Bloch,[27] and Whitehouse and Winson[209] recently showed that the fetal adrenal developed its capacity for cortisol synthesis at a relatively late stage. There has been some speculation over what role, if any, maternal ACTH, which is increased in pregnancy as we have pointed out earlier, plays in the development of fetal adrenal corticoidogenic function. Placental synthesis of ACTH is not at present held to be a fact and maternal ACTH is believed to pass across the placental barrier only with difficulty. In this respect, results of the experiments conducted by Christianson and Jones[41] on pregnant rats make the passage of maternal ACTH to the fetus doubtful (similar in scope to that of CG, discussed previously), and raise the question of whether the fetal adrenal, even at term, is mature enough to elaborate C-21 steroids. It is our view, nevertheless, that the fetal adrenal eventually reaches maturity at some stage of pregnancy, and that it has a normal capacity for synthesizing corticoids by the time of birth. It is possible that, while ACTH does not succeed in passing through the placental barrier, if at all, other than in minimal amounts, the fetal pituitary may stimulate adrenal function by means of its own ACTH. In the light of modern knowledge (see Chapter 8), on the other hand, vasopressin could also stimulate the fetal pituitary to produce adrenocortico-

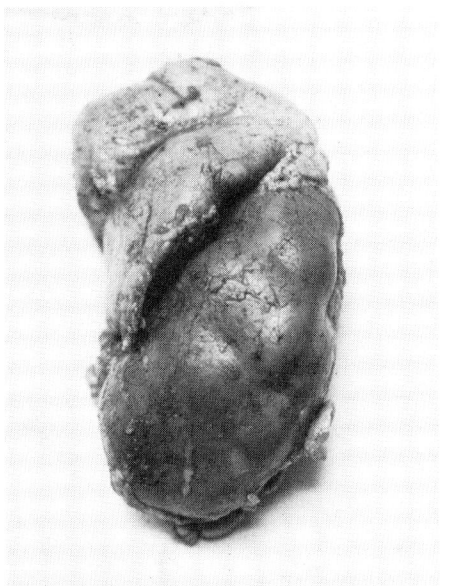

Figure 20–13. Adrenal cortex of a four month old fetus; note its exaggerated size in comparison to that of the kidney.

tropin. Increased vasopressin levels have been demonstrated in the maternal blood, and the molecular size of this hormone would make placental passage a distinct possibility.

During the last two months of intrauterine life, maturation of the metabolic cortex parallels the degree of metabolic autonomy attained by the fetus, commensurate with the rate at which the placenta involutes as a metabolic and reserve organ, and as the liver develops to take over the governing function hitherto discharged by the placenta.

20.2.3. FETO-PLACENTAL STEROID METABOLISM

We have already indicated (Chapter 19, Section 19.7.2) that placental steroid synthesis cannot be conceived as dissociated from fetal steroidogenesis, particularly insofar as *fetal adrenal function* is concerned. Based on a series of fundamental studies, Diczfalusy and his group[20, 24, 52, 53, 211, 212] have established the so-called "Stockholm concept," which can be summarized as follows: The placenta is a producer of *incomplete steroids*, its output depending almost entirely on the supply of steroids available in the *maternal* circulation and, *particularly, in the fetal circulation* (Fig. 20–15). The main estrogen precursors are 3-sulfates of various 3β-hydroxyandrosten-5-derivatives. The placenta does not contain the whole steroidogenic enzyme system, sharing it, as it does, with the fetus. While 3β-ol-dehydrogenase and δ-4-5-isomerase are mainly contained within the placenta, 17α-hydroxylase is present only in the fetal adrenal (and in part the fetal testis). Consequently, the placenta and the fetus together constitute a *functional unit*, conjointly synthesizing the major part of those estrogens, especially estriol, which are excreted in the urine of pregnant women. A comprehensive idea of how these transformations take place is diagrammed in Figure 20–15.

On reexamining Figure 20–15, it is apparent that the fetal adrenal is essential for the production and sulfation of dehydroepiandrosterone (DHEA). Probably, this type of esterification is aimed at sparing the fetal tissue from excessively rapid in situ utilization of DHEA, as well as from having estrogens accumulate within the fetal compartment. By virtue of its ability to deesterify DHEA, only the placenta utilizes the latter for estrogen synthesis.

Passage of estrogens to the fetus takes place through the amnion rather than the placenta (Katz et al.[114]). According to Villee and Loring,[204] fetal adrenal steroidogenesis differs from that occurring in the adult in that progesterone does not figure in it as an obligatory intermediary metabolite. Progesterone synthesis is a predominantly maternal function (see Fig. 20–15)[70, 91, 154] but, as the fetal adrenal matures progressively, its progestogen forming capacity grows commensurately.[162] However, the rate of progestogen synthesis by the fetal adrenal in the armadillo[26] as well as in the human[98] is elevated, suggesting that a distinct, nonprogesteronic precursor is involved in fetal adrenal corticoid synthesis.[60, 65, 170]

20.2.4. FETAL THYROID

The fetal thyroid shows signs of activity at a quite early stage (Fig. 20–11). Injection of ^{131}I into a chicken egg results in immediate concentration of radioactivity within the embryo's thyroid.[82, 187, 193] The fetus of rodents is similarly capable of trapping the ra-

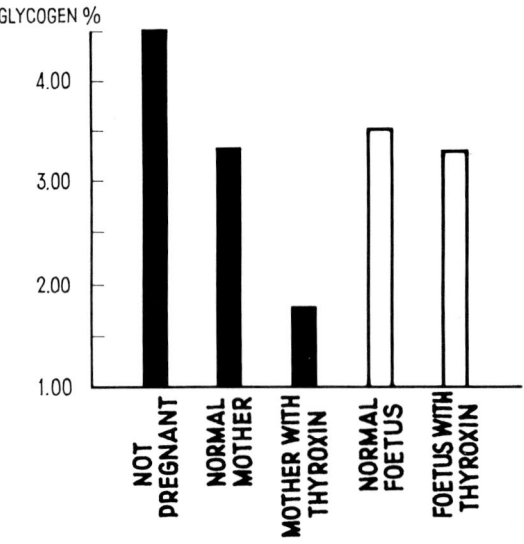

Figure 20–14. Hepatic glycogen in pregnant rats and their fetuses, with or without thyroxine administration. Thyroxine treatment accentuates maternal glycogenolysis, normally observed in pregnancy, while having no effect on fetal glycogenesis, which may be construed as evidence that thyroxine is rapidly inactivated by fetal body.

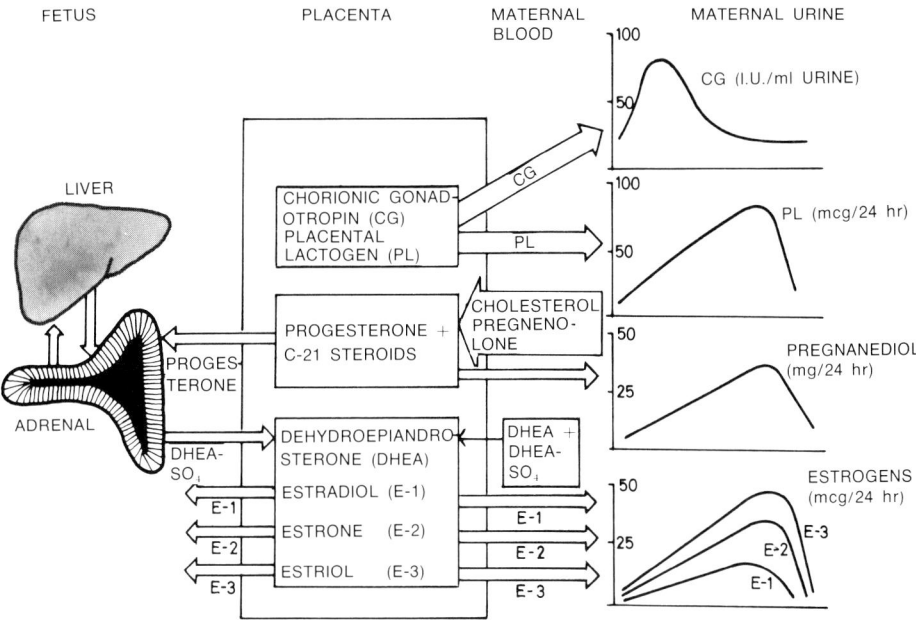

Figure 20-15. Diagrammatic representation of steroidogenesis in fetoplacental unit. (From Benirschke and Driscoll: *Handbuch der Speziellen Pathologischen Anatomie und Histologie*, Vol. 7, Part 5. New York, Springer, 1967.)

dioactive substance[106, 123, 198, 213] and Beierwaltes[18] reported the same findings in dogs. As regards the human fetus, Hodges and colleagues[101] and Shepard[175] have reported a *positive ^{131}I uptake rate beginning with the twelfth week of pregnancy*. It has further been determined (Olin et al.[144]) that thyroglobulin synthesis by the human fetal thyroid begins about the fifty-sixth day.

The relationship between this unquestionable fetal thyroid activity and the maternal compartment has not yet been sufficiently clarified. Propylthiouracil, injected into rats,[47, 48] or into women,[35] produces hypertrophy of the fetal thyroid. There is disagreement (Morreale and Escobar, personal communication) as to whether such a fetal goiter is hyper- or hypofunctional, although Beierwaltes[18] believes he has determined fetal thyroid hyperfunction by means of ^{131}I uptake measurements. This belief seems justified if one considers the case recorded by Fioretti and Carretti[68] of fetal thyroid hyperplasia in a stillborn fetus of a myxomatous mother. There are two possible explanations for this inverted functional relationship (see Section 20.3.1): (1) passage of *thyroxine* from the mother to the fetus, where it assumes the role of regulating the fetal pituitary-hypothalamic system, and (2) passage of *maternal thyrotropin* into the fetal compartment.

PASSAGE OF THYROXINE FROM THE MOTHER TO THE FETUS. The possibility that thyroxine passes across the placental barrier, perhaps with the exception of insignificant amounts, has been dismissed by us as unlikely. Nevertheless, passage of a variety of thyroid extracts has been proved to take place by Grumbach and Werner,[90] Roy and Kobayashi,[164] and Yamazaki and colleagues.[215] Postel[150] found that although thyroxine passed through the placental barrier with difficulty, *triiodothyronine* did so relatively promptly, and postulated that the question of passage might involve a "precursor" substance, a view later shared by Schultz and his co-workers.[172]

PASSAGE OF THYROTROPIN FROM THE MOTHER TO THE FETUS. Notwithstanding the fact that Bernheim and associates[23] and Romanoff and Lauffer[161] admitted that the placenta was permeable to TSH, we have repeatedly stated that, owing to the large molecular size of the proteins composing the adenohypophysial hormones (including that of insulin and HCG), we consider such passage difficult, if not impossible. Knobil and Josimovitch[119] failed to confirm thyrotropin passage through the placental barrier, which was confirmed by Geloso[76] and Nataf and his co-workers.[141] According to these authors, in vitro cultures of fetal tissue reveal active secretion independently of whether TSH is added to the culture media. It may be suspected that a different regulatory mechanism is at play for fetal thyroid hormone synthesis, distinct from that of the adult, which would explain the paradoxical reactions described by Morreale and Escobar.

20.2.5. PANCREAS

In 1911, Carlson and Drennan pancreatectomized adult dogs and found that the resulting pancreatoprival diabetes was much less severe in pregnant than in non-pregnant bitches. In addition, pancreatectomy at an early stage of pregnancy produced greater effects than when resection was performed at a late stage of pregnancy. During pregnancy, the animals remained in a compensated condition but developed typical diabetes after delivery. These findings suggest that by the time the fetal pancreas has developed, it secretes sufficient insulin to cross the placental barrier and to protect the mother from the adverse effects of having no pancreas.

However, there is considerable controversy over the question of placental passage of insulin. In 1936, this author performed the experiment reproduced in Figure 20–16, in which insulin was found not to cross the placental barrier but, on the contrary, to remain contained within the fetal circulation, attracting surplus maternal carbohydrates and utilizing them for the fetal body.[29] Subsequently, Knobil and Briggs,[118] Adam and colleagues,[3] and Mintz and co-workers[139] also subscribe to our view in denying passage of insulin through the placenta. However, just as in the case of the adenohypophysial protein hormones, passage of insulin cannot be ruled out in absolute terms. It is conceivable that a small portion may cross the placental barrier in spite of the molecular structures involved; however, what can be rejected a priori is free diffusion of insulin across the materno-fetal barrier. It should further be added that, on the basis of the recent findings by Freinkel and Goodner,[73, 80, 81] the placenta would appear to degrade insulin through a process of proteolysis.

20.2.6. PITUITARY

Histologically, the pituitary of various animal species has been described to undergo

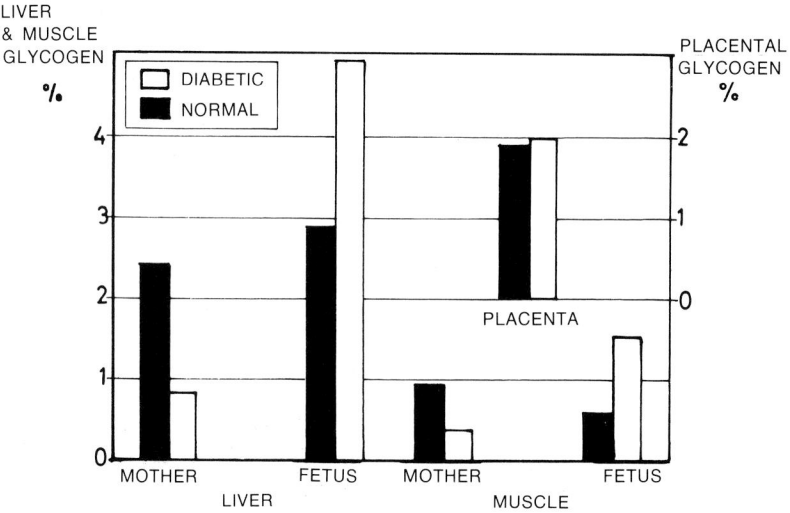

Figure 20–16. Experiment on normal control, female rabbit on eighteenth day of pregnancy and similar rabbit, partly pancreatectomized three days prior to experiment. Determination of hepatic and muscular glycogen content in mother and fetus reveals that fetuses of diabetic rabbits contain more glycogen than do control animals, while mother is depleted of glycogen. This demonstrates that fetal insulin does not cross the placental barrier, with the surplus maternal glucose being utilized by the fetal body.

differentiation at a relatively early stage of embryonal development. Hog embryos, for instance, develop anterior lobe intracellular granules at the 50 to 170 mm stage, according to Nelson and colleagues.

Discrepant results have been reported after removal of the fetal pituitary in different animals.[63, 103, 109] However, Knigge's experiments[117] with fetal pituitary transplants would seem to indicate that the fetal pituitary, in animals and man alike, possesses unequivocal activity. This is also the opinion held by Jost.[108] Similarly, Wells and Foote (see Chapter 15) have noted that decapitation of fetuses in well advanced gestation caused not only gonadal atrophy but atrophy of the adrenals and the thyroid as well.

Jailer and colleagues[107] and Bedoya and Maldonado,[17] as well as Milkovic and Milkovic,[138] have all shown that the pituitary-adrenal axis is not yet fully developed at the time of birth. Or, in other words, *the pituitary at birth does not respond to hypothalamic stimuli.* Apparently, this phenomenon results not from lack of endocrine properties of the pituitary but from *immaturity of the nervous system. As a result, the fact that the pituitary may not betray manifest endocrine activity during embryonal life does not mean that its parenchyma is immature, as might be suspected at first sight, but rather that this is due to lack of neurogenic stimuli which are necessary for the pituitary to function.*

Cornblath and his associates[43] have shown that growth hormone is produced by the fetal pituitary, a finding favoring the concept of possible independent activity of this gland during embryonal life.

20.2.7. PARATHYROID

The fetal parathyroids at term carry out an active function and are ready to assume the all-important task of regulating the calcium metabolism of the newborn. There is a reciprocal compensatory functional relationship between the fetal parathyroid and the homologous gland in the mother, much along the same lines as has been seen to occur in the thyroid, adrenal and pancreas.[1, 109] In the recent past, a highly interesting syndrome, consisting of maternal hyperparathyroidism in association with tetany in the newborn, has been described (Walton[207] and Van Arsdel[196]). This syndrome is an excellent example of how excessive functional activity by one of the mother's glands may produce atrophy of the corresponding fetal gland, and vice-versa.

20.2.8. FETAL THYMUS

The development of the thymus is one of the most interesting phenomena of fetal endocrinology. Though its full role is still poorly known, the thymus unquestionably acts as an antagonist of the gonad during embryonal development. Absence of the thymus in males, as distinct from females, is associated with elevated fetal mortality, as though the underlying cause involved intolerance to estrogen effect.[92] Kincl and his group[116] reported that thymic extracts prevented development of androgenic sterility in newborn rats. Bearn[12] stresses the antagonistic effect exerted on the thymus by the adrenal and by the pituitary. Anencephaly[28, 29, 65, 170] is well known to be associated with thymic hyperplasia and pituitary-adrenal aplasia at the same time. Similarly, Bearn[12] has seen thymic hyperplasia in rabbit embryos that had been either decapitated or adrenalectomized.

20.2.9. ENDOCRINE ROLE OF FETAL LIVER

In Figure 20–15, the fetal liver has been incorporated into the system of feto-placental steroid synthesis, in keeping with the concept developed by Diczfalusy and associates.[20, 24, 52, 53] Greig and MacHaughton[89] have shown that 92 per cent of a dose of C-14 labeled progesterone, injected into the umbilical cord, can be found in the liver. Wu and his colleagues[214] have equally well demonstrated that the liver of young fetuses synthesizes estrogens.

20.3. MATERNAL-FETAL ENDOCRINE INTERRELATIONSHIPS

Elsewhere[24] we have summarized the conditions that determine the interactions between the endocrine glands of the mother and those of the embryo. These can be formulated in the following way:

20.3.1. LAW OF COMPENSATORY ATROPHY

Introduction of a hormone into the body in excessive amounts is followed immediately by diminished activity of that pituitary trophic hormone which stimulates the secretion of the hormone in excess. Thus, for instance, injections of estrogen suppress FSH secretion; injections of cortisone lower ACTH; injections of thyroxine diminish TSH secretion.

20.3.2. MATURITY OF THE TARGET ORGANS

All the fetal endocrine glands are, to a greater or lesser extent, subject to the action of the mother's pituitary and placental hormones. Their response is commensurate to the degree of maturity attained by the corresponding gland. ACTH exerts a sufficiently potent stimulus from the first months of gestation; nevertheless, the fetal adrenals do not produce their own corticoids until after the twenty-sixth week because, up to that point, their fascicular zones have not reached the necessary degree of maturity.

20.3.3. PLACENTAL PERMEABILITY

The interrelationship between the maternal and the fetal glands just described is established in accordance with the rate of interchange taking place across the placental filter. Hormones of high molecular weight, for example, insulin and CG, may be detained on one side of the barrier or the other, failing to affect the body of the mother (insulin) or the fetus (CG).

Thus, the materno-fetal unit may not be qualified as an example of simple parabiosis; although it is in actuality a state of parabiosis, it might be more aptly called "*conditioned parabiosis.*" The conditioning factor here is the interposition of a placental membrane between the two circulations.

20.3.4. FETAL ENDOCRINOPATHIES

The compensatory nature of the endocrine changes occurring in the fetus allows the formulation of a final general principle: "*The emergence of any endocrinopathy in the mother results in the development of an opposite endocrinopathy in the fetus.*"

Examples of this have been mentioned previously, such as the fact that babies of hypercortical mothers are born with addisonism, that maternal thiouracil therapy produces fetal hyperthyroidism, and that maternal diabetes is associated with hyperinsulinism and hypoglycemia in the newborn. In short, the presence of a *congenital endocrinopathy* reflects a primary disorder in the pregnant woman.

The importance of this cannot be overemphasized, not only as regards the better understanding of the etiology of a given endocrinopathic symptomatology in infancy but also as regards the necessity of applying endocrine therapy judiciously. *The present-day availability of potent hormone preparations for therapeutic use commands utmost caution in their application during gestation, if we are to avert the danger of drug-induced endocrine embryopathies.*

REFERENCES

1. Aceto, T., Batt, R. E., Bruck, E., Schulz, R. B., and Perez, R.: *J. Clin. Endocr. Metab.*, 26:487, 1966.
2. Acevedo, H. F., et al.: *J. Clin. Endocr. Metab.*, 23:885, 1963.
3. Adam, A. J., et al.: *Diabetes*, 18:409, 1969.
4. Adams, E. C., and Hertig, A. T.: *J. Cell. Biol.*, 41:3, 1969.
5. Alexander, D. P., et al.: *Endocrinology*, 40:1, 1968.
6. Amoroso, E. C.: *Ann. d'Endocr.*, 16:435, 1955.
7. Anderson, L. L., Dick, G. W., Mori, H., Henricks, D. M., and Mellampy, R. M.: *J. Physiol.*, 124:87, 1966.
8. Baillie, A. H., Ferguson, M. M., and Hart, D. M. K.: *J. Clin. Endocr. Metab.*, 26:738, 1966.
9. Barber, H. R. K., Graber, E. A., and O'Rourke, J. J.: *Obstet. Gynec.*, 27:414, 1966.
10. Bartolomei, G., and Tronchetti, G.: *Ann. d'Endocr.*, 19:615, 1958.
11. Bayliss, R. I. S., et al.: *Lancet*, 1:62, 1955.
12. Bearn, J. G.: *Endocrinology*, 80:979, 1955.
13. Beaton, G. H., et al.: *Endocrinology*, 57:748, 1955.
14. Bech, K., Tygstrup, I., and Nerup, J.: *Acta Path. Microbiol. Scand.*, 76:391, 1967.
15. Beck, P.: *Diabetes*, 18:146, 1969.
16. Bedoya, J. M., and Rodriguez, M.: *Acta Gin.*, 2:499, 1951.
17. Bedoya, J. M., and Maldonado, M.: *Acta Gin.*, 6:65, 1955.
18. Beierwaltes, W. H.: *Endocrinology*, 80:545, 1967.

19. Beller, F. K., and Pollich, J. P.: *Arch. Gynäk.*, 196:136, 1961.
20. Bengtsson, G., Ullberg, S., Wiqvist, N., and Diczfalusy, E.: *Acta Endocr.*, 46:544, 1964.
21. Benson, R. C., et al.: *Obstet. Gynec.*, 14:11, 1959.
22. Bergman, P., et al.: *Acta Endocr.*, 35:293, 1960.
23. Bernheim, N., et al.: *Ann. d'Endocr.*, 18:10, 1957.
24. Bird, C. E., Wiqvist, N., Diczfalusy, E., and Solomon, S.: *J. Clin. Endocr. Metab.*, 26:1144, 1966.
25. Bloch, E., and Benirschke, K.: *Endocrinology*, 76:43, 1965.
26. Bloch, E., et al.: *Endocrinology*, 71:628, 1962.
27. Bloch, E.: *Steroids*, 13:589, 1965.
28. Botella, J.: *Arch. Gynäk.*, 183:73, 1953.
29. Botella, J.: *Obstetrical Endocrinology*. Springfield, Ill., Charles C Thomas, 1961.
30. Botte, V., and Chieffi, G.: *Arch. Ost. Gin.*, 72:434, 1967.
31. Bret, A. J., Coiffard, D., and Crimail, P.: *Rev. Franc. Gynec. Obstet.*, 55:669, 1960.
32. Brownley, H. C., Warren, J. E., and Parson, W.: *Amer. J. Obstet. Gynec.*, 80:628, 1960.
33. Bryans, F. E., and Beitler, A.: *Amer. J. Obstet. Gynec.*, 82:52, 1961.
34. Burger, A.: *Acta Endocr.*, 55:587, 1967.
35. Burrows, G. N.: *J. Clin. Endocr. Metab.*, 25:403, 1965.
36. Burt, R. L., and Pullian, R. E.: *Obstet. Gynec.*, 14:519, 1959.
37. Carpent, G., and Desclin, L.: *Ann. d'Endocr.*, 28:245, 1967.
38. Carr, E. A., et al.: *J. Clin. Endocr. Metab.*, 19:1, 1959.
39. Cassano, F., et al.: *Ann. Ost. Gin.*, 82:801, 1960.
40. Cavallero, C., Magrini, U., Dellepiane, M., and Ciselj, T.: *Ann. d'Endocr.*, 26:409, 1965.
41. Christianson, M., and Jones, I. C.: *J. Endocr.*, 15:17, 1957.
42. Contopoulos, A. N., and Simpson, M. E.: *Endocrinology*, 64:1023, 1959.
43. Cornblath, M., et al.: *J. Clin. Endocr. Metab.*, 25:209, 1965.
44. Corner, G. W.: *Contrib. Embryol.*, 31:117, 1945.
45. Csapo, A., and Lloyd-Jacob, M.: *Amer. J. Obstet. Gynec.*, 83:1073, 1962.
46. Curry, D. M., and Beaton, G. H.: *Endocrinology*, 63:155, 1958.
47. D'Angelo, S. A.: *Proc. Soc. Exper. Biol. Med.*, 121:555, 1966.
48. D'Angelo, S. A.: *Endocrinology*, 81:132, 1967.
49. Dässler, C. G., and Kyank, H.: *Gynaecologia*, 155:175, 1963.
50. Dässler, C. G.: *Acta Endocr.*, 49:283, 1965.
51. Davis, M. E., and Plotz, E. J.: *Obstet. Gynec. Survey*, 11:1, 1956.
52. Diczfalusy, E., et al.: *J. Clin. Endocr. Metab.*, 23:503, 1963.
53. Diczfalusy, E.: *Acta Gin.*, 16(Suppl.):7, 1965.
54. Dieckman, W. J., et al.: *Amer. J. Obstet. Gynec.*, 60:1043, 1960.
55. Doe, R. P., Dickinson, P., Zinne, H. H. M., and Seal, U. S.: *J. Clin. Endocr.*, 29:757, 1969.
56. Dokumow, S. I.: *Acta Endocr.*, 38:161, 1961.
57. Dowling, J. T., Freinkel, N., and Ingbar, S. H.: *J. Clin. Endocr. Metab.*, 21:779, 1961.
58. Dubreuil, G., and Marc-Riviere, M.: *Ann. d'Endocr.*, 11:62, 1950.
59. Dworkin, H. J., Jacquez, J. A., and Beierwaltes, W. H.: *J. Clin. Endocr. Metab.*, 26:1329, 1966.
60. Easterling, W., et al.: *Steroids*, 8:157, 1966.
61. Editorial: *Brit. Med. J.*, 2:861, 1955.
62. Eglin, J. M., and Jessiman, A. G.: *J. Clin. Endocr. Metab.*, 19:369, 1959.
63. Eguchi, Y.: *Endocrinology*, 71:31, 1962.
64. Elger, W.: *Arch. Anat. Microsc. Morphol. Exper.*, 55:657, 1966.
65. Emerman, S., Dancis, J., Levitz, M., Wiqvist, N., and Diczfalusy, E.: *J. Clin. Endocr. Metab.*, 25:178, 1965.
66. Estrada, W. J., et al.: *Amer. J. Obstet. Gynec.*, 78:1176, 1959.
67. Ferraris, G. M., and Scorba, A.: *Minerva Ginec.*, 7:308, 1955.
68. Fioretti, P., and Carretti, N.: *Riv. Ital. Ginec.*, 50:170, 1966.
69. Flickinger, G. L., Wu, C. H., and Touchstone, J. C.: *Acta Endocr.*, 54:30, 1967.
70. Francis, F. E., and Kinsella, R. A.: *J. Clin. Endocr. Metab.*, 26:128, 1966.
71. Frandsen, V. A., and Stakeman, L.: *Acta Endocr.*, 38:383, 1961.
72. Frazer, F. C., and Fainstat, T. D.: *Pediatrics*, 8:257, 1951.
73. Freinkel, N., and Goodner, C. J.: *Arch. Int. Med.*, 109:235, 1962.
74. Friedrich, R., Rippmann, E. T., and Kauffmann, V.: *Schw. Med. Wschr.*, 99:833, 1969.
75. Gala, R. R., and Westphal, U.: *Acta Endocr.*, 55:47, 1967.
76. Geloso, J. P.: *Ann. d'Endocr.*, 28(Suppl.):1, 1967.
77. Gemzell, C. A.: *J. Clin. Endocr. Metab.*, 13:898, 1963.
78. Gimlette, T. M. D., and Pifanelli, A.: *J. Clin. Path.*, 21:767, 1968.
79. Gitlin, D., Kumate, J., and Morales, C.: *J. Clin. Endocr. Metab.*, 25:1599, 1965.
80. Goodner, C. J., and Freinkel, N.: *Endocrinology*, 65:955, 1959.
81. Goodner, C. J., and Freinkel, N.: *Endocrinology*, 67:862, 1960.
82. Gorbman, A.: *Endocrinology*, 55:546, 1952.
83. Goss, D. A., and Lewis, J.: *J. Clin. Endocr. Metab.*, 23:986, 1963.
84. Govan, A. D. T.: *J. Endocr.*, 40:421, 1968.
85. Grattarola, R., and Li, C. H.: *Endocrinology*, 65:802, 1959.
86. Greenwald, G. S.: *Endocrinology*, 80:118, 1967.
87. Greenwald, G. S., and Johnson, D. C.: *Endocrinology*, 83:1052, 1968.
88. Greer, M.: *Endocrinology*, 65:178, 1959.
89. Greig, M., and MacNaughton, M. C.: *J. Endocr.*, 39:153, 1967.
90. Grumbach, M. M., and Werner, S. C.: *J. Clin. Endocr. Metab.*, 16:1392, 1956.
91. Harbert, G. M., Jr., et al.: *Obstet. Gynec.*, 23:413, 1964.
92. Harness, R. A., and Love, D. N.: *Acta Endocr.*, 51:526, 1966.
93. Harness, R. A., et al.: *Acta Endocr.*, 52:409, 1966.
94. Hausknecht, R. U.: *Amer. J. Obstet. Gynec.*, 97:1085, 1967.
95. Hawker, R. W.: *Endocrinology*, 52:117, 1953.

96. Heinemann, M., Johnson, C. E., and Mann, E. B.: *J. Clin. Invest.*, 27:91, 1948.
97. Hilliard, J., Spies, H. G., and Sawyer, C. H.: *Endocrinology*, 82:157, 1968.
98. Hillman, D. A., and Groud, C. J. P.: *J. Clin. Endocr. Metab.*, 25:243, 1965.
99. Hirschfeld, J., and Söderberg, U.: *Acta Endocr.*, 39:645, 1960.
100. Hirschowitz, S., and Berge, J.: *South Afr. J. Obstet. Gynec.*, 4:5, 1966.
101. Hodges, R. E., et al.: *J. Clin. Endocr. Metab.*, 15:661, 1965.
102. Hottinger, A.: *Schw. Med. Wschr.*, 89:419, 1959.
103. Hutchinson, D. L., Westover, D. L., and Will, D. W.: *Amer. J. Obstet. Gynec.*, 83:857, 1962.
104. Iino, S., and Greer, M. A.: *Endocrinology*, 68:253, 1961.
105. Israel, S. L., Stroup, P., Seligson, H., and Seligson, D.: *Obstet. Gynec.*, 14:68, 1959.
106. Jacobson, A. G., and Brent, R. L.: *Endocrinology*, 68:253, 1961.
107. Jailer, J. W., et al.: *J. Clin. Endocr. Metab.*, 11:187, 1951.
108. Jost, A.: In *Probleme der fetalen Endokrinologie*, ed. H. Nowakowsky. Berlin, Springer, 1957.
109. Jost, A., Pic, P., Maniey, J., and Legrand, C.: *Acta Endocr.*, 43:618, 1963.
110. Jungman, R. A., and Schweppe, J. S.: *J. Clin. Endocr.*, 28:1599, 1968.
111. Kalkhoff, R. D., Jacobson, M., and Lemper, D.: *J. Clin. Endocr.*, 30:24, 1970.
112. Kaplan, N. M.: *J. Clin. Endocr. Metab.*, 21:1139, 1961.
113. Kaplan, S. L., and Grumbach, M. M.: *J. Clin. Endocr. Metab.*, 25:1370, 1965.
114. Katz, S. R., Dancis, J., and Levitz, M.: *Endocrinology*, 76:722, 1965.
115. Kerr, G. R.: *J. Clin. Endocr. Metab.*, 22:137, 1962.
116. Kincl, F. A., Oriol, A., Folch-Pi, A., and Maqueo, M.: *Proc. Soc. Exper. Biol. Med.*, 120:252, 1965.
117. Knigge, K. M.: *Amer. J. Physiol.*, 202:387, 1962.
118. Knobil, E., and Briggs, F. N.: *Endocrinology*, 57:147, 1955.
119. Knobil, E., and Josimovitch, J. B.: *Ann. N.Y. Acad. Sci.*, 75:895, 1959.
120. Kostyo, J. L.: *Endocrinology*, 60:33, 1957.
121. Laidlaw, J. C., Cohen, M., and Gornall, A. G.: *J. Clin. Endocr. Metab.*, 18:222, 1958.
122. Lajos, L., et al.: *Gynaecologia*, 156:234, 1963.
123. Lampe, L., et al.: *Acta Physiol. Acad. Sci. Hung. (Budapest)*, 31:289, 1967.
124. Lanman, J. T., and Silverman, J. M.: *Endocrinology*, 60:437, 1957.
125. Lanman, J. T.: "Fetal Endocrinology in Late Pregnancy," in *Physiology of Prematurity*, ed. J. T. Lanman, Vol. I. New York, The Josiah Macy Foundation, 1957.
126. Lanman, J. T., and Dinerstein, J.: *Endocrinology*, 64:494, 1959.
127. Levine, S. E.: *Fed. Proceed.*, 22:T-260, 1963.
128. Lewis, A. A.: *J. Clin. Endocr. Metab.*, 13:769, 1963.
129. Lunaas, T., Baldwin, R. L., and Cupps, P. T.: *Acta Endocr.*, 58:521, 1968.
130. Lynch, M. G., et al.: *Amer. J. Obstet. Gynec.*, 77:335, 1959.
131. MacNaughton, M.: "Endocrinology of the Fetus," in *Fetus and Placenta*, ed. A. Klopper and E. Diczfalusy. Oxford, Blackwell, 1969.
132. Man, E. B., et al.: *J. Clin. Invest.*, 30:137, 1951.
133. Man, E. B., Reid, W. A., and Jones, W. S.: *Amer. J. Obstet. Gynec.*, 102:244, 1968.
134. Man, E. B., Reid, W. A., Hellegers, A. E., and Jones, W. S.: *Amer. J. Obstet. Gynec.*, 103:328, 1969.
135. Meinini, E., and Diczfalusy, E.: *Endocrinology*, 68:492, 1961.
136. Mikhail, G., Wiqvist, N., and Diczfalusy, E.: *Acta Endocr.*, 42:219, 1963.
137. Mikhail, G., Noall, M., and Allen, W. M.: *Endocrinology*, 69:504, 1961.
138. Milkovic, K., and Milkovic, S.: *Endocrinology*, 73:735, 1963.
139. Mintz, D. H., Chez, R. A., and Horger, E. O.: *J. Clin. Invest.*, 48:176, 1969.
140. Mowbray, R. R., and Tickner, A.: *Lancet*, 2:511, 1952.
141. Nataf, B. M., Rivera, E. M., and Chaikoff, I. L.: *Endocrinology*, 76:35, 1965.
142. Nelson, W. W., Forks, G., and Greene, R. R.: *Amer. J. Obstet. Gynec.*, 76:66, 1958.
143. Niemi, M., and Ikkonen, M.: *Nature*, 189:592, 1961.
144. Olin, P., Vecchio, G., Erkholm, R., and Almqvist, S.: *Endocrinology*, 86:1041, 1970.
145. Parker, R. M., and Beierwaltes, W. H.: *J. Clin. Endocr. Metab.*, 21:792, 1961.
146. Parache, J., Del Olmo, J., Alberto, J. C., Cherp, J., and Botella, J.: *Acta Gin.*, 21:569, 1970.
147. Pedersen, P. H., and Larsen, J. F.: *Acta Endocr.*, 58:481, 1968.
148. Phillip, E.: In *Probleme der fetalen Endokrinologie*, ed. H. Nowakowsky. Berlin, Springer, 1957.
149. Picard, C.: *Bull. Fed. Soc. Obst. Gyn. Lang. Franc.*, 29:447, 1968.
150. Postel, S.: *Endocrinology*, 60:53, 1957.
151. Poulton, B. R., and Reece, R. P.: *Endocrinology*, 61:217, 1957.
152. Rathmacher, R. P., et al.: *Endocrinology*, 81:430, 1967.
153. Rawlings, W. J.: *Brit. Med. J.*, 2:336, 1962.
154. Rawlings, W. J., and Krieger, V. I.: *Fertil. Steril.*, 15:173, 1964.
155. Rennels, E. G.: *Endocrinology*, 79:373, 1966.
156. Rivarola, M. A., Forest, M. G., and Migeon, C. J.: *J. Clin. Endocr. Metab.*, 28:34, 1968.
157. Robertson, H. A., and Falconer, J. R.: *J. Endocr.*, 22:133, 1961.
158. Robinson, K. W., Hawker, R. W., and Robertson, P. A.: *J. Clin. Endocr. Metab.*, 17:320, 1957.
159. Rodríguez-López, A.: *Acta Gin.*, 6:417, 1959.
160. Rodríguez-Soriano, J. A.: *Acta Gin.*, 3:9, 1952.
161. Romanoff, D. L., and Lauffer, H.: *Endocrinology*, 59:611, 1956.
162. Roos, T. B.: *Endocrinology*, 81:716, 1967.
163. Rosenthal, H. E., Slaunwhite, W. R., and Sandberg, A. A.: *J. Clin. Endocr.*, 29:352, 1969.
164. Roy, S. K., and Kobayashi, Y.: *Proc. Soc. Exper. Biol. Med.*, 110:699, 1962.
165. Russell, K. P., Tanaka, S., and Starr, P.: *Amer. J. Obstet. Gynec.*, 79:719, 1960.
166. Ryan, J. J.: *Acta Endocr.*, 44:81, 1963.
167. Schalch, D. S., and Reichlin, S.: *Endocrinology*, 79:275, 1966.
168. Schlegel, R. J., Farias, E., Russon, N. C., Moore, J. R., and Gardner, L. I.: *Endocrinology*, 81:565, 1967.

169. Schmidt, I. G., and Hoffmann, R. A.: *Endocrinology*, 55:125, 1954.
170. Schwers, J., Eriksson, G., and Diczfalusy, E.: *Acta Endocr.*, 49:65, 1965.
171. Schild, W., Jussen, A. W., and Schürhalz, K.: *Arch. Gynäk.*, 203:39, 1966.
172. Schultz, M. A., Forsander, J. B., Chez, R. A., and Hutchinson, D. L.: *Pediatrics*, 35:743, 1965.
173. Schwarz, B., and Talley, L.: *J. Reprod. Fertil.*, 15:39, 1968.
174. Serra, G. B., Perez-Palacios, G., and Jaffe, R. B.: *J. Clin. Endocr.*, 30:128, 1970.
175. Shepard, T. H.: *J. Clin. Endocr.*, 27:945, 1967.
176. Siersbaek-Nielsen, K., and Molholm-Hansen, J.: *Acta Endocr.*, 60:423, 1969.
177. Singh, B. P., and Morton, D. G.: *Amer. J. Obstet. Gynec.*, 72:607, 1956.
178. Smith, P. E.: *Endocrinology*, 56:271, 1955.
179. Spellacy, W. N., et al.: *Obstet. Gynec.*, 25:862, 1965.
180. Spellacy, W. N., and Buhi, W. C.: *Amer. J. Obstet. Gynec.*, 105:888, 1969.
181. Spellacy, W. N., Buhi, W. C., and Birk, A. S.: *Obstet. Gynec.*, 36:328, 1970.
182. Spies, H. G., Hilliard, J., and Sawyer, C. H.: *Endocrinology*, 83:354, 1968.
183. Staemmler, H. J.: *Arch. Gynäk.*, 182:706, 1952.
184. Steinbeck, A. W., and Thiele, H.: *Acta Endocr.*, 36:479, 1961.
185. Stempak, J. G.: *Endocrinology*, 70:443, 1962.
186. Stoffer, R. P., et al.: *Amer. J. Obstet. Gynec.*, 74:300, 1957.
187. Stoll, R., et al.: *Ann. d'Endocr.*, 17:15, 1956.
188. Surface, M., Campana, G., and Polvani, F.: *Ann. Ost. Gin.*, 89:687, 1967.
189. Swanson, H. E., and Ezrin, C.: *J. Clin. Endocr. Metab.*, 20:952, 1960.
190. Sybulsky, S., and Venning, E. H.: *Canad. J. Biochem.*, 39:203, 1961.
191. Tonutti, G.: In *Probleme der fetalen Endokrinologie*, ed. H. Nowakowsky. Berlin, Springer, 1957.
192. Trayner, I. M., et al.: *J. Endocr.*, 37:443, 1967.
193. Trunnell, J. B., and Wade, P.: *J. Clin. Endocr. Metab.*, 15:107, 1955.
194. Tuchmann-Duplessis, H.: *CIBA Colloquia on Ageing*, 2:161, 1956.
195. Tyson, J. E., Rabinovitz, D., and Merimee, T. J.: *Diabetes*, 17(Suppl. 1):347, 1968.
196. Van Arsdel, P. P.: *J. Clin. Endocr. Metab.*, 15:680, 1955.
197. Van Den Driesche, R.: In *Oxytocin*, ed. Caldeyro-Barcia and Heller. Oxford, Pergamon Press, 1961.
198. Van Heyningen, H.: *Endocrinology*, 69:720, 1961.
199. Varangot, H.: *Compt. Rend. Soc. Biol. (Paris)*, 149:1764, 1955.
200. Venning, E. H.: *Brit. Med. J.*, 2:1644, 1961.
201. Verne, J., and Herbert, S.: *Ann. d'Endocr.*, 17:413, 1956.
202. Villee, C. A., Engel, L. L., and Villee, D. B.: *Endocrinology*, 65:465, 1959.
203. Villee, C. A., and Loring, J. M.: *Endocrinology*, 72:824, 1963.
204. Villee, C. A., and Loring, J. M.: *J. Clin. Endocr. Metab.*, 25:307, 1965.
205. Wagner, G., Transbol, I., and Melchior, J. C.: *Acta Endocr.*, 47:549, 1964.
206. Walser, A.: *Praxis*, 58:325, 1969.
207. Walton, R. L.: *Pediatrics*, 13:227, 1954.
208. Werner, S. C.: *Amer. J. Obstet. Gynec.*, 75:1093, 1958.
209. Whitehouse, B. J., and Winson, G. P.: *Nature*, 221:1051, 1969.
210. Williams, B.: *Lancet*, 2:670, 1963.
211. Wilson, R., Eriksson, G., and Diczfalusy, E.: *Acta Endocr.*, 46:525, 1964.
212. Wilson, R., Bird, C. E., Wiqvist, N., Solomon, S., and Diczfalusy, E.: *J. Clin. Endocr. Metab.*, 26:115, 1966.
213. Woolman, S. H., and Zwilling, E.: *Endocrinology*, 52:526, 1953.
214. Wu, C. H., Flickinger, G. L., Archer, D. F., and Touchstone, J. C.: *Amer. J. Obstet. Gynec.*, 107:313, 1970.
215. Yamazaki, E., Noguchi, A., and Senigerland, D. W.: *J. Clin. Endocr. Metab.*, 20:794, 1960.
216. Yen, S. C. C., Saaman, N., and Pearson, O. H.: *J. Clin. Endocr.*, 27:1341, 1967.
217. Yen, S. S. C., Vela, P., and Tsai, C. C.: *J. Clin. Endocr.*, 31:29, 1970.
218. Yoshimi, T., Strott, C. A., Marshall, J. R., and Lipsett, M. B.: *J. Clin. Endocr.*, 29:225, 1969.
219. Zander, J.: *Arch. Gynäk.*, 198:112, 1963.
220. Zander, J., and Rünnebaum, B.: *Acta Endocr.*, 54:19, 1967.
221. Zuspan, P. F., Wahley, W. H., Nelson, G. H., and Ahlquist, R. P.: *Amer. J. Obst. Gynec.*, 95:284, 1966.
222. Zuspan, F. P.: *J. Clin. Endocr.*, 30:357, 1970.

Chapter 21
MAINTENANCE AND INTERRUPTION OF GESTATION

The hormonal correlations that characterize gestation have been studied in preceding chapters. In order to understand how these correlations are interrupted and labor is initiated, it will *first of all be necessary to examine which factors maintain gestation and which factors cause interruption of gestation.*

21.1. FACTORS RESPONSIBLE FOR MAINTAINING GESTATION

Were a foreign body, comparable in size to that of a few months old conceptus, introduced into the cavity of the uterus, it would provoke contractions and would be rapidly expelled. What prevents the same thing from occurring in gestation is a series of endocrine correlations that sustain pregnancy and maintain the fetus anchored in the uterus. The preservation of pregnancy requires at least these two elements: (a) *nutrition, available at all times, first to the embryo, then to the fetus,* and (b) *a myometrium maintained at rest, so as to allow the embryo's growth and intrauterine development.*

The first of the two requirements is provided for by the epithelial part of the uterus, *the decidua,* and modifications of the latter consequent to the rise of the placenta in the midst of it. The second condition is met by virtue of a *special kind of behavior of the myometrium.*

21.1.1. NUTRITION OF THE IMPLANTED EGG

The problems pertaining to implantation were examined in Chapter 19. Once the egg is implanted, its trophoblast begins to function and to secrete gonadotropic hormone which, by maintaining corpus luteum activity, *prolongs the progravid reaction* and induces the *formation of the decidua.* Concerning the nutritional requirements of the embryo, which are beyond the scope of this book, the reader is referred to recent sources on the subject.[134]

Broadly outlined, *hemotrophic nutrition* (see Chapter 19) begins with extravasation of blood around the egg (hemorrhage of implantation or placental sign) at the time of the first missed menstruation. Histiotrophic nutrition continues taking place alongside incipient hemotrophic nutrition until the end of the third month of gestation. *At that time, histiotrophic nutrition ceases, which marks the beginning of exclusive hemotrophic nutrition.*

Once histiotrophic nutrition has disappeared, neither the *maternal placenta,* that is, the decidua, nor the gland of internal secretion that helps maintain the decidua are any longer necessary. *Upon cessation of histiotrophic nutrition, the corpus luteum disappears.*[34, 132] In those animals in which nutrition is provided by the decidua throughout pregnancy (rodents, the sow), the presence of the corpus luteum is necessary for the entire duration of pregnancy.[35]

21.1.2. ACTIVE UTERINE GROWTH DURING GESTATION

Even though no longer elaborated by the corpus luteum, progesterone continues to be synthesized by the placenta for the duration of pregnancy (see Chapter 19). At first thought, progesterone production would appear to be redundant from the moment progestational action on the endometrium has ceased to be necessary. However, progesterone, which from that moment on is synthesized in primates by the placenta (and possibly also by the adrenal) and which continues to be elaborated by the corpus luteum in rodents, has still some important missions to accomplish in gestation. Those are principally two: (1) *to contribute toward uterine growth and vascularization*, and (2) *to maintain the uterine muscle fiber at rest, by counterbalancing estrogenic activity.*

During pregnancy, the myometrium grows actively, increasing approximately 20 times in size. This growth is a consequence of ovarian hormonal activity, pertaining to both estrogens and progestogens (Reynolds[105]). In the recent past, the action of steroids on uterine growth has been analyzed in detail by Velardo,[132, 133] Lerner[82] and Schofield.[114] *The main "metrotrophic" hormone is estradiol*, followed in order of decreasing activity by estrone and estriol. In weak dosages, progesterone inhibits the effect of estradiol. However, whenever acting in such high concentrations as it does in pregnancy, it potentiates the effects of estradiol.

According to Reynolds and Mackie,[106] uterine growth goes hand in hand with changes in shape of the uterus. At first, the uterus is distended passively and assumes a *spherical shape.* Later, active growth tends to impart to it a more *cylindrical shape.*

These changes in shape have very important *consequences for the vascular supply to the uterus.* Reynolds and Mackie[106] subscribe to the idea that the blood supply is compromised during the first phase and facilitated during the second, so that steroid-induced phenomena of active uterine growth may be concluded to *gradually improve uterine blood flow.*

The action of progesterone, exerted almost exclusively on the endometrium during the first trimester of human pregnancy, is exerted at the level of the myometrium during the following two trimesters. This action elicits essentially three well defined types of effects: (1) uterine growth, an effect in part shared with estrogens; (2) *state of rest for the muscle fibers*, and (3) state of *improved uterine vascularization*, as a result of the two preceding effects combined.

The way the vascular supply develops in the gravid uterus has been well known since the studies by Ramsey.[104] The gradual process of vascular development is a direct continuation of that observed during the progestational phase, induced by the action of progesterone. In rodents, progesterone increases vascularity in the gravid uterus markedly,[71, 115] and the same phenomenon occurs in simians and humans. The vessels thus developed, whose mission is obvious and is aimed at facilitating the nutritional supply to the fetus, are constricted whenever the uterus tenses up or contracts. *As a result, progesterone produces increased blood flow to the uterus by three convergent mechanisms:* (1) by inducing vascular development; (2) by exerting a growth-inducing effect on the uterine muscle, resulting in decreased myometrial distention; and (3) by inhibiting uterine contractions.

21.1.3. UTERINE-SEDATING ACTION BY PROGESTERONE

Progesterone sedates uterine contractions,[19, 34, 39, 105, 129] as we have already indicated in Chapter 3. The mode of action involved, based on the so-called "sodium pump," has by now been generally recognized, thanks to the work of Csapo[39, 40] which was subsequently confirmed by others (Needham and Williams,[97] Schofield[115]). The same sedating effect, though to a lesser extent, is also exerted by synthetic progestogens (Zarrow et al.[141]). The main action of progesterone consists in neutralizing the effect of oxytocin (Kumar et al.[80]) and is not an immediate one but rather of the delayed type, requiring a period of 24 hours to take place (Csapo and Lloyd-Jacob[41]).

Csapo[40] has shown that the source of progesterone during pregnancy in primates is the placenta. Progesterone of placental origin *acts locally* on the uterus in such a way that, as a result, the uterine segment corresponding to the placental insertion site contracts least, which is of great clinical importance during delivery. This type of local action by progesterone and progesterone analogues, which will be emphasized later, has also been confirmed by Jung,[74] Kumar and associates,[79] Schofield,[115] and Zarrow and colleagues.[141] *From the third month onward, the single most important factor involved in maintaining gestation is therefore the uterine-sedating action of progesterone.*

The mode of action of progestational hor-

TABLE 21-1. Mode of Progesterone Action in Maintaining Gestation

PHASE	TIME	ORIGIN OF PROGESTERONE	MODE OF ACTION
Preimplantation and previllous phase	From fertilization to fourteenth day postfertilization (twenty-eighth day of cycle)	Progestational corpus luteum	Stimulation of tubotrophic type of nutrition and progestational endometrial reaction
Phase of chorion	From fourteenth day to thirteenth week	Gestational (gravidic) corpus luteum	Decidual reaction, histiotrophic type nutrition
Phase of placenta	From thirteenth week to fortieth week	Placenta	Eccentric development of myometrium, uterine rest, vascularization

mone in human pregnancy has been outlined in Table 21-1.

21.2. FACTORS CAUSING INTERRUPTION OF GESTATION

Progesterone partakes actively in preserving gestation. *Lack of progesterone by itself may be considered enough to cause interruption of pregnancy.* However, let us now study those actions which produce uterine contractions and precipitate labor.

21.2.1. ESTROGENS

The stimulatory effect of estrogens on the uterus was discovered by Robson and was studied in humans by Reynolds.[105] Later, Martin,[90] Morrow[96] and Schofield[114] made an in-depth study of the pharmacologic uterine effects of estrogens in different animal species. In response to estrogen stimulation, intense spontaneous contractility has been shown to occur in the isolated human uterus at our laboratory[24,129] (Figs. 21-1 and 21-2). These experiments suggested that increasing amounts of estrogens near term induced a state of uterine hypersensitivity and rendered the uterus susceptible to stimuli precipitating labor. That this is actually the case has been shown by the fact that estrogens can be used to induce abortion in experimental animals (Greenwald[56]), even though it has not been possible to induce such abortions in humans. Naturally, many objections may be raised to the estrogenic theory. First is the failure to demonstrate an abortion-inducing or labor-activating effect of estrogens in the human species, and second is the fact that the highest concentrations of estrogens do not seem to occur at the time of labor.[66,90,114]

Different correlations exist in the cow (Holm and Galligan[67]), in which prolonged pregnancy is associated with excessive estrogen levels. Järvinen and co-workers[72] have demonstrated that estrogens in women intensified Braxton-Hicks contractions, whereas Martin-Pinto and colleagues[91] observed that previous estrogen therapy decreased the period of latency of the near-term isolated human uterus to oxytocin, which has been equally confirmed among our group by Terragno[129] and Gutiérrez. It would seem to us that the effect of estrogens in precipitating labor, rather than being the result of an absolute increase in total estrogens, stems from an increase in the free fraction at the expense of the conjugated (sulfate, glucuronate) fraction of estrogens, as has been recently demonstrated by Smith,[121] thereby confirming the studies of Cohen and Marrian, which were made as early as 1929.

Earlier ideas concerning the role played by estrogens in the myometrial response to oxytocin have been revised as a result of the recent studies on rats by Acker and Courrier,[1] on ewes by Roberts and Share,[109] and on strips of isolated human uterus by Martin-Pinto and co-workers.[92] In addition, Spratto and Miller[122] found that the myometrial catecholamine content was modified by the action of estrogens, and admitted that this might be the main mechanism of action involved.

Investigations by Csapo[40,41] have revealed, however, that estrogens counteract uterine-sedating activity of progesterone (see Chapters 2 and 3). It is possible, in fact,

Figure 21-1. A, Recording of in vitro contractions of strip of human nongravid uterus. B, Recording of strip of human gravid uterus obtained by cesarean section. Compare contractions of gravid uterus with those of nongravid uterus. Recordings were registered under identical experimental conditions.

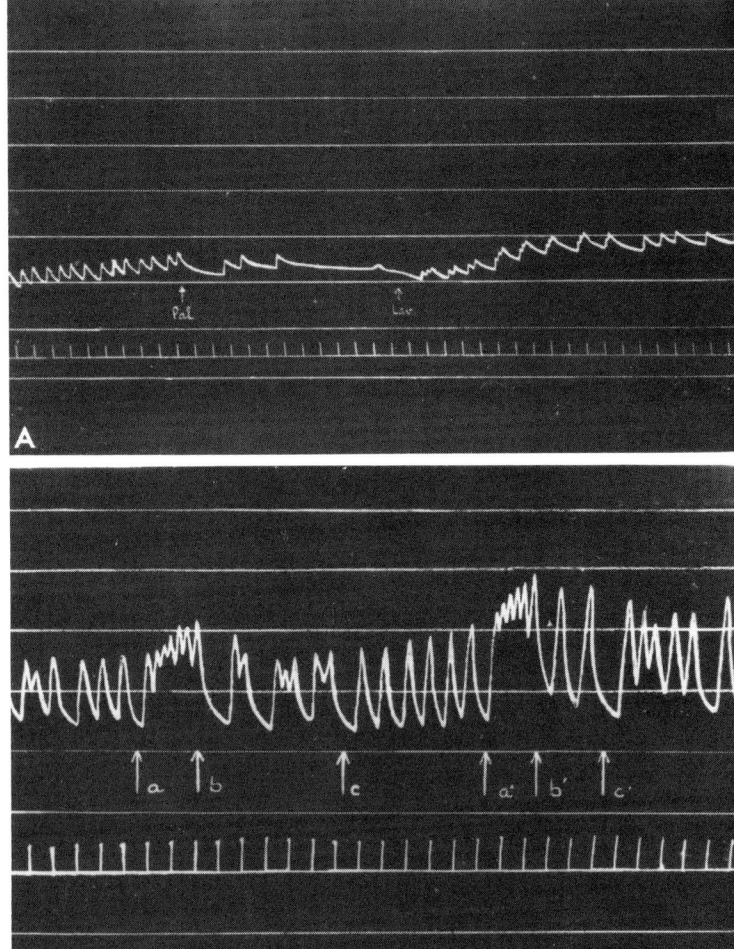

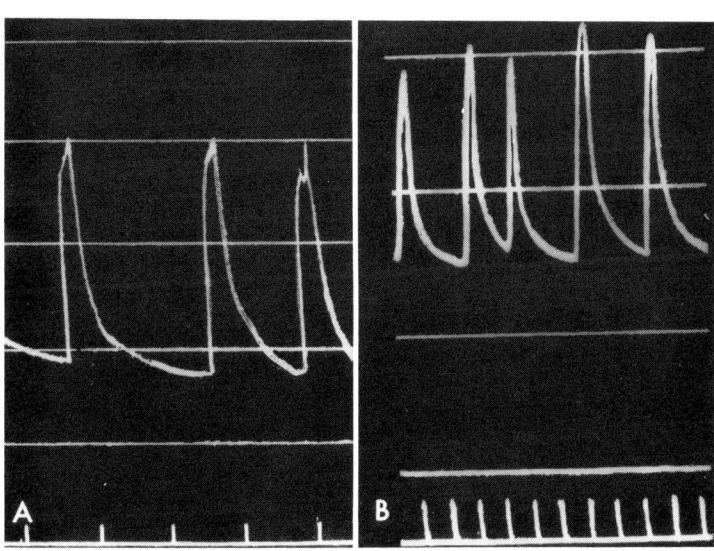

Figure 21-2. A, Spontaneous contractions in strip of isolated human uterus previously treated with estrogens. Slow rhythm (scale in minutes). B, Spontaneous contractions of human uterus under similar conditions. Accelerated rhythm. This represents a myomatous uterus with excessive ovarian estrogen production.

that elevated estrogen concentrations may cause labor indirectly by a similar mechanism. It is our opinion that the underlying mechanism is related to *imbalance between estrogen and progesterone levels.* Progesterone is known to accelerate the process of hepatic estrogen degradation, so that it may be speculated that an eventual decrease in progesterone level, apart from having an effect on the uterus, might entail an increase in estrogens and thereby further aggravate the existing imbalance, brought about in the first place by lowered progesterone. Llauro and his co-workers[85] made a comprehensive study of progesteronemia in the course of labor, reaching the conclusion that plasma progesterone levels were inversely related to the degree of intensity of contractions. Roberts and Share[109] found that progesterone injections lowered the rate of reflex oxytocin release in the ewe.

The role played by estrogens in pregnancy may be summarized as probably one of joint action with progesterone in maintaining gestation. Before labor, a drop in progesterone levels occurs, which offsets the existing balance between estrogen and progesterone activity and results in sensitization of the uterine fiber. In the process, the role of estrogens changes, as it were, from one of hormones concerned with *maintenance of gestation and synergistic action with progesterone* into one of substances *interrupting gestation and counteracting progesterone.*

21.2.2. NEUROHORMONES

Dixon and Marshall assumed oxytocin to be the uterine stimulant of choice in labor (see Chapter 8). Robinson, Robson and Ferguson believed instead that the precipitation of labor was a consequence of *uterine sensitization to oxytocin by estrogens.* Oxytocin was believed to be secreted at a continuous rate throughout gestation, and the reason why the above effect would not come about until the end of gestation was thought to be the result of uterine sensitization rather than rising oxytocin levels, as originally postulated. Csapo[39] and Reynolds[105] called attention to the circumstances surrounding the sensitizing effect of estrogens, maintaining that the latter occurred because estrogens modified the metabolism of the myometrium, rendering the muscle sensitive to all types of stimuli and increasing spontaneous contractility. It is therefore doubtful whether the presumptive sensitizing effect to oxytocin is a specific one.

Important as oxytocin may be, it is not essential for the initiation of labor. Over a period of 26 years, Marañón studied a woman with diabetes insipidus whose five pregnancies terminated in sluggish labor, although each delivery eventually occurred by natural route. However, the fact that labor may occur without oxytocin activity does not necessarily mean that oxytocin activity is absent in normal labor. Collin and Racadot[33] have found that the Gomori-positive substance in the neurohypophysis and in the hypothalamus decreased in the normal postpartum woman (see Chapter 8), while Suzor and colleagues[127] have reported increased blood oxytocin values during labor and in abortion. Fuchs[50] confirmed the presence of increased oxytocin levels in abortion in rabbits.

The bioassay procedures developed by Hawker and colleagues[58, 59, 60] and by Vorherr and his associates[135] are sensitive enough to detect minute amounts of oxytocin in the blood. By means of such methods, circulating oxytocin levels have been found to be very low near the end of pregnancy and to rise significantly only during labor, even then decreasing at intervals between contractions. Because oxytocin is rapidly inactivated and has a very short life span in blood,[108, 120] its action is believed to be the result of rapid discharges rather than sustained levels. This suggests that *the function of oxytocin is one of maintaining rather than triggering labor.*

21.2.3. THE PLACENTA

It has been suggested that the regressive changes, observed in the placenta toward the end of pregnancy, are possibly associated with the release of substances capable of stimulating uterine contractions. Attempts at extracting from the placenta substances with actions similar to those of oxytocin have not been successful, but various investigators have isolated other specific compounds possessing oxytocin-like activity.

ACETYLCHOLINE. This has been isolated from the placenta by several workers.[6, 7, 106, 119] However, it is important to point out that acetylcholine is encountered in the placenta in highest concentrations not during, but several weeks before, labor (Chan and Du Vegneaud[26]). Acetylcholine has been identified in the serum of pregnant women by Stroup[125] and by Eagle,[45] and has also been reported by Page and his co-workers[99] to be excreted in increased amounts in the urine. Choline and acetylcholine, at least in the human species, are known to stimulate uterine contractions and to act more effectively in the presence of estrogens.

HISTAMINE. The role of histamine in initiating labor and abortion had already been stressed in one of our earlier works.[16] The recent studies by Bjuro and his associates[15] underscore the significant role of histamine in stimulating uterine contractions, as well as the equilibrating role of *histaminase* activity.

EPINEPHRINE AND NOREPINEPHRINE. Israel and co-workers[71] and Ritzel and co-workers[107] have studied the effect of epinephrine on the human uterus. This effect is relaxing, anti-oxytocic in nature, in direct contrast to the effect of epinephrine on the rodent uterus. Investigations conducted at our laboratory by means of paralyzing the sympathetic lumbar chain with paravertebral infiltration of novocaine (Iglesias) or with sympathicolytic drugs (Pereira) showed that such procedures invariably produced uterine spasmolysis. More recently, however, the existence of an *epinephrine-norepinephrine antagonism* in this respect has been uncovered. Kaiser and Harris,[76] in 1950, and Garrett,[52] in 1954, described the *spasmolytic effect* of norepinephrine, which was later confirmed by Stroup[125] and, in a very complete and recent study, by Zuspan and his colleagues.[142] In the view of Stone and his co-workers,[124] incidentally shared by Zuspan's group, initiation of labor depends on the reciprocal equilibrium between epinephrine (uterine-sedating) and norepinephrine (uterine-exciting) activity in the pregnant woman's plasma.

Sabanah and associates[119] have drawn attention to the fact that an existing *equilibrium between acetylcholine and catecholamines* also plays a role in initiating labor. Spratto and Miller[122] observed that catecholamine levels increased under the influence of estrogens.

SEROTONIN. Berry and Hughes,[13] Israel and his co-workers[71] and Bengtsson and Csapo[9] have reported *elevated blood serotonin values during pregnancy*. The placental origin attributed to the latter would seem to us questionable. Nevertheless, serotonin exerts a potent oxytocin-like effect on the human uterus, as evidenced by the observations of Terragno[129] and Gutierrez (Figs. 21–3 and 21–4) at our clinic.

PROSTAGLANDINS. At best, prostaglandins deserve to be mentioned only briefly here. Although outside of pregnancy they play a significant role in uterine contractility, their obstetrical uterine activity is of little consequence. From the prostate, Bergström and Sjövall[11] have isolated a substance that stimulates uterine contractions. Sandberg and his colleagues[112] have described several similar substances possessing analogous activity, whose effects on the Fallopian tube and on the isolated uterus have been studied by Ingelman-Sundberg and co-workers[70] and by Sandberg and associates.[113] The chemical structure of different prostaglandins has been described by Bydgeman and his colleagues[20, 21] in great detail. A comprehensive review concerning the physiology of this group of substances has been published by Bergström[12] and by Pickles.[102] On the basis of modern investigations, the mode of action involved would appear to be confined to acetylcholine release, with associated changes in Na-K balance.[101]

It is probable that prostaglandins, as well as other, yet poorly known substances, play some role in initiating labor. What is unquestionable is the fact that both the pla-

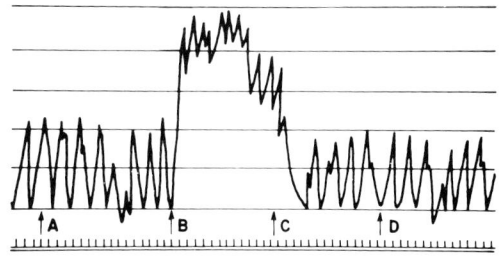

Figure 21–3. Contractions in strip of lower segment of gravid uterus, obtained by means of cesarean section. A, D, Spontaneous motility; B, addition of 50 mcg of serotonin to solution (50 ml); C, rinse. Time in minutes. (From Terragno: Thesis, University of Madrid, 1965.)

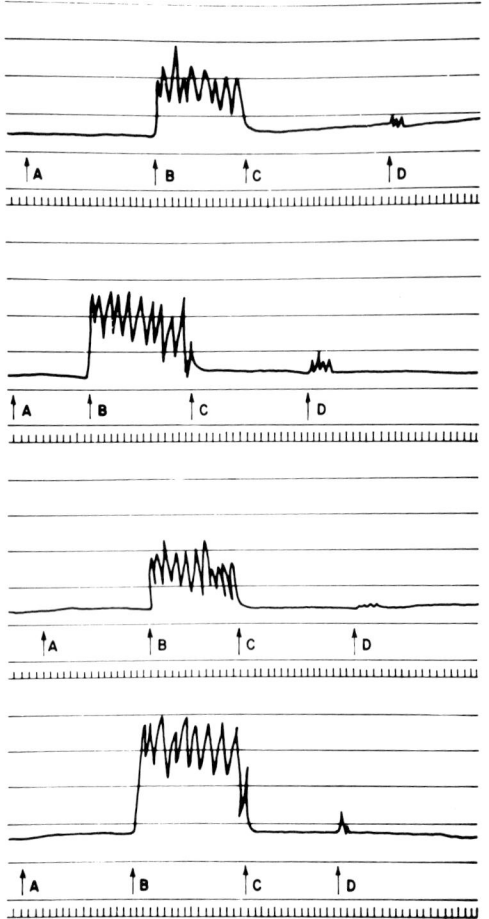

Figure 21-4. Experiment analogous to one in Figure 21-3. *B,* Addition of 20 mcg of serotonin to each strip; *C,* rinse. Time in minutes. There are no spontaneous contractions. Strips were obtained from lower uterine segment intrapartum. (From Terragno: Thesis, University of Madrid, 1965.)

centa and the uterine wall at term secrete a series of substances that are able to precipitate contractions.

21.3. EVOLUTION OF THE PLACENTA

The placenta, whose internal secretion was studied in Chapter 19, has so far been analyzed here in terms of a somewhat static organ. Far from being that, the placenta undergoes a *rapid process of evolution,* reproducing a vital cycle at a much more rapid rate than can be observed in any other organ of the body; witness the embryonal development, coming of age, aging and demise of this organ, all within a short span of nine months. *The placental aging process creates a serious conflict with regard to fetal nutrition, so much so that, were it not for immediate delivery, the critical point reached would be of such gravity as to seriously jeopardize the life of the fetus.*

In considering the causes of labor, it must not be forgotten that parturition is above all a teleologic necessity designed to avert intrauterine death of the fetus. Frequently, premature delivery is but a natural defense mechanism intended to cope with a serious threat to fetal life.

We shall study consecutively: (1) morphologic evolution of the placenta, and (2) uterine blood flow during gestation.

21.3.1. MORPHOLOGIC EVOLUTION OF THE PLACENTA

The fact that the human placenta is subject to continuous evolution during gestation has to be repeatedly stressed. The changes involved may be viewed as evidence of *gradual adaptation of the placenta to its function as a filter.* These changes affect essentially: (1) the size and surface of the villi; (2) the vascularization of the villi; and (3) the characteristics of epithelial lining.

SIZE AND SURFACE OF VILLI. If immature chorionic tissue, such as shown in Figure 21-5, is examined and compared with well formed, midterm placenta (Fig. 21-6), and the latter in turn with near-term placenta (Fig. 21-7), the most noticeable changes encountered consist in progressive diminution of the size of villi. The rate at which the villi decrease gradually in size has been measured by Botella and Clavero.[17, 18] At the same time, crowding of villi becomes increasingly apparent, leading to an increasingly larger surface area of interchange. In Figure 21-8, the placental stage of evolution at seven months is compared with that at nine months.

The curve in Figure 21-9 shows the rate at which the placental surface area increases, according to data obtained by Clavero and Botella.[29] By increasing its surface area considerably, the placenta adapts specially to processes of filtration (Huggett[69] and Clavero-Nuñez et al.[30, 31, 32]).

VASCULARIZATION OF VILLI. As shown by Huggett,[69] if rat embryos are destroyed before the chorion is transformed into placenta, the latter fails to develop. This is so because organization of chorionic villi depends on ingrowth of allantoic vessels. Penetration of these vessels into chorionic villi is the essential event in the process of chorionic transformation into placenta. Because the vessels are derived from the fetal mesenchyme, the phenomenon is also referred to as "fetalization" of villi (Thomsen and Hiersche[130]). The development of fetal vasculature in the course of gestation has been studied by Clavero[30] and subsequently by Crawford,[36] Paine[100] and Javert and Reiss.[73] The vessels not only increase in number but also assume a peripheral disposition in the villi (Figs. 21–8 and 21–10).

ALTERATIONS OF CHORIONIC LINING. As villi are progressively vascularized, the chorionic epithelium becomes thinner and thinner. Whereas the Langhans layer of a four month placenta is well defined, that of a term placenta has undergone complete atrophy, and even the syncytial layer has become flat and shrunken. As pointed out previously, the hemochorial placenta of primates is transformed into a hemoendothelial placenta, in which the blood circulating through the villous capillary bed is separated from the blood in the intervillous spaces merely by fetal capillary endothelium, since once the chorionic in-

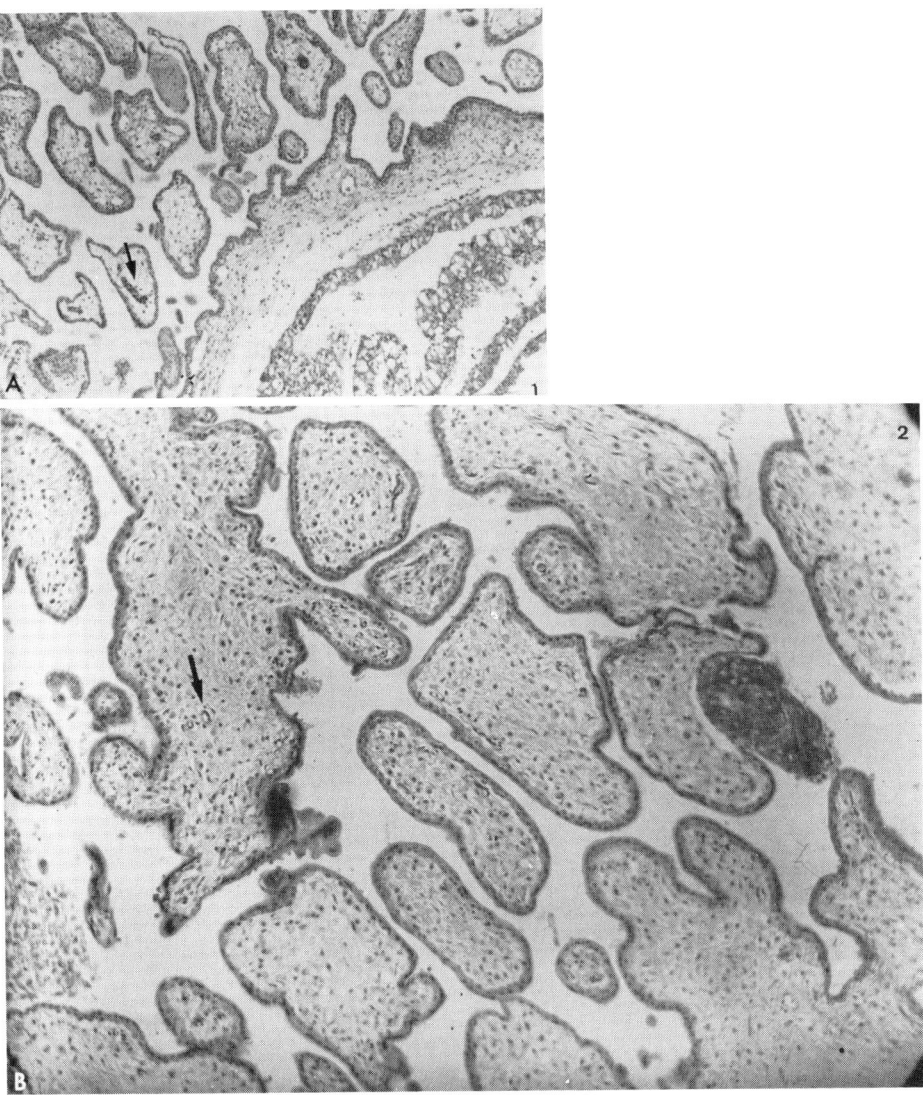

Figure 21–5. Histology of chorion frondosum in a six week old conceptus seen under low (50×) magnification (A) and medium (250×) magnification (B). Vascularization of villi is barely beginning at points indicated by arrows.

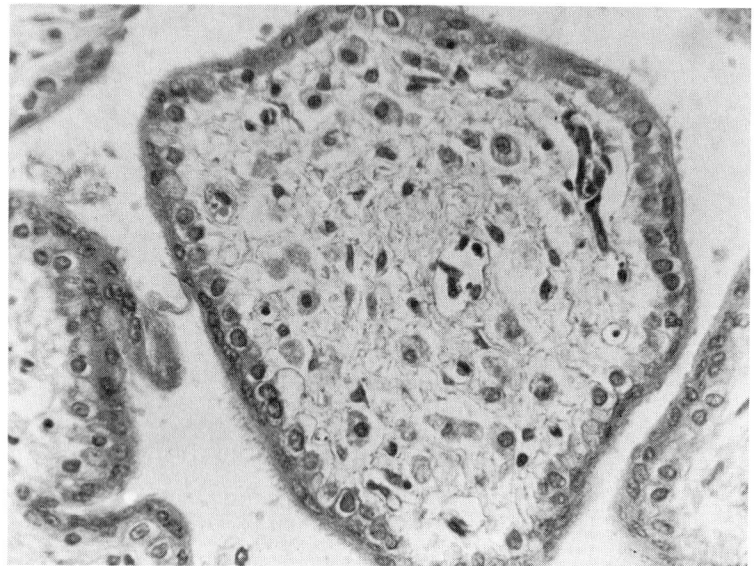

Figure 21-6. Histologic appearance of chorionic villus from 16 week abortus. Vessels are somewhat better developed than in Figure 21-5, though still centrally located (500×).

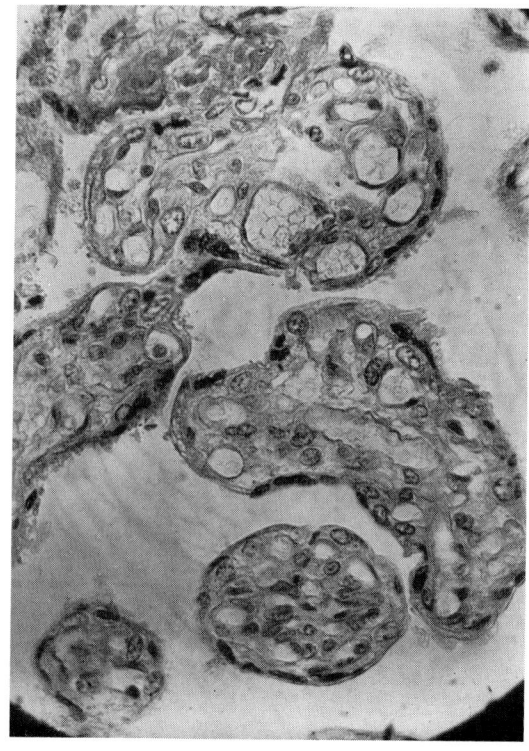

Figure 21-7. Chorionic villus in normal term placenta. Note decreased diameter when compared with Figures 21-5 and 21-6. Layer of Langerhans has disappeared; the syncytiotrophoblast is mostly flattened. There are more numerous and larger vessels, with marginal distribution.

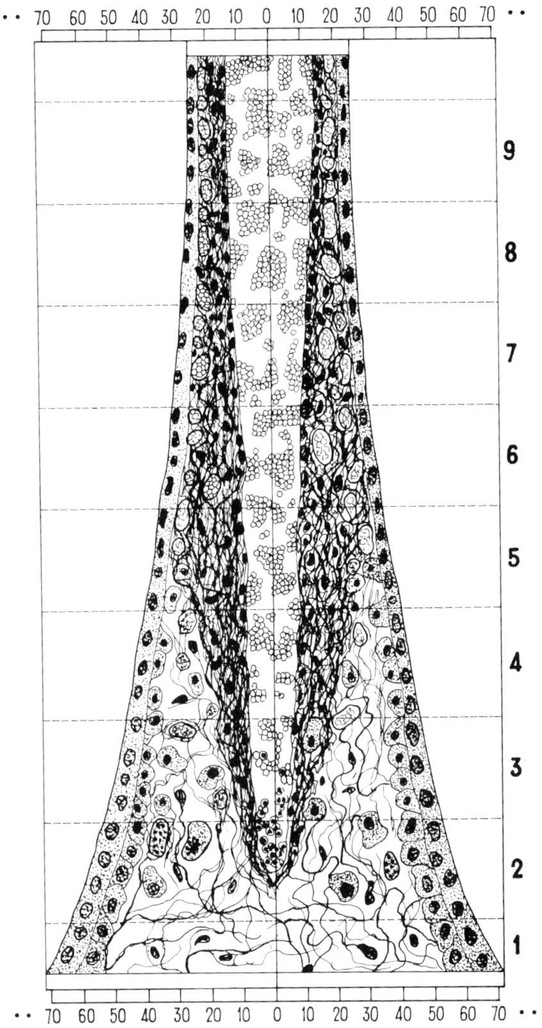

Figure 21-8. Diagrammatic representation of developing chorionic villus. Observe development of vascular supply, increasingly peripheral in distribution, the gradual atrophy of surface epithelium and the decreasing size of the villus. (From Botella-Llusiá: *Obstetrical Endocrinology.* Springfield, Ill., Charles C Thomas, 1961. After Hörman.)

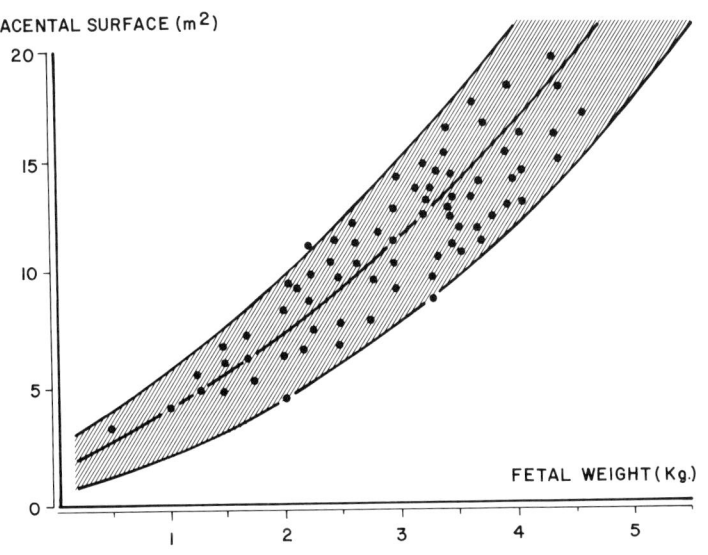

Figure 21-9. Rate of increase of placental surface in the course of normal gestation. (From Clavero-Nuñez and Botella-Llusiá: *Amer. J. Obstet. Gynec.*, 86:234, 1963.)

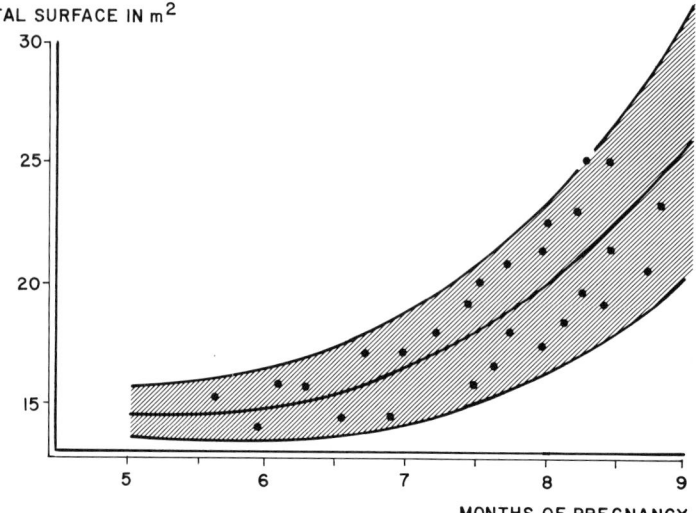

Figure 21-10. Rate of increase of surface area of villous capillary network in the course of normal gestation. (From Clavero-Nuñez and Jiménez-Ayala: *Acta Gin.*, 15:133, 1964.)

tegument has undergone atrophy, the fetal vessels are practically in contact with the intervillous spaces across a tenuous membrane. The histochemical changes pertaining to *placental senescence* and the associated atrophy of the epithelial lining have been studied by Clavero[30] and by Villee.[134] There is no doubt that chorionic tissue undergoes a process of true aging. Actively functioning components of the epithelium regress to the point where the placenta at term is structurally a vast fetal vascular network bathed in the blood of the intervillous spaces. The maternal placenta (decidua) has undergone atrophy long before, and what once was a nutritional maternal membrane is also converted to a mere vascular bed. Thus, *as a result of gestational evolution, the decidua and placenta of primates tend to be moulded into an eminently vascular organ whose active epithelial components undergo atrophy.*

21.3.2. UTERINE IRRIGATION DURING GESTATION

Commensurate with fetal vascular organization and proliferation, blood flow through the uterus increases to a considerable extent. Based on the study of anatomic preparations, Ramsey[104] reconstructed the progressive development of uterine vasculature. It is apparent that *progressive vascularization (fetalization) of placental villi occurs concomitantly with similarly progressive vascularization of the uterine bed.*

Uterine blood flow during gestation was studied by Barcroft[5] in the ewe in 1947. Interestingly, there is an evident increase in uterine vascular irrigation up to a certain point in gestation in sheep, after which the rate of irrigation begins to decrease gradually. Subsequently, MacClure-Browne and Veall[87] studied the blood flow of the human uterus indirectly. Their results indicated that blood flows through the human uterus at a rate of 600 ml per minute, which is roughly 20 to 25 per cent of the total circulating body volume per minute. In other words, about one fifth of the body's total blood volume flows through the gravid uterus per minute.

Recently, Clavero-Nuñez at our clinic measured the rate of uterine blood flow during pregnancy and in labor by means of radioactive xenon. His results, although differing slightly from those of MacClure-Browne and Veall, reveal that, at labor, a critical situation develops in uterine irrigation and that, in fact, delivery is tantamount to fetal "liberation" from a situation that is rapidly becoming untenable.

According to these studies, uterine blood flow may drop by 60 per cent or more in overmature pregnancies and in eclampsia. Obviously then, important a factor as uterine blood flow may be, it comes closer and closer to reaching a crisis as pregnancy advances.

21.3.3. PLACENTAL SENESCENCE AND THE MATERNO-FETAL CONFLICT

Figure 21-9 shows how the total villous surface of the human placenta increases in a progressive and noticeable way until a few weeks before labor. After that, the filtering surface may decrease significantly, even in normal pregnancy. If one considers that, after this point, the total placental surface no longer increases but may even decrease, and that villous filtering conditions (vascularization, permeability) are at the same time impaired, one easily sees that the nutritional condition of the human fetus at term becomes critical.

A really critical point is reached by the fortieth week of pregnancy, beyond which the fetus' nutritional conflicts, precipitated, on the one hand, by the vascular crisis and, on the other, by placental senescence, reach a maximum. Parturition ensues as a rescue operation at a time when fetal nutrition would otherwise no longer be possible.

21.4. INITIATION OF LABOR

21.4.1. "TIMING" IN PREGNANCY

Notwithstanding the great variety of explanations advanced, it is not known why human labor is initiated at 40 weeks from the time of cessation of menses.

Since ancient times, external, astral and meteorologic factors (such as the phases of the moon) have been invoked in the precipitation of labor. A return of sorts to some of these ancient ideas has been marked by modern admission that meteorologic factors, similar to those currently known to be involved in the development of eclampsia, may possibly be involved in labor. Whatever the case may be, gestation is undoubtedly adapted to an internal rhythm of its own. For that matter, all vital phenomena of the body are regulated by a "timing" mechanism or rhythm, which rhythms are measured in terms of *biologic weeks* (see Chapter 12). The biologic week has nothing to do with the calendar week. Although occasionally it may match the duration of the latter, it depends on the internal rhythm inherent in vital phenomena rather than on outside influences. The biologic week does not last for the same length of time in every person, although its duration fluctuates in the vicinity of seven days. A woman's inherent rhythm is translated into the menstrual cycle, which lasts for four biologic weeks. Because this week varies in length from woman to woman, the corresponding intermenstruum is equally of variable duration. Interestingly, the biologic week multiplied by four marks the menstrual rhythm, and 40 biologic weeks equal the duration of pregnancy.

As indicated in the preceding paragraph, an inevitable conflict in fetal nutrition develops near term. Labor supervenes whenever, depending on the "internal timing," the moment has come. *However, timing, or the inherent rhythm, of these events is not an arbitrary phenomenon but is adapted to the process of placental maturation and senescence and to the imperative needs of fetal nutrition.*

21.4.2. HYPERDISTENTION OF THE MYOMETRIUM

An important factor involved in the triggering mechanism of labor, which must be studied here before entering into purely endocrine considerations, is the effect of passive stretching of uterine fibers by progressive fetal growth. As a result of being stretched, the uterine fiber shows the effect reproduced in Figure 21-11: increased intensity of contractions. It is for this reason that in twin pregnancies, hydramnios, etc., labor is initiated earlier than normally.

A variable "mode of reacting" on the part of the myometrium has also been noted by Deis and Pickford.[43] Accordingly, there is a difference in the uterine muscle's response to sympathetic blocking agents (DH ergotamine, Bretilium) between the beginning of pregnancy and at the time of labor.

21.4.3. ENDOCRINE CAUSES OF LABOR

Estrogens and progesterone produce typical though antagonistic effects on the myometrium (Chapters 2 and 3). For instance, estrogenic hormone enhances the myometrial capacity to contract, whereas progesterone has a "sedating" effect. The oxytocin-like effect of estrogens, it is important to point out, stems primarily from enhancement of the uterine response to oxytocin. In

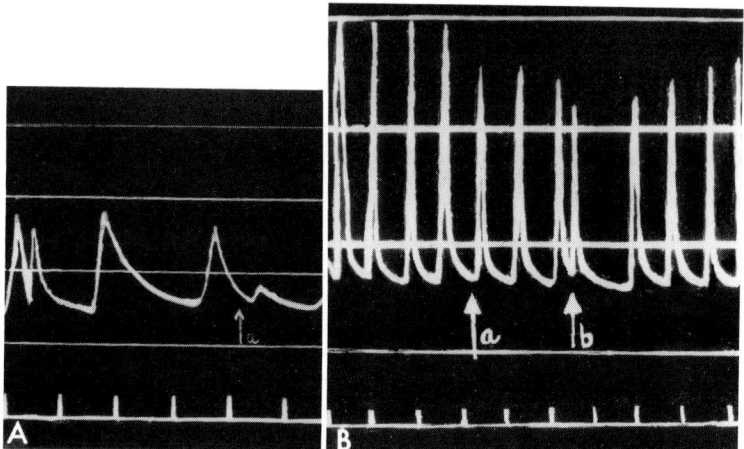

Figure 21-11. Effect of stretching on contractility of gravid uterine muscle fiber. *A*, Strip of gravid human uterus subjected in vitro to 5 g stress. *B*, Same fibers subjected to 15 g stress. (From Botella-Llusiá and Terragno: *Acta Gin.*, 16:656, 1965.)

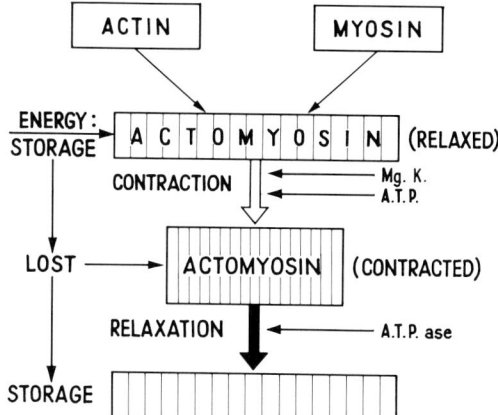

Figure 21-12. Behavior of actomyosin in energy cycle of gravid uterus. (From Botella-Llusiá: *Obstetrical Endocrinology.* Springfield, Ill., Charles C Thomas, 1961.)

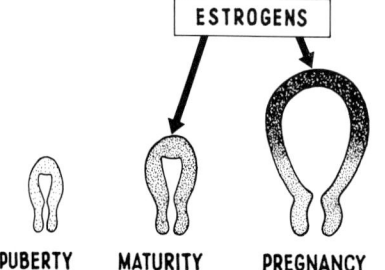
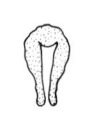

Figure 21-13. Scheme of the action of estrogens on actomyosin storage in the uterus during maturation and during pregnancy. (From Botella-Llusiá: *Obstetrical Endocrinology.* Springfield, Ill., Charles C Thomas, 1961.)

this way, control of uterine motility during pregnancy depends on the reciprocal ratio between estrogens and progesterone. Whenever estrogens predominate, the uterus tends to contract; whenever progesterone predominates, the uterus tends to stay at rest. Recently, the hypothesis postulating that estrogen-progesterone imbalance plays a role in initiating labor has received ample confirmation.[55, 84, 93, 103, 139]

In a previous section, we commented on the proved role of progestogens in protecting the myometrium of both animals and man from agents causing contraction,[41, 44, 71, 79, 80, 115, 140, 141] as well as from the counteracting effects of estrogens,[41, 73, 90] and we have stated that, in the final analysis, the initiation of labor depends on uterine contractile activity as determined by the existing *estrogen-progesterone equilibrium*. In prolonged pregnancies, high levels of progesteronemia are maintained (Holm and Short[66]), and exceptionally large amounts of pregnanediol are eliminated in the urine (Furuhjelm[51]).

In at least some animals, relaxin also exerts a protective function.[8, 9] In the ewe, increased activity of circulating relaxin delays labor,[57] whereas in castrated guinea pigs, abortion does not occur so long as sufficient doses of relaxin are administered (Deanesly and Zarrow[42]).

21.4.4. ROLE OF OXYTOCIN IN INITIATING LABOR

According to Cross,[37, 38] oxytocin is probably not the only excitant of contraction, and its function, instead of serving to *initiate* labor, is concerned with maintaining contractions once they have been set into motion by other excitants. As a result of measurements of intramammary pressure, Caldeyro-Barcia and Poseiro[22] maintain that oxytocinemia increases during the expulsion period. Hawker and his colleagues[60, 61] found no significant variations in oxytocin levels, but their method of estimation may be viewed as less sensitive than that employed by Caldeyro-Barcia and Poseiro. On the basis of overwhelming clinical evidence, available from intrapartum injections of oxytocin,[9, 14, 23, 49, 123] it must be admitted that labor is unquestionably promoted either because of an *actual* intrapartum increase in oxytocin levels, or because of a *potential* increase resulting from loss of oxytocinase activity (see below).

Numerous investigators[27, 28, 53, 54, 81, 95, 117, 118] have found increased plasma oxytocinase activity during pregnancy, and noted that the latter decreases during labor (see Section 21.4.9).

It is also possible that oxytocin *analogues*, such as *deamino-oxytocin*,[26, 47, 68] act as contraction-inducing agents whose effects are even more potent. Incidentally, Collin and Racadot[33] observed that, in animals in labor, the *Gomori-positive substance*—believed to be identical with oxytocin (see Chapter 9)—in the supraoptic and paraventricular hypothalamic nuclei was subject to rapid evacuation. In Chapter 8, we described the reflex of oxytocin secretion by the supraoptic and paraventricular hypothalamic nuclei initiated by stimulation of the uterine cervix. That reflex is also referred to as the *Ferguson-Harris reflex*. Its specificity, and the fact that it is not associated with vasopressin secretion other than by a central mechanism of stimulation, has been demonstrated by Aulserbrook and Holland.[4] Tindal and his colleagues[131] have reproduced this reflex by means of electric stimulation of the uterine cervix. Studied in the ewe, the Ferguson-Harris reflex was found by Roberts and Share[108, 109] to be suppressed by progesterone, enhanced by estrogens and, insofar as the amount of oxytocin secreted is concerned, associated with a much greater response during labor.

21.4.5. MODE OF ACTION OF OXYTOCIN

Oxytocin produces increased electric excitability of the uterus (Wiqvist[138]). Since increased excitability is conditioned by changes in electrolyte balance, the effects of oxytocin depend mainly on concentrations of potassium and calcium.[10] Changes in the concentrations of these cations are brought about by the "sodium pump" mechanism, described by Csapo[39] and explained in Chapter 3. Clinically, this has also been confirmed by Hawkins and Nixon.[62] Movement of sodium ion out of the cell and that of potassium causes alterations of membrane potential[89] and changes in the phospholipid content of the myocyte.[86] *Oxytocin thus acts by provoking a chain reaction in all those biochemical processes that produce contraction of the uterine smooth*

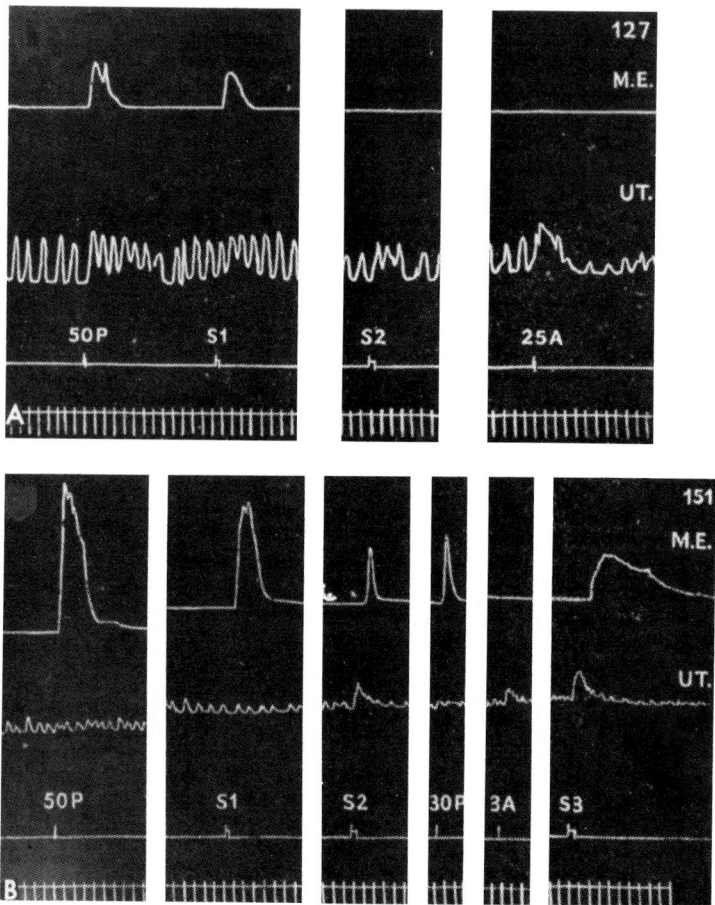

Figure 21–14. Stimulation of hypothalamus in female rabbit by means of stereotaxic devices. Simultaneous recording of uterine contractility and lactiferous duct contractility. *M.E.*, Mammary tracing; *UT*, uterine tracing. *A*, Rabbit, six days postpartum (50 P, 50,000 units of pitocin; S1, stimulation of supraoptic nucleus; S2, stimulation of lateral hypothalamic nucleus; 25A, 25 mcg epinephrine). Note that injection of pitocin causes simultaneous contractions in uterus and lactiferous ducts, as does stimulation of supraoptic nucleus. In contrast, stimulation of lateral hypothalamic nucleus (S2) elicits uterine contractions but no mammary ejection, indicating a direct neural type of action rather than Pituitrin-mediated effect. Injection of 25 micrograms of epinephrine (25A) produces the same effect. *B*, Rabbit, 45 days postpartum, in full lactation but with involuted uterus. The lactiferous ducts respond with great intensity to pitocin injection and to supraoptic nucleus stimulation, but the uterus is anergic. On the other hand, the uterus retains excitability to epinephrine and lateral nucleus stimulation. This proves that pituitary action fails not because the uterus is completely refractory but because it lacks adequate preparation (estrogen priming) to respond to pitocin. 3A, 3 mcg epinephrine; S3, stimulation of hypothalamic nucleus. (From Cross: *Brit. Med. J.*, 11:152, 1955.)

muscle fibers, once the electrolyte balance of the fibers has been previously adjusted by increased estrogen and decreased progesterone activity.

21.4.6. ROLE OF HYPOTHALAMUS IN CONTROLLING OXYTOCIN SECRETION

Advances made in the past few years on the physiology of the neurohypophysis have clarified many aspects of central nervous system control of labor in laboratory animals. Reynolds[105] was able to show that labor could be induced in denervated gravid rabbits by means of hypothalamic stimulation. Since what had been severed was the afferent nerve supply, the only logical explanation for that finding was to assume that the hypothalamus excited the neurohypophysis to secrete. Harris[63, 65] showed that dilatation of the uterine cervix in rabbits provoked labor (which clinical observations also reveal to be true in woman). A reflex mechanism therefore had to be considered, such as one mediated by the vegetative motor innervation of the uterus. However, Reynolds as well as Harris and Jacobson[64] succeeded in demonstrating that transection of the pituitary stalk suppressed this reflex mechanism. In addition, Harris was able to show that cervical dilatation caused increased oxytocinemia.[65] Similarly, Hawker et al.[58] found increased blood levels of oxytocin in the ewe following cervical dilatation. By means of neurostereotaxic techniques (Fig. 21–14), Cross[38] was able to pinpoint the nucleus that, when excited, elicited oxytocin secretion. This is the *paraventricular* nucleus (Fig. 21–15). Stimulating this nucleus provokes not only uterine contractions but also milk ejection from the nipple (see Chapter 22), an effect well known to be caused by oxytocin activity.

The paraventricular nucleus is a highly specific center of oxytocin secretion. Its stimulation fails to affect levels of vasopressor hormone (Cross[37]) or those of antidiuretic hormone (Olivecrona[98]).

The existence of a *neuroendocrine reflex* for the initiation of labor has thus been proved. The centripetal afferent limb of that reflex arc is the neurovegetative system, which is stimulated in a primordial way by *distention of the uterus* and by *cervical dilatation*. Suranyi and his colleagues[126] have found baroreceptor nerve endings in the uterine cervix. These endings excite the supraoptic nucleus in a more or less direct way. The supraoptic nucleus is highly specific and deserves the perhaps metaphorical name of "center of labor." The oxytocin secreted by it (see Chapter 7) gains access to

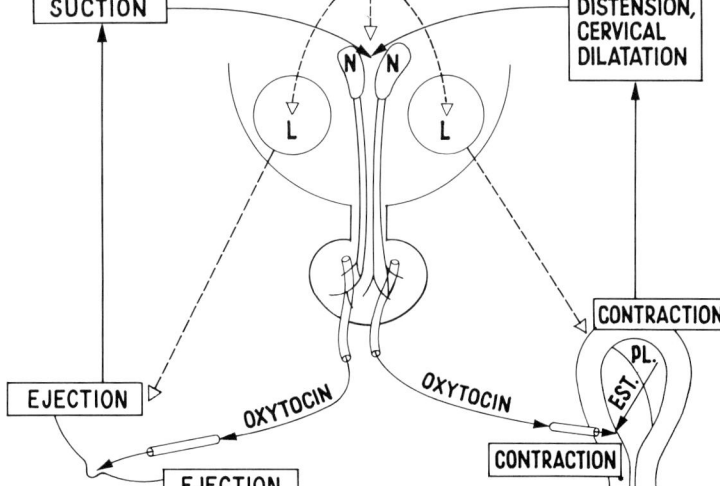

Figure 21–15. Diagram of pitocin effect on uterus and breast.

the bloodstream in the posterior lobe and is carried to the uterus, which it excites.

Labor can also be induced by excitation of the lateral hypothalamic nuclei, although the phenomenon occurs only in animals with intact uterine innervation and is not associated with any increase in oxytocin blood levels, so that it may be assumed to represent a *different*, nonneuroendocrine, but rather typically neural, *reflex* (Figs. 21-15 and 21-16).

As indicated in Figure 21-15, telencephalic influences as well as emotions may act on the nucleus of labor and either excite or paralyze uterine contractions. This would explain the influence of such emotions as fright, fear, etc., on the course of the obstetric process.

21.4.7. OTHER NEUROHORMONES IN LABOR

VASOPRESSIN. Although Cross[37, 38] asserts the specificity of the product the hypothalamic nuclei secrete as a result of cervical dilatation, it is also true that labor elicits *release of vasopressin* by adjacent nuclei, which is of importance in clinical obstetrics (see Chapter 42). In normal gestation and labor, such factors are inactivated by specific enzymes. Assali and associates,[2] Eglin and Jessiman,[46] Hawker,[58] Reynolds and Mackie,[106] and Roth and Slater[110] have all reported increased *vasopressinase activity*. However, in some cases the initiation of labor would appear to result from alterations of the toxemic type (see Chapter 44) rather than from vasopressin-vasopressinase interactions.

Investigations of the last few years prove that pituitary oxytocin is not the only factor involved in exciting uterine contractility and myometrial activity. As we have pointed out, estrogens exert a sensitizing effect, resulting in increased excitability, although the real decisive factor remains oxytocin.

In addition to the pituitary hormones, however, other oxytocic substances must be taken into account.

ACETYLCHOLINE. Acetylcholine synthesis by the placenta has been demonstrated, as well as an increased rate of such synthesis during the last minutes of gestation.[96] This is one of the mechanisms of placental autodeterminism in the genesis of labor. Acetylcholine not only acts as an excitant per se but also sensitizes the uterine fiber to pituitary hormone activity. It probably also acts by exciting the hypothalamus, thereby indirectly provoking oxytocin release. Near term, acetylcholine is present in increased amounts in the blood,[83] and is probably one of the factors that may account for the precipitation of labor in the absence of retropituitary function.

21.4.8. HISTAMINE

The presence of histamine in the placenta and in the uterine wall at the end of pregnancy has been demonstrated clearly and amply confirmed. Histamine is a potent excitant of uterine contractions. In some pathologic conditions of pregnancy, such as abortion, uteroplacental apoplexy and gestosis, it is of exceptional importance. The presence of histamine activity, in conjunction with acetylcholine activity, adequately explains why the retrohypophysis is not indispensable for the dynamics of labor.

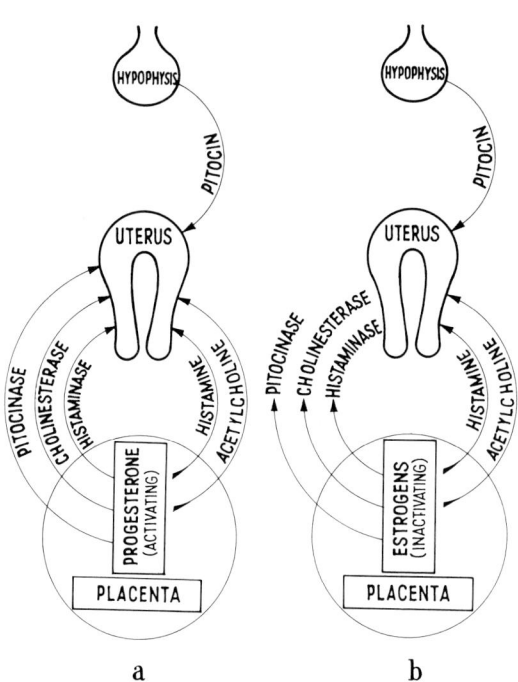

Figure 21-16. Initiation of labor. A, Placenta at term elaborates substances that inactivate physiologic stimulants of uterus. B, During labor, these enzymatic inactivators cease being effective because of placental senescence, allowing myometrial stimulants to initiate labor. (From Botella-Llusiá: *Obstetrical Endocrinology.* Springfield, Ill., Charles C Thomas, 1961.)

21.4.9. ANTIOXYTOCIC SUBSTANCES

As with oxytocin, other substances that are able to produce contractions are not encountered in the final days of gestation but have been demonstrated in the blood and urine long before the onset of labor.[59, 99] *However, their action fails to be exerted until the appropriate moment because it is inhibited or inactivated by specific enzymes* (see Fig. 21–14). The following enzymes are involved:

OXYTOCINASE. Bengtsson and Csapo[8] called attention to the complete lack of response to oxytocin by the gravid uterus and postulated that this resulted from the presence of oxytocinase, previously identified and described in the uteri of animals and man by Page and co-workers[99] and by Audrain and Clauser.[3] Carballo and Mendez-Bauer[25] isolated oxytocinase from the placenta, and Beller and Schnitz,[6] Mellander,[94] and particularly Semm,[116, 117] isolated it from the plasma. Semm made the observation that oxytocinase activity diminished at term and suggested that, as a result of no longer being inactivated, blood levels of oxytocin increased. Hyperdistention of the gravid uterus, it was found, led to increased oxytocinase activity.[75, 78] This is probably why Hawker and associates[60] were unable to find increased oxytocin blood levels during labor. Even assuming that such increased levels as were encountered with ultrasensitive methods by Caldeyro-Barcia and Poseiro[22] actually do occur, it is quite possible that similar elevations are of little importance and that the real reason for the existing excitation of the uterine fiber at labor should be sought instead in the *diminished rate of oxytocinase inactivation*.

In addition, Semm[118] demonstrated that oxytocinase was produced by the placenta and that the enzyme disappeared in toxemia, which might very well explain some important aspects of the physiology of toxemic disorders.

A high rate of plasma oxytocinase activity throughout gestation, that decreased during labor, was subsequently borne out as one of the possible basic mechanisms involved in the induction of labor by the studies of Chan and Warenburg,[28] Gilliland and Prout[54] and others. Mellander[95] reported increased oxytocinase activity in twin pregnancies and diminished activity in premature labor, which was also confirmed by Semm.[117] On the other hand, Lambrinopoulos[81] found that prolonged labor was associated with excessive oxytocinase activity, while Geldening and co-workers[53] found increased aminopeptidase activity in the serum in overmature pregnancies. Finally, the recent discovery by Chan and his associates[27] that *some penicillin derivatives possess antioxytocic activity* may prove of great clinical significance with respect to modern overuse of antibiotics.

CHOLINESTERASE. Demonstrated by Navratil a long time ago, the presence of cholinesterase has been fully confirmed in modern times.[124] The cholinesterase enzyme system acts by a yet incompletely known mechanism in opposing not only acetylcholine activity but also the action of all other oxytocic agents.

HISTAMINASE. The effects of antihistaminic agents on the clinical course of allergies in pregnancy are currently under study.

The antioxytocic enzyme system as a whole opposes the action of the aforementioned excitants of contraction and thereby discharges the function of protecting gestation prior to labor.

21.5. SUMMARY OF INTRAPARTUM CORRELATIONS

Based on the data presented, induction of labor can be inferred to be largely a process of hormonal correlation. As pregnancy develops, preparations for labor are made by three different mechanisms: (1) By means of progressively increasing pituitary and placental production of *substances possessing oxytocic activity:* oxytocin, acetylcholine and histamine. As gestation advances, these substances are found in increasing concentrations in the tissues and blood, reaching a peak during the final phases of pregnancy. (2) By means of a parallel increase in production of *estrogens and progesterone*, designed to stimulate the development of the muscle fiber and to enhance its capacity for energetic contractions. From a functional point of view, Braxton-Hicks contractions—the spontaneous contractions occurring during the last period of gestation—are but a reflection of the slow process of conditioning the muscle fiber. (3) By means of progressive *distention of the uterine muscle* which, in terms of contractility, is more efficient the more it is stretched.

Having described how the uterus is being prepared for labor, some consideration must be given to the factors which interrupt the balance of gestation. This balance is offset mainly by a double *feto-placental* and *feto-uterine* conflict. The first of these, that is, disharmony between fetal and placental growth, implicitly leads to degeneration and aging of the placenta. Aging of the placenta is characterized by loss of capacity for progesterone synthesis on the one hand, and loss of antioxytocic, antihistaminic and antiacetylcholinic power on the other. These functional placental disturbances entail *loss of the defense mechanism, hitherto present in gestation, against agents capable of exciting the gravid uterus.* This loss of inhibition occurs prior to labor. The induction of labor therefore results not from an increase in oxytocin substances but from a decrease in antioxytocic substances.

The second conflict, namely, that between the fetus and the uterus, also plays a primordial and interesting role. Because of the increasing rate of growth of the fetus, the uterus undergoes gradual distention. *This distention acts reflexly* through sensitive nerve endings in the uterine wall. *As a result, growing distention of the uterus causes increased production of oxytocin by a reflex mechanism and contributes, through a series of neuroendocrine mechanisms, toward precipitating labor in a definitive manner.*

21.6. REGRESSION OF GRAVIDIC CHANGES

In those animals in which the corpus luteum persists till the very end of gestation (e.g., the cow), oxytocin exerts luteolytic activity (Wilks et al.[137]). Wagner and coworkers[136] observed lack of LH and FSH release in the cow under the influence of oxytocin. At a later stage, as soon as the effects of the hormonal mechanism of labor disappear, gonadotropin levels are found to rise again[48] and ovarian activity as well as endometrial proliferation is resumed.[77]

REFERENCES

1. Acker, G., and Courrier, R.: *Compt. Rend. Acad. Sci. (Paris)*, 268:2196, 1969.
2. Assali, M. H., Dignam, W. J., and Longo, L.: *J. Clin. Endocr.*, 20:581, 1960.
3. Audrain, L., and Clauser, H.: *Biochim. Biophys. Acta*, 38:494, 1960.
4. Aulserbrook, L. H., and Holland, R. C.: *Amer. J. Physiol.*, 216:818, 1969.
5. Barcroft, J.: *Studies on Prenatal Life.* Oxford, University Press, 1946.
6. Beller, F. K., and Schnitz, H.: *Geburtsh. u. Frauenhk.*, 20:563, 1960.
7. Bengtsson, L. P.: *Amer. J. Obstet. Gynec.*, 74:484, 1957.
8. Bengtsson, L. P.: *Acta Obstet. Gynec. Scand.*, 41 (Suppl. 1):87, 1962.
9. Bengtsson, L. P., and Csapo, A.: *Amer. J. Obstet. Gynec.*, 83:1083, 1962.
10. Berger, E., and Marshall, J. M.: *Amer. J. Physiol.*, 201:931, 1961.
11. Bergström, S., and Sjövall, J.: *Acta Chemica Scand.*, 15:1701, 1960.
12. Bergström, S.: *Science*, 157:382, 1967.
13. Berry, K. W., and Hugs, M. L.: *Obstet. Gynec.*, 14:612, 1959.
14. Bishop, E. H.: *Obstet. Gynec.*, 11:290, 1958.
15. Bjuro, T., Lindberg, S., and Westling, H.: *Acta Obstet. Gynec. Scand.*, 40:152, 1961.
16. Botella, J.: *Rev. Esp. Farmacol.*, 2:899, 1941.
17. Botella, J., and Clavero, J. A.: *Acta Gin.*, 13:507, 1962.
18. Botella, J., and Clavero, J. A.: *Arch. Gynäk.*, 198:56, 1963.
19. Bruns, P. D., et al.: *Amer. J. Obstet. Gynec.*, 73:579, 1957.
20. Bydgeman, M., and Samuelson, B.: *Clin. Chim. Acta*, 13:465, 1966.
21. Bydgeman, M., et al.: *Amer. J. Obstet. Gynec.*, 106:567, 1970.
22. Caldeyro-Barcia, R., and Poseiro, J. J.: *Ann. N.Y. Acad. Sci.*, 73:813, 1959.
23. Caldeyro-Barcia, R., and Heller, H.: *Oxytocin.* Oxford, Pergamon Press, 1961.
24. Calvo de Mora, S.: *Acta Gin.*, 15:307, 1964.
25. Carballo, M. A., and Mendez-Bauer, C. J.: *Actas del II Congreso Uruguayo de Ginecología*, 2:308, 1957.
26. Chan, W. Y., and Du Vigneaud, V.: *Endocrinology*, 71:977, 1961.
27. Chan, W. Y., Fear, R., and Du Vigneaud, V.: *Endocrinology*, 81:1267, 1967.
28. Chan, W. Y., and Warenburg, M.: *Endocrinology*, 82:475, 1968.
29. Clavero, J. A., and Botella, J.: *Amer. J. Obstet. Gynec.*, 86:234, 1963.
30. Clavero, J. A.: *Acta Gin.*, 15:69, 133, 1964.
31. Clavero-Nuñez, J. A., et al.: *Acta Gin.*, 19:417, 1968.
32. Clavero-Nuñez, J. A., et al.: *Acta Gin.*, 20:617, 1969.
33. Collin, R., and Racadot, J.: *Ann. d'Endocr.*, 14:546. 1956.
34. Corner, G. W.: *Contrib. Embryol.*, 31:117, 1945.
35. Corner, G. W., and Csapo, A.: *Brit. Med. J.*, 1:687, 1953.
36. Crawford, J. W.: *Obstet. Gynec. Brit. Emp.*, 63:548, 1956.
37. Cross, B. A.: *Nature*, 173:450, 1954.
38. Cross, B. A.: *J. Endocr.*, 12:151, 1955.
39. Csapo, A.: *Rec. Progr. Horm. Res.*, 12:405, 1956.
40. Csapo, A.: *Ann. N.Y. Acad. Sci.*, 75:790, 1959.
41. Csapo, A., and Lloyd-Jacob, M. A.: *Nature*, 192:329, 1961.

42. Deanesly, R., and Zarrow, M. K.: *Endocrinology*, 73:522, 1963.
43. Deis, R. P., and Pickford, M.: *J. Physiol.*, 173:215, 1964.
44. Douglas, R. G., and Kramm, E. E.: *Amer. J. Obstet. Gynec.*, 73:1206, 1957.
45. Eagle, E.: *Amer. J. Obstet. Gynec.*, 42:262, 1941.
46. Eglin, J. M., and Jessiman, A. B.: *J. Clin. Endocr.*, 19:369, 1959.
47. Embrey, M. P.: *J. Endocr.*, 31:185, 1965.
48. Fayman, C., Ryan, R. J., Zwirek, S. J., and Rubin, M. E.: *J. Clin. Endocr.*, 28:1323, 1968.
49. Franklin, K. S., and Winstone, W. E.: *J. Physiol.*, 125:43, 1954.
50. Fuchs, A. R.: *J. Endocr.*, 30:217, 1964.
51. Furuhjelm, M.: *Acta Obstet. Gynec. Scand.*, 41:370, 1962.
52. Garrett, W. J.: *J. Obstet. Gynec. Brit. Emp.*, 61:586, 1954.
53. Geldening, M. G., Titus, M. A., Schroeder, S. A., Mohun, G., and Page, E. W.: *Amer. J. Obstet. Gynec.*, 92:814, 1965.
54. Gilliland, P. F., and Prout, T. E.: *Metabolism*, 14:918, 1965.
55. Goodlin, R. C.: *Amer. J. Obstet. Gynec.*, 107:429, 1970.
56. Greenwald, G. S.: *J. Endocr.*, 26:233, 1963.
57. Hall, K., Hoare, M., and Turner, C. B.: *J. Endocr.*, 25:271, 1962.
58. Hawker, R. W.: *Quart. J. Exper. Physiol.*, 41:301, 1956.
59. Hawker, R. W., and Robertson, P. A.: *Endocrinology*, 60:652, 1957.
60. Hawker, R. W., Roberts, V. S., and Walmstey, C. F.: *Endocrinology*, 64:309, 1959.
61. Hawker, R. W., Walmstey, C. F., Roberts, V. S., Blackshaw, J. K., and Downes, J. C.: *J. Clin. Endocr.*, 21:985, 1961.
62. Hawkins, D. F., and Nixon, W. C. W.: *J. Obstet. Gynec. Brit. Comm.*, 68:62, 1961.
63. Harris, G. W.: *Arch. Gynäk.*, 183:35, 1953.
64. Harris, G. W., and Jacobson, D.: *Proc. Roy. Soc. London, B*, 139:265, 1952.
65. Harris, G. W.: In *Hypothalamic Hypophyseal Interrelationships*, ed. Field, Guillemin and Carton. Springfield, Ill., Charles C Thomas, 1956.
66. Holm, L. W., and Short, R. V.: *J. Reprod. Fertil.*, 4:137, 1962.
67. Holm, L. W., and Galligan, S. J.: *Amer. J. Obstet. Gynec.*, 95:887, 1966.
68. Hope, D. B., and Du Vigneaud, V.: *J. Biol. Chem.*, 237:3146, 1963.
69. Huggett, A. G. S.: *Ann. N.Y. Acad. Sci.*, 75:873, 1959.
70. Ingelman-Sundberg, A., Sandberg, F., Ryden, G., and Joelson, I.: *Bull. Fed. Soc. Obstet. Gynec. L. Franç.*, 17:783, 1967.
71. Israel, S. L., et al.: *Obstet. Gynec.*, 13:672, 1959; 14:68, 1959.
72. Järvinen, P. A., Luukainen, T., and Väistö, L.: *Acta Obstet. Gynec. Scand.*, 44:258, 1965.
73. Javert, C. T., and Reiss, C.: *Surg. Gynec. Obstet.*, 94:256, 1952.
74. Jung, H.: *Arch. Gynäk.*, 198:145, 1963.
75. Jung, H., and Klock, F. K.: *Gynaecologia*, 167:28, 1969.
76. Kaiser, I. H., and Harris, J. S.: *Amer. J. Obstet. Gynec.*, 59:775, 1950.
77. Kava, H. W., Klinger, H. P., Molnar, J. J., and Romney, S. L.: *Amer. J. Obstet. Gynec.*, 102:122, 1968.
78. Klimek, R., Drewniak, K., and Bientarz, A.: *Amer. J. Obstet. Gynec.*, 105:427, 1969.
79. Kumar, D., Goodno, J. A., and Barnes, A. C.: *Nature*, 195:1204, 1962.
80. Kumar, D., Goodno, J. A., and Barnes, A. C.: *Amer. J. Obstet. Gynec.*, 84:1111, 1962.
81. Lambrinopoulos, T. C.: *Obstet. Gynec.*, 23:780, 1964.
82. Lerner, L. J.: *Ann. N.Y. Acad. Sci.*, 75:460, 1959.
83. Lewis, A. A. G.: *J. Clin. Endocr.*, 13:769, 1953.
84. Liggins, G. C., Kennedy, P. C., and Holm, L. W.: *Amer. J. Obstet. Gynec.*, 98:1080, 1967.
85. Llauro, J. L., Rünnebaum, B., and Zander, J.: *Amer. J. Obstet. Gynec.*, 101:867, 1968.
86. Luukainen, T. V., and Csapo, A.: *Fertil. Steril.*, 14:65, 1963.
87. MacClure-Browne, I. E., and Veall, N.: *J. Obstet. Gynec. Brit. Emp.*, 60:141, 1953.
88. Marañón, G.: *Brit. Med. J.*, 2:749, 1947.
89. Marshall, C. F., and Csapo, A.: *Endocrinology*, 68:107, 1961.
90. Martin, L.: *J. Endocr.*, 26:31, 1963.
91. Martin-Pinto, R., et al.: *Amer. J. Obstet. Gynec.*, 97:881, 1967.
92. Martin-Pinto, R., Lerner, U., Pontelli, H., and Rabow, W.: *Compt. Rend. Soc. Biol. (Paris)*, 162:228, 1968.
93. Martin-Pinto, R., Lerner, U., and Pontelli, H.: *Amer. J. Obstet. Gynec.*, 98:457, 1967.
94. Mellander, S. E. J.: *Nature*, 191:176, 1961.
95. Mellander, S. E. J.: *Acta Endocr.*, 48(Suppl.):96, 1965.
96. Morrow, H. S.: *Surg. Gynec. Obstet.*, 85:105, 1947.
97. Needham, D. M., and Williams, J. M.: *Biochem. J.*, 73:171, 1959.
98. Olivecrona, N.: *Nature*, 173:1001, 1953.
99. Page, E. W., Titus, M. A., Mohun, G., and Glendening, B. B.: *Amer. J. Obstet. Gynec.*, 82:1090, 1961.
100. Paine, C. G.: *Obstet. Gynec. Brit. Emp.*, 64:668, 1957.
101. Paton, D. M., and Daniel, E. E.: *Canad. J. Physiol.*, 45:795, 1967.
102. Pickles, V. R.: *Internat. J. Fertil.*, 12:335, 1967.
103. Rado, A., Crystle, C. D., and Townsley, J.: *J. Clin. Endocr.*, 30:497, 1970.
104. Ramsey, E. M.: *Ann. N.Y. Acad. Sci.*, 75:726, 1959.
105. Reynolds, S. R. M.: *Ann. N.Y. Acad. Sci.*, 75:691, 1959.
106. Reynolds, S. R. M., and Mackie, J. D.: *Proc. Soc. Exper. Biol. Med.*, 108:649, 1961.
107. Ritzel, G., Staub, H., and Huntzinger, W. A.: *Deutsch. Med. Wschr.*, 82:400, 1957.
108. Roberts, J. S., and Share, L.: *Endocrinology*, 83:272, 1968.
109. Roberts, J. S., and Share, L.: *Endocrinology*, 84:1076, 1969.
110. Roth, K., and Slater, S.: *Amer. J. Obstet. Gynec.*, 83:1325, 1962.
111. Ryden, G., and Sjoholm, I.: *Acta Obstet. Gynec. Scand.*, 48:Suppl. 3, 1969.
112. Sandberg, F., Ingelman-Sundberg, A., and Ryden, G.: *Acta Obstet. Gynec. Scand.*, 43:95, 1964.

113. Sandberg, F., Ingelman-Sundberg, A., and Ryden, G.: *Acta Obstet. Gynec. Scand.*, 44:585, 1965.
114. Schofield, B. M.: *J. Endocr.*, 25:95, 1962.
115. Schofield, B. M.: *J. Physiol.*, 166:191, 1963.
116. Semm, K.: *Zbl. Gynäk.*, 84:1665, 1962.
117. Semm, K.: *Arch. Gynäk.*, 198:149; 1963; 199:265, 1963.
118. Semm, K., and Bernhard, J.: *Arch. Gynäk.*, 199:271, 1963.
119. Sabanah, E. H., et al.: *Amer. J. Obstet. Gynec.*, 89:841, 1964.
120. Sjoholm, J., and Ryden, G.: *Acta Endocr.*, 61:432, 1969.
121. Smith, O. W.: *Acta Endocr.*, 51:Suppl. 104, 1965.
122. Spratto, G. R., and Miller, J. W.: *J. Pharmacol. Exper. Therap.*, 161:1, 1968.
123. Stewart, R. H., and Slezak, R. M.: *Obstet. Gynec.*, 11:295, 1958.
124. Stone, M. L., Piliero, S. J., Hammer, H., and Portnoy, A.: *Obstet. Gynec.*, 16:675, 1960.
125. Stroup, P.: *Amer. J. Obstet. Gynec.*, 84:595, 1962.
126. Suranyi, S., Kovacs, T., and Molnar, G.: *Ztschr. Geb. u. Gyn.*, 144:175, 1956.
127. Suzor, P., et al.: *Gynec. Obstet.*, 55:122, 1952.
128. Taleisnik, S., and Tomatis, M. D.: *Neuroendocrinology*, 3:303, 1968.
129. Terragno, N.: Thesis, University of Madrid, 1965.
130. Thomsen, K., and Hiersche, H. D.: "The Functional Morphology of the Placenta," in *Fetus and Placenta*, A. Klopper and E. Diczfalusy. Oxford, Blackwell, 1969.
131. Tindall, J. S., Knaggs, G. S., and Turvey, A.: *J. Endocr.*, 40:205, 1968.
132. Velardo, J. T.: *Anat. Rec.*, 130:444, 1958.
133. Velardo, J. T.: *Ann. N.Y. Acad. Sci.*, 75:441, 1959.
134. Villee, C. A.: In *The Placenta and Fetal Membranes*, Baltimore, Williams & Wilkins, 1960.
135. Vorherr, H., Kleeman, C. R., and Lehman, E.: *Endocrinology*, 81:711, 1967.
136. Wagner, W. C., Saatman, R., and Hansel, W.: *J. Reprod. Fertil.*, 18:501, 1969.
137. Wilks, J. W., Hansell, W., and Armstrong, D. T.: *Endocrinology*, 84:1032, 1969.
138. Wiqvist, H., et al.: *Acta Endocr.*, 41:161, 1962.
139. Yannone, M. E., MacCurdy, M. E., and Goldfien, A.: *Amer. J. Obstet. Gynec.*, 101:1058, 1968.
140. Zarrow, M. X., et al.: *Fertil. Steril.*, 11:370, 1960.
141. Zarrow, M. X., Anderson, W. C., and Callantyne, M. R.: *Nature*, 198:690, 1963.
142. Zuspan, F. P., Cibils, L. A., and Pose, S. V.: *Amer. J. Obstet. Gynec.*, 84:841, 1962.

Chapter 22
ENDOCRINE PHYSIOLOGY OF THE BREAST

22.1. INTRODUCTION

The breast is a characteristic organ of the mammalian group (*Mammalia*). Nevertheless, lactation is not necessarily confined to mammals. For example, the "crop gland" in some birds (pigeon) has a regulation identical to that of the mammalian breast.

The purpose of the breast is to produce milk for breast-feeding or lactation. In mammals, lactation is the final reproductive phase. Those mammalian species whose newborns require no maternal milk during the neonatal period are rare; perhaps the only mammalian species in which this is not an absolute prerequisite is the human species. The lactational turnover of nutrition from the mother to the suckling infant is enormous. The baby seal, for instance, gains about 45 kg during the suckling period. However, even more striking is the situation in mice, in which the entire litter gains approximately 50 gm in weight, while the mother herself only weighs 25 gm. The mouse thus gives away twice her own body weight in milk during lactation. Again, a good cow may yield 20,000 liters of milk a year, which is 45 times her own weight.

Regulation of lactation is automatic to the extent that it often overrules the nutritional requirements of the mother. It is entirely possible for the baby to deplete the mother nutritionally, accomplishing what has been known as an act of "metabolic cannibalism." Though as far as the human species is concerned, in civilized countries, except for rare instances, this does not develop, the occurrence of serious lactational malnutrition is still tragically common in poor and underdeveloped countries.

The most primitive mammals, or protheria, which are oviparous, have modified cutaneous glands secreting milk that is licked by the suckling as it drains off the mother's abdominal hair. There are no nipples. Metatheria, on the other hand, have distinct mammary glands located in a pouch; however, it is in eutheria in which mammary development is greatest.

Mammary development and function are both subject to endocrine regulation. At present, the mechanism involved in the physiology of the mammary gland of experimental animals, such as mice, rats, etc., is well known, although with respect to woman many issues still remain to be elucidated. The next section deals with the subject of mammary development and function as a whole, applying, wherever possible, pertinent data as of now available through comparative physiology.

For the sake of greater conciseness of our study, this chapter has been divided into five parts; (1) development of the breast (mammogenesis); (2) initiation of milk secretion (lactogenesis); (3) maintenance of milk secretion (lactopoiesis); (4) milk ejection; and (5) a brief study of the effects of lactation on the reproductive cycle.

22.2. MAMMOGENESIS

The breast is a *quaternary* sex character of woman, that is, a somatic character that *develops as an independent sex character only after puberty*. Later we shall study briefly breast development during the various phases of female sexual life and the different hormones influencing such development. It should be pointed out that the term *mammogenesis* refers to morphogenetic development only and not to functional breast development (*lactogenesis*), which will be discussed later.

22.2.1. FETAL DEVELOPMENT OF THE BREAST

To a large extent, fetal breast development takes place independently of hormone activity; however, the end of the first trimester of intrauterine life marks the beginning of obvious differences in development between the male and the female breast. Although it is influenced by circulating estrogens, the male breast is also influenced by a hormone derived from the fetal testis, probably testosterone. This phase of differentiation of the rudimentary breast into male and female types has lasting effects and is of decisive importance with regard to the development of congenital malformations and the eventual pathology of the breast.

22.2.2. MAMMARY DEVELOPMENT AFTER BIRTH

The process of breast development from fetal life to adulthood has been reviewed by Richardson[141] and by Linzell.[114] The assumption that the breast undergoes no development prior to *puberty* because of its *quaternary* sex character was shown to be erroneous. Though it is true that the active phase of mammary growth does not start until puberty, Raynaud[138] demonstrated the occurrence of constant and active growth of the breast during infancy. Classic studies by Flux[53] and Folley[55] had shown that *isometric growth* of the breast occurred in baby animals in relation to body surface. A second spurt of growth, known as allometric growth[56, 57] was shown to supervene during the prepuberal phase at a rate surpassing the body surface quotient, and to reflect the beginning of sex hormone activity. Damm and Turner[42] and Donovan and Jacobson,[48] as well as Tucker and Reece,[179] used histochemical reactions for deoxyribonucleic acid (DNA) as a means of determining mammary growth. Quantitatively, the presence of DNA is known to be related to the action of the mammogenic hormones and is not conspicuous during the phase of isometric growth, appearing only during the phase of prepuberal development and in relation to cyclic activity.

The process of puberal breast development is a continuous one and is carried over without interruption into adult life, including pregnancy and lactation (Figures 22–1 and 22–2).

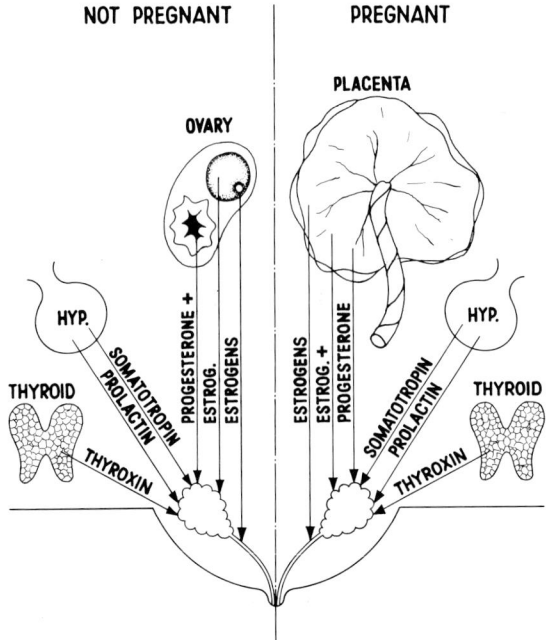

Figure 22–1. Scheme of actions promoting mammary growth in pregnant and nonpregnant woman.

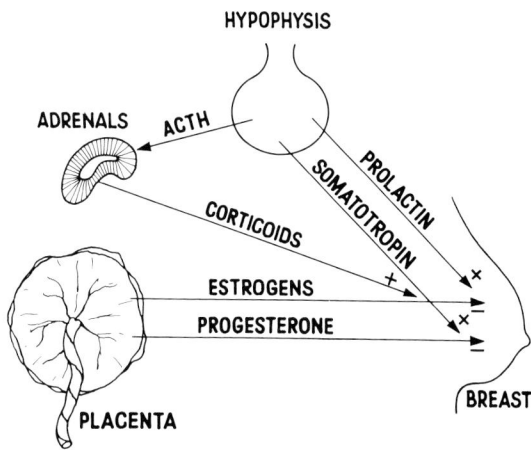

Figure 22-2. Diagram of hormones that regulate secretion of milk (galactogenesis). (From Botella-Llusiá: *Obstetric Endocrinology.* Springfield, Ill., Charles C Thomas, 1961.)

Histologically, the process is characterized first by growth of the lactiferous ducts and then, after attainment of sexual maturity (that is, as a result of the development of a sexual cycle with a corresponding progestational phase), by acinar growth as well.[141, 142] In this respect, though, there are considerable variations among different species. Acinar development is more pronounced in species having a long progestational phase, such as the primates, than in those in which progesterone merely plays a secondary role in the cycle.

22.2.3. EFFECTS OF CASTRATION ON THE BREAST

It is a well known fact that castration leads to atrophy of the mammary gland in animals as well as in women.[56, 141] Such atrophy is characterized by arrest of allometric growth. However, isometric growth continues if castration is performed during the prepuberal phase. It is only pertinent to point out that, in such rodents as rats and mice, total arrest of mammary development is not observed following castration unless the animals are in addition adrenalectomized[57] or hypophysectomized,[52, 53] which may be construed as evidence that, in the absence of ovarian function, the adrenal, the pituitary and, perhaps, the thyroid may—if but in part—stimulate mammary development.

This has led to the increasingly widely held view that *the ovary plays an important, though not exclusive, role in mammary growth.*

Anderson and Turner[5] reported disappearance of mammary DNA content following castration.

22.2.4. ACTION OF ESTROGENS

Both naturally occurring and synthetic estrogens exert a *proliferative* effect on the breast. The estrogenic effect seems to be associated, above all, with proliferation of the *lactiferous ducts*. In this respect, the studies conducted on rats and mice by Folley[55] and by Meites,[116] and later on women by Etienne,[50] are recognized as classics.

The effects of estrogenic activity have been analyzed with the DNA technique by Smith and Richterich.[162]

The question concerning the effects of estrogens on the *mammary acini* has been the object of more controversy. Folley,[56] for instance, had observed that, with the exception of some species, such as monkeys, estrogens failed to produce complete mammary development. A similar response to estrogens has been observed in bitches (Trentin et al.[176, 177]). In other animals (laboratory rodents), as well as in women, complete breast development, with proliferation of acini, cannot be achieved unless progesterone or some other hormones are administered in addition to estrogens. Benson and his associates[14] indicated that the effect of estrogens on the breast varied in relation to the animal's age, being most pronounced in young animals and decreasing thereafter with advancing age. A similar phenomenon probably also takes place in woman. Bernwordt and Turner[19] observed that estrogens failed to elicit a full proliferative effect on the mammary glands of thyroidectomized rats. The differences observed in this type of action are probably the result of varying degrees of mammary tissue *receptivity* to estrogens. Sander[151] demonstrated that uptake of tritiated estradiol by mammary tissue varied in relation with the animal's age[152] but was not affected by hypophysectomy.[153]

22.2.5. ACTION OF PROGESTERONE

Currently, there is general agreement that estrogens have a specific effect on the lactiferous ducts and only a partial effect on the acini of the human breast. It has been recognized that in order to achieve complete development of mammary lobules the action of progesterone in addition to that of estrogen is necessary (Cowie and Tindal,[35] Smith[161]). This law applies almost in general to the supplementary role progesterone plays in regard to the effect of estrogens on various target organs, particularly the endometrium and the myometrium. If hypophysectomized rats (Moon et al.[125]) are injected with both estrogen and progesterone the rate of the resulting mammary growth is much greater than that following injection of estrogen alone. Hahn and Turner,[90] as well as Benson and his associates[14] have shown that in castrated rats estrogen injections elevated the DNA content of lactiferous ducts only, whereas estrogen plus progesterone administration induced much more global development, resulting in elevated acinar DNA content as well.

According to Srivastava and Turner,[165] the same holds true for castrated male rats.

During pregnancy, the breast is subject to the effects of elevated amounts of estrogens in association with progesterone, which probably accounts for the remarkable degree of development reached by the breast during the gestational period. Richardson[141] and Folley[55] have sought to assess the optimal ratio between estrogens and progesterone that is capable of inducing maximal proliferative effects on the breast. The ratio found to be most effective is similar to that in which the two hormones are found to occur during advanced pregnancy. However, the combined stimulative action seems to have a limit beyond which no additional effect is produced by increasing dosages of either estrogens or progestogens. On the other hand, as regards both dosages and ratio between these two sex hormones, there seem to exist enormous variations among various kinds of animals, as revealed by the studies of Smith and Richterich,[162] and those of Speert,[163] on monkeys. Consequently, the problem is highly complicated by the fact that the two ovarian hormones, estrogens and progesterone, not only act on the breast at different levels but also elicit quite different responses in different species of animals.

One thing is clear: *progesterone activity is necessary for complete mammogenesis in laboratory rodents as well as in the human species.*

22.2.6. PITUITARY AND MAMMARY GROWTH

Turner and his co-workers[125, 126] had injected hypophysectomized animals with estrogens and progesterone, noticing that the effect was incomplete. Flux[54] had found that estrogens with an adequate dose of progesterone were sufficient to restore histologic normalcy of the mammary gland in castrated animals but not in animals that had undergone hypophysectomy and castration at the same time. Brookreson and Turner,[25] studying the DNA content as an index of the mammary growth rate, later reached identical conclusions. Tawalker and Meites,[169] on the contrary, reported that in both castrated and adrenalectomized rats, that is, rats totally lacking ovarian steroids, pituitary extract by itself was enough to induce mammary growth. On the basis of this, Turner and his associates postulated the existence of two separate pituitary mammogenic factors they thought were responsible for ductal and acinar development, respectively. This theory subsequently received considerable criticism. For one thing, purified pituitary extracts yield no principle with mammogenic action. For another, complete proliferation of the breast can be achieved by associating estrogens with progesterone, provided that injections are given either locally[55] or in elevated dosages.[33] The prevailing idea at present is that there are no pituitary mammogenic principles involved but that the influence of ovarian steroids on mammary tissue is controlled by somatotropin and prolactin activity (Hadfield and Young,[88] Thatcher and Tucker[171]). It was subsequently shown that injection of prolactin or somatotropin potentiated the local effect of estrogens on the breast (Damm and Turner,[43] Iversen[100]). These findings have been confirmed by Cowie and his colleagues[36] in recent times, and it is now generally acknowledged that, apart from their lactopoietic effects, which will be studied later, prolactin as well as growth hormone *potentiates, or strengthens*, the proliferative effect of estrogens and progesterone on the mammary gland.

22.2.7. ACTION OF ANDROGENS ON THE MAMMARY GLAND

Testosterone is generally admitted to inhibit mammogenesis. Using the DNA test, Turkington and Topper[182] observed an anti-estrogenic effect of androgens, with suppression of mammary proliferation.

However, there is considerable divergence of opinion in this respect. While verifying the anti-estrogenic effect, Bengtssson and Norgren[15] find that, on the other hand, the action of progesterone on the mammary acini is strengthened. Donovan and Jacobsohn[49] have observed acinar proliferation in hypophysectomized rats following injection of androgens. The action of androgens would appear to vary at different levels of the mammary gland, inducing proliferation only in the acinar components and, in addition, depending to a great extent on the individual's state of endocrine balance and condition of pituitary function.

22.2.8. OTHER HORMONES

ADRENAL CORTEX AND MAMMARY GROWTH. Adrenal cortical function is necessary for milk secretion, as we shall see later. Aside from this, Folley[56] and Cowie have shown that bilateral adrenalectomy produced mammary atrophy in rats. Marañón and Fernández-Noguera,[115] and subsequently Jull and co-workers,[105] demonstrated that corticoids, particularly if administered to old males, produced gynecomastia. On the other hand, Trentin and Turner[176] have found that the breasts of castrated female rats did not undergo complete atrophy unless both adrenals were removed. Recently Barnawell[12] confirmed the mammogenic effect of hydrocortisone on isolated breast tissue growth in culture media.

PLACENTA. Placental action on gravidic mammogenesis is very important. In the view of Folley[55] and Richardson,[141] estrogens and progesterone produced by the placenta are essential factors during pregnancy in bringing about prominent mammary gland development. In the course of the last years, however, the existence of a newly recognized hormonal principle, known as *placental lactogen*, has come to shed additional light on this problem.

The presence of some placental mammotrophic principle, similar to that of the pituitary, had already been assumed from the classical studies by Cerruti and Lyons.[27] Although of purely speculative nature, this assumption was also shared by Griffith and Turner.[71] It was subsequently possible to isolate a placental substance with somatotropin-like (viz., growth-promoting) properties[189] that also stimulated lactogenesis, apparently possessing prolactinic activity[147] at the same time. These findings were eventually substantiated by immunofluorescent studies.[147, 157, 189] By means of immunofluorescent techniques, Turkington and Topper[181] succeeded in determining the presence of significant gestational levels of that hormone, as well as finding an associated, unquestionable mammotrophic effect. Independently of its mammotrophic action in gestation, this substance seems to be involved in releasing colostric secretions, and shall be studied in more detail later.

THYROID. Thyroidectomy suppresses mammary development.[55, 56, 141, 145] Conversely, thyroxine therapy promotes breast development.[50, 71, 101, 126] Currently, the prevalent concept, supported by the work of Schmidt and Moger,[156] does not envision thyroxine as a direct morphogenetic factor but rather as one potentiating the effects of steroids on the breast. As a matter of fact, Anderson and Turner[3] showed that the amounts of estrogens and progesterone necessary to induce complete breast development in castrated and hypophysectomized animals were much smaller if either pituitary extract, or even a small quantity of thyroxine, was added to the steroid mixture. On the other hand, Jacobson[101] believed that the effect under consideration was entirely nonspecific, and solely due to the accelerated rate of tissue metabolism produced by thyroactive substances.

RELAXIN. Research by Wada and Turner[184, 185] emphasized the role of relaxin in stimulating mammogenic development in the rat and mouse and in increasing the presence of tissue DNA.

22.2.9. MAMMOGENESIS AT TERM AND DURING THE LACTATIONAL PERIOD

An initial type of secretion, *colostrum*, is already present in the breast by the end of pregnancy. However, during this phase, the DNA content is still rising (Tucker and Reece[180]). Griffith and Turner have shown that allometric mammary growth continues during the early stage of lactation.[71, 72] Equally, Berwordt and colleagues[20] found the same effect and ascribed it to mammotrophic activity—as distinct from galactopoietic activity—by somatotropin and prolactin. This proliferative effect on the breast during the last phase of gestation probably depends on placental lactogen activity rather than on the action of estrogens and progesterone.

The existence of at least five hormones possessing specific mammogenic action may be inferred from the foregoing data, and all of them are capable to some extent of stimulating DNA synthesis and allometric mammary growth per se. These are estrogens, progesterone, placental lactogen, somatotropin and prolactin. None of these alone appears to be able to act with full efficiency unless acting in concert with the others. In a nonspecific way, corticoids and thyroactive substances would also seem to play an important role. For two reasons, however, their actions cannot be conceived as purely mammogenic in nature: (1) It is possible that the action of corticoids may be an indirect one, mediated by steroid stimulation of the estrogenic or progestational type, a distinct possibility if one considers the close metabolic interrelationship of this group of compounds; (2) thyroxine possibly acts as a metabolic activator at the same end-organ level as do the foregoing hormones (Fig. 22–1).

22.3. INDUCTION OF MILK SECRETION (LACTOGENESIS)

In the preceding paragraphs, we intended to illustrate how the breast is prepared for secretion in the course of all processes of development, sexual maturation and pregnancy. Secretion takes place after parturition as a physiologic phenomenon with an abrupt onset. We shall study consecutively: (1) hormones that provoke lactogenesis; (2) dynamics of lactogenesis; and (3) neural influences involved in lactogenesis.

22.3.1. HORMONES THAT CONTROL LACTOGENESIS

In the first place, lactogenesis results from the action of one of the pituitary hormones, *prolactin*, which has already been studied in Chapter 7 (Section 7.6). Until recently, this product of the adenohypophysis had been considered to be the only factor responsible for lactation; it is now known that this is not the case, and that milk secretion is precipitated by the intervention of at least as many hormones as these: (1) prolactin, (2) somatotropin, (3) ACTH, (4) placental lactogen, (5) corticosteroids, (6) thyroactive substances, (7) insulin.

PROLACTIN. As pointed out in Chapter 7, Stricker and Grüter[167] had demonstrated that hypophysectomy suppressed lactation. As a result of having developed the pigeon crop bioassay, Riddle and Bates[143] were later able to isolate the active principle involved from the adenohypophysis of various species.

Among the various actions of prolactin (see Chapter 7), lactogenic activity is now known to be probably the least important of all (Folley[56]), whereas, on account of its more constant and fundamental actions exerted in maintaining the cyclic corpus luteum, prolactin perhaps deserves to be called the third gonadotropin or luteotropin.

For a long time, prolactin was considered to be the only lactotropic principle of the pituitary.[143] In the meantime, however, it has been shown to lack the capacity for producing complete lactation in hypophysectomized animals (Cowie et al.[34]), an effect in turn obtainable with injections of crude pituitary extracts (Cole and Hopkins[32]) or with mixtures of purified prolactin and somatotropin (Cowie and Tindal[35]). Nevertheless, total pituitary extracts, which are known to be devoid of prolactin, even in high dosages fail to provoke lactation.[1, 118] Cowie and associates[37] have shown that, if lactating rabbits are hypophysectomized, lactation is suspended after two to six days and can be restored with ovine or human prolactin but not with bovine prolactin. It is possible that some of the contradictory reports in the past concerning the action of prolactin on lactation in experimental animals are due to similar *differences in specificity*.[18]

Prolactin can be estimated by means of *bioassay*[107, 131] or *radioimmunoassay*[7, 133] procedures, as indicated in Chapter 7. The latter have the advantage of circumventing the above-mentioned problems of specificity. Variations in blood prolactin levels have been studied by Simkin and Goddart,[160] who reported marked elevations, above all during the first days of the lactational period.

In summary: *though admitted to specifically promote lactation, prolactin is not the only pituitary substance with lactogenic activity.*

SOMATOTROPIN. Some of the most valuable data concerning the effects of other pituitary hormones or lactation have been supplied by veterinarians. Pure prolactin preparations have been found to possess scanty lactogenic potency[54] in cows and goats, whereas when admixed with somatotropin or with total pituitary extracts, their value increases considerably. Bingtarningsih and associates[23] found that growth hormone had to be added to prolactin in order to achieve lactation in hypophysectomized rats. Their findings have been confirmed by various authors.[17, 64, 65] In the same way, the association of growth hormone with prolactin was found to be necessary in order to obtain prolonged lactation.[83, 118]

Apart from behaving as a mammogenic, that is, morphogenetic, factor, growth hormone may therefore be also considered as an important prosecretory element of the breast (Fig. 22–2).

ACTH. A number of investigators[35, 64, 65] hold that ACTH is necessary for the maintenance of lactation. Wagner and his associates[186] have noted that, while neither thyrotropin nor luteotropin activity was increased in lactating cows, ACTH levels were markedly elevated. Experiments conducted by Cotes and co-workers (Fig. 22–3), which we shall discuss in due time, raise serious doubts concerning these observations. It is more likely that effects ascribed to ACTH are mediated by the adrenal, since corticoids are known to be, in effect, indispensable for lactogenesis.

PLACENTAL LACTOGEN. In Chapter 19 (Section 19.5.5), we indicated that a new placental hormone, intermediate in action between somatotropin and prolactin, had been isolated recently by means of radioimmunologic techniques. This compound, discovered by Josimovitch and MacLaren,[104] who called it placental lactogen, was produced in vitro[86] by cultures of chorionic tissue, and was found to induce lactation in pregnant rabbits without interrupting pregnancy. Immunologically, it seemed to cross-react with human STH and was therefore believed to be closely related to the latter.[60] Turkington and Topper[181] studied human placental lactogen action on mouse mammary gland maintained in tissue culture and compared its activity with that of bovine prolactin. The prosecretory effects

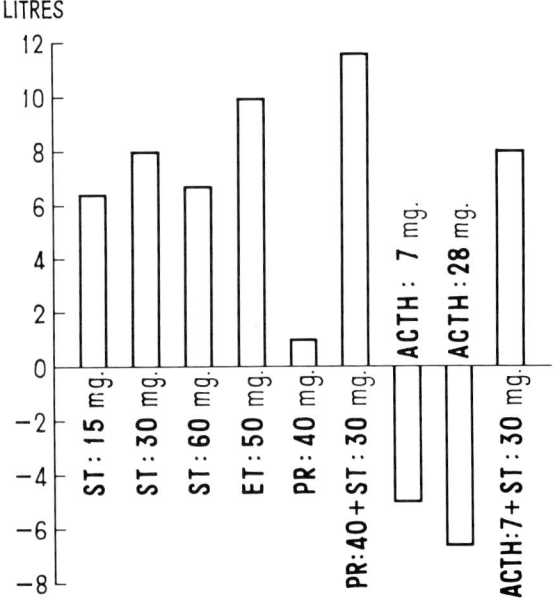

Figure 22–3. Effects of single injections of various pituitary principles on the amount of milk secreted in a 24 hour period by a group of cows. Ordinate shows increased (or decreased) production, as compared with average set arbitrarily as 0 liters. (From Cotes et al.: *Nature,* 164:992, 1949.)

of the two substances were found to be identical. Because the placenta has already been expelled by the time lactation is initiated, the role of placental lactogen is not known. Nonetheless, lactogen is believed to be implicated in the *preparation of the breast for secretion and the production of colostrum.*

CORTICOIDS. Many years ago, Nelson demonstrated that hypophysectomy abolished secretion in lactating rats and hence postulated the existence of a hormone, *corticolactin*. This has not been proved to exist. Nevertheless, the adrenal cortex exerts an unquestionable effect on milk secretion. Cortisone pretreatment of rats during pregnancy results in a significant increase of milk secretion after parturition.[103] Cortisone increases the secretion of colostrum in pregnant rats.[178] According to Meites and his associates,[117] cortisol acetate activity is synergistic with prolactin, potentiating the latter's lactation-inducing effect.[117] In contrast, Hahn and Turner[89] found that aldosterone lacked such action. Testosterone was found by Hamberger and others[91] to enhance lactation in rats, but the effect was abolished by adrenalectomy. Meites considers cortisone, cortisol and hydrocortisone to be necessary for the restitution of full milk-secreting capacity in animals hypophysectomized at a time of full secretory activity.[116] As a final note of interest, the action of hydrocortisone in inducing milk secretion in mammary tissue cultured in vitro has been demonstrated by Gala and Westphal[63] and by Barnawell[12] during the past few years.

By and large, all indications are that glucocorticoids exert important effects on lactation. Because of equally significant effects on maintenance of milk secretion or lactopoiesis, more shall be said about glucocorticoids later.

THYROACTIVE SUBSTANCES. Balmain and associates[11] reported that lactation was initiated in association with increased oxygen consumption by the breast. Potter and his co-workers[136] found that lactation in rats increased the animals' oxygen consumption and that such increase was simply the result of elevated breast tissue metabolism. Similarly, Iino and Greer[99] noted accumulation of radioactive iodine in the tissue of the lactating breast. Thyroid hyperfunction was estimated by Grosvenor and Turner[74] to be an indispensable condition for the development of milk secretion in rats. These same authors observed that, in addition to STH and prolactin, oxytocin and thyroxine injections were necessary to bring about normal secretion in hypophysectomized animals; these observations were later amply confirmed.[12, 20]

Thyroid function therefore seems to be indispensable for adequate function of milk secretion where the thyroid effect may be assumed to result from stimulation of metabolic activity of breast tissue.

INSULIN. Hellman[95] observed islet cell hyperplasia, particularly involving the beta cells, during prolonged lactation in rats. Berwordt and colleagues[20] consider insulin to be a necessary factor in maintaining mammary function. Since STH is known to have contra-insular or anti-insulinic activity, it is not apparent whether the changes occurring in the islets are reactive in nature or are a necessary corollary of mammary activity.

Thus, it is evident that normal function of a major part of the endocrine system is required to maintain lactation. Ablation of either a single or several glands of internal secretion has been found to lead to suppression of lactation to a variable extent. An important exception in this regard is the ovary, which, when suppressed, does just the opposite, that is, stimulates milk secretion.

22.3.2. DYNAMICS OF LACTOGENESIS

Milk secretion, consequently, results from the action on the breast by a specific hormone, prolactin, in indispensable association with the actions of a series of hormones we have already enumerated.

A remarkable feature about the action that precipitates milk secretion is the fact that it should not occur except at a quite particular time in life, remaining completely inhibited for the rest of life. It should therefore be useful to analyze the *dynamics of lactogenesis.*

The issues to be examined are: (1) preparation for lactation; (2) factors inhibiting lactation; (2) neural factors involved in initiating lactation; (4) pharmacology of prolactin release; (5) prolactin in pituitary tissue and in blood.

PREPARATION FOR LACTATION. There is evidence that throughout pregnancy lactation is being prepared for. First, there is the fact that the mammary gland is brought to its utmost development by the actions of estrogens, progesterone and placental lactogen, and probably also growth hormone; and second, there is the fact that throughout gestation, prolactin release is inhibited and prolactin accumulates gradually in the adenohypophysis (Grosvenor and Turner[79]). Currie and Dekansky,[41] Meites,[116] and, later, Hymer and colleagues,[98] as well as Nicoll and Meites,[132] Ratner and associates[139] and Chen and Meites,[29] demonstrated that the prolactin content of rat pituitary increased if the animal was treated with mixtures of ovarian hormones in variable amounts. Many years previously, on the contrary, Collip and Selye had shown that ovariectomy in pregnant, or at least pseudogravid, rats precipitated lactation, which was recently confirmed by Liu and Davis.[113]

Consequently, there seems to be no doubt that during pregnancy estrogens and placental progesterone, on the one hand, stimulate and promote gravidic mammogenesis to the utmost while also, on the other, inhibiting prolactin release and probably also producing a local inhibitory effect on the breast. In this way, the tensional load is being increasingly weighted in favor of milk secretion but stopping short of actual secretion.

FACTORS INHIBITING LACTATION. Secretion of all pituitary hormones, with the exception of prolactin, ceases in animal pituitary tissue transplanted beneath the renal capsule[9, 87] (see also Chapter 8). The same is true about pituitary tissue grown in culture, which was found to elaborate only prolactin.[108] Haun and Sawyer,[94] much to their surprise, found that destruction of the medial tuberal region of rabbits stimulated, rather than interrupted, lactation. The same phenomenon was later observed by Averill and Purves[10] in female rats. Electric stimulation of the hypothalamus failed to produce lactation (Kuroshima et al.[109]). It has similarly been determined that such substances as reserpine and perphenazine, which anesthetize the median eminence, stimulate lactation.[119, 124] Thus, we seem to be dealing with the opposite effect to that produced by the remaining releasing factors which, quite unlike the effect observed in this case,[9, 87] apparently are associated with a positive effect (Figs. 22–4 and 22–10).

In the course of the past few years, a *factor inhibiting prolactin release* (PIF, or prolactin inhibiting factor) was isolated from the median eminence. We owe the isolation and purification of this factor to the work of Arimura and colleagues,[8] Gala and Reece,[62] Kragt and Meites[108] and Schally and associates.[155] Grosvenor and co-workers[78] recently found that secretion of PIF by the rat hypothalamus was inhibited through the suckling reflex. The factor appears to occur in all mammals, but apparently it does not occur in birds, since a prolactin *releasing* factor (Lehrman[112]), presumably exerting the reverse effect of the mammalian factor, has been isolated from pigeons.

As a result, blood prolactin levels can be said to rise during the period of lactation because of disappearance of a prolactin inhibiting factor (PIF) which, under the effect of sex hormone stimulation, is produced by the hypothalamus throughout pregnancy. The end-organ role played by

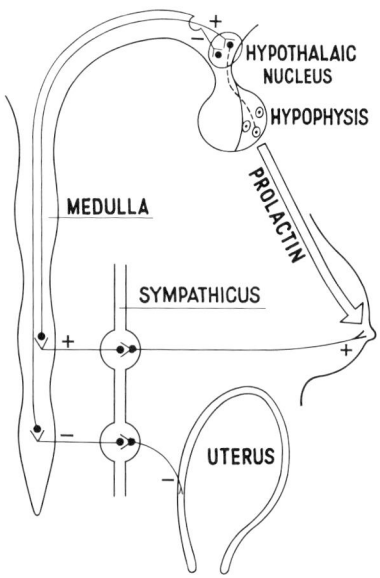

Figure 22–4. Diagrammatic representation of neural control of lactation. (From Botella-Llusiá: *Obstetric Endocrinology.* Springfield, Ill., Charles C Thomas, 1961.)

the sex nucleus of the hypothalamus in response to estrogen and progestogen activity is well known, and has been discussed in Chapter 8.

NEURAL FACTORS INVOLVED IN INITIATING LACTATION. As a result of investigations by Jacobson[101] and Desclin,[46] transection of the pituitary stalk has been known to cause suppression of lactation. Classically, it was held that, by severing the stalk, passage of chemical mediators eliciting prolactin release was interrupted. (Denamur and Martinet[44]). That this is not the case has been indicated in the preceding paragraph. It would therefore have to be assumed that suppression of lactation occurs either because the release of some other hormones that intervene in lactogenesis, such as somatotropin or ACTH, is inhibited by transection of the pituitary stalk, or else because oxytocin release is blocked in the process, oxytocin being necessary for the maintenance of lactation. In the opinion of Galle and his associates[66] the effects of transecting the pituitary stalk result from the second type of mechanism.

On the other hand, destruction of the hypothalamic median eminence produces a stimulatory effect on lactation (Haun and Sawyer,[94] Averill and Purves[10]). Galle's opinion has been substantiated by the finding that simple injection of oxytocin immediately restores lactation suppressed as a result of pituitary stalk severance.[59, 66] In contrast, Grosvenor[75] has shown that if the spinal cord instead of the pituitary stalk is transected in lactating rats, lactation is similarly suppressed—but it requires not just oxytocin but also prolactin for it to be restored.

Identical results were found with female rabbits by sectioning the cervical spine (Mena and Beyer[122]) and with female cats by injuring the afferent pathways to the median eminence (Beyer et al.[21]). A similar effect can be produced by means of dorsal ramisection (Beyer and Mena[22]). Early investigations had already demonstrated that suckling maintained lactation but had no effect on the denervated breast. Similarly, Meites and co-workers[119, 120] have been able to maintain lactation by means of stimulating the nipple and the uterine cervix electrically in rats separated from their litter.

All the established phenomena of this nature permit almost complete reconstruction of the neurohormonal reflex arc that is involved in precipitating milk secretion all the way from the initial impulse created at the nipple by a suckling. This, however, seems to suggest the negative possibility that the hypothalamic center may secrete some inhibitor, rather than stimulator, of prolactin release, that some other center may be involved in elaborating a factor directly releasing prolactin, or, alternatively, that the impulse created by suckling, which travels along the rami communicantes to the dorsal cord and from there to the hypothalamus, may act as a PIF inhibitor at the hypothalamic level. The PIF content of hypothalamic nuclei was measured in recent years by various investigators. Sar and Meites[154] found that the hypothalamic PIF content decreased following treatment with progesterone, testosterone and cortisol, which might explain the reason for the inhibitory effect of some of these steroids. A similar effect, causing a fall in prolactin release, is apparently produced by implantation of purified prolactin in the median eminence of lactating rats.[30, 187]

However, it must be pointed out that some authors assume oxytocin to act as a releasing factor for prolactin, which, if valid, would mean that oxytocin acts as a PIF antagonist at the adenohypophysial level (Huntingford[97]). Beyer and Mena[22] noticed an increase in oxytocin content of the hypothalamic lateral nuclei as a result of stimulating the nipple. They believe that, since transection of the stalk suspends lactation in animals, the substance reaching the pituitary and provoking release of prolactin must be oxytocin. Such a rationale is supported by the fact, demonstrated by Cowie and associates, that adenohypophysial cells in goats continue to secrete prolactin after the pituitary stalk is cut but can be depleted by a dose of 5 IU of oxytocin. In commenting on these findings, however, Ota and his co-workers[134] hold that oxytocin does not act as a releasing factor, although, if administered in conjunction with growth hormone, it is capable of maintaining already initiated lactation for a certain period of time.

In all likelihood, there are considerable differences in this respect from one species to another, and although oxytocin is generally thought not to be the specific releasing factor for prolactin, and although the mammalian median eminence is not believed to produce any chemical prolactin releasing agent, some role for oxytocin cannot be altogether ruled out in certain animal species.[80, 106, 120, 121, 146]

Illumination suppresses PIF production and increases prolactin secretion in female ducks,[67] a further point in evidence concerning the effect of environmental lighting on the median eminence (see Chapter 8).

PHARMACOLOGY OF PROLACTIN RELEASE. Lactation is affected by all substances that act on the hypothalamic nuclei. In 1958, Desclin[46] discovered that reserpine produced a stimulatory effect on prolactin secretion. The same phenomenon has later been reported by Lederer and De Meyer,[110, 111] Tindal,[172] Gala and Reece,[61] and Himwick.[96] Interestingly, though it is known to anesthetize the hypothalamic sex center and to provoke anestrus in rats, reserpine has been found to stimulate lactation, which may be construed as indirect evidence for the existence and inhibitory nature of PIF. In contrast, chlorpromazine as well as anesthesia[73] in general produces inhibition of lactation. Also tested in this regard were the actions of serotonin, found to stimulate lactation, and those of acetylcholine and epinephrine (Meites et al.[121]). Finally, concerning the pharmacologic action of oxytocin, we again stress the contradictory nature of available data.

PROLACTIN CONCENTRATION IN PITUITARY TISSUE AND IN THE BLOOD. Grosvenor and Turner,[81, 82] Simkin and Goddart,[160] and Steinetz[166] all measured prolactin concentrations in the blood. Prolactinemia rises during suckling and disappears under anesthesia. Grosvenor and Turner[79] have determined prolactin concentrations in rat pituitary, recording an increase during the period of lactation. Castration produces an increase in the prolactin content of the human pituitary (Currie and Dekansky[41]), whereas in rabbits transection of the pituitary stalk, as already indicated, results in increased prolactin content of the anterior lobe.[106]

22.4. MAINTENANCE OF LACTATION (LACTOPOIESIS)

Advances in veterinary and human clinical experience have established the fact that factors initiating lactation are different from those maintaining lactation. In animals producing milk for commercial sale, the lactopoietic factors are really the ones that count from the standpoint of output. In the human species, too, it is a common clinical observation that those women who begin postpartum lactation with a dramatic performance may soon lose their capacity to nurse, whereas, conversely, those starting sluggishly may later turn out to be excellent nursing mothers.

This is what draws the line between the concept of *lactopoiesis* and that of *lactogenesis*. The following aspects of lactopoiesis shall be studied: (1) hormonal factors, (2) neural factors, (3) metabolic and nutritional factors, and (4) psychogenic factors.

22.4.1. ENDOCRINE FACTORS OF LACTOPOIESIS

Unlike in lactogenesis, in which prolactin is the *specific* hormone, aside from such other essential substances as growth hormone, in lactopoiesis prolactin plays a secondary role. *Somatotropin* and *oxytocin* seem to be the two main catalysts involved in maintenance of secretion. We shall study consecutively prolactin, somatotropin and oxytocin.

PROLACTIN. Folley and Knaggs[55, 56, 57] were first to succeed in maintaining lactation in hypophysectomized animals by merely injecting growth hormone, or growth hormone with oxytocin, and by applying the suckling stimulus. The experiments conducted by Cotes on dairy cows (see Fig. 22–3) are revealing inasmuch as they prove that lactation can be maintained with growth hormone alone. Meites and Nicoll[118] observed an analogous phenomenon in the rat and underscored the role of cortisone.

It has been possible to maintain lactation in goats[64] and rats[65] without using prolactin. Similarly, Grosvenor and Turner[83, 84] have studied the pituitary prolactin content in lactating animals, finding the latter to be quite elevated at the onset of lactation but to decrease gradually, until it disappears completely, in prolonged lactation. The same authors[81] have studied blood prolactin concentrations in dairy animals, failing to find any correlation between daily milk production and prolactinemia.

SOMATOTROPIN. As far as maintenance of secretion is concerned, somatotropin seems to play a more significant role. The early initial investigations by Stricker and Grüter,[167] as well as those by Riddle and Bates,[143] had indicated that lactation was suspended following hypophysectomy not only in animals that had just begun lactating but also in those which had been lactating for a long period of time. More recent investigations[118, 119, 158] revealed that injections of growth hormone and oxytocin were enough to maintain milk secretion in lactating animals subjected to hypophysectomy. According to these studies, prolactin was not found to be indispensable in the presence of somatotropin activity. Cotes (see Fig. 22-3), and subsequently Cowie and Tindal,[35] demonstrated that cows injected with somatotropin consistently yielded a larger number of liters of milk per day.

The effect of somatotropin on lactation is to a great extent *species* dependent. In the cow, growth hormone exerts prolactinic activity,[51, 135] which in part, explains the previously mentioned experiments. Human somatotropin, in contrast, does not appear to possess any cross-activity. Spellacy and associates[164] found no increase in plasma STH levels in lactating women. Rimoin and his co-workers[144] do not believe human growth hormone to possess any lactogenic activity, nor to be indispensable for maintenance of lactation.

ACTH. According to Cowie and colleagues,[33, 34] unless hypophysioprival animals (rats) are injected with ACTH, lactation cannot be restored to normalcy in full measure. These findings have been confirmed by Folley[56] and by Shaw and his associates.[158] It is not known whether a direct type of action, or one mediated by the adrenal cortex, is involved.

CORTICOIDS. Cortisone, hydrocortisone and cortisol all enhance milk secretion in lactating animals (Ahren and Jacobson,[1] Johnson and Meites[103]). Aldosterone lacks any similar action.[35] The action by glucocorticoids, which may possibly also explain ACTH activity, seems to be linked to a *nonspecific* type of action: that involving biosynthesis of milk carbohydrates.

INSULIN. Normal regulation of carbohydrate metabolism appears to be directly dependent on the amount of milk produced. This is the unquestionable conclusion that must be drawn from the findings of Balmain and his co-workers,[11] later confirmed by Ahren[2] and Nicoll and Meites,[132] in which insulin was shown to be necessary for *lipogenesis* in in vitro incubated slices of breast tissue.

THYROXINE. Grosvenor and Turner[74] reported that L-thyroxine increased milk production in cows. Whether or not such action by thyroxine is specific is not known.

OXYTOCIN. As will be indicated in the next section, oxytocin is indispensable for mammary depletion. In its absence, milk outflow bogs down and the resulting stasis apparently causes a compensatory decrease in milk production. In one way or another, oxytocin activity is essential for maintenance of lactation. In hypophysectomized animals, lactation can be carried on only if oxytocin is injected in addition to STH (Rothchild and Quilligan[146]).

METABOLIC AND NUTRITIONAL FACTORS. From the preceding data, the importance of *regulating of the mammary function* is evident. The majority of hormonal effects with a bearing on lactopoiesis, which we have just outlined, are clearly regulatory in nature, involving either carbohydrate biosynthesis (STH, ACTH, corticoids) or lipogenesis (insulin, thyroxine). In animals, adequate nutrition (Grosvenor[76]), appetite and commensurate gain in weight (Denamur[45]), coupled with adequate water and mineral balances (Cross,[39] Anderson and Gale[4]), seem all to have a decisive influence on the amount of milk secreted.

In woman, these actions are of utmost

TABLE 22-1. Effect of Insulin on Lipogenesis in Slices of Mammary Gland, Incubated In Vitro with Carboxy-^{13}C-Me-^{3}H Acetate (0.02 M) Plus ^{14}C Glucose (0.3%, w/v)*

INSULIN	RADIOISOTOPE CONTENT OF FATTY ACIDS FORMED AFTER 3 HOURS INCUBATION, QUANTA OF ENERGY PER MINUTE CORRESPONDING TO EACH MILLIGRAM OF SUBSTANCE		
	Carbon-14 (Derived from Glucose)	Carbon-13 (Derived from Carboxyl)	Hydrogen-3 (Derived from Methyl)
No addition	381	0.054	95
Addition	805	0.140	202

*From Balmain et al.: *Biochem. J.*, 56:234, 1954.

importance. As reported in a recent bulletin of the WHO (World Health Organization, Report No. 365, 1965), starvation seriously affects the lactating population in underdeveloped countries, causing marked impairment of lactational function.

22.4.2. NEURAL FACTORS INVOLVED IN LACTOPOIESIS

The already mentioned endocrine and nutritional factors are necessary in order to maintain a sufficient rate and quality of secretion. They are, in effect, the *biochemical factors involved in milk synthesis.* However, the most essential factor contributing to maintenance of lactation is the *suckling stimulus.* Since ancient times, it has been a well known fact that when a child stops breast feeding, milk secretion disappears rapidly and the breast undergoes involution. Harris[92, 93] has demonstrated that although the lactiferous ducts are cut secretion is not interrupted provided the breast continues to be suckled. Similarly, suckling of the nipples on one side only is enough to prevent milk secretion from disappearing from the nipples that are not stimulated. Milk secretion can be triggered by stimulating either the nipple[92] or the uterine cervix[120] electrically. The reflex that maintains secretion is the same that initiates secretion, as pointed out earlier (Fig. 22–4).

The reflex under consideration is associated with an inhibitory type of action on the center of the median eminence, since the factor inhibiting lactation (PIF) is secreted by this zone, as we have already said. In Chapter 8, we also mentioned the fact that oxytocin, to which some degree of prolactin activity has been attributed, has nothing to do with this factor and is secreted not by the median eminence but by the supraoptic and paraventricular nuclei. Nevertheless, the action of oxytocin is essential for maintenance of lactation in hypophysioprival animals receiving growth hormone, while the role played in lactopoiesis by stimulation of the nipple or the uterine cervix, or both, must also be construed as giving support to the role of oxytocin.[140, 150]

This poorly understood phenomenon may be explained in two ways. On the one hand, as proposed by, among others, Reiher[140] and Sammelwits and his associates,[150] oxytocin may be able to elicit release of prolactin in some way, or, on the other hand, it may do so when acting in concert with growth hormone. However, the most widely accepted idea is that milk *stasis* in lactiferous ducts leads to *local impairment* of breast secretion. Under these circumstances, it would be the function of oxytocin to provoke expulsion or *ejection of milk.* Tindal and Yokohama[173] reported acinar milk stasis to be associated with disappearance of prolactin secretion.

22.5. MILK EJECTION

Richardson[142] found that *myoepithelial cells* were present in the acinar wall in the goat (see Figure 22–8), while Cross and his associates[40] similarly identified them in the acini of the sow. The workers associated with Caldeyro-Barcia (Sala and Althabe,[148, 149] Sica-Blanco et al.[159]) have successfully catheterized the human breast and measured intracanalicular pressure by means of a system of micromanometers (Fig. 22–5). Upon injection of oxytocin, the pressure was found to rise (Figs. 22–6 and 22–7), and contralateral suckling and cervical dilatation produced the same effect. These findings have been corroborated at our clinic by Dominguez and Pereira,[47] who were able to see how the uterus contracts coincidently with suckling (Fig. 22–8). Folley and Knaggs[57] found that levels of circulating oxytocin consistently rose in cows during milking, and that a similar elevation could be obtained by means of electric stimulation of the nipple or the uterine cervix.[58] Identical phenomena were later brought to light in laboratory rodents,[16, 174, 183] as well as in the human species.[31]

Moore and Zarrow[127] observed isometric contractions in isolated strips of goat mammary gland, as well as in human tissue; nasal sprays using oxytocin have already become a routine method for enhancing milk flow (Wenner,[188] Newborn and Egli[128]). In addition, considering the fact that suckling in rats has been found to cause discharge of Gomori-positive neurosecretory material from the supraoptic and paraventricular nuclei,[38, 93, 137] all indications are that suckling elicits discharge of oxytocin which, by acting on the myoepithelial cells

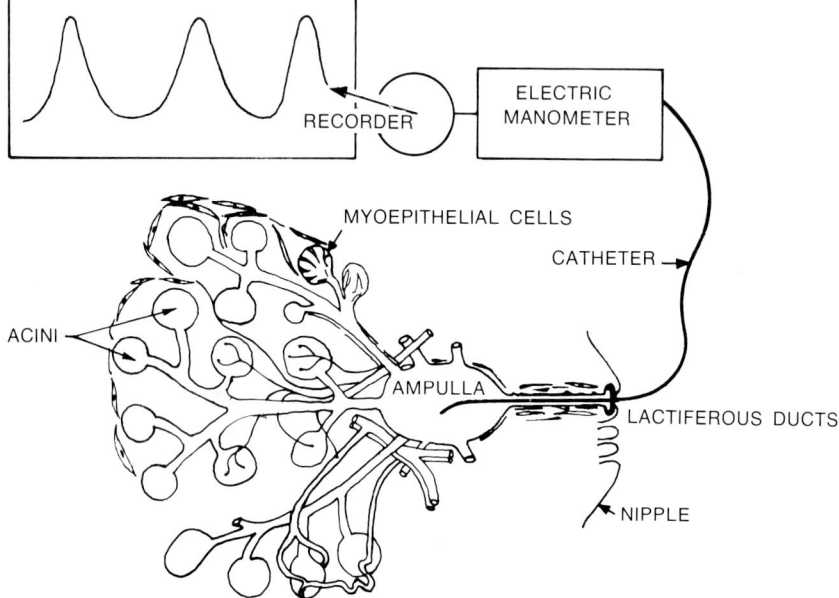

Figure 22-5. Method for recording intramammary pressure in woman, after Sica-Blanco and Sala. (Diagram courtesy of Dr. N. L. Sala. Thesis, University of Buenos Aires, 1961.)

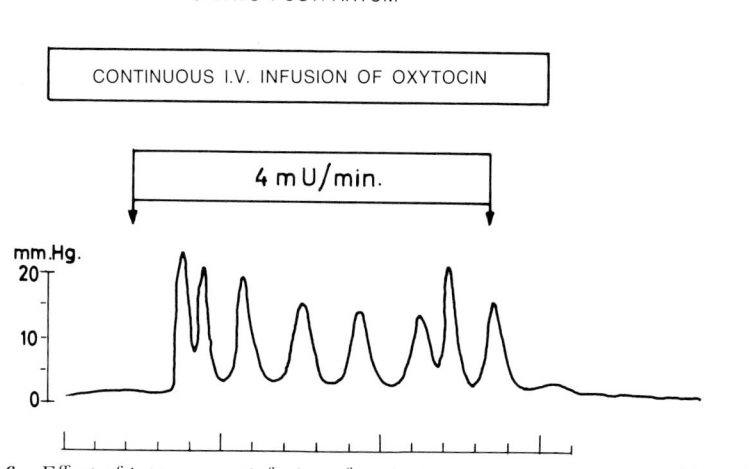

Figure 22-6. Effect of intravenous infusion of oxytocin on mammary pressure. (From Sala.[148])

Endocrine Physiology of the Breast

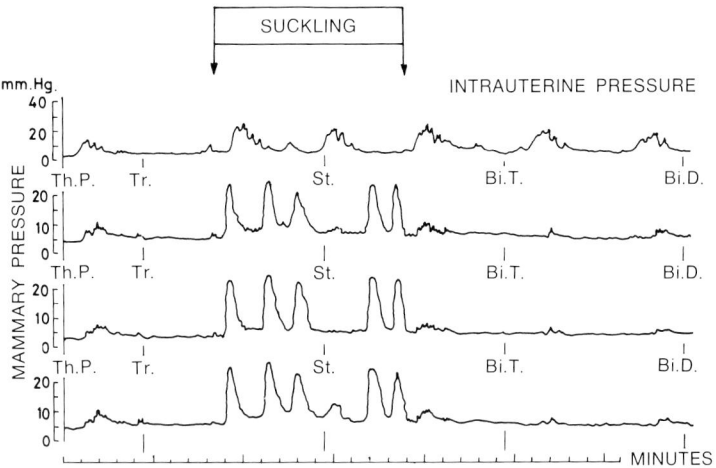

Figure 22-7. Effect of suckling on uterine contractions in puerpera. (From Sala.[148])

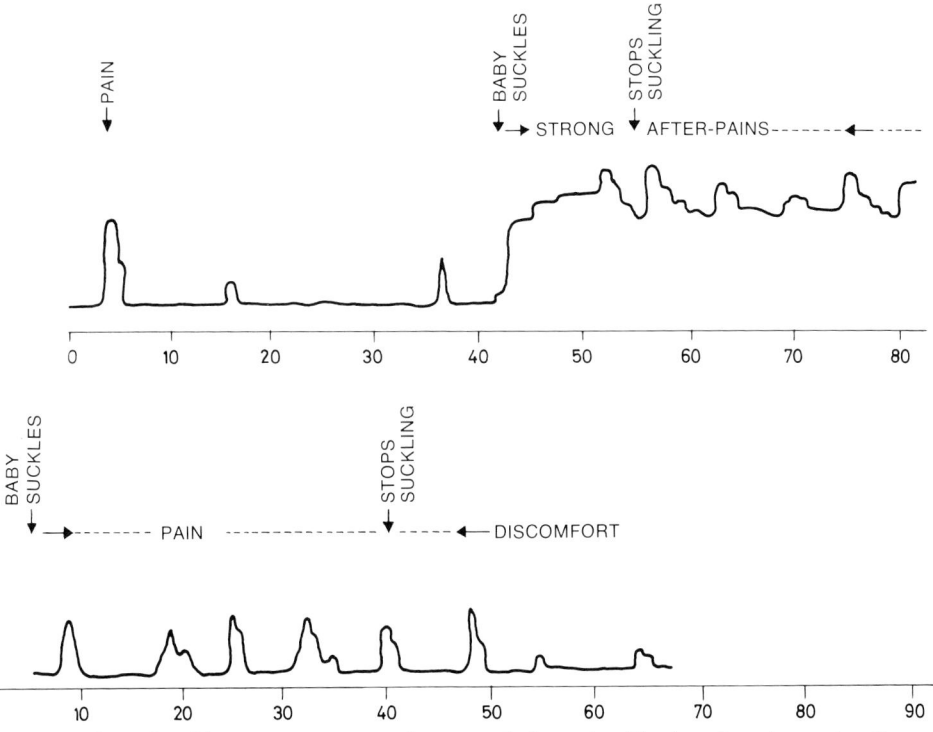

Figure 22-8. Effect of suckling on appearance of puerperal after-pains. Tracing of uterine contractions obtained by means of external tocography. Time in minutes. *A*, Severe puerperal after-pains. *B*, Contractions of less intensity. (From Domínguez and Pereira: *Acta Gin.*, 10:405, 1959.)

of the breast, produces contraction of the latter and, consequently, *milk ejection.*

Tindal and Yokohama[173] were able to abolish this neuroendocrine reflex by means of anesthesia, while Chan[28] obtained similar results with epinephrine. Electric stimulation of the supraoptic nucleus provokes milk ejection,[45, 47] whereas sectioning of the pituitary stalk inhibits the effects of both suckling[130] and electrical stimulation of the supraoptic nucleus.[46] Tindal and his associates[174] were later able to trace the pathways involved in the reflex from mammary nerve endings to the spinal ganglia and the medulla, and from there, over the lateral tegmentum between the geniculate bodies, to the paraventricular nucleus.

As pointed out previously, suckling not only affects oxytocin secretion but also acts on the median eminence, inhibiting PIF, as a result of which prolactin release is enhanced. However, this is not the only way the reflex of the suckling stimulus acts on the nucleus of the median eminence. Taleisnik and Tomatis[168] observed that the suckling reflex resulted in enhanced release of melanogenic hormone in rats, while Minaguchi and Meites,[123] also working with rats, noted decreased LHRF activity as a result of the same kind of nipple stimulation.

All the above findings bring out the fact that there is a reflex for milk ejection that is independent of, but travels parallel with, the reflex of prolactin secretion. It originates in the nipple (and the uterine cervix) and ascends along the nervous pathways to the supraoptic and paraventricular nuclei, where it elicits a discharge of oxytocin, causing milk ejection (Fig. 22-10).

Prolactin secretion is intimately related to this neuroendocrine reflex mechanism. Two parallel reflexes are involved. Moreover, Newton[130] has demonstrated that, concomitantly with an increase in oxytocin, an increase in prolactin activity also takes place.

The psychosomatic aspects of lactation have been well recognized in the human species but exist also in animals. Grosvenor and Mena[77] recently demonstrated that certain offensive odors, noises or flashing lights interrupted milk secretion in rats, just as sudden frightening, aggravating or grievous experiences can "cut short" milk secretion in women. A psychodynamic study of lactation in woman has been published by Newton and Newton,[129] while Grosvenor demonstrated that the mere fact of hearing the litter cry, even without seeing the babies, resulted in increased milk secretion in rats. In addition, it was shown that crowded conditions abolished lactation in mice.

All the foregoing facts are suggestive of close connections between the hypothalamic centers and psychic function, relationships which are tentatively summarized in Figure 22-10.

22.6. INFLUENCE OF LACTATION ON THE ENDOCRINE SYSTEM AND ON THE REPRODUCTIVE CYCLE

The impact of lactation on the endocrine glands, particularly the ovary, is quite considerable. In this respect, we shall examine consecutively the pituitary, the thyroid and the ovary.

22.6.1. PITUITARY AND LACTATION

During lactation, the pituitary undergoes histologically characteristic changes, reflected by increased numbers of acidophilic cells (Hymer et al.[98]) and loss of pregnancy

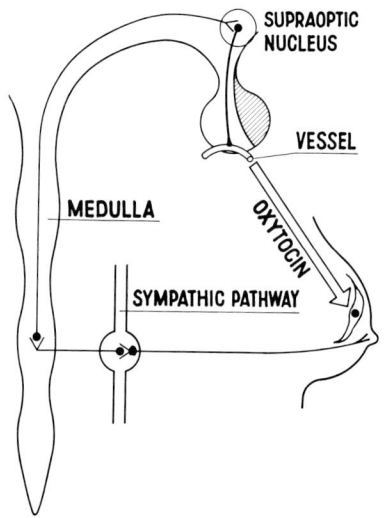

Figure 22-9. Diagram of neuroendocrine reflex of oxytocin release by suckling effect. (From Botella-Llusiá: *Obstetrical Endocrinology.* Springfield, Ill., Charles C Thomas, 1961.)

Endocrine Physiology of the Breast

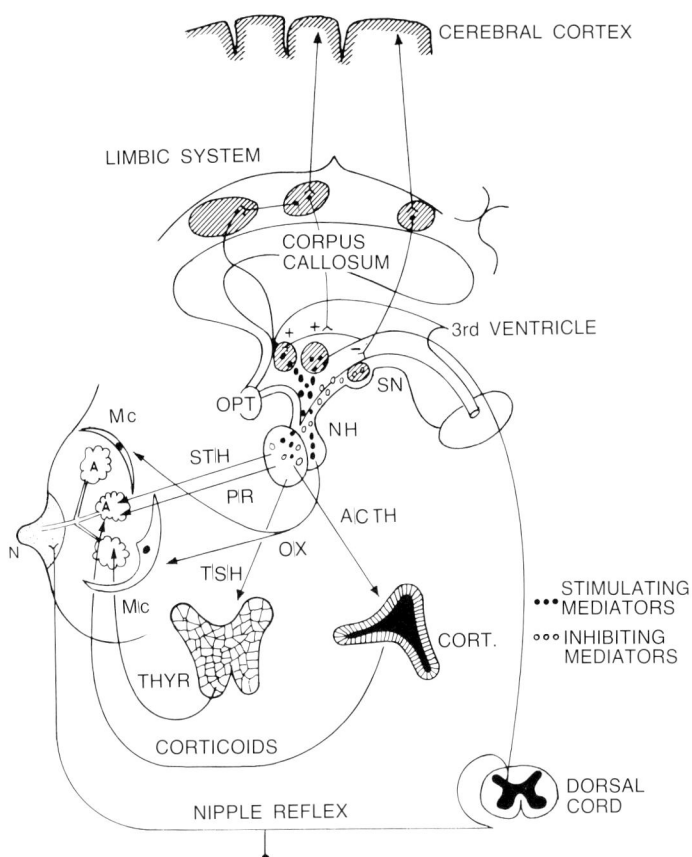

Figure 22–10. Endocrine regulation of milk secretion and milk ejection. Diagram also shows neural connections involved. ADH, Adenohypophysis; NH, neurohypophysis; SO, supraoptic nucleus; PV, paraventricular nucleus; OPT, optic chiasm; SN, sex nucleus of median eminence of tuber cinereum; STH, growth hormone; PR, prolactin; OX, oxytocin; TSH, thyrotropin; ACTH, adrenocorticotropin; A, mammary acini; N, nipple; Mc, myoepithelial cells. (From Botella-Llusiá and Clavero-Nuñez: *Fisiologia Femenina*, 9th ed. Barcelona, Editorial Científico Medica, 1971.)

cells (Cameron et al.[26]). At the same time, there is commensurate loss of gonadotropin releasing power (Greenwald,[70] Johnsen and Fuchs[102]). The latter phenomenon is particularly important in the Chiari-Frommell syndrome (see Chapter 45), in which there is amenorrhea, with paralysis of the sexual cycle and associated persistent galactorrhea.

22.6.2. THYROID AND LACTATION

Thyroid function in relation to lactation has already been discussed. Grosvenor and Turner,[80] who studied thyroid function in lactating rats, found evidence of thyroid hyperfunction.

22.6.3. OVARIAN CHANGES DURING LACTATION

The repercussions of lactation on ovarian function vary considerably from one animal species to another. In mice, there is persistence of large corpora lutea (Greenwald[69]), with a tendency toward formation of deciduomata. Such giant corpora lutea secrete excessive amounts of both estrogens and progesterone.[68] In rats, there is less tendency to deciduomata formation but persistence of corpora lutea and lack of ovulation[85, 97] are the norm. In bitches, on the other hand, corpora lutea persist but lack the capacity for progesterone synthesis (Telegdy et al.[170]). Corpora lutea are not formed either in simians or in women, although ovulation is interrupted and there is a decrease in gonadotropin secretion, particularly that of LH.

The difference observed between laboratory rodents and primates consists fundamentally in that the gravidic corpus luteum of the latter does not keep functioning until the end of gestation. Under such conditions, a discharge of prolactin cannot act on any preexisting corpus luteum, as is the case in rats and mice, in which the corpus luteum is kept in a functional state throughout gestation. Prolactin is capable of maintaining a corpus luteum already formed, but it cannot induce formation of a new one.

Much discussion has been devoted to the question of whether or not ovulation occurs during the lactational period in man. As a matter of fact, anovulatory cycles and even amenorrhea occur very frequently but depend on the degree of lactational function in each individual case. Suspension of the human ovarian cycle seems to depend, in this case, on paralysis of the hypothalamic sex centers.[14, 24] Paralyzation of this type, identical in nature to that observed in the Chiari-Frommell syndrome, may be conceived as one more example of the antagonistic activity of the sex center on lactation — and of lactation on the sex center — repeatedly mentioned before.

However, in many women lactation and ovulation can occur simultaneously, depending on the intensity of the neurohormonal phenomena of lactation which, being of lesser degree in these cases, tends to be associated with precarious lactation. What is unquestionable about such ovaries is that prolactin is unable to cause any effect comparable to that observed in rodents. As a result, everything hinges on how long the gravidic corpus luteum stays functional.

REFERENCES

1. Ahren, K., and Jacobson, D.: *Ann. d'Endocr.*, 17:547, 1966.
2. Ahren, K.: *Acta Endocr.*, 30:593, 1959.
3. Anderson, R. R., and Turner, C. W.: *Proc. Soc. Exper. Biol. Med.*, 113:308, 1963.
4. Anderson, B., and Gale, C. C.: *Proceed. II Int. Congr. Endocr.*, London, 1964. Excerpta Medica Congress Series, 1965.
5. Anderson, R. R., and Turner, C. W.: *Proc. Soc. Exper. Biol. Med.*, 113:333, 1963.
6. Apostolakis, M., Tehile, L., and Berle, P.: *Endokrinologie*, 54:145, 1969.
7. Arai, Y., and Lee, L. H.: *Endocrinology*, 81:1041, 1967.
8. Arimura, A., Saito, T., Müller, C. Y., Bowers, E. E., Savano, S., and Schally, A. V.: *Endocrinology*, 80:972, 1967.
9. Averill, R. L. W.: *Brit. Med. Bull.*, 22:261, 1966.
10. Averill, R. L. W., and Purves, H. D.: *J. Endocr.*, 26:463, 1963.
11. Balmain, J. H., Folley, S. J., and Glascock, R. F.: *Biochem. J.*, 56:342, 1954.
12. Barnawell, E. B.: *Endocrinology*, 80:1083, 1967.
13. Ben David, M., Dikstein, S., and Sulman, F. G.: *Proc. Soc. Exper. Biol. Med.*, 121:873, 1966.
14. Benson, G. K., Cowie, A. T., Cox, C. P., Folley, S. J., and Hosking, Z. D.: *J. Endocr.*, 31:157, 1965.
15. Bengtsson, B., and Norgren, A.: *Acta Endocr.*, 36:141, 1961.
16. Berde, B., and Cerletti, A.: *Acta Endocr.*, 34:543, 1960.
17. Berman, R., Bern, A. H., Nicoll, C. S., and Strohman, R. C.: *J. Exper. Zool.*, 156:353, 1964.
18. Bern, H. A., and Nicoll, C. S.: *Rec. Progr. Horm. Res.*, 24:681, 1968.
19. Berwordt, R. von, and Turner, C. W.: *Proc. Soc. Exper. Biol. Med.*, 103:356, 1960.
20. Berwordt, R. von, Moon, R. C., and Turner, C. W.: *Proc. Soc. Exper. Biol. Med.*, 104:530, 1960.
21. Beyer, C., Mena, F., Pacheco, P., and Alcaraz, M.: *Amer. J. Physiol.*, 202:465, 1962.
22. Beyer, C., and Mena, F.: *Amer. J. Physiol.*, 208:585, 1965.
23. Bingtarningsih, B., Lyons, W. R., Johnson, R. E., and Li, C. H.: *Endocrinology*, 61:540, 1958.
24. Botella-Llusiá, J.: *Obstetrical Endocrinology*. Springfield, Ill., Charles C Thomas, 1961.
25. Brookreson, A. D., and Turner, C. W.: *Proc. Soc. Exper. Biol. Med.*, 102:744, 1959.
26. Cameron, E., Foster, C. L., and Allanson, M.: *J. Reprod. Fertil.*, 12:199, 1966.
27. Cerruti, R. A., and Lyons, W. R.: *Endocrinology*, 67:884, 1960.
28. Chan, W. Y.: *J. Pharmacol. Exper. Therap.*, 147:48, 1965.
29. Chen, C. L., and Meites, J.: *Endocrinology*, 86:503, 1970.
30. Clemens, J. A., Sar, M., and Meites, J.: *Endocrinology*, 84:868, 1969.
31. Coch, J. A., Fielitz, C., Crovetto, J., Cabot, H. M., Coda, H., and Fraga, A.: *J. Clin. Endocr.*, 40:137, 1968.
32. Cole, R. D., and Hopkins, T. R.: *Endocrinology*, 71:395, 1962.
33. Cowie, A. T., Daniel, P. M., Knaggs, G. S., Pritchard, M. M. L., and Tindal, J. S.: *J. Endocr.*, 28:253, 1964.
34. Cowie, A. T., Knaggs, G. S., and Tindal, J. S.: *J. Endocr.*, 28:267, 1964.
35. Cowie, A. T., and Tindal, J. S.: *J. Endocr.*, 22:403, 1961.
36. Cowie, A. T., Tindal, J. S., and Yokohama, A.: *J. Endocr.*, 34:185, 1965.
37. Cowie, A. T., Hartman, P. E., and Turvey, A.: *J. Endocr.*, 43:651, 1969.
38. Cross, B. A.: *Brit. Med. Bull.*, 11:151, 1955.
39. Cross, B. A.: *Symp. Soc. Exper. Biol.*, 18:157, 1964.
40. Cross, B. A., Goodwin, R. F., and Silver, I. A.: *J. Endocr.*, 17:63, 1958.
41. Currie, A. R., and Dekansky, J. B.: *Acta Endocr.*, 36:185, 1961.
42. Damm, H. C., and Turner, C. W.: *Proc. Soc. Exper. Biol. Med.*, 98:192, 1958.
43. Damm, H. C., and Turner, C. W.: *Proc. Soc. Exper. Biol. Med.*, 99:471, 1958.
44. Denamur, R., and Martinet, J.: *Ann. d'Endocr.*, 22:755, 1961.
45. Denamur, R.: *Dairy Sci. Abstr.*, 27:193, 1965.
46. Desclin, J.: *Compt. Rend. Soc. Biol.*, 151:1774, 1958.
47. Domínguez, A., and Pereira, A.: *Acta Gin.*, 10:405, 1959.
48. Donovan, B. T., and Jacobsohn, D.: *Acta Endocr.*, 33:197, 1960.
49. Donovan, B. T., and Jacobsohn, D.: *Acta Endocr.*, 34:214, 1960.
50. Etienne, M.: *Ann. d'Endocr.*, 21:331, 1960.

51. Flaskamp, D., et al.: *Arch. Gynäk.*, 205:267, 1968.
52. Flux, D. S.: *J. Endocr.*, 11:233, 1954.
53. Flux, D. S.: *J. Endocr.*, 12:57, 1955.
54. Flux, D. S.: *J. Endocr.*, 17:300, 1958.
55. Folley, S. J.: *Brit. Med. Bull.*, 5:139, 1948.
56. Folley, S. J.: *Brit. Med. Bull.*, 11:147, 1955.
57. Folley, S. J., and Knaggs, G. S.: *J. Endocr.*, 34:197, 1965.
58. Folley, S. J., and Knaggs, G. S.: In *Advances in Oxytocin Research*, ed. J. H. B. Pinkerton. Oxford, The Pergamon Press, 1965.
59. Frascini, F., Martini, L., Motta, M., and Zanobini, A.: *Ann. d'Endocr.*, 22:782, 1961.
60. Friesen, H. G.: *Endocrinology*, 79:212, 1966.
61. Gala, R. R., and Reece, R. P.: *Endocrinology*, 72:649, 1963.
62. Gala, R. R., and Reece, R. P.: *Proc. Soc. Exper. Biol. Med.*, 117:833, 1964.
63. Gala, R. R., and Westphal, U.: *Endocrinology*, 76:1069, 1965.
64. Gale, C. C.: *Acta Physiol. Scand.*, 59:269, 1963.
65. Gale, C. C.: *Acta Physiol. Scand.*, 61:228, 1964.
66. Gale, C. C., Taleisnik, S., Friedmann, H. M., and MacCann, S. M.: *J. Endocr.*, 23:303, 1961.
67. Gourdji, D.: *Compt. Rend. Acad. Sci. (Paris)*, 264:1482, 1967.
68. Greenwald, G. S.: *J. Endocr.*, 17:17, 1958.
69. Greenwald, G. S.: *J. Endocr.*, 17:24, 1958.
70. Greenwald, G. S.: *Gen. Comp. Endocr.*, 2:453, 1962.
71. Griffith, D. R., and Turner, C. W.: *Proc. Soc. Exper. Biol. Med.*, 102:619, 1959.
72. Griffith, D. R., and Turner, C. W.: *Proc. Soc. Exper. Biol. Med.*, 106:873, 1961.
73. Grönroos, M., Kalliomaki, J. L., and Marjanen, P.: *Acta Endocr.*, 31:154, 1959.
74. Grosvenor, C. E., and Turner, C. W.: *Amer. J. Physiol.*, 200:483, 1961.
75. Grosvenor, C. E.: *Endocrinology*, 74:548, 1964.
76. Grosvenor, C. E.: *Proc. Soc. Exper. Biol. Med.*, 121:366, 1966.
77. Grosvenor, C. E., and Mena, F.: *Endocrinology*, 80:840, 1967.
78. Grosvenor, C. E., Mena, F., and Schaefgen, D. A.: *Endocrinology*, 81:449, 1967.
79. Grosvenor, C. E., and Turner, C. W.: *Proc. Soc. Exper. Biol. Med.*, 96:723, 1957.
80. Grosvenor, C. E., and Turner, C. W.: *Proc. Soc. Exper. Biol. Med.*, 99:517, 1958.
81. Grosvenor, C. E., and Turner, C. W.: *Endocrinology*, 63:535, 1958.
82. Grosvenor, C. E., and Turner, C. W.: *Proc. Soc. Exper. Biol. Med.*, 100:70, 1959.
83. Grosvenor, C. E., and Turner, C. W.: *Proc. Soc. Exper. Biol. Med.*, 100:158, 1959.
84. Grosvenor, C. E., and Turner, C. W.: *Proc. Soc. Exper. Biol. Med.*, 101:699, 1959.
85. Grota, L. J., and Eik-Nes, K. B.: *J. Reprod. Fertil.*, 13:83, 1967.
86. Grumbach, M. M., and Kaplan, S. L.: *Trans. N.Y. Acad. Sci.*, 27:167, 1964.
87. Guillemin, R.: *Ann. Rev. Physiol.*, 29:313, 1967.
88. Hadfield, G., and Young, S.: *Brit. J. Surg.*, 46:265, 1958.
89. Hahn, D. W., and Turner, C. W.: *Proc. Soc. Exper. Biol. Med.*, 121:1056, 1966.
90. Hahn, D. W., and Turner, C. W.: *Proc. Soc. Exper. Biol. Med.*, 122:183, 1966.
91. Hamberger, L., and Ahran, K.: *J. Endocr.*, 30:171, 1964.
92. Harris, G. W.: *Arch. Gynäk.*, 183:61, 1963.
93. Harris, G. W., and Jacobson, D.: *Proc. Roy. Soc., London (Ser. B)*, 139:265, 1953.
94. Haun, C. K., and Sawyer, C. H.: *Endocrinology*, 67:270, 1960.
95. Hellman, B.: *Acta Obstet. Gynec. Scand.*, 39:331, 1960.
96. Himwick, H. W. E.: *Science*, 127:59, 1958.
97. Huntingford, P. J.: *J. Obstet. Gynec. Brit. Comm.*, 70:929, 1963.
98. Hymer, W. C., MacShan, W. H., and Christiansen, R. G.: *Endocrinology*, 69:81, 1961.
99. Iino, S., and Greer, M. A.: *Endocrinology*, 68:253, 1961.
100. Iversen, S.: *J. Endocr.*, 17:99, 1958.
101. Jacobson, D.: *Acta Endocr.*, 35:107, 1960.
102. Johnsen, S. G., and Fuchs, F.: *Dan. Med. Bull. (Copenhagen)*, 8:145, 1961.
103. Johnson, R. M., and Meites, J.: *Endocrinology*, 63:291, 1958.
104. Josimovitch, J. B., and MacLaren, J.: *Endocrinology*, 71:209, 1962.
105. Jull, J. W., Bonser, G. M., and Dorsett, J. A.: *Brit. Med. J.*, 1:797, 1964.
106. Kanematsu, S., Hilliard, J., and Sawyer, C. H.: *Endocrinology*, 73:345, 1963.
107. Kovacic, N.: *J. Reprod. Fertil.*, 15:254, 1968.
108. Kragt, C. L., and Meites, J.: *Endocrinology*, 80:1170, 1967.
109. Kuroshima, A., Arimura, A., Bowers, C. Y., and Schally, A. V.: *Endocrinology*, 78:216, 1966.
110. Lederer, J., and De Meyer, R.: *Ann. d'Endocr.*, 20:377, 1959.
111. Lederer, J., and De Meyer, R.: *Ann. d'Endocr.*, 20:902, 1959.
112. Lehrman, D. S.: *Science*, 211:48, 1964.
113. Liu, T. M. Y., and Davis, J. W.: *Endocrinology*, 80:1043, 1967.
114. Linzell, J. L.: *Physiol. Rev.*, 39:354, 1959.
115. Marañón, G., and Fernández-Noguera, J.: *La Enfermedad de Addison*. Madrid, Espasa-Calpe, 1950.
116. Meites, J.: *Endocrinology*, 76:1220, 1965.
117. Meites, J., Hopkins, T. F., and Tawalker, P. K.: *Endocrinology*, 73:261, 1963.
118. Meites, J., and Nicoll, C. S.: *Endocrinology*, 65:572, 1959.
119. Meites, J., Nicoll, C. S., and Tawalker, P. K.: *Proc. Soc. Exper. Biol. Med.*, 101:563, 1959.
120. Meites, J., Nicoll, C. S., and Tawalker, P. K.: *Proc. Soc. Exper. Biol. Med.*, 102:127, 1959.
121. Meites, J., Nicoll, C. S., and Tawalker, P. K.: *Proc. Soc. Exper. Biol. Med.*, 104:192, 1960.
122. Mena, F., and Beyer, C.: *Amer. J. Physiol.*, 205:313, 1963.
123. Minaguchi, H., and Meites, J.: *Endocrinology*, 80:603, 1967.
124. Mishinsky, J., Lajtos, Z. H., and Sulman, F. G.: *Endocrinology*, 78:919, 1966.
125. Moon, R. C., Griffith, D. R., and Turner, W. C.: *Proc. Soc. Exper. Biol. Med.*, 101:788, 1959.
126. Moon, R. C., and Turner, W. C.: *Proc. Soc. Exper. Biol. Med.*, 101:332, 1959.
127. Moore, R. D., and Zarrow, M. X.: *Acta Endocr.*, 48:186, 1964.
128. Newborn, M., and Egli, G. E.: *Amer. J. Obstet. Gynec.*, 76:102, 1958.

129. Newton, M., and Newton, R. N.: *J. Paediatr.*, 33:698, 1948.
130. Newton, M.: In *The Mammary Gland*, ed. S. K. Kon and A. T. Cowie, Vol. I. New York, Academic Press, 1961.
131. Nicoll, C. S.: *Endocrinology*, 80:641, 1967.
132. Nicoll, C. S., and Meites, J.: *Endocrinology*, 72:544, 1963.
133. Niswender, G. D., Chen, C. L., and Midgley, A. R.: *Proc. Soc. Exper. Biol. Med.*, 130:793, 1969.
134. Ota, K. S., Shinde, Y., and Yokohama, A.: *Endocrinology*, 76:1, 1965.
135. Peckham, W. D., Hotchkiss, J., Knobil, E., and Nicoll, C. S.: *Endocrinology*, 82:1247, 1968.
136. Potter, G. D., Tong, W., and Chaikoff, I. L.: *J. Biol. Chem.*, 234:350, 1959.
137. Racadot, J.: *Ann. d'Endocr.*, 18:628, 1957.
138. Raynaud, A.: *Ann. d'Endocr.*, 17:580, 1956.
139. Ratner, A., Tawalker, P. K., and Meites, J.: *Proc. Soc. Exper. Biol. Med.*, 112:12, 1963.
140. Reiher, K. H.: *Geburtsh. u. Frauenhk.*, 22:885, 1962.
141. Richardson, K. C.: *Brit. Med. Bull.*, 5:174, 1948.
142. Richardson, K. C.: *J. Endocr.*, 9:170, 1953.
143. Riddle, O., and Bates, R. W.: In *Sex and Internal Secretions*, 2nd ed. Ed. E. T. Engle. Baltimore, Williams & Wilkins, 1939.
144. Rimoin, D. L., Holzman, G. B., and Merimee, T. J.: *J. Clin. Endocr.*, 28:1183, 1968.
145. Robinson, M.: *Brit. Med. Bull.*, 5:196, 1948.
146. Rothchild, I., and Quilligan, J.: *Endocrinology*, 67:122, 1960.
147. Saaman, N., Yen, S. C. C., Friesen, H., and Pearson, O. H.: *J. Clin. Endocr.*, 26:1303, 1966.
148. Sala, N. L.: *Fisiología y Farmacología de la Eyección Láctea*. Thesis, University of Buenos Aires, 1961.
149. Sala, N. O., and Althabe, O.: *Acta Physiol. Lat. Amer.*, 18:88, 1968.
150. Sammelwits, P. H., Aldred, J. P., and Nalbandov, A. V.: *J. Reprod. Fertil.*, 2:387, 1961.
151. Sander, S.: *Acta Physiol. Microbiol. Scand.*, 73:29, 1968.
152. Sander, S.: *Acta Endocr.*, 58:49, 1968.
153. Sander, S.: *Acta Endocr.*, 59:235, 1968.
154. Sar, M., and Meites, J.: *Proc. Soc. Exper. Biol. Med.*, 127:426, 1968.
155. Schally, A. V., Steelman, S. L., and Bowers, C. Y.: *Proc. Soc. Exper. Biol. Med.*, 119:208, 1965.
156. Schmidt, G. H., and Moger, W. H.: *Endocrinology*, 81:14, 1967.
157. Sciarra, J. J., Kaplan, S. L., and Grumbach, M. M.: *Nature*, 199:1005, 1963.
158. Shaw, J. C., Clung, A. C., and Bunding, L.: *Endocrinology*, 56:327, 1955.
159. Sica-Blanco, Y., Mendez-Bauer, C., Sala, N. L., Cabot, H. M., and Caldeyro-Barcia, R.: *Arch. de Ginec. Obstet. (Montevideo)*, 17:63, 1959.
160. Simkin, B., and Goddart, D.: *J. Clin. Endocr.*, 20:1095, 1960.
161. Smith, T. C.: *Endocrinology*, 57:33, 1955.
162. Smith, T. C., and Richterich, B.: *Endocrinology*, 65:51, 1959.
163. Speert, H.: *Contrib. Embryol.*, 32:11, 1948.
164. Spellacy, W. N., Buhi, W. C., and Birk, S. A.: *Amer. J. Obstet. Gynec.*, 107:244, 1970.
165. Srivastava, L. S., and Turner, C. W.: *Endocrinology*, 79:650, 1966.
166. Steinetz, B. G.: *Endocrinology*, 67:102, 1960.
167. Stricker, P., and Grüter, F.: *Compt. Rend. Soc. Biol. (Paris)*, 99:1978, 1928.
168. Taleisnik, S., and Tomatis, M. D.: *Neuroendocrinology*, 3:303, 1968.
169. Tawalker, P. K., and Meites, J.: *Proc. Soc. Exper. Biol. Med.*, 107:880, 1961.
170. Telegdy, G., Endröczi, E., and Lissak, L.: *Acta Endocr.*, 44:461, 1963.
171. Thatcher, W. W., and Tucker, H. A.: *Endocrinology*, 86:237, 1970.
172. Tindal, J. S.: *J. Endocr.*, 20:78, 1960.
173. Tindal, J. S., and Yokohama, A.: *Endocrinology*, 71:196, 1962.
174. Tindal, J. S., Beyer, C., and Sawyer, C. H.: *Endocrinology*, 72:720, 1963.
175. Tindal, J. S., Knaggs, G. S., and Turvey, A.: *J. Endocr.*, 43:663, 1969.
176. Trentin, J. J., and Turner, C. W.: *Endocrinology*, 41:127, 1947.
177. Trentin, J. J., De Vita, J., and Gardner, W. U.: *Anat. Rec.*, 113:162, 1962.
178. Tuchmann-Duplessis, H., and Mercier-Parot, L.: *Compt. Rend. Soc. Biol.*, 151:1125, 1957.
179. Tucker, H. A., and Reece, R. P.: *Proc. Soc. Exper. Biol. Med.*, 112:1002, 1963.
180. Tucker, H. A., and Reece, R. P.: *Proc. Soc. Exper. Biol. Med.*, 115:884, 1964.
181. Turkington, R. W., and Topper, Y. J.: *Endocrinology*, 79:175, 1966.
182. Turkington, R. W., and Topper, Y. J.: *Endocrinology*, 80:329, 1967.
183. Vorherr, H., Kleeman, C. R., and Lehman, E.: *Endocrinology*, 81:711, 1967.
184. Wada, H., and Turner, C. W.: *Proc. Soc. Exper. Biol. Med.*, 101:707, 1959.
185. Wada, H., and Turner, C. W.: *Proc. Soc. Exper. Biol. Med.*, 102:568, 1959.
186. Wagner, W. C., Saatman, R., and Hansel, W.: *J. Reprod. Fertil.*, 18:501, 1969.
187. Welsch, C. W., Sar, M., Clemens, J. A., and Meites, J.: *Proc. Soc. Exper. Biol. Med.*, 129:817, 1968.
188. Wenner, R.: *Schw. Med. Wschr.*, 89:441, 1959.
189. Yen, S. S. C., Saaman, N., and Pearson, O. H.: *J. Clin. Endocr.*, 27:1341, 1967.

Part Six
EXPLORATION OF THE ENDOCRINE PATIENT

At this point we begin the clinical part of the book. Before entering the study of the endocrine syndromes of woman, several chapters are to be devoted to exploratory techniques in endocrine gynecology. We wish to emphasize the importance of purely clinical methods as well as of morphological methods (cytology and endometrial biopsy), and to underline the fact that hormonologic methods, valuable as they are, by contrast occupy a secondary place in clinical practice and are, for the time being, methods designed for research.

Chapter 23
CLINICAL EXPLORATION IN FEMALE ENDOCRINOLOGY

This chapter is concerned with the subject of clinical exploration. Owing to the remarkable advances made over the past few years in the field of hormone assay, exfoliative cytology and endometrial biopsy, the study of such exploratory procedures has been deliberately segregated and deserves to be treated in separate chapters. Nevertheless, in addition to our main discussion of general clinical exploration, this chapter will incorporate several special forms of exploratory techniques, based on laboratory procedures, which, owing to various considerations, have been included here. Thus, we shall study consecutively: clinical history, physical examination, tests performed routinely, and, finally, cervical mucus, basal body temperature, peritoneoscopy and radiographic exploration.

23.1. CLINICAL HISTORY

Taking the clinical history of a female patient suffering from an endocrinopathy is not significantly different from what we may do in gathering the clinical history of any other female patient. Nevertheless, some ground rules must be observed and will be briefly reviewed.

After having secured information from the patient concerning the usual personal data, such as age, occupation, marital status, etc., some care must be exerted to explore any possible special circumstances. For instance, the place of the patient's habitual residence and related geographic conditions should be investigated. It has been shown, for example, that *Eskimo women do not menstruate during the six months' duration of the polar night*. Various authors have similarly underscored the *relationship existing between climate and menstrual changes*. In our experience, menstrual alterations may frequently occur in women who have changed their place of residence. Thus, it is not uncommon to observe, for instance, suspension of menstrual periods in travelers from America, particularly after a rapid trip, such as by plane, as a result of the geographic change to which they are subjected. It is not known whether the only factor involved is displacement across the surface of the globe, or whether such other factors as high altitude flight or psychic inhibition imposed by a strange environment are equally involved. It is very important, too, to recognize the importance of the environmental conditions surrounding the patient; for example, college age women may frequently be observed to develop amenorrhea in the course of intense studies associated with mental overtaxation. Hawkins has called attention to the fact that the incidence of dysmenorrhea and menstrual disturbances is much higher in large cities, such as New York, than it is in rural areas. General environmental influences of this kind may also be involved in the type of amenorrhea we frequently observed in maidservants that had just begun to cope with city life. For these reasons, a record of factors pertaining to occupation, habitual place of residence, travels and way of life is of extraordinary importance in compiling a patient's history.

Any piece of information concerning the

patient's *sex life* is also of great value. Related anamnestic data should, as much as possible, comprise conditions prior to menarche and the patient's state of health during infancy and her prepuberal years, since the occurrence of illness, weakness or any other type of disturbances between the ages of eight and 12 may decisively affect later sexual development. This observation has been particularly well borne out by the experiences of both the Spanish Civil War and World War II. In Spain as well as in various other countries at war, it has been observed that those girls who during the war or postwar period were between the ages of eight and 12 and were subjected to great deprivations, to starvation and to all kinds of anxiety eventually developed disturbances in their somatic and sexual development which were of such importance that in many instances the consequences entailed life-long sexual endocrinopathies.

As far as menarche is concerned, it is of great interest to explore the possibility that failure of menarche to appear may in some way be related to any of the previously mentioned geographical or war-related factors. Apart from just marking down the time at which menarche occurred, we must also insist on analyzing the circumstances under which the patient had entered her puberal phase: whether development was premature or delayed, whether or not menstruation was regular; in short, a detailed description of the manner in which sexual maturity came about.

A history of past *pregnancies*, if the woman is married, is indispensable. This is important not only from the gynecologic point of view but may also be informative from the endocrine point of view as well. *Toxemia* of pregnancy often reveals a background of adrenal or thyroid pathology. Similarly, *parturition* and the *puerperium* are events that favor the development of pituitary pathology, such as acromegaly, pituitary cachexia and Sheehan's syndrome. Woman's endocrine balance may likewise be affected by the psychosomatic effects of gestation. The syndrome of pelvic congestion, which appears in women shunning or dreading coitus, is well known. This aspect has been particularly stressed by Benedek and Rubenstein.[6]

A climacteric woman must also be questioned about her climacterium, as well as about any other pertinent details. As pointed out in Chapter 8, endocrine gynecology is closely related to the nervous system, so that this aspect deserves to be carefully evaluated.

Our next step must be directed toward the study of the patient's *family history*. Female endocrinopathies are associated with pronounced hereditary tendencies. Recurrence of congenital anomalies of the gonad or of menstrual pathology in the same family is a common observation. In this regard, it must be remembered that any observed menstrual disturbances may be of a different or even opposite type when occurring in the mother than when occurring in daughters or among various sisters. When one daughter presents, for instance, with oligomenorrhea and with a state of ovarian insufficiency, we may thus find a sister who has a hemorrhagic tendency and a syndrome of hyperestrinism. What here may seem to contradict the preceding statement is nevertheless a confirmatory finding, because the underlying background of such familial disturbances is always an endocrine pituitary or ovarian insufficiency that may give rise to different forms of manifestations. The patient should therefore be asked about her mother's as well as her sisters' menstrual peculiarities and about other related data.

Next in line is the *history of the patient's present illness*, in which all questions should be directed to details relevant to the present disease process. In female endocrinopathies in general, the patient usually relates to the history of her *menstrual process*. Marañón had quite pertinently brought up the question of subjective *overemphasis of menstrual symptomatology* on the part of female patients coming to the gynecologist or to the endocrinologist for a checkup. Not infrequently, a woman may fail to be aware of obvious serious obesity, of a lesion on the genitalia, or of the symptoms of significant adrenal insufficiency, and instead is greatly concerned about the fact that her menstrual periods may be more frequent or more widely spaced than usual. In this respect, we wish to quote a case of most serious adiposogenital dystrophy, resulting in death a few months after the patient was brought to our clinic. Nevertheless, her mother brought her solely on account of amenorrhea, presenting her more or less in the following vein: "It seems unbelievable that this most beautiful and well developed child should be so badly off as to have no periods." The beauty and extraordinary development the mother was referring to was no less than 120 kg (about 250 lb) of fat in a girl of 14.

Inquiries concerning the patient's *dietary intake* should not be omitted. The influence of diet on sexual life has already been discussed in Chapter 10 and shall again be taken up further ahead. It is important to remember that malnutrition may cause sexual alterations of consequence. Quite a few years ago, Gaethgens became aware that animals on a diminished diet showed lack of ovarian development. Similarly, Guilbert noted that a decrease in dietary proteins resulted in discontinuation of the menstrual cycle, while Stephens demonstrated that menstruation in malnourished individuals could be restored to normalcy by reestablishing a protein and vitamin rich diet. Although these issues will be stressed again in due time, the importance of analyzing the patient's diet must be kept in mind for the eventual evaluation of an endocrine case.

History taking should not be concluded without questioning the patient about a group of symptoms pertaining to general endocrinopathies, which must also be included here. Questions should be asked about the presence or absence of headaches, vertigo, fatigability, nervousness, dyspnea, palpitations, gain or loss of weight, increased or decreased libido, increased or decreased appetite, polydipsia, polyuria, and finally, not less important, the presence of leukorrhea.

23.2. PHYSICAL EXAMINATION OF THE ENDOCRINE PATIENT

23.2.1. INSPECTION

Inspection of the endocrine patient is of utmost importance, from both a local and general point of view.

GENERAL INSPECTION. A patient with a female endocrinopathy usually offers some alterations that are grossly visible. Since many details are likely to be overlooked by initial inspection with the patient fully dressed, it should be necessary, wherever possible, to inspect the patient fully undressed in spite of the natural bashfulness of many female patients. The different types of constitutional habitus should be recorded as outlined in Chapter 18. Women belonging to the *hypoplastic type of constitution* can be seen to be short in stature and to have an infantile somatic appearance. Their hair is silky and fine and their skin is thin. This hypoplastic type is often found in women with estrogenic insufficiency, particularly in those cases in which the clinical picture is the result of a primary pituitary lesion.

Occasionally, the patient is tall and lean (*asthenic*), with scanty fat panniculus, a very acute xyphoid angle and with all the characteristic features pertaining to the leptosomatic type. Within the framework of the asthenic constitutional habitus, female endocrinopathies are often associated with conditions of hyperestrinism, so that such women may be noted to have well developed breasts and other strongly pronounced female attributes.

Obese and stocky women usually belong to the *pyknic habitus*, which may be associated with hyperluteinism, adrenal cortical hyperplasia and other related conditions. In these cases, we may observe brachylineal obese females, with abundant fat panniculus and well developed breasts and hips. On the other hand, obesity sometimes coincides with hypogonadal conditions or with combined hypogonadal and hypopituitary conditions, in which case it is of the type that is associated with hypoplasia, such as is usually found in the adiposogenital syndrome.

Lastly, a considerable number of endocrine patients appear to be virilized. *Virilization* in woman is characterized by the appearance of a male type of hair distribution, a beard and moustache and hypertrichosis of the abdominal midline and thighs. The examiner must avoid the error of confusing *simple hypertrichosis*, that is, *overall hyperplasia of the pilar system*, with *hypertrichosis due to virilization*, in which hairiness, apart from being increased, has a *male type of distribution*. In order to diagnose a viriloid condition in a woman, we must therefore be guided by other symptoms of virilization in addition to hairiness, such as *shape of skeleton, distribution of fat panniculus, quality of voice*, etc.

Also of interest is the *eunuchoid habitus*, usually with very long arms and cubitus valgus, which, in contradistinction to the asthenic habitus, is associated with scanty or no breast development and lack of female configuration of the hips.

MORPHOGRAPHY. What further must not be omitted is *evaluation of bodily proportions*, which in some syndromes may facilitate *a priori* establishment of the diagnosis (gigantism, dwarfism) and, above all, the *biotypologic classification* of the individual.

However, because evaluation in this instance is "qualitative" in nature, the need has arisen for "quantitative" forms of expressing an individual's somatic features in order to establish precise clinical standards of comparison and classification. This has been accomplished by Decourt and Doumic[17] in a very simple manner, which is worth describing. Application of such standards is advisable above all in female sexual endocrinology. Called *morphography* by its authors, this method consists of the following steps:

Five parameters are arranged into columns (Fig. 23–1): (1) thoracic perimeter; (2) height of the greater trochanter of the femur; (3) stature; (4) bitrochanteric diameter (maximal width of hips); and (5) bideltoid or bihumeral diameter (maximal width of shoulders).

Different scales are available for male and female standards, as shown in Figure 23–2. These are arranged so as to give a horizontal line for what is arbitrarily considered a "normal" set of proportions in male or female, respectively.

In accordance with this basic scheme, the corresponding measurements in each individual case are recorded on the scale. Decourt[16, 18] has defined different morphographic types for puberty, Turner's syndrome, dwarfism, etc., as shown in Figure 23–3, which shall be discussed in detail in the corresponding chapters.

LOCAL INSPECTION. The different components of the genital apparatus must be inspected locally. For instance, a meticulous inspection of the breasts is of great endocrinologic interest. It should be noted whether these are enlarged or decreased in size, whether or not the areola is well formed and pigmented, as it is in pregnancy, and whether or not Montgomery's tubercles are apparent. Contrary to common belief, hyperpigmentation of the breast and prominence of Montgomery's tubercles are not exclusive in pregnancy but may be also observed in the presence of some luteinized tumors, choriocarcinoma, Cushing's disease and a few other conditions.

The vulvar region must also be inspected. Frequently, a typically male distribution of

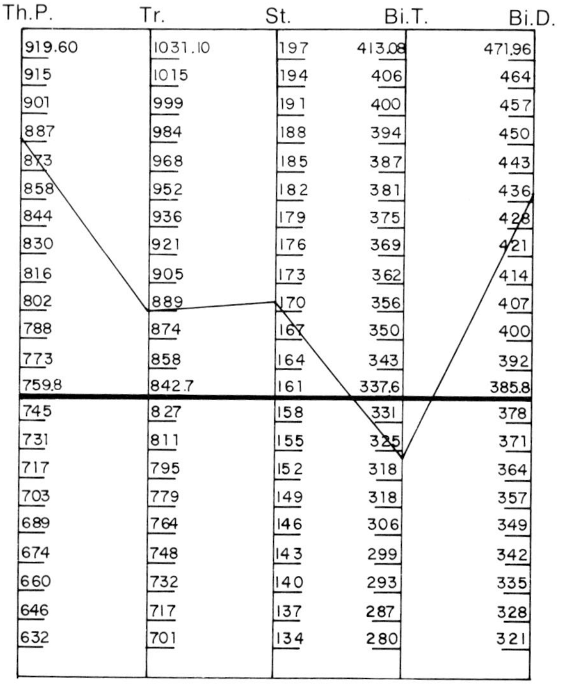

Figure 23–1. Morphography of normal woman in centimeters, using the female scale. Thick straight line represents average morphography of normal woman; thin line, average morphography of normal male. *Th.P.*, Thoracic perimeter; *Tr.*, height of greater trochanter; *St.*, stature; *Bi.T.*, bitrochanteric diameter; *Bi.D.*, bideltoid diameter (shoulder width). (From Decourt and Doumic: *Sem. Hôp. Paris*, 26:2457, 1950.)

Th.P.	Tr.	St.	Bi.T.	Bi.D.
919.60	1031.10	197	413.08	471.96
915	1015	194	406	464
901	999	191	400	457
887	984	188	394	450
873	968	185	387	443
858	952	182	381	436
844	936	179	375	428
830	921	176	369	421
816	905	173	362	414
802	889	170	356	407
788	874	167	350	400
773	858	164	343	392
759.8	842.7	161	337.6	385.8
745	827	158	331	378
731	811	155	325	371
717	795	152	318	364
703	779	149	318	357
689	764	146	306	349
674	748	143	299	342
660	732	140	293	335
646	717	137	287	328
632	701	134	280	321

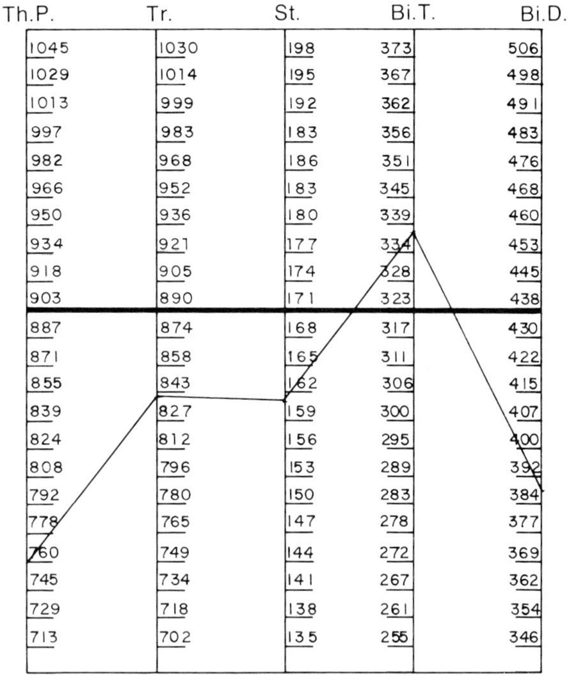

Clinical Exploration in Female Endocrinology 489

Th.P.	Tr.	St.	Bi.T.	Bi.D.
1045	1030	198	373	506
1029	1014	195	367	498
1013	999	192	362	491
997	983	183	356	483
982	968	186	351	476
966	952	183	345	468
950	936	180	339	460
934	921	177	334	453
918	905	174	328	445
903	890	171	323	438
887	874	168	317	430
871	858	165	311	422
855	843	162	306	415
839	827	159	300	407
824	812	156	295	400
808	796	153	289	392
792	780	150	283	384
778	765	147	278	377
760	749	144	272	369
745	734	141	267	362
729	718	138	261	354
713	702	135	255	346

Figure 23-2. Morphography of normal man in centimeters, using the male scale. Thick line, average normal male morphography; thin line, average female morphography compared to that of male. See Figure 23-1 for identification of parameters. (From Decourt and Doumic, *Sem. Hôp. Paris*, 26:2457, 1950.)

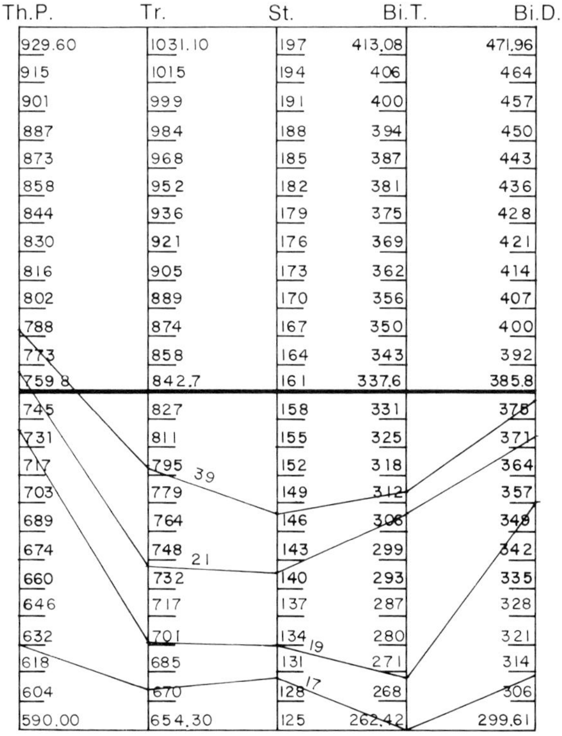

Th.P.	Tr.	St.	Bi.T.	Bi.D.
929.60	1031.10	197	413.08	471.96
915	1015	194	406	464
901	999	191	400	457
887	984	188	394	450
873	968	185	387	443
858	952	182	381	436
844	936	179	375	428
830	921	176	369	421
816	905	173	362	414
802	889	170	356	407
788	874	167	350	400
773	858	164	343	392
759.8	842.7	161	337.6	385.8
745	827	158	331	378
731	811	155	325	371
717	795	152	318	364
703	779	149	312	357
689	764	146	306	349
674	748	143	299	342
660	732	140	293	335
646	717	137	287	328
632	701	134	280	321
618	685	131	271	314
604	670	128	268	306
590.00	654.30	125	262.42	299.61

Figure 23-3. Instances of pathologic female morphography in four cases of Turner's syndrome. All four cases reveal decrease in stature, lowered height of trochanter and narrowed hips, with approximately normal shoulder width and thoracic perimeter. See Figure 23-1 for identification of parameters. (From Decourt: *Les etats intersexuels.* Paris, Maloine, 1962.)

hair may be found, with hypertrophy of the clitoris and with a masculine appearance and virilization of this region.

23.2.2. WEIGHT AND MEASUREMENTS

The weight, height and measurement of several body diameters, such as the bisacromial diameter, the bitrochanteric diameter, circumference of chest and abdomen, etc., are data that must not be omitted whenever exploring an endocrine patient. The standard measurements of normal woman, as reproduced in Figure 23-1, may serve as a criterion for such measurements. A *sudden gain in weight* is usually observed in women developing *edema*, particularly in toxemia of pregnancy, whereas a *slow increase in weight* is characteristic of obesity, such as is seen in adiposogenital dystrophy, castration and some forms of hypogonadism. On the other hand, *weight loss* may be seen in some cases of hyperestrinism, in hyperthyroidism and in certain endocrinopathies associated with cachexia.

As far as stature is concerned, this undergoes little or no modification in the adult woman, but young girls or adolescent patients may experience quite important changes. For instance, girls with a *late onset of puberty,* or with *eunuchoidism*, show *exaggerated growth* of the trunk and extremities between 15 and 18. On the contrary, girls suffering from *primary pituitary insufficiency* may present with *premature and almost absolute arrest of statural development* beginning with the prepuberal phase.

23.2.3. PALPATION

Palpation is of lesser importance in endocrine exploration. Nevertheless, large abdominal tumors can be readily palpated, and so can ovarian tumoral processes, such as functional tumors, cysts or other destructive tumors. Finally, it must be borne in mind that ascites associated with certain ovarian syndromes may also become perceptible by means of palpation. However, data obtained by palpation are of secondary importance compared to other endocrine aspects.

23.2.4. VAGINAL EXAMINATION

By comparison, vaginal examination is of extraordinary importance. By means of digital exploration, we may discover a series of data concerning the genital tract which are of diagnostic value in determining possible endocrinopathies.

First to be noted is the spaciousness of the vagina and the degree of turgescence of the vaginal mucosa. Underdeveloped vaginas, with scant rugosity and thin walls, are observed in all syndromes of hypofolliculinism, in what has commonly been termed *genital hypoplasia*. Such women are noted not only for their hypoplastic and thin-walled vaginas but also for evidence of commonly associated vaginitis and leukorrhea. Tactual examination of the uterus may permit estimation of its size as an important corollary. Thus, hypoestrinism invariably goes hand in hand with a diminished size of the uterus (*hypoplastic or infantile uterus*), and such a uterus is generally found in forceful anteflexion, giving rise to what is known by the name of *hooked uterus or cochleate uterus*. However, we must not commit the error of assuming that uterine hypoplasia is necessarily associated with hypoestrinism. Nogales and Botella[27] have found that a permanently hypoplastic uterus may be the consequence of genital tuberculosis, particularly uterine tuberculosis occurring during adolescence, even though ovarian function may subsequently be restored to normalcy. Similarly, de la Fuente[19] has produced statistical evidence that women with a so-called infantile uterus are capable of conceiving normally, which is against the concept of endocrine ovarian insufficiency.

A highly interesting pathognomonic sign with regard to uterine hypoplasia is *sinistroposition*, or deviation of a hypoplastic uterus to the left (Fig. 23-4), which has been described by Frank and has afterwards been confirmed, notably by our own studies.[9]

Occasionally, some female endocrinopathies are associated with an enlarged uterus and ample development of the vaginal mucosa and cavity. An increase in uterine size of purely endocrine origin may be encountered in association with Swiss-cheese endometrial hyperplasia, or hemorrhagic metropathy of Schroeder, but similar enlargement of the uterus, of indirect endo-

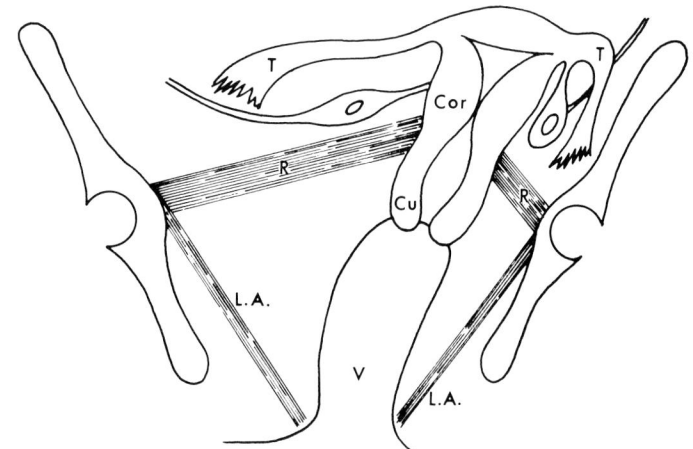

Figure 23-4. Sinistroposition of uterus. *Cor*, uterine body; *Cu*, cervix; *R*, uterine retinacula; *L.A.*, levator ani; *V*, vagina; *O*, ovary; *T*, tube.

crine origin, may be observed with endometriosis, myomas, and other neoformative conditions affecting the uterus, in which estrogens play a stimulative or predisposing role.

Vaginal examination may also facilitate palpation of the ovary. This organ may thus be found to be increased in size, or to reveal the presence of ovarian tumors which, particularly if functional, may be of great endocrine significance.

Sometimes a persistent follicle may be palpated in the ovary, and if a certain amount of pressure is applied between the explorer's abdominal and vaginal hands a follicle may even be perceived to rupture between the fingers. Whenever such an exploratory maneuver is performed, it is not unusual to witness a hemorrhagic episode, occurring four to six days afterwards, owing to hormone withdrawal. Alternatively, polycystic ovaries of the Stein syndrome are generally palpable through the abdominal integument, particularly in lean women with flaccid abdominal walls. A great deal more information can be extracted through tactual examination of the abdomen, although the ones already mentioned are the most important for the endocrinologist.

23.2.5. VAGINOSCOPY

Although vaginal examination by means of a speculum, of great importance in gynecology in general, may not necessarily contribute any significant data, it should be practiced nevertheless whenever possible. It is a means for obtaining vaginal exudates for cytologic examination as well as for the study of cervical mucus. The properties of the latter in relation to a possible functional disturbance are discussed later. By the same token, the thickness and turgescence of the vaginal mucosa reflect fairly accurately the functional state of the ovary. It is likewise not unusual to observe erosions around the external os (cervical erosions) in hyperestrogenic women. However, all such findings are usually of little help in establishing a functional diagnosis.

23.3. ROUTINE LABORATORY TESTS

23.3.1. MORPHOLOGIC EXAMINATION OF THE BLOOD

Examination of blood morphology is of marginal interest for the diagnosis of endocrine gynecopathies. A syndrome of anemia, which so far is of obscure etiology, associated with hypoestrinism, is occasionally observed in girls. Secondary anemia is encountered in cases of hyperestrinism associated with hemorrhagic syndromes. Anemia directly related to marrow hypoplasia may be observed in some states of juvenile ovarian insufficiency. This disorder, classically known as chlorosis, is currently in doubt as a clinical entity, although it is definitely seen in some patients. The presence of leukocytosis is recognized to be significant as an expression of endocrine disturbances in thyroid and adrenal syndromes, but it is seldom related to ovarian syndromes.

23.3.2. BLOOD CHEMISTRY

The study of blood chemistry is a most valuable tool in endocrine patients during gestation. It is also of interest in those conditions of sexual endocrinopathy which are associated with pituitary, thyroid, pancreatic or adrenal pathology. Only exceptionally, however, does it have any direct diagnostic value in ovarian endocrinopathy.

23.3.3. URINALYSIS

Urinalysis is also an indispensable element for diagnosis and in some cases may supply data of interest, such as glucosuria, false glucosuria, or lactosuria. Ketonuria frequently appears in some instances of hypoovarian function. Finally, the microscopic study of urinary sediment, which shall be dealt with later, is interesting from a cytological point of view.

23.3.4. BASAL METABOLISM

Measurement of the basal metabolic rate is a most important test in female endocrinology. It is of value not only from the standpoint of thyroid pathology but also from the standpoint of primary ovarian pathology. Low basal metabolic rates are not confined to hypothyroidism but also occur in the syndrome of primary hypoestrinism. In general, a low basal metabolic rate in a case of hypoestrinism may be assumed to be of primary pituitary origin. Similarly, alterations in basal metabolism may be observed in adrenal hypercortical syndromes, in cases of luteal dysfunction and in a number of conditions of endocrine pathology related to pregnancy, such as, for instance, habitual abortion.

23.3.5. THE THORN TEST

Application of this test is valuable in a great variety of conditions related to genital endocrinopathies. For instance, a high percentage of negative results obtained with this functional test, indicating pituitary-adrenal insufficiency, has been found to occur in pregnancy and labor (Sol and Merlo,[38] Bedoya and Maldonado[5]).

23.4. STUDY OF CERVICAL MUCUS

The amount of secretion and the physical properties of cervical mucus are related to estrogenic activity. The fact that secretion of cervical mucus is hormone dependent has been established in recent years by Botella and Nogales.[9] Among the properties of cervical mucus, *stringiness and crystallization* are most directly related to the level of estrogenic activity. Palmer[30] had noted that stringiness of cervical mucus increased about the fourteenth day of the cycle. He attributed that finding to the action of estrogens and included stringiness among the effects of estrogenic stimulation on cervical secretory activity. Earlier than this, in 1946, Papanicolaou had also observed stringiness and copiousness of mucus discharge in the vaginal exudate at the time of ovulation and interpreted those findings as positive signs of follicular rupture. Pommerenke[33] insisted upon the significance of cervical secretion of mucus as an index of adequate ovarian function and, in conjunction with Viergiver, studied the correlation between the amount and fluidity of the mucus, on the one hand, and basal body temperature, on the other, arriving at the conclusion that the two were related. At present, the prevailing idea is that both the amount and fluidity of cervical mucus depend on estrogenic activity. According to generally accepted ideas, estrogens are believed to enhance the amount and fluidity of mucus secretion, whereas progesterone has the opposite effect. Consequently, the physiologic findings in a normal cycle should consist in a gradual increase in amount and fluidity of cervical mucus up to the moment of ovulation and, once the corpus luteum is formed, in a decrease in the amount of mucus and, at the same time, an increase in the viscosity of the mucus.

Rydberg[35] found that one of the properties of cervical mucus was that of crystallizing in the form of fern leaves relating to the tetragonal system (Fig. 23–5). The formation of fern leaf patterns can be quite clearly observed whenever a drop of cer-

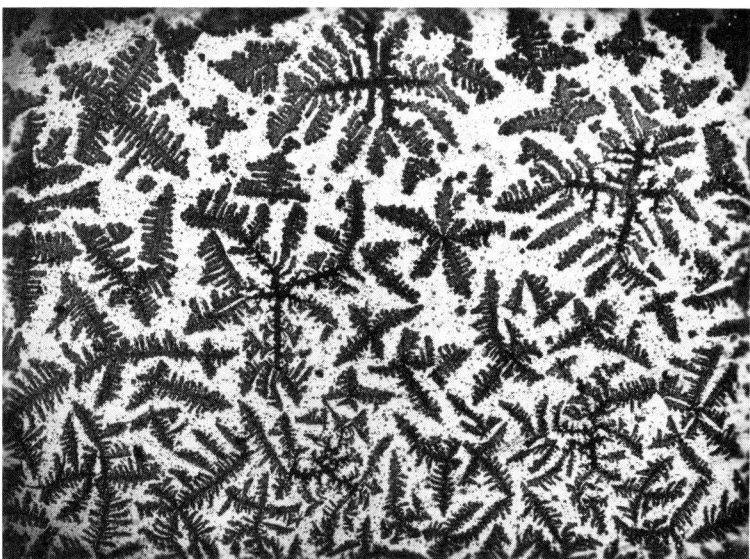

Figure 23-5. Crystallization of cervical mucus from thirteenth day of normal cycle. Crystallization occurs in the form of large fern leaves.

vical mucus is deposited on a cover slip and allowed to dry. Under these conditions, quite distinct images are obtained, which are easily reproducible and demonstrable. Campos da Paz[11] studied cervical crystallization in different gynecologic conditions and reached the conclusion that optimal crystallization of mucus was obtained precisely at the close of the proliferative phase, coincident with the time of ovulation. Accordingly, Roland[34] successfully applied this method as a test for human ovulation. Grünberger and Holkup[21] subsequently studied crystallization in many cases, concluding that it was an index not only of ovulation but also of overall adequate ovarian function. Research undertaken by de la Fuente and Gálvez,[20] by means of correlative studies of endometrial curettings and cervical crystallization, and subsequent studies by Urdan and Kurzon,[45] correlating crystallization with basal body temperature curves, have shown beyond any doubt that cervical crystallization is stimulated by the action of estrogens. It would thus appear that crystallization increases during the first half of the cycle, reaches a peak at ovulation and during the days following, then slowly declines as a result of the inhibitory effect of progesterone, and disappears by the third week of the cycle (see Chapter 13).

At our clinic, Montalvo and Castro performed a great deal of work in comparing endometrial histology, crystallization patterns and vaginal cytology. On the basis of these studies, the degree of crystallization of cervical mucus during the first half of the cycle can be inferred to be directly proportional to the level of estrogenic activity. During the second half of the cycle, however, crystallization is no longer proportional to estrogen levels because intervening progesterone activity, occurring in normal cycles, inhibits crystallization. On the other hand, in cases of anovulatory cycles or with follicular persistence, in which corpora lutea fail to develop, crystallization can be found to continue throughout the rest of the cycle. The amount, fluidity, stringiness and crystallization of cervical mucus may be viewed as parameters that are stimulated in parallel and that grow progressively during the proliferative or follicular phase until reaching a peak at the time of ovulation. To the clinician, estimation of this type of data constitutes a simple and easily explorable means of assessing estrogenic function. Thus, it can be stated that the presence of adequate estrogenic function, with normal ovulation, is associated with progressive crystallization of mucus up to the fourteenth or fifteenth day of the cycle; that deficient estrogenic function, with or without normal ovulation, is associated with lack of crystallization or with scanty crystallization during the first half of the cycle, and that a state of hyperestrinism, with follicular persistence or with a monophasic cycle, is associated with cervical crystallization throughout the cycle.

Because of these reasons, cervical crystallization has extraordinary significance as a means of estimating estrogenic function. Although not a quantitative test, it may nevertheless constitute a symptomatic and qualitative test of extraordinary interest that must be recommended here.

23.5. BASAL BODY TEMPERATURE

Basal body temperature charts have become a valuable adjunct for exploring ovarian endocrine function. It has been a good many years since Van der Velde noted cyclic oscillations of body temperature in women. Fraenkel became aware of the fact that premenstrual temperatures in women were half a degree above basal body temperatures, a finding later confirmed by Schröder (Fig. 23–6). However, these observations were largely ignored until the question of physiologic hyperthermia in young women was again brought up by specialists in tuberculosis. Beckmann[4] insisted that the premenstrual rise in body temperature, particularly in younger women, was of little diagnostic significance. It was not until 1940, however, that the cyclic nature of the temperature changes was recognized by Benedek and Rubenstein,[6] who emphasized that temperatures were low during the follicular phase whereas they rose during the secretory phase. These authors ascribed the differences in temperature to the occurrence of ovulation and believed that ovulation was associated with a drop of basal body temperature to subnormal levels. Palmer[30] applied knowledge of temperature curves to the study of disturbances of ovarian function and was able to show that women with anovulatory cycles experienced no rise in temperature during the second half of the cycle; this important finding was confirmed by Williams shortly thereafter.

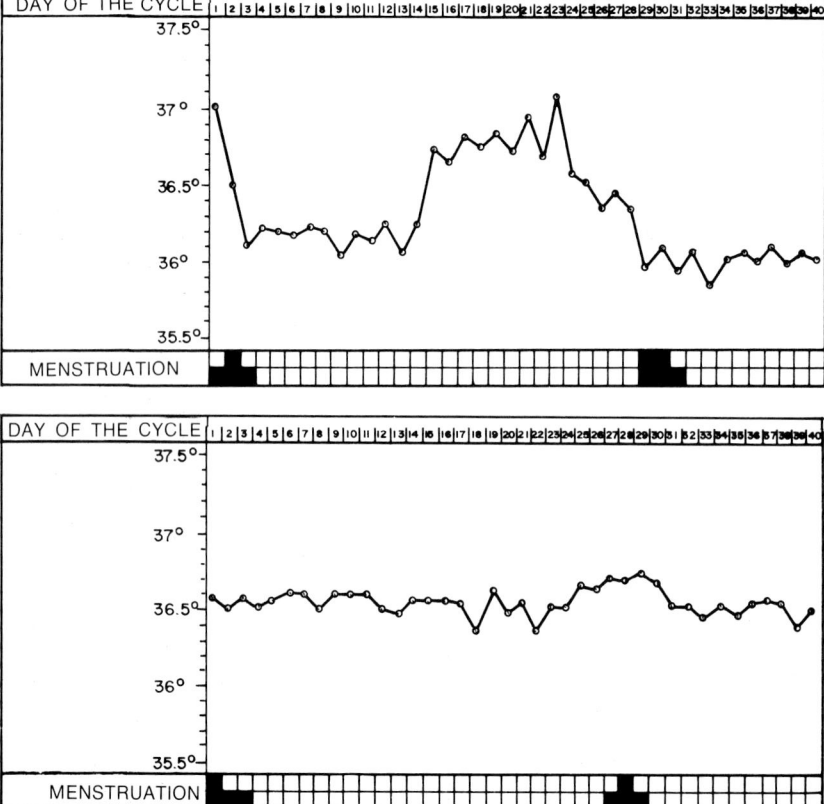

Figure 23–6. Biphasic (A) and monophasic curves (B) of basal body temperature.

Figure 23-7. Plot of basal body temperature in a cycle with luteal insufficiency resulting from hyposecretion of the corpus luteum.

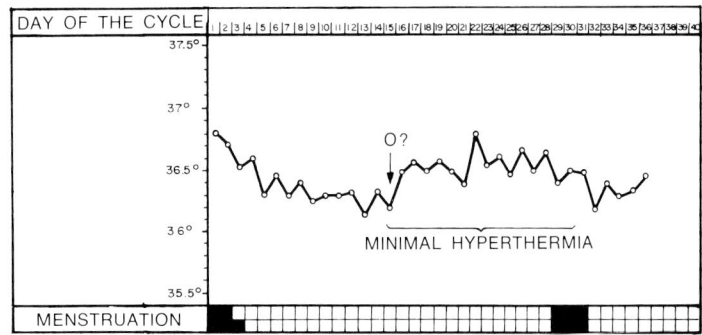

Various authors, but mainly Viergiver and Pommerenke, subsequently correlated the changes occurring in basal body temperature with those observed in the properties of cervical mucus, whereas Rubenstein correlated the changes with vaginal cytology. The cyclic changes observed in both curettings and cytology were found to run parallel with the curve of basal body temperature, and the course of the latter was found to clearly reflect the follicular and secretory phases of the cycle.

Nieburgs later showed that premenstrual elevations of basal body temperature, lasting approximately from ovulation to menstruation, resulted from the action of progesterone and could be reproduced by administering progesterone. In 1953, Williams[52] made a comprehensive study of basal body temperature and of its diagnostic value in the menstrual cycle. He concluded that premenstrual elevations of basal body temperature were a progesterone effect that was prolonged in cases of pregnancy. He further found that ovulation was not always accompanied by a drop to subnormal body temperature, as believed by Rubenstein, but could always be determined by the presence of a sudden upswing in the temperature curve. The basal body temperature curve is of great diagnostic value in the study of sterility and anomalies of the cycle, since it not only permits recognition of the presence or absence of a biphasic cycle but also facilitates determination of the duration of each phase of the cycle. In 1954, we applied the study of basal body temperature to the diagnosis of cycles with a short luteal phase[7] (Figs. 23-7 and 23-8).

As for the question of how to obtain basal body temperature charts, we proceed in the following simple way: the patient is asked to take her temperature every morning while still in bed, before breakfast. She is instructed to do so the first thing in the morning after awakening, without getting up. There seems to be no need for a special thermometer. Any good clinical thermometer will do but it is important to stress the requirement that all measurements should be performed with the same instrument to avoid errors based on differences in graduation. The thermometer can be inserted into the mouth, rectum, axilla or groin. We prefer the inguinal approach and recommend application of the thermometer to the right groin. Variations in temperature readings may also depend on the length of time during which the thermometer is applied, and therefore temperatures should be read

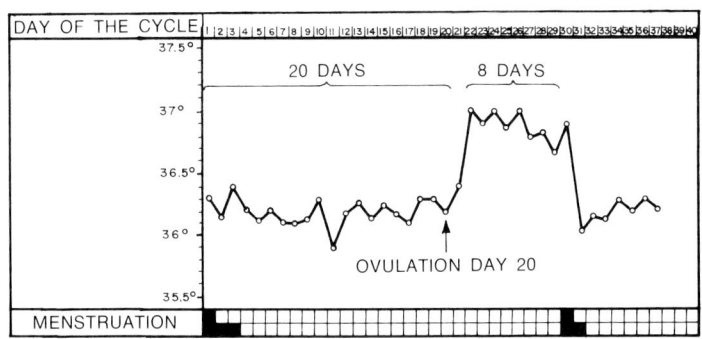

Figure 23-8. Plot of basal body temperature in a cycle with luteal insufficiency resulting from delayed ovulation, with short progestational phase.

after a fixed period of time, which we have set at five minutes. Finally, it should be pointed out that any sexual activity is bound to raise basal body temperatures, so that temperatures must be recorded after at least 10 hours of total sexual rest. If the above precautions are observed, basal body temperature plots are found to be fairly homogeneous, and the patient herself can chart the data obtained each day, making it into a graph and adding the number of days of menstruation and the corresponding dates of the month. Such graphs are very useful for the management of endocrine therapy, as shall be noted later.

23.6. PERITONEOSCOPY OR CULDOSCOPY

Peritoneoscopy can be performed through the abdominal wall (*transabdominal peritoneoscopy* or *celioscopy*) (Fig. 23-9) or through the posterior vaginal fornix (*transvaginal peritoneoscopy* or *culdoscopy*).

23.6.1. CULDOSCOPY

Decker[14] observed that the knee-chest position produced a negative intraabdominal pressure in the pelvic region, which he was able to measure. He made use of this phenomenon by inflating the space within the pelvis with gas. This was done by puncturing the posterior vaginal fornix and then setting the abdominal cavity in communication with the exterior or with a source of gas. Then, by introducing a telescope, he could readily visualize the pelvic organs.

Since 1944 or 1945, this method has gained wide acceptance, particularly in the United States (Decker,[14] Te Linde and Rutledge,[41] Abarbandel,[1] Teton[42]). Its application has also been introduced in Argentina by Peralta Romas,[32] and in France by Palmer and Palmer,[28] who, although they advocate abdominal laparoscopy, also practice culdoscopy. In Germany, Thomsen,[43] and in Scandinavia, Sjövall,[37] have found the procedure satisfactory. In Spain, to our knowledge, ours is the first instance of having applied this procedure for diagnostic purposes.[8]

TECHNIQUE. The routine we follow at present differs little from the original technique devised by Decker.

Preparation of the patient consists of an evacuant enema several hours before the procedure and sedation (injection of Escofedal) half an hour prior to culdoscopy, followed by bladder catheterization.

We use local anesthesia with 1 per cent novocaine, first raising a little wheal in the mucosa of the vaginal vault. To be sure, the sensitivity of the vaginal vault is of low order and we suspect that such puncture could be performed even without anesthesia.

Before applying anesthesia and performing the eventual puncture, the perineum must be depressed with a speculum as

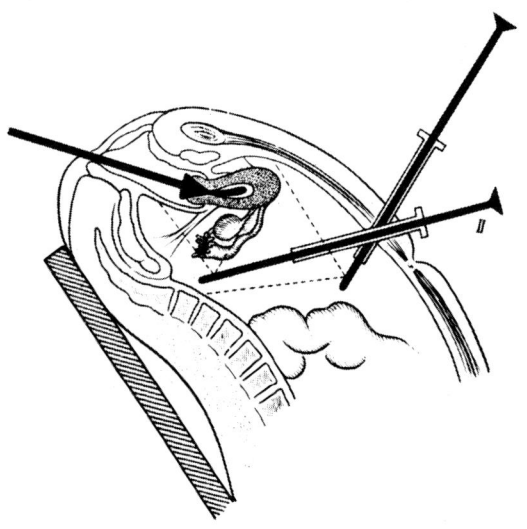

Figure 23-9. Transabdominal celioscopy. Position I of endoscope is used to visualize internal female genitalia from "above." In position II, the endoscope is introduced deeper and swung so as to disclose the posterior aspect of the genital tract and Douglas' pouch. A rigid cannula is used in catheterization so that the uterus may be displaced anteriorly. (From Palmer and Palmer.[28])

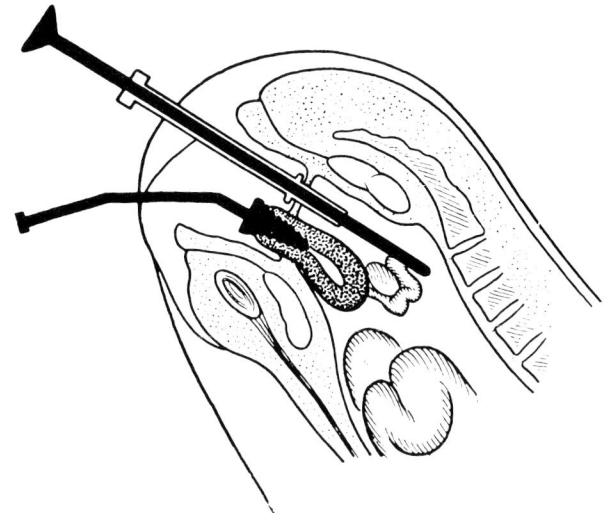

Figure 23-10. Technique of culdoscopy (transvaginal celioscopy or Douglascopy). (From Palmer and Palmer.[28])

much as possible, particularly by displacing the vaginal fundus, so as to stretch the vaginal vault and to separate the rectum from the vagina and the uterus. This facilitates puncturing and reduces the hazard of possibly injuring the rectum (Fig. 23-10).

In order to prevent the trocar from accidentally injuring a bowel loop during the procedure, the same syringe and needle that are used for local anesthesia are then used to inject 10 ml of air into the abdominal cavity through the wall of the posterior vaginal cul-de-sac. If the air can be injected with ease, it is assumed that the needle is in the peritoneal space. Once this is accomplished, puncture with the trocar is begun in a gentle, steady manner, and the trocar is introduced to the hilt. On removing the stylet, a whistling sound should be anticipated, reflecting *aspiration* of air as a result of negative intraabdominal pressure. Only then can one assume the trocar to have entered the peritoneal space correctly. In the absence of such a sign, puncture should be repeated.

Errors in selecting the puncture site may be incurred by choosing either too posterior a location (risk of injuring the rectum!) or, more frequently, too anterior a location, resulting in penetration into the posterior aspect of the uterine cervix.

The optical system is then introduced and exploration is begun in an orderly, systematic way, examining first the uterine fundus, then the ovaries, the tubes, the peritoneum, etc.

After completing the exploration, the abdomen is depressed with the cannula still in place so as to allow as much air as possible to escape, which averts most of the inconveniences associated with pneumoperitoneum.

As a rule, our patients are hospitalized for 24 hours. However, since no untoward effects have been noted in any of our cases, there seems to be no strong objection to letting the patient go home as soon as the exploration has been completed.

LIMITATIONS OF THE METHOD. This is undoubtedly a very useful exploratory procedure. Nevertheless, it has its limitations which prevent it from being applicable in every case.

It is contraindicated in: (1) adnexal as well as cervical and vulvovaginal acute infections; (2) space occupying lesions of Douglas' pouch: uterine tumors, ovarian tumors, extensive endometriosis, etc., or both active and residual inflammatory masses; (3) fixed retroversion of the uterus is an impediment; but not so mobile retroversion, which can be corrected in the knee-chest position. Other causes for contraindication are a Douglas' pouch hematocele and ectopic pregnancy, but not suspicion of uncomplicated ectopic pregnancy. Occasionally, too, Douglas' pouch may be blocked by loose adhesions in the form of a roof which go undetected during exploration but which make culdoscopy impossible; these are detected only in the course of the procedure if, after having performed a correct puncture, the pneumoperitoneum fails to develop.

In some cases, moreover, culdoscopy cannot be accomplished even though Douglas' pouch is free of obstacles because the peritoneum becomes detached from the vagina and is reflected ahead of the trocar and the optical instrument. This most often happens when the puncture site has been chosen too close to the uterine cervix (particularly by beginners, because of fear of puncturing the rectum). To avoid such a contingency, it is necessary to depress the perineum vigorously with the speculum and to place its tip as close to the sacrum as possible, then puncture away from the uterus. As already pointed out, we usually make a previous test run with the same needle that is used for anesthesia and with the syringe filled with air, by injecting some of the latter; thus the correct placing for the introduction of the trocar can be checked out.

It must also be stressed that culdoscopy is not a routine modality of exploration. Though it is relatively free of danger, it is not altogether harmless and, in addition, it constitutes an inconvenience to the patient. It must therefore be employed only when really necessary to clarify a diagnosis that otherwise would remain in doubt.

INDICATIONS. The main and most common indications, in our view, are:

1. A suspected adnexal infection the diagnosis of which cannot be arrived at by means of bimanual exploration, either because of adiposity or for other reasons. In our view, the most frequent indication for culdoscopy is pelvic pain, since quite often the diagnosis "nothing involving the genital apparatus" remains uncertain unless substantiated.

2. The differential diagnosis between a persistent follicle and other adnexal disturbances.

3. The study of the ovarian functional state, particularly as regards the presence or absence of corpora lutea.

4. The differential diagnosis between appendicitis and adnexitis.

5. Suspected endometriosis.

6. Suspected uncomplicated ectopic pregnancy.

7. Investigation of tubal permeability whenever the presence of a dye injected into the uterine cavity must be verified at the ampullary end of the tube (but this is not the most appropriate method available for this purpose).

USE OF CULDOSCOPY IN THE DIAGNOSIS OF ENDOCRINE GYNECOPATHY. In the field of endocrinology, culdoscopy has concrete applications, as mentioned above. It facilitates visualization of the ovaries and helps to establish a diagnosis as to the *functional state* of the ovary. The findings of endocrine interest in the ovary are, first, the presence of more or less mature follicles, second, the presence of a corpus luteum and, third, the appearance of persistent follicles, polymicrocystic ovaries or ovarian tumors.

Whenever culdoscopy is performed during the second half of the cycle, the presence of a corpus luteum should be verifiable; if no corpus luteum is found, an *anovulatory cycle* can be suspected. With this method, anovulation can be diagnosed with greater dependability than on the basis of endometrial curettings, since diagnosis with the latter is confined to determining the presence of a monophasic cycle, which can equally well occur in the presence of ovulation either because of failure of a corpus luteum to be formed (aluteinic ovulatory cycle) or, more likely, because the endometrial response to ovarian hormones is deficient. In contrast, direct examination of the ovary by means of culdoscopy precludes such equivocal findings. In the presence of a corpus luteum, there is no doubt that ovulation has taken place, more convincingly so if culdoscopy done shortly after ovulation still reveals a recognizable ovulatory stoma.

Nevertheless, what appears to be a clearcut matter may not always be so. A corpus luteum may not always be discernible by culdoscopy. On the one hand, it may be imperceivable because it is located in some part of the ovary that happens to face the parietal peritoneum opposite the ovarian surface visualized by the endoscope; on the other hand, even well formed corpora lutea may not be readily visible on the ovarian surface, particularly if culdoscopy is done during the third week of the cycle. It has been our experience that the more advanced the cycle, the more pigmented the corpus luteum becomes and the more visible it is against the background of the ovarian surface. Older corpora lutea therefore can be more readily visualized, which for practical purposes means that premenstrual culdoscopy, performed, say, between the twenty-third and twenty-seventh days, offers a far better chance for distinctly recognizing the presence of a corpus luteum.

Senarclens[36] performed routine culdoscopy on women he studied by means of both cytology and hormone assay. In his view, the exact stages of the patient's ovarian cycle cannot be assessed by means of culdoscopy in every case. When we compare the data obtained by culdoscopy with those obtained by biopsy or by pregnanediol determinations, the functional value of the latter two methods may be concluded to be superior to that of culdoscopy.

At our clinic,[10, 40] 47 apparently normal women with regular menstrual periods have been studied in a systematic manner. The following concomitant tests were performed on those 47 women: determination of urinary pregnanediol values, study of vaginal cytology, endometrial curettage supplemented by a number of histochemical stains, and culdoscopy. The results can be seen in Table 23–1.

Our studies concerning the potentialities of culdoscopy for the functional diagnosis have aroused considerable interest. Cohen[13] and Clyman,[12] as well as Palmer and De Brux,[31] have repeated these observations on a larger series of patients. Their results agree with those obtained by us. For all its apparent objectivity, culdoscopy frequently fails to establish the presence of a corpus luteum which in effect is there and is overlooked. This almost invariably is because in such cases the corpus luteum is located on the "eclipsed" face of the ovary. *Culdoscopy is limited to revealing only what the ovary can reveal of the surface that is visible.*

As shown in Table 23–1, the various exploratory methods do not correlate with each other in absolute terms. Endometrial curettage and cytology are the methods whose results are most consistently in agreement. Chemically determined pregnanediol levels correlate in a lesser number of cases, whereas culdoscopy only correlates in 36.3 per cent of the cases with results of curettage and cytology. Consequently, culdoscopy cannot be considered to be equally valuable in every case, which is the consensus reached at the symposium on endoscopy in 1964.[40]

Nevertheless, the variety of concrete and positive data it can reveal is of such magnitude that application of culdoscopy be-

TABLE 23–1. Correlation Between Celioscopic Exploration and Other Means of Assessing the Functional Condition of the Ovary*

	CELIOSCOPIC FINDINGS IN WOMEN WITH NORMAL OR APPARENTLY NORMAL CYCLES						
Day of Cycle	No. of Cases	Vaginal Cytology	Pregnanediol (24 hrs)	Basal Temperature	Celioscopy		Laparotomy
10–14	18	Estrogenic 10 Inconclusive 7	Negative 10 <5 mg. 5 >5 mg. 5	Low 16 Elevated 2	C.L. −17 C.L. +1 FOL. +15 FOL. −3		In three cases, evidence of recent ovulation with corpus luteum
21–24	29	Estrogenic 7 Folded 20 Inconclusive 2	Negative 10 <5 mg 8 >5 mg 16	Low 3 Elevated 21 Inconclusive 5	C.L. −9 C.L. +20 FOL. +7 FOL. −22		In three cases, evidence of anovulatory cycle

PERCENTAGES OF CORRELATION AND DISCREPANCY WITH DIFFERENT METHODS OF EXPLORATION†										
Endometrial Phase	No. of Cases	Vaginal Cytology		Pregnanediol (24 hrs)		Basal Temperature		Celioscopy		Laparotomy	
		C	D	C	D	C	D	C	D	C	D
Secretory	43	32	11	29	14	30	13	28	15	40	3
Proliferative	17	12	5	11	6	10	7	12	5	17	0
Total	60	4	15	40	20	40	20	40	20	70	3
Percentage of error		26.6		33.3		33.3		33.3			

*From J. Botella-Llusiá and S. Dexeus: *Actas del symposium internacional sobre la endoscopia ginecológica.* Palermo, Italy, November 14, 1964.
†C, Correlation; D, discrepancy.

comes a necessity in many cases of female endocrinopathy.

23.6.2. TRANSABDOMINAL CELIOSCOPY

Transabdominal celioscopy had been employed before culdoscopy was introduced. It was subsequently eclipsed by the transvaginal approach, but has lately regained the favor of many workers (Albano and Cittadini,[2] Palmer,[28,30] Thomsen[43] and Thoyer-Rozat[44]). Its main advantage would seem to consist in permitting a wider "panoramic" view of the genital tract and in offering a cleaner endoscopic image. It has an additional advantage in that it can be performed under general anesthesia, which is rendered difficult by the knee-chest position mandatory for culdoscopy.[40]

The performance of this modality of celioscopy requires the institution of a pneumoperitoneum at positive pressure, usually by means of carbon dioxide, known for its rapid rate of reabsorption.

Further progress has been achieved with the introduction of an endoscope for both the transabdominal and transvaginal approaches, provided with an extraabdominal quartz light source. By virtue of the better panoramic view it offers, which we have already mentioned, the transabdominal technique has been made use of increasingly over the past few years (Figs. 23-9, 23-11 and 23-12).

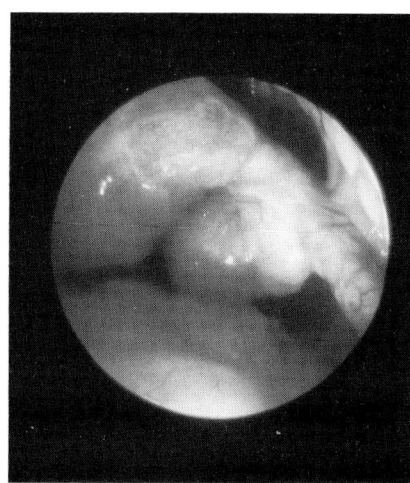

Figure 23-12. Ovary with corpus luteum obtained through transabdominal celioscopy. View corresponds to position II of the endoscope in Figure 23-9.

23.7. RADIOGRAPHIC EXPLORATION

Radiographic exploration certainly holds an important place in the study of sexual endocrinopathy. It comprises a series of diverse methods, each capable of yielding valuable data. These are: (1) hysterosalpingography; (2) gynecography; (3) radiographic exploration of the adrenals; (4) radiographic exploration of the pituitary; and (5) radiologic signs in certain endocrine gynecopathies.

23.7.1. HYSTEROSALPINGOGRAPHY

Hysterosalpingography is not an exploratory procedure of fundamental importance in gynecologic endocrinology, but it is of great value for the study of sterility and even in routine clinical gynecology. Nevertheless, certain data that can be obtained with it are of interest. For instance, the size of the uterine cavity can be estimated and from that the presence or absence of genital hypoplasia can be evaluated. Genital hypoplasia is known to be reflected by the presence of a uterine cervix disproportionately long in relation to the small uterine body.

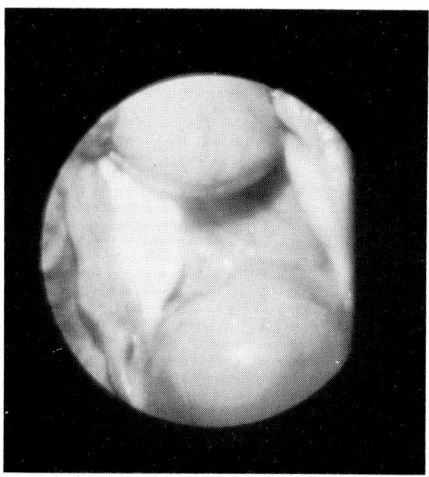

Figure 23-11. View obtained by transabdominal celioscopy revealing uterus, Fallopian tubes and normal ovaries. This view corresponds to position I of the endoscope in Figure 23-9.

Such altered proportions between the cervix and the uterine body can be readily recognized radiographically.[29] Similarly, any increase in size of the shadow of the uterine cavity can be monitored in the course of estrogen therapy in endocrinopathy. Finally, such other data concerning the Fallopian tube as displacement by an ovarian mass, etc., are also of interest, although they are of a secondary nature.

23.7.2. GYNECOGRAPHY

By the term gynecography, Stein[39] designated an exploratory procedure which consists in inducing a pneumoperitoneum with carbon dioxide in a woman in a forced knee-chest position. With or without the help of simultaneous hysterosalpingography (Figs. 23–13 and 23–15), this method may give quite distinct images, particularly as regards the contour of the uterus or that of the adnexa. The ovarian shadow can be visualized and it can be determined whether the ovaries are normal in size or enlarged (Fig. 23–14). The so-called Stein syndrome, consisting of enlarged polymicrocystic ovaries which, as shall be pointed out, are associated with certain endocrine alterations, can be diagnosed specifically with this method. It similarly facilitates the diagnosis of congenital ovarian atrophy (Turner's syndrome) (Kreel et al.[24]), streak ovaries, disjoined ovaries, persistent follicles and ovarian tumors.

23.7.3. PNEUMOKIDNEY

Exploration of any adrenal enlargement is of extraordinary importance in gynecologic endocrinology, since it may facilitate the diagnosis of adrenogenital syndrome. This procedure consists in injecting carbon dioxide into the perirenal compartment in order to obtain a roentgenographic outline of the triangular shadow of the adrenal. Such a pneumokidney may disclose the presence of cortical hyperplasia or tumors responsible for sexual symptomatology (viz., adrenogenital syndrome, Chapter 33).

23.7.4. ROENTGENOGRAPHIC EXPLORATION OF THE SELLA TURCICA

In some cases, roentgenographic exploration of the sella turcica is also of great interest. The sella turcica is increased in size as a result of tumors or of hyperplasia in cases of acromegaly. Considerable enlargement of the sella turcica may be observed in the syndrome of galactotropic hyperpituitarism, a typical endocrine genital syndrome. In contrast, a decrease in the size of the sella is typical of ovarian insufficiency of

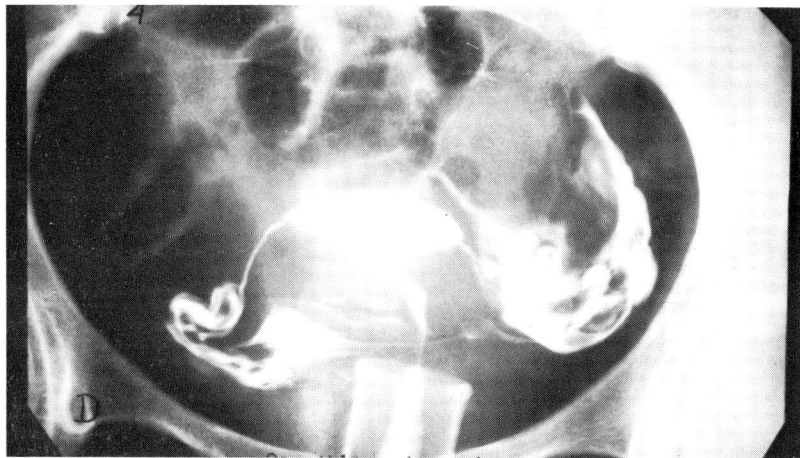

Figure 23–13. Hysterosalpingography in a case with normal uterus and tubes. Contrast medium filling both tubes is beginning to spill into peritoneal cavity, clearly outlining contour of both ovaries. Although this is not a direct endocrinologic type of exploratory procedure, one may obtain a number of indirect data of utmost endocrinologic interest.

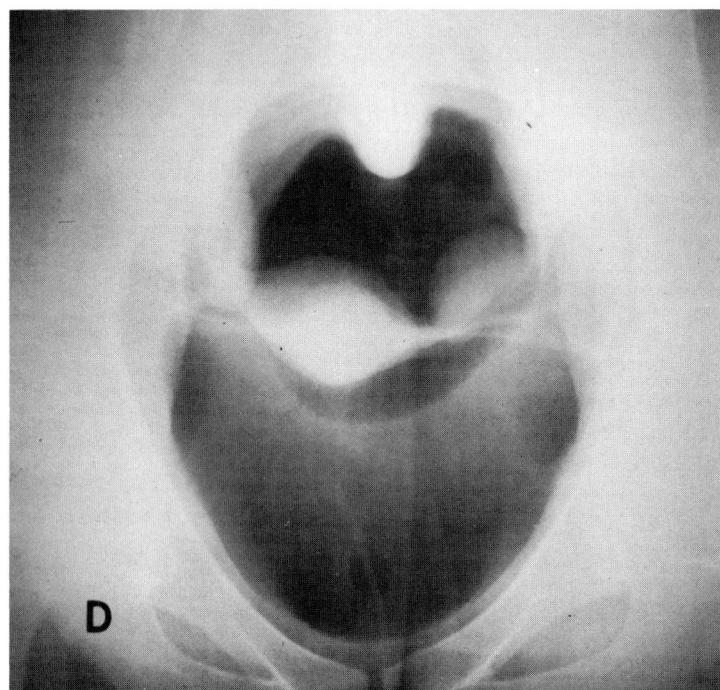

Figure 23-14. Gynecography, revealing contour of uterus and ovaries.

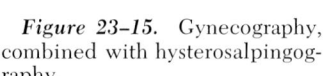

Figure 23-15. Gynecography, combined with hysterosalpingography.

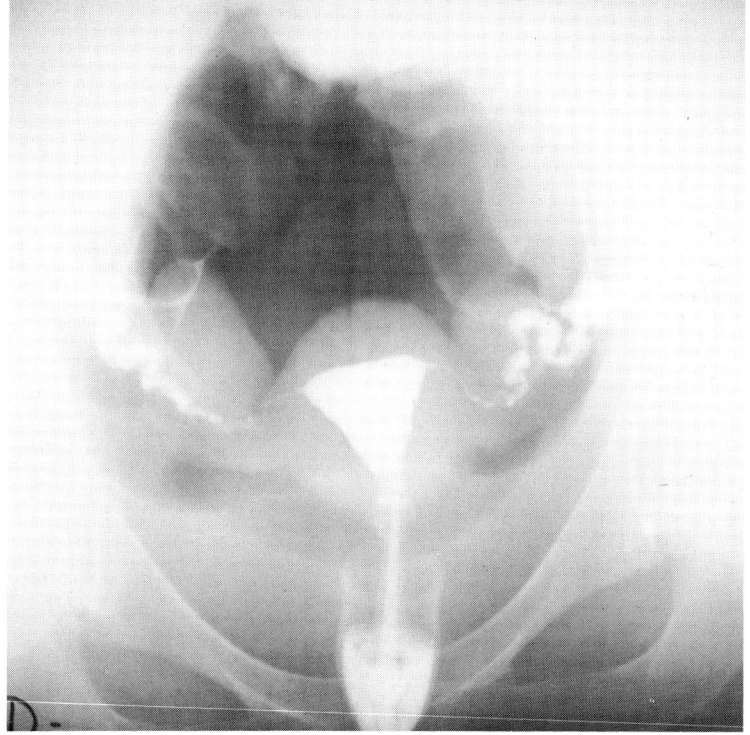

primary pituitary origin. Thus, primary hypoestrinism of pituitary origin is associated with a decreased size of the sella turcica which is characteristic enough to permit differentiation of this syndrome from that of ovarian insufficiency resulting from primary hypoplasia of the ovary (see Chapter 25).

23.7.5. RADIOLOGIC SIGNS IN SOME FORMS OF ENDOCRINE GYNECOPATHY

It would be beyond the scope of this book to examine the totality of skeletal signs appearing in all types of endocrinopathy, since even the most important ones pertaining to parathyroid pathology, dwarfism, gigantism, acromegaly, endocrine craniopathy and adrenal osteoporosis are too numerous to be described here. Nevertheless, it seems pertinent to insist on a number of special radiologic signs that should be explored in cases of *amenorrhea* insofar as these may reflect *gonadal dysgenesis* (see Chapter 27).

Although these are discussed in more detail elsewhere they may be briefly outlined here.

SIGN OF THE ANVIL-SHAPED TIBIA OF VAGUE,[46] also confirmed by Kosowicz,[22] which consists of a protruding medial tibial condyle, occasionally associated with exostosis that juts out over the diaphysis (Fig. 23-16).

SIGN OF THE FOURTH METACARPAL, described by Archibald and colleagues[3] and confirmed by Vague and associates,[7,48] which consists in a *shortening* of the fourth metacarpal bone so that a line drawn tangentially to the circumference of the heads of the fourth and fifth metacarpals, when extended, intersects the heads of the remaining metacarpal bones instead of passing distally to them as it does normally (Fig. 23-17).

SIGN OF THE CARPAL ANGLE OF KOSOWICZ.[23] This consists in a distal displacement of the pyramidal bone of the proximal carpal row, giving rise to a decreased angle of the ulno-radio-carpal joint line of less than 110 degrees as compared to 132 to 140 degrees normally (Fig. 23-18).

OSTEOPOROSIS. This condition occurs in postmenopausal women, described by Vanek,[49] which is also observed in primordial ovarian failure of all types.

Finally, there are a variety of roentgenographic data to which the reader is referred (Marañón,[25] Wilkins[51]).

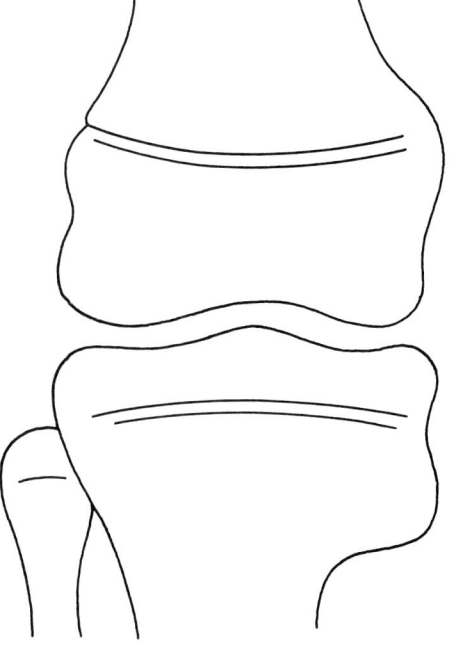

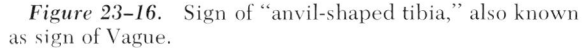
Figure 23–16. Sign of "anvil-shaped tibia," also known as sign of Vague.

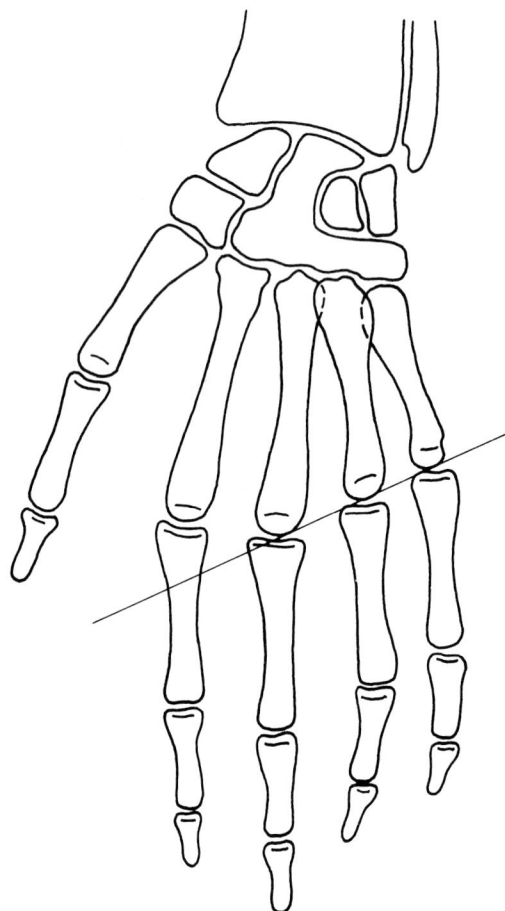

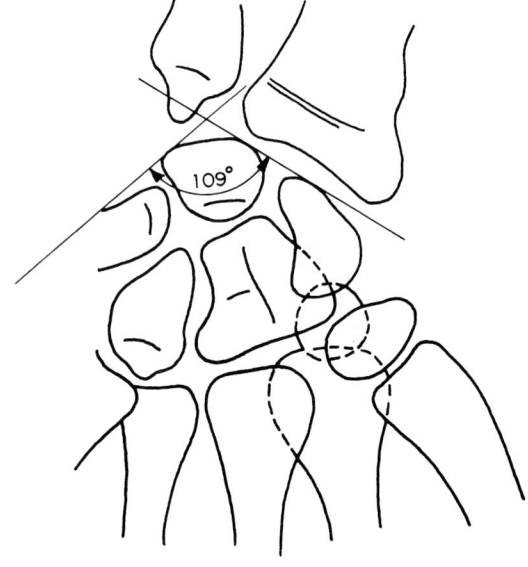

Figure 23-17. Sign of the short fourth metacarpal bone. A line drawn across the distal tips of the fifth and fourth metacarpal bones should not intersect the distal extremity of the third metacarpal and should cross the index finger at the level of the first interphalangeal joint.

Figure 23-18. Sign of the "carpal angle" of Kosowicz. Proximal displacement of the semilunar bone causes the carpal joint line of the wrist to form an angle of 100 to 110 degrees, whereas normally this angle should be at least 120 degrees.

REFERENCES

1. Abarbanel, A. R.: *Conferences du Congres Jubilaire International de Gynecologie*, Paris, 1951. Paris, L'Expansion Scientifique Française, 1951.
2. Albano, V., and Cittadini, E.: *La Celioscopia in Ginecologia*. Palermo, G. Denaro Editore, 1963.
3. Archibald, R. M., Finby, N., and De Vito, F.: *J. Clin. Endocr.*, 19:1312, 1959.
4. Beckmann, A.: *Ztschr. f. Tuberkulose*, 52:273, 1949.
5. Bedoya, J. M., and Maldonado, A.: *Acta Gin.*, 6:291, 1955.
6. Benedek, T., and Rubenstein, B. B.: *El Ciclo Sexual de la Mujer*. Buenos Aires, 1942.
7. Botella, J.: *Colloques sur la fonction luteale*, Vol. I. Paris, Masson & Cie., 1954.
8. Botella, J., Bedoya, J. M., and de la Fuente, F.: *Acta Gin.*, 3:481, 1952.
9. Botella, J., and Marín-Bonacher, E.: *Acta Gin.*, 4:29, 1956.
10. Botella, J., Caballero, A., Clavero, J. A., and Vilar, C. E.: *Esterilidad e infertilidad humanas*. Barcelona, Editorial Científico-Médica, 1967.
11. Campos da Paz, A.: *Amer. J. Obstet. Gynec.*, 61A:790, 1951.
12. Clyman, M.: *I. F. A. Panamerican Conference*, Miami, Jan. 14, 1960.
13. Cohen, M. R.: *Amer. J. Obstet. Gynec.*, 78:267, 1959.
14. Decker, A.: *Amer. J. Obstet. Gynec.*, 63:654, 1952.
15. Decker, A., and Decker, W. H.: *Practical Office Gynecology*. Philadelphia, F. A. Davis, 1956.
16. Decourt, J.: *Le morphogramme au cours de la puberté Femmine*, in *La Puberté et ses Troubles*. Paris, Masson & Cie., 1958.
17. Decourt, J., and Doumic, J. M.: *Sem. Hôp. Paris*, 26:2457, 1950.
18. Decourt, J., and Guinet, P.: *Les etats intersexuels*. Paris, Maloine, 1962.
19. Fuente, F. de la: *Actas de la Sociedad Española de Esterilidad*, 2:57, 1954.
20. Fuente, F. de la, and Gálvez, J.: *Actas de la Sociedad Española de Esterilidad*, 2:64, 1954.
21. Grünberger, V., and Holkup, H.: *Arch. Gynäk.*, 182:263, 1953.
22. Kosowicz, J.: *Acta Endocr.*, 31:321, 1959.
23. Kosowicz, J.: *J. Clin. Endocr.*, 22:949, 1962.
24. Kreel, L., Ginsburgh, J., and Green, M. F.: *Brit. Med. J.*, 1:682, 1969.
25. Marañón, G.: *El Crecimiento y sus Trastornos*. Madrid, Espasa Calpe, 1953.
26. Nicolino, J., Anselmi, E., and Vague, J.: *Sem. Hôp. Paris*, 36:2565, 1960.
27. Nogales, F., and Botella, J.: *Actas de la Sociedad Española de Esterilidad*, 3:126, 1955.
28. Palmer, R., and Palmer, E.: *Les Explorations Fonctionnelles Ginecologigues*. Paris, Masson & Cie., 1963.
29. Palmer, R., Cherigie, G., and Pulsford, J.: *Ann. Ost. Ginec. (Milan)*, 81:59, 1959.
30. Palmer, R.: *Bull. Acad. Chir.*, 86:659, 1960.
31. Palmer, R., and De Brux, J.: *Bull. Fed. Soc. Obstet. Gynec. L. Franç.*, 19:405, 1965.
32. Peralta Ramos, A. G.: *Amer. J. Obstet. Gynec.*, 61A:356, 1951.
33. Pommerenke, V. T.: *Amer. J. Obstet. Gynec.*, 52:1023, 1946.
34. Roland, M.: *Obstet. Gynec.*, 11:38, 1958.
35. Rydberg, E.: *Acta Obstet. Gynec. Scand.*, 28:172, 1948.
36. Senarclens, R. de: *Colloques sur la fonction luteale*, Vol. I. Paris, Masson & Cie., 1954.
37. Sjövall, A.: *Acta Obstet. Gynec. Scand.*, 30:288, 1950.
38. Sol, J. R. del, and Merlo, J. G.: *Acta Gin.*, 3:533, 1952.
39. Stein, I. F.: *Gynecography*, in *Progress in Gynecology*, ed. Sturgis-Meigs, 2nd ed. New York, Grune & Stratton, 1951.
40. Symposium Internacional sobre la Endoscopia Ginecológica, Palermo, Nov. 15, 1964.
41. Te Linde, R., and Rutledge, F.: *Amer. J. Obstet. Gynec.*, 55:102, 1948.
42. Teton, J. B.: *Amer. J. Obstet. Gynec.*, 60:665, 1950.
43. Thomsen, K.: *Geburtsh. u. Frauenhk.*, 11:587, 1951.
44. Thoyer-Rozat, J.: *La Coelioscope, Technique et Indications*. Paris, Masson & Cie., 1962.
45. Urdan, B. E., and Kurzon, A. M.: *Obstet. Gynec.*, 5:3, 1955.
46. Vague, J.: *La differentiation sexuelle et ses troubles*. Paris, Masson & Cie., 1953.
47. Vague, J., Nicolino, J., and Anselmi, E.: *Ann. d'Endocr.*, 22:40, 1961.
48. Vague, J., and Nicolino, J.: *Ann. d'Endocr.*, 24:482, 1963.
49. Vanek, R.: *Ann. d'Endocr.*, 21:899, 1960.
50. Vokaer, R.: *La fonction ovarienne et son exploration*. Paris, Masson & Cie., 1956.
51. Wilkins, L.: *The Diagnosis and Treatment of Endocrine Disorders in Childhood and Adolescence*. Springfield, Ill., Charles C Thomas, 1957.
52. Williams, W. W.: *Sterility*, 3rd ed. Springfield, Ill., Charles C Thomas, 1964.

Chapter 24

HORMONE ASSAY

The purpose of this chapter is limited to serving as a mere technical aid. It pretends in no way to be a summary of all currently available methods of hormone assay, nor is it designed to be a treatise on either the principles involved or the interpretation of the various types of hormone assay. It is intended solely to present a list of those methods which we believe can be recommended on account of their dependability and easy performance with regard to both diagnosis and research.

Two groups of new techniques have come to revolutionize the field of hormone assay: (1) *radioimmunoassay,* and (2) procedures devised to determine the specific binding proteins or *competing proteins.* Our experience with these new methods, with the exception of those estimating insulin, growth hormone and placental lactogen, has been limited and we shall therefore confine ourselves to only listing them briefly here.

24.1. CHEMICAL METHODS OF ESTIMATING URINARY STEROIDS

24.1.1. INTRODUCTION

Determination of steroids in urine and in other body fluids is based on two types of reactions: *group reactions,* that is, reactions given by the molecule as a whole, and *side chain reactions.* For instance, *estrogens* whose molecules possess a phenol ring give the so-called *phenolsteroid* reaction, based either on the Kober reagent or on special fluorescence induced with sulfuric acid. These reactions pertain to the molecule as a whole. In contrast, the reactions given by *pregnanediol* or by *corticoids* are determined by side chains. Thus, the ketoalcohol side chain at carbon 21 of corticoids can be degraded by periodic acid treatment to give formaldehyde and 17-ketosteroids. The resulting corticoids are known as *formaldehydogenic corticoids.* This is a typical side chain reaction. With other procedures, the oxygen of the ketone group at carbon 3 can be reduced; in such reactions, phosphomolybdic acid is reduced and corticoids are then estimated on the basis of the corticoid reducing capacity of the group on carbon atom 3. Thus, what is assayed in one type of reaction is the presence of the side chain, and in the other, the molecule as a whole. Neither type of reaction is entirely specific. Reactions in which the entire molecule is determined, such as is the case with *phenolsteroids,* are reactions which, to a greater or lesser extent, are associated with all of the unsaturated aromatic ring structures. On the other hand, side chain reactions may be observed with any group of molecules possessing similar side chains, e.g., any alcohol-ketone group can give the formaldehyde reaction. For this reason, the chemical methods upon which estimation of these hormones is based are *methods of limited specificity.* A higher degree of specificity is achieved by fractionation of urine and, following extraction, by further purification of the compounds to be estimated. For instance, corticoids are extracted after hydrolysis of urine and are fractionated by means of different procedures, using various solvents. As a result of this, a corticoid extract is obtained in which, *by virtue of the fact that it contains no compounds other than corticoids, the previously nonspecific reaction given by mixtures of organic compounds is converted to a specific reaction.*

Estrogens are assayed by means of hydrolysis plus extraction procedures, by which estrogens are separated from the rest of neutral steroids. A total estrogen extract is thus obtained, which can be titrated directly as a fraction by itself, referred to as "phenolsteroids" by, among others, Jayle and his colleagues.[49, 50] This total fraction can be further broken down into its three components, estrone, estradiol and estriol, each then being estimated independently. Quantitative estimation of either the total phenolsteroids or the three component fractions can be done by means of any of the following three methods: (1) colorimetry, based on the Kober reaction or on some similar reaction; (2) fluorimetry, based on fluorescence elicited from this type of compound by sulfuric or phosphoric acid; (3) spectrophotometry in the ultraviolet light range. In UV light, the absorption spectrum of these compounds displays a characteristic low in the 248 to 252 millimicron range and a characteristic absorption peak at 280 to 282 millimicrons, which are sufficiently distinctive for their identification.

Pregnanediol determinations are also based on extraction and fractionation using different solvents and by isolating a *glucuronic complex* through precipitation with barium chloride. Pregnanediol obtained through these methods is measured by means of weighing the precipitate, which has a characteristic melting point. Other methods for pregnanediol consist of acid hydrolysis followed by extraction of free pregnanediol with various solvents. Instead of the glucuronic complex, these methods lead to isolation of *free pregnanediol*. The latter can be precipitated and weighed, or can be measured colorimetrically by virtue of the yellowish-brown color complex it develops in the presence of sulfuric acid (Astwood reaction, Guterman reaction or Botella-Tornero reaction). Finally, free pregnanediol, obtained through acid hydrolysis and extraction, can be separated by means of column chromatography and subsequently determined either gravimetrically or colorimetrically. Similar principles are utilized in all the various methods currently employed for the determination of pregnanediol.

Free progesterone in urine and blood has recently been determined by Zander, using an original method. This method is based on extraction and fractionation with various solvents, followed by paper chromatography and by characterization of the chromatographically isolated compounds by means of photometry in the UV light range. The compounds thus characterized can be estimated quantitatively by ultraviolet spectrophotometry; finally, characterization of progesterone can be accomplished either by means of fluorescent color reactions or by spectrophotometry with infrared light. The last mentioned method was described by Zander and Simmer[117] in 1954.

17-Ketosteroids are determined by means of the *Zimmermann reaction*,[118] using metadinitrobenzene in almost all procedures. Following acid hydrolysis, the extraction procedure is carried out with carbon tetrachloride and the extract thus obtained is allowed to react with metadinitrobenzene in the presence of alkali. The resulting color reaction is measured colorimetrically in the 5200 Angstrom range.

24.1.2. DETERMINATION OF URINARY ESTROGENS, ACCORDING TO BROWN[16]

This method, described in 1955, allows separate determination of the three fractions (estradiol, estrone and estriol) in the low concentrations they are generally found in the urine of men and nonpregnant women. This method has been successful and has found universal acceptance.

PRINCIPLE INVOLVED. The Brown method consists in extracting estrogens by means of methylation, followed by chromatographic separation on alumina columns, elution, and colorimetric measurement using a modified Kober color method.

Reagents and Materials

(a) **REAGENTS.** *Ether*, washed with saturated $FeSO_4$ and distilled water, stored in dark bottles, and used within 24 hours of purification.

Petroleum ether (boiling point at 40 to 60° C) and *benzene*, redistilled and saturated with distilled water.

Ethanol (absolute), boiled and refluxed in the presence of NaOH pellets to remove aldehydes.

Boric acid (chemically pure); *dimethyl sulfate*, redistilled; *8 per cent $NaHCO_3$ solution in 20 per cent NaOH.*

Alumina (Savory & Moore, Ltd., London)

of mesh size 100/150 and activity II-III, deactivated with 9 to 10 per cent water to the activity specified later.

(b) COLOR REAGENTS. The estriol color reagent is prepared by dissolving *quinol* (20 g) in 1000 ml of 76 per cent (v/v) H_2SO_4, the estrone reagent by dissolving quinol (20 g) in 1000 ml of 66 per cent (v/v) H_2SO_4, and the estradiol reagent by dissolving quinol similarly in 60 per cent (v/v) H_2SO_4. The reagents should be used within 24 hours of preparation.

(c) STANDARD ESTROGEN SOLUTIONS. These are prepared in ethanol (5 mg/100 ml). Solutions are stored at 4° C and are stable indefinitely.

(d) APPARATUS. All glassware must be washed in distilled water, then in a chromic acid mixture, which must be rinsed off in running tap water, then with distilled water and finally with sodium sulfite to destroy traces of chromic acid, which would otherwise alter the results of the method, rinsing again with tap water and then with distilled water.

The spectrophotometer employed by Brown was a UNICAM S.P. 600 with 1 ml cuvettes. A Beckmann D.U., or any comparable model, can be used instead.

TECHNIQUE. The very exacting and complicated technique, described in a summary fashion, requires considerable training for trouble-free execution.

(a) COLLECTION OF URINE SPECIMENS. At least two or three determinations, each run in duplicate, should be performed at one time. Twenty-four hour specimens of urine are collected without preservative and stored in the refrigerator at 4° C. If the 24 hr volume is less than 1200 ml, the speci-

TABLE 24–1. Separation of Estrone, Estriol and Estradiol in the Form of Methyl Ethers by the Method of Brown

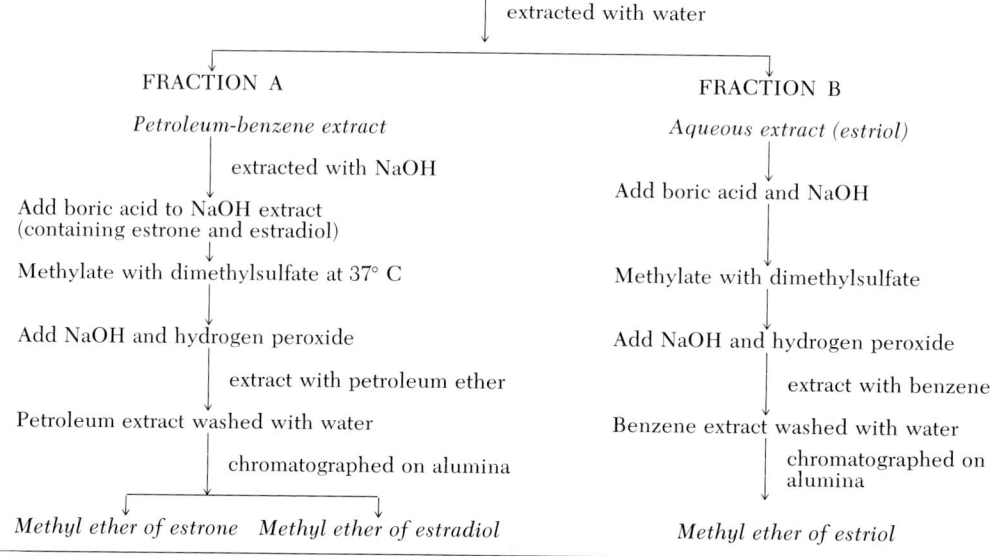

men is diluted to this volume with distilled water.

(b) HYDROLYSIS AND EXTRACTION. The flow sheet for the extraction is shown in Table 24–1. Part of the urine sample (200 ml) is placed in a reflux condensor with 30 ml of concentrated HCl (11 N) and the mixture is boiled for 60 minutes, then cooled abruptly under running tap water. The cooled mixture is extracted once with 200 ml and twice with 100 ml volumes of ether. The ether is then extracted with concentrated sodium carbonate solution, of pH 10.5, and then shaken thoroughly with 20 ml of 8 per cent NaOH. The carbonate layer is discarded but the NaOH layer is reserved and is neutralized with 80 ml of 8 per cent sodium bicarbonate to pH 10. The aqueous layer is then discarded. The ether layer is washed again with 20 ml of 8 per cent sodium bicarbonate and subsequently with 10 ml distilled water. After that, the water is drained off as completely as possible.

(c) EXTRACTION OF THE PHENOL FRACTION AND METHYLATION. The ether solution is evaporated to dryness in a water bath. The residue is dissolved in 1 ml ethanol and cooled. Benzene (25 ml) is added and the mixture is poured into a separating funnel containing petroleum ether. This solution is extracted with 25 ml volumes of water and then with 25 ml volumes of 1.6 per cent NaOH.

The *water extracts*, which contain the *estriol* fraction, are transferred into a stoppered Erlenmeyer flask containing 0.9 g of boric acid and 4 ml of 20 per cent NaOH.

The *NaOH extracts*, which contain the *estrone* and *estradiol* fractions, are added to a similar flask containing only 0.9 g boric acid. The two flasks are placed in a 37° C water bath and 1 ml dimethylsulfate is added to each. The dimethylsulfate must be handled *with extreme caution*, under a fume hood and by means of a *safety pipette*. The Erlenmeyer flasks are shaken until the solute dissolves completely and are kept at 37° C for 30 minutes. The procedure is repeated by adding 1 ml more dimethylsulfate, together with 2 ml 20 per cent NaOH to replace the alkali neutralized by the first 1 ml addition of dimethylsulfate. The flasks are shaken until all dimethylsulfate has dissolved; they are kept at 37° C for another 30 minutes and then are allowed to stand at room temperature overnight.

(d) REMOVAL OF IMPURITIES AND EXTRACTION OF METHYLATED ESTROGENS. Ten milliliters of 20 per cent NaOH and 2.5 ml of 30 per cent hydrogen peroxide are added to each Erlenmeyer flask, the contents of which are transferred to separatory funnels. The estrone-estradiol fraction (fraction A) is extracted with 25 ml of petroleum ether, and the estriol fraction (fraction B) is extracted with 25 ml of benzene. Both extracts are washed twice with 5 ml volumes of distilled water, and the water is drained off as completely as possible.

(e) CHROMATOGRAPHY. The column chromatography tubes must have an internal diameter of 13 mm, a capacity of 40 ml and a porous glass support (porosity No. 3) for the alumina column, and an interchangeable B-19 cone for connection with receiving flasks or tubes. Chromatograms are run in batches of six. The rate of flow of solvents must be adjusted to 1 drop/ 2 seconds (30 drops per minute). The column is prepared by partly filling the tube with benzene and adding 2 g of standardized alumina. The estriol fraction is applied to an alumina column prepared in benzene, whereas the estrone-estradiol fractions are applied to columns prepared in petroleum ether.

The *elution* is performed in the following manner:

Column A (Estrone-Estradiol)

(A) 12 ml of a mixture of 25 per cent benzene in petroleum ether.

(B) 15 ml of a mixture of 40 per cent benzene in petroleum ether.

(C) 12 ml of the same mixture of 40 per cent petroleum ether.

(D) 12 ml of pure benzene.

Column B (Estriol)

(A) 12 ml of a mixture of 1.4 per cent ethanol in benzene.

(B) 15 ml of a 2.5 per cent ethanol solution in benzene.

(f) ELUTION OF THE COLUMN. Details pertaining to the standardization of the alumina can be found in the original publication by Brown.[16] Provided the column is prepared well and the activity of the alumina is correct, estrone methyl ether begins to appear at the level of 16 to 20 ml of eluate. The estradiol must be recovered in the first 10 ml from the same column. Finally, estriol is eluted in the first 12 ml from column B.

(g) COLOR REACTION. Three milliliters

of the quinol reagent (see *Reagents*) are added to the estrogen fractions in Kober tubes, which are then heated for 30 minutes in a water bath. The tubes are shaken intermittently. They are then cooled in a bath of cold water and 1 ml of distilled water is added to each estriol tube, 0.5 ml to each estrone tube and 0.2 ml to each estradiol tube.

The tubes are shaken and reheated in the boiling water bath for 10 minutes. They are then cooled again as before and optical densities are read in the spectrophotometer at the following wavelengths:

Estrone and estriol = 480, 516 and 552 mμ
Estradiol = 480, 518 and 556 mμ

24.1.3. DETERMINATION OF URINARY ESTROGENS, ACCORDING TO ITTRICH[47]

The main drawback complicating estimation of estrogens is caused by the *presence of interfering chromogens*. The original methods of Jayle and his associates[49] and of Stevenson and Marrian[105] were beset with this problem. Brown's method, which has just been described, largely does away with this cause of error, which has been eliminated in the recent modifications by Hashimoto and Neeman[41] and by Schild.[99] But it is above all the technique proposed by Ittrich[47] which in a simple and reliable way estimates both total and fractional estrogen values in biologic specimens without the errors induced by the chromogenic supplement. The technique used by us is the original one, as it was described by the author in 1960, though important modifications have since been introduced by the application of *fluorimetry* (Roy,[94] Stoa and Thorsen[106]).

Principle Involved

The method employs a modified Kober reagent, and the color complex is extracted with a mixture of p-nitrophenol and chloroform. Values are read fluorimetrically for greater sensitivity, and a procedure of microextraction and hydrolysis renders the method suitable for work in the micromethod range.

Reagents

(a) ETHER, CHEMICALLY PURE, prepared in the same manner as in Brown's method (see page 507).

(b) PETROLEUM ETHER, of same specifications as in Brown's method.

(c) ETHANOL, ABSOLUTE, boiled with NaOH pellets and zinc powder in a reflux condenser.

(d) CHLOROFORM (analytic grade), thoroughly washed with water, desiccated over calcium chloride, filtered and distilled. One milliliter ethanol (solution c) is then added to each 100 ml. Store in dark bottle in cool place.

(e) SODIUM BICARBONATE, 8 per cent solution, as in Brown's method.

(f) HYDROQUINONE REAGENT. Concentrated H_2SO_4 (52 volumes for estrone and estradiol; 68 volumes for estriol) is added to 100 ml graduated flasks to complementary amounts of distilled water (extreme caution must be exerted in this procedure); 2 g hydroquinone is then added.

(g) PARA-NITROPHENOL SOLUTION. Two grams of para-nitrophenol (analytic grade) is dissolved in 100 ml chloroform and 1 ml ethanol (solution c) is added.

(h) STANDARD SOLUTIONS. Standardized solutions of crystallized estrogens are prepared by dissolving 1 mg of the corresponding hormone in 100 ml ethanol (solution c).

Technique in Urine Specimens

(a) EXTRACTION AND PURIFICATION

Hydrolysis. Ten milliliters of urine and 1.5 ml of concentrated HCl are boiled for 1 hour at 100° C, then cooled in a refrigerator.

Extraction. Extract by shaking in a separating funnel three consecutive times: first with 10 ml, second and third times with 5 ml volumes of ethyl ether.

Purification. Four milliliters of 8 per cent sodium bicarbonate and NaOH of pH 10.5 are added, then 3 ml of 8 per cent sodium carbonate. Mixtures are then washed twice with 2 ml distilled water.

Distillation of ether. The mixture is placed into the still with a sand bath and an electric heater and is distilled until the residue has separated.

Separation of the phenol fraction. The residue is dissolved in 5 ml benzol and 5 ml petroleum ether.

Extraction. Four, 3 and 2 ml of 1 per cent NaOH are added successively and the mixtures are shaken. The NaOH is neutralized by adding 1 ml of concentrated HCl for each 4.5 ml of alkali. Three additional extractions with 10, 5 and 2 ml volumes of ethanol follow.

The *residue is washed* three times with 2 ml volumes of distilled water.

After *evaporation in a vacuum*, the dried residue is ready for chromatographic estimation.

(b) CHROMATOGRAPHY

Composition of the column. Three grams of aluminum oxide, dissolved in equal volumes of benzol and carbon tetrachloride.

Elution. (1) Five milliliters of carbon tetrachloride, 5 ml benzol and 9 ml of 0.8 per cent solution of ethanol in benzol to eliminate impurities; (2) 10 ml of 0.8 per cent solution of ethanol in benzol = *estrone*; (3) 10 ml of 3 per cent solution of ethanol in benzol = *estradiol*; (4) 12 ml of 20 per cent solution of ethanol in benzol, plus 1 ml water = *estriol*.

(c) COLOR REACTION

The product of elution is *desiccated* in each of the three fractions b, c and d. Fraction a is discarded.

(d) MODIFIED KOBER REACTION

One milliliter *hydroquinone reagent* (solution f, page 510) is *added* to residue and kept in a boiling water bath at 100° C for 40 minutes and then cooled in ice for 3 minutes. Distilled water (1.4 ml) is added, remaining unmixed as a surface layer, and the solution is refrigerated for 5 minutes, shaken for 20 seconds and again refrigerated for 3 minutes. Two milliliters of the para-nitrophenol solution is then added (which, without mixing, settles at the bottom); this is followed by 3 minutes of refrigeration on ice, shaking for 20 seconds and centrifugation for 2 minutes, with separation of the upper phase.

Tubes are then *stored* on ice and in the dark prior to reading.

Spectrophotometry is performed at 500, 538 and 577 mµ wavelengths.

Preparation of standard curves. As with Brown's modality, these are prepared according to Allen's method.[5]

Readings can be taken either colorimetrically or fluorimetrically; the latter method is especially recommended because of its great accuracy.

24.1.4. ESTIMATION OF URINARY PREGNANEDIOL: OLD METHODS

Over the past 20 years, a large number of methods have been developed for the estimation of urinary pregnanediol. The principle involved in most of these is almost identical. The most commonly known methods are:

1. The original Venning-Browne gravimetric method in which, following extraction with butanol, the total complex of 21-glucuronates is precipitated.

2. The method of Allen,[5] a modification of the preceding one, in which the glucuronate complex is determined by colorimetric means.

3. A further gravimetric modification of the original method, developed by Kaufman and his associates,[61] which eliminates 20-ketosteroids from the glucuronic complex.

4. The method of Astwood and Jones, in which free pregnanediol is extracted by means of acid hydrolysis without esterification of glucuronic acid. This is an original but equally gravimetric method.

5. Guterman[39] discovered that free pregnanediol obtained through acid hydrolysis developed a characteristic yellow color with sulfuric acid, on which he based a simple qualitative method.

6. Guterman's qualitative method was subsequently adapted for quantitative measurements by Kullander[63] and by Botella and Tornero,[10] through estimating the resulting color complex photometrically. However, the method yields only approximate values since results comprise a considerable amount of nonspecific chromogens (up to 20 per cent, in our own experience).

7. After working extensively on the principle of acid hydrolysis, Marrian and his colleagues[73] have created a new method based on that principle. The procedure of Watteville and his associates[114] is similarly based on this principle, and so is Carda-Aparici's modification of the method (described later), which is recommended for its accuracy and simplicity.

8. Elberlein and Bongiovanni[28] have perfected a *paper chromatographic* method, suitable for research, the technique of which is described on the following pages.

Of all the up-to-date methods that have

been used for the determination of urinary pregnanediol, we recommend two, one for routine clinical work, the second for research, which we shall describe in detail later in this chapter.

24.1.5. CHROMATOGRAPHIC DETERMINATION OF PREGNANEDIOL, ACCORDING TO TOLLER AND CARDA

Principle Involved. Huber was first to introduce a modification as fundamental as column chromatography to existing methods for the determination of urinary pregnanediol; this was designed to yield pregnanediol in crystalline form. By and large, simple gravimetric determination of the crystals is a more accurate procedure than photocolorimetry. The method of Guterman and its modifications are adequate insofar as the techniques of extraction and subsequent removal of acids and phenol are concerned, but isolation and purification of pregnanediol can be performed more efficiently by means of chromatographic adsorption using an aluminum oxide column, which secures a larger yield of pregnanediol in pure crystalline form.

Watteville and his co-workers[114] introduced certain modifications into Huber's method and developed their well-known technique of chromatographic adsorption, which has currently gained wide acceptance. Toller later simplified the methods of Huber and Watteville considerably; Carda, in Spain, adapted the method in the following form:

Technique

(a) COLLECTION OF URINE SPECIMENS. As specified in previous methods.

(b) HYDROLYSIS AND EXTRACTION OF URINE. The entire 24 hr specimen of urine, or a filtered aliquot volume thereof, is poured into an Erlenmeyer flask with 50 ml of pure toluene. To minimize the hazards of the high flammability of toluene, the mixture is heated on an electric plate provided with a sand bath and a reflux cooling system. As soon as the boiling point is reached, concentrated HCl (analytic grade) is added in 1 ml volumes for each 10 ml of urine, and the mixture is boiled for 15 minutes in order to hydrolyze and extract the pregnanediol glucuronidate. The flask is then cooled under running tap water for 10 minutes.

After adding toluene and shaking the flask vigorously, the mixture is transferred to a cylindrical separating funnel with an upper stoppered opening. The residue remaining in the Erlenmeyer flask is washed twice with toluene to recover any trace of pregnanediol. Since two 10 ml volumes of toluene are used each time, the total volume of solvent in the funnel rises to 70 ml. The mixture is allowed to stand and the urine in the lower layer is decanted, so that the toluene separated from the urine remains in the separatory funnel. Ten grams of NaOH pellets are then added and the mixture is shaken energetically 50 to 60 times, then filtered through Schleicher paper No. 597. The funnel and filter are once more washed with 15 ml toluene each, as a result of which the total volume of toluene employed amounts to 100 ml. The filtrate is collected in an Erlenmeyer flask.

Ten milliliters of 2 per cent NaOH in methanol are now added, and the contents brought to boil over an electric plate and sand bath until they are reduced in volume to approximately 10 ml. The NaOH solution in methanol can be stored for up to a month in the refrigerator but only for 15 days at room temperature.

(c) CHROMATOGRAPHY AND ELUTION. A column is prepared with aluminum oxide, according to Brockman's method, 1 to 2 cm in height, using a buret or pipette, into which are laid first a cotton layer, then the aluminum oxide with benzene (as vehicle that is allowed to drain off), and two or three circles of filter paper adapted to the inside of the buret. The concentrated toluene filtrate with the added NaOH-methanol solution is filtered and allowed to percolate down the column. The pregnanediol content from the toluene extract remains adsorbed to the column, imparting to it an orange color. A few other steroid contaminants, as well as cholesterol, are also retained.

The column is then washed with pure benzene to dissolve any impurities of this type. For this purpose, it is enough to add 10 ml of benzene to the column.

The pregnanediol adsorbed to the column is eluted with a mixture of benzene and absolute ethanol in a proportion of 20 volumes of benzene to 1 volume of ethanol. Ten milliliters of this mixture is added and the eluate is collected in a Petri dish; the procedure is repeated three times, with the same volume of solvent, collecting the residue each time in the Petri dish.

The eluate is then desiccated in a vacuum or allowed to evaporate over a 48 hr period. The crystals of pregnanediol thus formed at the bottom of the Petri dish must be weighed, making allowance for the weight of the container. Filter paper can also be used instead of a Petri dish. The degree of purity of the crystals is finally assessed by determining their melting point, which should be 234° C.

24.1.6. PAPER CHROMATOGRAPHY FOR URINARY PREGNANEDIOL, ACCORDING TO ELBERLEIN AND BONGIOVANNI[28]

Principle Involved

A new method is described here for the determination of urinary pregnanediol, which utilizes enzymatic hydrolysis of pregnanediol glucuronidate, followed by ascending paper chromatography and spectrophotometry. Analysis of absorption spectra and recovery experiments, as well as analysis of controls, has established the sensitivity, specificity and accuracy of this method, which the authors, whose authority on the subject is recognized, recommend emphatically.

Method, Apparatus and Reagents

(a) A COMPACT PAPER HOLDER. This should be made of steel, without tin ingredients, as previously described by the authors. It consists of a cylindrical framework of specified dimensions, which allow the chromatography paper to be accommodated in the form of a cylinder fitting into the container.

(b) BETA-GLUCURONIDASE. A product known as "Ketodase," by Warner-Chilcott, is recommended.

(c) ACETATE BUFFER. This should be 1.0 M, pH 4.5.

(d) FAST-ACTING SOLVENT FOR CHROMATOGRAPHY. Equal volumes of methanol (Merck), ethyl acetate (Merck) and methylene chloride (also Merck) (this product must be distilled over sodium carbonate). The resulting mixture can be stored in a refrigerator for several months.

(e) SOLVENT SYSTEM FOR PAPER CHROMATOGRAPHY, described by the same authors, consisting of: isooctane (Eastman, Practical), distilled on sodium carbonate, 225 ml; toluene (Baker, redistilled), 275 ml; methanol, 400 ml; distilled water, 100 ml. After equilibration of this mixture at room temperature, it separates into two phases and can be stored in the refrigerator for three months.

(f) FILTER PAPER, WHATMAN NO. 2. Sheets measuring 18¼ by 22½ inches, divided lengthwise.

(g) SILICA GEL (Davison Chemical Co.). 200 g are stirred in 500 ml of distilled water twice with 200 ml volumes of 95 per cent ethanol and once with 100 ml of absolute ethanol. The washed silica gel is spread over a large sheet of filter paper and allowed to dry at room temperature for 6 to 12 hours, and is then stored in a desiccator. It can be preserved indefinitely.

(h) PHOSPHOMOLYBDIC ACID SOLUTION. Four grams of phosphomolybdic acid (Fisher, certified) is dissolved in 100 ml absolute ethanol. The solution can be stored in a tightly stoppered dark bottle at room temperature for up to three months.

(i) SULFURIC ACID MIXTURE. Fifty to 60 g of sodium bisulfite (reagent grade, Merck) is added carefully to 200 ml of concentrated sulfuric acid in a 1000 ml flask, stirring gently while fumes are being emitted, and then allowing the solution to cool. The acid is decanted into a small bottle, in which it can be kept at room temperature. With this mixture, pregnanediol absorption spectra in the 425 mμ range are more than twice as strong as when the sulfuric acid used has not been subjected to this treatment.

Hydrolysis

A 10 ml volume of urine from a 24 hr specimen, 1 ml of acetate buffer and 0.7 ml of ketodase (3500 units) are incubated at 37° C overnight for 12 to 18 hours.

After hydrolysis, the urine is extracted twice with 10 ml volumes of benzene, and the benzene is washed twice with 10 ml 1 N NaOH and twice again with 10 ml of distilled water. The benzene layer is separated and allowed to evaporate to dryness at 45 to 50° C under a soft stream of filtered air.

Paper Chromatography

(a) PREPARATION OF PAPER. A large sheet of Whatman No. 2 filter paper is divided lengthwise. Each of the two resulting sheets measures 9 1/8 by 22 1/2 inches. Three lines are drawn across the strips with a hard pencil at 2.5, 5 and 9 cm, respectively, from either end. The paper is folded along the midline so that the first line drawn faces the operation. Pencil marks are made at 1.8, 2.8, 6.4, 7.4, 11.0, 12.0, 15.6, 16.6, 20.2 and 21.2 cm from the left margin. Using a pair of scissors, cuts extending from the free margin to the first line at 2.5 cm are made at each mark. Parallel cuts are made 0.5 cm to the left of the first, 0.5 cm to the right of the second, 0.5 cm left of the third, and so on alternately, and the narrow ribbons that have been formed in this way are extended to the 5 cm line and cut out. If the sheet is now spread flat, it will be noticed that 5 rectangular application strips, each 1 cm wide and 5 cm long, have thus been created, the center of each strip being separated from the center of the one next to it by a distance of 4.6 cm. A sufficient number of papers are cut out in this manner and are stored in a place inaccessible to sunlight.

(b) APPLICATION OF EXTRACTS. The sheet is now inserted into the paper holder with the application strips facing down. A pure pregnanediol standard (15 to 25 mcg) is applied throughout the length of the left strip, and up to four extracts can be placed on the remaining strips. Extracts can be transferred quantitatively from a flask to the paper with methylene chloride in 3 to 4 minutes, using a Pasteur pipette and a hair dryer to facilitate rapid evaporation. The solvents of both the standard and the test extracts advance from the initial line to the third line at 9 cm after the addition of 10 ml rapid chromatographic solution through the basal trough of the paper holder. Passage of this solution takes 10 to 15 minutes. The remaining solvent is aspirated and the paper inside the holder is dried by applying hot air from the hair dryer for 5 minutes.

(c) CHROMATOGRAPHY AND ELUTION. The stationary phase of the solvent is added to the trough in the previously described manner and the paper holder is inserted. After overnight equilibration at room temperature, the mobile phase is added and allowed to act for 6 hours. After completion of the chromatographic procedure, the solvent remaining in the cylinder is aspirated, and the paper inside the holder is dried with a hair dryer. The chromatogram is then removed from the holder and laid lengthwise. Four vertical lines are drawn on it at 4.6, 9.2, 13.8 and 18.4 cm from the left margin. The strip on the far left, containing the standard, is cut out, fixed in 5 ml of the phosphomolybdic solution, and dried at 80° C, either in a small oven or under an infrared light source for 3 to 5 minutes. The solvent front is usually found 24 to 36 cm from the base line. After measuring the level of the standard, horizontal lines 1.5 cm above and below the standard are drawn. Each of the resulting rectangles, measuring 4.6 by 6.7 cm, are carefully cut out and divided into 16 small pieces, which are inserted into an 18×150 mm test tube and eluted with 5 ml methanol for at least 3 hours, or overnight. The methanol is then decanted into a 100 ml flask and the elution is repeated three times at 10 to 15 minute intervals to assure quantitative recovery. The combined methanol eluates (20 ml) are evaporated over a water bath or with a stream of filtered air.

(d) PURIFICATION OF EXTRACTS. Whenever washed filter paper is used, eluates from the dried paper are transferred into test tubes with distilled methylene chloride for the final steps. If, as in this instance, the filter paper has not been washed, it is necessary to remove impurities from the paper, which may be time consuming. For this purpose, an ordinary 10 ml syringe with a No. 22 to No. 25 size needle is used as a glass column. A plug of washed glass wool is placed at the bottom. Ten milliliters of 1 per cent ethanol in methylene chloride solution is added, followed by 3 g of washed silica gel; a plug of glass wool is used to cover the silica gel. The column is washed with 10 ml of the same solvent, and the paper eluate is transferred to the column; rinse the flask in which it had dried with five 2 ml volumes of the same solvent. The column is washed with 20 ml of a 2 per cent ethanol solution in methylene chloride, which is discarded, and the pregnanediol fraction is eluted with 20 ml of a 7.5 per cent solution of ethanol in methylene chloride. The terminal portion is collected in a test tube (10 × 150) and is dried in a water bath with the aid of an air stream for 15 to 20 minutes. Four eluates can be conveniently purified at once in 30 to 40 minutes.

(e) SPECTROPHOTOMETRY AND CALCULATIONS. A 2 ml volume of a bisulfite-sulfuric acid mixture is added to each test tube, as well as to the control tube containing 20 to 25 mg pregnanediol, and to the tube with the blank. The tubes are tapped gently to distribute the acid equally and are placed in a water bath for 4 minutes. After cooling to room temperature (15 to 20 minutes), the contents of each tube are transferred to 1.2 or 2.5 ml cuvettes and are read in a Beckmann D.U. spectrophotometer at 390, 425 and 460 mμ. Calculations are based on the following correction formula:

$$\text{O.D. corrected (425)} = \text{O.D. 425} - \frac{(\text{O.D. 390} + \text{O.D. 460})}{2}$$

24.1.7. MICROMETHOD OF ZANDER AND SIMMER[117] FOR THE DETERMINATION OF PROGESTERONE IN BLOOD AND TISSUES

In recent years, several methods have been developed for the chemical estimation of minute quantities of progesterone (Butt et al.,[19] Pearlman and Cerceo,[87] Short and Levett[102]), the most practical and widely used method being that of Zander and Simmer.[117]

These methods have somewhat overshadowed the classical Hooker-Forbes technique,[44, 45] a bioassay procedure described later in this chapter.

Principle Involved

The method is based on extraction of progesterone using various solvents, and isolation and characterization by means of paper chromatography. With 50 ml of blood, quantities as small as 0.05 microgram per ml can be measured. This is an extremely delicate method, still experimental in nature, and therefore it is described here only briefly.

Collection and Preparation of Blood Specimens

Fifty milliliters of citrated blood (10/1) is used. Centrifuge and separate plasma. Add mixture of 3 volumes absolute ethanol and 1 volume ethyl ether (for preparation of these two reagents, see Brown's method, page 507). The amount to be added is 250 ml, which is done quite slowly, while shaking the mixture, over a period of *one hour*.

Extraction of Progesterone

The alcohol-ether mixture is centrifuged and decanted carefully into a funnel with a stopcock. The residue is washed with 125 ml alcohol-ether for 1 hour. The alcohol-ether of the two washings is pooled and concentrated by evaporation to a volume of 5 ml. This residue is diluted in 40 ml distilled water.

It is then extracted three times with 20 ml volumes of ethyl acetate (reagent grade). Desiccate the product of three extractions (totalling 60 ml) with sodium sulfate. Filter.

Desiccate again in a vacuum until residue is dry.

Residue is dissolved in methanol (70 volumes methanol plus 30 volumes water), using five 2 ml volumes to give a total of 10 ml. Heat to 40° C to facilitate dissolution. Then allow to stand for 18 hours *at a temperature below 15° C*.

Centrifuge at less than 5° C for 10 minutes.

Decant and dilute with 20 ml distilled water. Extract three times, each with 30 ml volumes of petroleum ether. Desiccate in a vacuum until residue is dry. The residue is then dissolved in 1 ml methanol, which is divided into three portions: 0.25 ml, 0.5 ml and 0.25 ml. These are placed into 1 ml microbeakers and the methanol is carefully evaporated over a water bath. The residue is then dissolved in 0.2 ml methanol and four portions of the latter solution (three fractions of 0.08 ml and one of 0.04 ml) are carried *with a micropipette* to four prepared pieces of chromatography paper.

Paper Chromatography

The method consists of microchromatography with three types of solutions used in the washing step, one an 80 per cent solution of methanol-ligroine, another a 70 per cent methanol-n-hexane solution and the third an 80 per cent solution of methanol-petroleum ether. Because of the extremely small volume of reagents involved, localization and elution require special apparatus. Readings are taken in the UV light range with a Beckmann D.U. model.

24.1.8. DETERMINATION OF NEUTRAL 17-KETOSTEROIDS IN URINE, BASED ON THE PRINCIPLE OF ZIMMERMANN[118] AND ITS MODIFICATIONS

Zimmermann[118] introduced the metadinitrobenzene color reaction in the presence of alkali for the demonstration of neutral 17-ketosteroids. The method employed by us is that of Zimmermann, modified by Botella in 1958. A useful micromethod, allowing great economy in specimens, is that by Vestergaard.[112] Over the past few years, moreover, *chromatographic fractionation* of 17-ketosteroids has reached a degree of development permitting differentiation of adrenal and ovarian forms of virilism (see Chapter 39). From among the number of proposed methods, that by Kirschner and Lipsett,[62] using gas-liquid chromatography, and that by Seki and Matsumoto,[101] using paper chromatography, are outstanding.

Technique

(a) MODE OF COLLECTING URINE SPECIMENS. The patient is instructed to discard the urine first voided in the morning. From that time onwards, all urine voided until the following morning is to be collected, including that which is voided first on the following morning. Usually it is not necessary to add any preservative to the urine, except for special cases and during hot summer days. Formation of bothersome amounts of ammonium carbonate can be prevented by adding a heavy metal salt, e.g., copper sulfate, in a 1 mg per milliliter ratio.

(b) HYDROLYSIS AND EXTRACTION OF URINE. The great variety of extractive and hydrolytic procedures so far published have been a matter of great controversy. The method to be described here is based on the work by Robbie and Gibson and has proved to be convenient and rapid, as well as efficient when compared with other procedures.

Part of the urine (100 ml) is brought to boil in a funnel with reflux cooling. Ten milliliters of concentrated HCl is added as soon as the urine starts to boil, and boiling is continued for another 10 minutes. After that, the urine is cooled and, without removing it from the funnel, 30 ml of carbon tetrachloride is added through the reflux cooler, and the content is boiled for another 10 minutes. After cooling, the carbon tetrachloride layer is decanted and replaced by the same volume of fresh carbon tetrachloride and boiled again for 10 minutes. As before, the carbon tetrachloride is again decanted and added to the first extract.

The total carbon tetrachloride volume thus extracted from approximately 60 ml is washed successively with water (20 ml), $2 N$ NaOH (20 ml), water (20 ml) and again water (20 ml). Carbon tetrachloride washed four times in this way is then evaporated to dryness in a water bath with the aid of a vacuum pump to remove any traces of moisture. The dry residue is then dissolved in aldehyde-free absolute ethanol. The volume of ethanol varies according to whether a high or low yield of ketosteroids is anticipated. With normal urines, a 4 ml volume of ethanol should be sufficient. In cases of virilism, 8 ml volumes should be used, whereas, if very low values are anticipated, 2 ml or even 1 ml may be adequate. The ethanol extracts obtained are stable enough and do not decompose. However, they must be protected from evaporation by tightly stoppering the tubes containing them.

(c) COLORIMETRIC ESTIMATION: REAGENTS

Ethanol. The importance of using absolute alcohol of good quality cannot be overemphasized. Many commercial products of absolute alcohol are not adequate without previous purification and, unless guaranteed, must be purified in the following way:

Absolute alcohol is treated with 4 g per liter of metaphenylenediamine chloride and kept in darkness for a week, stirring it occasionally, then distilling it and discarding the first and last portions of the distillate. The alcohol thus obtained is entirely pure and is suited for the estimation of 17-ketosteroids.

Metadinitrobenzene. The compound must be pure and crystallized. Unless it is reagent grade, it may be purified in the following manner: 20 ml of the compound is dissolved in 750 ml 95 per cent ethanol. The solution is heated to 40° C and 100 ml of 2 N NaOH is added. After 5 minutes, the solution is cooled and 2500 ml water is added. The metadinitrobenzene now precipitates and can be collected through a Büchner funnel, washed through the funnel with water and then dried and twice recrystallized in 120 ml absolute ethanol. The crystal needles obtained should be almost colorless and have a melting point of 90.5° C.

The reagent consists of a 2 per cent metadinitrobenzene solution in absolute ethanol. Nine grams of chemically pure potassium hydroxide is dissolved by shaking in 50 ml absolute ethanol. The solution is filtered and its concentration is controlled by titrating with acid, using methyl orange as an indicator, within limits of 2.48 to 2.52 normal. The solution must be stored in a refrigerator and must be totally colorless, any trace of color in it being sufficient reason to discard it.

(d) Procedure. The following tubes are prepared.

(1) Blank: 0.2 ml ethanol, 0.2 ml metadinitrobenzene and 0.2 ml KOH.

(2) Urine extract: 0.2 ml urine extract, 0.2 ml metadinitrobenzene and 0.2 ml KOH.

(3) Standard: 0.2 ml standard solution, 0.2 ml metadinitrobenzene and 0.2 ml KOH. The standard solution is prepared with 0.1 mg androsterone, or dehydroepiandrosterone, dissolved in 0.2 ml absolute ethanol. It is convenient to weigh out 1 mg androsterone on an analytic balance and to dissolve it in 20 ml absolute ethanol.

The tubes are placed in a thermostat at 25° C for one hour. During the incubation period, the tubes must be protected from light; preferably, they should be kept in complete darkness. After one hour incubation, absolute ethanol (10 ml) is added to each tube, mixed and read on a photoelectric colorimeter by comparing standard, test and blank values.

Some urine extracts undergo intense red discoloration. Normally, however, the dilution is of such magnitude that this color interference is slight. On the other hand, whenever low ketosteroid values are measured, this factor must be taken into consideration. Colorimetric readings should be made using two different filters, green within 5200 Angstrom and blue-violet in the 4200 Angstrom range. Readings through both filters are necessary to correct for chromogen interference in the method described previously. There is a linear correlation between extinction value and amount of steroid present if the latter is less than 0.1 mg androsterone. With large concentrations of steroids, the calibration curves deviate from a straight line. With very high values, it is important to dilute the original urine extract and to repeat development of the color reaction. We have already pointed out in this context that the volume of solvent to be added to the urine extract varies with regard to anticipated values. Nevertheless, the procedure must be repeated if a given result proves to be in an unexpected range.

(e) Correction for chromogens. Apart from 17-ketosteroids, other substances develop color reactions with the reagents. The following formula has been suggested to correct extinction values obtained in the presence of interfering chromogens:

$$\text{Green corrected} = \frac{\text{green observed} - 0.6 \text{ v}}{0.73}$$

24.1.9. MICROMODIFICATION OF THE PRECEDING METHOD, BY VESTERGAARD[112]

Considering the prevailing tendency to reduce as much as possible the amount of urine necessary to perform these determinations, a micromethod based on the same principle as the preceding one, but requiring only 2 ml of urine, is described here. It is a very rapid procedure in which hydrolysis, extraction and washing are all performed in the same centrifuge tube.

Reagents

Ethyl ether (see page 507).

Absolute ethanol (purified by distillation with zinc powder and KOH).

Potassium hydroxide, 2.5 N and 1.25 N, alcoholic.

Metadinitrobenzene, 2 per cent alcoholic.

Dehydroepiandrosterone acetate standard, containing the equivalent of 50 mg androsterone per 100 ml.

Androsterone standard in alcoholic solution of identical concentration.

Collection of Urine Specimens

Measure amount of 24 hr specimen; determine specific gravity. A 2 ml volume is used for the test.

Special Glassware

Glass tubes of special construction are used throughout the procedure. They are made from pyrex centrifuge tubes (capacity about 12 ml) which are supplied with ground glass stoppers fitting tightly. Each tube is provided with a broad lip serving as a support for a rubber ring, so that pressure on the tube lips throughout centrifuging is exerted through rubber. All manipulations with these tubes are carried out by means of a syringe connected with a glass capillary.

Hydrolysis

A 2 ml volume of urine is placed into the tubes and 0.3 ml of concentrated HCl is added. The tubes are placed on a boiling water bath for 17 minutes and then cooled under tap water.

Extraction

Add 4 ml of ethyl ether with syringe pipette, extract in mechanical shaker for 1 minute, draw off urine and add 4 ml distilled water to ether extract. Decant (or draw off with pipette). Add 10 to 15 NaOH pellets, shake for 90 seconds. Filter through sintered glass filter (or paper) into test tubes. Wash three times with 1 ml volumes of ether. *Allow ether to evaporate.*

Zimmermann Reaction

Place control solutions of androsterone and dehydroepiandrosterone, 0.4 ml each, into tubes. Add to each tube the same amount of ether as in sample tubes and allow ether to evaporate at 50° C.

A 10 ml volume of KOH solution (see page 517) is placed into an Erlenmeyer flask (50 ml capacity) with 5.5 ml metadinitrobenzene solution. Using a micropipette filled with this solution, deliver 0.24 ml to each sample and control tube. The tubes are then stoppered and transferred to a water bath at 25° C for 1 hour in darkness. Then, 3.76 ml absolute ethanol is added and results are read in photocolorimeter (Beckmann) at 520 and 420 mμ.

Correction Formula for Nonspecific Chromogens

Vestergaard proposes the following empirical formula to correct for chromogen interference:

$$\text{Extinction 520 corrected} = \frac{2 \times \text{Extinction 520} - \text{Extinction 420}}{1.67}$$

24.2. BIOASSAY METHODS FOR SEX HORMONES IN BLOOD AND URINE

24.2.1. FUNDAMENTALS OF BIOASSAY OF ESTROGENS

A bioassay procedure for the estimation of estrogens was first utilized by Allen and Doisy, who used vaginal exfoliation in mice or rats as the basic criterion for the test (mouse or rat estrus test, see Chapter 2). Currently, however, exfoliative vaginal cytology has been dismissed as unreliable for bioassay purposes. The methods presently in use are the following:

1. Method of Astwood, based on measuring increments in weight of the uterine horn in spayed rats. This modality is still in use and, in 1963, was judged accurate by Thevenet and his co-workers.[107] Elftman[29] uses the same type of bioassay, but analyzes any changes at the level of the Golgi apparatus in endometrial cells.

2. Dorfman[27] assays the effects of estrogens on the chick oviduct, any weight increment in which is logarithmically proportional to the injected dosage.

3. The reaction of vaginal *canalization* following local injection of estrogens has been utilized by Littrell and Tom in the guinea pig, and by Lloyd and his asso-

ciates[71] in the rat as an ultrasensitive means for detecting estrogenic activity.

The last two methods, in conjunction with that of Dorfman, will be described here.

Juvenile female guinea pigs weighing 200 g are used. The vaginas of animals of this weight are still completely closed (Fig. 24-1, A). Also suitable for the test owing to their extraordinary sensitivity are adult guinea pigs, weighing 300 to 350 g, which have been spayed one month prior to the test. However, using juvenile guinea pigs bypasses the inconvenience of surgical castration. Any guinea pig weighing 200 g may be considered to be juvenile, so that by simply observing this criterion no further precautions are necessary.

The injection site must be selected in the vicinity of the vaginal orifice, using a thin needle which is inserted under skin quite superficially. The total dosage to be administered is divided equally into two halves, each to be injected at a point lateral to the hymenal membrane on both sides. The hymenal membrane of the guinea pig is crescent-shaped, as shown in Figure 24-1, and is injected through each extremity. When using blood or urine, the usual amount injected is 0.06 to 0.08 ml,

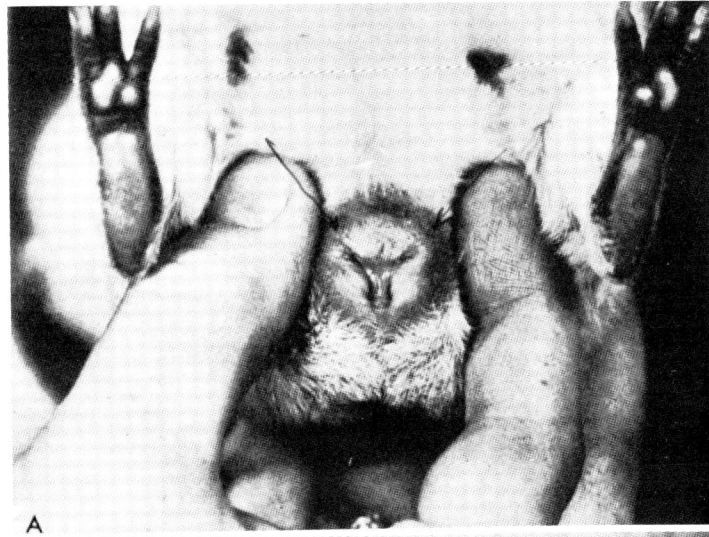
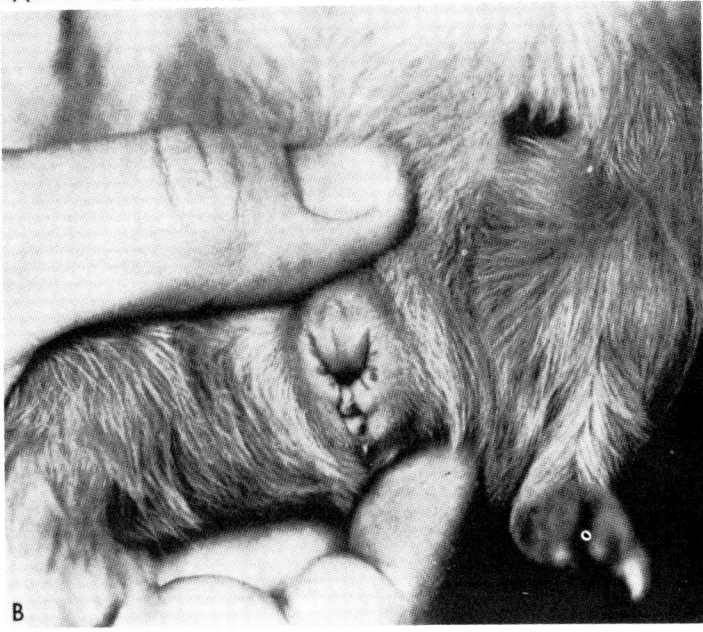

Figure 24-1. A, Perineum of juvenile female guinea pig, showing intact membrane and intact vulvar area (control animal). B, Vaginal patency in young guinea pig injected with estrogens. Positive reaction. (From Hartman, Littrell and Tom: *Endocrinology*, 39:120, 1946.)

hence 0.03 to 0.04 ml through each injection site.

The reaction to be observed occurs successively in the following order:

(1) Appearance of an intense white line, resembling the stigma of a maturing follicle, which forms at the midpoint of the crescent.

(2) Beginning of *vaginal patency,* first apparent as a small groove, associated with intense edema.

(3) Early vaginal patency, from an opening of the size of a pinhead, progressing to complete patency.

(4) Complete vaginal patency, achieved after 24 to 48 hours (average, 36 hours), from the time of injection (Fig. 24–1,*B*). The vagina remains patent for 9 to 20 days, after which the test can be repeated on the same animal only if it is castrated, since adulthood is reached in the meantime.

(5) Castrated animals may be employed in repeat tests, provided 20 days are allowed to lapse from one determination to the next.

Vaginal patency is achieved with as tiny quantities of estrogens as 0.0000004 mg. This is, if the test is performed with serial dilutions of the test fluid, the highest dilution eliciting a positive response corresponds to 4×10^{-7} mg estrogen. This allows determinations of minimal amounts of estrogens and hence quantitative bioassay not only of urinary but also of midcycle female serum or blood values.

For the exact quantitation of test substances, the authors recommend a scale of three control animals injected with 4, 8 and 12 ($\times 10^{-7}$) milligrams of estrogens.

24.2.2. MODIFICATION BY LLOYD, ROGERS AND WILLIAMS[71] OF THE PRECEDING METHOD, USING RATS

Immature female rats of the Sprague-Dawley strain are used. The animals must be three weeks old and weigh 21 to 25 g. A volume of 0.02 ml test substance is injected in two doses on either side of the vaginal introitus (0.01 ml each side). Whole blood, serum or urine may be used. The minimal amount of estrone capable of producing a response of vaginal patency is 0.00025 mg. This method can therefore be employed as a substitute for the preceding one.

For quantitative determinations, control animals are injected with 0.00025, 0.00050 and 0.00075 mg estrone standard and results are compared with those obtained in test animals.

The vagina opens at a slower rate than in guinea pigs. Generally, some patency is first recognized after five days, but complete patency is not seen before one week from the time of injection.

Compared with the guinea pig test, the rat bioassay is less sensitive. Larger dosages of estrogens and longer periods of time are necessary to elicit the desired effect of vaginal patency. One advantage of working with rats is that they are less expensive to maintain. The procedure is adequate for qualitative estimations, whereas for quantitative tests, guinea pigs are to be preferred.

24.2.3. BIOASSAY OF ESTROGENS BY THE CHICK OVIDUCT METHOD, ACCORDING TO DORFMAN[27]

Fundamentals

The method is based on treating pullets with estrogens for five consecutive days during the first 15 days of life and determining the oviduct response 24 hr after the last injection. The response of the chick oviduct to various estrogens is known to be very intense in accordance with the embryonal and youthful nature of that organ. The ratio of oviduct weight (in milligrams) to body weight (in grams), multiplied by 100, gives the so-called "oviduct potency ratio" which is logarithmically proportional to the level of concentration of stilbestrol injected (provided levels vary between 25 and 50 micrograms). This is a highly sensitive quantitative method.

Technique

White Leghorn pullets, one to three days after hatching, are used. Experiments may begin on the fourth to seventh day of life. The material to be studied is injected subcutaneously once daily for five days. Twenty-four hours after the last injection, the animals are sacrificed with chloroform and the oviduct is carefully dissected, washed, blotted with filter paper and weighed immediately to within 0.5 mg on a torsion balance. The results obtained give the ratio of the weight of the oviduct (in milligrams, multiplied by 100) to the body weight (in grams).

The total material administered the animal is dissolved in 0.5 ml of corn oil and 0.1 ml is injected daily. The unstimulated control group of animals receives a similar schedule of treatment, with only the corn oil, and the animals of the standard group receive standard estrone dissolved in corn oil. The method employed by the authors consisted in assaying an estrogen against itself, using the design previously described by Bliss in 1944. The following design is used to ascertain the potency ratio:

$$\frac{\text{High Dose (Standard)}}{\text{Low Dose (Standard)}} = \frac{\text{High Dose (Unknown)}}{\text{Low Dose (Unknown)}}$$

Estrone can be assayed by this method with sufficient accuracy, but considerable quantities of materials must be used. It takes a total of 20 pullets to determine estrone levels at concentrations not lower than 640 micrograms. On the other hand, using estradiol benzoate, the assay can achieve greater accuracy. With 20 pullets, quantities of 100 micrograms may be determined with standard errors of ±10 per cent. Folic acid deficiency in the animals must be avoided, since it was shown by Hertz to cause loss of response by the chick oviduct to estrogens.

24.2.4. BIOASSAY FOR MINUTE AMOUNTS OF PROGESTERONE, BY HOOKER AND FORBES[44]

Principle Involved

Hooker and Forbes,[44, 45] Flux,[32] and recently Leroy and associates[66] have utilized *the local effect* of progesterone on the endometrium as the basis for their bioassay techniques. The Hooker-Forbes technique avails itself of the apparently specific changes in stromal nuclei of the mouse endometrium elicited by locally introduced progestogens.

Technique

Adult female mice, which have previously been ovariectomized, are used. Ovariectomy is performed in the usual manner at least 16 days prior to the assay. The spayed mice are maintained on a routine diet and under routine laboratory conditions.

The test animal is anesthetized with sodium amytal supplemented with ether and is placed on its back on a special operating table for small animals. During laparotomy, one uterine horn is delivered through a mid-ventral incision and anchored by a needle passed through the mesometrium (Fig. 3-11, page 49). A tight ligature is placed near the cranial end of the horn. A second thread is placed approximately 5 mm caudad to the first, and a single loose overhand knot is tied. The ends of both ligatures are passed through two slots of a device such as that illustrated in the figure, and are clamped horizontally above the animal. By means of the threads the horn is elevated slightly above the abdominal wall and held securely. A special syringe for intrauterine injection is used, assuring injection of volumes less than 0.01 cc. This syringe consists of a micrometer caliper head mounted on a brass base to which a 0.5 ml tuberculin syringe is clamped. The syringe is readily dismountable; to fill it, the plunger is moved by advancing the micrometer bolt.

Prior to use, the apparatus is calibrated by filling the syringe with mercury and by delivering and weighing measured quantities. Disregarding the graduations on the syringe, the advancement of the micrometer bolt necessary to deliver the smallest volume required for injection (0.0003 ml) is ascertained.

After making sure that the needle is filled with fluid, the horn is grasped with a forceps about 3 mm caudal to the posterior ligature (see Fig. 3-11, page 49) and the needle, bevel up, is inserted into the uterine lumen immediately cranial to the forceps and pushed forward almost to the anterior ligature. The desired volume of fluid is then discharged into the horn and the needle is withdrawn. During withdrawal, tension is placed on the caudal thread sufficient to produce a sharp angle in the horn when the needle is removed. The tension is continuously maintained until the knot is drawn tight.

After cutting the threads close to their knots, the second horn is similarly injected, if desired, the organ is returned to the abdominal cavity, and the body wall is closed with silk sutures. For optimal results, the total volume injected must not exceed 0.0006 ml, since larger amounts were found to produce objectionable distension and to alter the results.

The optimal interval between intrauterine injection and autopsy was determined to be 48 hours. The segment of horn between the two ligatures is extirpated and the tissue fixed in Lavdowsky's fluid, which produces less shrinkage of nuclei than other fixatives. Paraffin sections 6 microns in thickness are stained with Harris's hematoxylin and eosin. The specific response to progesterone consists primarily of nuclear hypertrophy of endometrial stromal cells (see Fig. 3–12, page 50). Nuclei assume a smooth, slightly elongated, oval outline. Chromatin particles are fine and evenly distributed, and nucleoli are conspicuous. It is necessary to distinguish between stromal nuclei and nuclei pertaining to epithelial cells of the glands. The nuclei of the latter do not appear to be modified by progesterone.

24.2.5. MEASUREMENT OF STEROIDS BY MEANS OF SATURATION ANALYSIS

Modern investigations (Barakat and Elkins,[6] Baulieu et al.,[7] and Diczfalusy[25]) have established the fact that all steroids, estrogens, androgens, and progestogens, as well as corticoids, are transported by specific *binding proteins*. On the basis of this fact, Elkins and Newman[30] and Murphy[81] devised the so-called technique of *"saturation" analysis*, in which the steroid hormone to be assayed is combined with its specific binding protein, the unsaturated excess of which can be determined. This allows exact calculation of the concentration of the steroid hormone in question in urine, blood or any other body fluid. The method has been adapted for the determination of estrogens by Corker and Exley,[22] as well as by Mercier-Bodard and co-workers.[75] Progesterone can similarly be assayed by saturation techniques, thanks to procedures developed by Johansson and Wide[60] and by Lipsett and co-workers.[70] Moreover, Vermeulen and Verdonck[111] have applied the same principle to the assay of testosterone. Although our own experience with these techniques is limited, we believe that the assay of steroids will depend mainly on such procedures in the future.

24.2.6. OTHER MODERN METHODS FOR THE ESTIMATION OF STEROIDS

Scommegna[100] published a comprehensive review of recent advances made in the field of estrogen assay. Excellent results have been reported for *gas chromatography* (Nilson and Bengtsson[83]).

A further interesting development is the introduction, by Midgley and Niswender,[76] of radioimmunoassay procedures for the measurement of steroids, a technique previously employed only for protein hormones. A radioimmunoassay for estrogens has been recently developed by Abraham and co-workers.[1]

24.2.7. METHOD OF PHILPOT AND PHILPOT, MODIFIED BY MIYAKE AND PINCUS, FOR THE ESTIMATION OF CARBONIC ANHYDRASE IN ENDOMETRIAL EXTRACTS

An increase in the endometrial carbonic anhydrase content is one of the effects of progesterone (see Chapter 3, page 44). An accurate bioassay procedure in animals is based on this principle.

Necessary Reagents

1. Solution A-1 (saturated solution of sodium carbonate at 5°C).
2. Solution A-2 (27.3 volumes per cent of solution A-1).
3. Solution B (0.221 g of sodium bicarbonate in 1000 ml distilled water).
4. Bromothymol blue, 0.1 per cent aqueous solution.

Technique

1. Half fill 500 ml aspirator bottle with solution B (sodium bicarbonate).
2. Open CO_2 tank and start the bubbling in order to saturate solution B with CO_2 (about 1 bubble per second for 10 to 15 minutes).
3. Place 0.1 per cent bromothymol blue solution in the burette (5 ml).
4. Place 0.1 ml bromothymol solution in each test tube (1.5 × 15 cm).
5. Fill large burette (50 ml) with solution B, saturated with CO_2.

6. Place 5 ml of saturated solution B into each test tube.

7. Stopper each test tube immediately after step 6.

8. Transfer all test tubes to an ice bath.

9. Fill 100 ml graduated cylinder with 100 ml tap water. Adjust regulating tube at approximately 35 ml level.

10. Connect all tubing.

11. Prepare ice bath in 4000 ml beaker and start stirrer.

12. Place solution A-2 in 50 ml Erlenmeyer flask and immerse in ice bath.

13. Start preparation of control series (control tubes):

(a) Add distilled water to the test tube to total 5.6 ml volume.

(b) Add one drop of octyl alcohol.

(c) Place test tube in ice bath and bubble CO_2 through solution for 2 minutes.

(d) Add 0.5 ml of solution A-2 to test tube and at the same time start stopwatch.

(e) When initial blue color turns green-yellow, record the time.

(f) Repeat, adjusting regulator until reaction time is 65 to 75 seconds. This is the control reaction time.

14. Begin measurement of enzyme activity.

(a) Substitute distilled water in control tube with enzyme extract and proceed as in Step 13, (a) through (e).

(b) Adjust dilution of enzyme extract until reaction time is 25 to 30 seconds (one enzyme unit = 1 EU).

15. The enzyme unit per gram of wet tissue (EU/g) is calculated as follows:

$$EU/g = \frac{1000}{2\ CV}$$

where C = concentration of extract (mg/ml) and V = volume of extract which is required to shorten reaction time from 65 to 75 seconds to 25 to 30 seconds (ml/EU).

24.3 ESTIMATION OF GONADOTROPINS

Discussion of techniques for the estimation of protein hormones other than gonadotropins, such as placental lactogen (see method of Saxena et al.[97]) or prolactin (see method of Bryant and Greenwood[17]), has been omitted here.

The study of gonadotropins, which until recently had been measured by bioassay methods, has been greatly advanced over the past few years by the introduction of radioimmunoassay techniques. Nevertheless, as a result of comparative studies of bioassay and immunoassay procedures for gonadotropins, authoritative opinion on the subject (Albert[4]) still favors the use of bioassay procedures. Let us briefly examine first the bioassay and then the immunoassay techniques involved.

24.3.1. ESTIMATION OF CHORIONIC GONADOTROPIN, USING THE MALE OF RANA ESCULENTA

Principle Involved

Until somewhat over a decade ago, human chorionic gonadotropin was estimated with the method of Zondek, which required six rats, each weighing 30 to 35 g, to be injected with the test material over a period of two days. The presence of sufficient gonadotropin levels produced "estrus," resulting in the appearance of "squames" in vaginal smears. Hamburger modified this biologic test by using mice under similar circumstances.

It is quite obvious that in order to complete a successful assay with any of these methods, it may be necessary to employ a large series of animals which, apart from fulfilling the specifications of weight, must be ready for use on short notice.

Another drawback of these procedures is that they are time consuming. Thus, by the time it becomes apparent that a given test must be repeated, the test substance may no longer be usable and a fresh specimen may have to be obtained.

In contrast, the use of the male frog *Rana esculenta* offers several advantages, particularly as regards low cost and abundant supply. The reaction, if positive, becomes apparent quite rapidly and there are no known instances in which a reaction that at three hours was negative had later become positive. A new batch of animals may therefore be injected with smaller amounts of test fluid in the presence of a uniformly positive reaction and, by the same token, variable amounts of test fluid may be injected on an exploratory basis, allowing further study of negative or intermediate zone reactions.

24.3.2. TECHNIQUE

The test essentially consists in injecting decreasing amounts of the fluid to be assayed, until a previously observed positive reaction becomes negative.

The smallest amount still eliciting ejaculation of sperm in two or three male frogs is the equivalent of an *esculenta unit*. It goes without saying that the designation of such a unit varies somewhat according to geography, since different species of frogs are used by different authors.

Almost invariably, the test fluid consists of urine, which must be collected from an early morning specimen in a clean container devoid of any trace of alcohol.

If serum is to be used in the test, it should be prepared through centrifugation of a blood sample obtained by venous puncture.

Male frogs weighing 15 to 20 g are used. The type of syringe generally used for insulin injections may be employed (Fig. 24–2,A), starting with 1 ml of test fluid and gradually decreasing the amount injected. Amounts of test fluid smaller than can be measured with the syringe are diluted conveniently to a 50 per cent, 10 per cent, or even weaker solution.

A fine gauge needle must be used and inserted into the muscular mass of the hind legs before reaching the dorsal lymphatic sac to avoid reflux of test fluid from the puncture site (Fig. 24–2,B).

The test is read after three hours by aspirating the cloacal contents with a capillary pipette (Fig. 24–2,C) and depositing a drop of the removed fluid on a slide, prefer-

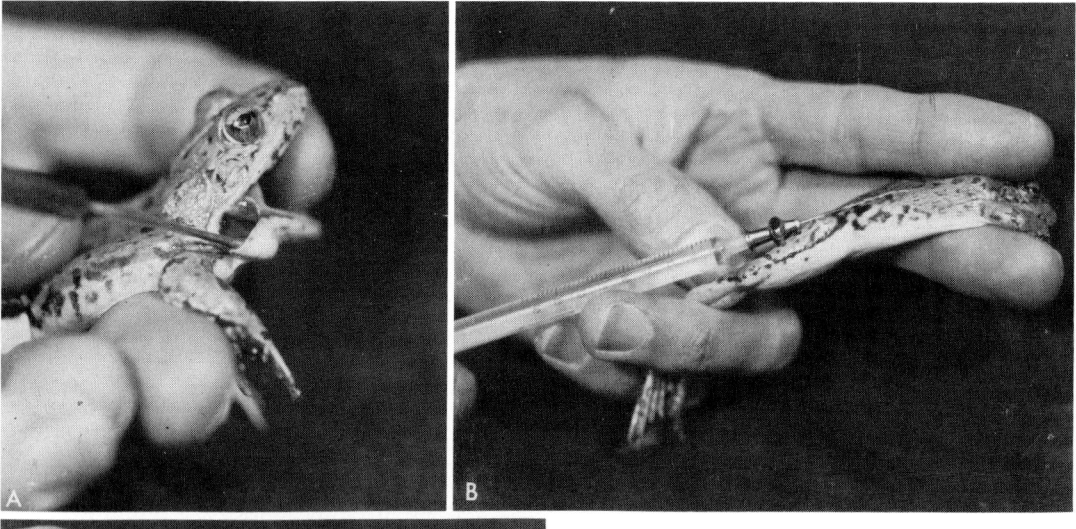

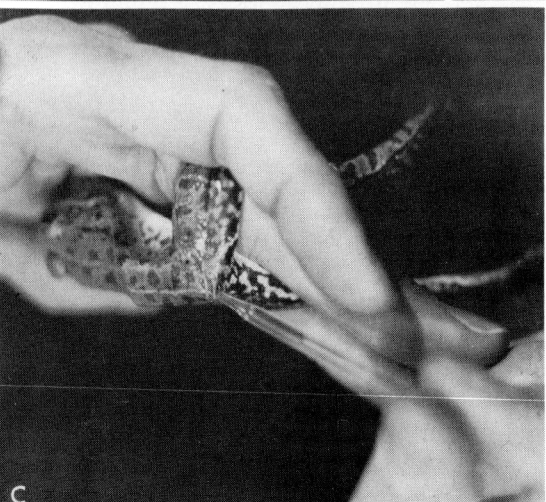

Figure 24–2. Rana esculenta test. A, Demonstration of sexual pouches (to verify male sex of animal). B, Injection of test urine into animal. C, Removal of cloacal fluid for analysis. (From Bedoya and Puras: Geburtsh. Frauenheilk., 10:509, 1950.)

ably with a recessed well, which is then examined under the microscope.

24.3.3. STANDARDIZATION

While for practical purposes it may be enough to know how many esculenta units are contained in a given specimen, it is nevertheless important to correlate results obtained with esculenta frogs with those obtained by other authors using different species of batrachians. For this reason, it must be known what the equivalent of one esculenta unit is in terms of international units of gonadotropins.

In order to establish the necessary correlation, we availed ourselves of frogs originating from the province of Segovia and weighing 15 grams, with as little variation as possible. All frogs had been captured recently and had never before been used for similar purposes.

A standard international preparation of human chorionic gonadotropin was prepared in 1 ml volumes of different strength dilutions, using the following stock solutions as starting points:

Solution a = One tablet (100 IU) HCG for each 5 ml (20 IU/ml).
Solution b = One tablet HCG for each 10 ml (10 IU/ml).
Solution c = One tablet HCG for each 20 ml (5 IU/ml).
Distilled water.

By mixing these solutions in known proportions, dilutions containing 1 to 18 IU per milliliter were obtained, and each of those dilutions were used for injecting a batch of 10 animals according to the usual technique, with the results read after 3 hours. In negative cases, results were confirmed several hours later.

The reaction was uniform and unequivocally positive in all animals that had received five or more international units of gonadotropins. This was construed to mean that, whenever chorionic gonadotropin is injected in sufficient dosages, and provided that the injection is performed in a correct way, it invariably causes the male *Rana esculenta* to ejaculate spermatozoa.

Accepting as minimal the dosage which produced ejaculation in two thirds of the batch of injected animals, this dose was found to correspond to 4 IU (causing ejaculation in 7 of 10 animals). Consequently, one esculenta unit was found to be equivalent to 4 IU of chorionic gonadotropin.

A few of the animals gave positive reactions with dosages below 2 or 3 IU, an expected and acceptable phenomenon within the range of possible variations of weight and sensitivity of the animals. None of the animals, however, reacted with dosages below 1 IU.

One further conclusion we were able to draw from this study was the fact that the esculenta unit was an arbitrary value that depends on the sensitivity of the animals. Over a period of one month, animals previously exposed to the test showed a marked decrease in sensitivity to gonadotropin, requiring a double dose of international units to produce a positive response. In these animals, one esculenta unit corresponded to approximately 8 IU.

Animals that are used repeatedly in the test may therefore be expected to give an irregular response that may lead to diagnostic error.

There is no doubt that a similar loss of sensitivity was the underlying cause leading us originally to establish an esculenta unit as the equivalent of 15 IU, since the above findings were not known to us at that time, and the frogs we were using for the biologic diagnosis of pregnancy were being reused repeatedly.

Although it has been studied extensively by empirical means, the *mechanism* involved in the reaction by male batrachians is poorly understood. It seems paradoxical that the generally gametokinetic activity of gonadotropin A (FSH) should provoke little or no spermiation in batrachians, whereas chorionic gonadotropin (LH, ICSH) should provoke energetic and specific ejection of spermatozoa. Significant contributions toward clarifying this question have been made by Burgos and Ladman,[18] by Garmier,[35] and by our own group[11] as well.

In effect, it has been shown that two different phenomena are involved in the testis of batrachians: (1) *spermatogenesis*, induced by FSH just as in mammals, and (2) *spermiation*, or release of preformed spermatozoa, consisting in the detachment of the latter from the Sertoli cells, to which they adhere intimately. The second mechanism is triggered by the urinary hormone of pregnancy (Fig. 24–3). A positive pregnancy reaction is therefore a mere *abrupt release of spermatozoa that are completely formed.*

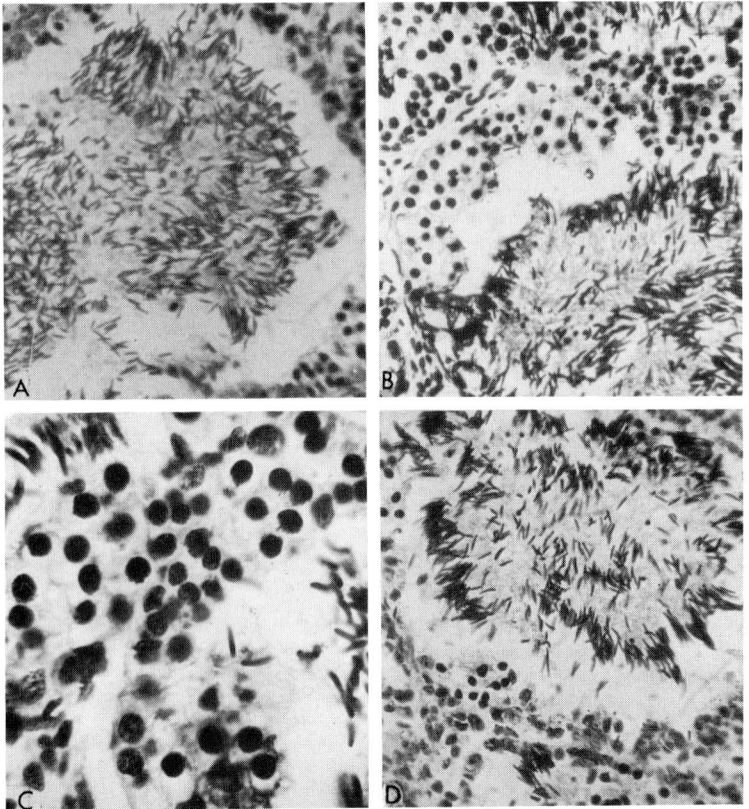

Figure 24–3. Spermiation in *Rana esculenta*. A, Testis in resting stage (450×); spermia are seen in great numbers, filling the lumen of tubules and adhering to Sertoli cells. B, Onset of spermiation: "release" of spermia (450×). C, Spermatogenesis, multiplication of germ cells (900×). D, Advanced phase of sperm release in a positive pregnancy test. Observe detachment of spermia from entire circumference of tubule and reduction in number of spermia within lumen (450×). (From Botella et al.[11])

This release takes place as a result of a process of lysis of the Sertoli cell cytoplasm, wherein depolymerization of mucopolysaccharides and glycogen, as shown by Botella and colleagues[11] and by Van Dongen, plays an important role.

24.3.4. BIOASSAY OF FSH, ACCORDING TO HEINRICHS AND EULENFELD[43]

Recent advances in hormone research produced a number of methods, considerably improving past bioassay techniques, for the estimation of pituitary gonadotropins at the low concentrations in which they occur in the urine of nonpregnant women. Though still considered as extremely laborious and difficult, these methods are finding greater and greater application in the field of endocrinology (castration, Turner's syndrome, etc.). Because of its accuracy, the method of Heinrichs and Eulenfeld, developed in 1960, deserves to be described in detail.

Principle Involved

This method is a modification of Albert's method, with a perfected extraction procedure for urine by means of kaolin. The commonly used end points for the assay are uterine or ovarian weight in mice or rats.

Technique

A 1000 ml volume of urine is obtained from a homogenous mixture of a 24 hr specimen and stored in a refrigerator at 4° C. Any urine containing albumin or blood is discarded.

ACIDIFICATION. Use acetic acid to pH 4.5.

ADDITION OF KAOLIN (20 g kaolin Merck, DAB 6). Shake for a few seconds.

FILTRATION. By means of a special pressure filtering apparatus (type MD 140-30, made by *Membranenfilter Gesellschaft*, Göttingen, Germany), the urine is filtered under 5 atm pressure from a nitrogen container. (A sheet of Schleicher and Schüll type 1575, or Whatman No. 50, filter paper is first placed at the bottom of the pressure chamber.) During filtration, the kaolin cake is retained in the pressure chamber.

EXTRACTION. Tap water, equal in volume to that of the original urine, acidified with acetic acid to pH 4.5, is added to the kaolin. The kaolin is then eluted with a 100 ml volume of ammonium hydroxide solution prepared by dissolving 1 volume of ammonium hydroxide (trademark Riedel, Haen, mol. wt. 17.03, analytic grade reagent) in 5 volumes water. The pH of this solution must be 12. The eluate is transferred to the pressure filtration chamber and, after adding 50 ml water, is again filtered at 15 atm. The filtrate, amounting to about 150 ml, is brought to pH 5.5 with acetic acid (9 to 11 ml), and 20 ml acetone is added to precipitate gonadotropins. The mixture is shaken for 5 minutes, refrigerated for 30 minutes and then centrifuged. The residue at the bottom of the centrifuge tube, containing the gonadotropins, is dried with P_2O_5 to constant weight in a desiccator.

BIOASSAY. The method of uterine weight, using intact infantile female mice, serves as the assay procedure. Selection of the animals is made on the basis of weight (8 to 11 grams) rather than age. The average uterine weight among 100 animals weighing between 8 and 11 g was found to be 5.4 mg.

The extracts obtained by desiccation are dissolved in 2 ml distilled water and injected in 0.5 ml aliquots intramuscularly each day for three days. Seventy-two hours after the first injection, the animals are sacrificed with ether. The uteri are removed, fixed in Bouin's fluid for 24 hrs, blotted on filter paper and weighed on a torsion balance.

The assay is always run in parallel with a known international standard (preparation HMG 20A, Organon). One international biologic unit is equivalent to 1 mg standard. At least 24 animals must be used in each assay.

24.3.5. BIOASSAY OF LUTEINIZING GONADOTROPIN (LH) BY THE OVARIAN ASCORBIC DEPLETION METHOD OF PARLOW[86]

Principle

The most sensitive methods for the detection of luteinizing activity in the ovary are based on the study of ovarian *metabolic processes*. Ellis[31] assessed the capacity of the ovary for trapping iodinated albumin as an index of luteinizing hormone activity. However, the most dependable test would seem to be one based on measuring ovarian ascorbic acid depletion. Parlow[86] discovered that, as in the adrenal following ACTH injection, tissue vitamin C content diminished or disappeared in the ovary after injection of LH. This reaction was not observed with other types of gonadotropins. Several different methods, based on Parlow's principle, have been described by such authors as MacCann and Taleisnik,[74] Ward and his colleagues,[113] and more recently, Sakiz and Guillemin.[96] The method of Sakiz and Guillemin may be summed up as follows.

Technique

Rats of the Sprague-Dawley strain, or the Holzman strain, are pretreated with two injections of 50 IU pregnant mare serum, the object of which is to accomplish priming of the ovary, inducing follicular maturation. A subsequent injection of LH produces depletion in the ovarian ascorbic acid content. The ovarian ascorbic acid content is determined by means of the method of Mildlin and Butler, based on decolorization of 2,6-dichlorophenol-indophenol in a solution of metaphosphoric acid. The test is quite specific for LH; neither FSH nor HCG produces any effect on the ovarian ascorbic acid content.

24.3.6. IMMUNOASSAY OF PROTEIN HORMONES

General Considerations

Exact knowledge of the chemistry of steroid hormones has resulted in the development of spectrophotometric methods, some of which have been described here. Over the past 20 years, these have immeasurably advanced the study of a large number of problems concerning the physiology and metabolism of this group of hormones. By comparison, the protein hormones of the pituitary, pancreas and other glands have so far been demonstrated only by bioassay procedures, and their study is lagging relatively far behind.

Therefore, development of *immunologic techniques* for the characterization and estimation of these substances constitutes a significant step forward.

Methods based on immunologic techniques have been described for *growth hormone*,[26, 33, 41, 44, 80] *prolactin*,[64] and, recently, *insulin*, (Goetz et al.[36]). Of all hormones, however, the gonadotropins have particularly been subject to study with these methods.

The immunologic properties of pituitary gonadotropins have been studied by Li[67] and by Moudgal and Li.[80] These workers' findings have made it possible to differentiate between the properties of LH and those of HCG, two hormones possessing great biologic similarities although they have been shown to be immunologically distinct entities. Similarly, Goss and his group,[37, 38] as well as Lunenfeld,[72] have subsequently devised a bioassay procedure for the characterization of FSH. Recently, further work in the field has resulted in a variety of bioassay procedures for all adenohypophysial hormones.

Undoubtedly, chorionic gonadotropin, both human and animal, has been studied most extensively. Human chorionic gonadotropin can be demonstrated by the immunologic technique devised by Wide and Gemzell,[115, 116] the basis of a large number of modifications. Wide and Gemzell's method, currently most widely used, is based on the *hemagglutination inhibition reaction*, while other bioassay methods resort to techniques involving *complement fixation* or *precipitin reactions*. Outstanding among these is the method developed by Islami and Fisher,[46] which permits execution of the Wide and Gemzell[115] reaction on a slide.

The accuracy of the latter method, as compared to that of biologic pregnancy tests, is considerable. In a publication by Plaza and Mesa[88] in 1963, in which the results of 2725 biologic pregnancy tests reported by various investigators are reviewed, the authors found the margin of error to be 1.6 per cent, whereas statistics by Smith[103] (1964) revealed a margin of error of 2 per cent. These figures would indicate that, as regards both accuracy and sensitivity, this technique for the estimation of human CG, and consequently for the detection of pregnancy, compares favorably with the previously described frog tests.

Method of Wide and Gemzell[116] for the Determination of HCG in Urine by a Hemagglutination Inhibition Reaction

1. GENERAL PRINCIPLES. If human chorionic gonadotropin is injected into a rabbit, it results in the production of a specific antibody. Should such an *antigonadotropin* be allowed to react with previously sensitized blood cells of another animal (Fig. 24-4), it would cause agglutination of blood cells. Agglutination may be seen with the naked eye, at the bottom of the tube, as a uniform red circle formed by agglutinated red cells (see Fig. 24-7).

If these agglutinated red cells are now placed in contact with a solution containing HCG, the protein hormone competes with the red cells for antigonadotropin and a reversal of agglutination occurs (Fig. 24-5). The patterns obtained in a reversal of agglutination and in a control suspension of previously stabilized red cells may be observed to be identical in both cases: a uniform red ring of blood cells (Fig. 24-7). This differs from the diffuse, irregular clumps of cells dispersed over the bottom of the tube seen prior to reversal.

If, on the other hand, a test fluid such as urine, containing no chorionic gonadotropin (Fig. 24-6) is allowed to react with the agglutinated red cells, there is no competition for antigonadotropins, which are therefore not released by the red cells as they are in the preceding instance, and the red cells consequently remain agglutinated. If the agglutination pattern is now compared with that in the control tube, a diffuse circle is seen in the former as compared with a button in the latter. The above discrepancy between the test and the control tube indicates a negative reaction, whereas lack of agglutination in both tubes constitutes a positive test (Fig. 24-7).

2. TECHNIQUE. Essentially two types of techniques are currently used in Spain: one utilizing Prepuerin by *Burroughs Wellcome & Co.*, and the other employing Pregnosticon by *Organon Oss*. The *modus operandi* is as follows:

A. Prepuerin. The reagent kit consists of:

(a) Lyophilized test suspension (erythrocytes sensitized to HCG).

(b) Lyophilized control suspension (nonsensitized, stabilized erythrocytes).

(c) Buffer, in tablets.

Hormone Assay

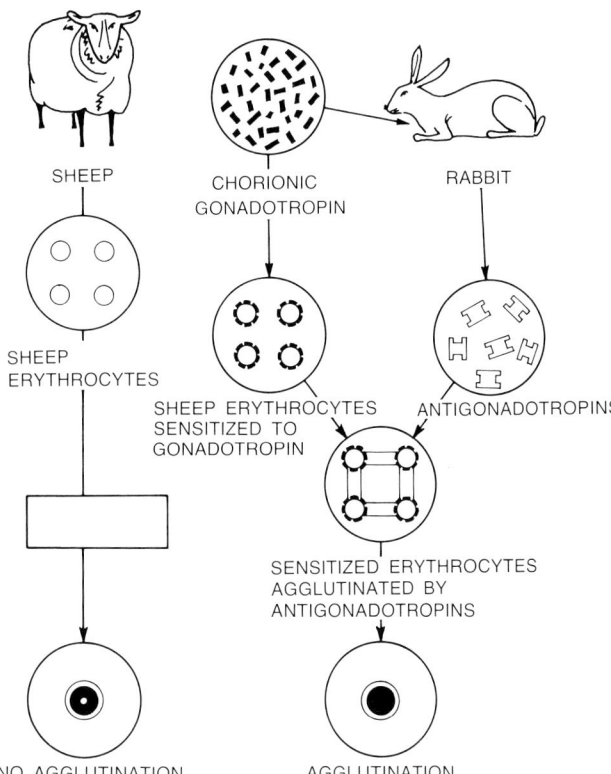

Figure 24-4. Agglutination of CG-sensitized sheep erythrocytes by serum of rabbit immunized with purified gonadotropin.

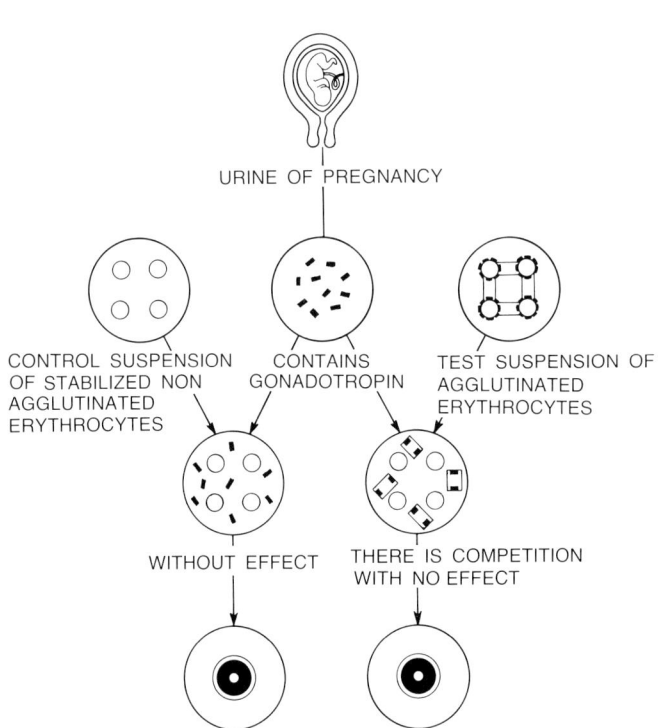

Figure 24-5. Inhibition of hemagglutination by chorionic gonadotropin contained in urine of pregnancy.

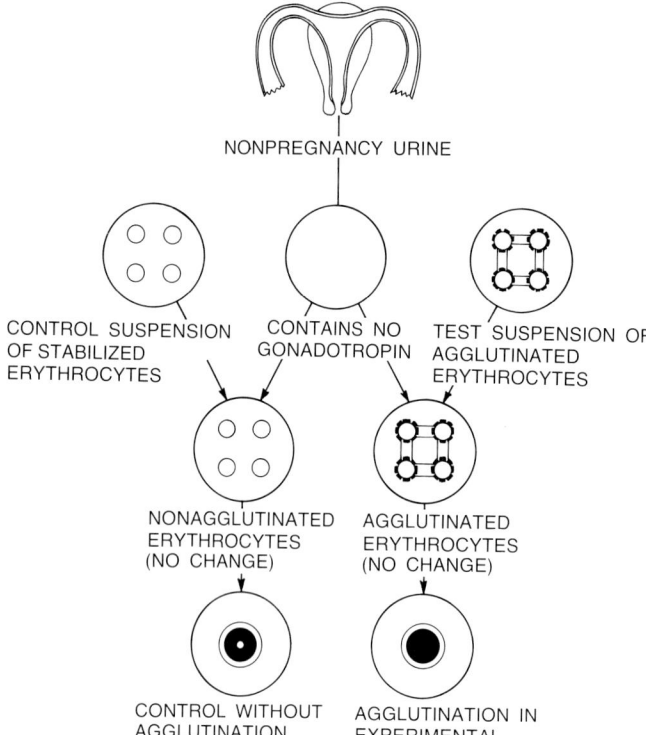

Figure 24-6. In the absence of urinary gonadotropin, there is no inhibition of hemagglutination.

The buffer solution is prepared first by dissolving one tablet in 4 ml hot distilled water, and then adding 16 ml cold distilled water. This solution is used to dissolve the lyophilized suspensions as well as to dilute the urine specimen, using two series of hemolysis tubes in a special rack with a mirror at the base, which facilitates reading of results. The serial dilutions of urine in buffer are: 1/5 in tube 1, 1/10 in tube 2, and 1/20 in tube 3 of each series. Tube 4 contains only 1 ml buffer without urine and serves as a control.

The final step consists in adding 0.1 ml of the "test suspension" to each of the tubes of the test series and 1 ml of the "control suspension" to each tube of the control series.

The rack must now be left undisturbed and kept from all vibrations. Results are read 6, 12 and 24 hours later. For a clear visual representation of the test results, see Figure 24-7.

B. Pregnosticon. The reagent kit of the pregnosticon test consists of:

(a) HCG immunized rabbit serum, lyophilized and supplied in ampules, which may be used as test tubes.

(b) Sensitized erythrocytes.
(c) Medium for erythrocyte suspension.
(d) Lyophilized urine, both positive (from pregnant women) and negative.

To ampule a, add 0.1 ml of filtrate of unknown urine and 0.4 ml of the red cell suspension, previously prepared by adding 4 ml of medium c to reagent b. The red cell suspension is stable for one week in the refrigerator. Control tubes are prepared with solution d in the same manner as in the Prepuerin test and results are read after 2, 6 and 12 hours.

24.3.7. RADIOIMMUNOASSAY

Radioimmunoassay techniques for protein hormones have undergone such remarkable development over the past years that any attempt to discuss them in detail would go far beyond the scope of this book.

It must be pointed out that separate and fully specific estimation of FSH, LH and chorionic gonadotropin (HPG) has currently become an accomplished fact. Recently,

Jaffe and Midgley,[48] as well as Raiti and Davis,[90] published very complete and comprehensive reviews on the subject.

RADIOIMMUNOASSAY OF FSH. A specific anti-FSH serum was obtained and titrated by Robyn and Diczfalusy[92] in 1968. Radioimmunoassay methods that make use of this specific serum, or of other similar preparations, have been described during the past two years by Albert and his associates,[3] Cargille and co-workers,[20] Mori[79] and Raiti and Blizzard.[89]

RADIOIMMUNOASSAY OF LH. Albert and co-workers[3] similarly described a radioestimation method for LH. Subsequently, other methods were developed by Franchimont,[34] Schams and Karg[98] and Thomas.[108]

RADIOIMMUNOASSAY OF CHORIONIC GONADOTROPIN. Ryan[95] described a radioimmunoassay procedure, based on alkaline extraction, that differs from Gemzell's original method.

24.4. FUNCTIONAL OR "DYNAMIC" TESTS IN EXPLORING THE ENDOCRINE SYSTEM

24.4.1. INTRODUCTION

A number of investigators[2,8] have voiced strong reservations concerning the semeiotic value of various hormone assays for the interpretation of endocrine conditions. The need arose therefore for exploring the reserve or function of the different endocrine glands by means of excitation or loading tests, referred to by Jayle[53-56] as *dynamic exploration tests*. Although many such tests have been devised for each and every endocrine gland, only those concerned with the glands of steroid production (adrenals, testis and ovary) deserve comment here. A recent review on the subject has been published by us.[13]

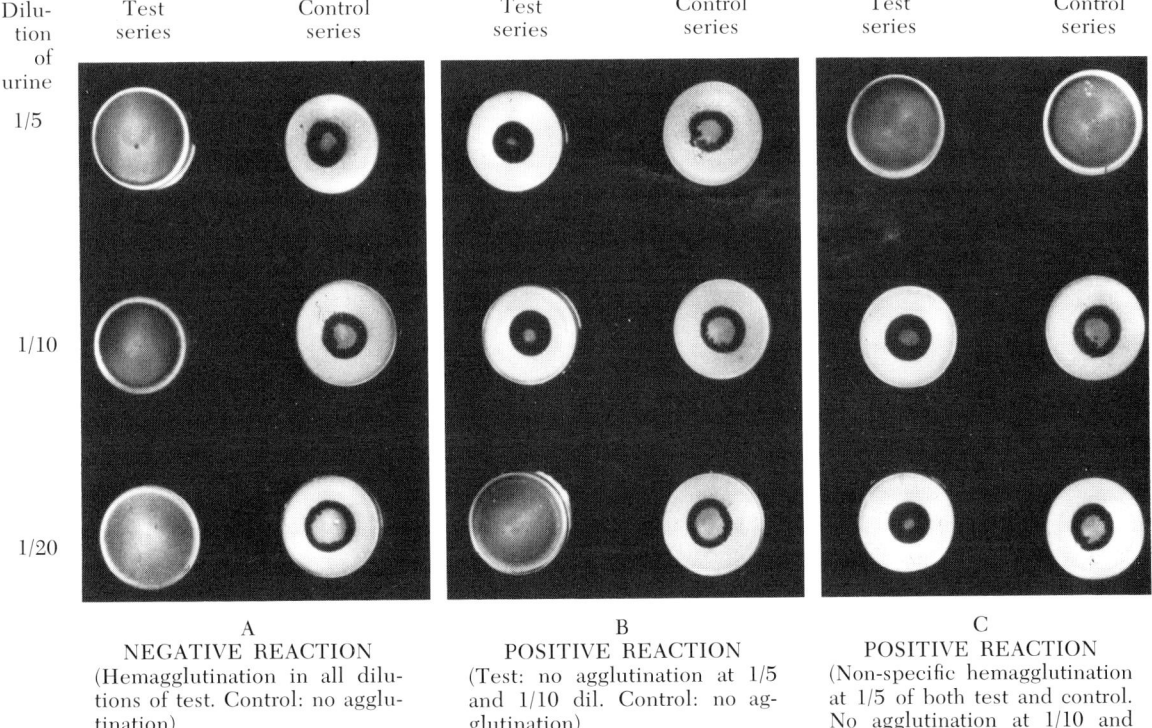

Figure 24-7. The Prepuerin test. (Courtesy of Burroughs, Wellcome & Company, Ltd.)

24.4.2. ADRENAL DYNAMIC TESTS

Thorn and Forsham[109] had earlier attempted to explore the function of the "pituitary-adrenal axis" with injections of epinephrine, and to assess the capacity of isolated adrenal cortex with injections of ACTH. Later, inhibition tests using *dexamethasone* and *metopirone* were introduced as substitutes for the Thorn test, without entirely replacing the latter.

In fact, these tests are not interchangeable. The Thorn test and a few subsequently proposed tests (Bricaire et al.[14, 15]) are stimulation tests *aimed at the diagnosis of hyperfunctional cortical conditions*, whereas the others are *suppression tests* intended for the diagnosis of *hypofunctional cortical situations*.

(A) Stimulation Tests

These are: the classic Thorn test and its modalities, using either epinephrine or ACTH, and the more recently introduced tests of Bricaire and co-workers, using ACTH and determination of Porter-Silber positive steroids.

Thorn Test

It is a well known fact that injection of a cortisone type hormone produces *eosinopenia* of sufficient severity to reduce the concentration of circulating eosinophils, on the average by 50 per cent. Thorn and Forsham[109] recommended a test wherein the adrenal cortex was stimulated to hyperactivity and its capacity for responding was measured in terms of the resulting eosinopenia. There are two ways of performing this functional or dynamic adrenal test: (1) by means of assessing *postepinephrine* eosinopenia, and (2) by means of inducing eosinopenia with an injection of ACTH.

(a) POSTEPINEPHRINE EOSINOPENIA. This is the most commonly followed routine of exploration in the Thorn test. It consists of injecting the patient with 0.25 milligrams of epinephrine and taking a white cell count before the test and 2 and 4 hours after the test. In a normal individual, the eosinophil count ought to drop to *half* the original figure. Lack of any reduction in the number of circulating eosinophils is interpreted as complete absence of cortical function, whereas a drop of less than 50 per cent indicates adrenal cortical insufficiency.

Epinephrine stimulates the center of the hypothalamic median eminence (see Chapter 8), producing local secretion of CRF (corticotropin releasing factor); the latter elicits release of ACTH by the adenohypophysis, which in turn stimulates the fascicular layer of the adrenal cortex to produce glucocorticoids, which are the responsible agents for the resulting eosinopenia. Consequently, this test *not only determines adrenal function but also explores the functional capacity of the entire hypothalamic-pituitary-adrenal axis*. Some of the modifications of this test are based on determining *lymphopenia* or a *rise in corticoid excretion*.

(b) POST-ACTH EOSINOPENIA. With the exception of injecting 25 mg of ACTH, the test is performed in the same manner. In this case, what is explored exclusively is adrenal reserve. Since the eosinopenic or lymphopenic response is subject to fluctuations and to changes involving the hematopoietic system, the newer dynamic tests are designed to determine urinary corticoid excretion values.

Modern Stimulation Tests

Jayle and his associates[49-57] recommended the injection of 25 to 50 mg ACTH in conjunction with urinary 17-hydroxycorticosteroid determinations, taken before and after the injection, as a dynamic test of adrenal function. Following the same line of reasoning, Bricaire and his colleagues[14, 15] in 1966 tested a new corticotropin compound, Ba-30, 920 by Ciba, and studied the resulting fluctuations in urinary 17-hydroxycorticosteroid levels.

(B) Suppression Tests

Although it is a convenient tool for detecting any deficit in cortical function, the Thorn test is not suitable for the demonstration of hypercorticism. For this condition, studies conducted by Liddle and his colleagues[68, 69] using the *dexamethasone test* are therefore of great significance.

Dexamethasone (9α-fluoro-16α-methylprednisolone) (Fig. 24–8) is a corticoid which possesses little glucocorticoid, but strong antirheumatic, activity and, above

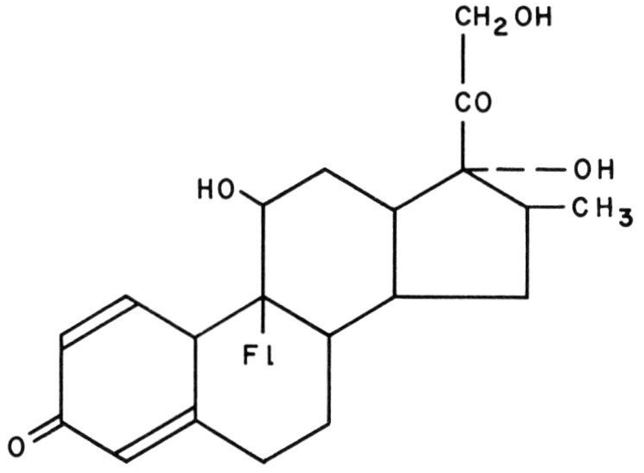

Hormone Assay

Figure 24–8. Dexamethasone (9α-fluoro-16α-methyl-prednisolone).

all, shows marked potency for suppressing ACTH release. This property is utilized for the study of *adrenocortical hyperfunction*. Liddle and his associates[69] estimated that the amount of 4 mg of the drug (divided into four daily doses of 0.5 mg for two days) was sufficient to suppress ACTH production and, consequently, excretion in the urine of 17-hydroxycorticosteroids (Porter-Silber positive steroids) in a normal individual (Fig. 24–9).

The test is performed as shown in Figure 24–9. 17-Hydroxycorticosteroid (17-HOCS) determinations are done at least twice before the test is begun. Dexamethasone (2 mg/day) is administered orally in four equally spaced fractions to assure adequate impregnation, and 17-HOCS determinations are performed daily over a period of six days.

Figure 24–9 illustrates a normal response. The shaded area includes the margin of standard deviation. The base line rate of 17-HOCS excretion must not drop below 3 mg/24 hr, nor must it exceed 11 mg/24 hr. On the second day of treatment, excretion rates decrease and may drop close to zero, only to return to basal levels by the sixth day. *In patients suffering from adrenocortical hyperfunction*, the results are totally negative, as shown in Figure 24–12. If this is the case, Liddle and co-workers[69] recommend the use of the *reinforced test* (Fig. 24–10) which consists in injecting 2 mg every six hours, for a total dose of *16 mg* in two days. If hypercorticism is of primordial pituitary origin (pituitary Cushing's disease; see Chapter 33), such a large dose is expected to cause a *better than 50 per cent reduction* in basal 17-HOCS values, whereas in the adrenal variety of Cushing's disease (adrenocortical tumor), the response is *zero*.

Subsequently, Nugent and associates,[84] in 1965, and Bricaire and colleagues,[14] in 1966, developed somewhat similar modifications of the dexamethasone method. Bricaire's group proposed a screening test in which the patient receives 1 mg dexamethasone at midnight and, 8 hours later, plasma *cortisol* values are measured by the fluorimetric method of Moor. Plasma cortisol levels of 10 mcg/100 ml are within normal limits, whereas levels between 10 and 25 mcg/100 ml indicate simple hypercorticism, and values above 25 mcg/100 ml indicate Cushing's disease.

(C) Metopyrone Test

In 1956, Rosenfeld and Bascom[93] synthesized *Amphenone* (Fig. 24–11), which was found to interfere with the activity of various steroidogenic enzymes (see Chapter 2). The pharmacologic properties of Amphenone were studied by Jenkins and his co-workers,[58] although the drug could not be applied in exploratory practice, owing to its high degree of toxicity. Subsequently, a group of workers at the Ciba laboratories (Chart and Sheppard[21]) synthesized Metopyrone, a derivative of Amphenone (Fig. 24–11) which, they were able to demonstrate, inhibited specifically 11β-hydroxylase activity, known to be indispen-

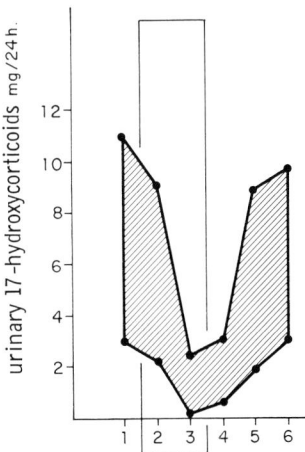

Figure 24–9. Dexamethasone test in a normal individual. Shaded area indicates limits of physiologic variations in 17-hydroxycorticoid levels. Note decrease caused by inhibition of ACTH release. (From Albeaux-Fernet: *L'année endocrinologique*. Paris, Masson & Cie., 1969.)

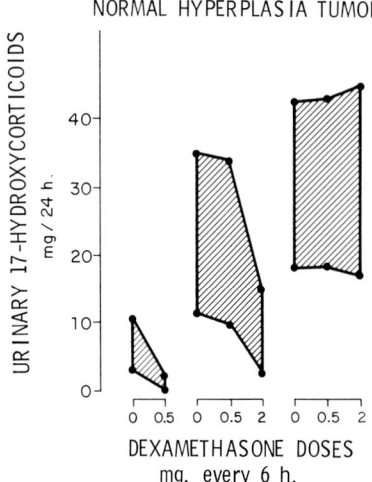

Figure 24-10. Dexamethasone test findings in normal individuals, in patients with simple adrenal hyperplasia and in patients with adrenal tumors. Abscissa indicates milligrams of dexamethasone injected. Normal individuals respond to a dose of 0.5 mg every 6 hrs. (2 mg/day) with a drop in 17-hydroxycorticoid values, whereas those with adrenal hyperplasia respond only to doses as large as 2 mg every 6 hrs (8 mg/day). In patients with adrenal tumors, on the other hand, even larger doses produce no drop in 17-HOCS levels. This test permits the differential diagnosis between Cushing's disease of pituitary origin and that of adrenal origin. (From Albeaux-Fernet: *L'année endocrinologique.* Paris, Masson & Cie., 1969.)

reserve of the pituitary. Thus, the test is primarily a measure of the capacity of the anterior lobe for secreting ACTH.

In practice, the test is performed in the following manner: Without prior therapy, urinary 17-HOCS rates are determined on two consecutive days, after which a total dose of 4.5 g of Metopyrone (Su 4.885, Ciba), divided into six doses of 750 mg, is administered over a period of 24 hr. Urinary 17-HOCS values are determined over a period of four more days (see graph in Figure 24-13).

In normal individuals (Fig. 24-13), the rate of 17-HOCS excretion starts rising by the evening of the first day of treatment, reaching a peak 24 hours later. According to Liddle,[68] peak values of 300 per cent are normally observed. In adrenal insufficiency (Addison's disease) and in pituitary insufficiency, the test gives negative results. Similarly, Soulariac and his associates[104] reported that the Metopyrone test was negative in hypophysectomized patients. Albeaux-Fernet[2] suggested that a second stimulation test was necessary to make the differential diagnosis in these cases. Metopyrone also affects the excretion rate of 17-ketosteroids and sodium, but these are of lesser practical significance than that of 17-hydroxycorticosteroids.

It is thus apparent that adrenal function

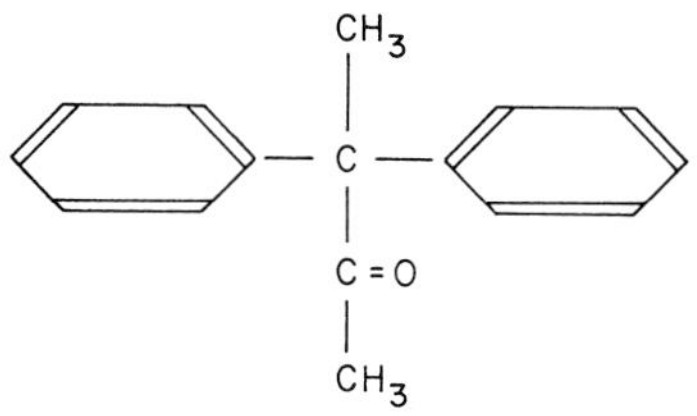

sable for the biogenesis of all corticosteroids (see Chapter 9). The mode of action of Metopyrone is shown diagrammatically in Figure 24-12. By inhibiting 11-hydroxylation, it blocks formation of cortisol, cortisone, corticosterone and aldosterone, arresting the process of adrenal steroidogenesis at the level of 17-hydroxycortexone and related cortexones. As a 17-HOCS, 17-hydroxycortexone gives the Porter-Silber reaction, although it possesses no corticoid action or ACTH-suppressing activity. These properties have been confirmed in human experiments by Liddle and associates.[68, 69] Thus, this test serves as an *indirect pituitary stimulation test,* since, as a result of the inhibition of cortisol and cortisone secretion, as well as the suppression of ACTH release, it triggers and increasingly stimulates formation of cortexones by a mechanism analogous to that involved in androgen production in the adrenogenital syndrome (see Chapter 33). Because 17-hydroxycortexone gives a positive Porter-Silber reaction, the quantity of urinary 17-HOCS is proportional to the endocrine

AMPHENONE

A

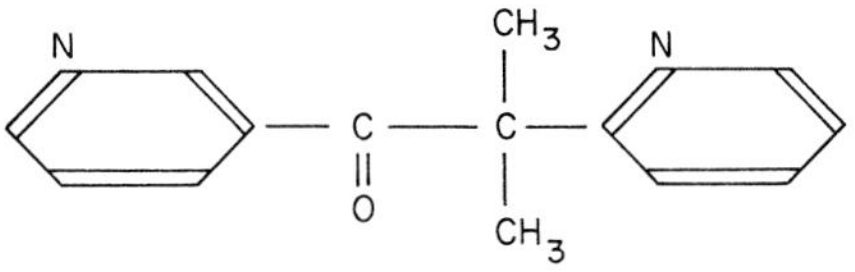

METOPYRONE (METOPYRAPONE) (SU 4885, CIBA)

B

Figure 24-11. Amphenone and Metopyrone (metyrapone).

Hormone Assay

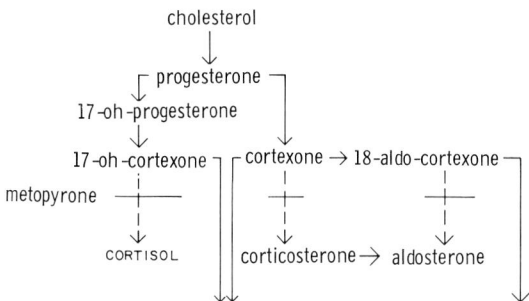

Figure 24–12. Inhibition of adrenal steroidogenesis by Metopyrone (metyrapone). This compound inhibits 17-hydroxylase activity, thereby blocking conversion of corresponding cortexones to cortisol, corticosterone and aldosterone. (From Albeaux-Fernet: *L'année endocrinologique*. Paris, Masson & Cie., 1969.)

may at present be explored in great depth by means of dynamic tests, both of the stimulation and of the suppression variety, which yield much more expressive data than can ever be gathered from interpreting excretion values of urinary steroids. Application of these tests in *endocrine gynecology* facilitates immeasurably the exploration of a number of adrenal endocrinopathies with sexual repercussions (Chapter 33).

24.4.3. TESTICULAR FUNCTION TESTS

Dynamic tests for the exploration of testicular function have so far found less applicability. Recently, Lederer and Bataille[65] investigated urinary 17-ketosteroid values following an overdose of chorionic gonadotropin. They used 15 IU chorionic gonadotropin and found that the fractions excreted in greatest quantities were androsterone and etiocholanone. Gilbert-Dreyfus, moreover, studied the response of plasma testosterone. It would seem to us indispensable that, for proper evaluation of this test, either urinary 17-ketosteroids be separated chromatographically, or plasma testosterone levels be determined simultaneously, since the adrenal fraction masks the results in simple determinations of total 17-ketosteroids following HCG loading. Our own studies[10, 11] revealed that chorionic gonadotropin stimulates formation of 17-ketosteroids (mainly etiocholanone and DHEA) at the level of the adrenal cortex.

These two tests only estimate the endocrine reserve of the testicular interstitium, that is, the Leydig system, but do not reflect testicular spermatogenetic capacity. Botella[12] recently studied the reserve of the Leydig system by means of injecting HCG in doses of 10,000 IU and determining the Botella-Casares (BC) index of spermatic progression before and after HCG loads, to which the patient was subjected in a chronic rather than acute type of experiment (see graph in Figure 24–14).

24.4.4. OVARIAN FUNCTION TESTS

These are of greatest interest to us. Championed by Jayle,[53, 54, 56] they have been mainly employed by French investigators (Palmer and Palmer[85]). We shall now discuss in sequence the dexamethasone test for female androgenism, several tests involving gonadotropin loading techniques, and the combined dexamethasone-gonadotropin test, currently of greater applicability.

Dexamethasone Test for Female Virilism

The significance of this test was pointed out by Jayle,[55] who found it *indispensable for the correct assessment of whether a given syndrome of virilism is of ovarian or adrenal origin*. As practiced by Jayle, the test is performed in a slightly different way from that described by us previously.

TECHNIQUE. Using a 24 hr specimen

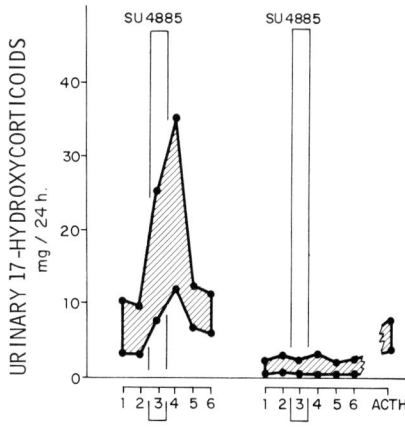

Figure 24–13. Metopyrone test. Left, Normal individual. Right, patient with adenohypophysial insufficiency. Because administration of ACTH results in an increase of 19-hydroxycorticoids in pituitary insufficiency, the latter condition can be distinguished from Addison's disease, in which such a rise does not take place. (From Jayle.)

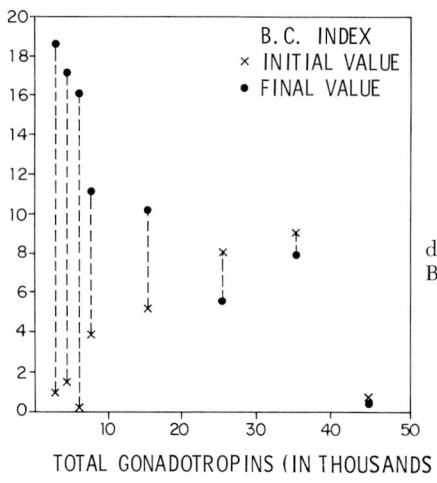

Figure 24–14. Response to administration of 1000 IU HMG daily in males with testicular spermatogenic insufficiency. (From Botella-Llusiá: *Acta Gin.*, 18:365, 1967.)

of urine, basal 17-HOCS values (Fig. 24–15), as well as chromatographic fractions of 17-ketosteroids (Fig. 24–15) are determined once or, preferably, twice. Then 3 mg of dexamethasone is administered daily in small dosages given every six hours for a total of 18 mg over a six-day period. Urinary creatinine values are also determined in order to avoid errors in re-collection. Upon completion of dexamethasone administration, determination of urinary steroid values is repeated. Results to be anticipated in a normal woman are shown in Figure 24–15.

Owing to suppression of pituitary function, there is a drop in 17-HOCS levels to 1 mg or below. In the absence of such a drop, it may be suspected that dexamethasone administration has not been effective, invalidating the test. The 17-ketosteroid fractions, corresponding to DHEA and 11-oxy-17-ketosteroids, are expected to be depressed to zero values. Only androsterone and etiocholanone are decreased to a lesser extent, if at all.

In cases of adrenal virilism (adrenogenital syndrome), basal values of DHEA and 11-oxy-17-ketosteroids are greatly elevated (two to five times normal) but, most significantly, these fractions drop completely or nearly completely after the test, reductions in values amounting to more than 75 per cent. Conversely, the initially elevated fractions in cases of ovarian virilism, such as Stein-Leventhal syndrome, are androsterone and etiocholanone, with values ranging from 7 to 15 mg/24 hr. These are not as high as the DHEA values observed in the adrenogenital syndrome but, unlike the latter, remain constant, or hardly show any alterations, after dexamethasone administration. This test is therefore quite conclusive in the differential diagnosis of virilism.

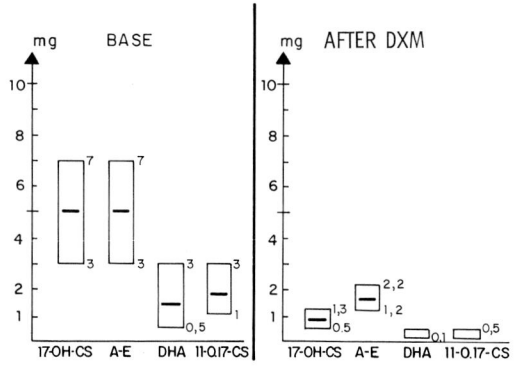

Figure 24–15. Dexamethasone (DXM) test in normal woman. 17-OH-CS, 17-Hydroxycorticoids; A-E, androgenic fraction, androsterone plus etiocholanone; DHA, dehydroepiandrosterone; 11-0.17-CS, 11-oxy-17-ketosteroids. (From Jayle.)

Gonadotropin Loading Tests

Administration of gonadotropin in the study of ovarian function is an excellent dynamic test. Either chorionic or pituitary gonadotropin may be used, although, as a rule, HCG is used. The resulting effects are studied on the basis of estrogen and pregnanediol excretion, or may be assessed at the end-organ level, by studying the endometrium, the cervix (cervical mucus) or, most commonly, the vaginal exudate.

CHORIONIC GONADOTROPIN. In 1956, Jayle and his associates[51] introduced the procedure of stimulating the ovary with 15,000 IU of CG and then estimating the functional capacity of the ovary on the basis of the total urinary phenolsteroid (total estrogen) output. He originally used 5000 IU of pregnant mare serum (PMS) three times daily, following by determination of total estrogens three days after the last injection. Elevations above 50 per cent were considered to reflect adequate ovarian function, whereas negative results were obtained in cases of sterility of ovarian origin (anovulatory cycle) and in various forms of primary ovarian amenorrhea. However, the test was found to be unable to discriminate between follicular and corpus luteum function.

Jayle later repeated the test in regard to both phenolsteroid and pregnanediol determinations. Subsequently, he abandoned the concept of using gonadotropin loading alone in favor of a combined approach, using both chorionic gonadotropin and dexamethasone, which we will describe later in this chapter.

PITUITARY GONADOTROPINS (HPG AND HMG). Crooke and his associates[23] applied HPG injections in association with fractional determination of estrogens (method of Brown, page 507) and estimation of pregnanediol before and after the test. Similarly, Diczfalusy and colleagues[24] have conducted a comparative study of the effects of HPG and HMG on the rate of estrogen and pregnanediol excretion. The action of gonadotropin stimulation on ovulatory function was studied by Cox and his co-workers[22a] who used Pergonal-500 in dosages of 150 IU HMG daily for three days, using a total of 450 IU, coupled with determinations of estrogen and pregnanediol excretion levels and basal body temperature. A modification of this technique has been proposed by Netter's group,[82] advocating injection of a total of 7500 IU HMG over three days, followed by 5000 IU of chorionic gonadotropin. Lately, a number of dynamic tests for ovarian function based on administration of HMG and HPG have been developed for the treatment of gonadal insufficiency (see Chapter 32).

GONADOTROPIN LOADING AND ITS EFFECT ON TARGET ORGANS. Examination of endometrial biopsies, physical properties of cervical mucus, basal body temperature and vaginal cytology following administration of CG, HPG or HMG also constitute informative modalities of ovarian function tests. A simple procedure proposed by Montalvo-Ruiz[78] allows satisfactory assessment of ovarian function in amenorrhea. It consists of daily injections of 1000 IU HMG for one week, followed by serial examination of vaginal cytology, in which the karyopyknotic index is used as a guide for evaluating the ovarian response.

Dynamic Test of Jayle, Using CG and Dexamethasone

Because the basal sex steroid excretion rate does not reflect faithfully enough the true functional state of the ovary, Jayle proposed and pioneered in the development of various methods for the estimation of ovarian function based on gonadotropin stimulation. In 1961, he developed a dynamic test combining stimulation with suppression,[52] which, in a subsequently perfected form,[53, 54, 55, 56] has served principally for the assessment of functional corpus luteum reserve and permitted the establishment of true "luteal insufficiency" on biochemical grounds. This test involves simultaneous suppression of the pituitary by means of dexamethasone and stimulation of the ovary by means of chorionic gonadotropin (Fig. 24–16).

TECHNIQUE. The basal body temperature chart is plotted from the first day of the cycle and, if possible, compared with that of preceding cycles. On the day the first thermal upswing is noted (Fig. 24–16), a 24 hr urine specimen is collected and total urinary 17-ketosteroids, as well as breakdown of the fractions pertaining to androsterone-etiocholanone, dehydroepiandrosterone and 11-oxy-17-ketosteroids, are determined. The estrogen fractions pertaining to estradiol, estrone and estriol are likewise determined. On the third day after

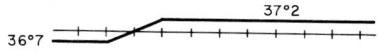

Figure 24-16. Diagrammatic outline of the test of Jayle. See Figure 24-15 for identification of abbreviations, with addition of: PG, pregnanediol; PGT, pregnanetriol; O_I, estrone; O_{II}, estradiol; O_{III}, estriol. For further details, see text.

TABLE 24-2. Types of Response Obtained in the CG + Dexamethasone Test*

RESPONSE	FRACTION A-E, (MG/24 HRS)	PREG-NANETRIOL (MG/24 HRS)	PREG-NANEDIOL (MG/24 HRS)	ESTRADIOL + ESTRONE (MCG/24 HRS)	ESTRIOL (MCG/24 HRS)
Normal	1.6 (1–2.2)	1.5 (1–2)	6.5 (5–9)	33 (25–40)	48 (30–60)
Castration hypopituitarism	0.3 (0–0.7)	0 (0)	0.2 (0–0.6)	3 (0–5)	7 (5–10)
Lutein-follicle insufficiency	1.5 (0.7–2)	0.9 (0.5–1.8)	3.1 (1–4.5)	18 (10–25)	25 (15–35)
Follicle insufficiency, pure	1.4 (1–2)	1.1 (1–1.8)	6.4 (5–8.3)	17 (10–20)	25 (20–30)
Luteal insufficiency, pure	1.7 (1.2–2)	1.2 (1–2)	3.3 (2–4.5)	31 (25–40)	41 (35–50)
Hyperandrogenism	3 (2.5–5.5)	1.6 (0.6–2.7)	5.7 (2–14.5)	34 (10–75)	50 (20–100)
Hyperestrinism	2 (1.6–2.4)	2 (1.5–2.4)	5.4 (0.5–9)	45 (30–60)	80 (40–100)

*After Jayle.

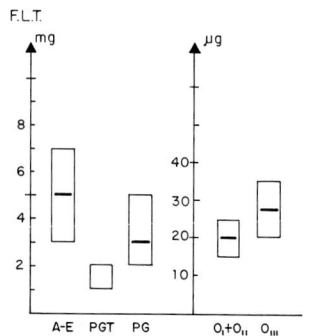
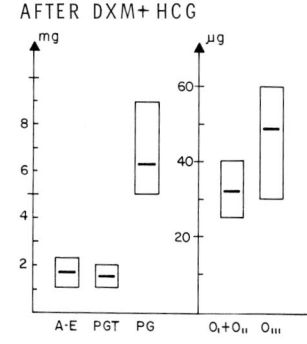

Figure 24-17. The dynamic test of Jayle in a normal woman. See Figures 24-15 and 24-16 for identification of abbreviations. For clarification, refer to text.

the thermal rise, 5000 IU of chorionic gonadotropin and 3 mg (distributed in four 0.75 mg dosages) of dexamethasone are administered. The same dosage of dexamethasone is maintained daily for six more days, whereas CG is given once every 48 hr for a total of 15,000 IU. The high dose of CG, according to the authors, is not hazardous and produces no disturbances. On the eighth day after the occurrence of the thermal elevation (the last day of dexamethasone administration, 24 hr after CG has been discontinued), another 24 hr urine specimen is collected and all the previously mentioned determinations, plus that of pregnanediol and pregnanetriol, are repeated.

Results representing a normal response in woman are shown in Figure 24–17. The androsterone-etiocholanone fraction of 17-ketosteroids is reduced to one third, pregnanetriol (adrenal origin) remains unaltered, pregnanediol increases by 100 per cent, and the estrone-estradiol fraction of estrogens is similarly increased by 100 per cent, whereas the estriol fraction, corresponding to corpus luteum estrogen synthesis, is increased by 200 per cent. These results *indicate the presence of a corpus luteum with adequate function.*

The data obtained from the exploration of various ovarian syndromes have been incorporated by Jayle into a synoptic representation (Table 24–2). Although, at present, the subclassification of so many syndromes that are seldom seen would seem to us excessively artificial, there is no doubt that the work under consideration constitutes the most significant attempt made to date to perform quantitative biochemical explorations of ovarian function in general and of luteal function in particular.

Notwithstanding our belief that the test is of primordial importance, to comment on each of the data contained in the table would involve an unwarranted digression, since the results have yet to be borne out by wider experience and by a large number of applications.

REFERENCES

1. Abraham, G. E., O'Dell, W. D., Edwards, R., and Purdy, J. M.: *Karolinska Symposia on Research Methods in Reproductive Endocrinology.* Vol. II, ed. E. Diczfalusy. Stockholm, Karolinska Sjukhuset, 1970.
2. Albeaux-Fernet, M.: *L'année endocrinologique*, 14:24, 1962.
3. Albert, A., Rosenberg, E., Ross, G. T., Paulsen, C. A., and Ryan, R. J.: *J. Clin. Endocr.*, 28:1214, 1968.
4. Albert, A.: *J. Clin. Endocr.*, 28:1683, 1968.
5. Allen, W. M.: *J. Clin. Endocr.*, 10:71, 1950.
6. Barakat, R. M., and Elkins, R. P.: *Lancet*, 2:25, 1961.
7. Baulieu, E., Raynaud, J. P., and Milgrom, E.: *Karolinska Symposia Res. Meth. Reprod. Endocr.*, 2:104, 1970.
8. Bedoya, J. M., and Plaza, F.: *Geburtsh. u. Frauenheilk.*, 10:509, 1950.
9. Botella, J.: *Arch. Gynäk.*, 183:73, 1953.
10. Botella, J., and Tornero, M. C.: *Rev. Diag. Biol.*, 1:99, 1951.
11. Botella, J., Plaza, F., and Del Sol, J. R.: *Studies on Fertility*, 8:58, 1956.
12. Botella, J.: *Acta Gin.*, 19:329, 1968.
13. Botella, J.: *Acta Gin.*, 19:485, 1968.
14. Bricaire, H., Moreau, L., Laudat, P., and Schoeller, P.: *Ann. d'Endocr.*, 27:173, 1966.
15. Bricaire, H., Leprat, J., Laudat, P., Lutton, J. P., Milgrom, E., and Laurent, D.: *Ann. d'Endocr.*, 28:66, 1967.
16. Brown, I. B.: *Biochem. J.*, 60:185, 1955.
17. Bryant, G. D., and Greenwood, F. C.: *Biochem. J.*, 109:831, 1968.
18. Burgos, M. H., and Ladman, A. J.: *Endocrinology*, 61:20, 1957.
19. Butt, W. R., et al.: *Biochem. J.*, 49:434, 1951.
20. Cargille, C. M., Robbard, D., and Ross, G. T.: *J. Clin. Endocr.*, 28:1276, 1968.
21. Chart, J. J., and Sheppard, H.: *J. Med. Pharm. Chem.*, 1:407, 1959.
22. Corker, C. S., and Exley, D.: *J. Endocr.*, 43:30, 1969.
22a. Cox, R. I., Cox, L. W., and Black, T. L.: *Lancet*, 2:888, 1966.
23. Crooke, A. C., Butt, W. R., and Bertrand, P. W.: *Acta Endocr.*, 53:Suppl. 111, 1966.
24. Diczfalusy, E., Johansson, E., Tillinger, K. G., and Bettendorf, G.: *Acta Endocr.*, 45(Suppl.): 90, 1964.
25. Diczfalusy, E. (ed.): "Steroid Assay by Protein Binding," *Karolinska Symposia Res. Meth. Reprod. Endocr.*, 2:359, Stockholm, Karolinska Sjukhuset, 1970.
26. Dominguez, J. M., and Pearson, O. A.: *J. Clin. Endocr. Metab.*, 22:865, 1962.
27. Dorfman, R. I.: *Endocrinology*, 42:85, 1948.
28. Elberlein, W. R., and Bongiovanni, A. M.: *J. Clin. Endocr. Metab.*, 17:1476, 1957.
29. Elftman, H.: *Proc. Soc. Exper. Biol. Med.*, 105:19, 1960.
30. Elkins, R., and Newman, B.: *Karolinska Symposia Res. Meth. Reprod. Endocr.*, 2:11, 1970.
31. Ellis, S.: *Endocrinology*, 68:334, 1961.
32. Flux, D. S.: *J. Endocr.*, 20:307, 1960.
33. Franchimont, P., and Salmon, J.: *Ann. d'Endocr.*, 23:556, 1962.
34. Franchimont, P.: *Ann. d'Endocr.*, 29:403, 1968.
35. Garmier, R.: *Rev. Franç. Gynec. Obstet.*, 55:407, 1960.
36. Goetz, F. C., et al.: *J. Clin. Endocr. Metab.*, 23:1237, 1963.
37. Goss, D. A., and Lewis, J.: *Endocrinology*, 74:83, 1964.

38. Goss, D. A., and Taymor, M. L.: *Endocrinology,* 71:321, 1962.
39. Guterman, H. S.: *J. Clin. Endocr. Metab.,* 15:407, 1955.
40. Guterman, H. S., and Schroeder, M.: *J. Lab. Clin. Med.,* 33:356, 1948.
41. Hashimoto, Y., and Neeman, M.: *J. Biol. Chem.,* 238:1273, 1963.
42. Hayashida, T.: *Ciba Colloq. Endocr.,* 14:338, 1962.
43. Heinrichs, H. D., and Eulenfeld, F.: *Acta Endocr.,* 34(Suppl.):53, 1960.
44. Hooker, C. W., and Forbes, T. R.: *Endocrinology,* 41:159, 1947.
45. Hooker, C. W., and Forbes, T. R.: *Endocrinology,* 45:71, 1949.
46. Islami, Z. S., et al.: *Amer. J. Obstet. Gynec.,* 83:586, 1964.
47. Ittrich, G.: *Acta Endocr.,* 35:34, 1960.
48. Jaffe, R. B., and Midgley, A. R.: *Obstet. Gynec. Surv.,* 24:200, 1969.
49. Jayle, M. F., et al.: *Ann. d'Endocr.,* 14:642, 1953.
50. Jayle, M. F., et al.: *Ann. d'Endocr.,* 22:798, 1961.
51. Jayle, M. F., et al.: *Compt. Rend. Soc. Biol. (Paris),* 150:1351, 1956.
52. Jayle, M. F., Veyrin-Forrier, F., Geller, S., and Emge, F.: *Gynec. Obstet.,* 60:381, 1961.
53. Jayle, M. F.: "L'epreuve de l'exploration dynamique de l'ovaire par les gonadotrophines," in *Les gonadotrophines en gynecologie.* Paris, Masson & Cie., 1962.
54. Jayle, M. F.: "L'exploration dynamique de la fonction luteale," in *Actas del VII Congreso de Endocrinólogos de Lengua Francesa,* Beirut, 1963. Paris, Masson & Cie., 1963.
55. Jayle, M. F.: Inhibition of the adrenal cortex by dexamethasone, *Proceed. I Internat. Congr. Steroids,* Vol. 2, Milan, 1964. New York, Academic Press, 1965.
56. Jayle, M. F.: "L'exploration dynamique de la fonction endocrinienne des ovaires," in *Colloque sur la fonction endocrinienne des ovaires,* ed. M. F. Jayle. Paris, Gauthier-Villars, 1967.
57. Jayle, M. F.: *Analyse des steroides hormonaux,* Vol. II. Paris, Masson & Cie., 1962.
58. Jenkins, W., et al.: *Science,* 128:478, 1958.
59. Johanson, A. J., Guyda, H., and Light, C.: *J. Pediat.,* 74:416, 1969.
60. Johansson, E. D. B., and Wide, L.: *Acta Endocr.,* 62:83, 1969.
61. Kaufmann, C., Westphal, U., and Zander, J.: *Arch. Gynäk.,* 179:247, 1961.
62. Kirschner, M. A., and Lippsett, M. B.: *J. Clin. Endocr. Metab.,* 23:255, 1963.
63. Kullander, S.: *J. Obstet. Gynec. Brit. Emp.,* 55:159, 1948.
64. Laron, Z., and Assi, S.: *Nature,* 197:299, 1963.
65. Lederer, J., and Bataille, J.: *Ann. d'Endocr.,* 28:111, 1967.
66. Leroy, F., Manavian, D., and Hubinot, P. O.: *J. Endocr.,* 39:227, 1967.
67. Li, C. H.: *Ciba Colloq. Endocr.,* 14:20, 1962.
68. Liddle, G. W.: *J. Clin. Endocr. Metab.,* 20:1539, 1960.
69. Liddle, G. W., et al.: *J. Clin. Endocr. Metab.,* 18:906, 1958; 19:875, 1959.
70. Lipsett, M. B., Doerr, P., and Bermudez, J. A.: *Karolinska Symposia Res. Meth. Reprod. Endocr.,* 2:155, 1970.
71. Lloyd, C. W., et al.: *Endocrinology,* 39:256, 1946.
72. Lunenfeld, B.: *J. Clin. Endocr. Metab.,* 21:478, 1961.
73. Marrian, G. F., Sommerville, I. F., and Keller, R. J.: *Lancet,* 1:89, 1948.
74. MacCann, S. M., and Taleisnik, S.: *Amer. J. Physiol.,* 199:847, 1960.
75. Mercier-Bodard, C., Alfsen, A., and Baulieu, E.: *Karolinska Symposia Res. Meth. Reprod. Endocr.,* 2:204, 1970.
76. Midgley, A. R., and Niswender, G. D.: *Karolinska Symposia Res. Meth. Reprod. Endocr.,* 2:320, 1970.
77. Miyake, T., and Pincus, G.: *Endocrinology,* 63:816, 1958.
78. Montalvo-Ruiz, L.: *Acta Gin.,* 19:297, 1968.
79. Mori, K. F.: *J. Endocr.,* 42:55, 1968.
80. Moudgal, N. R., and Li, C. H.: *Endocrinology,* 68:704, 1961.
81. Murphy, B. E. P.: *Karolinska Symposia Res. Meth. Reprod. Endocr.,* 2:37, 1970.
82. Netter, A., Salomon, Y., and Cabau, A.: *Ann. d'Endocr.,* 27:52, 1966.
83. Nilson, I., and Bengtsson, L. P.: *Acta Obstet. Gynec. Scand.,* 47:213, 1968.
84. Nugent, C. A., Nichols, T., and Tyler, F.: *Arch. Int. Med.,* 116:162, 1965.
85. Palmer, R., and Palmer, E.: *Les explorations fonctionelles gynecologiques.* Paris, Masson & Cie., 1963.
86. Parlow, A. F.: *Fed. Proceed.,* 17:402, 1958.
87. Pearlman, W. H., and Cerceo, E.: *Endocrinology,* 53:599, 1953.
88. Plaza, F., and Mesa, A.: *Arch. Fac. Med., Madrid,* 4:301, 1963.
89. Raiti, S., and Blizzard, L. M.: *J. Clin. Endocr.,* 28:1719, 1968.
90. Raiti, S., and Davis, W. T.: *Obstet. Gynec. Surv.,* 24:289, 1969.
91. Robyn, C., and Diczfalusy, E.: *Acta Endocr.,* 59:255, 1968.
92. Robyn, C., and Diczfalusy, E.: *Acta Endocr.,* 59:261, 1968.
93. Rosenfeld, G., and Bascom, W. D.: *J. Biol. Chem.,* 222:565, 1956.
94. Roy, E. J.: *J. Endocr.,* 25:361, 1962.
95. Ryan, R. J.: *J. Clin. Endocr.,* 28:866, 1968.
96. Sakiz, E., and Guillemin, R.: *Endocrinology,* 72:804, 1963.
97. Saxena, B., Demura, H., Gandy, H. M., and Peterson, R. E.: *J. Clin. Endocr.,* 28:519, 1968.
98. Schams, D., and Karg, H.: *Acta Endocr.,* 61:96, 1969.
99. Schild, W.: *Ztschr. Ges. Exper. Med.,* 135:13, 1961.
100. Scommegna, A.: *Obstet. Gynec. Surv.,* 24:387, 1969.
101. Seki, T., and Matsumoto, K.: *J. Chromatography,* 10:400, 1963.
102. Short, R. V., and Levett, I.: *J. Endocr.,* 25:239, 1962.
103. Smith, L. G.: *Amer. J. Obstet. Gynec.,* 89:583, 1964.
104. Souleriac, A., et al.: *Ann. d'Endocr.,* 28:101, 1967.

105. Stevenson, M. F., and Marrian, G. F.: *Biochem. J.*, 41:507, 1947.
106. Stoa, K. F., and Thorsen, T.: *Acta Endocr.*, 41:481, 1962.
107. Thevenet, M., Hanry, R., and Farmaniani, J.: *Ann. d'Endocr.*, 24:773, 1963.
108. Thomas, K.: *Bull. Roy. Soc. Belg. Gynec. Obstet.*, 38:449, 1968.
109. Thorn, G. W., and Forsham, P. H.: In *Progress in Endocrinology*, ed. S. Soskin. New York, Grune & Stratton, 1950.
110. Venning, E. H.: *Endocrinology*, 38:79, 1946.
111. Vermeulen, A., and Verdonck, L.: *Karolinska Symposia Res. Meth. Reprod. Endocr.*, 2:239, 1970.
112. Vestergaard, P.: *Acta Endocr.*, 8:193, 1951.
113. Ward, D. N., McGregor, R. F., and Putch, J. D.: *Endocrinology*, 71:474, 1962.
114. Watteville, H., et al.: *J. Clin. Endocr.*, 8:982, 1948.
115. Wide, D., and Gemzell, C. A.: *Acta Endocr.*, 39:539, 1962.
116. Wide, D., and Gemzell, C. A.: *Ciba Colloq. Endocr.*, 14:296, 1962.
117. Zander, J., and Simmer, H.: *Klin. Wschr.*, 32:529, 1954.
118. Zimmermann, W.: *Chemische Bestimmungsmethoden der Sexual-hormone*. Berlin, Springer, 1958.

Chapter 25
ENDOCRINE CYTOLOGY

Over the years, the number of procedures available for cytologic and histologic exploration has increased so dramatically that it seems impossible to even begin to summarize the wealth of accumulated data. The purpose of this chapter is to initiate the reader in this type of exploratory technique and to familiarize him with its diagnostic potentialities. While the preceding chapter dealt with estimating female endocrine function by measuring products of incretion in the blood and urine, the present chapter is concerned with analyzing cytologic effects in the very target organs subjected to hormone activity. Cytodiagnostic procedures may consequently be viewed as a form of *autobioassay* in which the effects of hormone action are studied directly in woman's cells.

25.1. VAGINAL CYTOLOGY

Although the study of vaginal cytology dates back to over a century ago, having been first described by Pouchet in 1847, later in more detail by Heape in 1894 and by Herwerden in 1906, practically all significant progress in this branch of gynecology has been realized in the course of the past 30 years. Currently, there are numerous journals and societies devoted exclusively to the study of the vast amount of knowledge accumulated in this field.

25.1.1. HISTORY

After the pioneering studies already referred to, the most significant breakthrough in the field was the work of Stockard and Papanicolaou who, in 1917, described the phenomenon of vaginal exfoliation in the guinea pig. In 1922, Long and Evans,[36] as well as Allen and Doisy,[1] described cyclic vaginal exfoliation in rats and mice and, based on those findings, developed their method for the assay of estrogenic hormone (see Chapter 2). Although the fact that vaginal exfoliation in rats, mice, rabbits, guinea pigs and monkeys is cyclic was confirmed in later years, attempts at discovering the cycle in the human vaginal mucosa were long unsuccessful. Dierks, in 1929, and Ramón-Vinós, in 1932, were first to detect the existence of a human vaginal cycle with some degree of certainty. In 1928, Ramírez[58] produced the first work in Spanish on human vaginal cytology and, three years later, Papanicolaou[48] published a monograph on female cytology that yet lacked any precise description of the cycle. In 1936, Papanicolaou and Shorr[49] described the changes characterizing menopause and castration and, two years later, each of the two authors published his own staining method, both of which are still very much in use as essential cytologic staining procedures. In 1939, Salmon and Frank[63] studied the effects of sex hormones on cytology and, during the same year, Murray[44] published the first detailed and complete description of the human vaginal cycle.

In 1941, Botella and Asin made a complete description of the different cell types found in vaginal smears. Among the various outstanding monographs published about that time, two by Papanicolaou and colleagues[50, 51] and four by Pundel[53, 54, 55, 56] deserve to be cited. Works by Zinser, Smolka and Soost, as well as articles in the journal *Acta Cytologica*, all dealing exclusively with the study of cytology, have appeared since and should be mentioned. In 1964, Montalvo[42] published his work on cytology, which is highly recommended.

In 1943, Papanicolaou and Traut[50] introduced a new discipline in vaginal cytology:

the diagnosis of cancer. Since that time, cytology has been divided into two branches: *endocrinologic* and *cancerologic* branches. Only the first is the object of our study, although the second has reached a much greater degree of development.

25.2. STAINING OF SMEARS

The number of procedures that have been developed for the staining of cytologic material is countless. However, two procedures deserve to be described: the Papanicolaou[49] and the Shorr[65] staining techniques. Also to be mentioned here is a procedure for examining smears by means of *phase contrast microscopy*. The nuclear stains have found their greatest application in cancer cytology. Other special staining procedures, such as stains for glycogen, which are useful in research, are of little practical value in routine cytodiagnostics. As shown by us, and confirmed by others, the *presence of glycogen in exfoliated cells is not a direct index of estrogenic activity*.

25.2.1. THE PAPANICOLAOU STAINING PROCEDURE

TECHNIQUE OF TAKING SMEARS. The general rules outlined for the collection of cytologic material are applicable to the Papanicolaou procedure as well as to most other staining procedures. For maximal readability, a smear must be uniformly spread, must not be too thick to avoid impenetrable clumping of cells, and must not be too diluted since excessive separation between cells renders counting them difficult. Because the upper third of the vagina is the region in which the mucosa exhibits the greatest range of cyclic variations in response to hormonal stimuli, the material to be examined should preferably be obtained at this level of the lateral fornix. Inclusion of cervical secretion should be avoided, and collection should be confined to vaginal exudate, which alone can reveal the reactions in the vaginal mucosa for diagnostic purposes.

The mode of obtaining smears varies, depending on whether cytologic study is intended for hormonal diagnosis or for the early detection of malignancy. The best means for the former, we emphasize, is a rubber bulb aspirator ("Papanicolaou pear"). With the speculum in place, any exudate over the lateral aspect of the vaginal fornix is aspirated. The contents of the "pear" are then projected directly onto a slide in a manner that sprays the material evenly and makes need for further spreading unnecessary.

Other authors recommend the use of a cotton swab applicator; however, this method seems to distort some cells and to give misleading results, and is not recommended. Similarly, Ayre[6] recommends the use of the spatula bearing his name. While this is a good procedure for obtaining abundant cellular material, it has a similar drawback in that it may cause folding of cells and erroneous interpretation as far as luteal smears are concerned. *Consequently, we advise the use of a Papanicolaou rubber pear for collection of exfoliated material for smears.*

FIXATION OF SMEARS. Smears must not be allowed to dry, but should be submerged in the fixative while still fresh, that is, immediately after collection. Adequate fixation is of *paramount importance* and can be achieved only if the fixative is permitted to act on a *freshly obtained specimen*. The fixative is composed of equal volumes of ether and 96 per cent ethyl alcohol. Unless applied immediately, the fixative does not prevent epithelial cells from losing their basophilia so that the ratio of acidophilic and basophilic cells (so important for the diagnosis) may thereby be altered. The fixative must be stored in tightly stoppered containers, since ether evaporates more rapidly than alcohol and the proportion in which the two are mixed will change. If reused repeatedly, the mixture should be filtered from time to time to eliminate contaminants, such as detached cells floating in the fixative, which render the fluid cloudy and may cause erroneous interpretation.

STAINING PROCEDURE

1. Ether-alcohol fixative, 15 min.
2. Pass through 70 and 50 per cent alcohol (five to six dips each).
3. Wash in distilled water.
4. Harris' hematoxylin for 6 min.
5. Wash in two changes of distilled water.
6. Dip two to three times in 0.5 per cent solution HCl.
7. Wash in running tap water.

8. Immerse in weak solution of lithium carbonate, 1 min.
9. Rinse in water.
10. Dehydrate through 50, 70, 80 and 96 per cent alcohol (four to six dips each).
11. Stain in Orange G solution for 3 min.
12. Rinse in two changes of 96 per cent alcohol.
13. Stain in EA 31 solution for 4 min.
14. Rinse in two changes of 96 per cent alcohol.
15. Dehydrate in absolute alcohol for 2 min., clear in xylol for 5 min. and mount.

Harris' hematoxylin is prepared according to the following formula:

HARRIS' HEMATOXYLIN

Stock solution:

Hematoxylin	1	gm
Absolute alcohol	10	ml
Aluminum ammonium sulfate	20	gm
Distilled water	200	ml
Mercuric oxide	0.5	gm
Glacial acetic acid	8	ml

Dissolve hematoxylin in absolute alcohol.
Dissolve aluminum ammonium sulfate in hot distilled water. Mix both solutions and bring rapidly to boiling (95° C).
Remove from heat source and add mercuric oxide. Cool in running tap water and, to the cold solution, add acetic acid. Store in tightly stoppered containers.

Working solution:
Two volumes of stock solution are mixed with one volume of saturated aluminum ammonium sulfate solution (15 gm in 100 ml distilled water and 4 ml glacial acetic acid); add crystals of aluminum ammonium sulfate in excess. Filter before use.

A schematic representation of the staining procedure is given in Figure 25-1.

25.2.2. SHORR'S STAINING PROCEDURE

Shorr's stain is simpler than Papanicolaou's and it generally gives less informative results. Smears are fixed as usual. Slides are run through the following staining steps:

1. Stain for 4 to 6 min. in Shorr's solution, which has the following composition: ethyl alcohol (50%), 100 ml; Biebrich scarlet, hydrosoluble, 0.5 gm; orange G, 0.25 gm; fast green FCF, 0.075 gm; phosphotungstic acid, 0.5 gm; phosphomolybdic acid, 0.5 gm; and glacial acetic acid, 1 ml.
2. Dip 10 times in 96 per cent alcohol.
3. Dip 10 times in absolute alcohol.
4. Clear in xylol for 30 sec. Mount in Canada balsam. A diagram of the setup used in Shorr's staining procedure is shown in Figure 25-2.

A modification of this procedure consists in using Harris' hematoxylin in combination with Shorr's solution. Following the usual fixation step, the smears are then carried through these steps:

1. Dip 10 times in 70 per cent alcohol.
2. Dip 10 times in distilled water.
3. Stain in Harris' hematoxylin for 2 min. (for preparation, see preceding section).
4. Wash gently in running tap water.
5. Lithium carbonate, dilute solution (equal volumes with distilled water).
6. Rinse in distilled water, 10 dips.
7. Dehydrate in 70 and 96 per cent alcohol (10 dips each).
8. Stain in Shorr's solution for 5 min.
9. Ten dips in 96 per cent alcohol.
10. Ten dips in absolute alcohol.
11. Xylol, 30 sec.
12. Mount in Canada balsam.

A diagrammatic outline of this procedure is given in Figure 25-3.

O'Morchoe's recent modification[46] of Shorr's staining solution has the following composition, which is recommended:

Biebrich scarlet, hydrosoluble	1.5	gm
Orange G	0.5	gm
Aniline blue, hydrosoluble	0.125	gm
Fast green	0.375	gm
Phosphotungstic acid	1.25	gm
Phosphomolybdic acid	1.25	gm
Absolute alcohol	250.00	ml
Distilled water	250.00	ml
Glacial acetic acid	5.00	ml

25.2.3. PHASE CONTRAST MICROSCOPY

Preparations to be viewed under phase optics must be fresh and unfixed, and are preserved in a special humid chamber. This method has lately reached fuller development and application, particularly in Germany. Among its advantages are speed

Endocrine Cytology

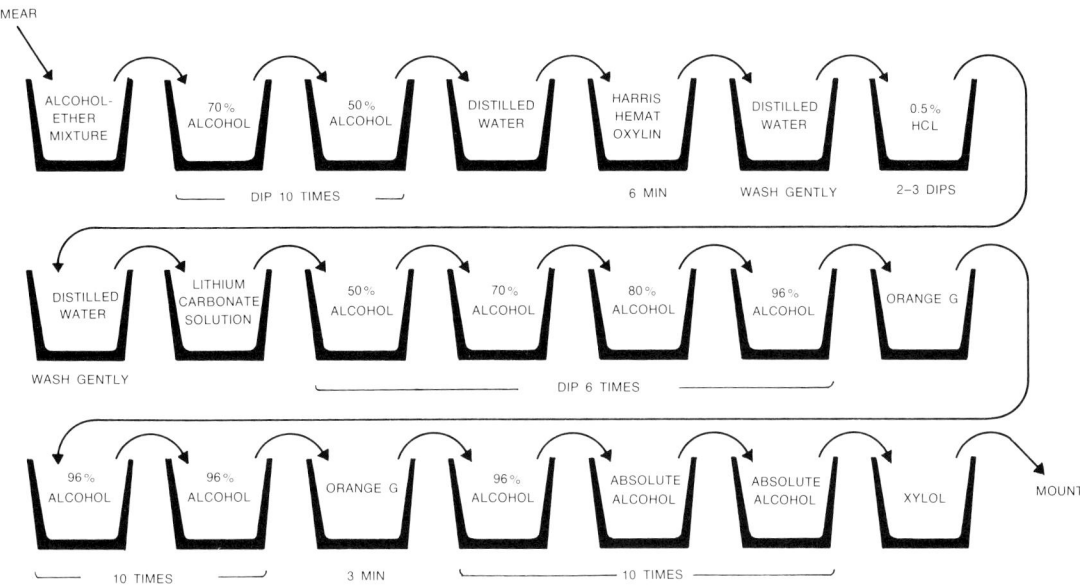

Figure 25–1. Papanicolaou staining technique, modified by Montalvo. (From Montalvo-Ruiz: *Citologia Vaginal, Cervical y Endometrial: Hormonal y Maligna.* Barcelona, Editorial Cientifico-Médica, 1964.)

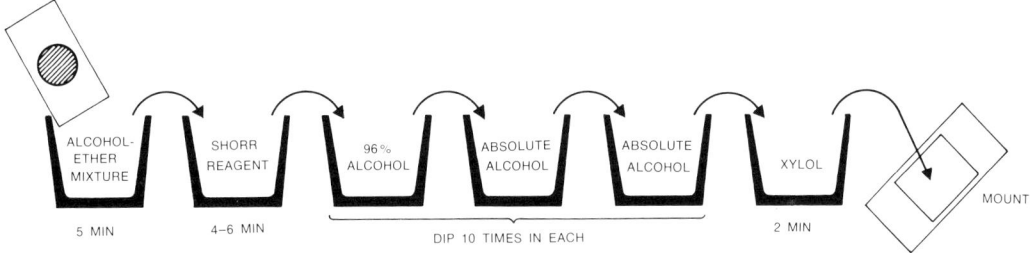

Figure 25–2. Setup for simple Shorr procedure.

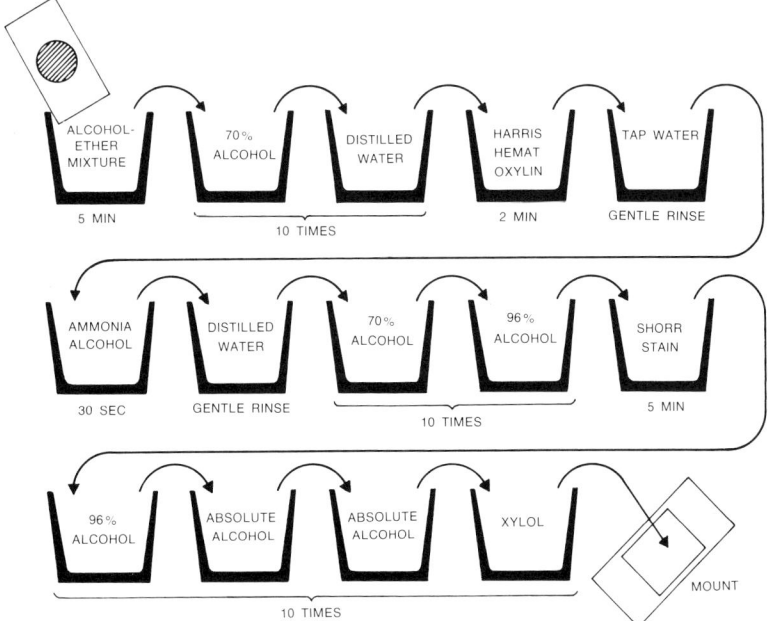

Figure 25–3. Setup for modified Shorr procedure.

and undistorted viewing of live cellular structures without fixation artifacts. Its drawbacks for endocrinologic diagnostic purposes are the difficulties of interpretation.

25.2.4. FLUORESCENT MICROSCOPY

This method, introduced by Bertalanffy and his co-workers,[8] is based on induced fluorescence using Acridine Orange and has found application mainly in the cytodiagnosis of cancer, although it has also been tested for use in hormone cytology by Wied and Manglano.[78] Though undoubtedly an interesting procedure, it offers no significant advantages over the classical Papanicolaou technique.

25.3. CHANGES OBSERVED IN VAGINAL CYTOLOGY

The following paragraphs are intended to summarize briefly the *normal cytologic findings* in the course of woman's prepuberal and sexual life. For greater detail, the reader is referred to any of the readily available modern monographs on the subject. Our present subject comprises the study of vaginal cytology (a) at birth and during childhood; (b) at puberty; (c) throughout the cycle; (d) in the course of pregnancy; and (e) at menopause and after menopause.

25.3.1. VAGINAL CYTOLOGY AT BIRTH AND DURING CHILDHOOD

As shown by various investigators (Tortora,[73] Ferin,[20, 21, 22] Pundel,[52, 53] and Montalvo and Slocker[41]), vaginal smears at birth are of the purely estrogenic variety, revealing an elevated karyopyknotic index and marked acidophilia.

It is of interest to note that, according to findings by Montalvo and Slocker[41] at our clinic, the appearance of glycogen in the vaginal epithelium of the newborn is usually delayed until the fifth day of life. Thus, the presence of glycogen in the baby girl does not parallel the peak of estrogenic exfoliation but, on the contrary, is coincident with the cessation of that event. A similar phenomenon has also been observed by Schramm,[64] whose findings indicate that the appearance of glycogen coincides with predominant occurrence of intermediate type cells. This apparent paradox has been clarified by the studies of Botella and associates,[14] who demonstrated that vaginal glycogen was deposited not in the superficial layers but in the intermediate layers of the epithelium. Consequently, abundance of glycogen in exfoliated cells does not occur in superficial type smears, that is to say, smears of the estrogenic type. For the same reason, as has already been pointed out, the presence of glycogen is no longer considered to be of cytodiagnostic significance in estimating ovarian function.

During childhood, smears may be either of the hypertrophic or of the totally atrophic type (Pundel,[52, 53] Allende et al.,[2] Montalvo[39]). There is no further increase in vaginal exfoliation until the onset of puberty.

25.3.2. VAGINAL CYTOLOGY AT PUBERTY

As pointed out previously (see Chapter 15), signs of hormone activity may be observed even *before the appearance of menarche*. Starting at the age of ten, and often earlier, the karyopyknotic index and the acidophilic index begin to increase gradually. Cyclic manifestations begin to appear at the age of 13 and are first irregular, eventually becoming normal, until the levels of normal woman are reached.

Because of the difficulties encountered in obtaining cytologic material from virgins, Lencioni and Staffieri[35] proposed the use of the *urocytogram*, a method with which they were able to diagnose an interesting case of precocious puberty. On the other hand, Sonek[66] employs a narrow cannula through which he introduces a slender cotton swab into the posterior vaginal fornix of girls or virgins. Montalvo[39] prefers the use of a cannula in conjunction with the Papanicolaou pear (see Section 25.2.1).

25.3.3. VAGINAL CYTOLOGY IN THE COURSE OF THE MENSTRUAL CYCLE

Murray,[44] in 1938, had already called attention to the occurrence of nuclear changes during the menstrual cycle. Subsequently, Allende and colleagues[2] and later Pundel[52] noted that the "nuclear index" underwent gradual changes until the time of ovulation. On studying the nuclei of exfoliated cells, a considerable proportion of them, particularly of those that are flattened and polygonal, may be seen to contain shrunken, *pyknotic* nuclei. *These karyopyknotic cells are known to reflect estrogenic activity and their number increases gradually over the entire proliferative phase* (Fig. 25-4). The term "karyopyknotic index" is meant to express the incidence of this type of cells among each hundred cells counted. Pundel[52] has shown that the karyopyknotic index increases up to the moment of ovulation and then begins to decline.

The curve of this index parallels that of the eosinophilic index, which in turn represents the incidence of cells with eosinophilic cytoplasm (in Papanicolaou and Shorr stains) for each hundred cells counted.

While acidophilia and pyknosis diminish during the second half of the cycle, a concomitant increase in cytoplasmic folding (folded cells) has been shown to occur due to progesterone activity by, among others, Allende and his colleagues,[2] Papanicolaou, Pundel, and Wied and associates.[76] Both an elevated *index of folded cells* and a high *index of clumped cells* are therefore characteristic of the last two weeks of the cycle. When no decrease in acidophilia and pyknosis occurs, and when in addition there is absence of folding and clumping of cells, it must be assumed that one is dealing with an *anovulatory cycle*. Mauro and co-workers[38] studied the cytology of the cycle in the simian *Macaca mulatta*, finding patterns identical with those in woman.

25.3.4. VAGINAL CYTOLOGY IN THE COURSE OF PREGNANCY

The description of "navicular cells" (Fig. 25-5) must be credited to Papanicolaou,

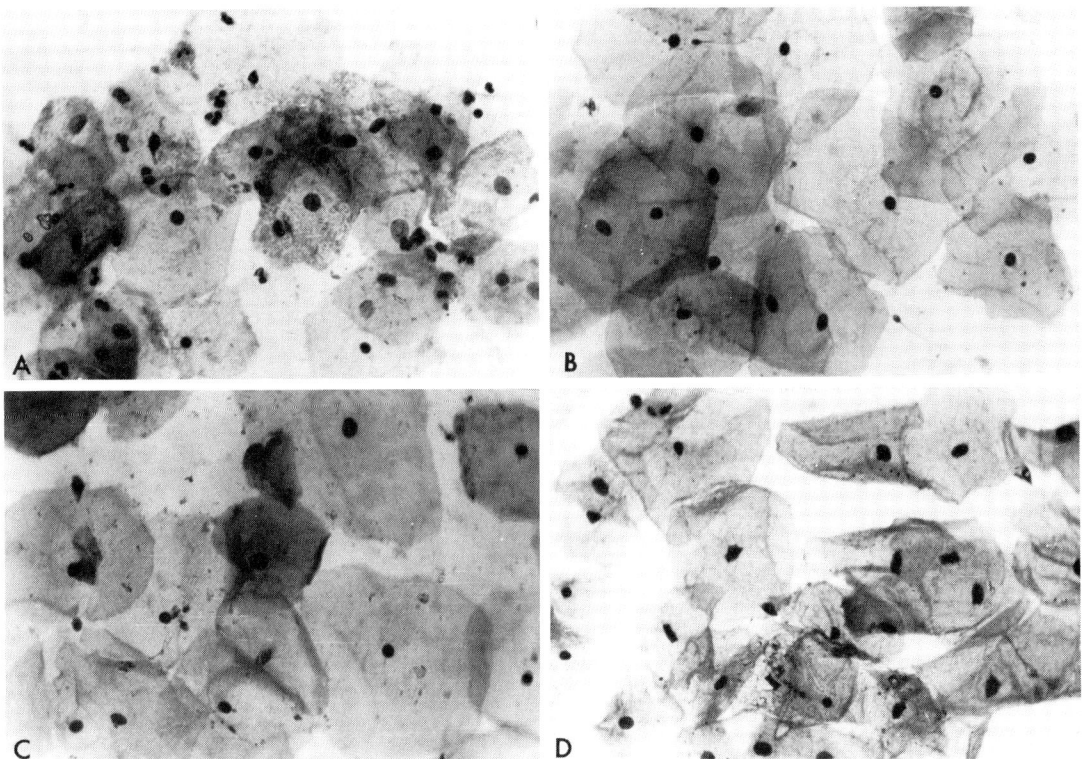

Figure 25-4. Vaginal cytology in the course of the cycle. Nullipara, age 28, with biphasic temperature curves and probable ovulation. *A*, Sixth day of the cycle. *B*, Twelfth day of the cycle. *C*, Fifteenth day of the cycle. *D*, Twentieth day of the cycle.

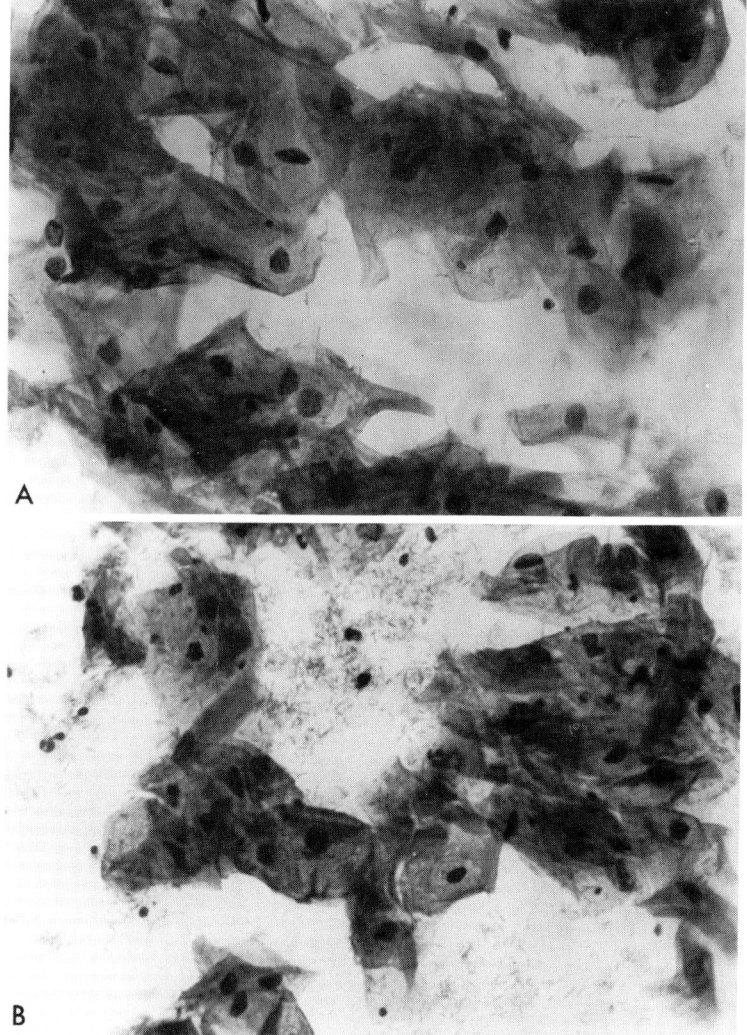

Figure 25-5. Vaginal cytology during pregnancy. A, Third month. B, Eighth month.

who, many years ago, had called attention to the occurrence in pregnancy of certain basophilic cells with peculiar boatlike shapes which he considered so distinctive that he went so far as to say that they were a diagnostic sign of pregnancy.

More recently, the cytology of pregnancy has been studied exhaustively by Pundel,[53] Gaudefroy,[25, 26] von Haam and Efstadion,[29] and other investigators. These changes were found to be characteristic and are represented in Figure 25-5. At the beginning of pregnancy, smears are of the same type as that seen during the luteal phase of the cycle, exhibiting a high incidence of folding and clumping and, at the same time, of pyknotic and acidophilic cells. After the fourth month, typical navicular cells appear in the smears and their presence persists throughout the rest of normal pregnancy until the eve of labor.

Cytology is an extremely fine index of gravidic pathology, according to Montalvo. An increased incidence of acidophils which, like pyknosis, can be induced by means of estrogen therapy, and a drop in percentage of navicular cells, must be considered as indicative of *threatened abortion*. Cytologic patterns of pregnancy were recently studied by Niklicek[45] and by Rezende and associates.[60] The urocytogram of pregnancy has been described by Lencioni and his co-workers.[34] Similar cytologic alterations may be observed *near parturition*, in *toxemia of pregnancy* and in other pathologic conditions of pregnancy, which will

Endocrine Cytology

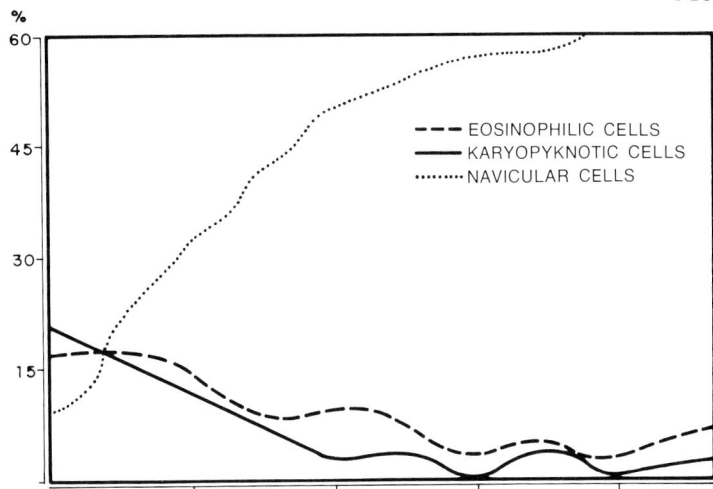

Figure 25-6. Percentage of karyopyknotic, acidophilic and navicular cells in the course of normal pregnancy.

be discussed in later chapters (see Chapter 39 and those following).

25.3.5. VAGINAL CYTOLOGY AT MENOPAUSE AND FOLLOWING CASTRATION

Menopause is characterized by regression of vaginal cell types. Since the work of Papanicolaou and Shorr,[49] the occurrence of *atrophic menopausal smears* has classically been admitted. Nevertheless, as was pointed out in Chapter 16, a large percentage of menopausal women do not present evidence of vaginal atrophy and continue to show more or less "estrogenic" smears.

The occurrence of significant estrogenic activity, with high eosinophilic and karyopyknotic indices during and after menopause, has also been described by Sora,[67] Berger and Keller,[7] Botella, Pundel,[57] and Montalvo, and most recently, by De Waard and associates,[18] and by Stone and co-workers.[69] These results are consistent with data obtained on the basis of estrogen determinations as well as examinations of endometrial biopsies, all indicating that, quite frequently, there is active estrogen production during this period of woman's life.

More or less complete atrophy usually develops following castration, but this is not necessarily permanent (Botella). Occasionally, "paradoxical" smears are encountered in which estrogenic activity is obvious.

25.4. EFFECTS OF SEX HORMONES ON VAGINAL CYTOLOGY

The problems arising from the effects of the sex steroids on cytology were examined in Chapters 2, 3 and 4. More than to anything else, vaginal cytology is susceptible to the *action of estrogens* in a highly specific way. Nevertheless, this specificity of response to estrogens, or for that matter to androgens, is far from being absolute. Although the essential factors involved in producing such effects have already been covered, a summary of the cytologic criteria for estimating sex hormone activity seems to be in order.

25.4.1. ESTROGENS

The main criterion for assessing evidence of estrogen effect on the vagina is an *elevated pyknotic index*. As a result of a comparative study on this and the acidophilic index, Pundel reached the conclusion that, although both can be considered as results of estrogen activity, the pyknotic index is the more specific. Ferin investigated the effects of estrogens on the vaginal cytology of castrated women; dosages of the order of 1 mg per day were found to be sufficient to produce elevations of both the pyknotic and acidophilic indices by 25 per cent. The correlation was similarly convincing when the cytologic findings were compared with results of other methods for the detection of estrogenic activity, such as estrogen assay (Guinot-Segui,[28] Tornero[72]) and endometrial curettage (Montalvo,[36] Botella[12]). It must be emphasized, however, that *glycogen contents* could not be correlated with estrogenic activity (Schramm,[64] Botella et al.[14]).

In recent years, the issue of estrogenic indices has been revived.[70] What criteria should be adopted for measuring the level of estrogenic activity in a given smear? Although Ferin[24] and Boschann[11] have expressed skepticism about the value of having such indices, Wied[79] recently defined several cellular indices as follows:

Karyopyknotic Index (percentage of squamous cells with nuclear pyknosis).

Eosinophilic Index (percentage of squamous cells with cytoplasmic eosinophilia).

Maturation Index (ratio of parabasal/intermediate/superficial cells).

Maturation Value (among 100 cells counted, a value of 1 is given to each superficial cell, 0.5 to each intermediate cell and 0 to each parabasal cell; a simple value below 50 is consistent with estrogenic deficit).

Montalvo[43] attaches little significance to the eosinophilic index because of *false cytoplasmic eosinophilia* resulting from drying artifacts in smears. Karyopyknosis is of much greater significance and ought to be determined by means of *phase contrast microscopy*.[42,79] In addition, Kobilkova[32] favors the use of *serial cytology*, a point of view that is supported by the comparative biochemical and cytologic studies by Boquoi and Hammerstein[9] and by MacRae.[37]

25.4.2. PROGESTOGENS

In addition to estrogenic cellular indices, Wachtel[75] and Wied[79] distinguish two types of progestogenic cellular indices:

Folding Index (percentage of cells with folded cell margins, or navicular cells).

Clumping Index (number of cell clumps among 100 cells counted; because cells in clumps cannot always be counted, this index is sometimes impossible to establish).

The cytohormonal effects of progestogens have been studied by Pundel, Ferin, Roth[61] and others, reaching identical conclusions.

Wied and his colleagues[76,77] deny having found any evidence of specificity concerning progestational activity. In castrated women who are injected with progestogens after having previously been primed with estrogens, a progestogen effect on the vaginal epithelium can be readily recognized. Obviously, *regression of estrogenic cytology is essentially a negative effect*. It permits assessment of luteal activity provided that progestogens have been given without any steroids other than estrogens. However, on the basis of a single smear, the presence of luteal activity cannot be affirmed either way. It is for this reason that similar cytologic patterns may be seen with androgen and corticoid therapy, and even in those cases in which the effects of an already suppressed estrogenic stimulus are in the process of wearing off. As opposed to this viewpoint, it may be argued that *progesterone in effect exerts a positive action on the vaginal wall*. Botella and associates[14] found that such action resulted in superficial modifications of the vaginal epithelium owing to deposition of significant amounts of a PAS-positive, amylase-resistant material, thought to be a mucopolysaccharide (see Chapter 3). It is the author's opinion that cellular folding during the luteal phase is *caused by the mucopolysaccharide content of the superficial cells and is precipitated by alcohol-ether fixation, commensurate in degree with the cellular mucin content*. In support of this line of reasoning is the fact that folding of cells is not observed in freshly collected material viewed under phase contrast.

If these findings are valid, then, it follows that folding of cells under the influence of progestational activity is by no means a negative effect but, on the contrary, *a positive effect that results directly from cytochemical activity of progesterone*. In agreement with Pundel[52] and Ferin,[23] this author therefore believes the effect of progesterone on vaginal cytology to be a specific one.

25.4.3. ANDROGENS

Contrary to Pundel's affirmation, we do not believe that androgens exert any specific effect in this regard. Though Boschann[10,11] and, later, Wied and associates[76,77] were able to describe androgenic effects in vaginal smears of postmenopausal and castrated woman, it is doubtful whether there is any valid criterion for judging the effects of endogenous androgens in a woman who is not receiving exogenous androgens.

25.4.4. CORTICOIDS, PITUITARY HORMONES

By virtue of their similarity to progesterone, all corticoids exert to some extent a progestational type effect on vaginal cytology. Montalvo[40] studied the effects of deoxycorticosterone, while Ferin[23] and Pundel[52] used cortisone. Finally, neither chorionic gonadotropin (Botella and Montalvo[13]) nor ACTH (Cianci and Benfatto[17]) would seem to affect vaginal cytology in any direct way.

25.5. ENDOCRINE CYTOLOGY OF THE URINARY BLADDER, ENDOMETRIUM AND ORAL MUCOSA

In sexual endocrinology, cytologic patterns are subject to cyclic fluctuations that are basically similar in any of the three organs under consideration. *This is to say that informative cytohormonal data may be provided by cytologic material originating in any of the above organs.*

25.5.1. BLADDER CYTOLOGY

As a result of the work of Del Castillo and his associates,[16] the diagnostic significance of the marked parallelism between *urothelial cytology* and sexual function has been well established. For practical reasons, its use has been advocated particularly *in pregnancy* (Álvarez-Bravo and González-Ramos,[3] Lencioni et al.[33, 34, 35]). Requesens[59] strongly favors this method whenever a vaginal approach is not feasible.

25.5.2. ENDOMETRIAL CYTOLOGY

Over the past few years, endometrial cytology has undergone rapid expansion. Montalvo and Hecht[30] conducted comparative studies of endometrial cytology and endometrial biopsy. De Amaral-Ferreira,[4] De Brux and Fromet-Dupré,[15] and Ishizuka and Shigenaga[31] have established the cytohormonal features of the proliferative phase, whereas Boschann[10, 11] described the secretory phase. Similarly, De Brux and Fromet-Dupré[15] achieved cytologic characterization of endometrial hyperplasia.

In practice, however, this method may be of limited value, since the obtaining of study material is just as tedious as that of biopsy material and the latter provides in addition much more accurate information for diagnostic purposes.

25.5.3. ORAL CYTOLOGY

Oral cytology has similarly been found to reflect the menstrual cycle and to be useful for cytohormonal diagnosis. Anderson and associates,[5] as well as Dokumov and Spasov,[19] have been using oral cytology for diagnostic endocrine evaluation with good results.

25.6. OTHER ENDOCRINE INDICATIONS FOR CYTOLOGY

Teter and Boczkowsky[71] rely heavily on cytology for the diagnosis of *gonadal dysgenesis*. Rubio and associates[62] and Wachtel[74] maintain that women with estrogenic cytology have a poorer oncologic prognosis (see Chapter 46). Steele and Breg[68] employ amniotic cytology for the diagnosis of gravidic problems.

REFERENCES

1. Allen, W. M., and Doisy, E. A.: *J.A.M.A.*, 81:819, 1923.
2. Allende, I. de, Shorr, E., and Hartman, C. G.: *Contrib. Embryol.*, 31:198, 1945.
3. Álvarez-Bravo, A., and González-Ramos, M.: *Obst. Gin. Mex.*, 11:321, 1956.
4. Amaral-Ferreira, C. de: *Acta Cytol.*, 2:603, 607, 1958.
5. Anderson, W. R., Belding, J., and Pixley, E.: *Acta Cytol.*, 13:81, 1969.
6. Ayre, E. A.: *Cancer Cytology of the Uterus.* New York, Grune & Stratton, 1951.
7. Berger, J., and Keller, M.: *Gynaecologia*, 137:250, 1954.
8. Bertalanffy, L. von, Masin, F., and Masin, M.: *Science*, 124:1024, 1956.

9. Boquoi, E., and Hammerstein, J.: *Acta Cytol.*, 13:332, 1969.
10. Boschann, H. W. von: *Acta Cytol.*, 2:602, 607, 1958.
11. Boschann, H. W.: *Acta Cytol.*, 12:93, 1968.
12. Botella, J.: *Colloques sur la fonction luteale.* Paris, Masson & Cie., 1954.
13. Botella, J., and Montalvo, L.: *Acta Endocr. Obst. Hisp. Lus.*, 2:81, 1949.
14. Botella, J., Nogales, F., and Montalvo, L.: *Acta Citol.*, 2:363, 1958.
15. Brux, A. de, and Frommet-Dupré, J.: *Acta Cytol.*, 2:613, 1958.
16. Castillo, E. B. del, Argonz, J., and Galli-Mainini, C.: *J. Clin. Endocr.*, 8:76, 1948.
17. Cianci, S., and Benfatto, G.: *Bol. Soc. Ital. Biol. Sper.*, 29:1225, 1953.
18. De Waard, F., and Banders van Halejwin, E. A.: *Acta Cytol.*, 13:675, 1969.
19. Dokumov, S. I., and Spasov, S. A.: *Acta Cytol.*, 14:31, 1970.
20. Ferin, J.: *Gynec. Obstet.*, 47:774, 1948.
21. Ferin, J.: *Ann. d'Endocr.*, 14:919, 1953.
22. Ferin, J.: *Colloques sur la fonction luteale.* Paris, Masson & Cie., 1954.
23. Ferin, J.: *Acta Cytol.*, 2:338, 1958.
24. Ferin, J.: *Acta Cytol.*, 12:97, 1968.
25. Gaudefroy, M.: *Acta Cytol.*, 3:218, 1959.
26. Gaudefroy, M.: *Acta Cytol.*, 3:228, 1959.
27. González-Ramos, M.: *Acta Cytol.*, 3:298, 1959.
28. Guinot-Segui, A.: *Acta Gin.*, 4:565, 1953.
29. Haam, E. von, and Efstadion, T. D.: *Acta Cytol.*, 3:209, 1959.
30. Hecht, E. L.: *Amer. J. Obstet. Gynec.*, 71:819, 1956.
31. Ishizuka, Y., and Shigenaga, Y.: *Acta Cytol.*, 12:146, 1968.
32. Kobilkova, J.: *Acta Cytol.*, 11:497, 1967.
33. Lencioni, J. L., Berli, R. R., and Staffieri, J. J.: *Ann. d'Endocr.*, 17:765, 1956.
34. Lencioni, L. J., Martinez-Amezaga, L. A., and Lo Blanco, V. S.: *Acta Cytol.*, 13:279, 1969.
35. Lencioni, L. J., and Staffieri, J. J.: *Acta Cytol.*, 13:382, 1969.
36. Long, J. A., and Evans, H. M.: *Mem. Univ. Calif.*, 6:1, 1922.
37. MacRae, D. J.: *Acta Cytol.*, 11:45, 1967.
38. Mauro, J., Serrone, D., Somsin, B., and Stein, A. A.: *Acta Cytol.*, 14:384, 1970.
39. Montalvo, L.: *Citologia Vaginal, Endocervical y Endometrial: Hormonal y Maligna*, 2nd ed. Barcelona, Editorial Científico-Médica, 1967.
40. Montalvo, L.: *Acta Gyn.*, 4:243, 1953.
41. Montalvo, L., and Slocker, C.: *Acta Gyn.*, 2:19, 1950.
42. Montalvo, L.: *Acta Cytol.*, 12:95, 1968.
43. Montalvo, L.: *Acta Cytol.*, 12:118, 1968.
44. Murray, E. G.: *Arch. Gynäk.*, 165:365, 1938.
45. Niklicek, O.: *Acta Cytol.*, 12:140, 1968.
46. O'Morchoe, P. J., and O'Morchoe, C. C. C.: *Acta Cytol.*, 11:145, 1967.
47. Papanicolaou, G. N.: *Proc. Soc. Exper. Biol. Med.*, 22:346, 1925.
48. Papanicolaou, G. N.: *Amer. J. Anat.*, 52:519, 1933.
49. Papanicolaou, G. N., and Shorr, E.: *Amer. J. Obstet. Gynec.*, 31:806, 1936.
50. Papanicolaou, G. N., and Traut, H. F.: *The Diagnosis of Uterine Cancer by Vaginal Smears.* New York, The Commonwealth Foundation, 1943.
51. Papanicolaou, G. N., Traut, H. F., and Marchetti, A. A.: *The Epithelia of Woman's Reproductive Organs.* New York, The Commonwealth Foundation, 1948.
52. Pundel, J. P.: *Les frottis vaginaux et cervicaux.* Paris, Masson & Cie, 1950.
53. Pundel, J. P.: *Acquisitions recentes en cytologie hormonale.* Paris, Masson & Cie., 1957.
54. Pundel, J. P.: *Acta Cytol.*, 1:62, 1957.
55. Pundel, J. P.: *Acta Cytol.*, 3:24, 1959.
56. Pundel, J. P., and Lichtfus, C.: *Acta Cytol.*, 3:246, 1959.
57. Pundel, J. P.: *Acta Cytol.*, 12:121, 1968.
58. Ramírez, E.: *Rev. Mex. Biol.*, 8:1, 1928.
59. Requesens, L. F.: *Actas Soc. Esp. Est. Esterilidad*, 6:191, 1958.
60. Rezende, J. de, et al.: *Acta Cytol.*, 14:78, 1970.
61. Roth, O. A.: In *Gynäkologische Zytologie*, ed. H. Runge. Leipzig, Theodor Steinkopff, 1934.
62. Rubio, C. A., Hvalec, S., and Pareja, A.: *Acta Cytol.*, 11:176, 1967.
63. Salmon, U. J., and Frank, R. T.: *Proc. Soc. Exper. Biol. Med.*, 33:612, 1933.
64. Schramm, B.: *Colloques sur la fonction luteale.* Paris, Masson & Cie., 1954.
65. Shorr, E.: *Science*, 91:321, 579, 1940.
66. Sonek, M.: *Acta Cytol.*, 11:41, 1967.
67. Sora, P.: *Minerva Gin.*, 6:20, 1954.
68. Steele, M. V., and Breg, W. R.: *Lancet*, 1:383, 1966.
69. Stone, D. F., Sedlis, A., Stone, M. L., and Turkel, W. V.: *Acta Cytol.*, 11:349, 1967.
70. Symposium: Hormonal Cytology. *Acta Cytol.*, 12:87, 1969.
71. Teter, J., and Boczkowsky, K.: *Acta Cytol.*, 11:449, 1967.
72. Tornero, M. C.: *Actas Soc. Esp. Est. Esterilidad*, 4:111, 1956.
73. Tortora, M.: *Arch. Ost. Gin. Ital.*, 41:290, 1946.
74. Wachtel, E.: *Acta Cytol.*, 11:35, 1967.
75. Wachtel, E.: *Acta Cytol.*, 12:101, 1968.
76. Wied, G. L., Del Sol, J. R., and Dargan, A. M.: *Amer. J. Obstet. Gynec.*, 75:98, 1958.
77. Wied, G. L., Del Sol, J. R., and Dargan, A. M.: *Amer. J. Obstet. Gynec.*, 75:289, 1958.
78. Wied, G. L., and Manglano, J. I.: *Acta Cytol.*, 6:554, 1962.
79. Wied, G. L.: *Acta Cytol.*, 12:87, 1968.

Chapter 26

ENDOMETRIAL BIOPSY AND ITS DIAGNOSTIC VALUE

26.1. INTRODUCTION

As an exploratory technique, endometrial biopsy has gained a place of preeminence in the course of the years. Its contributions to endocrine gynecology have indeed been remarkable. This chapter is devoted to a brief appraisal of the practical aspects of the technique and interpretation of *microcurettage*.

26.1.1. HISTORY

Although various investigators studied the morphology of the endometrial cycle even in the nineteenth century, it was not until Schröder[46] introduced "diagnostic curettage," facilitating the taking of a large number of specimens of endometrial tissue from all phases of the cycle, that this type of exploratory technique received a decisive impetus. Subsequently, the great impact produced by the work of Schröder's successor Meyer[34] led to the formulation of the doctrine of the "sexual endometrial cycle" in Germany 45 years ago.

However, *total curettage* is a surgical intervention in the full sense of the word, requiring dilatation of the cervix and, hence, anesthesia, and cannot be practiced prodigally. Although Tietze[48] and Anspach and Hoffman[1] had advocated the use of total curettage for purely diagnostic purposes, its use had not been generalized until the advent of a more innocuous and painless procedure, such as lineal curettage, or *microcurettage*, which could be applied to ambulatory patients. Only then did endometrial histopathology become a method of exploration that is currently within the competence of the practicing gynecologist

at large. The Reifferscheid,[44] Cotte[13] and Agüero types of curettes and the "aspiration biopsy" techniques, devised by Klinger and Burch[28] and by Novak,[42] were to constitute the most significant development to advance this method of exploration.

26.1.2. GENERAL PRINCIPLES OF ENDOMETRIAL BIOPSY AS A MEANS OF FUNCTIONAL DIAGNOSIS

The endometrium is remarkably sensitive to the influence of the sex hormones, responding specifically and swiftly to cyclic variations (see Chapter 13). During the first half of the cycle, it is subjected to the influence of estrogens, and during the second half it responds to progesterone. While a biopsy performed during the first two weeks may yield information relative to the degree of estrogenic response, in general, curettage is preferably scheduled for the second half of the intermenstruum, which more truly reflects the degree of luteal activity. Thus, whereas cytology is the test *par excellence* for estimating estrogenic activity, microcurettage provides the best criterion regarding progesterone activity.

26.2. TECHNIQUE OF MICROCURETTAGE

26.2.1. TYPES OF MICROCURETTAGE

At present, endometrial biopsy is performed essentially by two different methods, based on either *microcurettage* or *aspiration*. For the former, a curette of variable design is used, consisting basically of an intrauterine sound, 2 to 4 mm in caliber, provided at one end with a small receptacle which, when retracted, removes a few cubic millimeters of endometrial tissue. The curettes of Reifferscheid, Cote or Agüero are all representative of this type (Fig. 26–1).

The aspiration technique is carried out by means of a hollow cannula provided with a toothed or cutting end, the entire device connected to an aspirator or simply to a syringe. The models of Kurzrock, Khanpaa, Klinger, and Burch and Novak (Fig. 26–2) are representative of this modality.

26.2.2. PREPARATION OF INSTRUMENTS

It is convenient to prepare microcurettes of variable caliber (numbers 4, 5 and 6 correspond to the same calibers as Hegar's

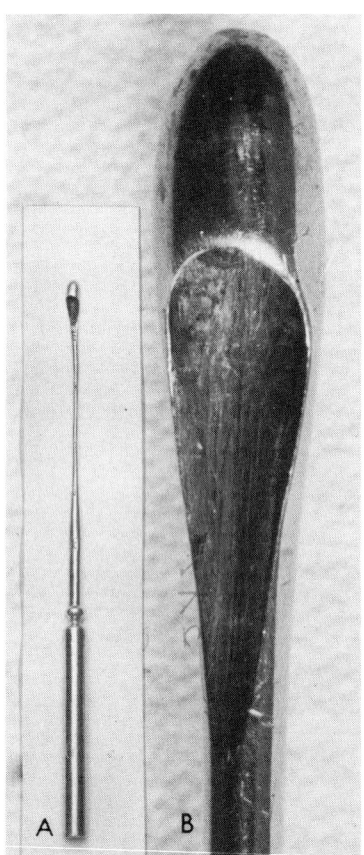

Figure 26–1. Reifferscheid curette, modified by Agüero, for endometrial biopsy. *A*, One third original size; *B*, four times original size.

dilators), so as to be able to adapt to the size of the cervical canal.

Apart from the microcurettes, a set of retractors, speculums, tentaculum clamps and forceps must be conveniently sterilized.

26.2.3. APPROPRIATE TIME FOR DOING THE PROCEDURE

Since microcurettage may be intended for different purposes, the appropriate time for the intervention must be selected accordingly. In general, the procedure is performed *pre-* or *intramenstrually*, except for unusual cases to be discussed later.

1. *Intramenstrual microcurettage* has the advantage that it cannot interrupt incipient gestation in any case and that, besides, the procedure is greatly facilitated by the fact that the cervix is already slightly dilated as a result of menstruation. Among its drawbacks is the major one of obtaining mostly necrotic endometrial tissue which is often inadequate for histologic interpretation.

2. *Premenstrual microcurettage* yields neat and clear histologic preparations but may cause greater discomfort to the patient, apart from exposing the patient to the risk of inadvertently interrupting an overlooked pregnancy, acquired in the course of the last cycle. The latter accident occurs less frequently than one might expect. Jackson[26] described 36 cases in which microcurettage was erroneously performed on pregnant women (with the pregnancies confirmed at a later stage), of which only five cases subsequently aborted. Nonetheless, unlikely as they are, such accidents may occur and must be averted by asking the patient to abstain from sex, as recommended by Novak,[42] from the eighth day of the cycle until the time of the test.

26.2.4. PREPARATION OF PATIENT AND SURGEON

Microcurettage does not require previous anesthesia and the procedure may be done on an ambulatory basis. A routine type of vaginal disinfection with iodine tincture is sufficient, taking the precaution of canceling the procedure should the patient show any signs of acute cervicitis.

As for the surgeon, sterilization of hands

Endometrial Biopsy and Its Diagnostic Value

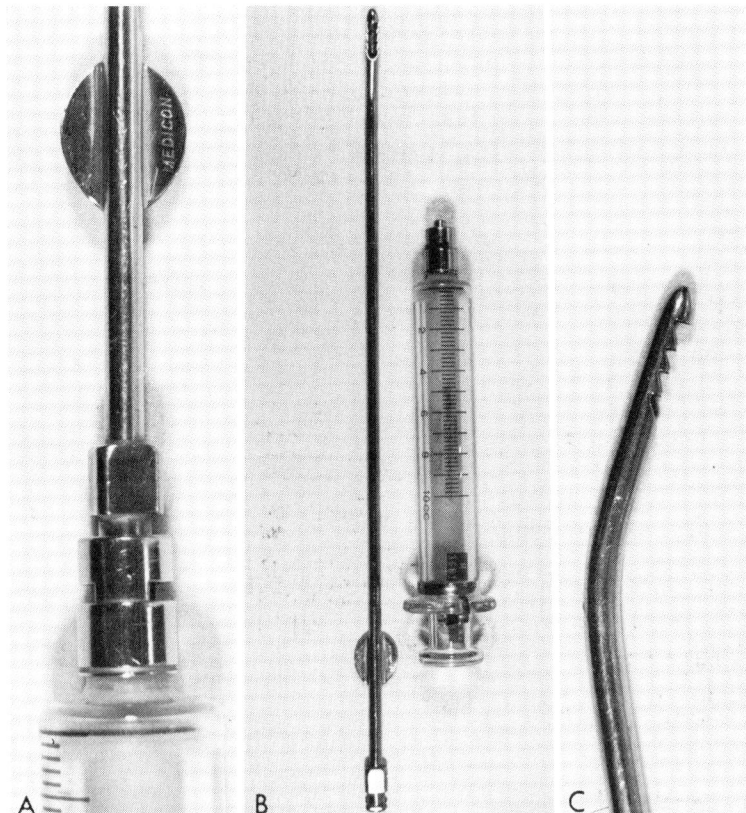

Figure 26-2. Burch aspiration cannula for endometrial biopsy. *A*, Connection between cannula and syringe, magnified one and a half times. *B*, View of complete set, consisting of cannula and aspiration syringe, half their natural size. *C*, Distal end of cannula, one and a half times its natural size.

is not necessary as long as contact with distal parts of instruments to be introduced is avoided.

Out of thousands of instances of ambulatory microcurettage performed at our clinic, we have never witnessed a single accident worth mentioning, nor has it ever been necessary to hospitalize the patient.

26.2.5. TECHNIQUE

Before taking the biopsy, it is advisable to perform a gynecologic exploration in order to assess the size and position of the uterus as well as the condition of the adnexa. After the woman is placed in dorsal recumbent position, the uterine cervix is visualized by means of the speculum or retractors. The cervix is painted with the disinfectant and then grasped with a tenaculum clamp and pulled downward and outward, thereby displacing the uterus into a more or less horizontal position. The microcurette is then gently inserted through the cervical os and endocervical canal until it reaches the fundus. The uterine index (cervical and body index) is determined by reading off the graduations marked on the curette. The cutting side of the curette is then turned against one of the surfaces of the cavity and, with gentle but steady pressure, pulled downward. This will cause a particle of endometrial tissue to be cut out and trapped in the receptacle at the terminal portion of the curette. Once this is achieved, application of pressure is discontinued and the curette is withdrawn carefully, procuring to keep the cutting edge away from the uterine wall, particularly while passing through the isthmus and endocervix, so as to avoid cutting any more particles from those regions, which might dislodge the already curetted tissue. Since the piece of mucosa removed by this instrument is quite tiny, it is advisable to repeat the procedure once more and to curette a piece from the opposite surface of the endometrial cavity and, if necessary, the same may be done from both cornua. The tenaculum and speculum or retractors are removed and this minor operation is thereby completed.

26.2.6. MICROCURETTAGE IN VIRGINS

It has been believed erroneously that microcurettage is impossible to perform in virgins. Only if the hymen is completely closed may it be entirely impossible, but the procedure can be performed in most cases provided the following precautions are taken: (a) use of virginal retractors, introduced with great care and delicacy; (b) downward traction of the cervix with a tenaculum hook that occupies less space than a Museaux clamp; (c) introduction of a microcurette of the smallest caliber (occasionally curettage must be combined with suction); (d) in many cases, the use of anesthesia becomes necessary in order to overcome the patient's anxiety and embarrassment, which may render the procedure difficult (pentothal or Evipan is adequate for that purpose); and (e) the patient's consent, or, in case of a minor, her parents' consent, in writing, must be obtained.

Microcurettage in virgins may often be irreplaceable and in spite of the minor difficulties involved, it should not be renounced if it is believed to be necessary. Recently, Slocker[47] at our clinic used hyaluronidase to relax the hymen for microcurettage.

26.2.7. COLLECTION OF SPECIMENS

The tissue is extracted from the receptacle of the microcurette with a needle and is placed into 95 per cent alcohol in a clean container, which is the fixative of choice if the staining reactions to be listed below will be used. Without describing the histologic techniques, these consist of the usual paraffin secretion, stained routinely with hematoxylin and eosin and with Best's carmine. We have added to these the stains for alkaline glycerophosphatase of Gomori and the periodic acid-Schiff method, according to Hotchkiss-McManus.

26.2.8. INDICATIONS

Indications for microcurettage are multiple and can be summed up in the following order:

1. Diagnosis of anovulatory cycle, particularly sterility.
2. Diagnosis of ovarian endocrine disorders.
3. Diagnosis of endometrial inflammatory disease.
4. Diagnosis of endometrial tumors, especially endometrial carcinoma.
5. Diagnosis of processes related to gestation (retained secundines, ectopic pregnancy).

26.3. INTERPRETATION

26.3.1. SECRETORY PHASE

As pointed out on previous occasions (Botella et al.[6]), microcurettage is one of the most reliable procedures for the diagnosis of anovulatory cycle. In order to establish the diagnosis by comparison, the entire secretory phase must be examined. A premenstrual, rather than intramenstrual, curettage is done and the diagnosis of anovulatory cycle is based on the presence of a proliferative endometrial pattern instead of the expected secretory phase. Naturally, the method is limited to ascertaining the presence of a biphasic uterine cycle, corresponding to an ovarian hormonal cycle with progesterone secretion. Therefore, any premenstrual finding of a proliferative pattern only justifies the assertion that the ovary in such a case does not secrete progesterone, but it does not permit conclusions as to whether or not ovulation has taken place.

The histologic features of secretory endometrium are shown in Figures 26–3 and 26–4. The essential criteria employed in interpreting the histologic findings are: presence of dilated glands, exhibiting rounded and tortuous contours, and filled with products of secretion. Detailed examination of gland epithelia reveals that their thickness is decreased and that the cells, arranged in a single layer, contain rounded nuclei, located midway between the basal membrane and the free surface in the lumen. Mitotic figures are invariably absent. The stroma is loose and edematous. Moricard[37] drew attention to what he considered were important diagnostic features of the secretory phase; these are *connective tissue spurs*, which are stromal prolongations insinuated between epithelial folds, as may be seen in Figure 26–4, and appearance of *periglandular vessels,* also

Endometrial Biopsy and Its Diagnostic Value 557

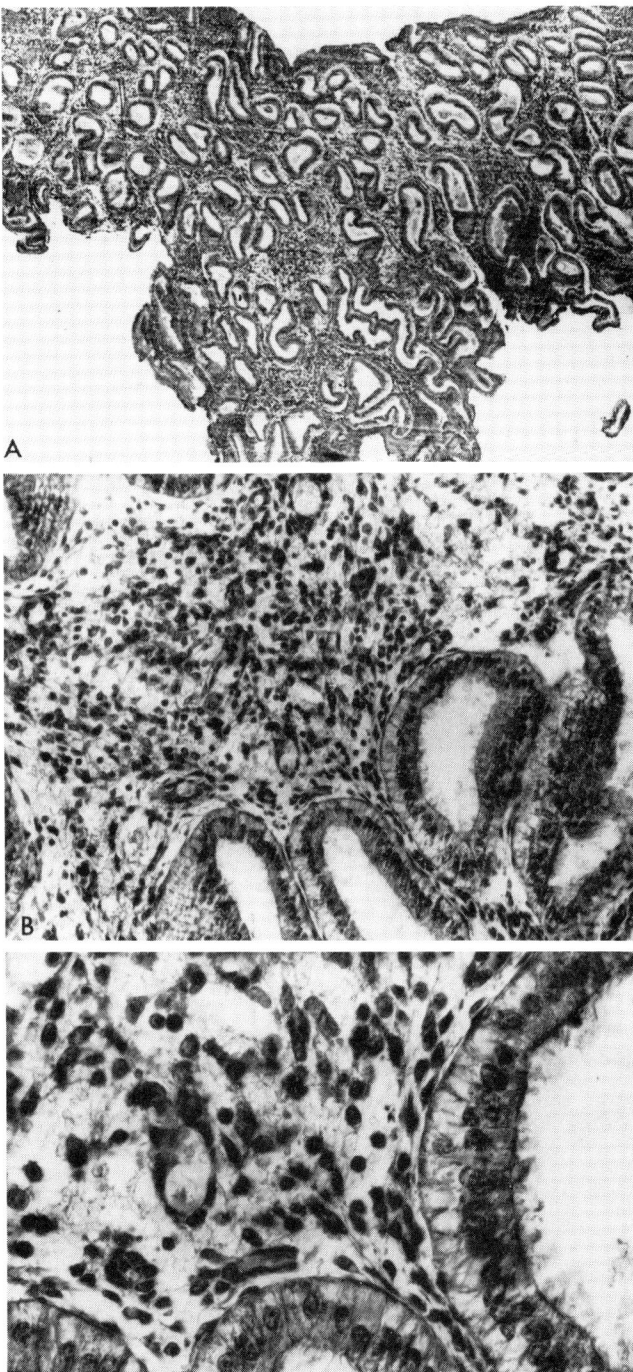

Figure 26-3. A, Early secretory pattern, eighteenth day of normal biphasic cycle, showing tortuous and dilated glands (35×). B, Nuclei are arranged in a single row in midportion of cells and no longer reveal mitotic activity (160×). C, Characteristic subnuclear vacuoles give positive reactions for glycogen in Best's carmine and PAS stained preparations (400×).

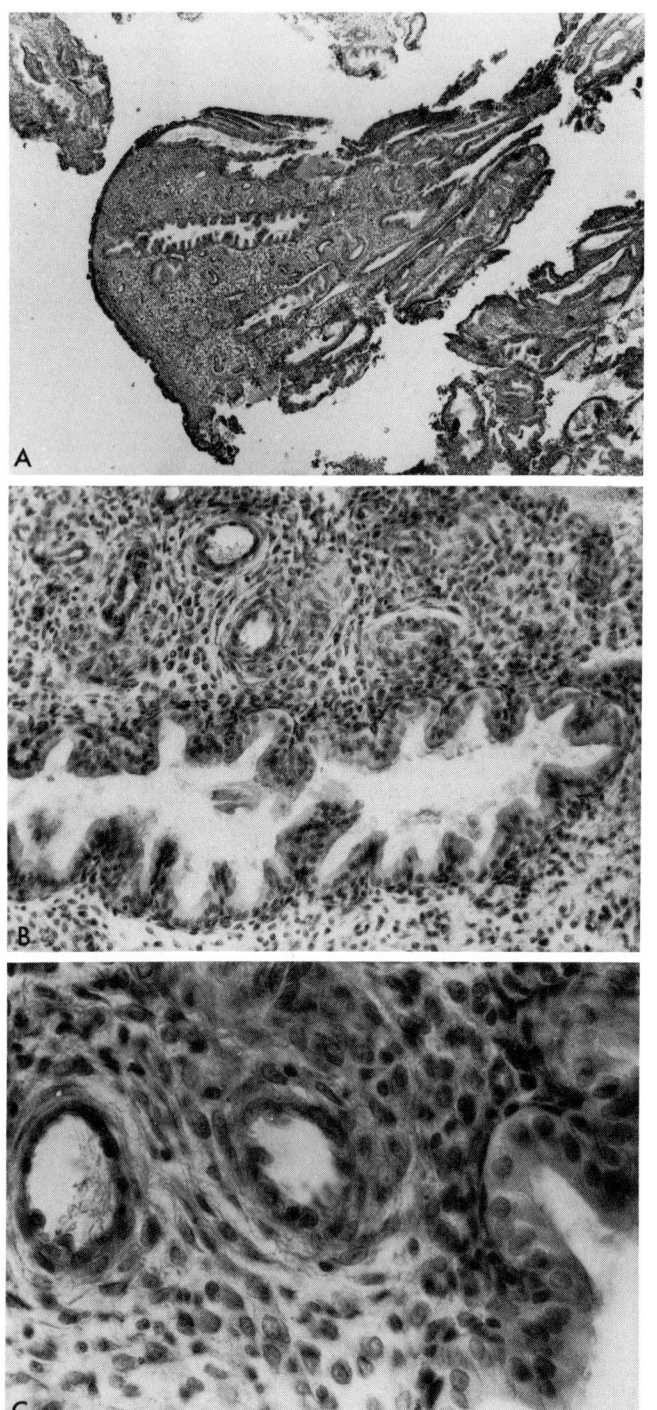

Figure 26–4. Advanced secretory phase. Biopsy taken on the twenty-sixth day of cycle in a woman with normal biphasic cycle. *A,* Wavy, festooned configuration of glands, revealing "connective tissue spurs" (35×). *B,* Although retaining single row alignment, nuclei have returned to basal location after disappearance of subnuclear vacuoles (160×). *C,* Stroma, somewhat more edematous than in Figure 26–3, reveals presence of numerous spiral vessels (400×).

described by Ferin[17] and by us,[8] which have been found to stand out much more distinctly in Gomori's stain than in routine hematoxylin-eosin stains.

The ancillary use of the Gomori technique and of stains for glycogen (Best's carmine and PAS) for the diagnosis of the secretory phase is discussed later in this chapter.

Dallenbach-Hellweg[14] and Wynn and Harris[49] have introduced the *electron microscope* as an aid in diagnosing functional endometrial disorders. Unlike histochemistry, which has proved its extraordinary value in solving diagnostic problems, ultrastructural techniques on this type of tissue are, in our view, still in the experimental stage.

26.3.2. ANOVULATORY CYCLE

The proliferative endometrial pattern found in premenstrual biopsies in cases of anovulatory cycle varies somewhat in relation to the degree of associated hyperestrinism. A distinction must be drawn between: (1) a monophasic cycle in which the endometrium exhibits an early proliferative phase, and (2) a monophasic cycle in which the endometrium reveals an advanced proliferative phase. The first of these two patterns (Fig. 26-5) is characterized by presence of scanty numbers of glands, with narrow lumina, but whose epithelium may be tall and composed of cells and nuclei at different levels, conveying the impression of multistratification

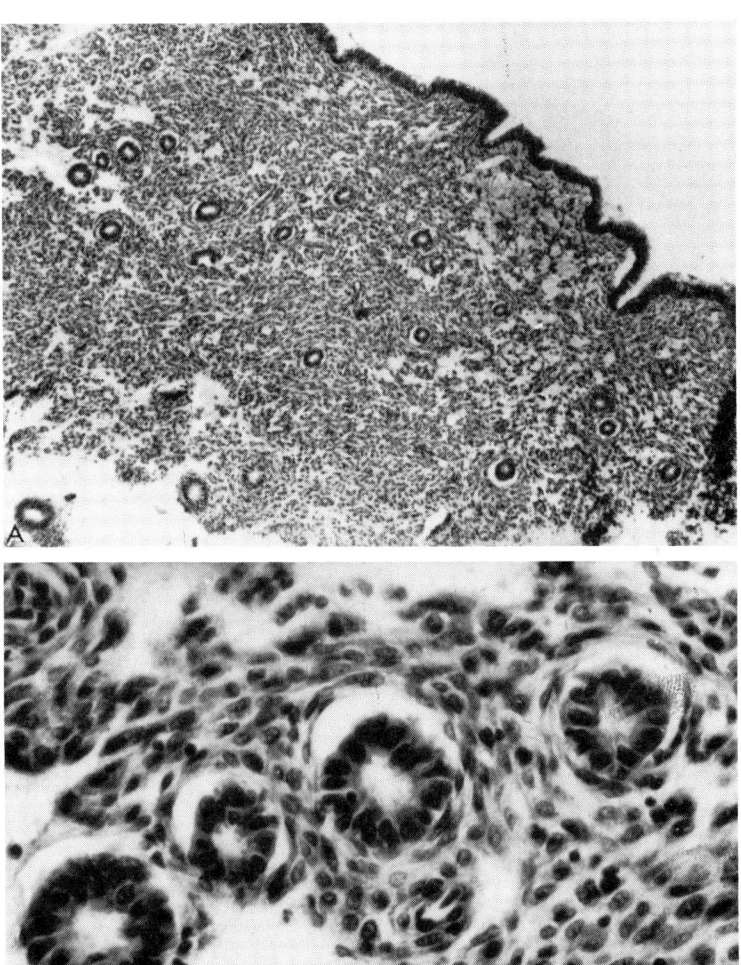

Figure 26-5. Endometrial biopsy obtained on the twenty-third day of cycle of a patient with monophasic cycle with endometrial hypoplasia. A, Mucosa reveals little evidence of proliferation (65×). B, Narrow glands lined with low epithelium and dense stroma without spiral vessels suggest scanty estrogenic stimulation (400×).

(pseudostratified epithelium). The stroma is markedly condensed and some areas resemble cellular fibrous tissue. The epithelial cells in the glands may show distinct mitotic figures.

In the advanced proliferative pattern, glands tend to be somewhat dilated, although epithelia usually retain their characteristics of tallness and pseudostratification (Fig. 26–6). Mitoses are present as a typical feature of epithelial proliferation. The stroma may be looser in texture and may occasionally display areas of slight edema. The differences between this pattern and that of moderate endometrial hyperplasia are minor.

In order to establish the diagnosis of anovulatory cycle it is often not enough to view routine H&E stained slides alone. This is particularly true about the so-called *"incomplete secretory phase"*; to solve such questionable cases, we use Best's carmine stain, a well-known technique, which should be applied whenever a patient is investigated for possible sterility. The type of data that can be provided by special stains, such as Best's carmine, PAS and alkaline phosphatase methods, insofar as they are contributory to more precise characterization of intermediate endometrial patterns of difficult interpretation (Botella[7]), is discussed in the last section of this chapter.

26.3.3. CONDITIONS OF HYPERESTRINISM

Irrespective of whether they are associated with bleeding or not, conditions of hyperestrinism are characterized by endometrial hyperplasia; the degree of hyperplasia may vary to a considerable extent. In its most discreet form, the findings may be indistinguishable from those of an anovulatory cycle. It must be added that most cases of hyperestrinism are caused by an anovulatory cycle in which the follicle persists because it fails to rupture.

One of the basic features of endometrial hyperplasia is dilatation of glands (Fig. 26–7). Within the gland spaces there may be found epithelial proliferations which in secretions appear to be independent islets. Buxton[11] and Ferin[18] dispute the diagnostic significance of such proliferations and suggest that they may be telescoping artifacts produced during the removal of endometrial tissue. Nevertheless, it is a matter of unquestionable observation that *this type of alteration is most likely to develop in cases of most severe endometrial hyperplasia*. In other cases, such proliferations are absent, while glands are cystically dilated, a type called "Swiss cheese endometrium" (Fig. 26–7). The epithelium in these cases is similar to that of the proliferative phase, although, as a result of dilatation of glands, it may be somewhat flattened. Numerous mitotic figures may be present, and their counts may be of prognostic significance (Kottmeier[29]). The stroma may be loose and, from time to time, quite edematous, which is known to be one of the typical actions of estrogens, causing an *edematogenic stromal effect*. Vessels are likewise dilated, a fact emphasized particularly by Falconer.[19] Finally, another typical feature, which consists of *focal squamous metaplasia of the epithelium*, may be observed in cases of extreme hyperestrinism.

26.3.4. HYPOESTRINISM

The endometrium shown in Figure 26–5 exemplifies a mild degree of hypoestrinism. In extreme cases, there is atrophy or hypoplasia of the endometrial mucosa. Characteristically, the first indication that one is dealing with hypoplasia is conveyed by the gross appearance of the scanty amount of tissue curetted. Microscopically, this tissue is made up of small islets of dense stroma containing an exiguous number of interspersed glands. The glands have narrow lumina and are lined with a low epithelium. They contain little cytoplasm and their dense nuclei tend to occur in clusters. However, they are not arranged at the same midcell level as in the typical secretory pattern but, despite the sparsity of the tissue as a whole, may be pseudostratified.

Quite often, such patterns of hypoplasia do not really reflect true states of hypoestrinism but represent instances of what we designated elsewhere as *mucosas without function*. Steitz and Masshof have recognized the existence of this type of endometrium as being at variance with the ovarian cycle, and Moricard[37] termed it *metrosis of receptivity*, attaching great significance to its occurrence. The same

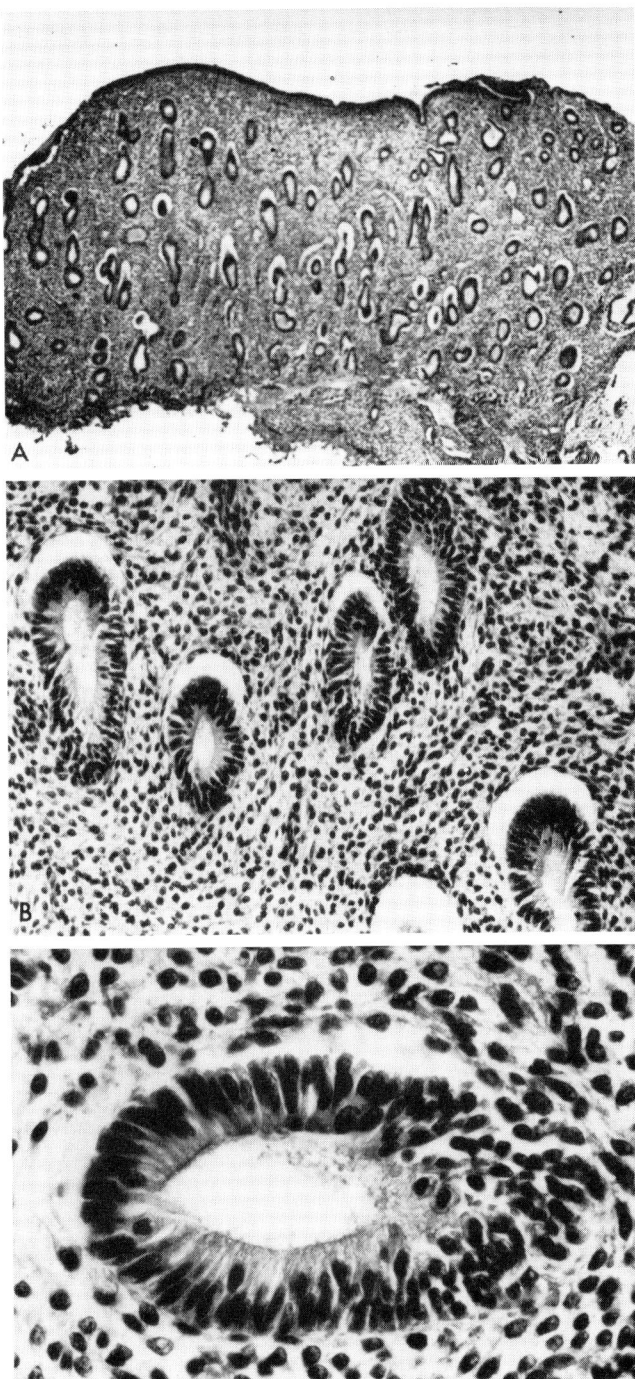

Figure 26-6. Endometrial biopsy taken on the twenty-third day of cycle of a patient with anovulatory monophasic cycle. *A,* Straight glands with tall epithelium and nuclei disposed at different levels (25×). *B,* Occasional mitotic figures (160×). *C,* Dense and cellular stroma reveals no spiral vessels (400×).

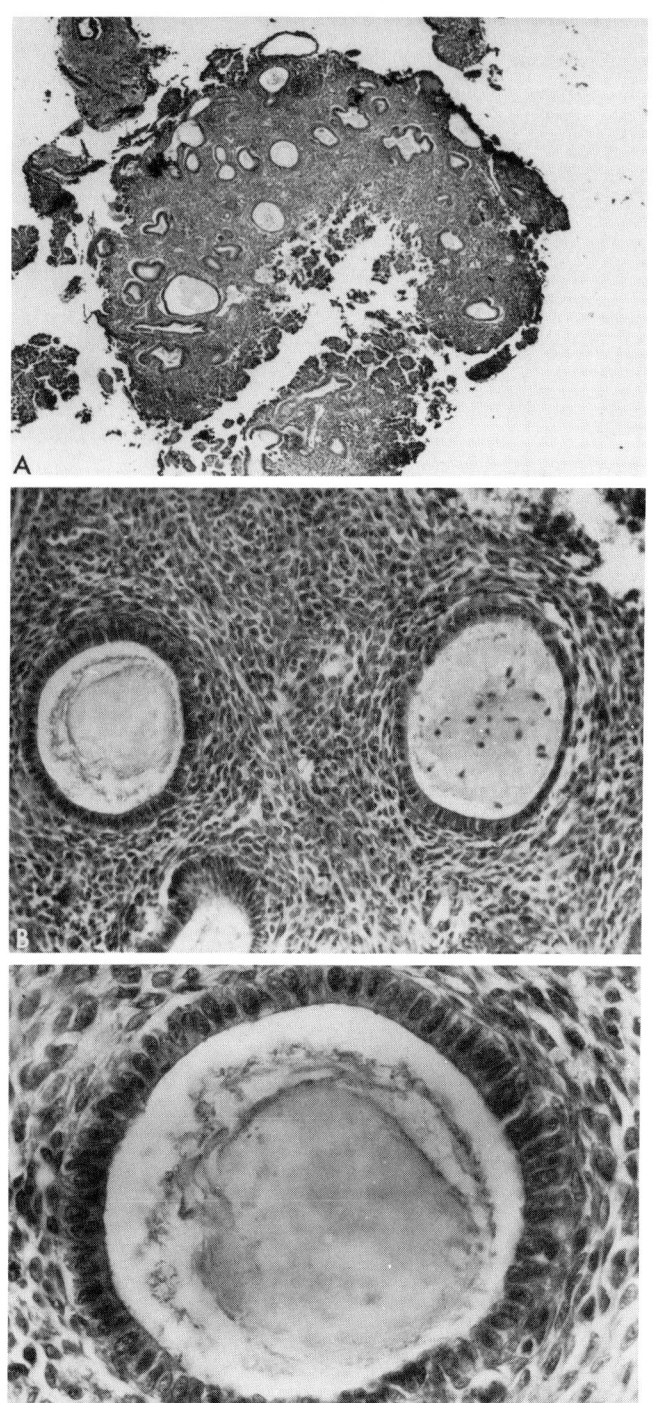

Figure 26-7. Biopsy obtained on the twenty-third day of the cycle of a patient with cystic endometrial hyperplasia of the "Swiss-cheese" type. Highly cellular, dense stroma containing dilated glands with epithelia of the proliferative type, under low (25×), intermediate (160×) and high (400×) magnifications.

features have been found to be present in many cases of tuberculous endometritis which have failed to heal completely (Nogales[39]) and these generally are associated with amenorrhea or oligomenorrhea, but may also coexist with normal menses (Marin[32, 33]).

26.3.5. IRREGULARITIES IN THE ENDOMETRIAL CYCLE

Lately, special attention has been devoted to the question of why the histologic response is often unequal in different areas of the endometrium. As a result, areas with a proliferative pattern may occur side by side with foci of secretory appearance. Called *irregular maturation of the endometrium*, this phenomenon has been described by Hoffmann and by Morillo. In histologic preparations of similar conditions, islets of typical proliferative endometrium can be recognized on a background of endometrium that is entirely of the secretory type.

A condition that is apparently related to the above is the so-called *irregular shedding of the endometrium*, described in recent years by Holmström[25] and by Brewer and Jones.[12] In this case, what appears to be a normal secretory endometrium is not shed all at once but is shed in zones and, moreover, incompletely, clinically giving rise to metrorrhagia.

26.3.6. ENDOMETRITIS

Microcurettage frequently reveals the presence of inflammatory changes. It is of interest to note that this is often the case when the clinical interpretation is one of functional disorder. Endometritis can be divided into three types: banal, postabortive and tuberculous.

BANAL ENDOMETRITIS. The incidence of banal endometritis in our study material is 5.72 per cent. The histologic picture ranges from a mild inflammatory cell infiltrate to purulent endometritis. Such endometria reveal essentially a dense stromal infiltration with polymorphonuclear leukocytes and plasma cells. Consequently, the stroma appears to be unusually cellular and numerous glands are distended by a purulent exudate, which also extends to the surface of the mucosa, giving rise to a patchy coat of pus and fibrin.

POSTABORTIVE ENDOMETRITIS. The incidence found by us is 2.38 per cent. In its most readily recognizable form, chorionic villi are conspicuous, although in long-standing cases of postabortive endometritis, remnants of the chorion may be difficult, if not impossible, to recognize. They usually reveal fibrosed remnants of necrotic villi, surrounded by involuting decidual cells and an inflammatory stroma with altered glands. Only the special phosphatase stain may occasionally reveal the true nature of such lesions.

TUBERCULOUS ENDOMETRITIS. Tuberculous endometritis has been intensively studied at our clinic, mainly by Nogales.[39] The frequency with which this type of endometritis has been found to be associated with sterility (10 per cent of all sterile patients; see Chapter 38) and with other apparently functional disturbances, such as amenorrhea, etc., is significant. It is obvious that these surprising findings yielded by endometrial curettage are of great diagnostic value in female genital tuberculosis, not only of the uterus but also of the adnexa, a fact emphasized by Bedoya.

More than anything else, the salient histologic feature is the presence of tubercles, with their usual composition of epithelioid cells, multinucleated giant cells and a surrounding lymphocytic infiltrate. They are seldom confluent and are usually noncaseous. Interestingly, a pseudohyperplastic endometrial pattern has recently been described by Nogales[39, 40] in association with tuberculosis, in which epithelial glandular growth has a "foamy" appearance and the interior of the glands is invaded by elements of the tubercle.

26.3.7. DIAGNOSIS OF NEOPLASIA, ESPECIALLY OF ADENOCARCINOMA OF THE BODY

Many times, curetted tissue permits the establishment of a definite diagnosis of endometrial carcinoma. However, it must be pointed out that not infrequently a tumor located in an inaccessible part of the cavity may be missed.

For this reason, it has been our contention (Botella and Nogales[9, 10]) that negative results obtained by microcurettage are without diagnostic significance. That is to say that, while the diagnosis obtained from endometrial biopsy revealing adenocarcinoma is certain, a "normal" result by no means rules out the presence of *carcinoma*. In cases of doubt concerning a "normal" diagnosis, it is advisable to practice total curettage and to process all the tissue.

26.3.8. DIAGNOSIS OF ABORTIVE RESTS AND OF ECTOPIC PREGNANCY

In most instances, the presence of placental tissue is diagnostic per se; however, in some cases, such as old abortions or abortions that occurred at a very early stage of pregnancy, the finding of chorionic tissue may come as a surprise. Suspected abortion is seldom a valid indication for performing microcurettage, although quite frequently the procedure will reveal evidence of unsuspected abortion (Marín and Botella[33]).

With ectopic pregnancy, microcurettage — if the procedure is performed with due precaution and avoids traumatization — will probably reveal the presence of decidual tissue and clarify the diagnosis. A characteristic feature of ectopic pregnancy is the appearance of "clear cells" in the endometrial glands (Arias-Stella phenomenon) (Fig. 26–8).

Although such conditions as endometritis, carcinoma, retained secundines and ectopic pregnancy are only remotely related to endocrine gynecology, these have been mentioned here both because they are incidental to many exploratory maneuvers initially undertaken in searching for sexual endocrinopathy, and because they represent important factors from the standpoint of *differential diagnosis*.

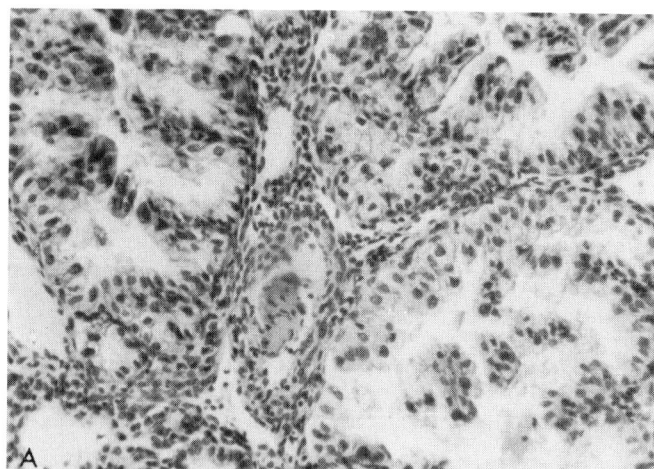
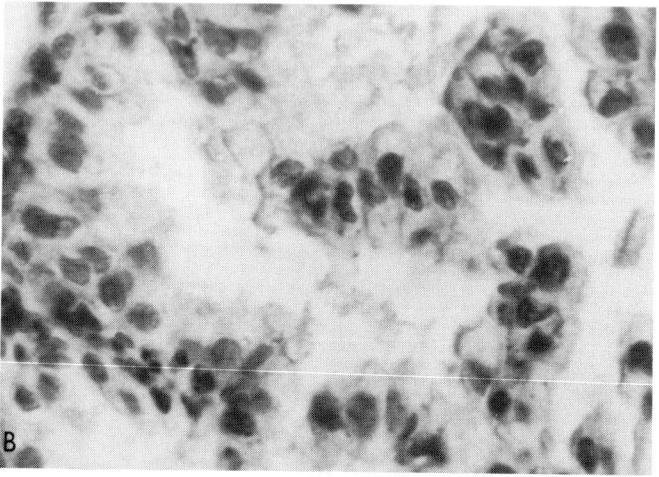

Figure 26–8. Arias-Stella reaction, pathognomonic with extrauterine pregnancy. A, 150×; B, 400×.

26.4. ENDOMETRIAL HISTOCHEMISTRY

The use of histochemical methods for the study of the endometrium, reviewed briefly in Chapter 12, has been gaining importance as regards both clinical diagnosis and practical application. Those interested in the subject may find valuable information in publications by, among others, Atkinson,[3,4] Dempsey and Wislocky,[15] Runge,[45] Ebner,[16] Ober[43] and Botella and Nogales.[9]

26.4.1. ALKALINE GLYCEROPHOSPHATASE

In 1941, Gomori[22] developed a simple and accurate method for histologic visualization of phosphatase activity. Since then, both alkaline and acid phosphatases have been detected in the human endometrium and described by various authors.[3,4,5,9,15] In a previous work, Nogales and Botella[41] studied in detail the characteristic features of phosphatase activity during the different days of the cycle in order to find out whether it had any practical application for the assessment of endometrial function. These changes are quite specific and may be described as follows:

FIRST WEEK OF THE CYCLE. Alkaline phosphatase, which reveals the most typical changes, may be found as early as the first postmenstrual day and is detected by the intense staining of the gland epithelia, without appearing in gland spaces or in vascular endothelia at this stage (Fig. 13-11).

SECOND WEEK OF THE CYCLE. Alkaline phosphatase activity in the glands continues to increase and becomes very intense also in the surface epithelium. Glands are beginning to undergo dilatation and slight phosphatase staining may be found in their lumina (Fig. 26-9).

THIRD WEEK OF CYCLE. Although phosphatase activity is induced by the action of estrogens on the endometrium (see Chapter 2), patterns observed during the third week are extremely interesting and enable us to satisfactorily diagnose the occurrence of ovulation and the formation of a corpus luteum. A characteristic feature of this period is *phosphatase depletion in gland epithelia* in conjunction with *intraglandular accumulation of phosphatase staining material*, consistent with displacement of enzyme activity from epithelia into gland lumina (Fig. 26-9).

FOURTH WEEK OF THE CYCLE. During the fourth week, not only has all phosphatase activity been eliminated from the gland epithelium but in addition positive staining material in the lumen has disappeared and gland spaces appear empty. The reaction, however, remains positive within the walls of *endometrial vessels*. As already indicated,[7,41] vascular phosphatase-positive effects are not brought about by progesterone activity but result from the fact that phosphatase activity is greatest in newly formed vessels, and since the characteristic feature of the fourth week is endometrial vascular proliferation, the vascular pattern is revealed conspicuously by the phosphatase method. Vascular phosphatase activity is actually present throughout the cycle, although for the reasons already mentioned it becomes more conspicuous toward the end of the cycle.

ENDOMETRIAL HYPERPLASIA. The histologic findings in endometrial hyperplasia are similar to those of the second week of the cycle. However, a note of difference is marked by the absence of phosphatase activity from epithelia of cystically dilated glands as opposed to noncystic glands, which show a strongly positive reaction. This seems to prove the fact that only the latter are subject to active proliferation (see Chapter 28).

ENDOMETRITIS. The phosphatase method is of great diagnostic help in the postabortive type of endometritis, as stated previously. Most interesting changes were observed and described with this method in tuberculous endometritis (Nogales[40]); however, their description here would be an unwarranted digression.

The great value of the Gomori reaction consists in permitting us to identify the particular time of the endometrial cycle with remarkable accuracy; it is therefore of great help for the diagnosis of insufficient or delayed progestational phases (Botella).

26.4.2. GLYCOGEN

Glycogen is stored in the endometrium for the purpose of providing the egg with a readily available source of energy. Undoubtedly, glycogen synthesis is the most

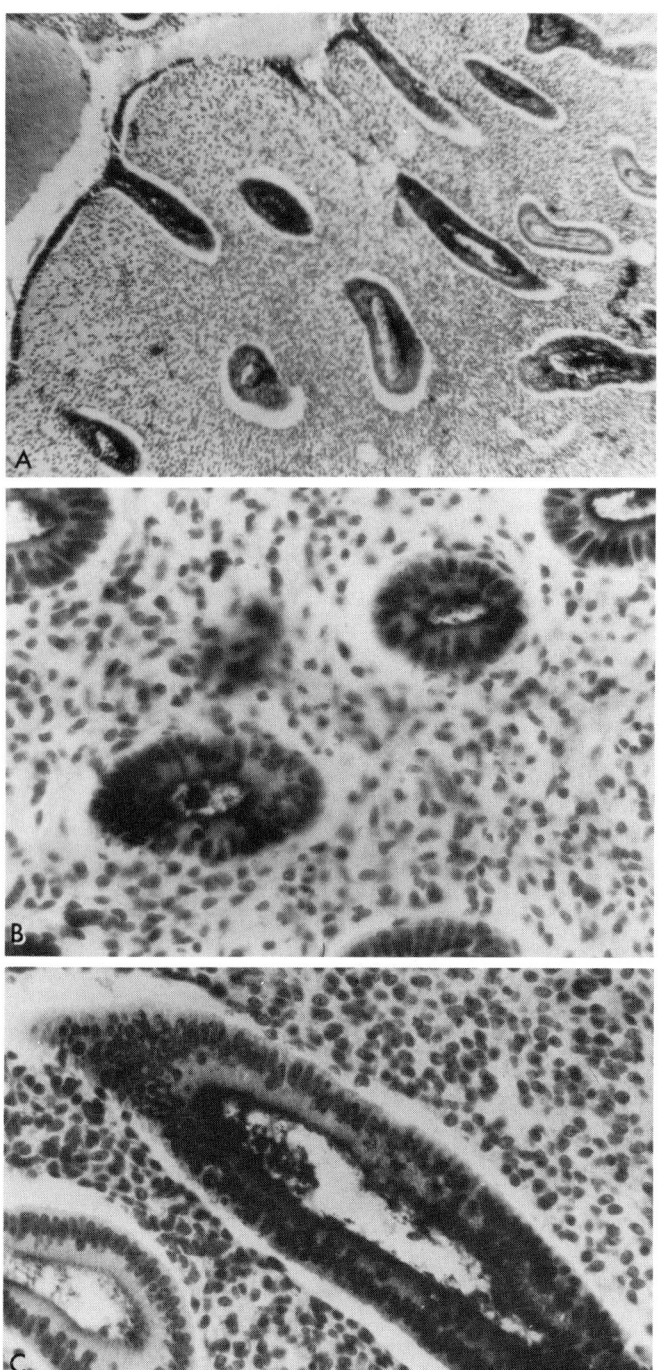

Figure 26-9. Endometrium during second week of cycle, stained for alkaline glycerophosphatase by the Gomori method. *A,* Low power view (100×), revealing positive staining reaction in glandular and surface epithelium. *B,* At higher magnification (420×), glands are still poorly dilated, the epithelium staining positive and beginning to eliminate some phosphatase into lumen. *C,* Greater dilatation of gland, with more pronounced phosphatase activity in lumen (420×).

important of all biochemical functions of the endometrium. In view of this, demonstration of this polysaccharide in the cells of endometrial glands and stroma is of utmost diagnostic importance.

METHODS. The presence of glycogen can be demonstrated by various methods. Moricard[38] used the iodine reaction. Ferin,[17] Hughes and colleagues,[23, 24] and Botella and Nogales[8, 9] have repeatedly used Best's carmine method. However, better results than those obtained with the two preceding methods are obtained with the periodic acid-Schiff (PAS) reaction, either in its original form or as modified by Runge[45] and Ebner[16] (Alsian blue–PAS), which presently constitute the most reliable procedures for the localization of glycogen deposits. Descriptions of the techniques involved may be found in modern manuals of staining technology (Pearse, Lison, etc.).

LOCALIZATION OF GLYCOGEN IN THE COURSE OF THE CYCLE. FIRST WEEK. Little glycogen is found in the endometrium during the first week; whenever it is detected in gland spaces, it seems to be a carry-over from the preceding cycle.

SECOND WEEK. Although the second week classically pertains to the follicular phase, glycogen begins to appear in glands before the end of the week. This is believed to result from the production of small amounts of progesterone by the mature follicle prior to ovulation (see Chapters 2 and 13).

THIRD WEEK. Glycogen is found accumulating in large amounts within the cells of endometrial gland epithelia. Commonly, beginning with the sixteenth day, increasingly abundant glycogen deposits are seen in the basal portions of the cells.

FOURTH WEEK. About the twentieth or twenty-first day, glands begin to undergo changes in shape, the thickness of lining epithelia declining and nuclei in columnar cells lining up at a suprabasal level. The *luminal* (supranuclear) portions of the cells are now observed to deposit glycogen in increasing amounts as the cycle progresses, and the glycogen eventually is seen emptying into the gland spaces, forming part of the secretory product.

By the time the *premenstrual* phase is reached, all glycogen is contained in the intraluminal gland secretion.

CORPUS LUTEUM INSUFFICIENCY. It must be emphasized that some endometria occasionally reveal an insufficient degree of secretory transformation. The significance of the associated glycopenia has been recently brought to light by a number of workers.[7, 11, 24] Nogales and Botella[41] have stressed the role of corpus luteum insufficiency as a cause of sterility.

26.4.3. MUCOPOLYSACCHARIDES

Mucopolysaccharides also show important fluctuations during the cycle and may be used as an ancillary means for the diagnosis of functional anomalies, particularly those involving the stroma. The question has been investigated by Merlo[36] at our clinic by plotting the incidence of both acid and neutral mucopolysaccharides in the course of normal cycles.

The staining procedures most often used are the simple PAS technique and, above all, the PAS–Alsian blue method in which neutral mucopolysaccharides stain pink and acid mucopolysaccharides stain blue or blue-violet. The findings are:

FIRST WEEK OF THE CYCLE. Glands are devoid of mucopolysaccharides. The stroma contains abundant acid mucopolysaccharides.

SECOND WEEK. There is a marked increase in stromal acid mucopolysaccharides, and isolated granules of neutral mucopolysaccharides begin to appear.

THIRD WEEK. Little mucopolysaccharide may be observed in the stroma, but neutral mucopolysaccharides appear in gland epithelia and smaller amounts of acid mucopolysaccharides within products of gland secretion.

FOURTH WEEK. A characteristic feature for this period is a marked increase in both acid and neutral mucopolysaccharides in the stroma. Acid mucopolysaccharides are found around spiral arterioles, while neutral mucopolysaccharides form intracellular inclusions, which are most pronounced whenever there is a decidual reaction.

As far as the glands are concerned, these are characteristically *filled with large amounts of acid mucopolysaccharides* during the fourth week. Together with existing variations in glycogen content, these reactions offer an informative guide for the characterization of the time of the cycle and for the evaluation of normal endometrial function.

26.4.4. OTHER HISTOCHEMICAL REACTIONS

In addition to the basic staining reactions we have just outlined, other methods are available that have so far been used for research.

RIBONUCLEIC ACID (RNA) AND DEOXYRIBONUCLEIC ACID (DNA). The presence of RNA is usually demonstrated with the methyl green–pyronine procedure (according to Brachet), whereas that of DNA is brought out by the Feulgen reaction. Both compounds can be assumed to reflect nuclear activity, viz., proliferation, and are increased during the first two weeks of the cycle and, particularly, in endometrial hyperplasia. Endometria have been studied with nuclear stains by Atkinson,[5] by Long and Doko[30] and, at our clinic, by Merlo.[35, 36]

SUCCINIC DEHYDROGENASE. Long and Doko[30] and MacKay and associates[31] have localized this enzyme mainly in the secretory phase.

PHOSPHORYLASE AND PHOSPHOAMIDASE. These enzymes, involved in polymerization of sugars that are glycogen precursors, have been demonstrated by Foraker and his group.[20, 21]

CHOLESTEROL. The presence of cholesterol and other lipids has been studied by Long and Doko,[30] MacKay and co-workers,[31] Atkinson,[4, 5] and others. Their peak incidence occurs during the progestational phase.

REFERENCES

1. Anspach, B. M., and Hoffman, J.: *Amer. J. Obstet. Gynec.*, 28:473, 1934.
2. Arias-Stella, J.: *Arch. Path.*, 60:49, 1955.
3. Atkinson, W. B., et al.: *Cancer*, 2:132, 1949.
4. Atkinson, W. B.: In *Menstruation and its Disorders*, ed. E. T. Engle. Springfield, Ill., Charles C Thomas, 1950.
5. Atkinson, W. B.: *Texas Rep. Biol. Med.*, 13:603, 1955.
6. Botella, J., Nogales, F., and Vilar, E.: *Gynaecologia*, 127:201, 1949.
7. Botella, J.: *Colloques sur la fonction luteale*. Paris, Masson & Cie., 1954.
8. Botella, J., and Nogales, F.: *Actas Soc. Esp. Est. Esterilidad*, 3:3, 1955.
9. Botella, J., and Nogales, F.: *Rev. Franç. Gynec.*, 52:411, 1957.
10. Botella, J.: *Internat. J. Fertil.*, 4:300, 1959.
11. Buxton, C. L.: In *Menstruation and its Disorders*, ed. E. T. Engle. Springfield, Ill., Charles C Thomas, 1950.
12. Brewer, C., and Jones, G. S.: *Amer. J. Obstet. Gynec.*, 55:18, 1948.
13. Cotte, G.: *Gynec. Obstet.*, 27:210, 1930.
14. Dallenbach-Hellweg, D.: *Endometrium*. Berlin, Springer, 1969.
15. Dempsey, E. W., and Wislocky, G. B.: *Amer. J. Anat.*, 80:1, 1947.
16. Ebner, H.: "Histotopochemie," in *Gynäkologische Zytologie*, ed. H. Runge. Leipzig, Theodor Steinkopff, 1954.
17. Ferin, J.: *Ann. d'Endocr.*, 11:179, 1950.
18. Ferin, J.: In *Colloques sur la fonction luteale*. Paris, Masson & Cie., 1954.
19. Falconer, B.: *Acta Obstet. Gynec. Scand.*, 27: Suppl. 5, 1947.
20. Foraker, A. G., Celli, P. A., and Denham, J. W.: *Cancer*, 7:100, 1954.
21. Foraker, A. G., and Zamarriyo, J.: *Acta Cytol.*, 6:365, 1962.
22. Gomori, G.: *Cell Comp. Physiol.*, 71:12, 1941.
23. Hughes, E. C.: *Amer. J. Obstet. Gynec.*, 49:10, 1945.
24. Hughes, E. C., Ness, A. W., and Lloyd, C. W.: *Amer. J. Obstet. Gynec.*, 50:1295, 1950.
25. Holmström, E. G.: *Amer. J. Obstet. Gynec.*, 53:727, 1947.
26. Jackson, M. H.: *J. Obstet. Gynec. Brit. Emp.*, 35:64, 1938.
27. Khanpää, A. W.: *Acta Obstet. Gynec. Scand.*, 19:1, 1949.
28. Klinger, H. H., and Burch, W. I.: *J.A.M.A.*, 99:559, 1932.
29. Kottmeier, H. L.: *Acta Obstet. Gynec. Scand.*, 27:Suppl. 6, 1947.
30. Long, M. L., and Doko, F.: *Ann. N.Y. Acad. Sci.*, 75:504, 1959.
31. McKay, P. E., et al.: *Obstet. Gynec.*, 8:140, 1956.
32. Marín, E.: *Actas Soc. Esp. Est. Esterilidad*, 1:345, 1954.
33. Marín, E., and Botella, J.: *Acta Gin.*, 2:257, 1951.
34. Meyer, R.: *Arch. Gynäk.*, 100:1, 1913.
35. Merlo, J. G.: *Acta Gin.*, 11:11, 1960.
36. Merlo, J. G.: *Acta Gin.*, 11:323, 1960.
37. Moricard, R.: *Gynec. Obstet.*, 43:36, 1948.
38. Moricard, R.: *Colloques sur la fonction luteale*. Paris, Masson & Cie., 1954.
39. Nogales, F.: *Acta Gin.*, 2:35, 1951.
40. Nogales, F.: *Arch. Gynäk.*, 186:371, 1955.
41. Nogales, F., and Botella, J.: *Acta Gin.*, 6:3, 1955.
42. Novak, E.: *Obstet. Gynec. Survey*, 5:297, 1950.
43. Ober, K. G.: *Klin. Wschr.*, 28:9, 1950.
44. Reifferscheid, W.: *Zbl. Gynäk.*, 65:760, 1941.
45. Runge, H.: "Die Bedeutung der histochemischen Methoden für die Gynäkologie," in *Klinische Fortschritte, Gynäkologie*, ed. T. Antoine. Vienna, Urban & Schwarzenberg, 1953.
46. Schröder, R.: *Arch. Gynäk.*, 98:81, 1912.
47. Slocker, C.: *Acta Gin.*, 5:251, 1954.
48. Tietze, K.: *Arch. Gynäk.*, 173:276, 1943.
49. Wynn, R. M., and Harris, J. A.: *Fertil. Steril.*, 18:632, 1967.

Part Seven
OVARIAN SYNDROMES

We are now in a position to undertake the clinical study of female endocrinopathies, availing ourselves of the exploratory procedures analyzed in the preceding chapters. Notwithstanding the current means at our disposal, a great deal of knowledge is still poorly defined and explanations for many aspects of clinical experience, even to a greater extent than in physiology, are necessarily confined to the realm of pure hypothesis.

Following the same sequence that was used in Part One, Part Seven begins with the pathology of internal ovarian secretions. The most relevant syndromes are those which are derived from disorders of estrogenic secretions, whether from omission (hypoestrinism) or from commission (hyperestrinism). In addition, a brief discussion is presented concerning the syndromes of the corpus luteum and those of ovarian androgenism. Part Seven is concluded with an endocrinologic analysis of ovarian tumors possessing incretory activity.

Chapter 27

HYPOESTRINISM

27.1. CLASSIFICATION OF OVARIAN FUNCTIONAL DISORDERS

In this part of the book, we begin our discussion of gynecologic endocrine disease. A total review in general of all endocrinopathies affecting woman need not be undertaken, since a large number of these do not affect the reproductive system in any specific way. Therefore, only those disturbances having a direct bearing on the genital system will be examined. On the other hand, this does not mean that our study must be confined to the gonads. Diseases of the pituitary, adrenal, thyroid, pancreas and, less frequently, other endocrine glands, may adversely affect ovarian function, giving rise to *pluriglandular genital syndromes*, with important repercussions on the sexual sphere. This and the next chapter are concerned with *ovarian endocrine pathology*. Four consecutive chapters dealing with various aspects of this subject are devoted to hypoestrinism, hyperestrinism, corpus luteum and virilization syndromes, and functioning ovarian tumors.

The question of how to classify ovarian functional disorders has long been a matter of controversy. For many years, the classification of ovarian functional disorders was *based on symptomatology*. Because menstrual symptoms tend to be the most prominent, *classification of menstrual anomalies overlapped to a great extent that of ovarian functional disorders*. Such criteria may still be prevalent in relatively up-to-date textbooks, although their fallacy had been underscored by Marañón[59] long ago. In the meantime, many important arguments may have been raised in addition to those offered by Marañón. In the first edition of this book, we indicated that amenorrhea was not necessarily determined by ovarian hypofunction but could be the result of continuous estrogen hypersecretion (hyperhormonal amenorrhea, see Chapter 28). Similarly, functional metrorrhagia and menorrhagia are not inevitably linked to hyperovarian function. So, for instance, a decrease in ovarian function has been found to be a common underlying cause for many forms of juvenile metropathy. The same arguments might even be compounded as regards functional alterations of the corpus luteum. Of late, Albright has proposed a classification of amenorrhea based on urinary excretion levels of FSH and estrogens, distinguishing as many as six different varieties. This may illustrate the complexities involved in classifying menstrual disturbances and the type of errors that may be incurred by classifying ovarian functional disorders solely on the merits of menstrual disturbances. We have therefore refrained from adopting any of the above-mentioned criteria and, in keeping with the usual classification system adopted for other glands of internal secretion, we shall divide ovarian functional disorders into those caused by hypofunction and those caused by hyperfunction.

However, *it must be realized that the ovarian gland is in fact a double gland*, made up of two endocrine units that are to a certain extent independent of each other, the follicle and the corpus luteum. Ovarian functional disorders must accordingly be divided not only into hypo- and hyperfunctional types but also into *follicle syndromes* and *corpus luteum syndromes*. In this context, the terms hypo- and hyperfolliculinic, employed by various authors, may eventually find wider acceptance. Aside from this, however, it must also be taken into consideration that the follicle is not the only source of estrogens and that other structures may be responsible for hypersecretion of estrogenic compounds, and may give rise to conditions that are indistinguishable from hyperfolliculinism. Particularly in recent years, much has been written about extraovarian sources of estrogens. The terms hypo- and hyperfolliculinic, too, lend themselves to misinterpretation, either as implying decrease or increase in follicular hormone, or as denoting hypo- or hyperfunction of the follicle. For this reason, we have adopted the designations *hypoestrinism* and *hyperestrinism* as most expressive of conditions involving either lack or excess of estrogen production, whether of ovarian or extraovarian origin.

Consequently, our classification of ovarian functional disorders comprises in the first place the *estrogenic syndromes*, hypoestrinism and hyperestrinism; in the second place, the *luteinic syndromes*, hypoluteinism and hyperluteinism; and in the third place, based on the premise that some ovarian cells are capable of elaborating androgens, so-called *ovarian hyperandrogenism*. This classification would be incomplete without the inclusion of *functioning ovarian tumors*, in some instances producers of estrogens, in others, producers of androgens or progesterone, though occasionally also responsible for elaborating hormones of extraovarian nature that may cause important endocrine disturbances. These must be included among the endocrine disorders of the ovary regardless of what type of hormone they may secrete.

Chapter 27 will be concerned with the study of syndromes of hypoestrinism, the other aspects being developed in subsequent chapters.

27.2. HYPOESTRINISM

27.2.1. DEFINITION

Hypoestrinism may be defined as a condition in which estrogens are not being produced in the ovary in adequate amounts. Theoretically, the occurrence of an extraovarian type of hypoestrinism is conceivable, since estrogens are known to be also elaborated by the adrenal and, possibly, by the placenta. However, deficient adrenal estrogen production may be significant from the clinical viewpoint only when occurring during embryonal life, and it is therefore discussed with disorders of sexual differentiation and development. On the other hand, deficient estrogen production by the placenta has yet to be shown to produce pathologic alterations in a conclusive manner, although its implication in abortion and, perhaps, in toxemia of pregnancy is suspected. This problem has been discussed in Chapter 13. Hence, in its present usage hypoestrinism connotes only deficient production of estrogens by the ovary.

Deficiencies in ovarian estrogenic secretion may be traced to many causes. First of all, they may stem from *primitive* secretory failure, that is, from the *absence of puberty*. Such an ovary has failed to mature by the time puberty is due, or has matured incompletely or partially, setting up a permanent ovarian deficit.

Obviously, such a situation may not have its origin in the ovary itself. Disturbances in other glands of internal secretion, principally the pituitary, may be responsible for lack of ovarian stimulation at the time of puberty, although the ovary itself may be normally developed. Conversely, the pituitary may be normal or even hyperfunctional, but a malformed or *locally altered* ovary may not have the capacity for estrogen synthesis and may give rise to hypoestrinism. Primitive hypoestrinism may therefore have either an *ovarian* or a *pituitary* origin. Occasionally, it may also have an *adrenal* or *thyroid* origin, though such instances are rare.

Secondary hypoestrinism is due to cessation of secretion by a well developed, previously normally secreting ovary. Here, too, *pluriglandular disorders*, that is, disturbances in other glands of internal secretion, may be involved (Chapters 31 and 34); moreover, as with primitive hypoestrinism, a *local ovarian cause*, such as destructive disease or premature aging, may be involved.

Finally, hypoestrinism also occurs after menopause and following surgical or radiologic castration (Chapter 37).

27.2.2. CLASSIFICATION OF HYPOESTRINISM

1. *Primitive hypoestrinism* (onset of manifestations at puberty)
   a. *Primitive ovarian hypoestrinism*
   b. *Primitive pituitary hypoestrinism*
2. *Secondary hypoestrinism* (onset of manifestations in adult life)

a. Endocrine alterations (to be studied in Chapters 31 and 34)
  b. Destructive ovarian processes (inflammation, tumors, etc.)
  c. Premature senility or ovarian atrophy
3. *Postmenopausal and postcastrational hypoestrinism* (discussed in Chapter 37)

27.3. PRIMITIVE HYPOESTRINISM

Apart from studying the ovarian and pituitary varieties of primitive hypoestrinism, we shall also discuss the thyroid and adrenal forms.

27.3.1. PRIMITIVE OVARIAN HYPOESTRINISM

The present trend in female endocrinology is to conceive of primitive ovarian failure within the context of *ovarian dysgenesis*, that is, resulting from faulty ovarian differentiation during embryonal life. While, according to this concept, all the previously mentioned conditions may be classified as *gonadal dysgenesis* and included among the anomalies of sexual determination (Chapter 35), we have classified as such only Turner's syndrome, which alone has been proved to be a true instance of gonadal dysgenesis. The "borderline" conditions are therefore included here and classified as: (1) *Ovarian agenesis (Wilkins-Fleischmann syndrome)*, (2) *ovarian hypogenesis or hypoplasia (Greenblatt's syndrome and Gordan's syndrome)*, and (3) *sex reversal and afunctional ovaries* (see Table 27-1). Unlike the editions of this book antedating 1956, this edition excludes Turner's syndrome from this chapter and places it among the congenital anomalies of the gonad; this division may be arbitrary, since it is recognized that the conditions discussed in the present chapter are equally congenital in nature and, by and large, correspond cytologically to gonadal dysgenesis.

Primitive ovarian hypoestrinism is a rare condition. Moraes-Ruehsen and Seegar-Jones[64] have used *dynamic tests* in their study of 300 cases of amenorrhea and found primitive ovarian failure in only 21 cases (7 per cent). Various authors (Brown et al.,[15] Hoffenberg et al.,[39] Overzier[72] and Vague et al.[84]) have found evidence that only 20 per cent of patients with Turner's syndrome show a chromosomal sex complement other than XO. We shall concern ourselves above all with those *syndromes of gonadal agenesis or hypogenesis in which the chromosomal constitution is XX*.

TRUE GONADAL AGENESIS. A case of true ovarian agenesis was described by Wilkins and Fleischmann[90] in 1944, although at that time the genetic nature of Turner's syndrome had not yet been recognized. As a result, we have since applied the term *Wilkins-Fleischmann syndrome* to true ovarian agenesis. In the course of the following years we had begun to suspect that such an entity was nonexistent until Overzier and Linden[73] produced evidence to the contrary. We therefore advocate the continued use of the term Wilkins-Fleischmann syndrome (Figs. 27-1 and 27-2).

OVARIAN HYPOGENESIS. Ovarian hypogenesis or hypoplasia is by far the most common condition in which an XX karyotype is associated with a *rudimentary ovary*. It is also known by the name of "Greenblatt's syndrome," after Greenblatt who described it in 1956 (Greenblatt et al.[35]). Apart from essential amenorrhea, an XX sex chromosome complement and rudimentary ovaries, which nevertheless may contain readily recognizable primordial follicles, this syndrome is characterized by tall stature, eunuchoidism, mild virilization and absence of skeletal anomalies. These features are illustrated in Figures 27-3 and 27-4. As in all of these cases, furthermore,

TABLE 27-1. Systematization of Primordial Ovarian Hypoestrinism

I. Genetic sex XO	True Turner's syndrome (80 per cent of cases); see Chapter 35
II. Genetic sex XY	Sex reversal syndrome; see Chapter 35
III. Genetic sex XX	A. *Total gonadal agenesis* (20 per cent of cases): Wilkins-Fleischmann syndrome
	B. *Congenital ovarian hypoplasia*
	(1) with normal stature: Greenblatt's syndrome
	(2) with short stature: Gordan's syndrome
	C. *Normally developed ovary, but without function* (possibly identical with "sex reversal" syndrome)

574   *Ovarian Syndromes*

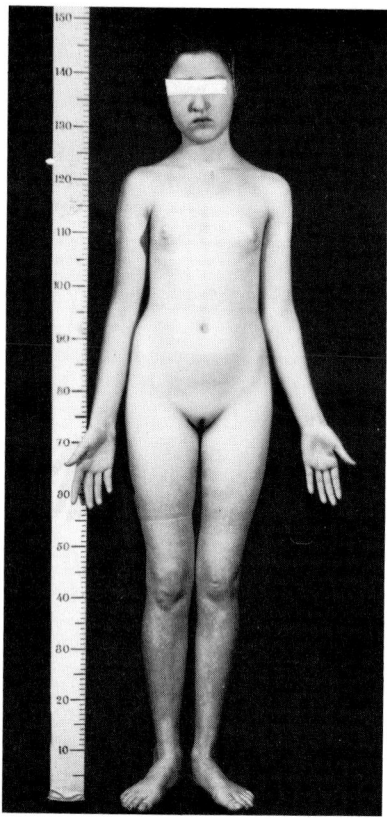

Figure 27–1. Wilkins-Fleischmann syndrome in woman, aged 21, with primary amenorrhea. There had been arrest of growth since age 13. Note short stature (145 cm), span equal to height, absence of breast development, atrichosis. Other observations: elevated gonadotropinuria (above 80 IU FSH per 1000 ml urine); estrogenuria, negative; vaginal cytology, atrophic. (Courtesy of Sopeña.)

Figure 27–2. Case similar to that in Figure 27–1. Woman, aged 23, with primary amenorrhea. Arrest of growth occurred at age 13, and there is defective distal ossification. Gonadotropinuria, 120 IU; negative estrogenuria; atrophic vaginal cytology. (Courtesy of Sopeña.)

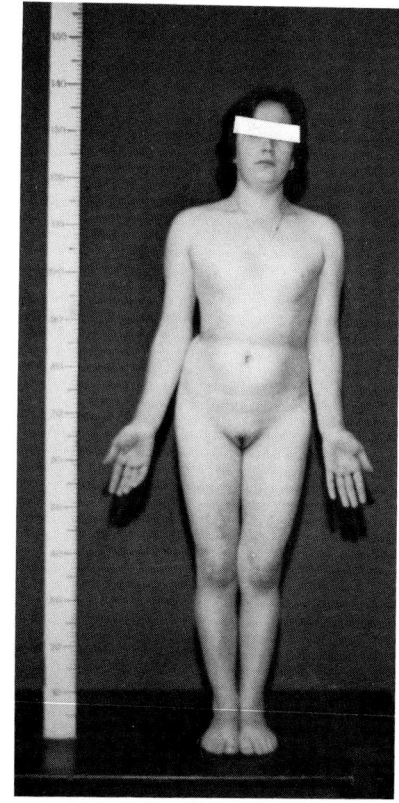

Hypoestrinism

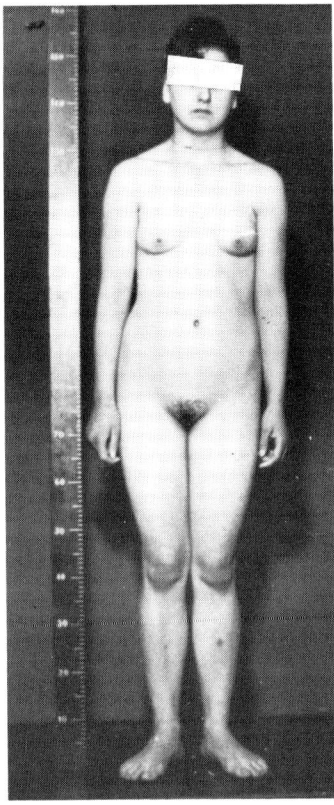

Figure 27-3. Syndrome of ovarian hypoplasia (Greenblatt's syndrome) in woman, aged 20. Normal stature, poor breast development and scanty pubic and axillary hair. Gonadotropin levels were not increased; positive estrogenuria (20 to 25 mcg per 1000 ml) was present; vaginal cytology was hypotrophic. (Courtesy of Sopeña.)

drome of Wilkins-Fleischmann has been described by Klotz and associates[50] in identical twins. It consisted in the presence of ovaries seemingly normal as to size and gross appearance but totally devoid of germinal elements and totally unresponsive to gonadotropin stimulation. A similar case has been found by Laitinen and Pesonen,[53] who observed a totally negative response to dexamethasone (see Chapter 24). Donaldson and his co-workers[22] prefer the use of the *insulin stimulation test*. If an increase in the titer of growth hormone in the peripheral blood is obtained as a result of insulin stimulation, it may be assumed with certainty that one is dealing with a primary hypoovarian condition of the Turner type or one of its analogues. It is hoped that much can be learned in the near future about ovarian agenesis or hypogenesis by the extended use of functional or dynamic tests.

vaginal cytology is typically *atrophic* (Fig. 27-5).

A condition differing somewhat from the Wilkins-Fleischmann syndrome was described by Gordan[33] in 1955. In this form there are similarly ovarian hypoplasia and a genetic sex of XX, but, in contrast, the patients present with short stature, virilism and abundance of ovarian hilar cells. Patients with short stature and XX chromosomal complements may well be included in this group, under the name of *"Gordan's syndrome."*

To avoid confusion, both the syndrome described by Lisser and associates[56] and that reported by Kerkhof and Stolte[45] have been omitted from the present review, since they appear to have been basically identical to the Wilkins-Fleischmann syndrome.

Another syndrome resembling the syn-

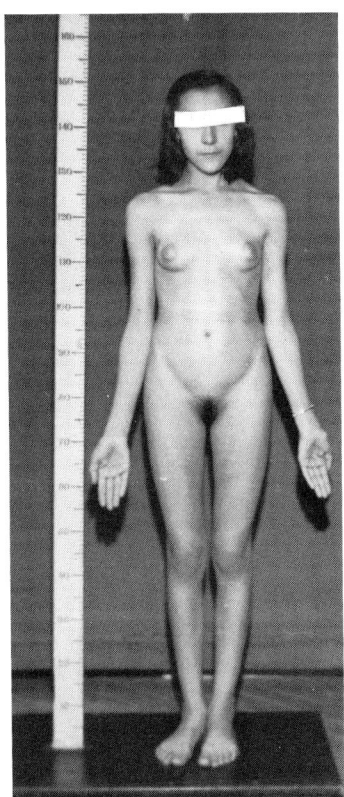

Figure 27-4. Case similar to that in Figure 27-3, in woman aged 20. Note short stature, small breasts, and scanty pubic and axillary hair. There is marked predominance of span (165 cm) over height (153 cm). Estrogens, 30 mcg; FSH, below 50 IU. (Courtesy of Sopeña.)

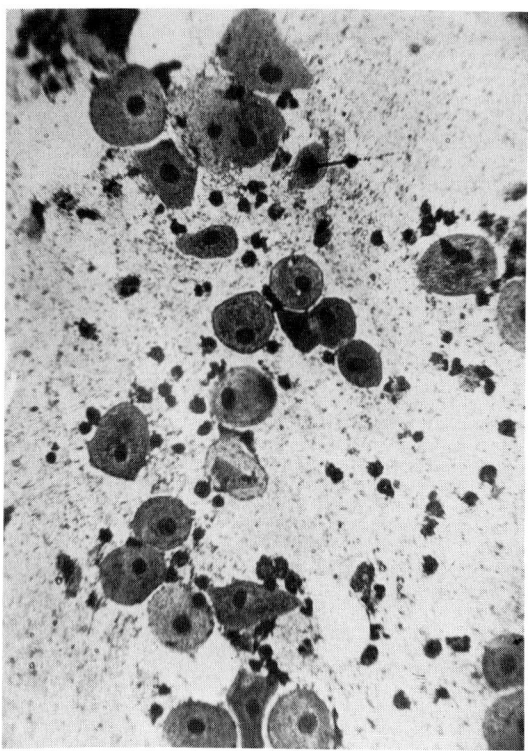

Figure 27–5. Atrophic vaginal smear, composed exclusively of basal and parabasal cells, from a case of ovarian agenesis.

CASES OF HYPOGENESIS WITH AN XY OR XO CHROMOSOMAL COMPLEMENT. Recently, Belausch and associates,[6] Klotz and co-workers,[50] and Morsier and Gautier[67] described an *olfactogenital syndrome* characterized by atrophy of the olfactory tract in association with nonfunctional ovaries and with lack of response to gonadotropin. This syndrome shall be discussed in more detail in Chapter 32.

27.3.2. SYMPTOMATOLOGY: GENERAL SIGNS

It has been emphasized repeatedly that these patients lack the characteristic features of Turner's syndrome. They do not show the short stature and the characteristic pterygium colli, and the presence of cubitus valgus is inconstant. On the other hand, they frequently present with signs of mild virilization, such as observed by Gordan and colleagues,[7,33] and occasionally with modest development of the breasts, such as observed in our own cases and in those of Sopeña[11,80] (Figs. 27–2 and 27–4).

Endocrinologically, these patients have gonadotropinuria[8,14] and their vaginal cytology is not of the completely atrophic type,[88,89] so that the impression conveyed is that either their rudimentary ovaries or perhaps their adrenals secrete estrogens in minimal amounts, sufficient to counteract marked pituitary hyperfunction as it is known to occur, for instance, in typical Turner's syndrome.

A series of diagnostic studies on two such patients, in which FSH and LH levels were determined and ovarian functional tests used, were recently conducted by Breckwoldt and Bettendorf,[14] Laitinen and Pesonen,[53] Netter and associates[69] and Vague and co-workers.[87]

Anatomically and pathologically, some ovarian tissue invariably is present. As a matter of fact, this is what distinguishes this group of syndromes: the presence of recognizable, though incompletely developed, ovarian tissue. Primordial follicles as well as oocytes were found to mature,[46] but the follicular apparatus is incapable of attaining full maturation and ovulation never occurs. The earliest phases of follicular development frequently lead to atresia, as is the case in infantile ovaries.[18]

Radiologically, the findings in these conditions are also of interest, although they are not exclusive of this group of syndromes and are observed equally in gonadal dysgenesis (see Chapter 23). These are: *Vague's sign,*[85,86] or sign of the anvil-shaped tibia (mentioned in Chapter 23, page 503); *sign of Kosowicz,*[51,52] or sign of the carpal angle, illustrated in Figure 27–6; and the *sign of the short fourth metacarpal bone,* described originally by Archibald,[4] which is of great diagnostic value (Fig. 27–7).

Concerning the question of *statural relationships,* Decourt's[19,20] morphography is highly informative and allows a clear distinction to be made between these syndromes, in which stature is normal, and Turner's syndrome, in which stature is short (Figs. 27–8 and 27–9).

These patients in addition develop characteristic *circulatory symptoms.* The phenomenon of acrocyanosis and cold extremities is almost invariably present. Hands tend to be cold, cyanotic and sweaty (genital hands of Marañón[59]). Similarly, acrocyanosis usually involves the feet and the calves. The appearance of the genital

Hypoestrinism

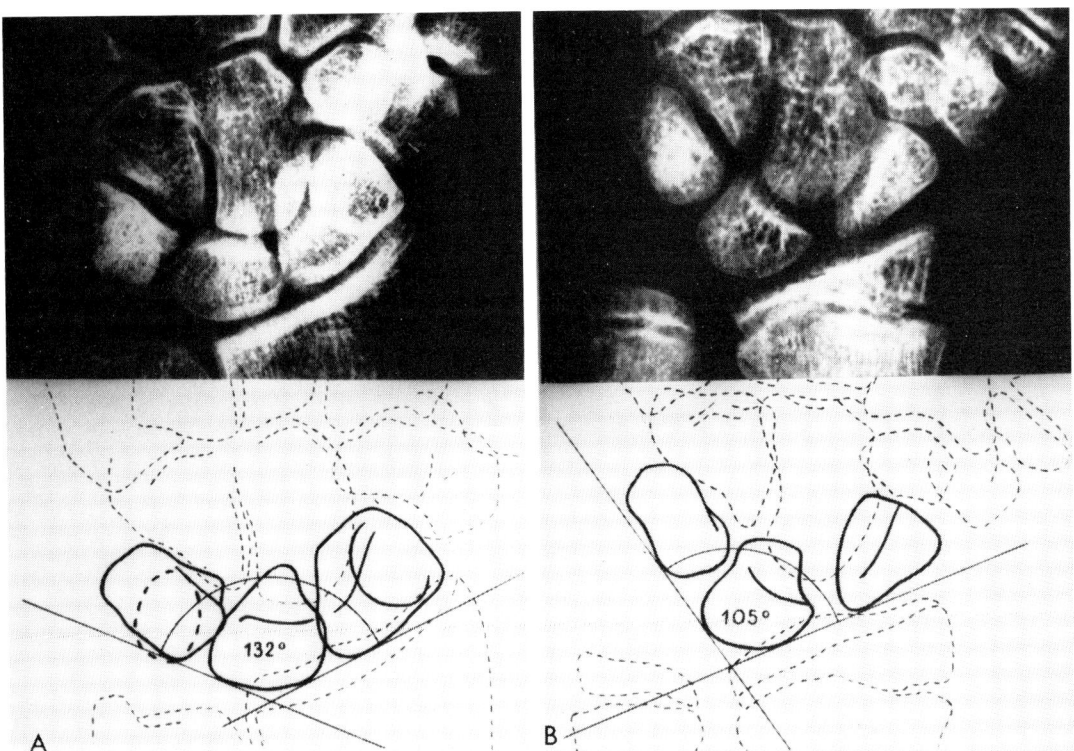

Figure 27-6. Sign of the carpal angle. *A*, Normal. *B*, Case of gonadal dysgenesis. Distal displacement of pyramidal bone results in a decreased angle of the ulnoradiocarpal joint line. (From Kosowicz: *J. Clin. Endocr. Metab.*, 22:949, 1962.)

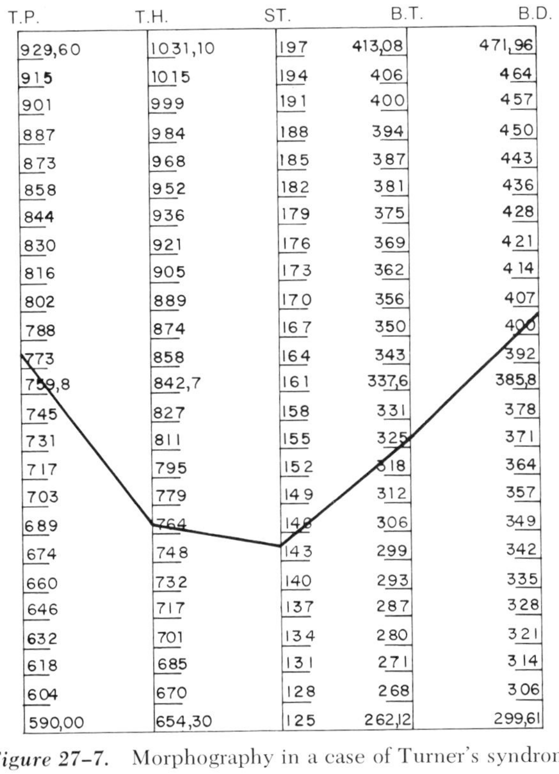

Figure 27-7. Morphography in a case of Turner's syndrome.

T.P.	T.H.	ST.	B.T.	B.D.
929,60	1031,10	197	413,08	471,95
915	1015	194	406	464
901	999	191	400	457
887	984	188	394	450
873	968	185	387	443
858	952	182	381	436
844	936	179	375	428
830	921	176	369	421
816	905	173	362	414
802	889	170	356	407
788	874	167	350	400
773	858	164	343	392
759,8	842,7	161	337,6	385,8
745	827	158	331	378
731	811	155	325	371
717	795	152	318	364
703	779	149	312	357
689	764	146	306	349
674	748	143	299	342
660	732	140	293	335
646	717	137	287	328
632	701	134	280	321
618	685	131	271	314
604	670	128	268	306
590,00	654,30	125	262,12	299,61

Figure 27-8. Morphography in a case of Wilkins-Fleischmann syndrome.

Figure 27-9. The hand in gonadal dysgenesis: sign of the short fourth metacarpal (see Chapter 23, page 503).

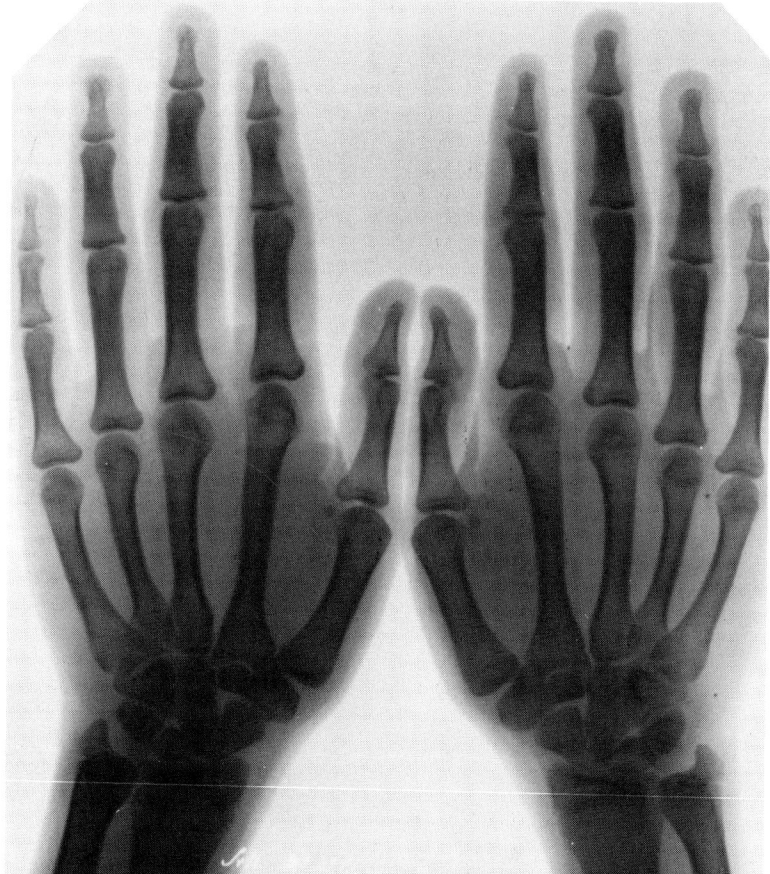

Hypoestrinism

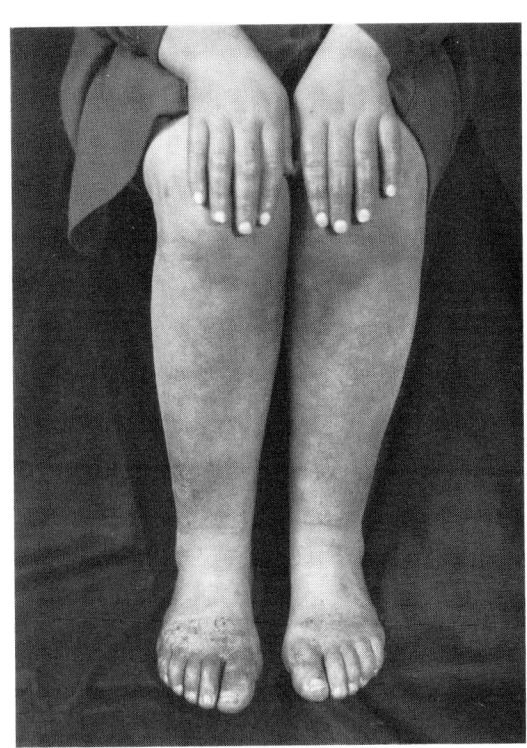

Figure 27-10. Dysgenetic hands and feet, with erythema pernio of the lower extremities.

foot parallels in every respect that of the genital hand, as is illustrated in Figure 27-10. Frequently, such associated circulatory disturbances give rise to the appearance of erythema pernio over the limbs. *Anemia* occasionally may also supervene.

Associated *cutaneous manifestations* may similarly be significant. Apart from erythema pernio, and the corresponding chilblains, this group of patients frequently suffers from *juvenile acne*, a true nightmare of many young girls, which fortunately responds very well to estrogen therapy.[1, 65]

27.3.3. LOCAL SYMPTOMS CONFINED TO THE GENITAL TRACT

Prominent among these is poor development of the uterus, sharing some features with the *infantile type of uterus*, characterized by disproportionate development of the cervix in relation to the uterine body (Fig. 27-11). Liu[57] emphasized the importance of *cervix-to-body ratios* for the diagnosis of constitutional hypoestrinism and for that purpose devised a hysterometer that can be used for measuring the cervical and endometrial cavities separately. Apart from appearing hypoplastic, the uterus generally tends to be deviated to the left, resulting in what we call *uterine sinistroposition* (Fig. 27-12), which has also been noted by Frank and by Martius.

Endometrial findings in these patients are typical. There is *endometrial hypoplasia*, which has also been frequently found by us in sterility and which microscopically shows a characteristic dense cellular stroma containing few extremely atrophic glands.

Menstrual symptoms consist of decreased menses. They may range from *essential amenorrhea* in the most severe cases to *retarded menarche* in more benign cases. Essential amenorrhea in these syndromes may be indistinguishable from retarded menarche at an early stage of puberty. Once menstruation develops, menses may be scanty, hypomenorrheic or oligomenorrheic, that is, of fewer days in duration and with lesser blood loss per day than normal. This type of constitutional *oligomenorrhea*, as a rule, persists for the rest of life and may be interspersed with more or less extended phases of temporary amenorrhea (amenorrheic bouts).

However, it would be erroneous to assume that all women with a hypoplastic

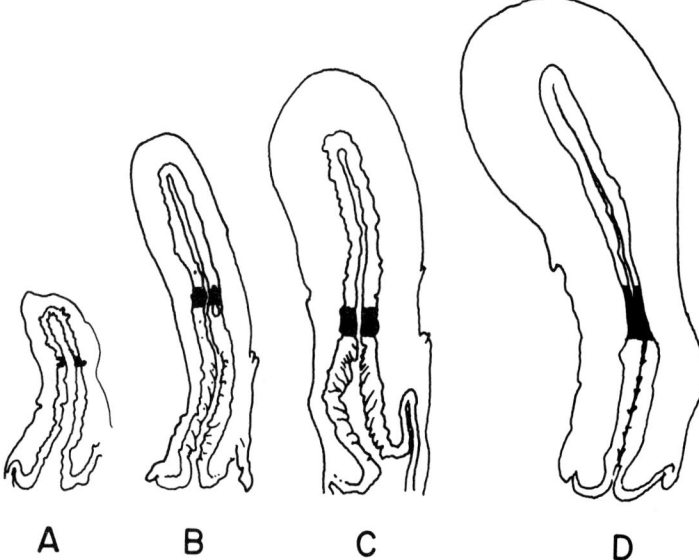

Figure 27–11. Evolution stages of uterus. *A*, Fetal uterus. *B*, Infantile uterus. *C*, Uterus of the prepuberal period. *D*, Adult uterus. Blackened segment marks the isthmus.

Figure 27–12. Gynecography in a case of primordial hypoestrinism from extreme ovarian hypoplasia (variant of Turner's syndrome). There is pronounced sinistroposition of the uterus, which is markedly decreased in size. Note also the hypoplastic tubes and streak ovaries.

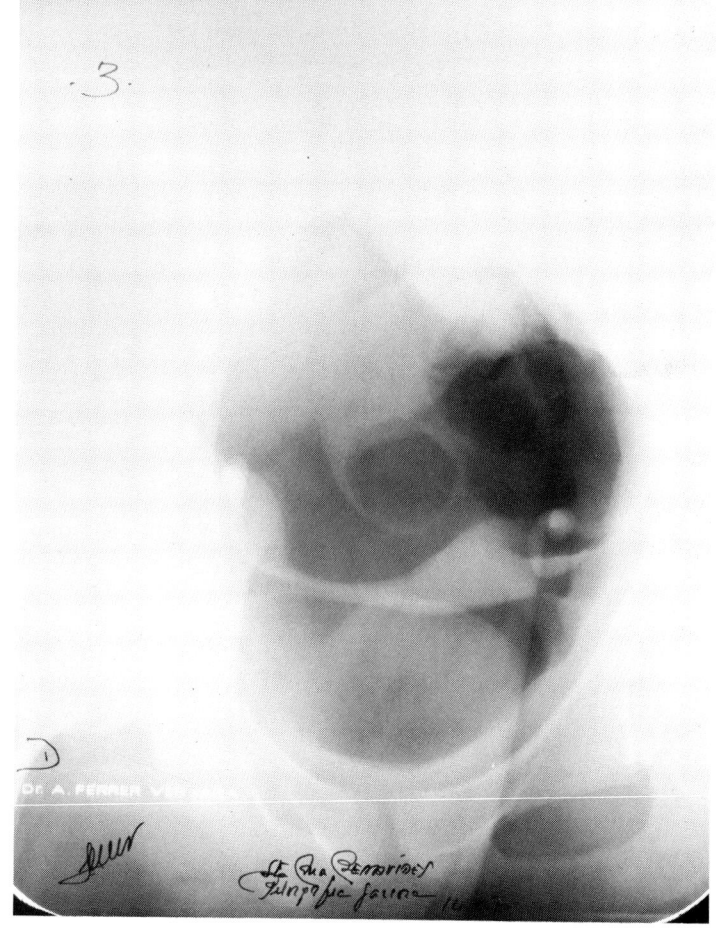

Hypoestrinism

ovarian syndrome and with hypoestrinism of ovarian origin necessarily exhibit disorders of diminished menstruation.[44, 45] In fact, it is not unusual to encounter women with hypoestrinism whose menstrual periods are more or less normal, in which case the diagnosis relies on somatic features and laboratory data rather than on the menstrual history. Similarly erroneous are commonly held beliefs that the terms "amenorrhea" and "oligomenorrhea" necessarily imply ovarian failure in every case. In a large series of endometrial curettings from our clinic (Fig. 27-13), Marín-Bonachera[60] found that the type of endometrial atrophy or hypoplasia that is suggestive of hypoestrinism could be recognized in 55 per cent of the cases. Amenorrhea was associated with a normal biphasic endometrial pattern in 20 per cent of the cases and, moreover, there was persistent proliferation, or hyperplasia indicative of hyperestrinism, in 13 per cent of the cases. In the light of these findings, amenorrhea is not synonymous with hypoestrinism. Evidently, suspension of menstruation is often the result of causes other than diminished ovarian function. Similar data have been compiled on women with scanty menses, of the constitutional oligomenorrheic type, shown in Figure 27-14, in which the discrepancies among the diverse causes of hypoestrinism are readily apparent. In spite of scanty menses, the endometria of such women most often appear normal even though revealing a similar incidence of either hyperplasia or hypoplasia. These findings can have only one meaning: that, contrary to prevalent notions that hypoestrinism with oligomenorrhea and hyperestrinism with hypermenorrhea are synonymous, both hypo- and hyperestrinism of similar degree may in fact cause diminished menses.

We have emphasized these expressive findings because they help to dispel the erroneous idea we upheld in the past in identifying menstrual disorders with ovarian disorders. As our knowledge of physiopathology in functional gynecology increases, it becomes more and more understandable why it is so difficult to achieve an etiopathogenic classification of menstrual disorders. We have therefore deliberately dispensed with describing such disorders in terms of clinical syndromes and, from now on, propose to use the terms amenorrhea, oligomenorrhea and menorrhagia when signifying only the symptoms of female endocrinopathies.

Insofar as the *endocrinology* of these conditions is concerned, it should be made clear that pituitary function in all cases is normal or, at most, only slightly increased. Whenever present, pituitary hyperfunction is not so marked as to result in a demon-

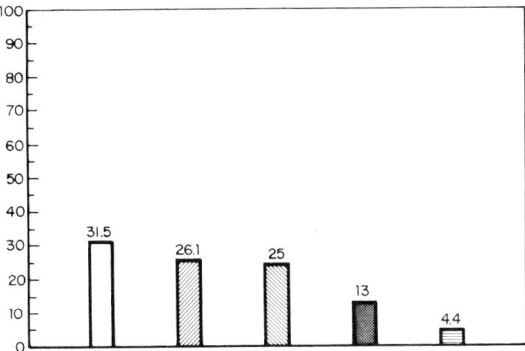

Figure 27-14. Endometrial findings in women with scanty menses. Notice that 31 per cent of endometria were normal and 26 per cent were hyperplastic. Only 25 per cent of oligomenorrheic women revealed hypoplastic or atrophic endometrial patterns. Hence, only 25 per cent of cases with oligomenorrhea revealed signs of hypoestrinism. (From Marín: *Acta Gin.*, 3:565, 1952.)

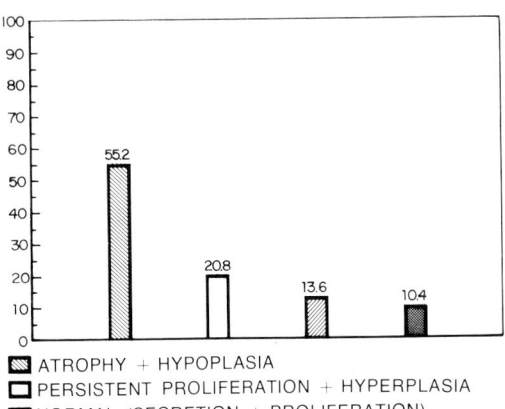

Figure 27-13. Endometrial patterns in amenorrhea. Note high incidence of normal or hyperplastic endometria. (From Marín: *Acta Gin.*, 3:565, 1952.)

strable rise in urinary FSH excretion, as it does in Turner's syndrome. Radiographically, the sella turcica appears within normal limits and is never enlarged. Determinations of urinary estrogens reveal values below normal. Interestingly, the finding of atrophy in endometrial curettings and vaginal cytology may occasionally not be associated with any comparable subnormal drop in urinary estrogen values. It seems justifiable to speculate that hypoestrinism in these cases is not absolute and is perhaps caused by defective metabolization of estrogens. In order to interpret such paradoxical findings, much more will have to be known about the intermediary metabolism of the compounds involved. Nevertheless, it may be asserted that the conditions under consideration are not always associated with decreased or absent urinary estrogen values.

Cytohormonal studies on *vaginal smears* may be extremely helpful in this group of patients (Wied[89]). As a rule, hypoestrogenic patients reveal predominance of basal and parabasal cells. As a result of estrogen therapy, the cellular formula changes correspondingly.

The foregoing paragraphs contain a rough outline of the syndrome of hypoestrinism resulting from constitutional ovarian hypoplasia. Actually, the described symptomatology is equally valid for any other form of hypoestrinism and shall be referred to repeatedly during the later description of primitive pituitary hypoestrinism as well as during the study of secondary hypoestrinism.

27.3.4. SEX REVERSAL

As in the preceding editions of this book, we include this syndrome here reluctantly because, by standards of purity of concept, "sex reversal" must really be considered as an anomaly of *sex determination*, that is to say, as an example of true gonadal dysgenesis (Chapters 35 and 36). In clinical experience, nonetheless, women suffering from this syndrome have manifestations of primitive ovarian insufficiency with hypoestrinism.

The description of the clinical picture is an outgrowth of recent advances made in the field of genetic sex. In 1956, Antliff and Young,[3] and in 1957, Engstrom and colleagues,[25] called attention to a condition in female patients in whom there were rudimentary to well developed but afunctional ovaries and *absence of Barr bodies* in somatic cells, the patients consequently presenting as genetic males. Klotz and his group[48, 49, 50] reported having observed identical cases in which the karyotype corresponded to XY or XO formulas.

Patients in this category usually have well developed ovaries (Fig. 27–15), but fail to reveal any evidence of follicular maturation. Although in isolated instances such women may have what appear to be normal menses, they are sterile and usually amenorrheic. FSH levels are elevated, as they are in all instances of primitive ovarian failure. Similar cases have been described by Ashley and Jones,[5] Hutchings,[40] Stoddard and Engstrom,[83] and Wilson and associates.[91]

Since the somatic sex in these individuals is male and the gonad is female, and there is no evidence of testicular rests or of any other attribute of hermaphroditism, it may be postulated that these are instances of genetic males who, through an error of gonocyte induction, develop ovaries instead of testes. The term "sex reversal" is based on this hypothesis.

Interestingly, such patients reveal no congenital ovarian malformations other than *disturbances in receptivity.*

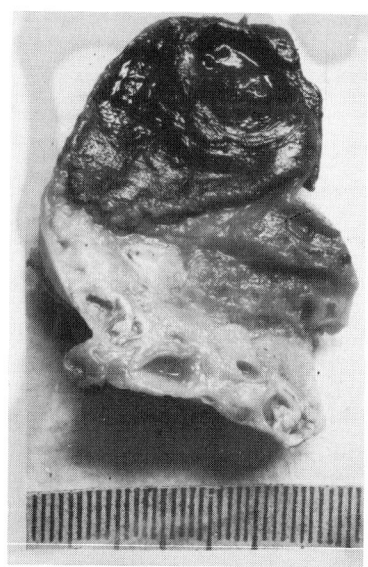

Figure 27–15. Ovary partly destroyed by hemorrhagic corpus luteum.

27.3.5. DISORDERS OF RECEPTIVITY TO ESTROGENS

Twenty-five years ago, Moricard[66] developed the concept of *metrosis of receptivity*, by which he understood the refractory condition of some endometria to respond to estrogenic stimuli. Brechner and associates[13] and Mobbs[63] later discovered the fact that tritiated estrogens would accumulate selectively in the endometrium, myometrium and vagina of various animals. Stander and Atramadal[81] confirmed this finding with regard to the mammary gland also. Furthermore, Puca and Bresciani,[76] Jensen and co-workers,[41] and Mercier-Bodard and associates[62] described a group of *estrogen binding proteins* in the blood and tissues. McGuire and Lisk[58] found that the mechanism of estrogen fixation was impaired in female rats that had been sterilized with testosterone. As a result, it is evident that *failure to respond to normal estrogen levels* may give rise to symptoms in all similar to those of hypoestrinism.

27.3.6. DISORDERS OF RECEPTIVITY TO GONADOTROPINS

While the preceding sections relate to situations in which, in the presence of hypoplastic uteri, vaginas and breasts, the ovaries are apparently normal, recent publications have described the occurrence of *ovaries that fail to respond to adequate stimulation by normal levels of gonadotropins*. In fact, such is precisely the situation that is found in gonadal dysgenesis, e.g., Turner's syndrome (see page 799), in which elevated levels of gonadotropins fail to elicit any response on the part of the ovaries. In occasional instances that are less dramatic than Turner's syndrome, the findings consist of afunctional ovaries in association with essential amenorrhea due to lack of receptivity to gonadotropins. Such cases have been referred to as "*Seegar-Jones syndrome.*"[78]

Klotz,[49] Goldrach[32] and Müller and co-workers,[68] whose recent reports deal with similar cases, found absence of sex chromatin in their patients; in a review of seven cases of nonfunctional ovaries, Klotz described anomalies of karyotype of the kind previously mentioned (XY and XO).

A vast new field of enormous potential has thereby been opened to research. It is quite probable that a whole range of "functional" ovarian failures are based not so much on functional as on chromosomal anomalies, and that, in the broadest sense of the term, these are really cases of gonadal dysgenesis disguised, as it were, under the appearance of simple estrogenic insufficiency.

The situation here is exactly the opposite of what is known to occur in Klinefelter's syndrome: in the latter case a genetic female develops as a male, possessing testes. Because of this analogy, we have informally called the condition "female Klinefelter" notwithstanding our awareness of the conceptual error involved, since an authentic Klinefelter is XXY, whereas the present analogue is XY. Nevertheless, the term appears to be expressive enough in describing the syndrome.

27.3.7. PRIMITIVE HYPOESTRINISM OF PITUITARY ORIGIN

ETIOLOGY. The clinical picture results from pituitary failure at puberty; pituitary stimulation of the gonads is absent in these girls at the time of sexual awakening, resulting in a persistent infantile condition. Despite the fact that the condition involves pituitary gonadotropin insufficiency, there is usually a background of other manifestations of hypopituitarism.

According to our present view, the majority of cases are actually hypothalamic rather than primitive pituitary syndromes. A great many instances of amenorrhea of this type, associated with hypogonadotropinuria,[14, 21, 53, 87] may really be neurogenic or even psychogenic in origin. Certain malnutritional types of amenorrhea must also be included in this section. Lerner and his associates[55] have shown that malnutrition in rats caused diminished gonadotropin secretion (or, possibly, release). This is probably also true in the human species.

A possible *autoimmune etiology* for the syndrome has also been considered. Brambilla and Sirtori,[12] as well as Landau and associates,[54] ascribe some forms of hypopituitarism to the occurrence of *antigonadotropins*.

The prognosis is good. The symptoms

first become apparent during the prepuberal period of girls with retarded sexual maturation. The syndrome runs a protracted course throughout puberty until the age of 18 or 20, when it may show signs of regression. Quite often, particularly under adequate therapy, complete cures may be accomplished, in which case there may be mild residual sexual hypoplasia that nevertheless is frequently compatible with normal menstrual function and even fertility.

CLINICAL FORMS. There are two types of clinical manifestations. In one, pituitary insufficiency becomes apparent prior to puberty because of *retarded growth*, resulting in girls who are short in stature, conspicuously shorter than those with the syndrome of primitive hypogonadism (Fig. 27–16). At the same time, hypopituitarism may also be suggested by evidence of a decrease in the size of the sella turcica (Fig. 27–17), in which there are fusion of the clinoid processes and a radiologic image of what has been designated as *sella turcica obtecta*. It may be of interest to point out that such pituitary glands, enclosed as they are within the restricted space of a sella turcica obtecta, may be but partially or temporarily, rather than totally, insufficient. Indeed, we believe these are instances of constitutional pituitary hypoplasia in which any signs of reestablishment of normal function, should they appear at a later stage, must be brought about by the stimulatory action that such pituitaries are subjected to by virtue of the compensatory effort of other glands of internal secretion.

The other clinical form presents with mild *obesity*. The nature of *temporary puberal obesity* of this kind is hard to analyze. Though seen more frequently in boys, it is also relatively common in girls. The question of whether such obesity is of hypothalamic or of purely pituitary, or perhaps gonadal, origin cannot at present be answered satisfactorily. We suspect a hypothalamic origin. At any rate, the obesity is transient in nature whenever pituitary function and menstruation follow the usual pattern—that is, whenever the onset of puberty is delayed, the patient eventually loses her excessive fat spontaneously. Since in the light of current knowledge of pituitary pathology it is doubtful that parenchymal insufficiency of this gland can cause obesity, it may be suspected that these cases result from extrapituitary hypogonadotropism of *hypothalamic origin*. In other words, delayed onset of puberty is due to delayed hypothalamic timing in relaying the order to secrete gonadotropins to the pituitary. For these reasons, the conditions in question might be considered as closely related to the "chronopathies." As a result, the two clinical types of puberal pituitary insufficiency just described may be viewed as etiologically distinct entities. One, characterized by short stature, may be postulated to be a true type of hypopituitarism, whereas the other, associated with obesity, may be postulated to be a form of hypopituitarism caused by delayed hypothalamic maturation. Of course, for the time being, this is all purely hypothetical, and it must be realized that the exact nature of the two clinical entities can only be elucidated by further studies.

SYMPTOMS. Apart from obesity and short stature, which were emphasized as the cardinal symptoms of each of the two

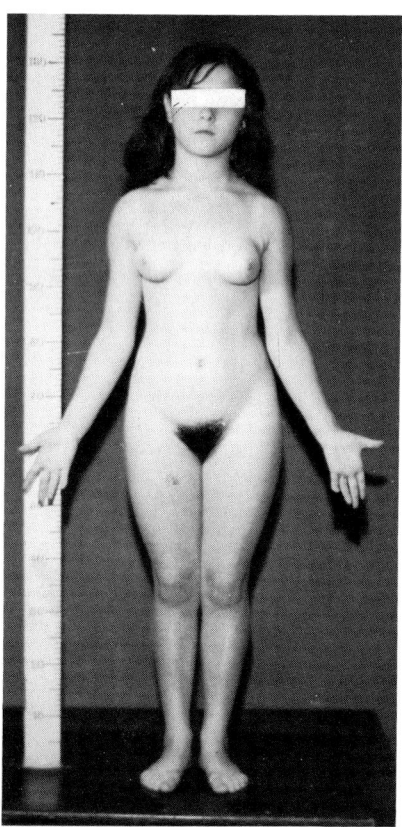

Figure 27–16. Biotype in estrogenic insufficiency of pituitary origin (delayed puberty). Girl, aged 17, with essential amenorrhea, short stature, and habitus of younger age group.

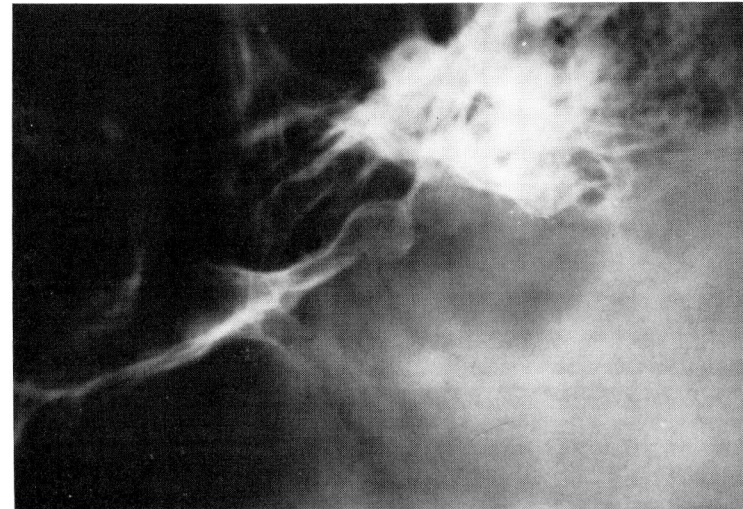

Figure 27-17. Sella turcica of patient in Figure 27-16. Fusion of clinoid processes gives rise to so-called sella turcica obtecta.

clinical forms described, the rest of the *symptomatology* is essentially similar to that described in the preceding section. The only distinctive features are the temporary nature of the clinical picture and the frequency with which menstruation is found to be unaffected.

Endocrinologically, the most significant finding is a decrease in urinary gonadotropin values. Whereas FSH is invariably more or less elevated in cases of primitive ovarian hypoestrinism, there is complete absence of urinary FSH in every case of pituitary hypoestrinism.

PITUITARY EUNUCHOIDISM. Grauer, Hurxthal and Simpson described a clinical entity characterized by isolated deficiency in pituitary gonadotropin activity, i.e., isolated hypogonadotropism, associated with eunuchoidism and showing a familial tendency. Particularly, this aspect of familial or hereditary tendency is of extraordinary interest. The syndrome occurs much more frequently in males than in females; several female cases were described by Biben and Gordan[7] recently. The three male siblings with eunuchoidism reported by Hurxthal revealed symptoms of pituitary insufficiency; however, none showed urinary gonadotropins. Because of the presence of eunuchoid features in these patients, the existence of concomitant hypopituitarism and hypogonadism is suspected. However, in the female patients that have so far been described, the ovaries appeared to be completely normal. Other than its familial incidence, a characteristic feature of this syndrome is its association with other congenital anomalies. The association of hypopituitarism with congenital anomalies, similarly with a familial tendency, is also known to occur in Laurence-Moon-Biedl's syndrome. This raises the question of whether pituitary eunuchoidism might not really be a discrete manifestation or an abortive form of Laurence-Moon-Biedl's syndrome. Concerning its etiology, Biben and Gordan[7] assume that it results from a chromosomal aberration involving X chromosome-linked aberrant genetic tendencies. Interesting in this respect is a case of female eunuchoidism, with an XYY karyotype, observed by Boczkowsky.[9] In fact, it seems likely that most cases of familial congenital anomalies that are associated with sexual disturbances, such as Laurence-Moon-Biedl's syndrome, pituitary eunuchoidism, and possibly some forms of Turner's syndromes, as well as male pseudohermaphroditism (see below), all have a common origin. Some of these questions shall be enlarged upon when discussing hermaphroditism.

Thus, it is evident that all those forms of primitive hypoestrinism in which gonadal failure is congenital, causing permanent amenorrhea or oligomenorrhea as well as sterility, may be divided, according to modern opinion, into two large groups: a group of primitive ovarian hypogonadism and a group of primitive pituitary hypogonadism. Whereas the disorders of the first group are congenital and thus are already present during embryonic life and during infancy, those of the second group are acquired at the time of puberal sexual awakening. In the absence of external manifestations relative to sexual activity, both groups present clinically with the spectrum of amenorrhea, sterility and primary genital infantilism. These syndromes may be divided into two large groups: the first revealing evidence of reactive hyperpituitarism, the other occurring concomitantly with hypopituitarism. Accordingly, FSH excretion in the first group is increased, and in the second is impaired or absent. Consequently, gonadal failure may similarly be classified as hypogonadotropic or hypergonadotropic in type. Although the latter terminology frequently appears in modern publications, it is our belief that clinical classifications should never be based on a single laboratory finding, let alone on laboratory tests as difficult and capricious as are those involved in estimating gonadotropic hormones.

27.3.8. FALSE PRIMITIVE HYPOESTRINISM

We have repeatedly described cases in which the clinical picture of *primitive amenorrhea* often led us to suspect Turner's syndrome, only to find, at laparotomy, evidence of *tuberculosis of the female genital tract*.[80] Adnexal inflammatory disease, in general, and tuberculous forms, in particular, are quite liable to produce amenorrhea in adult women. However, whenever affecting the patient prior to puberty, these inflammatory conditions jeopardize ovarian maturation, and the ovarian response to pituitary endocrine stimuli is impaired. Such cases *do not reveal the symptomatology of Turner's syndrome* and yet may not be easily distinguished from that syndrome. Despite primitive amenorrhea, the *breasts* and *pubic hair* are usually developed (Fig. 27–18). Urinary estrogen values are usually within normal limits, or slightly subnormal, but *vaginal cytology is not of the atrophic type and gonadotropin levels are not elevated.*

It is our opinion that the ovary in these cases functions normally. However, owing to premature tuberculous infection, the endometrium may have undergone *atrophy* and lost its capacity for responding to ovarian hormonal activity, so that menstruation does not occur. The occurrence

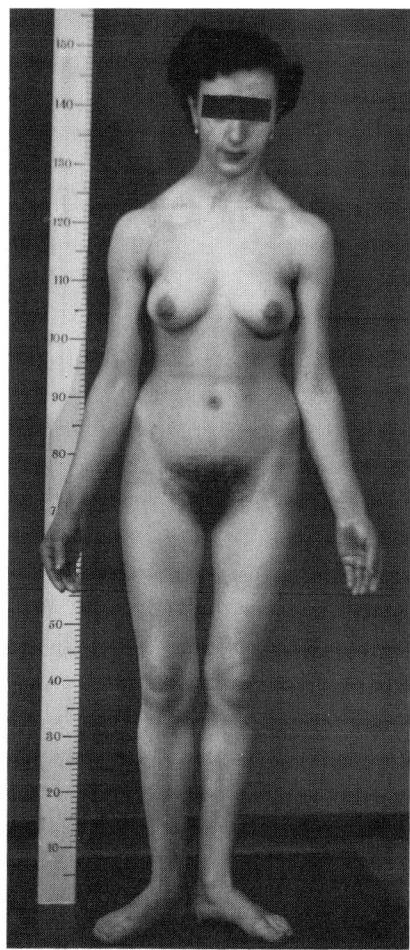

Figure 27–18. Primary amenorrhea from genital tuberculosis, acquired prior to puberty, in woman aged 20. Height, 153 cm; weight, 43 kg; metabolism, above 43 per cent; endometrium, atrophic; gonadotropins, 60 IU per 1000 ml urine; estrogens, 20 mcg; 17-ketosteroids, 6 mg; pregnanediol, negative; vaginal cytology, atrophic; exploratory laparotomy, peritoneal and adnexal tuberculosis.

of this syndrome is possibly more common than is admitted and still may well be the leading cause of primitive amenorrhea in our practice.

27.3.9. HYPOESTRINISM OF THYROID AND ADRENAL ORIGIN

As pointed out previously, thyroid function as well as adrenocortical function is fundamental for ovarian estrogen synthesis. Thyroid hypofunction results in poor development of the follicular apparatus and, consequently, in defective estrogen secretion.[26, 29, 37] Equally, each passing day enlarges our knowledge concerning the relationship which exists between adrenal function and ovulation.[18, 51] There is a growing awareness that lack of ovarian function in patients having apparently normal ovaries may not depend on a pituitary alteration but may reflect thyroid or adrenal endocrinopathy. Canu[16] pointed out the fact that secondary amenorrhea resulting from geographic factors, for instance, following a change in residence, frequently is observed in girls or women suffering from hypothyroidism. Whenever one is faced with the problem of assessing a nonfunctioning ovary, it may therefore be extremely difficult to determine whether lack of responsiveness to gonadotropic stimulation results from: (1) pituitary hypofunction, (2) thyroid or adrenal hypofunction, or (3) an unknown chromosomal aberration, of any of the types analyzed in the preceding section.

27.4. SECONDARY HYPOESTRINISM

In contradistinction to primary hypoestrinism, in which ovarian function is invariably impaired, owing to either ovarian or pituitary causes, the second variety of hypoestrinism has its onset at any time in life, in women who have previously had normal function. The early period of normalcy may occasionally carry those patients through several pregnancies and, thus, even women who had many children are not immune to developing late gonadal failure.

As a rule, little mention is made in modern literature of this secondary form of ovarian failure, which tends to be confused with amenorrhea. It has been made abundantly clear that amenorrhea is not necessarily a consequence of hypoestrinism, and the same assertion may be made even more forcefully as regards secondary hypoestrinism, the two entities running a parallel course in only a limited number of cases. In contrast, various anatomopathologic alterations of the ovaries, sometimes with evidence of major destruction of the ovarian parenchyma, may lead to partial or complete loss of ovarian function.

27.4.1. PATHOGENESIS OF SECONDARY HYPOESTRINISM

The term *pathogenic forms* refers to those fundamental anatomopathologic processes that may result in late ovarian failure. In the first edition of this book, the classification in Table 27-2 was offered.

ACUTE OOPHORITIS. Acute suppurative oophoritis may cause variable destruction of the ovarian parenchyma with abscess formation (Fig. 27-19). Although the regenerative capacity and resistance of the ovarian parenchyma is quite remarkable, as evidenced by the frequent occurrence of not only follicles but also corpora lutea in abscess walls, growth of functional elements is often inhibited in the vicinity of a suppurative process (see *adnexitic ovary*, page 605).

CHRONIC OOPHORITIS. Destruction of the ovarian parenchyma and resulting atrophy of its constituent elements is more common in chronic oophoritis. Figure 27-20 illustrates an old ovarian inflammatory process which had reduced the gland to an atretic mass, with practically no residual functional capacity. Although tuberculosis had been described as rarely involving the ovary and therefore seldom causing secondary ovarian deficiency, Kehrer and Wilkins and Fleischmann[90] reported cases of severe destructive tuberculosis of the ovary.

In addition, MacKiney and his colleagues have compiled a series of interesting statistics that show ovarian involvement by tuberculosis not as rare as generally thought.

TABLE 27-2. Pathogenic Forms in Secondary Hypoestrinism

1. *Inflammatory processes*
   a. Acute oophoritis
   b. Chronic oophoritis
   c. Actinomycosis, leprosy, etc.
   d. Leukemia, lymphocytic type (Paltauf-Sternberg)
2. *Degenerative and trophic processes*
   a. Parenchymal hemorrhage
   b. Diffuse amyloidosis
   c. Polymicrocystic degeneration of ovary
   d. Adnexitic ovary
3. *Tumors*
   a. Ovarian adenomas
   b. Primary carcinomas
   c. Metastatic carcinoma
   d. Sarcoma, fibroma
   e. Teratomas

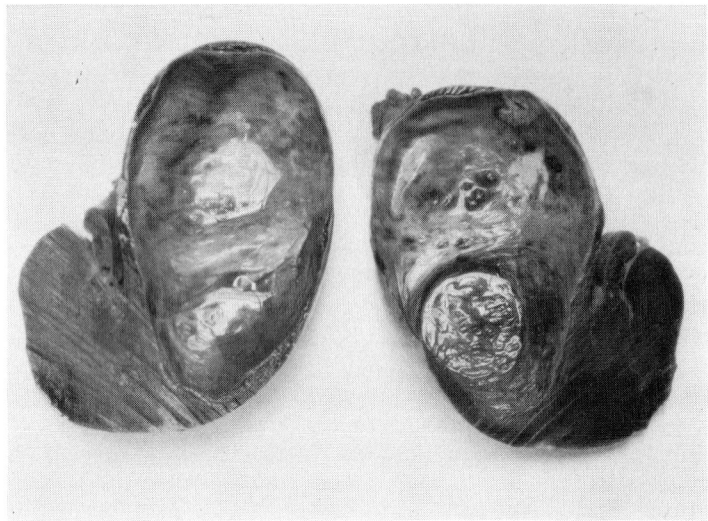

Figure 27-19. Ovarian abscess with interstitial parenchymal hemorrhage and destruction of gland.

ACTINOMYCOSIS AND LEPROSY. In 1934, Cornell collected 71 cases of ovarian actinomycosis, all of which were associated with destruction of ovarian parenchyma, secondary amenorrhea and atrophy of genitalia. A great many more cases have been collected since, and although actinomycosis of the female genital tract is a rare occurrence, it is now well known to produce secondary destruction of the ovary.

When involving the ovary, *leprosy* similarly leads to destruction of the gland, as has been known since the ancient descriptions of the disease by Adams (1807), Danielssen (1848), Couzier (1876), and a host of later reports.

Finally, *lymphocytic leukemia*, of the Paltauf-Sternberg type, and related conditions having a propensity to produce leukemic infiltrates in the ovarian medulla were mentioned by Geilpel (1920) and Brakeman (1923) among the causes for secondary amenorrhea and genital atrophy.

PARENCHYMAL HEMORRHAGE. Hemorrhage into the ovary is common and may cause extensive destruction, although seldom is the gland totally destroyed.

Perhaps most interesting of all secondary alterations of ovarian function is the *adnexitic ovary*, described by us in cooperation with Sopeña.[11, 80] We have applied the term *adnexitic ovarian syndrome* to a set of symptoms reflecting the functional alterations produced in ovaries by surrounding chronic pelvic inflammatory disease. By virtue of its thick tunica albuginea, the ovary is known to be more resistant to infection than the Fallopian tube, and functional alterations caused by such suppurative destructive processes as those previously described are not common. However, whenever an inflammatory process of sufficient magnitude occurs in the Fallopian tube, the adjacent ovary is altered. It is not known whether the resulting alterations result from impregnation with toxins or from circulatory

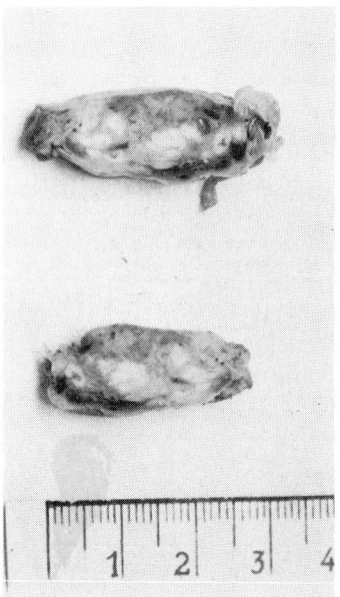

Figure 27-20. Adnexitic ovary with marked destruction and atresia of parenchyma, but without evidence of active residual inflammation.

Hypoestrinism

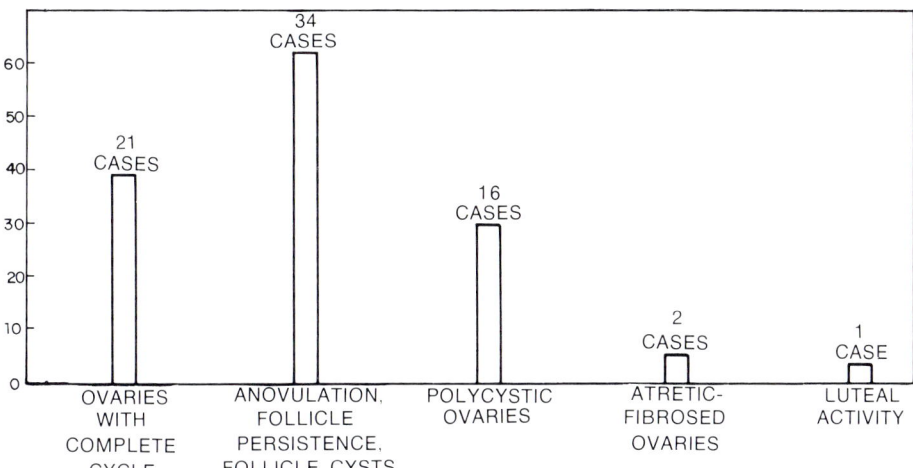

Figure 27-21. Ovarian findings in 74 cases of chronic adnexitis (adnexitic ovary). (From Sopeña: *Rev. Esp. Obst. Gin.*, 5:84, 1946.)

changes. The fact is that such ovaries, their function disturbed by nearby inflammation, give rise to extremely variable symptoms, ranging from hyperestrogenic dysfunction to ovarian atrophy, as shown in Figure 27-21. In the majority of cases, the adnexitic ovary is associated with follicular persistence or with anovulatory cycles (and is therefore again discussed as a potential cause of hyperestrinism). Occasionally, however, the adjacent inflammatory process is able to produce destruction or atresia of the ovarian parenchyma comparable in extent to that shown in Figure 27-22. In the case illustrated, a voluminous hydrosalpinx can be seen to have caused compression of ovarian parenchyma to the point of rendering the ovary almost afunctional.

POLYMICROCYSTIC DEGENERATION OF THE OVARY. This is, of course, a condition in which estrogen production is markedly reduced. Since such ovaries are known to *secrete* androgens in large amounts, this subject is taken up again in more detail in a later chapter (Chapter 29), dealing with ovarian hyperandrogenism. It must be admitted that not all cases of polymicrocystic degeneration are associated with hyperandrogenism and that there are some forms

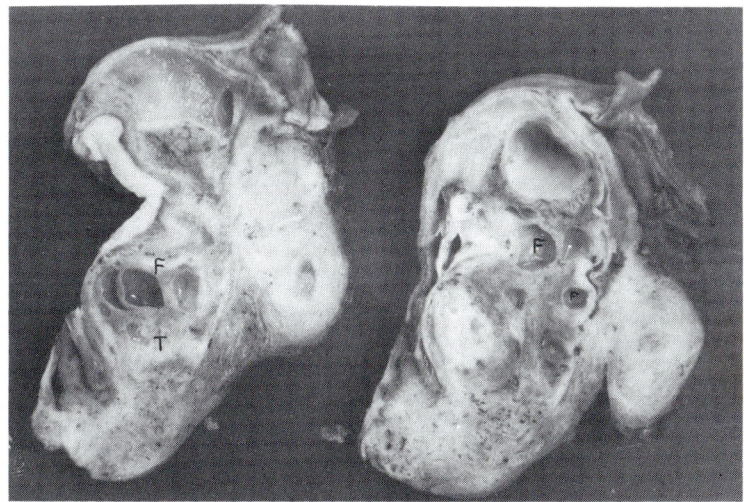

Figure 27-22. Extensive destruction of the ovarian parenchyma in adhesive chronic pelvic inflammatory disease. *F*, Follicle; *T*, hyperthecosis.

that are purely hypoestrogenic, which must all be included in this group.

OVARIAN TUMORS. These may involve more or less parenchyma, either by compression or by replacement or destruction. However, because the ovary has a considerable capacity to withstand neoplasia, only fast growing tumors, such as malignant blastomas and Krukenberg tumors, cause extensive and rapid enough destruction to produce impairment of ovarian function, with subsequent atrophy of genitalia.

HYPOTHALAMIC TYPE OF SECONDARY AMENORRHEA. Modern investigations indicate that secondary amenorrhea in the majority of cases is of psychosomatic origin. Such amenorrhea invariably has a hypothalamic background. Drew and Nicholson-Stifel,[23] in reporting the results of meticulous studies conducted on women entering religious life, emphasize the primordial role that deep-seated emotional stress, such as a change in mode of life necessitating a greater adaptive response, or physical separation from home, plays in suppressing menstruation.

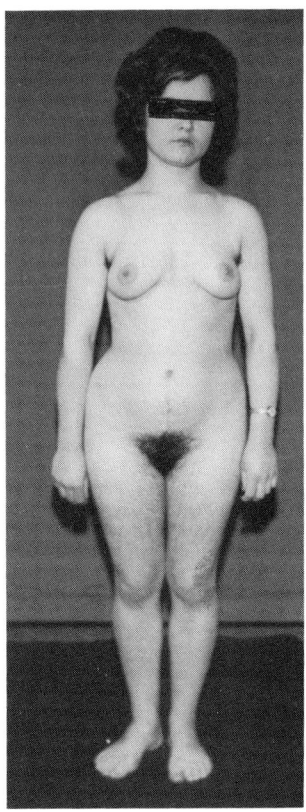

Figure 27-23. Biotype of patient suffering from secondary hypoestrinism.

27.4.2. SYMPTOMATOLOGY

This syndrome makes its appearance in a phase of life long after sexual differentiation has been completed. Alterations of the infantile type are therefore not encountered. On the contrary, the observed changes are of the regressive variety and may be categorized as representative of *premature pathologic menopause*. Premature regression of female sexuality may also be observed, indeed quite often, in pluriglandular syndromes in which ovarian regressive changes are subordinated to other alterations taking place in the rest of the genital apparatus. These alterations will be studied in Chapters 31 and 32.

The symptom most frequently prompting the patient to seek medical advice is *secondary amenorrhea*, or rather, progressive *oligomenorrhea*. Oligomenorrhea is accompanied by bouts of amenorrhea, which increase in frequency until there is essentially complete cessation of menstrual activity.

Physical examination in those patients is very informative (Fig. 27-23). Despite the presence of normal female morphology, the breasts appear flabby and, frequently, there is atrophy of the labia majora and minora, as well as loss of pubic hair.

Kinsell and his associates[47] drew attention to the frequency with which acne may be observed in these patients. *Circulatory symptoms* are also common and the history may elicit complaints of spells of burning sensations and shortness of breath. Occasionally, there is evidence of acrocyanosis with characteristic *genital hands*, although more rarely than in primitive hypoestrinism. In general, libido is greatly diminished and there is sterility of the secondary type. Owing to the known effects of estrogens on *calcium metabolism*, already discussed in Part One of this book, these patients may develop calcium deposits in the extremities, with spurious rheumatoid arthritis, as pointed out by Govaerts and associates.[34]

As to *symptoms* related to the *genitalia*, these are much more accessible to exploration and, perhaps, more conspicuous than they are in patients with primitive hypoestrinism. Atrophy of the labia majora and, to a lesser extent, of the vulva, is noticeable. The vaginal mucosa shows regressive changes, marked decrease in thickness and, cytologically, predominance of parabasal cells and leukocytes. Such vaginas show significantly reduced resistance to external injurious agents. As opposed to patients with primitive hypoestrinism, most of them virgins without evidence of either mechanical (coitus) or bacterial insults, the vaginas of secondary hypoestrinism often reveal *nonspecific vaginitis* that is difficult to treat. This type, rather than being caused by any specific virulent bacterial agent, is simply the result of lowered resistance of the vaginal mucosa in general to any microbial agent. Also common in these patients are ulcerative or trophic lesions of the vagina (ulcus rodens) which are equally related to the hypohormonal disorder.

Uterine disturbances are typical. The uterus is not always decreased in size, although if it is, the decrease is, for obvious reasons, not as marked as in primary hypoestrinism. Most of these patients are multiparous women, so that previous gravidic uterine hypertrophy does not lend itself to the same degree of complete regression as in the underdeveloped infantile uterus. The endometrial changes usually encountered (Fig. 27-24) are striking and consist of endometrial atrophy or of afunctional patterns in which the endometrial cycle seems to have been arrested. It must be remembered that, as a result of the original anatomopathologic lesion involved, the endometrial response to hormones may be lacking in many of these cases, so that the picture of hypoestrinism may be complicated by primary endometrial atrophy owing to lack of response to estrogens. This possibility was stressed particularly by Zondek and his associates[92] some time ago. Ryan and Engel[77] found that normal endometrial activity was a prerequisite for the reactivation of estrogens and that endometrial atrophy thus contributed to defective metabolization of estrogens, thereby giving rise to a vicious circle.

Aside from this, affected patients often reveal the presence of cervical erosions or ulcerations that show little tendency to heal. Concomitant with the already mentioned atrophy of breasts, these women in general undergo a process of gradual defeminization.

The *differential diagnosis* of some forms of amenorrhea may pose a problem. Thus, while primitive hypoestrinism is not easy to confuse with polyhormonal amenorrhea, secondary hypoestrinism is. It must therefore be insisted that the diagnosis of secondary hypoestrinism be made only after careful evaluation of all data, including history and presence of amenorrhea.

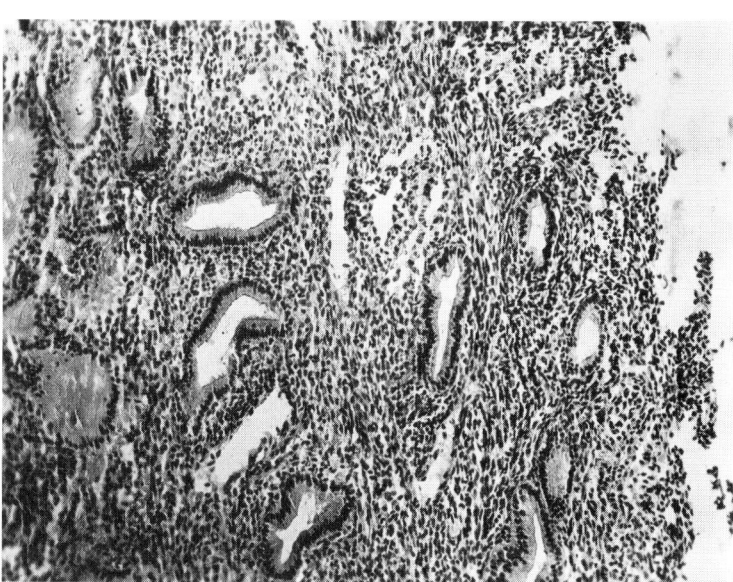

Figure 27-24. Hypoplastic endometrium in case of secondary hypoestrinism.

Di Paola[74] advocated the study of crystallization patterns of cervical mucus as a valuable adjunct in the differential diagnosis of hyperhormonal amenorrhea (abundant crystallization) and hypoestrogenic amenorrhea (absence of crystallization). By the same token, vaginal cytology is an index of utmost value. Whenever necessary, an endometrial biopsy may be performed. Nevertheless, we believe this condition to be a particular instance in which cervical mucus and cytohormonal studies may prove much more informative than microcurettage, since the endometrium may be involved by metrosis of receptivity, which is seldom the case with the vagina or uterine cervix.

The treatment of secondary hypoestrinism is discussed later as part of the treatment of all other syndromes of hypoestrinism.

27.5. TREATMENT OF HYPOESTRINISM

Therapy in hypoestrinism may follow two different norms: (1) *substitution therapy*, based on administering estrogen or, more commonly, both estrogen and progesterone, and (2) *stimulation therapy*, using such preparations of human origin as HPG (human pituitary gonadotropin) or HMG (human menopausal gonadotropin). Owing to lack of readily available HPG, HMG is the preparation most commonly employed in practice. *Clomiphene* has also been shown to give very good results.

Substitution therapy is mandatory in *primitive ovarian* disorders with hypergonadotropism, whereas stimulation therapy is preferably used in *hypopituitary* or hypophysiothalamic disorders which are associated with hypogonadotropism, as suggested in Table 27-3.

TABLE 27-3

FORM OF HYPOESTRINISM	HORMONE TYPE	TREATMENT
Primordial ovarian	Hypergonadotropic	Substitution
Pituitary or hypophysiothalamic	Hypogonadotropic	Stimulation

27.5.1. PRIMITIVE HYPOESTRINISM OF OVARIAN ORIGIN

For practical therapeutic purposes, hypoestrinism of primitive ovarian origin may be divided into two modalities: the first, occurring along with essential amenorrhea, which includes mainly Turner's syndrome; and the second, in which menstruation, though exiguous, is present and in which the cycle is more or less regular despite genital hypoplasia.

Treatment of the first modality is merely aimed at preventing the endocrine repercussions caused by estrogen deficiency whereas, with the second type, treatment is intended to reinforce the cycle in different organs of the genital tract.

In *Turner's syndrome and related conditions*, artificial induction of cycles by means of hormone therapy should not be contemplated. Although this might be achieved with elevated dosages of estrogens, used in conjunction with progesterone, the usefulness of such cycles would be questionable since they would be entirely artificial and extemporaneous. Because of this, the sole purpose of therapy in these cases is to administer sufficient amounts of estrogens to curb the pituitary and, by thus reducing the degree of hypergonadotropism, to palliate the patient's general malaise. The rationale of estrogen therapy in such patients is also strengthened by the fact that it protects the external genitalia from excessive atrophy (risks of vaginitis, vulvitis, trophic ulcers) and that it exerts a beneficial effect on the autonomous nervous system and on the peripheral circulation. Dosages to be employed are small and should not exceed 0.5 mg per day. Larger dosages may lead to a cumulative effect and induce iatrogenic hyperestrogenism and even enhance the chances for carcinogenesis, as has been suggested by Zondek and Rozin.[92] Therefore, injections of elevated dosages of estradiol or of synthetic estrogens (Chapter 2) have no practical application in these conditions. Three types of preparations may be indicated: (1) subcutaneous implantation of tablets; (2) injection of preparations of slow absorption; and (3) daily oral administration of tablets. At present, the most common therapy is based on *long-acting estrogen preparations*, usually consisting of various estradiol ethers,

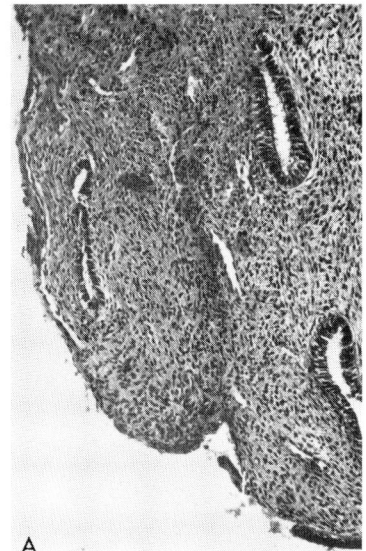
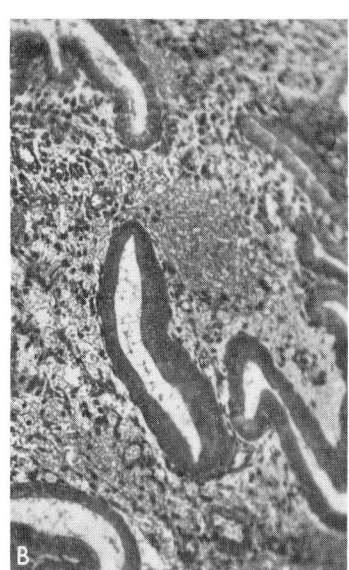

Figure 27-25. Effect of estrogen therapy on endometrial hypoplasia. A, Before treatment. Note isolated rudimentary glands and extremely dense stroma with scanty ground substance. B, After 2 months' course of treatment with monthly dose of 30 mg estradiol benzoate. Note enhanced gland development and comparatively looser texture of stroma.

whose action lasts from 14 to 28 days (Junkmann and Witzel[42, 43]). However, in Turner's syndrome and related conditions, the *usefulness of sustained administration of high dosages must be questioned*. It may seem to be more sensible to withhold therapy in patients feeling well or, at best, to give some oral preparations of estrogens *in weak dosages* to maintain a vegetative balance.

In cases of *constitutional hypoovarian function*, it is advisable to attempt to reestablish regular cycles. For this purpose, estrogens are recommended in dosages large enough to produce a normal proliferative phase in an otherwise atrophic endometrium (Fig. 27-25). Ferin[27, 28] must be credited for having established the necessary dosages by compiling pertinent data experimentally in castrated women. This dose was found to be 30 mg estradiol benzoate in an oily vehicle intramuscularly. However, it must be remembered that, depending on the route of administration and the type of compound used, important factors may be introduced that may modify effectiveness of therapy.

Quite understandably, therapy for these conditions can only be of the substitution type, since hypoplastic or primarily insufficient ovaries are unable to react to gonadotropin activity which, in the first place, is already increased as a result of a compensatory feedback mechanism. However, while this is true in theory, therapeutic administration of estrogen has been shown in practice to cause spontaneous initiation of regular menses in many women and to even produce lasting results after therapy is discontinued.

At present, therapy is based on either (1) *oral administration* of estrogens or (2) *parenteral administration of long-acting preparations (depot)*.

Oral preparations are usually diethylstilbestrol (0.5 mg/day), or preferably ethinyl estradiol or Mestranol (ethinyl estradiol-methyl-ether) in dosages ranging from 15 to 100 mcg a day (0.015 to 0.1 mg). High dosages, once recommended, are not necessary. To avert the possibility of withdrawal hemorrhage, dosages are tapered off gradually. In addition, it is important that these preparations be administered only during the first half of the cycle; otherwise, i.e., during the second half of the cycle, they must be combined with progesterone (Chlormadinone, Duphaston, Provera), in dosages of 1 to 3 mg.

Depot preparations are used with injections that combine estrogen (such as estradiol valerianate, 10 to 20 mg per cycle) with progesterone (such as 17α-hydroxyprogesterone caproate, 125 to 500 mg per cycle). Combined estrogen-progesterone therapy is aimed at preventing the production of iatrogenic hyperestrinism in those cases in which treatment is to be extended over periods of months or years. A new modality of depot preparations is based on the use of Quinestrol, which is a 3-cyclopentyl ether of ethinyl estradiol. The compound dissolves in body fat, where it is stored for longer periods of time[2, 61]; it is released slowly in the bile without being degraded,[82] which assures a long-lasting effect.

27.5.2. TREATMENT OF HYPOESTRINISM OF PITUITARY ORIGIN

Therapy of hypoestrinism of pituitary origin is based on three different approaches: (1) administration of gonadotropins, (2) excitation radiotherapy, and (3) cyclic injections of ovarian hormones. It must be admitted that the results obtained with these methods leave much to be desired.

INJECTION OF GONADOTROPINS. As just mentioned, the results obtained with combined injections of gonadotropins of pregnant mare serum and human chorionic gonadotropin have not measured up to expectations.[36, 38, 40, 55, 75] Gemzell and his associates[31] reported favorable results with injections of human gonadotropin (see Section 27.5.2).

EXCITATION RADIOTHERAPY. Found to be an effective tool, excitation radiotherapy is discussed in Chapter 40, which deals with the treatment of sterility of endocrine origin.

HUMAN GONADOTROPINS. The isolation and purification of human gonadotropins (HPG and HMG) (Chapter 7) constituted an important landmark in endocrine therapy. Purified homologous preparations do not provoke formation of *antigonadotropins* and are not subject to rapid deactivation from immune reaction, as is the case with heterologous preparations. The most commonly used hormone is HMG (Pergonal, Humegon), used mainly in the treatment of sterility and discussed in greater detail in Chapter 41. Cooke and associates,[17] as well as Furujhelm and co-workers,[30] employed it in the treatment of amenorrhea.

The use of *Clomiphen* is also discussed in Chapter 41. Botella[10] and Netter and his associates[70, 71] reported excellent results in the treatment of amenorrhea. The reader is referred to Chapter 41 for information on dosages.

27.5.3. INDUCED PSEUDOPREGNANCY

One of the most telling symptoms of hypoestrinism, particularly of the secondary variety, is the small size of the uterus ("infantile uterus") (see Fig. 27-11). For this condition, a course of treatment, called *artificial pseudopregnancy*, has been introduced,[34, 74] which consists in suppressing menstruation by means of *elevated dosages of progestogens*. Absence of menstruation over a period of two to three months leads to intrauterine conditions similar to those present in early pregnancy, with increased vascularization and hyperplasia of muscular elements. This is an efficient mode of therapy for the prevention of certain forms of abortion and sterility.

27.5.4. TREATMENT OF SECONDARY HYPOESTRINISM

Most of what has already been said relative to the treatment of primary benign hypoestrinism may be applied here equally well, with minor modifications. It is important to realize that the cycle in secondary hypoestrinism is often not modified ostensibly and that the patient's complaints include instead such disorders as menstrual irregularities, dysmenorrhea, hypomenorrhea or oligomenorrhea and, occasionally, vaginitis and leukorrhea, all secondary to hypoestrinism. Treatment of such conditions ought to be the same as that outlined previously, that is, estrogen and progesterone in intramuscular injections, combined over one cycle. For some attenuated forms of the syndrome, however, there is a distinct need for a simpler mode of therapy. We then resort to oral administration of estrogens and progesterone for alternate periods throughout the cycle. Oral estrogens are given in dosages of 1 to 3 mg per day, beginning with the first day and extending to the fourteenth day of the cycle, then administering 5 mg progesterone daily until the beginning of the next menstrual period. Because orally administered preparations are largely destroyed on their passage through the liver, we recommend the use of ethinyl estradiol as the estrogen (see Chapter 2), and of pregneninolone as the progestogen of choice (Chapter 3). In some instances, we have seen favorable results with long-acting preparations after injecting 20 to 30 mg estrogens on the first day of the cycle and 60 to 80 mg progestogen on the fourteenth day. Nevertheless, it must be pointed out that long-acting preparations produce anomalies in the appearance of menstrual periods. Also, because of the high dosages involved, it is often necessary to use only half the preparation, the rest of the expensive preparation often being wasted.

Finally, it should be mentioned that many cases of apparent hypoestrinism are *not worth while treating*. Particularly, women with scanty menses or with genital hyperinvolution in the wake of numerous pregnancies, if free from any other complaints requiring treatment, are best left alone. The same applies to cases of Turner's syndrome in which no secondary alterations of endocrine or neurovegetative nature are evident. Why should we insist on changing a precarious situation of compensation and balance reached by nature itself? *The practicing physician should also be well advised about the risks involved in using estrogens*, the carcinogenic effect of which, while obviously exaggerated in many recent publications, cannot be dismissed too lightly. Modern therapy, and endocrine therapy in particular, has been committing the sins of excess and abuse. Only too often, poorly understood conditions are treated with extremely elevated dosages of hormones, when the prudent attitude would be to abstain from any therapy altogether. In other instances, despite a correctly established diagnosis and indications for treatment, therapy may destroy whatever precarious balance may have been achieved by the body at great effort, and may cause more harm than good. It must therefore be borne in mind that endocrine therapy should be evaluated with utmost prudence, avoiding excessively elevated dosages of hormones, and, finally, one must realize that hormone therapy should not be instituted without prior judicious examination of the necessary indications.

REFERENCES

1. Allalouf, D. A., and Ber, A.: *Endocrinology*, 69:210, 1961.
2. Ansari, A. H.: *Fertil. Steril.*, 20:414, 1969.
3. Antliff, H. R., and Young, W. C.: *Endocrinology*, 59:74, 1956.
4. Archibald, R. M., Finby, N., and De Vito, F.: *J. Clin. Endocr.*, 19:1312, 1959.
5. Ashley, D. J. B., and Jones, C. H.: *Lancet*, 1:74, 1958.
6. Belausch, J., Musset, R., and Netter, A.: *Ann. d'Endocr.*, 26:267, 447, 1965.
7. Biben, R. L., and Gordan, G. S.: *J. Clin. Endocr.*, 15:391, 1955.
8. Björo, K.: *Acta Obstet. Gynec. Scand.*, 41:Suppl. 6, 1962.
9. Boczkowsky, K.: *J. Clin. Endocr.*, 30:111, 1970.
10. Botella, J.: *Enfermedades del Aparato Genital Femenino*, 9th ed. Barcelona, Editorial Científico-Médica, 1970.
11. Botella, J., and Sopeña, A.: *Acta Gin.*, 14:321, 1963.
12. Brambilla, F., and Sirtori, C. M.: *Fertil. Steril.*, 19:382, 1968.
13. Brecher, P. I., Vigersky, R., Wotiz, H. S., and Wotiz, H. H.: *Steroids*, 10:635, 1967.
14. Breckwoldt, M., and Bettendorf, G.: *Endokrinologie*, 50:162, 1966.
15. Brown, C. W. M., et al.: *Lancet*, 1:16, 1960.
16. Canu, M.: *Gynec. Prat.*, 19:125, 1968.
17. Cooke, A. C., Butt, W. R., and Bertrand, P. T.: *Lancet*, 2:514, 1966.
18. Curtis, E. M.: *Obstet. Gynec.*, 19:444, 1962.
19. Decourt, J.: In *Les troubles de la puberté féminine*. Paris, Masson & Cie., 1958.
20. Decourt, J., and Guinet, P.: *Les états intersexuels*. Paris, Maloine, 1962.
21. Dignam, W. J., Parlow, A. F., and Daane, T. A.: *Amer. J. Obstet. Gynec.*, 105:679, 1969.
22. Donaldson, C. L., Wegienka, L. C., Miller, D., and Forsham, P. H.: *J. Clin. Endocr. Metab.*, 28:383, 1968.
23. Drew, F. L., and Nicholson-Stifel, E.: *Obstet. Gynec.*, 32:47, 1968.
24. Dukes, P. P., and Goldwasser, E.: *Endocrinology*, 69:21, 1961.
25. Engstrom, W. W., Stoddard, F. J., and Bertram, E. G.: *J. Lab. Clin. Med.*, 50:811, 1957.
26. Eskin, B. A., Pratman, M. B., and Petit, M. D.: *Endocrinology*, 69:195, 1961.
27. Ferin, J.: *J. Clin. Endocr.*, 12:28, 1952.
28. Ferin, J.: In *Colloques sur la fonction luteale*. Paris, Masson & Cie., 1964.
29. Fisher, D. A., and Oddie, T. H.: *J. Clin. Endocr.*, 23:811, 1963.
30. Furujhelm, M., Lunell, L. O., and Odeblad, E.: *Acta Obstet. Gynec. Scand.*, 45:63, 1966.
31. Gemzell, C. A., Diczfalusy, E., and Tillinger, K. G.: *Acta Obstet. Gynec. Scand.*, 38:465, 1959.
32. Goldrach, C.: *Ann. d'Endocr.*, 22:536, 1961.
33. Gordan, G. S., et al.: *J. Clin. Endocr.*, 15:1, 1955.
34. Govaerts, J., D'Allemagne, M. J., and Melon, J.: *Endocrinology*, 48:433, 1951.
35. Greenblatt, R. B., Carmona, N., and Hingdon, L.: *J. Clin. Endocr.*, 16:235, 1956.
36. Greenblatt, R. B.: *J. Clin. Endocr.*, 18:227, 1958.
37. Grosvenor, C. E.: *Endocrinology*, 70:763, 1962.
38. Gurtman, A. I., et al.: *Obstet. Gynec.*, 10:261, 1957.
39. Hoffenberg, P., Jackson, W. P. U., and Müller, W. H.: *J. Clin. Endocr.*, 17:902, 1957.
40. Hutchings, J. J.: *J. Clin. Endocr.*, 19:375, 1959.

41. Jensen, E. V., Suzuki, T., and Numata, M.: *Steroids*, 13:417, 1969.
42. Junkmann, K.: *Rec. Progr. Horm. Res.*, 19:389, 1957.
43. Junkmann, K., and Witzel, H.: *Ztschr. Horm. Vit. Forsch.*, 9:97, 1957.
44. Kao, C. Y., and Gam, R. S.: *Amer. J. Physiol.*, 201:714, 1961.
45. Kerkhof, A. M., and Stolte, L. A.: *Acta Endocr.*, 21:106, 1956.
46. Kharmisheva, V. Y.: *Fed. Proceed.*, 22:314, 1963.
47. Kinsell, L. W., et al.: *J. Clin. Endocr.*, 13:809, 1953.
48. Klotz, H. P., et al.: *Ann. d'Endocr.*, 19:971, 1958.
49. Klotz, H. P.: *J. Clin. Endocr.*, 20:327, 1960.
50. Klotz, H. P., Nathan-Kahn, J., Jouin-Courrier, D., Bernard-Miller, S., and Jacob, A.: *Ann. d'Endocr.*, 27:161, 1966.
51. Kosowicz, J.: *Acta Endocr.*, 31:329, 1959.
52. Kosowicz, J.: *J. Clin. Endocr.*, 22:949, 1962.
53. Laitinen, O., and Pesonen, S.: *Acta Endocr.*, 50:524, 1965.
54. Landau, B., Landau, R., and Schwartz, A. D.: *J. Clin. Endocr. Metab.*, 25:339, 1965.
55. Lerner, L. J., et al.: *J. Clin. Endocr. Metab.*, 63:295, 1958.
56. Lisser, H., Curtis, L. E., Escamilla, R. F., and Goldberg, M. B.: *J. Clin. Endocr.*, 7:665, 1947.
57. Liu, F. T. Y.: *Amer. J. Physiol.*, 198:255, 1960.
58. MacGuire, J. L., and Lisk, R. D.: *Nature*, 221:1068, 1969.
59. Marañón, G.: *El Crecimiento y sus Trastornos.* Madrid, Espasa Calpe, 1953.
60. Marín-Bonachera, E.: *Acta Gin.*, 3:356, 1952.
61. Meli, A., Steinetz, B. G., and Giannina, T.: *Proc. Soc. Exper. Biol. Med.*, 127:1042, 1968.
62. Mercier-Bodard, C., Alfasen, A., and Baulieu, E. E.: *Karolinska Symposia Res. Meth. Reprod. Endocr.*, 2:204, 1970.
63. Mobbs, B. G.: *J. Endocr.*, 41:69, 1968.
64. Moraes-Ruehsen, M., and Seegar-Jones, G.: *Fertil. Steril.*, 18:440, 1967.
65. Morgan, C. F.: *Endocrinology*, 73:11, 1963.
66. Moricard, R.: *Gynec. Obstet.*, 43:36, 1948.
67. Morsier, G., and Gautier, G.: *Pathol. Biol.*, 11:1267, 1963.
68. Müller, P., et al.: *Rev. Franç. Gynec.*, 58:113, 1963.
69. Netter, A., et al.: *Ann. d'Endocr.*, 19:783, 1958.
70. Netter, A., and Lumbroso, P.: *Ann. d'Endocr.*, 19:1163, 1958.
71. Netter, A., et al.: *Ann. d'Endocr.*, 21:257, 1960.
72. Overzier, C.: *Schw. Med. Wschr.*, 87:285, 1957.
73. Overzier, C., and Linden, H.: *Gynaecologia*, 142:215, 1956.
74. Paola, G. di, and Lelio, M. de: *J. Clin. Endocr.*, 13:974, 1953.
75. Philipp, E.: *Acta Gin.*, 2:449, 1951.
76. Puca, A., and Bresciani, F.: *Nature*, 218:967, 1968.
77. Ryan, K. J., and Engel, L. L.: *Endocrinology*, 52:287, 1953.
78. Seegar-Jones, G., and Moraes-Ruehsen, M.: *Amer. J. Obstet. Gynec.*, 104:597, 1969.
79. Seegar-Jones, G., Moraes-Ruehsen, M., Johanson, J., Raiti, S., and Blizzard, R. M.: *Fertil. Steril.*, 20:14, 1969.
80. Sopeña, A.: *Sesiones de la Cátedra de Ginecología*, 1963–1964.
81. Stander, S., and Atramadal, A.: *Acta Endocr.*, 58:235, 1968.
82. Steinetz, B. G., Meli, A., Giannina, T., and Beach, V. L.: *Proc. Soc. Exper. Biol. Med.*, 124:1283, 1967.
83. Stoddard, F. J., and Engstrom, W. W.: *J. Clin. Endocr.*, 20:780, 1960.
84. Vague, J., et al.: *Ann. d'Endocr.*, 19:139, 1958.
85. Vague, J., Nicolino, J., and Anselmi, E.: *Ann. d'Endocr.*, 22:40, 1961.
86. Vague, J., and Nicolino, J.: *Ann. d'Endocr.*, 24:482, 1963.
87. Vague, J., et al.: *Ann. d'Endocr.*, 27:477, 1966.
88. Wachtel, E.: *Acta Cytol.*,
89. Wied, G. L.: *Obstet. Gynec.*, 9:646, 1957.
90. Wilkins, L., and Fleischmann, W.: *J. Clin. Endocr.*, 4:357, 1944.
91. Wilson, H., et al.: *J. Clin. Endocr.*, 20:534, 1960.
92. Zondek, B., Taff, R., and Rozin, S.: *J. Clin. Endocr.*, 10:615, 1950.

Chapter 28

HYPERESTRINISM

28.1. DEFINITION, INCIDENCE, CLASSIFICATION

The concept of *hyperestrinism* has been a matter of controversy. The most common definition given, that of "an abnormal endocrine condition characterized by excessive amounts of estrogens," leaves much to be desired in view of the fact that *pregnancy*, which is associated with highest levels of estrogens, cannot be qualified as hyperestrinism. Only *feminizing ovarian tumors* fall into this category, whereas a great many other syndromes associated with excessive estrogen levels are thus excluded from the above definition.

In view of this, a revised definition of hyperestrinism is desirable: *hyperestrinism is a clinical syndrome characterized by an abnormal end-organ response to increased estrogen levels or to prolonged action of normal estrogen levels.* Though longer and more complicated than the first one, this second definition reflects more accurately what is meant by hyperestrinism.

By the same token, such terms as hyperovarism or hyperfolliculinism, used to designate this syndrome (Gilbert-Dreyfus,[47] Ufer[126]), are inadequate. Hyperovarism implies ovarian hyperfunction affecting both estrogen and progesterone activity, apart from disregarding the fact that many cases of hyperestrinism may in fact be instances of ovarian insufficiency. On the other hand, hyperfolliculinism, meaning hyperfunction of the ovarian follicular apparatus, fails to express the true scope of the syndrome, since hyperestrinism may also be produced by *extraovarian causes*.

28.1.1. INCIDENCE

The true incidence of hyperestrinism is difficult to assess, since the diagnosis may depend on essentially different clinical criteria. Thus, for instance, while some authors (Beclère[6]) define hyperestrinism on the basis of increased urinary phenolsteroids, others, such as Ufer[126, 127] or Wied,[138] accept vaginal cytology as the guide to diagnosis. According to our own criteria, the diagnosis must be based on a correlation of all forms of exploration with the clinical manifestations and on defining the disease on the merits of all symptoms and exploratory data as a whole, rather than solely on any isolated feature.

In the final analysis, before classifying a given patient as hyperestrogenic, we are guided by endometrial histology, which is the criterion our data on incidence are based upon. In a recent review of 3000 endometrial biopsies performed at our clinic, including necessary histochemical studies, we found the incidence of hyperestrogenic patterns described in Table 28-1.[16]

TABLE 28-1. Incidence of Hyperestrinism in 3000 Endometrial Biopsies*

ENDOMETRIAL PATTERN (ON 23RD DAY OF CYCLE)	INTERPRETATION	NO. OF CASES	PERCENTAGE
Normal secretory	Normal	1351	45.03
Poorly secretory	Estrogen-progesterone imbalance	182	6.06
Hyperplastic secretory	Doubtful	119	3.96
Normal proliferative	Hyperestrinism of rhythm	303	10.10
Hyperplastic proliferative	Hyperestrinism, quantitative type	270	9.00
Hypoplastic proliferative	Hypoestrinism	221	7.36

*From Botella.[16]

The results reveal that severe forms of hyperestrinism, associated with endometrial hyperplasia, were present in only 9 per cent of the cases studied, which is nonetheless a significant incidence in the clinical practice of gynecology. An additional 10 per cent of cases consisted of instances of less apparent hyperestrinism, such as anovulatory cycles, which are equally capable of producing pathologic manifestations in the long run. In addition to these figures, it must be taken into account that hyperestrogenic conditions occur in a large number of cases with leiomyomas, endometriosis and malignancy.

28.1.2. CLASSIFICATION

Above all, we must make a distinction between *ovarian hyperestrinism*, produced by ovarian causes, and *extraovarian hyperestrinism*, produced by other causes. Ovarian hyperestrinism in turn may be of two different types. As already stated, hyperestrogenic effects may be the consequence of either brief activity of large quantities of estrogens or prolonged activity of not necessarily excessive amounts of estrogens. As a result, *hyperestrinism of quantity* must be distinguished from *hyperestrinism of rhythm*. Quantitative hyperestrinism occurs more frequently during the second half of the cycle as a result of excessive accumulation of estrogens produced in the course of the cycle. Thus, this type constitutes what various workers in recent years have qualified as *acute hyperestrinism*.

The chronic variety of quantitative hyperestrinism may be produced by estrogen-secreting ovarian tumors, such as, for example, granulosa cell tumors or thecomas. Hyperestrinism of rhythm is always of the chronic variety and is caused by those processes which, even though not generating estrogens in amounts above normal—owing to the continuous manner in which estrogens are secreted and, *above all, to the absence of corpus luteum formation*—lead to accumulation of estrogenic compounds without the damper activity of antagonists and thereby allow the establishment of unopposed continuous estrogen activity, which in the long run is bound to produce pathologic manifestations.

Extraovarian hyperestrinism is occasionally seen in the *adrenogenital syndrome* (see Chapter 37). The action of the adrenal cortex is known to be determined in most instances by simple hyperplasia or by the presence of adenomas or carcinomas. From a clinical standpoint, however, a more important entity is *hepatic hyperestrinism*, which occurs in hepatic insufficiency because of failure of the liver to deactivate estrogens. As already pointed out in Chapter 2, the liver is the organ mainly responsible for degrading circulating estrogens and for detoxifying the body of estrogens. Parenchymal lesions of the liver may therefore lead to pathologic accumulation of estrogens in the female as well as in the male. The most common liver conditions causing hepatic hyperestrinism result from toxic drug injury, for instance, the kind seen in experimental carbon tetrachloride intoxication, apart from, specifically, cirrhosis.

Intimately related to the preceding form is *nutritional hyperestrinism*, which is caused by dietary deficiency of various factors pertaining to the vitamin B complex, particularly vitamins B_1, B_2 and B_6. These vitamins are indispensable for hepatic biocatalysis of estrogens.

A further form, also of extraovarian origin, is *iatrogenic hyperestrinism*, a previously unknown entity, which has developed in recent years as a result of increasing incidence of abusive therapeutic practices, such as hormone-induced "shock" or faultily administered "attack" therapy. In many instances, it must be added, similar conditions are self-inflicted, usually occurring in women of the climacteric age who ingest ovarian extracts or hormones in order to rejuvenate themselves, or make use of estrogen-containing preparations for cosmetic purposes.

Finally, it must be borne in mind that more than one of the above etiologic factors may be involved at one time and that ovarian disorders may readily result in hyperestrinism or that estrogen intake may quite rapidly lead to intolerance to estrogens in any given patient with hepatic insufficiency.

The foregoing points of our discussion have been summarized in Table 28-2.

28.2. PATHOGENIC FORMS; OVARIAN HYPERESTRINISM

Under this heading, we shall study all those ovarian changes that are liable to

TABLE 28–2. Classification of Hyperestrinism

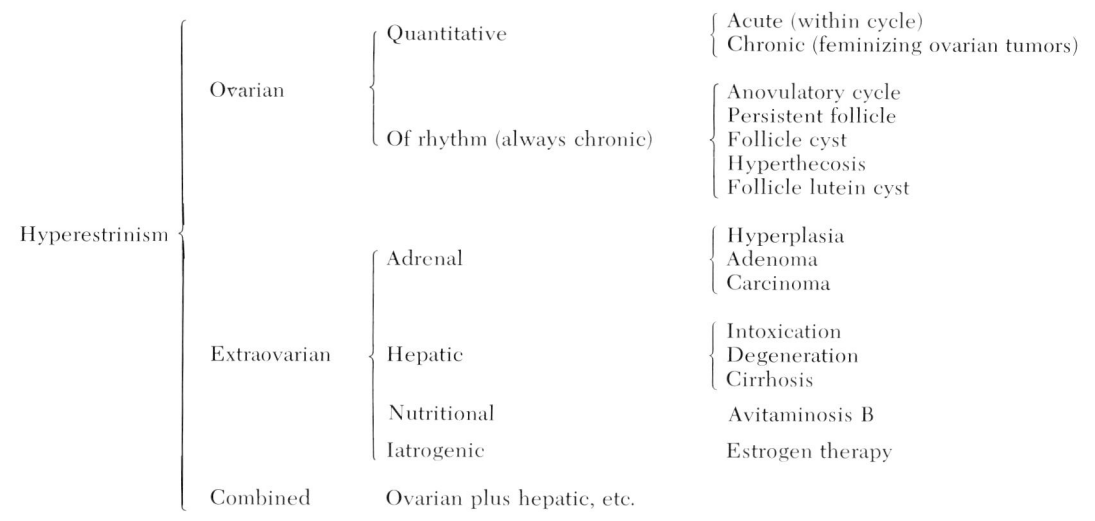

produce hyperestrinism. It must be remembered that such ovarian alterations as are capable of causing the syndrome may not necessarily be conspicuous, and that minor functional and structural changes in the ovary may be associated with significant elevations of estrogen levels. It must also be borne in mind that the main ovarian source of estrogens is the *theca interna* (Chapter 2). Consequently, all those ovarian formations that have a well developed theca interna are potential estrogen producers and may give rise to hyperestrinism. In a broader sense, the term ovarian hyperestrinism may be made synonymous with *thecal hyperplasia*. On the other hand, pathologic proliferations of the granulosa, though important as potential producers of hyperestrinism, by comparison play a secondary role.

The following sections are concerned with the examination of those ovarian alterations that, by virtue of associated hyperplasia of the theca or granulosa, or both, may account for excessive estrogen production.

28.2.1. FOLLICULAR PERSISTENCE

Simple follicular persistence, as a cause of hyperestrinism, is a relatively common finding. According to various authors, the incidence of this type of anovulatory manifestation ranges from 2 to 10 per cent of all gynecologic patients. By our own statistics, which we have already quoted, an anovulatory cycle occurs in approximately 15 per cent of sterile women. The significance of follicular persistence as a cause of hyperestrinism had been emphasized long ago and has since been insisted upon by Wahlen.[134] Wahlen called attention to the fact that cystic endometrial hyperplasia quite often was associated not with a single large persistent follicle, as had been suggested by Schröder, but instead with a constellation of smaller follicles, giving rise to a polycystic ovary.[104, 137] Bedoya and Gomez-Herrera have studied a series of women presenting with the anatomical findings of follicular persistence. Data compiled by them are shown in Figure 28–1.

Their findings seem to support the contention that small follicles may play an important role in the pathogenesis of hyperestrinism, as had previously been pointed out by Botella and Calvo-Marcos,[15] and subsequently by Vara and Nemineva.[131] Recently, Giorgy[48] showed that persistent follicles contained estrogens in higher concentrations than did mature follicles. Moreover, Hunter and Leathem[58] found that they contained more *histamine*.

An ovary under these conditions assumes the appearance of the so-called *polymicrocystic* ovary. In the past, we considered polymicrocystic ovaries as an entity distinct from simple follicular persistence; in reality they are not. There is much confusion in modern literature con-

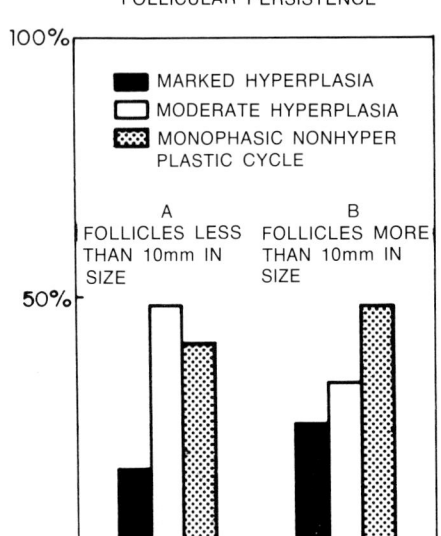

Figure 28-1. Effects on endometrium of follicular persistence.

cerning the question of "polycystic" ovaries and the Stein-Leventhal syndrome. *In our opinion, these are two different conditions.* In the first, the ovary has many follicles maturing simultaneously, without ever quite reaching full maturity, although their component elements are more or less normal, whereas the "polycystic" ovary of the Stein-Leventhal syndrome is associated with *hyperthecosis* and with altered steroidogenesis, marked by *increased production of androgens*. As a result, the latter syndrome must be classified as a form of hyperandrogenism (see Chapter 29, Section 29.3.4) rather than hyperestrinism. Singh[109] is of the same opinion.

28.2.2. POLYMICROCYSTIC OVARIES

The simple polymicrocystic ovary, as already indicated, may be confused with multiple small persisting follicles maturing simultaneously. As distinct from this, the *fibrous polymicrocystic ovary* is a pathologic entity which should be considered as an *androgenic rather than estrogenic ovary*,[79, 120] that is, as *a different endocrine and clinical entity*. In persistent follicles, in fact, estrogens are formed by a hyperplastic, well-preserved granulosa and by the adjacent theca. In polymicrocystic ovaries, in contrast, either the granulosa is atrophic or the young follicle is not yet capable of estrogen synthesis to any significant degree. *In such ovaries, the element responsible for increased estrogen production is the theca.* The polymicrocystic ovary must thus be viewed as a variant of *hyperthecosis.*

Histochemical studies by Sun and Rakoff[119] have suggested that the theca in polymicrocystic ovaries is the site of major estrogen synthesis.

As for the *etiology* the condition is now admitted to be caused by *lack of FSH secretion and increased LH (ICSH) secretion by the pituitary* (Ingersoll and MacArthur,[59, 80] Scommegna et al.,[104] Weisz and Lloyd[137]), as a result of which follicles fail to reach full maturity, whereas the theca undergoes *premature luteinization.* MacArthur and associates,[80] as well as Sommers and Wadam,[114] postulate that this is the result of a pituitary disorder of hypothalamic origin. The presence of concomitant adrenal hyperplasia, observed by Mellinger and his associates,[87] and of associated hyperthyroidism, reported by Scommegna and his colleagues,[104] also seems to support a pituitary hypothesis. In their studies of dexamethasone suppression and HCG stimulation tests, Lopez and his co-workers[77] found no increase in androgen production by polycystic ovaries of the "pure" type (see Section 28.2.1) but found instead evidence of increased estrogen synthesis, which permits classification of such ovaries among the forms of hyperestrinism. Miklosi[89] postulates that this is an *autoimmune disease*, caused by sensitization to one's own gonadotropins. Seegar-Jones and his associates[78] attribute the condition to a disorder of hypothalamic origin. In summary: *although it may be asserted that the "polycystic ovary" appears to be a disorder involving the hypophysiothalamic axis, too little is known at present with certainty concerning its etiology.*

It must be remembered that an increase in LH activity (see Chapter 4) provokes hyperplasia not only of thecal cells but also of the interstitial cells of the testis and of the cells in the sexual zone of the adrenal cortex, producing what may be considered as a "disease of a system." It is therefore not surprising that various authors[60, 94] should have reported the finding of *hilar cell hyperplasia* in polycystic ovaries, considering that hilar cells are homologues of

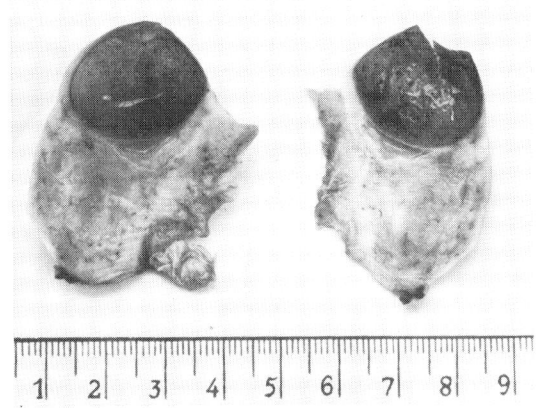

Figure 28-2. Ovary in a case of follicular persistence.

testicular Leydig cells and thus should be equally susceptible to LH activity.

An interesting finding in *hyperthecosis*, to be examined later, is the occurrence of *hyperandrogenism with or without associated hyperestrinism*, which is also known to occur in the adrenogenital syndrome.

Polymicrocystosis may occur in the absence of large persistent follicles (Fig. 28-3), or it may be associated with follicular persistence (Fig. 28-2). Although it may sometimes cause severe forms of hyperestrinism (Fig. 28-4), usually it does not.

28.2.3. THECAL HYPERPLASIA AND FIBROTHECAL MASSES

Hyperplasia of the theca interna, which produces estrogens,[108, 141] may be associated with hyperestrinism. Thecal hyperplasia may occur in two different forms: (1) *thecal hyperplasia in the young ovary*, in which the process is most often observed in the theca interna of atretic follicles, and (2) *thecal hyperplasia in the senescent ovary*, which assumes the form of widely scattered foci of fibrothecal proliferation that do not have any connection with the thecal elements of follicles, not even the atretic follicles. The finding of fibrothecal masses in association with hyperestrinism, particularly with hemorrhagic metropathy, is not unusual. Bedoya and Gómez-Herrera have recognized their presence in a considerable percentage of cases with hemorrhagic metropathy (Fig. 28-5), reporting an incidence of 22.5 per cent. Various workers who have studied thecal hyperplasia (Culiner and

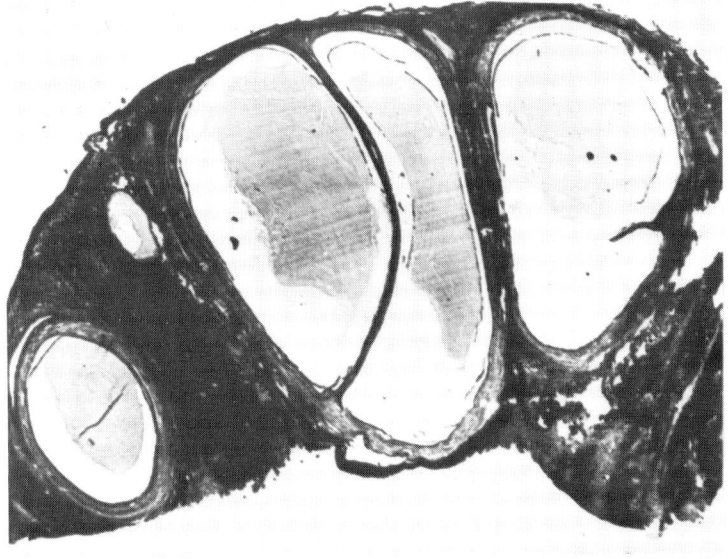

Figure 28-3. Section of ovary revealing persistence of large follicles.

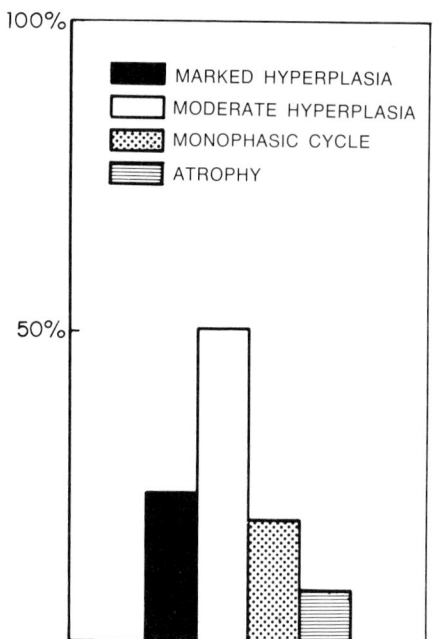

Figure 28-4. Endometrial changes associated with polycystic ovaries.

Figure 28-5. Ovarian findings in 100 cases of hemorrhagic metropathy resulting from cystic glandular hyperplasia of the endometrium. Most are caused by variable degrees of follicular persistence. A considerable number are the result of ovarian hyperthecosis, a significantly smaller number stem from polymicrocystic ovaries and an even smaller number from functional tumors. (From Bedoya and Gomez-Herrera.)

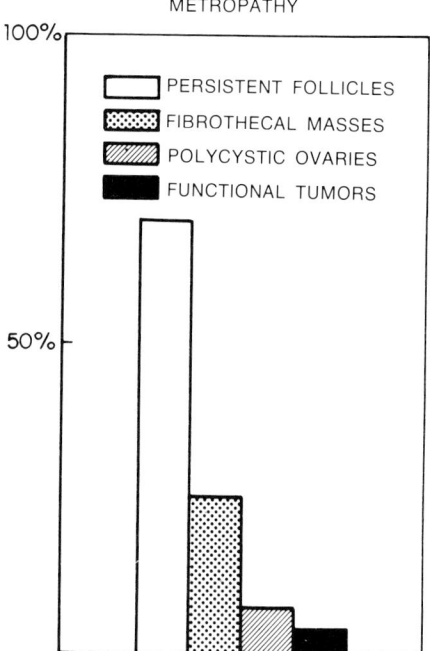

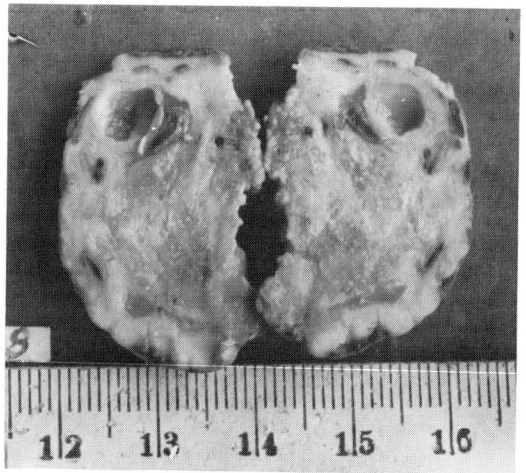

Figure 28-6. Fibrothecal masses (ovarian hyperthecosis).

Shippel[28]) indicate that the association with hemorrhagic metropathy is most commonly observed in the climacteric age group. It is usually most noticeable in the central portion of the ovary, where it assumes the disposition of diffuse fibrous masses (Fig. 28–6). The etiology is at present not clearly understood. Obviously, increased FSH activity is not involved. We are inclined to believe that such hyperplasia is caused by LH activity. Not infrequently, such foci of thecal proliferation may be observed to be luteinized. However, their functional capacity is not always clear, since, while they often produce estrogens, they occasionally appear to be definitely related to increased androgen production, as was demonstrated by Culiner and Shippel[28] (see Chapter 29).

Thecal hyperplasia of this type is responsible for the occurrence of *very late hyperestrinism* in some cases. We have seen such cases after the age of 65 in which the diagnosis was "functioning ovarian tumor," but in which only thecal hyperplasia was found at laparotomy. Bilde[11] relates an analogous case in which the patient was 78 years old.

Since hyperthecosis is frequently induced by pituitary activity, such as *increased levels of ICSH*, theca cell luteinization, as well as hilar cell hyperplasia,[76, 99] which are often found to be associated with hyperthecosis, may well have a common underlying cause.

28.2.4. FOLLICLE-LUTEIN CYSTS

Botella and Calvo-Marcos[15] frequently observed the presence of lutein cysts in association with uterine myomata (Fig. 28–9). Such cysts were persistent corpora lutea that histologically revealed regressive changes in the granulosa layer, with thecal hyperplasia (Fig. 28–10). The fact that such cysts should produce excessive amounts of estrogens rather than progesterone is not surprising in view of their histologic appearance. These cysts are discussed in Chapter 29, which is concerned with the pathology of the corpus luteum.

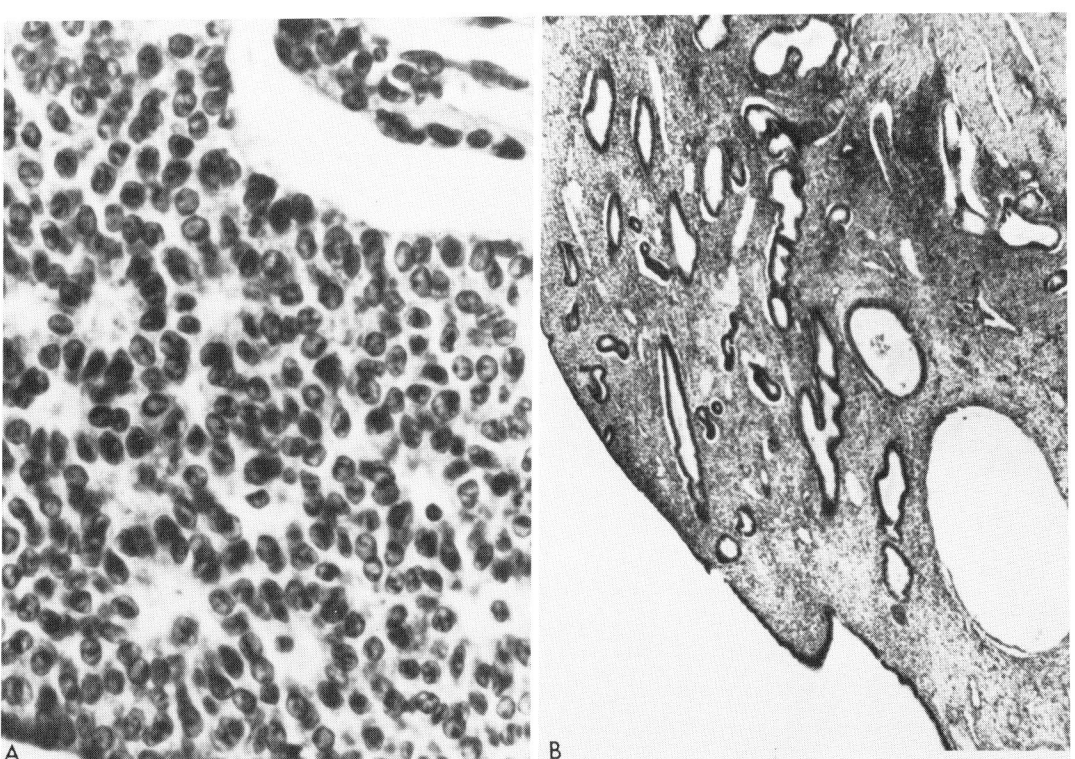

Figure 28–7. A, Granulosa cell tumor causing hyperestrinism (see Chapter 30). B, Endometrium of same case, revealing cystic glandular hyperplasia.

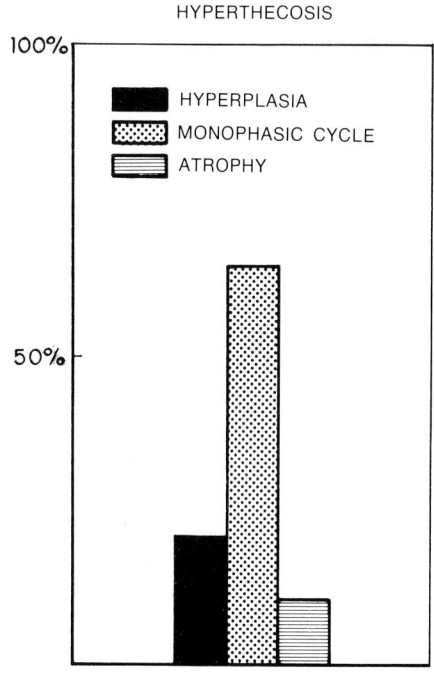

Figure 28-8. Endometrial findings in ovarian hyperthecosis with fibrothecal masses. Only a small number reveal endometrial atrophy, apparently representing cases in which fibrothecal tissue secretes no estrogens. Another, somewhat larger, group exhibits hyperplasia while in the majority of cases there is a persistent simple proliferative phase.

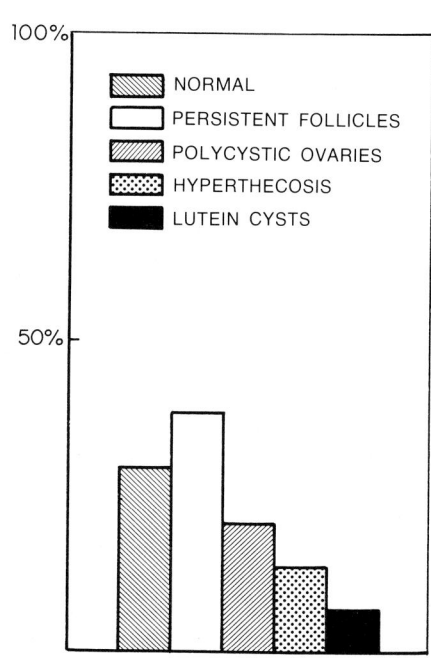

Figure 28-9. Ovarian findings in cases with uterine leiomyomas. Note possibly significant association with follicle-lutein cysts. (From Botella and Calvo-Marcos.[15])

Hyperestrinism

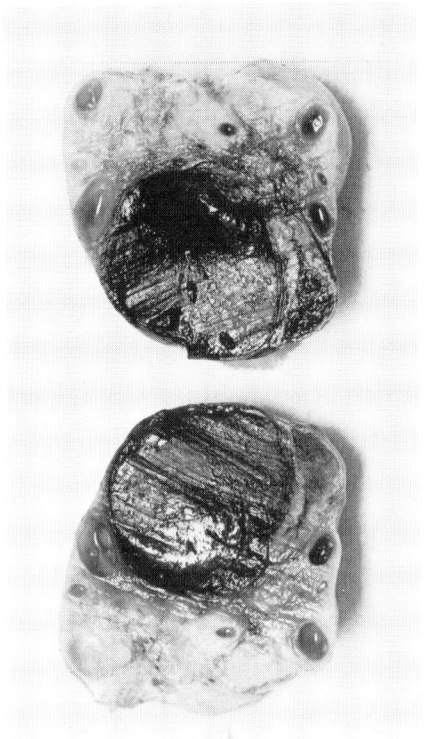

Figure 28-10. Cystic corpus luteum, producing predominantly estrogens.

28.2.5. ADNEXITIC OVARY

The adnexitic ovary syndrome, described by Sopeña,[112] had been mentioned in Chapter 27. It is found following a chronic inflammatory process of the adnexa, which, without infecting or destroying the ovary, nevertheless produces significant alterations in the vicinity of the ovary. As shown in Figure 27-20 in the preceding chapter, such adnexitic ovaries sometimes display impaired function with associated hypoestrinism and endometrial atrophy. More frequently, however, they may give rise to follicular persistence in association with the syndrome of hyperestrinism, usually moderate in degree. Figure 28-11 illustrates a case of bilateral chronic adnexitis, with extensive tuboovarian adhesions; one of the ovaries shows atresia and the presence of small follicles, whereas the other reveals a single persistent follicle of large size. The reason for follicular persistence in such ovaries is not quite clear. Sopeña[112] is of the opinion that these are brought about by reactive thickening of the albuginea in response to inflammation, whereby the resulting induration of the ovarian cortex renders rupture of follicles and ovulation difficult. Nevertheless, more recently we have been inclined to suspect that the condition resulted from pituitary influence, similar in kind, perhaps, to that previously described in connection with the etiology of follicular persistence. MacCarthy and his associates[81] dispute the presence of endocrine ovarian changes due to adnexitis.

Adnexitic ovaries may also frequently reveal the presence of granulosa-lutein cysts or of follicle cysts with hemorrhagic contents (Fig. 28-11). These structures may also be capable of causing hyperestrinism.

28.2.6. SYNDROME OF "THE REMAINING OVARY"

Following surgical extirpation of one ovary, the contralateral ovary usually develops follicular persistence in conjunction

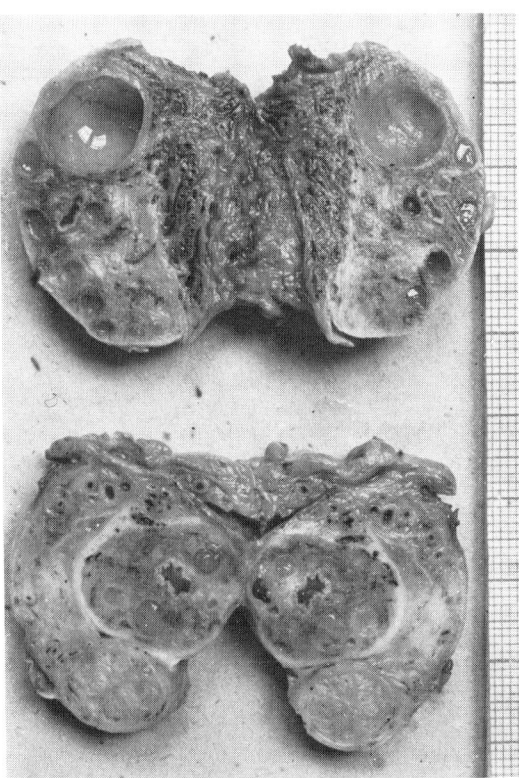

Figure 28-11. "Adnexitic ovary," with adhesive tuberculous salpingitis. Gonadal parenchyma is intact, although it reveals persistent follicles and multiple atretic follicles. No corpora lutea are noted. (From Sopeña.[112])

with a greater or lesser degree of hyperestrinism. This syndrome, of which the clinicians are well aware, has been called "syndrome of the remaining ovary."[112]

It has been known for a long time that unilateral ovarian ablation in rodents was associated with follicular hypermaturation in the remaining ovary.[46, 75, 76] Rats develop a maximal degree of follicular proliferation,[40] with abundant estrogen production and permanent estrus.[40, 136, 143] Since such a reaction does not occur in hypophysectomized animals,[27, 124] the phenomenon is thought to be caused by *compensatory pituitary hyperfunction* in response to the loss of half of the ovarian parenchyma. In support of this interpretation, too, is the finding that the contralateral ovarian reaction may be averted by means of oral contraceptives even in nonhypophysectomized animals. Nevertheless, the reaction may also depend in part on adrenal function, since adrenalectomy has been found to block the appearance of polymicrocystosis in semicastrated rats.[39] Thus, contralateral ovarian hypertrophy would seem to be attributable to a gonadotropin stimulus of utmost intensity, since neither FSH alone[136] nor combined FSH and LH administration[143] is capable of producing any higher degree of follicular proliferation in the remaining ovary of the rat.

A similar response has been observed in ewes,[92] golden hamsters,[53] sows[2] and monkeys.[123] The phenomenon has long been known to occur in women and has recently become the object of renewed interest through the work of Sopeña[112] and some of the later works of Funck-Brentano. The reactions observed appear to vary in different species. In rats, the corpus luteum persists following hysterectomy because the rat endometrium possesses *luteolytic capacity.*[7] This is not the case in either women or female monkeys whose corpora lutea undergo normal involution after hysterectomy.[7, 62] Uncini-Manganelli and Becca[128] point out the fact that, after a period of one year following hysterectomy, only the ovary of hysterectomized animals shows evidence of regressive changes, whereas the rest of the endocrine system, including the pituitary, remains unaffected. In one way or another, the ovarian cycle in women without uteri is profoundly affected. Dordelman and Wolker[33] found that, of 216 women examined before the operation, only 122 retained biphasic basal body temperature recordings following hysterectomy. The remaining 94 (43 per cent) had developed monophasic recordings, indicating that the absence of the uterus *resulted in an anovulatory cycle.* To us, this percentage appears to be both clinically and statistically significant.

It is not known why the presence of a more or less intact uterus should, to a certain extent, have a damping effect on the formation of polymicrocystic ovaries after hemicastration. Thus, in rats[21, 96] and ewes,[92] resection of one uterine horn in addition to that of one ovary even further enhances the hyperfollicular reaction in the remaining ovary. A similar effect apparently also occurs in women, since the extent of polycystic degeneration in the remaining ovary has been found to be greater if the uterus is also resected than if only one ovary, or one ovary and its tube, is removed.

As a result, the hyperfollicular ovarian reaction may be concluded to be of compensatory pituitary origin. However, the endocrine mechanism involved has not yet been fully elucidated.

28.2.7. THE OVARIAN SUBSTRATE OF ACUTE HYPERESTRINISM

Gilbert-Dreyfus[47] and Ufer[126] have described an acute form of hyperestrinism, a syndrome characterized by pathologic estrogen accumulation during the premenstrual phase which, without modifying the cycle and frequently without modifying menstruation other than in a minor way, causes the appearance of symptoms of estrogen intolerance during the last stage, or last week, of the cycle. The clinical symptomatology of this syndrome is described later in this chapter. Pathologic premenstrual accumulation of estrogens has been tentatively ascribed to various mechanisms, particularly to alterations in estrogen metabolism (discussed later in this chapter). However, certain ovarian findings observed by us would seem to provide reasonable evidence for an anatomic basis for this disorder. We are referring to ovaries in which mature follicles, fully functional, were found to coexist with an active corpus luteum. This type of delayed follicular maturation or, as it were, asynchronous ovulation within the cycle, has been described under the name of *paracyclic ovulation*, which has been mentioned in Chapter 11. The ovary in Figure 28–12, showing evidence of paracyclic ovulation, justifies the assumption that hyperestrinism may be associated with a normal secretory phase.

28.2.8. ETIOLOGY OF OVARIAN DISORDERS LEADING TO HYPERESTRINISM

A variety of causes appear to produce the disorder. In those cases in which hyperestrinism can be traced to hypertrophy of the follicular apparatus (anovulatory cycle, persistent follicles, etc.), the underlying cause seems to be increased FSH activity. On the contrary, in such conditions as hyperthecosis, follicle-lutein cysts and possibly also in a certain number of "remaining ovaries," the cause seems to be increased LH activity.

INCREASED FSH ACTIVITY. Dörner[38] has been able to induce hyperfolliculinism in rats by means of FSH injections. These findings are in agreement with the observations made by Varangot and associates[132] and by Staemmler[117] that the rate of FSH excretion was increased in human cases with follicular persistence.

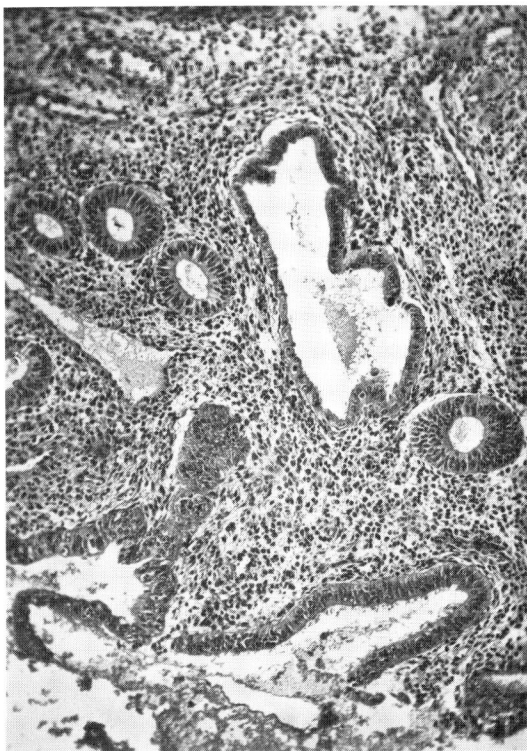

Figure 28–13. Mucosa in a case of irregular endometrial maturation, revealing partly secretory and partly proliferative pattern. Stroma is exclusively of the proliferative type.

INCREASED LH ACTIVITY. Döring[37] and Dörner[38] reported increased LH levels in conjunction with hyperthecosis. Numerous workers[8, 13, 45, 54] have been able to provoke hyperthecosis in ovaries of rodents by means of massive injections of LH.

HYPOTHALAMIC EFFECTS. A hitherto poorly known aspect of hyperestrinism has been a possible *hypothalamic effect as a causative agent*. Purshottan[99] noted that tranquilizers sometimes produced anovulatory cycles with hyperestrinism. Similar effects were observed by Barraclough and his colleagues[5] in rats whose hypothalamus had been paralyzed with testosterone. Finally, Desclin and his co-workers[31] achieved identical results by injuring the basal nuclei of the brain in the same species. The author postulates that destruction of the *tuber cinereum*, or paralyzation of the same center with testosterone or some anesthetic, produces suppression of the LH release mechanism, thereby causing lack of ovulation and, consequently, follicular persistence with an anovulatory cycle and even hyperestrinism.

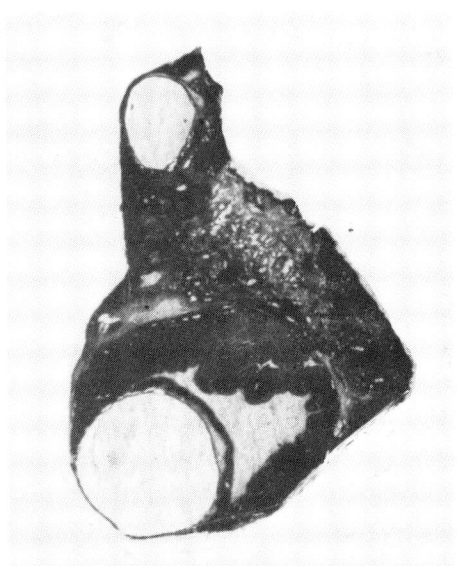

Figure 28–12. Coexistence of active corpus luteum with one mature and one persistent follicle.

28.2.9. FUNCTIONING OVARIAN TUMORS

Some of the functioning ovarian tumors, such as *thecomas* and *granulosa cell tumors*, may give rise to the severest forms of hyperestrinism that we have yet encountered. These two types of neoplasia have been classified by Novak among the group of *feminizing mesenchymomas*. They have been described by others to be almost invariably associated with endometrial hyperplasia and, in many instances, with myomas, adenomas or carcinomas. Although granulosa cell tumors and thecomas undoubtedly may possess the greatest hyperestrogenic potency (see Chapter 30, Section 30.2.3), it seems worthwhile to mention that there are also *feminizing varieties of Leydig cell tumors*.[72, 87a, 118a]

Thus, we are faced again with the problem of ambisexuality of such structures as Leydig cell tumors, adrenocortical hyperplasia, hyperthecosis, etc., which, for yet unknown reasons, may be masculinizing in one instance, and feminizing in another.

Further details concerning the endocrine aspects of functioning tumors of the ovary are discussed in Chapter 30.

28.3. EXTRAOVARIAN HYPERESTRINISM

Extraovarian hyperestrinism, as previously defined, may be caused by estrogens from sources other than the ovary — for instance, the adrenal — or it may result from failure of estrogen destruction, or from inadequate drug therapy. The two first forms of hyperestrinism, resulting from adrenal and hepatic insufficiency, respectively, may frequently be superimposed on ovarian forms. Many clinical syndromes of hyperestrinism may therefore have a double etiology: ovarian and extraovarian.

28.3.1. HYPERESTRINISM OF ADRENOCORTICAL ORIGIN

In the chapter on adrenal physiology (Chapter 9), we made it clear that the adrenal also elaborates estrogens. Although, under normal conditions, the amounts produced are small, they occasionally may give rise to hyperestrinism. This is particularly true in menopausal and postmenopausal women (see Chapter 39), in whom adrenal estrogenic activity may be suspected to be a contributing factor in the development, or at least the progressive growth, of some tumors (Botella[17]).

There is evidence that this happens in animals. Castration in female guinea pigs,[116] mice,[46, 52] hamsters[63, 135] and rats[49, 68] is followed by reactive adrenal hyperplasia of various types, sometimes even by tumors, that may all be associated with estrogen hypersecretion.

Houssay,[56] more than anyone else, and Little[76] have explored this question in

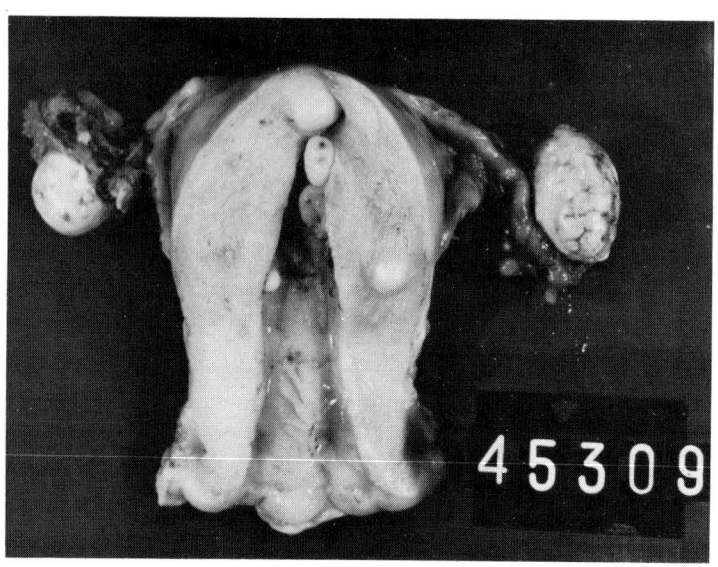

Figure 28–14. Surgical specimen in a case of ovarian thecoma, showing concurrent endometrial hyperplasia, endometrial polyps, multiple leiomyomas and adenomyosis, the last two involving the myometrium.

depth and demonstrated that castration in some strains of rats produced *adrenal estrogenic overcompensation*, which, in turn, caused the animals to go into a state of permanent estrus, rather than anestrus as is the norm, and which was in addition responsible for the development of various kinds of tumors, such as adenoma, myoma and fibroma of the uterus or the breast.

There are two sets of well defined circumstances under which *adrenal hyperestrinism* may occur in the human species: the first is represented in children by the appearance of the feminizing type of adrenogenital syndrome, described by Mellicow and Cahill,[86] or the type of adrenogenital syndrome that produces precocious puberty in girls (see Chapter 33); the second is the appearance of metropathy with endometrial hyperplasia in postmenopausal women in the absence of active ovarian function (Maurizio and Pasetto[85]). It is possible that certain genital cancers arising after the age of 55 may be related to estrogens elaborated by the adrenal, although we have been unable to find any evidence to that effect in our studies[17] (see also Chapter 46).

28.3.2. HEPATIC HYPERESTRINISM

The important role the liver plays in estrogen metabolism has been underlined in Chapter 2. The same relationships that were found to exist in experimental animals between estrogen activity and liver function were also shown to exist in human clinical experience. Pearlman and De Meio[95] and Pincus and his colleagues[98] were the first to call attention to conversion of estrone to estriol by the human liver. Zondek and Finkelstein[144] described the presence of a specific estrinase in the livers of man and animals and also in certain plants, such as potatoes, beets and some mushrooms. In addition to estrinase, Engel and Rosenberg[41] isolated from the liver an enzyme that attacked and degraded estradiol. Later studies by Roberts and Szego,[101] Pearlman and De Meio,[95] Stimmell and Steale,[118] Segaloff and colleagues,[106] and Ryan and Engel[102] have greatly clarified the existing relationship between liver function and estrogen metabolism. In this regard, the discovery of *an enterohepatic circulation of estrogens* (Hanahan et al.[54]) is of great interest. In addition, work with *ovarian transplants to the spleen* has revealed the fact that ovarian internal secretions were inactivated by the liver (Bernstorff[8]).

Clinically, hyperestrinism of hepatic origin is seen in the following cases: (1) hepatitis; (2) hepatosis; (3) liver cirrhosis; (4) nutritional deficiencies; and (5) hepatoovarian syndrome.

HEPATITIS. Sutherland and MacBride[126] indicated the existence of a relationship between hyperestrogenic hemorrhagic metropathy and certain forms of hepatitis. Szego[121] verified the same finding in animal experiments.

HEPATOSIS. Furlong[45] and Valcourt[129] and their associates have shown that carbon tetrachloride intoxication resulted in hyperestrinism of hepatic origin.

LIVER CIRRHOSIS. The appearance of *gynecomastia* in males suffering from liver cirrhosis is a well known clinical observation. Sopeña and Tornero,[113] as well as Lyngbye and Morgensen,[79] found increased estrogen excretion in advanced cirrhosis.

NUTRITIONAL DEFICIENCIES. This problem is perhaps of greatest importance and has been the object of repeated studies in the course of the past several years.[116, 120]

As far back as 1941, Biskind and Biskind[12] observed that deficiency of *various vitamin B group factors* resulted in loss of estrogen degrading capacity by the liver. Segaloff and associates[106] and Singher and co-workers[110] found that loss of estrogenolytic power was mainly the result of *pyridoxine, pantothenic acid and biotin deficiency*. Various authors[24, 68] subsequently confirmed these findings and, moreover, demonstrated the role played by *pteroylglutamic acid* in the degradation of estrogenic compounds.

Proteins (Van Der Linde and Westerfeld,[130] Vasington et al.[133]) and among them *casein* and the sulfur-containing amino acids and polypeptides (cystine, cysteine, glutathion) were also found to be involved.

HEPATOOVARIAN SYNDROME. Any hepatic pathology—but most commonly such benign forms as nutritional deficiency, hepatitis, etc.—may adversely affect the capacity of estrogen degradation in the climacteric female. Considering the fact that *both ovarian and extraovarian estro-*

gen production in this phase of life tends to be increased, it is easy to understand why even minor deficiencies in detoxification may be associated with moderate elevations of estrogen levels, giving rise to hyperestrinism through a combination of the two factors. The resulting clinical picture, by no means of rare occurrence, has been described by French authors (Huet et al.[57]) under the name of *hepatoovarian syndrome* and obviously plays an important role in functional disorders of the climacterium.

28.3.3. IATROGENIC HYPERESTRINISM

A number of authors[1, 15, 47, 49] have reported cases in which estrogen therapy had caused metrorrhagia or other disturbances of the estrogen-induced type. In our practice, we have come across this phenomenon with a certain frequency, particularly in women of the climacteric age group who ingested large amounts of the hormone, almost invariably self-prescribed, for the purpose of prolonging their femininity. Because corpus luteum formation is generally absent and, concomitantly, the basis for physiologic antagonism to estrogens is also lacking in this age group, development of hyperestrinism from estrogen therapy is all the more prevalent. On one occasion, we witnessed a hemorrhagic metropathy in a postmenopausal woman as a result of percutaneous absorption of a cosmetic ointment containing estrogens.

Without further explaining the details of this syndrome, we therefore again emphasize the risk involved in uncontrolled and injudicious estrogen therapy, particularly during menopause and afterwards.

28.4. CLINICAL FORMS OF HYPERESTRINISM

First of all, the clinical manifestations of hyperestrinism must be divided into two clinically different forms of the syndrome: acute hyperestrinism, occurring in the latter half of the cycle of women who are not exposed to prolonged effects of hyperestrinism, and chronic hyperestrinism, developed by women who are subjected to prolonged although not necessarily increased estrogen activity. The various manifestations pertaining to the second form must be studied as they occur not only within but also outside the confines of the genital apparatus.

28.4.1. ACUTE HYPERESTRINISM

For many years, it was our belief that hyperestrinism developed only in pathologically altered cycles and in the absence of corpus luteum formation. However, as a result of the clinical findings of various investigators, we have recently come to recognize a so-called *brief* or acute form of this syndrome, caused by simple accumulation of endogenous estrogens in the days preceding menstruation. The pathogenesis of this acute form of hyperestrinism is not yet very clear. In the view of some authors, it might be the result of asynchronous maturation of new follicles during the secretory phase, as shown in Figure 28–10. This would presumably involve pooling of all estrogenic products secreted by the new follicles with those produced by the corpus luteum itself so as to give high-crested estrogen waves during the second half of the intermenstruum, which were described by Beclère[6] and by Gilbert-Dreyfus.[47] In other instances, a defective liver mechanism of estrogen deactivation would have to be implicated. Whether resulting from impaired liver degradation,[8, 102, 118] or from lack of estrogen-antagonizing activity by an insufficient corpus luteum[126, 127, 136] — or perhaps as a result of a special state of end-organ *reactivity* to estrogens — all of the above mentioned factors could account for this condition of acute intolerance to estrogens, which is sometimes also linked to psychosomatic disturbances of various interpretation.[50]

Clinically, these women have normal menses, usually with slightly delayed onset (by not more than a few days). Bleeding is usually not more copious than in normal cycles, or, at best, is only slightly so. These patients present with *premenstrual dysmenorrhea*, the pain in the pelvic region gradually gaining in intensity until becoming almost unbearable on the day preceding menstruation. At the same time, *mastodynia* and *premenstrual edema* become manifest. The edema may be attributed to the water-retaining activity by estrogens, which was described in Chapter 2. Caroll[25] suggested that the appearance of premenstrual edema was a symptom of hyperestrinism. Changes in mood as well as sensations of abdominal fullness may also be of clinical significance.

Also of interest are the findings revealed by *vaginal cytology*. Ufer[126] and Wied[138] reported the presence of large numbers of estrogenic cells on a background of an otherwise secretory pattern with typical folded cells.

Gennes drew attention to another clinical form of acute hyperestrinism, which he called "syndrome of the fourteenth day." This consisted in sudden development of genital pain, feeling of fullness and breast pain, and occasionally, transient intermenstrual spotting. This clinical picture, essentially corresponding to what German authors called "Mittelschmerz," is assumed to be precipitated by an unusually high-peaked estrogen wave at the moment of ovulation.

At any rate, there is as yet no incontrovertible evidence as to whether this syndrome is due to hyperestrinism or simply reflects a peritoneal crisis resulting from violent follicular rupture.

28.4.2. HEMORRHAGIC METROPATHY

Many years ago, Schröder[103] described a clinical picture under the name of "hemorrhagic metropathy," which was characterized by follicular persistence, absence of ovulation and cystic glandular hyperplasia of the endometrium, eventually to be shed with abundant hemorrhage. This syndrome, by no means uncommon, had been accepted perhaps too unquestioningly as the underlying mechanism in virtually all types of functional bleeding. In recent years, however, it was found that functional bleeding in women did not always comport with such a model of persistent proliferation and hyperplasia, but rather was associated with various other types of functional disorders. As shown graphically in Figure 28–16, a review of functional bleeding, conducted by us in cooperation with Marín-Bonachera,[83] had revealed the typical findings of Schröder's hemorrhagic metropathy in somewhat less than 50 per cent of cases. At the same time, a considerable number of cases showed normal endometrial patterns without evidence of hyperplasia (20.9 per cent), whereas the remainder showed conditions ranging from endometritis, endometrial atrophy, neoplasia and unsuspected carcinoma, to a few cases with decidual reaction or incomplete endometrial maturation. As previously indicated (Fig. 28–1), not all cases with follicular persistence, not even all those with large follicles, were found to be associated with severe endometrial hyperplasia or with metrorrhagia. In many cases, follicular persistence was found to be associated with simple proliferative endometrial patterns, without hyperplasia, and with normal menses. Upon reexamining the graph in Figure 28–5, it may be noted that, notwithstanding the fact that most cases of hemorrhagic metropathy with cystic endometrial hyperplasia are associated with follicular persistence, the etiology in approximately

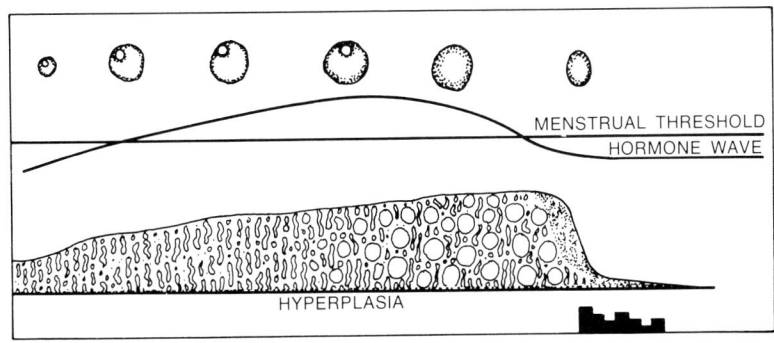

Figure 28–15. Hyperhormonal amenorrhea, followed by metrorrhagia; there is also follicular persistence.

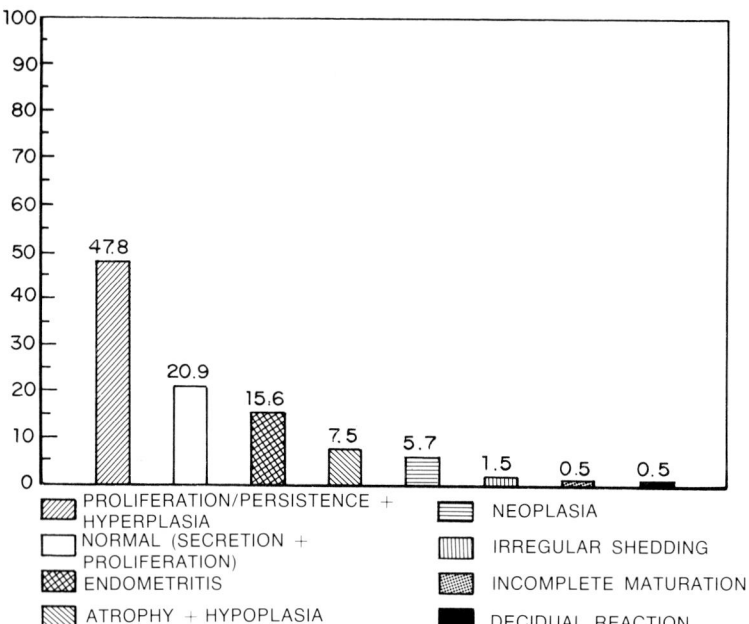

Figure 28–16. The causes of functional bleeding, clinically classified as "metropathy." Note that in minority of cases the cause is persistent hyperplasia or proliferation. (From Marín.[83])

one third of the cases seems to be related to hyperestrogenic ovarian functional disorders other than simple follicular persistence. Jacobs and Lindlay[61] and Southam[115] later published similar statistics. In other words, Schröder's syndrome reflects a commonly occurring interrelationship of follicular persistence, cystic glandular endometrial hyperplasia and menometrorrhagia, not all three signs necessarily being present at once. Follicular persistence may occur without hyperplasia or without bleeding and, similarly, hyperplasia may occur without follicular persistence or without bleeding. Finally, apparent functional bleeding in a female patient may be unrelated to any of the already described ovarian or uterine disorders.

A complete study of hemorrhagic metropathy from a clinical standpoint would involve many purely gynecologic considerations that go beyond the scope of female endocrinology as such and which therefore will not be discussed here. The clinical picture of hemorrhagic metropathy may be recognized in all age groups between puberty and the climacterium, allowing the following distinctions: *juvenile, adult and postmenopausal hemorrhagic metropathy.*

In some instances, particularly in functioning granulosa cell tumors, hemorrhagic metropathy may also develop many years after menopause and may be associated with reappearance of menstruation.

Hemorrhage may not always develop in a uniform manner. Most frequently, bleeding has a pseudomenstrual character and repeats itself at more or less regular intervals, but sometimes, especially in cases of follicular persistence with a prolonged cycle, bleeding episodes may alternate with periods of amenorrhea and are then the more copious the more extended the intervals are between them. In addition, the amount of blood lost varies from case to case. Generally, the duration of a single bleeding episode may extend over a greater number of days than usual: from six to 20 days, or even more, and the daily blood loss may also be considerably increased.

Furthermore, occasional bleeding disorders follow a pattern of multiple menstruations at short intervals or, in other instances, give rise to irregular episodes of frank metrorrhagia, with subintrant recurrences.

These manifestations are accompanied by extragenital symptoms, of which the most common ones are *mastodynia,* sometimes with breast engorgement or even *mastopathy* (discussed later), *premenstrual tension*, headaches, often tenacious in nature, and *edema*. The edema, as pointed out earlier, is of the hyperestrogenic type owing to water and sodium retention.

At physical examination, the external genitalia are usually found to be turgescent and sometimes slightly congested. As a rule, the uterus is considerably enlarged in a uniform way, without protrusions or irregularities unless, as may often be the case, the clinical picture is complicated by the presence of uterine leiomyomas. Adnexal findings vary greatly. In some cases, the ovaries are markedly enlarged (Fig. 28–17); in others, however, the only enlargement detected may be that of an ovary containing a persistent follicle.

Endocrinologic examination of the patient may reveal data of utmost significance. Temperature recordings are flattened permanently, which corresponds to absent corpus luteum function. *Vaginal cytology* is always of the hyperestrogenic type, with elevated acidophilic and karyopyknotic indices. However, such vaginal changes may be absent because of a sharp drop in estrogen levels at the time of hemorrhage or immediately afterwards.

Urinary estrogen values have been studied by a number of investigators, mainly by Beclère,[6] Brown,[19] Diczfalusy and Lauritzen[33] and Timonen.[125] An increase in urinary estrogens is not the most constant finding, although generally these are quite elevated. What, on the other hand, is a constant finding, as has been indicated by the foregoing authors and corroborated by our own experience, is the absence of urinary pregnanediol.

The most important data of diagnostic value are provided by the study of endometrial tissue. The endometrium may be found to reach enormous thickness and may display a "polypoid" tendency when viewed in a cross section of the uterus. Microscopically, the pattern of cystically dilated glands in the mucosa is typical (Figs. 28–18 and 28–21). Both glands and stroma are in the process of active proliferation and display numerous mitotic figures, particularly the former. Also frequently present in the stroma are areas of vascular thrombosis and necrosis. Histochemical studies of the endometrium have provided a note of added interest in recent years. Our own studies concerning the presence of *glycogen* revealed that glycogen was not deposited in endometrial hyperplasia, as opposed to malignant forms of hyperplasia or adenocarcinoma in which its presence may be an important detail allowing the differential diagnosis of some doubtful cases. In contrast to the absence of glycogen, endometrial hyperplasia gives intensely positive reactions for *alkaline glycerophosphatase*. The histologic appearance of a proliferative endometrium stained with the Gomori method is illustrated in Figure 26–9 in Chapter 26. It should be pointed out that the enzyme is demonstrated in proliferative glands only and is never visualized in cystic glands, which would seem to indicate that gland cystification is an end-stage phenomenon in endometrial growth.

Schröder[103] originally described three typical phases in the evolution of such endometria: a *phase of proliferation*, during which the patient experienced no bleeding and the endometrium proliferated until it

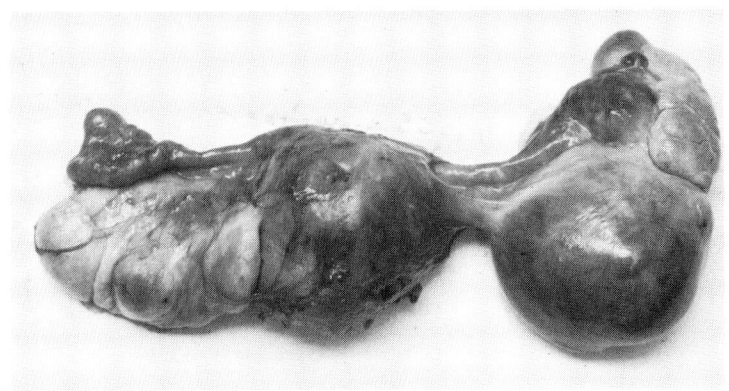

Figure 28–17. Bilateral enlargement of hyperestrogenic ovaries. There was also mild myometrial hyperplasia.

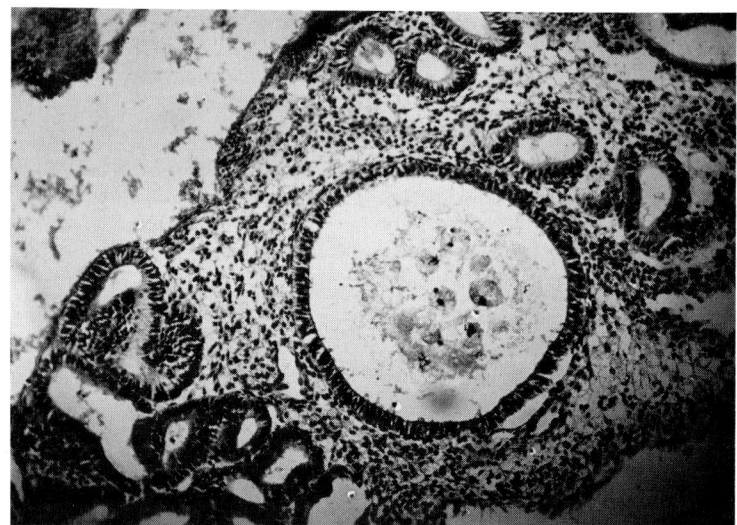

Figure 28-18. "Swiss cheese" hyperplasia.

reached its hyperplastic appearance; a *phase of necrosis,* in which hemorrhage supervened; and a *phase of regeneration,* following necrosis and hemorrhage. In reality, this sequence of events, which reflects an attempt to ascribe to the hyperplastic endometrium a cycle of the menstrual type, cannot be found in the majority of cases. It must also be realized that the rate of endometrial maturation in hemorrhagic metropathy is highly irregular and that while some zones within the endometrial cavity are at one of the three phases, other zones may be undergoing different phases of evolution. These three phases, therefore, can only serve as a guideline as far as endometrial evolution toward eventual hemorrhage is concerned.

28.4.3. HYPERESTROGENIC AMENORRHEA

The same description that was given for bleeding patterns in follicular persistence applies to hemorrhagic metropathy. Thus, it is clear that episodes of metrorrhagia alternate with amenorrhea. If the periods of amenorrhea are of extended duration,

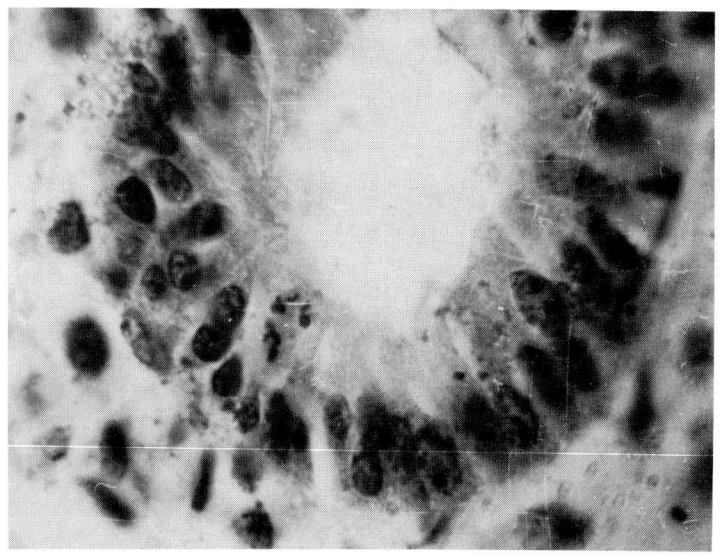

Figure 28-19. High power detail of a gland from a typical case of cystic endometrial hyperplasia. A tripolar mitotic figure is present in one cell.

the clinical presentation of cystic endometrial hyperplasia may be marked by apparent lack of menstruation, mimicked by a bout of amenorrhea of up to several months' duration. Zondek and Finkelstein[144] first described a form of amenorrhea that was associated with elevated urinary estrogen excretion, a finding that was subsequently confirmed by a number of authors.[47,66] However, the presence of cystic endometrial hyperplasia, or at least persistent endometrial proliferation, may give quite variable clinical symptoms. Most commonly, menstrual bleeding is increased either as simple hypermenorrhea or as very copious bleeding, reaching proportions of hemorrhagic metropathy. However, it may also be associated with amenorrhea, or even with normal menstruation despite the presence of marked endometrial hyperplasia in some cases. The occurrence of endometrial hyperplasia in women whose menstrual periods appear to be within normal limits has recently been emphasized by Falconer,[42] Kottmeier[70] and Wahlen.[134]

The finding of persistent proliferative patterns, or of endometrial hyperplasia, in amenorrhea is not exceptional either. Such periods of amenorrhea, as a rule, are not of long duration; they usually last from one to three months, until the persistent follicle or follicles involved undergo atresia and the resulting hormone withdrawal produces bleeding.

As in Chapter 27, the significance of this finding in exploring amenorrhea must again be stressed. On the other hand, the frequency with which increased urinary estrogens are also encountered in amenorrhea has been brought to light by Sopeña and Tornero[113] (see Table 28-3).

TABLE 28-3. Hyperhormonal Amenorrhea with Elevated Estrogens and Absent or Scanty Pregnanediol

CASE	AGE	ESTROGENS (MCG/24 HR)	PREGNANEDIOL (MG/24 HR)	UTERUS
1	33	200	Negative	Normal
2	42	400	8	Normal
3	38	250	Negative	Normal
4	29	150	1.23	Retroflexed
5	26	300	0.50	Retroflexed
6	42		2	Normal

28.4.4. FUNCTIONAL BLEEDING ASSOCIATED WITH ATYPICAL HYPERPLASIA

The term "atypical" has been used here not in a premalignant or malignant connotation but rather as denoting those partially hyperplastic endometrial patterns which histologically differ considerably from typical "Swiss cheese" hyperplasia of Schröder's syndrome, and which may give rise to functional bleeding of various types. Many kinds of endometria fall into this group, which is not necessarily associated with hyperestrinism. Nevertheless, they must be listed here inasmuch as they enter the differential diagnosis of classical metropathy. These are: (1) irregular endometrial maturation; (2) irregular endometrial shedding; (3) hyperplasia with secretion; and (4) endometrial squamous metaplasia.

IRREGULAR ENDOMETRIAL MATURATION. This term is used here to designate a phenomenon described in 1935 by Traut and Kuder, which is characterized by the simultaneous presence of areas with secretory appearance side by side with areas having a frank proliferative appearance. Isolated examples of endometria exhibiting such features are illustrated in Figures 28-13 and 28-20. Proliferative glands, some cystically dilated, may be observed to coexist with other glands exhibiting secretory changes. The secretory features are never quite pronounced and seem to correspond, at best, to those of an early secretory phase. In spite of that, we have recently been able to demonstrate the presence of glycogen in such secretory areas.[17] The etiology of such conditions remains obscure. Essentially, two different explanations have been advanced for the phenomenon of irregular maturation. Seitz[107] suggested patchy inflammation of the endometrium as a result of which some areas become refractory to the action of progesterone. Consequently, the situation would be analogous to *metrosis of receptivity*, as understood by Moricard.[93] On the other hand, American authors instead postulate a situation of imbalance between estrogen and progesterone synthesis, an opinion we have come to share, and therefore classify the disorder as a form of luteal insufficiency. This entity shall be discussed again within the context of corpus luteum syndromes.

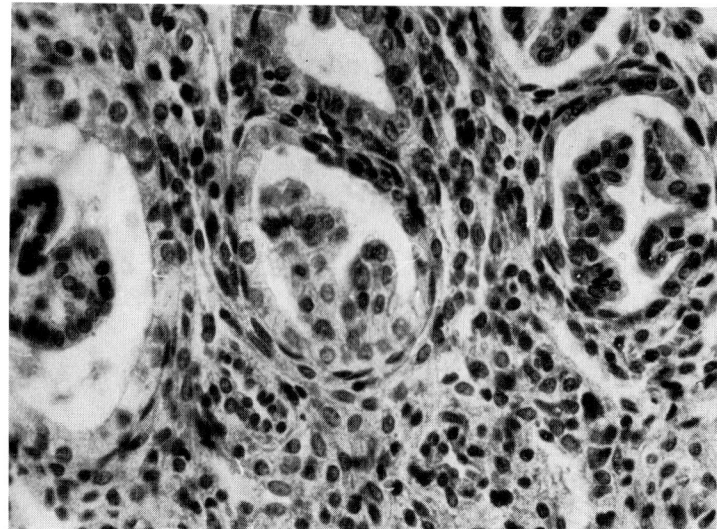

Figure 28-20. Atypical endometrial hyperplasia with intraglandular epithelial metaplasia.

IRREGULAR ENDOMETRIAL SHEDDING. Under the name of irregular shedding, MacKelvey and Samuels,[82] Holmstrom and MacLennan,[55] and Brewer and Jones[18] described a condition characterized by metrorrhagia, or copious menstrual bleeding, with passage of secretory endometrium. Since this condition has recently been shown to be caused by the persistence of the corpus luteum, with relative hyperluteinism, it will be treated with syndromes of the corpus luteum in Chapter 29. Figure 28-16 suggests the extent to which irregular endometrial shedding may play a part in the genesis of functional bleeding.

HYPERPLASIA WITH SECRETION. In recent years, the finding of endometrial hyperplasia associated with secretory changes has gained clinical significance. Its histopathology was described by Te Linde and Wharton.[123] We have also frequently come across this endometrial pattern in menorrhagia and in functional bleeding. Histologically, these exuberantly thickened endometria reveal (1) prominently developed glands which may be cystically dilated, their secretory pattern and glycogen content notwithstanding; (2) a stromal reaction, similarly hyperplastic in nature, with marked edema, indicative of a condition of hyperestrinism; and (3) a vascular reaction, with dilatation and thrombosis, as in simple hyperplasia. The etiology of this endometrial pattern probably consists of hyperestrinism in the presence of a normally developed corpus luteum, that is, an instance of acute hyperestrinism (see Figure 28-12).

Giorgy[48] studied the hormone content of ovaries both in irregular shedding and in hyperplasia with secretion and found that ovarian follicles in these conditions contained more progesterone than estrogen, which is just the opposite of what is found normally. Therefore, a great number of the underlying disturbances seem to result from *abnormal ovarian steroidogenesis*.

ENDOMETRIAL SQUAMOUS METAPLASIA. In severe forms of hyperestrinism, particularly in conjunction with feminizing ovarian tumors, the columnar gland epithelium may be transformed into a polystratified cuboidal epithelium which, although not identical to it, bears a striking resemblance to squamous epithelium (Fig. 28-20). The nature of this metaplasia is puzzling, since it may be associated with demonstrable glycogen deposits without any other evidence suggestive of progestinic effects. It probably represents incipient atypia in the course of transition to adenocarcinoma, as the latter also may reveal the presence of intracellular glycogen. The clinical presentation is similar to that of the common form of metropathia hemorrhagica.

28.4.5. ADENOMA, MYOMA, ENDOMETRIOSIS

The role of hyperestrogenism in the pathogenesis of *adenoma, myoma* and *en-*

Hyperestrinism

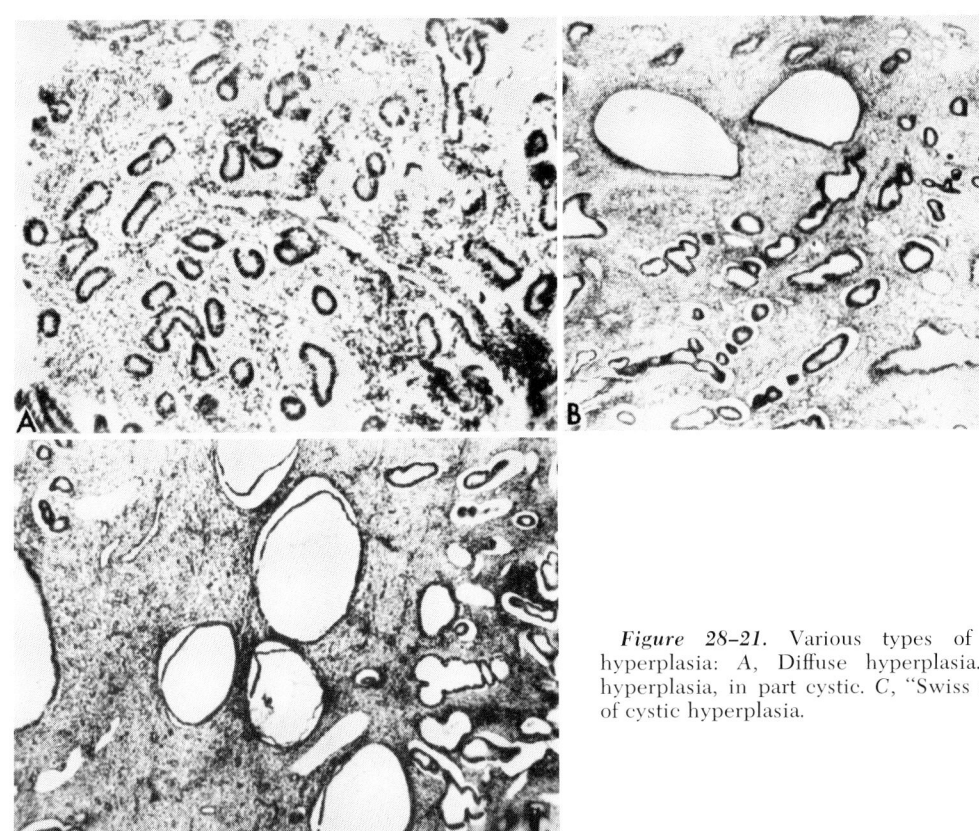

Figure 28–21. Various types of endometrial hyperplasia: *A*, Diffuse hyperplasia. *B*, Diffuse hyperplasia, in part cystic. *C*, "Swiss cheese" type of cystic hyperplasia.

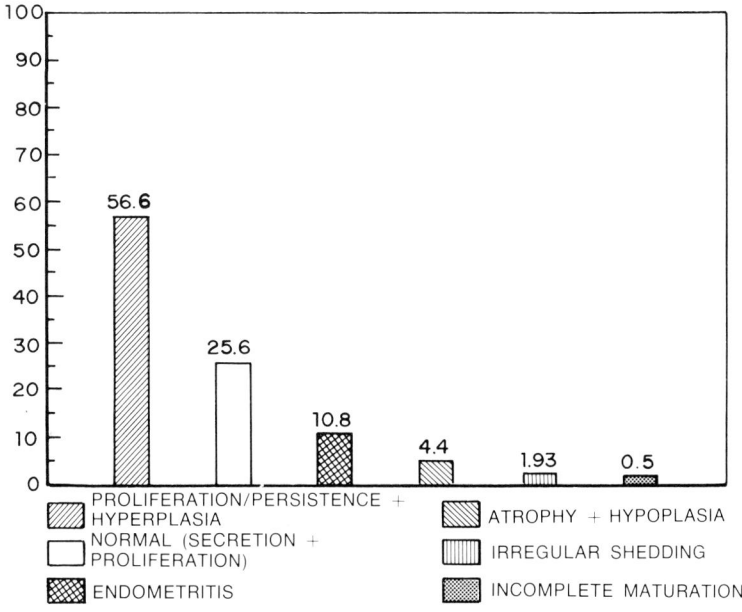

Figure 28–22. Endometrial findings in women with menorrhagia.

dometriosis has been suspected for a long time. These conditions are generated by concomitant genetic and hormonal causes. The genetic causes involved might be thought of as equivalent to Roux's so-called factors of determination, whereas the hormonal causes would correspond to factors of realization—in this particular instance, to estrogens. Various investigators[46, 56, 75] have succeeded in inducing, experimentally, the growth of endometrial adenoma, or uterine myoma and fibromyoma, in mice, rats and guinea pigs by means of injecting or implanting large amounts of estrogens. Similarly, ovaries with follicular persistence, or polymicrocystic ovaries, are often found in the presence of adenomas or myomas. Botella and Calvo-Marcos[15] have studied the relationship between hyperfollicular ovaries and uterine myomata. The data obtained by them are shown in Table 28-4.

In a later study, in co-operation with Nogales (unpublished observations), we have again reviewed a series of ovaries from cases with leiomyomas. We were impressed by the high incidence of multiple ovarian follicles and that of faultily developed corpora lutea, revealing abnormalities in the development of the granulosa lutein layer. It is our opinion that myomata are associated with hyperestrinism, which is the result of defective corpus luteum steroidogenesis rather than any of the other causes classically implicated.

The role of estrogens in the pathogenesis of *endometriosis* has first been suggested by the classic experiments of Harbitz. In these, endometriosis was produced by transplanting pieces of endometrium to rabbits and treating them with estrogens. In the absence of estrogen therapy, transplants did not "take" and endometriosis could not be induced experimentally. Bedoya, who conducted a study of ovaries in cases with endometriosis, observed that in a disproportionately high number of cases endometriosis occurred concomitantly with the type of ovaries that we described as excessive estrogen producers. Kistner[64, 65] and Scott and Wharton[105] also hold the view that development of endometriosis is determined by hyperestrogenism, basing their contention on the finding of hyperestrogenic ovarian changes in bearers of endometriosis.

28.4.6. ESTROGENS AND CARCINOMA

Even though this subject is to be examined in more detail in Chapter 46, it merits a few brief general considerations here. Estrogens would seem to behave as growth-promoting agents insofar as uterine and mammary carcinomas are concerned, although no direct carcinogenic effect has been proved in spite of numerous investigations undertaken for that purpose.

In contrast, *carcinoma of the uterine cervix* does not seem to be related to estrogens. As for *endometrial adenocarcinoma*, an unquestionable relationship appears to have been established with the demonstration that the incidence of carcinoma of the fundus in cases with granulosa cell tumors and thecomas was 20 times greater than in normal women as a group.[30] Nevertheless, our own studies failed to show any significant statistical differences between a group of 70 women with endometrial carcinoma and another group of 50 postmenopausal women of similar age insofar as either urinary estrogen concentrations or findings relative to endometrial patterns were concerned; nor were there any distinctive vaginal cytologic findings. This question will be taken up in greater detail in Chapter 46.

28.4.7. MAMMARY DYSPLASIA

Under the general term *mastopathy* or *mammary dysplasia*, we include a series of

TABLE 28-4. Ovarian Findings in Women with Myomas

TYPE OF OVARY	NO. OF CASES	PERCENTAGE
Group A: Ovaries with complete cycle	30	30
Group B: Anovulatory cycle, follicular persistence, follicle cysts	38	38
Group C: Polymicrocystic ovaries	18	18
Group D: Fibrous atretic ovaries	10	10
Group E: Follicle-lutein cysts	4	4
TOTAL	100	100

endocrine conditions, to some extent distinct from one another, in which the breast is the site of pathologic changes of proliferative nature, caused by estrogenic activity. The actions of estrogens on the physiology of the breast have been reviewed in Chapter 22; these are exerted, as mentioned, mainly at the level of the lactiferous ducts, in which they provoke a proliferative phase. By enhancing the above proliferative process, occasionally to pathologic proportions, the syndrome of hyperestrinism may give rise to a series of symptoms of different kinds. These may be grouped into three basic syndromes: *mastodynia, adenosis and fibrocystic disease of the breast.*

MASTODYNIA. By *mastodynia* we refer to a clinical entity involving persistent breast pain, exacerbated premenstrually and localized in an indurated area of the breast, that shows palpable, increased consistency. The dense tissue may be confined to a single segment of the gland, or it may involve the other gland and be bilateral. Despite the frequent occurrence of this disease, its clinical and pathologic parameters are ill-defined. The main symptoms include: *pain*, insidious in onset and gradually increasing in intensity, *premenstrual* manifestation and characteristic *breast engorgement*. Mastodynia occurs in young women with relative frequency, the majority of cases occurring between the ages of 35 and 40, with a peak incidence at age 37. The most common localization is the upper outer quadrant of the breast, but it may also occur around the periphery of the gland and quite particularly along the external margin of the breast.

The hyperestrogenic origin of mastodynia is nowadays fully recognized mainly through the endocrinologic studies of Bacigalupo and Schubert.[3]

A relationship between hyperestrinism and mastodynia was also recognized by Geschickter. However, it is of interest to point out that pregnanediol elimination in such patients is not increased so that enhanced estrogen activity is not matched by associated hyperluteinism. The condition might thus be compared with what we have defined as acute hyperestrinism. Premenstrual mastodynia is often part of the symptomatology in women suffering from acute hyperestrinism.

ADENOSIS. Adenosis is characterized by the appearance, in one or both breasts, of multiple nodules, ranging in size from 1 mm to 1 cm, most commonly distributed over the periphery of the upper or lower hemisphere. The breasts are usually not enlarged but are of a dense consistency, with a granular texture. Pain may develop in a similar way to mastodynia and may flare up premenstrually. Most of the patients involved are sterile and, although they also reveal a peak incidence between the ages of 35 and 40, the disease may also occur toward the end of sexual maturity.

This condition was originally described under the name "papillary cystadenoma" by Schimmelbusch, and was later called by other authors *nonencapsulated adenoma of the breast* or *chronic cystic mastitis*. In 1934, Lewis and Geschickter described the disease for the first time as a genuine adenosis or hyperplasia.

The most frequently occurring symptoms consist of numerous palpable granulations, rarely exceeding the size of a peanut, scattered peripherally over the upper outer portion of the breast. Pain is a less constant symptom than it is in mastodynia and so is premenstrual engorgement, which may be absent. The prognosis is more doubtful than in mastodynia; it may be difficult to distinguish between genuine mastodynia and an incubation stage of neoplasia. Among 79 cases of adenosis treated surgically by Geschickter, 49 were treated by performing mastectomy, while the remaining cases were treated by simple excision. Of 30 cases with simple excisions, three (10 per cent) eventually developed carcinoma. This raises serious questions concerning the prognosis of adenosis, as well as whether too conservative surgery does not pose additional risks for the patient. Endocrinologically, adenosis is attributable to hyperestrinism. However, unlike the case with mastodynia, hyperestrinism appears to be continuously present, so that the disease may be classified as a chronic form of hyperestrinism. Adenosis of the breast occurs frequently in combination with endometrial hyperplasia or with uterine myomas, as indicated in a large number of publications.

FIBROCYSTIC DISEASE OF THE BREAST. The condition is characterized by the appearance of isolated or multiple cysts ranging from 1 to 5 cm in greatest dimension. It occurs in breasts of women nearing menopause. Anatomic or surgical examination usually reveals the presence of thin-walled cysts, filled with translucent or whitish fluid. The cysts have a smooth lining, without papillarity. The breasts are usually enlarged and contain increased amounts of fibrous connective tissue in addition to the cystic structures. Solitary cysts are benign. The presence of many cysts, however, may arouse suspicion of dealing with malignancy. The age of the patients generally oscillates between 30 and 60, with a peak incidence at about the age of 45. The disease is the most common form of functional mastopathy and tends to occur in sterile women after a long life of nongravidity.

The principal symptom of this disease is the appearance of cysts. These commonly develop at a rapid rate, although subsequently remaining stationary for long periods of time. Unlike the case with the preceding conditions, the breasts are large and adipose. Cysts may be readily recognized by translumination. In general, breasts which are prone to develop cystic disease do not develop adenosis, so that a distinction may be made between two types of breasts: small and dense breasts with little fat, such as occur in young women, which tend to develop adenosis, and large and fatty breasts with a propensity for cystic disease, which occur in women of older age groups.

A subvariety of this disease is *polycystic disease*. Both the macrocystic and polymicrocystic forms tend to show a familial incidence and frequently occur in several sisters at the same time. It must not be forgotten, on the other hand, that cystic endometrial hyperplasia, uterine leiomyomata and endometriosis usually also show a distinct familial tendency. After all, the familial tendency is not to the development of these specific lesions but to the development of hyperestrinism.

pregnanediol titers, especially in cases of cystic disease. Urinary pregnanediol values have been found to be decreased, although not to any considerable extent, in adenosis, whereas they are usually within normal limits in mastodynia, a fact which, according to Geschickter, may be helpful in establishing the differential diagnosis. Brown,[19] as well as Diczfalusy and Lauritzen,[32] reported elevated estrogen values in these cases.

Results of hormone studies would appear to indicate that hyperestrinism is the underlying cause of mammary dysplasia. Various investigators have achieved experimental induction of mammary dysplastic conditions by means of estrogen therapy. As stated above—and as shall be reiterated in Chapter 46—administration of estrogens to animals with a known carcinogenic tendency may result in mammary malignancy. In animals with no known propensity to develop carcinoma, the various changes induced by estrogen therapy bear a resemblance histologically to the variegated forms of mammary dysplasia in women. Gardner[46] and Smith and associates[111] have been able to induce adenomatous proliferations in rat mammary glands by means of prolonged estrogen administration. After continuous estrogen treatment of mice, Burrows[20] similarly observed development of cystic mammary structures that were comparable to those occurring in woman. Women with polycystic ovaries or with follicular persistence are frequently known to have associated fibrocystic disease of the breast. In the light of present-day knowledge, therefore, the various forms of mammary dysplasia may be considered to be determined by the syndrome of hyperestrinism and to be common "fellow travelers" with all conditions of hyperestrinism in which the main manifestations are apparent in the genital tract proper.

28.4.8. ENDOCRINOLOGY OF FUNCTIONAL DISORDERS OF THE BREASTS

Studies of urinary estrogen and pregnanediol excretion among the different disorders under consideration revealed invariably elevated estrogen and low

28.5. DIAGNOSIS OF HYPERESTRINISM

The diagnosis is based on: (1) clinical data, discussed in preceding sections; (2) vaginal cytology; (3) endometrial biopsy; (4) assay of urinary and blood estrogen values; and (5) gonadotropin loading tests.

28.5.1. VAGINAL CYTOLOGY

The study of vaginal cytology is one of the most sensitive cytohormonal methods for evaluating estrogenic activity, and consequently it is the most useful for the diagnosis of hyperestrinism. The different *estrogenic indices* proposed for estimating the degree of estrogen saturation[14, 69, 90, 91, 139] were discussed briefly in Chapter 25 (Section 25.5.4). It is true that their value is relative. However, they acquire real significance in *"serial vaginal cytology,"* whereby the different indices are read on a daily basis, or, preferably, every 48 hours over a period of one or more cycles. What matters most in hyperestrinism is not the absolute estrogen level at any given moment, but the presence of *persistent estrogenic activity on a continuous basis*, which of course cannot be determined except through serial cytology.

28.5.2. ENDOMETRIAL BIOPSY

Endometrial biopsy is basically a qualitative method and is indicated in particular for the diagnosis of some clinical forms of hyperestrinism—for instance, cystic glandular hyperplasia of the endometrium.[16, 18, 42, 55, 120]

28.5.3. ASSAY OF ESTROGENS

A single high estrogen value in blood or urine is of limited value, for the aforesaid reasons. It is of greater interest to observe consistently elevated values or, even more significantly, to find evidence of estrogen-progesterone imbalance. For techniques for hormone assay, as well as for information on normal values, see Chapter 24.

Gonadotropin loading tests[78, 81] have little to offer. They help to discern whether a given luteal *deficit* is of primordial ovarian or of primordial pituitary origin. In this respect, it should be pointed out, *hyperestrinism* may be confused with *hypoluteinism*. It seems preferable to speak, as does Moricard, in terms of *estrogen-progesterone imbalance*.

28.6. TREATMENT OF HYPERESTRINISM

Instead of an absolute and pathologic increase in the activity of a single hormone, hyperestrinism must be considered as a state of imbalance between two groups of hormones. On one side of the balance are estrogens, responsible for stimulating the different segments of the female genital tract, and on the other side are progesterone, androgens and, in part, corticoids, which act as estrogen antagonists and counterbalance actions exerted on common target organs. The maintenance of reciprocal balance between the two groups of hormones, preventing either from gaining predominance, is what Lipschütz has denominated *steroid homeostasis*. By definition, hyperestrinism is nothing else than a break in the mechanism of steroid homeostasis in favor of estrogens. For practical purposes, it makes little difference whether the decrease occurs in the activity of estrogens or in that of the group of antagonistic hormones.

These factors should be borne in mind at all times in the treatment of hyperestrinism. The therapist's purpose must be not to *eliminate*, but rather to *antagonize*, estrogen activity by reestablishing homeostasis by artificial means. Accordingly, two main groups of hormones form the basis for the treatment of hyperestrinism: *progestogens* and *androgens*. Under certain circumstances, treatment with *gonadotropins* or with *vitamins* may also be effective. Not to be overlooked, hyperestrinism is also amenable to *radiologic* and *surgical* therapy.

28.6.1. TREATMENT WITH PROGESTOGENS

Progesterone was the first progestogen to be employed and enjoyed the most widespread use in the treatment of syndromes of hyperestrinism. Its application dates back to 1934, when, for the first time, Kauffmann noted transformation of cystic endometrial hyperplasia following injection of 60 mg of progesterone during the cycle. Kauffmann's estimates subsequently turned out to be too low. Ferin,[43, 44] who treated castrated women with both estrogens and progesterone, found that the necessary dosage ranged between 250 and 500 mg, a figure with which Kauffmann later agreed. Progesterone should be administered during the second half of the cycle.

In the course of the past years, progestogen therapy has made great advances. Two types of products have been marketed: *long-acting progestogens (progesterone caproate)* and *synthetic progestogens*, of great potency by the oral route.

Progesterone caproate (see Chapter 3) has been used extensively in recent years.[26, 58] Its action lasts from 12 to 14 days, so that a single injection is sufficient to cover the entire secretory phase of the cycle (Fig. 28-23). Thus, adequate therapy may be achieved with a single monthly injection of 250 mg.

It is equally important to recognize the need for maintaining the cycle at all cost. For this reason, treatment is supplemented with simultaneous estrogen therapy using estradiol derivatives, as indicated in Figure 28-25.

Synthetic progestogens, described in Chapter 3, are a whole series of compounds possessing potent progestational activity if taken orally. Their use has become universal in recent years.[4, 13, 29, 34, 44, 71, 98, 122, 142] Those used most commonly are *norethisterone*, chlormadinone and duphaston, administered in combination with an oral or percutaneous estrogen. An excellent modern review on therapy using synthetic progestogens has been published by Kistner.[67]

28.6.2. ANDROGENS

The use of androgens has been advocated in recent years. We have employed androgen therapy abundantly and recommended its use during the second half of the cycle, just as we have recommended progesterone, but in slightly higher dosages (up to 200 mg). On the other hand, Greenblatt[50] recommends that androgen therapy be instituted during the first half of the cycle, using 25 mg testosterone propionate injected every second day. Greenblatt proposes a total dose of 300 to 350 mg for the cycle, which, in our opinion, is perhaps too elevated. Androgen therapy may consist of testosterone dipropionate in the form of injectables in an oily vehicle, in dosages of 10 to 50 mg, or an average of 25 mg per injection. Oral preparations may also be used, especially *methyltestosterone*, sublingually, in dosages of 400 to 500 mg per cycle, also as suggested by Greenblatt.[49] Preparations in the form of suspensions of crystals or, preferably, emulsions, may also be used effectively. Emulsions are currently available in dosages of 50, 125 and 250 mg. As a rule, a 250 mg dose should be adequate for a month-long course of treatment of hemorrhagic metropathy. A compound specially recommended by Dorfman[35] is *ethyltestosterone*.

Special care must be exerted to avoid androgen overdosage, the dangers of which are twofold: *virilization* and *enhanced libido*. Virilization supervenes as a result of excessive androgen levels and is generally more pronounced in postmenopausal women. *Enhancement of libido* is due to a specific testosterone effect, which has been commented upon in Chapter 4. This poses no serious problems in the treatment of married women but may be an undesirable side effect in single women or in widows during therapy of, for instance, juvenile or postmenopausal metropathy. We therefore use androgen therapy in adult cases of hyperestrinism and prefer progesterone in the very young or in climacteric patients. Guidelines for androgen therapy are given schematically in Figure 28-24.

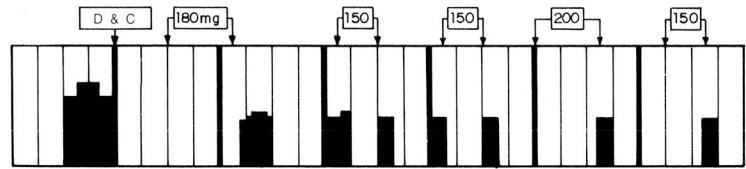

Figure 28-23. Menstrual chart in a patient with hemorrhagic metropathy, successfully treated with progesterone.

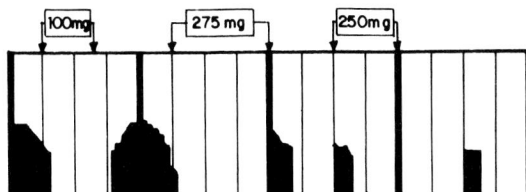

Figure 28-24. Menstrual chart in a case of hyperplastic metropathy treated with androgens.

28.6.3. TREATMENT WITH ESTROGENS

Treatment of hyperestrinism with the very causative agent of the disorder may appear to be reckless and paradoxical. Nevertheless, it must be borne in mind that menstruation is triggered by hormone withdrawal and that, as long as blood estrogen levels remain elevated, endometrial bleeding does not supervene. The conditions under which metrorrhagia may be induced in hyperestrinism require a drop in estrogen levels. In those cases in which elevated estrogen levels are maintained constant, such as occurs in prolonged follicular persistence, the clinical picture that develops is one of hyperhormonal amenorrhea, discussed earlier.

The idea of inhibiting or averting the occurrence of hemorrhage by means of estrogen administration came from Karnaky, who engaged in extensive studies of this form of therapy. Sutherland and MacBride[120] made an equally meritorious contribution in their comprehensive publications on the subject. Obviously, this is not the treatment of choice insofar as causal therapy and permanent cure of metrorrhagia are concerned: it is a palliative procedure, to be employed on an emergency basis until severe blood loss can be controlled. Regarding mode of administration of such paradoxical therapy, a stilbestrol type preparation may be used orally. Administration of 100 to 200 mg of diethylstilbestrol (that is, a rather high dose) produces a rapid hemostatic effect.

28.6.4. COMBINATIONS OF HORMONES

Combined hormone therapy of hyperfolliculinemia using progesterone and testosterone was recommended by Gilbert-Dreyfus[47] some time ago. Later, Greenblatt[51] also endorsed the use of such combinations. For this purpose, commercial preparations containing both testosterone (15 to 25 mg) and progesterone (10 mg) are available. A combination of this type enlists the antiestrogenic effects of both hormones but, by balancing them mutually, counters the virilizing and libido-stimulating effect of testosterone. The progesterone is intended to antagonize the virilizing effect of testosterone as well. This medication should similarly be used during the second half of the cycle, following the guidelines that were previously outlined for the isolated use of either progesterone or testosterone. It represents the ideal solution for the treatment of the *acute form of hyperestrinism*. In fact, we are convinced that, in cases of acute hyperestrinism, an elevated estrogen level occurs in the presence of normal or even subnormal levels of progesterone. This can only mean that production of luteal hormone is not impaired and yet the pathologic syndrome arises notwithstanding. To add more progesterone under these conditions seems useless, while to administer testosterone may lead to the already mentioned undesirable side effects. The progesterone-testosterone formula may be given in high dosages and produces rapid improvement of symptoms. Combined hormone therapy of this type has also been found to produce favorable effects on such disorders as premenstrual tension and headache, mastodynia, menstrual edema and other, similar disturbances.

28.6.5. TREATMENT OF HYPERHORMONAL AMENORRHEA

Hyperhormonal amenorrhea must not be treated with estrogens. Zondek and Finkelstein[144] proposed the so-called "two day treatment." The latter consists in administering two single doses of 2 mg of estradiol combined with 10 mg of progesterone (Fig. 28-25). Using this formula, Zondek and Finkelstein,[144] Ufer[126, 127] and Greenblatt[50] reported prompt appearance of menstruation. In discussing the mechanism of action involved, Ufer expresses the opinion that it should be attributed to a hormone with-

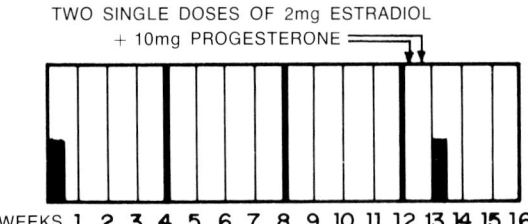

Figure 28–25. Menstrual chart in a case of secondary amenorrhea treated with the "two days'" treatment.

drawal effect provoked by estrogenolytic activity of progesterone. Seitz[107] had earlier made the observation that progesterone only acted in such cases by producing what he termed withdrawal hemorrhage.

28.6.6. ESTROGEN ANTAGONISTS

Under this heading, we have grouped a series of synthetic hormones or drugs, all exerting a damping effect on estrogen activity, which are effective therapeutic agents in the treatment of hyperestrinism. They may be divided into two groups: steroid and nonsteroid estrogen antagonists.

STEROID ESTROGEN ANTAGONISTS. Progestogens, androgens and some corticoids all possess antiestrogenic activity. Dorfman[36] tested a series of 17 steroids for antiestrogenic and antimammary tumor activity, expressing the results in terms of percentage of uterine inhibition, as follows:

	Per Cent
9α-Fluoro-11β,17α-dihydroxy-6α-methyl-1,4-pregnadiene-3,20-dione,17-acetate	61
5α-Androstane-11β,17β-diol	45
17β-Hydroxy-2α,17α-dimethyl-4,9 (11)-androstadiene-3-one	45
Androstadiene-3,17-dione	42
17-Methyl-5α-androstane-3β,11β,17-triol	42
Dehydro-17-methyltestosterone	35
Dehydrotestosterone propionate	32
17-Dimethyltestosterone	30
9α-Bromo-11-keto-17-methyltestosterone	27
Hydroxy-17-methylandrostane-3,11-dione	24
Hydroxy-4,17-dimethyltestosterone	20
Androsterone	16
9α-Fluoro-17β-hydroxy-17-methyl-5β-androstane-3,11-dione	12
Methyl-19-nortestosterone	10
11β-Hydroxy-6α-methylprogesterone	8
11-Keto-17-methyltestosterone	4
Hydroxyprogesterone	0

The first compound, also known as U-17323, is obviously the estrogen antagonist with most potent activity of all compounds tested. Next in order of potency are androstanediol and androstadiene, as well as all their derivatives.

NONSTEROID ESTROGEN ANTAGONISTS. The compound known by the name of chlorotrianisene or TACE (Fig. 28–26) is an estrogen that inhibits the pituitary. Its derivatives are both antiestrogenic agents and pituitary inhibitors. Two compounds have been used predominantly, for their antiestrogenic action: compound MER-25, also called *ethamoxytriphetol*, tested by Kistner[64, 65] and by Lerner and colleagues,[73] and MRL-41 (Clomiphene). The mechanism of antiestrogenic activity of MER-25 has been recently clarified by the studies of Callantyne and associates,[23] Meyerson and Lindstrom,[88] and Wyss and co-workers,[140] who all concur in pointing out that the action of *ethamoxytriphetol* is based on inhibition of *estrogenic receptors* at the tissue level. The second compound, MRL-41, which has the generic name *Clomiphene*, was introduced by Greenblatt and co-workers[51] and tested by a number of other investigators.[30] It is presently widely used as an ovulation-inducing agent and is discussed in more detail in Chapter 41, in conjunction with ovulation-stimulating activity.

The great similarity between the chemical structures of these two compounds may be noted in Figure 28–26, which probably explains the pharmacologic action common to both compounds.

Other estrogen antagonists are actinomycin D, whose action was discovered by Bialy and Pincus[10] and confirmed by Cliterhoe and Leathem[26] and by Rinard,[100] and a series of recently described synthetic compounds of which the two most important ones are 4-estrene-3-one-spiro-17α-tetrahydrofuran, synthesized and tested by Bialy and his co-workers,[9] and the compound known as 1-(2-p-α-paramethoxyphenyl-β-nitrostyryl-phenoxy-ethyl-pyrrolidine)-monocitrate, or CN-55945-27, synthesized by Callantyne and co-workers[22] and by Marshall and O'Brien.[84]

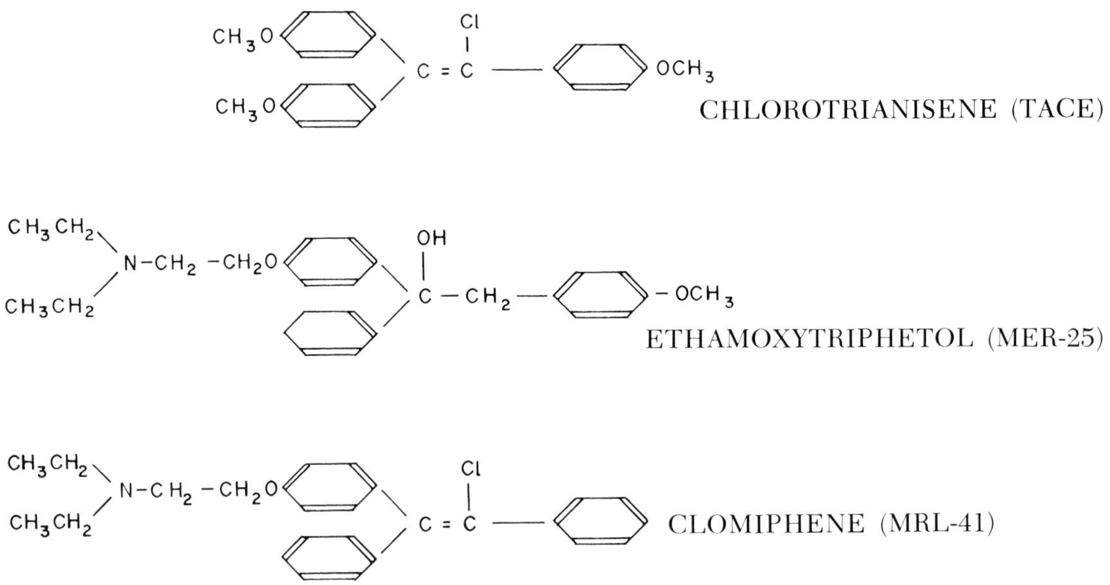

CHLOROTRIANISENE (TACE)

ETHAMOXYTRIPHETOL (MER-25)

CLOMIPHENE (MRL-41)

Figure 28-26. Structural analogies between chlortrianisene (TACE), ethamoxytriphetol (MER-25) and clomiphene (MRL-41).

28.6.7. RADIOTHERAPY AND SURGERY

Roentgen castration is a method of radiotherapy aimed at arresting ovarian maturation temporarily or permanently, resulting in suppression of follicular growth. Estrogen synthesis, however, is not consequently brought to a total standstill; nevertheless, since no continued growth of new follicular elements takes place, the possibility of follicular persistence is eliminated. The prominent role assigned to this method of castration in the past has given way to better developed and perfected methods of hormone therapy, which have greatly reduced the indications for this form of radiotherapy.

Another modality for treatment of only the symptoms, not the cause, of certain types of functional bleeding rests on *intracavitary use of radium*. This type of treatment has no endocrine basis and relies on a simple local effect.

The results of *surgical treatment* of hyperestrinism, utilizing total or partial wedge resection of one or both ovaries, are far from satisfactory. Earlier in this chapter, we indicated the mechanism by which, in fact, removal or destruction of part of the ovarian parenchyma entails a pituitary reaction resulting in hypermaturation of follicles. The successful production of polyfollicular ovaries achieved by Lipschütz in animals after partial ovarian resection was based on the same mechanism. A similar phenomenon sometimes occurs in women. Therefore, quantitative resection of a certain portion of ovarian tissue may produce not the desired reduction in estrogenic activity but instead the opposite effect.

REFERENCES

1. Allen, E. A., and Gardner, W. C.: *Cancer*, 1:359, 1951.
2. Anderson, L. L., Butcher, R. L., and Mellamby, R. M.: *Endocrinology*, 69:571, 1961.
3. Bacigalupo, C., and Schubert, K.: *Klin. Wschr.*, 38:804, 1960.
4. Barfield, W. E., and Greenblatt, R. B.: *Internat. J. Fertil.*, 8:641, 1963.
5. Barraclough, C. A., et al.: *Endocrinology*, 68:62, 1961.
6. Beclère, C.: *Acta Gin.*, 1:265, 1950.
7. Beling, C. G., Marcus, S. L., and Markham, S. M.: *J. Clin. Endocr.*, 30:30, 1970.
8. Bernstorff, E. C.: *Endocrinology*, 49:302, 1951.
9. Bialy, G., Merrill, A. P., and Pincus, G.: *Endocrinology*, 79:125, 1966.
10. Bialy, G., and Pincus, G.: *Endocrinology*, 78:286, 1966.
11. Bilde, T.: *Acta Obstet. Gynec. Scand.*, 46:429, 1967.
12. Biskind, M. S., and Biskind, G. R.: *Science*, 94:962, 1941.
13. Bolker, H. I., et al.: *Endocrinology*, 60:214, 1957.

14. Boschann, H. W.: *Acta Cytol.*, 12:93, 1968.
15. Botella, J., and Calvo-Marcos, M.: *Rev. Esp. Obstet. Ginec.*, 1:1, 1944.
16. Botella, J.: *Rev. Franç. d'Endocr. Clin. Nutr. Metab.*, 4:397, 1963.
17. Botella, J.: *Proceed. 1st Internat. Congr. Exfol. Cytol.* Philadelphia, J. B. Lippincott, 1962.
18. Brewer, H. C., and Jones, O. I.: *Amer. J. Obstet. Gynec.*, 55:18, 1958.
19. Brown, J. B.: *J. Endocr.*, 19:52, 1959.
20. Burrows, H.: *The Biological Actions of the Sex Hormones.* Cambridge, Cambridge University Press, 1945.
21. Butcher, R. L., Chu, K. Y., and Mellamby, R. M.: *Endocrinology*, 71:810, 1962.
22. Callantyne, M. R., et al.: *Endocrinology*, 79:153, 1966.
23. Callantyne, M. R., Clemens, L. E., and Shih, Y. H.: *Proc. Soc. Exper. Biol. Med.*, 128:382, 1968.
24. Campbell, R. M., and Kosterlitz, H. W.: *J. Physiol.*, 106:12, 1947.
25. Caroll, W. R.: *Endocrinology*, 36:266, 1945.
26. Cliterhoe, H. J., and Leathem, J. H.: *Endocrinology*, 76:127, 1965.
27. Cochrane, R. L., and Holmes, R. L.: *J. Endocr.*, 35:427, 1966.
28. Culiner, A., and Shippel, S.: *J. Obstet. Gynec. Brit. Emp.*, 56:439, 1959.
29. Davis, M. E., and Wied, G. L.: *J. Clin. Endocr.*, 17:1237, 1957.
30. Delson, B.: *Amer. J. Obstet. Gynec.*, 57:1120, 1949.
31. Desclin, L., Flament-Durand, J., and Gepts, W.: *Endocrinology*, 70:429, 1962.
32. Diczfalusy, E., and Lauritzen, C.: *Oestrogene beim Menschen.* Berlin, Springer, 1961.
33. Dordelman, P., and Wolker, H.: *Münch. Med. Wschr.*, 110:2061, 1968.
34. Dorfman, R. I.: *Endocrinology*, 68:43, 1961.
35. Dorfman, R. I., Kincl, F. A., and Ringold, H. J.: *Endocrinology*, 68:17, 1961.
36. Dorfman, R. I.: *Endocrinology*, 71:492, 1962.
37. Döring, G. K.: *Arch. Gynäk.*, 199:115, 1963.
38. Dörner, G.: *Zbl. Gynäk.*, 84:737, 1963.
39. Edgren, R. A., and Peterson, A. L.: *Acta Endocr.*, 47:485, 1964.
40. Edgren, R. A., Parlow, A. F., and Peterson, A. L.: *Endocrinology*, 76:97, 1965.
41. Engel, P., and Rosenberg, E.: *Endocrinology*, 37:45, 1945.
42. Falconer, B.: *Acta Obstet. Gynec. Scand.*, 26:453, 1946.
43. Ferin, J.: *Bull. Soc. Roy. Belg. Obstet. Gynec.*, 25:265, 1955.
44. Ferin, J., and Vanek, R.: *Ann. d'Endocr.*, 19:545, 1958.
45. Furlong, E., et al.: *Endocrinology*, 45:1, 1949.
46. Gardner, W. U.: *Cancer Res.*, 1:632, 1941.
47. Gilbert-Dreyfus, P.: *Med. Franç.*, 47:264, 1960.
48. Giorgy, E. P.: *J. Reprod. Fertil.*, 10:309, 1965.
49. Greenblatt, R. B., and Barfield, W. E.: *J. Clin. Clin. Endocr.*, 11:821, 1951.
50. Greenblatt, R. B.: *J. Clin. Endocr.*, 16:289, 1956.
51. Greenblatt, R. B., Roy, S., and Mahesh, V. B.: *Amer. J. Obstet. Gynec.*, 84:900, 1962.
52. Greenwald, G. S.: *J. Reprod. Fertil.*, 2:351, 1961.
53. Greenwald, G. S.: *Endocrinology*, 71:664, 1962.
54. Hanahan, D. J., et al.: *Endocrinology*, 53:163, 1953.
55. Holmstrom, G., and MacLennan, W. R.: *Amer. J. Obstet. Gynec.*, 53:727, 1947.
56. Houssay, B. A.: "Tumores Suprarrenales con Acción Estrogénica en los Animales Castrados," Geneva, *Proceed. II World Congr. Gyn. Obst.*, 1954. Ed. L. Georg, Geneva, 1955.
57. Huet, J. A., et al.: "Le Syndrome Hepato-Ovarien," *L'Expansion Scientifique Francaise.* Paris, 1949.
58. Hunter, F., and Leathem, J. H.: *Endocrinology*, 82:171, 1968.
59. Ingersoll, F. M., and MacArthur, J. W.: *Amer. J. Obstet. Gynec.*, 77:795, 1959.
60. Jackson, R. L., and Dockerty, M. B.: *Amer. J. Obstet. Gynec.*, 73:161, 1957.
61. Jacobs, W. M., and Lindlay, J. E.: *Amer. J. Obstet. Gynec.*, 71:1323, 1956.
62. Johanson, E. D. B., and Knobil, E.: *Endocrinology*, 84:464, 1969.
63. Keyes, R. H.: *Endocrinology*, 44:274, 1949.
64. Kistner, R. W.: *Amer. J. Obstet. Gynec.*, 75:264, 1958.
65. Kistner, R. W.: *Amer. J. Obstet. Gynec.*, 81:233, 1961.
66. Kistner, R. W., and Smith, O. W.: *Fertil. Steril.*, 12:121, 1961.
67. Kistner, R. W.: *The Use of Progestins in Obstetrics and Gynecology.* Chicago, Year Book Publishers, Inc., 1969.
68. Kline, I. T., and Dorfman, R. I.: *Endocrinology*, 48:345, 1951.
69. Kobilova, J.: *Acta Cytol.*, 11:497, 1967.
70. Kottmeier, H. L.: *Acta Obstet. Gynec. Scand.*, 27:Suppl. 5, 1948.
71. Kourides, I. A., and Kistner, R. W.: *Obstet. Gynec.*, 31:821, 1968.
72. Laufer, A., and Sulman, F. G.: *J. Clin. Endocr.*, 16:1151, 1956.
73. Lerner, L. J., Holthaus, F. J., and Thompson, F. J. A.: *Endocrinology*, 63:295, 1958.
74. Leventhal, M. L.: *Amer. J. Obstet. Gynec.*, 76:825, 1958.
75. Lipschütz, A. von: *Steroid Hormones and Tumours.* Baltimore, Williams & Wilkins Co., 1950.
76. Little, C. C.: *Amer. J. Obstet. Gynec.*, 61A:64, 1951.
77. Lopez, J. M., Migeon, C. J., and Seegar-Jones, G.: *Amer. J. Obstet. Gynec.*, 98:749, 1967.
78. Lopez, J. M., Migeon, C. J., and Seegar-Jones, G.: *Amer. J. Obstet. Gynec.*, 103:555, 1969.
79. Lyngbye, J., and Morgensen, E. F.: *Acta Endocr.*, 36:350, 1961.
80. MacArthur, J. W., et al.: *J. Clin. Endocr.*, 18:1202, 1958.
81. McCarthy, C. P., Mroueh, A., and Glass, R. H.: *Obstet. Gynec.*, 33:792, 1969.
82. MacKelvey, M. I., and Samuels, R. M.: *Amer. J. Obstet. Gynec.*, 53:627, 1947.
83. Marin-Bonachera, E.: *Acta Soc. Esp. Esterilidad*, 4:192, 1956.
84. Marshall, J. M., and O'Brien, O. P.: *Endocrinology*, 80:748, 1967.
85. Maurizio, E., and Pasetto, N.: "L'Hiperestrogenismo Extraovarico," in *Atti e Memorie della Società Italiana d'Endocrinologia.* Livorno, Editorial Belforte, 1955.
86. Mellicow, M. M., and Cahill, G. F.: *J. Clin. Endocr.*, 10:24, 1950.

87. Mellinger, R. C., et al.: *J. Clin. Endocr.*, 15:567, 1955.
87a. Merrill, J. A.: *Amer. J. Obstet. Gynec.*, 78:1258, 1959.
88. Meyerson, B. J., and Lindstrom, L.: *Acta Endocr.*, 59:41, 1968.
89. Miklosi, S. A., and MacCosker, P. J.: *J. Endocr.*, 39:361, 1967.
90. Montalvo, L.: *Acta Cytol.*, 12:95, 1968.
91. Montalvo, L.: *Acta Cytol.*, 12:118, 1968.
92. Moor, R. M., and Robson, L. E. A.: *J. Reprod. Fertil.*, 11:307, 1966.
93. Moricard, R., and Moricard, F.: *Gynec. Obstet.*, 47:131, 1950.
94. Morris, J. M., and Scully, R. E.: *Endocrine Pathology of the Ovary*. St. Louis, C. V. Mosby, 1958.
95. Pearlman, W. H., and De Meio, R. H.: *J. Biol. Chem.*, 179:141, 1949.
96. Perry, J. S., and Rowlands, I. W.: *J. Reprod. Fertil.*, 2:332, 1961.
97. Peterson, D. L., Edgren, R. A., and Jones, R. C.: *J. Endocr.*, 29:255, 1964.
98. Pincus, G., et al.: *Endocrinology*, 59:695, 1956.
99. Purshottan, W.: *Amer. J. Obstet. Gynec.*, 83:1405, 1962.
100. Rinard, G. A.: *Endocrinology*, 82:786, 1968.
101. Roberts, S., and Szego, C.: *Endocrinology*, 40:73, 1947.
102. Ryan, K. J., and Engel, L. L.: *Endocrinology*, 53:277, 1953.
103. Schröder, R.: *Arch. Gynäk.*, 104:27, 1915.
104. Scommegna, A., Del Castillo, E., Borushek, S., and Gold, J. J.: *Fertil. Steril.*, 16:571, 1965.
105. Scott, R. B., and Wharton, R. L.: *Amer. J. Obstet. Gynec.*, 84:867, 1962.
106. Segaloff, R., et al.: *J. Biol. Chem.*, 173:431, 1948.
107. Seitz, L.: *Arch. Gynäk.*, 173:376, 1942.
108. Short, R. V.: *J. Endocr.*, 24:59, 1962.
109. Singh, K. B.: *Amer. J. Obstet. Gynec.*, 103:1078, 1969.
110. Singher, H. O., et al.: *J. Biol. Chem.*, 154:79, 1944.
111. Smith, G. V., Smith, O. W., and Pincus, G.: *Amer. J. Physiol.*, 121:98, 1938.
112. Sopeña, A.: *Rev. Esp. Obstet. Gin.*, 5:1, 85, 165, 225, 229, 1946.
113. Sopeña, A., and Tornero, M. C.: *Actas Soc. Esp. Esterilidad*, 4:247, 1956.
114. Sommers, S. C., and Wadam, P. J.: *Amer. J. Obstet. Gynec.*, 72:160, 1956.
115. Southam, A. L.: *Ann. N.Y. Acad. Sci.*, 75:840, 1959.
116. Spiegel, A.: *Virchows Arch.*, 305:367, 1940.
117. Staemmler, H. J.: *Klin. Wschr.*, 38:940, 1960.
118. Stimmell, B. F., and Steale, C. F.: *J. Clin. Endocr.*, 12:489, 1952.
118a. Strong, J. A., et al.: *Lancet*, 2:955, 1956.
119. Sun, L. C. D., and Rakoff, A. E.: *J. Clin. Endocr.*, 16:971, 1956.
120. Sutherland, A. M., and MacBride, J. M.: *J. Obstet. Gynec. Brit. Emp.*, 61:238, 1964.
121. Szego, C.: *Endocrinology*, 57:541, 1955.
122. Taymor, M. L., and Sturgis, S. H.: *Amer. J. Obstet. Gynec.*, 79:316, 1960.
123. Te Linde, R. W., and Wharton, L. R.: *Amer. J. Obstet. Gynec.*, 80:844, 1960.
124. Telegdy, G., and Rubin, B. L.: *Steroids*, 8:441, 1966.
125. Timonen, S.: *Geburtsh. Frauenhk.*, 20:780, 1960.
126. Ufer, J.: *Acta Gin.*, 4:215, 1953.
127. Ufer, J.: *Hormontherapie in der Frauenheilkunde*. Berlin, Walter de Gruyter, 1959.
128. Uncini-Manganelli, C., and Becca, B.: *Riv. Ital. Ginec.*, 52:259, 1968.
129. Valcourt, A. J., et al.: *Endocrinology*, 57:692, 1955.
130. Van Der Linde, R., and Westerfeld, W. W.: *Endocrinology*, 47:265, 1950.
131. Vara, P., and Nemineva, K.: *Acta Obstet. Gynec. Scand.*, 31:94, 1952.
132. Varangot, J., Cedard, L., and Tchobrovsky, C.: *Ann. d'Endocr.*, 23:45, 1962.
133. Vasington, F. D., et al.: *Endocrinology*, 62:557, 1958.
134. Wahlen, T.: *Acta Obstet. Gynec. Scand.*, 29: Suppl. 6, 1949.
135. Watterville, H. de: *J. Clin. Endocr.*, 11:251, 1951.
136. Weifenbach, H.: *Acta Endocr.*, 50:7, 1965.
137. Weisz, J., and Lloyd, C. W.: *Endocrinology*, 77:735, 1965.
138. Wied, G. L.: *Acta Cytol.*, 2:269, 1958.
139. Wied, G. L.: *Acta Cytol.*, 12:87, 1968.
140. Wyss, R. H., Karsznia, R., Henrichs, L. R. W., and Herrmann, W. L.: *J. Clin. Endocr.*, 28:1824, 1968.
141. Yin, P. S., and Sommers, S. C.: *J. Clin. Endocr.*, 21:472, 1961.
142. Zander, J., et al.: *Geburtsh. u. Frauenhk.*, 23:871, 1963.
143. Zarrow, M. X., Sundram, S. K., and Stob, M.: *Proc. Soc. Exper. Biol. Med.*, 119:331, 1965.
144. Zondek, B., and Finkelstein, M.: *Endocrinology*, 36:291, 1945.

Chapter 29

CORPUS LUTEUM SYNDROMES, OVARIAN HYPERANDROGENISM

In this chapter are discussed two types of syndromes which, though differing significantly from each other, are to a certain degree related. The first group is caused by pathologic alterations of the corpus luteum which, rather than producing hyperluteinism, most often lead to ovarian dysfunction because of impaired luteal activity. The second group comprises those conditions in which ovarian androgen synthesis, occurring to a minor degree in normal ovaries, is pathologically enhanced. The subject of hyperluteinism and hyperandrogenism of ovarian origin, resulting from functioning tumors, is dealt with in Chapter 30.

29.1. LUTEAL INSUFFICIENCY

29.1.1. INTRODUCTION

Progestational insufficiency is by far the most important of all disorders of corpus luteum function. By progestational insufficiency we mean "defective function, as to intensity or duration, of the progestational corpus luteum." Two forms of luteal insufficiency are to be distinguished: that of the *progestational corpus* and that of the *gestational corpus.* As pointed out by us on various previous occasions, the form causing the most serious consequences for woman's fertility is not, as might be expected, that of the gestational corpus, i.e., insufficiency of the corpus luteum of pregnancy, but rather insufficiency of the mensual (progestational) corpus luteum.[15, 17, 19] During the second half of the menstrual cycle, no other endocrine gland is able to replace progesterone production by the progestational corpus luteum; in contrast, during pregnancy in primates,[10, 11, 17, 18] additional sources of progestogen production are provided by the young chorion and by the adrenal glands. This accounts for the fact, which although it was long known was confirmed only recently,[18, 161] that lutectomy during the first few months of gestation causes abortion in only about 15 per cent of the cases. On the other hand, deficient function of the progestational corpus is known to account for a good many cases of infertility and early as well as late abortion. Recent publications on the subject[16, 88, 96, 105] have come to confirm our observations and underline the clinical significance of this syndrome.

29.1.2. CONCEPT OF LUTEAL INSUFFICIENCY

Luteal insufficiency, as defined here, refers to deficient corpus luteum function in terms of *intensity* and *duration*. The reason for using intensity and duration as parameters is based on our past experience, through which we were able to discern two basic types of dysfunction. The development and regression of the progestational corpus luteum were studied by Brewer and Jones[22] and, later, by Noyes and Haman.[117] In a 28 day cycle, the acme of secretory activity should last from the sixteenth through the twenty-fourth day before declining. This phase is usually demarcated by a "plateau" in basal body temperature recordings. On studying temperature charts in cases with a diagnosis of progestational insufficiency, we observe that some plateaux were of normal height but were several days short in duration, whereas others had the normal span of eight to 10 days but were low in height. Graphs of this kind, however, would be worthless unless correlated with endometrial histology and with the rate of pregnanediol excretion. In the first type, pregnanediol excretion either started later or terminated earlier than normally, or both, while endometrial biopsies revealed a well developed, though chronologically delayed, secretory phase. For instance, endometria obtained on the twenty-third or twenty-fourth day of the cycle would show features of an eighteenth or nineteenth day endometrium, such as tall columnar cells with subnuclear glycogen, stainable glycerophosphatase within the gland spaces, etc. In the second variety, on the other hand, urinary pregnanediol was detected early but gave values below 3 mg per 24 hr, while the endometrium showed poor secretory transformation and secretory changes were inconspicuous although present from an early as the fifteenth or sixteenth day of the cycle. In addition, their glycogen content was scanty and showed gradations that imperceptibly blended into such other cases as would obviously qualify as "monophasic cycles."

Consequently, there are two fundamental varieties of luteal insufficiency: (1) that resulting from shortened phase, and (2) that resulting from weakened phase.

LUTEAL INSUFFICIENCY DUE TO SHORTENED PHASE. Shortening of the secretory phase may be the result of two different mechanisms: premature decay of the corpus or insufficient luteotrophic action. The latter has not yet been adequately studied but could explain why an initially well formed corpus luteum should degenerate prematurely. The luteotrophic principle of the anterior lobe of the pituitary is known to be identical to prolactin, so that luteal insufficiency, owing to short-lived or ephemeral corpus luteum function, may actually be caused by *prolactin insufficiency*. Regarding body temperature, two different types of curves may occur. The first is a curve matching the normal menstrual rhythm, that is, lasting for 28 days, but in which ovulation is delayed, taking place around the eighteenth or twentieth day, as shown in Figure 29-1. If the duration of the cycle in such cases is not shortened, it is because the proliferative phase lasts longer than normally. If the secretory phase of a case similar to that illustrated had a normal physiologic duration, the entire cycle would have to last longer. Thus, these are cycles in which the duration of the proliferative phase is lengthened by the same number of days by which the secretory phase is shortened. We chose to call such forms luteal insufficiency *with delayed ovulation*. There is another variety of shortened secretory phase which occurs in short cycles in which the proliferative phase is of normal duration but the secretory phase is reduced to as much as a bare four days. In the latter type of cycle, urinary pregnanediol occurs in approximately physiologic titers, but excretion is *confined to a much shorter period of time*. Such conditions may be categorized as having a secretory phase of normal intensity but of reduced duration.

So far as endometrial histology is con-

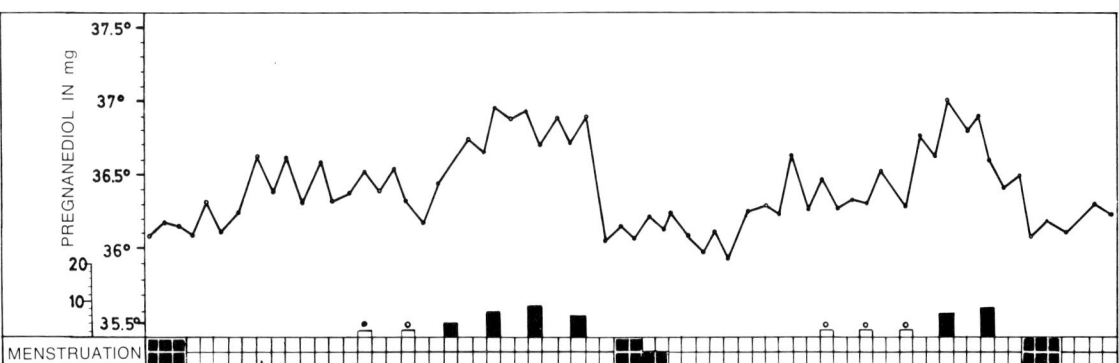

Figure 29–1. Basal body temperature recording and urinary pregnanediol values in luteal insufficiency resulting from shortened secretory phase.

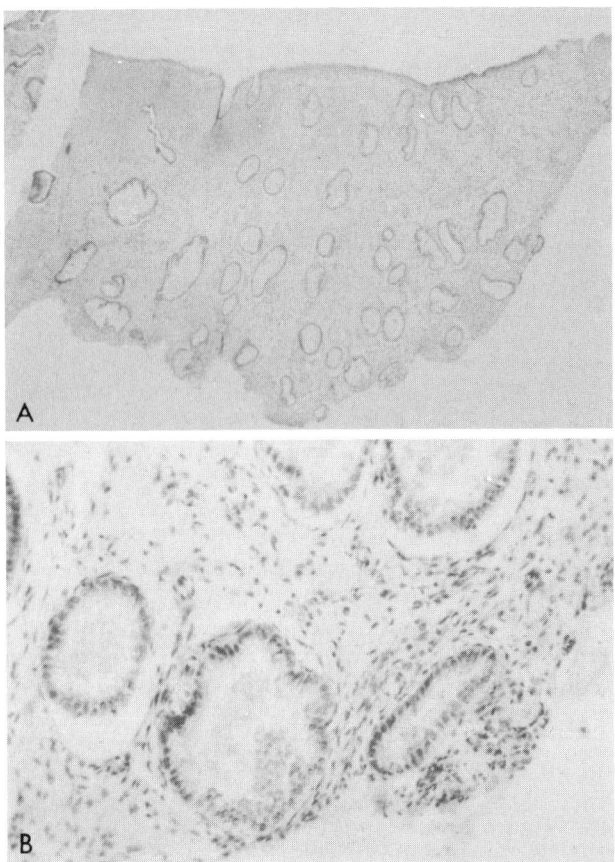

Figure 29-2. Progestational insufficiency. A, Endometrial biopsy taken on twenty-third day of cycle, showing marked glycopenia (Best's carmine stain, 35×). B, Detail from same specimen, at higher magnification (100×).

cerned (Fig. 29-2), the findings are distinctive in that, during the last week of the cycle, with menstruation imminent, the pattern is still only that of an early secretory phase. Phosphatase studies are usually very informative, revealing still positive reactions in gland lumina, whose contents normally would have turned negative by this time. Epithelia may still be tall columnar and reveal glycogen accumulations in the basal portions of cells.

LUTEAL INSUFFICIENCY DUE TO WEAKENED PHASE. A second variety of luteal insufficiency is found in women in whom corpus luteum function is of *normal duration* but secretory activity is *diminished in intensity*. The thermal chart characteristic of the latter modality is illustrated in Figure 29-3. It reveals that ovulation occurs in a normal way, with the thermal elevation taking place at the expected time, but that sometimes this elevation is so slight as to be questionable. At the same time, although urines become positive for pregnanediol at the right time, the observed values remain low. Montalvo,[106] at our clinic, found that vaginal cytologic findings in such patients showed scanty numbers of folded cells and bore cytohormonal resemblance to smears seen in follicular persistence.

Endometrial findings reveal a poorly developed secretory phase. The appearance of glands suggests low functional capacity owing to inadequate secretory transformation (Fig. 29-4). The finding that glycogen deposits are scanty in such deficiently transformed glands is of similar significance (Fig. 29-2). This modality thereby differs from the preceding one, since glycogen in the former is deposited in normal amounts and at the expected rate although afterwards it disappears at a markedly delayed rate.

Malkani,[98] as well as Botella in earlier works, described progestational endometrial insufficiency resulting from *endometritis*, which in fact is not an instance of corpus luteum dysfunction but represents a disorder at the end-organ level and should

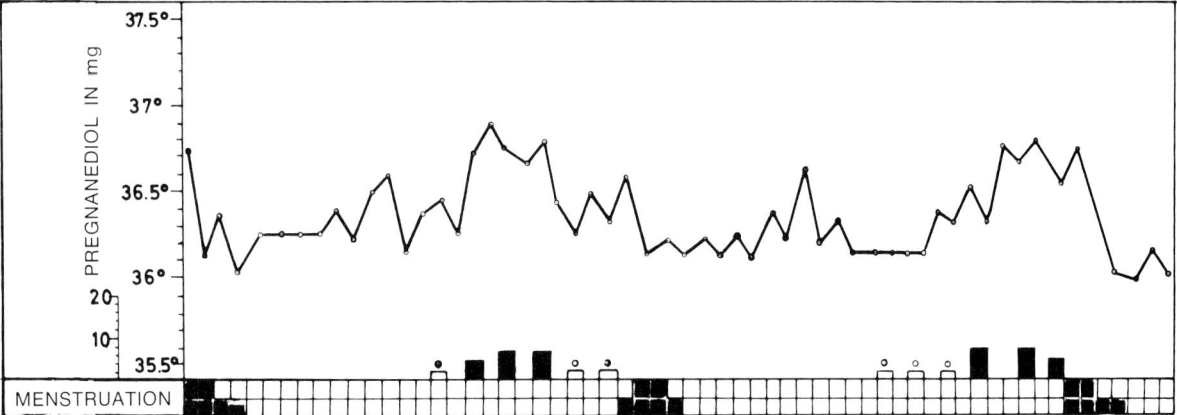

Figure 29–3. Luteal insufficiency with secretory phase of normal duration but decreased intensity: Pregnanediol excretion lasts as long as that of normal cycle but reveals low values.

not be included in the present category. Pertinent data concerning progestational insufficiency are summarized in Table 29–1.

29.1.3. INCIDENCE OF PROGESTATIONAL INSUFFICIENCY

Progestational insufficiency is a relatively common finding. Among our statistical data, compiled from 3000 endometrial biopsies from cases of sterility, which constitute the largest published series of its kind, we found 182 cases with this type of insufficiency, that is, a total incidence of 6.06 per cent (see Table 29–2).

Undoubtedly, the incidence of progestational insufficiency in the Madrid series is lower than that reported from any other part of the world, which to some extent may be

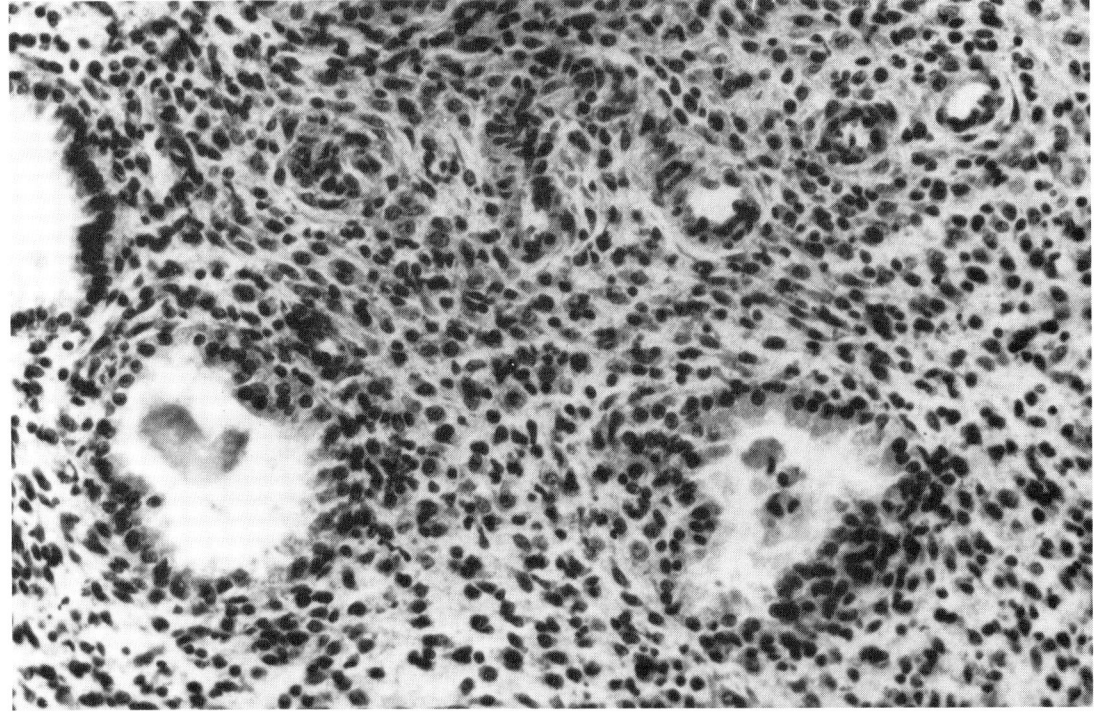

Figure 29–4. Endometrium in progestational insufficiency. Glands are poorly developed, although the stroma shows evidence of progestational changes, with ingrowth of spiral vessels.

TABLE 29-1. Progestational Insufficiency

SHORT PROGESTATIONAL PHASE	PROGESTATIONAL PHASE WITH ABSOLUTE INSUFFICIENCY
Corpus luteum: Decaying rapidly	*Corpus luteum:* Malformed
Etiology: Pituitary luteotrophic insufficiency	*Etiology:* Gonadotropin (LH) insufficiency
Temperature rise: Normal, few days' duration	*Temperature rise:* Low, of normal duration
Pregnanediol: Normal rate, few days' duration	*Pregnanediol:* Low
Endometrial pattern: Early secretory	*Endometrial pattern:* Insufficient secretory transformation

TABLE 29-2. Incidence of Progestational Insufficiency* Among Endometrial Biopsies from 3000 Cases of Infertility†

TYPE OF ENDOMETRIUM	NUMBER OF CASES	PERCENTAGE
Secretory:		
Normal	1351	45.03
Insufficient	182	6.06
Hyperplastic	119	3.96
Proliferative:		
Normal	303	10.10
Insufficient	221	7.36
Hyperplastic	270	9.00

*Incidence of progestational insufficiency: 6.06 per cent.
†From Botella-Llusiá.

due to the strict diagnostic criteria we used. Nevertheless, as shown in Table 29-3, our figures compare well with those reported by Noyes[117] and by Foss and his associates,[46] who are recognized authorities on the subject.

Thus, *progestational insufficiency affects approximately six in every 100 women coming for consultation because of infertility.*

The question naturally arises whether the changes observed in the secretory phase are by themselves responsible for infertility or whether they are incidental to different, more profound underlying causes. In order to provide an answer to this question, we undertook a study the results of which are listed in Table 29-4. From among our 182 instances of progestational insufficiency, we examined 60 cases in which complete data—i.e., so-called "minimal requirements," such as fertility studies on both marriage partners—were available. In 13 cases (21 per cent), infertility could have been accounted for by evidence of seminal changes in the male; 7 cases revealed tubal obstruction or serious tubal dysfunction. In addition to these, various clinical or uterine findings known to be of relative significance in infertility were found in 15 cases (25 per cent). In the remaining 25 couples, that is, 42 per cent of the entire series examined, there was no other detectable cause for infertility in either member other than the insufficient secretory endometrium found in the first instance, which thus had to be assumed to be solely responsible for the absence of pregnancy. When these figures are projected against the total number of infertile couples, it may be asserted that 2.5 per cent of all infertile marriages seem to owe their infertility to this type of alteration.

Various authors[25, 56, 98, 117] emphasize how difficult it is to attribute sterility in a given case to progestational insufficiency alone. To do so, not only must endometrial biopsy confirm the presence of defective endometrial development, but the latter finding

TABLE 29-3. Incidence of Progestational Insufficiency, According to Different Sources

AUTHOR	YEAR	NO. OF CASES EXAMINED	PROGESTATIONAL INSUFFICIENCY	PERCENTAGE
Palmer[119]	1950	99	28	28.2
Hughes, Van Nees and Lloyd[60]	1950	324	162	50.0
Kurzrock[77]	1951	2667	305	11.4
Noyes[117]	1953	2227	203	9.1
Gillam[50]	1955	134	18	14.3
Foss, Horne and Hertig[46]	1958	856	54	6.3
Cohen and Hankin[32]	1959	122	32	26.2
Botella[16]	1959	2000	119	5.2
Malkani[98]	1962	2556	439	17.2
Botella[21]	1963	3000	182	6.1

TABLE 29-4. Cases of Progestational Insufficiency and Other Possible Causes of Infertility in Either Mate

NO. OF CASES EXAMINED	MALE FACTORS	TUBAL FACTORS	CERVICAL OR UTERINE FACTORS	NO OTHER CAUSE FOR INFERTILITY
60	13 (21%)	7 (11%)	15 (25%)	25 (42%)

Incidence of progestational insufficiency: 6.06 per cent. Corrected incidence of progestational insufficiency as effective cause of infertility: 2.54 per cent.

must also be supported by ancillary means, such as urinary pregnanediol determinations and study of exfoliative cytology and basal body temperature curves. Even then, the diagnosis of progestational insufficiency established for one particular cycle cannot be interpreted as the patient's cause of infertility, since it may not be representative of all other cycles. It is mainly for reasons such as these, involving diagnostic considerations, that our figures concerning the incidence of progestational insufficiency as the sole cause of infertility may be below those reported by other authors.

29.1.4. ANATOMIC BASIS OF PROGESTATIONAL INSUFFICIENCY

There is as yet little known regarding which type of corpora lutea are indeed insufficient. While different anomalies in corpus luteum development may be recognized at laparotomy, it remains to be shown conclusively that such anomalies in effect correspond to the functional alterations just described.

A common finding relative to poorly developed corpora lutea, or *corpora lutea aberrantia*,[22, 25, 46, 51] is that they are frequently observed in hypoplastic or senile ovaries. In other instances, the corpus luteum is found to have been the site of hemorrhage (*hemorrhagic corpus luteum*) (Fig. 29-5). A more rare finding, described by Stieve,[152] is the luteinization of unruptured follicles, which necessarily must be assumed to be insufficient.

A further form of *relative insufficiency* of the luteal phase, in which hyperestrinism coexists with progesterone production, has been observed by us in ovaries revealing coincidence of corpora lutea with mature follicles, illustrated in Figure 29-6.

29.1.5. MECHANISM OF INFERTILITY DUE TO PROGESTATIONAL INSUFFICIENCY

Our criteria for progestational insufficiency have already been indicated to be based on delayed formation of the corpus luteum, or on a hypoplastic corpus, following otherwise normal ovulation that may lead to fertilization, rather than on total absence of luteinization, as may be the case in anovulatory cycles. *Infecundity*, in this case, is not caused by lack of fertilization but results from inability of the blastocyst

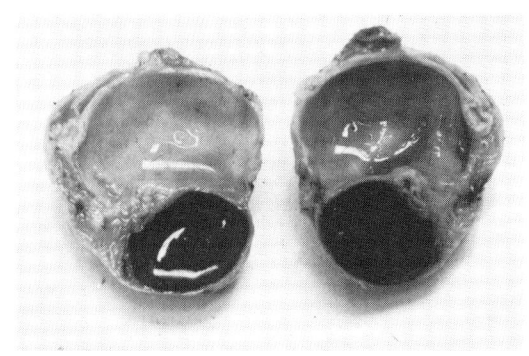

Figure 29-5. Hematoma of the corpus luteum, causing luteal insufficiency.

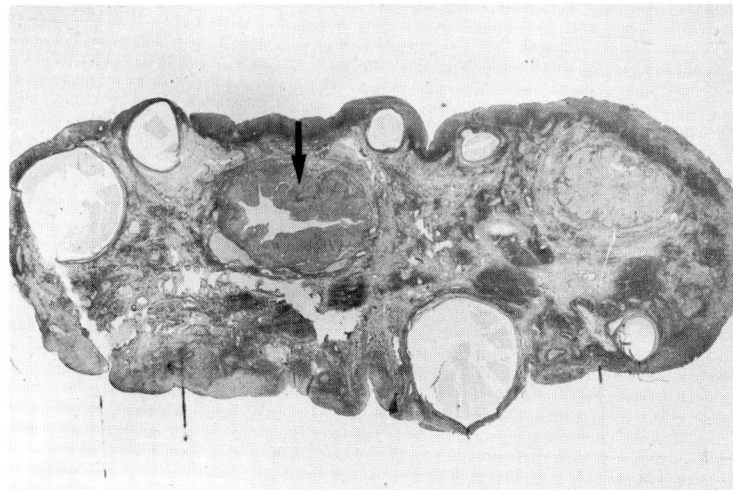

Figure 29–6. Ovary with several persistent follicles and corpus luteum in retrogression (arrow). There was evidence of anovulation in the last cycle and progestational insufficiency in preceding cycles.

to implant in the uterus.[15, 18] Recent studies concerning the mechanism of implantation[29, 36, 91, 101] have demonstrated that progesterone plays an essential role in the nidation of the mammalian egg. Studies on deferred implantation in some wild animals, such as the armadillo, deer, bison and marten,[29, 36, 101] have shown a definite correlation between progesterone levels and the number of blastocysts accepted by the endometrium.

In the human species, implantation is not governed by the law of "all or nothing." Undoubtedly, between the two extremes of failure of nidation and complete nidation, there is a whole range of intermediate situations involving *defective nidation,* the significance of which is to be emphasized later.

Suffice it to say here that implantation may fail to take place because of faulty endometrial transformation resulting from corpus luteum deficiency in an ovulatory cycle.

29.1.6. DIAGNOSIS OF PROGESTATIONAL INSUFFICIENCY

One issue, which in our opinion has not been sufficiently emphasized, concerns *the minimal requirements for diagnosing progestational insufficiency.* The finding of an occasional cycle revealing a somewhat less developed secretory phase may obviously not serve as sufficient ground for establishing the diagnosis.[25] Above all, it is necessary that evidence of corpus luteum insufficiency be confirmed in every cycle, or in most cycles, of a female patient.

In addition, it must be borne in mind that a defective endometrial pattern per se does not constitute conclusive evidence, since it may reflect a local defect as a result of which the endometrial response to progesterone is impaired.[15, 98] Besides, it is necessary for biopsies to be repeated on the same day of the cycle to avoid errors of interpretation as a result of differences in the range of secretory patterns occurring between beginning and end of each phase.[117]

In this respect, it must be remembered that there is a form of progestational insufficiency that is characterized only by a late start of the secretory phase, so that what may be a normal pattern on the eighteenth day may be a pathological one on the twenty-sixth day. Nor must the physician depend on endometrial biopsy as his sole guideline; pregnanediol determinations, cytology and study of body temperatures are also necessary. For the diagnosis of progestational insufficiency to be firmly established, the following requirements must be fulfilled:

1. Endometrial pattern characteristic of secretory phase insufficiency on the twenty-fourth or twenty-fifth day of the cycle.
2. If possible, complete histologic study, including Gomori's stain for alkaline glycerophosphatase and the PAS method for glycogen. Familiarity with the sequence of

endometrial changes revealed by the above histochemical reactions in the course of the normal cycle is of considerable help in establishing the diagnosis.

3. Basal body temperature recordings, which must reveal either of the two patterns outlined previously.

4. Serial determinations of urinary pregnanediol must reveal values below 4 mg per 24 hr or must be negative up to the nineteenth day.

5. Serial study of vaginal cytology which should reveal estrogen-progesterone imbalance in terms of a persistent high karyopyknotic index, rather than absence of folded cells, during the second half of the cycle.

6. The presence of all of the above changes must be ascertained not just in one isolated cycle but also in the course of several consecutive cycles, since the occurrence of interspersed anovulatory cycles is a characteristic feature of this syndrome.

29.1.7. PROGESTATIONAL INSUFFICIENCY AND EARLY ABORTION

Although the previously mentioned correlation between progesterone levels and number of implantations is not apparent in the human species because, as a rule, there is only one egg implanted (only exceptionally two or more), Hertig and his co-workers[55,56] have described instances of defective implantation resulting in abortion. These pathologic implantations were characterized by too superficial nidation and by the fact that they occurred in endometria with poor secretory transformation.

All these facts lead one to suspect that while severe secretory insufficiency of the endometrium may well be associated with infertility because of total lack of implantation, occasionally an egg may nevertheless succeed in implanting, only to be affected by the deficient endometrial environment, which by itself is abortive in nature and leads to death.

This suspicion may be supported by one particular finding, made repeatedly in several instances among our study material, which to our knowledge had not been sufficiently studied and explored in the past. This consisted in relatively frequent microscopic evidence of abortive rests in premenstrual biopsies from patients with infertility. The women involved, who were being explored for primary or secondary sterility, in each case denied having had a recent miscarriage. Biopsies, however, revealed the presence of unquestionable

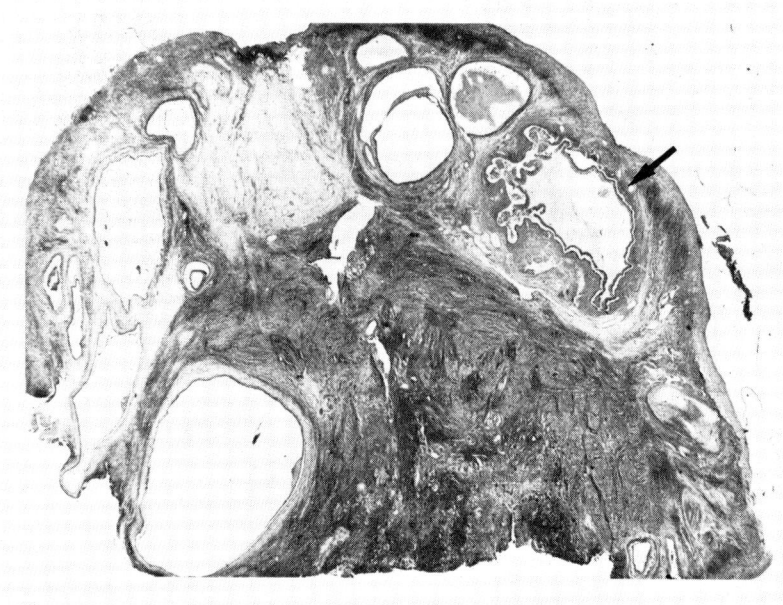

Figure 29-7. Ovary revealing numerous maturing follicles, as well as partially luteinized follicle undergoing atresia (arrow). Partial luteinization of this kind may be associated with mild progestational endometrial changes.

TABLE 29-5. Incidence of Ignored Early Abortion as Cause of Apparent Sterility in 3000 Infertile Women

ENDOMETRIAL FINDINGS	NO. OF CASES	PERCENTAGE
Abortive rests	40	1.33
In primary sterility	27	0.90
In secondary sterility	13	0.43
In villous stage	23	0.74
In previllous stage	8	0.28
Undetermined	9	0.29

chorionic tissue in endometria that otherwise were within normal limits and whose pattern corresponded to the day of the cycle on which they were obtained. Identical findings have been described by Marín and Botella[13, 99] under the designation "syndrome of ignored abortion as cause of apparent sterility in women," a term which, although somewhat lengthy, describes the syndrome fairly accurately. The incidence of this syndrome in our series of 3000 endometrial biopsies is given in Table 29-5.

The incidence of ignored abortion was 1.33 per cent. If one considers the fact that the finding in question is entirely fortuitous in any given cycle, this syndrome must necessarily be suspected to occur in many instances of infertility without being detected unless endometrial biopsies are taken during that particular cycle in which the incident happened to take place. It seems logical to assume that while a number of women undoubtedly have abortions that go undetected, such abortions must, as a rule, have occurred on repeated occasions for a woman to appear permanently infertile. This, to our view, means that infertility from early and subclinical abortion must have a much higher incidence than is presently suggested by available data. This point of view is supported by the observations of Hertig and his group,[46, 55, 56] who found that approximately 40 per cent of conceptuses, implanted in the uterus and discovered before the first missed menstruation, were potentially abortive. This means that *the abortivity of young embryos is of staggering proportions and eludes detection except for isolated instances.*

Prompted by our clinical findings, we have attempted to explore any possible existing relationship between ignored early abortion and progestational insufficiency. For that purpose we were guided by the previously outlined criteria concerning diagnosis, that is, that any insufficiency of this type could not be diagnosed unless found to be consistently present in several consecutive cycles. As a result, 20 of 40 patients, registered at our clinic for having previously revealed the above mentioned type of endometrial findings, were followed over several consecutive cycles by endometrial biopsies, pregnanediol determinations, serial study of vaginal cytology and meticulous plotting of temperature curves for up to six months. The results of this study are summarized in Table 29-6.

It may be noted that not only were hypoluteal cycles found to be surprisingly common but also, in addition, there were intercurrent anovulatory cycles. It was therefore apparent that these cycles comprised a whole range of transition forms between borderline hypoluteinism and the most complete form of hypoluteinism: aluteinism of the anovulatory cycle.

The total of the 80 cycles studied is broken down in Table 29-6. Sixty-three of these were either anovulatory or hypoluteal cycles, indicating an unusually high incidence (78 per cent) of progestational insufficiency in association with the syndrome of early abortion.

Thus, there is little doubt that the underlying cause for the syndrome of early abortion is progestational insufficiency which, by producing defective nidation, results in very early death of the embryo, the latter being, so to say, "swept away" with the first subsequent menstruation.

TABLE 29-6. Ignored Habitual Abortion: Follow-Up of Twenty Cases During Several Consecutive Cycles

TYPE OF CYCLE	CYCLE NUMBER					
	1	2	3	4	5	6
Normal	4	6	3	2	1	2
Progestational insufficiency	11	11	14	10	6	4
Anovulatory	2	3	1	0	0	1
Not studied	4	0	2	8	13	13
Per cent of normal	20	30	15	10	5	10

29.1.8. PROGESTATIONAL INSUFFICIENCY AND LATE ABORTION

The term "late abortion" is used here in contradistinction to the preceding type of abortion, but it actually refers to abortuses of two to three months' gestation, that is, *clinical* abortions in instances in which menstruation has been missed once or twice.

It must be added that what is under consideration here is not the functioning of the corpus luteum of pregnancy but that of the mensual or *progestational* corpus luteum. The changes occurring in the former in abortion have been studied in depth[9, 34, 41, 50, 93] and will not be entered into here. It is our belief that gestational luteal deficiencies play a much lesser role in the genesis of abortion than is generally thought and that whenever abortion supervenes, it is caused not by alterations in ovarian progestogen synthesis but rather by alterations in progestogen synthesis by the chorion. However, leaving the question of gestational disorders for future consideration, our present concern is to establish whether progestational insufficiency, by affecting the mode of implantation, is capable of causing late abortion.

MacBryde and Moyes[93] reported that, of a series of 175 women with habitual abortion, 67 per cent of patients had hypoluteal cycles. Pigeaud and his associates[123] found endometrial vascular sclerosis as the cause of repeated abortions and, similarly, in a follow-up of habitual abortions, Javert[64] found evidence of chronic changes in corpus luteum function. Botella[17, 18, 19] emphasized the frequency with which he observed anovulatory or hypoluteal cycles in women with habitual abortion. In Table 29-7, we have summarized our observations on a group of 50 habitual aborters, followed over a total of 117 cycles by means of the same exploratory methods that were used on the patients of Table 29-6. The results are quite similar to those obtained previously, revealing an incidence of between 75 and 92 per cent hypoluteal or anovulatory cycles. Thus, the incidence of progestational insufficiency and associated faulty implantation is equally high in late abortion.

Another study was undertaken to determine the significance of *hypoluteal etiology* as compared to other causes of abortion. An eliminatory study, similar to the one on infertility from hypoluteinism that is summarized in Table 29-4, was set up for that purpose. The problems encountered proved to be more difficult to solve, owing to the fact that the causes for habitual abortion are not so clear-cut or readily demonstrable as those producing infertility. Nevertheless, the results shown in Table 29-8 are fairly informative. On the basis of these data, it may be concluded that repeated abortions, even though occurring at a considerably advanced stage of gestation, have a hypoluteal etiology in no less than 20 per cent of cases.

Among the conditions playing an important role in endometrial implantation, the so-called "irritable uterus" syndrome must be mentioned as a frequent cause of abortion. According to the observations of Palmer,[119] this is similarly the result of luteal insufficiency.

As stated earlier, insufficiency of the corpus luteum of pregnancy, that is, *gestational insufficiency,* is not of great consequence in the production of abortion

TABLE 29-7. Clinically Noticeable Abortions: 50 Cases Studied During a Total of 117 Consecutive Cycles

TYPE OF CYCLE	CYCLE NUMBER					
	1	2	3	4	5	6
Normal	3	7	2	3	1	4
Progestational insufficiency	21	23	11	8	11	21
Anovulatory	0	1	0	1	0	0
Not studied	26	21	37	38	38	25
Per cent of normal	14	24	15	25	8	16

TABLE 29-8. Cases of Habitual Abortion in Which Other Possible Etiologic Factors Were Considered

NUMBER OF CASES	ANOMALOUS CAVITY°	ENDOCRINE ALTERATIONS†	OTHER CAUSES‡	NO OTHER ETIOLOGY
50	16 (32%)	15 (30%)	9 (18%)	10 (20%)

°Anomalous cavity: Incompetent cervix or bicornuate uterus.
†Endocrine alterations: Thyroidopathies, prediabetes and diabetes.
‡Other causes: Syphilis, toxoplasmosis, listeriosis, etc.

owing to the fact that, once gestation has been initiated, the young chorion and certainly also the adrenal cortex are capable of synthesizing progesterone. In contrast, *defective preparation of the endometrial bed* causes inadequate nidation, thus jeopardizing adequate trophoblastic function from the very outset, from both the endocrine and the nutritional points of view, and carrying the potential threat of abortion, which may supervene either at once, before the first menstruation is missed, or at a later stage, during the second or third month of gestation.

29.1.9. ETIOLOGY AND TREATMENT OF PROGESTATIONAL INSUFFICIENCY

ETIOLOGY. For the time being, studies aimed at clarifying the underlying etiology of this endocrine disorder have, to our knowledge, not yet been undertaken. While the foregoing discussion was concerned with the manner in which progestational insufficiency is diagnosed, the frequency with which it is observed and the disturbances it produces, data now available are unable to provide sufficient insight into the etiology of this endocrinopathy. In the absence of specific hormonal studies on the subject, whatever may be said concerning its etiology at the present time is necessarily speculative. We believe that the disorder is of pituitary or hypophysiothalamic origin and depends on failure of *luteotrophic hormone (LTH) secretion* rather than on FSH or LH deficiency, since the task of preserving the corpus luteum belongs to LTH.

The recent investigations by Perloff[120] and Staemmler,[148] on urinary gonadotropin determinations (FSH and LH), suggest the possibility that a deficit in either, particularly LH, might be involved in corpus luteum insufficiency. Similarly, using the dexamethasone-gonadotropin test (see Chapter 24), Laitinen and Pesonen[78] have found cases in which lack of gonadotropins was associated with poor formation of corpora lutea. Finally, Callard and Leathem,[27] Gospodarovicz[53] and Lindell[86] have all observed that, under various pathologic conditions, even well formed corpora lutea may fail to produce progesterone as a result of some alteration in their intimate mechanism of steroidogenesis.

TREATMENT OF PROGESTATIONAL INSUFFICIENCY. Obviously, so long as the etiology remains unknown, *therapy aimed at the causative factor* cannot be contemplated. Therapy therefore is confined to "hormonal substitution" and consists in administration of *progestogens* during the second half of the cycle, between days 14 and 28, in order to compensate for secretory corpus luteum failure and to facilitate adequate development of the progestational reaction in the endometrium. The *type of preparation* preferred by us is 17-hydroxyprogesterone caproate. We do not advise the use of norethisterone or of any of the synthetic progestogens that are active per os. This is because the latter type of progestins primarily induces stromal growth, while having little effect on the glands, whose secretion is extremely important for the implantation and nutrition of eggs in the morula stage.[36, 41] Another reason against the use of synthetic progestins is the fact that, whenever administered to women with delayed ovulation after the fourteenth day, these drugs may *inhibit ovulation.*

In this way, the daily absorption rate amounts to 15 or 20 mg, which corresponds roughly to the amount produced and metabolized by the body of normal progravid women.

Therapy of this type may be said to have generally favorable effects. Cohen and Hankin[32] reported that of 16 patients treated with caproate, four subsequently became pregnant, whereas no pregnancies developed in any of the 12 patients treated with norethisterone.

Although most of our own experience to date is with progesterone, that is, with *substitution therapy*, we now see great promise in *stimulation therapy*, which we have practiced in combination with HMG and HCG (Pergonal-Pribogonyl), or in combinations of Clomiphene with HCG.

29.2. HYPERLUTEINISM AND DYSLUTEINISM

Corpus luteum hyperfunction is much less common than luteal insufficiency. Genuine corpus luteum hyperfunction is observed only in extremely rare *ovarian luteomas*. Other than that, the different forms of luteal hyperfunction tend rapidly to acquire a degenerative character, which eventually converts initial hyperfunction into hypo- or dysfunction. It is mainly for this reason that the term *dysluteinism* is to be preferred to *hyperluteinism*.

The following conditions are to be examined: (1) follicle lutein cyst; (2) persistent corpus luteum; and (3) tumors of the corpus luteum.

29.2.1. FOLLICLE LUTEIN CYST

Abnormally elevated luteinizing activity is able to induce cystic development of the corpus luteum. It must be remembered, above all, that the cells of both the granulosa and the theca may be luteinized in response to LH activity. Therefore, the existence of two fundamental varieties of luteinized cysts may be admitted: the so-called luteinic cysts of the *granulosa* and cysts of the *theca*, more commonly known as *granulosa-lutein cysts* and *theca-lutein cysts*, respectively.

GRANULOSA-LUTEIN CYSTS. These are the more common variety of the two.[30] Distinction must be made between *cystic corpora lutea* and *genuine corpus luteum cysts*.

Cystic corpora lutea are often found in pregnancy and in general are not known to cause any severe endocrine disturbances.

In addition to these, Novak[116] distinguishes genuine corpus luteum cysts, which are commonly believed to be derived from a hematoma of the corpus luteum. During the hemorrhagic or vascularization phase of the corpus luteum, minor hemorrhage into the lumen occurs normally, but this is limited in extent. Sometimes, however, the cavity of the corpus is flooded with blood, giving rise to hematomas that may be of considerable size. Luteal cells are not subject to alterations and maintain their function during the early stages of development of this structure, but because the life span of luteal cells is limited, degenerative changes soon set in. As a result, fatty replacement and fibrosis develop, and the granulosa-lutein cells lose their function little by little; in contrast, the theca-lutein cells remain viable for long periods of time (Figs. 29–8 and 29–9). *As a result, a structure develops in which progesterone-producing luteal elements decline, whereas estrogen-producing thecal elements retain their activity.* The resulting cysts secrete predominantly estrogens, which justifies their name of follicle-lutein cysts, as they were designated by Novak[116] and later by Rowlands.[131]

Grossly, follicle-lutein cysts are cystic structures ranging from 2 to 7 cm in greatest dimension. Generally, their lining has a faint yellowish hue, and quite frequently they have a prominent vascular pattern which, being the residue of corpus luteum vascularization, distinguishes them from simple follicle cysts.

A common variety of follicle-lutein cysts are *corpus albicans cysts*, in which the luteinized layer has undergone complete hyalinization, giving rise to large corpora albicantia, whose cavities are distended with fluid.

Finally, brief mention should be made of those cystic follicles in which the granulosa layer has been luteinized in the absence of corpus luteum formation. This process is sometimes observed in persistent follicles by the time they begin to undergo atresia. The ovarian changes observed in the presence of hydatidiform mole and choriocarcinoma (see Chapter 44) are of the same type.

THECA-LUTEIN CYSTS. These cysts are usually seen in association with hydatidiform mole and choriocarcinoma, in which case they commonly occur as multiple cysts, whose walls reveal pronounced thecal luteinization. The process would seem to consist of exaggerated follicular atresia, with luteinization of thecal cells in such atretic corpora. The exact significance and nature of the theca-lutein cysts will be examined in the chapter on hydatidiform mole and choriocarcinoma (Chapter 43).

29.2.2. CORPUS LUTEUM PERSISTENCE

The phenomenon of corpus luteum persistence had been recognized many years ago. Persistent corpora lutea were studied by Meyer and, more recently, by Kayser.[70] These writers described the occurrence of *luteal persistence in prolonged amenorrhea*, in which the corpus luteum remained viable for several weeks. Obviously, such cases are rare. These authors considered them as fully functional, persistent corpora lutea, the occurrence of which is currently

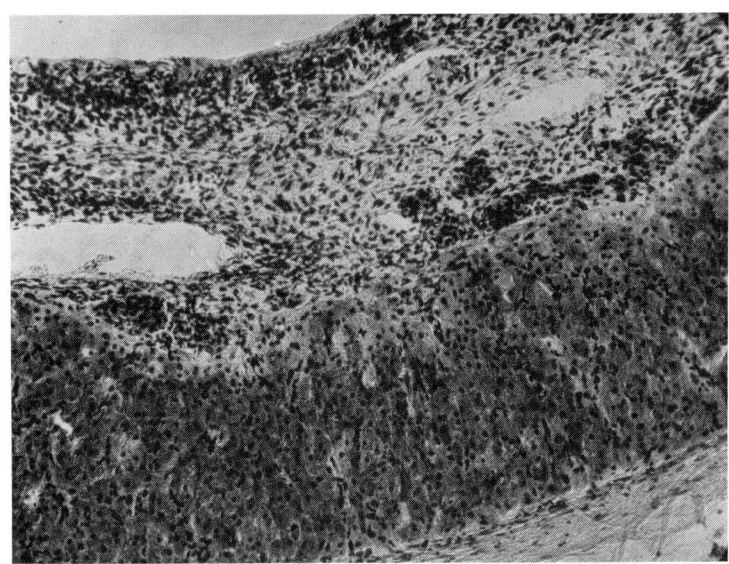

Figure 29–8. Wall of follicle-lutein cyst, with degenerative changes in granulosa layer and a hyperplastic, highly functional theca.

being disputed. What, on the other hand, has been described in recent years as an instance of luteal persistence is the entity known as *irregular endometrial shedding*, which is discussed below.

LUTEAL PERSISTENCE WITH AMENORRHEA. Instances of an occasional corpus luteum lasting for a month or longer and causing amenorrhea have been described. We have seen similar cases (see Fig. 29–10). The women involved appear to develop a condition resembling early gestation, with absent menses, usually not more than twice; enlarged and turgescent uterus; and frequently a voluminous corpus luteum that is readily palpable in one of the ovaries. In these cases, confusion with early pregnancy, or, more likely, with well tolerated ectopic pregnancy, is very possible. Kehere believed that this condition resulted from pituitary hypergonadotropism B, triggered by a persistent psychosexual stimulus. While the occurrence of luteal persistence in cases similar to that observed by us may be impossible to deny categorically, it must at least be admitted that such cases are extremely rare.

IRREGULAR ENDOMETRIAL SHEDDING. Under this term, various American authors described an entity characterized by functional uterine bleeding in the presence of a secretory endometrium. The pertinent findings were first described by Jones in 1938 and later studied in depth by Holmstrom and MacLennan,[58] MacKelvey[94] and Botella and associates.[20, 115]

Endometrial findings in these cases consist of secretory endometria with menstrual necrosis, as shown in Figure 29–11. For a case to be acceptable as an instance of irregular endometrial shedding, MacLennan[95] stipulates that the presence of secretory endometrium must be verified at least five days after the onset of menstruation. The mechanism of bleeding involved, according to MacKelvey,[94] is the prolongation of menstrual desquamation, which, as usual, begins in a certain endometrial area

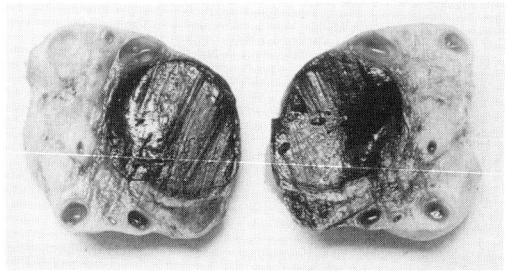

Figure 29–9. Ovary with corpus hemorrhagicum, associated with destruction of granulosa-lutein layer and preservation of luteinized theca.

Corpus Luteum Syndromes, Ovarian Hyperandrogenism

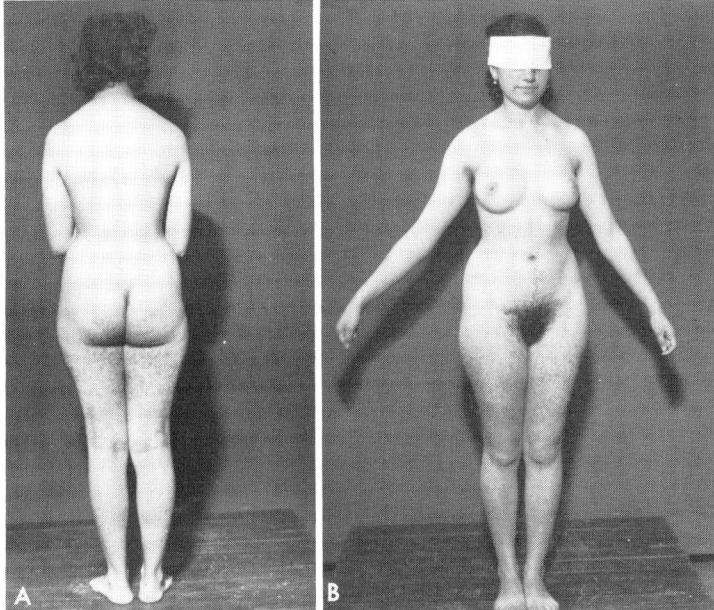

Figure 29-10. Luteal persistence with amenorrhea and moderate hirsutism of lower extremities.

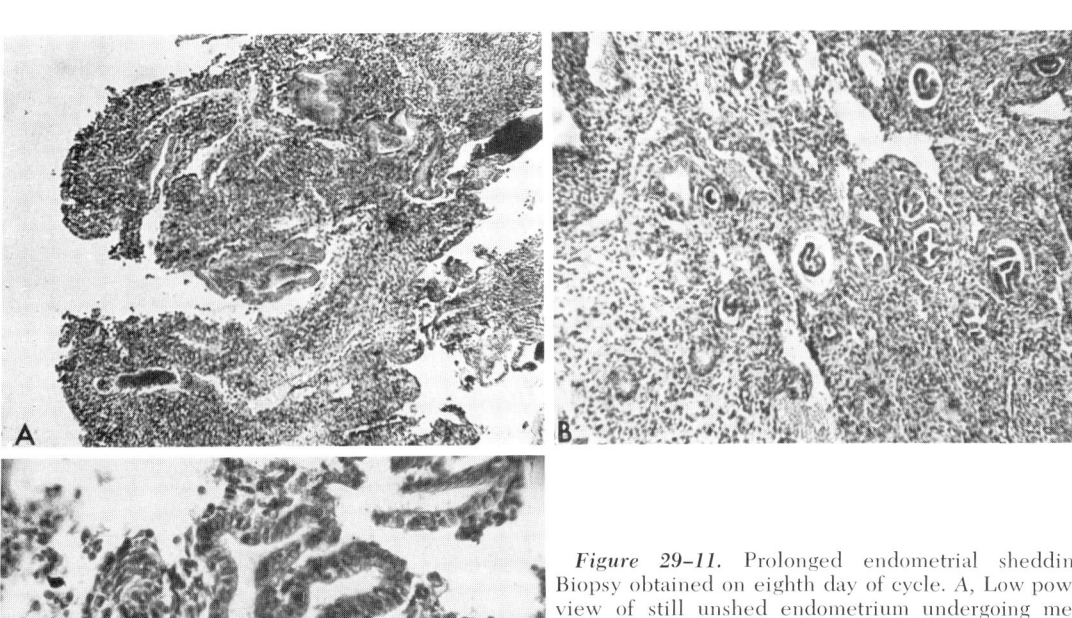

Figure 29-11. Prolonged endometrial shedding. Biopsy obtained on eighth day of cycle. *A*, Low power view of still unshed endometrium undergoing menstrual necrosis. *B*, Retraction of glands and evidence of menstrual necrosis in stroma. *C*, High power detail of menstrual necrosis. Findings in this instance indicate that the endometrial shedding process of the preceding cycle had not yet been completed on eighth day of present cycle.

but fails to take place simultaneously throughout the cavity, so that while one endometrial region has already been sloughed off and eliminated, another is still in the process of being shed, and as a result, bleeding occurs successively from various points of the uterine cavity, which thus take turns in producing menstrual hemorrhage.

The largest series reported to date was published by MacLennan[95] in 1952 and comprised 53 thoroughly studied cases of irregular shedding. According to this investigator, the findings provided by simple curettage are not enough to assume that one is dealing with irregular shedding and he presents documentary evidence based on total curettage or on sections of total hysterectomy specimens.

Some light on the etiology of this condition seems to have been shed in 1950, in clinical experimental studies conducted by Masters and Magallon.[100] These authors induced irregular endometrial shedding artificially in castrated and postmenopausal women by means of administering 25 mg progesterone daily for many days. It is a well known observation that progesterone administration in high dosages often leads to prolonged menstruation. From their observations, these authors concluded that irregular endometrial shedding was the result of corpus luteum persistence and, consequently, of absence of progesterone withdrawal.

Favoring this point of view is also the fact, recently noted by Sopeña and Tornero,[146] that women with copious but irregular menstrual bleeding frequently reveal very high urinary pregnanediol values, even during the days of menstruation (see Table 29-9). Similarly, Nogales,[114] at our clinic, often encountered secretory endometrium that was not yet completely shed during the first days of the cycle. The finding of viable remnants of secretory endometrium may extend beyond the first week of the cycle, sometimes to the beginning of the second week, to the tenth day, or even later. It is of interest to point out that, according to our own observations,[115] it is precisely under these circumstances that a definite association may be found between the presence of persistent secretory endometrium and high levels of pregnanediol excretion (Table 29-9), as well as elevated concentrations of endometrial glycogen (Botella and Tornero[14]). There-fore, all available data are in keeping with the views expressed by Masters and Magallon[100] to the effect that irregular endometrial desquamation is caused by lack of progesterone deprivation at the time of menstruation and is, consequently, a result of genuine hyperluteinism.

We have studied such endometria in a group of young women,[20, 147] performing the biopsies between the fourth day of the cycle and the tenth postmenstrual day. The results, listed in Table 29-10, comprise 220 observations and indicate a high incidence of persistent secretory endometrium beyond the fifth day of the cycle. Surprisingly, the menstrual picture in all 56 cases with positive findings revealed that more than half of the cases (55 per cent) experienced no significant menstrual alterations despite persistence of secretory endometria (Table 29-11). It would thus appear that *slow or irregular endometrial shedding does not invariably lead to functional bleeding.*

Currently, as indicated in Chapter 13, it is thought that menstrual endometrial shedding may be less complete and less total than originally assumed. Bartelmez admits that a secretory endometrium is subject to slow regression rather than shedding in many instances. According to Nogales, the result is a *process of regeneration superseding the previous cycle*, which our own finding would seem to confirm in 55 per cent of the cases. Bleeding episodes only appear in 30 per cent of those cases in which there is delayed shedding or regeneration during the preceding cycle. *Justifiably, then, irregular endometrial shedding may be concluded to be a form of functional bleeding associated with de-*

TABLE 29-9. Urinary Hormone Elimination in Women with Irregular Endometrial Shedding*

CASE	AGE	ESTROGENS (MCG)	PREGNANEDIOL (MG/24 HR)
1	43	200	7.0
2	38	250	20.5
3	28	100	18.4
4	29		2.9
5	21		29.02
6	36	100	5.23
7	37		5.20
8	40		2.4
9	42	250	20.5

*From Sopeña and Tornero.[146]

TABLE 29-10. Prolonged Endometrial Shedding*

ENDOMETRIAL FINDINGS	4TH DAY	5TH DAY	6TH DAY	7TH DAY	8TH DAY	9TH DAY	10TH DAY	TOTAL	PER CENT
Normal proliferation	13	17	19	17	24	30	34	154	70
Secretion	11	6	6	7	9	6	11	56	25.5
Hyperplasia or persistent proliferation	1	1	2	2	3	0	1	10	4.5

*From Botella and Marín.[20]

layed endometrial shedding, the underlying etiology of the delaying mechanism so far remaining obscure.

What undoubtedly lies at the root of the disorder is *prolonged longevity of the corpus luteum*,[94, 95, 117] the reason for which may be related to either abnormal hypothalamic stimuli or prolactin hyperactivity.[38, 133]

29.2.3. LUTEINIZED GRANULOSA CELL TUMORS AND LUTEOMAS

Related luteal syndromes are described in Chapter 30 (Section 30.2.6).

29.3. OVARIAN HYPERANDROGENISM

Although we have known for a good many years that substantial amounts of androgens were found in women, we had assumed that they were derived from physiologic adrenocortical activity. Expressed in terms of 17-ketosteroid levels, androgen excretion in normal woman ranges from 8 to 10 mg per 24 hr (see Chapter 4). Following castration in women, such androgen values not only do not fall but may actually rise, owing to the fact that castration results in hyperplasia of the adrenal cortex. In view of this fact, ovarian androgen biogenesis was once doubted to occur. What mainly led to awareness of ovarian androgenic function was evidence that virilism in some cases occurred in the absence of either the adrenal cortex or such functioning tumors as arrhenoblastoma. We were thus obliged to acknowledge the possibility of ovarian virilism without tumor. A search for the origin of ovarian virilism in apparently normal ovaries opened the way to the discovery that a series of ovarian interstitial elements was capable of elaborating androgens. Ovarian androgen synthesis appears to acquire greater significance in pathologic conditions than under normal conditions.

Recent studies[4, 5, 6, 96, 168] produced evidence that ovarian androgen biogenesis was the result of *metabolic disturbances in steroid synthesis*. Androgens are known to be precursors of estrogens (see Chapter 4), so that interference with the enzyme system of steroidogenesis can determine abnormally high production of androgens.

As to the site of interference of ovarian estrogen synthesis, resulting in pathologic androgen synthesis, two types of elements may be involved: (1) the *hilus cells*, true ovarian analogues of the Leydig cells, and (2) *hyperplastic thecal tissue*, whatever its nature.

29.3.1. PHYSIOPATHOLOGY OF OVARIAN ANDROGEN BIOGENESIS

Masculinization of ovarian origin was recognized by Hill in 1937, and by Deanesly

TABLE 29-11. Prolonged Endometrial Shedding: Duration of Menstrual Bleeding*

DURATION OF BLEEDING	4TH DAY	5TH DAY	6TH DAY	7TH DAY	8TH DAY	9TH DAY	10TH DAY	TOTAL	PER CENT
Eumenorrhea (4–5 days)	5	4	1	1	2	5	2	20	55.5
Hypomenorrhea (3 days or less)	2	1	1	1	–	–	–	5	13.9
Hypermenorrhea (6 days or longer)	–	2	2	4	1	1	1	11	30.6

*From Nogales, Marín, and Botella.[115]

in 1938. Ponse[128] investigated some forms of masculinization occurring in female guinea pigs either in relation to ovarian luteinization or as a result of administration of chorionic gonadotropin. Both the guinea pigs with luteinized ovaries and those injected with chorionic gonadotropin were found to have enhanced 17-ketosteroid excretion, similar in magnitude to the degree of masculinization. Similarly, if adrenalectomized female rats were injected with gonadotropins, their ovaries were noted to react by undergoing diffuse luteinization, particularly involving the theca, which was followed by signs of masculinization and growth of the clitoris.

By adopting hypertrophy of the clitoris as an index of masculinization, Ponse[128] was able to show that chorionic gonadotropin, when given to hypophysectomized animals, produced masculinization of utmost intensity. This, in Ponse's view, was due to the fact that chorionic gonadotropin produced thecal hyperplasia much more readily in hypophysectomized than in nonhypophysectomized animals, because regression of the granulosa in the former favored follicular atresia and, consequently, thecal luteinization.

Plate[124, 125] also stressed the role played by thecal hyperplasia in the production of hirsutism. As a result of the preceding observations, as well as of many other studies of clinical and experimental nature, too numerous to be discussed here, thecal hyperplasia with luteinization may be concluded to result in production of androgens by the ovary, and to be the cause of both experimental and clinical masculinization. In the light of these investigations, the source of ovarian androgenism must be assumed to be linked to the thecal reaction.

On the other hand, attention had long been called to the so-called *hilus cells* as an important source of ovarian androgen production. Their description dates back to Berger who, many years ago, described such cells as *parasympathicotropic cells,* without, however, recognizing their true significance. The same author, as well as Sternberg and his colleagues[151] and Van Campenhout,[162] later showed that the appearance of these cells in some forms of virilism was of great significance. Such cells are found in the region of the ovarian hilus (Figs. 29–12 and 29–13) in every woman, appearing particularly prominently toward the climacterium. With injections of chorionic gonadotropin in elevated dosages, amounting to 10,000 IU daily for several days, Sternberg and his associates[151] were able to induce hyperplasia of hilus elements.

In view of the fact that while hilus cells undergo hyperplasia, urinary 17-ketosteroids have been observed to rise commensurately, it has been inferred that the hyperandrogenic ovarian reaction is caused by LH stimulation of hilus elements. This hypothesis is supported by evidence, reported by Sternberg, that clinical cases of masculinization unquestioningly were re-

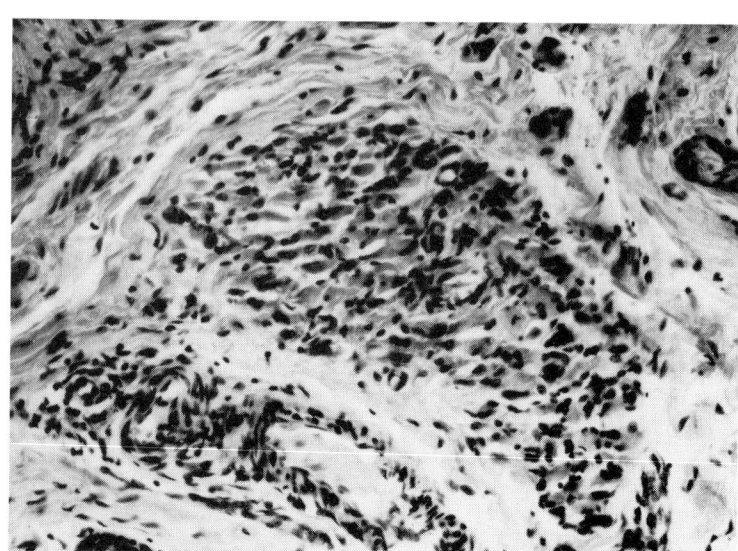

Figure 29–12. Hilus cell aggregate, at low magnification, in the ovary from a woman suffering from virilization.

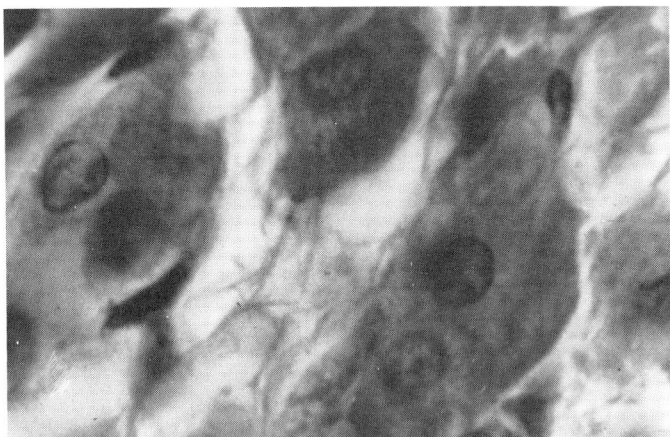

Figure 29-13. Hilus cells seen at high magnification. Note similarity to testicular Leydig cells.

lated to hilus cell hyperplasia. Similarly, hilus cell tumors causing masculinization have been reported by Sachs and Spiro,[132] as well as by Waugh and his associates.[164] As a result, it may be assumed that *at least two different structures in the ovary are capable of androgen synthesis under the influence of LH: on the one hand, the theca, and on the other, the hilus cells.*

It must be remembered that the adrenal cortex, as pointed out in Chapter 8, secretes androgens under the influence of chorionic gonadotropin. Whenever confronted with a case of virilization in woman in the absence of evidence of ovarian or adrenal tumor, the three following mechanisms must therefore be considered:

1. Secretion of androgens by a hyperplastic adrenal cortex (adrenal virilism, adrenogenital syndrome).

2. Production of androgens by the theca (ovarian hyperthecosis, Stein-Leventhal syndrome and related conditions).

3. Secretion of androgens by ovarian hilus elements (hilus cells).

What the three different modalities share is a common response to chorionic gonadotropin stimulation, which in all three instances provokes production of androgens, with associated increase in urinary 17-ketosteroid excretion and masculinization.

29.3.2. SYNDROME OF MASCULINIZATION DUE TO OVARIAN HILUS CELL ACTIVITY

Ovarian hilus cells are present in the form of microscopic nests located along the ovarian hilus and the adjacent mesoovarium (Figs. 29-12 and 29-13). There are great variations in the number and location of such cells although, as a rule, they are encountered in all ovaries, especially those of adult women.

A relatively constant relationship has been described between ovarian hilus cells and the abundant nonmyelinated nerve fibers of the mesoovarium. The cell nests are usually found in direct continuity with such fibers and are often enmeshed and grouped into nodules by surrounding nerve fibers. The significance of this peculiar relationship is not yet clearly understood, but it does give rise to configurations that are similar to those found in the male gonad.

Cytologically, ovarian hilus cells are identical to Leydig cells. They reveal a similar range of morphologic variations, particularly as regards nuclear and cytoplasmic details, including distribution of intracytoplasmic lipoids. Both types of cells contain a lipochrome pigment and, quite characteristically, so-called *Reinke crystalloids.*

Sternberg and his associates[151] reported five cases in which masculinization was associated with tumors of this cell type and added another six cases of simple hilus cell hyperplasia, in which masculinization was also manifest. Subsequent communications by Sachs and Spiro[132] and by Waugh and co-workers[164] seem to establish beyond any doubt that the cells under consideration are associated with a masculinizing effect.

As indicated in Chapter 30, ovarian "Leydig cell" tumors must be categorized as functioning tumors that are closely related to arrhenoblastomas. However, only a small number of tumors composed of this cell type have so far been reported, so that virilism is much more often encountered in the presence of hilus cell hyperplasia.

From the clinical point of view, virilization of this type usually occurs in adult women in their forties (Fig. 29–14). Facial hypertrichosis is a common finding while, at the same time, it is not unusual to observe loss of hair from the scalp. Menstrual periods may frequently be missed, the breasts may undergo atrophy and there may be an early onset of menopause. Urinary 17-ketosteroids, studied mainly by Segaloff and his associates,[136] were reported to be elevated, ranging between 15 and 40 mg per 24 hr, according to figures supplied by Sternberg and his co-workers[151] (Fig. 29–15).

For therapy for these conditions, some authors recommend oophorectomy, while others suggest high dosages of estrogens. However, these procedures have given poor results. Although oophorectomy removes the cause of ovarian virilism, the resulting castration is followed by adrenocortical hyperplasia, which in turn raises androgen production by that organ. Botella and Gomez-Maestro[12] showed that castration of women occasionally produced virilism through an adrenocortical reaction (see Chapter 38). Consequently, castration can be expected to give at best inconsistent results.

The treatment proposed and used by us with good results over the past years consists of so-called *ovarian demedullation.* It is based on a wedge resection of the ovary, a method which has given good results in the treatment of Stein-Leventhal's syndrome, by decreasing follicular atresia and thereby reducing hyperthecosis. While the purpose of wedge resection is to achieve remission of ovarian hyperandrogenism in terms of hyperthecosis, we use electro-cautery in addition to destroy the entire medullary and hilar region of the gland. Once this is accomplished, both ovaries are closed with fine catgut.

The results of this procedure are shown in Figure 29–15, revealing a significant reduction in previously elevated 17-ketosteroid levels in the urine of four women after treatment.

29.3.3. HYPERTHECOSIS

In 1942, Geist and Gaines called attention to a syndrome of virilization, with hirsutism and other masculinoid features, in women who had neither ovarian tumors nor adrenal changes to account for these manifestations but who, on the other hand, revealed evidence of thecal cell hyperplasia. In 1949, Culiner and Shippel[35] reported three cases presenting with virilization and polymicrocystic ovaries with numerous atretic follicles, accompanied by evidence of thecal hyperplasia. In 1950, Meaker[102] published a survey of 65 women who had presented with analogous symptoms in conjunction with thecal hyperplasia. Of these 65 women, 30 had revealed only amenorrhea and infertility, 22 had only infertility, and the rest also showed virilization. In 1951, Plate[124] collected three more cases of virilism with thecal hyperplasia. The hyperthecosis syndrome has many points in common with and is closely related to the Stein-Leventhal syndrome, which is described later.

The etiology of these conditions may be deduced from the previously mentioned observations by Ponse. It would seem that primary degeneration of elements in the

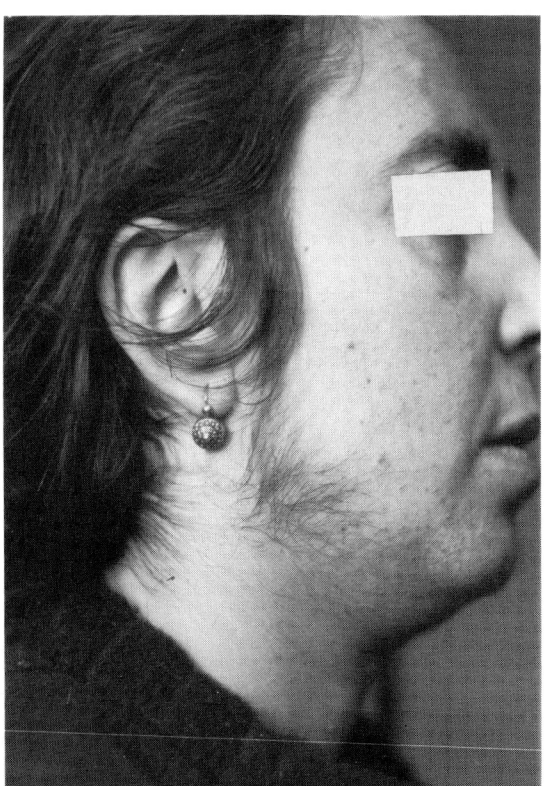

Figure 29–14. Hirsutism in Case 1 (M.G.A.) from Figure 29–15, resulting from hilus cell hyperplasia.

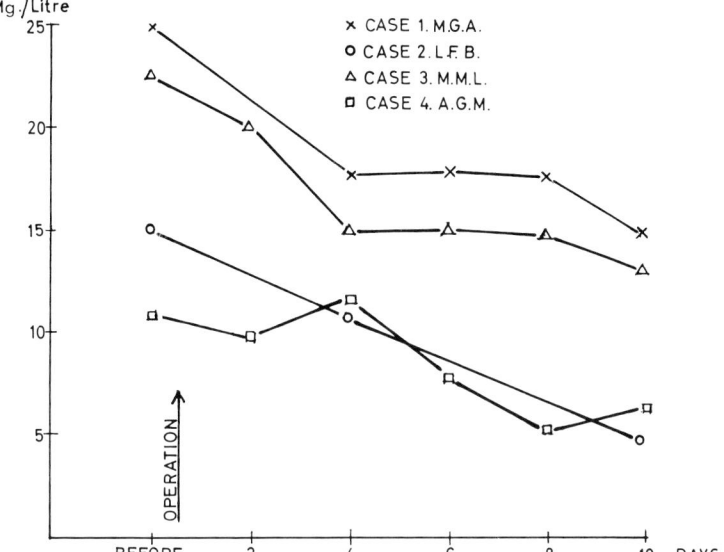

Figure 29-15. Twenty-four hour urinary excretion rates of total 17-ketosteroids in four cases with hilus cell hyperplasia. Operative procedure consisted of ovarian demedullation in all four women.

granulosa layer is in part responsible for the proliferative reactions in the theca, much like that occurring in physiologic follicular atresia. Degeneration of the characteristic elements in the granulosa, in turn, presumably causes a pituitary hyperreaction involving increased LH secretion. Exaggerated gonadotropic activity by the latter is thought to induce further hyperplasia and, more importantly, luteinization of the theca interna.

Clinically, virilism from hyperthecosis may develop fairly pronounced features that may occasionally be highly suggestive of the presence of a functioning tumor of the androgenic variety. Not infrequently, amenorrhea and, of course, infertility play a prominent role in the symptomatology of these women. In many respects, the condition resembles hilus cell hyperplasia, which has already been described, and, like the latter, affects predominantly mature women about the age of 40. The treatment proposed by us is likewise ovarian wedge resection plus destruction of the central and hilar portions of the ovary by means of electrocoagulation.

29.3.4. "ESSENTIAL" OVARIAN VIRILIZATION

In many instances, excessive production of androgens may be associated with ovaries revealing scanty, if any, pathologic changes. It must not be forgotten that androgens are intermediary metabolites of normal ovarian steroid synthesis[134] and that minor changes in enzyme activity may cause a shift in the synthetic pathway from estrogens to androgens. Oakey and Stitch[118] have noted that estrogen synthesis by atretic follicles may be arrested at the androgen stage. According to Lisse,[87] ovarian androgenization is not necessarily associated with predominance of any particular tissue element and may occur in ovaries that appear structurally normal.

29.3.5. STEIN-LEVENTHAL SYNDROME

DEFINITION. In 1936, Stein and Leventhal described a syndrome characterized by bulky polycystic ovaries, amenorrhea and infertility. Three years later, Stein and Cohen[149] described the corresponding ovarian histology as characterized by simultaneous maturation of many follicles that fail to reach full size, degeneration of the granulosa, absence of corpora lutea, and a peculiar type of fibrosis of the entire ovarian cortex, generally accompanied by *thecal hyperplasia*.

Plate[125, 126] distinguishes *two different types* of polymicrocystic ovaries: one, in which there is no evidence of thecal hyperplasia, *without hyperthecosis*, and another, in which hyperplasia of the follicle theca fully corresponds to the clinical picture described above as *hyperthecosis*.

Dokumov and Dashev,[39] as well as Sun and Rakoff,[154] studied the foci of fibrosis in such ovaries by histochemical means. Confirming the findings of Plate, they in fact observed thecal hyperplasia in many instances in which thecal cells contained abundant lipoid inclusions and gave a strongly positive reaction with Ashbel and Seligman's diazo method, which is a known histochemical reaction for 17-ketosteroids. The association of hyperthecosis with positive reactions for 17-ketosteroids and with unquestionable features of virilization (Fig. 29–20) was confirmed by Sun and Rakoff. In contrast, simple polymicrocystic ovaries are known to be associated only with infertility and amenorrhea, not with virilization.

A distinction can thus be drawn between two clinical entities: (1) *simple ovarian polymicrocystosis*, which is not hyperandrogenic and therefore is not included in the present study, and (2) *polymicrocystosis with hyperthecosis and virilization*.

In our opinion, there is much confusion concerning the definition of this syndrome, a fact also deplored by Goldzieher and Green,[51] Taymor and associates,[158] and Barnard and Audit.[7] Some authors (Decourt et al.,[37] Axelrod and Goldzieher,[4,5] Mahesh and Greenblatt[97]) refer to all conditions with polyfollicular ovaries as syndrome of "polycystic ovaries." As a result, many different ovarian conditions characterized by hyperestrinism (Chapter 28, Section 28.2.2) are included in the same category. We agree with Netter and his co-workers[108] and with Zander[169] that the term "Stein-Leventhal syndrome" should be confined to those cases which are characterized by: (1) *large, polycystic ovaries with thecal hyperplasia*, and (2) *virilization*, which we believe is of utmost importance.

From now on, all future reference to this syndrome shall be made in strict observance of these two criteria. Unless they are met, the term Stein-Leventhal syndrome will not be employed.

ETIOLOGY AND PATHOGENESIS. For many years, we had entertained the possibility that the Stein-Leventhal syndrome was of pituitary origin and that the underlying cause for all its characteristic disturbances was to be found in adenohypophysial hyperfunction (perhaps of hypothalamic origin), resulting in hypersecretion of LH.[42, 61, 71] Nevertheless, it has recently been demonstrated that pituitary dysfunction, though indeed present, was *secondary to a primordial ovarian disorder*. The ovarian disorder stems from *abnormal steroid metabolism*.

In 1961, Zander,[168] as well as Warren and Salhanick,[165] showed that the normal ovary was able to convert progesterone to 17-hydroxyprogesterone, and the latter, in turn, was converted to androstenedione, 19-hydroxyandrostenedione and estrone. In the Stein-Leventhal syndrome, the androstenedione-estrogen conversion step does not take place, owing to a block in 19-hydroxylation of androstenedione (Fig. 29–18).

The results of numerous investigations over the past years (Axelrod and Goldzieher,[5,6] Conti et al.,[33] Mahesh and Greenblatt,[97] Leventhal and Scommegna,[85] Noall and Kaufman,[113] Shearman and Gannon,[140] Staemmler and Sachs,[148] and Zander[168, 169]) are in general agreement that the syndrome may be produced by three different mechanisms, each involving a more or less complete block in ovarian steroidogenesis.

1. Lack of 3β-ol-dehydrogenase, as indicated in Figure 29–19, whereby progesterone synthesis is blocked and steroid metabolism is shunted toward production of dehydroepiandrosterone, with no possibility of further conversion resulting in an increase in urinary neutral 17-ketosteroids.

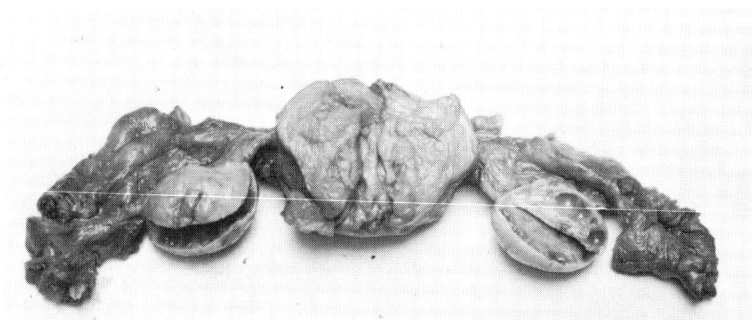

Figure 29–16. Subtotal hysterectomy specimen with slightly enlarged uterus and bilateral polycystic ovaries.

Figure 29-17. Ovary in typical Stein-Leventhal syndrome. *A*, Low power view of partly atretic follicle, hemmed in by thickened tunica albuginea (left). *B*, High power detail of albuginea, revealing presence of marked collagenosis.

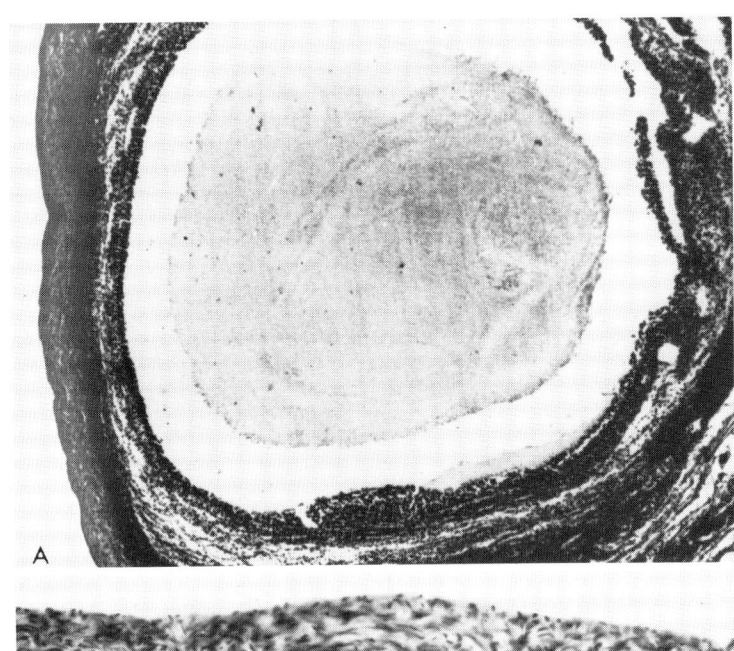
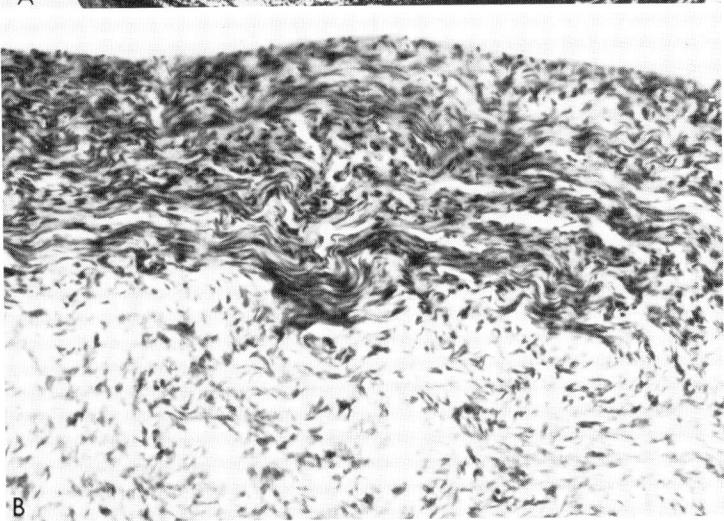

This mechanism has been stressed by Leventhal and Scommegna[85] and by Zander.[169]

2. The mechanism outlined on the left side in Figure 29-18, consisting of lack of 19-hydroxylase, which leads to interference with production of 19-hydroxyandrostenedione and 19-hydroxytestosterone. This, as shown, in turn results in accumulation of androsterone and testosterone and produces virilization of a much more pronounced degree than that of the preceding variety. This mechanism has been elucidated above all by Mahesh and Greenblatt,[97] Zander,[169] and Bruni and his associates.[23]

3. Finally, the mechanism outlined on the right in Figure 29-18, in which conversion of 19-hydroxy-derivatives to estrogen is blocked because of lack of *aromatization*, is believed to give rise to hypoestrogenic syndromes with virilization. This mechanism was described by Segre[137] and by Zander.[169]

All three mechanisms described may be assumed to be frequently associated with, or superimposed on, each other.

GENETIC FACTORS. The Stein-Leventhal syndrome might be included among the *genetically determined errors of metabolism*, were it not for lack of conclusive evidence that a genetic basis is involved. Short[142] postulates that the enzymatic defect is linked to an anomaly in one of the X chromosomes, whereas Netter and his associates have described four cases of Stein-Leventhal syndrome with abnormal karyotypes. In two of these, the defect consisted in *amputation of one arm of the X chromosome* (see Chapter 35), while the

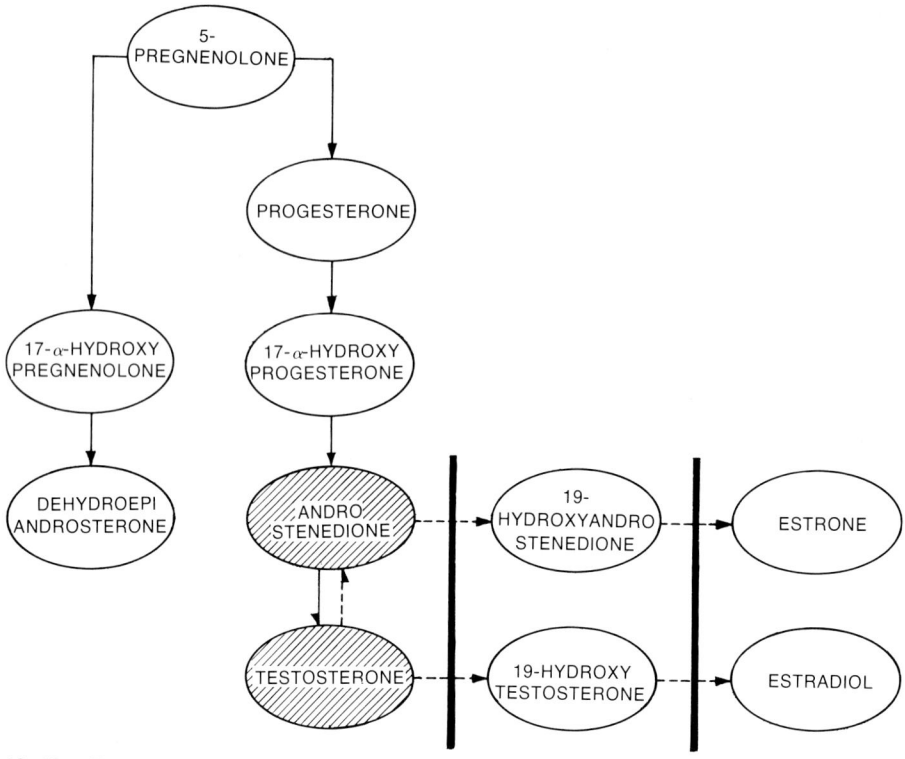

Figure 29-18. Diagram of androgen synthesis in Stein-Leventhal syndrome, type I: Inhibition of 19-hydroxylase. (From Zander.[169])

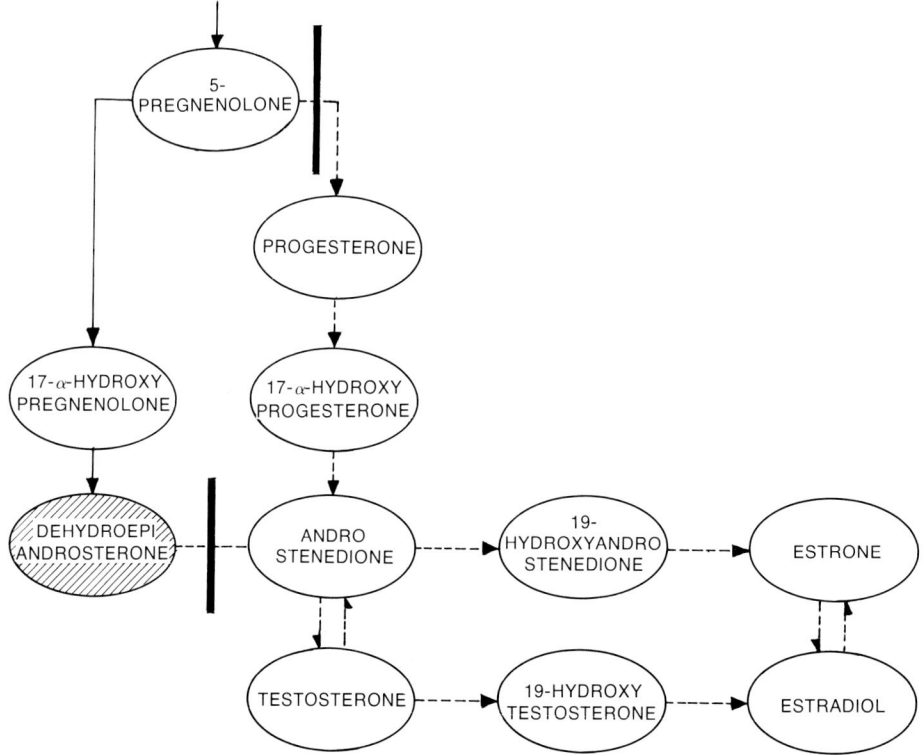

Figure 29-19. Diagram of androgen synthesis in Stein-Leventhal syndrome, type II: Inhibition of 3-β-ol-dehydrogenase. (From Zander.[169])

other two were XX/XXX mosaics. In our own patients with Stein-Leventhal syndrome, who so far number 15, we have never encountered any changes in karyotype; neither did Byrd and co-workers[26] in nine cases, or Knorr and co-workers,[74] in 16 cases. This of course does not mean that such anomalies might not exist. If they do, it is likely that the underlying enzymopathy is linked to a chromosomal aberration, a view held by Netter. In this respect, however, further study will be necessary before a definite answer can be provided.

ROLE OF PITUITARY AND HYPOTHALAMUS. It has been mentioned earlier how Plate[127] and Ingersoll and MacArthur[61] ascribed the etiology of Stein-Leventhal syndrome to increased LH activity, which they thought provoked both an adrenal reaction (described below) and ovarian hyperthecosis. A pathogenesis of this type might in addition explain why psychosomatic factors are frequently observed in this syndrome. Increased LH values have in effect been reported by some.[71,121,158,166] However, others[42,43] have reported an increase in FSH values. After suppressing the pituitary with cortisone[67] or with dexamethasone,[109] the patients have been found to improve clinically. In addition, slices from such ovaries incubated in vitro were found to be capable of a higher rate of androgen synthesis in the presence of LH.[80,81]

It might be argued, however, that the observed pituitary changes are in fact the result rather than the cause of excessive androgen activity. As indicated in Chapter 8 (Section 8.4.3), androgens exert a peculiar effect on the hypophysiothalamic system. If adult female rats are injected with testosterone,[44,129] cyclic activity is arrested and their ovaries develop large persistent follicles, identical to those found in anovulatory cycles, and the females become sterile. This effect, it was shown, is the result of suppression of cyclic LH secretion[163,166,170] and is also known to occur in the human species.[57,157] If a rat fetus or a suckling is given testosterone, or any other androgen, during the first five days of life, a single and relatively small dose[3,45,55,63,72,156] causes loss of hypothalamic secretory rhythmicity and the hypophysiothalamic system is converted to an organ without rhythm, *like that of the male*. This reaction can be induced in rats and guinea pigs,[54] but not in rabbits,[28] and probably also takes place in woman since she belongs to a species with a spontaneous, autonomous cycle. Further evidence implicating possible hypothalamic changes in the Stein-Leventhal syndrome is the fact that a similar syndrome can be induced in female rats by continuous exposure to illumination (Singh[143,144]), which at the same time would seem to suggest some form of pineal involvement.

All these facts suggest that the primary disorder may be enzymatic in nature and that accumulation of estrogens, resulting from enzymatic failure, may act secondarily on the hypothalamus by modifying the rhythmicity of LH secretion, which, in turn, would prevent a "preovulatory peak," and thus would represent the underlying cause of the anovulatory cycle with hyperthecosis. This hypothesis also leaves ample room for admitting that Stein-Leventhal syndrome might result from a congenital error of metabolism as well as for postulating a familial mode of transmission and a possible genetically determined origin.

ROLE OF ADRENAL CORTEX. The significance of the relatively common finding of polymicrocystic ovaries in association with the adrenogenital syndrome is discussed in Chapter 33. Conversely, the presence of *adrenal hyperplasia*[48,73,90,107,136] in the Stein-Leventhal syndrome is a matter of record. Perloff and Jacobson[121] have reported that even after castration women with the Stein-Leventhal syndrome respond to injections of chorionic gonadotropin with rising urinary 17-ketosteroid excretion. After a detailed study of the disease, Lanthier[81] raises the pertinent question of whether the urinary 17-ketosteroids in the Stein-Leventhal syndrome are of adrenal or of ovarian origin. Although some believe that the Stein-Leventhal syndrome and the adrenogenital syndrome are two distinct independent entities,[2,34,84] most workers in the field agree that the two conditions are related. Going even further, Pesonen and his associates[122] believe that what is involved is a systemic disorder common to both conditions, which makes its appearance simultaneously in both the ovaries and the adrenals, *as a result of a fundamental disturbance in steroid metabolism.*

There is a distinct possibility that, along with elevated LH activity, there may be an associated increase in ACTH activity and that both hormones may join forces in stimulating the adrenal cortex (see Chapter 9). Sommers and Wadam[145] have described pituitary basophilia in the Stein-Leventhal syndrome, while Mellinger and his colleagues[103] reported the association of Cushing's syndrome in one instance.

OVARIAN HISTOLOGY. The essential feature is the presence of numerous persistent follicles that are "*half-ripened,*" in association with thecal hyperplasia, or *hyperthecosis*. Leventhal,[83] Garry and Fienberg,[49] Ellet and Barnes[40] and Salhanick[133] all believe that the most characteristic feature of the syndrome is fibrosis (in the opinion of Leventhal, true *ovarian collagenosis*), which is the main etiologic factor involved, since all other changes are of secondary importance (Fig. 29-17). Perloff and co-workers,[120] as well as Jackson and Dockerty,[62] found that frequently such ovaries revealed *hilus cell hyperplasia*, the origin of which might possibly be attributed to increased LH activity. A comprehensive histochemical study of such ovaries has recently been published by Dokumov and Dashev.[38, 39]

Perloff and his co-workers,[120] as well as Botella,[21] have alluded to the fact that the most significant finding in ovaries of the Stein-Leventhal syndrome, in their opinion, is the presence of *fibrosis involving the albuginea*.

STEIN-LEVENTHAL SYNDROME AS AN AUTOIMMUNE DISEASE. From the very outset, it had been suspected that a disturbance in gonadotropin activity lay at the root of the Stein-Leventhal syndrome. Miklosi and MacKosker[104] assume an etiology based on autoimmunization to one's own FSH and LH. The histologic observations by De Brux and Gerbier[24] seem to support such a supposition, although for the time being there are no conclusive data to confirm an autoimmune etiology.

CLINICAL FINDINGS. Recently the syndrome has been the subject of renewed interest and of numerous reports.[40, 84, 108, 137] As a matter of fact, the condition is relatively common, though not as common as suggested by the frequency with which an unsubstantiated diagnosis of Stein-Leventhal syndrome may be made.

Among the principal symptoms are *amenorrhea* or *menstrual irregularities* and, rarely, *metrorrhagia*. The most constant symptom is *hirsutism* (Fig. 29-20), accompanied by enlarged clitoris and loss of libido.

Endometrial biopsy may give equivocal results[69, 108] either because advanced cases may reveal endometrial atrophy or hypoplasia, or because early cases may show variable hyperplastic changes that may account for occasional instances of associated functional bleeding. In the latter situation, the clinical findings may reveal virilized, infertile women, with enlarged uteri and ovaries. Invariably, of course, the cycle is *anovulatory*, which causes *infertility* in these women.

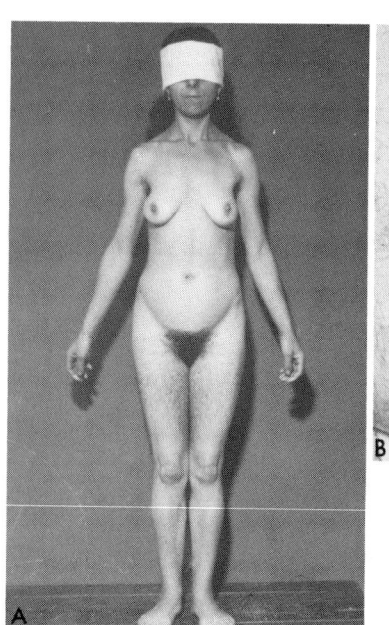
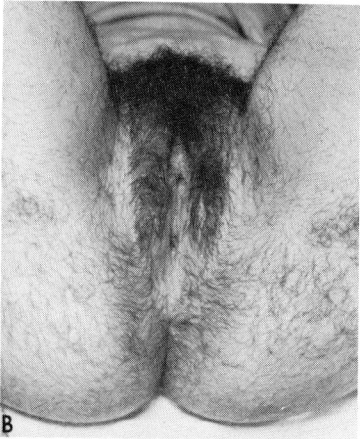

Figure 29-20. Somatic features and pudendal region of a woman with Stein-Leventhal syndrome. There are moderate hirsutism of pudendal region and lower extremities, elevated 17-ketosteroid levels, and infertility. In this instance, there is no evidence of obesity.

Corpus Luteum Syndromes, Ovarian Hyperandrogenism

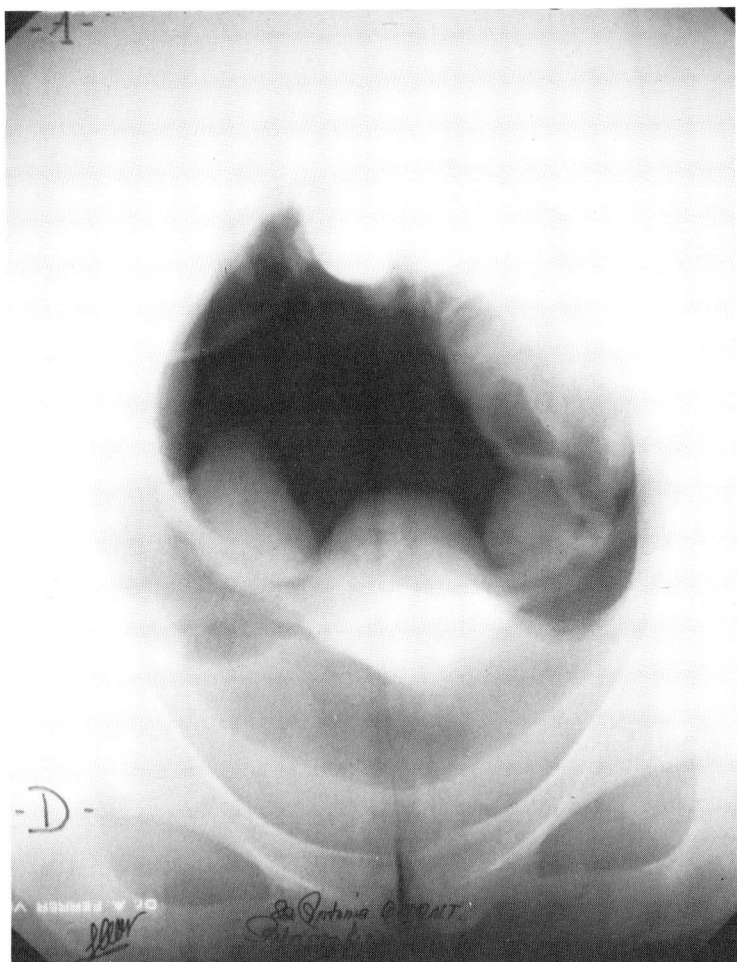

Figure 29-21. Gynecography in a case of Stein-Leventhal syndrome, revealing ovarian enlargement.

DIAGNOSIS. The diagnosis may be very difficult to establish with certainty. Stein[150] advises the use of pneumoperitoneum (gynecography) (Fig. 29–21). Landing[79] and Sturgis[153] believe that the diagnosis should be based on the presence of *hirsutism* and *increased rate of neutral 17-ketosteroid excretion*. The truth is, however, that sometimes 17-ketosteroid values may show only a minor increase, if any at all. A higher degree of diagnostic accuracy is provided by determinations of *testosterone* in the urine[88, 112] and in the plasma.[47, 59, 82, 155] It should also be pointed out that injections of LH produce an increase in neutral 17-ketosteroid excretion, which is an expressive diagnostic functional test. Finally, Jayle and his associates[65] and Koreman and his colleagues[76] use the *metopirone suppression test* for the differential diagnosis of adrenocortical hirsutism. As of late, the dexamethasone suppression and HCG stimulation tests,[66, 74] as well as the metopirone test,[139, 159] have repeatedly been recommended for the differentiation of ovarian virilism from adrenocortical virilism.

29.3.6. TREATMENT

Endocrine therapy with cortisone and cortisone derivatives, while giving excellent results in the adrenogenital syndrome (see Chapter 33), is ineffective in the Stein-Leventhal syndrome (Kologh et al.[75]). Yen and his associates[167] recently proposed treatment with *Clomiphene*. Though limited, our own experience with this drug has not been satisfactory. With the exception of one dissenting note from Perloff and his associates,[120] the general consensus is that the best treatment is ovarian wedge resection.[31, 111, 126, 130, 138, 141, 150] Trace and his colleagues[160] reported a decrease in urinary 17-ketosteroids following this procedure. Baulieu and associates[8] and Seeman and

Saracino[135] have demonstrated diminished androgen synthesis by ovarian tissue after this type of intervention. The mechanism of action involved is not known, and it is not understood why such a simple surgical act should modify ovarian steroidogenesis. According to data supplied by Leventhal, 65 per cent of women operated on in this way do eventually become pregnant, which, in our opinion, is perhaps an unusually high incidence. Evans and Riley[43] also reported good results in 25 cases that were operated on.

Our own experience gives less reason for optimism. Following ovarian wedge resection, 20 per cent of women with simple anovulatory cycles have been found by us to become pregnant (see Chapter 41). However, in cases of *genuine* Stein-Leventhal syndrome, the number of women experiencing clinical improvement amounted to less than 10 per cent, while very few were cured of hirsutism, usually the symptom of greatest concern to them.

Aware of the frequency with which Stein-Leventhal syndrome is associated with hilus cell hyperplasia, we advocate *ovarian demedullation* (see Section 29.3.2) at the same time that wedge resection is being performed. In the course of recent years, various authors (Allen and Woolf,[1] Kallio[68]) have come to follow the same line of reasoning.

29.3.7. THE STEIN-LEVENTHAL SYNDROME AND ITS BOUNDARIES

Before concluding, it seems pertinent to further demarcate the anatomopathologic concept of this syndrome from that of related conditions. At the present time, however, any kind of biochemical delimitation would appear to be premature.

1. *Stein-Leventhal syndrome and polymicrocystic ovaries*. In reality, not every ovary with *abundant, half-ripened follicles* is a "Stein-Leventhal ovary." Three varieties of polymicrocystosis must be distinguished:

a. Polymicrocystosis associated with estrogen production (see Chapter 28).

b. Inactive polymicrocystosis.

c. Polymicrocystosis associated with androgen production. (*This is the only variety pertaining to the Stein-Leventhal syndrome.*)

2. *Stein-Leventhal syndrome and hyperthecosis*. Hyperplastic thecal reactions may occur under many circumstances. In a *young woman*, hyperthecosis may coexist with half-ripened follicles or with atresia, whereas *in old women*, in whom the reservoir of available follicles is exhausted, hyperthecosis tends to be of the diffuse type, instead of being concentrated around follicles. In either case, the thecal reaction is a consequence of enhanced LH activity of pituitary origin, and may be categorized as follows:

a. Juvenile hyperthecosis (with follicles): Stein-Leventhal syndrome.

b. Senile hyperthecosis (without follicles):

(1) Central (ovarian fibrothecal masses)
(2) Cortical (cortical stromal hyperplasia).

As a consequence to our concept, it might be perhaps advisable to *abandon the term Stein-Leventhal syndrome* and adopt the more logical and comprehensive term *juvenile hyperthecosis*.

REFERENCES

1. Allen, W. M., and Woolf, R. B.: *Amer. J. Obstet. Gynec.*, 77:826, 1959.
2. Andrews, W. C., and Andrews, M. C.: *Amer. J. Obstet. Gynec.*, 80:632, 1960.
3. Aray, Y., and Gorski, R. A.: *Proc. Soc. Exper. Biol. Med.*, 127:590, 1968.
4. Axelrod, L. R., and Goldzieher, J. W.: *J. Clin. Endocr.*, 22:431, 1962.
5. Axelrod, L., and Goldzieher, J. W.: *J. Clin. Endocr. Metab.*, 22:537, 1962.
6. Axelrod, L., and Goldzieher, J. W.: *J. Clin. Endocr. Metab.*, 25:1275, 1965.
7. Barnard, I., and Audit, J. F.: *Gynec. Prat.*, 18:127, 1967.
8. Baulieu, E. E., Mauvais-Jarvis, D., and Corpechot, C.: *J. Clin. Endocr. Metab.*, 23:374, 1963.
9. Bengtson, L. P., and Fuchs, F.: *Acta Obstet. Gynec. Scand.*, 41:Suppl. 1, 117, 1962.
10. Botella, J.: *Acta Gin.*, 5:298, 1954.
11. Botella, J.: *Colloques sur la fonction luteale*, Vol. I. Paris, Masson & Cie., 1954.
12. Botella, J., and Gomez-Maestro, D. V.: *Arch. Med. Exper.*, 16:321, 1953.
13. Botella, J., and Marín, E.: *Actas Soc. Esp. Esteril.*, 4:29, 1956.
14. Botella, J., and Tornero, M. C.: *Actas Soc. Esp. Esteril.*, 4:293, 1956.
15. Botella, J.: *Proceed. II World Congress Fertil. Steril.*, Vol. I. Naples, 1956.
16. Botella, J.: *Proceed. III World Congress Fertil. Steril.*, Vol. I. Amsterdam, 1961.
17. Botella, J.: *Acta Gin.*, 10:317, 1959.
18. Botella, J.: *Internat. J. Fertil.*, 4:300, 1959.
19. Botella, J.: *Internat. J. Fertil.*, 7:147, 1962.
20. Botella, J., and Marín, E.: *Acta Gin.*, 9:1, 1958.
21. Botella, J.: *Acta Gin.*, 15:3, 1964.

22. Brewer, J. I., and Jones, H. O.: *Amer. J. Obstet. Gynec.*, 54:561, 1947.
23. Bruni, V., Cattaneo, A., and Forleo, R.: *Riv. Ost. Gin. Supl.*, 22:29, 1967.
24. Brux, J. de, and Gerbier, E.: *Gynec. Prat.*, 18:103, 1967.
25. Buxton, C. L., and Southam, A. L.: *Amer. J. Obstet. Gynec.*, 70:741, 1955.
26. Byrd, J. R., Mahesh, V. B., and Greenblatt, R. B.: *J. Clin. Endocr. Metab.*, 24:939, 1964.
27. Callard, G. V., and Leathem, J. H.: *Proc. Soc. Exper. Biol. Med.*, 118:996, 1965.
28. Campbell, H. J.: *J. Physiol.*, 181:368, 1965.
29. Canivenc, R.: In *Les fonctions de la nidation uterine et ses troubles*. Paris, Masson & Cie., 1960.
30. Cervino, J. M., et al.: *Ann. d'Endocr.*, 17:355, 1956.
31. Chamberlain, G., and Wood, C.: *Brit. Med. J.*, 1:63, 1963.
32. Cohen, M. R., and Hankin, H.: *Internat. J. Fertil.*, 4:58, 1959.
33. Conti, C., Sciarra, F., Concolino, G., and Sorcini, G.: *Europ. J. Steroids*, 2:45, 1967.
34. Cox, R. J., and Shearman, R. P.: *J. Clin. Endocr.*, 21:586, 1961.
35. Culiner, A., and Shippel, S.: *J. Obstet. Gynec. Brit. Emp.*, 56:439, 1949.
36. David, J. S. E., and Amoroso, E. C.: In *Les fonctions de la nidation uterine et ses troubles*. Paris, Masson & Cie., 1960.
37. Decourt, J., Jayle, M. F., and Mauvais-Jarvis, P.: *Presse Med.*, 70:365, 1962.
38. Dokumov, S. I., and Dashev, G. I.: *Amer. J. Obstet. Gynec.*, 86:183, 1963.
39. Dokumov, S. I., and Dashev, G. I.: *Amer. J. Obstet. Gynec.*, 91:185, 1965.
40. Ellett, R. P., and Barnes, D. D.: *Amer. J. Obstet. Gynec.*, 74:1201, 1957.
41. Eton, B., and Short, R. V.: *J. Obstet. Gynec. Brit. Emp.*, 67:587, 1960.
42. Evans, T. N., and Riley, G. M.: *Obstet. Gynec.*, 12:168, 1958.
43. Evans, T. N., and Riley, G. M.: *Amer. J. Obstet. Gynec.*, 80:873, 1960.
44. Feder, H. H., Phoenix, C. H., and Young, W. C.: *J. Endocr.*, 34:131, 1966.
45. Fels, E., Moghilewsky, J. A., and Libertun, C.: *Acta Physiol. Lat. Amer.*, 18:132, 1968.
46. Foss, B. A., Horne, H. W., and Hertig, A. T.: *Fertil. Steril.*, 9:193, 1958.
47. France, J. T., and Knox, B. S.: *Acta Endocr.*, 56:177, 1967.
48. Gallagher, T. F., et al.: *J. Clin. Invest.*, 37:794, 1958.
49. Garry, J., and Fienberg, R.: *Obstet. Gynec.*, 12:480, 1958.
50. Gillam, J. S.: *Fertil. Steril.*, 6:18, 1955.
51. Goldzieher, J. W., and Green, J. A.: *J. Clin. Endocr.*, 22:325, 1962.
52. Goldzieher, J. W., and Axelrod, L. R.: *J. Clin. Endocr.*, 22:425, 1962.
53. Gospodarovicz, D.: *Biochim. Biophys. Acta*, 100:618, 1965.
54. Goy, R. W., Bridson, W. E., and Young, W. C.: *J. Comp. Physiol.*, 57:166, 1964.
55. Hertig, A. T., Rock, J., and Adams, E. C.: *Amer. J. Anat.*, 98:435, 1956.
56. Hertig, A. T.: In *Les fonctions de la nidation uterine et ses troubles*. Paris, Masson & Cie., 1960.
57. Hoffmann, F., and Meger, C.: *Geburtsh. u Frauenhk.*, 25:1132, 1965.
58. Holmstrom, E. G., and MacLennan, E. C.: *Amer. J. Obstet. Gynec.*, 53:727, 1947.
59. Horton, R., and Neisler, J.: *J. Clin. Endocr. Metab.*, 28:479, 1968.
60. Hughes, E. C., Van Nees, A. W., and Lloyd, C. W.: *J. Clin. Endocr. Metab.*, 60:575, 1950.
61. Ingersoll, F. M., and MacArthur, J. W.: *J. Clin. Endocr. Metab.*, 77:759, 1959.
62. Jackson, R. L., and Dockerty, M. B.: *J. Clin. Endocr. Metab.*, 73:161, 1957.
63. Jacobson, D., and Norgren, A.: *Acta Endocr.*, 49:453, 1965.
64. Javert, C. T.: *Amer. J. Obstet. Gynec.*, 84:1149, 1962.
65. Jayle, M. F., et al.: *Acta Endocr.*, 36:371, 1961.
66. Jeffcoate, S. L., Brooks, R. V., and London, D. R.: *J. Endocr.*, 42:213, 1968.
67. Jefferies, W. M.: *J. Clin. Endocr.*, 22:255, 1962.
68. Kallio, H.: *Acta Obstet. Gynec. Scand.*, 40:16, 1961.
69. Kaufman, R. H., et al.: *Amer. J. Obstet. Gynec.*, 77:1271, 1959.
70. Kayser, K.: *Zbl. Gynäk.*, 57:266, 1963.
71. Keetel, W. C., Bradbury, J. T., and Stoddard, F. J.: *Amer. J. Obstet. Gynec.*, 73:954, 1957.
72. Kincl, F. A., et al.: *Acta Endocr.*, 49:193, 1965.
73. Klotz, H. P., Chimenes, H., and Nathan-Klein, J.: *Ann. d'Endocr.*, 24:662, 1963.
74. Knorr, K., Knorr-Gartner, H., and Uebele-Kalkhardt, B.: *Endokrinologie*, 54:364, 1969.
75. Kologh, S., et al.: *Ann. d'Endocr.*, 21:628, 1960.
76. Koreman, S. G., Kirschner, M. A., and Lipsett, M.: *J. Clin. Endocr. Metab.*, 25:798, 1965.
77. Kurzrock, R.: *Ann. Ost. Gin.*, 73:933, 1951.
78. Laitinen, O., and Pesonen, S.: *Acta Endocr.*, 50:524, 1965.
79. Landing, B. H.: *J. Clin. Endocr.*, 14:245, 1954.
80. Lanthier, A., and Sandor, T.: *Metabolism*, 9:861, 1960.
81. Lanthier, A.: *J. Clin. Endocr.*, 20:1587, 1960.
82. Lawrence, D. M.: *J. Obstet. Gynec. Brit. Comm.*, 75:922, 1968.
83. Leventhal, M. L.: *Amer. J. Obstet. Gynec.*, 76:825, 1958.
84. Leventhal, M. L.: *Amer. J. Obstet. Gynec.*, 84:164, 1962.
85. Leventhal, M. L., and Scommegna, A.: *Amer. J. Obstet. Gynec.*, 87:445, 1963.
86. Lindell, A.: *Acta Endocr.*, 47:277, 1964.
87. Lisse, K.: *Endokrinologie*, 53:78, 1968.
88. Lloyd, C. W., Lobotsky, J., Segre, E. J., and others: *J. Clin. Endocr. Metab.*, 26:314, 1966.
89. Lopez, J. M., Migeon, C. J., and Seegar-Jones, G.: *Amer. J. Obstet. Gynec.*, 98:749, 1967.
90. Lucis, O. J., Hobkirk, R., Hollenberg, C. H., MacDonald, S. A., and Blahey, P.: *Canad. Med. Ass. J.*, 94:1, 1966.
91. Lutwak-Mann, C.: In *Implantation of Ova*. Memoirs of the Society of Endocrinology, Cambridge University Press, 1959.
92. MacArthur, J. W., et al.: *J. Clin. Endocr.*, 18:1202, 1958.
93. MacBryde, W. C., and Moyes, J. M.: *Internat. J. Fertil.*, 4:323, 1959.
94. MacKelvey, J. L.: *Amer. J. Obstet. Gynec.*, 60:523, 1950.
95. MacLennan, C. E.: *Amer. J. Obstet. Gynec.*, 64:988, 1952.

96. Mahesh, V., Greenblatt, R. B., Aydar, C. K., and Roy, S.: *Fertil. Steril.*, 13:513, 1962.
97. Mahesh, V., and Greenblatt, R. B.: *J. Clin. Endocr.*, 22:441, 1962.
98. Malkani, D. K.: *Internat. J. Fertil.*, 7:53, 1962.
99. Marin, E., and Botella, J.: *Acta Gin.*, 4:339, 1953.
100. Masters, W. H., and Magallon, D. T.: *Amer. J. Obstet. Gynec.*, 59:970, 1950.
101. Mayer, G.: In *Les fonctions de la nidation uterine et ses troubles*. Paris, Masson & Cie., 1960.
102. Meaker, S. R.: *Fertil. Steril.*, 1:293, 1950.
103. Mellinger, R. C., et al.: *J. Clin. Endocr.*, 16:967, 1956.
104. Miklosi, S. A., and MacKosker, P. J.: *J. Endocr.*, 39:361, 1967.
105. Momigliano, E.: *Obstet. Gynec.*, 13:25, 1959.
106. Montalvo, L.: *Actas Soc. Esp. Esteril.*, 4:124, 1956.
107. Morris, J. M., and Scully, R. E.: *Endocrine Pathology of the Ovary*. St. Louis, C. V. Mosby Co., 1958.
108. Netter, A., et al.: *Rev. Franç. Gynec.*, 58:671, 1963.
109. Netter, A., Jayle, M. F., and Mauvais-Jarvis, P.: *Ann. d'Endocr.*, 21:590, 1960.
110. Netter, A., et al.: *Ann. d'Endocr.*, 22:548, 841, 1961.
111. Netter, A., and Thoret, Y.: *Gynec. Prat.*, 18:71, 1967.
112. Nichols, T., Nugent, C. A., and Tyler, F. A.: *J. Clin. Endocr. Metab.*, 26:79, 1966.
113. Noall, M. W., and Kaufman, R. H.: *Fertil Steril.*, 17:83, 1966.
114. Nogales, F.: *Actas Soc. Esp. Esteril.*, 4:173, 1956.
115. Nogales, F., Marin, E., and Botella, J.: *Actas Soc. Esp. Esteril.*, 6:133, 1958.
116. Novak, E.: *Obstetrical and Gynecological Pathology*, 2nd ed. Philadelphia, W. B. Saunders, 1947.
117. Noyes, R. W.: *Amer. J. Obstet. Gynec.*, 77:929, 1959.
118. Oakey, R. E., and Stitch, S. R.: *Acta Endocr.*, 58:407, 1968.
119. Palmer, R.: In *Les fonctions de la nidation uterine et ses troubles*. Paris, Masson & Cie., 1960.
120. Perloff, W. H., Steinberger, E., and Smith, K. E.: *Acta Gin.*, 16:475, 1965.
121. Perloff, W. H., and Jacobson, G.: *J. Clin. Endocr.*, 23:1177, 1963.
122. Pesonen, S., et al.: *Acta Endocr.*, 30:405, 1959.
123. Pigeaud, E., et al.: *Bull. Fed. Soc. Obstet. Gynec.*, 12:299, 1960.
124. Plate, W. P.: *Acta Endocr.*, 8:17, 1951.
125. Plate, W. P.: *Acta Endocr.*, 11:119, 1952.
126. Plate, W. P.: *Gynaecologia*, 150:267, 1960.
127. Plate, W. P.: *Arch. Gynäk.*, 198:473, 1963.
128. Ponse, K.: *Ann. d'Endocr.*, 16:89, 1955.
129. Ramirez, D., and MacCann, S. M.: *Endocrinology*, 76:412, 1965.
130. Roos, M., and Roos, J.: *Compt. Rend. Acad. Sci.*, 262:300, 1966.
131. Rowlands, I. W.: *J. Endocr.*, 19:81, 1959.
132. Sachs, B. A., and Spiro, D.: *J. Clin. Endocr.*, 11:878, 1951.
133. Salhanick, H. A.: *Amer. J. Obstet. Gynec.*, 84:162, 1962.
134. Schrieffers, H., and Schmidt, E.: *Hoppe-Seylers Ztschr. Physiol. Chem.*, 349:1085, 1968.
135. Seeman, A., and Saracino, R. T.: *Acta Endocr.*, 37:31, 1961.
136. Segaloff, A., et al.: *J. Clin. Endocr.*, 11:936, 1951.
137. Segre, E. J.: *Androgens, Virilization and the Hirsute Female*. Springfield, Ill., Charles C Thomas, 1967.
138. Severi, S., Sbiroli, C., Galli, A., and Forleo, R.: *Clin. Ost. Gin. (Roma)*, 70:493, 1968.
139. Sfikakis, A. P., Ikkos, D. G., and Diamantopoulos, K. N.: *J. Endocr.*, 39:61, 1967.
140. Shearman, R. P., Cox, R. I., and Gannon, A.: *Lancet*, 1:260, 1961.
141. Shearman, R. P., and Cox, R. I.: *Amer. J. Obstet. Gynec.*, 92:497, 1965.
142. Short, R. V.: *J. Endocr.*, 24:359, 1962.
143. Singh, K. B.: *Amer. J. Obstet. Gynec.*, 105:274, 1969.
144. Singh, K. B.: *Amer. J. Obstet. Gynec.*, 103:1078, 1969.
145. Sommers, S. C., and Wadam, P. J.: *Amer. J. Obstet. Gynec.*, 72:160, 1956.
146. Sopeña, A., and Tornero, M. C.: *Actas Soc. Exp. Esp. Esteril.*, 4:247, 1956.
147. Sopeña, A., and Botella, J.: *Acta Gin.*, 14:225, 1963.
148. Staemmler, H. J., and Sachs, L.: *Arch. Gynäk.*, 197:612, 1962.
149. Stein, I. F., and Cohen, M. R.: *Amer. J. Obstet. Gynec.*, 38:465, 1939.
150. Stein, I. F.: *Internat. J. Fertil.*, 7:123, 1962.
151. Sternberg, W. H., et al.: *J. Clin. Endocr.*, 13:139, 1953.
152. Stieve, H.: *Einfluss des Nervensystems auf Bau und Tätigkeit der Weiblichen Genitale*. Stuttgart, G. Thieme, 1952.
153. Sturgis, S. H.: *J. Clin. Endocr.*, 14:766, 1954.
154. Sun, L. C. D., and Rakoff, A. E.: *J. Clin. Endocr.*, 16:971, 1956.
155. Surace, M., and Polvani, F.: *Ann. Ost. Gin.*, 88:103, 1966.
156. Swanson, H. E., and Van Der Werff, J. J.: *Acta Endocr.*, 47:35, 1964.
157. Swanson, H. E., and Van Der Werff, J. J.: *Acta Endocr.*, 50:379, 1965.
158. Taymor, M., Clark, B. J., and Sturgis, S. H.: *Amer. J. Obstet. Gynec.*, 86:188, 1963.
159. Thomas, J. P.: *J. Clin. Endocr.*, 28:1781, 1968.
160. Trace, R. J., Keaty, E. C., and MacCall, M. L.: *Amer. J. Obstet. Gynec.*, 79:311, 1960.
161. Tulsky, A. S., and Koff, A. K.: *Fertil. Steril.*, 8:119, 1957.
162. Van Campenhout, E.: *Acta Anat.*, 4:73, 1947.
163. Van Rees, G. P., and Gans, E.: *Acta Endocr.*, 52:471, 1966.
164. Waugh, D., Venning, E. H., and MacEachern, D.: *J. Clin. Endocr.*, 4:486, 1944.
165. Warren, J. C., and Salhanick, H. A.: *J. Clin. Endocr.*, 21:1218, 1961.
166. Yen, S. S. C., Vela, P., and Rankin, J.: *J. Clin. Endocr.*, 30:435, 1970.
167. Yen, S. S. C., Vela, P., and Ryan, K. J.: *J. Clin. Endocr.*, 31:7, 1970.
168. Zander, J.: "In vitro Studien an Ovarien mit abnormaler Hormonbildung," in *Symposium über Krebsprobleme*. Berlin, Springer, 1961.
169. Zander, J.: *Rev. Franç. Endocr. Clin. Nutr. Metab.*, 4:409, 1963.
170. Zellmaker, G. H.: *Acta Endocr.*, 46:571, 1964.

Chapter 30
FUNCTIONAL TUMORS OF THE OVARY FROM THE ENDOCRINE POINT OF VIEW

30.1. GENERAL CONSIDERATIONS AND CLASSIFICATION

The vast volume of literature on the subject of ovarian hormone-producing tumors that has accumulated over the last years is indeed overwhelming. Several thousand cases are already on record, of which most are extensive case reports that had been published piecemeal. Not only is it impossible from a material standpoint to present a complete review of the literature, but also the greater part of the early data would be lacking in interest since they are no longer utilizable. In a textbook on endocrinology, our main interest must necessarily be oriented toward the purely endocrinologic aspects of these tumors, which is why the related genetic, clinical and surgical details can be reviewed here only cursorily.

In 1948, Novak[82] set up an *ovarian tumor registry* which after his death has been continued by his followers. It has since grown into a collection of several thousand conveniently ordered and classified tumors which, at present, constitutes the principal source of study material. Our own files contain several score of various types of tumors collected by us.

The most common variety are *granulosa cell tumors*, followed by *thecomas*, both types of tumors being relatively common, although they are often missed, particularly when of very small size. On the other hand, *masculinizing tumor* varieties are very rare. Among 64 functional ovarian tumors, Schneider[105] found 31 granulosa cell tumors, 24 thecomas, 8 hilus cell tumors and a single arrhenoblastoma.

As regards *classification* of functional ovarian tumors, we shall follow the same criteria that we enunciated in 1950 and modified slightly in 1967.[14] Accordingly, our classification is based on *histogenetic* considerations (Table 30–1). Because these tumors cannot be adequately characterized on the basis of morphologic studies alone, as recently acknowledged by Koss,[59] the only rational way of classifying them should be on their steroidogenic properties.

Only a limited number among the tumors listed in Table 30–1 may display functional activity. In the first place, there are the *mesenchymogenic tumors*, derived from the active or the sexual mesenchyme and, in the second place, there are *ovulogenic tumors* of teratoblastomatous nature that possess endocrine activity. Such tumors have been marked with an asterisk in the table; it is thus apparent that all the celomogenic, a large part of the ovulogenic and even some of the mesenchymogenic tumors lack hormonal activity.

While this classification is interesting from the vantage point of histogenesis, a simpler type of classification is preferable for endocrinologic purposes (see Table 30–2).

It may be noted that the terminology used for some entities in Table 30–2 does not agree with that used in Table 30–1. Thus,

TABLE 30-1. Classification of Ovarian Tumors†

OVARIAN ELEMENT	TUMOR PRODUCED

Germinal route (Gonocyte)	Germ cell tumors
	1. *Gonocytomas* (°)
	2. *Teratomas*
	  (a) Simple
	  (b) Complex
	3. *Teratoblastomas*
	  (a) Without endocrine activity
	  (b) Struma ovarii (°)
	  (c) Ovarian chorioepithelioma (°)

Coeloma (Pflüger's cords)	Coelomogenic tumors
	1. *Undifferentiated celoma* (nonmüllerian)
	  (a) Benign (Brenner tumor) (°)
	  (b) Malignant (primary carcinoma)
	2. *Differentiated celoma* (müllerian)
	  (a) Endosalpingioma
	  (b) Endometrioma
	  (c) Endocervicoma

Mesenchyme	Mesenchymogenic tumors
	1. *Inactive mesenchyme*
	  (a) Benign (fibroma)
	  (b) Malignant (sarcoma)
	2. *Active mesenchyme* (sexual)
	  (a) Feminizing (gynemesenchymomas)
	    (i) Granulosa cell tumor (°)
	    (ii) Thecoma (°)
	    (iii) Luteoma (°)
	  (b) Masculinizing (andromesenchymomas)
	    (i) Arrhenoblastoma (°)
	    (ii) Leydig cell tumor (°)
	  (c) Interrenal (interrenomesenchymomas) ovarian hypernephroma (°)

°Tumors marked with an asterisk may display hormonal activity.
†From Botella-Llusiá: *Enfermedades del Aparato Genital Femenino*, 7th ed. Barcelona, Científico-Médica, 1964.

for instance, luteomas, listed among gynemesenchymomas in the general classification, are categorized as gestagenic tumors. It shall be pointed out later that, its feminine lineage notwithstanding, this type of tumor may produce a virilizing effect as a result of a shunt in its metabolism. In the same way, the interrenomesenchymomas, or ovarian hypernephromas, are included in the same group by virtue of their predominantly masculinizing action. It must also be pointed out that these tumors structurally mimicking thyroid tissue only rarely display endocrine activity and are most often inert, so that while they are histologically classifiable as struma ovarii, they only seldom deserve this designation in terms of endocrine function.

30.2. FEMINIZING TUMORS

Included in this category are a group of tumors known as *granulosa cell tumors, thecomas and luteinized forms of either group*. As a whole, they actually represent a rather unique entity of tumor, called "*feminizing mesenchymomas*" by Novak[81] and "*gynemesenchymomas*" by ourselves. Structurally, these tumoral growths may reproduce the follicle both as regards the epithelial (granulosa) and the connective tissue (theca) components of the latter. Although they are usually not luteinized in the most commonly occurring varieties of such tumors, their cellular elements may undergo luteinization, just as the granulosa and theca may under physiologic conditions. Among the luteinized varieties, luteomas must be distinguished as standing apart because of their problematic luteal nature. We list them among the tumors of the masculinizing variety.

30.2.1. HISTOGENESIS

Meyer[76] assumed that these tumors arose in granulosa cell rests, present in mature follicles, which he called "Granulosabal-

TABLE 30-2. Endocrinologic Classification of Functional Ovarian Tumors

A. *Estrogenic tumors*
  1. Tumors of the granulosa
  2. Tumors of the theca
B. *Gestagenic tumors*
  1. Luteinized tumors of the granulosa and the theca
  2. Luteomas
C. *Masculinizing tumors*
  1. Testicular adenoma of Pick (arrhenoblastoma)
  2. Leydig cell tumor
  3. Ovarian hypernephroma (interrenomesenchymoma)
D. *Tumors with thyroid activity*
  1. Struma ovarii
E. *Tumors with gonadotropic activity*
  1. Ovarian chorioepithelioma

len." Such structures were believed to represent isolated islets of cells that had been pinched off in the process of follicle formation. Although such rests may actually be observed in the ovaries of children, Novak[82] and Schiller[103] reject this view. According to them, granulosa cells arise from the mesenchyme of embryonal ovaries. This point of view had also been accepted by Wainer and his associates[115] and by ourselves in classifying such tumors as mesenchymomas that are histogenetically derived from the sexual mesenchyme. Gonadal mesenchymal tissue has the potential for elaborating steroids, either estrogenic or androgenic in nature; the polarity and differentiation of the hormones secreted depend on the type of organizer stimulus the mesenchyme is submitted to during the embryonal phase of development. As indicated previously (see Chapter 6), the actions exerted by gonocytes and such chemical substances as cortexine and medullarine are able to sway the process of differentiation either way, that is, toward an ovary or toward a testis. The process of differentiation in this instance is determined not only by the character of the germ cells but also by the nature of endocrine differentiation of the mesenchyme. It may therefore be postulated that, as a result of any aberrant stimulatory influence during embryonal or adult life, altered mesenchymal development may give rise to tumors of the granulosa or theca cell type.

There are some interesting observations to support this point of view. Geist and his associates[37] have been able to induce granulosa cell and theca cell tumors experimentally in mice by means of x-rays. Li and co-workers,[62] as well as Lipschütz and Cerisola,[65] Jull and colleagues,[54] and Ely and colleagues,[25] have all observed tumors of similar appearance in transplants of rat ovary to the spleen. Evidently, all estrogens are degraded by the liver and, by ceasing to inhibit the pituitary, allow the latter to develop exaggerated gonadotropin activity, which induces transformation of ovarian tissue into a tumor of feminizing nature. As a result, it must be assumed that an unusually energetic gonadotropic stimulus, acting on the ovarian mesenchyme, is equally capable of shifting embryonal or undifferentiated mesenchymal growth in a feminizing direction. In further agreement with this assumption is the fact that Johnson and Witschi[51] likewise obtained growth of granulosa cell tumors experimentally in parabiotic rats when one of the parabionts was castrated. In this case, it must be assumed that pituitary hyperfunction, brought about by castration of one of the parabionts (see Chapter 17), exerted a tumorigenic effect on the ovaries of the other animal. *Consequently, everything would lead one to suggest a gonadotropic etiology for this type of tumor.* Nevertheless, considering the fact that identical results have been obtained by Lipschütz and his associates[64] with the administration of norethynodrel, which is a sterilizing steroid with a *pituitary-suppressing effect*, the true mechanism whereby such tumors are induced to grow is far from clear.

30.2.2. RELATIONSHIP BETWEEN TUMORS OF THE GRANULOSA AND THOSE OF THE THECA

For many years, the two varieties were described as independent entities, one as an epithelial tumor, the other as a connective tissue tumor.[3,4] Currently, the consensus is that they should be considered as *two similar and frequently associated forms of the same kind of mesenchymal tumor which, in the final analysis, is of connective tissue nature.* After all, there is no reason why the granulosa cell tumors and the thecomas should be viewed as two fundamentally different tumors. In 1947, Bedoya and Botella[11] described a granulosa cell tumor in which extensive areas were made up of a thecal component. Novak[81] proposed the designation *granulosa-theca tumor* for this type (Fig. 30–2). Nonetheless, from a histologic point of view, the predominance of either thecal or granulosa cells permits the description of these tumors as distinct granulosa cell tumors or thecomas, although it must be remembered that, from the endocrinologic and pathogenic point of view, the two varieties constitute a single entity.

30.2.3. GRANULOSA CELL TUMORS

These tumors occur in the ovary, usually are unilateral and range in size from that of a chick pea to that of a grapefruit. The tumors may be quite small in size, but they are then seldom detected. Macroscopically, they are usually rounded, ovoid or kidney-shaped. Their outer surface may be smooth and glistening, but sometimes it is lobulated. On sectioning, they are seen to be solid or may show small cystic cavities.

Microscopically, they may reveal a wide range of patterns, a fact mainly responsible for the confusion concerning nomenclature and classification (Figs. 30-1, 30-2 and 30-3). Whatever the structural features of these tumors, they all have one element in common: a small cuboidal cell type with scanty cytoplasm, relatively large nucleus and a striking resemblance to the cells of the granulosa layer. These cells are characteristic not only cytologically but also because they tend to be arranged in follicle-like configurations. This gives rise to cell clusters with tiny central cavities, called Call-Exner bodies (Figs. 30-1 and 30-3). Meyer[76] originally described several varieties of granulosa cell tumors according to predominantly macrofollicular, microfollicular, adenomatous and cylindromatous patterns. Basically, all are now believed to be mere variants of the same underlying structure.

Granulosa cell tumors may be benign or malignant. It is generally admitted that the so-called group of dysontogenetic ovarian tumors have a considerably lower potential for malignancy than the more common types of primary carcinomas. In spite of this, there are a number of granulosa cell tumors on record that recurred even after radical surgery. Their association with *precocious puberty* in young girls is discussed in Chapter 38 (Section 38.2.3). Recently, Zangeneh and Kelley[118] published a detailed review of the literature on the subject.

Granulosa cell tumors are frequently observed to run a malignant course. Dockerty and MacCarthy[19] reported that five of 30 cases (16.6 per cent) underwent malignant degeneration over a period of five years. Greene and Prencel[43] observed malignancy in seven of 38 cases (18.4 per cent), and Salerno[99] in nine of 28 cases (25 per cent). It may be roughly estimated that one in every five tumors is a malignant *granulosa cell carcinoma*.

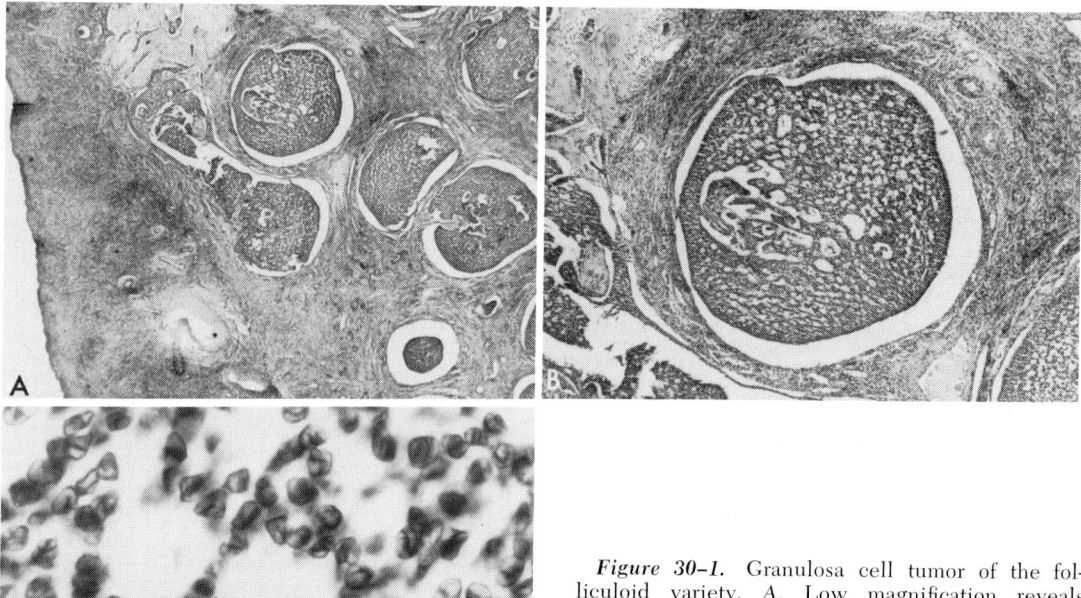

Figure 30-1. Granulosa cell tumor of the folliculoid variety. A, Low magnification reveals folliculoid structures (25×). B, Adenomatous appearance is seen at slightly higher magnification (75×). C, High power view (500×) of rosette-like arrangement of tumor cells (Call-Exner body).

Functional Tumors of the Ovary from the Endocrine Point of View

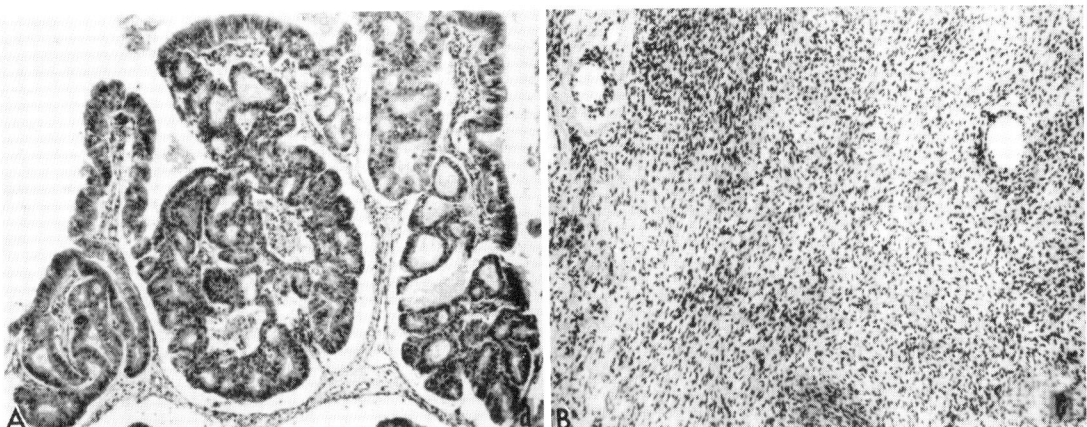

Figure 30–2. A, Adenomatous variety of granulosa cell tumor with a tendency to papillary growth pattern, supported by slender cores of vascularized connective tissue. B, Another area of same tumor, revealing extensive thecal component, partially luteinized and vascularized.

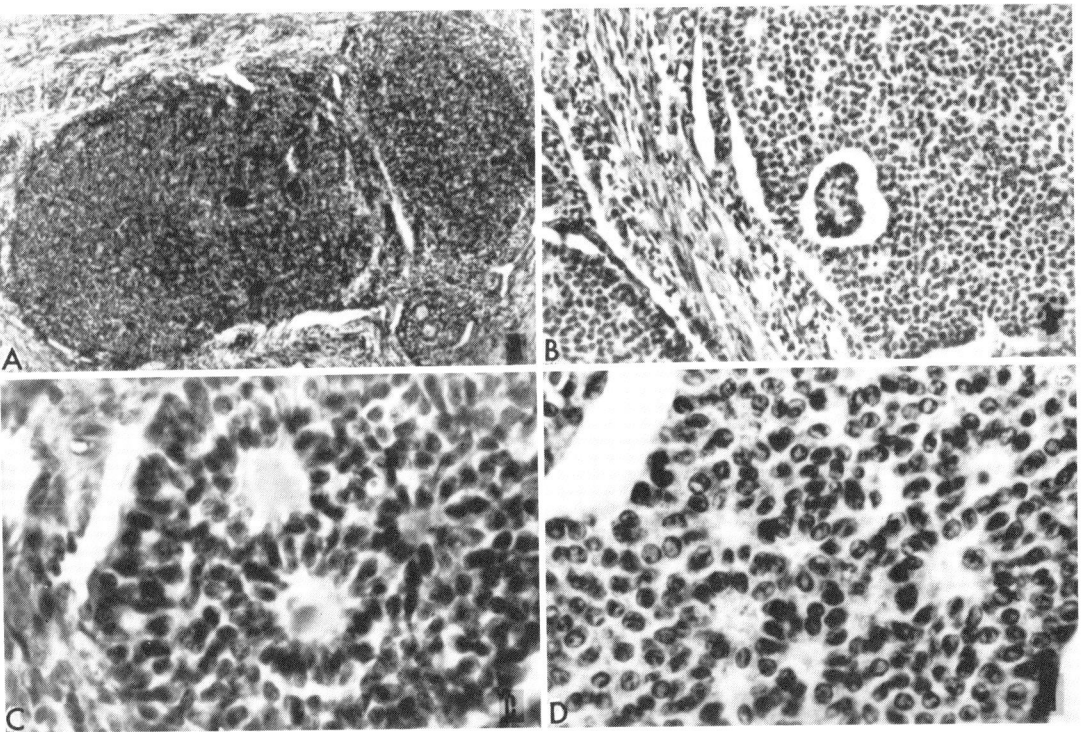

Figure 30–3. A, Nodular growth of granulosa cell tumor, with scanty intervening connective tissue stroma. B, Higher power reveals folliculoid growth pattern with stellate appearance. C, D, Call-Exner bodies at high magnification.

30.2.4. THECOMAS

Grossly, these tumors are similar in appearance to fibromas. They may be smaller than granulosa cell tumors, even of microscopic size, but they may nevertheless cause clinical symptoms (Figs. 30-4 and 30-5).

In a recent review, in cooperation with Nogales and Sánchez-Garrido,[13] we observed that two in 100 ovaries from women with endometrial adenocarcinoma contained tiny theca cell tumors that had been missed by the surgeon.

Microscopically, they commonly present a fibromatous growth pattern which characteristically is made up of fusiform cells lying in a more or less abundant ground substance (Fig. 30-5). In this respect, two fundamental varieties may be distinguished: a fibromatous variety, composed of elongated, spindle-shaped cells with small nuclei and abundant ground substance, and an "epithelioid" variety, made up of less fusiform, polyhedral-like cells which, although in general retaining their connective tissue appearance, are quite reminiscent of the characteristic epithelioid appearance of luteinized theca cells.

Thecomas, as pointed out by Traut and his associates,[111] are often found to contain frankly epithelial islets of the granulosa cell type. Studies by the same authors on the distribution of reticulin fibers in these tumors show no fundamental difference between one variety and the other. A great impetus to the study of the histochemical properties of these tumors has been given by the work of McKay and his associates.[69] According to Nogales, the demonstration of lipid (Fig. 30-6) and the study of reticulum by means of Del Rio-Hortega's impregnation method are two helpful aids in arriving at a definite diagnosis of thecoma.

Thecomas often occur in association with the Stein-Leventhal syndrome,[30] a fact suggesting that "hyperthecosis" in that syndrome (see Chapter 29) may favor development of such tumors. Thecomas are only exceptionally malignant. In a review of the world literature, Birkheiser[7] found only 12 malignant cases and even in some of these, malignancy could be questioned.

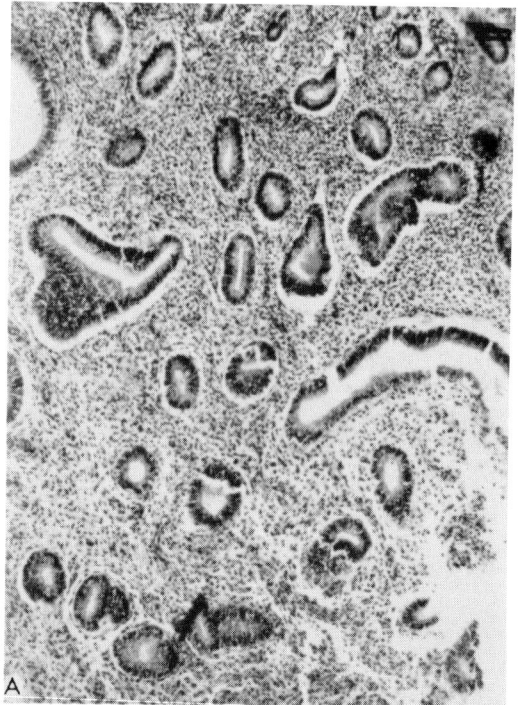
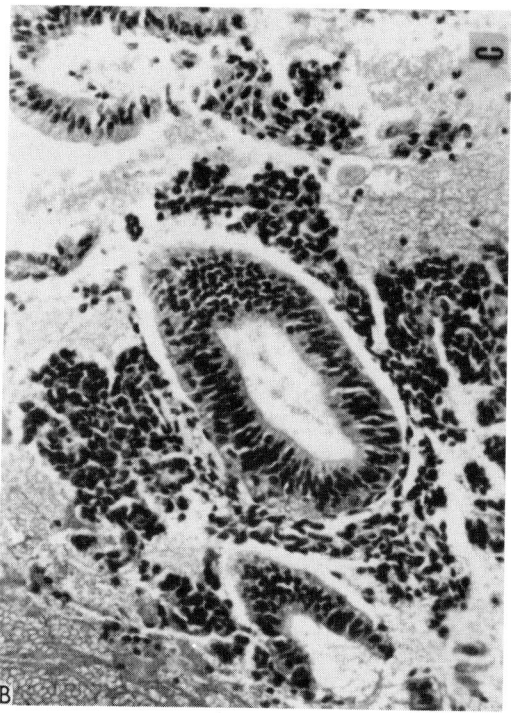

Figure 30-4. Endometrial hyperplasia associated with ovarian thecoma. A, Dense stroma (100×). B, Marked proliferation of gland epithelium (400×).

Functional Tumors of the Ovary from the Endocrine Point of View

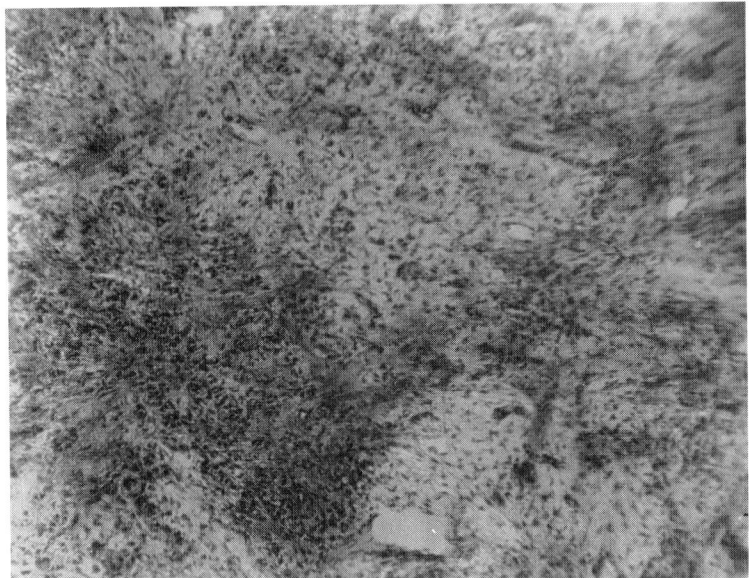

Figure 30–5. Histology of tumor causing endometrial findings shown in Figure 30–4.

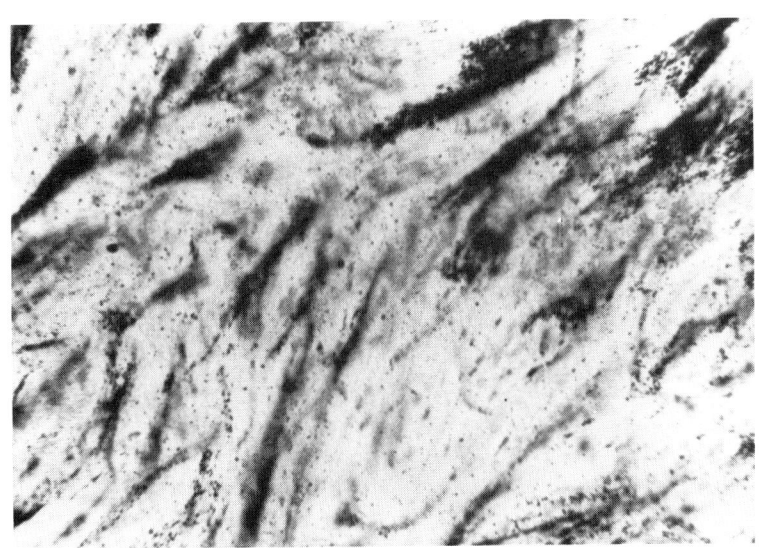

Figure 30–6. Thecoma stained with Sudan III.

30.2.5. ENDOCRINE PROPERTIES

Both granulosa cell tumors and thecomas may display endocrine activity and are *estrogen producers*. The clinical manifestations are consequently derived from secretion of estrogens, which is the most outstanding property of these tumors.

Estrogenic activity may become manifest in different ways, depending on what phase of life in which it appears. Accordingly, three main clinical forms may be distinguished: (1) *precocious puberty*, associated with tumors arising in the *prepuberal age group;* (2) *hyperestrinism*, with metropathia haemorrhagica, endometrial hyperplasia and, sometimes, mammary dysplasia, in association with tumors arising *during adult life;* (3) tumors arising *after menopause.* The manifestations are most characteristic in the third group; most feminizing tumors have been described in the postmenopausal age group not because they occur less frequently during the reproductive years but rather because they are more frequently detected after menopause, when the symptomatology they give rise to becomes most conspicuous. Symptoms include apparent reestablishment of menses or, more appropriately, what should be termed *pseudomenstrual periodic bleeding*. It may further involve general rejuvenation in the entire somatic appearance in postmenopausal women, as well as renewed turgescence of breasts.

Hormone studies on these patients were pioneered by Pincus[90] and by Jayle.[50] The rate of estrogenuria encountered greatly exceeded even the highest values found in any other syndrome of hyperestrinism. Urinary values amounting to as much as 1000 mcg per 24 hr were not unusual. Similar hyperestrogenic effects are found at the level of the target organs. *Vaginal cytology* shows a pronounced estrogen effect, with elevated karyopyknotic and acidophilic indices. In some cases, true *superficial cornification* of the vagina may be found (Pundel[93]). An almost constant endometrial finding of interest is *cystic glandular hyperplasia*, an example of which is shown in Figure 30–4.

Frequently associated with *hyperestrinism* are *leiomyomas*[4, 49] and, more significantly, *endometrial carcinoma*,[20, 35, 48] which is said to have a twenty-fold higher incidence in women with estrogenizing tumors.[13] This point will be reexamined in Chapter 46.

Recent studies concerning the *hormonal metabolism* of feminizing tumors reveal that a common feature to all such tumors is their capacity to synthesize estrogen from acetate or cholesterol or both. Marsh and his associates[72] incubated slices of granulosa cell tumors in the presence of C-14 labeled cholesterol and obtained radioactive estrogen. Griffiths and his colleagues[45] subsequently demonstrated formation of androstenedione and conversion of the latter to estrogen, and later also confirmed conversion of pregnenolone to estrogen. Goldberg and co-workers[40] isolated 3β-ol-dehydrogenase from such tumors, whereas Flickinger and his associates[31] discovered a pathway in estrogen synthesis involving dehydroepiandrosterone as the starting point, in a way quite similar to what is known to occur in placental estrogen synthesis. MacAuley and Weliky[68] incubated granulosa cell tumor tissue with tritiated pregnenolone and C-14 labeled progesterone. As a result, they found that the first substrate permitted estrogen synthesis whereas the second did not, which would indicate that tumor tissue is able to utilize only one of the two pathways available in normal estrogen formation (see Chapter 19, Section 19.8.1). One thing seems certain — namely, that while these tumors are estrogen producers, they do not exactly duplicate ovarian tissue in performance so that, from a biochemical standpoint, theirs is a pathological form of steroidogenesis.

30.2.6. LUTEINIZATION OF GRANULOSA AND THECA CELL TUMORS

It is of further histologic interest that the constituents of this type of tumors, both the granulosa cells and the theca cells, may occasionally undergo transformation into *typical lutein cells*. In general, this transformation is a development in the process of maturation of these tumors and therefore does not appear in actively proliferating tumors but rather in those with a low rate of growth. Luteinization may thus be considered as a *sign militating against malignancy*.

Occasionally tumors may reveal luteinization only in isolated foci and, even then, only of minimal degree. In some instances, luteinization may be of sufficient intensity for the tumor to be associated with signs of progesterone effect. Twombly[112] found increased urinary pregnanediol in a few such cases. We have seen a case with a luteinized thecoma in which the endometrium revealed typical secretory phase changes. Any evidence of progesterone effect on the endometrium is very seldom seen, since that would require a considerable degree of luteinization of the tumor. Whenever luteal transformation is extreme in extent, the tumor may, as will be indicated, display androgenic properties. Traut and his associates[111] stressed the difference between luteinized tumors and pseudoluteinized tumors. The first type are those in which evidence of progesterone effect is unquestionable. These are associated with demonstrably increased urinary pregnanediol levels and secretory endometria. On the other hand, pseudoluteinized tumors are those in which such effects cannot be recognized. We believe that, in most instances, tumors described as so-called luteomas are actually pseudoluteinized tumors.

30.2.7. TUMORS WITH OCCASIONAL FEMINIZING EFFECTS

New techniques for the determination of estrogens have made discovery of feminizing activity possible even in such tumors as were once believed to be inert. Flickinger and his associates[31] found both free and conjugated estrogens in the wall of an ovarian cystadenoma. Fox[34] found luteinized stromal cells in the walls of some cystadenomas, ascribing their presence to an estrogenic effect. In addition, Jopp[53] believes that Brenner tumors may be estrogen producers in view of the fact that they are frequently found in association with endometrial carcinoma. Eddie[22] showed that mucinous cystadenomas as well as both benign and malignant serous tumors were able to elicit estrogenic activity by the ovarian stroma.

30.3. MASCULINIZING TUMORS

While the preceding group of tumors (feminizing) is a relatively homogeneous group, comprising apparently a single entity, the masculinizing tumors have a quite different, often questionable or unknown, histogenesis; the only certain feature these tumors have in common is that they all produce masculinization.[67, 80] To classify these tumors more satisfactorily, further study is therefore necessary not just as regards their endocrinologic properties but also as regards their histogenesis.

The principal tumors found in this group are arrhenoblastomas, adrenal tumors or *hypernephromas*, so-called *masculinovoblastomas*, the more recently discovered Leydig or hilus cell tumors and, finally, we include here also luteomas, although the significance of so-called "luteomas" has not been fully clarified.

30.3.1. ARRHENOBLASTOMA

The term *arrhenoblastoma*, first used by Meyer,[76] is in fact applicable to the entire group of masculinizing tumors. However, by arrhenoblastoma, Meyer originally meant tumors arising from male-directed cells of testicular rests persisting in the ovary. By the same token, these tumors might be defined as *andromesenchymomas*, that is, tumors derived from proliferation of the masculinizing mesenchyme. Structurally, they tend to reproduce—though not in every detail—the architecture of the testis and may be considered as arising from heterologous ovarian rests.

GENESIS. The genesis of arrhenoblastoma, like that of any other tumor in this group, has been a matter of controversy. Schiller[103] postulated that differentiation of the ovarian mesenchyme in either a male or a female direction took place before the fifth week of embryonal life by virtue of the arrival at the gonadal primordium of certain migrant ameboid cells (the *gonocytes*), which are discussed in Chapter 15. Gonocytes are presumably carriers of chromosomal determination of sex and are consequently thought to be the equivalent of Speemann's organizers. Representing the "germinal route," gonocytes are postulated to influence the creation of either a male or a female gonad, in accordance with the sexual message carried by them. In other words, a testis would be generated whenever the gonocytes involved are carriers of male chromosomes and, conversely, gonocytes with female potentialities would be required to induce differentiation of an ovary.

Recent ideas concerning the development of the gonad were analyzed in Chapter 16. For further details, the reader is referred to that chapter.

INCIDENCE. Obviously, these tumors are rare. Most case reports are based on a single case and, up to 1945, Bedoya[3] had been able to collect only about 100 cases from the literature. The American Tumor Registry contains to date approximately 200 cases in all. However, calculating the incidence of arrhenoblastoma is complicated by the fact that different results are obtained depending on whether endocrinologic or histologic criteria are applied. If such tumors are defined on the basis of histologic patterns alone, as was recently done by Morris,[80] a higher incidence for arrhenoblastoma may be obtained, since small structures of testiculoid appearance are relatively common in the ovarian hilum. As far back as 1905, Pick described such hilar findings by the name of *testicular adenomas of the ovary*. The same author, however, recognized their inert nature in most instances. According to Novak and Mattingly,[83] apparent lack of activity by small adenomas of Pick results in part from the fact that their androgenic secretion is exiguous and is easily smothered or dominated by overall ovarian hormone activity.

However, there is another, more important reason for apparently scant or absent masculinizing activity by these tumors. Of all the ovarian structures, only the Leydig cells are thought to be a specific source of androgen, whereas Sertoli cells produce estrogens, as had been shown by Teilum.[108] As a result, it may be easy to understand why some adenomas of the testicular type should not be associated with masculinization and should even be responsible for feminizing effects, as in the case reported by Ehrlich,[23] in which a typical Sertoli cell adenoma in the ovary, in the absence of any apparent interstitial cell component, was associated with precocious puberty.

ANATOMIC PATHOLOGY. Arrhenoblastomas may have a complex histologic structure. It may comprise a wide range of histologic patterns, from the architecture of testicular tissue reproduced in a more or less typical manner, at one extreme, to extremely undifferentiated growth which may be confused with sarcoma, at the other (Fig. 30-7). What Pick described in 1905 was the highly differentiated form, which faithfully mimicks the architecture of the testis. The same form was described by Meyer as *adenoma tubulare testiculare* (Fig. 30-8). In rare instances, adenomas of this type may be in part carcinomatous, as found by Novak[81] in two cases.

Between the two extremes, there is an intermediate group characterized by tubular formations that are only vaguely reminiscent of testicular tubules. The cellular elements of the latter form may be arranged in a cylindroid or cylindromatous fashion, with zigzagging cords or columns. Interspersed among them may be aggregates of cells resembling Leydig cells; however, their presence is highly inconstant. Fat stains usually reveal the presence of lipids within the interstitial cells of the Leydig type, lending a special character to the tumor, which to some extent may be diagnostic of hormone activity.

An arrhenoblastoma of the intermediate type is shown in Figure 30-9, revealing some suggestion of pseudotubular pattern and the presence of Leydig type epithelioid cells between cell cords. In compari-

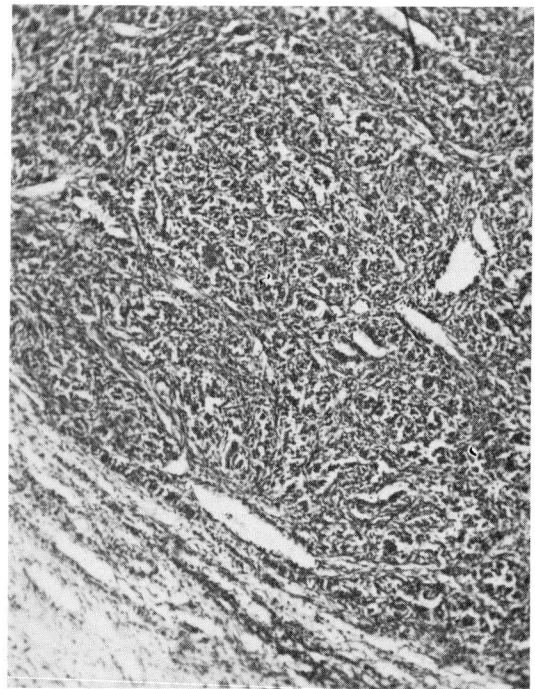

Figure 30-7. Highly undifferentiated arrhenoblastoma of ovary, resembling a sarcoma.

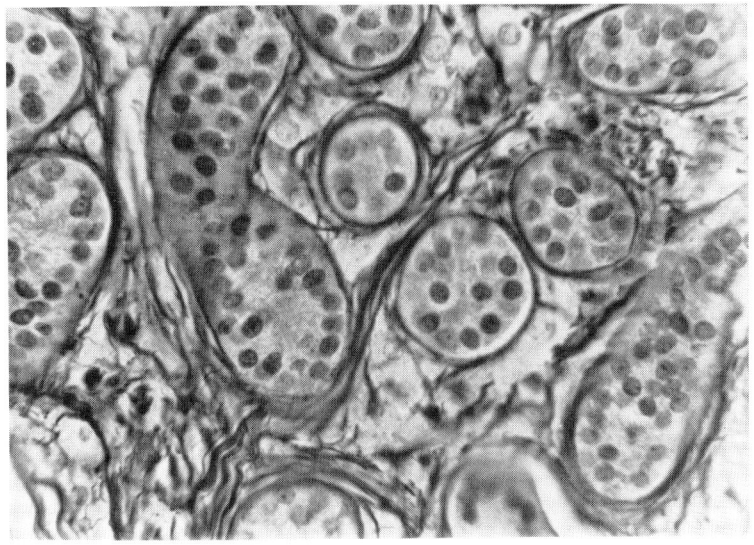

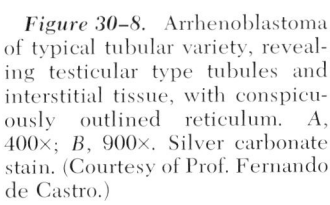

Figure 30–8. Arrhenoblastoma of typical tubular variety, revealing testicular type tubules and interstitial tissue, with conspicuously outlined reticulum. A, 400×; B, 900×. Silver carbonate stain. (Courtesy of Prof. Fernando de Castro.)

son, the tumor is markedly disorganized structurally and is rather suggestive of a connective tissue growth. However, as not shown by the illustration, the neoplasm was nodular and neatly demarcated by a fibrous capsule, which would indicate that the tumor is not a sarcoma or any other related variety of malignancy. It should be kept in mind that arrhenoblastoma is after all of mesenchymal derivation so that the common presence of semi-connective tissue foci in many of these tumors is not surprising.

CLINICAL CHARACTERISTICS. Asso-

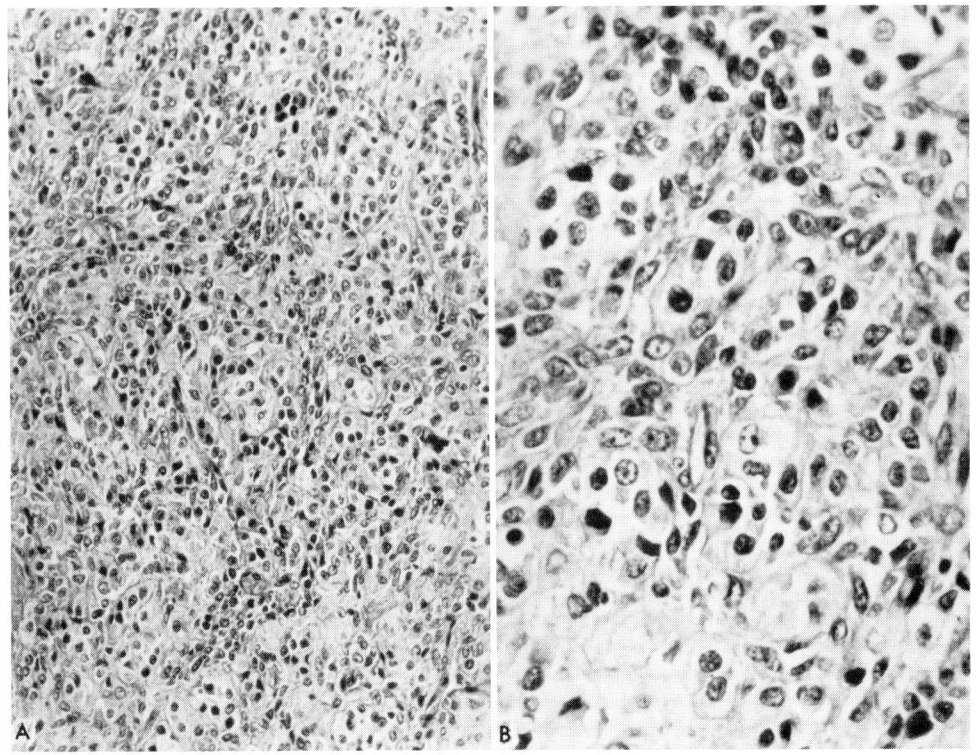

Figure 30–9. Arrhenoblastoma of the poorly differentiated type. A, 160×; B, 400×.

ciated symptoms may be either symptoms of negative or regressive effects or those attributable to positive effects of virilization. The first group comprises *all symptoms relative to regression of femininity*, such as increased slenderness, loss of scalp hair, flaccidity of breasts, amenorrhea and loss of typical female rounded contour. On the other hand, positive *symptoms of masculinization* are represented by hirsutism, growth of beard and moustache, enlarged clitoris and deepening of voice. To establish the diagnosis, however, evidence of virilization with hirsutism is not enough, since virilization may appear for different reasons, such as an adrenal disorder, and the presence of an ovarian tumor may be coincidental. As pointed out by Novak,[82] careful history taking may reveal that sometimes the patient with an ovarian tumor (nonvirilizing) has had symptoms of hypertrichosis ever since puberty. Such women may be constitutionally viriloid and the presence of an ovarian mass, e.g., a cyst or a persistent follicle, may be unrelated to their more or less apparent viriloid features which are life-long characteristics of such women. By the same token, it is necessary to make a clear distinction between different forms of hirsutism, that is, between increased piliation, which is common in dark complexioned women, and true virilization in which *hair distribution is of the male type* and does not merely represent a *general increase in hair growth*. The suspicion of dealing with an arrhenoblastoma must also be justified by evidence that, in addition to both virilization and an ovarian mass, there is a direct correlation between the appearance and growth of the mass and development of the symptomatology—in other words, evidence of abrupt masculinization.

ENDOCRINOLOGY. For obvious reasons, these tumors secrete small quantities of androgens.[51, 58] However, Graber and his associates,[42] who performed chromatographic fractionation of 17-ketosteroids, found the formula of 17-ketosteroids to be unaltered. Sandberg and colleagues,[100] as well as Savard and his co-workers,[102] have shown that tumor tissue incubated in vitro synthesized testosterone just as did normal testicular tissue.

Vague and colleagues[114] have isolated testosterone from arrhenoblastomas and have also observed an associated increase in plasma testosterone levels. Louros and his associates[67] and Radman and Bhagawan[94] have demonstrated that androgen synthesis by arrhenoblastomas is enhanced if the pituitary is suppressed either with dexamethasone or with large doses of chorionic gonadotropin, seemingly proving that steroidogenesis by these tumors is not ACTH dependent but is rather influenced by chorionic gonadotropin. Jones and co-workers[52] and Sandberg and co-workers[101] have studied the biochemical mechanism of androgen synthesis in arrhenoblastomas, and found that, as with feminizing tumors, tumor metabolism, in this instance, was not patterned on the model of androgen formation that was applicable to the normal testis.

30.3.2. ADRENAL TUMORS OF THE OVARY, OVARIAN HYPERNEPHROMAS OR INTERRENOMESENCHYMOMAS

This group of tumors is still the subject of much controversy. While the classical German school (Klaften,[56] Kleine,[57] Meyer,[76] Plate[91]) admitted this kind as unquestionably a distinct entity as a result of the presence of *Marchand's accessory adrenals* in the ovarian hilum, American scholars (Novak,[81] Marchetti and Lewis,[70] Rottino and MacGrath[97]), on the contrary, reject this interpretation and prefer the noncommittal term "clear cell tumors" (Figs. 30–10 and 30–11).

It would seem, however, that the individuality of this type of tumor has been recently recognized in America as well. Morris and Scully[78] acknowledge its distinctiveness and document their findings with convincing illustrations. Lately, Barody,[2] Griffin and Peerman,[44] and Pedowitz and Pommerance[88] have also reported well documented cases. Bjersing and his colleagues[9] have devised an ingenious method for the differential diagnosis of arrhenoblastoma and other masculinizing tumors, by means of the *suppression test*. As in the adrenogenital syndrome (see Chapter 33), this test consists in inhibiting ACTH secretion with either cortisone or dexamethasone, as a result of which urinary 17-ketosteroid excretion decreases if the tumor tissue is of adrenocortical nature and remains unaffected if it is an arrhenoblas-

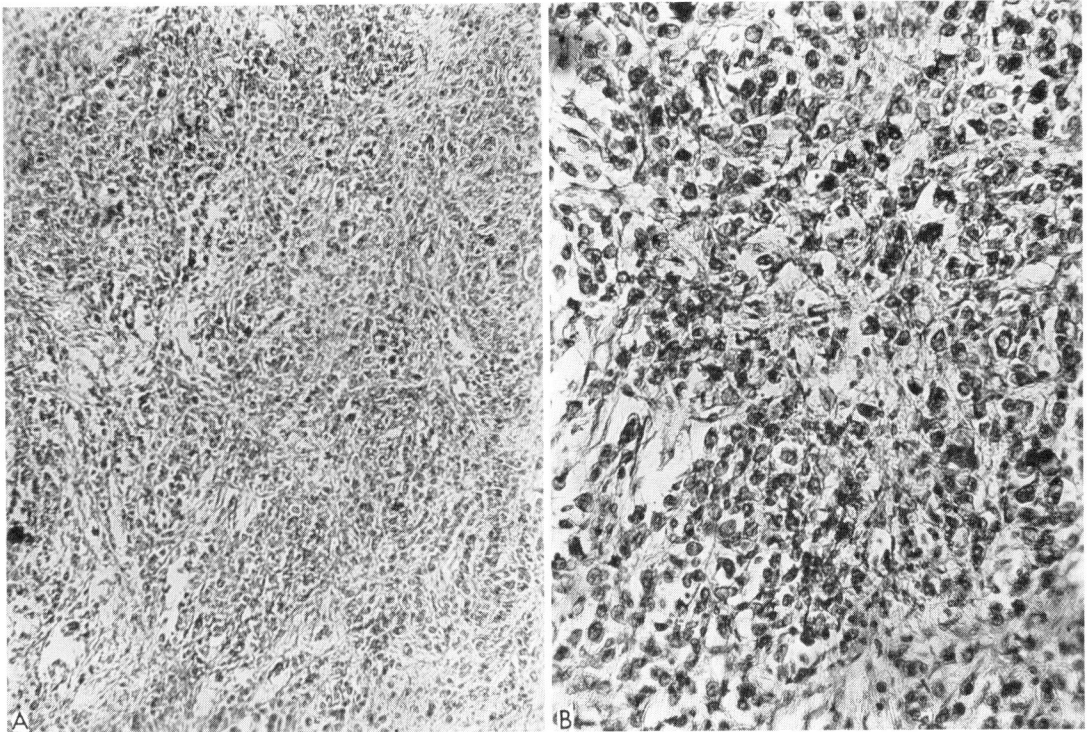

Figure 30–10. A, Ovarian clear cell tumor. It is doubtful whether this is a luteoma. B, High power detail.

toma or a similar kind of virilizing tumor. Further supportive evidence is provided by Pedowitz and Pommerance[88] who reported two cases of ovarian hypernephroma which produced Cushing's syndrome instead of virilization. Decisive evidence was finally brought to light by Sandberg and his associates[100] through hormone studies concerning the metabolism of tumor slices in vitro. In one instance of "clear cell tumor," they confirmed the presence of androgen biogenesis at the expense of cholesterol, pregnanolone and progesterone, following a pattern identical to that occurring in the adrenal but different from that occurring in the ovary. Rare as these tumors are, there seems to be no doubt that they faithfully reproduce neoplastic adrenal tissue, indistinguishable from adrenal adenomas, within the confines of the ovary.

The histogenetic explanation for these growths lies in the presence of interrenal inclusions in the hilum of the embryonal gonad, which may sometimes persist and which are then known as *Marchand's adrenals*. They are composed of the same type of tissue as that of the adrenal sexual zone, or the "third gonad" (see Chapter 9), to the extent that their pathologic proliferations may give actually rise to true instances of andrenogenital syndrome (see Chapter 33). However, just as the tissue involved in adrenal hyperplasia may pertain to the metabolic rather than the sexual zone and then produce effects characteristic of the former (for instance, causing Cushing's syndrome in association with adenomas or hyperplasia of the zona fasciculata), the ovary may also give rise to hypernephromas producing similar syndromes, as exemplified by the cases reported by Pedowitz and Pommerance.

The clinical manifestations associated with such tumors are discussed in Chapter 33, which deals with the adrenogenital syndrome and Cushing's syndrome.

30.3.3. MASCULINOVOBLASTOMA

This designation, which is really rather inadequate, has been commonly used for a group of tumors among which some authors

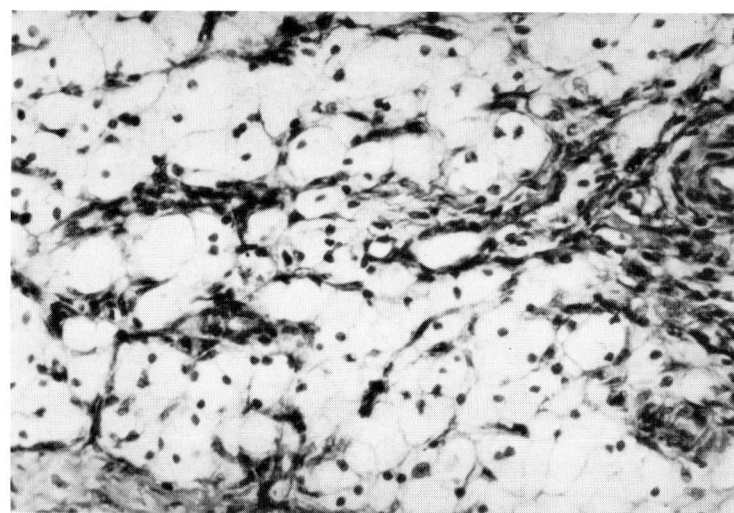

Figure 30–11. Adrenal tumor of the ovary (clear cell tumor).

include the already discussed varieties of hypernephroid tumors, as well as other tumors similar to both luteomas and arrhenoblastomas. In other words, this poorly defined category is a mixed bag of tumors obviously possessing masculinizing activity but defying definite histological classification. This includes, first of all, the "clear cell tumors" which are composed of cells with abundant cytoplasm and small nuclei, bearing considerable resemblance to either adrenal or luteal cells (see Fig. 30–10). Since no authoritative assessment of the histogenesis of this group of tumors seems to have been made, for the time being their designation by the term masculinovoblastoma may be justified. Some cases on which a complete hormone study had been performed were recently reported by Epstein and his co-workers[29] and by Bryston and associates.[15]

Some of the tumors among this group were once qualified as masculinizing luteomas, if for no other reason than because of existing similarities between their cell components and luteinized cells. By the same token, however, the similarity might be extended to include adrenal cells and Leydig cells as well. Novak does not admit this type of luteoma and believes that all such tumors should be included in the group presently under discussion, while reserving the term luteinic tumors exclusively for luteinized granulosa or theca cell tumors, which have been analyzed in the preceding sections. In addition, it must be remembered that luteinized thecal cells are currently recognized as potential androgen producers (see Chapter 29), so that any cells derived from the above luteal stock may also be endowed with androgenic activity. The tumor called by Lecène[61] "folliculome lipidique" might similarly be included in this category. Perhaps even some of the Leydig cell tumors, reported as such in the current literature, are, as Novak[82] says, incorrectly classified and should be placed here. Teilum[108] advocated the term "Leydig cell tumors" for this entire group of tumors, although Leydig cell tumors, as brought out in the next chapter, are, for other reasons, faily characteristic and can be readily separated from this group. As a result, luteomas and hypernephromas, as well as certain varieties of arrhenoblastomas and Leydig cell tumors, may be said to constitute, for the time being, an ill-defined group of tumors of which most examples reported in the world literature may be cases incorrectly classified. At present, there seems to be no good reason therefore for not accepting, at least provisionally, the qualitative terms "clear cell tumors" and "masculinovoblastoma." Besides, these tumors may be assumed to have a common histogenesis since they are known to arise from an essentially identical mesenchyme or interstitium. As pointed out by Rottino and MacGrath,[97] and subsequently by Marchetti and Lewis,[70] the proposed designation is purely nonspecific and provisional and does not preclude eventual reclassification of these tumors.

30.3.4. LEYDIG CELL TUMORS OF THE OVARY

The Leydig cell tumor of the ovary is one of the rarest virilizing tumors. The cell type of which it is composed, the hilus cell, originates in the hilar region of the ovary. Hilus cells were described as similar to the Leydig cell by Berger.[5] Because they have close relationships with sympathetic nerve fibers, the author also referred to them as sympathicotropic cells. Berger later demonstrated that either diffuse hyperplasia of hilus cells or adenomas composed of such cells could cause virilization. Although the literature was originally scanty, case reports have been recently reported with increasing frequency, so that it may be assumed that the tumor is not so rare that it is difficult to diagnose.

We are aware of about 16 well documented cases in the literature (those of Berger,[5] Waugh et al.,[117] four of Sternberg,[101] two of Ward et al.,[116] two of Merrill,[75] and those reported by Dreyfus, Sachs and Spiro,[98] Laufer and Sulman,[60] Dougherty et al.,[21] Birkheiser,[7] Eisenstadt and Petri,[24] German et al.,[38] and Vague et al.[113] To these, one might add those of Cosacesco and his associates[18] and Giordano and Haymond,[39] diagnosed by these authors as luteomas, but which in Berger's opinion are equally Leydig cell tumors.[5]

Like arrhenoblastomas, Leydig cell tumors may occasionally be associated with feminization. The reasons for such effects are even more difficult to explain in this instance, since the presence of a Sertoli cell component cannot be involved here. Feminizing Leydig cell tumors have been described by Teilum,[108] and subsequently also by Eisenstadt and Petri,[24] German and associates,[38] and Ward and colleagues.[116]

Clinically, the picture resembles that seen in the *adrenogenital syndrome*, except for those instances in which the tumor happens to display feminizing activity. The differential diagnosis, according to Sachs and Spiro,[98] is based on the *absence of increased 17-ketosteroid values* in the presence of Leydig cell tumors. The creatinine coefficient, an index of total functional body muscle mass, is considerably increased. The tumor is benign, the only reported fatality having occurred from an intercurrent carcinoma of the lung. Leydig cell tumors occur in the menopausal or postmenopausal age group as a rule.

Histologically, the growth pattern of ovarian Leydig cell tumors closely resembles that of Leydig cell tumors of the testis (Fig. 30–12). The neoplasm commonly arises in the ovarian hilum or in the mesovarium. Almost invariably, there is a close relationship between tumor cells and the nonmyelinated nerve fibers, as well as a rich vascular network. Like the Leydig cells of the testis, tumor cells vary greatly in size and shape. They are often polyhedral and occur in nests or columns. Their nuclei are vesicular, round or ovoid, containing few scattered chromatin clumps, with two or three nucleoli. Occasionally cells may be multinucleated. The eosinophilic and granular cytoplasm contains numerous vacuoles and lipoid inclusions.

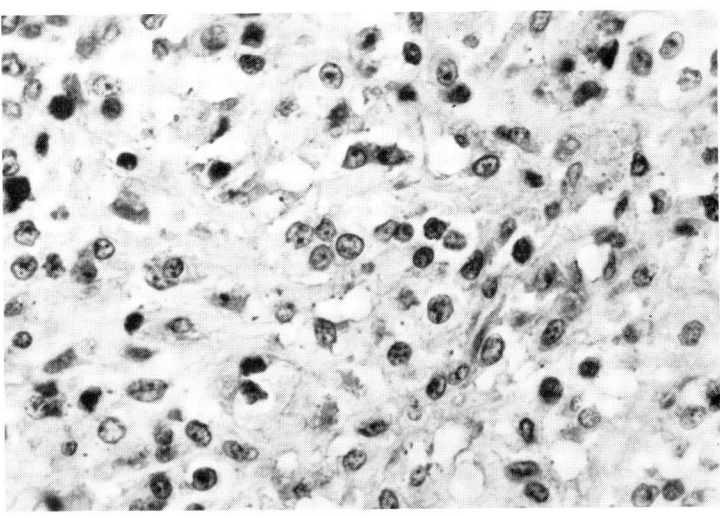

Figure 30–12. Leydig cell tumor of the ovary (hilus cell tumor).

A brown pigment may also be present and, most characteristically of all, there may be Reinke crystalloids. These are eosinophilic structures resembling small rectangular crystals. They are a distinctive feature of both normal and neoplastic Leydig cells and occur in both the testis and the ovary.

If one admits that ovarian hilus cells (see Chapter 4) are homologues of the interstitial cells of Leydig of the testis, the term *hilus cell tumor* may also be used for these tumors, since they may be assumed to result from neoplastic transformation of *hilus cell hyperplasia*, discussed in Chapter 29.

Hilus cell tumors have been recently described as an independent entity (Corral-Gallardo et al.,[17] Seliger et al.[106]). From a tumor of this type, Rosner and his associates[96a] isolated testosterone and found that testosterone synthesis also occurred in vitro.

30.3.5. GYNANDROBLASTOMA OF THE OVARY

The term gynandroblastoma refers to a combination tumor which is in part masculinizing, in part feminizing—that is, a neoplasm composed of both arrhenoblastoma and granulosa cell tumor. Such tumors are extremely rare, scarcely two dozen cases having been reported to date. The most interesting cases are those reported by Meyer,[76] Schiller,[104] Frankl,[36] Plate[92] and Emig and associates,[27] who list 23 cases up to 1959. In most of the cases reported, the tumors developed during the reproductive years and, notwithstanding the structural appearance of granulosa cell tumors, produced clinical features of virilization. With the exception of the case reported by Plate and one or two other unusual instances, no arrhenoblastomatous component was recognized histologically so that, had it not been for the associated paradoxical masculinizing effects, these tumors would have appeared as typical granulosa cell tumors. Such tumors have therefore also been called "virilizing granulosa cell tumors." However, this designation, as appropriately pointed out by Plate, is absurd, since the very nature of a granulosa cell tumor is incompatible with virilization. There is no doubt concerning the gynandromorphic nature of the tumor described by Plate, in which the feminizing portion of the tumor could be observed to form a distinct nodule surrounded by a virilizing component, as a result of which the ovarian tissue presented two quite independent tumoral growth patterns, in a kind of "neoplastic ovotestis."

30.3.6. LUTEOMA

Luteoma of the ovary is a highly debatable entity. The term has frequently been confused with hypernephroma as well as with some forms of arrhenoblastoma, while some authors apply it, as we have mentioned previously, to the miscellaneous group of masculinovoblastomas and to virilizing "clear cell tumors." First described as an entity in 1910 by Lecène,[61] who gave it the name of "folliculome lipidique," it was later studied by Cosacesco and his colleagues,[18] in 1931, and by Plate,[91] in 1933. During the following years, its individuality was denied by many. It was argued that the only indication of its luteal nature was the yellow color it displayed grossly, a color by no means confined to the corpus luteum but also characteristic of the adrenal, whose cells incidentally are similar to those of the corpus luteum. On the other hand, the most prominent clinical and pathologic features associated with these tumors was virilization, a paradoxical effect that seemed difficult to reconcile with the tumor's presumptive corpus luteum nature. However, in the course of the past years, mainly as a result of the studies by Ponse, Plate and Culiner, as well as numerous clinical and anatomopathological observations by Morris and Scully,[78] all of which have already been extensively commented upon in the preceding chapter, it has been learned that luteinization of the ovarian interstitial tissue may be associated with virilizing and androgenic activity. Moreover, the virilizing effects of large doses of progesterone on experimental animals are now well known; these were discussed in Chapter 3. Today, therefore, we no longer feel reluctance to admit that hyperluteinism may be associated with virilization. Various types of tumors histologically categorized as luteomas have in the meantime been studied from the standpoint of their steroidogenesis.[79, 84, 85, 96] Although some were found to synthesize progesterone, others were found to produce only androgens. In contrast, Lipsett and his associates[66] noted that, while failing to respond to ACTH, luteomas responded to LH stimulation with an elevated steroid output, which seems to demonstrate their ovarian, rather than adrenal, derivation.

On the other hand, the luteal nature of this type of tumor is in some cases quite evident whenever there is an associated *decidual reaction*. This decidual reaction observed in cases of luteoma by Novak[82] seems to be a good example. In 1944, Kepler and his colleagues[55] collected 14 cases of luteoma, up to that date one of the largest series known. They not only found unequivocal decidual reactions in the majority of cases but in addition isolated *pregnanediol* from the urine. Aside from this, the frequency with which such tumors are being reported at present would indicate a much higher clinical incidence for these tumors than one might anticipate if they were derived from such adrenal rests as are known by the name of "Marchand's accessory adrenals." Since the latter are thought to give rise to tumors of the adrenal variety, it would seem difficult to admit that luteomas might originate in a type of tissue whose occurrence is even rarer than that of the tumors themselves. The same would also seem to be a valid argument against any possible adrenal origin of these tumors. Ovarian hypernephromas have a much lower incidence. Twombly[112] described, in 1946, an interesting case of luteoma, with elevated pregnanediol excretion and with clinical symptoms of pseudopregnancy and decidual reaction. Although, in the cases reported by Anderson and his co-workers,[1] urinary pregnanediol values were elevated, no decidual reactions were found. Twombly believes that those tumors without any decidual reactions should be lumped together with the group of masculinovoblastomas and that only those tumors which are associated with a typical gravidic endometrial reaction should be considered as true adenomas of the corpus luteum. In that case, the world incidence of luteomas would be significantly reduced and only a few score of reported cases would qualify. The presence of urinary pregnanediol, in the opinion of Engel and co-workers,[28] is not a reliable finding. A careful study of urinary steroid excretion in one instance revealed considerable amounts of 17-ketosteroids but little pregnanediol. Regardless of whether or not the reported case was a true instance of luteoma, it must be added that the mere fact of pregnanediol excretion does not confirm the luteal—as opposed to a possible adrenocortical—nature of the tumor (Mason and Schneider[73]). It should be borne in mind that corticoids, as was pointed out in Chapter 9, may be eliminated in the urine as pregnanediol, so that any corticoid-producing tumors may be associated with increased pregnanedioluria. In addition, progesterone is also elaborated by the sexual zone of the adrenal. We have been able to find increased amounts of the urinary diol (see Chapter 32) in some cases of adrenogenital syndrome. This necessarily leads us to the conclusion that the finding of pregnanediol, or any other pregnane compound, in the urine does not indicate the nature of the tumor with the same degree of accuracy as does the finding of a *pseudogravid endometrial reaction*.

Conclusive proof is also provided by the fact that luteomas can be produced experimentally by means of the same procedures that are used to obtain experimentally induced granulosa cell tumors. Thus, for instance, Li and his associates,[62] Lipschütz and Cerisola,[65] and Ely and colleagues[25] have achieved experimental production of both luteomas and granulosa cell tumors in rat ovaries implanted in the spleen. In that way, estrogens generated by the ovary were inactivated on their passage through the portal system of the liver and, by not acting on the pituitary, gave free rein to unopposed gonadotropin activity, resulting in either temporary transformation of the FSH type or luteinization of the LH type of the granulosa. Under similar experimental conditions, the pituitary of castrated animals overstimulates the ovary to the extent that the latter is prone to develop either a granulosa cell adenoma or, through concomitant luteinization, a true luteoma. Such experimentally induced luteomas are the ultimate proof concerning the luteal nature of these tumors and confirm their factual existence. A similar experiment, in which radiotherapy was combined with gonadotropin injections and with splenic implantation, was later carried out by Biskind and Biskind,[8] with comparable results. Consequently, there can be no doubt that, even though it may be admitted that many cases reported in the literature as luteomas may not be genuine luteomas, this variety of ovarian tumor does exist, despite the difficulties that are often encountered in reaching a definite diagnosis.

Tumors of this nature have been studied at our laboratory by Nogales (Fig. 30–13).

30.3.7. TUMORS OCCASIONALLY ASSOCIATED WITH VIRILIZATION

This section includes some of the tumor varieties that are *not always functional* but, if so, usually are associated with a masculinizing effect.

BRENNER TUMORS. Brenner tumors have classically been described as nonfunctioning tumors. Recently, however, some cases have been reported to be associated with virilization (Besch,[6] Hamwi et al.,[47] Meining et al.,[74] Ming[77]). In vitro production of androgens by these tumors (Hamwi et al.) has been demonstrated.

GONOCYTOMAS. Teter[109] has grouped all dysgerminomas and seminomas in the literature under the common denominator of gonocytomas. According to Teter, these tumors arise as a result of pathologic proliferation of gonocytes which, in turn, induce secretory changes in the surrounding mesenchyme. He recognized four types, not all androgenic.[110] Types I and II are hormonally inert; type III is feminizing; and type IV is strongly virilizing. It is possible that some of the tumors reported as arrhenoblastomas are actually type IV gonocytomas. The tumor frequently develops in dysgenetic ovaries. We have observed one in an ovotestis of a true hermaphrodite (see Chapter 36).

KRUKENBERG TUMOR. Krukenberg tumors are well known to result from a carcinoma metastatic to the ovary, usually from a primary site in the gastrointestinal tract. These therefore have not been included in Table 30–1. Ober and his asso-

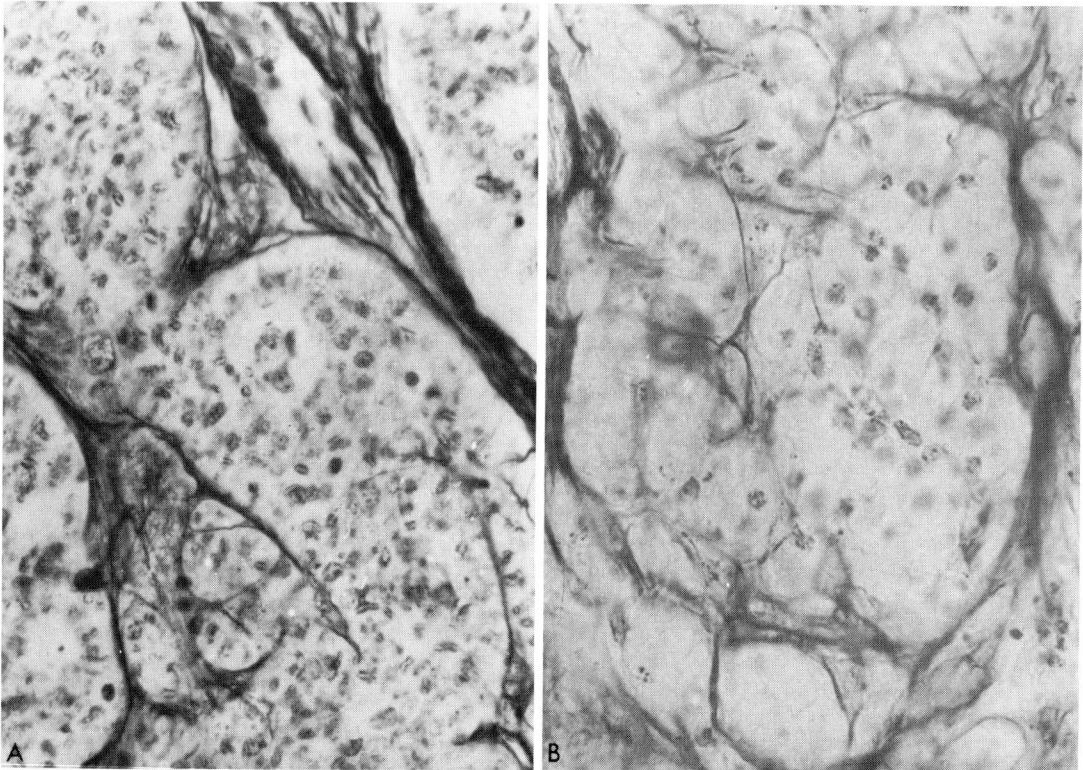

Figure 30–13. Luteoma seen with silver carbonate stain. A, Reticulin fibers visible around tightly packed granulosa-lutein cells. B, Another area of same tumor revealing loose arrangement of reticulum, with clear, lipid-laden tumor cells.

ciates[86] and Connor and his co-workers[16] have described cases associated with apparent virilization.

30.4. OTHER TUMORS WITH HORMONAL ACTIVITY

Tumors described under this heading are ovarian teratoblastomas that reproduce endocrine tissue structurally. Principally two types of neoplasia can be included in this category: *ovarian chorioepithelioma and struma ovarii.*

30.4.1. OVARIAN CHORIOEPITHELIOMA (CHORIOTERATOBLASTOMA)

Primary ovarian chorioepithelioma is a rare neoplasm. Klaften,[56] who had made a complete study of these tumors, admitted as such only those tumors which occurred in nulliparous women. In any woman who has had at least one known miscarriage, the finding of choriocarcinoma in the ovary may be the result of metastases from a uterine choriocarcinoma and thus be secondary in nature. In order to distinguish primary ovarian chorioepitheliomas from those which arise through neoplastic degeneration of the trophoblast of pregnancy or that of hydatidiform mole, Klaften proposes that the former be called *chorioteratoblastomas* and the latter *gestochorioepitheliomas*. Only about 25 or 26 cases of the first variety have been recorded in the literature. One of these was seen by us and reported in 1950.[12] It occurred in a 15 year old girl who, after normal puberty and with normal menstrual periods, developed menorrhagia and then metrorrhagia of increasing intensity. She presented signs of pregnancy, such as enlarged breasts, colostrous secretion, and hyperpigmentation of areolas and linea alba. These findings in conjunction with abdominal protuberance and a positive frog test, as well as metrorrhagia, suggested gestation with abortion. After the diagnosis was clarified, a voluminous mass was removed from the left ovary at laparotomy. Fifteen days later, the girl was reexamined at our clinic for further therapy. At that time, she revealed the presence of a vaginal metastasis which histologically was confirmed to be chorioepithelioma. The biologic pregnancy test was strongly positive, revealing excretion of half a million esculenta units per liter (1,000,000 IU). The patient was treated with radiotherapy, but died 20 days later from pulmonary metastases. The clinical histories of most of the reported cases reveal a similar course. In general, the patients involved are young girls in whom the tumor produces symptoms of pseudogestation by virtue of the high amounts of chorionic gonadotropins secreted by the neoplastic cells. It is of interest to note that some reports also describe the appearance of symptoms of *toxemia*, and *pyelitis*, which may be compared with toxemias of pregnancy and with gravidic pyelitis. That such reactions should occur in the absence of gestation is clear evidence of the hormonal origin of physiologic changes observed in pregnancy as well as of certain toxemias of pregnancy.

30.4.2. STRUMA OVARII

Struma ovarii is the presence of functioning thyroid tissue in an ovarian teratoblastoma. It is necessary here to separate this entity from those cases in which nonfunctional, or at least apparently nonfunctional, thyroid tissue is found within a dermoid cyst, viz., benign cystic teratoma. Bedoya,[3] at our clinic, reviewed cases of dermoid cysts containing inclusions of thyroid tissue. Such inclusions may be ascribed to the ability of such teratomas to reproduce structures of the branchial arches, which may happen to include a bud of thyroid gland. There are a relatively large number of publications reporting this type of finding (Fig. 30-14) while, on the contrary, the finding of teratoblastomas with functioning thyroid tissue is considerably rare. Prior to 1944, we had found only eight well documented cases of struma ovarii, of which the best studied cases were those reported by Emge.[26] In 1944, Gusberg and Danforth[46] described eight cases of struma ovarii, and since then other reports appeared with increasing frequency.[10] The data on which the functional capacity of the neoplastic thyroid tissue in such cases must be based are the following: (1) Increased

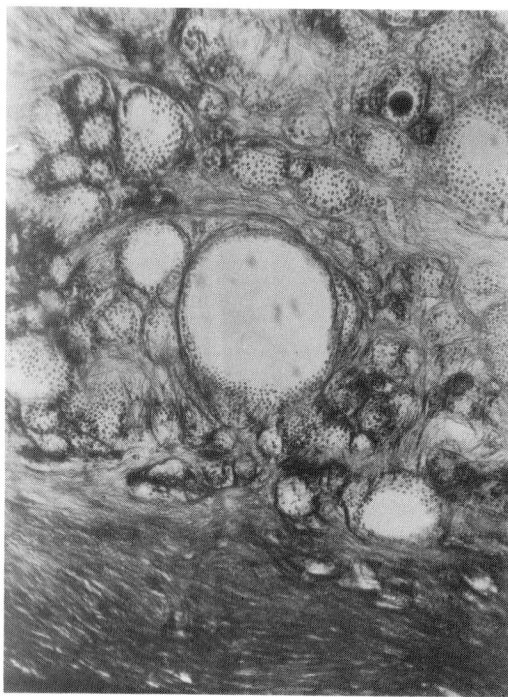

Figure 30-14. Thyroid tissue within the wall of a dermoid cyst. Follicle in upper right corner reveals presence of colloid material.

basal metabolic rate; (2) increased levels of circulating PBI, and (3) mainly, the capacity of the tissue under consideration for selectively trapping radioactive iodine (^{131}I). The last mentioned procedure has enabled Perlmutter and Mufson[89] to diagnose a case in which ^{131}I was found preoperatively in the ovary. Interestingly, this tumor at the same time produced thyrotoxicosis of ovarian origin, as well as compensatory atrophy of the cervical thyroid. Cases with similar findings most often occur in adult women between the ages of 30 and 50 and are characterized clinically by symptoms of thyrotoxicosis, weight loss, restlessness, hyperexcitability, hypermetabolism, tachycardia and exophthalmos. Thanks to the development of *scanning procedures* with ^{131}I, it has been possible in the last few years to discover cases of struma ovarii which would otherwise have been missed, since thyrotoxicosis is often absent owing to compensatory atrophy of the eutopic thyroid. What is remarkable in such cases is the fact that thyroid function may be transferred from the thyroid gland in the neck to the neoplastic ovarian thyroid tissue. Belonging to this variety are the cases reported by Foulkes and Fraser,[32] Fox and Clement,[33] González-Angulo,[41] Marcus and Marcus[71] and Paoletti.[87] Patients of this kind must be evaluated carefully before proceeding to remove the involved ovary because of the danger of producing strumiprival cachexia.

As a final comment, it should be mentioned that Ramagopal and Stanbury[95] found that the different iodine fractions characteristic of thyroid function were equally present in the tissue of struma ovarii.

REFERENCES

1. Anderson, A. F., Hain, A. M., and Patterson, J.: *J. Path. Bact.*, 55:341, 1943.
2. Barody, A. J.: *Amer. J. Obstet. Gynec.*, 82:721, 1961.
3. Bedoya, J. M.: *Los tumores funcionantes del ovario.* Madrid, Morata, 1946.
4. Bedoya, J. M.: *Tumores Ováricos.* Madrid, Editorial Acta Ginecologica, 1950.
5. Berger, L.: *Rev. Canad. Biol.*, 1:359, 1942.
6. Besch, P. K.: *Amer. J. Obstet. Gynec.*, 86:1021, 1963.
7. Birkheiser, S. W.: *Amer. J. Obstet. Gynec.*, 73:429, 1957.
8. Biskind, G. R., and Biskind, M. S.: *Amer. J. Clin. Path.*, 19:501, 1949.
9. Bjersing, L., Skanse, O., and Gennell, S.: *Acta Obstet. Gynec. Scand.*, 40:26, 1962.
10. Bortolozi, G.: *Ann. Ost. Gin. (Milano)*, 89:310, 1967.
11. Botella, J., and Bedoya, J. M.: *Obst. Gin. Lat. Amer.*, 5:165, 1947.
12. Botella, J., Nogales, F., Sopeña, A., and Carazo, J.: *Gynec. Obstet.*, 49:220, 1950.
13. Botella, J., Sánchez-Garrido, J., and Nogales, F.: *Acta Gin.*, 15:1964.
14. Botella, J.: *Acta Gin.*, 18:61, 1967.
15. Bryston, M. J., et al.: *J. Clin. Endocr.*, 22:773, 1962.
16. Connor, T. B., et al.: *J. Clin. Endocr. Metab.*, 28:198, 1968.
17. Corral-Gallardo, J., et al.: *Acta Endocr.*, 52:425, 1966.
18. Cosacesco, A., et al.: *Presse Med.*, 39:1264, 1931.
19. Dockerty, M. B., and MacCarthy, G.: *Amer. J. Obstet. Gynec.*, 37:424, 1939.
20. Dockerty, M. B., and Mussey, E.: *Amer. J. Obstet. Gynec.*, 61:147, 1951.
21. Dougherty, C. M., Thompson, W. B., and MacCall, M. L.: *Amer. J. Obstet. Gynec.*, 76:653, 1958.
22. Eddie, D. A. S.: *J. Obstet. Gynec. Brit. Comm.*, 73:283, 1967.
23. Ehrlich, E. N., et al.: *J. Clin. Endocr.*, 23:358, 1963.
24. Eisenstadt, J. B., and Petri, J. L.: *J. Clin. Endocr.*, 18:834, 1958.

25. Ely, C. A., Tuercke, R., and Chen, B. L.: *Cancer Res.*, 26:1441, 1966.
26. Emge, L. A.: *Amer. J. Obstet. Gynec.*, 40:738, 1940.
27. Emig, O. R., Hertig, A. T., and Rowe, F. J.: *Obstet. Gynec.*, 13:135, 1959.
28. Engel, L. L., Dorfman, R. I., and Abarbanel, A. R.: *J. Clin. Endocr.*, 13:903, 1953.
29. Epstein, J. A., et al.: *Amer. J. Obstet. Gynec.*, 74:982, 1957.
30. Evans, T. N., and Riley, G. M.: *Obstet. Gynec.*, 18:52, 1961.
31. Flickinger, G. L., Miravec, T., and Touchstone, J. C.: *J. Clin. Endocr. Metab.*, 25:1231, 1965.
32. Foulkes, J. F., and Fraser, T. R.: *J. Obstet. Gynec. Brit. Emp.*, 61:668, 1954.
33. Fox, Y. F., and Clement, K. W.: *Ann. Surg.*, 133:253, 1951.
34. Fox, H.: *Cancer*, 18:1041, 1965.
35. Frachtman, K. G.: *Amer. J. Obstet. Gynec.*, 81:770, 1961.
36. Frankl, O.: *Zbl. Gynäk.*, 61:85, 1937.
37. Geist, S. H., Gaines, J. A., and Pollack, A. D.: *Amer. J. Obstet. Gynec.*, 38:786, 1939.
38. German, C., et al.: *J. Clin. Endocr.*, 21:91, 1962.
39. Giordano, A. S., and Haymond, J.: *Amer. J. Clin. Path.*, 12:28, 1944.
40. Goldberg, B., Seegar-Jones, G. E., and Woodruff, J. D.: *Amer. J. Obstet. Gynec.*, 86:1003, 1963.
41. González-Angulo, A., et al.: *Obstet. Gynec.*, 21:567, 1963.
42. Graber, E. A., O'Rourke, J. J., and Sturman, M.: *Amer. J. Obstet. Gynec.*, 81:773, 1961.
43. Greene, J. W., and Prencel, R. W.: *Obstet. Gynec.*, 18:191, 1961.
44. Griffin, N. B., and Peerman, C. G.: *Obstet. Gynec.*, 21:215, 1963.
45. Griffiths, K., Grant, J. K., and Symington, T.: *J. Endocr.*, 30:247, 1964.
46. Gusberg, S. B., and Danforth, D. N.: *Amer. J. Obstet. Gynec.*, 48:537, 1944.
47. Hamwi, G. J., et al.: *Amer. J. Obstet. Gynec.*, 86:1015, 1963.
48. Ingraham, E., Black, E., and Rutledge, E.: *Amer. J. Obstet. Gynec.*, 48:760, 1944.
49. Ingraham, E., and Novak, E.: *Amer. J. Obstet. Gynec.*, 61:774, 1951.
50. Jayle, M. F.: *Conf. Congr. Internat. Jub. Soc. Fr. Gynec.* Paris, L'Expansion Scientifique Française, 1951.
51. Johnson, D. C., and Witschi, E.: *Cancer Res.*, 21:783, 1961.
52. Jones, G. S., Goldberg, B., and Woodruff, D. J.: *Obstet. Gynec.*, 29:328, 1967.
53. Jopp, H.: *Gynaecologia*, 161:25, 1966.
54. Jull, W., Streeter, D. J., and Sutherland, L.: *J. Nat. Cancer Inst.*, 37:409, 1966.
55. Kepler, R. I., Dockerty, M. B., and Priestley, G. B.: *Amer. J. Obstet. Gynec.*, 47:43, 1944.
56. Klaften, E.: *Arch. Gynäk.*, 158:130, 1934.
57. Kleine, H. O.: *Zbl. Gynäk.*, 63:2249, 1939.
58. Knight, W. R.: *Amer. J. Obstet. Gynec.*, 56:311, 1948.
59. Koss, L. G., et al.: *Cancer*, 23:1245, 1969.
60. Laufer, A. L., and Sulman, F. G.: *J. Clin. Endocr.*, 16:1151, 1956.
61. Lecène, P.: Quoted by Moulonguet, *Les diagnostics anatomocliniques*, Vol. II. Paris, Masson & Cie., 1932.
62. Li, M. H., Gardner, W. W., and Kaplan, H. S.: *J. Nat. Cancer Inst.*, 8:91, 1947.
63. Lipschütz, A. von: *Steroid Hormones and Tumors.* Baltimore, Williams & Wilkins, 1950.
64. Lipschütz, A. von, Iglesias, R., and Salinas, S.: *Nature*, 196:946, 1962.
65. Lipschütz, A. von, and Cerisola, H.: *Nature*, 193:145, 1962.
66. Lipsett, M. B., Kirschner, M. A., Wilson, H., and Bardin, C. W.: *J. Clin. Endocr.*, 30:336, 1970.
67. Louros, N. C., Batrinos, M. L., and Carcatzoulis, S.: *J. Clin. Endocr. Metab.*, 26:645, 1966.
68. MacAuley, M. A., and Weliky, I.: *J. Clin. Endocr.*, 28:819, 1968.
69. McKay, D. C., Robinson, D., and Hertig, A. T.: *Amer. J. Obstet. Gynec.*, 58:625, 1950.
70. Marchetti, A. A., and Lewis, L. G.: *Amer. J. Obstet. Gynec.*, 63:294, 1952.
71. Marcus, C. C., and Marcus, S. L.: *Amer. J. Obstet. Gynec.*, 81:752, 1961.
72. Marsh, J. M., et al.: *J. Clin. Endocr.*, 22:1196, 1962.
73. Mason, H. L., and Schneider, J. J.: *J. Biol. Chem.*, 184:593, 1950.
74. Meining, R. L., et al.: *Amer. J. Obstet. Gynec.*, 87:463, 1963.
75. Merrill, J. A.: *Amer. J. Obstet. Gynec.*, 78:1258, 1959.
76. Meyer, R.: *Amer. J. Obstet. Gynec.*, 22:697, 1931.
77. Ming, S. C.: *Amer. J. Obstet. Gynec.*, 84:666, 1962.
78. Morris, J. M. L., and Scully, R. E.: *Endocrine Pathology of the Ovary.* St. Louis, C. V. Mosby, 1958.
79. Morrow, L. B., Thompson, R. J., and Mellinger, R. C.: *J. Clin. Endocr.*, 28:1756, 1968.
80. Morris, E. H.: *Cancer*, 22:1, 1958.
81. Novak, E.: *Obstetrical and Gynecological Pathology*, 2nd ed. Philadelphia, W. B. Saunders, 1947.
82. Novak, E.: *Obstet. Gynec.*, 1:3, 1953.
83. Novak, E. R., and Mattingly, R. F.: *Obstet. Gynec.*, 15:425, 1960.
84. O'Malley, B. W., Lipsett, M. B., and Jackson, M. A.: *J. Clin. Endocr.*, 27:311, 1967.
85. Oakley, N. W., and Beilby, J. O. W.: *Proc. Roy. Soc. Med. (London)*, 62:40, 1969.
86. Ober, W. B., et al.: *Amer. J. Obstet. Gynec.*, 84:739, 1962.
87. Paoletti, I.: *Riv. Ital. Ginec.*, 45:70, 1962.
88. Pedowitz, P., and Pommerance, W.: *Obstet. Gynec.*, 19:183, 1962.
89. Perlmutter, M., and Mufson, M.: *J. Clin. Endocr.*, 11:621, 1951.
90. Pincus, G.: *The Hormones*, Vol. II. New York, Academic Press, 1958.
91. Plate, W. P.: *Gynec. Obstet.*, 28:42, 1933.
92. Plate, W. P.: *J. Obstet. Gynec. Brit. Emp.*, 45:254, 1938.
93. Pundel, J. P.: *Les frottis vaginaux et cervicaux.* Paris-Liege, Masson-Desoer, 1950.
94. Radman, H. M., and Bhagawan, B. S.: *Amer. J. Obstet. Gynec.*, 106:1187, 1970.
95. Ramagopal, E., and Stanbury, J. B.: *J. Clin. Endocr. Metab.*, 25:256, 1965.
96. Rice, B. F., and Segaloff, A.: *Acta Endocr.*, 54:568, 1967.

96a. Rosner, J. M., et al.: *Amer. J. Med. Sci.*, 37:638, 1964.
97. Rottino, A., and MacGrath, J. F.: *Arch. Int. Med.*, 63:686, 1939.
98. Sachs, B. A., and Spiro, D.: *J. Clin. Endocr.*, 11:878, 1951.
99. Salerno, L. J.: *Amer. J. Obstet. Gynec.*, 84:731, 1962.
100. Sandberg, A. A., et al.: *J. Clin. Endocr.*, 22:929, 1962.
101. Sandberg, E. C., Jenkins, R. C., and Trifon, H. M.: *Steroids*, 8:237, 1966.
102. Savard, K., et al.: *J. Clin. Endocr.*, 21:165, 1961.
103. Schiller, W.: *Klinik und Pathologie der Granulosazelltumoren*. Wien, W. Maudrich, 1934.
104. Schiller, W.: In *Progress in Gynecology*, 2nd ed. Ed. Meigs and Sturgis. New York, Grune & Stratton, 1950.
105. Schneider, G. T.: *Amer. J. Obstet. Gynec.*, 79:921, 1960.
106. Seliger, W. G., Blair, A. J., and Mossman, H. W.: *Amer. J. Anat.*, 118:615, 1966.
107. Sternberg, W. H.: *Amer. J. Path.*, 25:493, 1949.
108. Teilum, G.: *Acta Path. Scand.*, 23:248, 1946.
109. Teter, J.: *Gynaecologia*, 150:84, 1960.
110. Teter, J.: *Amer. J. Obstet. Gynec.*, 84:722, 1962.
111. Traut, H. F., Kuder, A., and Cadden, J. F.: *Amer. J. Obstet. Gynec.*, 38:798, 1939.
112. Twombly, G. H.: *Amer. J. Obstet. Gynec.*, 51:832, 1946.
113. Vague, J., et al.: *Ann. d'Endocr.*, 21:437, 1960.
114. Vague, J., et al.: *Ann. d'Endocr.*, 25:334, 1964.
115. Wainer, N. E., et al.: *Amer. J. Obstet. Gynec.*, 97:971, 1960.
116. Ward, J. A., et al.: *J. Clin. Endocr.*, 20:1622, 1960.
117. Waugh, D., Venning, E. H., and MacEachern, D.: *J. Clin. Endocr.*, 9:486, 1949.
118. Zangeneh, F., and Kelley, V. C.: *Amer. J. Dis. Child.*, 115:494, 1968.

Part Eight

ENDOCRINE SYNDROMES INVOLVING SEXUAL FUNCTION

Just as the endocrine glands (pituitary, adrenals, thyroid, etc.) govern sexual physiology, so pathologic processes affecting these glands produce sexual endocrine syndromes. Following the same order of sequence that has been used in the description of normal function, we will now describe the endocrinopathies of the pituitary, adrenals, thyroid, parathyroid and pancreas and the effects they have on sexual function. One chapter (Chapter 32) is devoted to the subject of neurogenic syndromes with genital repercussions.

Chapter 31
PITUITARY ENDOCRINOPATHY IN RELATION TO SEX

It would go beyond the scope of a textbook on female endocrinology to study pituitary endocrine pathology in all its aspects. The different pituitary endocrinopathies shall be reviewed here briefly insofar as they have a bearing on the endocrinology of the sexual sphere.

The question of pituitary pathology has been undergoing a thorough revision. Many outdated concepts have been reformulated and others are expected to be modified in the near future. Deserving special mention is the fact that *a large number of diseases that had been thought to be of purely pituitary origin have been recognized to be the result of hypothalamic disturbances.* In many respects, hypothalamic disorders predominate over pituitary disorders in producing the syndromes of this group (Everett[28]).

31.1. CLASSIFICATION

Pituitary disorders are classifiable as either endocrinopathies of the gland itself or as hypothalamic-pituitary diseases. The first are confined to simple alterations of the gland itself, whereas the second are caused by involvement of the gray nuclei at the base of the brain. Because the posterior lobe, or neurohypophysis, must be spoken of, in the light of present-day knowledge, as a dependency or prolongation of the hypothalamus, strictly speaking pituitary disorders are those which involve only anterior lobe function. By definition, all hypophysiopathies involving the posterior lobe are considered to be primary hypothalamic disorders. The many other disease processes involving the anterior lobe that have a mixed pituitary and hypothalamic genesis shall be dealt with as a separate group. Also, the study of sexual syndromes of neurogenic origin has been left to Chapter 32, which is concerned with hypothalamic pituitary syndromes and related conditions. The present chapter therefore deals exclusively with pure hypophysiopathies.

In the study of pituitary pathology, we recognize syndromes that result either from *hypofunction* or from *hyperfunction.* Among the former, we must include *absolute hypopituitarism,* as it is known to occur in Simmond's disease, as well as some forms of *relative hypopituitarism,* some of which are of great significance in the sexual sphere. Significantly, recently there has been a tendency to deemphasize the importance of Simmond's syndrome. As pointed out by Perkins and Rynearson,[60] most of the syndromes described as pituitary cachexia are in fact manifestations of hypothalamic disease. Within the context of hypopituitarism, much greater weight is being attached to lesser degrees of hypofunction which involve isolated segments of the endocrine system, such as the gonads, thyroid, or adrenals. The first of such partial types of insufficiency in particular is of great interest for the present study.

Where hyperpituitarism is concerned, not only *gigantism, acromegaly* and *pituitary basophilism* must be included, as is customarily done in endocrinology textbooks, but also some *partial forms of hyperpituitarism,* causing disorders in reproductive function. Special syndromes of this type include *gonadotropic hyperpituitarism* and *lactotropic hyperpituitarism,* the significance of which in gynecologic endocrinology will be stressed in due time.

TABLE 31-1. Classification of Pituitary Endocrinopathies

I Hypopituitarism	A. Absolute	Simmond's syndrome Sheehan's syndrome
	B. Relative	Gonadotropic hypopituitarism Corticotropic hypopituitarism Thyrotropic hypopituitarism
II Hyperpituitarism	A. Somatotropic (gigantism and acromegaly) B. Corticotropic (Cushing's disease) C. Gonadotropic D. Lactotropic	
III Hypothalamic-pituitary disorders	A. Adiposogenital syndrome B. Pituitary precocious puberty C. Pituitary obesity D. Chromophobe adenoma E. Diabetes insipidus F. Craniopharyngioma G. Anorexia nervosa	These are covered in Chapter 32

Finally, a third group comprises *hypothalamic-pituitary disorders*, the most prominent among which are Froehlich's syndrome, pituitary precocious puberty, pituitary obesity, chromophobe adenoma, craniopharyngioma, diabetes insipidus and anorexia nervosa, all of which are studied in Chapter 32.

31.2. HYPOPITUITARISM: ABSOLUTE HYPOPITUITARISM

Instances of absolute hypopituitarism occur less commonly than was once believed. Various investigators, such as Escamilla and Lisser,[27] Sheehan and Summers,[69] as well as Perkins and Rynearson,[60] dispute the relative significance of total hypopituitarism which, rather than representing instances of actual pituitary disease or pituitary cachexia, most often are related to other conditions, such as anorexia nervosa or large chromophobe adenomas (Nieman et al.[59]). Canong and Hume,[17] working with dogs, and Elkington and his associates,[26] working with women, have studied the effect of hypophysectomy on various endocrine functions. In fact, the hypophysioprival dog develops signs of gonadal insufficiency quite early, takes somewhat longer to develop thyroid insufficiency and attains hypocorticism only at a very late stage. This seems to indicate that *panhypopituitarism requires a long period of time or very extensive pituitary lesions in order to develop*. This is why instances of partial hypopituitarism occur more commonly.

Thus, from among the vast number of such cases reported, Escamilla and Lisser only accept about 100 cases as true instances of Simmond's cachexia. Consequently, the incidence of this disease would seem to be much lower than originally assumed.

Two main syndromes fall into this category, viz., pituitary cachexia, or *Simmond's disease,* and puerperal pituitary necrosis, or *Sheehan's disease.*

31.2.1. SIMMOND'S DISEASE

Simmond's syndrome (Simmond's disease) has frequently been cited as a perfect example of a condition reproducing the clinical picture of experimental hypophysectomy as a result of natural causes. It results from total loss of anterior lobe function, characterized by functional failure of all corresponding target organs: the adrenals, the gonads and the thyroid. Symptomatology therefore consists of secondary amenorrhea, genital atrophy, hypothermia, hypometabolism, emaciation and cachexia, hypocorticism and premature aging.

ETIOLOGY. Among the etiologic factors that may be directly involved are the following processes: embolism or thrombosis of one of the arteries to the anterior pituitary lobe; idiopathic atrophy of the gland from unknown causes; compression of the pituitary stalk by a suprasellar or intrasellar cyst; chromophobe adenoma; metastatic malignancy, tuberculosis, syphilis and xanthomatosis. Such lesions may have an acute, subacute or chronic course. Among acute processes, *pituitary necrosis* from ischemia occurs most frequently. The extent of necrosis depends on the magnitude of the circulatory damage involved. Besides postpartum necrosis of the pituitary, which is to be examined later, the most common cause of pituitary necrosis is *embolism*. Intrapituitary *hemorrhage* occurring as a complication of *cranial hypertension* has been found less frequently. Among subacute lesions, inflammatory processes with a tendency to *abscess* or *granuloma* formation are the principal offenders. Such is the case with tuberculosis, syphilis or actinomycosis. Finally, chronic lesions occur less commonly and are usually produced either by tumors or by atrophy and fibrosis of the gland of the so-called *idiopathic* type. Among the tumors leading to pituitary destruction, the most common ones are simple cysts, cholesteatomas or tumors of adenomatous or angiomatous nature. Occasionally, cysts of Rathke's pouch or craniopharyngiomas may cause compression of the sella, resulting in loss of pituitary function.

Almost 50 per cent of cases of Simmond's disease develop immediately *after delivery*, as reported by Escamilla and Lisser,[27] and most patients have a history of *atonic bleeding* during parturition. In general, the disease occurs more often in multiparous than in nulliparous women. This has led some authors, such as Simpson[71] and Hamblen,[42] to attribute the origin of the disease to exhaustion of the pituitary as a consequence of numerous pregnancies, In Chapter 20, the important changes the pituitary undergoes in the course of pregnancy and during lactation were described. The process of regression of those changes, particularly if taking place in glands exhausted by a sustained reproductive effort, could lead to idiopathic atrophy, which is one of the most common factors involved in the development of this disease. A loss of up to 50 per cent of the gland's parenchyma is expected to be tolerated without producing symptoms. Symptoms presumably appear whenever more than 60 per cent of the gland parenchyma is destroyed. Pertinent aspects of the disease are further analyzed under the discussion of Sheehan's syndrome.

ANATOMIC PATHOLOGY. The single most frequent finding is that of *atrophy and fibrosis*. Sometimes, degeneration of the hypothalamus and tuber cinereum is observed at the same time (Simpson[71]). Cases in which there is loss of basophilic as well as eosinophilic cells may also be observed although, as noted by Sheehan, chromophobe cells are retained by the residual pituitary parenchyma. Nonetheless, Herrick[43] calls attention to the fact that there may be extensive destruction involving several cell lines in the majority of cases, suggesting a *selective etiologic factor*, the nature of which is unknown. Instances in which some cell lines in the destroyed pituitary survive are relatively common. It remains to be seen whether there might be any relationship between this disease and some forms of hyperpituitarism that are associated with predominance of one cell line and atrophy of the rest.

Concomitant with pituitary atrophy, there is atrophy of the various glands of internal secretion. In woman, the ovaries appear to be reduced to rudimentary and atrophic structures. In the male, the testes are noticeably reduced in size. The thyroid, as well as the adrenals, similarly undergoes atrophy. In addition, such other organs as the liver, spleen, kidneys and heart also decrease in size, giving rise to the phenomenon of *splanchnomicria*. The heart also undergoes brown atrophy concomitantly with total disappearance of adipose tissue throughout the body.

CLINICAL PICTURE. The disease may develop at any time in life, but it usually makes its appearance in the later years of reproductive maturity, between the ages of 35 and 45. Brasel and his associates,[11] however, have described a form of "juvenile panhypopituitarism." Ellis[25] insists that the occurrence of the disease in infancy is exceedingly rare.

The onset of the disease is usually sudden but, as pointed out previously, may be insidious, permitting division of the disease into *acute, subacute and chronic forms*. Accordingly, the course of the disease may be rapid or, on the contrary, may have a very protracted evolution. Instances of up to 44 years' survival have been recorded. Most conspicuous of all symptoms is the associated *emaciation and cachexia*. Some patients may ultimately weigh as little as 34 kg. The skin becomes dry and paper-thin. Fingernails become brittle and sometimes are lost altogether. There is hair loss from the scalp and from the axillary and pubic regions. Dental deterioration and loss of teeth is common. Naturally, all the above changes impart to the patient the appearance of *premature senility.* At the same time, *subnormal temperatures* and *hypotension* are observed, as a rule. The basal metabolic rate may reach extremely low figures, such as minus 50 or below. In addition to the above, there may be lethargy, stupor, disorientation and lack of interest in environmental events. Marked hypoglycemia may also be present (Wadsworth[78]).

In the sexual sphere, there is amenorrhea, loss of libido and extreme atrophy of both external and internal genital organs. The uterus undergoes atrophy and is reduced to a rudimentary size, the ovaries likewise shrink and breasts usually waste away completely. The diagnosis is not difficult to make but requires the usual amount of clinical experience in ruling out anorexia nervosa, which is discussed in Chapter 32. The differential diagnosis of the two conditions is outlined in Table 31–2.

Fraser and Smith[35, 72] have also emphasized the importance of 17-ketosteroid determinations in order to be able to differentiate between the two diseases. In Simmond's disease, 17-ketosteroid levels have been reported to be remarkably decreased.

TREATMENT. Present forms of treatment give poor results. Nearly all patients with true Simmond's disease die despite therapy. Cases in which cures or turns to the better have been reported are suspected of being cases of anorexia nervosa. Anteropituitary extracts leave much to be desired and do not achieve complete or sustained substitution of normal pituitary function. Attempts have been made to remedy the lack of pituitary stimulation by means of administering the various hormones that are produced by the target glands, especially sex hormones, corticoids and thyroid hormone. With such methods, a measure of success, although temporary in nature, has been reported As an ancillary means of therapy, a high-calorie diet is instituted, containing abundant carbohydrates and vitamins, taken in small volumes that are compatible with associated splanchnomicria. Five to 10 gm of NaCl a day is given in order to compensate for adrenocortical insufficiency; this is accompanied by injections of corticoids and testosterone, and supplemented with thyroid tablets. Relatively good results were recently reported with the use of ACTH, as indicated by Sexton and his associates.[65] At any rate, adrenocorticotropin therapy cannot solve all the problems of this disease and, despite continued maintenance, cannot avert progressive devitalization and ultimate death of the patient.

31.2.2. POSTPARTUM NECROSIS OF THE PITUITARY, OR SHEEHAN'S SYNDROME

Sheehan's syndrome, described in the preceding section, occurs frequently during the puerperium. Cases of pituitary cachexia appearing during this phase of woman's sexual life had been described since ancient times. Sheehan[66] deserves credit not for having discovered the syndrome itself but for having discovered the *important role postpartum necrosis plays in its genesis.* He thus described a new nosologic entity, characterized by pituitary insufficiency at the beginning of the puerperium and caused by necrosis of the pituitary gland.

ETIOLOGY. Pregnancy is well known to be associated with pituitary hyperfunction and hypertrophy (Chapter 20). In addition to enhanced function and an increase in number of cells, the pituitary of pregnancy

TABLE 31–2. Differential Diagnosis of Simmond's Disease and Anorexia Nervosa

SIMMOND'S DISEASE	ANOREXIA NERVOSA
Cachexia	Cachexia
Weight loss	Weight loss
Genital atrophy	Genital atrophy
Marked decrease in basal metabolic rate	Marked decrease in basal metabolic rate
Very frequent asthenia	Less frequent asthenia
Hypotension	Hypotension
Onset related to pregnancy, delivery or infection	Onset independent of pregnancy, delivery or infection
Alteration of sella turcica	No alteration of sella turcica
Loss of axillary and pubic hair	No loss of axillary or pubic hair
Premature senility	No premature senility
Breast atrophy	No breast atrophy
Pallor	No pallor
Eosinophilia	Absence of eosinophilia
Lack of favorable response to therapy	Favorable response to therapy
Mortality rate, 97%	Almost no mortality

also reveals a markedly enriched vascularization. Sheehan showed that after delivery there was an abrupt reduction in the blood supply to the anterior lobe. Diminution in blood supply occurs as a physiologic phenomenon, initiating postpartum regression of the pituitary. Should severe intrapartum bleeding result in a sudden drop of blood pressure and produce vascular depletion, a lasting state of ischemia may develop in the pituitary which, when superimposed on the regressive changes already in progress, may cause more or less extensive necrosis. Although necrosis from ischemia seems to be the most commonly involved mechanism, Sheehan and Murdock,[68] and subsequently Cook and his associates,[20] described such other etiologic factors as pituitary thrombosis, metastatic pituitary abscesses and, moreover, destructive embolic processes involving the nearby hypothalamus. Though such processes are thought to be related above all to postpartum infections, Schneider[63] recently focused attention on the significance of *afibrinogenemia* as a causative factor in cerebral and pituitary microembolism, which may lead to eventual necrosis. This may well be the reason why a number of patients with toxemia of pregnancy and with uteroplacental apoplexy were described to develop postpartum pituitary necrosis.

ANATOMIC PATHOLOGY. As early as 1932, Smith[72] found that postpartum pituitary necrosis occurred much more frequently than suggested clinically; severe enough symptoms of pituitary insufficiency were observed in only 30 per cent of the cases, whereas in the remaining 70 per cent such symptoms failed to become apparent. This is undoubtedly due to the fact that a large portion of the gland parenchyma must be rendered useless before the gland's capacity for compensation fails.

Instances of silent pituitary necrosis have later also been described by Worms and Delanter,[84] as well as by a number of other investigators. As already indicated, the most common underlying lesion is necrosis, but embolism and metastatic abscesses may also be involved.

CLINICAL PICTURE. In general, the clinical symptoms are ushered in by complete failure of lactation. Gálvez and Sánchez-Agesta,[36] who recently described a case of Sheehan's syndrome, emphasize that this is a very early and valuable symptom. In addition to *agalactia*, there is severe wasting and marked asthenia, as well as a frankly negative Thorn test. It is a well known fact that parturition acts as a stress agent and causes accentuation of the eosinopenic response to epinephrine. However, Del Sol and Merlo,[73] at our clinic, had shown how a certain percentage of postpartum women gave negative results in the test of eosinopenia.

Such patients may well represent cases of so-called dormant Sheehan's syndrome, benign forms of which are probably much more common than generally believed. To be sure, a large proportion of women who suddenly become worse after delivery, who cannot breast-feed and who appear tired and listless, may well be mere instances of functional pituitary impairment to a greater or lesser extent.

By contrast, *severe forms* of the disease reveal quite manifest symptomatology. They present with amenorrhea, sometimes of long standing, with *uterine and genital hyperinvolution*, atrophic vaginal cytology, endometrial atrophy and absence of urinary sex hormone excretion. Urinary 17-ketosteroids and 11-oxysteroid levels may be reduced to zero. There is usually a history of *rapid weight loss*, thinning of axillary and pubic hair and a rapid fall in basal metabolic rate to figures of minus 40 or below. Symptoms of weight loss and hair loss have also been observed in recent studies by Teter and his associates,[77] who reported 20 cases, and by Ioanitiu and his colleagues,[44] who presented 26 more cases of their own. A characteristic form of mental sluggishness may become apparent, the skin usually becomes cold and dry, and, little by little, the typical picture of the previously described Simmond's disease sets in. We believe that no less than 50 per cent of the cases described in the early literature as pituitary cachexia were actually instances of this syndrome.

The *differential diagnosis* is mainly between this disease and some forms of hypercorticism. Kecskes and his associates[47] propose the ACTH test as a means of distinguishing between the two. Under certain circumstances, the symptoms of the disease may also be confused with those caused by some hypothalamic disorders (Whitehead[82]).

TREATMENT. Therapy yields results only in benign cases. First of all, a diet of high caloric intake, containing abundant carbohydrates, is instituted and given in small and frequent meals. At the same time, ACTH is administered, preferably in *depot* form for slow absorption. Some women may also require repeated blood transfusions in addition to intravenous administration of ascorbic acid and intramuscular injections of 100 to 200 mg tocopherol every second day. In recent years, injections of human gonadotropin (see Gemzell[38]) have produced good results, particularly when combined with synthetic ACTH (Synachten[44, 77]).

31.3. RELATIVE HYPOPITUITARISM

The term relative hypopituitarism is used in contradistinction to absolute hypopituitarism or panhypopituitarism, which has just been described. It is caused by diminished activity of one or several active pituitary principles while, in general, global pituitary function is maintained and, therefore, only isolated sectors of the economy are adversely affected. Basically, four varieties of partial hypopituitarism may be distinguished, involving respectively gonadotropin secretion, corticotropin secretion, thyroid stimulation and deficient production of growth hormone resulting in dwarfism. In theory, galactotropic hypopituitarism as well as a few other, less common, manifestations of pituitary insufficiency may also exist; however, in practice, the clinical individuality of such conditions has not been proved.

31.3.1. GONADOTROPIC HYPOPITUITARISM

Gonadotropic hypopituitarism constitutes a very common and highly interesting disease entity within the framework of female endocrinology (see Chapter 27). Although discussed in brief previously certain aspects of this type of hypopituitarism should be reiterated, particularly as regards its manifestations in conjunction with well defined pituitary pathology.

ETIOLOGY. The etiology remains a matter of conjecture. However, some authors (Buchanan and Balwey,[14] Buxton[15]) maintain that certain pituitary cells, most commonly eosinophils, *undergo systematic atrophy according to a definite pattern.* In addition, Shelton[70] and Wohl and Larsen[83] have also indicated that eosinophils in the pituitary may be congenitally absent or may be lost through infarction, calcification, syphilis or tuberculosis. The basophilic cell lines appear to be more resistant to injury, although instances of selective disappearance of basophilic cells have been reported by, among others, Elden and Rummer.[24]

Gonadotropic hypopituitarism occurs mainly in young girls and appears around puberty or up to the age of 30. Cases with a later onset are exceptional.

CLINICAL PICTURE. The genital manifestations of gonadotropic insufficiency may assume three different forms, depending on whether they become apparent before puberty, during adolescence or during maturity. When they appear *during the prepuberal phase* they give rise to a picture

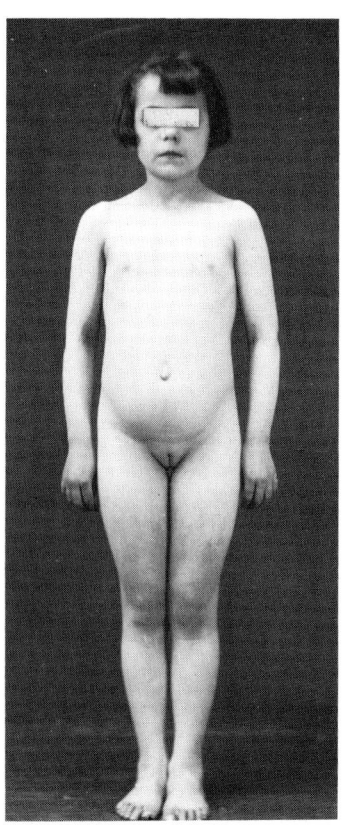

Figure 31-1. Case of pituitary dwarfism with hypogenitalism, in a girl aged 17. Height, 135 cm. There was essential amenorrhea. Note infantile habitus and complete absence of pubic hair and breasts.

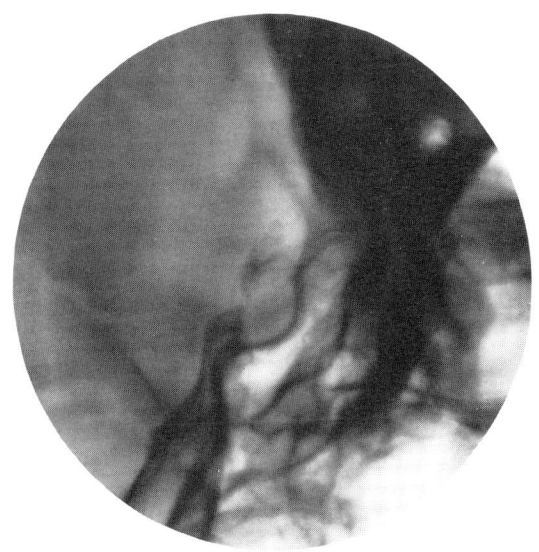

Figure 31–2. Sella turcica in a case of hypopituitarism similar to that in Figure 31–1. Note fusion of clinoid processes, giving rise to image of sella turcica obtecta.

of delayed puberty, which may eventually continue in the form of essential amenorrhea of pituitary origin. Whenever this form of hypogonadotropism is of the pure variety, there is no associated dwarfism. However, partial involvement of somatotropic function is quite frequent, and in this case there is genital infantilism with retarded growth, which may be characteristic of this syndrome. The case of the 17 year old girl in Figure 31–1, with complete infantile habitus and stature and with essential amenorrhea, exemplifies this condition. Breast development in such cases is conspicuous by its absence, as may be complete absence of axillary and pubic hair. Mentation may be retarded. The genital apparatus of the girl shown was unusually atrophic and infantile. Occasionally, the internal genitalia can hardly be perceived by palpation. Pituitary roentgenography, as may be seen in Figures 31–2 and 31–3, reveals an exceptionally small sella turcica, in which the clinoid processes merge into a kind of roof over the pituitary, giving an image that has been called *sella turcica obtecta*. As a rule, affected girls live their entire lives with essential amenorrhea and in a state of prolonged infantilism, although occasionally, not altogether surprisingly, the clinical picture may change and there may be a late appearance of menses. However, these women are invariably, to a greater or lesser extent, hypoestrogenic.

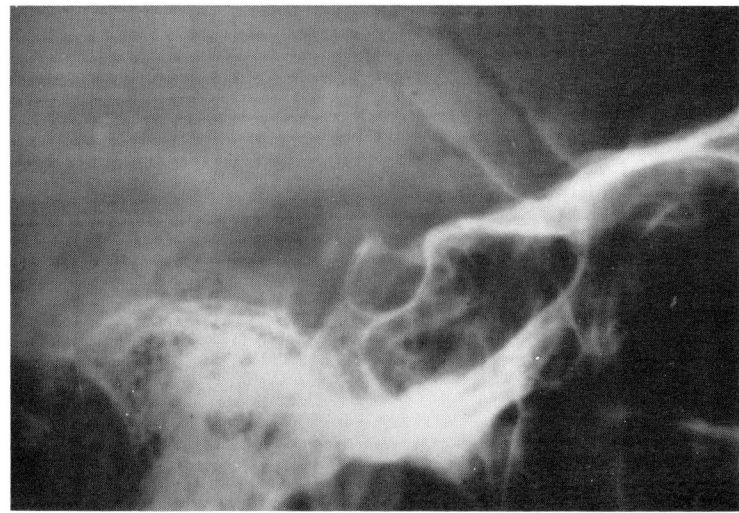

Figure 31–3. Sella turcica obtecta in a case of gonadotropic hypopituitarism with short stature.

Manifestations of pituitary insufficiency of the *juvenile or adult types* consist of secondary amenorrhea or secondary oligomenorrhea, without alterations in growth (Figs. 31–4 and 31–5). Nevertheless, genital symptoms are markedly pronounced. The uterus reveals involutional changes. Breasts are atrophied and flabby. Pubic and axillary hair is lost and the entire clinical picture may be accompanied by a state of general depression of vegetative functions, with emaciation, anorexia and asthenia. Not infrequently, the same clinical picture may develop in a secondary way after a prolonged period of lactation. In women with unduly protracted lactation, a transient form of pituitary atrophy may become apparent, similar in origin to serious forms of panhypopituitarism, but usually remaining at a low level of intensity. This gives rise to the clinical picture of genital subinvolution after lactation, associated with endometrial atrophy and usually with complete absence of ovarian maturation. We have called attention to the fact that such women often show absence of ovarian maturation while maintaining corpora lutea (Fig. 31–6). As pointed out in Chapter 22, this might be explained on the basis of the luteotrophic, and at the same time, follicle-suppressing, activity of prolactin. If sustained, prolactin secretion is thought to be responsible for the preservation of corpora lutea while also causing arrest in follicular maturation and follicular atrophy. This may represent an intermediate state between partial gonadotropic hypopituitarism and partial lactotropic hyperpituitarism, the two conditions frequently occurring as a combined form, which is discussed in the last section of this chapter.

The *short stature* displayed by these patients may obviously be accounted for by lack of growth hormone occurring simultaneously with gonadotropin insufficiency. Solomon and Greep[74] focus attention on the pathogenic mechanism that causes arrest of growth. To them, what causes arrest of development is not loss of STH secretion but *lack of thyrotropic hormone, resulting in hypothyroidism* and dwarfism. The relationship of hypothyroidism to short stature is taken up again in Chapter 33.

Moldawer and his associates[58] performed FSH and STH determinations in blood and urine of such patients, reporting low values for both.

TREATMENT. We have obtained good results in girls with delayed puberty and hypopituitarism by means of *diathermia to the base of the brain*. In other cases, radiotherapeutic stimulation of the pituitary with Kaplan's technique may be indicated.

Over the past few years, the use of human gonadotropins (HPG and HMG) has yielded excellent results in the experience of Gemzell[38] and Bettendorf (see Chapter 7). Since the disorder is related to anovulatory cycles, it shall be discussed in greater detail in Chapter 41, dealing with the subject of endocrine sterility. With a method of treatment using both menopausal gonadotropins (HMG) and chorionic gonadotropins (HCG), Mancini[54] reported good results in hypophysectomized males who had had testicular atrophy. It should be added that Flowers and his associates[32] have obtained good results by treating gonadotropic hypopituitarism with the pseudopregnancy treatment.

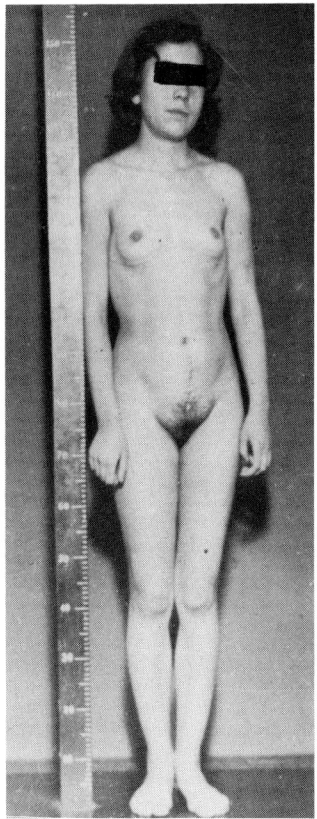

Figure 31–4. Patient (aged 22) suffering from gonadotropic hypopituitarism with retarded puberty, emaciation and eunuchoidism.

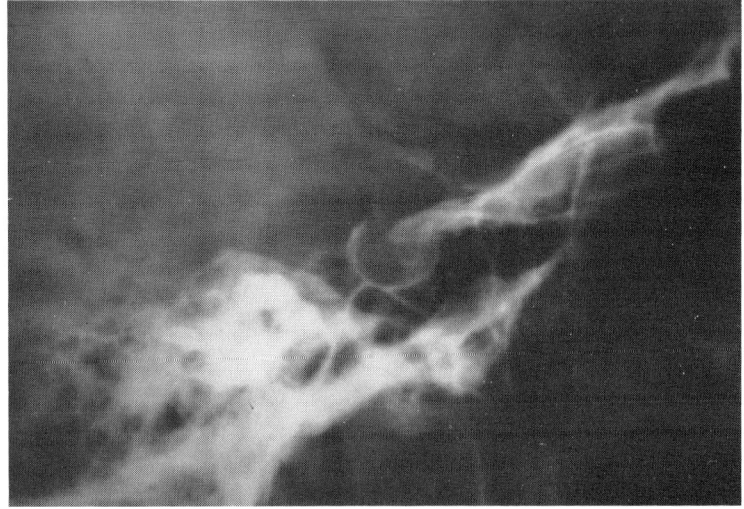

Figure 31–5. Sella turcica, reduced in size though not of the obtecta type, in a syndrome of gonadotropic hypopituitarism with tall stature and eunuchoidism.

There exists a long list of mild varieties of *pituitary insufficiency, subclinical in nature,* which no doubt produce anovulatory cycles, follicular persistence, or similar alterations. The relationship between pituitary function and the etiology of disturbances of follicular maturation has been discussed in Chapter 28.

31.3.2. OTHER FORMS OF RELATIVE HYPOPITUITARISM

Other forms of relative hypopituitarism are hardly significant enough to deserve being discussed at length, since their repercussions on the sexual sphere are much more peripheral in nature than those produced by gonadotropic insufficiency. Foremost among these is *corticotropic hypopituitarism.* It generally appears in young women in whom there is failure of ACTH secretion, resulting in adrenocortical insufficiency. The existence of this type of adrenocortical insufficiency of pituitary origin has been denied or, at least, admitted only with reservations by some authors (Marañón[55]). However, it has been observed by us with relative frequency in

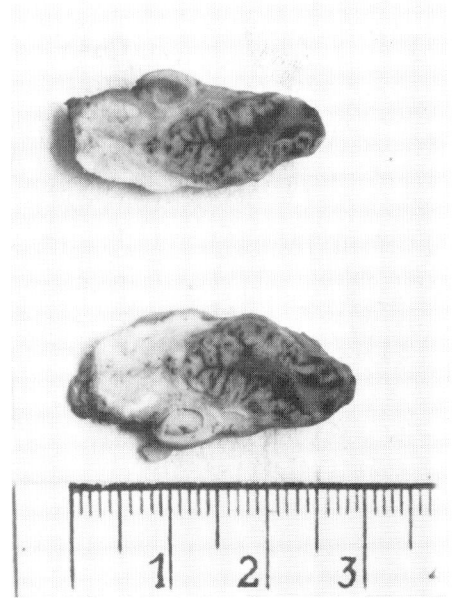

Figure 31–6. Secondary amenorrhea of pituitary origin. In addition to endometrial atrophy, one ovary (both halves of which are shown here) is atrophic but contains an apparently well developed persistent corpus luteum. In contrast, there is no evidence of follicular maturation, but there are numerous corpora albicantia.

gynecologic and, above all, obstetric conditions. This is precisely the type of insufficiency that causes *adrenal failure during the first trimester of gestation*, intimately implicated in the etiology of hyperemesis gravidarum (Botella[8]).

As for *thyrotropic hypopituitarism*, this is of interest whenever occurring in combination with gonadotropic hypopituitarism. In Figure 31-1, we presented a case of a hypogenital dwarf. In Figures 31-7, and 31-8 we present a hypogenital cretin. The girl shown had symptoms of panhypopituitarism but, more than anything else, showed evidence of delayed sexual development, delayed somatic growth and manifest thyroid insufficiency, with a markedly decreased basal metabolism. Cases of this kind are interesting because in the background of every instance of partial gonadotropic hypopituitarism there is thyroid insufficiency. In view of the importance of thyroid function for the development of the female gonad and for fertility (see Chapter 10), it is not surprising that sexual development in these girls, in whom thyroid insufficiency is a constant accompaniment of genital insufficiency unless receiving thyroid therapy, should be defective and should, particularly in the late stages, result in sterility. In Chapter 39, dealing with the endocrinology of these problems, related questions will be analyzed more thoroughly.

The majority of girls with delayed puberty of pituitary origin are short in stature. The question of short stature in relation to hypo-ovarianism has been brought up in Chapter 28, at which time we expressed our reservations concerning the possibility that simple ovarian agenesis might cause developmental arrest. What is beyond any doubt, however, is the fact that essential amenorrhea of pituitary origin is nearly always associated with dwarfism or, at least, with noticeable shortening in stature. This makes one wonder whether all cases of essential amenorrhea associated with both genital and somatic manifestations are not, after all, pituitary rather than ovarian in origin.

A series of minor forms of gonadotropic hypopituitarism interfere with normal ovarian function and are probably the underlying cause of mild estrogenic insufficiency, already studied in Chapter 26, and, particularly, that of *anovulation* and *luteal insufficiency* (see Chapter 29). Since the latter play an extremely important role in infertility, they are reexamined in Chapter 41. The diagram of Figure 31-9 offers an explanation for pituitary involvement in the genesis of these conditions.

31.4. HYPERPITUITARISM

Unlike pituitary insufficiency states, all forms of hyperpituitarism are *partial functional disorders*. We know of no condition in which all functions of the gland are equally elevated. As a matter of fact, pituitary hyperfunction as such does not exist. What does exist are different degrees of *dyspituitarism*, in which some functions fail while others are enhanced. A most representative form of hyperpituitarism is observed with pituitary adenomas. After conducting a comprehensive survey of pituitary adenomas reported in the litera-

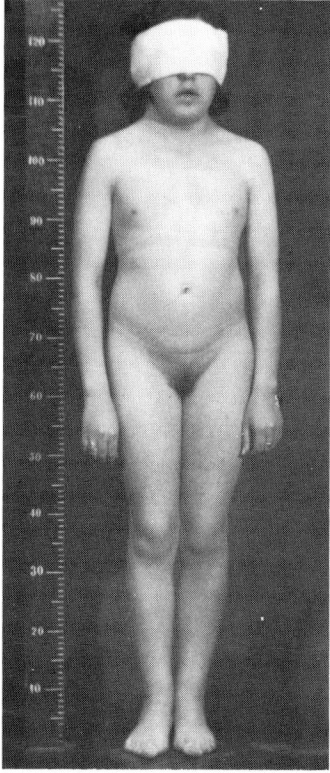

Figure 31-7. Case of gonadotropic hypopituitarism associated with thyrotropic hypopituitarism, in a girl aged 16. Height, 123 cm; totally infantile habitus. Note absence of pubic hair, lack of mammary development, and characteristic features of cretinism.

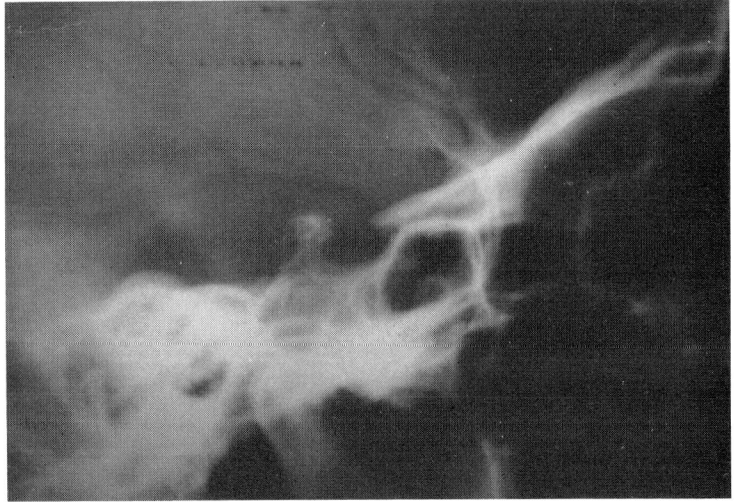

Figure 31-8. Sella turcica, reduced in size but not of the obtecta type, in same case as in Figure 31-7.

ture, Klinefelter[50] calls attention to the fact that most are chromophobe adenomas, that is, functionally inert tumors. Following in order of decreasing frequency are eosinophilic adenomas (25 per cent of the cases, often equally nonfunctional, although approximately half of them, viz., 12.5 per cent of all pituitary adenomas, produce the typical picture of *acromegaly*), and basophilic adenomas (only 3 per cent of all pituitary adenomas). In contrast to the first two the great majority of basophilic adenomas are functional, producing *Cushing's syndrome*.

This section deals successively with two syndromes, acromegaly and Cushing's syndrome, produced by eosinophilic and basophilic adenomas, respectively. It also reviews two minor forms of hyperpituitarism which are specifically linked to sexual function: *gonadotropic hyperpituitarism* and *lactotropic hyperpituitarism*.

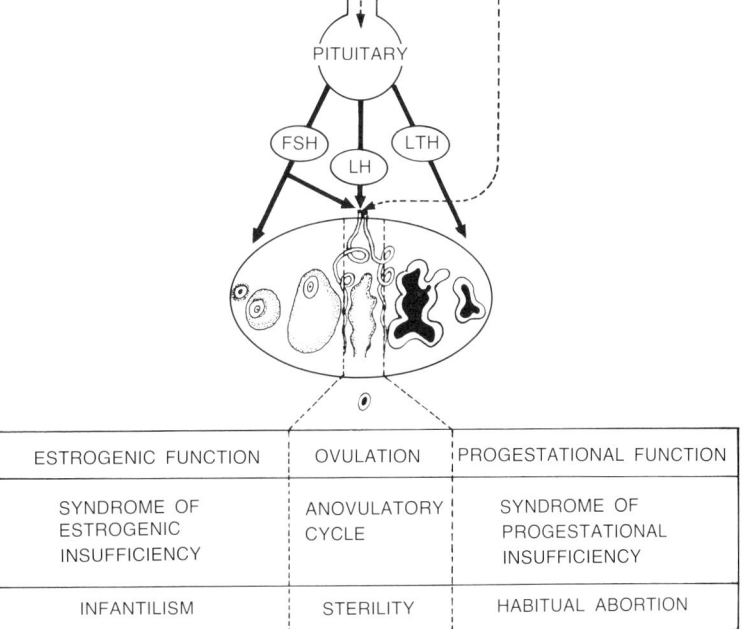

Figure 31-9. Diagram of gonadotropic insufficiency with threefold effect on ovary: estrogen insufficiency (primarily resulting from lack of FSH), anovulatory cycle (primarily resulting from lack of LH) and luteal insufficiency (from lack of LTH).

Consequently, it may be said that each active principle of the anterior lobe, with the exception of thyrotropic hormone, has a corresponding form of partial hyperpituitarism. The question of whether a similar form of thyrotropic hyperpituitarism is involved in hyperthyroidism is a matter of dispute and is not considered here because it bears no direct relationship to reproductive function.

31.4.1. SOMATOTROPIC HYPERPITUITARISM (GIGANTISM AND ACROMEGALY)

These disorders are now known to be produced by eosinophilic hyperplasia or by eosinophilic adenoma. The development of either *acromegaly* in some cases or *gigantism* in others depends on the moment of onset of pituitary hyperfunctional activity. Gigantism develops whenever hyperfunction appears before epiphysial closure of long bones is completed, whereas acromegaly develops after closure, when bones can no longer grow in length. The syndrome of acromegaly is therefore more commonly found in association with sexual-endocrine conditions and is characterized by above normal development of the terminal or acral portions of the bony skeleton, such as hands, feet, chin and nose. Acromegaly is usually associated with degenerative changes in the muscles, hypertrophy of the skin, hyperplasia of the connective tissue and, at the same time, exaggerated visceral development.

ETIOLOGY. The most common cause of gigantism is adenomatous hyperplasia of the eosinophilic cell components of the pituitary gland. However, paradoxical cases associated with sarcoma, carcinoma or syphilis have also been described. Adenomas probably arise from epithelial rests scattered over various segments of the pharyngeal vault or spenoid sinuses rather than from hyperplastic elements of fully developed glands.

ANATOMIC PATHOLOGY. The pituitary is usually noted to be markedly enlarged. While the presence of an eosinophilic adenoma in the strict sense of the word cannot always be confirmed, most cases reveal adenomatous hyperplasia. The areas involved are almost exclusively made up of eosinophilic cells, all other cell types having crowded out. A direct relationship has been observed between the total number of eosinophilic cells and the severity of symptoms. Usually, adrenal hyperplasia and, particularly, thyroid hyperplasia are also noted in these patients. Often, the thymus persists with diffuse hyperplasia of lymphoid elements. An additional feature of interest is an increase in the size of the liver, heart, lungs and remaining viscera. Similarly, the bowel may often grow to twice its normal length. The bony skeleton, too, reveals considerable alterations. The flat bones of the skull are markedly thickened, and the zygomatic arches and malar bones, as well as the mandible, are prominently developed and protuberant. Exostoses frequently are present. Vertebral changes, such as atrophy or compression, are also relatively common.

CLINICAL PICTURE. Clinically, acromegaly is observed in women more frequently than in men. In addition, it is more often seen in women of the reproductive age and bears a relation to the number of previous pregnancies. Almost all cases occur in the third decade of life. After the age of 40, the appearance of acromegaly is exceptional. The pure form of acromegaly is relatively common. On the other hand, pure nonacromegalic forms of gigantism are rare, since all pituitary giants as a rule reveal associated acromegaly. In general, acromegaly develops insidiously, the earliest manifestations consisting of muscle pain, fatigue, somnolence and nervous symptoms. *Headaches* and *ocular disturbances* appear usually early in the course of the disease. Characteristic growth of the bones of the extremities and overgrowth of salient facial bones, such as chin and nose, lead to *gradual disfigurement of the facies*. In addition to *increased size of hands and feet*, and enlargement of aforementioned bony regions, splanchnomegaly, macroglossia and profound psychic alterations deserve special mention. Occasionally, these patients develop genuine manic psychoses during the advanced stages of their disease. Also of great importance are *alterations affecting sexual function*. What calls attention *during the early stages of the disease* is *evidence of considerable enhancement of libido*, which later gives way to a state of total indifference and to *sexual atrophy*. At first, *menstrual irregularities* are common and metrorrhagia is not a rare phenomenon. Eventually, however, menstrual activity ceases and *premature menopause* ensues. Markedly regressive changes affecting the genital organs, vagina, uterus and ovaries appear in every case. The occurrence of *polycystic ovaries* has been described in some cases and has been related to the presence of increased gonadotropin A activity during the early phase of the disease. Sommers and Wadam[75] reported having encountered polycystic ovaries with hyperthecosis, similar to Stein-Leventhal ovaries, in acromegalic women. Finkler[31] reported the presence of persistent follicles and considerably increased urinary FSH excretion as an almost constant finding. Acromegaly may sometimes appear in the course of pregnancy, giving rise to complications which will be examined later.

Lactation in acromegaly is usually observed to be enhanced to the extent that some cases have been described to be associated with galactorrhea. This disorder is intimately linked to so-called galactotropic hyperpituitarism, also to be discussed later.

From the endocrine standpoint, the frequent occurrence of diabetes and hyperthyroidism in such cases must be emphasized. The early stages of acromegaly are invariably associated with partial pituitary hyperfunction insofar as FSH is concerned. Abelove and co-workers[1] have reported hyperelimination of FSH in the early stages of the disease. However, in the advanced stages of the disease, complete absence of gonadotropins and the presence of secondary genital atrophy seem to be the rule. Nevertheless, it is true that complete sexual endocrine studies concerning acromegaly have to date not been made public. Most of the data available in the literature are fragmentary and deserve little credence. This prevents us from defining the endocrine sexual condition of these patients with any degree of certainty other than to say that, in general, after a seemingly hyperfunctional early stage, there tends to be a rapid downhill turn to hypofunction.

ACROMEGALY AND PREGNANCY. Only seldom is pregnancy complicated by acromegaly. In the past, such cases were described by Kehrer[48] and, more recently by Finkler[30, 31] and by Abelove and his co-workers.[1] According to the last-mentioned authors, only 34 cases had been reported in the literature. The disease becomes clinically apparent in the course of gestation in young women. It should be pointed out that a certain degree of acromegaloid tendency is present even in normal pregnancy, which explains why acromegalic features are often recognized first in pregnancy. Gravidic acromegaly may therefore be viewed as an exaggeration of the transient physiologic process of acromegalization in every pregnant woman. The question of increased growth hormone activity during pregnancy has been commented upon in Chapter 20. Its probable physiologic role is to stimulate intrauterine fetal development. There is evidence that, during pregnancy, the pituitary is subject to temporary proliferation of eosinophilic cells, a subject we have discussed in some of our earlier publications. The case reported by Abelove is of particular interest because it had been followed over a period of many years, through three generations. Acromegaly did not produce sterility, nor did it seriously interfere with the evolution of pregnancy. Except for some tendency to polymenorrhea the patient showed an essentially normal menstrual pattern. The case reported by Finkler, with a similar follow-up after pregnancy, eventually revealed development of secondary sterility, associated with polycystic ovaries and copious menstrual periods. We have had the opportunity to observe the evolution of a benign pituitary tumor associated with acromegaly. The patient involved was a grand multipara, in her ninth pregnancy, who had first revealed symptoms of pituitary disease during her fifth pregnancy; these took the form of severe headaches, enlarged sella turcica and decreased visual fields. Facial acromegalization was slight but nevertheless clearly perceptible. This patient's fertility was unaffected, although her symptoms would invariably flare up during the first months of each pregnancy and then abate during the third trimester. The patient was under orders to avoid lactation in view of past experience indicating that lactation had an adverse effect on the clinical course of her disease. Our ideas concerning acromegaly and pregnancy may thus be summarized by saying that acromegaly, in its benign form, does not interfere with fertility and may be compatible with pregnancy. On the other hand, the etiology of the ailment in some cases may be related to pregnancy itself, as suggested by the not uncommon occurrence of acromegaly in women with multiple pregnancies and repeated lactation. Finally, it should be noted that although pregnancy does not significantly aggravate the course of the disease, lactation seems to be associated with a definitely adverse effect on symptomatology.

TREATMENT. Understandably, the treatment of acromegaly is unsatisfactory. *Irradiation* of the pituitary is still used and may give good results in some cases, in keeping with the findings of Davidoff[23] that 60 to 70 per cent of eosinophilic adenomas are radiosensitive. This view is shared by Goldzieher,[40] based on long experience with radiotherapy of eosinophilic adenoma.

Surgical management of serious forms of the disease, using hypophysectomy, has also been attempted. It goes without saying that this is an extreme measure that should be resorted to only when all other therapeutic means have failed. As far as endocrine therapy is concerned, the best results to date have been obtained with estrogens, mainly *stilbestrol*. In cases of pregnancy with acromegaly, the symptoms may improve after administration of large dosages of stilbestrol, 250 to 300 mg a day.

31.4.2. CORTICOTROPIC HYPERPITUITARISM (CUSHING'S SYNDROME)

In 1932, Cushing[22] described a syndrome characterized by obesity, amenorrhea, hypertrichosis, plethora and diabetes (Figs. 31–11 and 31–12). Cushing believed that the clinical picture described by him was caused by a *basophilic adenoma* of the pituitary. However, analogous cases were soon reported in which the pituitary turned out to be normal (Assmann[4]). In 1939, Crooke and Callow[21] were first to report cases of Cushing's syndrome caused by a malignant tumor of the adrenal cortex. Goldberg,[39] Cluxton and associates,[19] and Walters and Sprague[79] subsequently described several clinical cases in which the same syndrome was the result of either adenoma or carcinoma of the adrenal cortex. In 1950, Gebauer and Linke[37] reported four cases, of which two were due to pituitary basophilism, whereas the other two were associated with benign neoplasms of the adrenal cortex. It is now known, thanks to the investigations of mainly Albright[2] and Jailer and associates,[45] that the essential factor involved in Cushing's syndrome is *excessive production of glucocorticoids* by the adrenal cortex rather than the presence of a basophilic adenoma in the pituitary. As indicated in Chapter 9, glucocorticoids are secreted by the zona fasciculata. The endocrine disorder under consideration may therefore be attributed to pituitary basophilism in general but specifically to *hyperfunction of the zona fasciculata*.

ETIOLOGY. Pituitary basophils are known to elaborate, among other hormones, adrenocorticotropin (ACTH) (see Chapter 5). Basophilic adenomas of the pituitary may be associated with hypersecretion of this trophic hormone and, consequently, produce a stimulatory effect on the adrenal cortex. Hypercorticism due to basophilic adenoma does not affect all segments of the adrenal equally. In Chapter 9, adrenocortical function has been shown to be discharged by two functionally different portions, viz., the *metabolic cortex*, made up of the zona fasciculata and glomerulosa, and the *sexual cortex*, made up of the zona reticularis. The sexual cortex, or zona reticularis, as we had shown,[10] is mainly stimulated by gonadotropic hormone, whereas the zona fasciculata is specifically stimulated by *corticotropin* activity. As a result, the etiology of Cushing's disease may be determined by one of the following two mechanisms: (1) pituitary basophilism, associated with excessive ACTH activity and with reactive fascicular hyperplasia, and (2) an adrenocortical adenoma or adrenocortical hyperplasia, not subordinated to pituitary control. Naturally, in the first case, there is *bilateral hyperplasia* with comparable involvement of both glands, whereas in the second case, the *lesion* may be, and usually is, *unilateral*, and may range from simple adenomatous hyperplasia to cortical adenoma, or even carcinoma. The tumor-induced variety of Cushing's syndrome is reexamined in Chapter 32. As has been very aptly pointed out by Albright,[2] this variety of Cushing's syndrome is, in a way, the opposite of the adrenogenital syndrome. The clinical and physiopathological differences between the two conditions were outlined by us in 1953.[10] More than anything else, Cushing's syndrome is characterized by *adrenocortical hyperfunction that is metabolic in nature,* whereas the adrenogenital syndrome, as we shall see later, is characterized by *adrenocortical dysfunction of sexual activity.* It is evident that some cases represent combination forms of adrenogenital syndrome and Cushing's disease to the point that, as we shall point out, hirsutism in the latter may be in part attributable to an associated form of adrenogenital syndrome.

Kepler and his associates,[49] as well as Wilson and colleagues,[81] drew attention to the fact that mineralocorticoid involvement in the syndrome was not a consistent finding. Produced by the zona glomerulosa, mineralocorticoids are as a rule responsible for the hypertension, edema and changes in electrolyte balance that are usually observed in the course of the disease. However, such changes are not invariably present. As revealed by recent studies (see Chapter 9), rather than stimulating the adrenal cortex as a whole, ACTH ostensibly stimulates only the zona fasciculata; the zona reticularis and zona glomerulosa are only slightly, if at all, affected. Thus, whereas adrenocortical tumors are to a variable extent able to secrete a complex blend of mineralo-and glucocorticoids, in contrast, adrenocortical hyperplasia caused by pituitary basophilism is only seldom associated with symptoms characteristic of zona glomerulosa hyperfunction.

The diagram in Figure 31–12 shows how cortical hyperfunction from ACTH hyperactivity from pituitary basophilism affects the zona fasciculata and zona reticulata in equal measure, producing a parallel increase in corticoids as well as in 17-ketosteroids. The glomerulosa, which is not responsive to pituitary stimulation, does not undergo hyperplasia. By contrast, tumors involving the outermost portions of the adrenal cortex leave the reticular zone intact and cause hyperfunction with increased glucocorticoid and mineralocorticoid production. As a result, the clinical picture first described by Cushing is currently known to represent *two different entities:* one caused by genuine pituitary basophilism, and the other, caused by adrenocortical tumor. In the first, the pituitary is the site of the primary disorder, whereas the adrenal represents only reactive hyperplasia. In the second, pituitary function is within normal limits or is occasionally involved by *compensatory* atrophy of basophilic elements, whereas the adrenal cortex is the site of primary hyperplasia, neoplastic in nature. Consequently, the paradigm in Table 31–3 may be set up.

ANATOMIC PATHOLOGY. It is difficult to evaluate the true incidence of basophilic adenoma of the pituitary. There is no sharp demarcation line between basophilic hyperplasia and basophilic adenoma. Basophilic hyperplasia is probably caused by hypothalamic stimuli of yet undetermined nature, which would lead one to assume the existence of *central forms* of Cushing's disease.

Basophilic adenomas are benign. They may be single or multiple. They are usually quite small and generally produce only minor enlargement of the sella turcica, without associated neurologic symptoms, thereby differing from the normally much larger chromophobe adenomas. At necropsy, in addition, a number of undeniable basophilic adenomas have been encountered that had produced no endocrine symptoms and had to be considered as functionally inert.

As for the remainder of endocrine glands, it goes without saying that the adrenals reveal hyperplasia with considerable enlargement. The thymus is similarly enlarged and reveals lymphoid hyperplasia. The gonads are usually atrophied although, as indicated by us originally,[7] they may show evidence of transient hyperfunction. In the first edition of this book,[7] the ovary in Cushing's disease is pictured as revealing evidence of having undergone extensive luteinization. This, coupled with the fact that various investigators have reported

TABLE 31–3. Cushing's Disease

PITUITARY FORM	ADRENAL FORM
Basophilic adenoma of the pituitary	Adenoma or carcinoma of the zona fasciculata and sometimes zona glomerulosa
Adrenal hyperplasia	Adrenal neoplasia
Pituitary hyperplasia or neoplasia	Pituitary atrophy
Increase mainly in glucocorticoids and 17-ketosteroids	Increase in mineralocorticoids and glucocorticoids
No increase in mineralocorticoids	No increase in 17-ketosteroids
Metabolic symptoms superimposed on sexual symptoms	Exclusively metabolic symptoms

hyperexcretion of gonadotropins in some forms of Cushing's disease, has led us to the assumption that the ovary first undergoes hyperluteinization and is ultimately reduced to atresia as a result of excessive gonadotropin activity.

Primordial adrenal forms of this disease are predominantly due to adrenal tumors, 70 per cent of which are benign adenomas and 30 per cent adrenocortical carcinomas. These forms are not associated with either thymic hyperplasia or hyperplasia of the lymphoid tissue, and the pituitary undergoes reactive atrophy. Pituitary atrophy of this kind has been explained by Selye[64] as resulting from a compensatory mechanism. Naturally, only the basophilic system is affected, other aspects of pituitary physiology remaining spared. In cases with adrenocortical tumors, the presence of genital atrophy may be the result of a similar pituitary mechanism. Nevertheless, it must be remembered that cortisone by itself is capable of causing atrophy of the genital apparatus.

CLINICAL PICTURE. As originally described by Cushing[22] and later by Albright[2] and by Blackman,[6] the clinical symptomatology of this disease is well known. The last two authors, particularly, must be credited for having recognized and separated two distinct causal mechanisms and the corresponding two sets of different clinical manifestations. Characteristically, there is obesity involving the *upper half of the body*, particularly the face, shoulders and back, while sparing the body below the waist, including hips and lower extremities. The face reveals features of plethora, with acrocyanosis and with ecchymoses of pur-

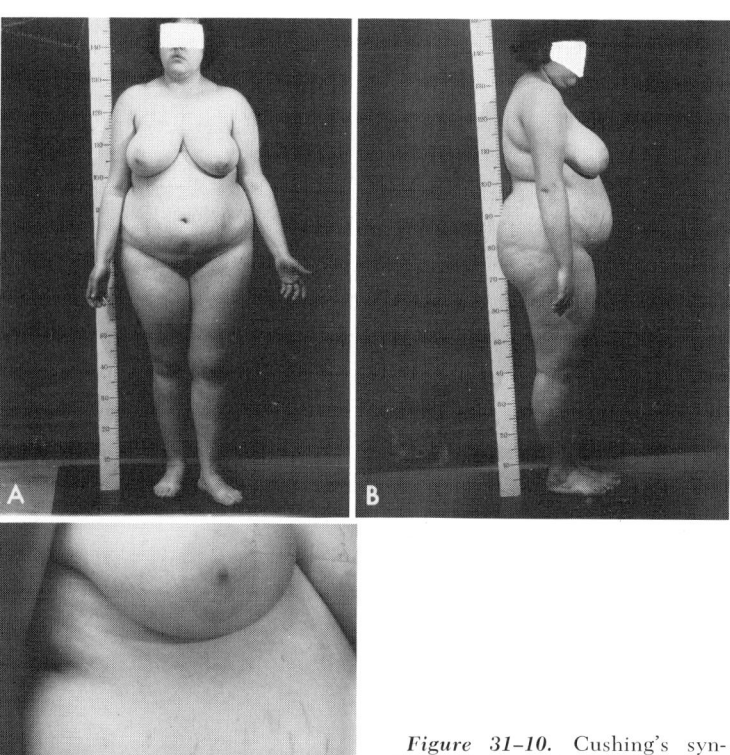

Figure 31-10. Cushing's syndrome. *A*, Frontal view. *B*, In profile. *C*, Detail of abdominal striae.

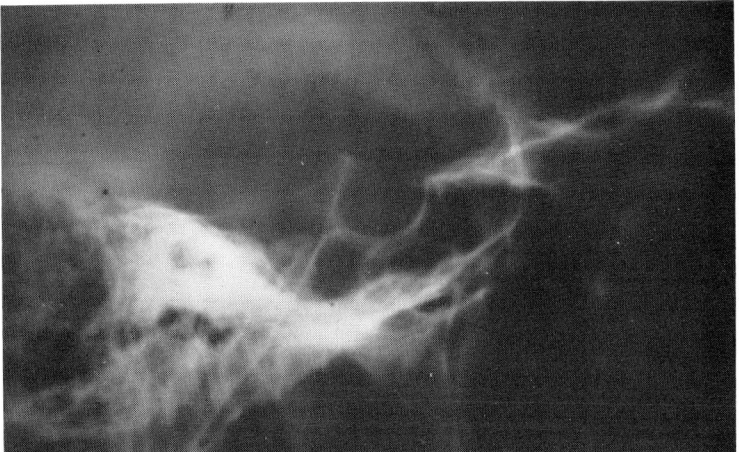

Figure 31-11. Enlarged sella turcica in same case of Cushing's syndrome as shown in Figure 31-10.

puric appearance. Similar ecchymoses are often encountered over other parts of the body, particularly over the abdomen, where there may also appear striae similar to those observed in primigravidas (Fig. 31-10). Much has been written about the origin of such striations as compared to gravidic striae, which are attributed to adrenal hyperfunction of pregnancy. An interesting observation in these patients may be a shortening of stature, which has been found to be related to *osteoporosis* of the vertebral column, resulting in a shorter spine and producing kyphosis. Other bones of the trunk, such as the ribs and the pelvis, and more seldom those of the skull, may also be involved by osteoporosis. The development of fat pads over the shoulders and the back of the neck, in conjunction with a bulging back owing to kyphosis, lends to these patients a characteristic *buffalo type* stance. There is hypertension and, in most cases, also marked cholesterolemia. These patients also develop albuminuria, cylindruria and marked glucosuria, as well as lowered glucose tolerance. Hematologically, most cases reveal polycythemia, less frequently leukocytosis. The disease involves predominantly females, 72 per cent of the cases occurring in women. Its onset becomes apparent at any time between the age of 30 and the climacterium. The onset is usually marked by cessation of menses and, in some cases, although not in all, by the appearance of hirsutism of the male type. It is, however, interesting to note that a few rare instances of prepuberal onset of Cushing's disease (Mellicow and Cahill[56]) were associated with precocious puberty. According to West and his associates,[80] this is the result of *increased production of estrogens*, particularly in young women and in girls, frequently leading to precocious puberty.

Greenblatt[41] called attention to the existence of two different clinical forms of the disease. In the syndrome resulting from pituitary basophilism, the extent of 17-ketosteroid hyperexcretion is matched by the degree of virilization present. On the other hand, the syndrome due to adrenal neoplasia is of a much purer type and produces no symptoms of hirsutism. At the same time, it produces a clinical picture of obesity, diabetes and hypertension of considerably greater intensity than that produced by the pure pituitary form. The clinical findings have been summarized diagrammatically in Figure 31-12.

TREATMENT. The treatment for each of the two forms is different. Irradiation is used mainly in cases with pituitary basophilism. With the latter, Freyberg and coworkers,[29] and Bromley,[13] have reported convincing results. To be effective, radiation therapy of the pituitary must be of sufficient intensity and duration. On the other hand, it must be recognized that many instances have been reported over the years in which radiation therapy turned out to be a failure. This seems to substantiate recently advanced ideas that this syndrome, too, may be in part of adrenal origin. Gebauer and Linke[37] have obtained satisfactory results with surgery in two cases of cortical origin. Obviously, a surgical approach requires absolute certainty that the disease is the result of an adrenal

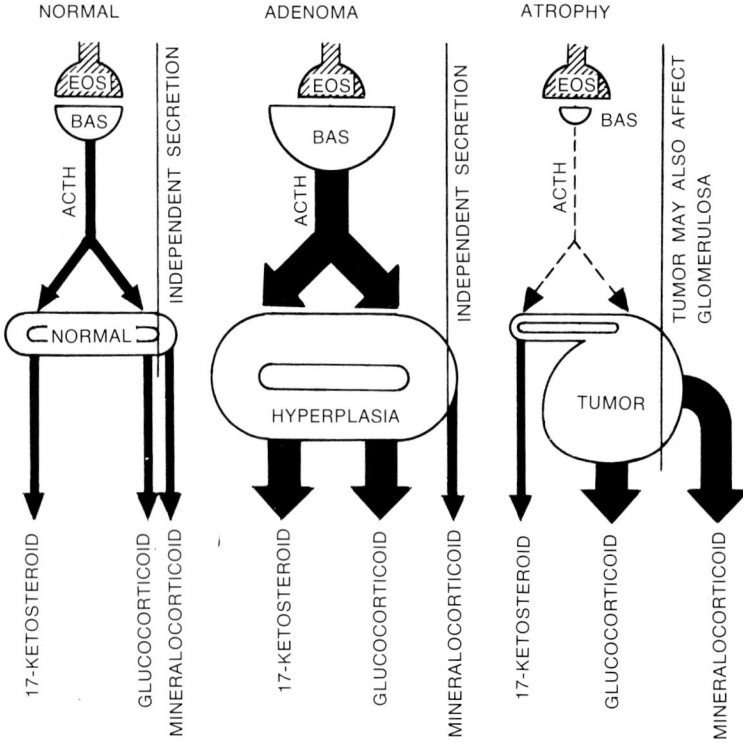

Figure 31-12. Diagram of endocrine conditions in Cushing's syndrome of pituitary origin (center), compared to those of Cushing's syndrome resulting from tumor (right). Note that both differ from normal conditions (left). (From Albright; modified slightly by Botella).

tumor and not of pituitary hyperplasia. A noteworthy case was reported by Byron and Pearl,[16] in which an adrenal tumor was surgically removed in a woman with Cushing's disease, with subsequent reappearance of menstruation and recovery of fertility, followed by several pregnancies.

The choice between irradiation of the pituitary and adrenal surgery must be made in each case individually and depends on whether the presence of an adrenal tumor can be demonstrated conclusively.

Such data as are listed in Table 31-3 may facilitate differentiation between the adrenal and pituitary forms of Cushing's disease. In addition, valuable information may be gained with pneumokidney, which may serve as a guideline in attempting to determine whether or not an adrenal neoplasm is the causative agent. Further data of value for the differential diagnosis may be obtained by means of the pituitary suppression test using *dexamethasone* (see Chapter 41).

31.4.3. GONADOTROPIC HYPERPITUITARISM

Quite seldom mentioned in textbooks of endocrinology except by Kehrer,[48] gonadotropic hyperpituitarism is an entity more common than is generally believed. Gonadotropic hyperpituitarism may develop under physiologic, or almost physiologic, conditions, especially during menopause. Such is the case in castrated women. As pointed out previously, it is characterized by elevated FSH excretion and usually less elevated LH excretion. A pathologic condition, featuring high rates of gonadotropin excretion and mild enlargement of the sella turcica, has been described, chiefly by Kehrer.[48] These alterations are associated with increased FSH activity, giving rise to polycystic ovaries.

ETIOLOGY. Such forms of partial hyperpituitarism are the result of disturbances affecting the sexual center of the hypothalamus rather than of alterations of the pituitary gland itself. These endocrine syndromes are therefore of *neurogenic origin*, both as regards the one presently under discussion and the syndrome of galactotropic hyperpituitarism, which is to be studied in a subsequent paragraph. Similar cases of gonadotropin hyperpituitarism have been described in women under conditions of psychosexual stimulation, or in those who engage in the practice of coitus interruptus or other aberrant practices leading to the syndrome of pelvic congestion (Taylor,[76] Castaño,[18] Botella[9]). This form of pituitary hyperfunction is not invariably associated with a permanent enlargement of the anterior lobe that will allow roentgenologic detection. However, we have observed some cases, such as that illustrated in Figure 31–13, which revealed mild but nevertheless distinctly appreciable sellar enlargement. Gonadotropin excretion is considerably increased insofar as FSH is concerned, with values found ranging from 100 to 500 IU in 24 hr, but an increase in luteinizing hormone (LH) excretion was also demonstrated recently.

CLINICAL FEATURES. The clinical manifestations of this form of gonadotropic hyperpituitarism are not uniform. Nevertheless, the most constant symptoms are follicular persistence or follicle-lutein persistence, associated with amenorrhea. By and large, *Zondek's syndrome*, or polyhormonal amenorrhea, and *Stein's syndrome*, from polymicrocystic ovaries, are both the result of the same form of hypergonadotropism. Under some circumstances, this type of enhanced gonadotropin activity leads to simultaneous maturation and atresia of numerous follicles, in conjunction with *hyperthecosis*. In these instances, amenorrhea is associated with signs of virilization. In Stein's syndrome, in which virilization occurs, the essential factor involved is always hyperpituitarism. The pathogenesis of the *adrenogenital syndrome*, at least in some cases, is linked to gonadotropic hyperpituitarism, as we shall point out in Chapter 32.

The condition usually develops during the fourth decade in women who have no past history of genital symptoms other than decreased fertility. The beginning of the clinical picture frequently sets in with delayed but abundant menstrual bleeding and with gradually developing episodes of amenorrhea that increase in duration and eventually end in lasting amenorrhea. Such amenorrhea is of the hyperhormonal type, without evidence of uterine atrophy but, on the contrary, a usually large and succulent uterus, without associated vaginal atrophy and with a consistent estrogenic pattern in exfoliative cytology. These women usually reveal enhanced libido and occasionally also signs of moderate virilization, with increased hairiness over the abdomen and lower extremities. The importance of this picture in the genesis of the adrenogenital syndrome is again stressed in the next chapter.

TREATMENT. Although estrogens in general have a stimulatory effect on pituitary LH release (see Chapter 6), they would seem rather to inhibit pituitaries of this type, in which the mechanism of rhythmicity is disturbed. We have registered good results by treating such cases with stilbestrol. We recommend the use of moderate dosages, of the order of 0.1 to 0.5 mg a day. To attempt reestablishment of cyclic pituitary function, known to be disturbed in the majority of cases, it may be

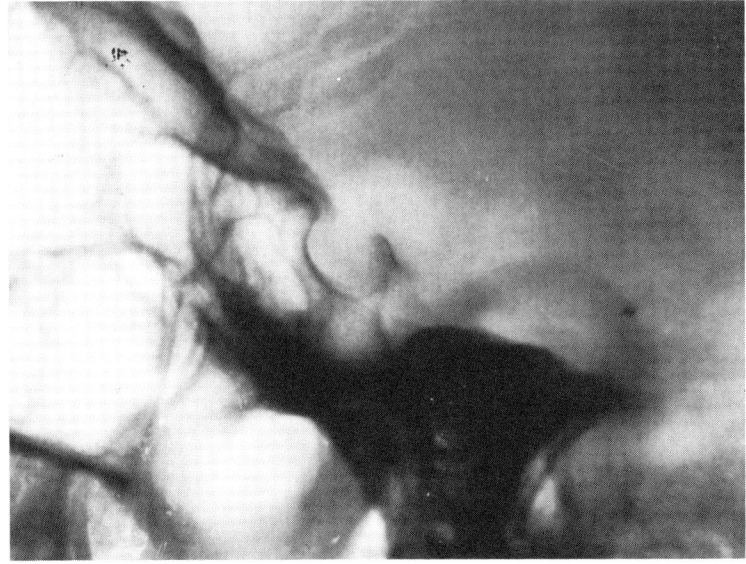

Figure 31–13. Gonadotropic hyperpituitarism. Slightly enlarged sella.

convenient to alternately administer stilbestrol and anhydrohydroxyprogesterone according to a rhythmic schedule. In some cases, pituitary radiation therapy may be indicated (Kaplan[46]).

31.4.4. GALACTOTROPIC HYPERPITUITARISM

In 1942, Schachter[62] described a clinical entity characterized by galactorrhea and amenorrhea. This picture, which has been repeatedly observed by us also, was described in detail by Mendel[57] in 1946. Forbes and his associates,[33, 34] who also described the same clinical picture, at the same time noted enlargement of the sella turcica, increased prolactin excretion, loss of gonadotropin activity and genital atrophy. In 1953, Argonz and Del Castillo[3] collected four cases of this entity, according to them consisting of: (1) hyperestrinism; (2) galactorrhea, and (3) hypogonadotropinuria. Enlargement of the sella turcica was found by them not to be a constant sign. Forbes and his co-workers,[33] who compiled 15 cases, described the same symptoms, but drew attention to the presence of sellar enlargement. The latter authors stress the importance of differentiating this syndrome from acromegaly which, as was pointed out by us previously, usually appears during gestation or during the puerperium and is similarly characterized by lactational potency. Whenever arising in the wake of prolonged lactation, this syndrome acquires special features, which are known by the name of *Chiari-Frommell syndrome* (Chapter 45).

There are two classical descriptions in the literature, one by Chiari-Frommell, according to which the disease is a consequence of gestation and, as already pointed out, is almost always associated with prolonged lactation; the other was described by Argonz and Del Castillo[3] or by Albright and Forbes,[2] which corresponds to a form of the disease that occurs without relation to pregnancy. As a matter of fact, it is the latter variety with which we are concerned here, since the Chiari-Frommell syndrome is discussed in Chapter 45, in connection with the endocrine pathology of gestation. Scaglione[61] believes that both varieties are one and the same.

Frequently, this syndrome is associated with discrete symptoms of acromegaly (Bricaire et al.,[12] MacCullagh et al.[53]), or with diabetes insipidus (Zecca and Passarelli[85]).

ETIOLOGY. The etiology of the syndrome of galactotropic hyperpituitarism is determined by a *lesion in the sex center of the median eminence*. By means of releasing factors, the sex center stimulates, as we have explained in Chapters 8 and 22, all adenohypophysial incretions with the exception of prolactin which instead is inhibited by a special factor, PIF (prolactin inhibiting factor). For this reason, pituitary transplants to any site other than their origin (such as spleen, anterior chamber of the eye) cease secreting all adenohypophysial hormones with the exception of prolactin which, for a change, they produce in excessive amounts. It has thus been learned that the syndrome is generated by destructive processes affecting the sex center and that, in the resulting absence of gonadotropin releasing factors (FSHRF and LHRF), this gives rise to amenorrhea and to ovarian atrophy, whereas, as a result of absent PIF activity, the adenohypophysis produces prolactin.

This syndrome has mainly been described in connection with tumors of the floor of the third ventricle (craniopharyngiomas, etc.) (Chapter 2, Section 2.3.3), as well as with embolism or degenerative processes (Chapter 32, Section 32.4.5). We have witnessed a case of an American patient who had sustained a severe fracture of the base of the skull in a car accident. A similar case was subsequently described by Linquette and co-workers.[52] Lavric,[51] on the other hand, described a case in which the etiology was believed to be related to polycystic ovaries of the Stein-Leventhal type. At the same time, a purely *psychogenic* origin, based on simple functional inhibition of the sex center, cannot be dismissed. *In summary: the syndrome of galactotropic hyperpituitarism stems from inhibition of the sex center of the median eminence of the tuber cinereum.*

CLINICAL PICTURE. The disease is characterized by a triad of symptoms consisting of *amenorrhea, galactorrhea and hyposecretion of both gonadotropins and estrogens*. We believe that sellar enlargement is a frequent finding (Fig. 31–14), although it cannot be considered as absolutely constant. In addition, the women involved

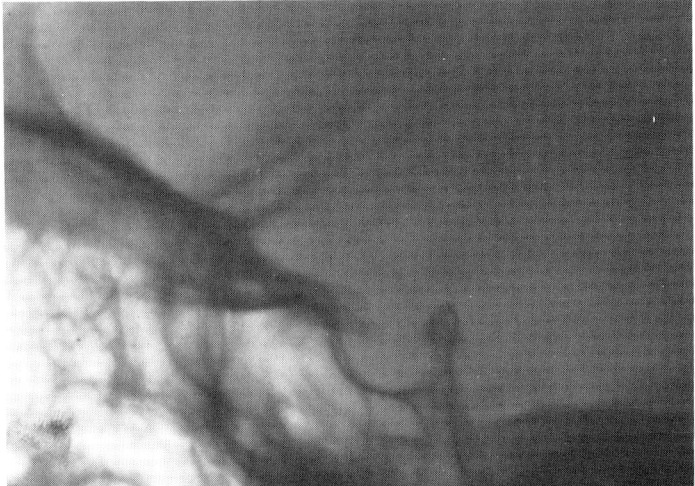

Figure 31-14. Galactotropic hyperpituitarism: Markedly enlarged sella turcica.

generally reveal atrophy of external genitalia, which is in contrast to superhormonal breast development. Almost invariably, the patient's chief complaint is related to the unpleasant symptom of galactorrhea, causing continuous, or almost continuous, soaking of wearing apparel. One of the women observed by us had such excessive milk secretion that, in order to rid herself of her problem, she felt she had no remedy other than to volunteer as a wetnurse.

TREATMENT. We have always treated such patients with estrogen. We start treatment with 1 to 5 mg stilbestrol daily by mouth until galactorrhea stops. It should be made clear to the patient that any attempt to discharge the breasts must be avoided, even though this may seem to be the only way to obtain some relief. Barbiturates (Nembutal, Prominal), in usual dosages, are given simultaneously to reduce hypothalamic hyperexcitability and, thereby, to suppress the secretory reflex arc. Once these procedures have secured cessation of milk hypersecretion, steps are then taken to restore the menstrual cycle. For this purpose, after the patient has received 1 to 5 mg estrogen for at least 12 days, a preparation combining estrogen and progesterone (in a ratio of 1 mg estrogen to 10 mg progesterone) is injected for four consecutive days. With this, and eventually with the help of prostigmine, the first menstruation is induced. As soon as this is achieved, a hormonal cycle must be instituted with a daily dose of 1 mg stilbestrol orally during the first two weeks of the cycle, followed by 0.5 mg stilbestrol in combination with 10 mg progesterone daily for the second half of the cycle. This bihormonal cyclic treatment is carried on for three or four months. Therapy for shorter periods of time often results in recurrence of the syndrome.

The hypothalamic-pituitary syndromes, to which allusion is made in the third section of the table on classification, mainly the adiposogenital syndrome, pituitary precocious puberty and related conditions, are in fact diseases of neurogenic origin with repercussions on sexual life. They are therefore discussed in the corresponding chapter on sexual syndromes of neurogenic origin (Chapter 32).

REFERENCES

1. Abelove, W. A., Rupp, J. J., and Paschkiss, K. E.: *J. Clin. Endocr.*, 14:32, 1954.
2. Albright, F.: *The Harvey Lectures*, 38:123, 1942.
3. Argonz, J., and Del Castillo, E. B.: *J. Clin. Endocr.*, 13:79, 1953.
4. Assmann, K.: *Klin. Wschr.*, 14:1663, 1935.
5. Bettendorf, G., et al.: *Gynaecologia*, 163:134, 1967.
6. Blackman, B. I.: *Bull. Johns Hopkins Hosp.*, 78:180, 1946.
7. Botella, J.: *Endocrinologia de la Mujer*, 1st ed. Madrid, Aguado, 1942.
8. Botella, J.: *Patologia Obstétrica*, 7th ed. Barcelona, Editorial Científico-Médica, 1966.
9. Botella, J.: *Enfermedades del Aparato Genital Femenino*, 8th ed. Barcelona, Editorial Científico-Médica, 1967.
10. Botella, J.: *Arch. Gynäk.*, 183:73, 1953.
11. Brasel, J. A., Wright, J. C., Wilkins, L., and Blizzarel, R. M.: *Amer. J. Med.*, 38:384, 1965.
12. Bricaire, H., et al.: *Ann. d'Endocr.*, 20:719, 1959.

13. Bromley, B. J. F.: *Brit. J. Radiol.*, 9:818, 1936.
14. Buchanan, J. A., and Balwey, H. A.: *Endocrinology*, 24:365, 1939.
15. Buxton, S. J. D.: *Brit. J. Surg.*, 27:181, 1939.
16. Byron, C. S., and Pearl, H.: *Fertil. Steril.*, 5:455, 1954.
17. Canong, W. F., and Hume, D. M.: *Endocrinology*, 59:293, 1956.
18. Castaño, C. A.: *Acta Gin.*, 4:1, 1953.
19. Cluxton, H., et al.: *J. Clin. Endocr.*, 5:61, 1949.
20. Cook, J. E., Ben, W. B., Franklin, M., and Embick, J. F.: *Arch. Int. Med.*, 87:517, 1951.
21. Crooke, A. L., and Callow, R. K.: *Quart. J. Med.*, 8:233, 1939.
22. Cushing, H.: *Intracranial Tumours*. Springfield, Ill., Charles C Thomas, 1932.
23. Davidoff, L. M.: *Bull. N.Y. Acad. Med.*, 16:222, 1940.
24. Elden, C. A., and Rummer, A. J.: *J. Clin. Endocr.*, 3:596, 1943.
25. Ellis, R. W. B.: *Practitioner*, 142:463, 1939.
26. Elkington, S. G., Buckell, M., and Jenkins, J. S.: *Acta Endocr.*, 55:146, 1967.
27. Escamilla, R. F., and Lisser, H.: *J. Clin. Endocr.*, 2:65, 1942.
28. Everett, J. W.: *Physiol. Rev.*, 44:373, 1964.
29. Freyberg, R. H. P., Barker, L. H., Newburg, P. S., and Coller, F. A.: *Arch. Int. Med.*, 58:187, 1936.
30. Finkler, R. S.: *J. Clin. Endocr.*, 14:1245, 1954.
31. Finkler, R. S.: *Internat. J. Fertil.*, 5:79, 1960.
32. Flowers, C. E., Vorys, N., Stevens, V., Miller, A. T., and Jensen, L.: *Amer. J. Obstet. Gynec.*, 96:784, 1967.
33. Forbes, A. P., Henneman, P. H., Griswold, G. C., and Albright, F.: *J. Clin. Endocr.*, 11:265, 1951.
34. Forbes, A. P., Henneman, P. H., Griswold, G. C., and Albright, F.: *J. Clin. Endocr.*, 11:749, 1951.
35. Fraser, R. W., and Smith, P. A.: *Quart. J. Med.*, 10:297, 1941.
36. Gálvez, J., and Sánchez-Agesta, A.: *Acta Gin.*, 5:551, 1954.
37. Gebauer, A., and Linke, A.: *Deutsch. Med. Wschr.*, 75:932, 1950.
38. Gemzell, C. A.: *Acta Gin.*, 18:595, 1967.
39. Goldberg, M.: *Med. Staff Proc. Univ. Calif. Hosp.*, 1:6, 1949.
40. Goldzieher, M. A.: *Clinics*, 1:1069, 1943.
41. Greenblatt, R. B.: *J. Clin. Endocr.*, 14:961, 1954.
42. Hamblen, E. C.: *Endocrinology of Women*. Springfield, Ill., Charles C Thomas, 1945.
43. Herrick, W. W.: *The Pituitary Gland*. Williams & Wilkins, Baltimore, 1938.
44. Ioanitiu, D., Alavez, E., and Serban, A. M. D.: *Rev. Roum. Endocr.*, 4:135, 1967.
45. Jailer, J. W., Longson, D., and Christy, N. P.: *J. Clin. Endocr.*, 16:1277, 1956.
46. Kaplan, I.: *Amer. J. Roentgenol.*, 49:370, 1948.
47. Kecskes, L., Gati, I., Keller, L., and Loch, E.: *Gynaecologia*, 156:229, 1963.
48. Kehrer, E.: *Endokrinologie für den Frauenarzt*. Stuttgart, F. Enke, 1937.
49. Kepler, E. J., et al.: *Rec. Progr. Horm. Res.*, 2:345, 1948.
50. Klinefelter, H. F.: *J. Clin. Endocr.*, 14:756, 1954.
51. Lavric, M. V.: *Amer. J. Obstet. Gynec.*, 104:814, 1969.
52. Linquette, M., Dupont-Lecomte, J., and Gasnault, J. T.: *Lille Medical*, 13:873, 1968.
53. MacCullagh, E. D., Allivisatos, J. G., and Schaffenberg, C. H.: *J. Clin. Endocr.*, 16:397, 1957.
54. Mancini, R. E.: *Acta Gin.*, 18:651, 1967.
55. Marañón, G.: *Ginecología Endocrina*. Madrid, Espasa Calpe, 1935.
56. Mellicow, M. C., and Cahill, G. F.: *J. Clin. Endocr.*, 10:27, 1950.
57. Mendel, E. B.: *Amer. J. Obstet. Gynec.*, 51:889, 1946.
58. Moldawer, M. P., Albright, F., Benedict, P. H., Forbes, A. P., and Henneman, P. H.: *J. Clin. Endocr.*, 18:1, 1958.
59. Nieman, E. A., Landon, J., and Wynn, V.: *Quart. J. Med.*, 36:357, 1957.
60. Perkins, R. F., and Rynearson, E. H.: *J. Clin. Endocr.*, 12:574, 1952.
61. Scaglione, V.: *Ann. Ost. Gin. (Milano)*, 89:248, 1967.
62. Schachter, M.: *Journ. Med. Lyon*, 23:17, 1942.
63. Schneider, C. L.: *J. Obstet. Gynec. Brit. Emp.*, 58:358, 1951.
64. Selye, H.: *Endocrinología*. Barcelona, Salvat, 1952.
65. Sexton, D. L., Morton, F. F., and Sexton, J.: *J. Clin. Endocr.*, 10:1417, 1950.
66. Sheehan, H. L.: *J. Path. Bact.*, 45:187, 1937.
67. Sheehan, H. L.: *Quart. J. Med.*, 8:272, 1938.
68. Sheehan, H. L., and Murdock, R.: *J. Obstet. Gynec. Brit. Emp.*, 45:456, 1938.
69. Sheehan, H. L., and Summers, V. K.: *Quart. J. Med.*, 18:319, 1949.
70. Shelton, E. K.: *The Pituitary Gland*. Baltimore, William & Wilkins Co., 1938.
71. Simpson, S. L.: *Major Endocrine Disorders*. London, John Bale, 1938.
72. Smith, P. H.: *Anat. Rec.*, 52:191, 1932.
73. Sol, R. del, and Merlo, J. G.: *Acta Gin.*, 3:533, 1952.
74. Solomon, J., and Greep, R. O.: *Endocrinology*, 65:158, 1959.
75. Sommers, S. C., and Wadam, P. J.: *Amer. J. Obstet. Gynec.*, 72:160, 1956.
76. Taylor, H. C.: *Amer. J. Obstet. Gynec.*, 57:211, 237, 254, 1949.
77. Teter, J., Wecewcz, G., and Ladygin, E.: *Rev. Franc. Endocr. Clin.*, 8:19, 1967.
78. Wadsworth, R. C., and MacKeown, C.: *Arch. Neurol. Psych.*, 46:277, 1941.
79. Walters, W., and Sprague, R. G.: *J.A.M.A.*, 141:653, 1949.
80. West, C. D., Damast, B., and Pearson, O. H.: *J. Clin. Endocr.*, 18:15, 1958.
81. Wilson, M., Romer, M. A., and Kepler, E. J.: *J. Clin. Invest.*, 19:701, 1940.
82. Whitehead, R.: *J. Path. Bact.*, 86:55, 1963.
83. Wohl, M. G., and Larson, E.: *Med. Clin. N. Amer.*, 26:1657, 1942.
84. Worms, G., and Delanter, D.: *Rev. Neurol. Psych.*, 2:261, 1955.
85. Zecca, D., and Passarelli, C.: *Anali Ost. Gin. (Milano)*, 89:263, 1967.

Chapter 32
SEXUAL SYNDROMES OF NEUROGENIC ORIGIN

After having for many years embraced the theory of exclusive hormonal regulation of sexual function, we now once more recognize the significant role played by the nervous system in correlating reproductive processes. A series of facts of everyday occurrence, as well as a wealth of clinical data, have all made it imperative to admit that the nervous system greatly influences the female sexual cycle. The past few years have brought to light a number of physiologic data that explain such intervention by the nervous system. The relationships existing between the nervous system, principally the hypothalamus, and sexual physiology have been discussed in Chapter 8. The present chapter is concerned with clinical syndromes of evidently neurogenic origin and, in addition, with examining such female endocrinopathic processes as may be related to psychosomatic disorders. Consequently, we shall study the following topics: (1) hypothalamic syndromes; (2) sexual syndromes of psychogenic origin, and (3) the psychosomatic origin of some disturbances of the cycle.

32.1. HYPOTHALAMIC SYNDROMES

The hypothalamus is known to be functionally linked to the pituitary to such an extent that, rather than speaking of two separate functions, the two must be thought of as one functional unit. This helps to explain why pathologic processes injuring or otherwise affecting the hypothalamus produce endocrine syndromes with pituitary participation and, furthermore, why such syndromes largely involve sexual function. Among hypothalamic syndromes manifestly involving reproductive function, the following must be described: (1) Froehlich's syndrome, (2) Lawrence-Moon-Biedl syndrome, (3) hypothalamic obesity, (4) hypothalamic sexual precocity, (5) "hypothalamic syndrome," to a large extent related to the preceding conditions, (6) diabetes insipidus, and (7) hypothalamic tumors.

32.1.1. ADIPOSOGENITAL SYNDROME OF FROEHLICH

Known by the name of *adiposogenital* syndrome, or *adipose hypogenitalism*, the syndrome described by Froehlich has the following characteristic features: *obesity, delayed sexual development and delayed skeletal development*. For many years, it was believed to result from pituitary insufficiency. As far back as 1917, Marañón and Pintos[57] described a case of secondary adiposogenital syndrome in a soldier who had sustained a cranial gunshot wound during the war in Africa. Autopsy revealed that the bullet had come to lodge, not in the pituitary, but in the *tuber cinereum*, after severing the stalk but without affecting the structure of the pituitary. By 1942, Wohl and Larson[98] admitted the neurogenic nature of this syndrome without reservations.

These early findings are in agreement with modern knowledge concerning the hypothalamic sex center (see Chapter 8). Accordingly, Froehlich's syndrome must be viewed as a hypothalamic disturbance simultaneously producing inhibition of the sex center of the *tuber cinereum* (Everett[29]) and a similarly hypothalamus-dependent alteration in lipid metabolism. Barraclough and Sawyer[8, 9, 10] (using rats), Clegg and associates[20] (sheep), daily and Ganong[21] (dogs), and Gloor,[37] Green,[39] and Herrmann and Lemarchands[44] (man), have all confirmed the finding that lesions affecting the cerebral cortex or the medulla had no effect on ovarian function while, in contrast, ovarian function was extremely sensitive to even the slightest disturbances involving the area lying between the *tuber cinereum* and the *mammillary bodies*.

The limits of this lesion have not yet been fully demarcated. On the one hand, a quite similar syndrome has been described under the name of Lawrence-Moon-Biedl syndrome; on the other hand, under the name of "thalamic syndrome," various authors have grouped certain lesions of the hypothalamus that are associated with alterations in sexual function, sometimes producing hypergenitalism (precocious puberty), sometimes leading to obesity and hypogenitalism. As a result, the adiposogenital syndrome may be viewed as synonymous with the so-called *hypogenital form of the thalamic syndrome*. In addition, hypothalamic obesity, associated with minimal or no sexual alterations, has been described as an independent clinical entity.

As a matter of fact, *all the foregoing conditions merely constitute different forms of the same disease process*. The latter involves *partial or total destruction of certain areas of the hypothalamus* which, depending on whether the main damage is located in centers of sexual activity or affects those of metabolism, may give rise to predominance of hypogenitalism over obesity or vice versa. As an alternative, the initial form of the lesion not uncommonly causes irritation rather than destruction of the hypothalamic sex centers and thus gives rise to the syndrome of precocious puberty. The present section is concerned with the description of typical Froehlich's syndrome and offers a short independent comment about each of the different modalities that have been described in the hypothalamic syndrome.

ETIOLOGY. The hypothalamic nature of the lesions is today universally accepted. The type of lesions described are mainly those suprasellar or extrasellar lesions that cause destruction of the connections between the hypothalamus and the pituitary. In this respect, it is of interest to mention that Wilkins and Fleischman[97] reported the finding of *suprasellar* calcifications, detectable on skull x-rays, as a possible etiologic factor (Fig. 32–1). Tumors involving the hypothalamus, such as craniopharyngiomas or pituitary chromophobe adenomas, have similarly been described as capable of producing the syndrome. Finally, the adiposogenital syndrome has been reported to occur frequently in the wake of encephalitis (Ford and Guild[32]).

Bleuler[17] stressed the *psychogenic etiology* of some forms of obesity with hypogenitalism. Such forms might be qualified as instances of *psychogenic Froehlich's syndrome*. Equally possible is a *traumatic*

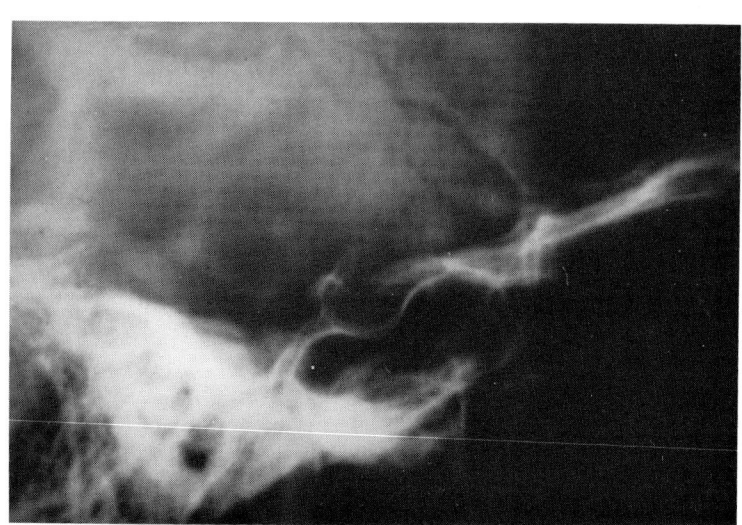

Figure 32–1. Suprasellar calcification in a case of Froehlich's syndrome.

etiology, of which the case reported by Marañón and Pintos[57] is a beautiful example.

CLINICAL PICTURE. Depending on the time in life at which it arises, the disease may present with different clinical manifestations, permitting the description of childhood forms, juvenile forms and adult forms. Symptoms may be grouped into *sexual, metabolic and skeletal types.* Sexual symptoms consist of retarded development of the genital apparatus, delayed puberty and oligomenorrhea or amenorrhea. Metabolic symptoms are a consequence of the characteristic obesity, which involves particularly the pelvic belt, lower part of the abdomen and legs. In addition, these patients also present with *retarded skeletal development*, genu valgum and usually short stature. It is *during childhood* that clinical manifestations are most striking. Not only is obesity pronounced but also retarded genital development is all the more noticeable. Excessive fat accumulates in the lower half of the body, the infraumbilical portion of the abdomen, the hips and the buttocks. The skin is delicate and may be likened to a thin sheet of alabaster. Hands are stocky and short, of the characteristic hypogenital type. A typical genu valgum becomes apparent and so does hypotrichosis. The onset of puberty is invariably delayed (Fig. 32–2).

If such hypogenital children do grow, they develop a characteristic psychology during the period of puberty. They become shy and, as a result, their sexual instinct is frequently modified. Occasionally, overcompensation for their genital complex causes them to become aggressive, antisocial or pretentiously hypersexual. In addition to their symptoms of obesity and hypogonadism, other hypothalamic symptoms may be present, such as polydipsia, polyuria, gastrointestinal disturbances and, sometimes, headaches and visual disturbances.

The *juvenile form* is characterized by scanty menses, primary or secondary amenorrhea and sometimes extended periods of amenorrhea in those young women who have not ceased menstruating altogether. Skeletal alterations are less prominent than when symptomatology develops in infancy.

In the adult form, the feature that develops most rapidly is obesity. Not uncommonly, obesity starts as a by-product of either pregnancy or the climacterium (Fig. 32–3). The most commonly observed symptom may be secondary amenorrhea, whereas infertility and oligomenorrhea may appear in milder forms. Loss of body hair is common. The syndrome in its late form never develops in a sudden manner. In general, it is preceded by a hypogenital condition and a tendency toward overweight, constitutionally present since childhood. In summary, then, *this syndrome may be stated to invariably have its origin in infancy, notwithstanding the fact that it sometimes remains dormant until its full development during adulthood.*

TREATMENT. Results are unsatisfactory. The use of pituitary extracts, serum gonadotropins and sex hormones has been advocated with a view to remedying the hypogenital condition. Obesity may be controlled by dietary means and thyroid therapy, as well as by diuretics. However, it must be realized that any treatment of this kind is merely symptomatic and that while it may achieve weight loss and resumption of menstrual activity, as well as increased menstrual bleeding in nonamenorrheic women, its discontinuation or interruption leads to reappearance of symptomatology.

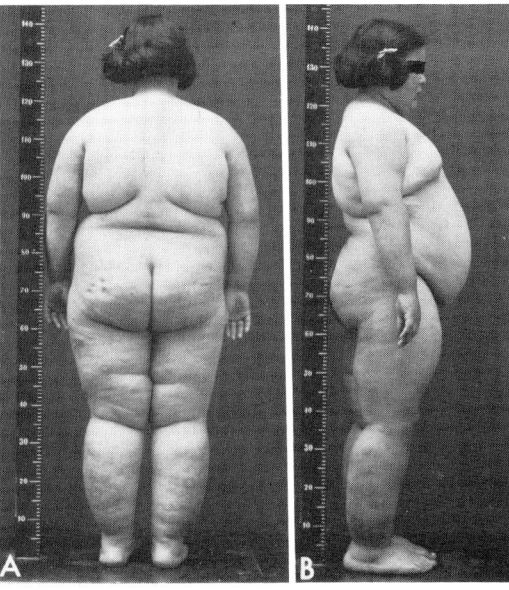

Figure 32–2. Adiposogenital syndrome of Froehlich, in a girl aged 14. *A*, Posterior view of the patient. *B*, Lateral view.

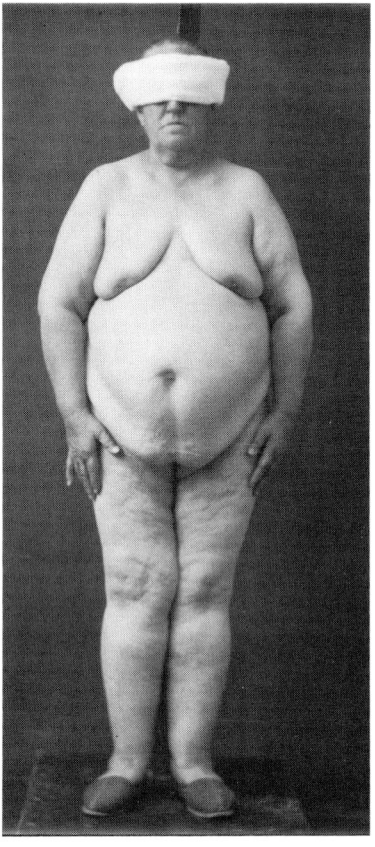

Figure 32-3. Case of Froehlich's adiposogenital syndrome, occurring in an adult.

32.1.2. LAWRENCE-MOON-BIEDL SYNDROME

The Lawrence-Moon-Biedl syndrome is actually a variant of the adiposogenital syndrome which, in addition to obesity and hypogonadism, is associated with *congenital anomalies,* such as polydactylia or syndactylia, retinitis pigmentosa and, usually, mental retardation. Since Warkany and his associates[95] made the observation that the family pedigrees of such patients usually disclosed a variety of congenital anomalies, it has been assumed that, from a hereditary standpoint, these patients usually are heavily stigmatized individuals in whom *some of the many congenital anomalies involved happened to produce a hypothalamic lesion that caused the Lawrence-Moon-Biedl syndrome. Consequently, the essential underlying factor is the presence of congenital anomalies, whereas obesity and hypogonadism are merely incidental consequences of one of* the many congenital malformations involved.

The present trend is to admit that hypogonadism in this syndrome may be primary in nature, owing to some ovarian congenital anomaly. Oettle and his associates[66] classify this syndrome among the forms of *gonadal dysgenesis* and see it as merely an instance of gonadal dysgenesis that is associated with the syndrome of hypothalamic obesity. This point of view currently has many advocates. A series of six autopsied cases collected by Anderson[2] revealed a surprising lack of anatomopathologic uniformity of the lesions involved, which is in keeping with current notions concerning the disease. The disorder most frequently reported in this syndrome is delayed genital development, with ovarian insufficiency, which may reflect the fact that most clinicians consider the presence of hypogonadism essential in any given case before accepting the diagnosis of Lawrence-Moon-Biedl syndrome. On the other hand, the association of simple obesity with congenital anomalies has also been frequently described and must be considered as *a variant of the syndrome without gonadal involvement.*

Although the clinical picture was originally thought to be consistent with hypopituitarism, it is a fact that, as in Froehlich's syndrome, the hypopituitarism involved is always secondary to an essential hypothalamic lesion.

Some later studies concentrated on the state of the gonads in this syndrome. Roth[77] showed the presence of decreased gonadotropin A (FSH) in the urine of female patients. Estrogens and 17-ketosteroids were similarly found to be decreased (Reinfranck and Nichols[73]). The gonads in three cases reported by Anderson were examined anatomically and revealed absent ovarian maturation in females and presence of testicular atrophy in males, Francke reviewed the autopsy findings in three female patients and found that two had normal ovaries in the resting stage, without evidence of maturation, and absence of pituitary gonadotropin activity. Thus, these two cases qualified as instances of primordial pituitary hypogonadism with normal ovaries. In the third case, however, the rudimentary nature of the gonads was consistent with the diagnosis of ovarian agenesis or hypogenesis and was associated with increased urinary gonadotropin values, thus presenting a picture not unlike that of Turner's syndrome. As a result of such findings, Francke,[33] Varney and his associates,[91] as well as Heller and Nelson,[43] expressed the belief that hypogonadism in Lawrence-Moon-Biedl's syndrome did not necessarily have a hypothalamic-pituitary etiology resulting from a hypothalamic disorder *but might, in some cases, be due to congenital ovarian malformations, giving rise to conditions similar to Turner's syndrome* and, hence, representing cases of ovarian hypogenitalism. As a result, our present concept of Lawrence-Moon-Biedl's syndrome should be modified and the syndrome should be redefined as characterized by congenital anomalies, obesity and hypogonadism, with the proviso, however, that hypogonadism may have either a hypothalamic-pituitary or a primordial ovarian origin.

32.1.3. HYPOTHALAMIC OBESITY

What is understood by hypothalamic, or cerebral, obesity is rapid accumulation of fat in conjunction with various intracranial disorders, most commonly diabetes insipidus, but sometimes also other hypothalamic symptoms. The type of obesity involved seems to be closely related to that seen in Froehlich's syndrome, probably with the only difference that, unlike in Froehlich's syndrome, sexual function is not involved. Wohl and Larson[98] have described the occurrence of obesity in association with lesions affecting the pituitary region, the infundibulum, the paraventricular nuclei or the floor of the third ventricle. As with Froehlich's disease, it may occur in the wake of encephalitis, and here too the pituitary may be spared by the primary process (Fig. 32–4). By and large, the disease may be described as resulting from destruction of the "fat center," or center of metabolic regulation, located in the floor of the third ventricle. In this respect, Barborka[5] long ago alluded to the role played by hypothalamic function in the development of obesity. Because of the nearness of the center for diuresis, this syndrome often occurs concurrently with diabetes insipidus.

The most common way the disease appears is following encephalitis. Hamblen[40] described the case of a 14 year old boy who, following epidemic encephalitis, developed the syndrome after gaining 50 kg in weight over a period of nine months. By definition, rather than by its very nature, the syndrome has no associated sexual manifestations. Whenever obesity occurs in conjunction with hypogonadism, it necessarily becomes a case of adiposogenital syndrome. Thus, the picture we are presently discussing, which might conveniently be called "Froehlich's syndrome without hypogenitalism," is offered here as a contribution to a clearer understanding of the essence of this type of hypothalamic syndrome.

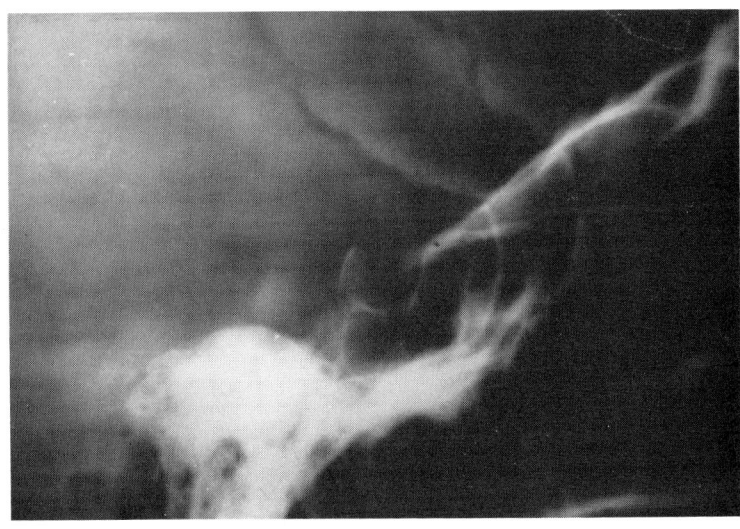

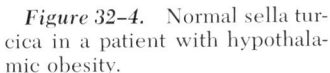
Figure 32–4. Normal sella turcica in a patient with hypothalamic obesity.

32.1.4. HYPOTHALAMIC SEXUAL PRECOCITY

Different etiologies of precocious puberty as a whole are discussed in Chapter 38. Among these are *hypothalamic lesions* that may cause premature sexual maturation in the absence of any endocrine lesions. We therefore use the term hypothalamic precocious puberty for those conditions in which, owing to the presence of hypothalamic lesions, female sexual maturation is advanced in time. The nature of the lesions may be extremely variable. The following different causes have been described: (1) hydrocephalus from obstruction of the aqueduct of Sylvius; (2) epidemic encephalitis; (3) tuberculomas or syphilitic gummas; (4) postencephalomyelitic disorders; (5) degenerative encephalopathies; (6) tumors involving the third ventricle; (7) hyperplasia of the *tuber cinereum;* (8) tumors of the pituitary stalk with extension to the third ventricle, and (9) pinealomas or pineal teratomas causing compression or irritation of the third ventricle. We have already explained in Chapter 31 how precocious puberty could be induced by pineal tumors not only through destruction of the pineal itself but also through irritation of the hypothalamus.

The common denominator in all these diseases is the presence of some lesion or disturbance in the hypothalamus. In the past, the cause of precocious puberty was attributed to hypothalamic tumors on the assumption that they produced hyperpituitarism in some indirect way. Any such hypothesis concerning the etiology of the disease was totally repudiated by the observations of Ford and Guild[32] that *at no time did precocious puberty occur in conjunction with pituitary hyperfunction in any of the cases studied.* According to these authors, moreover, epiphysial precocious puberty similarly was not due to loss of pineal function but had the same etiology as the hypothalamic type of precocious puberty. *Undoubtedly, some inhibitory center for gonadotropin secretion by the pituitary must exist in the hypothalamus that holds gonadotropin activity in check during childhood. Destruction of such a center presumably triggers off puberty.*

The condition is more common in males than it is in females. However, Hamblen described two well documented female cases. The condition usually occurs in girls between the ages of five and 10 who, in the course of convalescence from encephalitis, present with strikingly rapid development of breasts and external genitalia, as well as with premature menarche. Contrary to what is seen in cases of precocious puberty of adrenal origin (that is, rather than revealing any evidence of associated mental precocity), these patients show a characteristic involutional torpor in addition to other postencephalitic symptoms. Precocious somatic development occurring simultaneously with precocity of sexual development has also been reported in cases of gigantoid growth without associated eunuchoid features.

The disease is still poorly understood and what remains to be studied is the hypothalamic origin of most mechanisms involved in accelerating puberty and growth, whose relationship to chronopathies and to hypothalamic physiology has not yet been elucidated. In Spain, Matos and co-workers[61] reported a case of precocious puberty in a two year old girl who revealed severe hypoplasia of cerebral hemispheres that did not affect either the basal nuclei or the diencephalon. The pronounced degree of obesity observed in this case was probably also of centrogenic origin.

More shall be said on the subject of hypothalamic precocious puberty in Chapter 38.

32.1.5. HYPOTHALAMIC SYNDROME

Considerable significance has recently been attached to what Bauer[12] had denominated "hypothalamic syndrome." In 60 cases studied by him in that category, he found localized neoplastic, inflammatory or degenerative lesions in the region of the *tuber cinereum, mamillary bodies and infundibulum.* The tumors most frequently found were craniopharyngiomas and astrocytomas. Among inflammatory lesions, encephalomeningitis and encephalitis ranked highest in number while, among the rare group of degenerative lesions, sclerosis and arteriosclerosis were most common. Whenever the hypothalamus is destroyed by any of the above processes, the earliest symptoms to appear are sexual ones. They precede the appearance of vegetative symptoms which are followed, at a much later stage, by the appearance of local neurologic or neuro-ophthalmic symptoms.

The sexual symptoms of the hypothalamic syndrome may assume two different forms. The most commonly observed type, the syndrome of *hypothalamic precocious puberty*, differs in appearance from that of precocious puberty due to tumors or destruction of the pineal. It was first recognized in 1929 by Spatz,[83] who called it the hypothalamic form of precocious puberty. It was later studied by Papez and Ecker,[67] Seckel and associates,[80] and Bronstein.[18] Less commonly observed than the hypothalamic form of precocious puberty is Froehlich's syndrome, which has the same etiology. It is characterized by hypogonadism, which is usually more pronounced in males than in females because of involvement of seminiferous tubules in the former. In females, it occurs less frequently and is associated with amenorrhea. In either sex, it produces a marked degree of obesity. Cases of this type have been described by Moore and Cushing,[63] by Leghorn[54] and by Anderson.[2] In addition to genital atrophy and obesity, some cases are observed to be associated with vegetative symptoms, such as somnolence and diabetes insipidus. Perhaps the case reported many years ago by Marañón and Pintos,[57] in which an African war casualty revealed a bullet lodged in the brain that had destroyed the pituitary stalk and part of the hypothalamus, should be included among these forms of hypothalamic syndrome. The clinical symptoms in this patient consisted of obesity, diabetes insipidus and genital atrophy, with loss of libido.

The mechanism whereby some cases develop precocious puberty while others develop genital atrophy is unknown. The occurrence of genital atrophy might be easily accounted for on the basis of well-known subordination of pituitary function to hypothalamic centers, so that destruction of the latter would explain development of pituitary atrophy or inactivity. On the other hand, the opposite phenomenon, viz., premature awakening of the pituitary gland, can only be explained if the tumor, or other pathologic alteration involved, initially produced irritation rather than destruction. It is possible that a number of cases starting as precocious puberty terminate secondarily in genital atrophy, much as occurs in the adrenogenital syndrome (see Chapter 33).

32.1.6. OLFACTOGENITAL SYNDROME

Belaisch and his colleagues,[13, 14] as well as Morsier and Gautier,[64] described a syndrome characterized by *anosmia* and *amenorrhea* resulting from combined atrophy of the first cranial pair and the sex center. Such an entity might also be included in the present group of syndromes.

32.1.7. DIABETES INSIPIDUS

Just as the preceding conditions, diabetes insipidus is due to lesions affecting the hypothalamus. In this instance, however, the lesions have been localized somewhat more accurately: they occur in the *supraoptic nuclei* as well as in the *supraoptic hypophysial tract*. In light of Bargmann's investigations,[6, 7] mentioned in Chapter 8, the supraoptic nucleus is known to contain incretory cells that are provided with processes extending to the posterior lobe of the pituitary. All along the course of these processes, the secretory products from the cells of the supraoptic nucleus are delivered to the bloodstream. Since the secretory product is none other than the retrohypophysial antidiuretic substance, destruction of the supraoptic nucleus or of its connections with the posterior lobe results in lack of antidiuretic hormone and consequently in loss of hypothalamic-pituitary control over diuresis.

A variety of lesions have been implicated in the etiology of diabetes insipidus: tumors, inflammatory processes, encephalitis, basal meningitis, syphilis, fractures, xanthomatosis and pellagra. Of all of these, the last two are the most common causes of the disease: xanthomatosis appearing in 60 per cent of the cases, pellagra in 25 per cent, together accounting for 85 per cent of all cases (Lichtwitz[55]).

Although the cardinal feature of the disease is *polyuria*, the presence of *sexual symptoms* may occasionally also be noted. Clinical cases of *polyuria with hypogenitalism*, with or without associated obesity, have been described. Similarly, a case of precocious puberty with polyuria was reported by Ford and Guild.[32]

The disease is compatible with intercurrent pregnancy, since neither menstruation nor fertility is significantly affected in the majority of cases. Instances of gestation with diabetes insipidus have been reported by Hart and Breitman[41] and, subsequently, by Marañón.[58,59] A case reported by Marañón is of particular interest because the patient had been followed for diabetes insipidus for 26 years, during which time she had five pregnancies, each with a normal course during which diuresis was not affected but labor was complicated by marked atony of contractions, requiring frequent application of forceps.

Martinez-Diaz[60] later reviewed six similar cases from the Marañón Clinic, finding that delayed labor with weak contractions was a common feature in each of the cases. This seems to be a clear indication that labor can be realized despite lesions of the supraoptic or paraventricular nuclei—because, as postulated in Chapter 21, oxytocin is probably not the only hormone with myometrium-exciting activity—although any alterations in the above centers have a profound effect on the mechanics and rhythm of labor.

32.1.8. PITUITARY TUMORS AND THE HYPOTHALAMIC SYNDROME

The significant role played by pituitary tumors in the production of thalamic syndromes has been emphasized in previous paragraphs. Two types of tumors are most frequently found in this region: *chromophobe adenomas* and *craniopharyngiomas*. Although the first actually originate in the pituitary and the second arise from Rathke's pouch or from the pituitary stalk, most of the symptomatology produced by such tumors results from compression of or alterations in the hypothalamus rather than from destruction of the pituitary gland. In addition, the syndrome may also be caused by *tumors of the nasopharyngeal cavity*, as shown in Figure 32–5, illustrating the case of 33 year old woman who had been studied by us in cooperation with Sopeña. With the exception of obesity and amenorrhea, the remaining pituitary controlling functions were found to be preserved. *Chromophobe adenomas* seldom produce symptoms before puberty. The symptomatology that develops after puberty is accompanied by important neurologic signs (compression, hemianopia, symptoms of cranial pair involvement) and by pronounced symptoms of hypogenitalism. Hypogenitalism in these cases is often associated with obesity and with polyuria, which would seem to indicate that we are in fact dealing with an entity similar to Froehlich's syndrome rather than genuine primitive hypopituitarism.

As for *craniopharyngiomas*, that is, tumors of the craniopharyngeal duct or Rathke's pouch, these usually occur during, or slightly before, puberty. Apart from such neurologic symptoms as visual disturbances, hemianopia, headache, somnolence and disturbances of thermoregulation, they present with typical pituitary symptoms, such as dwarfism, obesity, hypogonadism and polyuria. Considering the coexistence of polyuria and obesity in this syndrome, it may clearly be understood why these are hypothalamic rather than pituitary symptoms. Nevertheless, occasional instances have been reported in which craniopharyngiomas were instrumental in destroying most of the anterior lobe of the pituitary gland, producing states of emaciation and cachexia not unlike those seen in panhypopituitarism. It is thus apparent that, while these two types of tumors frequently cause the hypothalamic syndrome, they may in some cases be linked to syndromes of the primitive pituitary type. Because their occurrence as causative agents of sexual alterations is uncommon, they have been only briefly cited here.

32.1.9. SYNOPSIS OF SEXUAL HYPOTHALAMIC SYNDROMES

It may be inferred from what has just been said in the foregoing paragraphs that the study of hypothalamic syndromes is just in its beginnings. By virtue of being provided with centers that control pituitary activity, the hypothalamus obviously takes direct part in sexual activity, metabolism, water exchange and other vegetative functions. Hypothalamic lesions are therefore necessarily associated with modifications of sexual function, with obesity, with diabetes insipidus and with other disturbances. However, the exact locations of the various regulatory centers for pituitary activity are still poorly known, making classification of the various syndromes along topographical lines impossible. Those hypothalamic

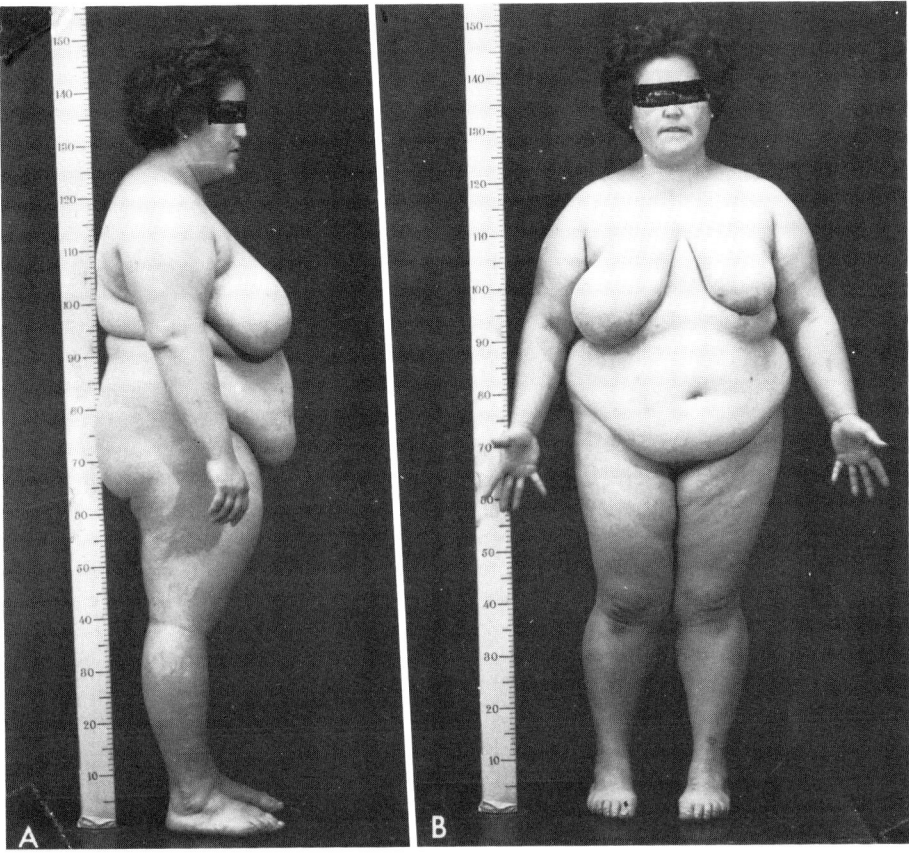

Figure 32-5. Case of a 33 year old patient with a tumor originating in nasopharyngeal cavity. Involvement of tuber cinereum caused secondary amenorrhea and obesity.

functions that seem to be most frequently affected by lesions involving this region of the brain pertain to sexual function, regulation of metabolism and regulation of water exchange. As a result, combinations of hypogonadism and obesity, obesity and diabetes insipidus, and hypogonadism and diabetes insipidus may be inferred to occur in variable gradations depending on the extent of involvement of the various centers. It would therefore seem appropriate to speak in terms of just one *hypothalamic syndrome*, within the framework of which Froehlich's syndrome, diabetes insipidus and obesity are mere partial aspects, combinable in different proportions. Special mention must be made of precocious puberty of encephalic origin. To our view, as well as to that of a number of modern authors,[12, 31, 32, 33] *pineal precocious puberty and hypothalamic precocious puberty are probably one and the same syndrome.* We believe that the hypothalamus must be the site of some center responsible for sexual maturation or, in more precise terms, some center that stimulates both somatic development and pituitary growth hormone secretion, while at the same time inhibiting pituitary gonadotropin secretion. The hormonal changes observed to occur in the pituitary at the onset of puberty are presumably caused by hypothalamic action. The chemical mediators capable of inhibiting gonadotropin secretion, as well as those others capable of stimulating gonadotropin synthesis, must therefore be assumed to originate in the hypothalamus, each being derived from different centers. Destruction of the gonadotropin synthesis stimulating center would be expected to cause hypogonadism; destruction of gonadotropin inhibiting centers, on the other hand, would provoke precocious puberty. Hypothalamic-hypophysial inhibition of sexuality may be conceived as having in part a pineal origin. According to such a concept, *the pineal may be conceived as a neuroendocrine gland, or nerve center, designed to inhibit sexual maturation, rather than as a simple endocrine gland.* Initiation of sexuality through loss of inhibitory impulses might be brought about not just by destruction of the pineal or by destruction of pineal-hypothalamic connections, but certainly also by destruction of the hypothalamic inhibitory center of sex. *In our opinion, therefore, both hypothalamic-pituitary precocious puberty and pineal precocious puberty are but partial aspects of the same clinical entity.*

32.2. SEXUAL SYNDROMES OF PSYCHOGENIC ORIGIN

The syndromes studied in the preceding paragraphs are syndromes in which psychogenic factors do not intervene or do so in a secondary way. In contrast, the two clinical entities about to be discussed are rooted in emotional disturbances and their origin is related to the cerebral cortex so that they fully qualify to be the object of study of *psychosomatic gynecology.* The two most essential disturbances of this kind are psychogenic amenorrhea and anorexia nervosa.

32.2.1. PSYCHOGENIC AMENORRHEA

In 1943, Klinefelter and his associates[48,49] called attention to a clinical syndrome in which amenorrhea developed from emotional causes. Amenorrhea of this type occurred in nurses and students who happened to be away from home for the first time. This symptom was also observed in immigrants or in patients with sexual maladjustment problems, or in women afraid of becoming pregnant. In all such cases, amenorrhea was believed to result from inhibition of the hypothalamus. Reifenstein and his associates[71,72] subsequently studied such cases and arrived at the conclusion that what was involved was a *psychogenic stimulus causing inhibition of hypothalamic function.* As a result of hypothalamic inhibition, release of gonadotropic hormone by the anterior lobe of the pituitary is blocked. Lack of gonadotropin activity determines paralysis of the ovarian cycle and absence of maturation. Unlike the situation in menopause, however, lack of ovarian maturation here does not result in hyperproduction of gonadotropin, owing to the fact that the physiologic stimulus for gonadotropin secretion is inhibited at the hypothalamic level. Amenorrhea of this type differs from primary ovarian amenorrhea in that, notwithstanding the presence of hypoestrinism, there is no hypergonadotropinism.[4]

Psychogenic amenorrhea may also be observed among maidservants for the same reasons it has previously been mentioned to develop in nurses and students away from home. Environmental changes in women would seem to result at times in hypothalamic sexual inhibition.

Apart from often requiring the help of a psychiatrist to adequately control the emotional factors involved, *treatment* of psychogenic amenorrhea must be aimed at changing the patient's life style and at creating favorable environmental conditions; endocrine therapy may consist of small amounts of estrogens administered continuously over a period of several months, for instance, 0.1 mg diethyl stilbestrol per day orally for three or four months.

Generally, the response to this type of therapy is menstrual bleeding twice a month, which indicates the presence of ovulation hemorrhage. If such treatment is carried on, double menstruation disappears and menstrual periods become normalized (Reifenstein[71]).

Goldzieher and Goldzieher,[38] Plotz and Wildbrand,[68] and Lancet and Joel[53] have reported cases of *psychogenic amenorrhea resistant to hormone therapy.* These cases were characterized by secondary amenorrhea, normal vaginal cytology and normal endometrial histology, as well as a normal steroid excretion pattern during the cycle. It would seem that such cases might be identified with what German authors call *low wave cycle,* viz., cases in which cyclic ovarian events take place but menstruation does not materialize. Their pathogenesis remains obscure. No doubt, a neural mechanism of the vasoconstrictive type is necessary for menstruation to occur. Psychogenic inhibition of the menstrual mechanism is probably not mediated by the pituitary but is suspected to act directly at the uterine level. Along similar lines, Stieve[86, 87] believes that most observed instances of psychogenic menstrual inhibition involve a local neural mechanism whereby local neurogenic factors necessary for menstruation to appear are inhibited (Fig. 32–6).

32.2.2. ANOREXIA NERVOSA

Anorexia nervosa is a clinical entity characterized by progressive weight loss, generally affecting females, less commonly males, at about the age of puberty. The clinical picture reveals symptoms similar to those of Simmond's disease, among which the principal ones are *cachexia* and sexual regression with *amenorrhea and hypogenitalism.*

This condition was described originally before the end of the nineteenth century as a purely nervous disorder, but after the discovery of pituitary cachexia in 1914 by Simmonds, such cases were frequently confused with Simmonds' disease. However, modern findings have demonstrated that anorexia nervosa has nothing to do with Simmonds' disease and that its *etiology is a neurogenic one and not a pituitary one.*

Heim[42] and Gagel[35] have studied cases with the above-mentioned clinical picture and attributed to them a hypothalamic etiology. On the other hand, a purely psychogenic origin is presently being espoused by Escamilla and Lisser,[28] Durand[26] and Kuhn.[51] The last two authors have undertaken a *psychoanalytic study* of patients suffering from mental anorexia and found a psychogenic cause for the disease in each case. The patients involved are usually pubescent girls with exaggerated ascetic tendencies who, owing to familial psychotrauma, have been led to consider food as a lowly and animal-like necessity. Within the setting of their sublimated life values, they strive to circumvent anything that might represent vegetative function. By the same token, they may sometimes be observed to refuse food so as to avoid breast development or the appearance of menstruation. The background of this disorder must thus be viewed as essentially set up by the *patient's own antisexual and antilife tendency*. Bleuler[17] calls attention to the fact that such patients usually are beset by *family problems*, such as squabbles with their parents, financial difficulties, etc. Bleuler also emphasizes the schizophrenic background of such girls.

The case illustrated in Figure 32–7, observed by Sopeña and ourselves, was a 22 year old oligophrenic girl with secondary amenorrhea since the age of 18, weight loss and mammary atrophy, but with normal gonadotropinuria (10 IU/24 hr), normal estrogenuria (100 mcg of Kober positive steroids in 24 hr) and normal vaginal cytology throughout the cycle. The sella turcica appeared to be normal (Fig. 32–8), which indicated that the pituitary was not demonstrably involved.

The main symptoms of the disease have been described by Benedetti,[15] by Nonnenbruch and Feuchtinger[65] and by Decourt and his associates.[26] Sometimes, the disorder may be coupled with *serious psychogenic alterations;* on other occasions, it may reveal a relationship to lipodystrophy, in which case the disease begins with extreme leanness, only later to lapse into exaggerated obesity, as observed in a case

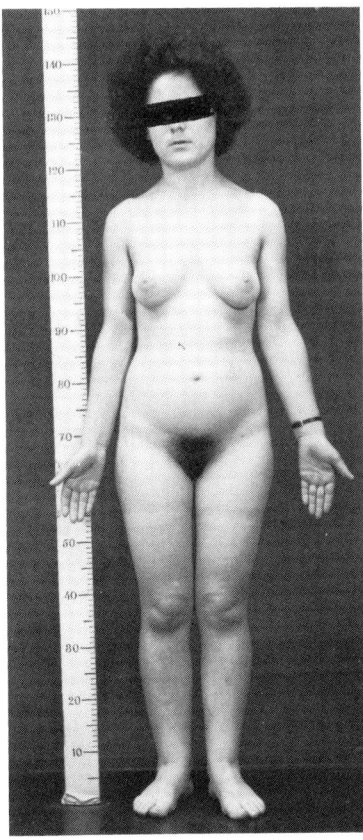

Figure 32–6. Psychogenic amenorrhea in a 22 year old patient with essential epilepsy. Ovarian findings were within normal limits.

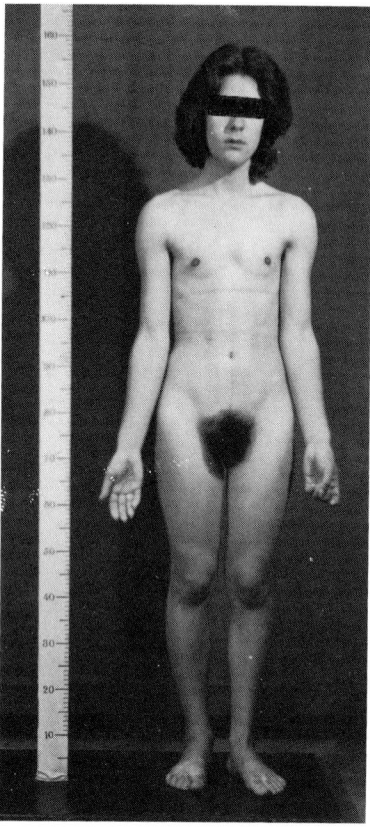

Figure 32-7. Anorexia nervosa and oligophrenia. Normal ovarian function was present and there was secondary amenorrhea of four years' duration.

reported by Waring and Ingraham.[94] In addition, Hertz[45] described symptoms of associated *adrenal insufficiency*, although, unlike those occurring in Simmonds' cachexia, he did *not* consider them to be *specific*. He saw them rather as a result of the condition of starvation that is typical of such patients.

The illness occurs much more rarely in males. In the latter instance, the symptomatology described above may be occasionally associated with Klinefelter's syndrome.[49]

Hormone assay studies on the urine of female patients have been reported by Venning and Browne[93] and, subsequently, by Shadaksharappa and his associates.[82] Urinary FSH excretion has been found to be within normal limits and urinary 17-ketosteroids, as well as corticoids, have similarly been found to be normal. In some serious forms of the condition there may be diminished excretion of hormones, but similar findings have been observed in all starvation syndromes. The basal metabolism of such patients was studied by Bartels,[11] who reported low rates. He believed that decreased metabolism was the result of pituitary hypofunction. In our own opinion, however, it stems from *centrogenous inhibition of metabolism*.

The credit for having distinguished anorexia nervosa from Simmonds' disease goes above all to Proger[69] and to Escamilla and Lisser.[28] These authors particularly stressed the fact that *endocrine alterations were absent in anorexia nervosa or, if present, were secondary to the patient's state of malnutrition*. Favoring this point of view are the observations of Reiss[74] on a case of anorexia nervosa with hyperpituitarism.

Although severe malnutrition may give rise to complications, the illness, according to Kay,[47] has a benign *prognosis* and does not, *per se*, lead to death. The condition differs from Simmonds' disease in that it does not show a progressive course and may regress. Anorexia nervosa is compared with Simmonds' disease in Table 32-1.

Treatment ought to be based, *in the first place*, on a psychiatric approach. Although favorable results have been reported with the use of sex hormones, gonadotropins, thyroid extracts and ACTH, such results may be attributed to *effects of suggestion* to which such patients are susceptible rather than to any positive therapeutic action. Consequently, this type of patient should be referred to a psychoanalyst for

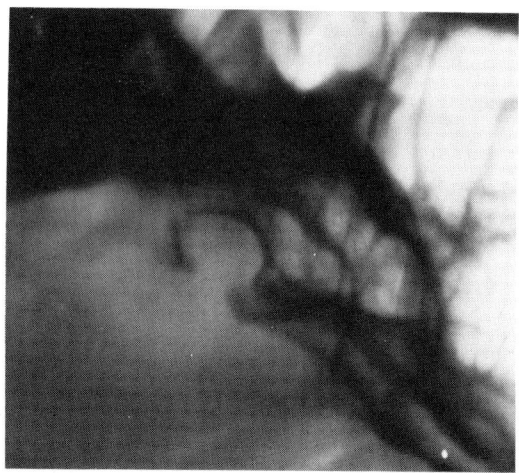

Figure 32-8. Normal sella turcica in a case of anorexia nervosa.

TABLE 32–1. Differential Diagnosis of Anorexia Nervosa and Simmonds' Disease

SIMMONDS' DISEASE	ANOREXIA NERVOSA
Similarities	
Cachexia	
Loss of sexual function	
Decreased basal metabolism	
Decreased blood pressure	
Differences	
Postpartum onset in about 50% of cases	Never associated with postpartum onset
Frequent changes in sella turcica	No changes in sella turcica
No response to therapy	Marked improvement with adequate therapy
Complete loss of body hair	Insignificant hair loss
Breast atrophy	No breast atrophy
Pallor	No pallor
Eosinophilia	No eosinophilia

adequate exploration of her problems and institution of appropriate therapy. Some authors advocate the use of electroshock, a measure we consider to be excessive in view of the only moderately serious nature of the illness.

In 1950, Decourt and his associates[22] studied 32 cases of anorexia nervosa, or what they called *mental anorexia*. As far as sexual disturbances are concerned, they pointed out that amenorrhea occurred quite early and could not be viewed as a mere consequence of malnutrition. It had to be interpreted as a disturbance of neuro-endocrine function, resulting in depression of sex hormone secretion. A biochemical study of amenorrhea in 15 of their patients was done and revealed the presence of ovarian insufficiency involving both estradiol and progesterone secretion. However, urinary FSH titers were found to be normal in most of the cases (Abate et al.,[1] Starkey and Lee[84]). The physiopathologic interpretation of these findings enabled the above authors to assert that inhibition of sexual function was not mediated by a pituitary mechanism—something we pointed out previously—but was brought about by *direct neurogenic inhibition* of ovarian as well as uterine function. In this regard, our ideas are similar to those of Stieve[86,87] who maintains that most of the neurogenic disturbances of the cycle are not the result of hypothalamic-pituitary involvement but of direct neurogenic action on ovarian function and on menstruation.

32.2.3. PSYCHOGENIC OBESITY AND FROEHLICH'S SYNDROME OF PSYCHOGENIC ORIGIN

Several authors, among them principally Nonnenbruch and Feuchtinger[65] and Waring and Ingraham,[94] have emphasized the frequent occurrence of centrogenous syndromes in which they observed the early leanness to evolve into late-stage obesity. Bleuler[17] similarly described syndromes of adiposity of psychogenic origin. This type of adiposity apparently develops in girls around puberty and consists in *central stimulation of appetite*, resulting in *bulimia* and leading to *purely exogenous obesity*. Despite the fact that they apparently differ from anorexia nervosa, both conditions are characterized by hypogenitalism with delayed puberty and oligomenorrhea, as well as genital infantilism and, in some cases, also essential amenorrhea. The fact that the two opposite disorders may appear during different life phases in the same patient would indicate that *there is probably a psychic area for the regulation of appetite which, when disturbed, may lead to either loss of or exaggerated increase in appetite and that, in the course of life, such disorders may transform from the one extreme to the other*. For these reasons, instead of speaking of nervous anorexia or bulimia, it would be more appropriate to speak of *centrogenous disturbances of appetite, associated with inhibition of sexual function*.

32.2.4. PSYCHOGENIC CHIARI-FROMMELL SYNDROME

Rankin and co-workers[70] reported 17 cases of Chiari-Frommell syndrome in which there were no demonstrable lesions in the nervous system. They qualified the disease as psychogenic in origin and achieved good results by treating the patients with Clomiphene.

32.3. CENTRAL INFLUENCES ON THE SEXUAL CYCLE AND ITS ANOMALIES

Although in the preceding sections we have examined the existing relationship between endocrine syndromes of neural origin and the sexual sphere, nothing has been said about the anomalies involving menstruation that are the result, not of endocrine, but of neural influences. This is a highly important aspect of modern gynecology, particularly insofar as the application of psychosomatic studies to this specialty is concerned. We intend to make but a brief review of the main problems to be encountered. We shall study successively: (1) neural influences in the genesis of hypoestrinism; (2) neural influences in the development of hyperestrinism; (3) menstrual alterations of centrogenous origin, and (4) endocrine disorders in the syndrome of pelvic congestion.

32.3.1. NEURAL INFLUENCES IN SYNDROMES OF HYPOESTRINISM

As a matter of fact, all conditions of hypogenital dystrophy analyzed in the present chapter, such as Froehlich's syndrome and related conditions, psychogenous amenorrhea, etc., are proof of the *depressive effect exerted by certain neural stimuli on ovarian function* and constitute more or less direct examples of *hypoestrinism of centrogenous origin*. While a great many instances of psychogenous amenorrhea occur in the presence of normal endocrine function, evidence has been forthcoming in recent years to the effect that unquestionably cases of hypoestrinism may result from psychic shock. In general, such cases occur in girls who have a previous history of constitutional hypoestrinism and a known tendency to ovarian hypofunction ("weak cycles" of Seitz[81]).

Rogers,[76] as well as Kroger and Fried,[50] offer abundant evidence on patients with psychogenic hypoestrinism who have been successfully treated by means of psychotherapy. The reason for the development of psychogenic hypoestrinism, as revealed by the studies of Klinefelter and associates,[48, 49] Freemont-Smith and Meigs[34] and, above all, Stieve,[86, 87] seems to lie in *lack of FSH production by the anterior lobe of the pituitary*. According to these authors, a concomitant reduction in, or abolition of, luteinizing hormone secretion might also be involved. Such gonadotropin inhibition may be understood in terms of the previously mentioned influence exerted by the *hypothalamic sex center*. Inhibition of the hypothalamus is known to provoke suspension of cyclic activity in animals,[8, 9, 29, 36] as well as amenorrhea with loss of libido in women.[37, 96] *Darkness* has been found to be another factor inhibiting gonadotropic activity in animals[30] and probably also in man.[10, 20]

The mechanism involved in *neurogenic hypoestrinism* is thought to work through several stages: secretory ovarian insufficiency stems from hypogonadotropism, the latter in turn resulting from default of hypothalamic stimulation which, in the first instance, follows cortical inhibition (Fig. 32–12). As very aptly pointed out by Kroger and Fried,[50] the mechanism involved in producing ovarian insufficiency cannot be exclusively explained on the basis of neuroendocrine correlations but may be admitted to involve direct and exclusive neural action. The presence of nerve endings in the ovary which, when excited, may stimulate ovarian function (Reynolds[75]) may be construed as evidence that secretory inhibition of the ovary may be at the root of functional ovarian failure.

32.3.2. HYPERESTRINISM

The opposite situation, too, may stem from psychogenic causes. Rogers[76] has indicated frequent occurrence of functional bleeding of psychogenic origin, whereas Bleuler[17] and Kroger and Fried[50] emphasized the significance of premenstrual tension. Functional bleeding is thought to be caused by the chronic variety of hyperestrinism, whereas premenstrual tension presumably results from the acute form of hyperestrinism. The mechanism whereby such states are produced might be mediated by the action of pituitary secretion. Hypothalamic excitation of centrogenous origin may give rise to increased FSH activity and to development of persistent follicles. As pointed out earlier, Freemont-Smith and Meigs[34] had emphasized the presence of reduced luteinizing hormone activity. This would presumably lead to persistent follicles with symptoms of hyperestrinism. Acute hyperestrinism during the second half of the cycle, as the causative agent of premenstrual tension (see Chapter 28), might stem from acute excitation of FSH secretion during the premenstrual phase.

Sexual Syndromes of Neurogenic Origin

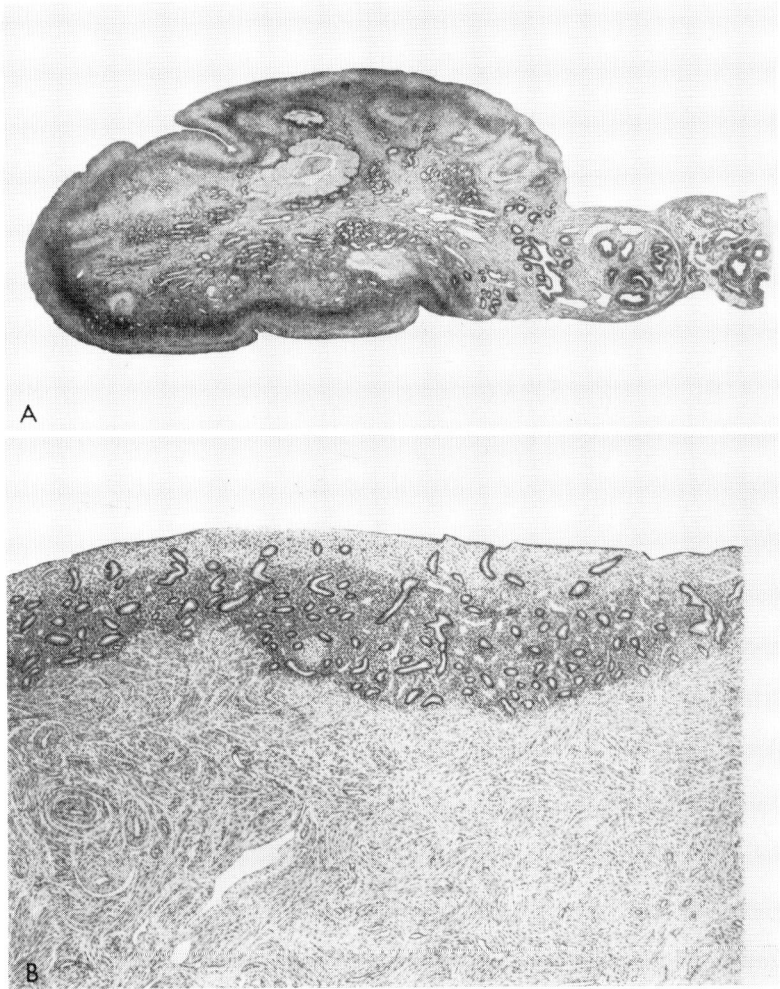

Figure 32–9. A, Section of ovary from a patient with psychosomatic amenorrhea. B, Section of endometrium from same patient. Note complete absence of ovarian maturation and presence of endometrial atrophy. (From Stieve: *Der Einfluss des Nervensystems auf Bau und Tätigkeit der Geschlechtsorgane des Menschen.* Stuttgart, G. Thieme, 1952.)

It must not be forgotten that Stieve[86, 87] attached great significance to the role played by ovarian nerve endings in the maturation process of the follicle and in ovulation. Similarly, Reynolds[75] has demonstrated the presence of spiral arterioles in the ovary, the constriction of which results in rupture of the follicle. Lack of an adequate neurogenic stimulus might conceivably inhibit ovulation and cause follicular persistence (Figs. 32–10 and 32–11). In Figure 32–12, we present a schematic outline of the neurogenic mechanism involved in the production of either hyper- or hypoestrinism. The significance of hypothalamic influence on *premenstrual tension* deserves to be mentioned. Miller-De Paiva and his co-workers[62] have shown that women suffering from premenstrual tension and edema have *increased antidiuretic hormone levels* in the blood. It is possible that the hypothalamic discharges involved are the result of psychogenic causes.

32.3.3. ANOMALIES IN THE MENSTRUAL RHYTHM FROM NEUROGENIC CAUSES

It is a matter of common observation that menstruation may be modified as a consequence of psychic trauma. Thus, for example, menstrual bleeding may frequently

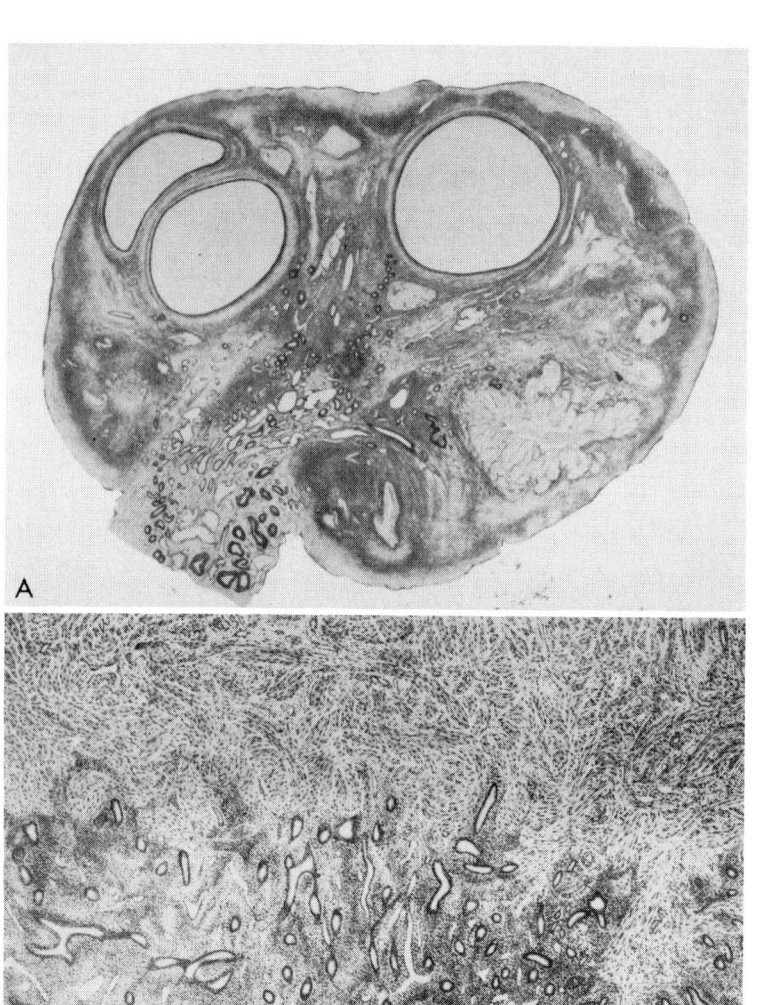

Figure 32-10. A, Section of right ovary from a 27 year old woman who developed amenorrhea for 42 days as a result of an emotional problem. Note maturing, nonfunctioning follicles. B, Nonfunctional endometrium, from same patient, in resting stage, indicating that ovarian follicles are nonfunctional. (From *Der Einfluss des Nervensystems auf Bau und Tätigkeit der Geschlechtsorgane des Menschen.* Stuttgart, G. Thieme, 1952.)

Sexual Syndromes of Neurogenic Origin

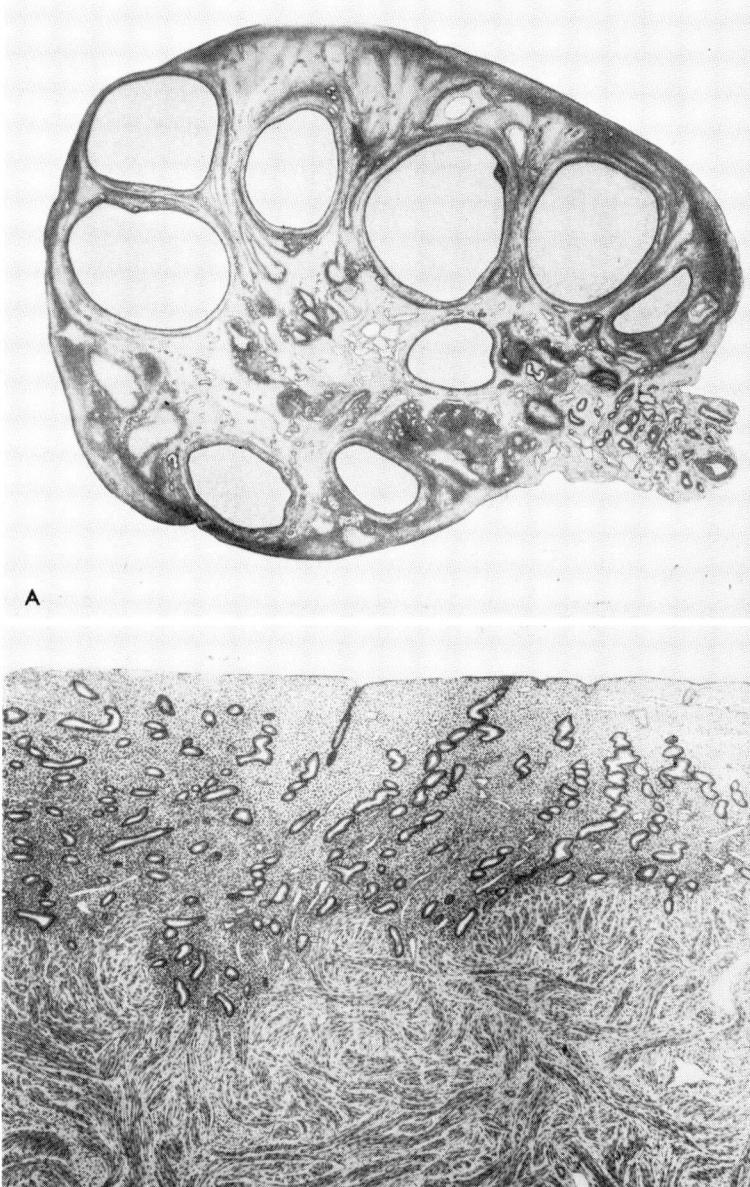

Figure 32–11. A, Section of right ovary from woman with absent menses for 58 days as a result of emotional upset. B, Endometrium from same patient, revealing proliferative phase, indicative of ovarian follicular function. (From Stieve: *Der Einfluss des Nervensystems auf Bau und Tätigkeit der Geschlechtorgane des Menschen.* Stuttgart, G. Thieme, 1952.)

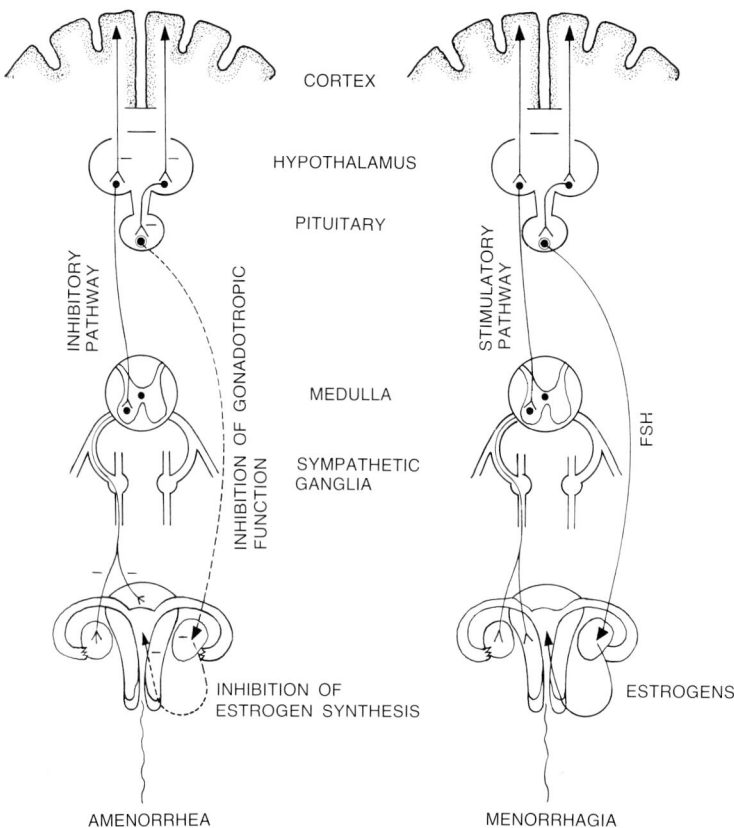

Figure 32-12. Mechanism involved in producing amenorrhea (left) or menorrhagia (right) of cerebral origin. Note the existence of a direct inhibitory-stimulatory neural pathway, passing from the cerebral cortex through the hypothalamus to the medulla, from where it reaches the uterus and ovary via sympathetic ganglia. Whenever these fibers carry inhibitory impulses they may cause amenorrhea of primary uterine or primary ovarian nature. Conversely, the same pathway may be utilized to produce local stimulation of the uterus and the ovaries (at right). There exists also a neuroendocrine pathway capable of both exciting and inhibiting pituitary gonadotropin function. At left, an inhibitory effect is exerted on the hypothalamic nuclei. These nuclei, in turn, may inhibit pituitary gonadotropin activity. At right, an adjacent center may produce stimulation in a similar way.

occur precipitantly in unusually bashful women as well as in newly-wed women coming for consultation. Instances of arrested or temporarily delayed menses, or occasionally even permanent amenorrhea, as a result of war, bombings or large-scale disasters have been recorded (Figs. 32–13, 32–14 and 32–15). Similarly, women in jail or in confinement are subject to changes in menstrual patterns. A modality of neurogenic amenorrhea is what we termed *maidservant amenorrhea,* which frequently occurs in girls who have abandoned their villages in search for a job in the city. Similar episodes are known to occur in college and boarding school students or in those who are faced with worrisome examinations. All these circumstances, which are common knowledge, explain by themselves the neurogenic etiology of the conditions under consideration as entirely independent of such factors as nutrition or changes in climate or life style, which might equally well account for them. Bleuler[17] classifies those circumstances capable of producing amenorrhea or menstrual abnormalities as follows:

(1) Mass catastrophes, earthquakes, explosions, fires, mass exodus, bombardments, factory explosions, threat of war, etc.; (2) wounds or trauma causing anxiety or fear; (3) grief caused by a sudden death, particularly that of a family member; (4) rape under duress; (5) suggestions of hypnosis; (6) sexual anxiety, for instance on the wedding night; (7) change in activity or place of residence; (8) fear of examinations; (9) fear of war; (10) urgent desire to become

pregnant, resulting either in amenorrhea by suggestion or in pseudopregnancy.

As a matter of fact, the foregoing list of causative factors is much too incomplete, and a vast array of circumstances might be added that may cause women to experience no less anxiety or fear.

Seitz[81] drew attention to the fact that not all women responded equally to psychologic trauma. Stieve[87] was able to show that, among girls or women in jail, under detention or in concentration camps, some presented with amenorrhea or with serious menstrual disorders, such as excessive bleeding, whereas others under the same circumstances of anxiety or nutritional deprivation revealed no alterations. In this respect, women may be categorized, according to Seitz, into *stable-cycled, labile-cycled and weak-cycled*. In the first category, external circumstances do not modify menstruation or do so to a minimal extent. In the second, menstruation is modified but is not discontinued, whereas in the third, menstruation ceases and gives way to amenorrhea.

It is noteworthy that such alterations are not always associated with changes in ovarian internal secretion. For instance, psychogenic amenorrhea has often been found not to coincide with hypoestrinism but to coexist with normal vaginal cytology and with endometria revealing persistent proliferative patterns. In that case, basal body temperature curves were found to be flat (Fig. 32–16). Thus, there are cases of true hyperhormonal amenorrhea, as defined by Zondek.[100] The ease with which amenorrhea with follicular persistence may be induced by psychogenic stimuli was emphasized by the same authors. Certainly, what in such cases seems to be involved is inhibition of the same type of neural stimulus that causes follicular rupture.

Under certain circumstances, amenorrhea may also be observed to occur in the presence of a *biphasic cycle* and alternating proliferative and secretory endometrial patterns, as well as with *characteristic biphasic temperature* curves (Fig. 32–17). Such circumstances may develop as a result of a neurogenic stimulus having an inhibitory effect on menstruation but not on the ovarian cycle. Menstrual vascular phenomena would seem to be lacking here, owing to inhibition by a neurogenic stimulus. This form of amenorrhea may be viewed as the opposite of the hyperhormonal form. While in hyperhormonal amenorrhea with persistent proliferative

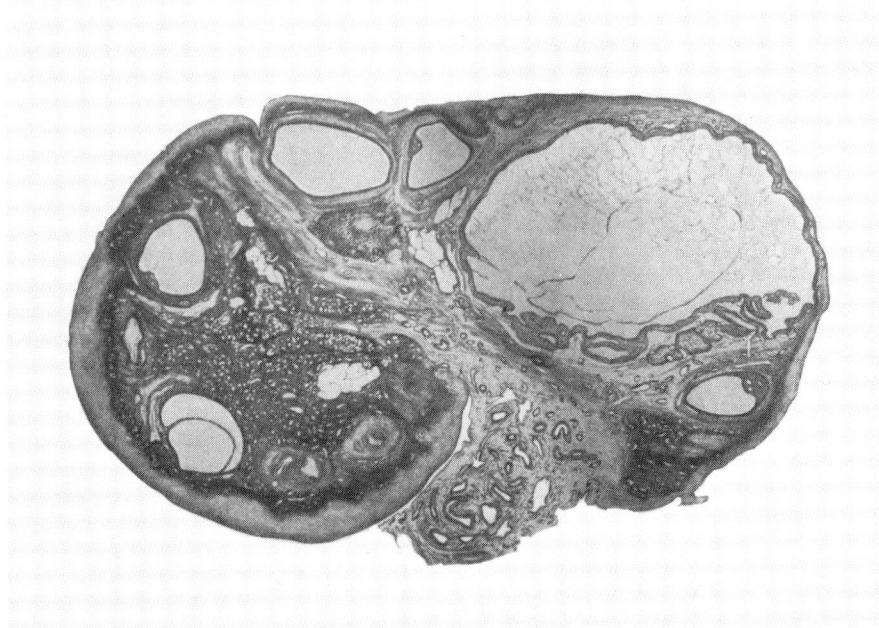

Figure 32–13. Ovary on the twenty-ninth day of the cycle in a woman who had experienced severe emotional upset. Note presence of ruptured follicle without luteinization. (From Stieve: *Der Einfluss des Nervensystems auf Bau und Tätigkeit der Geschlechtorgane des Menschen.* Stuttgart, G. Thieme, 1952.)

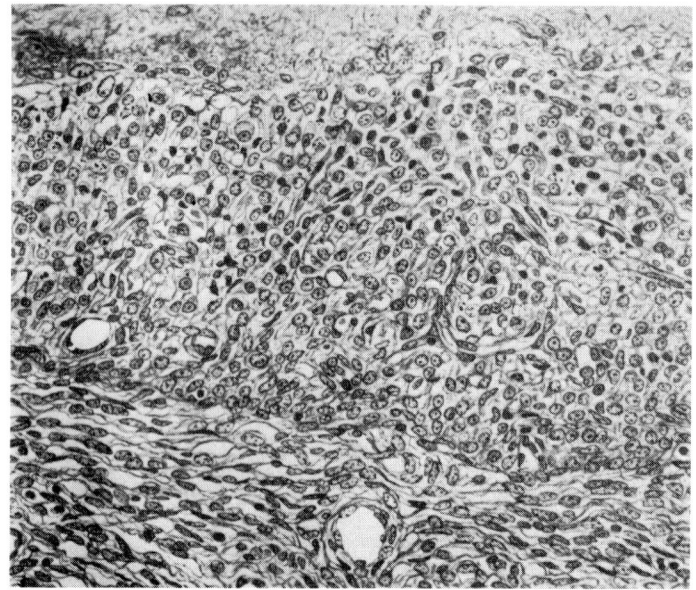

Figure 32-14. Section through the wall of ruptured follicle from Figure 32-13, revealing mild luteinization of the granulosa, which, however, is totally incomplete and insufficient. (From Stieve: *Der Einfluss des Nervensystems auf Bau und Tätigkeit der Geschlechtorgane des Menschen.* Stuttgart, G. Thieme, 1952.)

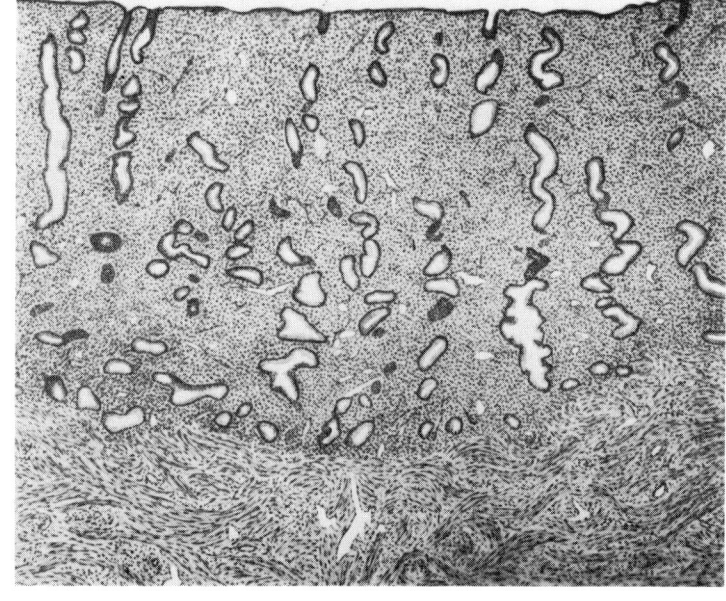

Figure 32-15. Proliferative endometrium from same patient as in Figures 32-13 and 32-14, betraying sham nature of apparently luteinized granulosa.

Sexual Syndromes of Neurogenic Origin

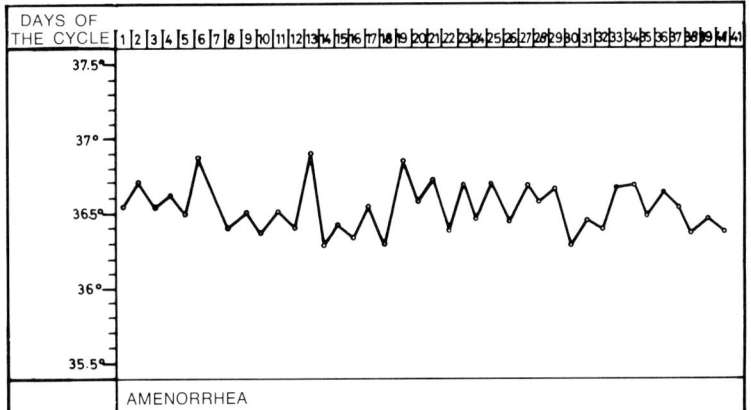

Figure 32-16. Neurogenic amenorrhea of hyperhormonal type, with flat basal body temperature curve.

phase, the inhibitory neurogenic phenomenon would appear to act on the ovary by suppressing ovulation, in psychogenic amenorrhea with low wave cycles, the inhibitory stimulus would act on the uterus by inhibiting menstruation. Two types of thermal curves characteristic of these circumstances have been recorded in Figures 32-16 and 32-17. In addition, Figure 32-18 offers a diagram of the pathology involved in the foregoing conditions.

Occasionally, *early menstruation,* with or without hypermenorrhea, may also be observed. Anomalies with augmented menstruation are caused by inversion of the same mechanism. Just as an inhibitory stimulus may cause suspension of ovulation, so a triggering stimulus may cause ovulation to occur ahead of time. Stieve[87] called this *paracyclic ovulation.* Such ovulation takes place outside the timetable of the cycle and is, so to say, out of step with the cycle's rhythm. According to Stieve, this is due to follicular rupture by an abrupt neural stimulus. The phenomenon is a physiologic event in the female rabbit and occurs whenever the animal mates with a male. Studies on rabbits have produced evidence, as mentioned in Chapters 6 and 8, that follicular rupture is carried out by neural stimulation of the anterior lobe of the pituitary, producing increased gonadotropin activity, which ultimately provokes rupture of the follicle. This means that the phenomenon of neurogenic follicular rupture in the rabbit occurs via a neuroendocrine mechanism. In contrast, the mechanism in woman, according to Stieve, would seem to be somewhat different and follicular rupture would appear to take place through *direct neural action on the ovary.* We thus come back to accepting the ancient hypothesis of Pflüger, which postulated that follicular rupture was conditioned by a neural stimulus. Whereas in some instances early menstruation may be due to

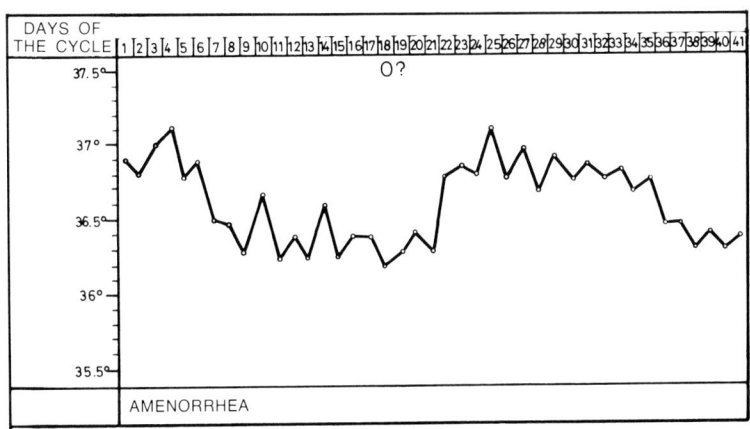

Figure 32-17. Neurogenic amenorrhea in a low wave type of cycle, with biphasic temperature curve on which probable day of ovulation is indicated.

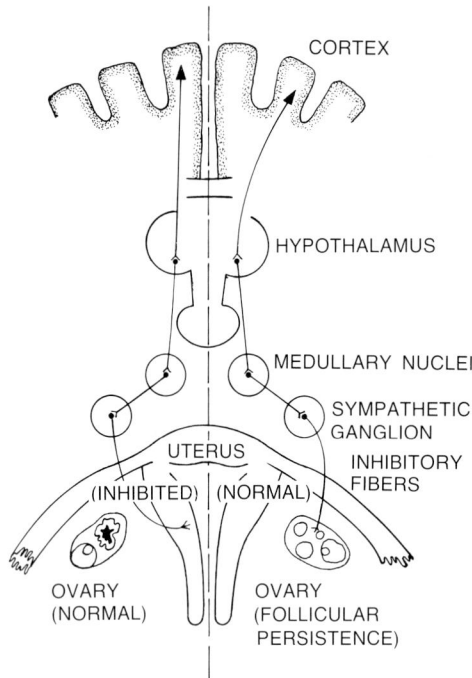

Figure 32-18. Schematic representation of neural pathway inhibiting ovaries and uterus, respectively. At left, inhibitory stimulus originating in cortex reaches, by way of hypothalamus and medullary nuclei, a sympathetic ganglion from which inhibitory fibers proceed to their destination in the endometrium. Amenorrhea produced in this instance is associated with a normal cycle, similar to that shown in Figure 32-17. At right, ovary is inhibited via hypothalamus, medullary nuclei and sympathetic ganglion. The last gives off inhibitory fibers to ovary, which may cause follicular persistence of the type illustrated in Figure 32-2.

paracyclic ovulation, other instances of premature menstruation are not accompanied by any changes in the ovarian cycle, the follicle-corpus luteum sequence taking place in a completely normal way. In these cases, the process is thought to be initiated by a neurogenic stimulus, which produces endometrial vasospasm and advances menstruation by a vascular mechanism, as we indicated previously in Chapter 13. A diagrammatic representation of such events is shown in Figure 32-18.

Neurogenic inhibition of the cycle may thus be subject to two different points of attack, *ovarian* and *uterine,* as shown in Figure 32-18. Whenever the point of attack is ovarian, follicular rupture does not occur or, if it does, there is no luteinization, as indicated in Figure 32-13. Ovaries that are inhibited in this way produce an anovulatory or, at least, an aluteal cycle by a neurogenic mechanism. Thus, amenorrhea of the polyfollicular or hyperhormonal type is produced in conjunction with a temperature recording similar to that shown in Figure 32-16.

On the other hand, whenever the point of attack is via the uterus, the ovary does not function normally and the temperature curve is like that shown in Figure 32-17, while amenorrhea is caused by lack of uterine response.

In the course of the past few years, a form of amenorrhea has been described that is attributed to disturbances of the amygdaloid nucleus. The prevailing impression today is that the amygdaloid nucleus regulates the activity of the hypothalamic sex center.[27, 90, 92]

Consequently, it may be said that, as far as amenorrhea due to psychic trauma is concerned, the point of attack of neurogenic inhibition in those instances with a normal ovarian cycle is the uterus, whereas in those that have a monophasic cycle the point of attack of neurogenic inhibition is the ovary.

32.3.4. SYNDROME OF PELVIC CONGESTION

The syndrome described under the name of pelvic congestion is characterized by a permanent condition of hyperemia of the genital organs as well as other, adjacent pelvic organs, usually accompanied by retroversioflexion, pelvic varicocele, cortical ovarian sclerosis and multiple aches of poorly defined nature. This syndrome has been described by Castaño[19] and has been thoroughly studied and analyzed by Taylor.[88] As shown by Taylor and Duncan,[89] the *psychosomatic origin* of the syndrome is unquestionable. It generally appears in young single women suffering from inadequate psychosexual stimuli, or in married women, particularly when they engage in such contraceptive measures as *coitus interruptus.* The mode of production of this condition, whose clinical description is beyond the scope of a textbook of endocrinology, is the following: a psychosexual stimulus causes psychogenous excitation of the hypothalamic sex center. Excitation of the sex center gives rise to *hypersecretion of gonadotropins, resulting in enhance-*

ment of ovarian function, which causes *pelvic congestion* and local changes, producing pain. The discomfort caused by the syndrome of pelvic congestion is similar to that caused by acute hyperestrinism, which was studied in Chapter 28. In either case, it is due to *persistent high estrogen levels during the second half of the cycle*. Consequently, it may be said that pelvic congestion is caused by a state of acute hyperestrinism of psychogenic nature.

32.3.5. EFFECTS OF DRUGS ON HYPOTHALAMIC SEX REGULATION

Great significance has been recently attached to the actions of some drugs on the hypothalamic sex center. This subject has been dealt with partially in Chapter 8 (Section 8.0.0). Although most of the information available on the subject is derived from animal experiments, it may be relevant to point out here the importance this modality may have for the treatment of some human syndromes.

PENTOTHAL. Pentothal inhibits ovulation in rats by anesthetizing the nucleus of the median eminence. Zeilmaker and Moll[99] have in addition shown that progestogens, too, exerted an anesthetic action at the same level.

RESERPINE. Labhsetwar[52] showed that Reserpine also anesthetized the hypothalamic sex center and decreased gonadotropinemia in rats. A similar anesthetic effect is produced by progestins, although by a different mechanism.

DOPAMINE. Kamberi and co-workers[46] have found that Dopamine, on the contrary, raised production of FSH releasing factor at the sex center level.

CATECHOLAMINES. Most related research has been done in the field of catecholamines. An increase in norepinephrine concentration of the anterior hypothalamus has been found to cause decreased pituitary function.[23] Possibly this is the reason for the phenomenon observed by Donoso and Stefano,[24] in which the norepinephrine concentration of the hypothalamic sex center of the rat was found to be increased following castration. The same authors[25] subsequently showed that the increase of norepinephrine following castration did not occur in adjacent regions but was specifically confined to the sex center. Lippmann and associates,[56] Sandler,[78] and Birge and co-workers[16] all believe that, by acting on the hypothalamic sex center, catecholamines inhibit the release of LH. Stefano and Donoso[85] found evidence of cyclic changes in the hypothalamic content of norepinephrine, whereas Schneider and MacCann[79] showed that, conversely, Dopamine produced an increase in LHRF. Although these are all still in the experimental stage, the above investigations are of interest since the pharmacologic actions they explore hold promise for possible future application in the syndromes studied in this chapter.

REFERENCES

1. Abate, C., Ferramosca, B., and Bernardi, P.: *Arch. Maragliano Pathol. Clin.*, 23:357, 1967.
2. Anderson, N. L.: *J. Clin. Endocr.*, 1:905, 1941.
3. Anderson, E.: *Amer. J. Proctol. Dis. Dig. Tract.*, 1:41, 1950.
4. Andreoli, C.: *Gynaecologia*, 150:12, 1960.
5. Barborka, C. J.: *Med. Clin. N. Amer.*, 21:23, 1937.
6. Bargmann, W.: *Arch. Gynäk.*, 183:21, 1953.
7. Bargmann, W.: *Das Zwischenhirn-Hypophysensystem.* Berlin, Springer-Verlag, 1954.
8. Barraclough, C.: *Anat. Rec.*, 127:262, 1957.
9. Barraclough, C., and Sawyer, C. H.: *Endocrinology*, 61:341, 1957.
10. Barraclough, C., and Sawyer, C. H.: *Endocrinology*, 65:563, 1959.
11. Bartels, E. D.: *Acta Med. Scand.*, 124:185, 1946.
12. Bauer, H. G.: *J. Clin. Endocr.*, 14:13, 1954.
13. Belaisch, J., Musset, R., and Netter, A.: *Ann. d'Endocr.*, 26:447, 1965.
14. Belaisch, J., Musset, R., and Netter, A.: *Ann. d'Endocr.*, 26:267, 1965.
15. Benedetti, G.: *Schw. Med. Wschr.*, 80:1129, 1950.
16. Birge, C. A., Jacobs, L. S., Hammer, C. T., and Daughaday, W. H.: *Endocrinology*, 86:120, 1970.
17. Bleuler, M.: *Endokrinologische Psychiatrie.* Stuttgart, G. Thieme, 1955.
18. Bronstein, I. P.: *Amer. J. Dis. Child.*, 64:211, 1952.
19. Castaño, C. A.: *Acta Gin.*, 4:1, 1953.
20. Clegg, M. T., et al.: *Endocrinology*, 62:790, 1958.
21. Daily, W. J. R., and Ganong, W. F.: *Endocrinology*, 42:442, 1958.
22. Decourt, J., Jayle, M. F., and Lavergne, G. H.: *Ann. d'Endocr.*, 11:571, 1950.
23. Deutsch, S. F.: *Psychosomatics*, 9:127, 1968.
24. Donoso, A. O., and Stefano, F. J. E.: *Experientia*, 23:665, 1967.
25. Donoso, A. O., Stefano, F. J. E., Bicardi, A. M., and Okier, J.: *Amer. J. Physiol.*, 212:737, 1967.
26. Durand, C. H.: *Praxis (Bern)*, 41:1038, 1952.

27. Elefteriou, B. E., Zolovick, A. J., and Norman, R. L.: *J. Endocr.*, 38:469, 1967.
28. Escamilla, R. F., and Lisser, H.: *J. Clin. Endocr.*, 12:65, 1952.
29. Everett, J. W.: *Physiol. Rev.*, 44:373, 1964.
30. Fiske, V. M., and Greep, R. O.: *Endocrinology*, 64:175, 1959.
31. Ford, F. R.: *Diseases of the Nervous System in Infancy.* Springfield, Ill., Charles C Thomas, 1937.
32. Ford, F. R., and Guild, H.: *Bull. Johns Hopkins Hosp.*, 60:192, 1937.
33. Francke, C.: *J. Clin. Endocr.*, 10:108, 1950.
34. Freemont-Smith, M., and Meigs, J. V.: *Amer. J. Obstet. Gynec.*, 55:1037, 1948.
35. Gagel, O.: *Wien. Arch. Klin. Med.*, 85:217, 1941.
36. Gale, C.: *Fed. Proceed.*, 18:50, 1959.
37. Gloor, P.: "Telencephalic Influences upon the Hypothalamus," in *Hypothalamic-Hypophyseal Interrelationships*, ed. W. S. Fields. Springfield, Ill., Charles C Thomas, 1956.
38. Goldzieher, M. A., and Goldzieher, J. W.: *J. Clin. Endocr.*, 12:42, 1952.
39. Green, J. D.: "Neural Pathways to the Hypophysis," in *Hypothalamic-Hypophyseal Interrelationships*, ed. W. S. Fields. Springfield, Ill., Charles C Thomas, 1956.
40. Hamblen, E. C.: *Endocrinology of Woman.* Springfield, Ill., Charles C Thomas, 1945.
41. Hart, S. D., and Breitman, H. B.: *Amer. J. Obstet. Gynec.*, 41:527, 1941.
42. Heim, F.: *Endokrinologie*, 28:28, 1951.
43. Heller, G. C., and Nelson, W. O.: *J. Clin. Endocr.*, 8:345, 1948.
44. Herrmann, H., and Lemarchands, H.: *Ann. d'Endocr.*, 17:689, 1956.
45. Hertz, H.: *Acta Med. Scand.*, 142:523, 1952.
46. Kamberi, I. A., Schneider, H. P. G., and MacCann, S. M.: *Endocrinology*, 86:278, 1970.
47. Kay, D. W. K.: *Proc. Roy. Soc. London (B)*, 146:669, 1953.
48. Klinefelter, H. F., Reifenstein, E. C., and Griswold, G. C.: *J. Clin. Endocr.*, 3:259, 1943.
49. Klinefelter, H. F., Reifenstein, E. C., and Albright, F.: *J. Clin. Endocr.*, 2:615, 1942.
50. Kroger, W. S., and Fried, S. C.: *Amer. J. Obstet. Gynec.*, 59:328, 1950.
51. Kuhn, R.: *Nervenarzt*, 24:191, 1953.
52. Labhsetwar, A. P.: *Endocrinology*, 81:357, 1967.
53. Lancet, M., and Joel, C. A.: *J. Clin. Endocr.*, 16:909, 1956.
54. Leghorn, H. H.: *Quart. J. Med.*, 7:183, 1948.
55. Lichtwitz, L.: *Bull. N.Y. Acad. Sci.*, 15:773, 1939.
56. Lippmann, W., Leonardi, R., Ball, J., and Coppola, J. A.: *J. Pharmacol. Exper. Therap.*, 156:250, 1967.
57. Marañón, G., and Pintos, J.: *Nouvelle iconographie de la salpêtrière*, 27:185, 1917.
58. Marañón, G.: *Brit. Med. J.*, 2:769, 1947.
59. Marañón, G.: *Bol. Inst. Pat. Med.*, 12:33, 1957.
60. Martínez-Díaz, J., and Llanos-Alcázar, L.: *Bol. Inst. Pat. Med.*, 15:47, 1960.
61. Matos, J., Blanco-Soler, C., and Ley, E.: *Acta Pediátrica*, 117:703, 1952.
62. Miller-de Paiva, L., Henriques, O. B., and Henriques, S. B.: *J. Clin. Endocr.*, 16:894, 1956.
63. Moore, R. A., and Cushing, H.: *Arch. Neurol.*, 34:828, 1935.
64. Morsier, G., and Gautier, G.: *Pathol. Biol.*, 11:1267, 1963.
65. Nonnenbruch, W., and Feuchtinger, O.: *Deutsch. Med. Wschr.*, 2:1845, 1942.
66. Oettle, A. G., Rabinovitch, D., and Seftel, H. C.: *J. Clin. Endocr.*, 20:683, 1960.
67. Papez, J. W., and Ecker, A.: *J. Neuropathol. Exper. Neurol.*, 6:151, 1947.
68. Plotz, J., and Wildbrand, U.: *Zblt. Gynäk.*, 67:866, 1953.
69. Proger, S.: *J.A.M.A.*, 114:1973, 1940.
70. Rankin, J. S., Goldfarb, A. F., and Rakoff, A. E.: *Obstet. Gynec.*, 33:1, 1969.
71. Reifenstein, E. C.: *Med. Clin. N. Amer.*, 30:1103, 1946.
72. Reifenstein, E. C., Forbes, A. P., and Albright, F.: *J. Clin. Invest.*, 24:416, 1945.
73. Reinfranck, R. F., and Nichols, F. L.: *J. Clin. Endocr.*, 24:48, 1964.
74. Reiss, M.: *J. Ment. Soc. London*, 89:270, 1943.
75. Reynolds, S. R. M.: *Physiology of the Uterus.* New York, Hoeber, 1949.
76. Rogers, F. S.: *Amer. J. Obstet. Gynec.*, 59:321, 1950.
77. Roth, A. A.: *J. Urol.*, 57:427, 1947.
78. Sandler, R.: *Endocrinology*, 83:1383, 1968.
79. Schneider, H. P. G., and MacCann, S. M.: *Endocrinology*, 87:249, 1970.
80. Seckel, L. P., Scott, W. W., and Bendit, E. P.: *Amer. J. Dis. Child.*, 78:484, 1949.
81. Seitz, L.: In *Biologie und Pathologie des Weibes*, Vol. I, ed. L. Seitz. Amreich, 1939.
82. Shadaksharappa, K., et al.: *J. Clin. Endocr.*, 11:383, 1951.
83. Spatz, B.: *Deutsch. Med. Wschr.*, 2:1929, 1956.
84. Starkey, T. A., and Lee, R. A.: *Amer. J. Obstet. Gynec.*, 105:374, 1969.
85. Stefano, F. J. E., and Donoso, A. O.: *Endocrinology*, 81:1405, 1967.
86. Stieve, H.: *Arch. Gynäk.*, 183:178, 1953.
87. Stieve, H.: *Der Einfluss des Nervensystems auf Bau und Tätigkeit der Geschlechtsorgane des Menschen.* Stuttgart, G. Thieme, 1952.
88. Taylor, H. C.: *Amer. J. Obstet. Gynec.*, 57:211, 637, 654, 1949.
89. Taylor, H. C., and Duncan, C. H.: *Amer. J. Obstet. Gynec.*, 64:1, 1952.
90. Tejasen, T., and Everett, J. W.: *Endocrinology*, 81:1387, 1967.
91. Varney, R. F., Kenyon, A. T., and Koch, F. C.: *J. Clin. Endocr.*, 2:137, 1942.
92. Velasco, M. E., and Taleisnik, S.: *Endocrinology*, 84:2, 1969.
93. Venning, E. H., and Browne, J. S. L.: *J. Clin. Endocr.*, 9:79, 1949.
94. Waring, P. R., and Ingraham, J. T.: *Lancet*, 2:55, 1950.
95. Warkany, J., et al.: *Amer. J. Dis. Child.*, 60:1147, 1940.
96. Waxenberg, S. E., Drellich, M. G., and Sutherland, A. M.: *J. Clin. Endocr.*, 19:193, 1959.
97. Wilkins, L., and Fleischman, W.: *J. Clin. Endocr.*, 4:306, 1944.
98. Wohl, M. C., and Larson, E.: *Med. Clin. N. Amer.*, 26:1657, 1952.
99. Zeilmaker, G. H., and Moll, J.: *Acta Endocr.*, 55:378, 1967.
100. Zondek, H., et al.: *Brit. Med. J.*, 2:340, 1959.

Chapter 33
ADRENAL ENDOCRINOPATHIES IN RELATION TO SEX

33.1. GENERAL CONSIDERATIONS

In Chapter 9, we described the physiology of the adrenal cortex in relation to sexual function, with special reference to our own investigations which have enabled us to assert the existence of an *accessory sex gland* in midst of the adrenal cortex. The "sexual adrenal," or "third gonad," is of extraordinary interest in the physiology of woman, particularly in its pathologic potential. The adrenal sexual syndromes *must be considered as part of the pathology of the endocrine-sexual system* rather than as diseases of one gland having more or less direct repercussions on the gonads. Apart from the endocrine sexual syndromes of the cortex, there are other syndromes that result from pathologic alterations of the "metabolic cortex," of which the most genuine representatives are Cushing's disease and Addison's disease. Just as in describing adrenal physiology we separate the *metabolic cortex* as an entity opposed to the *sexual cortex*, here too, we shall have to distinguish between *metabolic syndromes* and *sexual syndromes* in cortical pathology.

The adrenal sexual syndromes share certain general characteristics and their properties are related to the physiologic laws governing adrenal function. Among these are: (1) the bisexual character of the syndromes; (2) the dependence on pituitary physiology; (3) the independence of the adrenal sexual syndrome from the adrenal metabolic syndrome; and (4) evolutionary character of the syndrome in relation to the laws of sexual development.

33.1.1. BISEXUAL CHARACTER OF ADRENAL SEXUAL SYNDROMES

The sexual adrenal cortex functions in an identical way in both male and female. This means that any syndromes arising from malfunctioning may affect both sexes equally. During the embryonic era, the fetal sexual zone stimulates development of corresponding homologous sex characters of either the male or the female sex. Pathologic alterations of the adrenal during embryonal development may therefore result in sexual anomalies in boys as well as in girls.

The sexual portion of the adult adrenal cortex is able to produce both androgens and estrogens. The reason why there should be predominance of feminizing secretion in one case and of masculinizing secretion in another is yet unknown. However, in adult individuals, pathologic hyperplasia of adrenal tissue may be equally responsible for virilizing syndromes in females and feminizing syndromes in males. In addition, exaggerated feminizing symptomatology in females as well as exaggerated masculinizing symptoms in males may also occur, although they are much more difficult to discern. It would consequently be erroneous to describe the pathologic syndromes of the adrenal cortex as invariably leading to virilism, an error we shall try to dispel in our discussion of clinical descriptions of these pathologic conditions.

33.1.2. DEPENDENCY ON PITUITARY PATHOLOGY

The adequate stimulus for growth of the cortex, principally the zona fasciculata, originates in the pituitary and consists of *adrenocorticotropic* hormone (ACTH) activity. The corresponding stimulus for the sexual cortex, as already indicated in some of our earlier communications,[23,25] is also derived from the pituitary and is mediated by *luteinizing gonadotropin* (LH) which here, more than in any other situation, deserves the name interstitial cell stimulating hormone. The role played by this mechanism in compensating for conditions of gonadal insufficiency has been discussed by us elsewhere.[25] *Under certain conditions, the origin of hyperfunctional syndromes of the sexual cortex must be admitted to be caused by a compensatory mechanism mediated by the pituitary.*

33.1.3. COEXISTENCE WITH OTHER ADRENAL SYNDROMES

Since one of the essential features of sexual zone physiology is *independence from the metabolic cortex, cortical sexual syndromes may occur independently of cortical metabolic syndromes.* This may be observed to be the case above all in Cushing's disease, in which association of metabolic symptoms with sexual symptoms may occur, but the latter may also be absent altogether.

Various authors have similarly described instances in which *adrenogenital syndrome was associated with Addison's disease,* which in terms of function must be interpreted as resulting from coincident hypoplasia of one zone of the cortex and hyperplasia of the other. In addition, instances of Cushing's syndrome in association with total genital atrophy have also been described in large numbers. As a result, the following possible combinations may occur: (1) syndrome of adrenal sexual hyperfunction in the presence of normal metabolic zone function; (2) syndrome identical to the preceding but for atrophy of the metabolic zone; and (3) syndrome of the sexual zone in the presence of metabolic zone hyperplasia, giving rise to *panhypercorticism.*

The capacity of an individual's target organs to respond to sex hormones is inversely related to the individual's age. Accordingly, those adrenal sexual syndromes that have a premature onset are associated with much more intense manifestations than late forms. For instance, *congenital adrenogenital syndrome*, developing before birth, gives rise to pseudohermaphroditism. However, if it supervenes during infancy, it provokes precocious puberty followed by virilization, whereas with advancing age it produces increasingly fewer stigmata in female carriers. Similarly, insufficiency of the adrenal sexual zone is associated with barely perceptible symptomatology unless it is of the congenital type. This means that *adrenal sexual syndromes manifest themselves more intensely the more precociously they develop.*

33.2. ADRENOGENITAL SYNDROME

A clinical group of syndromes, known also as the *adrenogenital syndrome* (Wintersteiner), *interrenogenital syndrome* (Neumann), or *interrenal-genital syndrome* (Poll), is characterized by *sexual alterations in conjunction with adrenal cortical dysfunction.*

In its most dramatic forms, the dysfunction is caused by a *functional neoplasm*, generally a malignant tumor. However, such cases are rare and the syndrome is more often found to be caused by either *hyperplasia* or *adenoma* of the adrenal cortex. The cortex in fact partakes in the genesis of the syndrome not as a whole but only through the activity of the *reticular*, or *sexual, zone*. We shall later examine the question of which special characteristics of this zone are involved that allow it to be differentiated from the remaining histologic components of the interrenal system.

33.2.1. INCIDENCE

The syndrome is not a common one, although it has recently been reported with increasing frequency and may thus be assumed to be less rare than suggested by the number of reports in the past. In a review of the world literature from 1800 to 1946, we have been able to collect only 200 cases.[23] Since 1946 to date, however, this syndrome has been reported with increasing frequency. The number of reports over the past 10 years alone almost surpasses the number of cases reported during all of the past century and a half. Of course, several factors contribute to the increased frequency with which adrenogenital syndrome is presently diagnosed. First, since the syndrome is by now a well established entity, it is not easily overlooked by the diagnostician. Second, radiologic methods based on the use of *pneumokidney* have greatly facilitated the study of the adrenal shadow. Third, hormone studies and dynamic tests (see Chapter 24) have increasingly been used. Last, modern women are increasingly more aware of cosmetic and esthetic values, which prompt them to seek medical advice in the presence of pathologic hair growth, something intentionally concealed or glossed over in the past as of little significance.

In its fully developed form, the syndrome is characteristic and unmistakable, whereas attenuated forms may be confused with or superimposed on other virilizing syndromes.

The syndrome affects both sexes, more frequently women. In our series collected prior to 1945, approximately 85 per cent of the cases had occurred in women. Now, however, the syndrome is being discovered in men more frequently than in the past, so that the overall incidence according to sex may be estimated at approximately 30 per cent males to 70 per cent females.

33.2.2. ETIOLOGY

Classic studies[23, 27] admitted that the etiology of the adrenogenital syndrome was hyperplasia of the innermost zone of the adrenal cortex, that is, *hyperplasia of the sexual zone* (see Chapter 9). However, studies in recent years by American biochemists[20, 21] have brought to light important aspects of the *enzymatic etiology* involved in this process. Neither set of explanations contradicts the other and, probably, hyperplasia of the "third gonad" is nothing else than the *morphologic expression of a biochemical disorder*. In view of this, we shall first explain the classic hyperplasia theory, followed by discussion of the enzymatic etiology, and concluding by expounding our own ideas concerning compatibility of the two theories.

HYPERPLASIA OF THE SEXUAL ADRENAL. As was pointed out in Chapter 9, the doctrine of the *third gonad* admits the presence of an independent gland within the adrenal cortex, identifiable with the paleocortex or primitive fetal cortex, which later undergoes almost complete atrophy, only to reemerge during certain periods of life or under pathologic circumstances, specifically the adrenogenital syndrome and related conditions.

Histologically, the sexual zone is characterized by a "reticular" type structure, leading itself to confusion with the reticular zone,[23, 24, 122] and is further defined, from a histochemical standpoint, by sudanophobia, strong affinity for the reagent of Vines (Ponceau fuchsin), and an Ashbel-Seligman's diazo reaction for carbonyl groups. These histological and histochemical features are all the more pronounced in the hyperplastic cortex of the adrenogenital syndrome. In such instances, the "reticular" pattern of the tissue is quite manifest (Fig. 33–12), the reaction of Vines is strongly positive (as first demonstrated by Vines and confirmed by Botella and Cano[24]), and the diazo reaction of Seligman and Ashbel[104] is equally positive.

At present, the reason for such pathologic proliferations in this type of tissue is not known. It is evident that nearly all virilizing conditions are associated with increased LH activity (Botella and Cano[24]), which may account for the common finding of hyperthecosis and hilus cell hyperplasia in female virilism as well as in the adrenogenital syndrome. Not without interest in this respect is the suggestive theory enunciated by Chang and Witschi,[31] according to which the sexual changes might be induced by *aberrant gonocytes* present in the adrenal anlage.

While the theory of aberrant gonocytes may explain the occurrence of congenital forms, it would hardly offer a satisfactory explanation for the acquired forms of the disease. The latter would seem to result instead from an exaggerated pituitary effect on the adrenal cortex. In some animals, such as goats (Altman et al.[4]) and mice (Nandi et al.[89]), as well as rats (see Chapter 9), castration induces reactive adrenal hyperplasia, occasionally of sufficient intensity to produce true instances of adrenogenital syndrome.

The well known causes for adrenogenital syndrome are most commonly *hyperplasia*, rarely *tumor*. In the first instance, hyperplasia is inducible by pituitary hormone activity. In the second, tumors are postulated to arise from the previously mentioned aberrant gonocytes.

ENZYMATIC ALTERATIONS. The subject of *adrenal steroidogenesis* was reviewed briefly in Chapter 9. Via squalene and cholesterol, and under the influence of ACTH, progesterone is synthesized from pregnenolone. Since pregnenolone catabolism proceeds toward the 17-ketosteroid series, most of the 17-ketosteroids in adrenal metabolism are derived from the degradation of this progesteroid, except for a fraction originating in the conversion process of progesterone to dehydroepiandrosterone (see Chapter 9). Ultimate conversion of progesterone to corticoids depends on hydroxylation of carbon atoms 11, 17 and 21. *Three hydroxylases, 11-, 17-, and 21-hydroxylase, are all necessary for the progesterone-corticoid conversion process.* Bongiovanni and his colleagues[21] deserve credit for having demonstrated that *failure of 21-hydroxylase activity* is responsible for the adrenogenital syndrome, following a mechanism which is outlined in Figure 33-1.

After careful reexamination of Figures 9-13 and 9-14 in Chapter 9, it should become apparent why 21-hydroxylation is essential for the conversion of hydroxyprogesterone to cortisol, since biogenesis of both cortisol and cortisone is blocked in the absence of this enzyme. Due to the fact that both cortisol and cortisone are adequate suppressors of pituitary ACTH production, loss of 21-hydroxylation capacity entails ACTH overproduction, and hence more pregnenolone, more progesterone and more hydroxyprogesterone are generated at the expense of cholesterol and squalene, resulting in increased rates of 17-ketosteroid production and thus in *virilization*.

Bradbury and Slate,[26] Jailer and his

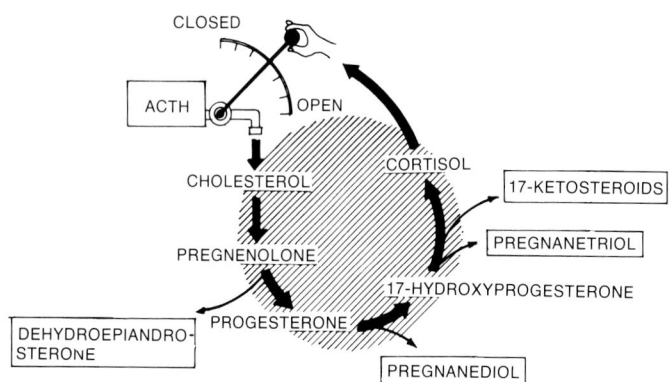

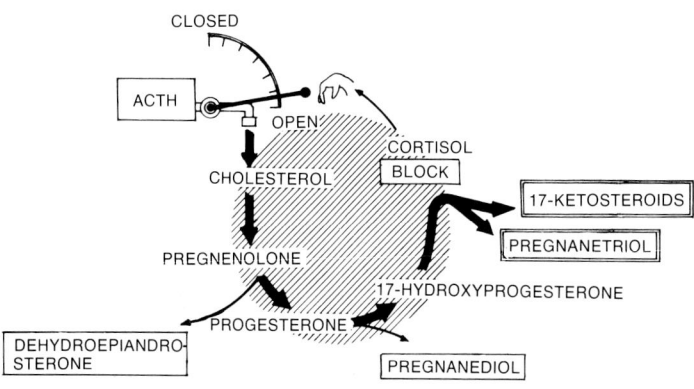

Figure 33-1. A, Regulation of steroid metabolism in the normal adrenal. ACTH stimulates conversion of cholesterol to pregnenolone, progesterone and, finally, cortisol. The last suppresses pituitary ACTH production, as a result of which a form of autoregulation is established in adrenal metabolism. B, Pathway typical of adrenogenital syndrome. As a result of 21-hydroxylase deficiency, 17-hydroxyprogesterone fails to be converted to cortisol. Lack of cortisol causes ACTH hyperproduction, thereby speeding up formation of intermediary catabolites, mainly 17-ketosteroids, and consequently giving rise to virilization. (After Bradbury.[26])

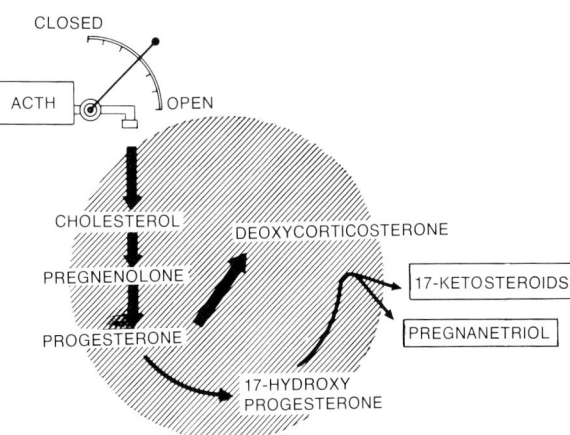

Figure 33–2. One of the varieties of adrenogenital syndrome. Progesterone metabolism is diverted to deoxycorticosterone production. The pathway is identical to that shown in Figure 33–1, except for accumulation of DOCA, which, in addition to virilism, produces hypertension and salt retention. (From Wilkins.[125])

colleagues,[63] Wilkins[125] and, more recently, Blunck and Bierich[19] showed that this was not the only enzymatic mechanism involved in blocking cortical steroidogenesis and that, consequently, other types of adrenogenital syndrome existed. Loss of 11-hydroxylase activity also causes lack of cortisone synthesis although, in the latter instance, there is associated accumulation of deoxycorticosterone (Figure 33–2). Such instances are associated with hypertension, representing a special clinical variety of the syndrome. Goldman and Winter[50] achieved inhibition of 11-hydroxylase activity by means of metopyrone and showed the feasibility of experimentally induced adrenogenital syndrome. Camacho and his co-workers[29] postulated four possible types of enzymopathy to be involved in the adrenogenital syndrome, resulting respectively from 21-hydroxylase, 11-hydroxylase, 3β-ol-dehydrogenase and 17α-hydroxylase deficiency.

In addition, Elberlein and Bongiovanni[41] have demonstrated that adrenal tumors lacked 3β-ol-dehydrogenase, the enzyme capable of converting pregnenolone to progesterone. This was found to result equally in lack of cortisol and cortisone production but, this time without progesterone production and, instead, with accumulation of pregnenolone, which was excreted in the form of urinary dehydroepiandrosterone. Thus, here too, accumulation of 17-ketosteroid produces virilization by the mechanism indicated in Figure 33–3. The occurrence of 3β-ol-dehydrogenase deficiency in adrenogenital syndrome was recently described by Goldman and colleagues,[49, 50, 51] Göbel[46] and Jenkins.[64]

The foregoing doctrine has been generally supported by the findings of Bergstrand and Gemzell,[18] Berardinelli and his colleagues,[16] and Bentinck and associates,[17] based on the study of cultures of hyperplastic adrenal tissue, as well as by investigations of Loras and Migeon[80] and those of Pierson,[98] on tissue cultures of adrenal carcinoma. The mechanism of pathogenesis advanced postulates that virilization in this instance is coincident with *lack of corticoids*, giving rise to a combination form of *adrenogenital syndrome and Addison's disease*,[77, 114, 125] a possibility first raised by us in 1946.[23]

ENZYMATIC THEORY AND THEORY OF THE SEXUAL ADRENAL. To interpret the etiology of adrenogenital syndrome by either theory is essentially a matter of resorting to either a unitarian or dualistic concept of adrenocortical function, as was pointed out in Chapter 9 (page 179). The mere fact that some steroids in the cortex may be converted to others does not mean that the steroids involved may not be transferred or circulated from one cortical zone to another. Accordingly, preliminary conversion steps (synthesis of squalene groups, cholesterol-pregnenolone conversion) are thought to take place in the zona reticularis. The action by 3β-ol-dehydrogenase, necessary for the conversion of pregnenolone to progesterone, is presumably also exerted in that zone. In contrast, 21-hydroxylase is believed to pertain to the cells of the zona fasciculata. Favoring the latter point of view is the finding that 21-hydroxylase is concentrated exclusively in the zona fasciculata of the normal adrenal (Chen et al.,[32, 120] Ayres et al.[9]). Stachenko and Giroud[111] put forward compelling

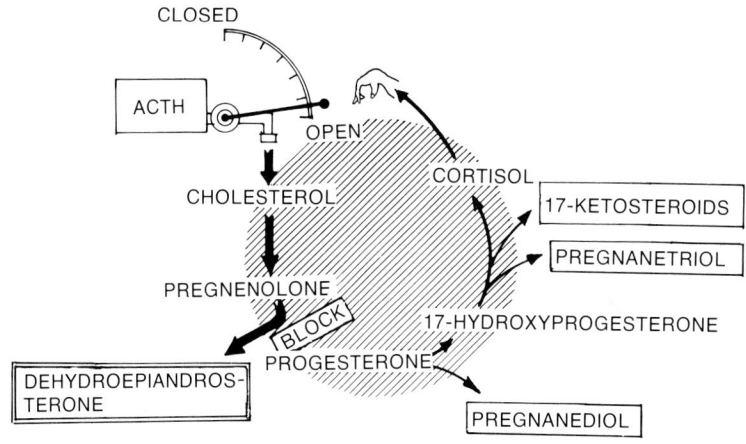

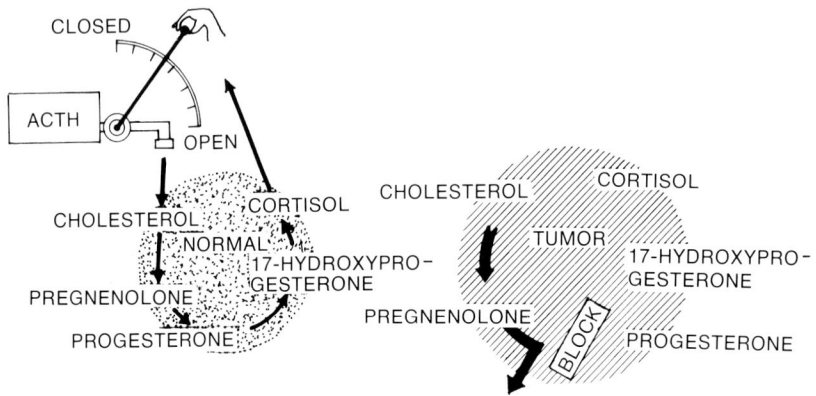

Figure 33–3. A, Another modality of adrenogenital syndrome. The blockade develops in the chain of conversion steps from pregnenolone to progesterone as a result of lack of 3β-ol-dehydrogenase. As a consequence, excessive amounts of dehydroepiandrosterone are produced, giving rise to virilization. The remainder of the effects involved are the same as those in Figure 33–1, B. Because this form of metabolic disorder occurs predominantly in the presence of tumors, urinary dehydroepiandrosterone is present in the tumor-induced variety of adrenogenital syndrome but not in cases of adrenogenital syndrome resulting from hyperplasia. B, Since tumors generally arise unilaterally, the contralateral adrenal functions normally and produces cortisol, thereby maintaining ACTH secretion in balance. This is why adrenal tumors are not associated with any increase in ACTH levels, although the involved adrenal produces no cortisol. (From Bradbury.[26])

arguments in favor of cortical zonation based on differences in enzyme activity of each layer.

Adrenal histology may then be admitted to be in general agreement with the histochemical findings. Except for rare instances in which it is associated with Cushing's disease, the adrenogenital syndrome is associated with atrophy of the zona fasciculata (see Figures 33–11, 33–12 and 33–14) and with *hyperplasia of the zona reticularis.* As pointed out previously, this finding is accompanied by differences in distribution of sudanophilic and fuchsinophilic material, as well as by a characteristic zonal distribution of the diazoreaction. Thus, everything seems to indicate that the tissue we are dealing with is in fact identical in composition to that making up the fetal adrenal cortex, or paleocortex, called by us the sexual adrenal (see Chapter 9). Atrophy of the fasciculata with hyperplasia of the reticularis coincides with accumulation of metabolic products generated by the latter (17-ketosteroids, pregnenolone, progesterone) and with lack of corticoids (cortisol, cortisone) normally generated by the fasciculata. The concurrence of Addison's syndrome with adrenogenital syndrome, observed on numerous occasions (to be discussed later), is thus precisely due to the conditions described.

This is why it must be admitted that the *adrenogenital syndrome* is caused by atrophy of the zona fasciculata, together with a loss of enzyme activity (*21-hydroxylation*) (see Fig. 33–1). This assertion is in full harmony with both theories.

Varied as some of the interpretations may be, the facts we have described remain the same. It seems certain that just as the unitarian and the pluralistic theories can be brought to harmonize, the two divergent etiologies proposed for the adrenogenital syndrome, either through hyperplasia of the "third gonad" or through lack of 21-hydroxylase, are not in conflict with each other either.

11-Hydroxylase failure, resulting in accumulation of deoxycorticosterone in cases noted also for sodium retention and hypertension, probably does not prevent the zona fasciculata from developing, at least partially. Some forms represent simultaneous reticular and fascicular hyperplasia, or what we previously referred to as "Cushing's plus adrenogenital syndrome." So far as tumors are concerned, it would seem to us that the disorder is even more complete in nature, to the extent that enzyme activity is curtailed even in the zona reticularis. Neoplastic tissue fails to synthesize corticoids from a very early stage of steroidogenesis, so that even progesterone synthesis cannot be accomplished. Nevertheless, since the process of steroidogenesis reaches at least the pregnenolone step, catabolites of the latter (which are androgenic) also lead to virilization.

A final hypothesis concerning the "congenital form" of the syndrome: this is the most severe form, which may give rise to true pseudohermaphroditism. It is only natural that this should be so since, as it is, the fetal zona fasciculata is barely developed and the existing cortex is made up of the "paleocortex," which has a much greater tendency to form 17-ketosteroids and to block the first stages of steroid metabolism. The underlying disorder is probably similar in nature to that involved in tumors, that is to say, that there is not only lack of 11- and 21-hydroxylase activity but also lack of 3β-ol-dehydrogenase activity which, as with tumors, leads to virilization of much greater intensity.

33.2.3. GENETICS OF ADRENOGENITAL SYNDROME

Chromosomal studies have been undertaken on such patients following the same line of thinking that sought to implicate some form of *chromosomopathy* in the etiology of the congenital enzyme disorder observed in Stein-Leventhal's syndrome (Chapter 29, page 649). In 1970, Edwards and his colleagues[40] reported a case of adrenogenital syndrome with an XO/XX/XXX mosaicism. It must be stressed, however, that similar findings are exceptional; nevertheless, the familial—and to some extent, hereditary—character of the syndrome has been emphasized by, among many others, Minozzi and his associates.[87] It is therefore

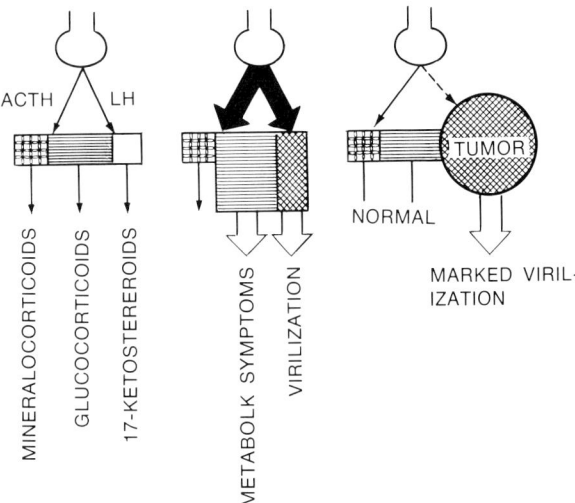

Figure 33–4. The two possible etiologies of the adrenogenital syndrome. Left (normal), pituitary control over 17-ketosteroid-producing zona reticularis and over glucocorticoid-producing zona fasciculata. Middle, pituitary hyperfunction determines both virilization and metabolic symptoms whenever both ACTH and LH are involved. Right, adrenal tumor giving rise to marked virilization in the absence of any pituitary reaction.

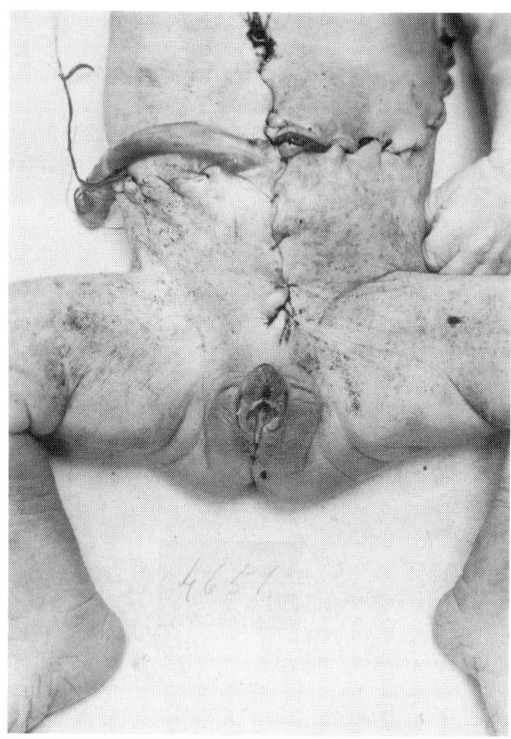

Figure 33–5. Case of congenital adrenogenital syndrome. Stillborn female fetus, revealing marked hypertrophy of clitoris.

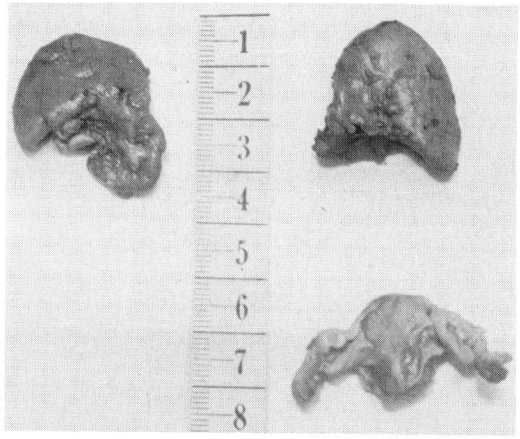

Figure 33–6. Gross appearance of adrenals and genital tract in the fetus of Figure 33–5. Note pronounced adrenal hyperplasia and apparently normal development of genital apparatus, uterus, tubes and ovaries.

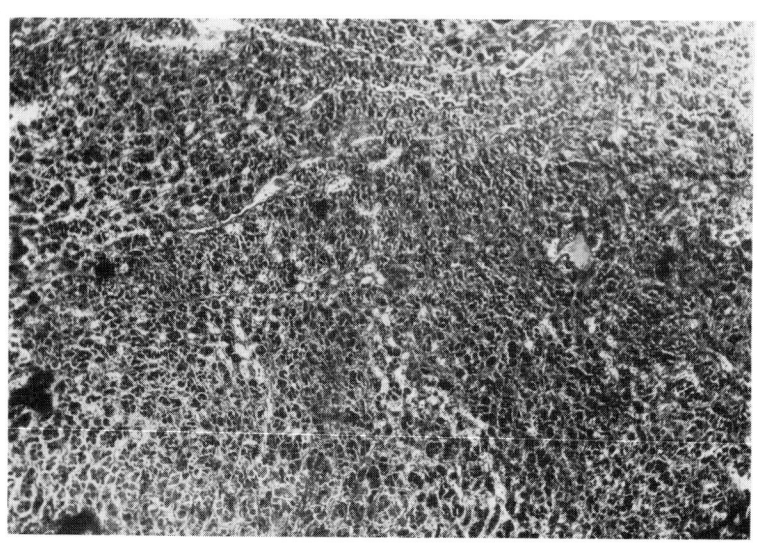

Figure 33–7. Severe adenomatous hyperplasia of zona reticularis in the adrenal of case presented in Figures 33–5 and 33–6. Note fuchsinophilic inclusions, which appear black.

possible that, other than some *chromopathy*, the syndrome may be due to some *genopathy*.

33.2.4. ANATOMIC PATHOLOGY

ADRENAL. The disorder is caused either by simple hyperplasia or by adenoma, occasionally even carcinoma, involving the sexual zone of the adrenal cortex. The sexual nature of the tissue involved becomes apparent in proliferations of both the hyperplastic and the neoplastic types. Histologically, *the characteristic component consists of fuchsinophilic tissue*, already described in Chapter 9. After studying the surgically removed adrenals of 33 patients of the surgeon Broster[27] in 1938, Vines[122] described their histopathology. In each case, the tissue was composed of cells with abundant cytoplasm containing inclusions, stainable with Fuchsin Xyledene Ponceau according to a method devised by Vines. Found by us to be a constant feature of the adrenal sexual zone under physiologic conditions,[22, 23] this type of

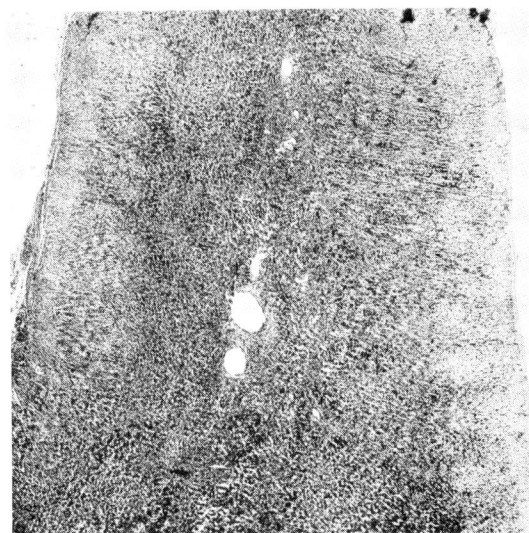

Figure 33–9. Hyperplasia of fuchsinophilic zone in adrenal from patient in Figure 33–8. There is marked overgrowth of fuchsinophilic zone at the expense of the medulla and a large part of zona fasciculata.

tissue fuchsinophilia is a characteristic property of sex hormone secreting adrenal cells. As may be noted in Figures 33–7 and 33–13, illustrating surgically removed specimens from patients with adrenogenital syndrome operated on and studied at our clinic, *this stain is positive in every case of adrenogenital syndrome to the extent that, whenever found in a surgical specimen, it may be construed as the single most reliable criterion for diagnosis*. This type of tissue may be present in variable amounts, ranging from large tumors to small foci of hyperplasia. Most commonly, however, the adrenals are only slightly enlarged (Figs. 33–11 and 33–17). Occasionally, hyperplasia of the sexual zone may be of such magnitude that it completely smothers the zona fasciculata, conveying the misleading impression of medullary hyperplasia and cortical atrophy on gross inspection of cross-sected specimens. Histologic examination reveals that the medulla is similarly encroached upon by the proliferative process in the reticularis, inwardly crowding the chromaffin tissue, and outwardly causing flattening of the fascicular layer (Fig. 33–12).

The finding fully explains the clinical picture *combining the symptoms of adrenogenital syndrome with those of addisonism*, mentioned previously.

In addition, the active element in such

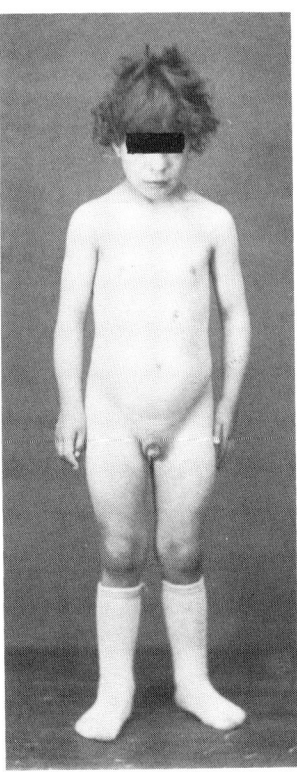

Figure 33–8. Infantile form of adrenogenital syndrome. Five year old girl with symptoms of precocious puberty, but with peniform growth of clitoris.

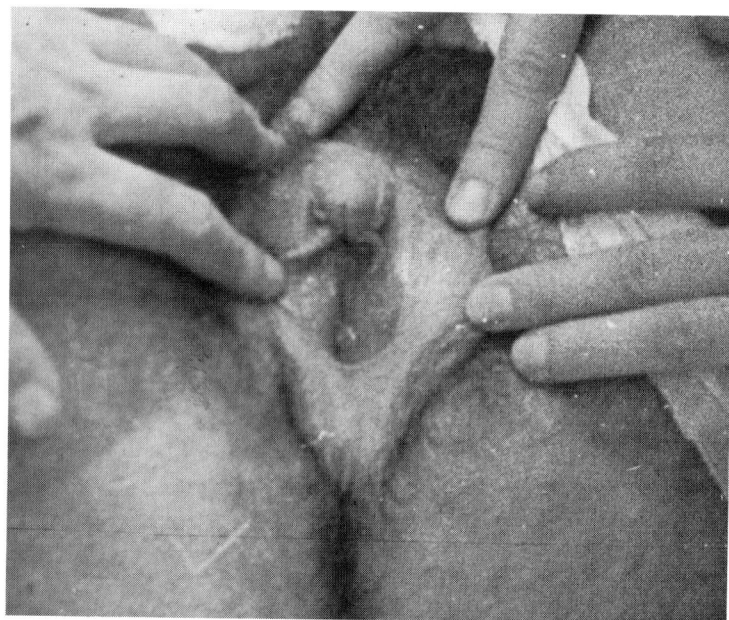

Figure 33–10. Pudendal region with pronounced hypertrophy of the clitoris in a juvenile case of adrenogenital syndrome.

Figure 33–11. Gross appearance of left adrenal removed from patient in Figure 33–10. Note narrow outline of zona fasciculata (light) and marked hyperplasia of zona reticularis (dark).

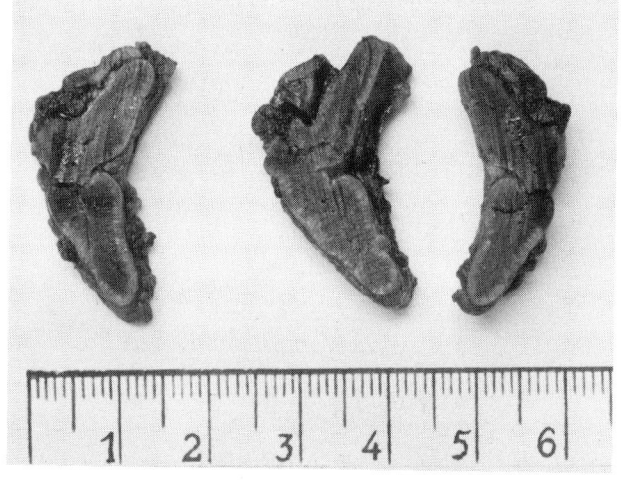

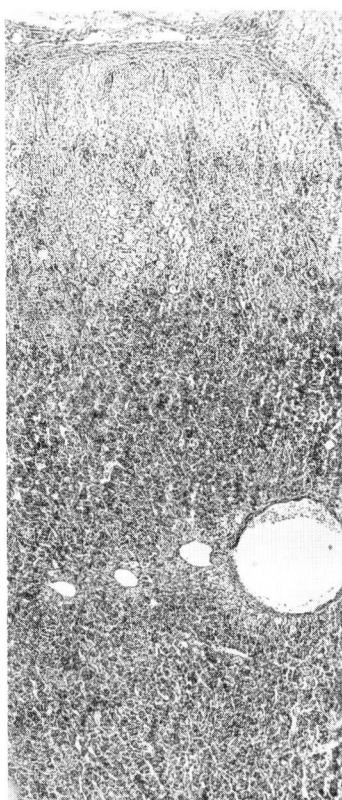

Figure 33–12. Microscopic view of adrenal from Figure 33–11. Medulla has disappeared and there is outward compression of fasciculata. Reticularis is markedly hyperplastic, with abundant fuchsinophilic inclusions.

proliferations has been characterized through staining reactions for carbonyl groups or for 17-ketosteroids by Seligman and Ashbel.[104] Besides giving positive staining reactions with fuchsin and with Ashbel's method, this tissue has also been found to contain *birefringent lipoids* in abundance, as shown by Howard and Benua.[59] In addition, the tissue is noted for its sudanophobia, so that the sexual zone in pathologic hyperplasia remains unstained while the metabolic zone stains intensely with Sudan III or Sudan IV, as shown in Figure 33–14.

OVARY. Ovarian changes are always present and, interestingly, reveal either *hyperthecosis* or *hilus cell proliferation*, or both, thereby duplicating certain changes seen in Stein-Leventhal ovaries, a fact pointed out by us in 1946[22] and recently emphasized by Kowal and his associates.[72] Ovarian changes of this type were also described by Landing,[76] Hooft and colleagues[58] and Milcou and colleagues.[86] In addition, Perloff[96] called attention to the fact that infertility from anovulation was common in mild forms of this syndrome and was, of course, the rule in advanced forms of the disease.

As of late, a different etiology has been proposed for the occurrence of anovulatory cycles and polycystic ovaries in adrenogenital syndrome.

As indicated earlier, in Chapter 29 (Section 29.3.5), hypothalamic impregnation with androgens, especially in baby animals or humans, causes "hypothalamic sterilization" with loss of LH release. Androgens elaborated in cases of adrenogenital syndrome, particularly those of the congenital or juvenile varieties, are currently believed to cause similar hypothalamic impregnation, resulting in *anovulation*.

FEMALE GENITAL TRACT. The extent to which the tubes, uterus and vagina are involved essentially depends on whether the syndrome develops at a premature or at a late phase. The process of fusion of the müllerian ducts may be found to be completely arrested in congenital cases. We have observed a case of a bicornuate uterus and sometimes also cases of rudimentary bicornuate uteri. In such cases, development of the genital tract has been arrested in a highly undifferentiated phase, corresponding to the first months of fetal life. However, whenever the syndrome has its onset in adult life, sometimes as late as menopause, very few manifestations, other than perhaps some functional impairment, may be recognized in the genital tract.

33.2.5. ENDOCRINOLOGY

The question of hormone production by either hyperplastic or neoplastic tissue is a highly interesting one. Here we shall give a brief summary of hormone elimination in such patients.

17-KETOSTEROIDS. Studies of urinary 17-ketosteroids in these patients have been undertaken by many workers (Bayer and Koets,[12] Gebauer and Linke,[45] Herweg et al.,[57] Kepler and Mason[67]). Our own findings in adrenogenital syndrome revealed similarly elevated 17-ketosteroid titers. In the case illustrated in Figure 33–15, daily excretion rates reached 110 mg, as compared to usual daily rates of 30 to 40 mg. Lloyd

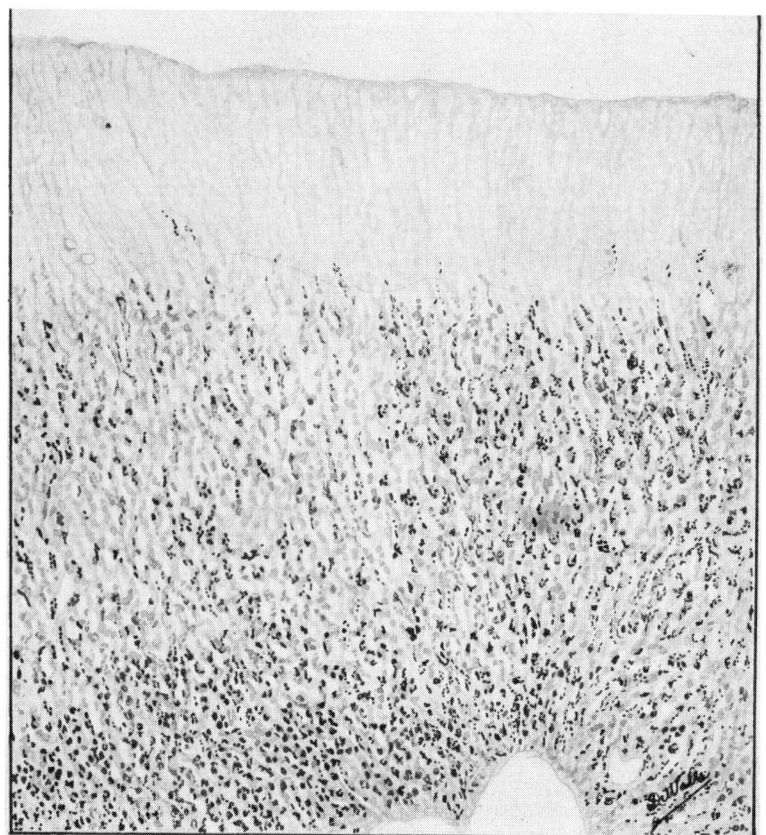

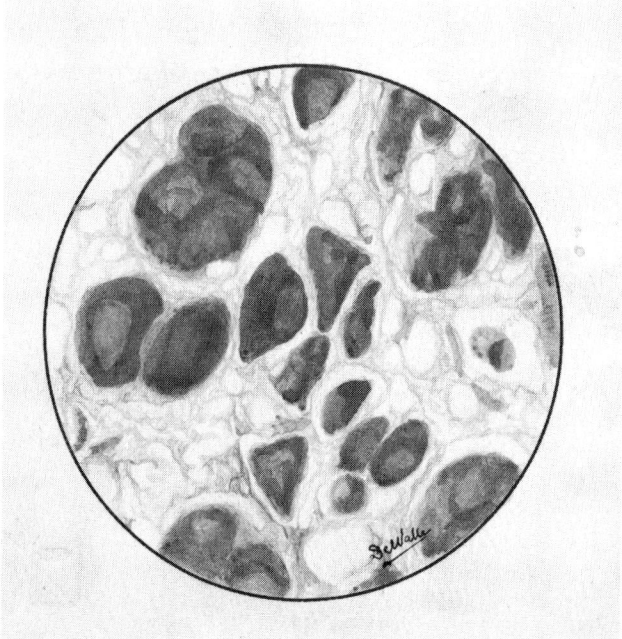

Figure 33-13. Direct reproduction of fuchsinophilic inclusions in Figures 33-11 and 33-12.

Adrenal Endocrinopathies in Relation to Sex

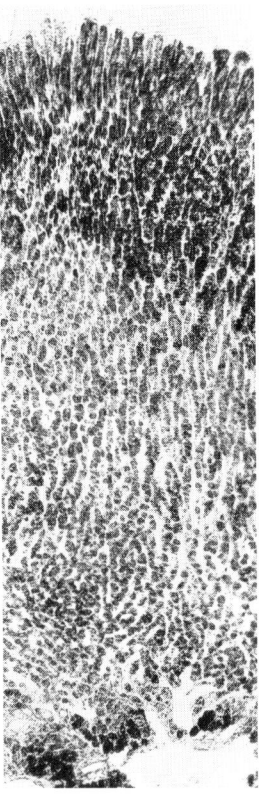

Figure 33–14. Section of adrenal from case in Figures 33–10 through 33–13, stained with Sudan III. Note that the sudanophilic zone (comprising the fasciculata and the glomerulosa) is significantly narrowed and displaced outward by sudanophobic zone (sexual zone).

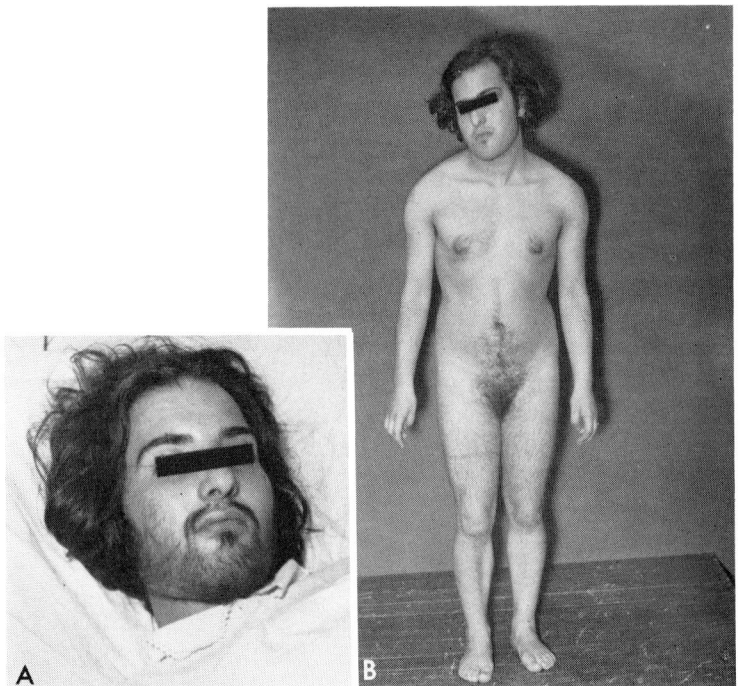

Figure 33–15. Case of adrenogenital syndrome with extreme virilization in a girl aged 18. Notice musculature and somatic build of entirely virile configuration.

and his associates[79] reported values of 82 mg/24 hr in a patient with adrenogenital syndrome, whereas in a patient with associated Cushing's syndrome, that is, a case of panhypercorticism, values found for corticosteroids were of the order of 36 mg. This would seem to indicate that 17-ketosteroid excretion is liable to undergo a much greater increase than corticosteroid excretion, even in those cases in which both cortical zones are involved. Azerad and his associates[10] have reported the values found in Table 33–1 for steroid excretion in two cases of adrenogenital syndrome.

Using a chromatographic procedure, Diamond and Young[36] have achieved the isolation of as many as 22 steroid fractions. In their view, chromatography of 17-ketosteroids is an important element in diagnosing adrenogenital syndrome. Other forms of virilism reveal different chromatographic patterns, a point particularly stressed by Azerad and co-workers.[10]

Since 1945, special significance has been attached to the presence of dehydroepiandrosterone, a special compound within the 17-ketosteroid series, found to be specifically increased in adrenal tumors but not in simple hyperplasia, as shown by Neelsen and associates[90] and by Crooke and Callow.[33] Based on these findings, Patterson,[95] in 1947, introduced a color reaction for dehydroepiandrosterone. It is easy to perform on urine and allows the diagnosis of adrenal tumor while ruling out virilism either from hyperplasia or from other causes. In 1950, Allen and his co-workers[3] improved this procedure.

TABLE 33–1. Excretion Rates of Urinary Steroids in Two Cases of Adrenogenital Syndrome

STEROID	FIRST CASE	SECOND CASE	NORMAL VALUES
G.B.S.	6.3 mg	22.4 mg	9 to 12 mg
G.C.	26.2 mg	7.0 mg	15 to 24 mg
S.B.S.	10.0 mg	36.4 mg	6 to 9 mg
Pregnanediol	0.33 mg	1.79 mg	6 to 9 mg

*From Azerad, Beaulieu and Jayle: *Ann. d'Endocr.*, sur deux cas d'hypercorticisme; intérêt de l'exploration polystéroidique urinaire. 14:505, 1953, Masson et Cie, Paris.

G.B.S. = Gluco-butyl-soluble steroids.
G.C. = Gluco-conjugated steroids.
S.B.S. = 3-Ketosteroids.

The question of why dehydroepiandrosterone occurs in large amounts in adrenal tumors while it is scant or absent in adrenal hyperplasia had not been satisfactorily explained until recently. The works of Elberlein and Bongiovanni[20, 21, 41] provided the necessary clarification, which is in full agreement with our previously explained ideas concerning the etiology of the disease. In hyperplasia, steroidogenesis is disturbed, owing to lack of 21-hydroxylation, which blocks formation of cortisone-cortisol but not that of progesterone. Upon reexamining Figures 33–1, 33–2 and 33–3, we can understand why the 17-ketosteroid fraction resulting from blocked cortisol and cortisone synthesis is mainly made up of androsterone and cholanolone, whereas deficient 3β-dehydrogenation, the characteristic disorder occurring in tumors, is associated with absent progesterone synthesis and with the appearance of dehydroepiandrosterone as a catabolite. Camacho and Migeon[28] have besides found an increase in plasma and urine *testosterone* levels. Axelrod and Goldzieher[8] reported abundant elimination of testosterone in cases of congenital adrenogenital syndrome. Finally, a new androgenic steroid compound, 16-androstenol, has been isolated by Gower and Stern[53] from the urine of women with adrenogenital syndrome.

ESTROGENS. As early as 1932, Bennett[15] demonstrated the existence of increased amounts of folliculin in the urine of a case of adrenogenital syndrome with precocious puberty. Frank[43] similarly found elevated values of that hormone in male cases of adrenogenital syndrome. Later, Sprague and co-workers,[110] as well as Kolff and Tyook,[71] found elevated urinary estrogens and, similarly, Azerad and associates[10] reported elevated values for phenolsteroids. Increased rates of estrogen excretion in adrenogenital syndrome are not unanimously accepted by all investigators. Thus, Lloyd and his co-workers[79] failed to find any urinary estrogens in a patient with adrenogenital syndrome. It seems quite possible that androgenic and estrogenic secretions vary considerably from case to case.[79]

Mellicow and Cahill[84] and, later, Keller[65, 66] also reported cases of adrenogenital syndrome with *elevated estrogen* levels. Wotiz and his co-workers[130] similarly reported an increase in estrogen levels, mainly *estriol*.

Adrenal Endocrinopathies in Relation to Sex

Nonetheless, the rate of estrogen production does not appear to be invariably increased, which is the main reason why, as shall be made clear when discussing the clinical features of the disease, most cases of adrenogenital syndrome are associated with virilization, although some may also reveal feminizing effects.[11, 29, 119] This probably depends on the level at which steroidogenesis is blocked, as indicated in Figure 33–1 and those that follow.

PREGNANEDIOL AND PREGNANETRIOL. Pregnanediol has been observed in the urine of two of our female patients with adrenogenital syndrome. The patient shown in Figure 33–15 revealed values ranging between 30 and 50 mg a day, while for the patient represented in Figure 33–16, the rate of excretion averaged 20 mg daily. Other investigators reporting increased pregnanediol excretion in adrenogenital syndrome have been Hain,[55] Lloyd and co-workers[79] and Allen and co-workers.[3] Values reported by most authors fluctuate between 20 and 40 mg/24 hr, that is, close to values eliminated by a pregnant woman.

In perfusion experiments on adrenals from patients with adrenogenital syndrome, Zander[132] observed much larger amounts of *progesterone* than are found in normal adrenals. His findings were indirectly confirmed by the studies of Axelrod and Goldzieher,[7] and by those of Pierson,[98] using ACTH.

Not only progesterone but also *17-hydroxyprogesterone* reaches the bloodstream in excessive amounts, as illustrated in the diagram of Figure 33–1. This accounts for the presence of urinary *pregnanetriol*, a catabolite of 17-hydroxyprogesterone. Bongiovanni,[20] Fukushima and colleagues,[44] Zander and Müller[131] and Kinoshita and associates[69] have detected large amounts of the triol in this syndrome. However, the examples offered in Figures 33–1, 33–2 and 33–3 indicate that pregnanetriol is only increased in typical forms of adrenogenital syndrome, that is, in those varieties caused by lack of 21-hydroxylase activity but not in those other forms in which 17-hydroxyprogesterone formation is also blocked.

GONADOTROPINS. Increased values of luteinizing hormone (LH) seem to be a constant finding in most cases. We were able to make this finding in a case described as far back as 1945.[23] Similar findings have been reported by Devis[35] and by Chalmers,[30] both in 1949. The role of gonadotropin in the genesis of the syndrome and in the production of adrenal hyperplasia

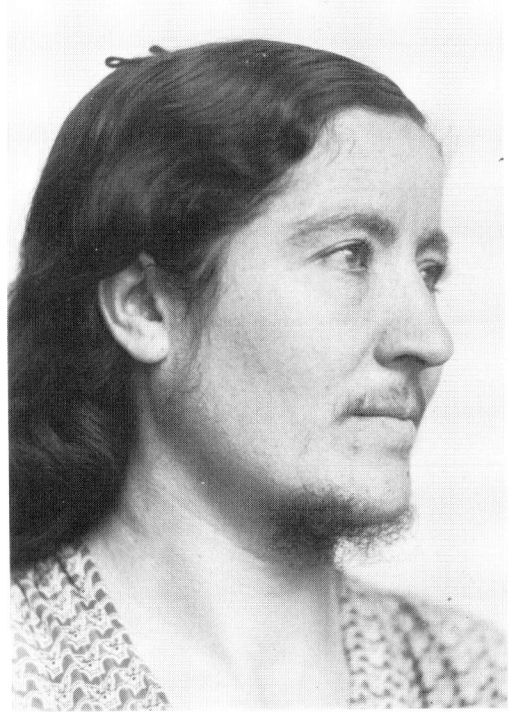

Figure 33–16. Adrenogenital syndrome in a 32 year old woman.

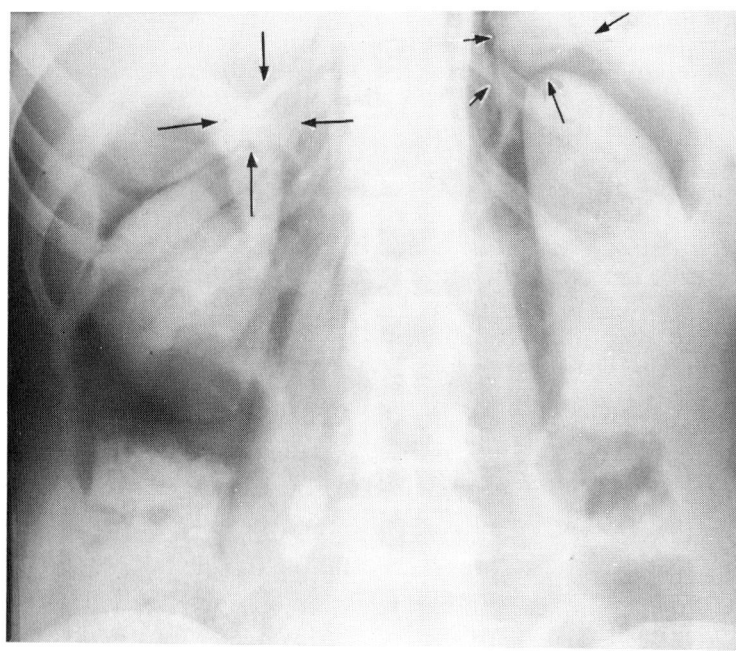

Figure 33-17. Pneumokidney in patient shown in Figure 33-16. Both adrenals are enlarged, particularly the one on the right side.

has been emphasized in our earlier publications on the subject, as well as in those by Chang and Witschi[31] and those by Printer.[100]

CORTICOSTEROIDS AND ADRENOCORTICOTROPIN. These, it should be mentioned in closing, are usually not elevated, with the exception of those instances of adrenogenital syndrome that are associated with Cushing's disease.[71, 72]

33.2.6. CLINICAL FORMS OF ADRENOGENITAL SYNDROME

The adrenogenital syndrome appears under a variety of clinical forms. It may involve both sexes. Regardless of sex, it may have either a predominantly virilizing or a predominantly feminizing character, the first being by far the more common.

BISEXUAL CHARACTER OF THE SYNDROME. The adrenogenital syndrome of classical description has been presumed to be exclusively feminizing, whereas the generally widespread view among clinicians is that the presence of an adrenal tumor is tantamount to virilization. The bisexual character of cortical secretion was stressed in Chapter 9. From among 227 cases collected by us from the world literature in 1946, we found that 193 (85 per cent) occurred in women while 34 (15 per cent) occurred in men. Among the female patients, 154 (79 per cent) cases presented signs of virilization, while 39 (21 per cent) cases showed evidence of hyperfeminization, with precocious puberty or exacerbation of menstrual periods. In the male series, 21 cases (61.7 per cent) revealed evidence of feminization, such as gynecomastia, decreased size of penis and loss of libido, but 13 cases (38.3 per cent) showed symptoms consistent with enhanced virility in addition to hypertrichosis.

This enables us to draw the following comparative summary concerning the occurrence of the syndrome in either males or females:
1. Occurrence in females (common):
   a. Virilization; increased 17-ketosteroids (common).
   b. Hyperfeminization: increased estrogens (rare).
2. Occurrence in males (less common):
   a. Feminization; increased estrogens (common).
   b. Hypervirilization; increased 17-ketosteroids (rare).

ISOSEXUAL ADRENOGENITAL SYNDROME. By definition, this syndrome produces no deviation of sex toward the opposite sex in either females or males. It is often not recognized at all. As a matter of fact, it is highly unlikely that any male with hypertrichosis, premature baldness and enhanced libido might be suspected of having adrenal hyperplasia, and most hairy and hypergenital males probably fail to arouse any suspicion in that respect (Klotz[70]). For the same reason, only parallel studies of both urinary 17-ketosteroids and estrogens have made it possible recently to identify those cases of hyperestrinism in women who revealed mild virilization with elevated urinary 17-ketosteroids at the same time that they revealed a hyperplastic uterus and bleeding disorders (Quint et al.[101]). It might thus become necessary to describe a *virilizing variety of metropathia haemorrhagica*, the origin of which may be largely sought in unrecognized adrenal hyperplasia, although similar effects may undeniably also be associated with ovarian hyperthecosis (see Chapter 29).

FEMINIZING ADRENOGENITAL SYNDROME IN MALES. In our monograph of 1946, we already indicated the occurrence of cases of adrenogenital syndrome in males, associated with feminization, gynecomastia and loss of libido. Over the past years, the number of reports of similar cases have multiplied.[11, 29, 66, 75, 84, 102, 103, 106, 108, 119, 123, 128] They may occur in the congenital forms of the syndrome, as reported by Camacho and associates[29] and by Mellikow and Cahill,[84] as well as in cases appearing during the puberal period (Snaith[108]) or in mature age (West et al.[128]), but they occur most commonly in males of the advanced age group owing to *adrenal carcinoma* (cases reported by Keller,[66] Rappaport et al.,[102] Siquier et al.[106] and Wallach et al.[123]). A review of all cases reported to date may be found in Wallach's work[123] and in an editorial.[39]

Hormone studies in these cases[66, 94, 101, 108] invariably revealed moderately increased estrogens. 17-Ketosteroid excretion may not be increased; in Slaunwhite and Buchwald's case,[107] chromatography revealed absence of androsterone, a rise in estrogens and evidence that 90 per cent of the 17-ketosteroids were made up of etiocholanolone, a compound with scant, if any, androgenic potency.

FETAL ADRENOGENITAL SYNDROME. The adrenogenital syndrome of the fetal stage is caused by *congenital hyperplasia of the sexual cortex*. What is involved is hyperfunctional activity by the temporary cortex, or "paleocortex," described in Chapter 9. Alterations of this type in the embryonic adrenal are responsible for the most severe kind of changes in the genital tract and, in girls, give rise to *female pseudohermaphroditism,* a condition in which, in the presence of normally developed ovaries, there is a male directed deviation in the development of either the internal genitalia (*internal female pseudohermaphroditism*) or the external genitalia (*external female pseudohermaphroditism*), or both.

Cases of external pseudohermaphroditism, an example of which is shown in Figure 33–5, occur more commonly. The case illustrated is that of a female fetus with hypertrophy of the clitoris and a rudimentary vagina. At autopsy, there was found considerable hyperplasia of both adrenals (Fig. 33–6); however, the internal genitalia showed no apparent changes. The uterus and the ovaries were found to be normally developed. Microscopic examination of the adrenals revealed the presence of *fuchsinophilic adenomatous hyperplasia* of the zona reticularis (Fig. 33–7). This case is a typical example of congenital adrenogenital syndrome of the virilizing variety, with production of external female pseudohermaphroditism. The cases presented in Figures 33–8 to 33–13 are examples of prepuberal appearance of the syndrome, which at laparotomy revealed bicornuate uteri, indicating actual fetal development of the syndrome, with a subsequent period of latency.

Pseudohermaphroditic female fetuses of this type reveal hypertrichosis in the form of abundant lanugo. Like lanugo, hypertrichosis of this kind is an ephemeral phenomenon. Nevertheless, such fetuses are born with stigmata of virilization and with pseudohermaphroditism. In some cases—for instance those described by Tilp and by Bayer and Lang, as well as those later described by Mellikow and Cahill[84] and, recently, by Mattox and coworkers[82]—apart from pseudohermaphroditism and more or less apparent hirsutism, there may be *fetal gigantism with excessive development of stature and of the thymus.*

Adrenal atrophy, as we shall see later, may cause hyperplasia of the thymus. It is possible that hyperplasia of the thymus in the cases previously reported was the consequence of corticogenic insufficiency. Fetal gigantism, in turn, might be due to hyperplasia of the thymus.

Vague and his associates[119] reported three cases of congenital syndrome in which they were able to demonstrate a congenital defect in 21-hydroxylase activity. This raises the question of whether the adrenogenital syndrome may not, after all, be the result of an *inborn error of metabolism*.

ADRENOGENITAL SYNDROME OF THE INFANTILE STAGE. This is the most common clinical form. The single most complete series of such cases, to our knowledge, is that published by Mellikow and Cahill,[84] although older descriptions may be found in the doctoral thesis of Gallais, as well as in the works of Matthias and Neumann. Here, too, the syndrome appears in females more often than it does in males. Among 62 cases compiled by us in the past, only 12 had occurred in males, as compared to 50 in females. It is of interest to point out that girls usually present with the syndrome of *transient hyperfeminization* or *precocious puberty*, which was present in 36 of the 50 cases studied. The clinical picture is characterized mainly by premature somatic and sexual development in girls. There is precocious puberty, with onset of menses between the ages of five and 10. At the same time, there is marked development of breasts and impressive somatic growth. This transient phase of sexual and bodily precocity, which is usually associated to a considerable extent with *mental precocity*, is rapidly followed by sexual inversion, with the appearance of hypertrichosis, mainly along the midabdominal line. The musculature becomes as powerful as that of a boy. The clitoris undergoes hypertrophy and the prematurely developed breasts undergo retrogression, whereas menstruation gives way to secondary amenorrhea. Many instances of precocious puberty, initially attributed to a pineal or encephalic origin, eventually degenerate into similar forms of secondary virilism, which bear out the adrenal etiology of the syndrome. Male instances of precocious puberty are also known to occur; for instance, a patient described by Player and Lisser, a four year old boy, had a deep voice, a beard, great muscular strength and great mental alertness. He exhibited libido and erections and behaved in front of women as would be expected from a young man of the age of 18. In some instances, although less infrequently, precocious puberty may occur without heterosexual changes, in which case girls retain their feminine features. Such cases of *isosexual precocious puberty* have been described in conjunction with adrenocortical tumors in both males and females. These may have to be classified among the varieties of adrenogenital syndrome that are virilizing in males and feminizing in females. In accordance with the remarks made above, the occurrence of similar cases may be anticipated. Quite commonly, what at an early age may begin as a simple cortical hyperplasia frequently gradually changes into a *malignant tumor*. The incidence of malignancy in the adrenogenital syndrome of the infantile age group is highest of all. Fifty per cent of the cases reported in the literature showed evidence of malignancy or developed malignancy eventually.

Figure 33-8 illustrates a case of adrenogenital syndrome in a five year old girl. Despite marked peniform development of the clitoris, there was no evidence of precocious puberty. The girl revealed adrenal enlargement in pneumoroentgenograms, and the presence of adrenal hyperplasia was later confirmed at autopsy (Fig. 33-9). Microscopically, there was evidence of abundant fuchsinophilic elements, but no evidence of neoplasia.

In summary, adrenogenital syndrome of infancy commonly displays precocious puberty with male directed sexual changes. In boys, symptoms are confined to premature sexual maturity. In girls, following an ephemeral phase of premature femininity, sex evolves inexorably toward an intersex state.

JUVENILE TYPE OF ADRENOGENITAL SYNDROME. The disease seems to occur less commonly between the ages of 15 and 25. Menstruation develops in a normal way and there is no precocious puberty. Following normal menarche, menstrual periods gradually become unevenly spaced until disappearing completely, after which signs of virilization set in. At this stage, the most conspicuous symptoms are extraordinary growth of axillary and abdominal hair as well as incipient hypertrichosis of the face. Muscular development and an athletic constitution have often been described as prominent features of this period. Many cases of juvenile adrenogenital syndrome with virilization have been reported in female athletes who won tournaments and championships.

We have had the opportunity to study two cases of adrenogenital syndrome occurring in the juvenile age group. One was a girl of 15, the other a girl of 18. In the first case, we were inclined to believe that the disease was of fetal onset but remained latent or with minimal symptomatology until the time of adolescence. There was essential amenorrhea. In contrast, the second patient had a normal puberty and secondarily developed virilization. Virilization was apparent in both cases, particularly in the second, in which the patient had grown a heavy beard and mustache of entirely masculine appearance. Muscular development was pronounced in both cases, both girls being reputed to be as strong as a man. As for such features as body contour, musculature, distribution of fat panniculus and hair, all were entirely of the male type. The voice was harsh and low pitched, of typical male resonance in both cases. Urinary 17-ketosteroids were elevated, amounting to 100 mg/24 hr in the second case. It is also relevant to mention that both cases were found to have elevated titers of urinary pregnanediol excretion.

ADULT TYPE OF ADRENOGENITAL SYNDROME. Prior to 1946, the number of cases of interrenalism of the adult age group (past 25 years of age) stood at 92. The number has since grown manifold mainly as a result of improved methods of diagnosis and of the fact that more attention is now being directed to this kind of clinical picture. In its most typical form, the syndrome appears in women with previously normal reproductive function through development of *amenorrhea*. At the same time, *obesity of the characteristic muscular type* makes itself manifest. Sometime afterwards, *the voice becomes hoarse* and a male type of hair growth develops all over the body, including growth of a beard and mustache. Frequently, the onset of virilization is noted to occur in the wake of pregnancy. In the case shown in Figure 33–16, hirsutism began during pregnancy and became accentuated postpartum, leading subsequently to a full-blown state of virilism. *Hypercorticism of the feminizing variety* in women is a rare phenomenon. Nevertheless, we have observed one case in which the presence of a moderate degree of hypercorticism was associated with hypertrichosis of the pubic region and thighs in the presence of a perfectly feminine type, with exaggerated breast development and female morphology. This patient had presented with metropathia haemorrhagica and revealed high levels of urinary estrogens and 17-ketosteroids (21 mg/24 hr). However, it must be recognized that the isosexual variety of adrenogenital syndrome in this age group is less common than it is in younger groups. As a rule, *the virilizing character of the adrenogenital syndrome may be said to become more pronounced with increasing age*. Not only does the degree of virilization tend to depend on the duration of the disease, as is the case, for instance, in precocious puberty, but it also depends on the time of appearance of the disease, *the tendency to virilization becoming greater the later the onset of the disease*.

ADRENOGENITAL SYNDROME AND GESTATION. The concomitant occurrence of adrenogenital syndrome with gestation[58, 93] has been reported in some cases. Adrenal virilism apparently did not impair normal fecundity in such cases. Although this is undoubtedly rare, a notable example of such an exceptional case has been recorded in one of the masterpieces of Spanish art: *La mujer barbuda (The Bearded Woman)* by Ribera, a painting that may presently be found in the Lerma collection at Toledo (Fig. 33–18). The model posing for the painter was a married woman, mother of eight, who had grown a striking beard, reproduced with great realism by El Españoleto. The painting depicts the woman as she was about to breast-feed her baby and, according to the legend inscribed at the foot of the painting, she had previously breast-fed all her other children without loss of nursing capacity. This was not a fictitious product of the artist's imagination but, on the contrary, a faithful reproduction of a strange but entirely possible event, done at the request of the viceroy of Naples. After all, the fact that that woman presented normal lactation is not surprising if one remembers, as pointed out in Chapter 22, that adrenocortical function is an important prerequisite for the normal process of milk secretion. On the other hand, such patients are also prone to develop abortion, as reported by Southren and associates.[109] In

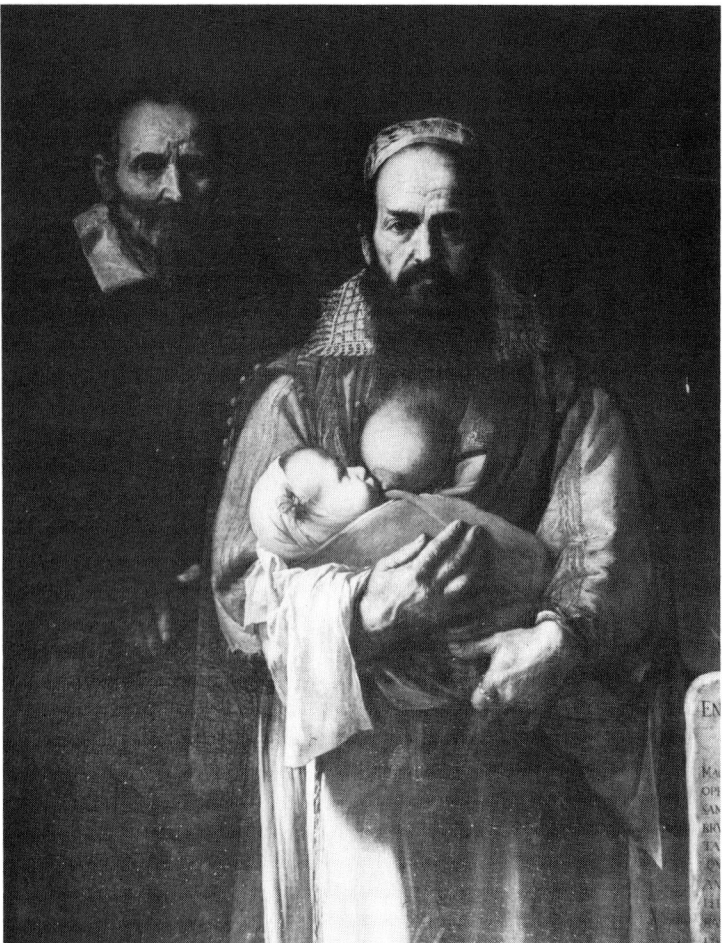

Figure 33-18. La mujer barbuda *(The Bearded Woman).* Painting by Ribera, in Lerma collection, Toledo.

Chapter 42, we list adrenal hyperplasia among the various etiologies that have been described as causing abortion. In addition, Perloff[96] has indicated that *infertility resulting from an anovulatory cycle* may often be associated with a moderate degree of hypercorticism. This additional aspect of the syndrome is examined in Chapter 41.

PSYCHIC CHANGES IN ADRENOGENITAL SYNDROME. The fact that the sexual instinct is quite independent of hormone activity has been well established in the literature of modern endocrinology. Thus, patients with arrhenoblastomas or even with true hermaphroditism present well established tendencies toward one sex and reveal no homosexuality. Similarly, none of the cases of adrenogenital syndrome that we have studied involved features of homosexuality. Some time ago, Allen and his associates suggested that adrenal proliferative processes led to alterations of the sexual instinct. We have been unable to confirm these findings. On the contrary, patients suffering from adrenogenital syndrome were found to experience interesting psychic alterations that were unrelated to sex. Hypercorticism during the fetal and infantile phases manifests itself by precocious mental development which, in the infantile form, leads to precocious libido, although without deviation of the sex instinct. In the adult type of adrenogenital syndrome, maniacal or demented conditions are frequently observed. It may therefore be asserted that while adrenogenital syndrome may be associated with psychic alterations these usually do not involve the sex instinct.

33.2.7. ADRENAL CARCINOMA

The endocrine mechanism involved in virilization due to carcinoma is somewhat different from that involved in simple hyperplasia. This does not preclude the possibility that the syndrome may also be associated with a feminizing effect. The most dramatic type of symptomatology in adrenogenital syndrome is usually produced by carcinomas (Fig. 33-19). As shall be indicated, the diagnosis can be made by means of the Allen-Patterson reaction or by means of pneumoroentgenography. Not unless 17-ketosteroid excretion rates are above 60 mg/24 hr, however, is any suspicion of tumor justified. *Treatment must always be surgical*, although, unfortunately, recurrences are almost the rule.

33.2.8. DIAGNOSIS

The problems encountered in diagnosing adrenogenital syndrome have recently been simplified by the introduction of new exploratory procedures, particularly pneumoroentgenography and methods for the determination of urinary steroids. *The clinical diagnosis of adrenal tumor* is based on the manner in which symptoms have developed. Pronounced virilism beginning early in life is always suspected of having an adrenal origin. Virilism of ovarian origin, such as occurs in hyperthecosis, in hilus cell hyperplasia or in virilizing ovarian tumors, is nearly always found in mature age and never occurs in either the infantile or juvenile age groups. In addition, the adrenogenital syndrome is often associated with increased muscular strength and with symptoms of metabolic hypercorticism. However, this fact should not be considered as holding true in all cases, since a great many cases of adrenogenital syndrome reported recently have been found to be associated with Addison's disease.[2, 3, 75, 107, 124] One way or another, adrenal manifestations of either hyperfunction or insufficiency accompany nearly every case of adrenogenital syndrome to some extent.

The diagnosis may be made more accurately by using the pneumokidney technique to visualize the area of the adrenal (Fig. 33-17). Injection of carbon dioxide into the perirenal space, followed by roentgenography, facilitates visualization of the adrenal as a triangular or semilunar shadow, located at the upper pole of the kidney. Adrenal hyperplasia by itself produces significant enlargement of the shadow, which can be readily appreciated, and tumors give an even larger image. A detailed description concerning the use of pneumokidney in adrenogenital syndrome may be found in publications by Dogliotti and La Croix[38] as well as Maurer.[83]

Urinary steroid excretion is also characteristic. As already stated above, 17-ketosteroid titers appear to be quite elevated. Amounts of 20 to 60 mg of 17-ketosteroids per 24 hours are average values in adrenal hyperplasia, while figures beyond 60 mg are frankly suspicious of tumor. Estrogen levels are found to be elevated in every case, even when associated with virilism. It would thus appear that predominance of viriliza-

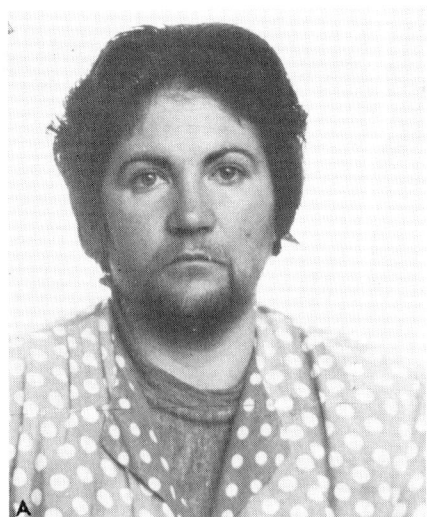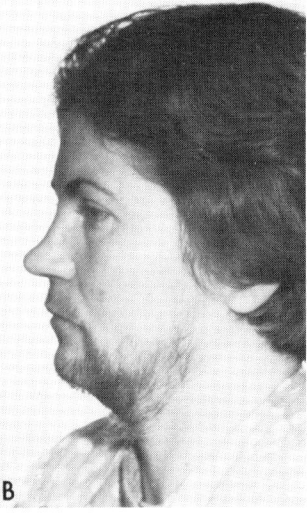

Figure 33-19. Woman, aged 36, para 2, abortions 2, with amenorrhea and progressive hirsutism for two years. 17-Ketosteroid levels, 80 mg/24 hr. Positive reaction of Allen-Patterson. Laparotomy: adrenal carcinoma.

tion over feminization, or vice versa, does not depend so much on exclusively male or female hormone production as instead on simple predominance of either estrogenic or androgenic activity in a situation in which both hormones are present in increased amounts.

Pregnanediol is also frequently elevated, as it was in all cases studied by us in which diol measurements were performed.

The distinction between adrenal tumors and simple adrenal hyperplasia is presently possible by means of the reaction of Patterson[95] or its modification by Allen and his co-workers.[3] *Urinary pregnanetriol* determinations may also be used to study such cases. Finally, according to some authors, such as Lieberman and his co-workers, the diagnosis of adrenogenital syndrome can best be assured on the basis of the steroid formula obtained by chromatography of urinary 17-ketosteroids.

33.2.9. TREATMENT OF ADRENOGENITAL SYNDROME

Treatment of adrenogenital syndrome may be of two types: surgical and hormonal.

SURGICAL TREATMENT. In our original surgical approach, we did not dare to remove but one adrenal,[23] following the norm established by Broster,[27] which was later also supported by Mellikow and Cahill.[84] Unilateral adrenalectomy usually produced an initial favorable response, although soon the contralateral adrenal would undergo hyperplasia and the syndrome would reappear. Thus, for example, in the patient in Figure 33–15, the initial level of 110 mg of total 17-ketosteroids dropped to 38 mg; although none of the subsequent values went below that figure, after several months values returned to as high as 60 mg and the patient had failed to show any improvement in the meantime. Marañón reported a case in which the patient was permanently cured after resection of a unilateral benign tumor. Also, Paiva and his associates[93] reported two similar cases with good results. In patients with malignant tumors, which predominate in the tumor group, unilateral resection produces great improvement, but a relapse of the syndrome may be anticipated owing to usual tumor recurrences, although the contralateral adrenal may remain intact.

A great advance in therapy has been marked by the introduction by Huggins[60] of bilateral adrenalectomy, followed by maintenance corticoid administration, a procedure which has found widespread acceptance.[11, 36, 74, 127] However, mainly for two reasons, this procedure has limited applications: first, because in cases of hyperplasia, endocrine therapy is more effective (see below), and second, because in cases of tumors, which are almost always malignant, the neoplasm is usually not bilateral.

HORMONE THERAPY. With the introduction of *pituitary-suppressive hormone therapy*, radical surgical management now no longer appears to be justified.

In 1949, Lewis and co-workers[77] used methyltestosterone or vinyltestosterone in an attempt to achieve pituitary suppression in cases of adrenogenital syndrome. Although they observed an evident drop in LH production, it did not appear to be of sufficient intensity to affect the clinical picture. Nor were results any better when paraoxypropiophenone was used. On the other hand, much better results were obtained with *cortisone*. In 1950, Wilkins[125, 126] treated a patient with adrenogenital syndrome with cortisone and observed a decrease in the rate of 17-ketosterone excretion. In 1952, the same author[126] attributed the effect of cortisone to pituitary suppression (Fig. 33–20).

Since then, satisfactory results with cortisone therapy, or with therapy based on cortisone derivatives (prednisone, prednisolone, dexamethasone, fluorocortisone, etc.), have been reported by Albright and associates,[1, 2] Venning and colleagues,[121] Migeon and Gardner,[85] Kupperman and associates,[73] Goldberg,[47] Alvarez and Smith,[5] and Goldman and Yacovac.[48]

Bradbury and Slate[26] showed that the mechanism of cortisone action consisted in replacing precisely that steroid whose lack lay at the root of the syndrome. In Figure 33–20, we offer an explanation as to why, in view of the fact that adrenogenital syndrome is caused by a *block in corticoid synthesis*, the only way of eliminating compensatory ACTH hyperactivity is by replacing cortisone, which is lacking.

Concerning dosages, Bradbury advocates the use of 100 mg daily as a starting dose, followed by empirical determination of the dose necessary to keep urinary 17-ketosteroid excretion below 10 mg/24 hr. This

Adrenal Endocrinopathies in Relation to Sex

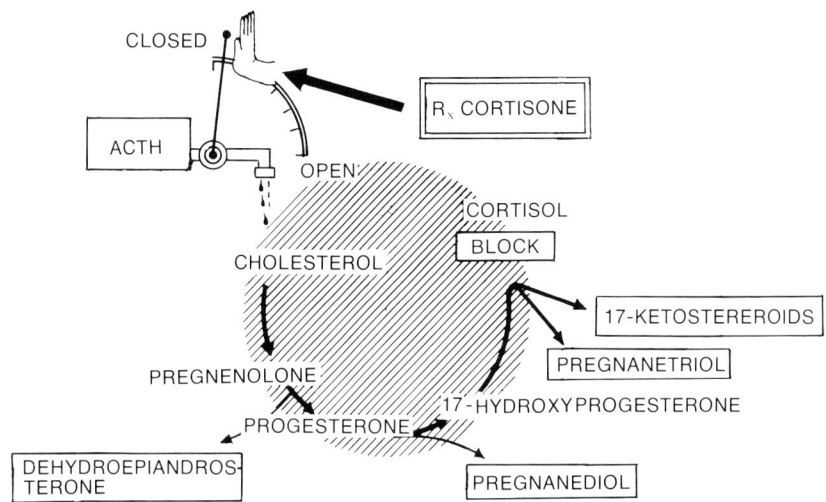

Figure 33–20. Effect of cortisone treatment in adrenogenital syndrome. Cortisone inhibits ACTH secretion and therefore reduces production of 17-ketosteroids and depresses pathologic metabolism of hyperplastic adrenal. Compare with Figure 33–3 to understand why cortisone is ineffective in cases of adrenogenital syndrome resulting from tumor.

dose has been found to usually oscillate within the daily 20 to 25 mg range.

One of the most brilliant examples of how successful cortisone therapy may be has been reported by Wilson and Keating,[129] who not only saw reversion of virilism and *return of menstrual periods* but also witnessed a *pregnancy with full term delivery.* We must admit that our own experience has not been equally encouraging.

In principle, endocrine therapy is contraindicated whenever there are indications for surgery. It is not indicated in cases of adrenal tumors, in which it is not effective, since the action involved is exerted via the pituitary. It is therefore effective only in cases of hyperplasia that have a primary pituitary etiology. Table 33–2 presents the differential features between the two forms.

33.3. OTHER SYNDROMES OF HYPERCORTICISM RELATED TO ADRENOGENITAL SYNDROME

Intimately related to the adrenogenital syndrome are other forms of hypercorticism, mainly *Cushing's syndrome,* which has already been mentioned in Chapter 32, and *Achard-Thiers syndrome,* called *diabetes of bearded women.*

33.3.1. CUSHING'S SYNDROME

The descriptions we offered in Chapter 32 absolve us from having to repeat the clinical description of this endocrine entity. The essential feature of Cushing's syn-

TABLE 33–2

HYPERPLASIA	TUMOR
Slow evolution	Rapid evolution
Increased LH	LH not increased
Urinary 17-ketosteroids not above 60 mg./day	Urinary 17-ketosteroids above 60 mg./day
Pneumoroentgenography: moderate bilateral adrenal enlargement	Pneumoroentgenography: considerable enlargement of one adrenal
Negative Patterson reaction	Positive Patterson reaction
Endocrine therapy	Surgical therapy

drome has been shown in recent years to be the *production of glucocorticoids by the adrenocortical zona fasciculata*. As with adrenogenital syndrome, Cushing's syndrome may be caused either by *hyperplasia* or by *tumor*. Where hyperplasia is involved, it is always secondary to *pituitary basophilism*, that is, to increased production of adrenocorticotropic hormone. Whenever the disease is caused by tumor, it is a *primary adrenal disorder*, brought about by autochthonous forces, without involvement of any pituitary reaction. As we know them from clinical descriptions, the symptoms of Cushing's disease are not related directly to pituitary basophilism but rather are related to hyperfunction of the metabolic adrenal cortex.[54, 61, 99] To a certain degree, Cushing's syndrome is opposed to adrenogenital syndrome, much in the same way that the metabolic zone of the adrenal cortex counteracts the sexual cortex, described by us as third gonad. To emphasize the existing differences as well as analogies between Cushing's disease and adrenogenital syndrome, we have listed the relevant facts in Table 33-3.

Despite the apparent independence of the two forms of hypercorticism, sexual and metabolic, in some instances the two forms may be combined. In this respect, we have already alluded to the frequent observation of obesity and gigantism occurring in children simultaneously with adrenogenital syndrome, which are nothing else than incipient manifestations of Cushing's disease. The fact that Cushing's disease may frequently be associated with features of virilization (Fig. 33-21) has similarly been pointed out in Chapter 32.

33.3.2. ACHARD-THIERS SYNDROME

In 1921, two French authors described under the name of *diabetes of bearded women* (diabète des femmes à barbe) a clinical entity characterized by virilism, with growth of a beard, obesity, hypertension and diabetes (Fig. 33-22). Evidently, what they described is a fairly harmonious combination of Cushing's syndrome and adrenogenital syndrome. Consequently, the syndrome must be assumed to involve a condition of *panhypercorticism*. Similar cases of virilism with diabetes had already been described in 1920 by Kraus and were later reported mainly by Shepardson and Shapiro,[105] Kepler and Mason[67] and Goldzieher.[52] There is as yet no consensus regarding the genesis of the syndrome. It was originally thought to be of either pituitary or metabolic origin. Over the past years, instead, the opinion of Goldzieher according to which the condition results from a form of total hypercorticism, has gained increasing acceptance. This opinion is shared by us. In fact, we believe that the name of diabetes of bearded women served in the past to include all cases that were intermediate forms between Cushing's syndrome and adrenogenital syndrome.

33.3.3. ADRENOGENITAL SYNDROME AND ADDISON'S DISEASE

Representing a form of hypercorticism, adrenogenital syndrome is actually the opposite of Addison's disease which, on the

TABLE 33-3. Differential Diagnosis Between Adrenocortical Syndrome and Cushing's Syndrome

ADRENOGENITAL SYNDROME	CUSHING'S SYNDROME
Produced by pathologic proliferation of the *sexual cortex*	Produced by pathologic proliferation of the *metabolic cortex*
Hyperproduction of 17-ketosteroids, estrogens and progesterone	Hyperproduction of corticoids, sometimes also 17-ketosteroids and other mineralocorticoids
Fuchsinophilia and sudanophobia of tissue involved	Sudanophilia and fuchsinophobia of tissue involved, whether hyperplastic or neoplastic.
Growth stimulated by luteinizing hormone (LH)	Growth stimulated by corticotropin (ACTH)
Produces sexual symptoms, no metabolic symptoms	Produces metabolic symptoms, no sexual symptoms

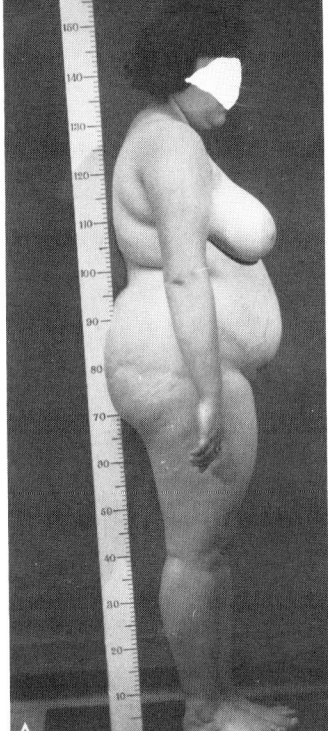
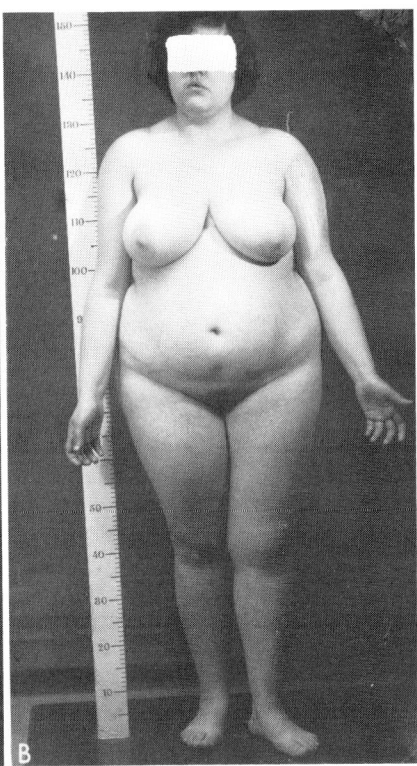

Figure 33-21. Cushing's syndrome in 27 year old woman, who had suffered from amenorrhea for five years. There was also progressively worsening obesity with striations, and hypertension. 17-Ketosteroid levels, 30 mg/24 hr; 11-oxysteroids, 18 mg/24 hr.

contrary, is due to cortical insufficiency. Nevertheless, existing dissociation between sexual zone and metabolic zone function makes it possible to anticipate the occurrence of conditions in which metabolic hypofunction may be combined with sexual hyperfunction, or vice versa. Such would seem to be the case, observed by some, in which exuberant proliferation of the sexual cortex stifles growth of the zona fasciculata, giving rise to adrenogenital syndrome in conjunction with Addison's disease. Figure 33-11 exemplifies a case in which the fascicular layer is smothered by hyperplasia of the sexual zone. Similarly, the surgeon Broster[27] had already called attention to the fact that many of his patients tended to develop acute hypocorticism. Instances in which hirsutism concurred with adrenal insufficiency were reported by Wilkins[126, 127] and by Thelander.[114] Finally, Camacho and co-workers[29] reported a case of adrenogenital syndrome that was associated with marked cortical hyperplasia, in which nevertheless death occurred under conditions of acute adrenocortical insufficiency.

Autopsy findings in such cases have been described by Lewis and his associates.[77, 78] Apart from hyperplasia of the zona reticularis, these usually consisted of flattening and destruction of the zona fasciculata.

What originally may have seemed to be an incomprehensible anomaly turned out to be an almost natural phenomenon in light of its enzymatic etiology. Indeed, it would only be natural that, if the syndrome is caused by a block in cortisol production, it should be similar to Addison's syndrome. *This condition results from insufficiency of the "metabolic cortex" in conjunction with hyperplasia of the "sexual zone."*

33.3.4. FALSE CONGENITAL ADRENOGENITAL SYNDROME

In reality, this entity does not belong here except for purposes of *differential diagnosis*. It consists of virilization of fetuses as a result of administration of nortestosterone-derived progestogens[62, 91, 112, 127] to their mothers during the first three months of gestation. This problem has been dealt with in Chapter 3. Figure 33-23 illustrates a case in which an erroneous diagnosis led to corticoid therapy, resulting in iatrogenic Cush-

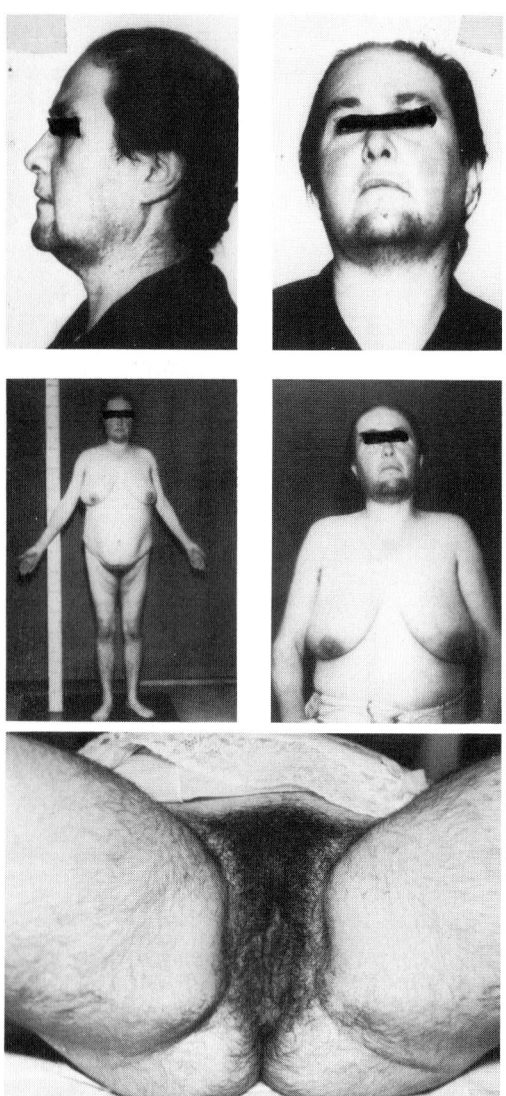

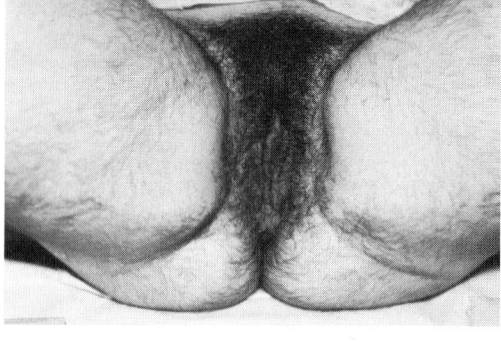

Figure 33–22. Woman, aged 40, suffering from virilization, secondary amenorrhea, and insulin-resistant diabetes (syndrome of Achard-Thiers).

Figure 33–23. Six month old girl whose mother was treated with 19-norpregneninolone during pregnancy because of threatened abortion. At birth, virilism was erroneously diagnosed as congenital adrenogenital syndrome. Treatment with hydrocortisone produced cushingoid obesity, iatrogenic in nature.

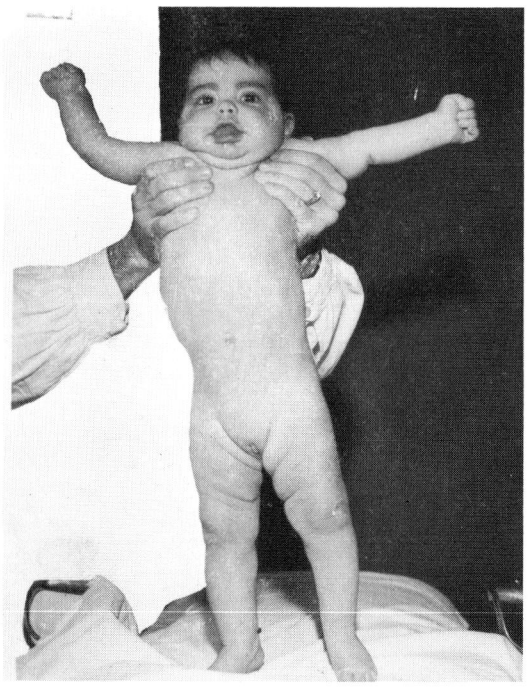

ing's syndrome. *Our purpose here is to warn of the danger of such mistaken diagnosis.*

33.4. CORTICAL INSUFFICIENCY OF THE SEXUAL ZONE

The metabolic adrenal has long been considered as the only representative of physiologic adrenal function. Although hyperfunctional syndromes of the sexual adrenal have been known to occur for some time, the question of hypofunction involving the same segment of the gland has been completely ignored. For many years, the clinician has known of the existence of metabolic adrenal insufficiency or Addison's disease. The disorder was once thought to be almost invariably due to tuberculous destruction of the cortex, involving the glomerular, fascicular and, of course, the reticular zones. Notwithstanding destruction of the three zones of the adrenal cortex, including the sexual zone, the resulting clinical picture seldom involves sexual symptomatology. This results from the fact that the disease usually supervenes during adult life, when the third gonad no longer plays any role in regulating sexual processes, and any resulting nonfunction of the sexual adrenal therefore produces no manifestations. Insufficiency of the sexual adrenal becomes apparent only during phases of third gonad activity, such as the period of embryonal development, and during puberty, pregnancy, castration and the climacterium. Of all moments at which cortical insufficiency may become manifest, the embryonal period is of greatest significance. Defective development of the sexual adrenal, or paleocortex, during the embryonic era gives rise to a syndrome of faulty differentiation of sex, designated by us *syndrome of congenital cortical insufficiency.*

33.4.1. SYNDROME OF CONGENITAL CORTICAL INSUFFICIENCY

It had long been suspected that the adrenal cortex and the thymus in anencephalic fetuses were the sites of some anomalies. In 1942, Botella[22] described four cases of anencephaly, all revealing atrophy of the adrenal cortex and hyperplasia of the thymus. In 1951, Decio and Centaro[34] published a detailed description of the endocrine system in anencephaly. In it, the *adrenal* was described as undergoing atrophy, which was all the more pronounced in degree the closer the fetus was to term. The *adrenal medulla* similarly was found to be very scant or absent. The *pancreas, thymus and testes* were generally within normal limits, whereas *ovarian development was delayed.* Hyperplasia of the thymus was so conspicuous that the gland was often twice its normal size. Finally, the anterior pituitary was well developed, while the neurohypophysis and the hypothalamus revealed significant changes.

A year later, Török[115] reported similar findings in the endocrine system of 20 cases of anencephaly. In 1953, Herlant[56] published a careful study of the pituitary in one case. The adenohypophysis was well preserved although some cell lines had disappeared. The neurohypophysis had failed to develop and hypothalamic centers alike were rudimentary. The adrenal cortex and the ovaries showed hypoplasia, whereas the thyroid appeared within normal limits. The occurrence of thymic hyperplasia and adrenocortical atrophy in such cases was subsequently confirmed by Biressi and his associates[18a] who, in addition, reported evidence of increased thyroid function.

Nichols and colleagues,[92] in 1956, denied the occurrence of adrenal atrophy in anencephaly. In three cases of anencephalic fetuses studied, he found that adrenals were normal. Shortly thereafter, Benirschke[14] was able to clarify the apparent contradiction. In young fetuses, the adrenals undergo atrophy and are impaired, particularly from the twentieth week onwards, and even more so after the twenty-eighth week. It would thus appear that the adrenals in anencephalic fetuses first develop in a normal fashion but then, from the fifth month until term, are subject to atrophy.

Bearn[13] disputed the origin of thymic hyperplasia. In his view, it was secondary to adrenal atrophy, since intact adrenal function seemed to be a necessary prerequisite for thymic involution.

Studies aimed at elucidating the cause of adrenal atrophy, which according to all indications is not primary but secondary in nature, have been undertaken by Kind[68] Anderson and associates,[6] and Tuchmann-Duplessis and Laroche.[116] The last-mentioned workers first demonstrated that the anterior pituitary was well developed whereas the hypothalamohypophysial connections were altered. Subsequently, Tuchmann-Duplessis and his group[117] were able to show that the secretory granules of the neurohypophysis were absent. In a later study,[118] in which they compared the findings in 19 anencephalic cases with those found in cases of hydrocephalus, they were able to implicate lack of ACTH as the cause of adrenal atrophy in anencephalous fetuses. Lack of ACTH activity stems in turn from lack of neurosecretion necessary to provoke ACTH release by the anterior lobe. ACTH is well known to be required for the maintenance of overall adrenal trophism and, hence, in its absence, the adrenal undergoes atrophy.

One more question concerning the endocrine problems related to anencephaly remains to be examined. Urinary 17-ketosteroids during the last months of gestation are generally assumed to be derived from the fetal adrenal. DiGeorge and his coworkers[37] have shown that 17-ketosteroid elimination in pregnancies of anencephalic fetuses was normal but that plasma 17-ketosteroid levels in newborn anencephalous fetuses might be elevated. The apparent paradox was attributed by the authors to increased placental production of 17-ketosteroids.

Frandsen and Stakeman[42] showed that the excretion of large amounts of estrogens toward the end of pregnancy was also largely of fetal adrenal origin. Concerning the anencephalous fetuses studied, they found that urinary estrogen values in their mothers were within normal limits. Because these findings did not correlate well with evidence of adrenal atrophy, MacDonald and Siiteri[81] studied placental function in cases of anencephaly. As a result, it was found that placental estrogen synthesis was enhanced, thus compensating for loss of adrenal estrogen synthesis. This phenomenon is similar to that observed by DiGeorge and his associates with regard to 17-ketosteroids. Ten Berge[113] studied placental endocrine function in several cases of anencephaly. In each case, the placenta produced excessive amounts of estrogens.

Furthermore, Zander and his colleagues[133] studied adrenal progesterone metabolism in anencephalous fetuses, finding significant changes and reporting that most progesterone produced in these cases was of placental rather than adrenal origin.

It may be concluded that the discrepancy observed between adrenal atrophy in anencephaly and seemingly unaltered steroidogenesis in pregnancies with anencephaly is only apparent. The reason for the apparent paradox lies in a compensatory increase in placental steroidogenesis in cases with anencephaly.

Experimentally, Van Wyk and his colleagues[120] achieved similar results by transecting the pituitary stalks in live embryonal rats.

Some investigators have indicated the existence of a certain degree of genital infantilism in children and youngsters with congenital or constitutional cortical hypoplasia. In reports by Kyle and O'Donovan,[74] as well as by Albright and colleagues,[1,2] both published in 1950, such an assessment was based on the finding of low urinary 17-ketosteroid values in cases of genital infantilism. Moeri,[88] who in 1951 confirmed the findings reported by us in 1942, similarly maintains that defective embryonal development of the sexual cortex may be the cause of congenital anomalies affecting the genital tract.

33.4.2. SEXUAL CORTICAL INSUFFICIENCY DURING PUBERTY

Albright and associates[1] believe that the adrenal cortex of puberty plays an important role in the appearance of *pubic hair*. In their view, cases of ovarian insufficiency without sexual cortical insufficiency reveal no lack of either pubic or axillary hair development. In cases with the syndrome of primary ovarian insufficiency, Philipp[97] found very low 17-ketosteroid values and attributed that finding to the presence of *constitutional adrenocortical insufficiency*. It seems therefore likely that the adrenal cortex of puberty cooperates with the gonad in the development of maturity and, particularly, in inducing characteristic sexual hair growth. If associated with gonadal insufficiency during puberty, adrenal insufficiency could possibly inhibit hair growth and, at the same time, might well be responsible for low urinary 17-ketosteroid values observed in such cases.

33.4.3. DURING PREGNANCY

The adrenal cortex plays an important role during pregnancy (see Chapter 19) in substituting for corpus luteum function, particularly during the critical transition period between corpus luteum decay and development of progestogen synthesizing function by the placenta. It thus serves as an important relay necessary for preventing interruption of progesterone production. This aspect shall be emphasized in Chapter 42, which is concerned with the genesis of abortion. *Insufficiency of the sexual adrenal cortex may obviously be the cause of early abortion.*

33.4.4. DURING THE CLIMACTERIUM AND IN CASTRATION

The sexual zone is responsible for estrogen secretion after cessation of ovarian activity. This type of estrogenic compensation is established to offset the effects of postmenopausal estrogen deficiency. It is a well known fact that the behavior of estrogens during the climacterium is subject to great individual variations. As pointed out in Chapter 18, some women reveal marked postmenopausal disorders, with endometrial and vaginal atrophy, while others show viable endometrial patterns and adequate proliferative activity of the vaginal epithelium long after menopause. Such differences may be ascribed to variations in adrenal function. It may be asserted that *adrenal sexual insufficiency causes aggravation of postmenopausal symptomatology.*

REFERENCES

1. Albright, F., Forbes, A. P., and Griswold, C. G.: *J. Clin. Endocr.*, 10:230, 1950.
2. Albright, F., Fraser, R., and Smith, P. H.: *Amer. J. Med. Sci.*, 204:625, 1942.
3. Allen, W. M., Hayward, S. J., and Pinto, A.: *J. Clin. Endocr.*, 10:54, 1950.
4. Altman, N. H., Street, C. S., and Terner, J. Y.: *Amer. J. Veter. Res.*, 30:583, 1969.
5. Alvarez, R. R., and Smith, E. K.: *Obstet. Gynec.*, 9:426, 1957.
6. Anderson, A. B. M., Turnbull, A. C., and Laurence, K. M.: *J. Obstet. Gynec. Brit. Comm.*, 76:196, 1969.
7. Axelrod, L. R., and Goldzieher, J. W.: *J. Clin. Endocr. Metab.*, 20:238, 1960.
8. Axelrod, L. R., and Goldzieher, J. W.: *Acta Endocr.*, 56:543, 1967.
9. Ayres, P. J., et al.: *Biochem. J.*, 65:22, 1957.
10. Azerad, E., Baulieu, E., and Jayle, M. F.: *Ann. d'Endocr.*, 14:505, 1953.
11. Bacon, F. E., and Lowrey, G. H.: *J. Clin. Endocr.*, 25:1403, 1965.
12. Bayer, L. M., and Koets, D.: *Amer. J. Med. Sci.*, 222:13, 1951.
13. Bearn, J.: *Proc. Soc. Exper. Biol. Med.*, 122:273, 1951.
14. Benirschke, K.: *Obstet. Gynec.*, 8:412, 1956.
15. Bennett, S. H.: *Amer. J. Anat.*, 67:151, 1940.
16. Berardinelli, W., et al.: *J. Clin. Endocr. Metab.*, 16:674, 1956.
17. Bentinck, R. C., Lisser, H., and Reilly, W. A.: *J. Clin. Endocr. Metab.*, 16:412, 1956.
18. Bergstrand, C. G., and Gemzell, C. A.: *J. Clin. Endocr. Metab.*, 17:871, 1957.
18a. Biressi, P. C., Scorta, A., and Parito, G.: *Folia Endocr.*, 15:74, 1962.
19. Blunck, W., and Bierich, J. R.: *Acta Paediat. Scand.*, 57:157, 1968.
20. Bongiovanni, A. M.: *Bull. Johns Hopkins Hosp.*, 92:244, 1953.
21. Bongiovanni, A. M., Elberlein, W. R., and Cara, J.: *J. Clin. Endocr. Metab.*, 14:409, 1954.
22. Botella, J.: *Arch. Esp. Morfol.*, 2:151, 1942.
23. Botella, J.: "La Tercera Gonada," *Suprarrenales y Función Sexual.* Madrid, Morata, 1946.
24. Botella, J., and Cano, A.: *Gynaecologia*, 124:166, 1947.
25. Botella, J.: *Arch. Gynäk*, 183:73, 1953.
26. Bradbury, J. T., and Slate, W. G.: *J. Clin. Endocr. Metab.*, 15:1291, 1955.
27. Broster, L. R.: *Adrenal Cortex and Intersexuality.* London, Chapman & Hall, 1938.
28. Camacho, A. M., and Migeon, C. J.: *J. Clin. Endocr. Metab.*, 26:893, 1966.
29. Camacho, A. M., Kowarsky, A., Migeon, C. J., and Brough, J.: *J. Clin. Endocr. Metab.*, 28:153, 1968.
30. Chalmers, W.: *J. Clin. Endocr.*, 9:941, 1949.
31. Chang, C. Y., and Witschi, E.: *Endocrinology*, 56:597, 1955.
32. Chen, P. S., et al.: *Proc. Soc. Exp. Biol. Med.*, 97:683, 1958.
33. Crooke, A. C., and Callow, R. K.: *Quart. J. Med.*, 32:233, 1939.
34. Decio, C., and Centaro, A.: *Rev. Ost. Gin. (Firenze)*, 6:236, 1951.
35. Devis, R.: *Ann. d'Endocr.*, 10:173, 1949.
36. Diamond, M., and Young, W. C.: *Endocrinology*, 73:429, 1963.
37. DiGeorge, A. M., Arey, J. B., and Bongiovanni, A. M.: *J. Clin. Endocr. Metab.*, 16:1281, 1956.
38. Dogliotti, G. C., and Lacroix, L.: *Recent Progr. Med.*, 42:337, 1967.
39. Editorial: *Presse Medicale*, 2:2359, 1961.
40. Edwards, J. A., Vance, V. K., Cohen, M. M., and Schussler, G. C.: *J. Clin. Endocr.*, 30:666, 1970.
41. Elberlein, W. R., and Bongiovanni, A. M.: *J. Clin. Endocr. Metab.*, 15:1531, 1955.

42. Frandsen, V. A., and Stakeman, G.: *Acta Endocr.*, 47:265, 1964.
43. Frank, R. T.: *Proc. Soc. Exp. Biol. Med.*, 31:1204, 1934.
44. Fukushima, D. K., Bradlow, H. L., Hellman, L., and Gallagher, F. T.: *J. Clin. Endocr. Metab.*, 23:266, 1966.
45. Gebauer, A., and Linke, A.: *Deutsch. Med. Wschr.*, 75:932, 1960.
46. Göbel, P.: *Endokrinologie*, 52:289, 1967.
47. Goldberg, M. B.: *J. Clin. Endocr. Metab.*, 14:389, 1954.
48. Goldman, A. S., and Yacovac, W. C.: *Proc. Soc. Exp. Biol. Med.*, 122:1214, 1966.
49. Goldman, A. S.: *J. Clin. Endocr.*, 28:231, 1968.
50. Goldman, A. S., and Winter, J. D. S.: *J. Clin. Endocr.*, 27:1717, 1967.
51. Goldman, A. S.: *Endocrinology*, 85:325, 1969.
52. Goldzieher, M.: *The Adrenal Glands*. Philadelphia, Davies & Co., 1944.
53. Gower, D. B., and Stern, M. I.: *Acta Endocr.*, 60:265, 1969.
54. Gray, C. H., et al.: *J. Clin. Endocr. Metab.*, 16:473, 1956.
55. Hain, A. M.: *J. Path. Bact.*, 59:267, 1947.
56. Herlant, M.: *Ann. d'Endocr.*, 14:889, 1953.
57. Herweg, J. C., Ackermann, L. W., and Allen, W. M.: *J. Clin. Endocr.*, 6:275, 1946.
58. Hooft, C., et al.: *Ann. d'Endocr.*, 17:1, 1956.
59. Howard, E., and Benua, R. S.: *J. Anat.*, 42:157, 1950.
60. Huggins, C.: *J. Urol.*, 68:875, 1952.
61. Ianacone, A., Gabrilove, J. L., Sohval, A. R., and Soffer, L. J.: *New Eng. J. Med.*, 261:775, 1959.
62. Jacobson, B. D.: *Amer. J. Obstet. Gynec.*, 84:962, 1962.
63. Jailer, J. W., Gold, J. W., and Cahill, G. F.: *Amer. J. Obstet. Gynec.*, 67:201, 1954.
64. Jenkins, J. S.: *Biochemical Aspects of the Adrenal Cortex*. London, Arnold, 1968.
65. Keller, M.: *J. Clin. Endocr. Metab.*, 16:1074, 1956.
66. Keller, M.: *Gynaecologia*, 156:259, 1963.
67. Kepler, E. J., and Mason, H. L.: *J. Clin. Endocr.*, 7:553, 1947.
68. Kind, C.: *Helv. Paediat. Acta.*, 17:224, 1962.
69. Kinoshita, K., Isurugi, K., Kunamoto, Y., and Takayasu, H.: *J. Clin. Endocr. Metab.*, 26:1219, 1966.
70. Klotz, P.: *Ann. d'Endocr.*, 22:506, 1961.
71. Kolff, W. J., and Tyook, K. B.: *J. Clin. Endocr.*, 10:270, 1950.
72. Kowal, J., Perloff, W. H., and Soffer, L. J.: *Acta Endocr.*, 44:15, 1963.
73. Kupperman, H. S., Finkler, R., and Burger, J.: *J. Clin. Endocr.*, 12:948, 1952.
74. Kyle, L. H., and Donovan, T. F.: *J. Clin. Endocr.*, 10:370, 1950.
75. Landau, R. L., et al.: *J. Clin. Endocr. Metab.*, 14:1097, 1954.
76. Landing, B. H.: *J. Clin. Endocr. Metab.*, 14:425, 1954.
77. Lewis, R. A., Klein, R., and Wilkins, L.: *J. Clin. Endocr.*, 10:703, 1950.
78. Lewis, R. A., and Rosemberg, E.: *Endocrinology*, 45:564, 1949.
79. Lloyd, C. W., et al.: *J. Clin. Endocr.*, 11:871, 1951.
80. Loras, B., and Migeon, C. J.: *Steroids*, 7:459, 1966.
81. MacDonald, P. C., and Siiteri, P. K.: *J. Clin. Invest.*, 44:465, 1965.
82. Mattox, V. R., et al.: *J. Clin. Endocr. Metab.*, 24:517, 1964.
83. Maurer, H. J.: *Ztschr. Urol.*, 62:481, 1969.
84. Mellikow, M. C., and Cahill, G. F.: *J. Clin. Endocr.*, 10:24, 1950.
85. Migeon, C. J., and Gardner, L. I.: *J. Clin. Endocr.*, 12:1513, 1952.
86. Milcou, S. M., et al.: *Sem. Hôp. Paris*, 36:244, 1960.
87. Minozzi, M., et al.: *Folia Endocr.*, 19:690, 1966.
88. Moeri, E.: *Acta Endocrinol.*, 8:259, 1951.
89. Nandi, J., Bern, H. A., Biglieri, E. G., and Pieprzyk, J. K.: *Endocrinology*, 80:576, 1967.
90. Neelsen, A. A., Pedersen-Bjergaard, T. K., and Tonesser, M.: *Acta Endocr.*, 1:41, 1948.
91. Neumann, F., and Junkmann, K.: *Endocrinology*, 73:33, 1963.
92. Nichols, J., Lescure, O. L., and Migeon, C. J.: *J. Clin. Endocr. Metab.*, 18:444, 1958.
93. Paiva, I. M., Lobo, J. J., and Silva, M.: *J. Clin. Endocr.*, 11:330, 1951.
94. Pasqualini, J., and Jaule, M. F.: *Clin. Chim. Acta.*, 8:283, 1963.
95. Patterson, J.: *Lancet*, 2:580, 1947.
96. Perloff, W. H.: *Internat. J. Fertil.*, 6:21, 1961.
97. Philipp, E.: *Acta Gin.*, 2:49, 1951.
98. Pierson, R. W.: *Endocrinology*, 81:693, 1967.
99. Prezio, J. A., et al.: *J. Clin. Endocr. Metab.*, 24:481, 1964.
100. Printer, K. D.: *J. Obstet. Gynec. Brit. Emp.*, 70:303, 1963.
101. Quint, B. C., Parker, R. T., and Hamblen, E. C.: *Amer. J. Obstet. Gynec.*, 73:206, 1957.
102. Rappaport, R., et al.: *Sem. Hôp. Paris*, 39:637, 1963.
103. Rose, E., et al.: *J. Clin. Endocr.*, 11:798, 1951.
104. Seligman, A. M., and Ashbel, R.: *Endocrinology*, 48:110, 1951.
105. Shepardson, A. C., and Shapiro, E.: *Endocrinology*, 24:237, 1939.
106. Siquier, F., et al.: *Sem. Hôp. Paris*, 39:362, 1963.
107. Slaunwhite, W. R., and Buchwald, K. W.: *J. Clin. Endocr. Metab.*, 20:787, 1960.
108. Snaith, A. H.: *J. Clin. Endocr. Metab.*, 18:318, 1958.
109. Southren, L. A., et al.: *J. Clin. Endocr. Metab.*, 21:675, 1961.
110. Sprague, R. G., et al.: *J. Clin. Endocr.*, 10:289, 1950.
111. Stachenko, J., and Giroud, C. J. P.: *Endocrinology*, 64:443, 1959.
112. Suchowsky, G. K., and Junkmann, C.: *Endocrinology*, 68:340, 1961.
113. Ten Berge, B. S.: *Bull. Roy. Soc. Belg. Gyn. Obst.*, 35:137, 1965.
114. Thelander, H. E.: *J. Paediat.*, 29:213, 1946.
115. Török, J.: *Acta Morphol. (Budapest)*, 1:231, 1952.
116. Tuchmann-Duplessis, H., and Laroche, J.: *Compt. Rend. Soc. Biol.*, 152:300, 1958.
117. Tuchmann-Duplessis, H., and Gabe, M.: *Bull. Acad. Nat. Med. Paris*, 144:102, 1960.
118. Tuchmann-Duplessis, H., and Mercier-Parot, L.: *Compt. Rend. Soc. Biol.*, 157:977, 1963.
119. Vague, J., et al.: *Ann. d'Endocr.*, 28:603, 1967.

120. Van Wyk, J. J., et al.: *J. Clin. Endocr. Metab.*, 20:157, 1960.
121. Venning, E. H., et al.: *J. Clin. Endocr.*, 12:1409, 1952.
122. Vines, H. W. C.: In Broster, L. R.: *Adrenal Cortex and Intersexuality*. London, Chapman & Hall, 1938.
123. Wallach, S., et al.: *J. Clin. Endocr. Metab.*, 17:495, 1957.
124. White, F. P., and Sutton, L. E.: *J. Clin. Endocr.*, 11:1395, 1951.
125. Wilkins, L.: *J. Clin. Endocr.*, 12:277, 1952.
126. Wilkins, L.: *Ann. d'Endocr.*, 19:841, 1958.
127. Wilkins, L.: *J.A.M.A.*, 172:1028, 1960.
128. West, C. D., et al.: *J. Clin. Endocr. Metab.*, 24:567, 1964.
129. Wilson, R. B., and Keating, F. R.: *Amer. J. Obstet. Gynec.*, 76:388, 1958.
130. Wotiz, H. H., Chatoraj, S. C., and Gabrilove, J. L.: *J. Clin. Endocr. Metab.*, 28:192, 1968.
131. Zander, J., and Müller, H. A.: *Geburtsh. Frauenhk.*, 13:16, 1963.
132. Zander, J.: *Klin. Wschr.*, 38:5, 1960.
133. Zander, J., Holtzmann, K., and Bengtsson, L. P.: *Acta Obstet. Gynec. Scand.*, 44:204, 1965.

Chapter 34
ENDOCRINE SYNDROMES OF OTHER GLANDS IN RELATION TO SEX

Although the existing physiologic relationships between various endocrine glands and the ovary were covered in Chapters 7, 9 and 10 in Part One of this book, we discussed only the physiologic aspects involved and have not dealt with clinical problems. It is fitting now for us to examine those clinical syndromes that result from altered internal secretions by glands other than the adrenal and the pituitary. Whereas pituitary and adrenocortical endocrinopathies produce quite ostensible and manifest repercussions in sexual function, this is not true as concerns the other glands of internal secretion which have less constant and rather ill-defined relationships to sexual syndromes. In this chapter, the relationship between endocrine-sexual states and syndromes caused by thyroid, pineal, thymic, pancreatic and parathyroid dysfunction will be discussed. Reference to the adrenal medulla has been omitted, since the syndromes related to it have little bearing on the regulation of sexual function.

34.1. THYROID SYNDROMES

The thyroid, together with the adrenal and the pituitary, is one of the accessory glands of sex. Although the significance of thyroid function insofar as control of sexual activity is concerned has been stressed by, among others, Siegert,[78] the relationship between thyroid syndromes and sexual states is not as direct as it is in the case of the pituitary or adrenal cortex.

34.1.1. GENERALITIES

The possible existence of some ovarian-thyroid synergism had been indicated by various investigators (Botella et al.[16]) many years ago. The question of ovarian-thyroid correlations was later reviewed by Young and his associates[93] and by Krohn and Zuckermann.[52]

The ovary would seem to exert a *stimulatory* effect on the thyroid. In 1936, we found that if rats on a thyroid resting diet were injected with estrogens they developed marked proliferation and subsequent hyperfunction of the gland[16] (see Chapter 10). These observations of ours were later confirmed by Calapa[21] and by Gillman and Gilbert.[40] Gillman and Gilbert demonstrated the stimulatory effect of estrogens on the thyroid of female monkeys. Desclin[25] also corroborated the finding of enlargement and increased functional complexity of the thyroid gland under the influence of estrogens. A complete review of the subject was made in Chapter 2. A great deal of modern research has confirmed the fact that ^{131}I uptake, PBI and thyroxine-binding globulin values are all increased under the action of estrogens, the thyrotropic effect of which can no longer be doubted.

In contrast, progestogens seem to have a damping effect on thyroid function, as found by us in 1935[16] and confirmed by Eskin and associates[29] in 1961. According to Hollander and his colleagues,[47] norethisterone and norethynodrel also inhibit thyroid function.

In the same way, thyroid incretion has a stimulating effect on the ovary. By injecting female rabbits with thyroxine, Maqsood[63] was able to accelerate sexual maturation and provoke ovarian development with hyperluteinization. Stein and Foreman[83] found that thyroxine had a specific mitogenic action on the ovary. Again, Soliman and Reineke[81a] noted how thyroprotein produced ovarian enlargement and accelerated puberty in rats. There may be some argument as to whether this action is a direct one or is mediated by the pituitary. As a result of thorough studies on female monkeys, Gillman and Gilbert[40] believe that the action involved is twofold, on the one hand stimulating luteal hormone secretion, and on the other, having a direct trophic effect on ovarian tissue.

More recently, Adams and Leathem[2] observed that rat ovaries in propylthiouracil-induced hypothyroidism underwent degenerative changes of the type found in the Stein-Leventhal syndrome. This question has been studied in detail in Chapter 10.

Our early ideas postulating that estrogens stimulated whereas progesterone inhibited thyroid function have been confirmed by the recent observations of Man and his associates,[62] as well as by those of Portioli and colleagues,[73] that estrogenic activity resulted in a rise in TBG (thyroxine-binding globulin) values. On the other hand, Brown-Grant[19] found that progesterone reduced ^{131}I uptake by the thyroid. The foregoing findings confirm the stimulatory effect of estrogens and the inhibitory effect of progesterone. Also recently, Nesbitt and his associates,[70] as well as Talanti,[85] have demonstrated that thyroidectomy, or thyroid suppression by means of thiouracil, was followed by lack of ovarian maturation. Recent investigations thus seem to uphold the old hypothesis of ovarian-thyroid synergism, as advanced by Marañón and defended by ourselves.

The effects thyroxine exerts on morphogenetic processes and on embryonic development are well known (see Chapter 10). Some time ago, Koneff and his associates[51] emphasized the role of thyroid function in embryonic morphogenesis. Adams and Bull[1] reported that thyrosuppressive drugs caused abortion. Thyroid hormone would thus seem to be necessary for the development of embryos, so that lack of it leads to the embryo's death, followed by abortion in animals as well as in woman.

Another indirect sex-related thyroid effect is the action of thyrocalcitonin in preventing postmenopausal osteoporosis. Recent investigations[6, 50, 74] underscore the fact that diminished ovarian function during the climacteric period depresses thyroid function, reduces thyrocalcitonin production and contributes to the osteoporosis so often afflicting postmenopausal women.

In summary, it may be said that: (1) *thyroid function is stimulated by estrogens.* (2) *The ovary is stimulated in a similar way by the thyroid.* (3) *Thyroid hormone, being necessary for embryonic development, is indispensable for the normal course and development of pregnancy.* (4) It must not be forgotten that thyroid function is controlled by pituitary thyrotropic hormone which, together with other pituitary functions, is influenced by sex hormone activity.

34.1.2. HYPOTHYROID SYNDROMES

The principal thyroid syndromes to be considered here are: (1) Thyroid cretinism and dwarfism, (2) myxedema, (3) strumiprival cachexia, (4) hypothyroidism induced by antithyroid drugs.

CRETINISM. Congenital thyroid hypofunction is well known to appear in an endemic or sporadic fashion. Usually, though not invariably, it is associated with cretinism and infantilism (Fig. 34–1).

MYXEDEMA. Myxedema is due to thyroid insufficiency acquired at any time in life. While there is a constitutional type of myxedema, characterized by thyroid hypoplasia or, as called by Kocher, *thyropenia*, myxedema is most often the result of secondary thyroid atrophy developing in the course of life. Myxedema may develop in the infantile or puberal period (*juvenile myxedema*), or it may appear in adults (*adult myxedema*).

STRUMIPRIVAL CACHEXIA. This is a condition that develops following surgical extirpation of the thyroid, whenever the amount of functioning tissue left behind is insufficient.

SUBCLINICAL FORMS OF HYPOTHYROIDISM. These are of special interest in gynecology, since they may only become apparent because of habitual abortion, infertility and occasionally amenorrhea, without causing any other symptoms or any noticeable physical changes (Fig. 34–2).

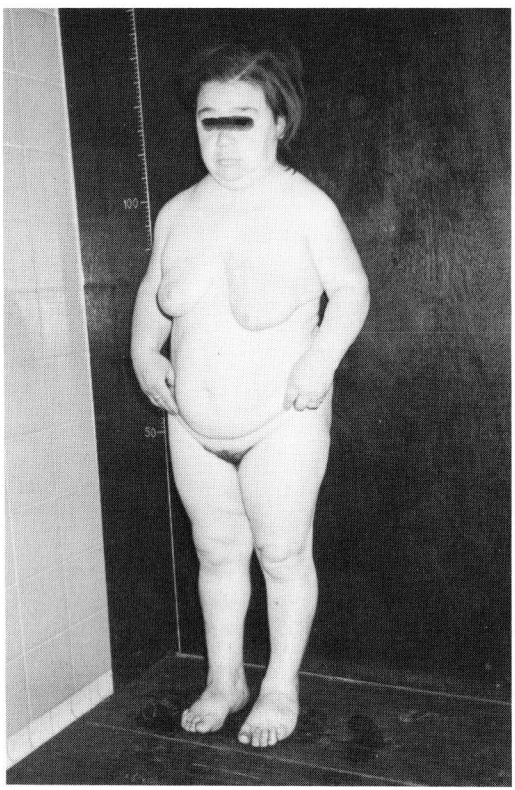

Figure 34-1. Cretin, with dwarfism. Aged 30; height, 130 cm. Essential amenorrhea, with pubic and axillary hair growth and breast development.

SECONDARY THYROID ATROPHY. Finally, attention must be focused on *secondary thyroid atrophy*, observed with increasing frequency in modern clinical experience, which is caused by abusive use of antithyroid drugs (thiouracil) or by overdosification of radioisotopes (^{131}I).

It is of interest to note that 80 per cent of all thyroid syndromes occur in women, according to data supplied by Eiselsberg,[27] whereas according to Luca,[59] the figure is even higher (90 per cent). Myxedema occurs much less commonly in males. Whenever hypothyroidism develops in childhood, the main symptoms comprise *arrest of somatic development*, as well as *arrest of mental development*, disproportionate and flat-boned skeleton, broad, flattened nasal bone, saccular edema of lower eyelids, stocky and short neck, short hands and, on X-rays, incomplete development of ossification centers.

Thyroid lesions developing in adulthood are associated with *hypothyroid adiposity*, weight gain, and abundant fat panniculus, particularly in the vulvar, supraclavicular and iliac regions. Nonpitting edema appears above all in the eyelids, nose and lips, and the patients show a *moon face*.

Apart from the characteristic changes just mentioned, important manifestations become apparent in relation to *sexual function*. First of all, the patients display either primary or secondary hypoplasia of the genital apparatus, with ovarian atrophy, and consequently present the picture of *hypogenitalism with amenorrhea*. In some cases, the symptoms are more discrete and only oligo- or hypomenorrhea is noted. One of the foremost complaints in such cases is *infertility*. Thyroid-related infertility had already been recognized by authorities in this field, and the thyroid is currently considered to be of great significance in the pathogenesis of infertility (Williams,[91] Botella[14]). Hypothyroid females are prone to have *abortions* (Slater et al.[80]), owing to loss of the morphogenetic action by thyroxine on the embryo (see Chapter 10). The role of hypothyroidism in the genesis of infertility and abortion shall be dealt with more extensively in Chapters 40 and 41.

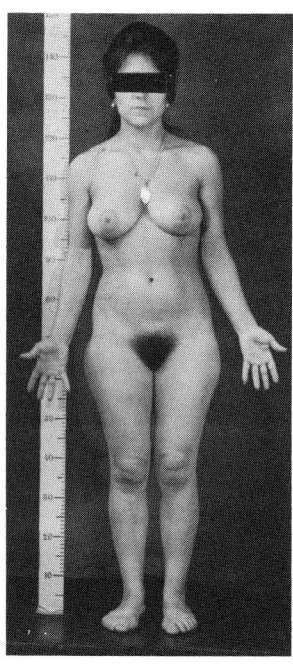

Figure 34-2. Woman, aged 26, with secondary amenorrhea of two years' duration. Basal metabolic rate, −28. Patient was treated exclusively with thyroid extract, with reestablishment of menses. There were no somatic alterations, nor were there any other symptoms.

Endocrine Syndromes of Other Glands in Relation to Sex

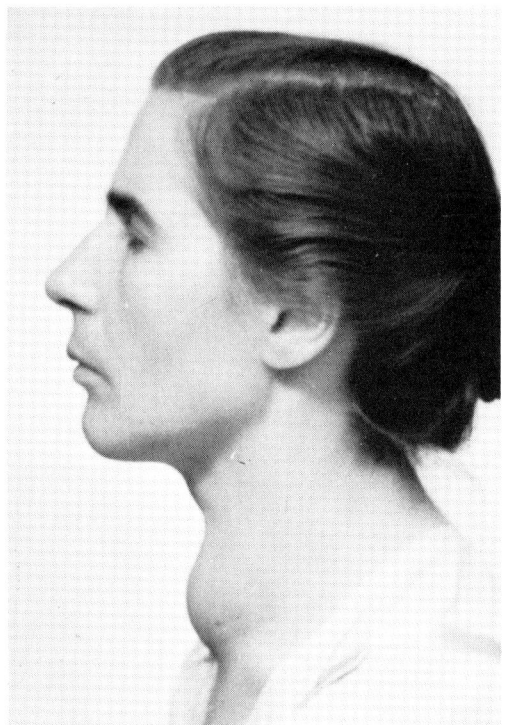

Figure 34-3. Goiter presenting without thyrotoxicosis or exophthalmos in a woman, aged 33, with secondary amenorrhea. Patient had been married for five years and suffered from infertility.

Important advances have also been made in exploring the question of sexual disturbances as a consequence of hypothyroidism. Mavromati[65] studied *menstrual patterns* in women with thyroid insufficiency. Such patients usually suffer from amenorrhea or hypomenorrhea and reveal endometrial hypoplasia, as well as changes in follicular maturation and corpus luteum formation. In most instances, particularly in young patients, thyroid therapy results in total reestablishment of cyclic ovarian function, with regular menstruation. Aeppli[3] conducted serial cytologic studies on seven hypothyroid women presenting with a history of hypomenorrhea and infertility. Contrary to what might be expected, vaginal cytology failed to reveal any evidence of hypoestrinism, suggesting instead persistence of follicular phase activity, with increased numbers of estrogenic cells and absence of luteal elements. Similar findings have been reported by Gillman and Gilbert,[40] who had studied the effects of thyroidectomy on estrus and menstruation in female monkeys. They further found that thyroidectomized animals often revealed persistent follicles and endometrial patterns consistent with cystic glandular hyperplasia. They concluded that the principal action of thyroid hormone on the ovaries consisted in stimulating luteinization. The trophic stimulus by thyroxine, as already mentioned in the preceding paragraph, seems to be necessary for normal corpus luteum development. This is also supported by Aeppli's findings that hypothyroidism was cytologically associated with persistent follicular smears.

Thorsöe[87] and Lupulesco and his colleagues[60] studied the ovarian histology of women who either had been thyroidectomized or had degenerative goiters. They found a high incidence of large polycystic ovaries similar to those seen in Stein-Leventhal syndrome, which is in agreement with the already mentioned observations in rats by Adams and Leathem, and which is also in keeping with the occurrence of anovulatory cycles, as reported by others.

In the studies by Lederer[56] concerning estrogen elimination in cases of hypothyroidism, it has been further noted that conditions of either hyperestrinism or hypoestrinism may be present. The association of *hypothyroidism with hypoestrinism* is predominantly observed in the older age groups, especially in menopausal women. *In contrast, young women usually present with evidence of associated hyperestrinism* from lack of corpus luteum formation, related to thyroid deficiency. However, it must be borne in mind that, rather than being absolute, this is a *relative form of hyperestrinism*, or hyperestrinism of rhythm, such as occurs whenever, in the absence of increased estrogen production, there is loss of corpus luteum function.

While studying the mechanism involved in infertility of hypothyroid origin, Dickerson[26] became aware of the unusually high incidence of either anovulatory or aluteal cycles, which, in his view, were the main reason for infertility in these conditions. The fact that some cases should reveal ovarian atrophy while others should be associated with follicular persistence or with aluteinism is not, in our opinion, a contradictory finding. After all, what we are dealing with is *variations in degree of ovarian insufficiency. The corpus luteum is the most complex and difficult of all structures for the ovary to produce.* In the presence of even the slightest degree of functional deficit of the female gonad, the first thing to become apparent is inability to achieve luteinization. Only if the degree of gonadal insufficiency reaches major proportions does lack of maturation become noticeable and atrophy of the gland evident. The action exerted by the thyroid on the ovary, we therefore believe, is relatively nonspecific in nature, causing loss of ability to form corpora lutea in mild forms of thyroid deficiency as compared to complete loss of ovarian maturation in severe forms. This explains why minor degrees of thyroid insufficiency are associated with infertility due to anovulation, without ostensible menstrual manifestations, whereas serious thyroid insufficiency causes amenorrhea and leads to a complete developmental arrest of the genital apparatus.

34.1.3. HYPERTHYROIDISM

The principal clinical forms of hyperthyroidism are Basedow's disease, basedowoid or thyrotoxic conditions and hyperthyroid emaciation. A feature common to all foregoing conditions is the fact that *they affect females far more frequently than males*. According to different statistical data (Kehrer[49]), between 85 and 92 per cent of all cases occur in women. The majority of cases appear during the reproductive span between ages 20 and 40.

As far back as 1929, Lisser called attention to the occurrence of menstrual irregularities in hyperthyroid women. The disorder most frequently observed was proio- and hypermenorrheic menstruation. Zondek and Koehler[94] later described the occurrence of metrorrhagia. On the other hand, Kehrer[49] reported complete absence of menstruation in cases of Basedow's disease. Lederer,[56] whose subsequent studies were concerned with the same question, found that, while menstrual bleeding was aggravated in benign conditions of hyperthyroidism, patients with severe cases of thyrotoxicosis developed amenorrhea. Consequently, it may be stated that *conditions with minor degrees of hyperthyroidism are associated with prolonged and profuse menstrual bleeding, whereas serious cases of hyperthyroidism present with amenorrhea*.

It seems relevant to point out that Larson and his colleagues[55] observed *gynecomastia* in hyperthyroid males; this may be construed as indicative of the fact that the estrogenizing action by thyroid hormone is exerted on the male as well as on the female. Long ago, Marañón had spoken of the "feminizing" action of the thyroid.

Dyspareunia, frigidity and sex instinct deviation are common findings in hyperthyroid women. Even though classical writers attributed similar aberrant psychosexual tendencies to hyperthyroidism itself and to its influence on the nervous system, these tendencies currently are believed to reflect *primary neurogenic* alterations that, while modifying the sexual instinct, at the same time provoke central stimulation of the thyroid (centrogenous Basedow's disease).

In addition, hyperthyroidism may be the consequence of enhanced psychosexual excitation by way of the ovary. The hyperthyrogenous action by estrogens has already been mentioned earlier in this chapter, as well as in Chapter 10. In some cases of permanent psychosexual excitation, such as those produced by pelvic congestion, the presence of either constant or sporadic hyperestrinism may lead to thyroid stimulation. Gianaroli and Civicchi[39] have studied vaginal cytology in syndromes of hyperthyroidism and were able to observe variations in estrogen levels by means of this indirect procedure. Although some hyperthyroid women, to be sure, reveal elevated estrogenic activity, what is apparently observed much more often is a tendency to a continuous, rather than quantitative increase, in estrogen secretion, coupled with a loss of ovarian cyclicity. We therefore believe that many instances of metrorrhagia or menorrhagia in hyperthyroid women actually stem from *alterations of the cycle* rather than from any absolute increase in estrogen levels.

Another, at least indirect, link between thyroid function and the ovary may be suggested by the finding of *uterine myomas*. The coincidence of myomas with hyperthyroidism has been observed with relative frequency (Botella[13]). It has been advanced as a clinical argument favoring the existence of a follicular-thyroid synergism. In fact, as has already been pointed out in Chapter 28, myomas are known to be, if not always, at least quite often related to conditions of hyperestrogenism. To us, the hyperthyroidism observed in cases of myomata is the result of thyroid stimulation from excessive estrogenic activity.

A very important clinical aspect of thyroid disease in relation to sex is development of hyperthyroidism during the climacterium (Marañón[64]). *Climacteric hyperthyroidism* has often been quoted as evidence against the existence of such a follicle-thyroid synergism. However, modern knowledge concerning the nature of endocrine changes during the era of sexual decline would indicate just the opposite, namely, that far from militating against it, this finding constitutes proof in favor of the synergism concept. In our own experience, indeed, women in the postmenopausal age group have a high incidence of hyperestrinism, if not of quantity, at least of rhythm. This question has already been discussed in Chapter 17. The endocrine processes related to the pathologic climacterium are still to be analyzed (Chapter 39).

34.1.4. THYROIDOPATHIES AND GESTATION

The present problem will have to be examined in a little more detail in connection with infertility and abortion (Chapters 41 and 42). Disturbances of thyroid function (hypo- or hyperfunction) may seriously interfere with gestation.

HYPOTHYROIDISM. Hypothyroid women are often *sterile*. Many cases of infertility respond favorably to thyroid therapy,[12, 14, 91] even though the diagnosis of hypothyroidism may not have been substantiated by laboratory means. In addition, as many abortions are produced[49, 78] as cases that respond to thyroid treatment. A further frequent complication of hypothyroidism may be late, even intrapartum, fetal death.

HYPERTHYROIDISM. On the other hand, hyperthyroidism seems to be better tolerated in pregnancy. Pregnant women show heightened tolerance to thyroxine,[4, 6, 48] probably because of increased fetal requirements for thyroid hormone (considering morphogenetic embryonal activity) and possibly also because the high state of readiness of the remainder of the incretory system compensates for and balances out any increase in thyroid function. This question has been discussed in Chapter 20. Seitz and Engelhorn (see Chapter 10) believed that hyperthyroidism was aggravated by gestation, but Marañón insisted that the contrary was true. Based on our own experience, we concur with the latter. Upon becoming pregnant—which they do with much greater facility than hypothyroid women—hyperthyroid women usually experience initial difficulties, owing to nausea, vomiting, malaise, serious asthenia and acidosis. However, once they pass the critical phase in the third or fourth month, they may be expected to improve steadily, so that, by term, they usually feel better than ever. The postpartum nearly always marks the beginning of a relapse.

Active thyroid substances pass through the placental barrier (see Chapter 20), as has been shown over and over again by, among others, Roy and Kobayashi[76] and Hamburg and his associates.[44] Quite recently, however, Fisher and his colleagues,[33] though admitting that this was true, voiced the belief that passage of such substances was hindered by increased amounts of thyroxine-binding globulin in the maternal blood if thyroid hormone was injected into the mother. However, in most cases of gestation with hyperthyroidism, this globulin factor hindering free thyroxine passage does not exist, so that the fetal blood may to a considerable extent be flooded with thyroxine.

The existence of a *conditional state of parabiosis* between the maternal and fetal bodies has been pointed out in Chapter 20. Herbst and Selenkow[45] believe that in these cases atrophy of the fetal thyroid is a possibility and may be aggravated by therapeutic administration of thiouracil to the mother. Thiouracil is known to cross the placental barrier. For this reason, the most prudent course of action is *not to administer thiouracil to a pregnant woman under any circumstances*, but rather to apply mild thyroid therapy to the newborn.

34.2. PINEAL SYNDROMES

Much about the pineal is still obscure. Even its incretory character is doubted by many. In view of its poorly known physiology and, in the absence of any demonstrable incretion peculiar to that gland, the physiopathologic relationship between the pineal and sexual function is questionable, and available data are contradictory.

34.2.1. GENERAL CONSIDERATIONS

Our present concept of pineal physiology is based on studying (1) the effects of pinealectomy, (2) the effects produced either by pineal transplants or by injections of pineal extracts, and (3) the symptomatology associated with pineal tumors. All three criteria are extremely unreliable. Pinealectomy is a traumatizing and difficult intervention which cannot be performed without, at the same time, irritating adjacent areas of the base of the brain that have important links with the pituitary and, thereby, to the endocrine system. As a result, many of the observed effects of pinealectomy may actually be the result of injury to the gray nuclei of the base of the brain.

Insofar as injections of pineal extracts are concerned, such extracts have been obtained under the most variable experimental conditions and are neither chemically pure nor otherwise specific substances, so that it is no wonder that the effects obtained with them should differ from case to case. Finally, pineal tumors not only may involve the gland itself by destroying it but, at the same time, may irritate, compress or destroy adjacent areas of the hypothalamus, thereby modifying pituitary function. While there is no lack of authors who have disclaimed all reports of an endocrine character of the epiphysis, others believe that the pineal may generate some intermediary or neuromimetic substance, by virtue of which it may control the physiology of other basal nuclei and even that of the pituitary. In the absence of details concerning the existing relationship between the pineal and the hypothalamus, and so long as it cannot be conclusively established whether the pineal has any direct or indirect influence on hypothalamic function, it may be impossible to elucidate the true relationship, if any, between the pineal gland and sexual function.

The effects of experimental pinealectomy on rats has been studied by Simonet and associates,[79] who reported the appearance of precocious puberty and ovarian luteinization. Milco and Pitis[66] found that pinealectomy produced hyperproduction of gonadotropic hormone by the pituitary, postulating that the intervention produced precocious puberty by causing hypothalamo-pituitary stimulation. Similarly, Moszkowska[69] noted that pineal resection in rats provoked a state of permanent estrous activity, but that the same result could be obtained by hypothalamic puncture. These investigations seemed to suggest the possibility that precocious puberty and gonadotropin hypersecretion, observed in animals following pineal resection, were due to some indirect mechanism involving hypothalamo-pituitary excitation. It must be borne in mind that the most common cause of precocious puberty is the presence of the hypothalamic syndrome. *The question of whether a hypothalamic syndrome may be triggered off by loss of pineal inhibition or whether, on the contrary, it is precipitated by mechanical irritation associated with pinealectomy and with pineal tumors cannot be answered at present.*

The inhibitory action on sex by the pineal seems to rest on firmer grounds, insofar as results obtained with experimental injections of pineal extracts are concerned. In 1935, Engel[28] injected rats with pineal extracts and observed delayed onset of puberty. Similar changes were observed in the experimental studies of Moszkowska[69] and those of Thieblot and his associates.[86] Nonetheless, the assumption that pineal extracts inhibit sexual activity is not unanimously admitted. Thus, Bors and Ralston,[11] in 1951, concluded that the only specific action of pineal extracts consisted in dilating frog melanophores, a finding that later became the basis for the only bioassay of its kind available for the purpose. Similarly, Loewenstein,[58] in 1952, demonstrated that pineal extracts exerted a parasympathomimetic effect, which was confirmed more recently (Anton et al.,[4] Reiss et al.,[75] Wurtman et al.[92]). *The two effects just mentioned, the melanogenous and parasympathomimetic effects, put pineal extracts into a category close to such neuromimetic substances as those secreted by the hypothalamic gray nuclei*, which are currently known to constitute the basis of neurohypophysial secretion. The pineal substance is probably a neural incretion rather than a hormone. The action of this incretion might well be that of inhibiting the hypothalamic sex centers. Though plausible, this hypothesis is far from having been substantiated.

In summary, it may be said that *the effects of the pineal on sex do not appear to be those of a true pineal hormone but rather seem to involve a yet obscure relationship* between the pineal gland and the hypothalamic gray nuclei, which in turn control ovarian activity by way of the pituitary.

34.2.2. PINEAL TUMORS

The main anatomopathologic alterations affecting the pineal occur during *infancy* and are caused by teratomas, gliomas, melanomas, pinealomas, inflammatory granulomas (such as tuberculomas or gummas), and, more rarely, carcinomas. Similar conditions in the pineal of adults occur only exceptionally, mainly because, after puberty, the gland is subject to retrogression. The reverse of what happens in thyroid endocrinopathies may be seen here: pineal tumors are much more common in boys than in girls. Berblinger[7] reported an incidence of 91.5 per cent for boys as compared to 8.5 per cent for girls. In boys, the effects produced by such tumors on sexual development have been known since ancient times. Boys present with *macrogenitosomia praecox*, with enlargement of penis. Girls develop unusually early menstruation. At the same time, somatic and mental precocity becomes apparent and unusually early appearance of puberty leads to development of tertiary sex characters. In this instance, development of *precocious puberty* mimics in every respect physiologic puberty, passing through the same stages in an accelerated fashion. It has been pointed out that there is a correlation between the onset of the syndrome of precocious puberty and the extent of pineal destruction caused by the tumor. It may be impossible to discern whether such pineal tumors produce precocious puberty simply by virtue of destruction of the pineal and therefore pineal sexual inhibition, or whether they act by irritating other regions (for instance, the hypothalamus). The syndrome of hypothalamic precocious puberty is well known and, in terms of etiology, cannot be differentiated from pineal precocious puberty. Kalm and Magoun[48] hold the view that the symptoms observed with pinealomas are not to be attributed to destruction of the gland itself but rather to excitation of the hypothalamus.

Pende[71] described the syndrome of *pineal calcification*, detectable roentgenographically, which is associated with enhanced libido and pituitary excitation. On the basis of studies concerning the presence of 17-ketosteroids in boys with various pineal symptoms, it seems likely, as proposed by Capretti and associates,[22] that pineal destruction is indeed associated with loss of an important factor inhibiting the onset of puberty but that, at the same time, precocious puberty may equally well be precipitated by either tumors or pathologic brain processes other than pineal tumors. Only further study and the acquisition of more precise clinical experience may one day solve the problem of exact differentiation between strictly pineal forms of precocious puberty and other types of precocious puberty of neurogenic origin, which are to be examined in the following chapter.

In summary, it may be said that pathologic syndromes of the pineal are essentially caused by tumors, occurring mainly in infancy and much more commonly in males than in females. These tumors frequently are associated with precocious puberty, with macrogenitosomia, which, *though apparently due to pineal destruction and loss of some endocrine factor capable of inhibiting sexual maturation, cannot be fully attributed to any single cause and may be related to hypothalamic excitation by the pathologic process.*

34.3. THYMIC SYNDROMES

Although the question of whether or not the thymus is an endocrine gland has not been fully settled either way, some pathologic syndromes pertaining to that organ have been described in relation to genital endocrinology. These include primarily thymic hyperplasia and myasthenia gravis.

34.3.1. GENERALITIES

In Chapter 10, brief mention has been made concerning the significance of the thymus and the possibility that its incretions may be antagonistic to sexual function. By studying the effects of estrogens on the thymus experimentally, Foglia and Martin-Pinto[34, 35] found that estrogens produced thymic atrophy. Because no similar effect could be observed in hypophysectomized animals, the above authors assumed that they were dealing with a correlative effect mediated by the pituitary. Subsequently,

Comsa[23] confirmed the findings of the two Argentine investigators. Certain pituitary principles were found to accelerate the process of thymic involution. Gregoire[43] showed that prolactin produced involution of the thymus and postulated that the mechanism involved some pituitary effect whereby the temporary thymic hyperplasia occurring during gestation was caused to regress slowly postpartum. In addition to prolactin, Brolin and Arturson[18] observed that gonadotropins also produced an inhibitory effect on the thymus.

Finocchio[31] studied the effect of thymic extracts on the ovary. Animals subjected to the action of thymic extracts showed complete loss of ovarian maturation. This seemed to confirm ancient speculation to the effect that thymic hormone, or whatever active principle may be involved, inhibited gonadal maturation.

Some time ago, Bomskov[9] claimed to have discovered the presence of a *thymotropic hormone* in the anterior lobe of the pituitary. Such a hormone was allegedly similar, or perhaps identical, to the growth promoting principle. According to Bomskov, the action of the anterior pituitary on growth was mediated by the thymus rather than being exerted directly. This line of reasoning was based mainly on the fact that cessation of physical growth in both humans and animals was concomitant with the phase of thymic involution. *Nevertheless, no thymotropic hormone has to date been identified.*

It may be of interest to mention that thymic function seems to be enhanced during pregnancy. According to Bomskov, the explanation for this phenomenon should be sought in enhanced growth hormone activity known to take place in every pregnancy. Probably, some kind of antagonism exists between pituitary and adrenal function on the one hand and thymic activity on the other. As already indicated by us, *hyperplasia of the thymus* is a constant finding in the syndrome of *congenital adrenocortical insufficiency* occurring in anencephalous fetuses. The occurrence of thymic hyperplasia in anencephaly was later confirmed by Decio and Centaro[24] as well as by Török.[88]

Briefly, it may be said that the thymus seems to counteract pituitary gonadotropin activity as well as both gonadal and adrenal function, although it would seem to display a certain degree of synergism with the pituitary somatotropic principle. Even though concordant, all of the foregoing data are extremely uncertain and will have to be substantiated in the near future.

34.3.2. ANATOMIC PATHOLOGY

The anatomic pathology of the thymus comprises congenital anomalies, hyperplasia and tumors.

CONGENITAL ANOMALIES. Congenital anomalies have been described by Gilmour[41] and consist of either total congenital absence of the thymus or absence of one of the thymic lobes. Other congenital anomalies consist of retrosternal descent of the gland or inclusions of thymic lobules within the thyroid gland.

HYPERPLASIA. Hyperplasia or simple enlargement of the thymus may be found in *status thymicolymphaticus* or in *myasthenia gravis*. Thymic enlargement, reactive in nature, may also be found in Addison's disease, in congenital cortical insufficiency (as pointed out earlier), in hyperthyroidism, in acromegaly and following castration. Mitchell and Rittershafer[67] have called attention to the occurrence of transient thymic hyperplasia following castration.

TUMORS. A total of 208 tumors of the thymus had been reported prior to 1929 and compiled in a statistical review by Blalock and his co-workers.[8] Skill in diagnosing thymic tumors has since grown considerably to the extent that it is now estimated that one in each 500 to 600 autopsies reveals a thymic tumor. The malignant tumors are either lymphosarcomas or carcinomas. Lymphosarcoma is the most common tumor involving the thymus. It appears primarily during infancy. Its peak incidence is between the ages of 10 and 14, and it occurs much more commonly in boys than in girls. It may give rise to metastases to the lungs, mediastinum and the cervical lymph nodes. Carcinoma of the thymus, on the other hand, is a tumor that appears in the older age groups. It too is more common in males than in females. It leads to invasion of contiguous structures. The term *thymoma* has been variably employed by some authors as synonymous for both lymphosarcoma and carcinoma of the thymus.

Benign tumors of the thymus are quite rare.

34.3.3. THYMIC HYPERPLASIA AND STATUS THYMICOLYMPHATICUS

Clinically, thymic hyperplasia and status thymicolymphaticus are characterized mainly by thymic enlargement, which may be associated with dyspnea, cyanosis and dysphagia. These conditions have a familial background or, at least, a *familial predisposition*. As with thymic tumors, their incidence in males is twice as high as that in females. Apart from enlargement of the gland, with signs of compression, other symptoms may include pallor, muscular flaccidity and lowered resistence to infection. Affected individuals may develop lymphocytosis and frequently present with eczema and with allergies. At the same time, there may be *lymphoid hyperplasia*, particularly involving the cervical lymph nodes and the spleen. Furthermore, such patients reveal a grave tendency to *sudden death* from external agents, such as trauma, infections, anesthesia or intoxication. In a word, there is an exaggerated decrease in their resistance to stress. In terms of sexual development, both boys and girls with status thymicolymphaticus present delayed puberty and the latter invariably have *amenorrhea*. In some cases, status thymicolymphaticus appears to be associated with *congenital malformations of the genital apparatus*, as has been indicated in Chapter 33.

34.3.4. MYASTHENIA GRAVIS

Myasthenia gravis is characterized by an extraordinary tendency to muscular fatigability, associated with lymphocytic infiltration of muscles and with lymphoid hyperplasia, in conjunction with increased size or persistence of the thymus.

The disease occurs with maximal frequency between the ages of 20 and 50, that is, during sexual maturity, and shows an approximately equal distribution between the sexes. The etiology of the disease, which consists of thymic hyperplasia or thymic tumors, is completely unknown. As a possible pathogenic explanation, it has been postulated that the thymus secreted a substance of the curare type which, however, could not be isolated from any of the patients suffering from myasthenia gravis (MacEachern[61]). Although generally the disease is characterized by hyperplasia or tumors involving the thymus, there may be cases of myasthenia gravis in which the gland reveals no significant changes.

The *clinical course* is characterized by an insidious onset of the disease. Frequently, the symptoms become apparent in the course of an infectious process or during the puerperium. A form of myasthenia gravis has been described that appears during pregnancy and is caused, in the view of various authors, by gravidic hyperplasia of the thymus. Indeed, during pregnancy, as we have already pointed out, the thymus grows in size and in function, only to regress during the postpartum period. In the absence of postpartum retrogression, persistence of thymic enlargement may well be the cause of the gravidic form of myasthenia gravis, or, more correctly speaking, the postgravidic form of the disease (MacEachern[61]). However, an interesting observation has been reported by Viets and his associates,[89] who described pregnancy in women with pre-existing myasthenia, and who found that their gestation was neither complicated nor aggravated by the condition. This might well be explained on the basis of the physiologic enhancement thymic function is subject to during pregnancy, leaving the possibility that excessive thymic incretions may be utilized by the fetus.

34.4. PANCREATIC SYNDROMES

Unlike the thyroid and adrenal, the pancreas has never been considered as an accessory gland of sex. Nor has it, for that matter, been suspected of inhibiting sex, as have the pineal and the thymus. From a physiologic standpoint, there seems to be hardly any relationship between the ovary and the pancreas.

34.4.1. GENERAL CONSIDERATIONS

In the first part of this book, dealing with physiology, the existing relationship between sex hormones and carbohydrate metabolism was discussed. An accelerating effect on carbohydrate catabolism by estrogens had been described by us[15] and later confirmed by Bullough.[20] Estrogens stimulate growth of certain epithelia by increasing their mitotic index and by enhancing oxygen consumption as well as glycolytic properties. Continuous estrogen administration to experimental animals is conducive to hydrocarbon breakdown with glycopenia. In this respect, it seems reasonable to admit that estrogens possess diabetogenic activity and that ovarian activity may aggravate diabetes. This has been observed to be true in some cases. Thus, for example, Morton and MacGavack[68] described instances of diabetes that developed concomitantly with puberty. As a rule, however, the situation is quite different. In women, diabetes usually appears *after menopause*, coincident with cessation of estrogenic activity. An antidiabetic effect by estrogens has been demonstrated by Foglia and Rodríguez,[36] who observed that experimental diabetes in castrated animals may be mitigated by means of ovarian transplants. Similarly, in cooperation with Rodríguez,[37] the same authors observed that castration predisposed females to experimental diabetes and that estrogens counteracted this effect. Later Foglia and his associates[34, 35] established the antidiabetogenic effect of estrogens. On the clinical level, Hoet[46] also found that estrogens contributed to prevention of dysglycemia in pregnancy and alleviated diabetes in pregnancy.

Borghelli[10] likewise attests to the fact that diabetes usually runs a benign course in the female as a result of compensatory estrogenic activity and that, once the latter is gone at menopause, the disease usually is aggravated.

Basabe and his co-workers[5] studied the effect of estrogens on insulinemia and reported a rise in the latter, that is, enhancement of pancreatic response by estrogens. At any rate, the relationship between ovarian function and the pancreas is a complicated one, since a diabetogenic effect by sex hormone activity can only occasionally be demonstrated. The question shall be reexamined in greater detail in Chapter 47.

34.4.2. DIABETES MELLITUS

Diabetes mellitus is a well known metabolic disease characterized by hypoinsulinism and inability to utilize circulating glucose. The pituitary has been found to play a fundamental role in the etiology of the disease, as has been shown by, among others, the pioneering work of Houssay. In addition, hyperthyroidism may also be a basic etiologic factor. Therefore, the relationship between diabetes and sex has to be viewed with respect to the thyroid and the anterior lobe of the pituitary.

The disease may occur equally frequently in childhood as in adult life. When diabetes appears in childhood, which it does with some frequency in the most serious forms of the disease, it may be associated with *delayed puberty*, as reported by Boyd and his associates[17] (Fig. 34-4). Girls with this condition have their first menstrual period between the ages of 18 and 20, or occasionally may present with *essential amenorrhea*. Juvenile diabetes, associated with oligo- or amenorrhea, produces a tendency to *marked obesity*, in the opinion of Fischer

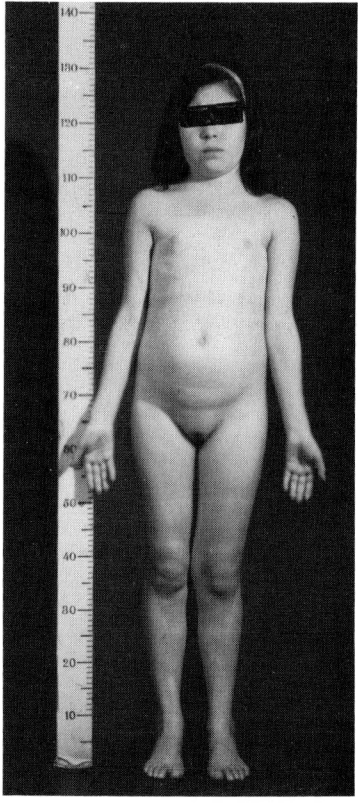

Figure 34-4. Diabetic impuberism and dwarfism in a girl, aged 19, with untreated diabetes, who suffered primary amenorrhea. There were axillary and pubic atrichosis and lack of mammary development. The patient showed spectacular improvement with insulin therapy: appearance of menses, with somatic and mental signs of puberty, as well as growth in stature.

and Florman.[32] Diabetes of adult onset may also produce amenorrhea (Kehrer[49]). During the premenstrual phase, there is usually an associated propensity to acidosis and coma, as shown by Cramer.

The incidence of infertility in diabetic women is considerable. The question of serious complications, to which diabetes may occasionally give rise in gestation, shall be discussed in Chapter 42. It shall also be pointed out there that the incidence of *toxemia of pregnancy* is considerably higher in diabetes.

Moreover, a high percentage of diabetes in females (50 to 55 per cent) develops during the *climacterium*. The reason for climacteric diabetes appears to be pituitary hyperfunction, as pointed out previously. Shipley and Danley[77] believe that female diabetes results from pituitary causes in a much greater proportion than male diabetes and, similarly, they attribute the frequent occurrence of amenorrhea and infertility in female diabetes to a pituitary origin.

To summarize, it may be said that diabetes in girls tends to produce essential amenorrhea and obesity, whereas, in adult women, it tends to provoke menstrual disorders, infertility and serious complications of pregnancy. Finally, in the climacterium, diabetes is common and results from pituitary dysfunction associated with that period.

34.5. PARATHYROID SYNDROMES

The principle parathyroid syndromes are hyperparathyroidism and hypoparathyroidism. These syndromes have little bearing on sexual function, although some sexual alterations have been described in association with parathyroid disorders.

In *parathyroprival tetany*, formerly a frequent complication of thyroid surgery, cases of amenorrhea and genital atrophy have been reported. Latent tetany may become manifest during menstruation, owing to fluctuations in calcemia occurring at that time of the cycle. Gravidic tetany will not be discussed here because there is considerable doubt as to whether its etiology is directly related to parathyroid function. *Hyperparathyroidism*, or von Recklinghausen's disease, occurs in combination with precocious puberty. This aspect, as well as its appearance as a complicating factor of pregnancy, has been described by Springham and Geist.[82] As we shall again stress in Chapter 39, the occurrence of postmenopausal osteoporosis is a common phenomenon although its relationship to parathyroid function is questionable.

Alterations of the cycle in women suffering from hypoparathyroidism have been reported by Graham and his associates[42] in 1964. Similarly, Liu[57] showed that parathyroid insufficiency or ablation of the glands produced important changes in uterine dynamics, resulting in spastic contractions.

During pregnancy, parathyroprival tetany is a much more serious and common event (Strozier and Bohmfalk[84]) and, although it has been asserted that the placental barrier is not permeable to parathyroid hormone,[53] it is a fact that children born to mothers who had gravidic tetany also suffer from tetany (Smith and Zike[81]). As a final comment, it is of interest to note that children born to *diabetic mothers* may reveal hypoparathyroidism (Kunstaedter et al.[54]), the reason for which is still unknown.

Klein and co-workers[50] maintain that parathyroid function plays a major role in the genesis of osteoporotic disturbances in connection with the cessation of ovarian function during the climacterium. Parathyroid hormone and thyrocalcitonin counteract each other insofar as calcium mobilization from the bone matrix is concerned.

34.6. ALTERATIONS IN SEXUAL FUNCTION IN DEFICIENCY SYNDROMES

Alterations in sexual function in deficiency diseases have long been known to occur. Among these, the most common are instances of amenorrhea in persons with malnutrition, the prototype of which is *starvation amenorrhea*. A detailed description of this condition, also known as wartime amenorrhea, is beyond the scope of this work. It is extremely difficult to tell when a given case of amenorrhea of this type may stem from psychogenic causes, as was often noted to be the case during World War II, or when it is caused by lack of food. Based on a study of postwar material in Germany, Wallau[90] noted that functional amenorrhea in peacetime made up 0.8 per cent of the clinical inventory but occurred three times as often during both the war and postwar periods, constituting 2.8 per cent of all patients coming for consultation. Most often, this type of amenorrhea is seen in young patients under the age of 30. The etiology seems to be a complex one and involves multiple nutritional factors. Plotz[72] called attention to the significance of *hypoproteinemia* and *amino acid deficiency* in nutrition. These occur more often in pyknic women than in asthenic women, an indication that women of this biotype are more susceptible in this respect.

Wallau,[90] who studied endometria in cases of amenorrhea of this type, found endometrial atrophy in 18 per cent, proliferative endometria in 46 per cent and secretory endometria of normal appearance in 55 per cent of the cases. This would seem to indicate that not all cases of amenorrhea have a purely endocrine etiology and that a *neurogenic component* may be involved in some of them.

Other disorders that may occur in deficiency states are *genital hypoplasia* and *infertility*. Kehrer[49] had emphasized the frequent appearance of amenorrhea and infertility in girls between or past the ages of 12 to 16 who had been exposed to nutritional deprivation. We have likewise mentioned this point[11] in calling attention to the fact that in the past we had observed many infertile women who, during the Spanish Civil War, had been subjected to adverse nutritional conditions.

In some cases, however, the underlying cause for such juvenile alterations in sexual function may be clearly traced to causes other than nutritional deficiency, particularly to *psychogenic trauma*, caused by such events as detention, imprisonment or death of a parent. This, once again, illustrates the difficulty in discerning a psychogenic component from a nutritional component in these patients.

Gaethgens[38] and Winkler and Binder have focused attention on the possibility that *hyperestrogenism* may be produced by nutritional changes. It is our belief that vitamin C, and possibly also vitamin E, deficiency may cause *defective ovarian maturation* (see Chapter 11) and give rise to follicular persistence with hyperestrinism.

Finally, impaired blood supply in malnutrition may similarly cause sexual alterations. In a case reported by Ezes,[30] a girl with congenital ovarian hypoplasia and essential amenorrhea suffered from a serious mitral valve defect. Upon completion of successful valvuloplasty, the surprising postoperative development was ovarian maturation with development of menses.

REFERENCES

1. Adams, A. E., and Bull, A. L.: *Anat. Rec.*, 104:421, 1949.
2. Adams, W. C., and Leathem, J. A.: *Endocrinology*, 75:138, 1964.
3. Aeppli, H.: *Gynaecologia*, 137:238, 1954.
4. Anton, T. A., Escobar, A., and Anton, S. M.: *Bol. Inst. Est. Med. Biol. (Buenos Aires)*, 20:281, 1962.
5. Basabe, J. C., Chieri, R. A., and Foglia, V. G.: *Proc. Soc. Exp. Biol. Med.*, 130:1159, 1969.
6. Baud, C. A., Stebenthal, J., and Langer, B.: *Schw. Med. Wschr.*, 99:657, 1969.
7. Berblinger, W.: In *Handbuch der Speziellen Pathologischen Anatomie und Histologie*, ed. Heinke-Lubarsch, Vol. VIII. Berlin, Springer, 1926.
8. Blalock, A., Mason, M. F., Morgan, H. J., and River, S. S.: *Amer. J. Surg.*, 110:554, 1939.
9. Bomskov, C.: *Ergeb. d. Inn. Med.*, 62:301, 1942.
10. Burghelli, R. F., et al.: *Diabetes*, 12:231, 1963.
11. Bors, O., and Ralston, W. C.: *Proc. Soc. Exp. Biol. Med.*, 77:807, 1951.
12. Botella, J.: *Endocrinologia de la Mujer*, 1st ed. Madrid, Aguado, 1942.
13. Botella, J.: *El Mioma del Útero, un Estudio Patogénico y Clínico*. Barcelona, J. Janés, 1949.
14. Botella, J.: *Acta Gin.*, 14:1963.
15. Botella, J., Amilibia, E., and Mendizábal, M. M.: *Arch. Gynäk.*, 159:447, 453, 1935.
16. Botella, J., Amilibia, E., and Mendizábal, M. M.: *Klin. Wschr.*, 15:1001, 1936.
17. Boyd, J. D., Jackson, R. L., and Allen, J. H.: *J.A.M.A.*, 118:694, 1942.
18. Brolin, S. E., and Arturson, C.: *Acta Endocr.*, 8:72, 1951.
19. Brown-Grant, K.: *J. Physiol.*, 190:101, 1967.
20. Bullough, W. S.: *Ciba Colloquia on Endocrinology*, 6:278, 1953.
21. Calapa, F.: *Minerva Ginec.*, 2:251, 1950.
22. Capretti, G., and Tusini, G.: *Ref. Excerpta Medica, Sect. III (Endocrinology)*, 6:93, 1953.
23. Comsa, J.: *Physiol. Comp. (Amsterdam)*, 3:128, 1953.
24. Decio, C., and Centaro, A.: *Riv. Ost. Gin. (Firenze)*, 6:326, 1951.
25. Desclin, L.: *Compt. Rend. Sci. Biol. (Paris)*, 146:781, 1952.
26. Dickerson, D. L.: *West. J. Surg.*, 55:342, 1947.
27. Eiselsberg, V.: *Arch. Klin. Chir.*, 49:207, 1895.
28. Engel, P.: *Z. Exper. Med.*, 96:328, 1935.
29. Eskin, B. A., Dratman, M. B., and Petitt, M. D.: *Endocrinology*, 69:195, 1961.
30. Ezes, H.: *Ann. d'Endocr.*, 11:619, 1950.
31. Finocchio, D.: *Giornale Ost. Gin.*, 12:113, 1948.
32. Fischer, A. E., and Florman, A. L.: *Amer. J. Dis. Child.*, 65:73, 1942.

33. Fisher, D. A., Lehman, H., and Lackey, C.: *J. Clin. Endocr.*, 24:393, 1964.
34. Foglia, W. G.: *Compt. Rend. Soc. Biol.*, 144:424, 1950.
35. Foglia, W. G., and Martin-Pinto, R.: *Rev. Soc. Arg. Biol.*, 28:43, 1952.
36. Foglia, V. G., and Rodríguez, R. R.: *Anales Fac. Med. Montevideo*, 35:785, 1950.
37. Foglia, V. G., Schuster, W., and Rodríguez, R. R.: *Endocrinology*, 41:428, 1947.
38. Gaethgens, G.: *Mangelernährung und Generationsvorgänge im weiblichen Organismus.* Leipzig, G. Thieme, 1943.
39. Gianaroli, I., and Vivicchi, L.: *Riv. Ital. Ginec.*, 35:266, 1952.
40. Gillman, J., and Gilbert, G.: *J. Obstet. Gynec. Brit. Emp.*, 60:445, 1953.
41. Gilmour, J. R.: *J. Path. Bact.*, 52:213, 1941.
42. Graham, W. P., et al.: *J. Clin. Endocr.*, 24:512, 1964.
43. Gregoire, G.: *J. Endocr.*, 5:115, 1947.
44. Hamburg, M., Sobel, E. H., Koblin, R., and Rinestone, A.: *Anat. Rec.*, 144:219, 1962.
45. Herbst, A. L., and Selenkow, H. A.: *Obstet. Gynec.*, 21:543, 1963.
46. Hoet, J. P.: *Ciba Colloquia on Endocrinology*, 6:330, 1953.
47. Hollander, C. S., et al.: *New Eng. J. Med.*, 269:501, 1963.
48. Kalm, H., and Magoun, R.: *Deutsch. Ztschr. Nervenheilk.*, 164:453, 1950.
49. Kehrer, E.: *Endokrinologie f.d. Frauenarzt.* Stuttgart, F. Enke, 1937.
50. Klein, D. C., Mori, H., and Talmage, R.: *Proc. Soc. Exp. Biol. Med.*, 124:627, 1967.
51. Koneff, A. A., et al.: *Endocrinology*, 45:242, 1949.
52. Krohn, P. L., and Zuckermann, S.: *Amer. J. Physiol.*, 151:429, 1953.
53. Krukowsky, M., and Lehr, D.: *Arch. Internat. Pharmacodyn.*, 146:245, 1963.
54. Kundstaedter, R. H., et al.: *Amer. J. Dis. Child.*, 105:498, 1963.
55. Larson, O., Sundbom, C., and Astedt, B.: *Acta Endocr.*, 44:133, 1963.
56. Lederer, J.: *Rev. Lyonnaise de Méd.*, 2:119, 1953.
57. Liu, F. T. Y.: *Amer. J. Physiol.*, 25:457, 1963.
58. Loewenstein, M. G.: *Exper. Med. Surg.*, 10:135, 1952.
59. Luca, F. De: *Folia Endocr.*, 16:141, 1963.
60. Lupulesco, A., et al.: *Endokrinologie*, 44:335, 1963.
61. MacEachern, D.: *Medicine*, 22:1, 1943.
62. Man, E. B., Reid, W. A., Hellegers, A. E., and Jones, W. S.: *Amer. J. Obstet. Gynec.*, 103:338, 1969.
63. Maqsood, M.: *Nature*, 166:692, 1950.
64. Marañón, G.: *El Climacterio de la Mujer y del Hombre.* Madrid, Espasa Calpe, 1936.
65. Mavromati, L.: *Rev. Franç. Gynec.*, 44:321, 1949.
66. Milco, S., and Pitis, M.: *Ref. Excerpta Medica, Sect. III (Endocrinology)*, 2:329, 1949.
67. Mitchell, A. B., and Rittershafer, C. R.: *Practice of Paediatrics.* Philadelphia, W. F. Prior & Co., 1942.
68. Morton, J. H., and MacGavack, T. H.: *Ann. Int. Med.*, 25:154, 1946.
69. Moszkowska, A.: *Compt. Rend. Soc. Biol. (Paris)*, 147:1983, 1953.
70. Nesbitt, R. E. L., Ardul-Karim, R. W., Prior, J. T., Shelley, T. F., and Rourke, J. E.: *Fertil. Steril.*, 18:739, 1967.
71. Pende, N.: *Folia Endocr.*, 6:191, 1953.
72. Plotz, E. J.: *Klin. Wschr.*, 28:102, 1952.
73. Portioli, I., Avanzini, L., Merialdi, A., and Rochi, F.: *Monit. Ost. Gin. Endocr. Metab.*, 39:589, 1968.
74. Raisz, L. G., and Niemann, I.: *Mature*, 214:486, 1967.
75. Reiss, M., et al.: *J. Endocr.*, 27:107, 1963.
76. Roy, S. K., and Kobayashi, Y.: *Proc. Soc. Exp. Biol. Med.*, 110:699, 1942.
77. Shipley, E. G., and Danley, R. S.: *Amer. J. Physiol.*, 150:84, 1947.
78. Siegert, H.: In *Biologie und Pathologie des Weibes*, ed. L. Seitz and I. Amreich. Vienna, Urban und Schwarzenberg, 1953.
79. Simonnet, H., Thieblot, L., and Melik, K.: *Ann. d'Endocr.*, 12:202, 1951.
80. Slater, S., et al.: *Fertil. Steril.*, 11:221, 1960.
81. Smith, J. R., and Zike, K.: *Amer. J. Dis. Child.*, 105:182, 1963.
81a. Soliman, F. A., and Reineke, E. P.: *Amer. J. Physiol.*, 168:400, 1952.
82. Springham, C. L., and Geist, S. H.: *J.A.M.A.*, 113:2387, 1939.
83. Stein, K. F., and Foreman, D.: *Anat. Rec.*, 105:643, 1949.
84. Strozier, J. E., and Bohmfalk, J. M.: *Amer. J. Obstet. Gynec.*, 85:541, 1963.
85. Talanti, S.: *Acta Physiol. Scand.*, 70:80, 1967.
86. Thieblot, L., Novadascher, J., and Le-Bars, H.: *Ann. d'Endocr.*, 10:192, 1949.
87. Thorsöe, H.: *Acta Endocr.*, 40:161, 1962.
88. Török, J.: *Ref. Excerpta Medica, Sect. III (Endocrinology)*, 6:318, 1953.
89. Viets, H., Schwab, R. S., and Brazier, M. A. B.: *J.A.M.A.*, 119:236, 1942.
90. Wallau, I.: *Arch. Gynäk.*, 176:320, 1948.
91. Williams, W. W.: *Sterility, a Diagnostic Survey of the Infertile Couple*, 2nd ed. Springfield, Mass., Walter Williams, 1964.
92. Wurtman, R. J., Axelrod, J., and Barchas, J. D.: *J. Clin. Endocr.*, 24:299, 1964.
93. Young, W. C., Rayner, B., Peterson, R. R., and Brown, N.: *Endocrinology*, 51:12, 1952.
94. Zondek, H., and Koehler, G.: In *Handbuch der norm. u. pathol. Physiol.*, ed. Bethe and Bergmann, Vol. 16. Berlin, Springer, 1930.

Part Nine
PATHOLOGY OF THE EVOLUTION OF SEX

In our review of the pathology of sex we shall follow the same order we used for the physiology in Part One of this book. We shall now analyze those pathologic alterations that may affect the *evolution of sex*, beginning with anomalies of sexual determination, followed by endocrine disorders of embryonic and puberal development and concluding with pathologic menopause and virilization.

Chapter 35
PATHOLOGY OF SEXUAL DETERMINATION: CYTOGENETIC MECHANISM

by Prof. J. A. CLAVERO-NUÑEZ
Department of Obstetrics and Gynecology,
Medical Faculty of the University of Madrid

35.1. DETERMINATION AND DIFFERENTIATION OF SEX

In Chapter 14, we made ample reference to the origin and determination of sex and pointed out that, in the human species, to which we shall confine ourselves henceforward exclusively, dimorphism is achieved potentially at the moment of fertilization, by virtue of the chromosomal formula resulting from the fusion of the spermatozoon with the ovum. Hence the concept of "chromosomal sex," capable by itself of inducing gonadal development. The specific inductors are thought to be the gonocytes of Fischel, representatives of Politzer's[57] *germinal route*. Upon reaching the undifferentiated, or hermaphroditic, gonad of a 7 mm embryo, they presumably initiate the complex mechanism of evolution in either a male or a female direction, depending on the karyotype they happen to be carrying.

In an 18 to 20 mm embryo, a slight difference between what is to be an ovary and what is to be a testis can already be discerned (Grosser,[23] Watzka[64]). However, from then onwards, a new series of "inductors," the hormones, begin influencing the evolution of sex. While *sex determination* is an instantaneous process, predetermined and of chromosomal origin, the *evolution* of sex is a life long process, notwithstanding the fact that sex is distinctly *differentiated* already in the fetus, a differentiation which reaches its peak in the years following puberty. Thus, the development of sex (differentiation and evolution) depends on endocrine stimuli leading, under normal conditions, to perfect harmony between genotype (chromosomal sex) and phenotype (somatic or gonadal sex). Under anomalous conditions, however, they act on the gonads and on the autosomes in general, leading to genuine pseudohermaphroditism. Naturally, the sooner such circumstances develop, the more serious are the results they may give rise to.

35.2. CHROMOSOMOPATHIES AND ENDOCRINOPATHIES

The inference one may draw from the foregoing statements is that a number of sexual alterations must depend on chromosomopathies (*pathologic sex determination*), while others are due to endocrinopathies (*pathologic sex development*). An etiologic distinction of this type, however, cannot be translated into practice as, unfortunately, the two nosologic groups involved are clinically indistinguishable. As a matter of fact, it is possible on the one hand that some genes are pathogenic without modifying chromosomal morphology, so that some of what are believed to be hormone-induced alterations are actually due to pathology of sex determination. On the other hand, it is also likely that both specific and nonspecific factors may injure the gonocytes or the rudimentary gonad, thereby giving rise to conditions not reflected by the karyotype, yet closely related to the process of sex determination.

These and similar difficulties, we believe, may be avoided by referring to such anomalies as anomalies involving the germinal route directly or indirectly and by establishing the classification found in Table 35-1, which is based on such an etiopathogenic criterion.

By making "alterations of the germinal route" synonymous with "pathology of sex determination," we should then be able to distinguish them easily from those other anomalies that result from dysendocrisiasis. The study of that second type of *alteration in sexual development* shall be dealt with in Chapter 37.

35.2.1. ANOMALIES OF THE GERMINAL ROUTE

A double pathogenic mechanism may cause the following alterations: (1) anomalies inherent in gonocytes, or *intrinsic anomalies of the germinal route*, and (2) anomalies resulting from pathogenic influences of the environment on the germinal route, or *extrinsic anomalies*, such as may be due to destruction of gonocytes or destruction of the primitive gonad.

Some of the *intrinsic anomalies* result from the presence of pathologic genes on chromosomes that appear intact. These are termed *genopathies*, as distinct from such other aberrations as are recognizable in chromosome structure (karyotype) and are termed *chromosomopathies*.

Genopathies, then, are those alterations that stem from obvious genetic failure in sex determination which, either in the presence of a distinctly female (XX) karyotype, give rise to serious sexual anomalies (e.g., pure XX gonadal dysgenesis), or in the presence of a male karyotype (XY), cause such individuals to develop as women (e.g., testicular feminization or sex reversal). *Characteristically, none in this type of syndrome reveals any recognizable changes either in the number or shape of chromosomes, notwithstanding the discrepancy between genotype and phenotype.*

In *chromosomopathies*, on the other hand, the underlying genetic disturbances are ostensibly apparent in the chromosomal makeup and can be recognized by studying the karyotype, either because of *quantitative changes* (more or less than 46 chromosomes), or because of *qualitative changes* (chromosomes differing in morphology from the standard set by the Denver classification). It is of special interest to describe both types of changes in gonosomes, or sex chromosomes, insofar as they are related to sex pathology; however, it must be remembered that there is no such clear-cut separation between autosomes and hetero- or gonosomes as had been supposed in the past, since soma, psyche and sex are the result of a balanced interplay of all genes integrating the 23 pairs of chromosomes in the human karyotype, although sexuality certainly is represented mainly by gonosomes.

Considerable progress in solving the question of heterochromosomal aberrations has been marked by the introduction of techniques using tritiated thymidine in conjunction with autoradiography,[3, 20, 61] allowing differentiation of "hot" X chromosomes from "cold" Y chromosomes. Until recently, there was no method available capable of selectively identifying the Y chromosome. However, by means of quinacrine chlorhydrate or quinacrine mustard, George[22] and

TABLE 35-1. Classification of Anomalies of Sexual Development

Sexual alterations	Due to germinal route anomalies	Intrinsic	Chromosomopathies	In autosomes
				In gonosomes
			Genopathies	
		Extrinsic (destruction of gonads or gonocytes)		
	Due to hormone effect on germinal route (to be discussed in Chapter 37, *Anomalies of Sex Differentiation*)			

Pearson and his colleagues[51] have been able to identify the Y chromosome. This is an important achievement inasmuch as it permits the demonstration of an XYY composition in a certain type of case.

Although most of our attention will be directed to the question of heterochromosome pathology, we shall also examine briefly the pathology of autosomes, since it is known that in 21-trisomy (mongolism or Down's syndrome) as well as in other *autosomopathies*, not only the patient's morphology is affected but so are his psyche (mental retardation) and sexuality (frequent sterility or production of teratological embryos or fetuses).

Extrinsic anomalies of the germinal route are the result of absence of gonocytes (perhaps this is what occurs in Overzier and Linden's cases of agonadism[48]) or destruction of the rudimentary gonad. The latter situation has been experimentally reproduced in rabbits by Jost,[33] demonstrating the existence of a dominant or basic sex in all animal species, the tendency to which becomes morphologically apparent whenever there is any gonadal disturbance. The concept of gonadal dysgenesis is based on this mechanism.

35.3. CYTOGENETICS OF CHROMOSOMOPATHIES

Two types of alterations, as mentioned above, may be recognized in chromosomopathies: (1) *quantitative* aberrations, in which the number of chromosomes differs from the normal number of 46, and (2) *qualitative* changes, in which the structure of some chromosomes differs from what is considered the norm. These two groups may occur singly but may occasionally also occur in combinations, giving rise to a third, *mixed type*, in which not only may there be more or fewer chromosomes than normal but one or several may also be atypical in shape.

Individuals bearing such altered karyotypes are called *pure or monodiagrammatic* carriers if all their cells display the same karyotype. But it may happen that some *cell groups* or *clones* differ from the rest by virtue of mutation or nondisjunction. As a result, different chromosomal patterns may concur in the same individual, a situation called *mosaicism*.

Chromosomal alterations may be divided into four main categories, which we shall describe briefly: (1) numerical aberrations, (2) structural aberrations, (3) mixed alterations, and (4) mosaicism.

35.3.1. NUMERICAL ABERRATIONS

Changes in the normal diploid number of chromosomes (46 in the human species) may be of two types, *euploidy* and *aneuploidy*.

Euploidy refers to a condition in which a cell contains one or several complete *sets* of chromosomes, each set of 46 chromosomes containing two sex chromosomes and 44 autosomes. A haploid or monoploid cell is one containing 23 chromosomes, the same number that is contained by sex cells. A normal or diploid cell has 46 chromosomes, a triploid cell 69, a tetraploid cell 92, etc.

Triploidy, tetraploidy and higher multiple forms are called *polyploidy*. This numerical aberration is the result of mitosis in which division of the cytoplasm does not take place (endomitosis). Polyploidy may also result either from C-mitotic duplication* or from endoreduplication.

Aneuploidy is characterized by an irregular number of chromosomes that do not occur in physiologic proportions (i.e., loss or gain of isolated chromosomes). Loss of one or several chromosomes results in *hypoploidy*, that is, less than 46 chromosomes, whereas *hyperploidy* is characterized by the presence of one or several chromosomes in excess of the normal diploid number.

In order to explain the loss of a chromosome (which is known as *monosomy* of the pair in which the loss occurred), or gain of additional chromosomes (trisomy, tetrasomy, etc., or in general terms, *polysomy*), we must resort to the mechanism of *nondisjunction*, described by Bridges[5] in 1913. Bridges observed that during *meiosis*, or reduction division, of oocytes of *Drosophila melanogaster*, both X chromosomes (or neither) would occasionally migrate to one ovular cell instead of being distributed equally between the two daughter cells. Nondisjunction also occurs during meiosis in spermatogenesis,

---

*C-mitotic duplication results from faulty spindle function, giving rise to "restitution nuclei."

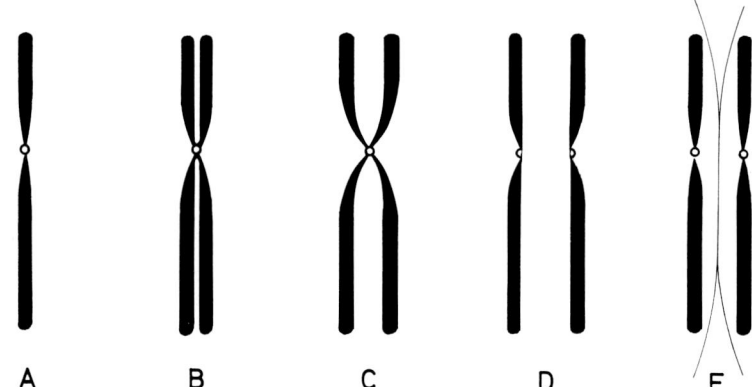

Figure 35-1. Schematic representation of mitosis of a single chromosome: *A*, prophase; *B*, late prophase; *C*, metaphase; *D*, anaphase; *E*, telophase.

as well as during *mitotic division of both germ cells and somatic cells.* Thus, *nondisjunction may be defined as the phenomenon whereby two daughter cells from any type of division end up with unequal numbers of chromosomes.*

The various *phases of normal mitosis* are represented in Figure 35-1, indicating that characteristic duplication of each chromosome in metaphase results in *two chromatids* joined at the centromere. The diagram in Figure 35-2 shows that *the centromere breaks during anaphase*, that the two chromatids separate from each other and that *the nuclear membrane, lost during metaphase, is rebuilt during telophase*, producing two daughter cells with a chromosomal constitution identical to that of the parent cell. As shown in Figure 35-3, nondisjunction involves displacement of both chromatids to one of the daughter cells.

In order to understand the genesis of zygotes affected by quantitative chromosomal anomalies, we must begin by analyzing the possible aberrations occurring in gametes from which they are derived. We shall therefore describe the mechanism of nondisjunction, first with regard to oogenesis and then with regard to spermatogenesis, taking into account that nondisjunction may occur during either the first or second — or at both — divisions.

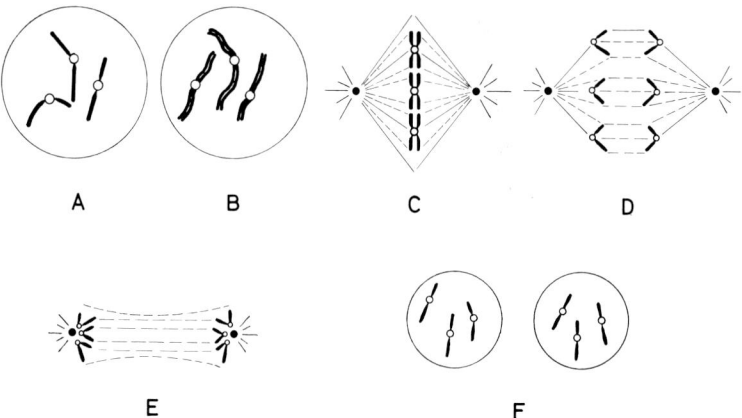

Figure 35-2. Representation of normal metaphase in a hypothetical nucleus with three chromosomes. *A*, Prophase. *B*, Late prophase: Beginning of separation of chromatids in each chromosome. *C*, Metaphase: Upon dissolution of nuclear membrane, centrioles have moved toward opposite poles of chromatin spindle, the three chromosomes occupying an equatorial plane that passes through centromere and lining up with chromatids parallel to this plane. *D*, Early anaphase: Chromosomes divide in equatorial plane and start migrating toward opposite poles. Anaphase terminates in *E*, phase of daughter stars. *F*, Telophase: Reconstruction of nuclear membrane, with disappearance of centrioles, giving rise to two daughter cells identical to parent cell (*A*).

Pathology of Sexual Determination: Cytogenetic Mechanism

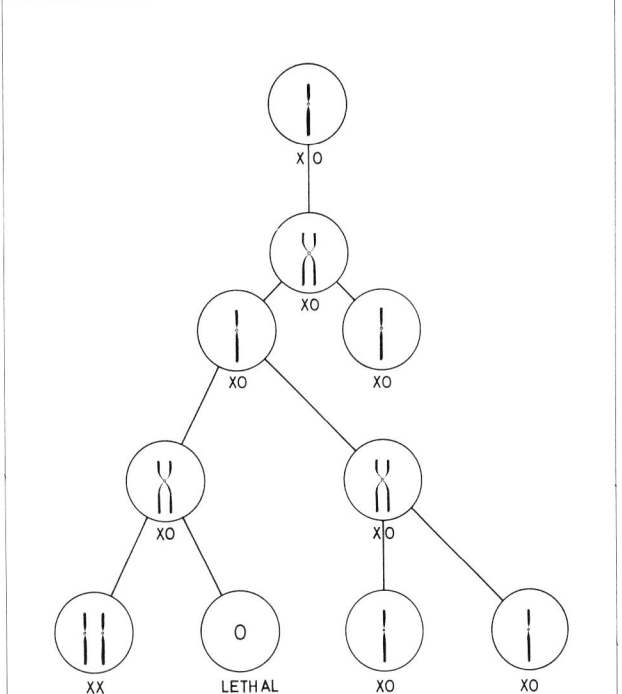

Figure 35-3. Simplified sequence of events in nondisjunction of chromosomes in mitosis. Normal division of XO-bearing cell gives rise to two analogues. One of the daughter cells gives rise to aberrant cells by a mechanism of "nondisjunction"; the other continues to reproduce in a normal way to illustrate difference.

35.3.2. NONDISJUNCTION IN OOGENESIS

Normal oogenesis was explained in Chapter 14 (Fig. 14-2). There, it was pointed out that mitosis of each oogonium produces two primary oocytes possessing the same number of chromosomes, and that these in turn generate secondary oocytes with half the number of chromosomes (haploid number) by reduction division. Secondary oocytes then undergo a process of maturation to give definitive ovules.

When the process of nondisjunction occurs during the first mitotic division (Fig. 35-4), the primary oocytes will have either none, one, three or four X chromosomes; when nondisjunction occurs in meiosis, the resulting secondary oocytes (would-be ovules through simple maturation) have none, one or two X chromosomes.

If nondisjunction occurs in meiosis, that is, the second division (Fig. 35-5), only ovules with two X chromosomes will be formed. Finally, considering the possibility that the process may involve both divisions alike (Fig. 35-6), the ovules resulting from such double anomaly would have none, one, three or four X chromosomes.

Thus, in theory at least, it is conceivable

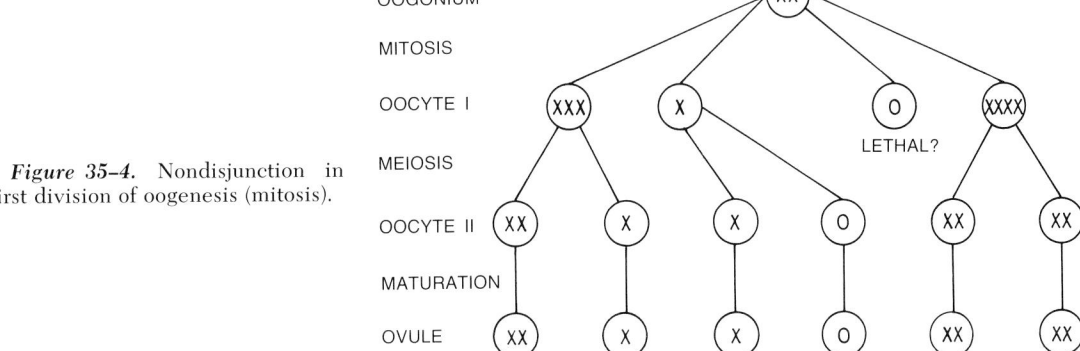

Figure 35-4. Nondisjunction in first division of oogenesis (mitosis).

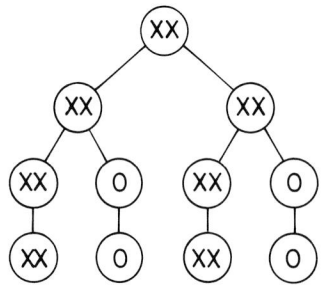

Figure 35–5. Nondisjunction in second division of oogenesis (meiosis).

to find ovules without an X gonosome or with one, two, three or four gonosomes, which may be fertilized either by normal spermatozoa or by anomalous spermatozoa resulting from a synonymous mechanism (see below).

35.3.3. NONDISJUNCTION IN SPERMATOGENESIS

Following the same rationale that applies to oogenesis, nondisjunction may occur in spermatogenesis during both cell divisions (which according to Boveri precede the maturation process of definitive spermatozoa), either singly or consecutively.

The mathematic possibilities that may obtain are represented diagrammatically in Figures 35–7, 35–8 and 35–9, clearly indicating the set of theoretically possible combinations. Nine different types of spermatozoa may result in this manner: one without any gonosome, two with one (X or Y), three with two (XX, XY or YY), two with three (XXY or XYY) and one with four (XXYY) gonosomes.

35.3.4. THE RESULTING ZYGOTES

Fertilization of ovules by spermatozoa, as just indicated, may generate the 21 different types of zygotes shown in Figure 35–10 from which, for the sake of greater clarity, all duplicate zygotes have been omitted. Some of the zygotes (or rather persons) with the quantitative gonosomopathies shown have actually been discovered and described in the literature, e.g., XO, XXX, XXXX, XXXXX, XYY, XXY, XXXY, XXXXY, XXYY, in addition to, naturally, the normal karyotypes for either sex (XX, XY). The rest (with 11 remaining to be discovered) are thought either to be statistically much less common or to represent instances incompatible with life, but their eventual discovery still remains a distinct possibility.

Figure 35–11 represents the theoretic origin of each of the 21 zygotes; it should be noted that the chances for them to occur do not depend on the number of mechanisms available for their production but rather on the likelihood that such gametes may be engendered in the first place and then be fertilized.

The *quantitative gonosomopathies*, just outlined, give rise to fairly well defined clinical syndromes. For instance, in women, *monosomies X (XO)* correspond to genuine Turner's syndrome. *Polysomies X* (XXX and XXXX known to occur) were originally called "super-females" (Jacobs et al.[30]), by analogy to some super-females of *Drosophila*, as reported by Morgan and his associates[46] in 1925. However, since such individuals actually turned out to be far from superior, the more descriptive term "triple-X females" or "tetra-X females," proposed by Stewart and Sanderson,[58] has been generally accepted. Males having an extra Y chromosome (XYY and XXYY) also were once referred to as "super-males," but these are now considered to belong to the large group of Klinefelter syndrome, cytogenetically defined as *polysomy X* (XXY, XXXY, XXXXY).

35.4. NUMERICAL ABERRATIONS OF AUTOSOMES

The mechanism of nondisjunction, as described for sex chromosomes, applies equally well to each of the 22 somatic chromosomes, theoretically giving rise to myriads of possible *quantitative autosomopathies*. These are not described here since, with the exception of those known to cause teratologic fetuses or to be associated with genital anomalies, their repercussions on sex determination are minimal. Perhaps the best studied instances of autosomal trisomy are of least interest in this respect, since *"mongoloids,"* or persons with Down's syndrome, usually present with normal sexuality, overshadowed as it may be by their somatic and, above all, mental changes (Penrose[52]). Lejeune and

Pathology of Sexual Determination: Cytogenetic Mechanism 781

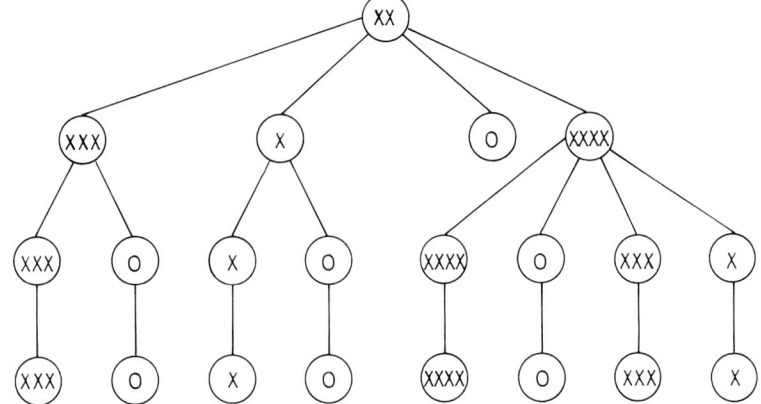

Figure 35-6. Nondisjunction in both divisions of oogenesis.

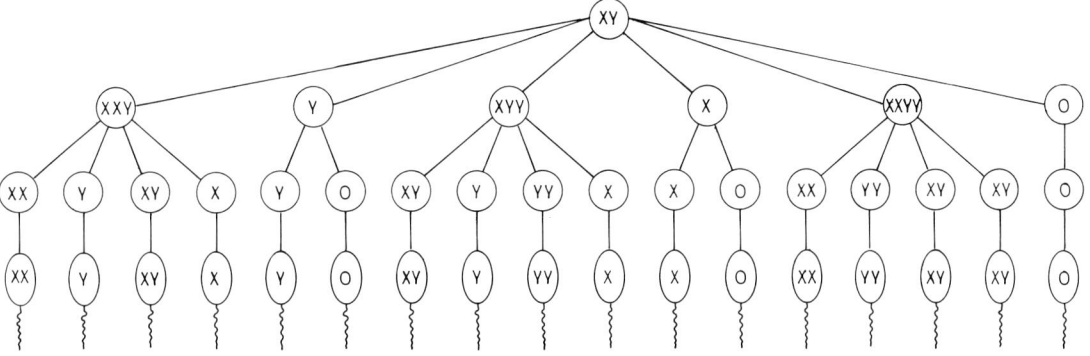

Figure 35-7. Nondisjunction in first division of spermatogenesis.

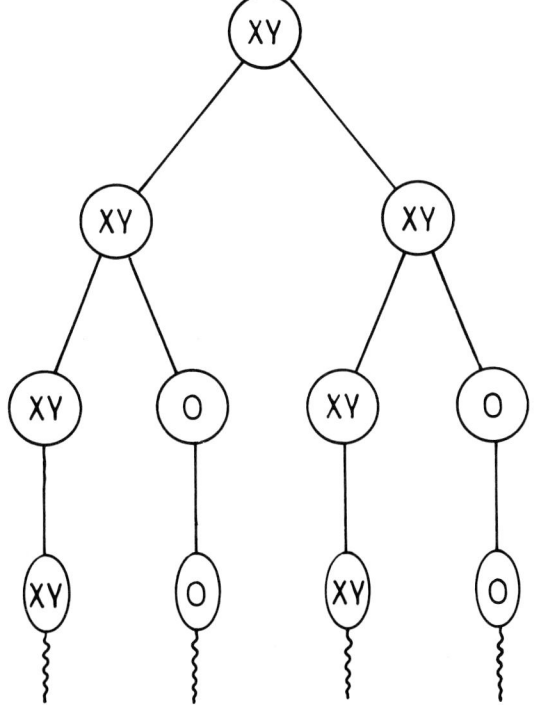

Figure 35-8. Nondisjunction in second division of spermatogenesis.

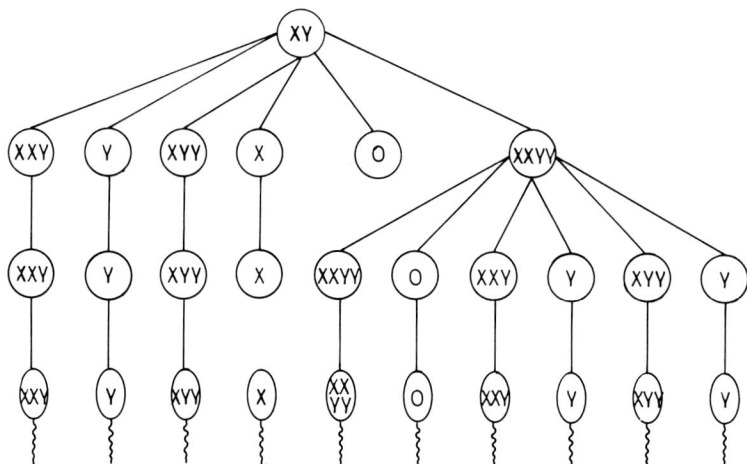

Figure 35-9. Nondisjunction in both divisions of spermatogenesis.

his associates[40] were the first to show that such individuals consistently revealed an extra chromosome, analogous to pair 21, occasionally appearing to be almost identical to the Y chromosome, in which case it was denominated the Philadelphia chromosome (or PH-1) (Nowell and Hungerford,[47] Baikie et al.,[1] Tough et al.,[59] Hall[24]). At any rate, neither Down's syndrome, its frequent occurrence notwithstanding, nor 22-trisomy occasionally encountered in Sturge-Weber's syndrome (Fraccaro[17]), is of particular interest to us. On the other hand, trisomies involving pair 18 (Edwars et al.,[13] Patau et al.,[49]) are frequently compatible with reproduction, though resulting in teratologic fetuses or in abortion, and those affecting pairs 13 to 15, found by Carr[6] in newborn infants with malformations, and by Delhanty and associates[9] in abortuses. Finally, serious gonadal alterations of the dysgenetic variety seem to be associated with aberrations involving pairs 6 to 12 (El Alfi et al.[15]).

The possibility of *quantitative autosomal aberrations coexisting with gonosomal aberrations* in the cells of the same individual has been confirmed clinically in females who were found to have *triple-X Down's syndrome* (trisomies involving pairs X and 21) by Uchida and associates[62, 63] and by Day and his colleagues,[8] as well as in males found to have *Down's syndrome with Klinefelter's syndrome* (Ford et al.,[16] Harnden et al.,[26] Lanman et al.,[38] Lehmann and Forssman,[39] Huxtinx et al.[29]).

	SPERMATOZOA								
	O	X	XX	Y	XY	XXY	YY	XYY	XXYY
O	O	XO	XX	YO	XY	XXY	YY	XYY	XXYY
X									
XX		XXX			XXXY			XXXYY	
XXX									
XXXX	XXXX	XXXXX	XXXXXX	XXXXY	XXXXXY	XXXXXXY	XXXXYY	XXXXYY	XXXXXYY

OVA (left axis), POSSIBLE ZYGOTES (bottom)

Figure 35-10. Theoretical range of possible zygotes resulting from fusion of gametes. For the sake of greater clarity, only those 21 that are not duplicates are represented.

Pathology of Sexual Determination: Cytogenetic Mechanism 783

Figure 35–11. Theoretical range of possible zygotes that can be produced by fertilization of ova and spermatozoa that are either normal or affected by nondisjunction in one or both divisions.

35.5. QUALITATIVE ALTERATIONS

This term refers to all chromosomopathies involving the structure of one or more of the 23 pairs that make up the karyotype, usually resulting in clinical congenital or hereditary anomalies. Anomalies affecting a single gene are not included here (since they constitute instances of *genopathies* rather than chromosomopathies). *The aberrations we include in this group consist of irregularities associated with disruption of normal correlations among the genes composing a chromosome, as a result of either translocation or deletion.*

In a diagrammatic fashion, a chromosome may be conceived as composed of a series of genes, "hooked up" in their *loci* (sites corresponding to each gene within the chromosome), which during prophase are aligned like the links of a chain, interrupted only at the point of the centromere which, like a brooch, keeps the long and short portions of the chain together. Accordingly, qualitative alterations may involve: (1) a single chromosome, or (2) two chromosomes. The same mechanisms may sometimes be involved in both types of alterations.

35.5.1. WITHIN THE SAME CHROMOSOME

According to Harnden,[27] a chromosome may be involved by the following anomalies:
1. Inversion
   a. Paracentric
   b. Pericentric
2. Translocation of genes, or shift of locus
3. Deletion, or loss of a gene
4. Ring chromosome formation
5. Isochromosome formation

INVERSION. Inversion consists of loss of sequential order involving a certain number of genes so that their loci occur in reversed order within one segment of the chromosome. If the centromere is not involved, this is called *paracentric* inversion (Fig. 35–12), whereas if it includes the centromere it is called *pericentric* inversion (Fig. 35–13).

TRANSLOCATION. Translocation of genes or exchange in position (Fig. 35–14) is brought about by a more complex phenomenon than the preceding one since it requires three breakages in one chromosome (not just simple breakage as in inversion), as a result of which one segment is reinserted in an anomalous position.

If any of these fragments, or for that mat-

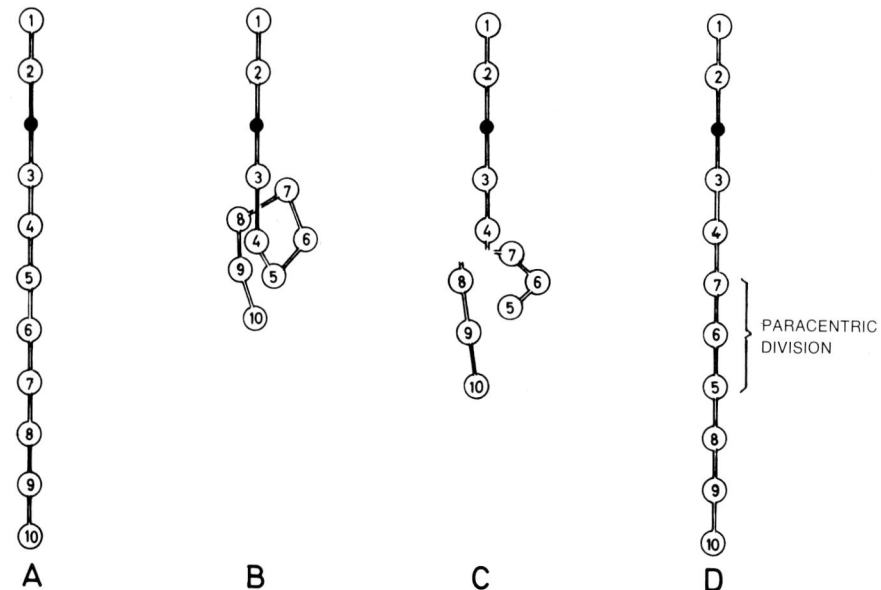

Figure 35–12. Paracentric inversion: Torsion, followed by detachment of fragment and subsequent reunion with same chromosome, gives rise to a phenomenon called *paracentric* inversion whenever the centromere is not involved.

Pathology of Sexual Determination: Cytogenetic Mechanism

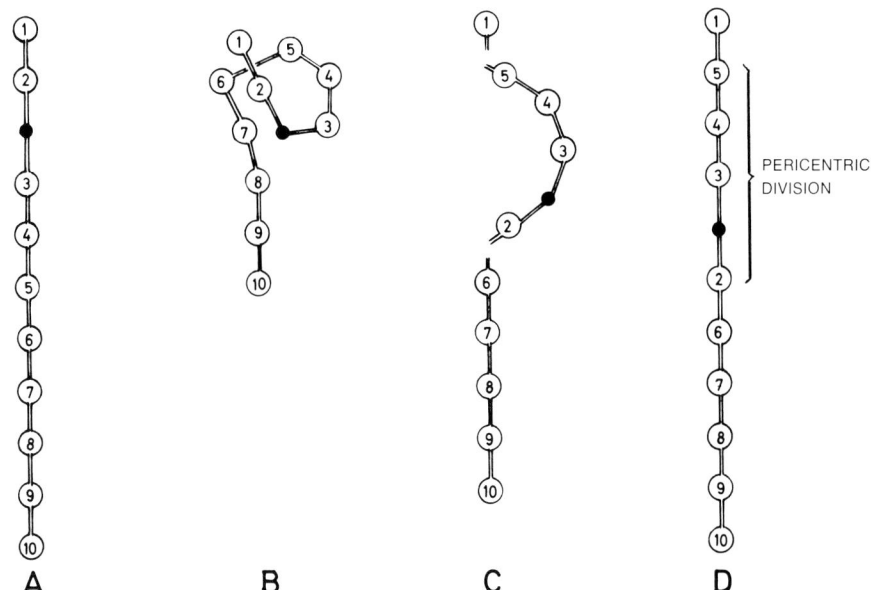

Figure 35–13. Pericentric inversion: Mechanism analogous to that shown in Figure 35–12, except for involvement of centromere, thereby resulting in *pericentric* inversion of genes.

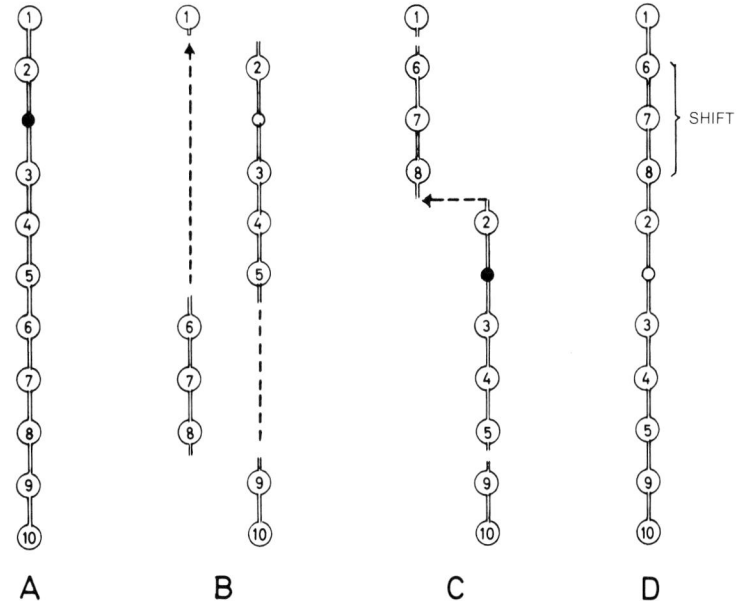

Figure 35–14. Shift of locus or *translocation* of genes within one chromosome: Triple breakage of chromosome *A* results in four fragments (*B*), migrating in direction of arrows (*B*, *C*), giving rise to change shown in *D*.

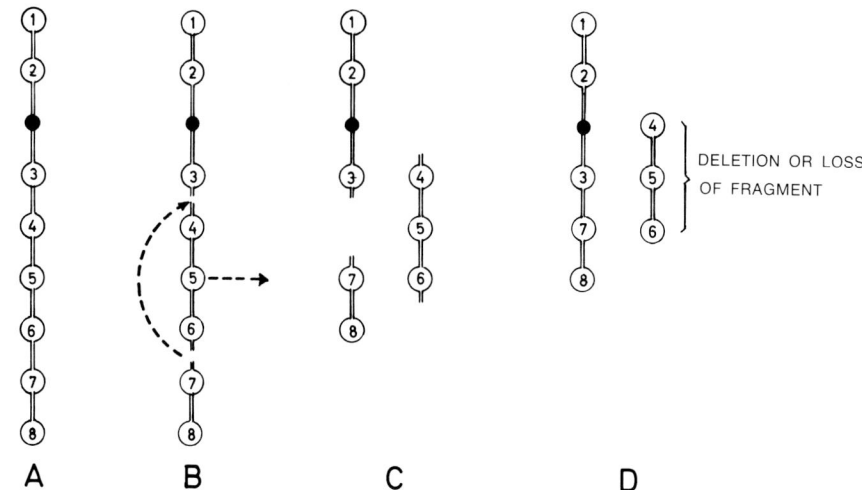

Figure 35-15. *Deletion* or loss of a fragment. *B, C,* Breakage and displacement of fragment. Two broken ends of chromosome reunite, giving rise to "deletion."

ter the fragment involved in inversion, is not reunited with the primitive chain, the resulting loss of part of a chromosome is referred to as *deletion* (Fig. 35-15). Such a fragment, unless reattached to another chromosome (*translocation by assimilation of a fragment*), tends to disappear, owing to lack of a centromere.

A special instance of deletion may give rise to a *ring chromosome* (Fig. 35-16). It begins as an inversion involving the centromere, followed by loss of the noninverted segment and by reunion of the two ends of the bent segment.

An *isochromosome* (Fig. 35-17) is a chromosome whose arms are equal in length and originates by a defect in the equatorial arrangement of chromosomes during mitosis, whereby one chromosome assumes an orientation perpendicular to the equatorial plane (Fig. 35-18). During anaphase, its long arms are pulled away to one would-be nucleus while its short arms become part of the other. In theory, it is conceivable for a single chromosome to give two isochromosomes, one *with long arms*, the other *with short arms*; however, in reality, this does not happen, because the centromere cannot

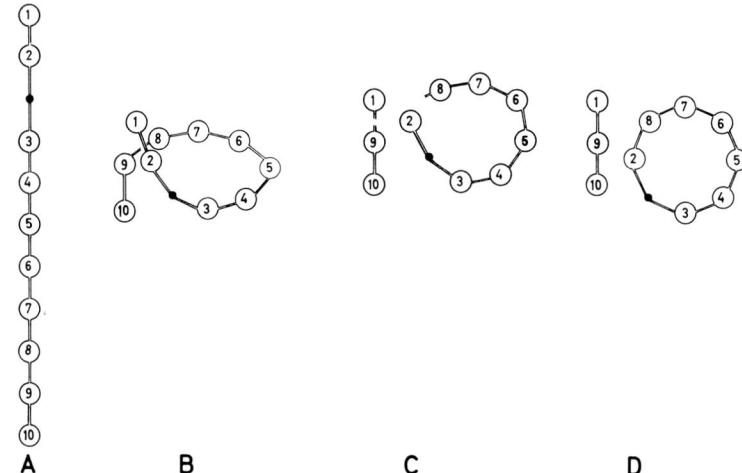

Figure 35-16. Formation of *ring chromosome*. *B,* Inversion involving centromere. *C,* Breakage. *D,* Reunion of broken ends gives rise to ring chromosome.

Pathology of Sexual Determination: Cytogenetic Mechanism 787

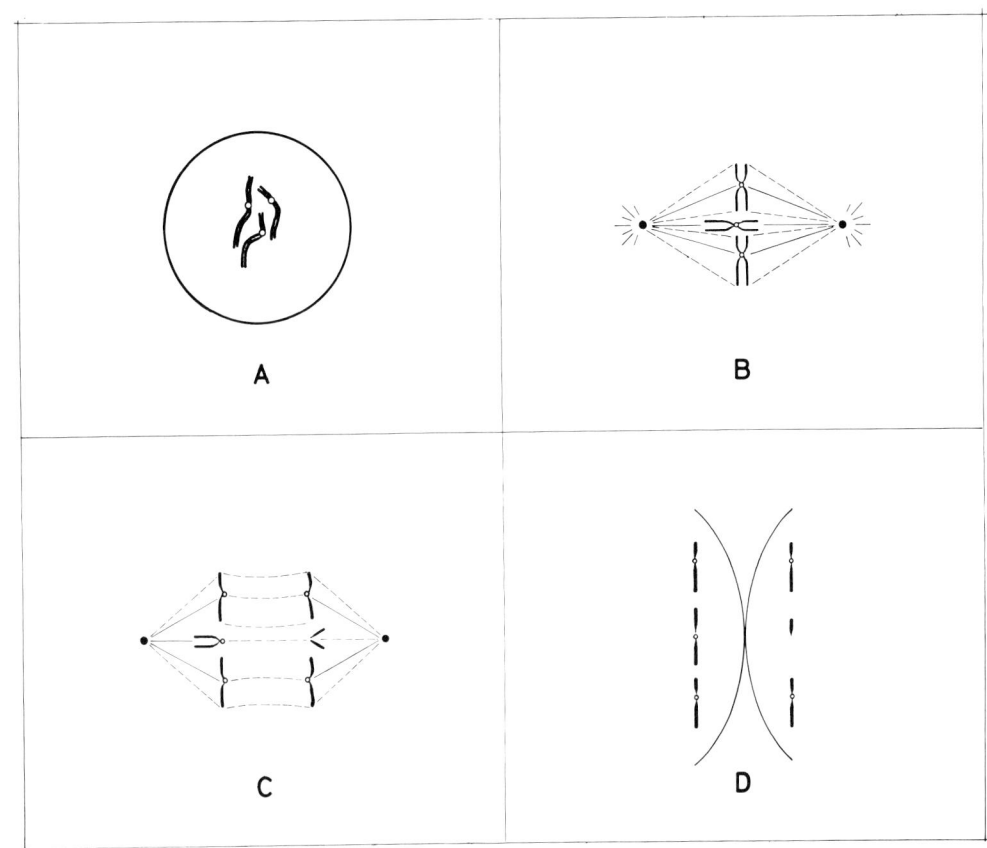

Figure 35-17. Formation of *isochromosome* during mitosis. A, Chromosomes condense. B, One chromosome assumes orientation perpendicular to equatorial plane, which is tangential to its centromere. C, During metaphase, the long arms of the chromosome with its centromere are pulled away to one centriole, while the short arms move to the other centriole. D, During telophase, one cell receives an isochromosome with two long arms, the other cell a fragment that tends to disappear.

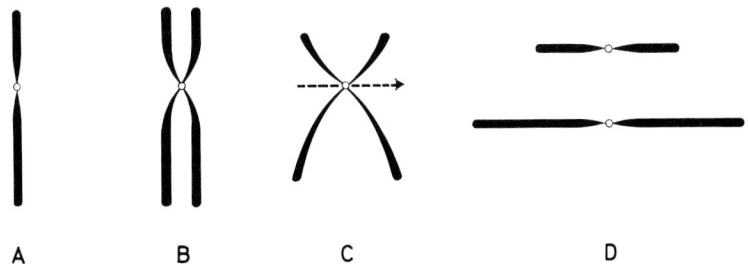

Figure 35-18. Diagrammatic representation of formation of one long-armed and one short-armed isochromosome from a single chromosome. This possibility exists only in theory, since the centromere remains attached in its totality to the set of arms forming the isochromosome, the other arms being abortive in nature.

be split and is retained in its entirety by one of the parts, the other part becoming abortive.

Because of their clinical significance, a brief comment must be made concerning ring chromosomes, deletions and isochromosomes. A *ring chromosome* may appear as the only aberration in a nucleus or it may be associated with other aberrations, such as translocation (Kempt et al.,[36] Genest et al.[21]), or there may be several types of coincident aberrations in the same cell (Lindsten and Tillinger[41]. Regardless of how it appears, the presence of a ring chromosome, as a rule, is linked with serious *morphologic and psychic alterations* and may even be responsible for *teratologic fetuses* Bain and Gauld[2]). Recently, Katayama and Matsukawa[34] described the presence of ring chromosomes as characteristic of certain types of breast cancer.

DELETION. Possibly the most significant aberration occurring in this group is deletion of an X chromosome, instances of which have been described by Jacobs and his associates,[31] and Harnden and Jacobs,[28] and Polani[54, 55] in chromatin positive women, some presenting with *essential amenorrhea*, others with frank *gonadal dysgenesis*. Despite its rare occurrence, this type of aberration would therefore seem to be of great significance in the pathology of sex determination.

In addition, the X chromosome, too, is most prone to produce *isochromosomes*, the most commonly described variety being the long-armed type. As shall be seen in Chapter 36, carriers suffer from *gonadal dysgenesis* (Fraccaro et al.[18]), a syndrome in which this aberration plays an etiologic role. In some instances, isochromosomes have been reported to involve other pairs, such as the sixth pair in mentally defective persons with characteristic facial features (Edwars and Clarke[14]), as well as group 21–22 in individuals appearing to be mongoloids (Fraccaro et al.[19]). Autosomal isochromosomes are also predominantly of the long-armed variety. Their genetic significance lies in duplication of genes of the long arms and deletion of those of the short arms, which represents a high order of chromosomal atypia. Autosomal deletions are very common. Meisner and his associates[43] recently described the so-called Philadelphia chromosome (or PH-1), resulting from deletion occurring in the G series of chromosomes (series 21–22, according to Denver classification).

35.5.2. *QUALITATIVE ALTERATIONS INVOLVING TWO CHROMOSOMES: TRANSLOCATIONS*

The exchange of genetic material taking place between two chromosomes is known by the name of *translocation*, which represents an event of cytogenetic importance. During the pachytene phase of meiosis, physiologic crossing over of genetic material occurs at points of contact, called *chiasmata*, between paired homologous chromosomes, which are the connecting bridges between the symmetrical loci of paternal and maternal chromosomes (it should be remembered that each pair has one component derived from the father, the other from the mother). *This is how genetic material is exchanged that will differentiate the gametes of the offspring from those of the parents.*

However, apart from physiologic crossing-over in meiosis (consequently, confined to gametogenesis) occurring in an equitable and symmetrical fashion (genes transferred are homologous and equal in number), all other forms of transfer of genetic material are known to be pathologic or, more or less, pathogenic. These may be classified as follows: (1) interchange of genetic material between two chromosomes, (2) assimilation of one fragment, and (3) assimilation of a chromosome.

Interchange of genetic material may occur in the form of an exchange of fragments between two heterologous chromosomes (Fig. 35–19) or between two homologous chromosomes, in the latter instance referred to as *duplication* if the genes involved are also homologous (Fig. 35–20). Incorporation of the centromere among the exchanged genetic material may give rise to a *dicentric chromosome*.

However, *duplication* most often results from *assimilation* of a broken-off fragment owing to deletion in the other chromosome of the pair. If the assimilated fragment has not originated in a homologue, the result is assimilation without duplication.

In addition, *assimilation of an entire chromosome* (Fig. 35–21) may take place between components of the same pair, re-

Pathology of Sexual Determination: Cytogenetic Mechanism   789

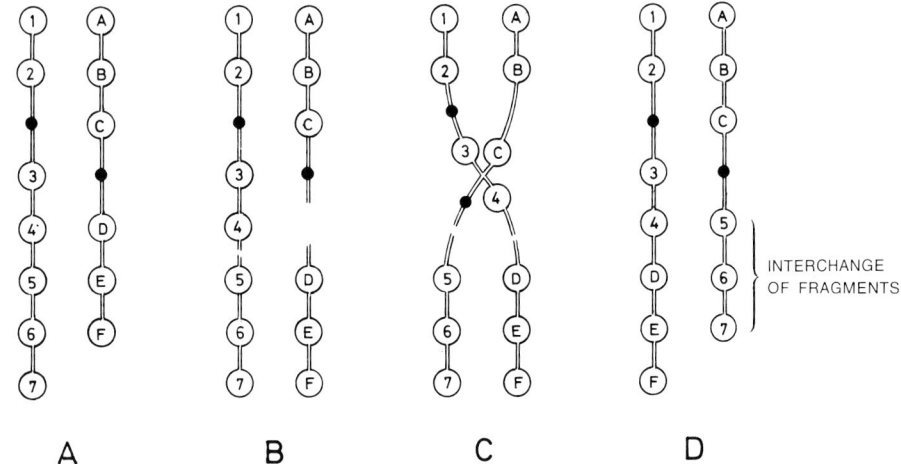

Figure 35-19. Interchange of fragments by translocation between two heterologous chromosomes.

sulting in the appearance of a *false isochromosome*, or between components of different pairs, giving rise to *false quantitative aberrations*, in which the karyotype reveals a missing chromosome that is actually incorporated in another chromosome.

A great many clinical instances of chromosomal aberrations resulting from translocation have been described to date. Interesting among these are *habitual abortion*, due to assimilation of a fragment between pairs 13–15 (Jacobsen[32]), also called *partial trisomy*, the occurrence of *habitual fetal death*, as a result of translocation in groups 21–22 and 17–18 (Lozzio and Valencia[42]), and the origin of *teratologic fetuses* from

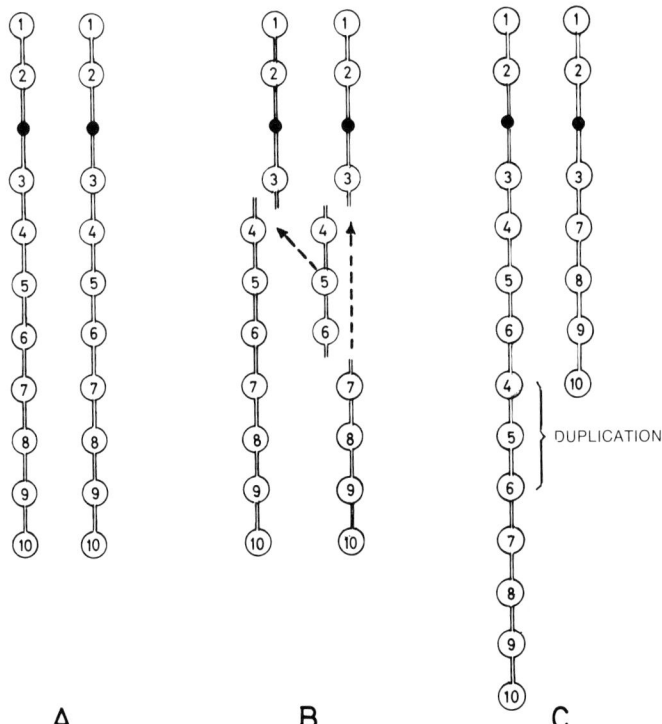

Figure 35-20. Genetic duplication by translocation between two homologous chromosomes.

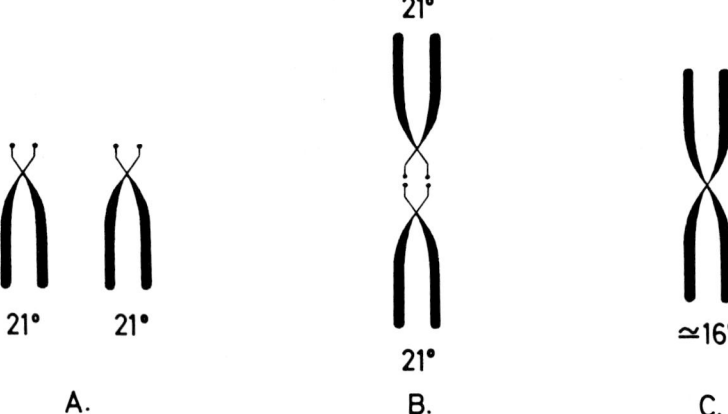

Figure 35–21. Assimilation of integral chromosome by total translocation of two homologous chromosomes. The result is a false isochromosome constituting a qualitative type of alteration. The resulting karyotype has one chromosome less (false quantitative alteration).

any type of translocation mechanism (Patau[50]). The diagnosis is most important from a clinical standpoint, since carriers appear to be phenotypically normal, as known from the early descriptions of Polani and his associates[56] and Penrose and co-workers,[53] and are capable of reproduction (Hamerton et al.[25]).

Sometimes, translocation carriers may reveal somatic anomalies of various types, such as *features reminiscent of Down's syndrome* (associated with assimilation of one group 13–15 chromosome by another chromosome, as described by Mercer and co-workers[44]); *polydysspondylism*, resulting from complete assimilation of chromosome 22 with another of pair 13 (Turpin et al.[60]); *mental retardation* in analogous cases (Moorhead et al.[45]); or *arachnodactylia and genital infantilism* in males with X-trisomy, in which two components are fused (Elves and Israels[15a]).

35.5.3. MIXED ALTERATIONS

Some nuclei may reveal both qualitative and quantitative chromosomopathies at the same time. *Translocation with assimilation of an entire chromosome* occupies an intermediate position between these and the ones studied previously. In the latter instance, the loss of a chromosome is more apparent than real because the genetic material corresponding to 46 chromosomes is actually represented by the 45 chromosomes present in the karyotype; however, since carriers of such translocations acquire different characteristics, these cases may be viewed as aberrations of the mixed type (Fig. 35–21). In any case, the anomalies involved play a secondary role in sex determination, being important only insofar as pathology of reproduction is concerned.

In contrast, *loss of one X gonosome with isochromosome formation in the other* is one more factor in the etiology of Turner's syndrome, to be amply discussed in the following chapter.

Other mixed types of aberrations are extremely rare and difficult to interpret. The last group of chromosomal aberrations to be discussed here is *mosaicism*.

35.5.4. MOSAICISM

Mosaicism refers to the presence of cells with different chromosomal constitutions, or karyotypes, in the same individual. Each genetically distinct cell line, of which there may be two or more, is called a *clone*.

Mosaicism results from nondisjunction occurring in the zygote or embryo phase rather than during gametogenesis, as it has been described here among monodiagrammatic qualitative alterations. For all tissues to reveal equally evidence of mosaicism, nondisjunction must occur at a very early stage, during the first cleavage stages of the morula. This type of mosaicism, referred to also as *zygotic mosaicism*, must be distinguished from those forms in which the aberration can be detected only in some tissues.

In the latter, nondisjunction occurs at a later stage, either in the embryo (*developmental mosaicism*) or in the fetus, or even as late as extrauterine life (*proliferative mosaicism*).

The effects such alterations have on carriers are decreasingly less significant the later in the course of life they develop, except for those instances in which such alterations supervene in cells with preexisting pathology. In this case, mosaicism is of little or no consequence as it often merely marks the return to normalcy of the involved cells. Such is the case in the *XXY/XX Klinefelter syndrome* whenever, even in advanced age, the loss of the Y chromosome is first noted to occur in one type of tissue (generally, the bone marrow). Since the cells of the tissue involved are less abnormal than the XXY cells, they are believed to possess greater capacity for reproduction as well as enhanced vitality, so that they soon assert themselves and may eventually replace the originally established (and originally the only) XXY cell line.

Similarly, instances of *XO/XX mosaicism, with Turner's syndrome*, are believed to arise from primitive XO cells which, by a process of nondisjunction, have assimilated two X chromosomes (Fis. 35–20); this would explain why the occurrence of normal cell clones has little or no modifying effect on the clinical picture of Turner's syndrome. In instances of *XX/XO mosaicism without Turner's syndrome*, on the other hand, even though associated with gonadal dysgenesis, the starting cells are most likely normal XX cells and the extent to which they are affected depends on the time of appearance of, and the type of tissue involved by, the process. According to Kava and Klinger,[35] mosaicism may also be associated with various forms of sterility.

Evidently, developmental and proliferative mosaicism is of less clinical significance than zygotic mosaicism which, by affecting all tissues of the body, *involves the germinal route*, an essential factor in the *pathology of sex determination*. The study of the gonad, or more specifically, the study of germ cells and gametes, is of primordial importance. Unfortunately, this is not always possible, owing to technical difficulties involved in culturing gonadal tissue, without mentioning the deontologic problems encountered in practicing systematic laparotomies in every woman explored for sexual disturbances. In the vast majority of cases of hermaphroditism described, we can therefore not dismiss the possibility that the karyotype obtained from the peripheral blood, bone marrow or skin may actually be different from that conditioning development of the same patient's ovarian or testicular tissues. The same criterion may be extended to the entire pathology of sex. Nevertheless, it is only logical to assume that whenever there is evidence of altered sex determination there must be genetic alterations present in other tissues as well, since regardless of whether it is initiated through pathologic gametes (quantitative as well as some qualitative chromosomopathies) or from anomalies arising during the earliest stages of embryonal development (mosaicism as well as qualitative aberrations), the disorder is almost certain to involve the immense majority of organic tissues.

In conclusion, as practiced today on the basis of karyotype determinations, the pathology of sex determination is always of diagnostic value in cases with positive findings; however, in the presence of suggestive clinical findings, a negative result does not have a definitive value because it does not rule out a possible mosaicism.

35.6. VARIATIONS IN THE OCCURRENCE OF THE SEX CHROMATIN

The sex chromatin, or Barr body, has been described in Chapter 14 (Section 14.8), where its diagnostic significance has been emphasized. Although its immutability in the course of life and during the cycle had been taken for an established fact, this has been proved not to be the case. Chu and his colleagues,[7] as well as Klinger,[37] have shown that a variety of factors may modify the sex chromatin. One of these is estrogens (Dokumov and Spasov[10]). Another highly important factor is the sexual cycle itself, during which statistically significant variations in frequency of the Barr body have been demonstrated.[4, 10, 11]

REFERENCES

1. Baikie, A. G., Court Brown, W. M., Buckton, K. E., Harden, D. G., and Jacobs, P. A.: *Nature*, 188:165, 1960.
2. Bain, A. D., and Gauld, I. K.: *Lancet*, 2:304, 1963.
3. Bartalos, M., and Baramki, T. A.: "Medical Cy-

togenetics." Baltimore, Williams & Wilkins, 1967.
4. Blanco del Campo, M., and Ramirez, O.: *Acta cytol.*, 9:251, 1965.
5. Bridges, C. B.; *J. Exp. Zool.*, 15:587, 1913.
6. Carr, D. H.: *Lancet*, 2:603, 1963.
7. Chu, E. W., Malmgren, R. A., and Kazan, E.: *Acta Cytol.*, 13:72, 1969.
8. Day, R. W., Wright, S. W., Koons, A., and Quigley, M.: *Lancet*, 2:154, 1963.
9. Delhanty, J. A. D., Ellis, J. R., and Rowley, P. T.: *Lancet*, 1:1286, 1961.
10. Dokumov, S. I., and Spasov, S. A.: *Ztschr. f. Geb. u. Gynäk.*, 169:85, 1968.
11. Dokumov, S. I., and Spasov, S. A.: *Acta Cytol.*, 12:131, 1968.
12. Dolan, B. E.: *Acta Cytol.*, 12:128, 1968.
13. Edwards, J. H., Harnden, D. G., Cameron, A. H., Crosse, V. M., and Wolfe, O. H.: *Lancet*, 1:787, 1960.
14. Edwards, J. H., and Clarke, G.: *Human Chromosome Newsletter*, No. 2, 1960.
15. El-Alfi, O. M., Powell, H. C., and Biesele, J. S.: *Lancet*, 1:700, 1963.
15a. Elves, M. W., and Israels, M. C. G.: *Lancet*, 2:909, 1962.
16. Ford, C. E., Jones, K. W., Miller, O. J., Mittwoch, V., Ridler, M., Penrose, L. W., and Shapiro, A.: *Lancet*, 1:709, 1959.
17. Fraccaro, M.: In Hamerton's *Chromosomes in Medicine*. London, Publ. Medical Advisory Committee of the National Spastics Society, 1962.
18. Fraccaro, M., Ikkos, D., Lindsten, J., Luft, R., and Kaijser, K.: *Lancet*, 2:1144, 1960.
19. Fraccaro, M., Kaijser, K., and Lindsten, J.: *Lancet*, 1:724, 1960.
20. Ganner, W. E.: *Wien. Klin. Wschr.*, 80:755, 1968.
21. Genest, P., Leclerc, R., and Auger, C.: *Lancet*, 1:1426, 1963.
22. George, K. P.: *Nature*, 226:80, 1970.
23. Grosser, O.: In *Biologie und Pathologie des Weibes*, Vol. I/I. Berlin, Urban and Sachwallenber, 1953.
24. Hall, B.: *Lancet*, 1:558, 1963.
25. Hamerton, J. L., Cowie, V. A., Giannelli, F., Briggs, S. M., and Polani, P. E.: *Lancet*, 2:956, 1961.
26. Harnden, D. G., Miller, O. J., and Penrose, L. S.: *Ann. Hum. Genet.*, 24:165, 1960.
27. Harnden, D. G.: In Hamerton's *Chromosomes in Medicine*. London, Publ. Medical Advisory Committee of the National Spastics Society, 1962.
28. Harnden, D. G., and Jacobs, P. A.: *Brit. Med. Bull.*, 17:206, 1961.
29. Huxtinx, T. W. Y., Eberle, P., Geerss, S. J., Tenbrink, J., and Wolting, L. M.: *Ann. Hum. Genet.*, 25:111, 1961.
30. Jacobs, P. A., Baikie, A. G., Court Brown, W. M., McGregor, T. N., McLean, N., and Harnden, D. G.: *Lancet*, 2:423, 1959.
31. Jacobs, P. A., Harnden, D. G., Court Brown, W. M., Goldstein, J., Close, H. G., McGregor, T. N., MacLean, N., and Strong, J. A.: *Lancet*, 1:1213, 1960.
32. Jacobsen, P., Dupont, A., and Mikkelsen, H.: *Lancet*, 2:584, 1963.
33. Jost, A.: *Rec. Progr. Horm. Res.*, 8:397, 1953.
34. Katayama, K. P., and Matsukawa, T.: *Acta Cytol.*, 12:159, 1968.
35. Kava, H. W., and Klinger, H. P.: *Fertil. Steril.*, 19:835, 1968.
36. Kempt, N. H., Lucas, M. K., and Ellis, J. R.: *Heredity*, 181:123, 1963.
37. Klinger, H. P.: *Ann. N.Y. Acad. Sci.*, 142:718, 1967.
38. Lanman, J. T., Sklarin, B. S., Cooper, H. L., and Hirschhorn, R.: *New Eng. J. Med.*, 263:887, 1960.
39. Lehmann, O., and Forssman, H.: *Acta Paediatr. Uppsala*, 49:536, 1960.
40. Lejeune, J., Gautier, M., and Turpin, R.: *Compt. Rend. Acad. Sci. (Paris)*, 248:1721, 1959.
41. Lindsten, J., and Tillinger, K. G.: *Lancet*, 1:593, 1962.
42. Lozzio, C. B., and Valencia, J. I.: *Lancet*, 1:1106, 1963.
43. Meisner, L., Inhorn, S. L., and Nielsen, P.: *Acta Cytol.*, 14:192, 1970.
44. Mercer, P. D., and Darakjian, G.: *Lancet*, 2:784, 1962.
45. Moorhead, P. S., Mellman, W. J., and Wenar, C.: *Amer. J. Human Genet.*, 13:32, 1961.
46. Morgan, T. H., Bridges, C. B., and Sturtevant, A. H.: *Genetics*, 2:1, 1925.
47. Nowell, P. G., and Hungerford, D. A.: *J. Nat. Cancer Inst.*, 25:85, 1960.
48. Overzier, C., and Linden, H.: *Gynaecologia*, 142:215, 1956.
49. Patau, K., Smith, D. W., Therman, E., Inhorn, S. L., and Wagner, H. P.: *Lancet*, 1:790, 1960.
50. Patau, K.: *Proceedings of the 11th International Congress on Genetics*, New York, July 14–19, 1963.
51. Pearson, P. L., Bobrow, M., and Vosa, G. G.: *Nature*, 226:78, 1970.
52. Penrose, L. S.: *Brit. Med. Bull.*, 17:184, 1961.
53. Penrose, L. S., Ellis, J. R., and Delhanty, J. A. D.: *Lancet*, 2:409, 1960.
54. Polani, P. E.: *Brit. Med. Bull.*, 17:200, 1961.
55. Polani, P. E.: In Hamerton's *Chromosomes in Medicine*. London, Publ. Medical Advisory Committee of the National Spastics Society, 1962.
56. Polani, P. E., Briggs, S. H., Ford, C. E., Clarke, C. M., and Berg, J. M.: *Lancet*, 1:721, 1960.
57. Politzer, G.: *Zschr. Anat.*, 100:331, 1933.
58. Stewart, J. S. S., and Sanderson, A.: *Lancet*, 2:21, 1960.
59. Tough, I. M., Court-Brown, W. M., Baikie, A. G., Buckton, K. E., Harnden, D. G., Jacobs, P. A., King, M. J., and McBride, J. A.: *Lancet*, 1:411, 1961.
60. Turpin, R., Lejeune, J., LaFourcade, J., and Gauthier, M.: *Compt. Rend. Acad. Sci (Paris)*, 248:3636, 1959.
61. Turpin, R., and Lejeune, J.: *Les chromosomes humains*, Paris, Gauthier-Villars, 1965.
62. Uchida, I. A., and Bowman, J. M.: *Lancet*, 2:1094, 1961.
63. Uchida, I. A., Lewis, J. A., Bowman, J. M., and Wang, H. C.: *J. Pediat.*, 60:498, 1962.
64. Watzka, M.: In Overzier's *La Intersexualidad*. Barcelona, Editorial Científico-Médica, 1963.

Chapter 36

PATHOLOGY OF SEX DETERMINATION: MAJOR GYNECOLOGIC SYNDROMES

By Prof. J. A. CLAVERO-NUÑEZ
Department of Obstetrics and Gynecology,
Medical Faculty of the University of Madrid

36.1. GENERALITIES

In Chapter 14, we have seen how important the role played by gonocytes is for sex determination and, naturally, for the ulterior development of sex. In Chapter 35, we have analyzed the mechanisms involved in the production of chromosomal aberrations. Now, the gynecologic syndromes caused by the latter remain to be described. It should be made clear that the so-called *intersexual states* are difficult to categorize for reasons to be stated later. Along general lines, however, they may be divided into: (a) those resulting from genetic causes, and (b) those from hormonal causes. The first are associated with failure in the mechanism of sex determination, so that the *gonads fail to develop sufficiently* and the resulting anomalous production of sex hormones gives rise to the intersexual state under consideration.

Intersexuality of primitive endocrine origin stems from failure in the mechanism of sexual differentiation. This may occur in the presence of *adequate gonadal development* with sufficient hormone production. The hormones produced, however, are counteracted by the action of another endocrine gland that results in intersexuality, as occurs, for instance, in the adrenogenital syndrome, in which the adrenal produces large amounts of androgens in female fetuses, which are thus subject to virilization at an early phase of intrauterine life.

It is not easy to separate clinically the "genetically" determined forms of intersexuality from the "hormonally" induced forms. Theoretically, the former should be associated with anomalies in the karyotype. However, this may not always be the case for any of the following reasons: (1) the aberration in question may not alter the shape of the chromosomes, as pointed out in Chapter 35. (2) In cases with mosaicism, the pathologic cell line may not occur in the type of tissue examined, bearing in mind that routine techniques for the study of the karyotype use blood, skin, etc., but do not comprise the study of germ cells. (3) In individuals with mosaicism, the pathologic clone of cells may in time have disappeared, owing to degeneration. It is an established fact that abnormal cell lines have less viability than normal ones, so that the former may gradually become extinct because they are outgrown by normal clones. Such changes do not necessarily take many years to be expressed in the karyotype and may be completed even during intrauterine life. (4) Finally, the genetic sex may have been correctly established but the primitive gonad may fail to respond to adequate stimuli. This category may be broadened to include those instances in which the gonad is presumably destroyed during the initial stages of normal gonocyte induced differentiation, as would seem to be the case in some forms of gonadal agenesis.

Thus, the current discipline of cytogenetics has significant limitations that ought to be recognized. Nonetheless, the mere fact that it cannot clarify the clinical diagnosis in every case does not detract from its value. The wealth of data accumulated through cytogenetics over the last 10 years has advanced knowledge of intersexuality more than any other technique has been able to do during all of the present century. It may be said that while cytogenetics is a complementary method of extraordinary value, it is by no means exclusive for the study of intersexuality. Among the other means available, histology remains the most outstanding method and is still the basis for the systematization of intersexuality.

Indeed, the difference between "genetic" intersexuality and "hormonal" intersexuality lies in the degree of gonadal differentiation. This chapter will be confined to the first category according to the following somatic classification: (1) *Phenotypically female* individuals who during childhood are not suspected to be intersexes but who after puberty fail to develop tertiary or quaternary female sex characteristics and/or present with amenorrhea or sterility. Their intersexuality is "functional" rather than "morphologic" in character. (2) *Phenotypic males* who are hypogenital and do not achieve complete sexual development. As in the preceding group, intersexuality is of the functional variety. (3) *Syndromes with intersexual phenotypes:* these may be individuals possessing both ovaries and testes at the same time (true hermaphrodites, exposed to both androgenic and estrogenic influences), or possessing but one type of gonad (pseudohermaphrodites). For clinical purposes, false hermaphrodites acquire the sex determined by their gonads rather than that indicated by their phenotype. A male pseudohermaphrodite, for instance, is one who, while looking like a woman, possesses testes. The intersexual character of the third group is predominantly based on morphology although it may also be functional in nature.

The most important examples of *phenotypically female intersex* are cases of so-called "gonadal dysgenesis," and only those among the first group of the preceding classification will be discussed here. The second group *(male hypogonadism)* has been excluded from this study, which deals solely with "gynecologic syndromes." The Klinefelter syndrome has been mentioned elsewhere (page 583).

In practice, *female pseudohermaphroditism* from genetic causes is confused with gonadal dysgenesis associated with virilization and will therefore be included in our first group. The most important group of genetically determined *male pseudohermaphroditism* is represented by the "syndrome of testicular feminization." True hermaphroditism is thought to be invariably caused by a genetic error, though frequently one that is not reflected by the karyotype. The three main syndromes to be studied here are: (1) gonadal dysgenesis, (2) testicular feminization, and (3) true hermaphroditism.

36.2. GONADAL DYSGENESIS: CONCEPT

The term gonadal dysgenesis may lend itself to a misleading concept of the syndrome under consideration. In fact, a gonad (whether ovary or testis) may be poorly developed, yet not necessarily associated with gonadal dysgenesis. As pointed out in the preceding paragraph, any type of alteration in sex determination may result in gonads that are more or less rudimentary, yet of the three main gynecologic syndromes with such gonads, only one is clinically referred to as "gonadal dysgenesis."

Hauser[55] defines gonadal dysgenesis as "a pathologic syndrome characterized by lack of germ cells in patients with external as well as internal (tubes, uterus, vagina) features of the female sex." This definition is conditioned by two fundamental prerequisites: (a) that there be no germ cells in the gonads, and (b) that both external and internal genitalia be female in nature.

The first prerequisite precludes any true hermaphroditism in which, as we shall see, the gonads and particularly the germ cells are fairly well differentiated. The second eliminates all cases of male pseudohermaphroditism resulting from testicular feminization despite the fact most of the time the rudimentary gonads lack germ cells, since those individuals never possess either a uterus or a Fallopian tube (müllerian organ).

Evidently, Hauser's definition encompasses a well defined syndrome which nevertheless allows room for quite a number of different clinical and histologic variants. In the first place, *morphologically* these may or may not be associated with dwarfism. The sexogenic mechanism may on the one hand be accompanied by typical malformations (Turner's syndrome), and on the other hand it may not be accompanied by any (pure sexogenic dwarfism). Occasionally, individuals with dysgenesis with normal stature may achieve complete sexual development, which is then referred to as "pure gonadal dysgenesis," according to Hoffenberg and Jackson.[58] Numerous intermediate forms may likewise occur and, to compound the diversity, any such case may be associated with virilization, giving rise to genetically determined instances of female pseudohermaphroditism.

The *histologic findings* in the gonads may not always reveal rudimentary ovaries. The gonads may reveal a variety of histologic patterns, ranging from undifferentiated, very rudimentary to fairly well developed ones (cases of hermaphroditism). As far as gonadal dysgenesis is concerned, the gonads found may mimick ovaries, testes or tumors. It is interesting to point out that, regardless of whichever of the three possibilities may be involved, the result is a syndrome that fits perfectly into Hauser's classification.

The polymorphous picture presented by dysgenesis morphologically and histologically is matched by the corresponding karyotype: from a *genetic* standpoint, there is likewise no uniformity. In Table 36–1, we present the various forms that may be encountered in practice.

How does a dysgenetic ovary or testis ever give rise to a syndrome of this type? Simply because after having undergone differentiation and functional maturation, the gonad is an inert organ lacking incretory power, regardless of what its histologic structure may be (see Chapter 14). How do different karyotypes give rise to dysgenetic gonads? This question may best be answered by another question: what was the karyotype of the deceased gonocytes? Rather than a genetic study of the body itself, the important thing is to find out why the germinal route in a given case has failed to induce gonadal differentiation. However, as a result of the disappearance of the germinal route, we shall actually never be able to learn how the syndrome has originated. The etiology of the disease lies in the germinal route, and only when the latter happens to have the same genetic formula as the rest of the body can the karyotype be of definitive value. This is why the same entity may occur in association with both normal and various types of abnormal karyotypes.

The cytogenetic limitations alluded to above make it necessary to view the karyotype as a mere ancillary technique in the study of intersex and not as the ultimate answer, as has been presumed by some. For the time being, anatomic pathology remains indispensable for the diagnosis of the different forms of intersex, although the information provided by the karyotype has immeasurably contributed toward the understanding of the diagnostic problems involved. The following paragraphs will attempt to outline the correlation between the karyotype of the various forms of gonadal dysgenesis and the clinical manifestations they may give rise to.

36.3. KARYOTYPE IN GONADAL DYSGENESIS

Based on the different karyotypes so far found to be involved in this syndrome, we may offer the classification presented in Table 36–1.

TABLE 36–1. Genetic Classification of Female Gonadal Dysgenesis

I. Normal karyotype (pure gonadal dysgenesis)	*In agreement with phenotype* (XX dysgenesis) *In disagreement with phenotype* (XY dysgenesis)
II. Abnormal karyotype	Single: XO (dysgenesis with 45 chromosomes); Xx (dysgenesis by deletion); Dysgenesis from X isochromosome; Superfemales: XXX (triple-X), XXXX (tetra-X) *Mosaicism*, combining above with XY, XYY

36.3.1. XX CONSTITUTION

Dysgenesis with an XX sex chromosome complement has been reported to occur in women with normal stature, well developed secondary sex characteristics, without evidence of congenital anomalies or mental retardation. This apparently represents the minimal degree of clinical repercussion produced by the syndrome, as typically exemplified by the case described by Hauser[55] in 1960. Cases reported by Jacobs and associates[66] in 1961, in a review of the karyotype found in association with primary amenorrhea, as well as by Clavero-Núñez,[23] who had studied the same subject in 1964, are examples favoring the concept of limited somatic involvement, although this may not be a constant finding. Theoretically, it is conceivable that all instances of pure gonadal dysgenesis are associated with phenotypically normal individuals, whereas those revealing somatic involvement may represent instances of undetected mosaicism. In a study of the karyotypes in 31 cases of gonadal dysgenesis published by Greenblatt and his colleagues,[44] several cases showed an XX sex chromosome complement. Schlegel and associates[107] described a case, admirably worked up by means of biopsies from multiple types of tissues, including the gonads, in which the only karyotype identified had an XX constitution.

36.3.2. XY CONSTITUTION

The discovery of an *XY sex chromosome constitution in gonadal dysgenesis* initially caused sensation since the Y chromosome had been generally believed to be inevitably associated with male directed development of the gonad. Following the finding that some rudimentary testes may be associated with karyotypes from which the Y chromosome was missing (see page 806, *Male Pseudohermaphroditism with Complete Feminization*), the concept of "crossed differentiation" was evolved which postulated that, under special conditions, a given genotype could induce development of the phenotype of the opposite sex. The possibility of dealing with an X gonosome deletion simulating a Y chromosome was initially considered. At present, however, there is no doubt as to the outspoken male significance of the Y component. As indicated previously, inversion of sex may be caused by destruction of the gonad, by loss of gonocyte differentiating potency or by an abnormal response to normal induction on the part of the gonad.

Prior to the clinical introduction of the analysis of the karyotype, instances of gonadal dysgenesis were reported to have occurred in women usually presenting with short stature, eunuchoid habitus or other somatic stigmata, though not infrequently they had a positive menstrual history (Overzier,[94] Hoffenberg and Jackson,[59] Greenblatt,[42, 43] Hutchins,[62] Stoddard and Engstrom[116]). The last mentioned authors introduced the term "sex reversal," based on the fact that even in the presence of a Y chromosome ovaries, uterus, Fallopian tubes and somatic female features can develop.

In 1959, Harnden and Stewart[53] reported the first instance of this type of dysgenesis in a sex chromatin negative woman with amenorrhea, dwarfism and an XY karyotype. Except for the fact that the patient had not been explored surgically, this would have been a conclusively proved case. Subsequently, surgically proved cases were reported by Grouchy and associates[45] in 1960, and by de la Chapelle[27] in 1962, which conclusively demonstrated the clinical occurrence of the syndrome. Cases of gonadal dysgenesis with an XY chromosomal complement were later also described in Italy by Pasetto and co-workers[96] and in Spain by Pujol-Amat and associates.[101]

36.3.3. XO CONSTITUTION

Among the vast group of patients with gonadal dysgenesis presenting with changes in the karyotype, we shall first consider *XO individuals with 45 chromosomes*, since this is what is most commonly found in *Turner's syndrome*, although not all cases of XO dysgenesis are associated with Turner's syndrome, nor are all cases of Turner's syndrome associated with an XO karyotype. Obviously, the classic syndrome as described by Turner in 1938[121] may or may not be associated with chromosomal changes which, if present, may reveal various types of constitutions, most frequently XO. While somatic anomalies rarely, if ever, appear in patients with an XX constitution, and occur to some extent in those with an XY constitution, persons with an XO constitution are invariably subject to develop profound corporal stigmata, to the extent that the latter were first mentioned when Turner's syndrome was discovered. On the other hand, as we have already indicated, an XO constitution is not invariably associated with gonadal dysgenesis, since in 1960 Bahner and his associates[5] published a report of a case of XO constitution associated with proven fertility and, a year later, Russell and co-workers[105] reported another case with a known history of menstruation and possible fertility. Nevertheless, we believe that these are exceptional cases (perhaps instances of unrecognized mosaicism) and that the XO karyotype is inherently associated with Turner's syndrome rather than dysgenesis.

36.3.4. MOSAICISM AND "MIXED" TYPES OF DYSGENESIS

Instances of dysgenesis with an XO/XX mosaicism have been described by Carr and his colleagues[19] and by Kowalyszyn.[78] Another case of mixed XO/XY gonadal dysgenesis was reported by Hung and co-workers.[60] Finally, MacDonough and his associates[83] described a case of dysgenesis with an XO/XXX mosaicism.

36.3.5. XX CONSTITUTION

Deletion of the X chromosome (Xx) (see Chapter 35) produces a form of gonadal dysgenesis that clinically resembles the "pure" forms, that is, those with an XX or XY constitution. The first typical case involving this variety was reported by Jacobs and colleagues[64] in 1960, the existence of which was to be confirmed by similar cases reported by Harnden and Jacobs[52] and by Polani[98, 99] a year later. More recently, Bovicelli[16] described another case and Kosowicz and co-workers[77] reported two cases of unilateral mixed dysgenesis in which only one gonad was involved, one in an XX patient with 46 chromosomes, the other in an XO/XX mosaic with 45 and 46 chromosomes respectively.

36.3.6. X ISOCHROMOSOME

An *X isochromosome* may occur as the only gonosome representative (a case reported by Moncada and Sopeña[87]) or in association with a normal X chromosome (Fraccaro et al.,[35] Jacobs et al.,[66] Hamerton et al.,[50] and Polani[98]). In the first instance, the patient reveals somatic alterations of the type found in Turner's syndrome; in the second, the somatic features of pure gonadal dysgenesis.

Since so far no isochromosome for the short arm of the X chromosome has been identified, any future reference to this special form of gonosome involves its long-armed type.

36.3.7. POLY-X FEMALES

"Superfemales" are women carrying three or more X chromosomes. The first cases of *triple-X* women were reported by Jacobs and co-workers[65] in 1959, whereas in 1961, two *tetra-X* females, both affected by mental deficiency, were described by Carr and his colleagues,[18] and a *penta-X* female was described by Kesaree and Wolley.[74] A number of poly-X females have since been reported although not all of the cases may have been well documented and some may possibly represent instances of pair 6 trisomy (see Chapter 12). Only by the presence of extra Barr bodies or, more specifically, the demonstration of X chromosome activity by means of radioactive tritium, may the presence of gonosomal trisomy in such cases be established more conclusively.

Triple-X individuals may be completely normal women although they have occasionally been found to be affected by mental deficiency, secondary amenorrhea and/or sterility. These symptoms become more pronounced as the number of X chromosomes increases, though interestingly they affect the soma and psyche to a greater extent than the gonads. Occasional rare cases may develop gonadal dysgenesis, conveying the impression of representing instances of inadvertent mosaicism rather than true "triple-X females." Barr and co-workers[8] have published a comprehensive review of all triple-X women reported in the literature, collecting a total of 143 cases, to which they added 12 cases of pure triple-X and one case of their own of XXX/xx mosaicism. Interestingly, Laszlo and Györy[79] called attention to the prevalence of hypomastia in association with triple-X karyotypes, of which they described six cases.

36.3.8. MOSAICISM

The form of *mosaicism* so far found to be most commonly associated with gonadal dysgenesis appears to be the combination XO/XX, which was first described by Ford et al.,[33] Tjio et al.,[120] and Fraccaro et al.,[36] and of which we reported two cases (Moncada and Sopeña[87]). In 1961, Jacobs and coworkers[66] found an XO/XXX karyotype in a case of dysgenesis without Turner's syndrome; in the series published by the same authors in a study on essential amenorrhea, there also appear two cases of dysgenesis, one with an XO/XY, the other with an XO/XYY mosaicism. Another case was reported the same year by Grumbach and his colleagues,[46] with an XO/XX/XXX constitution. Apart from what may be inferred to have been a case of an XO/XY/XXY sex chromosomal complement in the previously mentioned report by Jacobs, Forteza and his associates[34] recently published a report of an XX/XY mosaic.

Phenotypically, the clinical picture presented by the group of mosaicism varies greatly, ranging from Turner's syndrome in some XO/XY patients to what may be considered almost normal women, apparently in accordance with the following guidelines: (1) XO/XY cases are sex chromatin negative and are associated with Turner's syndrome; (2) XO/XX cases may be either Barr body negative, in which case they are associated with Turner's syndrome, or they may be sex chromatin positive, in the latter case with less apparent somatic stigmata; (3) the addition of a Y gonosome, or of an XY group, is associated with a delay in female-directed gonadal and somatic development (having at least a "neutralizing," if not outright masculinizing, effect); (4) the addition of either an X gonosome or an XX group advances gonadal as well as somatic evolution in the direction of normal woman and, despite persisting gonadal dysgenesis, the ovary tends to become better differentiated and the phenotype better developed.

Some of these guidelines are applicable to all cases of gonadal dysgenesis, although they cannot be viewed as absolute rules, as shall be pointed out later in discussing the clinical picture of the syndrome. In general, however, using normal XX woman as the prototype, dysgenesis (in terms of increasingly more rudimentary ovarian histologic features), as well as the changes affecting the phenotype and often also the psyche, becomes more significant in the following order: (1) Superfemales, (2) deletion of an X chromosome, (3) isochromosome in conjunction with a normal X chromosome, (4) mosaicism with various X chromosome groupings, (5) pure gonadal dysgenesis, (6) mosaicism with a single X group, (7) mosaicism without an XX group, (8) X-isochromosome in dysgenesis with 45 chromosomes, and (9) gonadal dysgenesis with 45 chromosomes.

36.4. CLINICAL PICTURE OF THE VARIOUS TYPES OF GONADAL DYSGENESIS

"Female gonadal dysgenesis" refers to a syndrome defined by the presence of congenital ovarian atrophy (streak ovaries or absent ovaries), associated or unassociated with: (1) Short stature, (2) limited development of remaining sex characters (small uterus, absence of pubic hair, absence of breast development), (3) congenital anomalies (short or webbed neck, or pterygium colli), and (4) other osseous or hormonal changes (osteoporosis, increased FSH and decreased estrogen values). Any type of clinical classification of the syndrome must be based on the various forms under which dysgenesis manifests itself: the clinical picture is expressed to the utmost whenever there is concurrence of all (and sometimes others) of the symptoms outlined above, which is then referred to as ovarian dysgenesis with Turner's syndrome. Based on a review of all cases of ovarian dysgenesis with or without Turner's syndrome published up to 1961, Polani[99] proposed the classification shown in Table 36-2.

Hauser[55] distinguishes four different variants of gonadal dysgenesis: (1) Swyer's syndrome, or pure gonadal dysgenesis, analogous to pure gonadal dysgenesis in the preceding classification (normal stature, without malformations, generally chromatin positive). (2) Rössle's syndrome, with short stature, no webbing of neck, sometimes as-

TABLE 36-2. Classification of Ovarian Dysgenesis (According to Polani)

- True dysgenesis
  - Webbed neck (and often other anomalies) and short stature (less than 147 cm) = Turner's syndrome
  - Without webbed neck
    - Short stature (sometimes with other anomalies)
    - Normal stature without any anomalies = pure gonadal dysgenesis
  - Pseudohermaphroditism with or without webbed neck
- False dysgenesis
  - Features of Turner's syndrome but with normal ovaries = Ullrich's syndrome

sociated with other malformations, constituting what is known as "sexogenous dwarfism." (3) Bonnevie-Ullrich syndrome, analogous to Turner's syndrome, but differing from the latter in that it occurs in earliest infancy. Not all infants falling into this group present dysgenetic gonads. They are generally chromatin negative. (4) Turner's syndrome, as originally defined by Turner (infantilism, congenital webbed neck and *cubitus valgus*). Generally, chromatin negative and with an XO karyotype. It should be made clear, however, that not all cases of Turner's syndrome, as defined by the above criteria, are necessarily associated with gonadal dysgenesis.

These four clinical variants may occur either in a pure form or in association, to a variable extent, with one of the following features, which may render their diagnosis difficult:

1. Abnormal rates of gonadotropin excretion, a characteristic feature of Turner's syndrome.
2. Virilization (phallic hypertrophy), resulting either from hilus cell hyperplasia or from virilizing adrenal hyperplasia.
3. Feminization: development of secondary and tertiary sex characteristics owing to hyperplasia or tumors involving either theca cell or adrenal cell elements.
4. Combination with other disease entities, such as, for example, Albright's dystrophy or Laurence-Moon-Biedl syndrome.

We believe that this classification is a satisfactory one because, in outlining the symptomatology of Turner's syndrome, it is flexible enough to allow for some symptoms to be added or excluded and at the same time reflects the fact that the complexity of the clinical manifestations is caused by the same underlying disorder of *sex determination*, invariably leading to more or less rudimentary gonadal development which, depending on the extent of nosologic significance of the disorder involved, may be associated or unassociated with somatic, mental or endocrine anomalies.

We shall first describe Turner's syndrome as the fundamental type within the framework of gonadal dysgenesis so as to be able to point out the differences existing between it and the syndromes of Bonnevie-Ullrich, Swyer and Rössle, whether in their pure or associated forms, by continuously drawing parallels between them and their etiology.

36.4.1. TURNER'S SYNDROME

CONCEPT. Since its original description in 1938 by Turner,[121] the syndrome characterized by the triad of infantilism, webbed neck and cubitus valgus has been known by the name of Turner's syndrome. As aptly pointed out by Hauser, the subsequent addition of all kinds of other symptoms or, on the other hand, the downgrading of the significance of some of those pertaining to the classical triad, e.g., pterygium colli, has created a series of clinical pictures based on erroneous criteria as to what constitutes the syndrome and, above all, has caused enormous confusion in terminology. As originally described, the syndrome does not specifically require the presence of gonadal dysgenesis, currently known to be prevalent in most cases, nor does it set any requirements for hormone levels. In 1942, the condition was described as associated with elevated gonadotropin and low estrogen levels by Albright and his associates[1] and by Varney and co-workers[124] and, later, by Del Castillo and colleagues[20,21] in one of the most comprehensive reviews on the subject published to date. These authors also noted a delay in ossification and often the presence of generalized osteoporosis, interpreted as resulting from estrogen deficiency. The same conclusion was reached by Albright and associates,[1] who found that osteoporosis in gonadal dysgenesis was comparable to postmenopausal osteoporosis. On this point, however, there is little agreement, since several authors believe that the osseous changes are those of osteogenesis imperfecta and are simply one more manifestation of associated congenital anomalies (Elliot et al.[31]).

The discovery of the sex chromatin, or Barr body, has established the fact that the majority of cases of Turner's syndrome have male patterns, that is, are chromatin negative. In 1955, Grumbach and his associates[47] found that 80 per cent of the individuals involved were chromatin negative as compared to 20 per cent of chromatin positive cases.

The eventual application of karyotype analysis revealed that most patients had 45 chromosomes, with 44 normal autosomes and only one gonosome: an X chromosome. However, this was soon found not to be the only type of constitution in Turner's syndrome. In addition to normal constitutions reported, some cases revealed sex chromosome complements consisting of an X isochromosome or of XO/XY, XO/XYY or XO/XX mosaicisms (this is one of the reasons why the term Turner's syndrome cannot be used as a synonym for gonadal dysgenesis).

As a result of the fact that the first cases studied by Albright, Varney, Wilkins and Del Castillo under the name of Turner's syndrome happened to be all associated with gonadal dysgenesis, however, a tendency has developed to use the term gonadal dysgenesis interchangeably with Turner's syndrome. On the other extreme, this has also caused misuse of the term Turner's syndrome when applied to such conditions as Ullrich's syndrome, in which women with the Turner triad retain normal ovaries. In our opinion, it seems logical to keep the term Turner's syndrome in honor of its author by making the distinction, however, whether or not such patients suffer from associated gonadal dysgenesis.

Serment and his colleagues[111] divide Turner's syndrome into three categories: (1) dysgenesis with typical Turner's syndrome, (2) pseudoturner, with normal stature and without skeletal anomalies, and (3) simple ovarian hypoplasia. Zarate and his associates[131] described a case that was phenotypically a Turner's syndrome with an XO karyotype but had developed ovaries, puberty and menstruation.

ETIOLOGY. Having thus outlined the features of Turner's syndrome, we shall exclude the entity known by the misnomer of Ullrich's syndrome[123] and refer specifically to variants involving gonadal dysgenesis. Among the various etiologic factors involved in Turner's syndrome, we shall be particularly concerned with one that is perhaps the most common and the most extensively studied factor.

The clinical occurrence of ovarian agenesis in contrast to the nonoccurrence of testicular agenesis, or, in other words, the fact that congenital absence of ovaries in females is known to occur whereas congenital absence of testes in males is not, can be explained on the basis of the experiments of Jost and his associates,[69-73] as well as those of Raynaud and Frilley[102] and Wells.[128, 129] Jost's and Raynaud's groups worked with rabbit embryos whereas Wells used birds. These workers observed that if embryos were castrated (surgically by Jost and by means of x-rays by Raynaud) before they reached a certain stage of development, they consistently turned out to be females at birth. Thus, for instance, female rabbit fetuses castrated before the nineteenth day (by performing cesarean sections on the mothers, followed by reinsertion of the fetuses) were found to subsequently develop normal genital tracts, with the exception perhaps of some decrease in size of organs at the time of birth. Also, male fetuses castrated under the same circumstances rapidly underwent retrogression of the wolffian ducts while the müllerian ducts completed their development, giving rise to females with ovarian agenesis. If the same operation was performed after the nineteenth day, organs derived from the wolffian structures showed development to a variable degree in direct proportion to the period of time by which castration had been delayed, whereas the organs derived from the müllerian ducts showed inverse ratios of underdevelopment or involution, giving rise to intersexual individuals. Jost asserted that failure of the male genital duct to develop followed a certain pattern of gradation, with stepwise downward involvement, whereby the urogenital sinus was last to achieve its characteristic features. If embryonic genital ducts were cultured in vitro (De La Balze et al.[6]) or transplanted to the anterior chamber of the eye (Bronski[17]), only the müllerian structures developed, which confirmed the fact that, apart from the significant hormonal effect exerted by the mother on the fetus through the placenta, a prominent role was played by the "dominant sex" or "basic sex" (see Chapter 14), whereby the presence of any anomalies in sex determination or in sexual development invariably resulted in the reproduction of one particular sex, which in rabbits as well as in humans was the female sex.

The critical period during which the fetal testis seems to exert a decisive influence on wolffian duct development (in the same animal) has been found to fall between the twenty-second and twenty-fourth days. The author explains the changes observed during subsequent days as resulting from the sex differentiating influence of some testicular substance, specifically produced during that period, which spreads locally along the genital tract more readily than it does by the bloodstream. As a result, the effect of this substance is postulated to be greater when acting on fetuses in situ than when injected. A possibility likewise to be considered is that, in accordance with the hypothesis of Jost and Wells, androgenic hormone may occur in some yet unknown protein-bound form, possessing enhanced potency of action, in a similar way to what is known to occur with the substance called "medullarine."

In addition, Jost noted that the action exerted by this hormone was a local one to the extent that, in unilateral castration, wolffian development was inhibited only on the castrated side, while remaining unaffected on the noncastrated side, apparently indicating a very low degree of diffusibility.

Jost's really ingenious experiments may explain the occurrence of variants of Turner's syndrome in which gonadal dysgenesis is produced by premature destruction of the fetal gonad rather than by any gonosomopathy. Nevertheless, this must be a remote possibility, since such features have not yet been confirmed in any of the cases so far reported. It seems more likely that XO carrying gonocytes lack differentiation-inducing potency, as a result of which the gonads remain in such a rudimentary state that they give rise to the symptomatology of ovarian agenesis. If the X gonosome is derived from the mother, it may be heteropyknotic and result in a chromatin positive individual, whereas gonosomes of paternal derivation invariably result in chromatin negative individuals.

XO/XY or XO/XYY mosaicisms similarly lack potency to induce a gonad to differentiate into an ovary; depending on the number of XO or XY gonocytes involved, the resulting gonad will be either like that of the preceding group or, owing to XY predominance, will tend to become a testis, so that the clinical picture given by the same karyotype may vary considerably.

In a similar way, XO/XX mosaicism may be associated either with dominance by XO gonocytes (gonadal agenesis) or with dominance by a variable number of XX chromosomes, which leads to conditions ranging from ovarian syndrome with Turner's syndrome to dysgenesis without associated malformations since, by definition, the underlying *primum movens*, in this instance, is a gonosomopathy.

CLINICAL FEATURES OF TURNER'S SYNDROME. Within the vast group of patients presenting clinically the classical Turner triad, we shall, as in the preceding section, consider only those associated with gonadal dysgenesis.

The syndrome is observed in the young age group, between the age of 8 and adulthood. It is hard to recognize before 8 years of age because it is indistinguishable from Bonnevie-Ullrich syndrome at that age or because it is not suspected in families in which short stature is common. These girls do not arouse medical attention until puberty, when one of the constant symptoms, namely, essential amenorrhea, becomes manifest. By that time, moreover, evidence of their stunted growth may be unmistakable (less than 147.5 cm among the English population, according to Polani) and their short and webbed neck, low insertion of the ears and, at the same time, their progeria, may lend to them the appearance of what Del Castillo and De La Balze refer to as the "sphinx-like look" (Fig. 36–1). Their chests are usually shield-like and devoid of female mammary development and their arms reveal typical *cubitus valgus*. The axillary and pubic hair is scanty (or absent) and the vulva as well as the entire body retains many more infantile features than corresponds to the patient's age. The intelligence quotient is usually decreased, not infrequently to the point of oligophrenia. Associated color blindness, otherwise known to affect

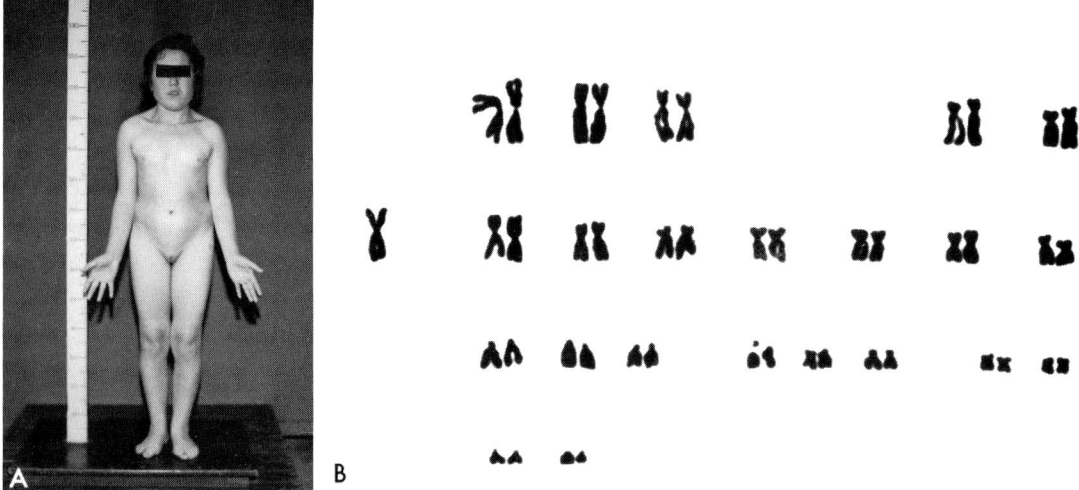

Figure 36-1. Gonadal dysgenesis with Turner's syndrome. A, Characteristic phenotype, which is explained in text. Woman, aged 20, with mental retardation, enlarged sella turcica, failure of cartilages to undergo ossification, atrophic vaginal cytology, negative estrogenuria, gonadotropin levels of 4 rat units per day, 17-ketosteroid levels of 3 mg per 24 hr. Patient had hypoplastic internal genital and müllerian tract, with a gonad resembling a "rudimentary testis." Cells were chromatin-negative. B, Karyotype (XO/45).

women very rarely, is a common finding and may be accompanied by other congenital anomalies involving vision (cataract, tunnel vision and strabismus) or other organs and systems, such as talipes cavus, Madelung's deformity, cervical rib, oligo- and arachnodactyly and, especially, coarctation of the aorta.

An interesting feature of these patients, described in great detail by Teter and Boczkowski[119] and by Taylor and his associates,[117] is the high incidence of tumors involving the genital tract (gonocytomas, gonadoblastomas). In addition, Henkin[56] found that anosmia, in addition to color blindness, was a frequently associated anomaly involving the sensory organs.

Among the findings mentioned by us previously were: (1) osteogenesis imperfecta, occasionally occurring in conjunction with osteoporosis, (2) low estrogen levels, and (3) elevated gonadotropin levels. The first two are thought to be responsible for the development of dwarfism, which cannot be attributed to pituitary insufficiency in view of both the elevated gonadotropin levels and evidence of increased growth hormone activity in such patients (Fraccaro et al.[37]). On the other hand, these symptoms may possibly also be linked to gonosomopathy. Teter and Boczkowski[119] emphasize the diagnostic value of cytology. In typical Turner's syndrome of the pure variety, they always find atrophic smears, as compared to slightly estrogenic smears in cases of pure gonadal dysgenesis (XY or "mixed" variety).

The 17-ketosteroid and, to a greater extent, the pregnanediol levels are low. Roentgenologically, the sella turcica may be normal or may reflect mild pituitary enlargement of the type observed in individuals who have undergone castration. The basal metabolic rate may be variable although, in general, it would appear to be increased in chromatin positive and diminished in chromatin negative cases. These patients frequently may suffer from essential hypertension, apparently unrelated to the anomalies that may involve their circulatory systems.

The *internal genital organs* may assume two different forms: (1) *streak gonads* (Fig. 36-2), with well developed Fallopian tubes and uterus, and (2) absence of gonads and müllerian tract. Naturally, between these two extremes, intermediate forms of all types may occur. Histologically, the cardinal feature of gonadal dysgenesis is the absence of germ cells from the ovarian stroma, which is very dense and represents the cortex. The medullary portion may reveal the presence of tubular structures, and the hilar area may show groups of epithelioid cells that are highly reminiscent of Leydig cells

Figure 36–2. Laparotomy findings in a patient with Turner's syndrome, revealing two hypoplastic tubes, uterine agenesis and rudimentary ovaries, which are reduced to two fibrous streaks (arrows).

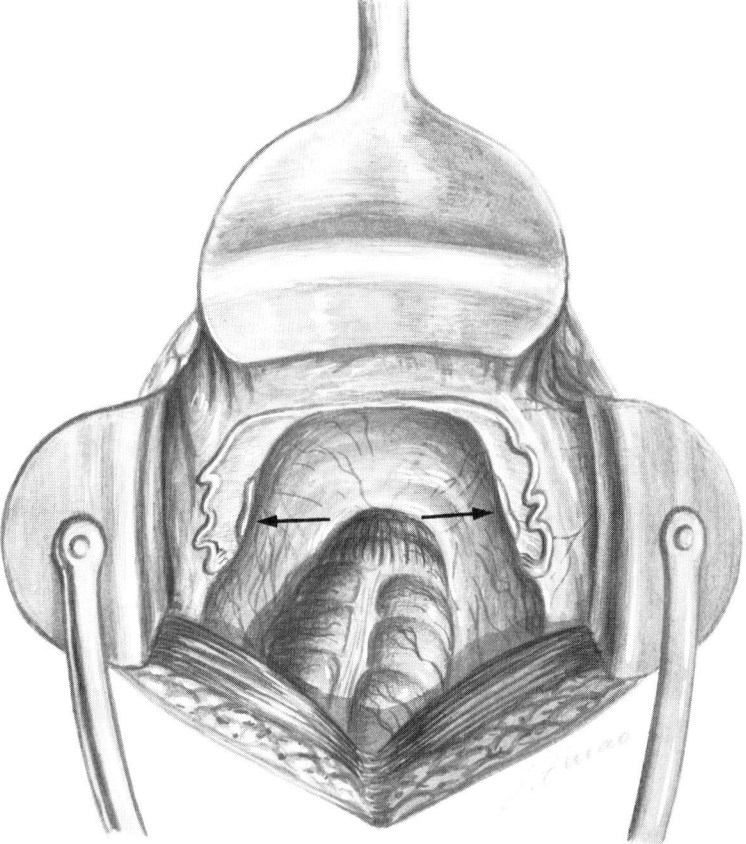

and are actually nothing else than rests of the mesonephric mesenchyma.

DIAGNOSIS OF TURNER'S SYNDROME. The typical somatic features and clinical data enumerated in our description of the symptomatology are expressive enough to alert the physician to the possibility of dealing with gonadal dysgenesis with Turner's syndrome; culdoscopy or transabdominal celioscopy allows us to arrive at an almost conclusive diagnosis, particularly in chromatin negative patients, which is corroborated by evidence of gonosomal anomalies in the karyotype. By and large, a biopsy of the rudimentary gonad is essential in establishing the diagnosis with certainty, since *dysgenesis is defined on purely histologic grounds.*

TREATMENT. Little can be done to cure Turner's syndrome. Nevertheless, some treatment aimed at stimulating general growth may be undertaken with high dosages of either estrogens or androgens. Estrogen therapy gives better results in this respect, as it alleviates some of the symptomatology usually appearing about the time of puberty, which Albright refers to as "prepuberal climacterium."

SUMMARY. Turner's syndrome with gonadal dysgenesis is caused by a gonosomopathy, the associated symptomatology depending on the importance of the chromosomal aberrations. Most often, these are XO individuals with deficient differentiating power of gonocytes, giving rise to highly variable pathology that may be associated with a wide range of symptoms. However, these patients may also be XX/XO mosaics, in which case the ovary may be more or less developed and, depending on the number of XX gonocytes present, some of the stigmata may be alleviated. Finally, similarly depending on the proportion in which each component is represented among the germ cells, XO/XY or XO/XYY karyotypes are associated either with analogous ovarian findings or with rudimentary testes, in the latter instance giving rise to intersexuality pertaining to the group of pseudohermaphroditism (Fig. 36–5). These will be covered after we have briefly reviewed the major differences between Turner's syndrome and the remaining variants of gonadal dysgenesis.

36.4.2. BONNEVIE-ULLRICH SYNDROME

This is very similar to Turner's syndrome from which, by most accounts, it differs only chronologically, being considered as Turner's syndrome in infants. Apparently, it is associated consistently with congenital lymphedema, involvement of cranial nerves, redundant skin, and auricular deformities. As with Turner's syndrome, it may or may not be associated with gonadal dysgenesis. So far, no definite differences between the karyotypes of the two conditions have been established.

36.4.3. RÖSSLE'S SYNDROME

This is defined as gonadal dysgenesis with stunted growth but unassociated with Turner stigmata. It may, however, be associated with some or all of the symptoms secondarily added to Turner's syndrome (Fig. 36–3). Since its etiology is a gonosomopathy, most commonly consisting of XO/XX/XXX, XO/XXX, XO/XX or X isochromosome/X constitutions (Fig. 36–3), it may be assumed that the lesser degree of dysgenetic pathology results from a greater share of XX gonocytes in these patients than in simple XO patients. Most of the variants previously qualified as of the "mixed" type may be included in this syndrome.

36.4.4. SWYER'S SYNDROME

This is an eponym for pure gonadal dysgenesis, which is characterized by the presence of dysgenesis without any associated somatic stigmata. As with the preceding variants, essential amenorrhea occurs as a rule, although it is not unusual to observe the appearance of menstrual bleeding episodes following hormone therapy, which would seem to indicate a considerable degree of uterine development in some cases. Some of the symptoms found in Turner's syndrome, other than those of the classical triad, may also occur. Since the karyotype usually reveals a normal XX or XY sex chromosome complement, it may be inferred that these cases may arise, in the first instance, as a consequence of partly destroyed ovaries in the manner of Jost, or the

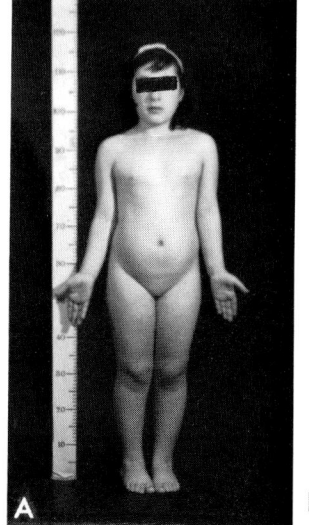
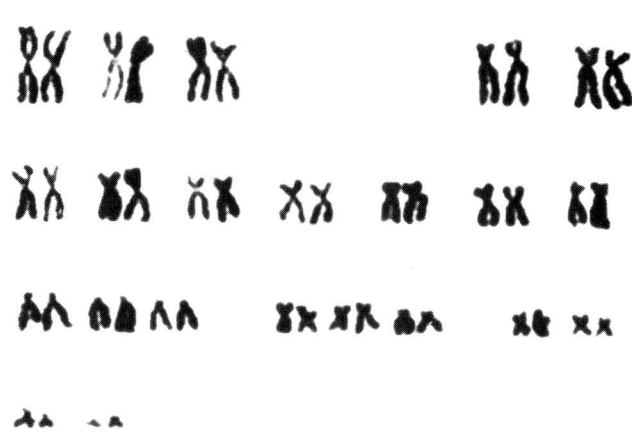

Figure 36–3. Gonadal dysgenesis with "sexogenous" dwarfism, or Rössle's syndrome. Girl, aged 12, with normal intelligence; height 118 cm.: Although this condition is reminiscent of Turner's syndrome, the face has normal features and there is no webbing of the neck. Other features: chromatin-negative cells, internal genitalia consisting of hypoplastic müllerian tract and two streak gonads, which are microscopically similar to "rudimentary testes." Karyotype reveals dysgenesis with 45 chromosomes, in which the special feature is the pressure of an aberrant X chromosome consisting of a long-armed "isochromosome."

loss of gonocyte-differentiating potency owing to a mutant gene, or an anomalous response of the gonad in the presence of normal gonocytes. Literally the same may be said concerning the second eventuality, by adding, however, the possibility that a yet unknown mechanism (perhaps involving mutation) may give rise to cross differentiation characteristic of "sex reversal."

36.5 PSEUDOHERMAPHRODITISM: SYNDROME OF TESTICULAR FEMINIZATION

36.5.1. CONCEPT

Among those individuals who present with pseudohermaphroditism conditioned by an aberration in sex determination, we shall establish a clinical gradation encompassing all variants from those closest to "asexuality" (which, as we have seen, seems to be constituted by chromatin negative variants of Turner's syndrome) to those revealing either perfect somatic feminization or perfect somatic masculinization. *The difference between gonadal dysgenesis and the kind of conditions under consideration lies in the fact the gonads in the former agree with the phenotype although not necessarily with the genotype or karyotype of the patient (sex reversal), whereas pseudohermaphrodites develop the opposite phenotype in relation to their gonads.*

Almost constantly, these patients have to a variable extent rudimentary gonads which lack germ cells. Even by histologic standards, therefore, they may be categorized as consistent with gonadal dysgenesis. How-

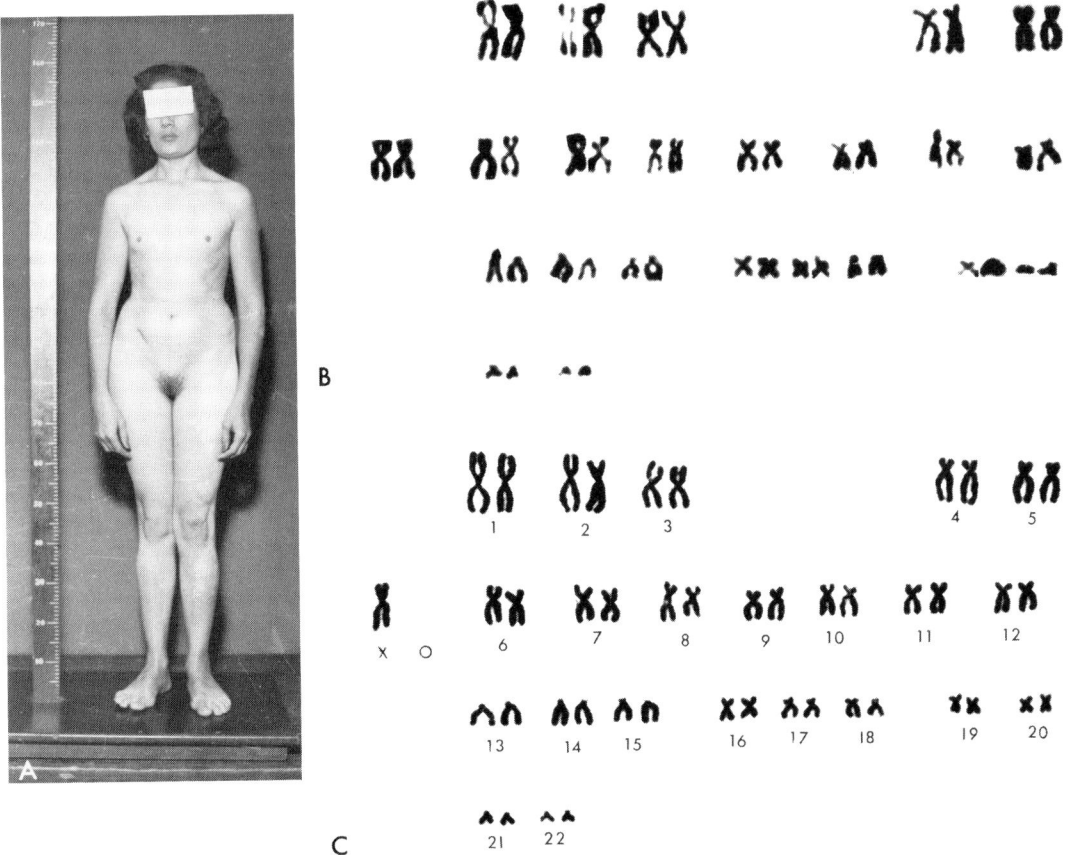

Figure 36-4. Gonadal dysgenesis without Turner's syndrome. A, Woman, aged 22; height, 162 cm. The only somatic feature of note is mammary aplasia. Findings include: radiographically normal sella turcica; hypoestrogenic vaginal smears with cytolysis; estrogenuria, 42 mcg; pregnanediol, negative; 17-ketosteroids, 3.5 mg per 24 hr; gonadotropins, 5 rat units per day; chromatin negative; hypoplastic internal genitalia with rudimentary ovaries. B, C, Karyotype reveals a mosaic pattern, composed of 46 normal chromosomes (XX), and 45 normal chromosomes (XO).

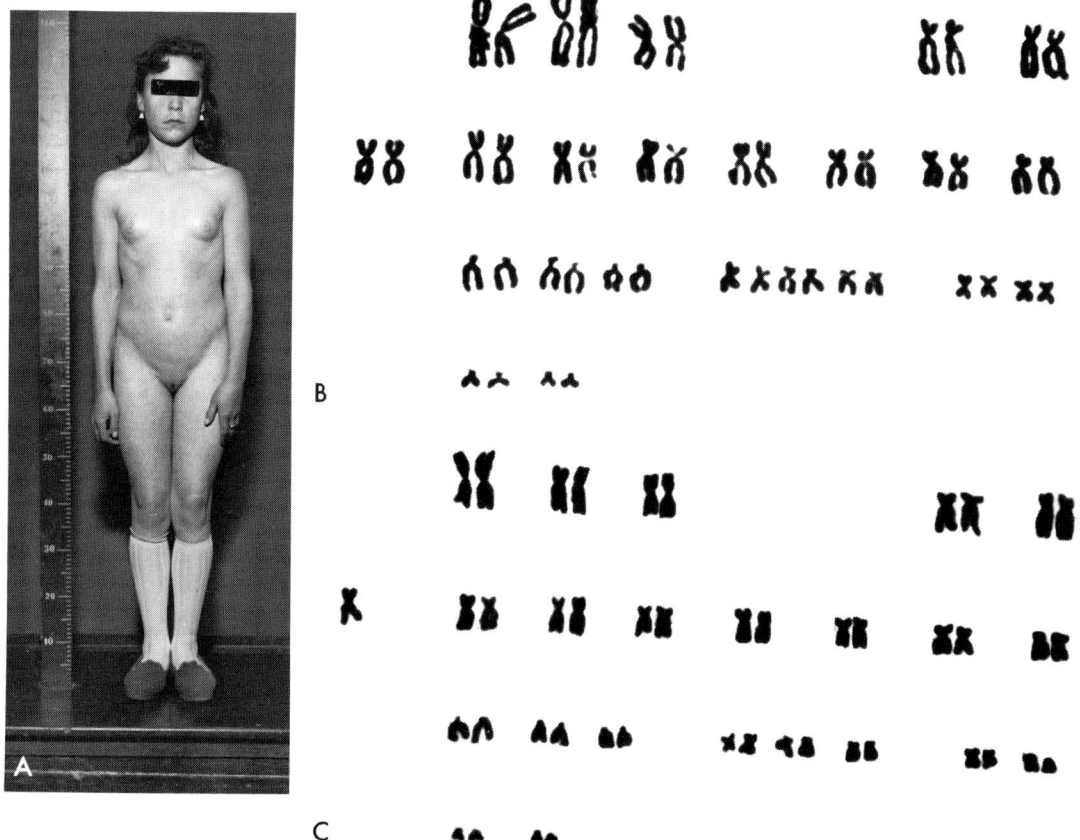

Figure 36–5. A, Gonadal dysgenesis without Turner's syndrome, similar to case in Figure 36–4, except for developmental arrest (149 cm) and absence of body hair. As in the other cases presented here, there was *amenorrhea*. The internal genitalia were very hypoplastic and the gonad was a rudimentary testis. Therefore, this represents a case of testicular (not ovarian) dysgenesis, with incomplete feminization. Karyotype revealed XO/XX mosaicism. *B*, XO cell line. *C*, XX cell line.

ever, because of the concept by now almost universally accepted, we reserve the latter designation to cases in which the gonads as well as the phenotype are of the same sex, poorly developed as such gonadal or phenotypic sex may be.

By convention, if not in fact, pseudohermaphroditism has thus been separated from other forms of gonadal dysgenesis. The sex of the gonad being by definition the opposite of the sex corresponding to the phenotype, we speak of either *testicular feminization* or *ovarian masculinization*, depending on the existing combination. However, it is a clinical fact that the former is always the result of aberrations in sex determination owing to the existence of a dominant or basic sex, whereas the latter is above all a common consequence of *pathology* of sex differentiation. As presently conceived, the syndrome of testicular feminization comprises a series of clinical features and chromosomal formulas that may be classified in accordance with either concept, as outlined in the preceding section.

36.5.2. THE KARYOTYPE IN TESTICULAR FEMINIZATION

In 1952, Botella and Nogales[14] described a syndrome characterized by *"male pseudohermaphroditism (presence of ectopic testes) with complete feminization."* Subsequent publications by Botella and Nogales[15] and by Morris[89] gave clinical support to this entity, for which Morris introduced the name testicular feminization. Although this term has been widely publicized, it incurs the error of confusing "a part for the whole." The designation suggested by Botella and Nogales would appear more appropriate since it implicitly recognizes the occurrence of other, less complete forms of testicular feminization.

The study of the gonads in intersexuality over the past years has disclosed the fact that *a number of intersexual states are actually associated with feminizing testes*. In many instances, feminization may not be as complete as that described originally and some cases may even reveal phenotypes quite similar to those observed in Turner's syndrome.

Karyotype analysis on patients with complete feminization by, among others, Stewart,[115] Jacobs and co-workers,[67] Lejeune and colleagues,[81] Puck and colleagues,[100] Grumbach,[48] and Chu and associates,[28] verified the fact that such individuals invariably had a normal male constitution, that is, 44 autosomes and an XY pair of gonosomes, without any structural chromosomal anomalies. The eight cases reported in 1961 by Alexander and Ferguson-Smith,[2] all conforming with the above findings, served to generalize the notion that every case of testicular feminization is associated with the same karyotype. This was further strengthened by the reports of Bartlett and his colleagues,[7] who found XY karyotypes in three members of the same family, and by Boczkowski,[13] who found XY karyotypes in eight families with testicular feminization.

Insofar as variants with complete feminization are concerned, the validity of an XY sex chromosomal constitution could be verified in three of our cases, one of which is illustrated in Figure 36–6. However, it is by no means certain that the same rule is obeyed in all cases, as the degree of associated feminization may vary. In 1961, Oikawa and Brizzard[93] reported a case of a female with a phenotype resembling that of Turner's syndrome, in which laparotomy revealed the presence of a streak gonad that histologically turned out to be a testis with-

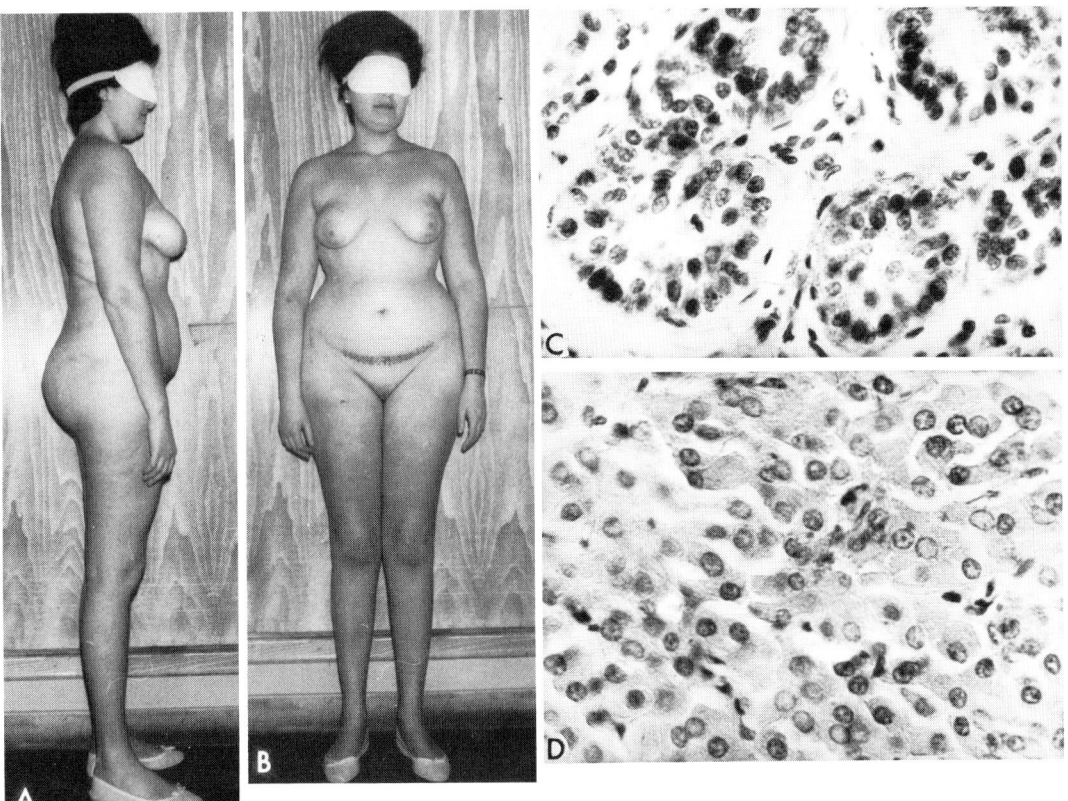

Figure 36–6. Case of testicular feminization. *A*, lateral view; *B*, frontal view. Note excellent breast development and distinctly feminine physique with, however, complete absence of pubic and axillary hair. Internal genitalia were absent as well, but there was a well developed vagina. Rudimentary testes were removed from each groin. *C*, Immature seminiferous tubules. *D*, Interstitial cells of the Leydig type in one of the testes. The genetic sex was male (XY), with 46 chromosomes.

out germ cells. The karyotype consisted of 46 chromosomes with a sex pair made up of one normal and one isochromosome X chromosomes. During the same year, Shah and his associates[112] described another case of male pseudohermaphroditism in which he could not identify any Y chromosome. Both of these cases may be interpreted as true instances of "sex reversal," in which the type of gonad is determined by the genotype of the opposite sex.

Bloise and his colleagues[12] studied a female with multiple congenital malformations, with intraabdominal embryonic testicular tissue and with an XO karyotype. Atkins and Engel[4] reported a case of a woman who was short in stature and had an elongated clitoris, underdeveloped internal genitalia and a single gonad that turned out to be an ectopic testis. The patient was chromatin negative and karyotype analysis revealed an XO/XX mosaicism. Fraccaro and his colleagues[38] reported a 61 year old woman, tall in stature, with essential amenorrhea (associated with Rössle's syndrome), with a peniform clitoris and a small uterus. She was not explored surgically, but her karyotype showed an XO/Xy/XXXy sex chromosome constitutuon, in which the small y represents deletion of a Y chromosome, or possibly an isochromosome for its short arms. Miles and his associates[90] described a girl with a phallus and very small internal female genital organs, in which the gonads were testes. She was chromatin negative with an XO/XxY karyotype, with the x denoting deletion of the X chromosome. Schuster and Motulsky[109] described a woman with a phallus and without a vagina, in whom the only internal genitalia consisted of two tubes, one containing a male gonad. Her sex chromosome complement was XX/XY/XO. Willemse and associates[130] described an XO/XY mosaicism in a woman with a uterus, with tubes, and with testes without spermatogenesis. Lewis and his coworkers[82] published a case of an XO/XY mosaicism in a male with a bifid penis and hypospadias and with an ectopic testis that harbored a seminoma. A second surgical intervention revealed a uterus (with an endometrial adenocarcinoma) and Fallopian tubes without evidence of ovarian tissue.

In view of the various genotypes described so far, the following schematic classification of the karyotype in testicular feminization may be suggested: (1) without Y gonosome (sex reversal), and (2) with Y gonosome, which in turn may give (a) pure XY forms or (b) mosaicisms.

36.5.3. CLINICAL PICTURE OF TESTICULAR FEMINIZATION

That some women may have testes has been a well known fact ever since 1905, when Pick[97] described three cases of this type. Other subsequent publications on the subject, apart from those of Botella and Nogales and of Morris mentioned previously, are those of Blairbell,[10] Wagner,[125] Goldberg and Maxwell,[40] Ward-MacQuaid and Lennon,[121] and Schneider and his colleagues.[125]

The clinical manifestations presented by these patients may range from complete feminization (Figs. 36-6, 36-7 and 36-8) to features simulating Turner's syndrome. This, as well as the fact that the karyotypes involved may range equally from XO to XY constitutions in the pure forms, and in addition consist of mosaicisms, enables us to establish a *new etiologic conception* which, like that suggested for gonadal dysgenesis, leaves ample room for possible new discoveries in the field of cytogenetics and endocrinology.

While discussing ovarian dysgenesis with Turner's syndrome, we have indicated that the ovaries in some XO individuals were often quite similar to rudimentary testes, revealing the presence of glandular formations in the medulla and the presence of Leydig-like cells in the hilar region. In some instances, it may be extremely difficult to decide whether the organ examined is a male or a female gonad, whereas in other cases (Nogales et al.[92]) the pathologist reports the presence of testicular tissue. We consider the last mentioned instances as transition forms leading from ovarian dysgenesis to testicular dysgenesis.

We offer the following explanation: XO germ cells for practical purposes lack differentiating potency although they may, within quite narrow limits, induce some differentiation. Thus, while it would appear that such differentiation most frequently proceeds in a female direction, perhaps owing to sex dominance, it unquestionably also may proceed in a male direction, with little or no difference in the resulting clinical picture. Possibly the origin of the X gonosome may also play a role in tipping

Pathology of Sex Determination: Major Gynecologic Syndromes

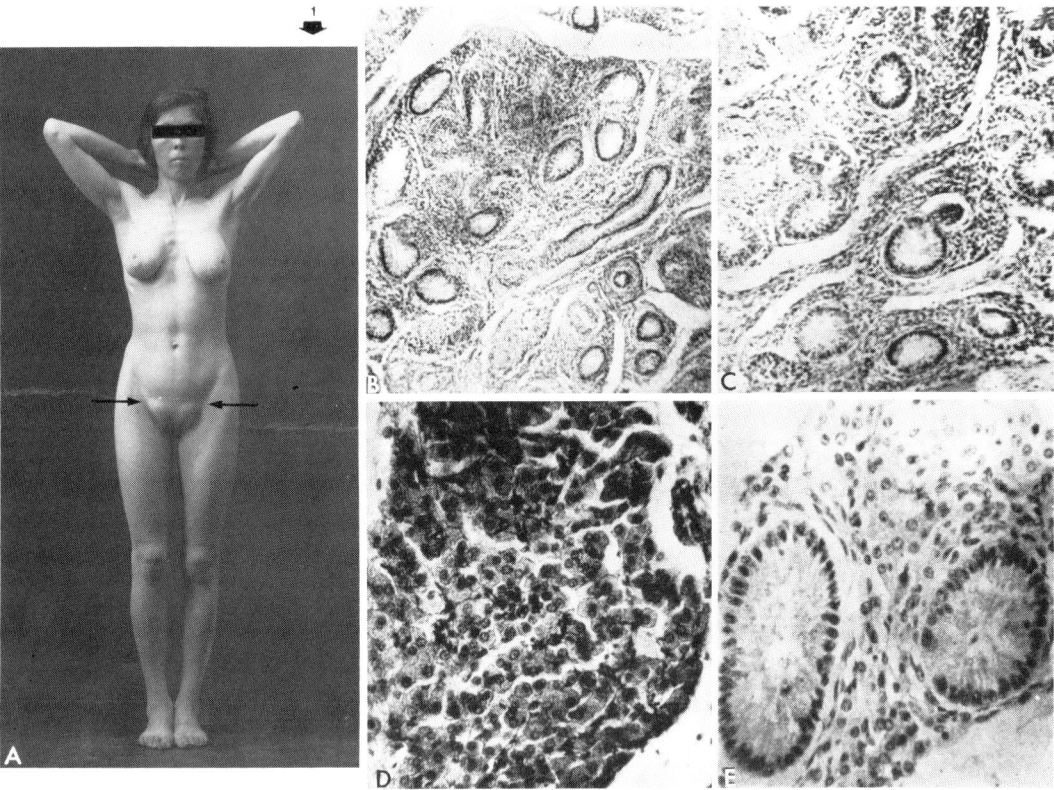

Figure 36-7. Testicular feminization in a 32 year old married woman maintaining normal marital relations, who suffered from essential amenorrhea and sterility. *A,* Somatic features are associated with normal breast development and feminine morphology, absence of pubic and axillary hair and obvious bilateral inguinal swelling. *B, C,* Sections of rudimentary testes with scanty seminiferous tubules and abundant interstitial tissue. *D,* Area composed of Leydig cells. *E,* High power appearance of seminiferous tubules, revealing lack of either maturation or spermatogenesis.

the balance either way. The result may be Turner's syndrome with gonadal dysgenesis, but involving in one instance ovarian dysgenesis and in the other testicular dysgenesis with feminization. The fact that those patients with 46 (or more) chromosomes do not have any Y chromosome cannot be explained otherwise than by invoking the mechanism of "sex reversal," as has been done in the pure XY type of ovarian dysgenesis. We shall therefore not repeat the possible genetic mechanisms involved. Accordingly, the occurrence of XO/XX, X isochromosome/X chromosome, etc., would be nothing else but the extreme manifestations of the same process: discrepancy between genetic sex and gonadal sex or sex inversion. A distinction must be made in women with Y chromosomes between those that are mosaics and those that are not. The karyotype serving as the model for the latter consists of an XO/XY constitution, since all

other modifications act etiologically in a similar way. Referring in general to all carriers of this constitution, whatever the syndrome it may be associated with, Dewhurst[29] compares the situation with the rabbit experiments of Jost. Failure in the development of a testis results in a primitive gonad that is similar to an ovary. However, if the failure is of lesser magnitude, the resulting gonad will be more or less like a testis, giving rise to the phenomenon of virilization. Thus, starting from a poor endowment of XY gonocytes, gonadal development first proceeds toward a rudimentary testis, insufficient to induce male-directed differentiation of the phenotype, which turns out to be female by virtue of sexual dominance, although with superimposed virilization. As a result, these individuals frequently develop a peniform clitoris, absence of vagina, and so forth. The presence of pronounced virilization may give rise to

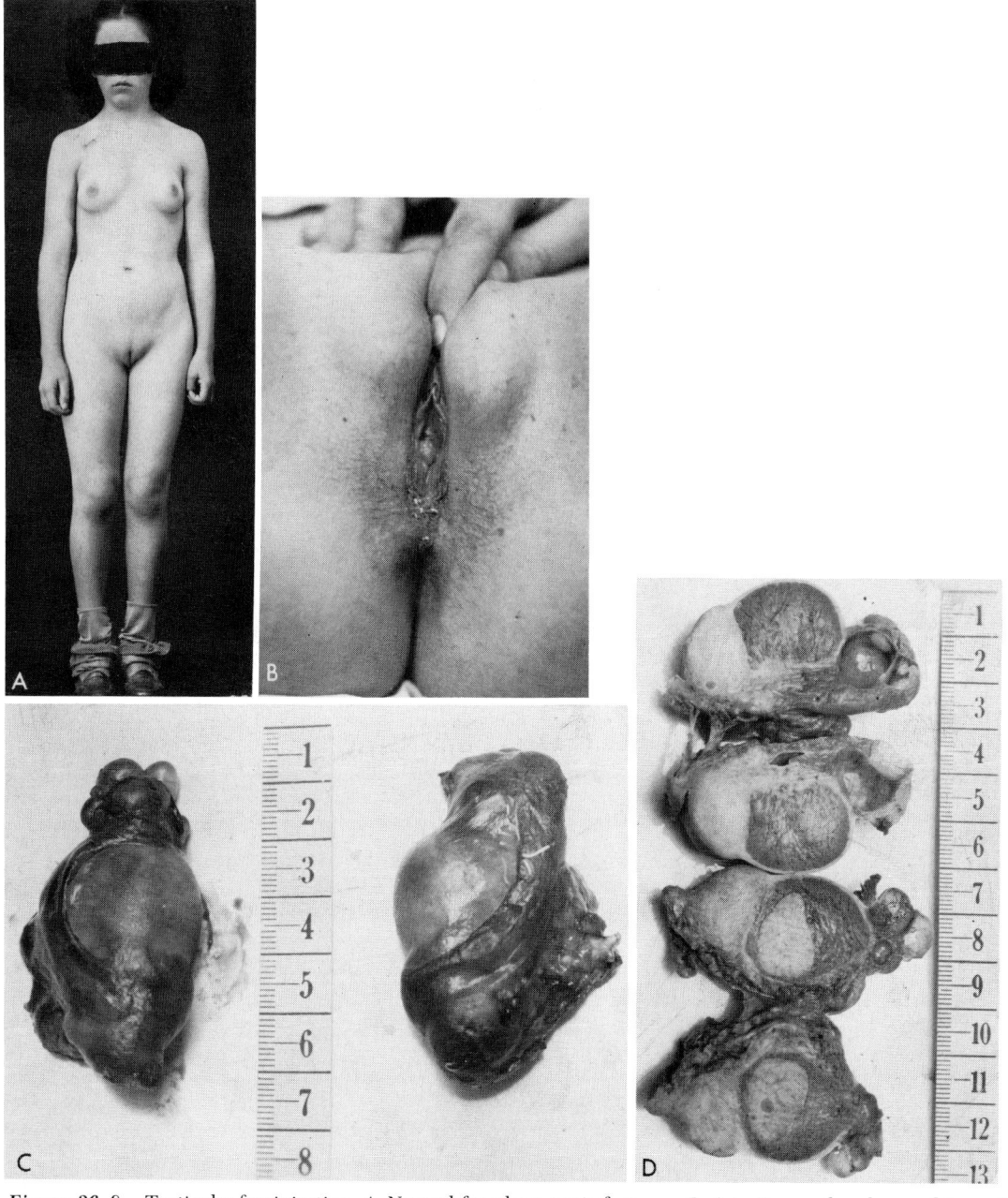

Figure 36–8. Testicular feminization. *A*, Normal female somatic features. *B*, A testis may be observed in each groin; vulva and vaginal introitus of distinctly female appearance. *C*, Gross appearance of both excised testes, with adnexa. *D*, Cut surface of testes, one of which displays a characteristic adenoma as a well circumscribed whitish mass.

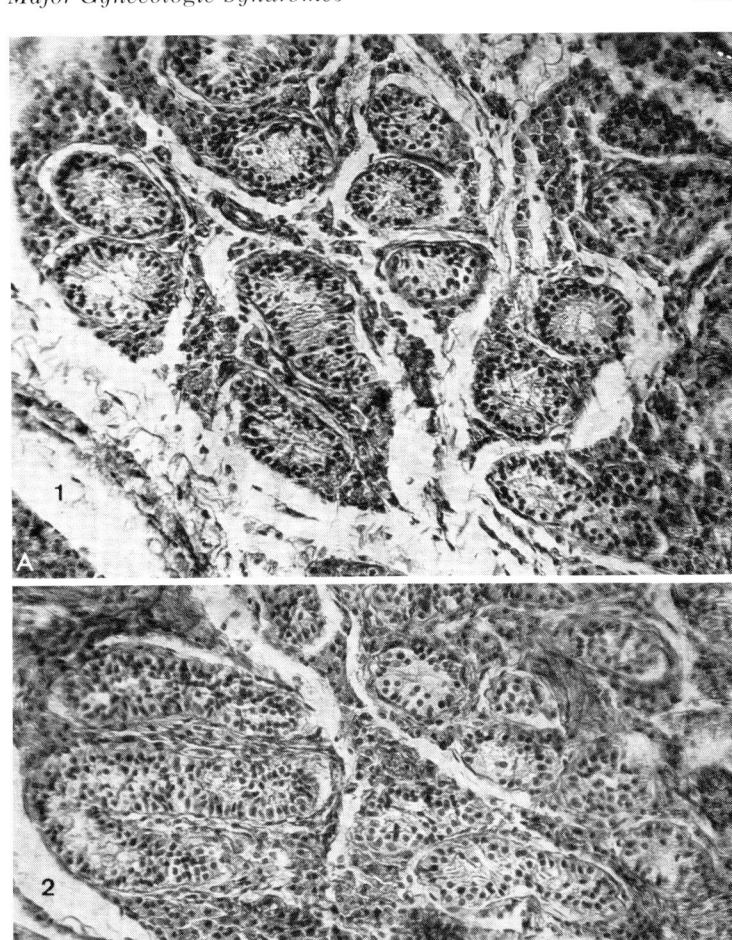

Figure 36–9. Histologic appearance of inguinal testis from patient shown in Figure 36–8. A, Area with few tubules and abundant interstitial tissue, structurally consistent with the usual pattern found in immature and ectopic testes. B, Area with abundant tubular structures, with interstitial tissue, consistent with an "adenoma of Pick."

cases similar to that reported by Lewis, in which there was a bifid penis, hypospadias, a testis with a seminoma, Fallopian tubes and a uterus with adenocarcinoma.[82]

While sex dominance may explain *incomplete feminization*, generally associated with virilization, the syndrome of *complete feminization* is more difficult to explain. Estrogen levels are within normal limits or frankly above normal. Hormone activity then must be considered as mainly responsible for the harmonious corporal development of these patients. Estrogens are derived from the testis, so that castration results in climacteric phenomena analogous to those observed in normal postmenopausal women. According to Botella and Nogales, a constant finding in such gonads is hyperplasia of Leydig cells, described as early as 1905 by Pick.[97] The estrogenic nature of the secretion elaborated by such gonads is at present well known. It is currently equally well recognized that Sertoli cell adenomas, and even the testis itself under physiologic conditions, may exert a feminizing effect on the male. Feminization would therefore seem to be the result of a humoral effect, superimposed on the gentic process, although it is not yet known why this should occur specifically with XY karyotypes without evidence of associated adenoma. Recently, some cases were reported in which testicular feminization was associated with partial feminization (Baron et al.,[7] Ionescu et al.[63]). The case illustrated by us in Figure 36-6 also corresponded to this type.

36.5.4. SYMPTOMATOLOGY

Incomplete feminization may assume clinical features quite reminiscent of those seen in gonadal dysgenesis. In fact, these are cases of testicular dysgenesis. As indicated repeatedly, the syndrome of male pseudohermaphroditism ranges from one extreme in which it overlaps Turner's syndrome to complete testicular feminization, at the other extreme (Botella-Morris syndrome). Table 36-3 briefly summarizes the possibilities. It should be stressed that male pseudohermaphrodites with a male phenotype possess either a uterus, or Fallopian tubes, or both, whereas those with normal stature and those with Pick's adenoma never actually undergo full feminization, as exemplified by our XXXY patient, who was found to have no vagina.

Thus, with the exception of pure XY type of feminization, all other variants present features overlapping those seen in ovarian dysgenesis. We shall therefore not refer to them other than emphasizing the importance of performing histologic examinations of the gonads in all cases of dysgenesis.

Complete feminization may produce no symptomatology of consequence other than essential amenorrhea, which is usually the chief complaint of such patients. In addition, what generally calls attention is absence of axillary and pubic hair, as well as the presence of "inguinal hernias" (Figs. 36-7 and 36-8), representing ectopic testes. These patients tend to be tall and slender, with delicate skin, excellent breast development of female appearance, normal or somewhat above normal intelligence and typical, occasionally slightly enhanced, female libido. A familial tendency, with the syndrome occurring in several siblings at the same time, has been known since the turn of the century. External genitalia appear normally developed, *internal genitalia* being absent, the vagina typically ending blindly. It should be remembered that incomplete feminization, as we have pointed out, is often associated with the presence of uterine development which, in contrast, is not the case in these patients. The length of the vagina is usually an index of estrogenic testicular function; the shorter the vagina the greater the estrogenic deficit. Hormone levels may be within normal limits, but tend to be elevated in cases with excellent feminization or lowered in less developed phenotypes (with absence of vagina, etc.). Androgen levels are usually noncontributory. Rates of excretion of 17-ketosteroids and FSH may be increased. The occurrence of associated osteoporosis or congenital anomalies is very rare. Vaginal cytology may vary in relation to estrogenic activity. These patients are invariably chromatin negative and, as pointed out previously, reveal a male karyotype, which indicates that these are actually males and not females.

Nevertheless, once the *diagnosis* has been arrived at on the basis of the described symptoms, the important point in *therapy* is to avoid questioning the patient's sex. Since both the phenotypic sex and the sex of rearing are in general distinctly feminine, nothing can be achieved by attempting to change this. On the other hand, it remains to be seen whether prevailing notions and definitions of sex may not continue being revised, as they have in the past, so that those conditions may be assessed in a different way in the future as, for instance, is now being done with female patients with Turner's syndrome.

Aside from such psychologic considerations, the foremost question to be solved is whether or not the ectopic gonads should be extirpated. In the first place, because of the

TABLE 36-3. Classification of the Feminizing Variety of Male Pseudohermaphroditism

Clinical forms:	With Turner's syndrome	Short stature	Normal stature
Associated with:	→	Virilization	Adenoma of Pick
May give rise to:		Pseudohermaphroditism with male phenotype	Complete feminization

inconveniences they cause and, in the second, owing to their known tendency to undergo malignant degeneration (Jones and Scott,[68] among others), their removal is always recommended. Whenever we are faced with a problem of inguinal masses and "gonadal dysgenesis" we can actually never be quite sure what type of "disease entity" we are dealing with unless extirpation is also done for diagnostic purposes. Following removal of the gonads, substitution therapy becomes a necessity as a result of the fact that disturbances of the climacteric type are bound to supervene much in the same way as they are after extirpating the gonads in normal women.

36.5.5. TESTICULAR FEMINIZATION AS A DISORDER INVOLVING TARGET ORGANS

In Chapter 4 (Section 4.6.3), we have seen how testosterone, along with other steroids, does not act on the end organs except in presence of a binding protein capable of fixing these steroids to the cells. Southren and his colleagues[113] have demonstrated specific fixation of testosterone to end organ tissue. Roy and Laumas[104] duplicated these experiments with tritiated testosterone. Attention has been called to the presence of testosterone 5α-reduction in the tissues of normal males, whereas patients with the syndrome of testicular feminization lack this action (Mauvais-Jarvis et al.[86]). At the same time, studies of in vitro steroidogenesis by tissue from feminizing testes conducted by Ghnassia[39] and Charreau and Villee[22] demonstrated that, contrary to previous assumptions, the testes from such patients normally secreted androgens rather than estrogens. As a result, Rivarola and his colleagues[103] and, subsequently, Masica and associates[85] postulated that testicular feminization was not the result of any primary disorder of the gonad but represented a defect of testosterone action at the level of target tissues. Consequently, not only are the tissues during embryonal life postulated to be insensitive to testosterone activity, allowing female-directed evolution, but also the testes fail to descend because androgens fail to have an effect on the *gubernaculum testis*. The ectopic testis usually reveals a rudimentary structure not unlike that described in the syndrome of testicular feminization and equally prone to be associated with gonadal dysgenesis.

36.5.6. SUMMARY

Testicular feminization comprises a series of syndromes characterized by testicular dysgenesis with feminization of the patient, clinically ranging from features of Turner's syndrome (transition forms of ovarian dysgenesis) to *complete feminization*. In general, cases with *incomplete feminization* reveal the presence of a uterus and tubes in association with virilization (hypertrophy of the clitoris), and their karyotypes either lack the Y gonosome (undifferentiated XO gonocytes or XX gonocytes with "sex reversal") or reveal a mosaicism (with moderate predominance of XY gonocytes). In either case, gonosomal participation in the etiology can be explained on the basis of "basic sex dominance" or on the genetic existence of "sex inversion."

As for *complete feminization*, all present indications are that the karyotype has a distinctly male sex chromosome complement (XY) and that development of perfect female phenotypes seems to be related to the estrogenic function of Pick's adenoma, whose hormone effect is thought to add up to the influence of the dominant sex. At present, it is not known why this chromosomal constitution should be commonly associated with Leydig cell hyperplasia.

36.6. TRUE HERMAPHRODITISM

36.6.1. CONCEPT

The occurrence of male individuals with complete feminization whose testes contain an area (adenoma of Pick) which, notwithstanding its distinctly male histology, physiologically functions as a female gonad brings us to a new syndrome, that of *true hermaphroditism, defined as those states in which ovarian tissue coexists with testicular tissue in the same individual.* Since the demarcation of ovarian dysgenesis from either testicular feminization or true hermaphroditism is based on purely histologic grounds, only a biopsy of the gonad in question can dispel any doubts as to the true nature of the syndrome explored, although both the phenotypic sex and chromosomal sex may be superimposed on any of the different clinical pictures we have so far described.

36.6.2. ETIOLOGY

The etiology of true hermaphroditism seems to be related to anomalies in sex determination which are in part analogous to those we have described in connection with the preceding syndromes. The concurrence of gonads of both sexes seems to suggest that development of the syndrome is linked to differentiation of XX and XY gonosomes. As we shall indicate later, these types of constitution have been demonstrated in some cases; however, it has been impossible to identify their presence in the majority of cases.

In order to establish a relationship between the phenotype, karyotype and gonadal sex we shall be obliged to invoke the oft repeated cytogenetic mechanisms whereby the same genotype may develop different kinds of phenotypes and gonads, depending on the predominance of those gonocytes that are least abnormal. In hermaphrodites, some gonocytes favor development of ovarian tissue, some that of testicular tissue, but the eventual appearance of the phenotype depends on the predominance of one type of tissue, because gonadal function is always hormonally adequate in true hermaphrodites unlike in the preceding syndromes, in which gonadal dysgenesis (either ovarian or testicular) involves absence of both germ cells and endocrine function. An exception to this rule is complete feminization, which we consider as a gradation step to true hermaphroditism.

Starting from the premise that we are dealing with a defect of sex determination resulting simultaneously in both male- and female-directed development of the gonads, it would be difficult to understand how either loss of gonocyte-differentiating potency or destruction of gonads could have anything to do with the disorder, which leaves us with some gonosomopathy as the only other possible alternative. Although gonosomes would be assumed to possess bivalent determining power, the development of one kind of tissue would always predominate over the other. This predominance is reflected in the phenotype of the patient, who owes his somatic features to his incretory system.

While hermaphrodites display a higher level of hormone production than do patients with gonadal dysgenesis (ovarian or testicular dysgenesis with feminization), their reproductive function is similarly developed to a greater extent although, despite the occasional presence of maturing germ cells in their gonads, they are invariably sterile. Hermaphrodites may then be viewed as individuals suffering from a gonosomopathy causing a kind of "gonadal dysgenesis" that is characterized by: (1) presence of both ovarian and testicular tissue, and (2) subnormal vegetative and generative function, which is nevertheless developed to a greater degree than that found in cases qualified by histologic criteria as true gonadal dysgenesis. In other words, they represent instances of gonadal dysgenesis (underdeveloped gonads) when speaking broadly on other than histologic terms.

36.6.3 KARYOTYPE IN TRUE HERMAPHRODITISM

The first cases reported between 1959 and 1960 seemed to be consistently associated with a female XX pattern (Harnden and Armstrong,[54] Hungerford et al.,[61] De Assis et al.,[3] Makino and Sasaki,[84] and Gordon et al.[41]). In the course of the same years, other constitutions began to be described: a mosaicism without a Y chromosome (XX/XXX) (Ferguson-Smith et al.[32]); a male karyotype (XY) (Sandberg et al.[106] and Grumbach[48]); and an XO/XY mosaic (Blank et al.,[11] Hirschhorn et al.,[57] Miller et al.[91]). The list of gonosomopathies described has since grown. In 1961, Conen and his associates[25] described an XO/Xy (deletion of Y) mosaic, and in 1962, Waxman and coworkers[127] described an XX/XY and Turpin and his colleagues[122] an XX/XXY karyotype, the latter analogous to one of the cases observed by us (Moncada et al.[88]).

To correlate these constitutions with the corresponding phenotypes poses a greater problem than in gonadal dysgenesis, although the genetic norm whereby XX groups cause feminization and XY groups cause masculinization seems to hold true. The clinical repercussions flowing from this fact are the almost constant emergence of manifestations of intersexuality, so that male phenotypes are associated with female internal genitalia in addition to breast development and the presence of vaginas, whereas female phenotypes reveal clitoral hypertrophy, inguinal gonads and other symptoms of virilization. A case of XY/XX/XXY hermaphroditism was described by Klay and his associates[75] and, subsequently, another with an XX/XY sex chromosomal complement by Park and his colleagues.[95]

36.6.4. CLINICAL PICTURE

The highly variable clinical picture of intersexual states ranges from complete feminization to complete masculinization, although it hardly ever occurs in either extreme form. Feminization in males and virilization in females, as well as a large variety of ectopic gonads (so-called inguinal hernias) descended into the inguinal canal have been described. The vagina is almost always present although it may occasionally remain invisible because of opening into a more or less internal urogenital sinus. The uterus may be bicornuate or monocornuate. In some cases, one gonad may be an ovary, the other a testis, with the Fallopian tubes and even the uterine body missing on the involved side. In cases with ovotestes, the female organs may have undergone atrophy commensurate in extent to the significance of testicular function. Individuals with well developed uteri may experience menstrual bleeding through the vagina. Bleeding may also occur through the penis in those cases in which the urogenital sinus extends into the urethra, ending in hypospadias.

Based on gonadal histology, the classification proposed by Klebs[76] about a century ago remains valid (with minor modifications). It distinguishes three categories of true hermaphroditism: I. *Lateral hermaphroditism*, with a testis on one side and an ovary on the other. II. *Bilateral hermaphroditism*, with two variants: (a) bilateral ovotestes, and (b) bilateral ovaries and testes. III. *Unilateral hermaphroditism*, with six variants: (a) ovary and ovotestis, (b) ovary and bilateral testes, (c) ovary and two ovotestes, (d) testis and ovotestis (for some, this constitutes an independent class IV), (e) ovotestis on one side and absence of gonads on other (class V, according to others), and (f) ovotestis on one side and other side not explored (class VI, according to others).

In view of the importance of these cases, we subsequently present three of our own patients (from the department of Prof. Botella), which may serve to illustrate the clinical course most commonly encountered.

CASE I. Case of true lateral hermaphroditism, illustrated in Figure 36–10. A 19 year old farmer presented himself at the clinic because of hypospadias, empty scrotum on the right side and gynecomastia. Physical examination revealed feminoid features, with well developed breasts and characteristic roundness of body contour. Although there was a suggestion of whiskers at the site of the beard, the skin over the rest of the body was hairless. The external gentalia consisted of two scrotal sacs, the right one empty, the left one containing a small infantile-sized testis. The penis had associated hypospadias. The patient gave a history of having bled through the urethral orifice. A detailed anamnesis indicated the occurrence of true menstruation in the past. Urethral cytology was of the vaginal type, consistent with cyclic changes. At laparotomy, there was seen complete absence of internal genitalia on the left side. On the right, a uterus unicornis opened behind the bladder into a rudimentary vagina, with a single right-sided round ligament, ovary and Fallopian tube. The uterus, tube and ovary were removed (Fig. 36–10,C). A cross section of the small Fallopian tube is shown in Figure 36–10,D, revealing normal features. The ovary contained a corpus luteum (Fig. 36–11,A), corresponding chronologically to the last days (twenty-seventh and twenty-eighth) of the cycle. It is noteworthy to mention that the last menstrual bleeding episode had taken place about three weeks earlier. Histologically, the endometrium was interpreted as in a poorly developed secretory phase (Fig. 36–11,B).

The study of urinary hormones by means of bioassay revealed between 30 and 50 rat units of estrogens per liter and between 25 and 50 international units of androgens per liter. Multiple urinary pregnanediol determinations were carried out in relation to the cycle. On admission, the patient experienced an episode of minor menstrual bleeding, three days following which the test for pregnanediol was negative. At the time of surgery, during which a corpus luteum was found, urinary pregnanediol was excreted at the rate of 10 mg per liter of urine. Vaginal cytology revealed concomitant cyclic changes. There seemed to be no doubt that the ovary in this patient was functioning

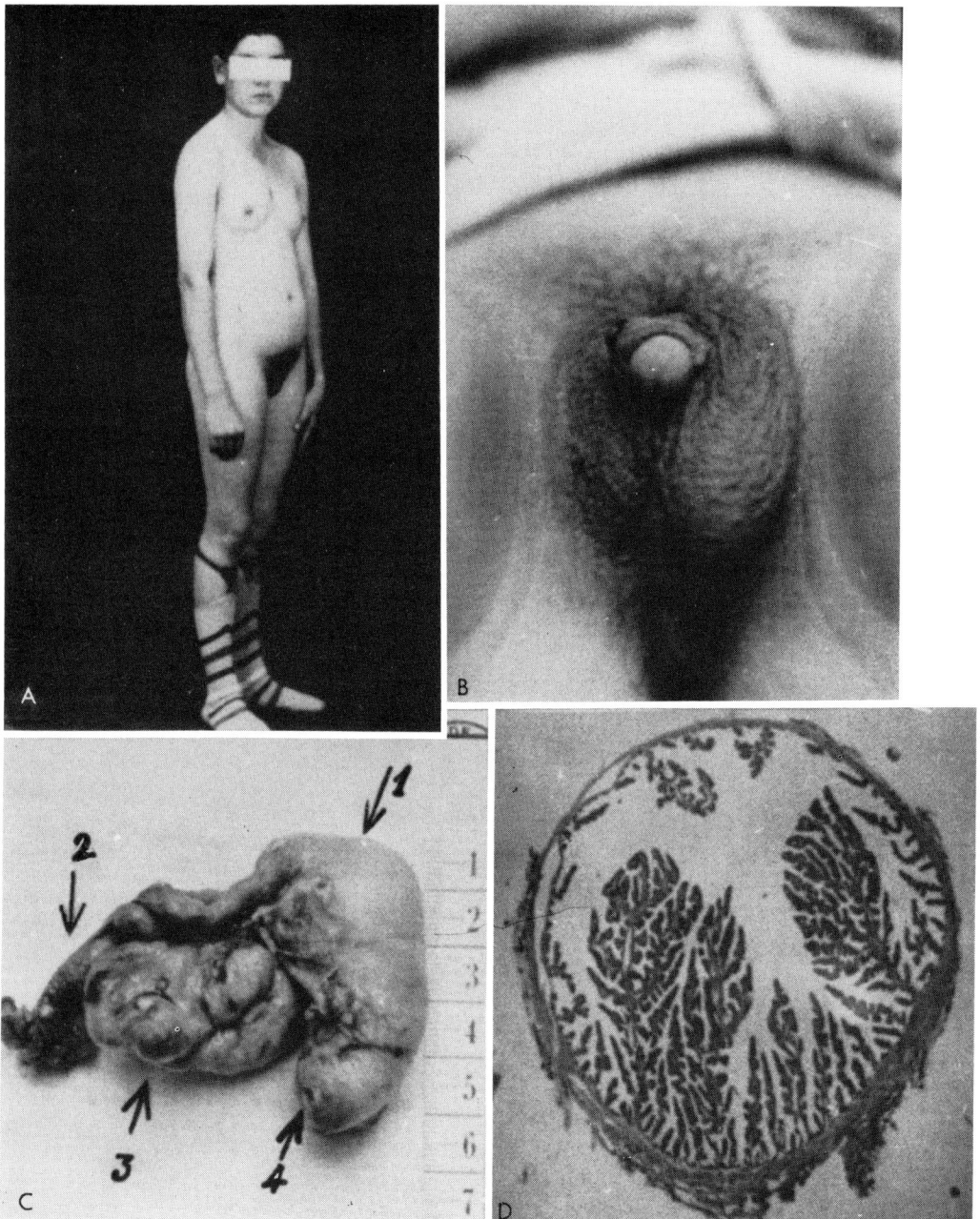

Figure 36-10. Case of true lateral hermaphroditism. *A*, Somatic features of patient. *B*, External genitalia with hypospadiac penis and empty scrotum on the right side. Left scrotum contains normal testis. *C*, Gross appearance of surgical specimen from the right side: 1, uterus; 2, Fallopian tube; 3, ovary; 4, uterine cervix. *D*, Section of Fallopian tube. (From Botella et al.: *Acta Gin.*, 1:85, 1950.)

normally and that both the Fallopian tubes and uterine findings were consistent with a normal female physiology.

The small testicle contained in the left scrotum was later explored surgically by Prof. A. de la Peña. Upon opening the scrotal sac, the testis appeared grossly normal and a biopsy taken at that time subsequently showed the histologic features of an immature, infantile-type testis. The findings in this case are of interest because they revealed a right sided female sex, developed to a considerable degree of complexity, and a left sided male sex, poorly developed and regressive in nature.

CASE II. A 31 year old woman with a

Pathology of Sex Determination: Major Gynecologic Syndromes

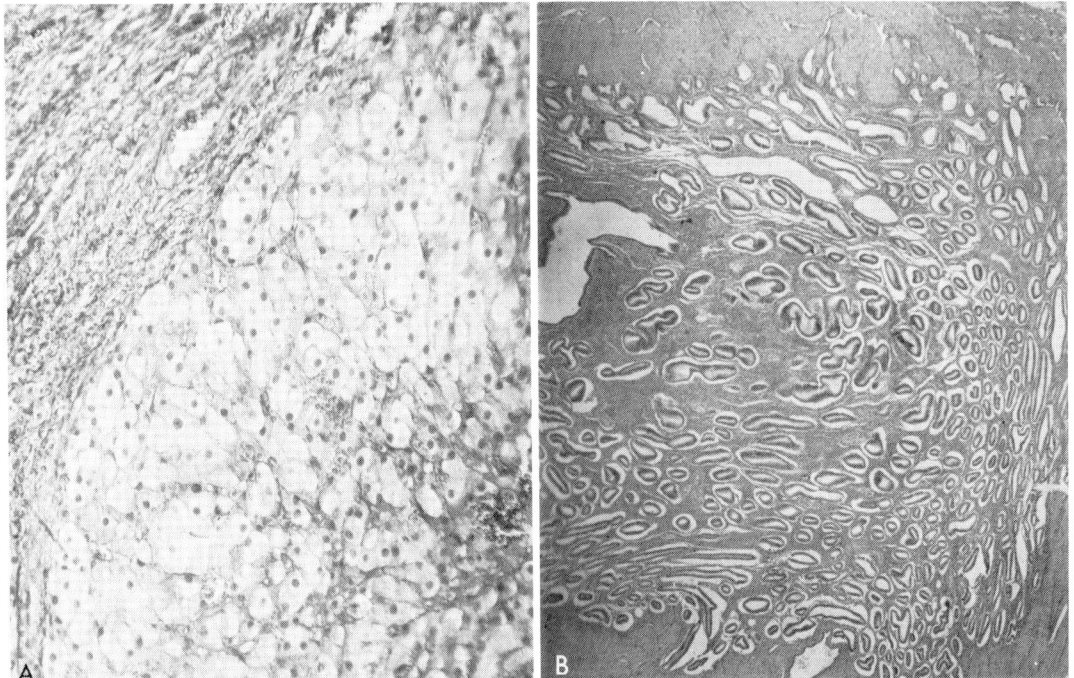

Figure 36-11. Histologic findings in the specimen shown in Figure 36-10,C. A, Corpus luteum in ovary. B, Endometrium revealing incipient secretory pattern.

perfectly feminine physique, although with slightly masculinoid facial features. Menarche at the age of 13, followed by a regular menstrual pattern of bleeding for 5 days every 28 days (5-28 type). Since the age of 17, she had experienced occasional bouts of amenorrhea, but never with complete interruption of menses. The external genitalia were of viriloid appearance. There was no scrotum; the vaginal introitus, however, was quite rudimentary, although independent of the urethral meatus. She presented a phallus-shaped clitoris, capable of erection. At laparotomy, she revealed a poorly developed, though symmetrically proportioned uterus, small Fallopian tubes of otherwise normal appearance and a left ovary, equally of normal appearance, which was removed and proved to be an ovotestis. The ovarian portion consisted mainly of a large follicle, with a well preserved granulosa layer, and an area containing several corpora albicantia. The testicular portion was made up of rudimentary cords of seminiferous tubules. In addition to the foregoing representative components of the ovotestis, the adnexal portion of the gland revealed both epididymal and tubal rests, as well as a canal-like structure that was interpreted as a müllerian vestige.

This case is also of interest because the genetic sex, as revealed by the study of the Barr body and the karyotype (XX), was found to be clearly female. Respecting the psychological tendencies of this patient, whose sexual identity was distinctly feminine, the surgical treatment consisted of resection of the penile clitoris and of reconstruction of the vaginal introitus so as to create a more permeable vagina and to impart a female configuration to the external genitalia, in agreement with the patient's chromosomal and psychosexual orientation, thereby facilitating her social adjustment.

CASE III. A case of bilateral ovotestes, observed and published in 1960 (Fig. 36-12). The patient was a 16 year old girl complaining of essential amenorrhea and bilateral inguinal swellings. The initial impression was that of dealing with a syndrome of "complete feminization"; however, on physical examination the patient displayed a well developed female physique and external genitalia in which the salient feature was a peniform clitoris, a finding indicative by itself of hermaphroditism rather than complete feminization, since it is uncommon in the latter. The basal metabolic rate and hematologic findings were within normal limits. Roentgenographic studies of the sella turcica and metacarpal bones showed no significant findings.

The genetic sex was female in the skin and vaginal and buccal mucosa as well as in the blood. Descending urography revealed normal structures bilaterally. Hormone studies revealed fluctuating, though balanced, estrogen and androgen levels; vaginal cytology was of the intermediate type (probably reflecting an androgen effect).

Gynecologic examination revealed a permeable vaginal introitus and a vagina ending blindly; there were no palpable internal genitalia.

A laparotomy was performed through the Pfannenstiel approach and disclosed complete absence of either male or female internal genitalia. However, both inguinal canals, which were accessible from the abdominal incision, revealed two masses of testiculoid appearance and topography (Fig. 36-12,C), which were removed and turned out to be ovotestes on histologic examination (Fig. 36-13).

The ovarian portion of the ovotestis consisted of immature follicles, some in the process of maturing, with well developed theca and granulosa layers. There were also numerous corpora atretica and albicantia. The testicular portion was quite heteroge-

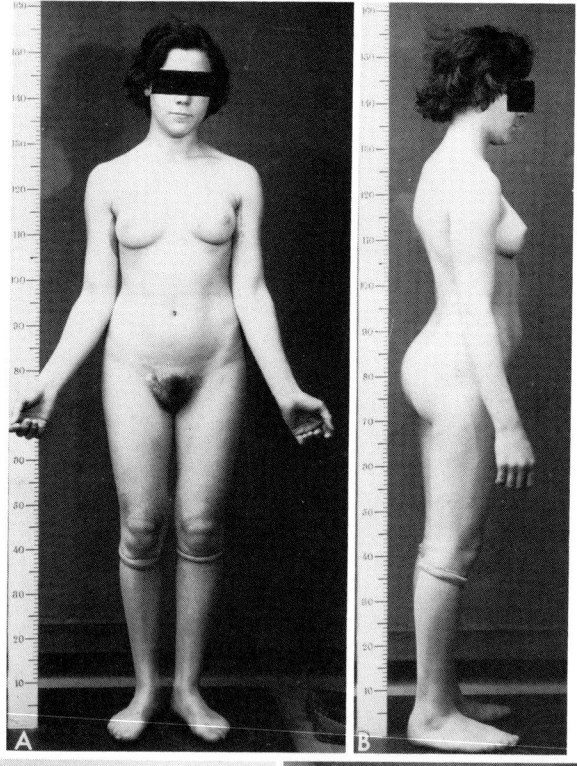
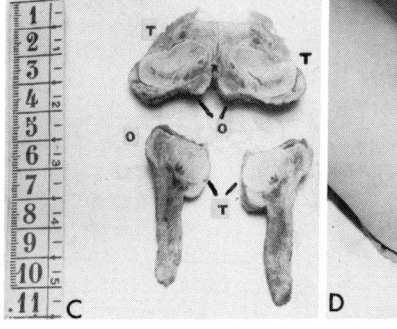
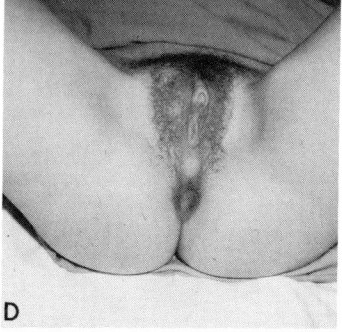

Figure 36–12. Case of true hermaphroditism. *A, B*, Girl with feminine physique. *C*, Tumoral masses removed from each inguinal canal. The inguinal masses were each made up of ovarian (O) and testicular (T) portions, and were besides provided with a pedicle containing both wolffian and müllerian structures. *D*, Pudendal region, with hypertrophy of clitoris. (From Botella et al.: *Acta Gin.*, 12:139, 1961.)

Pathology of Sex Determination: Major Gynecologic Syndromes

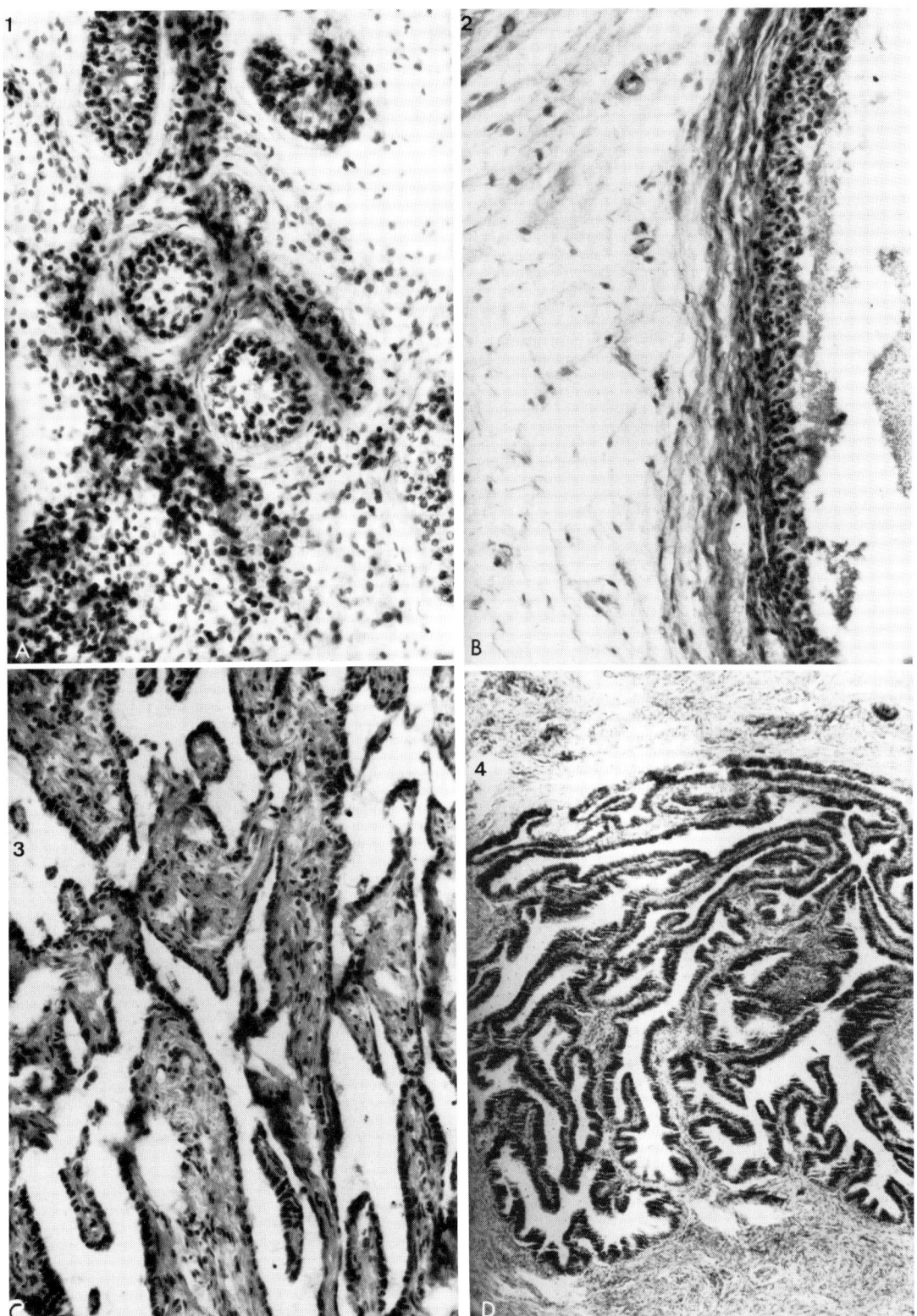

Figure 36–13. Histology of ovotestis from Figure 36–12. *A*, Testicular portion of ovotestis. *B*, Ovarian portion, showing wall of graafian follicle. *C*, Epididymal rudiments. *D*, Tubal rudiments.

neous, partly composed of seminiferous tubules of normal though immature appearance (as usually seen in children and in cryptorchidism). Some areas consisted of aberrant tubules similar to those found in Pick's adenoma and, finally, there was an area with a histologic pattern suggestive of dysgerminoma, apparently in an incipient phase of growth.

Both the pedicle and the hilar region of the ambiguous gland showed rudimentary tubular structures as well as mesonephric rests reminiscent of epididymis and vas deferens (Fig. 36–13).

The postoperative course was uneventful and the patient retained her female sexual attributes.

Her karyotype was obtained in 1963 during a follow-up examination. As shown in Figure 36–14, it consisted of an XX/XXY mosaicism and was described in detail elsewhere.[88]

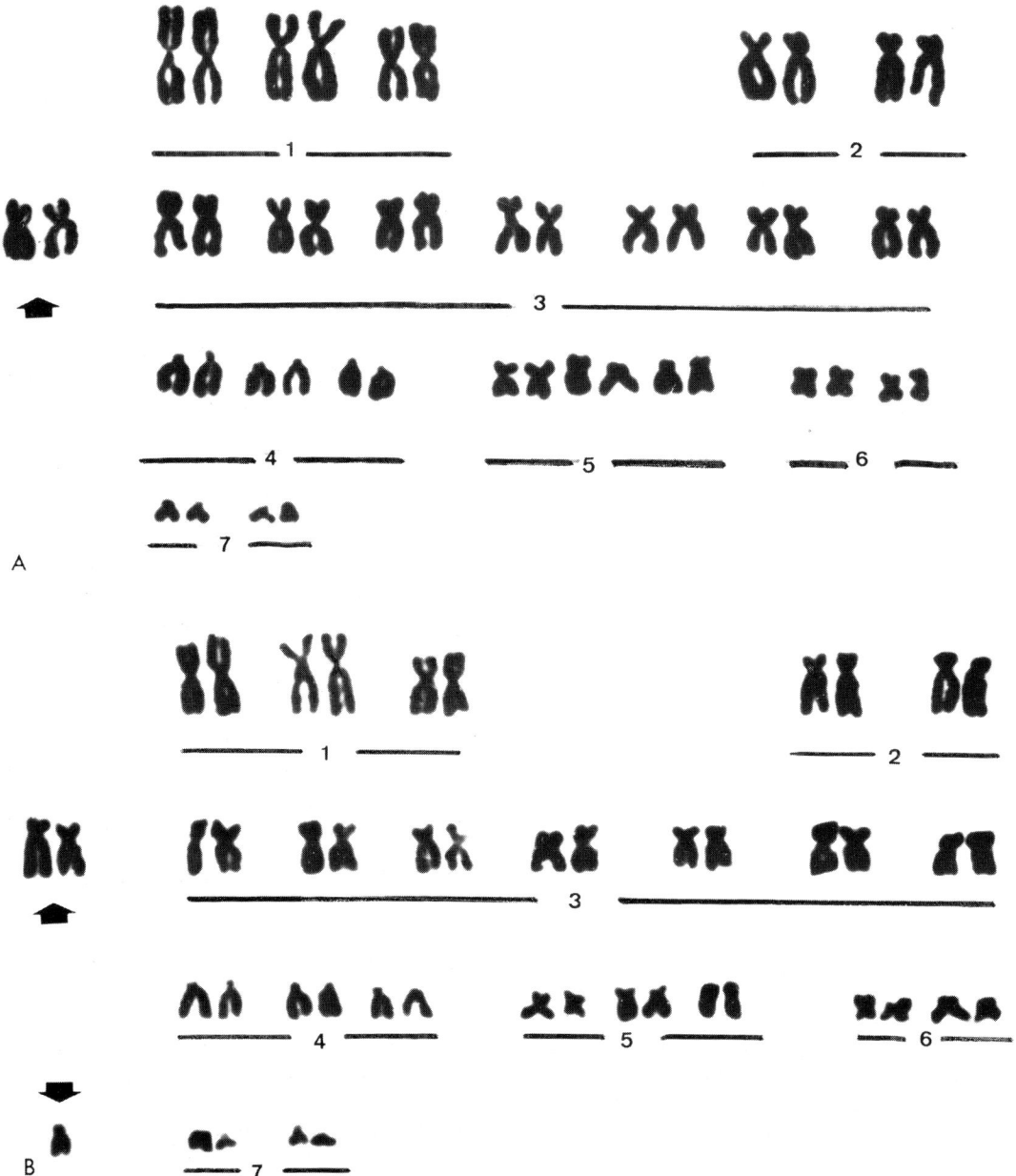

Figure 36–14. Karyotype of patient shown in Figure 36–12, consisting of double cell line mosaicism of 46(XX) and 47(XXY).

36.6.5. PSYCHOLOGY AND THERAPEUTIC MANAGEMENT

If the endocrine balance is an intermediate one between female and male, the psychology might similarly be expected to be an ambiguous one. The occurrence of homosexuality in these individuals has occasionally been emphasized. Two of the cases studied by us at first sight seemed to involve homosexual tendencies. However, after a thorough psychodynamic and psychoanalytic study, the above impression proved to be a superficial and unfounded one. Although the sexual instinct in both cases was ill-defined, this was the result of doubts about their own nature and of the fact that these patients were incapable of having relations normal for their sex. Upon analyzing their most intimate tendencies, however, the first patient, reared socially as a boy, had a definite masculine orientation, aspiring to dress as a male, to have a beard and mustache, and to marry, whereas the second, who believed herself to be a girl, likewise had the normal feminine desire to become engaged and to marry. This reaffirms us in our long-held belief that, although apparently influencing the sexual instincts in animals to a certain extent, sex hormones play a minor role, if any, in human sexual orientation, a product of educational standards and imaginative concepts of a higher order. These individuals develop the sexual tendencies of the sex they believe to belong to and in which they have been reared. True hermaphrodites, reared in the belief that they are women, develop a female sexual identity even though they may be aware of their features of masculinism and the discrepancies in their external genitalia. Conversely, those persons whose sex of rearing is male develop a male identity and a male type of libido despite the realization of their inferiority for coitus and normal sexual relations.

In a recent publication, Ten Berge[118] raises the question of how to manage such cases. As the most important requirement, he suggests that the patient's social sex be respected wherever possible and that no doubts be raised in the patient's mind concerning the sex he believes he is. We have defended similar views on previous occasions. The individual's social sex should be left unchanged, according to Hamblen[49] and Hampson and his associates,[51] so long as it coincides with the best possibilities for matrimonial and genetic function. Seegar-Jones[110] emphasizes the importance of diagnosing such anomalies in the newborn. He believes that determinations of urinary 17-ketosteroid levels and buccal Barr body counts should be enough to gain preliminary information concerning possible problems of this kind that may serve as the basis for not only the early medical but also the sociological and psychological management of the patient.

In the presence of adequate sexual function, there is no reason why intersexuals should not marry. Neither the cell nucleus nor the gonad constitutes one's sex; sex is defined, in the final analysis, by the appearance presented by an individual in the eyes of the other members of his own and the opposite sex, and the idea he has of himself. If the appearance is feminine and the sexual impulses have developed accordingly, the patient should be maintained in the same social sex and the true nature of the disorder should be withheld from her. The important guideline is to avoid creating a maladjusted being, in conflict with his own instincts and with society. In the first of the three cases presented, we left the patient as a male, because he had been reared as a man. We learned afterwards that he was doing well as a farmer. In the second case, we resected the phallus and reconstructed a wider vagina, and the patient returned several times to reiterate her gratitude. In the third case, castration was performed (mainly because such gonads often become cancerous), and the individual was left as a woman, able to marry and to lead a normal matrimonial life. As pointed out previously, we had adopted similar criteria for the syndrome of "complete feminization." Deontologically, we believe to have commited no error, since what defines sex in accordance with both divine and human law are both the external configuration and the instincts, whereas it has nowhere been established that sex must be defined precisely by the gonad, let alone by any XX or XY chromosomes. To us, a woman is an individual possessing the shape of woman and a feminine psychology who, by virtue of having a vagina, can cohabit as woman; on these accounts, any coincident male features do not void the validity of matrimony. To bar an individual from matrimony (which requires an exact explanation of his true plight), to change one's social sex or give publicity to such situations in any way, seems to us a monstrous thing, which might only drive an individual to suicide, or cause sexual deviation or other drastic reaction. Here, the physician's tact and professional secrecy become decisive qualities.

REFERENCES

1. Albright, F., Smith, P. E., and Fraser, R. A.: *Amer. J. Med. Sci.*, 204:625, 1942.
2. Alexander, D. S., and Ferguson-Smith, M. A.: *Pediatrics*, 28:758, 1961.
3. Assis, L. M. de, Epps, D. R., and Bottura, C.: *Lancet*, 2:129, 1960.
4. Atkins, L., and Engel, E.: *Lancet*, 2:20, 1962.
5. Bahner, F., Schwarz, G., Harnden, D. G., Jacobs, P. A., Hienz, H. A., and Walker, K.: *Lancet*, 2:100, 1960.
6. Balze, F. A. de la, et al.: *J. Clin. Endocr.*, 20:286, 1960.
7. Baron, J., Hauser, G. A., and Jirasek, J. E.: *Gynaecologia*, 163:14, 1967.
8. Barr, M. L., Sergovich, F. R., Carr, D. R., and Shaver, E. L.: *Canad. Med. Ass. J.*, 101:247, 1969.
9. Bartlett, D. J., Grant, J. K., Pugh, M. A., and Aherne, H.: *J. Obst. Brit. Comm.*, 75:199, 1968.
10. Blairbell, W.: *The Sex Complex*. New York, 1916.
11. Blank, C. E., Bishop, A., and Caley, J. P.: *Lancet*, 2:1450, 1960.
12. Bloise, W., Assis, L. M. de, Bottura, C., and Ferrari, I.: *Lancet*, 2:1059, 1960.
13. Boczkowski, K.: *J. Med. Genet.*, 5:181, 1968.
14. Botella, J., and Nogales, F.: *Acta Gin.*, 3:319, 1952.
15. Botella, J., and Nogales, F.: *Arch. Gynäk.*, 182:675, 1953.
16. Bovicelli, L.: *Riv. Ital. Ginec.*, 52:83, 1968.
17. Bronski, M.: *Proc. Soc. Exper. Biol. Med.*, 75:426, 1950.
18. Carr, D. H., Barr, M. L., and Plunkett, E. R.: *Canad. Med. Ass. J.*, 84:131, 1961.
19. Carr, D. H., Haggar, R. A., and Hart, A. G.: *Amer. J. Clin. Pathol.*, 49:521, 1968.
20. Castillo, E. B. del, Balza, F. A. de la, and Argonz, J.: *J. Clin. Endocr.*, 7:385, 1947.
21. Castillo, E. B. del, and Argonz, J.: *Ann. d'Endocr.*, 12:121, 1951.
22. Charreau, E., and Villee, C. A.: *J. Clin. Endocr.*, 28:1741, 1968.
23. Clavero-Núñez, J. A.: *Acta Gin.*, 7:397, 1964.
24. Clavero-Núñez, J. A., Botella, J., and Nogales, F.: *Acta Gin.*, 7:389, 1964.
25. Clavero-Núñez, J. A.: In *Esterilidad e Infertilidad Matrimonial*. Barcelona, Editorial Clientífico-Médica, 1967.
26. Conen, P. E., Bailey, J. D., Allemang, W. H., Thompson, D. W., and Ezrin, C.: *Lancet*, 2:294, 1961.
27. Chapelle, A. de la: *Acta Endocr. (Copenhaven)*, Suppl. 65, 1962.
28. Chu, E. H. Y., Grumbach, M. M., and Morishima, A.: *J. Clin. Endocr.*, 20:1608, 1960.
29. Dewhurst, C. J.: *Lancet*, 2:783, 1962.
30. Edwards, J. A., Vance, V. K., Cohen, M. M., and Schussler, G. C.: *J. Clin. Endocr.*, 30:666, 1970.
31. Elliot, G. A., Sandler, M. B., and Rabinowitz, D.: *J. Clin. Endocr.*, 19:995, 1959.
32. Ferguson-Smith, M. A., Johnston, A. W., and Weinberg, A. N.: *Lancet*, 2:126, 1960.
33. Ford, C. E., Jones, K. W., Polani, P. E., Almeda, J. C. de, and Briggs, J. H.: *Lancet*, 1:711, 1959.
34. Forteza, G., Baguena, R., and Bonilla, R.: *Rev. Esp. Obst. Gin.*, 127:13, 1963.
35. Fraccaro, M., Ikkos, D., Lindsten, J., Luft, R., and Kaijser, K.: *Lancet*, 2:114, 1960.
36. Fraccaro, M., Kaijser, K., and Lindsten, J.: *Lancet*, 1:886, 1959.
37. Fraccaro, M., Kaijser, K., and Lindsten, J.: *Acta Endocr. (Copenhaven)*, 34:496, 1960.
38. Fraccaro, M., Bott, M. G., Salzano, F. M., Ross, R. W., and Cranston, W. I.: *Lancet*, 1:1379, 1962.
39. Ghnassia, J. P.: *Ann. d'Endocr.*, 28:368, 1967.
40. Goldwerg, M. B., and Marxwell, A. F.: *J. Clin. Endocr.*, 8:367, 1948.
41. Gordon, R. R., O'Gorman, F. J. P., Dewhurst, C. J., and Blank, C. E.: *Lancet*, 2:736, 1960.
42. Greenblatt, R. B., Vazquez, E., and Acosta, O. M.: *Obstet. Gynec.*, 9:258, 1957.
43. Greenblatt, R. B.: *J. Clin. Endocr.*, 18:227, 1958.
44. Greenblatt, R. B., Byrd, R. J., McDonough, P. G., and Mahesh, V. B.: *Amer. J. Obstet. Gynec.*, 98:151, 1967.
45. Grouchy, J. de, Cottin, S., Lamy, N., Netter, A., Nett-Lambert, A., Trevoux, R., and Dalzant, G.: *Rev. Franç et Clin. Biol.*, 5:377, 1960.
46. Grumbach, M. M., Morishima, A., and Chu, E. H. Y.: *Excerpta Med. Intern. Congress Series*, 32:99, 1961.
47. Grumbach, M. M., Van Wick, J. J., and Wilkins, L.: *Excerpta Med. Intern. Congress Series*, 15:845, 1161, 1965.
48. Grumbach, M. M.: In *Clinical Endocrinology*, Vol. I, ed. E. B. Astwood. New York, Grune & Stratton, 1960.
49. Hamblen, E. C.: *Amer. J. Obstet. Gynec.*, 74:1228, 1957.
50. Hamerton, J. L., Jagiello, G. M., and Kirman, B. H.: *Brit. Med. J.*, 1:220, 1962.
51. Hampson, J. G., Money, J., and Hampson, J. L.: *J. Clin. Endocr.*, 16:547, 1956.
52. Harnden, D. G., and Jacobs, P. A.: *Brit. Med. Bull.*, 17:206, 1961.
53. Harnden, D. G., and Stewart, J. S. S.: *Brit. Med. Bull.*, 2:1285, 1959.
54. Harnden, D. G., and Armstrong, C. N.: *Brit. Med. Bull.*, 2:1287, 1959.
55. Hauser, G. A.: "Disgenesia Gonadal," In Overzier's *La Intersexualidad*. Barcelona, Editorial Científico-Médica, 1963.
56. Henkin, R. I.: *J. Clin. Endocr.*, 27:1346, 1967.
57. Hirschhorn, K., Decker, W. H., and Cooper, H. L.: *New Eng. J. Med.*, 263:1044, 1960.
58. Hoffenberg, R., and Jackson, W. P. U.: *Brit. Med. J.*, 1:1281, 1957.
59. Hoffenberg, R., and Jackson, W. P. U.: *J. Clin. Endocr.*, 17:902, 1957.
60. Hung, W., et al.: *Obstet. Gynec.*, 36:373, 1970.
61. Hungerford, D. A., Donnelley, A. J., Nowell, P. C., and Beck, S.: *Amer. J. Human Genet.*, 11:215, 1959.
62. Hutchins, J. J.: *Amer. J. Human Genet.*, 11:375, 1959.
63. Ionescu, B., et al.: *Ann. d'Endocr.*, 28:189, 1967.

64. Jacobs, P. A., Harnden, H. G., Court-Brown, W. M., Goldstein, J., Close, H. G., MacGregor, T. N., MacLean, N., and Strong, J. A.: Lancet, 1:1213, 1960.
65. Jacobs, P. A., Baikie, A. G., Court-Brown, W. M., MacGregor, Y. N., MacLean, N., and Harnden, D. G.: Lancet, 2:423, 1959.
66. Jacobs, P. A., Harnden, D. G., Buckton, K. A., Court-Brown, W. M., King, M., MacBride, J. A., MacGregor, T. N., and MacLean, N.: Lancet, 2:83, 1961.
67. Jacobs, P. A., Baikie, A. G., Court-Brown, W. M., Forrest, H., Roy, J. R., Stewart, J. S. S., and Lennox, B.: Lancet, 2:591, 1959.
68. Jones, H. W., and Scott, W. W.: In *Hermaphroditism, Genital Abnormalities and Related Endocrine Disorders*. Baltimore, Williams & Wilkins Co., 1958.
69. Jost, A., and Colange, R. A.: Comp. Rend. Soc. Biol., 143:140, 1949.
70. Jost, A., and Bozit, B.: Comp. Rend. Soc. Biol., 145:647, 1951.
71. Jost, A.: Rec. Progr. Horm. Res., 8:378, 1953.
72. Jost, A.: Comp. Rend. Soc. Biol., 147:1930, 1953.
73. Jost, A.: Ann. d'Endocr., 17:479, 1956.
74. Kesaree, N., and Wolley, P. V.: J. Pediat., 63:1099, 1963.
75. Klay, L. J., Sparkes, R. S., and Lagasse, L. D.: Amer. J. Obstet. Gynec., 99:495, 1967.
76. Klebs, E.: In *Handbuch der Pathologischen Anatomie*, 3. Berlin, Lig., 1870.
77. Kosowicz, J., Bialecki, M., Wojtowicz, M., and Sobieszcyk, S.: Amer. J. Obstet. Gynec., 105:1116, 1969.
78. Kowalyszyn, P. J.: Obstet. Gin. Lat. Amer., 25:488, 1967.
79. Laszlo, J., and Györy, G.: Zbl. Gynäk., 89:1499, 1967.
80. Laszlo, J., and Györy, G.: Zbl. Gynäk., 91:1001, 1969.
81. Lejeune, J., Turpin, R., and Gautier, M.: C. R. Acad. Sci. (Paris), 250:618, 1960.
82. Lewis, F. J. W., Mitchell, J. P., and Foss, G. L.: Lancet, 1:221, 1963.
83. MacDonough, P. G., Byrd, J. R., and Mahesh, V. B.: Fertil. Steril., 20:451, 1969.
84. Makino, S., and Sasaki, M.: Proc. Imp. Acad. Japan, 36:156, 1960.
85. Masica, D. N., Money, J., Erhardt, A. A., and Lewis, V. G.: John Hopkins Hosp. Med. J., 124:34, 1969.
86. Mauvais-Jarvis, P., Bercovici, J. P., and Gauthier, F.: J. Clin. Endocr., 29:417, 1969.
87. Moncada, E., and Sopeña, A.: Acta Gin., 6:351, 1964.
88. Moncada, E., Clavero-Núñez, J. A., Nogales, F., Sopeña, A., and Botella, J.: Acta Gin., 6:339, 1964.
89. Morris, J. M. C. L.: Amer. J. Obstet. Gynec., 65:1192, 1953.
90. Miles, Ch. P., Luzzatti, L., Storey, S. D., and Peterson, C. D.: Lancet, 2:455, 1962.
91. Miller, O. J., Breg, R., and Jailer, J. W.: Human Chromosome Newsletter, i:6, 1960.
92. Nogales, F., Botella, J., and Sopeña, J.: *Histología de las Disgenesias Gonadales*. San Feliu de Guixols, VI Reunión de Ginecólogos Españoles, 1964.
93. Oikawa, K., and Brizzard, R. M.: New Eng. J. Med., 264:1009, 1961.
94. Overzier, C.: Schw. Med. Wschr., 87:285, 1957.
95. Park, I. J., et al.: Obstet. Gynec., 36:377, 1970.
96. Pasetto, N., Montanino, G., Ferrante, E., and Vignetti, P.: Gynec. Obstet., 66:259, 1967.
97. Pick, L.: Arch. Gynäk., 76:191, 1905.
98. Polani, P. E.: In Hamerton's *Chromosomes in Medicine*, ed. The National Spastics Society. London, W. Heineman, 1962.
99. Polani, P. E.: Brit. Med. Bull., 17:200, 1961.
100. Puck, T. T., Robinson, A., and Tjio, J. A.: Proc. Soc. Exper. Biol. (New York), 103:192, 1960.
101. Pujol-Amat, P., et al.: Amer. J. Obstet. Gynec., 106:736, 1970.
102. Raynaud, A., and Frilley, M.: Ann. d'Endocr., 8:400, 1947.
103. Rivarola, M. A., Saez, J. M., Meyer, W. J., Kenny, F. M., and Migeon, C. J.: J. Clin. Endocr., 27:371, 1967.
104. Roy, S. K., and Laumas, K. R.: Acta Endocr., 61:629, 1964.
105. Russell, W. L., Russell, L. B., and Gower, J. S.: Proc. Nat. Acad. Sci. (Washington), 45:554, 1959.
106. Sandberg, A. A., Koepf, G. F., Crosswhite, L. H., and Hauschka, T.: Amer. J. Human Genet., 12:231, 1960.
107. Schlegel, R. J., Neu, R. L., Carneiro-Leon, J., and Gardner, L. I.: j. Clin. Endocr., 27:1588, 1967.
108. Schneider, B. W., Ommen, R. A. van, and Hoerr, S. O.: J. Clin. Endocr., 12:423, 1952.
109. Schuster, J., and Motulsky, A. G.: Lancet, 1:1074, 1962.
110. Seegar-Jones, G.: Ann. N.Y. Acad. Sci., 142:729, 1967.
111. Serment, H., et al.: Rev. Fr. Endocr. Clin., 7:641, 1966.
112. Shah, P. N., Naik, S. N., Mahajan, D. K., Dave, M. J., and Paymaster, J. C.: Brit. Med. J., 2:474, 1961.
113. Southren, A. L., Gordon, G. G., Tochimoto, S., Pinzon, G., Lane, D. R., and Stypulowsky, W.: J. Clin. Endocr., 27:686, 1967.
114. Stanesco, V., Maximilian, C., Florea, I., and Ciovirnache, M.: Ann. d'Endocr., 29:449, 1968.
115. Stewart, J. S. S.: Brit. Med. J., 2:592, 1959.
116. Stoddard, F. D., and Engstrom, W. W.: J. Clin. Endocr., 20:780, 1960.
117. Taylor, H., Barter, R. H., and Jacobson, R. D.: Amer. J. Obstet. Gynec., 96:816, 1966.
118. Ten Berge, S.: Gynaecologia, 149:112, 1960.
119. Teter, J., and Boczkowski, K.: Acta Cytol., 11:449, 1967.
120. Tjio, J. H., Puck, T. T., and Robinson, A.: Proc. Nat. Acad. Sci., 45:1008, 1959.
121. Turner, H. H.: Endocrinology, 23:566, 1938.
122. Turpin, R., LeJeune, J., and Breton, A.: Comp. Rend. Acad. Sci. (Paris), 255:3088, 1962.
123. Ullrich, O.: Zschr. Kinderhk., 49:271, 1930.
124. Varney, R. F., Kenyen, A. T., and Kock, F. C.: J. Clin. Endocr., 2:137, 1942.
125. Wagner, G. A.: Zbl. Gynäk., 51:1304, 1927.
126. Ward-MacQuaid, J. W., and Lennon, G. G.: Surg. Gynec. Obstet., 90:96, 1950.
127. Waxman, S. H., Kelley, V. C., Gartler, S. M., and Burt, B.: Lancet, 1:161, 1962.
128. Wells, L. J.: Anat. Rec., 97:409, 1947.
129. Wells, L. J.: Arc. d'Anat. Microscop., 39:409, 1950.
130. Willemse, C. H., Brink, J. M. van, and Los, P. L.: Lancet, 1:488, 1962.
131. Zarate, A., et al.: Obstet. Gynec., 33:818, 1969.

Chapter 37
ANOMALIES IN SEXUAL DIFFERENTIATION

37.1. GENERALITIES

Congenital anomalies of the genital tract resulting from disorders in *sex determination* were examined in Chapter 36. Because the process of sex determination is genetically determined, these anomalies have a *genetic* etiology. We shall now study the question of aberrations in *sexual differentiation* which instead is a process of hormonal morphogenesis, *so that the disorders to be studied presently all have an endocrine etiology.*

To a large extent, anomalies of endocrine origin have a *familial* incidence, and some have been found to be associated with an abnormal karyotype. The genetic factor here apparently is responsible for the endocrine changes that in turn produce the congenital malformations. An excellent review on the subject has been published recently.[49] Lubbs and Ruddle[32] reported having found changes in the karyotype of a large number of newborn infants presenting with defects in genital differentiation.

In Chapter 15 (Section 15.2), we made the point that the agents of sexual differentiation are the hormones of the gonads. Androgens induce development of wolffian ducts and atrophy of müllerian ducts, whereas estrogens have exactly the opposite effect. However, one of the essential principles involved in embryogeny is that of *active stimulation*. Failure of the müllerian duct to develop is not enough by itself to result in wolffian duct development. In the absence of estrogens, there is no müllerian development, but this does not necessarily lead to growth of wolffian duct structures, unless androgenic activity happens to be enhanced. Consequently, wolffian duct development requires not only absence of estrogenic activity but at the same time the presence of masculinizing principles in high concentration.

In the course of this chapter, we shall successively examine those disorders involving the genital tract of *genetic females* that result either from absence of estrogenic and androgenic activity or from absence of the first while the second is increased. In the first instance, the resulting anomalies appear to stem from lack of development of the female genital apparatus, whereas the second instance gives rise to female pseudohermaphroditism. To these two groups, we must add such *iatrogenic* sexual alterations on the fetus as are observed to occur in association with harmful androgen therapy of pregnant women carrying female fetuses.

37.2. ENDOCRINE BASIS OF CONGENITAL ANOMALIES AFFECTING THE FEMALE GENITAL TRACT

Lack of fetal or fetoplacental estrogenic secretion[17, 18, 42, 43] causes defects in the development and fusion of the müllerian ducts or may result in defective formation of the cloacal organs.[51, 59] These two groups of disorders shall be studied successively.

At present, there is abundant experimental evidence that androgens and estrogens provide the impulse for the development of the wolffian and müllerian systems, respectively. In birds, the hormonal influence on the development of the corresponding genital tracts was first stressed by Dantschakova,[12, 13] by Willier and his associates[58] and by Wolff and colleagues.[61] Thanks mainly to the investigations conducted by Witschi,[60] similar phenomena are known to occur also in batrachians and newts.

Insofar as mammals are concerned, a similar concept was reached later and has by now been completely confirmed. As a result of the studies conducted mainly by Greene and his colleagues[17, 18] and by Moore,[35] it has been shown that when high dosages of estrogens are injected into the mother they produce pathologic development of the wolffian ducts even in genetic females and, conversely, that addition of large amounts of estrogens may induce müllerian development even in genetic males. The subsequent investigations by Jost[30] have in addition brought to light the role played by androgens elaborated by the fetal testis itself in the development of the male embryo. A detailed experimental study concerning the effects produced by hormones injected into embryos has been published by Wells and Van Waagenen,[55] while Burns[7] has come up with evidence of similar effects in the opossum. A special contribution toward clarifying the effects involved has been made by Price and Pannabecker,[42] who studied the actions of estrogens and androgens on the müllerian and wolffian organs in vitro. Thus, there is at present no doubt that *the respective male and female genital tracts develop under the influence of the specific hormones of the corresponding gonads.*

As has been shown by Jost,[30] testicular incretion is necessary for wolffian tract development, whereas ovarian passivity is known to permit development of the müllerian ducts. In this respect, a great deal of modern research attests to the existence of endocrine activity in the fetal testis (see Chapter 20, Section 20.2.1). For instance, the fetal testes of rabbits have been found to display 3β-ol-dehydrogenase activity[4] as early as the twentieth day of pregnancy while, in the human testis, this enzyme has been detected during the third month of intrauterine life.[47] As a result, the testis is capable of direct testosterone synthesis from cholesterol during its earliest phase of development.[48] The ovary, on the contrary, lacks such properties.[1, 4, 31] Incidentally, administration of the antiandrogenic compound cyproterone to pregnant rats has been found to cause the male litter to be born as *pseudohermaphrodites*.[14]

A review of the various disorders of sexual differentiation reveals that they fall into two large categories: first, a group in which the observed alterations stem from simple arrest in the development of the corresponding male or female genital tracts. Naturally, since this work purposes to study the endocrinology of woman, only anomalies of the female genital apparatus shall be considered here.

Into the second group, we might include those cases in which, apart from a more or less underdeveloped female genital tract, either there appear male structures in the form of vestigial wolffian organs or there is evidence of male cloacal organs. The first form of congenital anomalies might be termed *"anomalies of differentiation of isosexual character."* The second modality might be called *"alterations of differentiation of heterosexual character,"* or *"pseudohermaphroditism."* These two main groups are examined in the following paragraphs.

37.3. ISOSEXUAL CONGENITAL ANOMALIES OF THE FEMALE GENITAL TRACT

Under this heading, two large groups of anomalies are encountered: (a) anomalies in the development and fusion of the müllerian ducts, and (b) anomalies in the development of the cloacal organs.

37.3.1. LACK OF DIFFERENTIATION AND DEVELOPMENT OF THE MÜLLERIAN SYSTEM

ETIOLOGY. During the embryonal development of the female genital tract, the ducts of Müller undergo midline fusion, and through canalization give rise to the Fallopian tubes, the uterus and the vagina as hollow organs. Concerning the embryology of the vagina, the classic investigations by Meyer and Scheid[34] had shown that the vaginal epithelium was derived from the urogenital sinus. While the vagina is histologically a cloacal organ, organologically speaking it is produced by the fusion of the müllerian ducts and is therefore a coelomic organ. During the embryonic stage müllerian duct development is controlled by the action of estrogens. So much has been demonstrated beyond doubt by the studies of Greene and his colleagues[18] as well as those of Raynaud[45] and Burns.[7] These investigators were able to show that estrogens injected into embryonic animals produced rapid development of the müllerian ducts. Similarly, Forbes had shown that estrogens were capable of inducing growth in rests of the müllerian duct in males. Subsequently, Raynaud and Frilley[46] demonstrated that estrogens inhibited the development of the wolffian duct. These findings were confirmed by Strickler.[50] There can therefore be no doubt at present that *developmental anomalies of the müllerian ducts result from failure in intrauterine estrogen production.*

Recently, Clark and Gorski[9] found that an *estrogen-binding protein* (see Chapter 2, Section 2.5.6) was present in the uteri of rat embryos. In their opinion, a variety of müllerian malformations may be caused by *defects in end-organ receptivity* rather than by estrogen deficiency per se. This opens an interesting and new perspective in the pathogenesis of congenital anomalies of the uterus, Fallopian tubes and vagina.

In our own opinion, moreover, the *adrenal cortex of the fetus* (see Chapter 9, Section 9.6) must be considered as an important source of steroids, androgens as well as estrogens, capable of providing the stimulus in each instance for both the wolffian ducts and the müllerian ducts respectively. We have further postulated that the presence of an adrenal "intermediate zone" or "sexual zone" is of utmost significance during the embryonal era, and have denominated the latter the "primitive cortex," or "paleocortex." The specific mission of this structure is to stimulate development of the müllerian ducts in females and that of the wolffian ducts in male embryos. A possible adrenal participation must therefore be considered in the etiology of such disorders as duplication or atresia of the female genital tract. Whenever the presence of congenital cortical insufficiency is detected it is, as pointed out previously (Chapter 33), invariably found to coexist with developmental anomalies of the gonads. We have also noted that uterine duplication in several cases studied by us was invariably associated with low 17-ketosteroid values. This has been confirmed by Philipp[41] and has led him to concur with us that the third gonad played an important role in the development and in the fusion of the müllerian ducts and that its failure resulted in failure of the latter to develop.

In Figure 37-1, a case of a double uterus is presented in which there were bilateral underdeveloped ovaries revealing a number of congenital malformations, as well as two small ovarian adenomas. The rate of urinary 17-ketosteroid excretion in that patient was 1.5 mg per 24 hr. The roentgenologic findings in similar cases of uterine duplication, observed by Philipp and suspected to be equally of adrenal etiology, are shown in Figures 37-2 and 37-3, kindly provided to us by Prof. Philipp. Because the clinical study of such malformations belongs to textbooks on gynecology, here we shall merely present their endocrine aspects. It may be assumed that malforma-

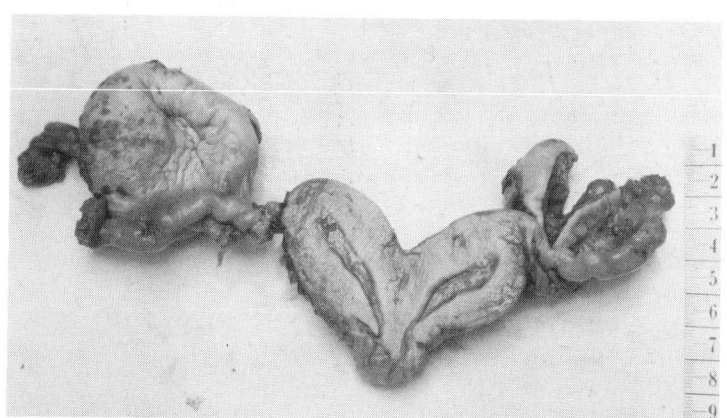

Figure 37-1. Double uterus with bilateral ovarian adenomas and disturbances in ovarian differentiation (rate of urinary 17-ketosteroid excretion, 1.5 mg per 24 hr).

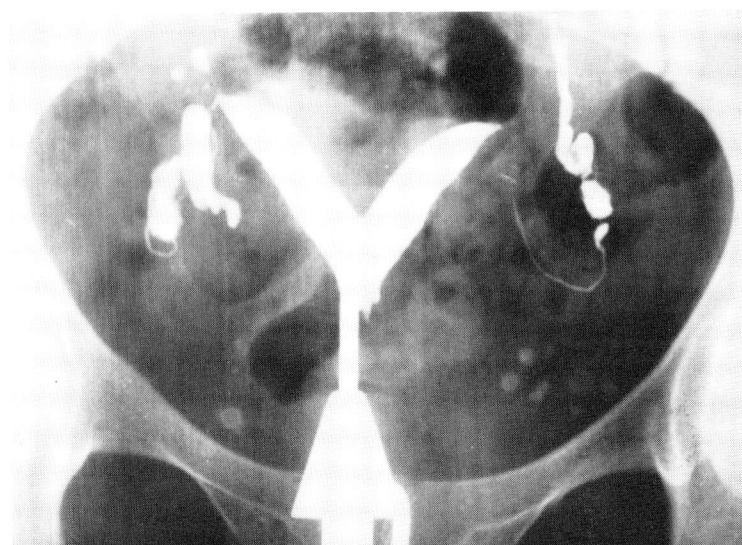

Figure 37–2. Uterus didelphys in a case with the syndrome of congenital ovarian hypoplasia. (Courtesy of Prof. Philipp.)

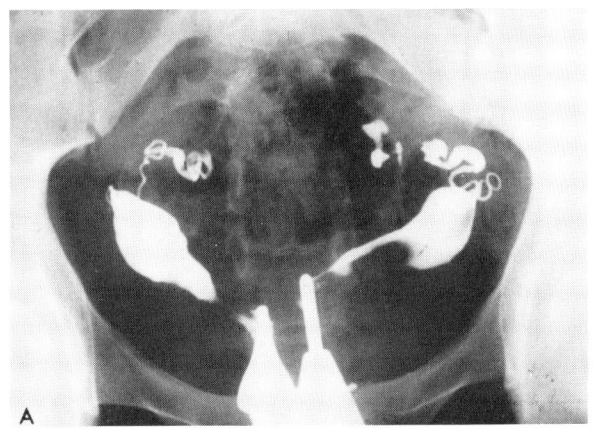

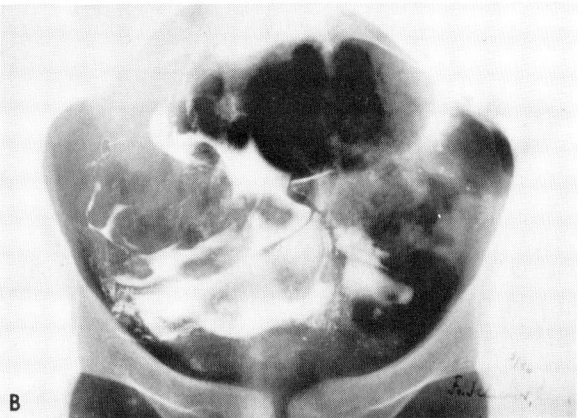

Figure 37–3. Uterus bicollis bicornis. A, Both hemiuteri and Fallopian tubes filled with contrast medium. B, Passage of medium into peritoneal cavity (positive test of Colle). (Courtesy of Prof. Philipp.)

tions of the genital apparatus owing to lack of differentiation of the müllerian ducts are a consequence of *embryonic dysendocrinia,* essentially brought about by deficient estrogen secretion, or what might be termed *hypoestrinism of embryonal life.* Embryonal hypoestrinism, in our opinion, *results from failure of adrenal function rather than failure of as yet nonexistent ovarian secretion.* The syndrome of congenital adrenal insufficiency, discussed in a previous chapter, is an experiment by nature itself, proving the correctness of this assertion. Congenital cortical insufficiency probably occurs much more frequently than is generally believed. In fact, such anomalies are extremely difficult to discover because this type of insufficiency produces no clinical symptomatology during adult life, since what is involved is the paleocortex, a zone destined to undergo atrophy and to play no role in adult life. They only come to light when, as a result of some organic malformation, for instance anencephaly, the fetus dies and an autopsy is performed.

ANATOMIC PATHOLOGY. It is not our purpose to engage in a complete review of all anatomic varieties occurring among congenital anomalies of the müllerian ducts due to hormonal causes. These may be systematized as follows: (1) Anomalies stemming from lack of fusion between the müllerian ducts, such as double uterus, uterus didelphys, septate uterus and various combinations of the latter with double or septate vaginas; (2) Lack of canalization of the müllerian ducts, which may occur at any level—the lower vaginal portion (vestibular atresia, vaginal atresia), the entire vagina (complete vaginal atresia), the uterus (uterine atresia) or the Fallopian tubes. Generally, this type of atresia is associated with duplication, since the disorder in differentiation affects both processes, fusion and canalization, so that interruptions of the müllerian tract may be observed to coexist bilaterally. Such is the case of the so-called syndrome of *semiatretic double uterus,* in which one of the uterine cavities communicates with the vagina, whereas the other has no communications and is the site of a *hematometra.* In gynatresia of the complete variety, such as occurs in cases of imperforate hymen, in vaginal atresia or in uterine atresia of a single uterus, the resulting *amenorrhea* may be confused with endocrine disorders, a fact which must be considered in the differential diagnosis.

In addition, anomalies with duplication are frequently associated with *unilateral renal agenesis,* an example of which is shown in Figure 37–4. Needham[39] and Musset and co-workers[38] explain this phenomenon as resulting from the fact that the mesonephros acts as an organogenic inducer of the metanephros and that transmission of mesonephric organizer substances to the metanephric anlage takes place through the wolffian ducts in the male embryo and through the müllerian ducts in the female embryo. Therefore, atresia of the müllerian ducts is believed to cause unilateral lack of development of the metanephric anlage. The correctness of this theory is borne out by the occurrence of such cases as that shown in Figure 37–4, in which there was a missing left kidney in conjunction with a double uterus that also revealed semiatresia on the left side.

37.3.2. ANOMALIES IN DIFFERENTIATION OF THE UROGENITAL SINUS

The external female genital organs are derived from the cloaca and from the urogenital sinus. Estrogens also induce female-directed differentiation in these organs, but *to a lesser degree in comparison to male-directed differentiation.* This means that while arrest in the development of these structures in the male embryo may give rise to highly interesting congenital anomalies, the same type of developmental arrest in the female causes minor, often barely perceptible, disorders. *The cloacal organs therefore play an insignificant role in congenital anomalies resulting from simple developmental arrest. In contrast, they play a role of extraordinary importance in congenital anomalies of heterosexual character, viz., in pseudohermaphroditism.*

The most common anomalies occurring in the cloacal region of woman as a result of developmental defects—that is, anomalies that are *isosexual* in character—are the following ones: (a) congenital absence of vagina (Figure 37–5), partial or complete; (b) imperforate hymen; (c) preternatural anus; (d) female hypospadias; and (e) double or septate vagina.

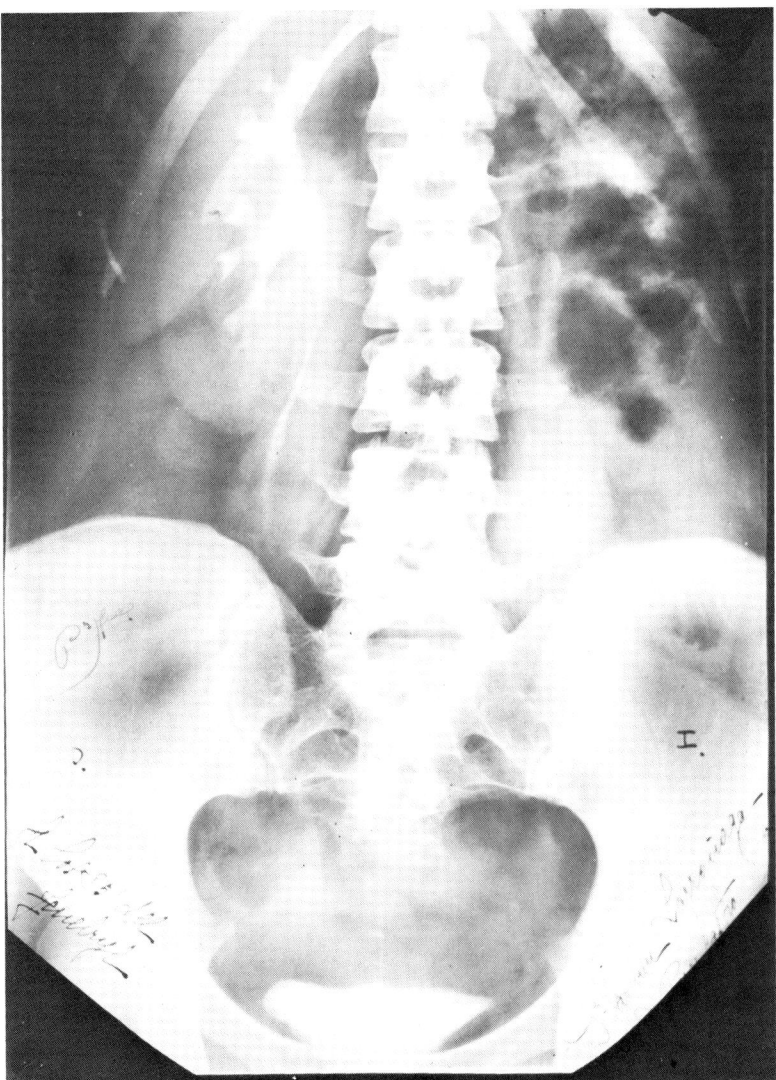

Figure 37-4. Left renal agenesis in a case of congenital ipsilateral atresia of müllerian duct.

Through the investigations of some embryologists (Harrison,[22] Price and Pannabecker[42]), it has been known that, notwithstanding its cloacal lining, the vagina is organogenically a müllerian organ. As a result, its absence or its duplication has in general a pathogenesis similar to that involved in lack of fusion or lack of development of the müllerian ducts, both studied in the preceding section. Various workers (Moore et al.,[37] Wells,[54] Price and Pannabecker,[42, 43] Greene,[17] and others) have shown that the processes of both development and fusion of the müllerian ducts are subject to estrogenic activity. This being so, it is plausible to surmise that lack of development of these structures results from lack of estrogenic activity. Of course, in view of the nowadays generally accepted fact that estrogenic stimulation, necessary for differentiation of the female genital canal, is derived from the placenta, it would be hard to concede that absence of estrogens plays any part in autogenesis. By admitting our hypothesis concerning the role of adrenocortical function in female genital organogenesis (see Chapter 15, Section 15.3.2, and also preceding section), this type of developmental arrest would be easy to explain. Jones and Scott[29] have described numerous cases of congenital absence of the vagina in which the uterus had failed to develop, remaining as a bicornuate rudimentary structure, whereas the ovaries were functioning normally (Figures 37–5 and 37–6). Similar findings have been reported by Bryan and his associates[6] and MacIndoe.[33] It seems worth while calling attention to the fact that only quite rarely (in 4 to 10 per cent of the cases, according to the above-mentioned sources), congenital absence of the vagina is associated with a normal functioning uterus, which is the major reason why hematometra seldom ever develops. This indicates that congenital absence of the organ, as pointed out previously, results from a systematic alteration of the müllerian ducts.

As regards the purely cloacal type of anomalies (preternatural anus, hypospadias, imperforate hymen), these are frequently associated with hypodevelopmental alterations of the rest of the genitalia. It must be borne in mind that, unlike the wolffian ducts, which are sensitive to the differentiating action of androgens, and the müllerian ducts, which are influenced by estrogens, the cloacal region, as shown by Price and Pannabecker[42] as well as by Zuckermann,[63] is susceptible to the actions of both androgens and estrogens to a similar degree. Thus, pathologic differentiation of this region is easily induced by the effect of heterosexual activity. Philipp[41] postulates that any type of arrest in female embryonal development is the result of the virilizing influence of the embryonal adrenal. The truth is that most instances of pseudohermaphroditism are associated with arrest in the development of these organs in addition to modifications of the viriloid type. This may be an argument favoring the above point of view. Nevertheless, one cannot completely dismiss the possibility that local tissue injury might lead to the arrest of isosexual development of the vaginal and cloacal organs without induction of male-directed development. This point of view has also been upheld by Wells and Van Waagenen[55] as well as by Burns.[7]

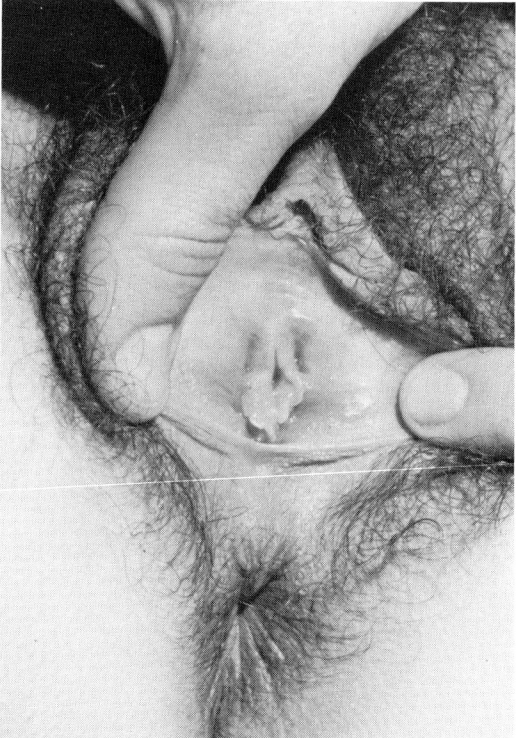

Figure 37–5. Congenital absence of vagina. Ovary had good function; vaginal cytology was normal, revealing cyclic changes, but there was absence of menstrual molimen.

Anomalies in Sexual Differentiation

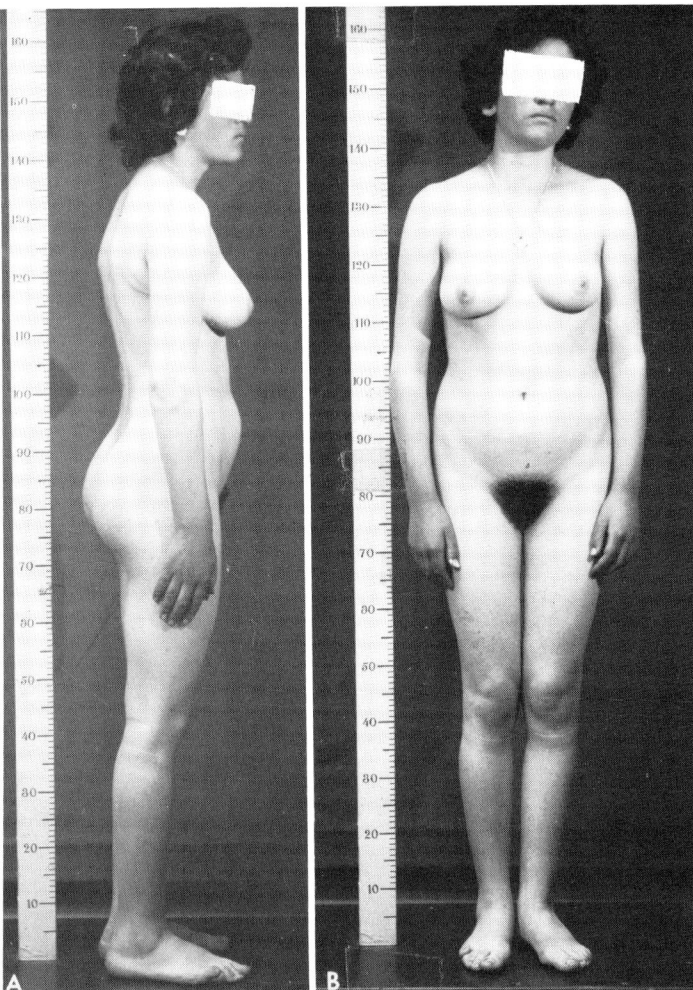

Figure 37-6. Biotypology of patient from preceding figure. At laparotomy, two ovaries with adequate function and a rudimentary bicornuate uterus were observed.

37.4. PSEUDOHERMAPHRODITISM (HETEROSEXUAL ABERRATIONS IN GENITAL DIFFERENTIATION)

According to prevailing ideas, *pseudohermaphroditism is believed to be the result of endocrine action during the developmental phase of the genital apparatus.* Following similar criteria, cases of pseudohermaphroditism may be divided into those in which müllerian or wolffian organs are involved (internal pseudohermaphroditism) and those in which cloacal organs are involved (external pseudohermaphroditism). The latter type may be encountered more frequently: the cloaca has been shown to be more susceptible to heterosexual stimuli than the corresponding ducts (Price and Pannabecker,[42, 43] Zuckermann[63]). Clinically, the two forms of pseudohermaphroditism most often observed are the *"congenital adrenogenital syndrome"* (see Chapter 33) and the syndrome of *"male pseudohermaphroditism with complete feminization"* (Chapter 36). Since both have already been dealt with in detail, we shall mention only briefly a few unusual cases of pseudohermaphroditism that have not been included in previous descriptions.

37.4.1. MALE PSEUDOHERMAPHRODITISM

Although by definition the subject of male pseudohermaphroditism is beyond the scope of this book, it is included here because, as in the syndrome of "complete feminization" described in the preceding chapter, affected individuals are often of gynecologic interest clinically despite the fact that their gonadal and genetic sex is male.

Jones and Scott[29] offer the following classification of male pseudohermaphrodites:

1. Male pseudohermaphrodites with ambiguous, or predominantly male, external genitalia, passing for women. No mammary development.
   a. With rudimentary or nonexistent müllerian ducts.
   b. With well-developed müllerian structures.
2. Male pseudohermaphrodites with female external genitalia and breast development, passing for women. There is no müllerian development.

The second category corresponds to the syndrome of "total feminization" of Botella and Nogales, or the "syndrome of testicular feminization" of other authors, and was covered extensively in Chapter 36, supplemented with the presentation of several of our cases. The first category (1a) is exemplified in Figure 37-7. The case is that of two siblings, 18 and 16 years of age, respectively, placed as maidservants in a household and who had always been taken for females, figuring as such in the civilian registry. Both revealed the presence of penile hypospadias, associated in one case with bilateral cryptorchidism, in the other with only left-sided cryptorchidism. At laparotomy, they revealed the presence of poorly developed male internal sex organs as well as rudimentary Fallopian tubes in the internal portion of the inguinal canal.

The endocrine explanation for these cases in the light of the investigations of Wolff and Gingingler,[61] Moore,[36] Greene[17,18] and Price and Pannabecker[42,43] lies evidently in hyperfeminization during gestation, possibly owing to placental or adrenal estrogenic hypersecretion. The presence of *cryptorchidism* is thought to have produced a decrease (or abolition in the bilateral case) in testosterone secretion, resulting in a feminoid, or at least hypovirile, appearance of the two individuals since puberty.

37.4.2. FEMALE PSEUDOHERMAPHRODITISM

Most commonly, pseudohermaphroditism with ovaries is determined by the

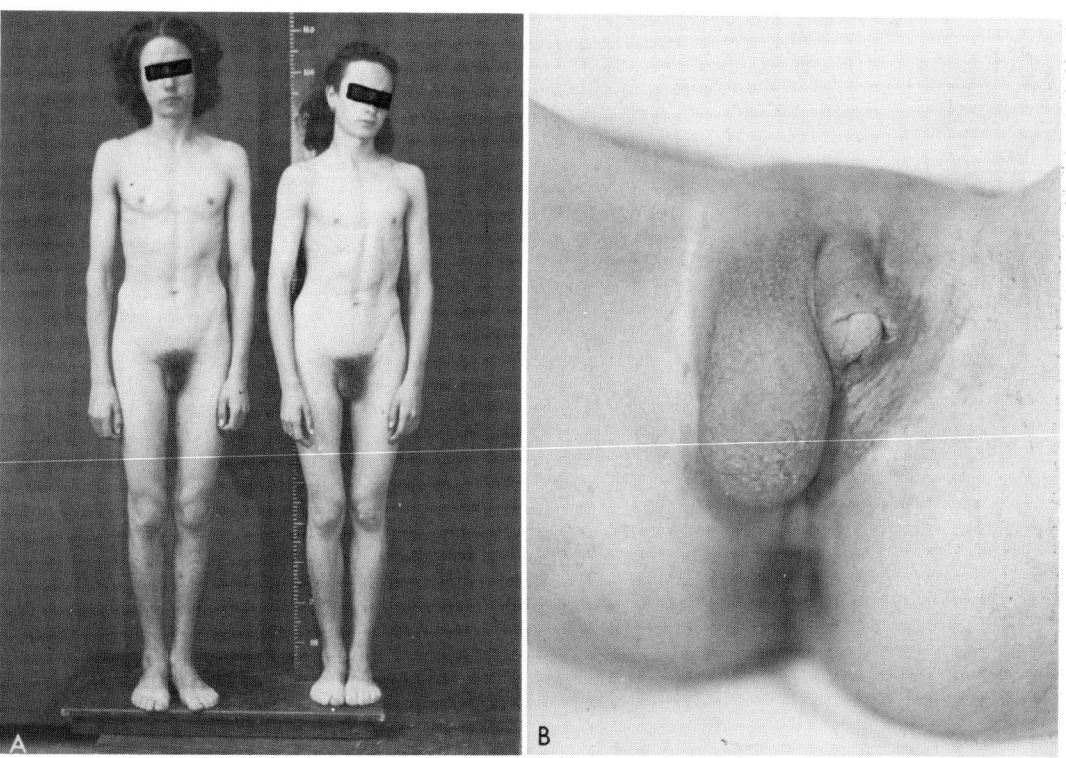

Figure 37-7. A, Male pseudohermaphroditism in two siblings. B, Perineal region of individual on the right: hypospadias, labioscrotal fold with rudimentary vagina, one scrotal sac with testis, the other empty.

congenital adrenogenital syndrome, which has already been discussed in Chapter 33. The varieties to be studied here are those which occur in the absence of adrenal hyperplasia: the syndrome that is called by Overzier "female pseudohermaphroditism without cortical hyperfunction," and by Jones and Scott[29] "nonvirilized female hermaphroditism." Typical examples of the latter are cases reported by Haynes and colleagues[24] in 1945, and those by Chanis[8] (1942); Brentnall[5] (1945); Cotte[10] (1947), two cases; Wilkins and colleagues[56] (1950); Zander and Müller[62] (1953); Papadatos and Klein[44] (1954), two cases; Hoffmann and associates[25] (1955); Hayles and Nolan[23] (1957); and five more cases collected by Jones and Scott,[29] in 1958. And this, by no means, is the list of world cases but a mere list of the best known and most widely publicized cases. These women have ovaries and often well developed Fallopian tubes and uteri. The presence of a phallus is noted at birth. It tends to grow during the years of puberty. In addition, there are vaginal atrophy and a scrotoid appearance of the labia majora (Figure 37-8). There is usually no hirsutism, but if there is, it is mild. Instances of *external* female pseudohermaphroditism of this type may be explained on the basis of androgenic hyperfunction during the fetal era and sensitivity to androgens of the female cloaca equal to that of the male cloaca. It is evident that the etiology of these cases can be traced to hyperandrogenism during the embryonal era, generally of adrenal origin.

Female pseudohermaphroditism with virilization is believed to be always of adrenogenital origin; however, we were able to observe a case of a 22 year old woman, with marked hirsutism, phalloid clitoris, absence of mammary development and well developed vagina and uterus. There was no adrenal hyperplasia.

It is of interest to mention that these cases show low 17-ketosteroid values and can thereby be differentiated from cases of adrenal origin.

37.5. PSEUDOHERMAPHRODITISM IN THE NEWBORN INDUCED BY TREATMENT OF THE MOTHER WITH ANDROGENIC SUBSTANCES DURING GESTATION

As pointed out in Chapter 15, in birds or reptiles whose eggs are treated with androgens,[13, 58, 59, 61] or in pregnant women who receive androgens during pregnancy,[17, 18, 37, 45] all fetuses with a female genetic sex undergo a process of masculinization. However, as a result of the widespread use of intensive hormone therapy, what up to now may have been only an experimental observation has unfortunately begun to occur clinically. The compounds most frequently leading to virilization are *testosterone and its derivatives*, and the new *synthetic progestins*; paradoxically, however, fetal virilization may be observed even following simple treatment with *progesterone* or with *estrogens*.

Experimental confirmation has been

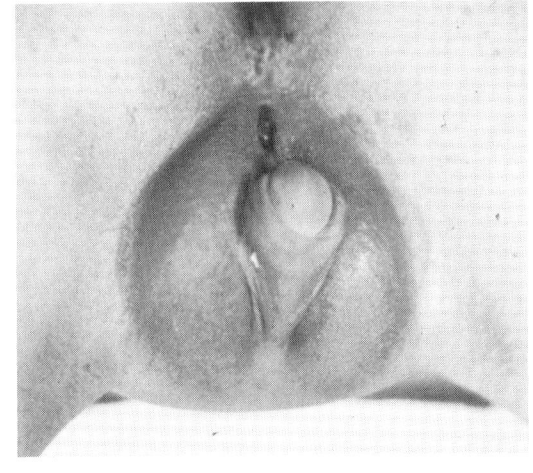

Figure 37-8. Female pseudohermaphroditism, with male appearance of external genitalia but without somatic masculinization. Vagina is permeable to a depth of 6 cm; labia majora of scrotal appearance but empty; there is a peniform clitoris, as well as uterus, tubes and ovaries.

provided by modern cases in which these effects were observed in newborn infants after administration of androgenic substances to their mothers during pregnancy. A case reported by Brentnall and another by Cotte are highly informative in that such effects were observed *in the presence of arrhenoblastomas in the mothers' ovaries, complicating gestation.*

37.5.1. ANDROGENS

Androgens are used only as an exception during pregnancy. Two such exceptional circumstances are: (1) malignant tumors of the breast, and (2) the use of anabolizing derivatives of androgens, such as, for example, methyltestosterone. Virilization stemming from testosterone administration has been described by Hoffmann and co-workers,[25] Bongiovanni and MacPadden,[3] Zander and Müller,[62] Goldman and Bongiovanni,[16] and Hayles and Nolan,[23] among many others. Androgenizing effects were observed with dosages ranging from 10 to 100 mg daily.

The anabolizing action of androgens has been employed by Zander and Müller (methyltestosterone) and by Vandekerckhove[53] (methylandrostendiol).

37.5.2. PROGESTOGENS

Synthetic progestogens, derivatives of 19-nortestosterone, have been found to have definite androgenizing effects on the fetus if employed during pregnancy. Because their administration is easy and their effects are potent, they have been and still are being recommended for the treatment of threatened abortion. Forbes and Coulombre[15] have assayed the metabolism of *norethisterone,* finding that it gravitated toward the 17-ketosteroid series rather than toward pregnanediol. Cases of neonatal pseudohermaphroditism following the administration of that compound have been reported by Grumbach and associates,[20] Hayles and Nolan,[23] Jacobson[26] and, above all, Wilkins and his colleagues,[56] who collected a most comprehensive series by means of a circular survey.

The effect of *19-methylnortestosterone* are even more harmful, as attested by the case reports of Grumbach and Ducharme,[21] Wilkins and associates,[56, 57] Hayles and Nolan,[23] and Neumann and Junkmann.[40] Similarly, *norethynodrel,* intended in one instance to effect sterilization in a woman who turned out to be already pregnant, inadvertently produced pseudohermaphroditism in a case reported by Grumbach and Barr.[19]

As far as dosages are concerned, these are quite variable, but as little as 10 mg of norpregneninolone and 30 mg of pregneninolone a day were found to be sufficient to cause virilization.

Progesterone is also able to exert a virilizing effect, though only exceptionally, as observed in cases collected by Hayles and Nolan,[23] Jones,[28] and Wilkins.[57] However, in the opinion of Suchowsky and Junkmann,[51, 52] who tested this compound in

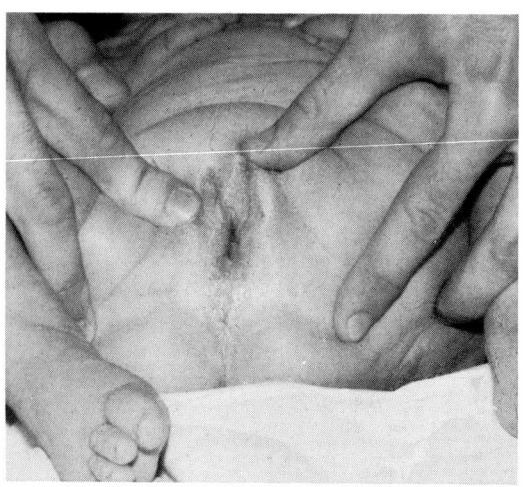

Figure 37-9. Six month old female with virilization induced by treatment of mother with large doses of norethisterone during pregnancy.

all its forms on experimental animals, there is no evidence to rule out the possibility that individual and isolated instances may have been cases of congenital adrenogenital syndrome (see Chapter 33) in which the administration of progesterone was incidental.

According to Courrier and Jost,[11] *pregneninolone* has also an androgenizing effect on gestation in rats.

37.5.3. ESTROGENS

Fetal virilization stemming from maternal estrogen treatment during gestation is unusual, but has been recorded in female mice by Jean[27] and in three women receiving stilbestrol in dosages of 10 to 25 mg (Bongiovanni et al.[2, 3]). Considering that the dosages quoted are similar to those frequently used in treating women with a whole range of gestational pathology, this may serve as a serious warning.

Estrogens do not exert the same effects at all times of gestation. Almost without exception, pseudohermaphroditism developed in those cases in which the androgenizing action had been exerted between the fifth and fifteenth weeks. Instances of drug-induced virilization in which therapy was started after the fifteenth week are most exceptional.

What might be termed *"syndrome of iatrogenic pseudohermaphroditism"* poses one of the most serious problems of modern day therapeutics, namely, the danger inherent in excessive or uncontrolled administration of drugs. At present, this is particularly true of those hormones that are employed as "shock" and "massive therapy" without regard to their oftentimes harmful effects. The practicing physician should be made increasingly aware of the damage that may result.

REFERENCES

1. Baker, G., and Franchi, L. L.: *Chromosoma*, 22:258, 1967.
2. Bongiovanni, A. M., Di Georgio, A. M., and Grumbach, M. M.: *J. Clin. Endocr.*, 19:1004, 1959.
3. Bongiovanni, A. M., and MacPadden, A. J.: *Fertil. Steril.*, 11:181, 1960.
4. Botte, V., and Chieffi, G.: *Arch. Ost. Gin.*, 72:434, 1967.
5. Brentnall, C. P.: *J. Obstet. Gynec. Brit. Emp.*, 52:235, 1945.
6. Bryan, A. L., Nigro, J. A., and Conseller, V. S.: *Surg. Gynec. Obstet.*, 88:79, 1949.
7. Burns, R. K.: *Amer. J. Anat.*, 98:35, 1956.
8. Chanis, D.: *J. Urol.*, 42:508, 1952.
9. Clark, J. H., and Gorski, J.: *Science*, 169:76, 1970.
10. Cotte, F. I.: *J. Mount Sinai Hosp.*, 14:170, 1947.
11. Courrier, R., and Jost, A.: *Compt. Rend. Soc. Biol. (Paris)*, 136:395, 1942.
12. Dantschakova, V.: *Compt. Rend. Soc. Biol. (Paris)*, 124:195, 1937.
13. Dantschakova, V.: *Der Aufbau der Geschlechte beim Höheren Wirbeltiere*, Jena, Gustav Fischer, 1941.
14. Elger, W.: *Arch. Anat. Microscop. Morphol. Exper.*, 55:657, 1966.
15. Forbes, T. R., and Coulombre, A. J.: *Proc. Soc. Exper. Biol. Med.*, 109:642, 1962.
16. Goldman, A. S., and Bongiovanni, A. M.: *Ann. N.Y. Acad. Sci.*, 142:755, 1967.
17. Greene, R. R.: *Biol. Symposia*, 9:105, 1942.
18. Greene, R. R., Burill, M. W., and Ivy, C. A.: *Science*, 88:130, 1938.
19. Grumbach, M. M., and Barr, M. L.: *Rec. Progr. Horm. Res.*, 14:255, 1958.
20. Grumbach, M. M., Ducharme, J. R., and Moloshok, R. E.: *J. Clin. Endocr.*, 19:1369, 1959.
21. Grumbach, M. M., and Ducharme, J. R.: *Fertil. Steril.*, 11:157, 1960.
22. Harrison, R. G.: *Textbook of Human Embryology*, Oxford, Butterworth, 1959.
23. Hayles, A. B., and Nolan, R. B.: *Proc. Staff Meet. Mayo Clin.*, 33:197, 1958.
24. Haynes, E., Thomas, H. A., and Wheeler, M. S.: *Anat. Rec.*, 154:307, 1941.
25. Hoffmann, F., Overzier, C., and Uhde, G.: *Geburtsh. u. Frauenhk.*, 15:1061, 1955.
26. Jacobson, B. D.: *Amer. J. Obstet. Gynec.*, 84:962, 1962.
27. Jean, C.: *Arch. Anat. Microscop. Morphol. Exper.*, 57:191, 1968.
28. Jones, H. W.: *Obstet. Gynec. Surv.*, 12:433, 1957.
29. Jones, H. W., and Scott, W. W.: *Hermaphroditism, Genital Anomalies and Related Endocrine Disease*, Baltimore, Williams & Wilkins, 1958.
30. Jost, A.: In *Ciba Collaquia on Ageing*, 2:18, 1956.
31. Jungman, R. A., and Schweppe, J. S.: *J. Clin. Endocr.*, 28:1599, 1968.
32. Lubbs, H. A., and Ruddle, F. H.: *Science*, 169:495, 1970.
33. MacIndoe, A.: *Brit. J. Plast. Surg.*, 2:254, 1950.
34. Meyer, R., and Scheid, H.: *Geburtsh. u. Frauenhk.*, 19:783, 1959.
35. Moore, C. R.: *J. Clin. Endocr.*, 10:231, 1950.
36. Moore, C. R.: In *La différenciation sexuelle chez les vertebrés*, ed. R. Courrier. Paris, Masson & Cie., 1951.
37. Moore, K. L., Graham, M. A., and Barr, M. L.: *Surg. Gynec. Obstet.*, 96:641, 1956.
38. Musset, R., Miller, P., Netter, A., and Solal, R.: *Gynec. Obstet.*, 66:145, 1967.
39. Needham, J.: *Biochemistry and Morphogenesis*. Cambridge University Press, 1942.
40. Neumann, F., and Junkmann, K.: *Endocrinology*, 73:33, 1963.
41. Philipp, E.: *Acta Gin.*, 3:1, 1952.
42. Price, D., and Pannabecker, R. R.: In *Le sexe*, ed. R. Courrier. Paris, Masson & Cie., 1960.
43. Price, D., and Pannabecker, R. R.: In *Ciba Colloquia on Ageing*, 2:3, 1958.

44. Papadatos, C., and Klein, R.: *J. Paediat.*, 45:662, 1954.
45. Raynaud, D.: In *Le sexe*, ed. R. Courrier. Paris, Masson & Cie, 1960.
46. Raynaud, D., and Friley, M.: *Ann. d'Endocr.*, 11:32, 1950.
47. Schlegel, R. J., Farias, E., Russon, N. C., Moore, J. R., and Gardner, L. I.: *Endocrinology*, 81:565, 1967.
48. Serra, G. B., Perez-Palacios, G., and Jaffe, R. B.: *J. Clin. Endocr.*, 30:128, 1970.
49. Simpson, J. L., and Christakos, A. C.: *Obstet. Gynec. Surv.*, 24:580, 1969.
50. Strickler, H. S.: *Endocrinology*, 42:230, 1948.
51. Suchowsky, G., and Junkmann, K.: *Geburtsh. u. Frauenhk.*, 20:1019, 1960.
52. Suchowsky, G., and Junkmann, K.: *Endocrinology*, 68:340, 1961.
53. Vandekerckhove, D.: *Ann. d'Endocr.*, 15:513, 1954.
54. Wells, L. J.: In *La différenciation sexuelle chez les vertébrés*, ed. R. Courrier. Paris, Masson & Cie., 1950.
55. Wells, L. J., and Van Waagenen, G.: *Contrib. Embryol.*, 35:175, 1954.
56. Wilkins, L., et al.: *J. Clin. Endocr.*, 18:559, 1958.
57. Wilkins, L.: *J.A.M.A.*, 172:1016, 1960.
58. Willier, B. H., Gallagher, T. F., and Koch, F. C.: *Anat. Rec.*, 61:Suppl. 50, 1935.
59. Witschi, E.: *Contrib. Embryol.*, 32:1, 1948.
60. Witschi, E.: *Le sexe*, ed. R. Courrier. Paris, Masson & Cie., 1960.
61. Wolff, E., and Ginglinger, A.: *Compt. Rend. Soc. Biol. (Paris)*, 132:909, 1935.
62. Zander, J., and Müller, H. A.: *Geburtsh. u. Frauenhk.*, 13:216, 1953.
63. Zuckermann, Sir Solly: In *La différenciation sexuelle chez les vertébrés*, ed. R. Courrier. Parris, Masson & Cie., 1950.

Chapter 38
ENDOCRINE PATHOLOGY OF PUBERTY

38.1. GENERAL CONSIDERATIONS

The subject of physiologic puberty was studied in Chapter 16, which deals with the mode of appearance of puberty and with the associated endocrine and genital processes. The present chapter deals in sequence with *precocious puberty,* by which we mean the appearance of sexual awakening before the age of 10, with *late puberty,* or the appearance of sexual maturation after the age of 20 and, finally, with the *menstrual pathology* of puberty, with special emphasis on *juvenile metropathy* and *juvenile dysmenorrhea* or menstrual molimen.

38.2. PRECOCIOUS PUBERTY

By precocious puberty we understand not only the premature appearance of menses but also the somatic, sexual and mental maturation in the process of which a girl is converted to a young woman prematurely. Precocious puberty may appear at any time during infancy, as early as 1 year of age, but most commonly it appears between the ages of five and 10. In Spain, the average age at menarche is 13. Menarche occurring between the ages of 10 and 13 is advanced in time but does not really constitute true precocious puberty.

38.2.1. ETIOLOGY AND CLASSIFICATION

The mechanism involved in bringing about puberty has been diagrammed in Figure 38–1, in keeping with the principles outlined in Chapter 16. Puberty, which essentially represents the emergence of cyclic ovarian and uterine activity, is determined by the action of pituitary gonadotropins, first by FSH and somewhat later by LH, exerted on the ovary, and by the action of ovarian hormones, the production of which is stimulated by the uterine gonadotropin effects. Pituitary secretion is controlled by the hypothalamus, *which in turn is committed to a double stimulatory and inhibitory function.* It is *inhibitory* during infancy, as long as lack of releasing factors causes the gonadotropins to be "locked" in the anterior lobe of the pituitary; and it becomes *stimulatory* beginning with the prepuberal phase, during which awakening of the hypothalamic sex nuclei determines first the initiation of FSH and then that of LH release. *Thus, puberty must be considered as essentially a hypothalamic phenomenon.*[5, 7, 80, 101]

Carraro and his associates[19] showed that, by virtue of its anesthetizing effect on the hypothalamus, reserpine caused delayed puberty in rats. On the other hand, it was also shown (Relkin[81]) that destruction of the rostral hypothalamic nuclei in the same species resulted in the disappearance of puberty.

The role of the *pineal* in sexual maturation was analyzed in Chapters 10 and 16, in which we stated that its influence is an inhibitory one. It should be mentioned, moreover, that the cerebral cortex is in intimate contact with the pineal and the hypothalamus and that these organs are connected by numerous fibers. These interrelationships can be drawn as in the diagram in Figure 38–1, in which, in addition to the neurohypophysial elements, we have

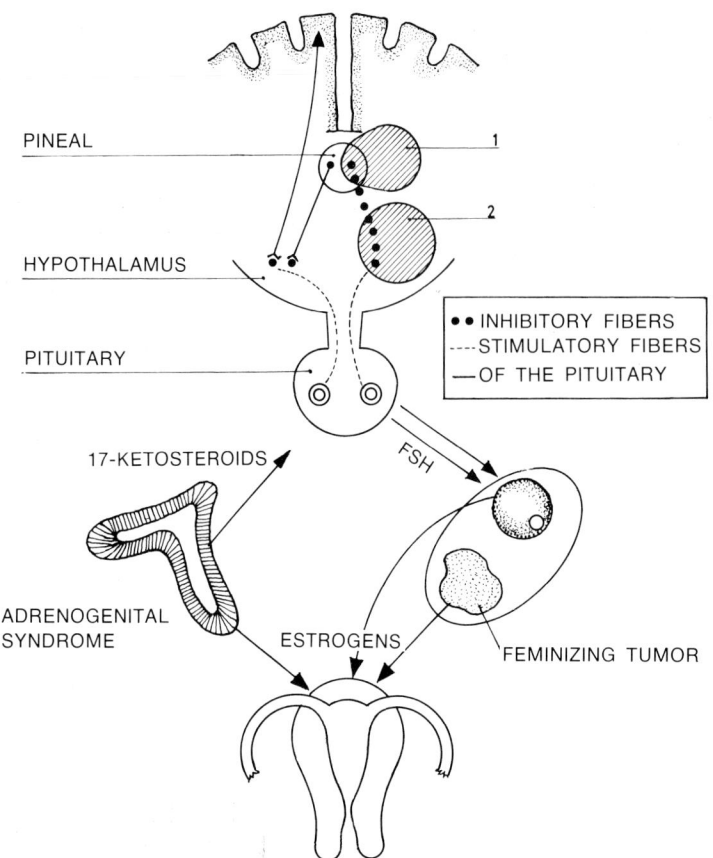

Figure 38-1. Schematic representation of the various endocrine and neurogenic mechanisms producing precocious puberty. 1, Pineal tumor destructive of inhibitory system. 2, Tumor or hypothalamic lesion destructive of inhibitory center at hypothalamic level.

included the *adrenal* and the *ovary* as possibly being instrumental in causing the pathologic changes conducive to precocious puberty.

Consequently, precocious puberty may be classified in the following manner:

Types of precocious puberty:
1. Constitutional
2. Gonadal
3. Adrenal
4. Hypothalamic
5. Pineal
6. Cerebral

Jolly[46] proposes a classification which, though not identical, is more or less similar (Table 38-1).

38.2.2. CONSTITUTIONAL PRECOCIOUS PUBERTY

Sexual and somatic precocity *without any demonstrable organic background* is usually considered to be of constitutional origin and is attributed to hereditary peculiarities. Instances of this type have been described by Lloyd.[58] According to the theory of Goldschmidt, explained in Chapter 15, it has been postulated that constitutional sexual precocity might be due to an excessive number of dominant sexual genes. Russell and Sachs[87] and Jolly[46] reported the occurrence of constitutional precocious puberty in members of the same family. Nevertheless, this type of precocious puberty *sine lesione* may be questioned, as those cases described may possibly have been instances in which the true causes involved were overlooked.

Jolly[46] called attention to the much higher incidence of this type of precocious puberty in girls than in boys (see Table 38-1).

38.2.3. PRECOCIOUS PUBERTY OF GONADAL ORIGIN

This type of puberty is encountered particularly in association with *granulosa cell tumors*. For the syndrome to develop, it is necessary that the tumor arise during the early years of childhood, which is not common. Thus, among the 250 cases of granulosa cell tumor collected from the world literature by Bland and Goldstein,[15] only seven had occurred before the age of 10 and produced precocious puberty. Klaften[52] and Varangot,[105] as well as Bland and Goldstein, all described cases with essentially similar features. These were unilateral ovarian tumors, often diagnosed as malignant (granulosa cell carcinoma), occurring in girls who presented with precocious puberty, menstruation and breast development. A case of granulosa cell carcinoma studied at our laboratory, which incidentally was associated with the earliest onset of precocity on record (age, five months), is shown in Figure 38-2.

Subsequently, Forlini,[33] Tweedie,[104] Lull,[60] Dancaster and colleagues,[27] and Niswander and Courey[74] reported additional cases. A review of all cases reported has recently been published by Zangeneh and Kelley.[113]

A quite similar but benign group of tumors are *thecomas*. The case reports of Betson and Eicher[14] and Coppeledge and Hasty[24] fall into this latter category.

Dokumov and Dekov[28] presented a case of feminizing ovarian tumor associated with precocious puberty which was unusual in that the neoplasm turned out to be a *feminizing hilus cell tumor*. We have already called attention to the fact that feminizing varieties of Leydig cell tumors (hilus cell tumors) have recently been reported with relative frequency (see Chapter 30).

A circumstance not recognized until recently is the finding that gonadal precocious puberty may also be caused by *dysgerminoma*. Although the occurrence of these tumors in infancy is relatively common, until recently their possible estrogenic effects were unknown. As pointed out in Chapter 30, however, they may sometimes display androgenizing activity. On the other hand, more rarely they may produce feminization or, when occurring in infancy, precocious puberty. Cases of this type have been published by Giusti[37] and by Teter,[102] both in 1962.

Instances of ovarian precocious puberty caused by *infantile polymicrocystic ovaries* have been described (Steiner and Hadawi[100]). In our opinion, these are instances of precocious puberty of hypothalamic origin in which effect has been mistaken for cause. This variety of precocious puberty is of entirely isosexual character, which means that, other than being advanced, the maturation process in those females is reproduced in a physiologic manner. Such girls develop breasts as well as pubic and axillary hair prematurely, although in a totally feminine fashion. They are mentally alert and tend to reveal a not-

TABLE 38-1. Forms of Precocious Puberty Among 69 Cases Described by Jolly*

ETIOLOGY	VARIETY	FEMALES	MALES
A. *Constitutional*		31	3
B. *Cerebral*	1. Tumor	1	4
	2. Meningitis	2	0
	3. Tuberous sclerosis	1	0
	4. Congenital anomalies	1	0
C. *Adrenal*	1. Hyperfunction, hyperplasia	0	6
	2. Carcinoma	1	2
D. *Gonadal*	1. Granulosa cell tumor	1	0
	2. Leydig cell tumor of testis	0	2
E. *Miscellaneous*	1. Female pseudohermaphroditism	7	0
	2. Albright's syndrome	0	0
	3. Hepatoblastoma	0	1
	4. Unknown	5	0
	Total	50	19

*From Jolly, H., SEXUAL PRECOCITY, 1966. Courtesy of Charles C Thomas, Publisher, Springfield, Illinois.

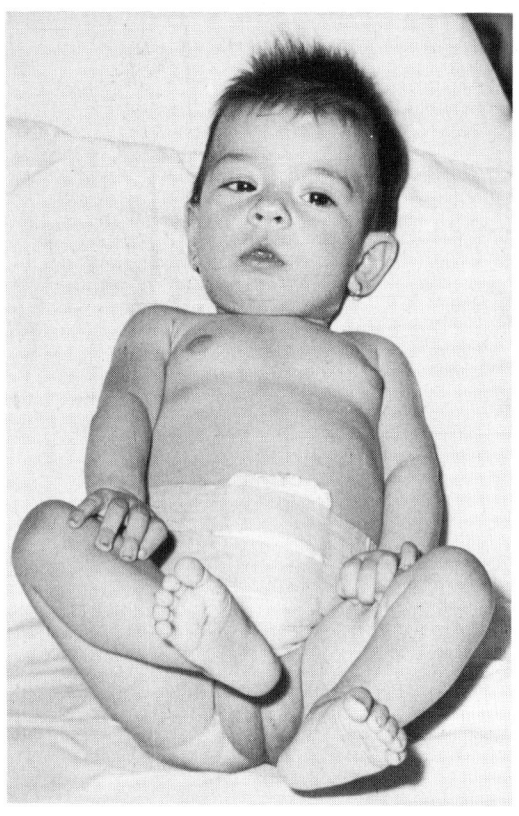

Figure 38-2. Case of precocious puberty in a six month old girl owing to a granulosa cell tumor. (Courtesy of Drs. Navarro and Nogales.)

iceable aversion to playing with other girls, preferring the chores of grown-ups. The premature appearance of libido has been reported in some instances.

38.2.4. PRECOCIOUS PUBERTY OF ADRENAL ORIGIN

Whenever hyperplasia and benign or malignant tumors of the adrenal cortex occur in infancy, they produce precocious puberty with precocious menarche (see Chapter 33), which is then followed by *rapid evolution toward the male sex.* Such girls thus change into tomboys and menstruation disappears secondarily. A sequence of events of this kind goes by the name of *heterosexual precocious puberty,* to be distinguished from isosexual precocious puberty, which results from granulosa cell tumors. In the form under discussion, the episode of *transient premature feminization is but an intermediate step toward definitive virilization,* that is, a particular instance of Marañón's theory[63] of sexual evolution. Before converting into a masculinized individual, such girls first pass through a period of ephemeral femininity.

The physiopathologic mechanism of this disorder is the following one: In most instances, the adrenal cortex is known to secrete androgens and estrogens simultaneously. Because the estrogenic effectors, viz., the müllerian organs, as well as the female somatic features, are more susceptible to hormone action than their male counterparts, the body first responds to the estrogenic stimulation. However, since the proportion of androgens secreted always surpasses that of estrogens, androgenic stimulation secondarily reaches predominance over estrogenic stimulation, until eventually it prevails completely.

The adrenogenital syndrome is not always of the predominantly virilizing variety, as repeatedly stressed in Chapter 33. Although they are extremely rare, cases of isosexual precocious puberty of adrenal origin are also known to occur. These represent instances of adrenogenital syndrome with predominant estrogen production. Clinically, such cases of feminizing adrenogeni-

Endocrine Pathology of Puberty

tal syndrome associated with precocious puberty have been described by Simpson[93] and designated by the generic term of "gynism." In these instances, hyperplasia or tumors of the adrenal were observed to determine purely female isosexual puberty, of the type induced by granulosa cell tumors.

On the other hand, Davis and Rakoff[26] reported a case of a girl with heterosexual precocious puberty and secondary virilization owing to an ectopic adrenal tumor of the ovary (ovarian hypernephroma).

Mellicow and Cahill[66] published about 20 cases of heterosexual precocious puberty of adrenal origin. Hormone studies concerning rates of urinary steroid excretion have been reported by Shadaksharappa and associates,[92] Lloyd and co-workers,[58, 59] Thompsett[103] and, later, by Visser and Degenhart.[106] Shadaksharappa and his colleagues found that urinary estrogen excretion in

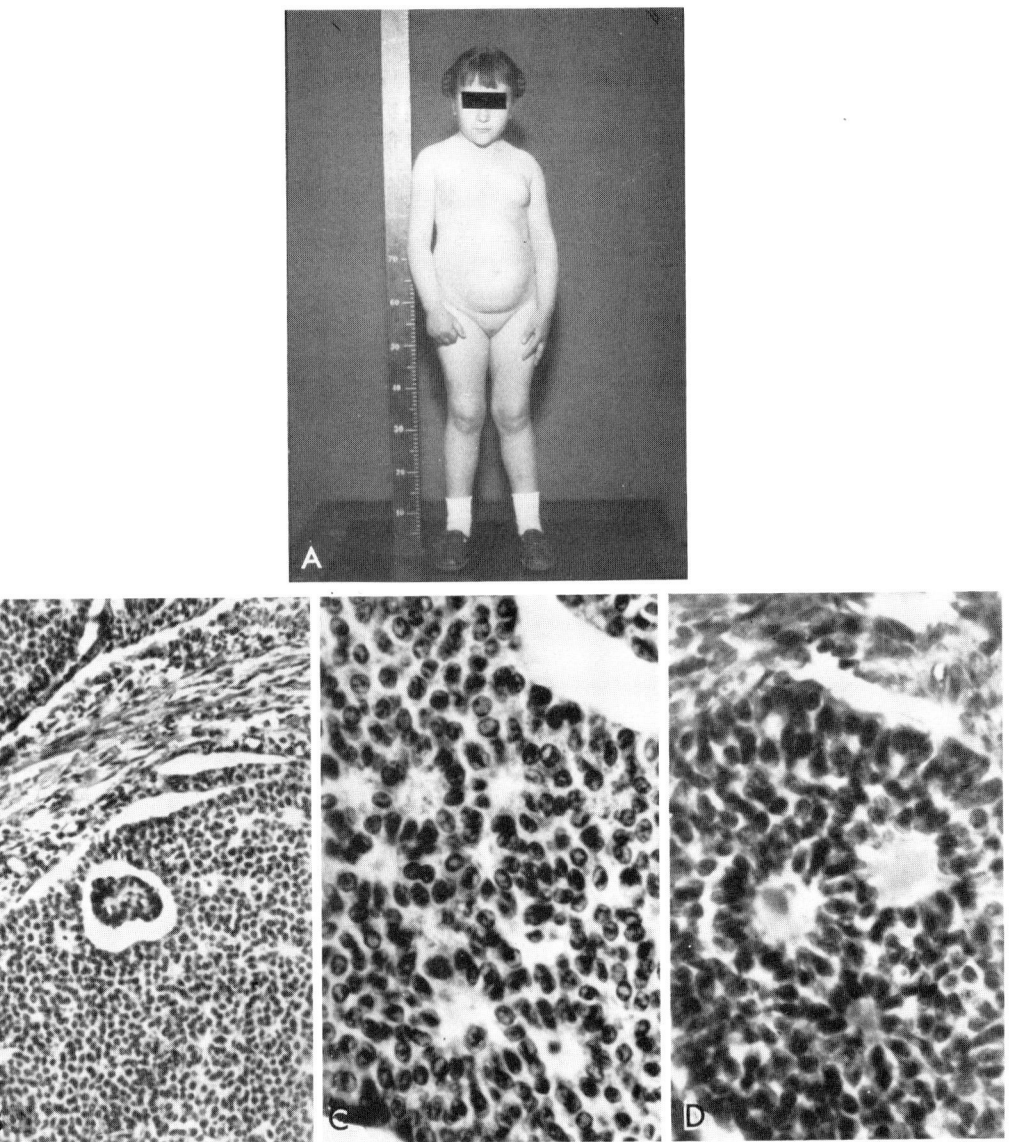

Figure 38–3. Case of precocious puberty owing to granulosa cell tumor in a seven year old girl. A, Physical appearance of patient. Note incipient breast development, although there is no pubic or axillary hair. Menstruation started at the age of six. B, Granulosa cell tumor of right ovary at intermediate magnification. C, D, Tumor at higher magnification, revealing typical "follicular" growth pattern, with Call-Exner bodies.

a case of isosexual precocious puberty amounted to 750 to 900 mcg per 24 hr, an enormous amount that accounts for premature maturation of the genital apparatus, whereas 17-ketosteroid values were in the order of 6 to 9 mg. In contrast, the values reported by Lloyd[59] in a case of heterosexual precocious puberty were 69 to 82 mg for 17-ketosteroids, and 96 mg for pregnanediol, with only scant amounts of estrogens. Thompsett maintains that the urinary steroid levels in these cases constitute a faithful index of the iso- or heterosexual nature of the syndrome, since in the former situation estrogens are high while 17-ketosteroids are low, whereas the reverse occurs in the latter modality. According to Conly and associates,[23] the most common tendency observed is for isosexual precocious puberty to be followed by virilization. These hormone findings not only reveal the etiologic mechanism involved in this form of precocious puberty but also prove that the iso- or heterosexual character of the disorder depends entirely *on the reciprocal ratio between the male and female principles secreted.*

38.2.5. HYPOTHALAMIC PRECOCIOUS PUBERTY

The term *hypothalamic precocious puberty* is used here in preference to *pituitary precocious puberty*, since we do not know of any purely pituitary condition capable of causing the disorder. At present, there is no doubt that precocious puberty is produced by hypothalamic disturbances secondarily involving FSH hypersecretion by the adenohypophysis which, other than that, retains its normal function. Bauer[8] compiled 60 cases of neoplastic or chronic inflammatory lesions affecting the hypothalamus, for which autopsy findings were also available. Among these, 24 (19 males, 5 females) had a history of precocious puberty. Hypothalamic precocious puberty, it has been observed by other workers, predominantly occurs in males, only seldom affecting females. Bauer points out that the fundamental precondition for precocious puberty of hypothalamic origin to develop is the presence of a normally functioning pituitary. In those cases of hypothalamic tumors or lesions in which the pituitary was also involved, premature sexual maturation invariably failed to materialize. The kind of lesions that are able to precipitate maturation are essentially such processes as tumors of the hypothalamus, astrocytomas or pinealomas extending to the hypothalamus, craniopharyngiomas, cysts, tuberculomas, syphilis and abscesses.

Papez and Ecker[75] described a case of hypothalamic infundibuloma which produced precocious puberty. Seckel and his associates[89, 90] reported six cases with various types of tumors, among which astrocytomas predominated. An astrocytoma was the cause of precocious puberty in the case reported by Weinberger and Grant, whereas that of MacCullagh and his associates[61] resulted from a glioma of the *tuber cinereum*. Though in the case of Elwers and Critchlow[29] there was no lesion in the floor of the third ventricle, there was extensive degeneration of the *amygdaloid nucleus*.

Jolly[46] refers to this form as the "cerebral" form and includes it among what in our classification corresponds to the last category. He states he has never observed any tumor that would selectively modify the hypothalamic sex center. If present, such modifications occur more commonly in males than in females (see Table 38–1). Ernould and his colleagues[30] described a destructive tumor involving the mamillary bodies that produced precocious puberty. The general impression is that any simple destructive process involving the sex center is capable of triggering the onset of puberty. This is also true of experimental animals.[7, 80]

Concerning the question of how hypothalamic tumors induce precocious puberty, Harris[40a] believes that the mechanism involved consists in *chronic irritation of the hypothalamic sex center*. Nevertheless, it may be hard to conceive how this kind of effect could be elicited by widely destructive tumors. We are inclined to agree with Morley[71] that the mode of production of precocious puberty involves *destruction of some inhibitory center for sexual maturation, that is, a center inhibiting pituitary FSH secretion.* The hypothalamus controls the process that adjusts infantile pituitary function to puberal pituitary function, involving the conversion of a somatotropin-producing pituitary to a gonadotropin-producing pituitary. *It is obvious that this mission cannot be accomplished unless there is some center capable of not only stimulating but also suppressing positive gonadotropin activity* (Fig. 38–1).

38.2.6. PRECOCIOUS PUBERTY OF PINEAL ORIGIN

Since 1898, when the first case of precocious puberty from pineal tumor was described, 475 cases have been reported in the literature; these were compiled by Kitay[51] and by Heubner[43] up to 1954. Of these 475 cases, 178 fell into the age group between one and 16 years of age, of which 145 were males and only 33 females. Those findings seem to bear out our previous statement, namely, that both the hypothalamic and pituitary varieties of precocious puberty occur much more commonly in males. Among the 178 cases occurring between the ages of one and 16 years, only 42 had a history of precocious puberty, which means that *only one fourth of all pineal tumors occurring in both boys and girls produced precocious puberty.* A review of the literature suggests two possible explanations for the existing relationship between this type of tumor and precocious puberty. According to some, precocious puberty stems from decreased secretion of a presumptive pineal hormone whose inhibitory effect on growth has been commented on in Chapter 10. However, this hypothesis has been accepted by us with some reservations, considering the fact that no conclusive evidence has so far been produced to confirm the endocrine character of the pineal. A second hypothesis, subscribed to by the majority of investigators (Talbot,[101] Wortham,[109] Russell and Sachs[87]), holds that pineal tumors may produce precocious puberty by virtue of indirectly stimulating the pituitary, as a result of either compression of the gland or production of pituitary hyperemia. Lastly, a third hypothesis, proposed by Morely,[71] admits the existence of *hypothalamic centers inhibiting pituitary gonadotropin secretion*, along lines identical to those referred to in the preceding section, and postulates that *compression of these inhibitory centers by adjacent pinealomas is the determinant of precocious puberty.*

On the basis of a review of the material published in the world literature with special reference to the degree of destruction found in the pineal gland and surrounding areas, Kitay[51] and Heubner[43] maintained that precocious puberty in patients with pineal tumors was not determined by compression of either the pituitary or the hypothalamus. Although hypothalamic compression could not be entirely ruled out as a possible etiologic factor, isolated destruction of the pineal by itself, without hypothalamic involvement, was in the author's view enough to produce the appearance of precocious puberty. Without supplying conclusive arguments, the author further suggested the possibility that, rather than representing an inhibitory endocrine gland, the pineal was in fact a *nerve center inhibiting the hypothalamus.* This hypothesis conflicts with the preceding one. Nevertheless, following the recent discovery of an *inhibitory sex center* in the anterior hypothalamus by Poll,[77] it may lend support to the ideas of Morley.

Shortly after Kitay's findings became known, Jolly[46] rejected any role the pineal might have in producing puberty. The table listing his cases (Table 38–1) reveals that not only cerebral tumors (of quite varied localization and anatomic pathology) but even such processes as *meningitis* or degenerative and congenital diseases involving the brain may cause precocious puberty. No such lesions were found to attack the pineal gland selectively.

As pointed out in Chapter 10, however, the endocrine role of the pineal has been reaffirmed in the last years by virtue of the discovery, isolation and purification of *melatonin*,[2, 21, 35, 36, 45, 47, 76, 110, 111] a pineal polypeptide, whose specific action consists in suppressing FSH release by way of the hypothalamic sex center. Consequently, the mode of action of the pineal by means of this incretion appears to be to inhibit the sex center from producing FSHRF (and possibly LHRF).

An important aspect of precocious puberty of pineal origin is the relationship between pineal function and *environmental lighting.* Darkness has been found to be responsible for pineal hypofunction.[72, 82] Perhaps, this is why *blindness in girls* is usually associated with *precocious puberty.*[114]

38.2.7. ALBRIGHT'S SYNDROME

In 1938, Albright and his co-workers[3] described a syndrome characterized by polyostotic fibrous dysplasia, *café-au-lait* spots and precocious puberty. In 1947, the same authors published a more comprehensive review of such cases. Apparently, the syndrome of *polyostotic fibrous dysplasia*, as also indicated by Bernardinelli,[11] develops in many instances without associated pigmentary lesions or precocious puberty, so that the fundamental feature of the syndrome in effect is fibrous dysplasia affecting multiple bones. Although frequently a part of the clinical picture, precocious puberty is not a constant development in the syndrome. In addition, Wortham[109] described some cases of polyostotic fibrous dysplasia, pigmentation and precocious puberty occurring in conjunction with acromegaly. Wortham suggests a possible explanation for this syndrome which has not yet been fully clarified. Accordingly, *the original Albright's syndrome is postulated to involve development of basal cranial exostoses, leading to irritation or injury of the hypothalamus which may result in precocious puberty*. Hence, the implication is that precocious puberty of this type is of hypothalamic origin secondary to osseous lesions.

38.2.8. CEREBRAL TYPE OF PRECOCIOUS PUBERTY

Precocious puberty may in some cases be a consequence of brain injury resulting from encephalitis, influenza, infectious diseases, internal hydrocephalus, etc. The case reported by Matos and his associates has already been referred to in Chapter 32; in that case, precocious puberty appeared as a result of nearly complete destruction of the telencephalon. As noted above, Jolly[46] similarly described cases produced by meningitis, congenital cerebral anomalies and degenerative diseases of the cerebral cortex. Encephalographic alterations have been found in some cases of precocious puberty both in animals[97] and in women.[57] Various authors postulated that some forms of precocious puberty were due to *cerebral psychosexual stimuli in cases of infantile dementia*. As it is, these cases require much more research in order to elucidate their etiologic peculiarities.

38.2.9. HORMONAL MECHANISM INVOLVED IN PRECOCIOUS PUBERTY

Regardless of what its etiology may be, precocious puberty in every case is determined by increased estrogen activity, which in turn results from *hyperproduction of gonadotropins*. In various animals, such as rats[1,10] and monkeys,[6] gonadotropin injections provoke precocious puberty. A premature increase in gonadotropin activity as the cause of precocious puberty in human clinical experience has been reported by Raiti and associates,[78] Rifkind and co-workers,[83] and Yen and Vicic.[113] Although the initial increase involves FSH activity,[54] precocious puberty may also be produced by increased LH levels.[40,112]

38.3. DELAYED PUBERTY

Since the timing of puberty in the female is of indeterminate nature, the menarche is used as the point of reference for *delayed puberty*, in those girls whose menarche appears after the age of 15. It is impossible to demarcate delayed puberty in the presence of essential amenorrhea although, in principle, menarche may be expected to occur between the ages of 15 and 20. Therefore, any woman who has failed to menstruate before the age of 20 may be considered as *definitely amenorrheic*.

The etiology of delayed puberty is largely confused with that of primitive hypoestrinism, the subject of which has been discussed in Chapter 27. Therefore, we shall but summarily list the various forms of this puberal disorder by describing the following varieties: (1) constitutional delayed puberty; (2) delayed puberty from localized uterine disorders; (3) delayed puberty of ovarian origin; (4) delayed puberty of pituitary origin; (5) hypothalamic delayed puberty; and (6) cerebral type of delayed puberty. As may be noted, the present etiologic classification, except for the constitutional form whose etiology is unknown, follows the same order in which we discussed the neuroendocrine mechanism that initiates menstruation.

Endocrine Pathology of Puberty

being a well known function of the adrenal cortex (Greenblatt,[39] Zurbrügg and Gardner[116]), puberal adrenal insufficiency determines delayed *development of pubic hair* (Fig. 38–7). This topic was discussed in more detail in Chapter 16.

38.3.8 ANDROGENIC TYPE OF DELAYED PUBERTY

In previous chapters (Chapters 8, 28), we have emphasized the inhibitory effect of androgens on the maturation of the female hypothalamus.[7, 38, 50, 85, 107] It has been repeatedly postulated that androgenism may be the underlying cause of delayed puberty, essential amenorrhea and sterility (see Chapter 28). The same mechanism has been invoked[39] for anovulation and amenorrhea in the Stein-Leventhal syndrome. Delayed puberty with elevated 17-ketosteroid values has been reported by a number of investigators (Kitay,[51] Jolly,[46] Seckel[90]). It seems plausible to speculate that hyperandrogenism of adrenal or ovarian origin might delay the onset of female puberty. Lately, this idea seems to be gaining in acceptance. Davidson[25] found that the administration of cyproterone (an antiandrogen) induced precocious puberty, while estrogenic implants would produce the same effect.[64, 73, 79, 95] Thus, all indications are that androgens act in a physiologic way as *moderators* of puberty and that their excessive activity may delay the onset of puberty.

38.3.9 OTHER FORMS OF DELAYED PUBERTY

To be included here is *Pendl's syndrome* or the *constitutional hyperthymic syndrome*, which, though involving boys more commonly, may occasionally be seen in girls.

Also to be cited here is delayed puberty resulting from *deficiency states*. It has been pointed out previously (see Chapters 11 and 34) that girls exposed to malnutrition during and after a time of war, in Spain as well as in the rest of Europe, later frequently

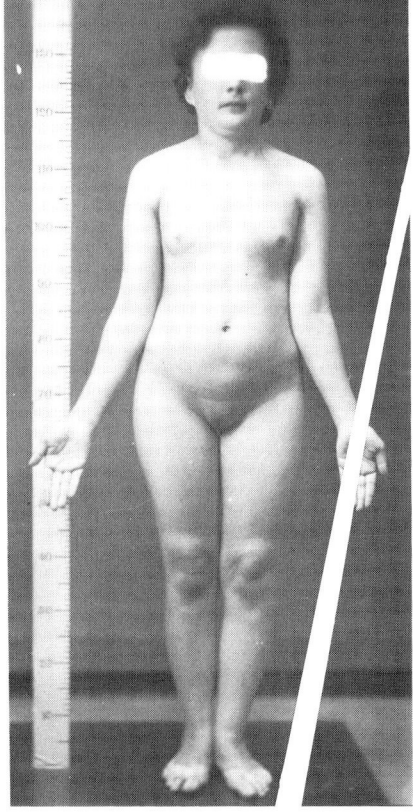

Figure 38–7. Woman, aged 20, with absence of pubic and axillary hair and essential amenorrhea. Serial vaginal cytology revealed atrophic smears. Negative estrogenuria; FSH, 90 rat units per 24 hr. (This case is physically reminiscent of Turner's syndrome.)

developed hypoestrinism or infertility problems. This group of patients is particularly prone to develop delayed puberty.

In this regard, the role played by hypoproteinemia[49] is of special interest.

In addition, the onset of puberty is delayed in all those *diseases of later childhood* that cause general physical debility with a slowdown in physical development. This is only natural since sexual function is a "superfluous" or "luxury" function, so that under precarious vegetative conditions, any organism must be anticipated not to restore reproductive function until more essential problems have been overcome. It is common knowledge to every general practitioner that delayed puberty in a girl is often remedied by simple administration of tonics and reconstituents.

38.4. MENSTRUAL DISORDERS OF PUBERTY AND ADOLESCENCE; JUVENILE METROPATHY

Regardless of whether it is normal, advanced or delayed, once it is begun menstruation may be beset by disturbances that are typical of the puberal age. One of these is *juvenile functional bleeding* or *juvenile metropathy;* another is *dysmenorrhea* or *menstrual molimen.*

Juvenile metropathy is a disorder characterized by irregular periods accompanied by menstrual hemorrhage, which may be serious. It is impossible to establish any single model on which juvenile metropathy may be patterned. Sometimes menstruation would appear on the expected date but would be unusually copious (hypermenorrhea), or sometimes bleeding would be irregular, without any cyclic rhythm or fixed duration, presenting a picture much like that of functional bleeding. Quite often, too, periods of metrorrhagia alternate with periods of normal menstruation, and even with very prolonged intermenstrual intervals, metrorrhagia then recurring after what appears to be a transient phase of amenorrhea.

38.4.1. ETIOLOGY

The physiologic occurrence in puberty of *anovulatory cycles* has been recorded by various authors (Mikulicz-Radecky and Kausch,[68] Clauberg and Breipohl,[22] Fluhman[31]) and has been mentioned in Chapter 16. The onset of menstruation does not take place in a sudden manner; at an early time of life, a monophasic cycle is established first, which only later gives rise to the appearance of a normal biphasic cycle. In most instances, juvenile metropathy is therefore an anovulatory type of menstruation in which hemorrhage develops as a result of a disturbance of follicular maturation. As has already been pointed out, putuitary factors are of utmost importance in the majority of cases, probably as a result of disharmony between the rates of FSH and LH secretion. Granted that psychosomatic influences, as it is now admitted, play a role in the genesis of metropathia haemorrhagica in adult women, many of the juvenile disorders may likewise be assumed to be of central neurogenic rather than primitive pituitary origin.

However, it must be realized that many instances of juvenile metropathy may be functional only in appearance and that the true underlying cause may be organic. The most important etiologic factor in that category is represented by *endometrial tuberculosis*, which quite frequently occurs under the guise of a metropathy resistant to hormone therapy.

Existing *therapeutic difficulties may be compounded by diagnostic difficulties* encountered in performing exploratory endometrial biopsies in virgins.

It must equally be remembered that *blood dyscrasias* are fairly common in the juvenile age group and that some instances of juvenile metropathy may have neither a functional nor an organic uterine etiology but may result entirely from disorders in blood coagulation. By and large, however, the etiology most frequently is anovulatory bleeding.

38.4.2. CLINICAL PICTURE

Juvenile metrorrhagia does not always appear with the same symptomatology. *Essentially, three different modes of appearance may be distinguished.* First, *menstruation may be delayed*, appearing every two or three months, in which case bleeding is quite copious at the moment of appearance. Alternate phases of metrorrhagia and amenorrhea may thus occur. Such cases are due to persistence of large follicles in the ovary and bleeding commonly has a hormonal etiology determined by hyperestrinism.

The second variety is one in which, after several more or less regular menstrual periods, the latter become gradually more and more abundant until eventually occurring as true *hemorrhagic episodes of long duration*, completely disrupting the menstrual cycle. Hemorrhage in this instance similarly results from follicular persistance, in association, however, with the development of secondary endometrial disorders, such as necrosis or incomplete shedding. In the last variety, *menstruation is regular* but bleeding is more abundant than usual.

Hamblen[41] also distinguishes those cases of juvenile metrorrhagia which appear late in adolescence. Such cases commonly are associated with a poor general condition of the patient, occasionally with severe anemia and malnutrition. *An important feature about these women is almost complete absence of dysmenorrhea*, a fact seemingly favoring the hypothesis that juvenile dysmenorrhea requires the presence of a corpus luteum.

38.4.3 DIAGNOSIS

Particularly since the introduction of *hyaluronidase* for the dilatation of the hymen (Slocker[94]), it has been possible to perform endometrial biopsies by means of small microcurettes in some cases. Whenever this type of exploratory procedure cannot be accomplished, a vaginal smear may permit evaluation of possible hyperestrinism by means of the Papanicolaou technique. In the opinion of Lencioni and Stafieri[56] and Sonek,[98] cytology is an excellent means for diagnosing some endocrine disturbances of puberty.

Pregnanediol determinations may also yield valuable data, since pregnanedioluria is known to be nil or extremely low in cases of juvenile metropathy. The consensus concerning low urinary pregnanediol is more unanimous as regards these cases than other forms of functional bleeding in adult women.

38.4.4. TREATMENT

Owing to certain peculiarities, the treatment of juvenile metropathy differs from that of metropathia haemorrhagica, discussed in Chapter 28. In the first place, *androgens must not be employed* in this form of metropathy. This is because androgens induce virilization in youngsters much more readily than in adult women as a result of the greater susceptibility of young tissues to hormonal influences and, as a matter of even greater concern, because androgenic activity enhances libido which, while of little consequence in married women, may be fraught with unpleasant consequences for single women.

Therefore, treatment should be based on *progesterone*, following the same guidelines for progesterone therapy that we have outlined previously. Gonadotropins also have an important place in the treatment of juvenile metropathy. Because in most cases the deficiency of pituitary function is temporary in nature, combined administration of serum gonadotropins and chorionic gonadotropins yields satisfactory results. The need for psychotherapy in many of these cases must not be overlooked, and attention should be directed equally to the patient's nutritional requirements, administering, if necessary, reconstituents and particularly ascorbic acid in liberal amounts.

Runge[86] attached great importance to a symptomatic form of therapy, based on *splenic radiotherapy*. The administration of an excitation dose of 150 to 200 r deep to the splenic region apparently enhances the process of blood coagulation, which is usually diminished in this condition. Good results with splenic radiotherapy were obtained at our clinic by Bedoya and Funcasta.[9]

38.5. DYSMENORRHEA OR MENSTRUAL MOLIMEN

The fact that menstruation may be associated with systemic repercussions has been common knowledge since time immemorial. Highly varied in nature, such repercussions are a reminder of the extent to which the entire body partakes in the menstrual crisis. In general, the sum total of menstrual disturbances has been designated by the generic name *molimina menstrualia*. But in some women, particularly during puberty, these disturbances may be of such intensity as to *constitute a genuine pathologic condition*. It may then be justifiably referred to as a "menstrual disease," a term proposed by us.

There is no general agreement as to whether these manifestations should be considered as normal and constant events or as definitely pathologic symptoms affecting but a minor group of patients. The truth is that there is a whole range of intermediate disturbances between girls menstruating with absolute regularity and normalcy, without the slightest evidence of pathology, and those in whom menstrual disorders are so severe as to deserve the denomination of a true menstrual disease.

38.5.1 SYMPTOMATOLOGY

The main symptoms are: (1) uterine pain; (2) premenstrual tension; (3) premenstrual edema; (4) nervous disorders, including headaches; (5) extragenital bleeding, and (6) hematologic disorders.

UTERINE PAIN. Menstrual uterine pain is a gynecologic problem with too many ramifications to allow a clinical description and etiologic analysis in this place. However, it should be made clear that the modern trend is to view essential dysmenorrhea as due to *vasospastic disorders* stemming from vasoconstriction of the uterine vessels. Smith and Smith[96] attribute it to the action of *menotoxins* and claim to have been able to reproduce uterine pain experimentally by injecting toxic extracts of the endometrial mucosa. This type of pain does not occur in women whose uteri have been removed, even though the ovaries are left behind and function normally. It equally fails to develop whenever the endometrium has been destroyed or has undergone atrophy although the myometrium remains intact.

PREMENSTRUAL TENSION. This term was applied for the first time by Frank[34] to designate a condition characterized the exaggeration of normal menstrual molimen and by congestion of all genital organs. It is accompanied by hyperexcitability, restlessness, emotional disturbances, insomnia, depression, vertigo, headache, fatigue and painful engorgement of the breasts. Its etiology is by no means clear though it has been suggested to be mainly related to excessive estrogenic activity.

MENSTRUAL EDEMA. A number of authors have called attention to the occurrence of edema in some women several days before and during menstruation. According to the explanation offered, edema would seem to be related to sodium retention, which is an indirect effect of excessive estrogen activity (see Chapter 2).

NERVOUS DISORDERS, ESPECIALLY HEADACHES. Most of the workers who have studied the problem, for instance Frank[34] and Reynolds and associates, believe that nervous instability, appreering as a by-product of premenstrual tension or sometimes as an independent symptom, is due to peculiarities of the nervous system in particularly unstable and neurotic women. The most dramatic symptom of all is *headache*, particularly if it is of the hemicrania type. Smith and Smith also attributed this syndrome to the toxic effect of products derived from the endometrium.

EXTRAGENITAL BLEEDING. This type of bleeding, also designated by the inadequate term "vicarious menstruation," seems to occur regularly in the menstrual molimen in some normally menstruating girls and occasionally also in amenorrheic women (from whom the term originally gave rise). Capillary fragility has been found to increase during the days preceding menstruation as well as during menstruation, which accounts for the bleeding tendency. Smith and Smith[96] have found that animals intoxicated by extracts of premenstrual endometrium developed vascular lesions and coagulability disorders quite similar to those just mentioned. In addition, it must be borne in mind that menotoxins exert a fibrinolytic effect, which is why menstrual blood, as it is well known, is incoagulable.

In view of the foregoing considerations, extragenital bleeding episodes, sometimes coinciding with menstrual molimen, must be ascribed to the effect of menotoxins on the vascular system and, above all, on the clotting mechanism.

In addition to the foregoing disorders, these women show a marked *tendency to hyperthermia*, usually resulting in a premenstrual rise in basal body temperature. As indicated in Chapter 13, this type of hyperthermia stems from the effects of progesterone.

38.5.2. ETIOLOGY

In attempting to summarize what has so far been said concerning the general symptomatology accompanying menstruation, it must be stressed that while these findings are by no means constant a good many girls present a fairly well defined clinical picture. The disturbance may be defined as a true "menstrual disease" which generally persists for as long as the girl has not completely matured.

On the basis of the previously offered isolated considerations concerning its pathogenesis, the menstrual disease may be inferred to be caused by the concurrence of two etiologic factors: (a) the effect of *menotoxins*, and (b) the effect of *abnormal estrogen metabolism*. We shall examine them consecutively.

MENOTOXINS. The symptoms of "menstrual disease" thus seem to be almost certainly nothing else than symptoms caused by menotoxin intoxication. Ever since ancient times, a stigma of impurity has been attached to the days of the menses. As folklore would have it, flowers would wither when touched by menstruating women, and other, similar things of ill-omen were common in legends. As a matter of fact, Bourget[18] demonstrated the presence of elevated concentrations of toxic substances in menstrual blood as early as 1900. During the same year, Gauthier, who similarly studied the composition of menstrual blood, found in it iodine and arsenic, to which he attributed its by that time already recognized toxic effects. In 1937, Mommsen and Sachs[69] observed that a few drops of menstrual blood were able to inhibit growth of certain plants and yeast cultures. Smith and Smith[96] isolated a toxic substance from menstrual blood that contained estrogens in its composition, which they believed resulted from the union of two molecules of estrone with a protein moiety. Menkin[67] also isolated a menotoxin from menstrual blood and was able to demonstrate that its properties were similar to those of another substance, called by him "necrosin," that he had found in the pleural exudate of a dog injected with turpentine.

In 1943, Smith and Smith[96] isolated the toxic substance from endometrial particles present in the menstrual blood. This menotoxin is mainly present in menstrual blood. If such blood is spun down and its three constituents—endometrial particles, red cells and plasma—separated, it may in fact be shown that the red cells contain no toxin; the plasma contains some, whereas the endometrial tissue particles contain the highest concentration. During menstruation, this substance may likewise be shown to occur in the saliva, venous blood, urine and sweat of women. This in a way may lend some credibility to ancient myths that contact with the hands of women during those days could cause flowers to wither.

According to Higgins and associates,[44] the toxic substance is endowed with proteolytic activity and is responsible for the strong toxic effect of menstrual blood and for the somewhat weaker effect of venous blood from menstruating women (Macht[62]). Some comment has previously been made concerning its chemical composition. Macht believes that it is a cholesterol derivative arising through transformation of sex hormones. Smith and Smith found that it is a globulin with estrogens attached to it in the previously indicated manner.

ANTIMENOTOXIN. Smith and Smith found that during the days of the menstrual period the circulating blood contained a substance that acted as an antibody to menotoxin. The antigenic properties of menotoxin have been experimentally demonstrated by the usual immunologic techniques. Menkin's necrosin has similar antigenic properties and the identity of the two substances has been confirmed immunologically.

ESTROPROTEIN. The antitoxic substance, a specific antibody to menotoxin, seems to be bound to a pseudoglobulin. Whether or not it may produce characteristic menstrual fibrinolysis depends on the ratios of the two bound substances.

These studies have a close bearing on the findings reported by Roberts and Szego[84] according to which active estrogens in the circulation are bound to a protein complex, or "estroprotein," which is a beta globulin linked to Kohn's fraction III-0. It is evident that the production of menotoxin in the menstrual uterus is not a haphazard occurrence but corresponds to a *phase in the intermediary metabolism of estrogens*, one of whose main steps is known to take place in the uterus, although its true significance is still shrouded in obscurity.

It is also of interest to note that Schiller and Pincus[88] and Smith and Smith[96] have shown experimentally that menotoxin produced pituitary stimulation in laboratory animals. Animals treated with menotoxin were found to be subject to reactive luteinization and adrenocortical hyperplasia.

PREMENSTRUAL HYPERESTRINISM. In

Chapter 28, we described transient premenstrual hyperestrinism, or *acute hyperestrinism*.

A series of menstrual symptoms, such as dysmenorrhea, premenstrual tension and premenstrual mastalgia, are undoubtedly the result of accumulation of estrogenic compounds premenstrually, which has a much greater tendency to occur in young women than in mature women. The symptom most directly attributable to the accumulation of these hormones is above all that of menstrual edema, reflecting the well-known estrogen effect on water retention by the tissues (Taylor, Warner, Welsh).

INFLUENCE OF ESTROGEN DETOXIFICATION. A question of extraordinary interest has been raised by the observation of various authors that estrogens disappear from the circulation with unusual speed on the eve of menstruation. It has been thought that this abrupt disappearance was caused by the intervention of the liver in their elimination and degradation (Schiller and Pincus[88]). Smith and Smith[96] have also called attention to the role played by the corpus luteum hormone in the estradiol-estriol conversion process, both estrogens being amenable to hepatic degradation and to renal clearance. Estrogen accumulation in the blood in pathologic amounts premenstrually, which appears to be responsible for some of the symptoms of "menstrual disease," might also be related to slow removal of circulating estrogens by the liver. Of interest in this respect is the fact that the common childhood tendency to hepatic insufficiency is usually corrected with the passage of years.

38.5.3. TREATMENT

At present, little can really be said in this respect. Most textbooks quote therapeutic results obtained with the ovarian hormones estrogens and progesterone. In our own clinical experience, these compounds very seldom produce any appreciable relief in women presenting with the symptomatology of "menstrual disease." The reason these two substances are not indicated therapeutically is obvious. Estrogens by themselves are precisely responsible for some of the menstrual symptoms. Any curative effect they may have is hard to reconcile with their known participation in the etiology of the disorder. On the other hand, it is true that owing to its estrogen-antagonizing effect, progesterone might seem to be indicated. However, as pointed out previously, menotoxins are produced more abundantly in secretory endometria, that is, under the influence of the corpus luteum hormone. As a result, by increasing the production of menotoxins, progesterone is counterproductive in the treatment of the disorder.

Some progress in the treatment of dysmenorrhea has been marked by the recent introduction of *contraceptive drugs* (see Chapter 47). Particularly commendable from among this group of drugs are preparations offering "combined therapy," in which a progestogen is associated with a small dose of estrogen (Anovial, Anovlar, Metrulen-M, Enovid, Lyndiol, Anacycline). These preparations have a triple effect: (1) they suppress ovulation temporarily, which is important, because, as pointed out repeatedly, essential dysmenorrhea does not usually occur in monophasic cycles; (2) by virtue of their progestogen content, they produce myometrial relaxation, doing away with painful uterine spasms; (3) they produce endometrial atrophy (iatrogenic endometrium), thereby contributing to decreased menotoxin formation.

It must be remembered that dysmenorrhea in many young women may be of *psychosomatic origin* and therefore amenable to *psychotherapy*.

REFERENCES

1. Abrams, C. A. L., Grumbach, M. M., Dyrenfurth, I., and Van de Wiele, R. L.: *J. Clin. Endocr.*, 27:467, 1967.
2. Adams, W. C., Wan, L., and Sohler, A.: *J. Endocr.*, 31:295, 1965.
3. Albright, F., et al.: *Endocrinology*, 22:411, 1938.
4. Albright, F., and Halsted, J. A.: *New Eng. J. Med.*, 212:250, 1955.
5. Amoroso, E. C.: *Brit. Med. Bull.*, 11:117, 1955.
6. Arslan, M., Wolf, R. C., Meyer, R. K., and Prasad, M. R. N.: *J. Reprod. Fertil.*, 17:119, 1968.
7. Barraclough, C. A.: *Endocrinology*, 68:62, 1961.
8. Bauer, H. G.: *J. Clin. Endocr.*, 14:13, 1954.
9. Bedoya, J. M., and Funcasta, C. G.: *Rev. Esp. Obst. Gin.*, 2:381, 1945.
10. Belterman, R., and Stegner, H. E.: *Acta Endocr.*, 57:279, 1968.
11. Berardinelli, W.: *J. Clin. Endocr.*, 10:1499, 1950.
12. Bergman, P.: *Obstet. Gynec.*, 19:1, 1962.
13. Bertaggia, A.: *Pediatria* (Napoli), 76:579, 1968.
14. Betson, J. R., and Eicher, D. M.: *Obstet. Gynec.*, 22:219, 1963.

15. Bland, I. B., and Goldstein, L.: *Surg. Gynec. Obstet.*, 61:250, 1935.
16. Bleuler, L.: *Endokrinologische Psychiatrie.* Stuttgart, G. Thieme, 1955.
17. Boczkowski, K., et al.: *Amer. J. Obstet. Gynec.*, 104:594, 1969.
18. Bourget, R.: *Compt. Rend. Acad. Sci.*, 112:493, 1900.
19. Carraro, A., Corbin, A., Fraschini, F., and Martini, L.: *J. Endocr.*, 32:387, 1965.
20. Chiang, W. T.: *Amer. J. Obstet. Gynec.*, 103:1173, 1969.
21. Chu, E. W., Wurtman, F. J., and Axelrod, J.: *Endocrinology*, 75:238, 1964.
22. Clauberg, C., and Breipohl, C.: *Zbl. Gynäk.*, 59:1948, 1935.
23. Conly, P. W., Sandberg, D. H., and Cleveland, W. W.: *J. Pediatr.*, 71:506, 1967.
24. Coppeledge, W. W., and Hasty, L. B.: *Amer. J. Obstet. Gynec.*, 80:637, 1960.
25. Davidson, J. M.: *J. Reprod. Fertil., Suppl.*, 2:103, 1967.
26. Davis, D. M., and Rakoff, A. E.: Quoted by Hoffmann in *Female Endocrinology*, p. 604. Philadelphia, W. B. Saunders, 1944.
27. Dancaster, C. P., Bruk, I., and Jackson, W. P. U.: *Brit. Med. J.*, 1:26, 1960.
28. Dokumov, S., and Dekov, D.: *J. Clin. Endocr.*, 23:1262, 1963.
29. Elwers, M., and Critchlow, V.: *Amer. J. Physiol.*, 198:387, 1960.
30. Ernould, H. J., Thibault, A., and Dechamps, G.: *Ann. d'Endocr.*, 26:281, 1965.
31. Fluhman, C. F.: *Management of Sex Disorders.* Philadelphia, W. B. Saunders, 1956.
32. Ford, F. R.: *Diseases of the Nervous System in Infancy, Childhood and Adolescence.* Springfield, Ill., Charles C Thomas, 1952.
33. Forlini, G.: *Atti Soc. Ital. Ginec.*, 37:392, 1942.
34. Frank, R. T.: *J.A.M.A.*, 97:165, 1931.
35. Fraschini, F., Mess, B., and Martini, L.: *Endocrinology*, 82:919, 1968.
36. Gittes, R. F., and Chu, E. W.: *Endocrinology*, 77:1061, 1965.
37. Giusti, G.: *Obstet. Gynec.*, 20:755, 1962.
38. Gorski, R., and Wagner, J. W.: *Endocrinology*, 76:226, 1965.
39. Greenblatt, R. B.: *The Hirsute Female.* Springfield, Ill., Charles C Thomas, 1963.
40. Grunewald, C., and Heugel, M.: *Presse Med.*, 77:295, 1969.
40a. Harris, G. W.: *Arch Gynäk.*, 183:98, 1953.
41. Hamblen, E. C.: *Endocrinology of Woman.* Springfield, Ill., Charles C Thomas, 1945.
42. Hauser, G. W., et al.: *Gynaecologia*, 152:279, 1961.
43. Heubner, R.: In *The Pineal Gland*, ed. J. I. Kitay and M. D. Altschule. Cambridge, Mass., Harvard University Press, 1954.
44. Higgins, H., Vail, V. C., and Davis, M. R.: *Amer. J. Obstet. Gynec.*, 46:78, 1943.
45. Hoffmann, R. A., and Reiter, R. J.: *Science*, 148:1609, 1965.
46. Jolly, H. *Sexual Precocity.* Springfield, Ill., Charles C Thomas, 1955.
47. Jouan, P., Garreau, A., and Samperez, S.: *Ann. d'Endocr.*, 26:535, 1965.
47a. Kammlade, W. G., Welch, J. A., Nalbandov, A. V., and Norton, H. W.: *J. Amer. Med. Sci.*, 11:646, 1952.
48. Kelly, L. W.: *J. Clin. Endocr.*, 63:50, 1963.
49. Kennedy, G. C., and Mitra, J.: *J. Physiol.*, 166:408, 1963.
50. Kennedy, G. C.: *J. Physiol.*, 172:393, 1964.
51. Kitay, I.: *J. Clin. Endocr.*, 14:622, 1954.
52. Klaften, E.: *Zbl. Gynäk.*, 58:204, 1934.
53. Krohn, P. L.: *Schw. Med. Wschr.*, 87:417, 1957.
54. Kulin, H. E., Rifkind, A. B., Ross, G. T., and Odell, W. D.: *J. Clin. Endocr.*, 27:1123, 1967.
55. Laszlo, J., and Györy, G.: *Zbl. Gynäk.*, 91:1001, 1969.
56. Lencioni, L. J., and Stafieri, J. J.: *Acta Cytol.*, 13:382, 1969.
57. Liu, N., Grumbach, M. M., Napoli, R. A., and Morishima, A.: *J. Clin. Endocr. Metab.*, 25:1296, 1965.
58. Lloyd, C. W., et al.: *J. Clin. Endocr.*, 11:857, 1951.
59. Lloyd, C. W.,: *J. Clin. Endocr.*, 15:1518, 1955.
60. Lull, C. F.: *Amer. J. Obstet. Gynec.*, 41:445, 1941.
61. MacCullagh, E. D., Rosemberg, H. S., and Norman, N.: *J. Clin. Endocr.*, 20:1286, 1960.
62. Macht, D. E.: *Amer. J. Med. Sci.*, 206:281, 1943.
63. Marañón, G.: *El Crecimiento y sus Trastornos.* Madrid, Espasa Calpe, 1954.
64. Martinovich, P. N., Ianesevich, O. K., and Martinovich, J. V.: *Nature*, 217:866, 1968.
65. Mayer, A.: *Folia Clinica Internat.*, 1:12, 1951.
66. Mellicow, M. A., and Cahill, G. F.: *J. Clin. Endocr.*, 10:24, 1950.
67. Menkin, M.: *Science*, 97:165, 1943.
68. Mikulicz-Radecky, F. Von, and Kausch, G.: *Zbl. Gynäk.*, 59:2296, 1935.
69. Mommsen, H., and Sachs, F.: *Münch. Med. Wschr.*, 1:208, 1937.
70. Moricard, F.: *Hormonologie Sexuelle Humaine.* Paris, Masson et Cie., 1943.
71. Morley, T. P.: *J. Clin. Endocr.*, 14:1, 1954.
72. Moszkowska, A., and Scemmama, A.: *Compt. Rend. Soc. Biol. (Paris)*, 162:636, 1968.
73. Motta, M., Fraschini, F., Giuliani, G., and Martini, L.: *Endocrinology*, 83:1101, 1968.
74. Niswander, K. R., and Courey, N. G.: *Obstet. Gynec.*, 26:381, 1965.
75. Papez, J. W., and Ecker, A.: *J. Neuropathol. Exper. Neurol.*, 6:15, 1947.
76. Pavel, S.: *Endocrinology*, 77:812, 1965.
77. Poll, J. L., et al.: In *Hypothalamic Hypophysial Interrelationships*, ed. S. Fields, R. Guillemin and C. A. Carton. Springfield, Ill., Charles C Thomas, 1956.
78. Raiti, S., Light, C., and Blizzard, R. M.: *J. Clin. Endocr.*, 29:884, 1969.
79. Ramaley, J. A., and Gorski, R. A.: *Acta Endocr.*, 56:661, 1967.
80. Ramirez, D. V., and MacCann, S. M.: *Endocrinology*, 72:452, 1963.
81. Relkin, R.: *Endocrinology*, 82:865, 1968.
82. Relkin, R.: *Endocrinology*, 82:1249, 1968.
83. Rifkind, A. B., Kulin, H. E., and Ross, R. T.: *J. Clin. Invest.*, 46:1925, 1967.
84. Roberts, S., and Szego, C. N.: *Endocrinology*, 39:182, 1946.
85. Rosner, J., Pomeau-Dellile, G., Tramezzani, J. H., and Cardinali, D.: *Compt. Rend. Acad. Sci. (Paris)*, 261:1113, 1965.
86. Runge, H.: *Geburtsh. u. Frauenhk.*, 2:495, 1940.
87. Russell, W. D., and Sachs, E.: *Arch. Pathol.*, 35:869, 1943.
88. Schiller, S., and Pincus, G.: *J. Clin. Endocr.*, 4:203, 1944.

89. Seckel, H., Scott, P. G., and Benditt, E. P.: *Amer. J. Dis. Child.*, 78:484, 1949.
90. Seckel, H. P. G.: *Amer. J. Dis. Child.*, 79:278, 1950.
91. Seegar-Jones, G. E., and Acosta, A. A.: *Amer. J. Obstet. Gynec.*, 84:701, 1962.
92. Shadaksharappa, K., et al.: *J. Clin. Endocr.*, 11:1383, 1951.
93. Simpson, S. L.: *J. Clin. Endocr.*, 11:778, 1951.
94. Slocker, C.: *Acta Gin.*, 5:251, 1954.
95. Smith, E. R., and Davidson, J. M.: *Endocrinology*, 82:100, 1968.
96. Smith, O. W., and Smith, G. V.: *Amer. J. Obstet. Gynec.*, 55:285, 1947.
97. Smith, E. R., and Davidson, J. M.: *Endocrinology*, 82:100, 1968.
98. Sonek, M.: *Acta Cytol.*, 11:41, 1967.
99. Srebnik, H. H., and Nelson, M. M.: *Endocrinology*, 70:723, 1962.
100. Steiner, M. M., and Hadawi, A. S.: *Amer. J. Dis. Child.*, 108:28, 1964.
101. Talbot, N. B.: *Functional Endocrinology from Birth through Adolescence.* Cambridge, Mass., Harvard University Press, 1952.
102. Teter, J.: *Endokr. Polska*, 13:365, 1962.
103. Thompsett, S. L.: *J. Clin. Endocr.*, 11:61, 1961.
104. Tweedie, F. J.: *Amer. J. Obstet. Gynec.*, 75:964, 1958.
105. Varangot, J.: Thesis, Paris, 1937.
106. Visser, H. K. A., and Degenhart, H. J.: *Helv. Paed. Acta*, 21:409, 1966.
107. Wagner, J. W., Erwin, W., and Critchlow, V.: *Endocrinology*, 79:1135, 1066.
108. Wilkins, L.: *Diagnosis and Treatment of Endocrine Disorders in Childhood and Adolescence,* 2nd ed. Springfield, Ill., Charles C Thomas, 1957.
109. Wortham, J. T.: *J. Clin. Endocr.*, 12:975, 1952.
110. Wurtman, R. J., Axelrod, J., and Chu, E. W.: *Science*, 141:277, 1963.
111. Wurtman, R. J., Axelrod, J., and Chu, E. W.: *Endocrinology*, 76:798, 1965.
112. Yen, S. S. C., Vicic, W. J., and Kearchner, D. V.: *J. Clin. Endocr.*, 29:382, 1969.
113. Yen, S. S. C., and Vicic, W. J.: *Amer. J. Obstet. Gynec.*, 106:247, 1970.
114. Zacharias, L., and Wurtman, R. J.: *Science*, 144:1154, 1964.
115. Zangeneh, F., and Kelley, V. C.: *Amer. J. Dis. Child.*, 115:494, 1968.
116. Zurbrugg, R. P., and Gardner, L. I.: *J. Clin. Endocr.*, 63:704, 1963.

Chapter 39
PATHOLOGY OF THE FEMALE CLIMACTERIC

39.1. GENERALITIES

The circumstances surrounding involution in woman were studied in Chapter 17. It is extremely difficult to draw the line between what is normal and what is pathological during that phase of life. Every woman experiences more or less pronounced disturbances which, without necessarily being abnormal, may prompt her to consult a physician. A whole range of gradations exists between those women experiencing simple physiologic or habitual disturbances and those actually developing true endocrine pathology in connection with sexual decline. Marañón,[67] Riley[91] and Sharman[95] stress the frequency with which sexual decline occurs in women beyond strictly physiologic limits. The concept of normalcy ought to be extended to include women with even minor complaints. Those who experience no symptoms whatsoever and would otherwise be unaware of having reached the end of their reproductive life, were it not for the cessation of menses, are exceptions, although, on the other hand, those women in whom menopausal disorders reach the proportions of an incapacitating disease are exceptions, too.

In a survey conducted on 1000 menopausal women in 1953 by the Council of the Medical Women's Association of England,[31] it was found that 84 per cent had noticeable disorders, but in only 10 per cent of the cases were these of sufficient severity to prevent the patients from leading normal lives. In this chapter, we shall refer exclusively to those more or less 10 per cent of women in whom the clinical symptoms of the climacteric are significant and provoke alterations consistent with *true disease*.

39.1.1. THE CLIMACTERIC AGE

It would be impossible to set any fixed date, not even any predetermined period of time, for the appearance of the climacterium. In Chapter 17, we alluded to the age of 42 as heralding the onset of the climacterium and to 52 as the age of its termination. Naturally, these dates are subject to considerable variations, but the term *precocious menopause* may be applied to those cases in which menopause occurs before the age of 42, whereas, conversely, *delayed menopause* refers to menopause occurring after the age of 52. The term *menopause* rather than *climacterium* has been used deliberately because the concepts of precocity or retardation in relation to the climacteric are much more difficult to establish than in relation to menopause. In the broadest sense of the word, the climacteric spans over 10 years of a woman's life, and it is impossible to pinpoint the beginning of the first and the disappearance of the last of the disturbances.

Any anticipation or delay in the appearance of menopause may result from a variety of etiologic factors. Basically, the following entities may be involved in the genesis of these chronologic variations: (1) constitutional factors; (2) ovarian factors; (3) pituitary factors; (4) adrenal and thyroid factors; (5) past history of pregnancies; (6) acquired diseases; and (7) influence of nutrition and way of life.

39.1.2. CONSTITUTION AND MENOPAUSE

The constitutional influence on the precocious or on the delayed appearance of menopause may be inferred from the fact that occasionally all female members in a family may reveal abnormal timing in the onset of menopause. It is a matter of common observation that the phenomenon may repeat itself in several sisters and may be passed on from the mother to her daughters. The relationship between the date of menarche and that of menopause is also influenced by constitutional factors to the extent that it may be asserted in general that women with early menarche reach menopause prematurely, while those with delayed menarche keep menstruating longer. The explanation for this phenomenon, emphasized particularly by Marañón,[67] is based on the fact that the ovarian reserve of oogonia is limited (see Chapter 12). With just one follicle being "set into motion" in each cycle, and the destruction by atresia of a large proportion of eggs in the long run, the sooner the ovary begins to mature the sooner it will exhaust its reserve of oocytes and, consequently, the sooner will cyclic generative processes cease. However, the objection that must be raised to this oversimplification is that the rate at which atresia occurs and the proportion of follicles involved naturally are not identical in every ovary, so that precocious menopause does not, in absolute terms, invariably correlate with early puberty.

Although anomalies in the karyotype must be included among the constitutional causes, Zarate and his colleagues[112] have been unable to find any changes in the karyotypes of eight women studied for precocious puberty.

39.1.3. OVARIAN FACTORS

The ovarian etiology of precocious menopause seems to be certain. Along general lines, it may be said that an advanced onset of menopause is related to an accelerated rate of ovarian atresia. Thus, those ovaries in which atresia proceeds at a rapid rate are always associated with the occurrence of early menopause. Ovarian atresia is facilitated by a series of processes involving the ovary, such as *sclerocystic degeneration, hyperthecosis,* and, in some instances, *pluriglandular disorders.* In Chapters 31 and 34, we noted that a number of pituitary, adrenal and thyroid disorders lead to rapid atresia of the ovary and determine secondary amenorrhea. As a matter of fact, permanent secondary amenorrhea is liable to be confused with precocious menopause in practice for the same reasons that essential amenorrhea is quite often mistaken for delayed menarche. The available number of primordial follicles is the essential factor underlying the tendency of the ovary to undergo atresia. Ovaries containing a large number of such elements have a greater available reserve and are capable of enduring atresia-inducing stimuli for longer periods of time. Although, in general, the combined oocyte count for both ovaries is usually put at 400,000, this figure is a mere approximation. Evidently, depending on the degree of differentiation of the elements in question, their number may just as well be much higher as much lower than that. Thus, for instance, in *ovarian hypogenesis,* that is, the syndrome of *primitive ovarian hypoestrinism,* we have frequently observed the appearance of precocious menopause. We believe that this merely reflects premature exhaustion of a defectively differentiated ovary.

In the final analysis, however, the role played by *harmonious ovarian maturation* as well as by *orderly and systematic recurrence of the cycle* seems to surpass in significance the absolute efficiency of the ovary as a gland and the duration of ovarian activity. It has been observed that women with grand multiparity usually experience menopause later than others and this must first of all be attributed to the fact that increased fertility is accompanied by constancy in the ovulatory cycles, with one by one maturation of follicles. In contrast, in women with anovulatory cycles, the follicles mature in a disorderly way, several at a time, and are used up at a faster rate. Possibly, too, certain endocrine factors, such as thyroid and adrenal factors, whose trophic effects on the ovary are unquestionable, may contribute to ovarian longevity, provided their action is balanced.

39.1.4. PITUITARY FACTORS

While the pituitary is universally referred to as the gland of puberty, few workers seem to realize the *fundamental role played by pituitary hyperfunction in the initiation of the climacterium.* As a rule, pituitary hyperfunction, analyzed previously in Chapter 17, may be observed in climacteric women. This hyperfunction is associated with excessive secretion of gonadotropins, which are responsible for the acceleration of ovarian function and the untimely exhaustion of the ovary in the preclimacteric phase. We have already indicated (see Chapter 28) how the degree of intensity of stimulation the pituitary exerts on the ovary is related to the amount of functioning ovarian parenchyma. In the course of life, the ovarian parenchyma is being worn down quantitatively, which determines an ever-increasing pituitary feedback. This reactive pituitary feedback consists of two components: *increased FSH activity*, tending to provoke disorderly maturation of follicles and accounting for the occurrence of relative hyperestrinism in the climacteric (to be discussed later). *LH activity* is also increased, which leads to luteinization of the follicular theca and to premature follicular atresia, contributing to a faster rate of ovarian involution. *Luteinic involution of the climacteric ovary* manifests itself by hyperthecosis which, as pointed out previously, is of pituitary origin. Thus, while the pituitary exerts a stimulatory effect on the puberal gonad, in terms of enhancing sexual maturity, it similarly stimulates the climacteric gonad but, because the latter is subject to more rapid exhaustion, its effect on the activity of the female gland in the latter instance is more negative in nature. *It may then be stated that a stimulatory factor, produced by the pituitary and necessary for sexual maturation to be achieved at puberty, is also instrumental in bringing about the appearance of the climacterium.* Relative hyperpituitarism during this phase of life, therefore, leads to a premature onset of menopause. Conversely, a delayed onset of menopause is usually observed in those women whose pituitary function has been depressed or, at best, maintained at a balanced level. Therefore, in the event of prolonged maintenance of sexuality, persistence of female cyclic activity ought not to be attributed to any glandular type of hyperfunction but rather to, so to speak, more economic utilization of available reserves of the genital apparatus.

39.1.5. THYROID AND ADRENAL FACTORS

It is a fact of fairly common clinical observation, emphasized by Marañón and Siegert,[96] that hyperthyroid women usually reach menopause tardily. This, of course, does not apply to cases of serious hyperthyroidism or thyrotoxicosis, in which sexual function may be modified prematurely, but rather to constitutional states of mild hyperfunction. Thyroid function, as indicated in Chapters 10 and 34, seems to involve *trophic* stimulation of the ovary. Rather than exerting any specific action on the female gonad, thyroid hormone seems to have a protective effect on the vital elements of the ovary, contributing to the preservation of the viability of ovules and granulosa cells. In this sense, *adequate thyroid function is thought to maintain the essential elements of the follicle and to prevent their premature atresia*. This is the explanation — in our view a plausible one — that may be offered for the commonly observed clinical phenomenon of late menopause.

Insofar as *adrenal function* is concerned, the latter seems to play no role whatsoever in prolonging menopause, although the vicarious action by adrenocortical sex hormones may avert or delay the development of climacteric symptomatology. In other words, *adequate adrenocortical function has no influence on the duration of menstruation and on the timing of menopause but is consistent with maintaining adequate estrogen levels into more advanced age.*

39.1.6. HISTORY OF PAST PREGNANCIES

The history of previous pregnancies is definitely related to the chronology of menopause (Sharman[95]). It is a commonly held, though *entirely erroneous*, idea that menopause sets in prematurely in those women who have had many children. While this may be so occasionally, it happens only exceptionally and is a result of the development of endocrine complications as a result of gestation, such as postpartum atrophy of the pituitary, or *Sheehan's syndrome* (see Chapter 31), which in its latent or attenuated forms may cause permanent loss of menstrual function after childbirth. But usually what happens is just the opposite. From our own statistics, it appears that the average age at which menopause occurs in multiparous women is 49, whereas in grand multiparas it is 51.5 years. To us, this seems to bear out what we have already stated concerning the predominance of regular ovulatory cycles in those women with a high degree of fertility. Their ovulatory cycles mean economy of oogonia, only one maturing every 28 days, and therefore maintaining ovarian activity longer. But it must be remembered that follicles do not mature, nor do they become atretic, during the interval of nine months of normal gestation. Each gestation therefore represents a long period of time during which progressive ovarian attrition is brought to a standstill. When the several gestations are added up, this may mean a considerable length of time during which the ovary does not, so to say, wear itself out and stops the process of bringing out new oogonia for maturation.

However, it is probable that the most fundamental explanation for the phenomenon is just the reverse, and that what actually occurs is that those ovaries endowed with great vitality and in an excellent state of trophism remain viable for long periods of time and that *enhanced fertility as well as delayed menopause might be the expression of an excellent state of functional gonadal development.*

39.1.7. OTHER FACTORS INFLUENCING THE CHRONOLOGY OF MENOPAUSE

A detailed analysis of all factors related to the duration of reproductive life, such as intercurrent disease, nutrition and a person's way of life, cannot be undertaken here without engaging in unwarranted digression. It is commonly held that a life of toil, with many deliveries and poor hygiene, is conducive to premature menopause. Of course, the development of secondary amenorrhea may be mistaken for early menopause but, in general, ovarian longevity is largely independent of these factors. A good example of this is the peasant woman from the village who, for all her external appearance of premature aging, continues menstruating into advanced age, despite her many pregnancies, her life of hard work and, quite frequently, the unhygienic conditions of her nutrition and environment.

39.2. ENDOCRINE CHANGES OF PATHOLOGIC CLIMACTERIUM

In addition to the ovary, the pituitary, the adrenal and the thyroid are all implicated in the endocrine mechanism of the normal climacterium, as has been pointed out in Chapter 17. Changes involving these organs may therefore lead to pathologic changes of the climacteric, which shall be studied in sequence.

39.2.1. OVARIAN PATHOLOGY OF THE CLIMACTERIC

In Chapter 17, we pointed out that it is erroneous to assume that the climacteric represents cessation of ovarian estrogen secretion. Indeed, in the *pathologic climacterium*, we frequently encounter the *syndrome of climacteric hyperestrinism*, which is but an exaggeration of the normal state. The diagnostic procedures for postclimacteric estrogen persistence and the occurrence of eventual hyperestrinism are three: (1) hormone assay; (2) vaginal cytology, and (3) histologic examination of endometrial and ovarian tissue.

ESTROGEN ASSAY. Zondek has called attention to the fact that the transition period between peak ovarian function and its extinction is marked by a phase of estrogenic predominance. Bonfirraro and Sensi[14] have found that only 71 per cent of premenopausal women over the age of 40 ovulate. A recent study by the World Health Organization yielded the figures presented in Table 39–1. It reveals that starting with the age of 40, the incidence of ovulatory cycles rapidly diminishes while that of progestational insufficiency and anovulatory cycles increases. Jayle and associates[50] and Brown[22] (see Fig. 39–4) found elevated urinary levels of phenol steroids in menopausal women. Estrogen elevation paralleled the intensity of menopausal complaints. Similar findings were made at our clinic by Sopeña and Tornero.[97] In addition, contemporary literature contains the contributions on the subject by Randall and colleagues[89] and, above all, by Mac Bryde.[62] The latter author reported that estradiol, estrone and estriol values in menopausal women were as elevated as those found in young women during the resting phase of the cycle. Carcatzoulis,[26] as well as Botella,[18, 20] studied postmenopausal estrogen levels in women more than three years after the last period and found that, although these hormones were lowered to almost trace levels in about two thirds of the women, the remaining third of the patients revealed persistence of *pathologic hyperestrogenism*, which shall be studied in this chapter as one of the most important manifestations of the abnormal climacterium.

Two further studies have contributed significantly to the understanding of menopausal ovarian function. Using the saturation test as an index of estrogenic deficit, Subrizi and his associates[102] demonstrated relatively elevated estrogen blood levels in many postmenopausal women. Mattingly and Huang[71] incubated slices of menopausal ovaries in vitro, reporting normal rates of estrogen synthesis for the ovarian stroma.

VAGINAL CYTOLOGY. Limburg[58] found evidence of estrogenic activity in the smears of 25 per cent of postclimacteric women. This was subsequently confirmed by Struthers,[101] who reported the occurrence of markedly estrogenic smears in 53 per cent of postmenopausal women. Wied[110] and Boschann,[16] as well as Montalvo,[73] later corroborated the high incidence of persistent estrogenic cytology in postmenopausal women. According to Stoll and Ledermair,[99] this may be observed in 20 per cent of the cases, whereas our own findings,[18, 20] as well as those of Osmond-Clarke and Murray[82] and von Haam,[42] would indicate that at least 30 per cent of all postmenopausal women reveal cytologic patterns suggestive of hyperestrogenism, or at least of persistent estrogenic activity. Matsukawa[72] and Folsome and associates[38] reported estrogenic smears in senile women, in one case, in an 81 year old woman.[38]

Pertinent cytologic findings thus seem to confirm the frequent (though not constant) occurrence of climacteric and postclimacteric estrogenism.

Interestingly, Berger,[12] Wied[110] and Boschann[16] indicated that this type of estrogenic activity could also be observed in the smears from castrated women, from which they inferred that the estrogens involved were of adrenal origin. The occurrence of hyperestrogenic smears in postmenopausal women has subsequently been demonstrated by a number of investigators.[65, 88, 100, 107]

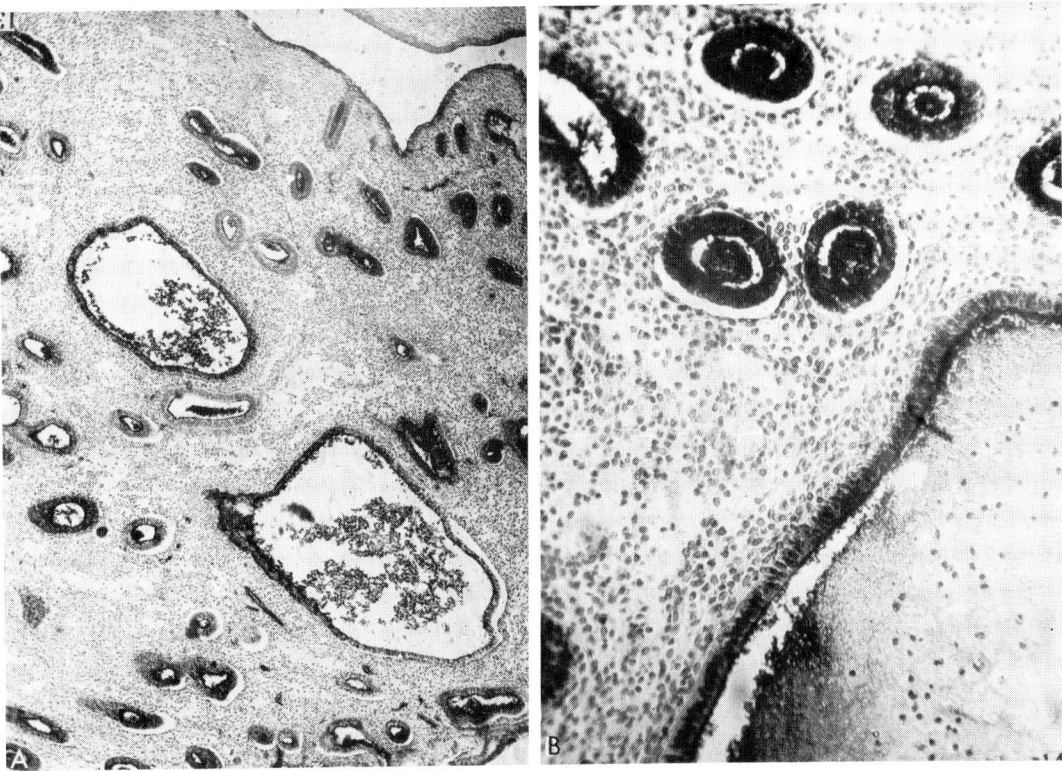

Figure 39–1. Endometrial hyperplasia of the cystic glandular type in a postmenopausal woman, using Gomori's stain for alkaline glycerophosphatase. *A*, Low magnification. *B*, Higher magnification. Note that the gland epithelia give a positive reaction, indicating that hyperplasia in this instance is of the "active," functional variety.

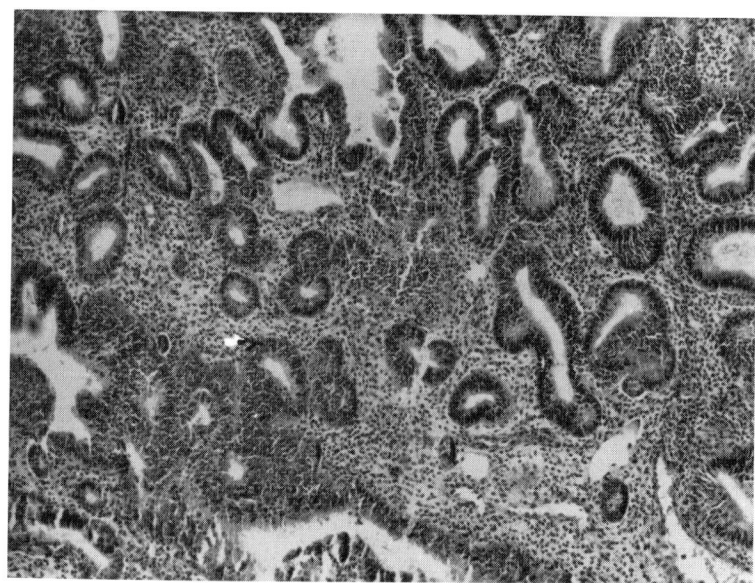

Figure 39-2. "Atypical" endometrial hyperplasia in a postclimacteric woman. Note polystratification of nuclei in gland epithelia, irregular contour of glands and scantiness of stroma. Hyperplasia in this instance appears to be degenerative in nature and not of the estrogenic variety.

ENDOMETRIAL FINDINGS. Should the preceding data not be convincing enough to establish the existence of postmenopausal estrogenism, Nogales,[77] in 1948, had also demonstrated the occurrence of proliferative patterns in at least 39 per cent of normal postmenopausal endometria. Although Novak[79] believes that such endometria are actually without function, Nogales' observations have been confirmed by Mac Bryde[63] and by Sutherland and Mac Bryde.[103] In our own studies[18] in 1962, we came up with evidence that about one third of all endometria revealed signs of proliferative activity in the postmenopausal age group. The same conclusions were reached by Herreros-Mediavilla, who completed his doctoral thesis at our clinic. His data indicate the occurrence of endometrial hyperplasia and persistent proliferation which may be asserted to be, if not constant, certainly a common finding even in women after the age of 50, along with a high incidence of active endometrial hyperplasia, indicative of *postmenopausal hyperestrinism.*

This naturally raises the question of what might be the origin of this paradoxical hyperestrogenism in postmenopausal women. Three main etiologic considerations may be offered: (1) an *ovarian*, (2) an *adrenal*, and (3) a *hepatic* origin.

OVARIAN ORIGIN. It had classically been admitted that all forms of postmenopausal hyperestrogenism were caused by feminizing ovarian tumors. The occurrence of menopausal or postmenopausal endometrial hyperplasia in association with thecoma has been particularly emphasized by Mussey and co-workers,[74] Husslein,[47] Craig[33] and Novak[81]; on the other hand, Diddle[35] and Sutherland and Mac Bryde,[103] in 1954, studied the relationship between postmenopausal hyperestrogenism and *granulosa*

TABLE 39-1. Endometrial Findings in Normal Women Before and After Menopause

TYPE OF ENDOMETRIUM	PREMENOPAUSAL	POSTMENOPAUSAL (YEARS AFTER)		
		0 to 3	4 to 6	More than 6
Normal secretory pattern	24.59%	22.10%	15.66%	8.57%
Insufficient secretory pattern	18.03	14.04	8.33	14.00
Monophasic cycle	18.03	21.12	16.66	14.28
Hyperplasia	16.39	9.09	20.08	21.42
Irregular maturation	18.03	18.08	25.00	7.14
Atrophy and hypoplasia	4.27	15.06	20.00	33.56

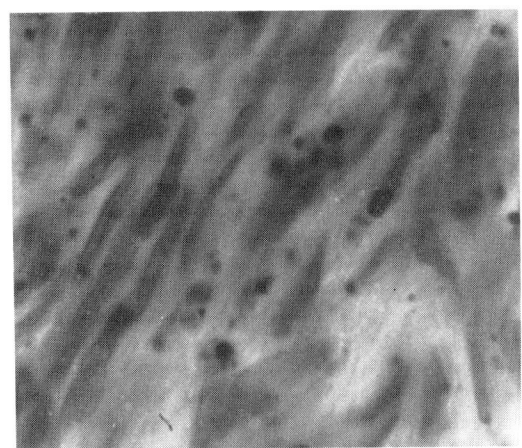

Figure 39–3. Small ovarian thecoma discovered in a woman with climacteric hyperestrinism. Lipid inclusions are noted in cells of connective tissue appearance. Sudan III stain.

cell tumors. They recorded 126 cases of endometrial hyperplasia among 1,000 cases with a history of postmenopausal bleeding, using as a criterion for the postmenopausal state at least one year of amenorrhea. Of those 126 cases, only 5 were found to be associated with either a granulosa or a theca cell tumor (Fig. 39–3).

In most instances of climacteric endometrial hyperplasia, the lesions found in the ovary are not so conspicuous as to reveal either type of tumor. This however does not preclude the possibility that some of these disorders may have an ovarian origin. In the first place, some workers believe that climacteric hyperproduction of estrogens is attributable either to *central hyperthecosis* (Fig. 39–4) or to *predominance of hilus cells.* Husslein[47] is inclined to ascribe this type of endometrial hyperplasia to an increase in the number of hilus cells, while Jones and Te Linde[51] believe that hilus

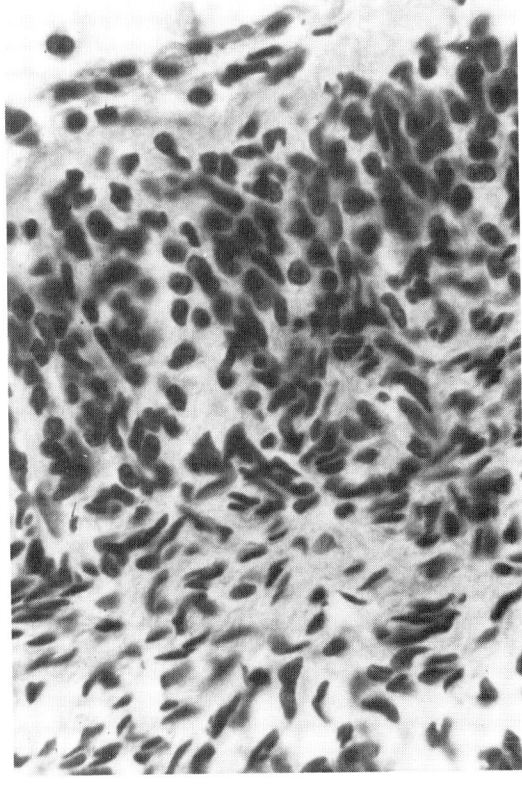

Figure 39–4. Hyperthecosis in a woman with climacteric hyperestrinism.

cells have estrogenic properties. Plate,[87] on the contrary, believes that hyperestrogenism may be due to an accelerated rate of ovarian atresia in conjunction with thecal hyperplasia. Recently, the possibility that *stromal cortical hyperplasia* may be the causative agent of hyperestrogenism has also been entertained. This possibility will be further discussed in Chapter 46. At this point, however, it should be remembered that, as we have stated in Chapter 28, hyperestrogenism is not so much a consequence of an overall increase in the amount of circulating estrogens as rather the result of a *continuous type of estrogenic activity without intervening luteal phases*. Indeed, it is well known that estrogen production ceases long before corpus luteum activity disappears during the climacterium. Consequently, certain structures in such ovaries, generally endowed with scant residual capacity for estrogen synthesis, may, in the absence of any intercurrent process of luteinization, nevertheless give rise to continuous *production of small amounts of estrogens which, by virtue of a cumulative effect, may lead to hyperestrogenism*. In this respect, it ought to be borne in mind that the body's estrogen tolerance during this period of life varies from one person to another to a great extent, probably owing to such factors as *estrogen metabolism* and *liver function*.

ADRENAL HYPERESTROGENISM. The significance of adrenal estrogen biogenesis during the menopause has been emphasized in several locations of this book (Chapters 9, 17 and 33). One of the fundamental functions of the "third gonad" is that of supplementing the ovary in its final phases of activity, or after that activity has ceased altogether. Castrated women continue eliminating estrogens in their urine (see also Chapter 17), sometimes in considerable amounts (Brown,[21] Bulbrook and Greenwood,[23] Botella[19]). Figure 39-5 graphically summarizes the data obtained by the first two authors, which correlate well with each other as well as with our own findings, indicating that a large portion of the estrogens produced during the menopause, if indeed not all, is of adrenal origin. There seems to be no valid reason why the adrenal origin of certain forms of climacteric hyperestrogenism should be refuted. Plate[87] reported the case of a 72 year old woman who was curetted because of severe metrorrhagia.

Her endometrium revealed marked hyperplasia and evidence of estrogen effect. Because the bleeding would not stop, a hysterectomy was performed, at which time the source of the estrogen effect was not found in the ovaries. After castration, the continuing high rate of urinary estrogen excretion proved that those estrogens were derived not from the ovary but from the adrenal cortex. The physiologic occurrence of climacteric hypercorticism has been described by Augustin and Maniculesco.[10] In animals, castration causes an increase in the rate of adrenal steroidogenesis (Nandi et al.[75]). Altman and his colleagues[7] reported a high incidence of hyperfunctional adrenocortical adenomas in castrated goats. Hence, we seem to be dealing with adrenal *overcompensation*, provoked by castration, a true "reactive adrenogenital syndrome." It is almost certain that this reaction is triggered by an increase in *gonadotropin activity* (to be discussed later).

The fact that, in rats, this reaction can be induced only in a particular strain seems to suggest involvement of a hereditary factor. It may similarly be assumed that a genetic

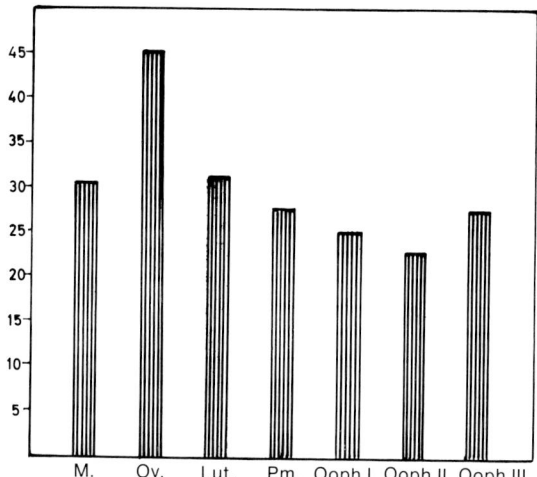

Figure 39-5. Combined data on elimination of total estrogens (micrograms per 24 hr) in normal, menopausal and castrated women. *M*, Normal woman during menstrual phase; *Ov.*, normal woman at time of ovulation; *Lut.*, normal woman during luteal phase; *Pm.*, post-menopausal woman (After Brown: *Lancet*, 1:320, 1955). *Ooph. I*, Woman oophorectomized before menopause; *Ooph. II*, woman oophorectomized after menopause (After Bulbrook et al.: *Brit. Med. J.*, 1:7, 1958). Note that excretion rates are considerably elevated, even after castration and in the climacteric. The fact that the latter two values are identical seems to indicate that postmenopausal estrogen production is largely of adrenal origin.

or constitutional factor is required in the human species for the climacteric crisis to result in hyperestrogenism. This, in our opinion, may be the reason why the reaction varies so markedly from one woman to another.

Nevertheless, the source of estrogens is not always to be sought for in the adrenal. In Chapter 2, other extraovarian and extraadrenal sources of estrogens were mentioned in connection with simultaneous castration and adrenalectomy. The same sources must be considered in clinical patients: we shall point out in Chapter 46 that, in the treatment of breast cancer, in order to achieve cessation of estrogen production, the pituitary must be suppressed, since not even adrenalectomy combined with castration brings about complete abolition of estrogenuria (Bulbrook and Greenwood[23]).

HEPATIC FACTORS. The role played by the liver in adequate estrogen inactivation was explained in Chapter 2. During this phase of life, impaired liver function occurs much more commonly in women than in men. As a result, several authors have described a *hepatoovarian syndrome*, which is particularly likely to occur during the climacterium. Obviously, any number of minor episodes of estrogen hyperproduction that in a woman with a normal endogenous metabolism would fail to have any effect on the target organs may lead to a cumulative action in the presence of hepatic insufficiency and engenders a picture of hyperestrogenism, the etiology of which is similar to that occurring in males with cirrhosis. In Chapter 28, we have already indicated how instances of functional bleeding have been described in association with various conditions of hepatic insufficiency and with cirrhosis in the female.

Hellman and his co-workers[44] studied the metabolism of tritiated estradiol in cases of destructive jaundice. As with other instances of hepatic insufficiency, they found that estrogenolysis was reduced in these cases.

Estrogenic insufficiency states undoubtedly also occur in the climacterium. Such cases of estrogenic insufficiency are in fact more common than instances of hyperestrogenism and therefore represent the physiologic norm for the menopausal ovary. The entity of climacteric hyperestrogenism described here is by no means a constant finding; it is simply a frequent finding.

Normally, ovarian function ceases during the climacterium, resulting in a reduction of estrogen production. Any pathologic increase in estrogen production must be considered as a frankly pathologic disorder.

39.2.2. PITUITARY PATHOLOGY IN THE CLIMACTERIUM

The regulatory and inhibitory role of estrogens in normal pituitary function was stressed in Chapters 6 and 7. Cessation of cyclic ovarian activity during menopause results in pituitary imbalance, characterized by hyperfunctional activity. *Climacteric hyperpituitarism* is a normal event, attributable to physiologic conditions of the climacteric (see Chapter 17). Occasionally, however, this type of hyperfunction may exceed its normal limits and turn into a *pathologic form of hyperfunction*. In the latter instance, it entails hyperproduction of: (1) *gonadotropins*, (2) *thyrotropin*, (3) *adrenocorticotropin*, and (4) *diabetogenic hormone*.

While the first form of dysfunction is related to vasomotor type of manifestations, making up most of the symptomatology of the pathologic climacteric, the second is related to climacteric hyperthyroidism (to be discussed later), the third to the genesis of certain forms of hypercorticism occurring during this phase of life and, finally, the fourth is related to the frequent occurrence of diabetes at this critical age. We shall examine each consecutively.

CLIMACTERIC HYPERGONADOTROPISM. It was stated in Chapter 17 that castration was followed by increased gonadotropin excretion in animals.[62, 84] Although originally this increase had been thought to involve FSH alone in both animals[84] and women,[3, 15, 85] later studies showed that LH was also excreted in greater amounts.[3, 9, 22, 28] Albert[3] established that FSH values were 10 times normal, whereas LH excretion rose to only 5 times its normal value. Apostolakis and Loraine[9] maintain that the increases are more than 20 and 10 times, respectively. Using the ascorbic acid depletion test (see Chapters 7 and 24), Parlow[84] found that LH excretion also was consistently elevated in castrated animals. While these data refer to urinary findings, MacArthur and his associates[61] have been able to demonstrate a rise in *plasma* gonadotropin levels as well.

The pituitary gonadotropin content, estimated by Cozens and Nelson[32] in castrated animals, and by Witschi[111] and Ryan[92] in postmenopausal women, has been found to be similarly increased.

The high level of gonadotropin activity during the female climacterium is of great interest. First, because the intensity with which climacteric pathologic phenomena (hot flushes, etc.) manifest themselves has been suggested to be related to gonadotropin levels (Fluhman), an opinion not shared by all (Riley[91]); *secondly*, because this type of gonadotropin activity explains the occasional occurrence of hyperestrogenic ovarian reactions; and *thirdly*, because it also clarifies the compensatory adrenal reaction wherein, as mentioned previously (Chapter 9), gonadotropin activity is the appropriate stimulant of the adrenocortical *sexual zone*.

The associated increase in LH activity is equally significant, since LH is active at the level of the adrenocortical sexual zone. In addition, any possible ovarian hyperproduction of estrogens during this phase of life depends on thecal or interstitial activity rather than on follicular function, in which case the action of LH is instrumental.

CLIMACTERIC HYPERTHYROIDISM. Loeser[60] and Siegert[96] reported increased values of *thyrotropic hormone* in the blood and urine of climacteric women. The significance of increased thyrotropin levels in relation to possible development of pathologic hyperthyroidism of the climacterium shall be examined later. The high rate of thyrotropin production would appear to result from lack of estrogens.

HYPERSECRETION OF ACTH. Various authors[35, 52] have postulated that ACTH was produced in excessive amounts during the climacterium. ACTH hyperproduction supposedly causes such isolated instances of hypercorticism as are occasionally seen in postmenopausal women. Without denying the possible significance of this disorder, we have rarely observed it. It is true that hypercortical reactions do occur in the climacterium. However, more than anything else, such reactions are due to the third gonad, that is, the sexual adrenal, whose specific stimulant, as indicated above, is LH. We therefore believe that the reason for the occurrence of climacteric hypercorticism, which is a sexual and not metabolic form of hypercorticism, lies in the increased activity of LH.

CLIMACTERIC DIABETES. Diabetes in women most commonly appears during the climacterium. Almost always, this is a "pituitary" form of diabetes.

39.2.3. CLIMACTERIC HYPERCORTICISM

Many years ago, Marañón[66, 67] stressed the significance of hypercortical reactions during the climacterium. In later years, we came up with abundant evidence supporting the occurrence of this type of hypercorticism.[17] The hypercortical origin of *climacteric virilism* will be stressed later in this chapter. Together with Santos-Ruiz and Gómez-Maestro[93] in 1950, we studied 17-ketosteroid excretion in climacteric women. The results obtained by us are shown in Table 39–2.

It is apparent that the climacterium is associated with hyperelimination of 17-ketosteroids, which is also observed after castration, but which disappears in a few years. Borth and associates[15] reported similar findings. Obviously, climacteric hypercorticism involves the sexual zone and is responsible for a rise in urinary 17-ketosteroid excretion. A parallel rise in estrogen excretion apparently also occurs.

In summary, the climacteric may be asserted to be marked by an adrenal reaction involving the sexual zone, associated with increased fuchsinophilic deposits in that zone as well as with elevated urinary excretion of 17-ketosteroids and estrogens of adrenal origin. Under normal circumstances, this reaction is purely compensatory in nature; however, it may occasionally exceed its normal limits and then lead to a condition of climacteric virilism. The adrenal metabolic zone, in comparison,

TABLE 39–2. Excretion of Neutral 17-Ketosteroids During the Female Climacterium

TYPE OF PATIENT	NO. OF CASES	MEAN 17-KETO-STEROID EXCRETION (mg/24 hr)
Normal women	4	5.68
Climacteric women	6	9.33
Postclimacteric women	6	4.28
Surgically castrated women	6	7.18

does not appear to undergo any structural or hyperfunctional changes during this phase of life.

39.2.4. CLIMACTERIC HYPERTHYROIDISM

It is evident that a number of the most conspicuous climacteric changes, such as nervous and psychological instability, emotional frame of mind, tachycardia, tremors and vasomotor manifestations, are highly reminiscent of hyperthyroidism. Siegert[96] demonstrated an increase in thyroid function during the climacteric and was able to detect a parallel increase in the levels of circulating thyrotropin. A rise in the basal metabolic rate in climacteric women was shown by Marañón,[67] while increased PBI values have been recorded by other investigators. However, a distinction should be made between the mild hyperfunctional thyroid reactions occurring in the normal climacterium and pathologic instances of *true hyperthyroidism*, presenting as the predominant symptom. Riley[91] recently studied various function tests (PBI, thyroxine-binding globulin, ^{131}I uptake) of the climacteric thyroid, failing to find any evidence of enhanced functional activity in the majority of cases. We believe that, while constituting far less than a constant finding, thyroid hyperfunction nevertheless does occur. The syndrome of "climacteric hyperthyroidism" of Marañón is uncommon (probably occurring in not more than 5 to 6 per cent of all cases) but, in our opinion, it does occur.

39.2.5. PANCREATIC DISTURBANCES AND THE CLIMACTERIUM

The development of diabetes during the climacterium has been emphasized by various authors (Cosnier[30]). The probable role of a pituitary mechanism in this diabetic tendency has already been indicated. Cantilo[25] and Lawrence and Madres[57] stressed the role of estrogens in controlling pituitary diabetogenic hyperfunction and in alleviating the symptoms of climacteric diabetes. The administration of small or intermediate dosages of natural or synthetic estrogens to women who developed glycosuria or diabetes during the climacterium leads to improvement of symptoms. In some cases, the administration of estrogens alone may be enough to treat this type of disorder without further need for insulin therapy.

39.3. SYMPTOMATOLOGY OF THE PATHOLOGIC CLIMACTERIC

The large variety of clinical phenomena occurring in climacteric women may be arranged into several major groups: (1) sexual symptoms; (2) circulatory symptoms; (3) digestive and metabolic symptoms; (4) nervous symptoms; (5) obesity; (6) virilism; and (7) osteoporosis.

39.3.1. SEXUAL SYMPTOMS; CLIMACTERIC AND POSTCLIMACTERIC METROPATHY

The physiologic involution of the genital organs during the climacterium was described in Chapter 17. Since our present purpose is to deal only with pathologic symptoms of the climacterium, we shall omit any reference to ordinary involutional symptomatology and instead analyze in greater detail the hemorrhagic disorders that may occur as a consequence of climacteric hyperestrogenism.

Just as endometrial hyperplasia, at least of a moderate degree, is found to involve the endometria of approximately 30 per cent of all postmenopausal women, so the occurrence of *functional bleeding* is a relatively common finding after a certain period of time has elapsed from the last menstrual period. The latter constitutes what we call *postclimacteric metropathia haemorrhagica*. Contrary to earlier assumptions, it would be erroneous to believe that this form of postclimacteric bleeding is invariably associated with malignant lesions. Marin-Bonachera,[69] at our clinic, compiled the statistical data concerning postclimacteric metropathy that are shown in Figure 39–6. These disclose that only 22.5 per cent of the cases that present with bleeding more than five years after their last menstrual period are associated with malignant tumors. The remaining 77.5 per cent of the cases comprised endometria that were hyper-

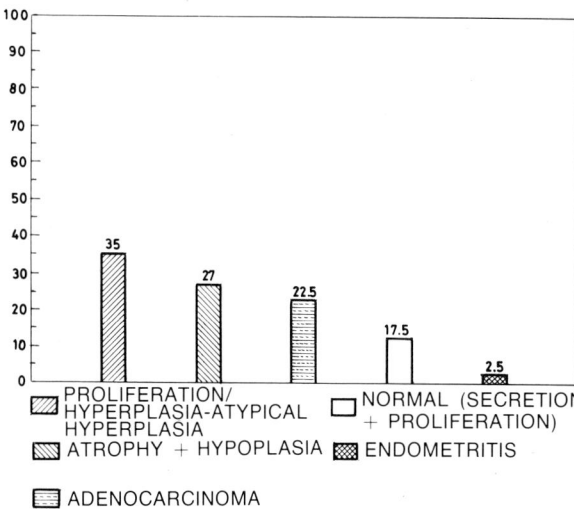

Figure 39–6. Endometrial findings in postmenopausal metropathia hemorrhagica. Noteworthy is the high incidence of endometrial hyperplasia at this phase of sexual life, when ovarian activity is extinct. (Cases observed at our clinic and collected by Marin.)

plastic as well as hypoplastic or normal in appearance, in which bleeding was unrelated to the phase of the cycle. In addition, a few rare cases revealed evidence of endometritis. Sutherland and Mac Bryde[103] reviewed 1000 cases of postclimacteric metropathy by means of endometrial biopsies. Their incidence of malignancy was 27.8 per cent, which does not differ significantly from that found by Marin-Bonachera at our clinic. Lajos[56] more recently reported 12 cases of metropathy of this type. Pacheco and Kempers[83] found that of 220 women with postmenopausal bleeding, 23 per cent had endometrial polyps, 16 per cent carcinoma and 20 per cent atrophy, whereas the remaining 41 per cent had various forms of persistent proliferation or hyperplasia. Their findings are also quite similar to those obtained by Marin-Bonachera. Copenhaver[29] arrived at similar conclusions in a smaller series of cases (27). Thus, there seems to be sufficient evidence that endometrial hyperplasia with bleeding is a common finding in postmenopausal and senile women.

As indicated in Figure 39–6, most of the cases of postmenopausal bleeding (comprising 35 per cent of all cases) consist of hyperplasia and therefore have the same etiology as metropathy in adult women in general. Essentially similar data have been reported by Wagner,[109] Jones and Cantor,[52] Payne and associates,[86] and, recently, Novak.[81] It is also evident that not all cases of postclimacteric and senile metropathy result from hyperplasia but that in a considerable percentage of cases, bleeding occurs in the presence of atrophic or strictly normal endometria. Whenever hyperplasia is involved, its hyperestrogenic origin *may or may not reside in the ovary*, as pointed out above. Not infrequently, however, it may be observed that some women present with an enlarged uterus, with evidence of metropathy owing to endometrial glandular hyperplasia and with a persistent follicle in one of the ovaries several years after they stopped menstruating. This means that anatomical findings identical to those seen in the classical Schröder's syndrome may be observed fairly long after the disappearance of menstrual activity. Sharman[95] and, among ourselves, Nogales have called attention to the occurrence of *late pregnancies*, not in the postmenopause stage but close to the menopause, that terminated in *abortion*. Abortion in those instances may be overlooked most often or may be confused with some of the "ailments" common to that age group. This is a relatively new discovery in clinical practice, to which more attention will have to be paid in the future.

A frequent complaint of menopausal women concerns *pathologic leukorrhea* (Kretzmar and Stoddard,[54] Sharman[95]), which is a consequence of atrophy, occurring in those 66 per cent of women who do not have persistent estrogenic vaginal smears.

39.3.2. CIRCULATORY SYMPTOMS

The phenomenon known as *"hot flushes"* or *"hot flashes"* is one of the most constant and most characteristic symptoms of the climacterium. The patient suddenly becomes aware of a feeling of warmth surging to her neck and head, and she blushes intensely. This feeling is rapidly followed by profuse sweating, pallor and chills. Paroxysms of this type are frequently accompanied by such feelings as weakness, anxiety, oppression, vertigo and, occasionally, nausea and vomiting. The attack may last from a few seconds to several minutes. In benign cases, hot flushes and sweating occur only every now and then in the evening, and only whenever there is an exceptional cause for emotional excitation. In the more severe forms, however, they may supervene in very short intervals, during the day as well as in the evening. These crises may precede, coincide with, or follow menopause and may continue to occur for long periods of time postmenopausally as the only symptom of the climacterium. We have already indicated that such vasomotor disturbances are essentially caused by a yet poorly known effect of pituitary gonadotropins on the vascular apparatus, more specifically, *on the neural control mechanism regulating the vascular apparatus*. Whatever the exact mode of action may be, *it has been possible to establish an exact correlation between the severity of climacteric vasomotor symptoms and the rate of urinary gonadotropin excretion* (Guirdham and Hopkins[39]).

Other circulatory manifestations may affect the rhythm of the heart beat as well as the blood pressure. *Cardiac arrhythmias*, such as simple tachycardia or paroxysmal tachycardia and, less often, bradycardia, may develop with no apparent anatomical changes or organic lesions. Sometimes they necessarily accompany vasomotor phenomena, whereas at other times they occur as independent symptoms. Irregularities in the cardiac rhythm may be benign in nature though in some cases they may be so accentuated and severe that the patient must be referred to a cardiologist.

Although in general the *blood pressure* tends to rise, the characteristic changes involving blood pressure are variability and instability rather than any absolute elevation. Physical exertion, the processes of digestion and nervous upsets tend to raise blood pressure to a much greater extent at this stage than at any other time in life.

The painful crises affecting the small and large arteries and veins, known by the name of *vasalgia*, may also be observed, and seem to be the consequence of vasospasms associated with climacteric circulatory phenomena. Another recently described complication of menopause is atherosclerosis, involving most particularly the coronary vessels and leading to myocardial infarctions. This disease is well known to affect males much more commonly than females, a fact specifically attributable to the preventive role of estrogens. In this regard, a number of authors[27, 34, 98, 104] over the past years have recommended the systematic employment of estrogens for the prevention of this kind of complications. We shall later (Section 39.4.2) raise some criticism concerning estrogen therapy.

Although most often the crises under consideration are of the pseudoangina type, a general tendency to arteriosclerosis (Novak and Williams[80]), and coronary sclerosis in particular (Berkson et al.[13]), has been recognized in postmenopausal women.

39.3.3. DIGESTIVE AND METABOLIC SYMPTOMS

Occasionally, there is loss of appetite, presence of colicky abdominal pain, tenacious constipation or, on the contrary, diarrhea and gastrointestinal disturbances; often *flatulence* also develops.

An important metabolic symptom in these patients is a rise in the *basal metabolic rate* and *weight loss* whenever there are associated climacteric hyperthyroid reactions. These symptoms are associated with tachycardia and nervous hyperexcitability and may give rise to a *false Basedow's syndrome* of menopause.

Another prominent metabolic symptom is *diabetes*. Marañón had called attention to the fact that 69 per cent of the diabetic women in his files developed their first symptoms between the ages of 40 and 50. The onset of diabetes often appears to be associated with emotional disturbances, enhanced emotivity playing no negligible role in the genesis of the disorder. *Despite the arguments invoked in favor of a pituitary basis for the genesis of climacteric diabetes and in spite of the possibly secondary role played by emotivity, there is evidence to the effect that diabetes develops only in those climacteric women who are especially predisposed.* In other words, the genesis of the disorders affecting the pancreas and carbohydrate metabolism in conjunction with the climacteric crisis has three different etiologic elements: (1) the predisposing role of hereditary factors; (2) diabetogenic hyperfunction of the climacteric pituitary, and (3) the role of emotivity and neurovegetative instability, so common during this phase of life.

39.3.4. NERVOUS SYMPTOMS

Comprising some of the most common disorders of the pathologic climacteric, the nervous symptoms consist of *neuralgia, anesthesia, paresthesia* or *hyperesthesia* of the skin or mucous membranes. They may also consist of *aching of muscles, bones and joints, sphincter spasms, generalized (or, more commonly, localized) itching, tingling, insomnia, somnolence, and other sensory disturbances.*

Obviously, these constitute a whole gamut of diverse disorders that in large part depend on the *neurological constitution of each particular patient.*

The *joint pains* affecting especially the arms and legs in the absence of any anatomic changes, and without interfering with normal joint motion, are important and characteristic complaints of this phase of life.

Paresthesias and *hyperesthesias* may be localized or generalized. The local forms may affect any part of the body; most commonly, however, they are restricted to the extremities, mainly the fingers and toes. In notable cases, even the slightest form of pressure, such as, for instance, the weight of a blanket, may elicit painful sensations.

Vulvar pruritus appears most often during the climacteric and postclimacteric phase and may represent a highly troublesome symptom for the gynecologist to cope with.

Headaches are usually observed in women who had shown a lifelong propensity to suffer from headaches. However, these grow in intensity and frequency with the onset of the climacterium. Occasionally such headaches are associated with temporary elevations of blood pressure or with nausea and vomiting. Some women complain of neuralgias in the muscles at the nape of the neck concomitant with headaches.

Some climacteric women also complain of *vertigo*, usually presenting in association with other vasomotor disturbances but occasionally occuring independently. It is usually accompanied by tachycardia and humming in the ears. *Insomnia* is a most common complaint. The patient may find it hard to fall asleep and may stay awake for hours or even all night. Sometimes, insomnia is caused by the tingling, pruritus or hyperesthesia, but it may occur without any exogenous type of irritation. Although it is more common in the male than in the female sex, the complaint of nervous fatigue and mental exhaustion may be often heard on the part of these women. Occasionally, this condition may reach the point of mental depression, or *climacteric melancholia,* which in the opinion of Marañón[67] is a characteristic development in these women. MacCandless[64] emphasizes the need for differentiating those instances of true depressive states owing to climacteric influences from other conditions in which preexisting psychoneurosis becomes manifest through anxiety over possible loss of sexual activity.

39.3.5. OBESITY

The coincidence of obesity with the climacterium has been mentioned by various authors.[38, 48, 81] As aptly pointed out by Marañón,[66] it is not so much a question of *climacteric obesity* occurring in the climacteric as rather a *question of which of the many forms obesity may assume during the climacteric stage*. In fact, we may distinguish three basic types of obesity during reproductive decline: (1) exogenous obesity; (2) plethoric obesity, and (3) hypogenital type of obesity.

EXOGENOUS OBESITY. Many women in the climacteric age group gain weight as a result of their way of life and change in eating habits. This is a fairly common phenomenon in Spain, particularly in the country and among well-to-do families. Women at this age may indulge in eating as a way of distraction. Fatty meals and, occasionally, a craving for pastry, along with a sedentary way of life, are conducive to obesity at this stage of life much more readily than at any other time, particularly in those women who have lost interest in remaining slender and maintaining shapeliness.

Probably the sedentary habits and pattern of overeating become more pronounced during this phase of life because of subconscious emotional problems that are *intimately related to the psychopathology of sexual decline.*

PLETHORIC OBESITY. Upon reaching the climacterium, some women develop a plethoric type of obesity, with predominant accumulation of fat over the upper half of the body, a ruddy complexion and often manifestations of hypertension as well as *hypercorticism.* This variety of obesity is characteristic of women with a pyknic habitus as pointed out by Marañón.[67] This obesity must be ascribed to a condition of hypercorticism and quite often is associated with genital hyperfunction, occurring precisely in those women that develop postclimacteric metropathia haemorrhagica. It may be asserted in quite general terms that there exists a type of climacteric woman characterized by a tendency to hypercorticism, hypertension, plethoric obesity and development of hyperestrogenism.

HYPOGENITAL TYPE OF OBESITY. The opposite type of obesity with regard to the plethoric type is one which occurs in women with no apparent tendency to either hypertension or hypercorticism. These are women in whom the genital apparatus is markedly inactive and undergoes complete atrophy and involution. This type of obesity is associated with a *whitish skin* which to a certain extent resembles that seen in Froehlich's disease. A typical feature of the hypogenital type of obesity is that adipose tissue tends to accumulate below the waistline, particularly around the hips and thighs, giving rise to what has been called *lipodystrophy of Barraquer.* Such patients are also prone to develop *lipomas* or *pseudolipomas,* usually in the region of the pelvic girdle.

Marañón[67] also pointed out that the disorder might coexist with the syndrome of Dercum, or painful adiposity of menopause, of which we, however, have so far failed to observe any instances.

39.3.6. CLIMACTERIC VIRILISM

The appearance of virilizing symptoms during the climacteric has been commented upon by a great many authors.[1, 17, 48, 87] In keeping with the theory of sexual evolution,[59] explained in Chapter 18, *every woman passes through a transient phase of virilization around the time of her sexual decline.* Usually, however, this type of virilization is very mild and barely manifests itself (Fig. 39–7). There may be slight hypertrichosis of the upper lip and at the site of the sideburns, a slight hardening of the features, sometimes a drop in the timbre of the voice, and in particular, an increase in the rate of urinary 17-ketosteroid excretion occurs as a silent witness of this transient virilization during sexual decline.

Occasionally, however, the climacteric is complicated by a syndrome of serious virilization. *Climacteric virilization* usually supervenes in women with obesity of the plethoric type and with a pyknic habitus, strongly suggestive of hypercorticism. Because of this, Marañón had assumed this type of climacteric virilization to be of *hypercortical origin* and to reflect adrenal hyperfunction. Nevertheless, our own observations permit us to maintain that climacteric virilism may be of *two different origins: on the one hand, of purely adrenal origin, and on the other, of ovarian origin.*

VIRILISM OF OVARIAN ORIGIN RESULTING FROM HILUS CELL PROLIFERATION.

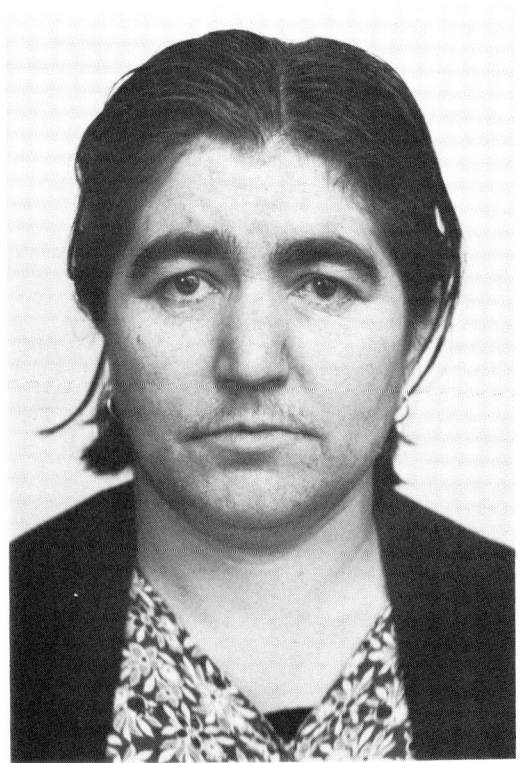

Figure 39–7. Mild climacteric virilism.

Occurs among climacteric women with a certain degree of frequency. Because of the absence of secretory activity on the part of the essential elements of the climacteric ovary, hilus cells tend to undergo a process of unchecked proliferation. Meyer assumed that the presence of mature follicles inhibited proliferation of any heterologous rests in the ovary. On the other hand, such heterologous rests are believed to be not only set free from the inhibitory influence of follicular maturation but moreover to be stimulated as a result of increased gonadotropin activity occurring during this phase of sexual life. The case of a 45 year old woman with early menopause and moderate virilization caused by hilus cell proliferation, demonstrated at laparotomy, is shown in Figure 39-8. In a similar way, ovarian *hyperthecosis* may play a role in causing temporary virilization in such patients.

THE ADRENAL FORMS OF CLIMACTERIC VIRILISM are usually pronounced. They apparently represent true instances of *climacteric adrenogenital syndrome*, whose genesis is facilitated by two factors: (a) a tendency of the sexual zone to undergo compensatory hyperplasia, and (b) an increase in pituitary LH production. They resemble the experimental cases in rats reported by Little and Houssay (see Chapter 9), in which adrenogenital syndrome was induced by means of castration.

39.3.7. CLIMACTERIC OSTEOPOROSIS

In Chapter 2, estrogens were stated to modify *calcium metabolism*, by increasing calcium fixation by the bone matrix. Clinically, this is proven by the occurrence of climacteric osteoporosis, an entity described as far back as 1885 by Pommer but not generally recognized until the publication of Albright's works[4, 5, 6] on the subject in 1941. According to the latter, the disappearance of ovarian function in the late climacteric phase (late postmenopausal phase) leads to progressive decalcification of bone, noticeably evident in the *thinning of bone trabeculae* in the vertebral bodies (Vanek[106]). Contrary to classical assumptions, the reduction in calcium fixation is *secondary* to reduction of available bone matrix which, by decreasing in volume, is able to fix less calcium and less phosphorus.

The available mass of bone matrix is the result of the bone modeling process, balanced between *osteoblastic* (deposition of osteoid) and *osteoclastic* (resorptive) activity. The interplay between these two kinds of activities is regulated by a series of factors (Fig. 39-9). *Estrogens, androgens, thyroid hormone* and *growth hormone* all have a proliferative effect on the osteoblasts, thereby *increasing the amount of bone matrix*. In contrast, *parathyroid hormone* and *glucocorticoids* exert a stimulatory effect on the osteoclasts and thus lead to osteoporosis. This is the underlying cause of osteoporosis in hyperparathyroidism as well as in Cushing's disease. To this, we must add the fact, demonstrated by Eisenberg and Gordan[36] as well as by Nordin and Smith,[78] that both estrogens and androgens inhibit this stimulatory effect on the osteoclasts. All factors stimulating osteoblastic activity simultaneously raise the level of *alkaline phosphatase* in the blood, which consequently assumes a diagnostic value, whereas those factors stimulating osteoclastic activity pro-

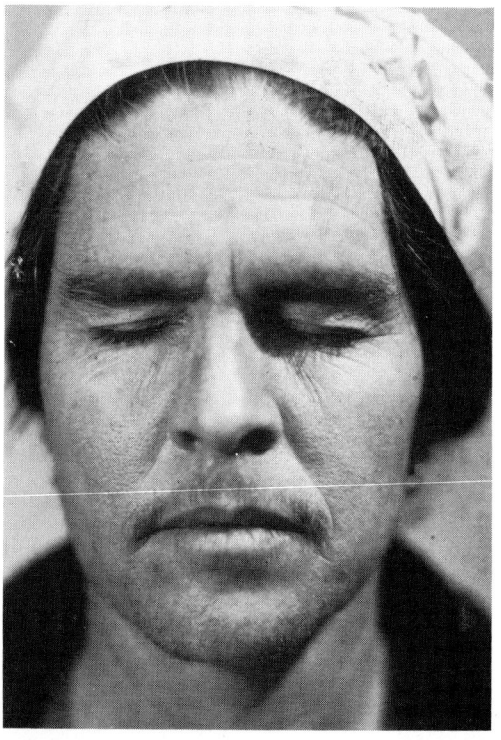

Figure 39-8. Climacteric virilism caused by proliferation of ovarian hilus cells; this was cured by means of ovarian demedullation.

Pathology of the Female Climacteric 873

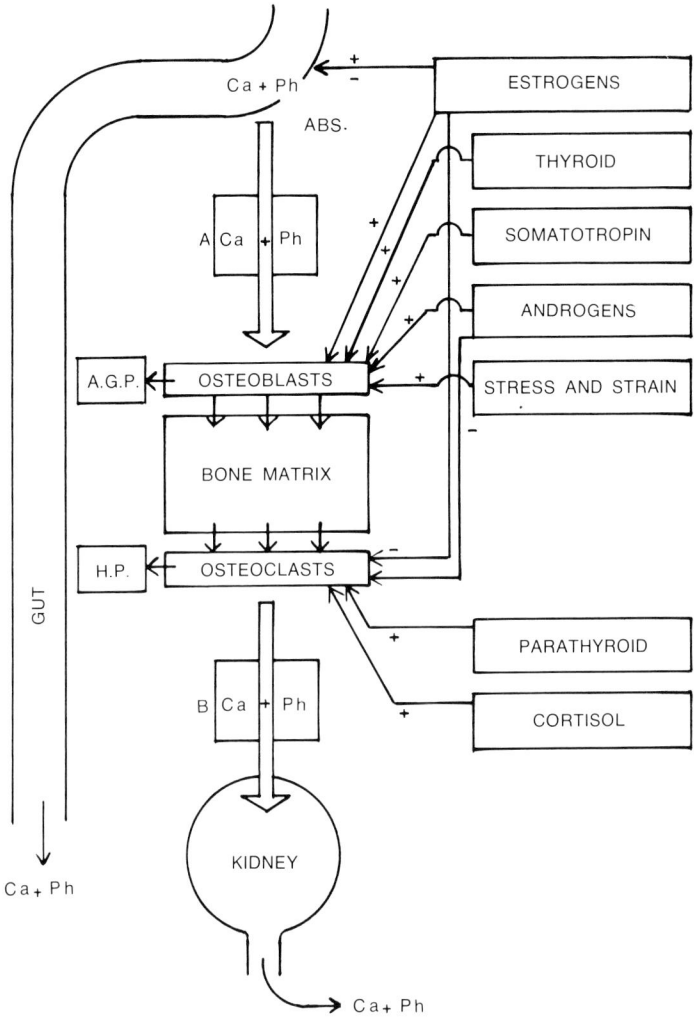

Figure 39-9. Mechanism of production of climacteric osteoporosis. Estrogens simultaneously exert an effect on the process of calcification in three ways: (1) by stimulating the absorption of calcium and phosphorus, (2) by stimulating the activity of osteoblasts and (3) by inhibiting the activity of osteoclasts. The actions of other hormones, such as thyroid hormone, growth hormone, corticoids and parathyroid hormone, have also been indicated. The presence of alkaline glycerophosphatase (A.G.P.) in the plasma is indicative of increased osteoblastic activity, whereas presence of hydroxyproline (H.P.) indicates an increase in osteoclastic activity.

duce a rise in *hydroxyproline* values. A method for the determination of hydroxyproline was recently introduced by Nordin and Smith[78] and by Ingiulla and associates,[49] and has greatly contributed toward clarifying the etiology of many cases, by permitting us to establish whether osteoporosis in a given case results from diminished osteoblastic activity or, conversely, from an increase in the rate of destructive osteoclastic activity. In addition, one more factor that enhances osteoblastic activity and, thereby, increases bone matrix formation, is what is known as "stress and strain," resulting in a constant effort to produce new osteoid in direct dependence on nutritional factors, most specifically, the level of *proteinemia*. As a result, besides indirectly involving protein anabolism, "stress and strain" induces increased calcium fixation by the bone. This is an additional reason why androgens, nitrogenizing anabolizing agents that they are, contribute to growth of bone matrix.

The complex pathogenic mechanism involved in osteoporosis has been diagrammed in Figure 39-9, which in addition also indicates how calcium and phosphorus are absorbed by the gut *under the influence of estrogens* and how the calcium and phosphorous derived from osteoclastic activity are eliminated by the kidney.

Over the past few years, the study of radioactive calcium and strontium balance (Eisenberg and Gordan,[36] Haas et al.,[43] Nordin[78]) has demonstrated that the Albright's hypothesis was not entirely correct. Apparently, the primary event taking place in osteoporosis is not the decrease in available bone matrix and in the rate of calcium fixation by bone but, on the contrary, *loss of calcium by the kidney*, followed by hypocalcemia. According to the foregoing investigations, the reduction in the amount of bone matrix and in calcium fixation occurs as a *compensatory phenomenon*. Regardless of whether the primary event takes place at the calcemic or, on the contrary, at the bone matrix level, the diagram shown in Figure 39-9 explains why postmenopausal reduction in estrogenic activity leads to osteoporosis, one of the most common complications of late menopause, provided of course that it is patterned on the hypoestrogenic model (Henneman[45]), which, as we have indicated above, does not invariably occur.

39.4. TREATMENT

Therapy of the various clinical forms of the pathologic climacteric necessarily pursues quite different ends. Basically, we distinguish two different aspects: (1) treatment of pathologic climacteric manifestations resulting from lack of estrogens, and (2) treatment of climacteric hyperestrogenism. It is easy to understand why therapy in each case should be totally different. What we are to treat in the first instance consists essentially in hypoestrinism, whereas the problem in the second is a condition of hyperestrinism. The vast majority of the pathologic disorders of the critical age respond to the first modality of treatment. The second modality of therapy is only employed in the much less frequently occurring—nevertheless clinically more striking—cases of climacteric hyperestrinism.

As a matter of fact, the treatment of the first form is aimed not at substituting the existing lack of estrogens but rather at *suppressing pituitary hyperfunction*, owing to loss of ovarian activity. Accordingly, we shall describe: (1) treatment of the pathologic climacterium based on pituitary suppression, and (2) treatment of the manifestations of hyperestrogenism of the climacterium.

39.4.1. PITUITARY SUPPRESSION

Pituitary hyperactivity in this instance is the consequence of a compensatory reaction resulting from estrogen deficiency. Consequently, estrogen therapy constitutes a form of pituitary suppressive treatment. However, because estrogens in some cases may produce harmful effects, other means for suppressing pituitary activity may also be employed: androgens or androgen derivatives, as well as combinations of hormones with pituitary suppressive drugs.

ESTROGENS. Treatment of the pathologic symptoms of the climacteric with estrogens is the oldest form of treatment in use. It is still advocated by Greenblatt and Barfield,[40] Reich and co-workers,[90] Masters and Magallon[70] and Gurtman and associates.[41] Its main drawback is that it may very easily lead to *iatrogenic hyperestrinism* at this phase of life (see Chapter 28), which is why other forms of treatment have been developed, based on androgens and hormone combinations.

Because of the preventive effect continuous administration of small dosages of estrogens has against osteoporosis and arteriosclerosis, Davis[34] advocates *continuous administration of estrogens* to postmenopausal women. We have already indicated that a number of authors[27, 48, 104] recommend systematic estrogen therapy in the menopause for the prevention of vascular sclerosis, myocardial infarction and osteoporosis. This procedure has been supported by Zuspan[113] and by Baton,[11] who advise the use of the long-acting estrogen preparation quinestrol. We have adopted a critical attitude.[20,104] As we have already pointed out, we believe that a large proportion of postmenopausal women are hyperestrogenic to begin with and that indiscriminate estrogen therapy may produce hyperestrinism and metrorrhagia, or even arouse a possible latent endometrial carcinoma. We therefore advise that estrogen administration be performed *under strict cytologic control*. The same opinion has been voiced by Buzzoni and co-workers[24] and by Sedlis and his associates.[94]

ANDROGENS. Androgens have been tested successfully in postmenopausal women by various investigators (Masters and Magallon,[60] Nathanson and Towne[76]). The rationale for the favorable results observed lies in the fact that testosterone as well as testosterone derivatives *similarly exert a pituitary-suppressive effect*. Nevertheless, androgen therapy in female patients may be associated with two types of undesirable side-effects: (1) it may lead to virilization, particularly if employed for extended periods of time, and (2) it enhances libido, which in unmarried women may have unpleasant consequences. A search for androgen derivatives with limited virilizing potency but good antipituitary action has led to the use of such compounds as *methyltestosterone* and *androstenediol*, employed by Borth and colleagues,[15] Cantilo,[25] Kurzrook and Rothbart,[55] Margolese[68] and Greenblatt and Barfield,[40] and currently enjoying great popularity. In addition to pituitary suppression, androgens in general, and methyltestosterone in particular, exert a favorable *anabolizing effect* in some cases. Last but not least, the *antitumorigenic action* of androgens, particularly valuable at this stage of life, must not be forgotten (see Chapter 46).

ESTROGENS-ANDROGENS. The administration of *mixtures of estrogens and androgens* or, less frequently, combinations of *androgens with progesterone*, is based on the same principle. Loeser,[60] Ufer,[105] and Hirshland and Hill[46] stress the efficacy of this type of therapy. Estrogens, on the one hand, suppress the pituitary, avert excessive involution of the genital tract and prevent the development of pruritus, senile vaginitis, kraurosis; androgens, on the other, also suppress the pituitary, but in addition counteract the effect of estrogens and prevent the development of neoplasia, functional bleeding, and so forth.

There is no general agreement as to the ratio in which these hormones should be used. For instance, Geist and Salmon have proposed a ratio of 10 mg androgen to 1 mg estrogen. On the other hand, Greenblatt, as well as Ufer, believe that such a ratio contains too much estrogens and advise a ratio of 25 mg to 1 mg. Watteville and Lunenfeld[108] have recommended the use of sublingual tablets (linguets) containing 0.01 mg ethinylestradiol and 5 mg methyltestosterone. Hirshland and Hill[46] have proposed the use of 90 mg testosterone enanthate associated with 4 mg estradiol valerianate in single monthly dosages. This last ratio, which appears to have been adopted by most manufacturers of these products, resorts to preparations that rely almost exclusively on the action of androgens, except for minute amounts of estrogens that are sufficient to inhibit both virilization and enhancement of libido.

PITUITARY SUPPRESSING DRUGS. Greenblatt and Barfield[40] have employed dexamethasone; subsequently, Ferriman and Purdie[37] successfully tested the preparation ICI 33828 (Dithiocarbamoylhydrazine). Either preparation may be indicated in cases of pronounced hyperpituitarism.

PROGESTOGENS. While progesterone itself is of no value in the treatment of menopausal disorders (Riley[91]), *oral progestogens* have been used extensively over the past years, apparently with satisfactory results (Appleby,[8] Riley[91]).

39.4.2. TREATMENT OF CLIMACTERIC HYPERESTRINISM

This does not differ from the treatment of hyperestrinism in general, as outlined in Chapter 28. It may be pointed out, however, that particularly good results have been reported by treating such women with *roentgen castration*. Kepp[53] published an excellent review concerning indications and dosages for this form of therapy for climacteric women.

39.4.3. OUTLINE OF TREATMENT

Much discussion has been devoted to the question of whether or not it is advisable to treat this type of patients with *estrogens* systematically (Davis[34]). The majority of authors do not agree with the criteria for indiscriminate estrogen therapy (Ingiulla and Gasparri,[48] Jones and Te Linde,[51] Sharman[95]). We have proposed the outline in Table 39-3 for therapy.

In treating the pathologic climacterium, we place particular emphasis on the *need for carefully evaluating each case on its own merits* rather than on adhering to any pre-set routine.

TABLE 39-3. Treatment of Climacteric Disorders

TYPE OF PATIENT	CYTOLOGY	ESTROGENS	17-KETOSTEROIDS	TREATMENT
Normoestrogenic	Intermediate	Normal*	Normal	Pituitary suppressors, vegetative equilibrators
Hypoestrogenic	Atrophic	Low	Normal	Estrogens†
Hyperestrogenic	Karyopyknotic	Elevated*	Normal	Androgens, progestogens, or both
Hyperandrogenic	Intermediate	Normal or low	Elevated	Estrogens and corticoids (or Dexamethasone)

*Within the limits of the lowered values corresponding to this phase of life.
†Controlled on the basis of vaginal cytology by discontinuing treatment as soon as cells become karyopyknotic (index over 10 per cent).

39.4.4. SUMMARY

Marañón[67] stated that *"each woman developed her own distinctive form of climacteric according to her endocrine constitution."* To this we might add that the *treatment must vary correspondingly*, depending on the form of climacterium to be dealt with. The term "critical age" is fully justified. Indeed, what is involved is one of the most outstanding biologic crises of woman, which is when she ought to be studied and treated most carefully.

REFERENCES

1. Albert, A., et al.: *J. Clin. Endocr.*, 18:843, 1958.
2. Albert, A., et al.: *J. Clin. Endocr.*, 21:839, 1961.
3. Albert, A.: *J. Clin. Endocr. Metab.*, 25:1119, 1965.
4. Albright, F., Smith, P. H., and Richardson, A. M.: *J.A.M.A.*, 116:2465, 1941.
5. Albright, F.: *Rec. Progr. Horm. Res.*, 1:293, 1947.
6. Albright, F.: *Ann. Int. Med.*, 27:861, 1947.
7. Altman, N. H., Strett, C. S., and Terner, J. Y.: *Amer. J. Vet. Res.*, 30:383, 1969.
8. Appleby, B.: *Lancet*, 226:407, 1962.
9. Apostolakis, M., and Loraine, J. A.: *J. Clin. Endocr.*, 20:1437, 1960.
10. Augustin, M., and Manciulesco, D.: *Rev. Fr. Endocr. Clin.*, 10:101, 1969.
11. Beaton, D.: *Brit. J. Clin. Practice*, 21:241, 1967.
12. Berger, J.: *Acta Cytol.*, 1:78, 1957.
13. Berkson, D. M., et al.: *Clin. Obstet. Gynec.*, 7:504, 1964.
14. Bonfirraro, G., and Sensi, G.: *Riv. Ost. Gin. (Firenze)*, 21:668, 1966.
15. Borth, R., Linder, A., and Riondel, A.: *Acta Endocr.*, 25:33, 1957.
16. Boschann, H. W.: *Acta Cytol.*, 1:77, 1957; 2:611, 1958.
17. Botella, J.: *Compt. Rend. Soc. Fr. Gynec.*, 19:17, 1949.
18. Botella, J.: *Proceed. 1st Internat. Congr. Exfol. Cytol.*, Philadelphia, J. B. Lippincott, 1961.
19. Botella, J.: *Arch. Fac. Med. (Madrid)*, 3:307, 1963.
20. Botella, J.: *J. Reprod. Med.*, 1:221, 1968.
21. Brown, J. B.: *Lancet*, 1:320, 1955.
22. Brown, P. S.: *J. Endocr.*, 25:427, 1963.
23. Bulbrook, R. D., and Greenwood, R. C.: *Brit. Med. J.*, 1:662, 1957.
24. Buzzoni, P., Curiel, P., and Noci, L.: *Riv. Ost. Gin. (Firenze)*, 23:457, 1968.
25. Cantilo, E.: *Endocrinology*, 28:20, 1941.
26. Carcatzoulis, S.: *Presse Med.*, 2:2375, 1961.
27. Castallo, M. A.: *Pennsylvania Med.*, 70:80, 1967.
28. Coble, Y. D., Kohler, P., Cargille, C. M., and Ross, G. T.: *J. Clin. Invest.*, 48:359, 1969.
29. Copenhaver, E. H.: *Geriatrics*, 23:128, 1968.
30. Cosnier, J.: *Ann. d'Endocr.*, 17:695, 1956.
31. Council of the Medical Women's Association of England: *Lancet*, 1:106, 1953.
32. Cozens, D. A., and Nelson, M. M.: *Endocrinology*, 68:767, 1961.
33. Craig, J. M.: *Amer. J. Obstet. Gynec.*, 97:100, 1967.
34. Davis, M. E.: *Clin. Obstet. Gynec.*, 7:558, 1964.
35. Diddle, A. W.: *Cancer*, 5:215, 1952.
36. Eisenberg, E., and Gordan, G. S.: *J. Clin. Invest.*, 40:1089, 1961.
37. Ferriman, D., and Purdie, A. W.: *J. Endocr.*, 31:173, 1965.
38. Folsome, C. E., Napp, E. E., and Tanz, A.: *J.A.M.A.*, 161:1447, 1956.
39. Guirdham, A., and Hopkins, P.: *Brit. Med. J.*, 5344:1543, 1963.
40. Greenblatt, R. B., and Barfield, W. E.: *Amer. J. Obstet. Gynec.*, 63:1, 1953.
41. Gurtman, A. I., et al.: *Obstet. Gynec.*, 10:261, 1957.
42. Haam, E. von: *Acta Cytol.*, 4:37, 1960.
43. Haas, A. G., Canary, J. J., Kyle, L. H., Meyer, R. J., and Schaaf, M.: *J. Clin. Endocr. Metab.*, 23:605, 1963.
44. Hellman, L. M., Zumoff, B., Fishman, J., and Gallagher, T. F.: *J. Clin. Endocr.*, 30:161, 1970.
45. Hennemann, P. H.: *Clin. Obstet. Gynec.*, 7:531, 1964.
46. Hirshland, H., and Hill, J.: *Amer. J. Obstet. Gynec.*, 86:177, 1963.
47. Husslein, H.: *Med. Klin.*, 3:86, 1948.
48. Ingiulla, W., and Gasparri, F.: *La Sindrome Menopausale*, presented at the "Congresso de la Societa Italiana di Ost. e Gin." Torino, Italy, 1965.
49. Ingiulla, W., Matteini, M., Sibilla, A., Bianchi,

G. F., and Sensi, G.: *Sul Problema della Osteoporose della Postmenopausa,* presented at the "Congress de la Societa Italiana di Ost. e Gin." Torino, Italy, 1965.
50. Jayle, M. F., et al.: *Ann. d'Endocr.,* 13:589, 1952.
51. Jones, E. S., and Te Linde, R. W.: *Amer. J. Obstet. Gynec.,* 57:854, 1949.
52. Jones, D. B., and Cantor, E. B.: *Amer. J. Obstet. Gynec.,* 62:365, 1951.
53. Kepp, R. K.: *Gynäkologische Strahlentherapie.* Stuttgart, G. Thieme, 1952.
54. Kretzmar, W. A., and Stoddard, F. J.: *Clin. Obstet. Gynec.,* 7:451, 1964.
55. Kurzrook, L., and Rothbart, H.: *Amer. J. Surg.,* 56:636, 1941.
56. Lajos, L.: *J. Obstet. Gynec. Brit. Comm.,* 70:1016, 1963.
57. Lawrence, R. D., and Madres, K.: *Lancet,* 1:601, 1941.
58. Limburg, H.: *Arch. Gynäk.,* 180:260, 1951.
59. Little, C. E.: *Amer. J. Obst. & Gyn.,* 61A:64, 1950.
60. Loeser, A. A.: *Gynec. Prat.,* 2:2, 1951.
61. MacArthur, J. W., et al.: *J. Clin. Endocr.,* 18:460, 1958; 24:425, 1964.
62. MacBryde, J. M.: *J. Clin. Endocr.,* 17:1440, 1957.
63. MacBryde, J. M.: *J. Obstet. Gynec. Brit. Emp.,* 61:691, 1954.
64. MacCandless, F. D.: *Clin. Obstet. Gynec.,* 7:489, 1964.
65. Magee, P. T.: *Acta Cytol.,* 11:179, 1967.
66. Marañón, G.: *La Evolución de la Sexualidad y los Estados Intersexuales.* Madrid, Morata, 1927.
67. Marañón, G.: *El Climaterio de la Mujer y del Hombre.* Madrid, Espasa Calpe, 1937.
68. Margolese, S.: *J. Clin. Endocr.,* 4:393, 1944.
69. Marín-Bonachera, E.: *Acta Gin.,* 3:557, 1952.
70. Masters, W. H., and Magallon, D. T., *J. Clin. Endocr.,* 10:384, 1950.
71. Mattingly, R. F., and Huang, W. Y.: *Amer. J. Obstet. Gynec.,* 103:679, 1969.
72. Matsukawa, T.: *Obstet. Gynec.,* 16:407, 1960.
73. Montalvo, L.: *Acta Cytol.,* 4:145, 1960.
74. Mussey, F., Dockerty, M. B., and Masson, J. C.: *Proc. Staff Meet. Mayo Clin.,* 23:63, 1947.
75. Nandi, J., Bern, H. A., Biglieri, E. G., and Pieprzyk, J. K.: *Endocrinology,* 80:576, 1967.
76. Nathanson, R. I., and Towne, G.: *Endocrinology,* 25:745, 1949.
77. Nogales, F.: *Arch. Med. Exper.,* 11:729, 1948.
78. Nordin, B. E. C., and Smith, D. A.: *Triangulo,* 6:287, 1964.
79. Novak, E.: *J. Obstet. Gynec. Brit. Emp.,* 55:725, 1948.
80. Novak, E. R., and Williams, J. T.: *Amer. J. Obstet. Gynec.,* 80:863, 1960.
81. Novak, E. R.: *Clin. Obstet. Gynec.,* 7:464, 1964.
82. Osmond-Clarke, F., and Murray, M.: *Brit. Med. J.,* 1:307, 1958.
83. Pacheco, J. C., and Kempers, R. D.: *Obstet. Gynec.,* 32:40, 1968.
84. Parlow, A. F.: *Endocrinology,* 74:102, 1964.
85. Paulsen, C. A., et al.: *J. Clin. Endocr.,* 15:846, 1955.
86. Payne, F. L., Wright, R. C., and Flatterman, M. N.: *Amer. J. Obstet. Gynec.,* 77:1216, 1959.
87. Plate, W. P.: *Arch. Gynäk.,* 198:453, 1963.
88. Pundel, J. P.: *Acta Cytol.,* 12:121, 1968.
89. Randall, C. L., Birtch, P. K., and Harkins, J. L.: *Amer. J. Obstet. Gynec.,* 74:719, 1957.
90. Reich, W. J., et al.: *Amer. J. Obstet. Gynec.,* 64:174, 1952.
91. Riley, G. M.: *Clin. Obstet. Gynec.,* 7:432, 1964.
92. Ryan, R. J.: *J. Clin. Endocr.,* 22:300, 1962.
93. Santos-Ruiz, A., Gómez-Maestro, D. V., and Botella, J.: *Arch. Med. Exper.,* 14/2:79, 1951.
94. Sedlis, A., Turkell, W. V., and Stone, D. F.: *Bull. N. Y. Acad. Med.,* 45:271, 1969.
95. Sharman, A.: "The Menopause," in *The Ovary,* Vol. I, ed. Sir Solly Zuckermann. New York, Academic Press, 1962.
96. Siegert, G.: In *Biologie und Pathologie des Weibes,* Vol. 1, 2nd ed., ed. Sietz and Amreich. Vienna, Urban & Schwarzenberg, 1953.
97. Sopena, A., and Tornero, M. C.: *Actas de la Socdad. Esp. Esterilidad,* 3:247, 1956.
98. Spritz, N.: *Modern Treat.,* 5:587, 1968.
99. Stoll, P., and Ledermair, O.: *Geburtsh. u. Frauenhk.,* 20:263, 1960.
100. Stone, D. F., Sedlis, A., Stone, M. L., and Turkell, W. V.: *Acta Cytol.,* 11:349, 1967.
101. Struthers, R. A.: *Brit. Med. J.,* 1:1331, 1956.
102. Subrizi, D. A., Curiel, P., and Gentili, G.: *Riv. Ost. Gin (Firenze),* 22:484, 1967.
103. Sutherland, A. M., and MacBryde, J. M.: *J. Obstet. Gynec. Brit. Emp.,* 61:238, 1954.
104. *Symposium:* "Clinical Use of Estrogens in the Menopause." *Lying-in (Chicago),* 1:221, 1968.
105. Ufer, J.: *Acta Gin.,* 4:215, 1953.
106. Vanek, R.: *Ann. d'Endocr.,* 21:899, 1962.
107. Waard, F. de, and Van Halewin, B.: *Acta Cytol.,* 13:675, 1969.
108. Watteville, H. de, and Lunenfeld, B.: *Schw. Med. Wschr.,* 83:14, 1953.
109. Wagner, H.: *Arch. Gynäk.,* 177:460, 1950.
110. Wied, G. L.: *Acta Cytol.,* 1:75, 1957.
111. Witschi, E.: "Bioassay for FSH in Human Hypophyses," in *Human Pituitary Gonadotropins,* ed. A. Albert. Springfield, Ill., Charles C Thomas, 1961.
112. Zarate, A., Karchmer, S., Gomez, E., and Castelazo-Ayala, L.: *Amer. J. Obstet. Gynec.,* 106:110, 1970.
113. Zuspan, F. P.: *J. Reprod. Med.,* 1:221, 1968.

Chapter 40

VIRILISM

40.1. DEFINITION

"Virilism" has been defined variously: to some, it means the sum total of *somatic manifestations* that make a woman acquire the physical and mental features characteristic of the male sex. To others, it simply means an endocrine condition—*abnormal accumulation of androgens in the female body* (Jailer and Holub[45]). Our definition of virilism has been formulated in different terms. By *primary sex characters* we mean those attributes that involve the gonads. *Secondary sex characters* are those pertaining to the genital apparatus of the female and the male, and *tertiary sex characters* are those somatic and mental features other than the gonads or the corresponding genital tract that make it possible to distinguish a man from a woman (see Chapter 18). Tertiary sex characters develop in both sexes beginning with puberty and, in addition to physical attributes, involve functional and psychological differences.

We define virilism as the appearance of male tertiary sex characters in woman.

The tertiary sex characters of concern involve: (1) Configuration of the skeleton; (2) external somatic shape and distribution of the fat panniculus; (3) distribution of hair growth peculiar to each sex; (4) development of the breasts in the female and lack of secretory development in the male; (5) greater development of the larynx in the male; (6) sex-linked variations affecting some parts of the various systems (larger size of the male adrenal cortex, distinctive characteristics of the digestive tract, sex-linked differences between a number of endocrine glands, degrees of lability of the vascular system, etc.); (7) psychological differences between the two sexes, including differences in libido.

As regards the distribution of hair growth, which is one of the most constant signs of virilism, it should be pointed out that *simple exaggerated development of body hair is not diagnostic of virilization*. This point has been emphasized by Jailer and Holub,[45] Gilbert-Dreyfus and colleagues,[25] Greenblatt,[30] and Hamilton and Terada,[33] and has been recently stressed by us.[10] *The mere presence of marked hirsutism in a woman is not sufficient reason to speak of virilism. In addition, such hair growth must present a male pattern of distribution and be associated with other intersexual features.* Unless these criteria are met, virilism may be falsely diagnosed in women with *simple hirsutism. This may be particularly true in Mediterranean peoples, in whom body hair is more ostensible.*

Over the past years, a growing tendency has developed to *consider virilism as exclusively an endocrine condition*. To be sure, the principal causes for virilism involve changes in internal secretions, but it must not be forgotten that some *genetic tendency* toward intersexuality may transform a woman into a mannish individual in the presence of only minor deviations in her endocrine balance. Hence, there is need for recognizing a *constitutional* or *genetic type of virilism* in addition to the *endocrine type of virilism*.

In reality, what happens is that the terms "virilism" and "hirsutism" are used interchangeably. Greenblatt,[30] Hamilton and Terada,[33] and Segre[90] insist on this point, which is considered by us to be of utmost importance. A woman may have abundant hair and not be virilized, particularly if her hair maintains a feminine type of distribution or is of the fine downy variety which, while quite visible in brunettes, may be overlooked in blond women. By the same token, a woman may have relatively sparse body hair and still have pronounced male features (deep voice, masculine skeletal form, enlarged clitoris). Finally, there are forms of hirsutism, such as the type of juvenile hirsutism that is associated with *hypothyroidism* (Perloff[79]), that have nothing to do with virilism.

Consequently, hirsutism may be dissociated from virilism, a fact that ought to be borne in mind.

For many years, the origin of virilism has been attributed exclusively to the adrenal or to masculinizing tumors of the ovary. As a result of relatively recent findings, it has been shown that *apparently normal ovaries may exercise androgenic function,* from which it may be inferred that certain types of ovarian virilism may occur in the absence of any apparent ovarian lesions.

No less significant for the differential diagnosis of the diverse forms of virilism are the recently developed exploratory techniques, particularly the assay for urinary steroids. Apart from that, we must mention the increasingly significant use of corticoids in the treatment of these disorders.

40.2. ANDROGENS IN FEMALE PHYSIOLOGY

This subject was already discussed in Chapter 4. The most essential points will be recapitulated here.

For many years, the occurrence of androgens in the female body was believed to constitute a kind of *atavistic trait* or an *error of nature,* but this hypothesis can no longer be sustained.

40.2.1. EFFECTS OF ANDROGENS

Androgens exert well-defined physiologic actions in the female body. Among these are:

1. Mahesh,[67] Zander[98] and others (see Chapters 2 and 3) have established in a convincing manner the fact that androgens are *intermediary metabolites* in the biogenesis of ovarian and adrenocortical hormones and therefore are found in both the female ovary and adrenal under physiologic conditions.

2. Androgens counterbalance certain excessive estrogen effects, thereby partaking in *steroid homeostasis* (see Chapters 4 and 28).

3. Androgens stimulate protein anabolism and take part in regulating protein metabolism.

4. Androgens are adequate stimulants of the *libido in the female.*

5. At puberty, *pubic and axillary hair* fail to develop without androgenic activity.

40.2.2. ANDROGEN SYNTHESIS BY THE FEMALE BODY UNDER NORMAL CONDITIONS

IN THE ADRENAL. Androgen synthesis by the female adrenal has been demonstrated by Botella[8] both experimentally and clinically (see Chapter 9). It plays an important role especially during pregnancy, the climacteric and following castration (Botella[9]), as well as following injections of chorionic gonadotropin (Botella,[9] Plate[80]).

IN THE OVARY. Androgen biogenesis by the normal ovary, once a matter of controversy, has now been accepted without reservation. In 1923, Berger[7] equated the hilus cells of the ovary (sympathicotrophic cells, or "Hiluszellen") with the testicular Leydig cells, later demonstrating their androgen synthetic action. Hill demonstrated the virilizing effect of ovarian transplants to the ear in female rabbits. Ponse[81] came up with valuable evidence favoring ovarian androgen biogenesis. As in the adrenal cortex, androgen biogenesis in the ovary has been found to be excited by chorionic gonadotropin. Various ovarian structures involved in androgen biosynthesis include (a) the *hilus cells,* or sympathicotrophic cells of Berger (Berger,[7] Botella[9]); (b) the *hyperplastic theca cells* (Ponse,[81] Plate[80]); (c) the *luteinized cells* of thecal origin in diffuse ovarian luteinization[27] or in lutein cysts[14]; (d) *the atretic follicles.* Oakey and Stitch[77] demonstrated that estrogen synthesis was incomplete in atretic follicles and in ill-developed graafian follicles and that the majority of steroid compounds failed to be converted beyond the preceding androgenic stage. Kirschner and associates[52] found that, because of estrogen deficiency, LH release was not inhibited in those women who, as a result, produced increasingly larger amounts of "incomplete" steroids.

40.3. "PHYSIOLOGIC VIRILIZATION"

The existence of androgenic secretion in normal woman accounts for the occurence of *transient states of virilization* during certain periods of life. Such circumstances arise mainly during the *female climacteric*. Many years ago, Marañón[68] had enunciated his doctrine of "evolution of sexuality." Marañón held that womanhood was not a definitive state of differentiation but an intermediary stage between childhood and manhood. Accordingly, a man was believed to pass through a fleeting, transitory period of feminization during puberty as an obligatory step on his way from childhood to manhood. In contrast, woman, in whom puberty began without any heterosexual changes, showed a tendency to undergo virilization during her climacterium. Marañón thus described the entity of *climacteric virilization* which we were later able to show[10] corresponded to a period of elevated urinary 17-ketosteroid excretion. It was our assumption[9] that the observed reaction was the result of *climacteric adrenocortical hyperfunction*. Using intravenous ACTH perfusion, Decourt and his co-workers[17] confirmed the presence of functional hyperactivity of the adrenal cortex during this period of life.

The evolutive tendency of the female sex toward masculinization and toward "climacteric virilism" seems to be a general biologic phenomenon. In the lower animal species, this evolution of the sexes is very clearly manifest, *not only in terms of chemistry, as in the human species, but also in terms of somatic features*. Accordingly, the species may be divided into *protandric species*, in which an initially male individual evolves into a female, and *protogynic species*, which includes man, in which initial differentiation is female-oriented whereas late evolution proceeds in a male direction (see Chapters 15 and 18).

The presence of either protogynic or protandric tendencies in a given species is not determined by chance but depends on the configuration and distribution of the *sex chromatin* (Chapter 14). The monogametic sex, viz., the sex in which the sex chromosomes are identical, is always the first to undergo differentiation. Thus, in the human species, in which chromatosexual symmetry occurs in the female sex (the monogametic sex), the female sex is first to be differentiated, whereas, on the contrary, the male sex (the digametic sex, with dissimilar sex chromosomes) constitutes the end-stage of evolution.

In human clinical experience, virilization in the female occurs much more frequently than does feminization in the male. More than to anything else, this must be attributed to the fact that the process of female-male oriented conversion coincides with the physiologic direction, whereas any transformation in the opposite way is contrary to the norms of physiologic evolution of the human species. *To a certain extent, the tendency to virilization in woman is a physiologic phenomenon.*

The occurrence of *virilization during pregnancy* was described recently (Alexander and Beresford,[1] Klotz,[53] Friedman et al.[24]). In gestation, particularly close to term, 17-ketosteroid levels are elevated (Jayle[47]). Insofar as 17-ketosteroid production is concerned, the gravidic adrenal does not seem to be unusually hyperfunctional (Botella et al.[11]). This is why we conclude that whenever a tendency to virilization becomes apparent during pregnancy, the presence of increased androgens must be attributed to either the maternal ovary or to the fetal glands. By developing the so-called "interstitial gland" to a significant degree close to term, the ovary seems to become an androgen-producing organ. However, it must be remembered that considerable amounts of 17-ketosteroids are elaborated by the adrenals as well as the testes of a male fetus, which gain access to the circulation and the urine of the mother prior to birth.

No relationship between the degree of virilism occurring during gestation and the sex of the fetus has ever been demonstrated.

40.4. CLASSIFICATION AND CLINICAL FORMS OF VIRILIZATION

Both the female adrenal and the fetal ovary are known to be capable of synthesizing androgens. Consequently, it seems feasible to classify virilism into an *ovarian* and an *adrenal* form. From the clinical standpoint, it is also convenient to distinguish between constitutional virilism and virilism stemming from pluriglandular disorders (of pituitary origin). Finally, certain minor forms of virilism related to cyclic activity ought to be included here as well. As a result, the following will be distinguished: (1) minor forms of virilism; (2) virilism of adrenal origin; (3) virilism of ovarian origin; (4) pituitary virilism, and (5) constitutional virilism.

40.4.1. MINOR FORMS OF VIRILISM

Netter and associates[72] described *women with amenorrhea*, without external signs of virilization, in whom urine polysteroid determinations revealed increased 17-ketosteroid values. The pathogenesis of amenorrhea in these cases was attributable to androgen hyperproduction by the hilar region of the ovary, in view of the fact that chromatography of 17-ketosteroids isolated from the urine showed the latter to be predominantly of ovarian rather than adrenal origin (see below). We have also seen cases of amenorrhea with elevated 17-ketosteroids and little tendency to virilization.

Sendrail and his co-workers[91] described a "premenstrual syndrome," accompanied by hyperandrogenism. Somatic virilization in these cases was rare but urinary 17-ketosteroids were increased and chromatographic fractionation revealed that these also were ovarian androgens.

Currently, the minor forms of virilism are suspected to be determined by some *ovarian metabolic disorder*. In Chapter 29, we explained why the Stein-Leventhal syndrome is attributed to *ovarian enzyme deficiency*. Mahesh[67] believes that, even though ovarian morphology is characteristic in this syndrome, similar enzymatic changes may be involved, causing defective estrogen and progesterone synthesis and excessive elaboration of androgens. Two different types of enzyme changes are thought to be involved: (1) lack of Δ4-androstenedione aromatization, and (2) lack of 3β-ol-dehydrogenase.

40.4.2. VIRILIZATION OF ADRENAL ORIGIN

Until about 20 years ago, virilization of adrenal origin, commonly known as *adrenogenital syndrome* (see Chapter 33), had been thought to be a rare disease. Up to 1946, we were able to collect only 200 cases from the world literature. Since then, however, innumerable cases have been reported.

As already indicated (Chapter 33), the disease is produced by *hyperfunction not of the adrenal cortex but only of the sexual zone*. It corresponds to what we elsewhere have called *hyperfunction of the third gonad*.

Like the Stein-Leventhal syndrome, at least in its nontumoral forms, the adrenogenital syndrome is an *enzymopathy*, which has led a number of workers[6, 32, 43] to suspect that the two syndromes may in fact often occur together.

The fully developed forms of the syndrome were described in Chapter 33. However, in addition, there are a good many larvated forms that are associated with only mild virilism.

Houssay and Higgins[40] were able to induce the adrenogenital syndrome experimentally by castrating female mice. The adrenal hyperplastic response resulted from reactive pituitary gonadotropin activity characteristic of castration. Botella[9] and Plate[80] have been able to confirm the stimulatory effect of chorionic gonadotropin on the human adrenal.

The *primitive adrenal* form is produced by tumors (nearly always adrenal carcinoma) that are independent of pituitary action. The two forms may be differentiated by the Allen reaction (see Chapter 33, Section 33.2.7) and by their different response to cortisone (Wilkins et al., Kupperman et al.[56] Segaloff[89]). The adrenogenital syndrome of pituitary origin improves with cortisone and cortisone derivatives, whereas the primitive adrenal form remains unaffected.

The adrenogenital syndrome is not invariably associated with virilization. In about 20 per cent of cases, usually in young males, there are associated features of feminization. *The earlier the disease appears in women the more pronounced is the associated virilizing effect.* The highest degree of virilization is encountered in the congenital forms, giving rise to the well-known syndrome of pseudohermaphroditism (see Chapters 33 and 37).

The disorder betrays a certain *constitutional and familial tendency* (Jailer and Holub[45]) and not uncommonly is associated with mental disorders, such as were reported by Allen and associates[2] some time ago (1938) and subsequently confirmed by Segre.[90]

Also very interesting are recent *metabolic studies* on the disease, which have been summarized in Chapter 33. It is noteworthy in the first place that Bradbury and Slate[13] found evidence of large amounts of *dehydroepiandrosterone* produced by the affected adrenals. This finding, by now confirmed by a number of investigators, allows establishment of a fairly reliable *differential diagnosis of adrenal virilism as distinct from other forms of virilism.*

In 1952, Jailer and van de Wiele,[44] and later Benedict and associates,[6] Mahesh[67] and Zander,[98] brought to light the fact that, from the metabolic standpoint, the adrenogenital syndrome is essentially characterized by the adrenal's inability to hydroxylate positions 11 and 21 in the structural formulas of steroids. This entails hyperproduction of 17-hydroxyprogesterone, an incomplete steroid, thus engendered instead of 17-hydroxycorticosterone (compound F). As pointed out above, 17-hydroxyprogesterone is easily converted to 17-ketosteroids in the body. The catabolism of this compound gives rise to not only androgens but also *pregnanediol*, discovered in 1938 by Marrian in the urine of patients with the adrenogenital syndrome.

The build-up of 17-hydroxyprogesterone appears to be linked to an abnormally developed zona reticularis and to the deposition in the latter of a carbonylic, fuchsinophilic substance. In 95 per cent of cases of adrenogenital syndrome in which the adrenals were examined histologically, reticular hyperplasia was found to be associated with abundance of fuchsinophilic cells.

All of this, explained in detail in Chapter 33, is repeated here for no other reason than that of drawing a parallel between virilizing adrenal syndromes and virilizing ovarian syndromes. In either case, interruption of steroidogenesis, although occurring at different times, produces the same result: a build-up of androgenic substances of the neutral 17-ketosteroid type. This happens because the androgens involved are relatively simple and are early metabolites of steroid metabolism. In summary, *virilism may then be said to be always a consequence of a failure in the biogenesis of the terminal steroids: estrogens, progesterone and corticoids.*

The principal modes of production of virilism are either adrenal or ovarian, although it is evident that any minor alterations in the intermediary metabolism, involving a block in steroid synthesis, inevitably result in androgenism, however minor in degree.

40.4.3. OVARIAN VIRILISM

Just as the adrenal form of virilism may be produced by adrenal hyperplasia or by tumors, ovarian virilism, until recently believed to be only the result of masculinizing tumors of the ovary, actually also involves a frequent *hyperplastic* origin.

The most classic *masculinizing ovarian tumors* described (see Chapter 30) are *arrhenoblastomas* or Pick's adenomas (Novak,[75] Radman and Bhagavan[82]).

Leydig cell tumors (Waugh et al.,[94] Sachs and Spiro[86]) have been described in recent years, although they occur less frequently than arrhenoblastomas. Like the tumors of the adrenal which are able to cause virilization, these are *essentially virilizing tumors.* They reproduce testicular structures involved in testosterone production and are classified among the vast group of well-known *functioning tumors of the ovary.*

Over the past years, a new variety of virilizing ovarian tumor has been described. It is the *lipoid cell tumor,* of which several new case reports have recently been published.[55, 61, 71, 78]

Deserving special mention is the luteoma, which has been dealt with in Chapter 30. It has now been proved to produce a virilizing effect, a phenomenon until recently poorly understood. Modern studies concerning steroidogenesis confirm the indirect virilizing action of progesterone. Rice and Segaloff[85] have shown that, apart from secreting progesterone, luteomas produce large amounts of androgens. Neumann and his colleagues[73] have demonstrated that the virilizing action by luteomas is likewise susceptible to suppression with the antiandrogen cyproterone. It should be further mentioned that ovarian luteomas during pregnancy cause fetal virilization because they produce large amounts of dehydroepiandrosterone sulfate as well as testosterone (O'Malley et al.[76]).

At present, however, great significance is being attached to *the androgenic effect of simple ovarian hyperplasia.* The main ovarian structures capable of secreting the male hormone have been mentioned above.

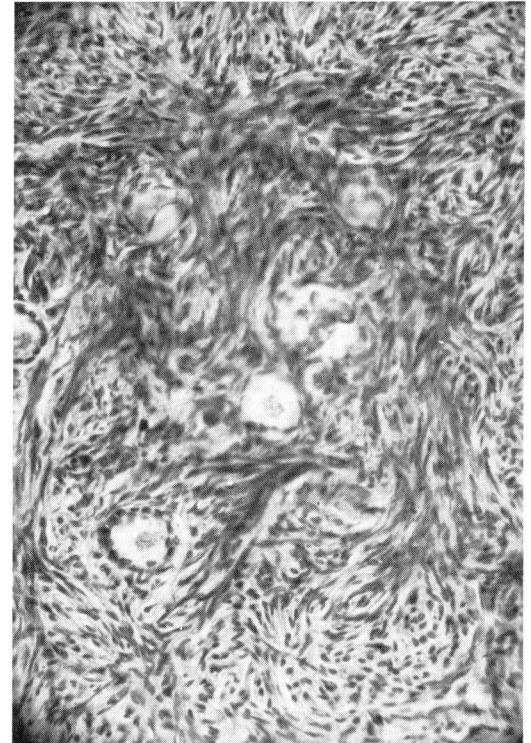

Figure 40-1. Hyperthecosis or theca cell hyperplasia; note large number of primordial follicles engulfed by fibrous cortical stroma.

Thus, both *theca cell hyperplasia* (Plate,[80] Holmer[37]) (Fig. 40-1) and *Berger cell hyperplasia* (Berger,[7] Hooft et al.,[38] Remouchamps and Ghijsbrecht[84]) (Figs. 40-2 and 40-3) are known to be capable of producing virilism. Virilization has also been described as caused by *diffuse ovarian luteinization* (Westman[95]). We have already indicated (Section 40.2.2) that the *corpus luteum* may exert an androgenic effect under pathologic conditions. Basically, three types of conditions are involved: (1) Diffuse interstitial luteinization (Gospodarowicz[27]); (2) degenerated lutein cysts (Callard and Leathem[14]); (3) luteomas (Plate[80]). However, the most important of all such apparently harmless androgenic ovarian formations occurs in the *Stein-Leventhal syndrome* (see Chapter 29 and figure 40-4). As is well known, this syndrome is associated with ovarian fibrosis in the presence of follicles that do not reach full maturity and impart to the ovary its *microcystic* appearance. In the opinion of Plate and Westman, all such ovaries present with thecal hyperplasia, so that virilism in these instances is attributable to *hyperthecosis*.

As a result of the introduction of *chromatographic fractionation for 17-ketosteroids*, the ovarian forms of virilization can now be distinguished from the adrenal forms of virilization. In the former, *androsterone* predominates in the urine, whereas in the latter *dehydroepiandrosterone* is predominant and can be separated from the former chromatographically.

Nevertheless, there are indications that the androgens eliminated in the urine of women with ovarian disorders of this type have a biologic action much greater than those obtained from patients with the adrenogenital syndrome. In fact, it has been observed that the rate of 17-ketosteroid excretion in the adrenogenital syndrome is always proportionately much higher than in ovarian virilism. Some forms of ovarian virilism have been described in which 17-ketosteroid excretion was not elevated. Significantly, too, urinary 17-ketosteroid excretion in cases with ovarian virilism cannot be modified by cortisone therapy.

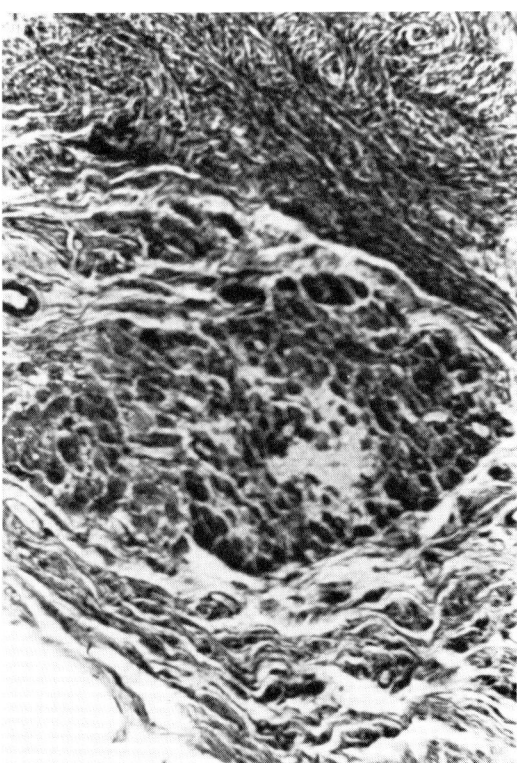

Figure 40-2. Hyperplasia of virilizing hilus cells (Berger cell hyperplasia).

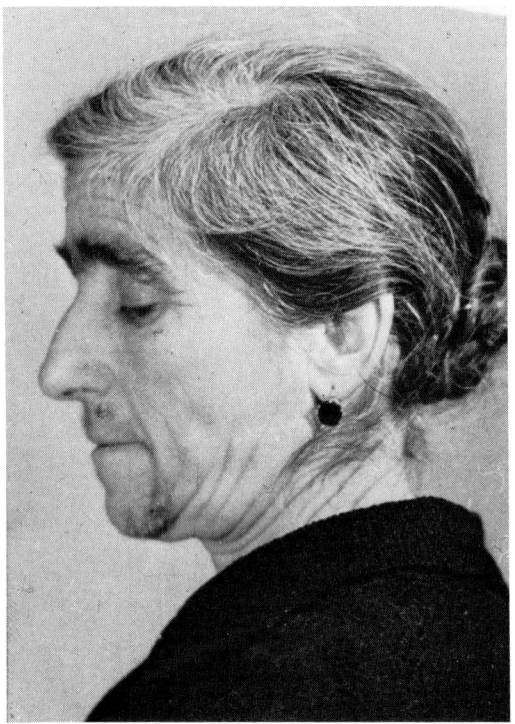

Figure 40-3. Climacteric virilism caused by Berger cell hyperplasia of the type shown in Figure 40-2.

common property of secreting androgens and being stimulated in its function by luteinizing gonadotropin (LH), as well as being localized in either the adrenal interstitial zone or the ovarian hilar or interstitial zone. This raises the legitimate question of whether virilism in the majority of cases, with the exception of those produced by tumors, may not be mere *systemic diseases* after all.

40.4.4. PITUITARY VIRILISM

The majority of cases in which endocrine virilism is attributed to activity of glands other than the ovary or the adrenal cortex have either been erroneously interpreted or been misdiagnosed cases which in the final analysis turned out to be pluriglandular disorders, with either the ovary or the adrenal playing the principal role.

Such is the case in *Cushing's syndrome:* according to Liddle,[60] only 25 per cent of patients with this disease develop virilism, in the latter instance owing to adrenal hyperplasia.

In recent years, the significance of ovarian virilism as compared to adrenal virilism has been considerably exaggerated. The truth is that despite modern procedures for the biochemical exploration of this group of patients, it is difficult to ascertain whether any given syndrome is a pure ovarian or a pure adrenal variety. Only those cases can be clearly defined in which autopsy studies or surgical specimens of both adrenal and ovarian tissues are available. However, the surprising finding in those cases in which anatomical studies of this kind have been done is the *frequent occurrence of associated adrenal hyperplasia and hyperthecosis.* We were able to demonstrate this association in a case observed in 1946. Similar findings were later reported by Scully[88] and by Hooft and associates[38] in 1956. It must not be forgotten that the adrenal sexogenous tissue and the ovarian interstitial androgenic tissue are both *derived from a common retrocoelomic mesenchyme* which in the embryo has the potentiality for engendering alike the gonad and the interrenal gland. *The sexual mesenchyme may therefore be said to have the*

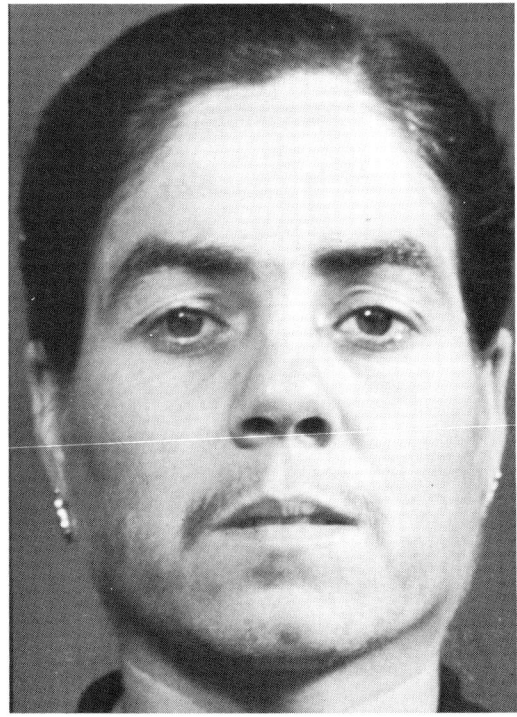

Figure 40-4. Virilism in the Stein-Leventhal syndrome.

Virilism

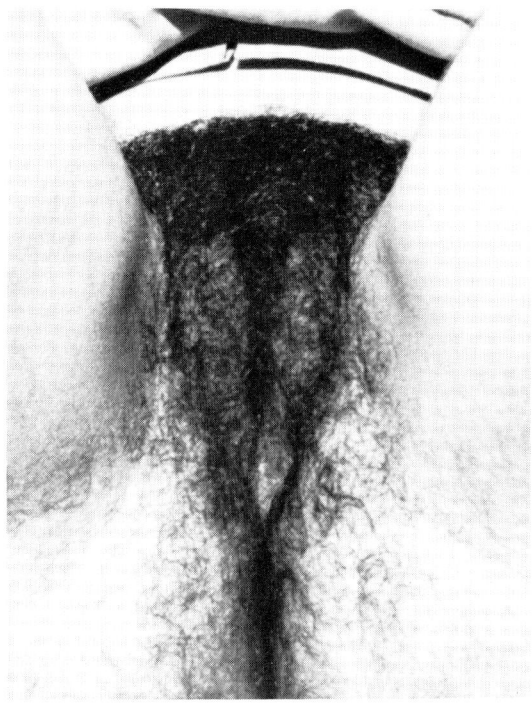

Figure 40-5. Hypertrichosis of the vulvoperineal region in a case of virilization.

The syndrome of Achard-Thiers, as stated previously, may in the final analysis be reduced to a variant of the adrenogenital syndrome; the type of virilization it produces similarly appears to be of adrenocortical origin (Greenblatt et al.[31]).

40.4.5. CONSTITUTIONAL VIRILISM

There exists, of course, a form of genuine virilism, that is, a form of *constitutional androgenism*. It is probably associated with sex chromosomal aberrations. However, such cases are extremely rare. Probably the majority of cases described as examples of constitutional virilism are simple cases of *hirsutism* rather than *virilism*.

40.5. EXPLORATION OF VIRILISM

Deliberately omitted here are data concerning clinical exploration, biotypologic measurement[21, 23] and other general details, which do not need to be enlarged upon. Over the past years, *biochemical means for exploring virilism* have achieved great importance. The study of steroid excretion in the various forms of masculinization has contributed a great amount of detail concerning their genesis and the question of how to differentiate the various clinical forms from each other.

40.5.1. DIRECT DIAGNOSIS

The diagnosis of virilism is basically made by *simple inspection*. Useful in this respect are the techniques proposed by Hamilton and Terada,[33] or by Ferriman and Gallway,[21] designed for the quantitative determination of body hair growth. To be sure, it is necessary to ascertain that one is dealing with true virilism and not with mere hirsutism. This means that, in addition to the amount of hair present, other features of virilization must be recognized (the quality of the voice, the presence of clitoral hypertrophy [Fig. 40-6], type of hair distribution,

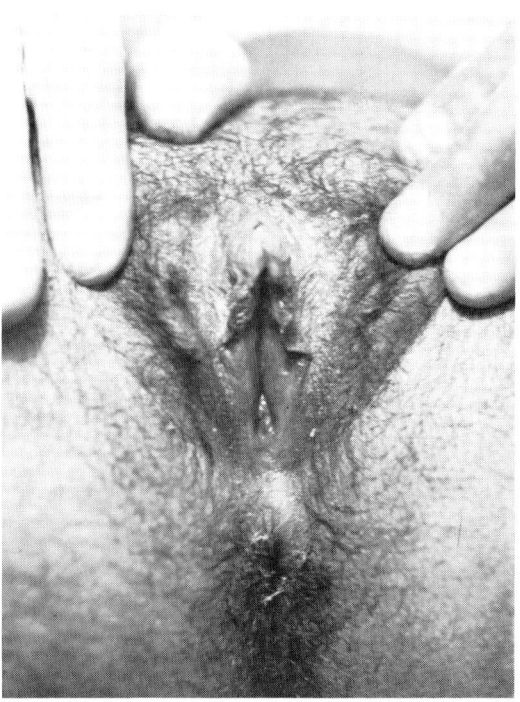

Figure 40-6. Clitoral hypertrophy in a case of virilism.

shape of skeleton, etc.). However, parameters of really great interest are provided by the *determination of urinary 17-ketosteroids and functional loading tests.*

URINARY 17-KETOSTEROIDS. Jailer and colleagues,[43,44] as well as Jayle and his associates,[4,48] have shown the significance of urinary 17-ketosteroid determinations. In normal women, values range from 5 to 13 mg/24 hr. Figures ranging from 15 to 20 mg/24 hr are found in mild forms of ovarian virilism, in the Stein-Leventhal syndrome and in Berger cell hyperplasia. Sometimes even virilizing ovarian tumors give rise to only slightly increased values. On the other hand, the adrenogenital syndrome is characterized by values of the order of 30 to 40 mg, while in cases of adrenal tumor, amounts as high as 90, 100 or higher are not unusual. Patterson and later Allen and associates[2] developed a color reaction for *dehydroepiandrosterone* (Allen-Patterson reaction) which is considered specific for adrenal tumors, not so much because these tumors are the only producers of this steroid, which characteristically is involved in all forms of virilization, but more importantly because only in adrenal tumors is it secreted in sufficient quantities to give the urinary color reaction. Recently, James and colleagues,[46] Lloyd[63] and Mahesh[67] criticized the practice of estimating total 17-ketosteroid values, since only too often the values obtained are not a faithful index of virilism. In the first place, not all 17-ketosteroids have a virilizing effect, nor do they all possess the same androgenic potency; in the second place, the reciprocal proportions in which these androgens occur in the different syndromes are variable, so that in some cases low values of highly androgenic 17-ketosteroids may produce pronounced virilization, while in other cases there may be large amounts of substances with lesser or no androgenicity, in which virilization therefore is absent or minimal. In general, ovarian syndromes may be said to be associated with the elimination of small amounts of highly androgenic steroids, while the elimination of large amounts of mildly androgenic steroids occurs in the adrenal syndromes. Audit and Boussemart,[3] Levesque and colleagues,[59] Netter and associates,[72] and Stein and associates[92] therefore advocate the use of *chromatographic fractionation of urinary 17-ketosteroids* (see Chapter 24), which has the advantage of facilitating the differential diagnosis.

TESTOSTERONE IN THE URINE AND PLASMA. In recent works, attention has been called to the significance of *testosteronuria* in the diagnosis of this type of virilism. Testosterone values are increased to a comparatively greater extent than are 17-ketosteroids, which explains why some women with low rates of 17-ketosteroid excretion may nevertheless be subject to pronounced virilization. The question of urinary testosterone excretion in virilism has been studied by Gobel and Teurer,[26] France and Knox,[23] Ismail and associates[41] and Lawrence.[58]

Plasma testosterone levels have been investigated by Bardin and Lipsett[5] and by Horton and Neisler.[39]

LOADING TESTS. We have devised a test based on chorionic gonadotropin loading, preceded and followed by estimation of urinary 17-ketosteroids. We found elevation of these compounds in cases of hyperadrenocorticism. Later, however, Plate[80] noted the same reaction and considered it to be expressive of an ovarian response to gonadotropin. In 1955, De Court and his co-workers[16,17] introduced a test based on intravenous infusion of ACTH and estimation of urinary 17-ketosteroids. This test is based on the same principle as ours but seems to be more specific and is positive only in cases of adrenal virilism.

Lately, similar loading tests have been developed in large numbers and seem to have gained greater importance. Lloyd[62,63] has made a detailed study of them. An increase in 17-ketosteroid values after the infusion of 25 mg ACTH is considered as positive evidence that the androgens are of adrenal origin. If, conversely, the increase is produced by the administration of gonadotropin, the test is interpreted as indicative of the ovarian origin of the disorder. Pituitary suppression can also be achieved with *dexamethasone* (Dignam et al.,[18] Jeffcoate et al.,[49] Lopez et al.[64]). Should a 1 mg dose of this substance cause a reduction in the rate of 17-ketosteroid excretion, the test is positive for adrenal virilism. In Chapter 24, an extensive commentary has been devoted to the *dynamic tests of the endocrine system*, some of which are designed to distinguish ovarian virilism from adrenal virilism. Laitinen and Pesonen[57] employ this test specifically for the differential diagnosis between hyperestrogenic amenorrhea and amenorrhea owing to hyperandrogenism.

OTHER DIAGNOSTIC MEANS. Several partial aspects involved in the exploration of this type of patient, as, for instance, the value of practising adrenal *pneumoradiographies*, deserve some comment. A method of this type was recently perfected by Dogliotti and Lacroix[19] and by Maurer[69] for the diagnosis of adrenal hyperplasia. Gilbert-Dreyfus and his colleagues were able to localize an adrenal tumor by means of *aortography*.

The question of whether any specific type of cells reflecting an androgenic effect characterize *vaginal cytology*, as assumed by Bourg,[12] has been a matter of controversy. Opinion on this issue remains divided, but it is our belief that, even though the existence of cells reflecting androgenic effect may be admitted, the criteria by which they may be recognized are unreliable.

Over the past years, much emphasis has been laid on the value of *gynecography* and *culdoscopy*, particularly as concerns the diagnosis of the Stein-Leventhal syndrome.

40.5.2. DIFFERENTIAL DIAGNOSIS OF VIRILISM

By using as a diagnostic aid the clinical exploratory data and the hormone studies indicated in the preceding section, it is possible to establish the differential diagnosis of the various forms of virilism. For this purpose, one may also resort to the various functional tests mentioned, as well as to the study of the response to cortisone treatment.

In Table 40-1, a comparison has been drawn between ovarian and adrenal virilism and between those data that may be helpful for the differential diagnosis of the two forms.

Of considerable interest, too, is the differential diagnosis of *primitive adrenal* and *primitive pituitary* cases of adrenogenital syndrome. A scheme intended to facilitate this differentiation is given in Table 40-2.

40.6. ANDROGENIC AMENORRHEA AND INFERTILITY

As we have indicated previously (see Chapters 9, 28, and 38), androgen injections into prepuberal female rats cause permanent anestrus, probably as a result of impregnation of the hypothalamic sex center which thus ceases to exhibit cyclic activity.[28, 42, 51, 83, 93, 99] It seems likely that this phenomenon also obtains in the human species. In the adrenogenital syndrome, with markedly elevated androgen levels, amenorrhea is a constant finding and the ovaries are polycystic,[66] giving the impression that the cycle has been paralyzed. Korenman and his associates[54] have shown that whenever androgen production in the adrenogenital syndrome is suppressed with dexamethasone, ovulation is reestablished. Hoffmann and Meger[35] injected testosterone into human ovaries locally and noted suspension of ovulation. Similarly, a number of recent reports[15, 20, 34] refer to the finding of suspended cycles and infertility as a result of administration of high dosages of androgens in both women and female experimental animals.

TABLE 40-1. Comparison Between the Ovarian and the Adrenal Forms of Virilism

OVARIAN VIRILISM	ADRENAL VIRILISM (ADRENOGENITAL SYNDROME)
Mild virilization	Marked virilization
Onset late in adult age or at menopause	Onset early in childhood or at puberty
17-ketosteroid excretion below 20 mg/24 hr	17-ketosteroid excretion above 20 mg/24 hr
Predominantly androsterone excretion	Predominantly dehydroepiandrosterone excretion
Injection of LH raises urinary 17-ketosteroid values	Injection of ACTH provokes major 17-ketosteroid elevation
Cortisone does not lower 17-ketosteroid elimination	Cortisone reduces 17-ketosteroid elimination

TABLE 40-2. Comparison Between Adrenogenital Syndrome of Pituitary Origin and That of Primitive Adrenal Origin

PITUITARY VARIETY	ADRENAL VARIETY
Mild clinical manifestations; benign forms of the syndrome	Severe clinical manifestations; accentuated forms of the syndrome
Bilateral *adrenal hyperplasia*	Unilateral *adrenal tumor*
Less than 60 mg 17-ketosteroids/24 hr	More than 60 mg 17-ketosteroids/24 hr
Negative Allen-Patterson reaction	Positive Allen-Patterson reaction
Urinary hyperexcretion of LH and ACTH	Absence of pituitary hormones in the urine
Frequently associated with Cushing's syndrome or with other hypercortical metabolic manifestations	Not associated with Cushing's syndrome; on the other hand, may give rise to manifestations of addisonism
Treatment with cortisone or cortisone derivatives effective; adrenalectomy not helpful	Treatment with cortisone is ineffective; adrenalectomy is indicated

Although not yet fully confirmed, the impression is nowadays prevalent that many cases of amenorrhea and infertility, particularly when associated with virilization, sometimes quite mild in degree, result from excessive androgenic activity. In this respect, the dynamic tests hold great promise for the diagnosis and so do corticoids for therapy, a point explained in Chapter 41.

40.7. TREATMENT

The treatment of virilism varies according to whether the case involved pertains to the ovarian or to the adrenal variety. Each of these forms is amenable to either *hormone therapy or surgery*. In addition, some consideration may also be given to some forms of symptomatic therapy, such as epilation.

40.7.1. TREATMENT OF ADRENAL VIRILISM

The treatment of the adrenogenital syndrome of primitive adrenal origin is entirely different from that used for the primitive pituitary form. (Table 40-2.)

The primitive adrenal form is amenable to *surgery*. Indeed, the tumors involved are frequently malignant, growing in total independence of pituitary control, and their evolution is not susceptible to hormonal influences. In most instances, such tumors are unilateral and can be excised with satisfactory results where virilism is concerned. Because they are frequently malignant, the prognosis insofar as function is concerned may be good, whereas it is poor with regard to effecting a permanent cure, since the malignancy usually recurs in time and eventually causes the patient's death.

In contrast, those cases which result from nontumoral adrenal hyperplasia lend themselves to *endocrine therapy*. In 1950, Wilkins and his colleagues[96] observed that cortisone caused a noticeable decrease in androgen secretion in patients with adrenal hyperplasia. Later these results were confirmed (Greenblatt,[29] Jayle et al.,[48] Jores,[50] Louchart and Jailer[65]). In Chapter 33, the mode of action of cortisone has already been explained. Later, too, attempts were made to suppress androgenic activity by means of cortisone derivatives, such as tetrahydrocortisone, metacortandracin and 9α-fluorocortisone. The results reported were equally satisfactory.

Not only cortisone but other, more potent and more effective corticoids have a capacity for suppressing ACTH production, which is the basis for this type of treatment. Thus, *fluorocortisone, prednisone* and *dexamethasone*, particularly the last, are highly effective in controlling adrenal virilism.

Cortisone therapy is ineffective in the pure adrenal form (owing to tumor), whereas surgery usually fails in cases of hyperplasia of pituitary origin. In such cases, removal of one adrenal produces compensatory hypertrophy of the other as a result of pituitary reaction, so that after a temporary and partial improvement following surgery, the syndrome of virilism develops anew, often with greater intensity than before (Botella[10]). In a few exceptionally severe cases, bilateral adrenalectomy may be attempted and the patient may be kept alive by means of corticoids and a salt diet, but this treatment seems to be unnecessarily drastic, particularly in view of the effectiveness of cortisone derivatives.

40.7.2. TREATMENT OF OVARIAN FORMS OF VIRILISM

Cases of *virilizing tumors of the ovary* (arrhenoblastomas, luteomas, Leydig cell tumors, etc.) can all be managed by *surgical therapy*. In the majority of cases, the tumors are unilateral and benign, in which case surgery may give spectacular results as far as the disappearance of hirsutism is concerned.

Cases of *nontumoral ovarian virilism* are equally susceptible to surgical management. Whereas according to Perloff[79] the symptomatology in the latter may improve with prednisone therapy, we have not been able to confirm this, and other ovarian hormones, advocated by Mellinger and Smith[70] do not give consistent results. These ovaries are difficult to modify in structure and function by any endocrine means. This is why various surgical procedures, of which wedge resection currently enjoys greatest popularity, have been proposed for the management of such dysfunctional ovaries.

Based on the premise that most of the hyperthecal and hilus cell proliferations are located in the central and hilar region of the ovary, we have developed the procedure called *ovarian demedullation* (1956) which consists of a central incision, made in the ovary down to the hilus, and electrocoagulation of all medullary and hilar structures. Afterwards the two halves of the ovary are sutured together in the same way as in a wedge resection.

The degree of virilism may reach quite variable proportions: from mild hypertrichosis in some cases to the striking virilism of the adrenogenital syndrome, there may be a whole range of imperceptible gradations. As noted previously, women have a physiologic tendency to undergo virilization and androgens are but a normal component of their endocrine balance. Therefore, *no exact limits can be set for what is yet normal and what has become pathological.* By the same token, evidently virile features in many women may go hand in hand with almost normal femininity. This is particularly true of modern woman who, despite her open tendency to imitate male usages and manners, keeps exerting her attraction to the full measure.

40.7.3. TREATMENT WITH ANTIANDROGENS

The antiandrogenic action of the progestogen derivative cyproterone acetate[87, 97] has been explained in Chapter 4. Its mode of action appears to consist in competing with testosterone at the target or end organ level (Neumann[74]). In experimental animals, at least, cyproterone in addition inhibits testosterone synthesis.[22, 36] This substance, which is still in an experimental testing stage, has not yet been fully applied to clinical use.

REFERENCES

1. Alexander, W. S., and Beresford, O. D.: *J. Obstet. Gynec. Brit. Emp.*, 60:252, 1953.
2. Allen, W. M., Hayward, S. J., and Pinto, A.: *J. Clin. Endocr.*, 10:54, 1950.
3. Audit, J., and Boussemart, E.: *Presse Med.*, 12:1112, 1954.
4. Azerad, E., Baulieu, E., and Jayle, M. F.: *Ann. d'Endocr.*, 14:505, 1953.
5. Bardin, C. W., and Lipsett, M. B.: *J. Clin. Invest.*, 45:891, 1967.
6. Benedict, P. H., et al.: *Fertil. Steril.*, 13:380, 1962.
7. Berger, L.: *Rev. Canad. Biol.*, 1:539, 1942.
8. Botella, J.: *Gynaecologia*, 133:80, 1952.
9. Botella, J.: *Arch. Gynäk.*, 183:73, 1953.
10. Botella, J.: *Encyclopedie Medico-Chirugicale, Gynecologie*, 146:D-10, 1957.
11. Botella, J., Tornero, M. C., and Fernández-Sánchez, L.: *Riv. Ost. Gin.*, 37:57, 121, 1955.
12. Bourg, R.: *Bruxelles Med.*, 34:1189, 1955.
13. Bradbury, J. T., and Slate, W. G.: *J. Clin. Endocr.*, 15:1291, 1955.
14. Callard, G. V., and Leathem, H. J.: *Proc. Soc. Exper. Biol. Med.*, 118:996, 1965.
15. Campbell, H. J.: *J. Physiol.*, 181:368, 1965.
16. DeCourt, J., Jayle, M. F., Crepy, O., and Judas, O.: *Ann. d'Endocr.*, 13:333, 589, 1952.
17. DeCourt, J., Jayle, M. F., Michard, J. P., and Baulieu, E.: *Ann. d'Endocr.*, 17:508, 1956.
18. Dignam, W. J., et al.: *Acta Endocr.*, 45:254, 1964.
19. Dogliotti, G. C., and Lacroix, L.: *Recenti Progr. Med. (Rome)*, 42:337, 1967.
20. Feder, H. H., Phoenix, C. H., and Young, W. C.: *J. Endocr.*, 34:131, 1966.
21. Ferriman, D., and Gallway, J. D.: *J. Clin. Endocr.*, 21:1440, 1961.
22. Forsberg, J. G., and Jacobson, D.: *J. Endocr.*, 44:461, 1969.
23. France, J., and Knox, B. S.: *Acta Endocr.*, 56:177, 1967.
24. Friedman, I. S., Mackles, A., and Daichman, I.: *J. Clin. Endocr.*, 15:1281, 1955.
25. Gilbert-Dreyfus, M., Zara, M., and Alexander, C.: *Sem. Hôp. (Paris)*, 27:32, 1398, 1951.
26. Gobel, P., and Teurer, G.; *Med. Welt (Stuttgart)*, 2:2268, 1968.
27. Gospodarovicz, D.: *Biochim. Biophys. Acta*, 100:618, 1965.
28. Goy, R. W., Bridson, W. E., and Young, W. C.: *J. Comp. Physiol. Psychol.*, 57:166, 1964.
29. Greenblatt, R. B. (ed.).: *The Hirsute Female*,

p. 211. Springfield, Ill., Charles C Thomas, 1963.
30. Greenblatt, R. B. (ed.): *The Hirsute Female*, p. 3. Springfield, Ill., Charles C Thomas, 1963.
31. Greenblatt, R. B., Dominguez, C. J., and Mahesh, V. B.: In *The Hirsute Female*, ed. R. B. Greenblatt. Springfield, Ill., Charles C Thomas, 1963.
32. Hamblen, E. C.: In *The Hirsute Female*, ed. R. B. Greenblatt. Springfield, Ill., Charles C Thomas, 1963.
33. Hamilton, J. B., and Terada, H.: In *The Hirsute Female*, ed. R. B. Greenblatt. Springfield, Ill., Charles C Thomas, 1963.
34. Harris, G. W., and Levine, S.: *J. Physiol.*, 181:379, 1965.
35. Hoffmann, F., and Meger, C.: *Geburtsh. u. Frauenhk.*, 25:1132, 1965.
36. Hoffman, W., and Breuer, H.: *Acta Endocr.*, 57:623, 1968.
37. Holmer, A. J. M.: *Acta Physiol. Pharmac. Neerl.*, 2:145, 1951.
38. Hooft, C., et al.: *Ann. d'Endocr.*, 17:1, 1956.
39. Horton, R., and Neisler, J.: *J. Clin. Endocr.*, 28:479, 1968.
40. Houssay, A. B., and Higgins, G. M.: *Proc. Staff. Meet. Mayo Clin.*, 26:323, 1951.
41. Ismail, A. A. A., Davidson, D. W., Kirkham, K. E., and Loraine, J. A.: *Acta Endocr.*, 61:283, 1969.
42. Jacobson, D., and Norgren, A.: *Acta Endocr.*, 49:453, 1965.
43. Jailer, J. W., Louchart, J., and Cahill, G. F.: *J. Clin. Invest.*, 31:880, 1952.
44. Jailer, J. W., and Van de Wiele, R. L.: *Gynaecologia*, 138:276, 1954.
45. Jailer, J. W., and Holub, D. A.: In *The Hirsute Female*, ed. R. B. Greenblatt. Springfield, Ill., Charles C Thomas, 1963.
46. James, V. H. T., Peart, W. S., and Iles, S. D.: *J. Endocr.*, 24:463, 1962.
47. Jayle, M. F.: *Ann. d'Endocr.*, 12:404, 1951.
48. Jayle, M. F., Crepy, O., DeCourt, J., and Baulieu, E.: *Ann. d'Endocr.*, 14:78, 1953.
49. Jeffcoate, S. L., Brooks, R. V., and London, D. R.: *J. Endocr.*, 42:213, 1968.
50. Jores, A.: *Ann. d'Endocr.*, 14:239, 1953.
51. Kincl, F. A., et al.: *Acta Endocr.*, 49:193, 1965.
52. Kirschner, M. A., Bardin, W. A., Hembree, W. C., and Ross, G. T.: *J. Clin. Endocr.*, 30:727, 1970.
53. Klotz, H. P.: *Ann. d'Endocr.*, 16:542, 1955.
54. Korenman, S. G., Kirschner, M. A., and Lipsett, M.: *J. Clin. Endocr. Metab.*, 25:798, 1965.
55. Koss, L. G., et al.: *Cancer*, 23:1245, 1969.
56. Kuppermann, H. S., et al.; *J. Clin. Endocr.*, 15:911, 1955.
57. Laitinen, O., and Pesonen, S.: *Acta Endocr.*, 50:254, 1965.
58. Lawrence, D. M.: *J. Obstet. Gynec. Brit. Comm.*, 75:922, 1968.
59. Levesque, J., et al.: *Ann. d'Endocr.*, 14:668, 1953.
60. Liddle, C. W.: In *The Hirsute Female*, ed. R. B. Greenblatt. Springfield, Ill., Charles C Thomas, 1963.
61. Lipsett, M. B., Kirschner, M. A., Wilson, H., and Bardin, W. A.: *J. Clin. Endocr.*, 30:336, 1970.
62. Lloyd, C. W., et al.: *J. Clin. Endocr.*, 23:413, 1963.
63. Lloyd, C. W.: In *The Hirsute Female*, ed. R. B. Greenblatt. Springfield, Ill., Charles C Thomas, 1963.
64. Lopez, J. M., Migeon, C. J., and Seegar-Jones, G.: *Amer. J. Obstet. Gynec.*, 98:749, 1967.
65. Louchart, J., and Jailer, J. W.: *Ann. d'Endocr.*, 14:97, 1953.
66. Lucis, O. J., et al.: *Canad. Med. Ass. J.*, 94:1, 1966.
67. Mahesh, V. B.: In *The Hirsute Female*, ed. R. B. Greenblatt. Springfield, Ill., Charles C Thomas, 1963.
68. Marañón, G.: *La Evolución de la Sexualidad y los Estados Intersexuales*. Madrid, Morata, 1927.
69. Maurer, H. J.: *Ztschr. f. Urol.*, 62:481, 1969.
70. Mellinger, R. C., and Smith, R. W.: *J. Clin. Endocr.*, 21:931, 1961.
71. Morrow, L. B., Thompson, R. J., and Mellinger, R. C.: *J. Clin. Endocr.*, 28:1756, 1956.
72. Netter, A., et al.: *Ann. d'Endocr.*, 15:559, 1954.
73. Neumann, F., Steinbeck, H., and Von Bernswordt-Wallrabe, R.: *Endokrinologie*, 52:54, 1967.
74. Neumann, F.: *Research in Reproduction*, ed. R. G. Edwards. Cambridge, Mass., Cambridge University Press, 2:3, 1970.
75. Novak, E. R.: In *The Hirsute Female*, ed. R. B. Greenblatt. Springfield, Ill., Charles C Thomas, 1963.
76. O'Malley, B. L., Lipsett, M. B., and Jackson, M. A.: *J. Clin. Endocr.*, 27:311, 1967.
77. Oakey, R. E., and Stitch, S. R.: *Acta Endocr.*, 58:407, 1968.
78. Oakey, R. E., and Beilby, J. O. W.: *Proc. Roy. Soc. Med.*, 62:40, 1969.
79. Perloff, W. H.: *J.A.M.A.*, 157:651, 1955.
80. Plate, W. P.: *Acta Endocr.*, 8:17, 1951.
81. Ponse, K.: *La fonction androgène de l'ovaire chez l'Animal*. Paris, Masson & Cie., 1955.
82. Radman, H. N., and Bhagavan, B. S.: *Amer. J. Obstet. Gynec.*, 106:1187, 1970.
83. Ramirez, D., and MacCann, S. M.: *Endocrinology*, 76:412, 1965.
84. Remouchamps, L., and Ghijsbrecht, P. F.: *Ann. d'Endocr.*, 15:229, 1954.
85. Rice, B. F., and Segaloff, A.: *Acta Endocr.*, 54:568, 1967.
86. Sachs, B. A., and Spiro, D.: *J. Clin. Endocr.*, 11:878, 1951.
87. Schneider, H. P., Staemmler, H. J., Sachs, L., and Schwarze, M.: *Arch. Gynäk.*, 206:64, 1968.
88. Scully, R. E.: *Amer. J. Obstet. Gynec.*, 65:1248, 1953.
89. Segaloff, A.: *J. Clin. Endocr.*, 15:142, 373, 1955.
90. Segre, E. J.: *Androgens, Virilization and the Hirsute Female*. Springfield, Ill., Charles C Thomas, 1967.
91. Sendrail, M., Gleizes, L., and Barraud, M.: *Ann. d'Endocr.*, 14:696, 1953.
92. Stein, A. A., et al.: *Amer. J. Obstet. Gynec.*, 86:360, 1963.
93. Swanson, H. E., and Van der Werff, J. J.: *Acta Endocr.*, 47:37, 1964.
94. Waugh, D., Venning, E. H., and MacEachern, D.: *J. Clin. Endocr.*, 9:486, 1949.
95. Westman, A.: *Acta Obstet. Gynec. Scand.*, 34:92, 1955.
96. Wilkins, L., Lewis, R. A., Klein, R., and Rosemberg, E.: *Bull. Johns Hopkins Hosp.*, 86:249, 1950.
97. Wollman, A. L., and Hamilton, J. B.: *Endocrinology*, 82:868, 1968.
98. Zander, J.: *J. d'Endocr. Clin. Nutr. Metab.*, 4:410, 1963.
99. Zellmaker, G. H.: *Acta Endocr.*, 46:571, 1964.

Part Ten
ENDOCRINE PATHOLOGY OF GESTATION

This part, dealing with the endocrine pathology of gestation, is perhaps the most incomplete section of the book. We are still very far from having mastered all hormonal aspects of infertility and abortion. Large gaps also remain in the endocrinologic study of toxemia of pregnancy, diabetes, and endocrine pathology of the mother and the newborn, and, no less important, a great deal still remains to be learned about those changes that can advance or delay labor, or that can induce pathologic alterations in milk secretion. These are all questions of great interest that have barely begun to be touched upon. At least a sketchy outline of each will be made in the chapters that follow. Among the first to be included here is the question of sterility. Since sterility involves pathology of fertilization, and since fertilization is the first act in gestation, we believe that Part Ten is the most suitable place to deal with the subject of *endocrine sterility*.

Chapter 41
ENDOCRINE FACTORS IN FEMALE STERILITY

A complete study of sterility exceeds the limits of this work. Nor can we engage here in any detailed analysis of the numerous related endocrine problems. Any one seeking more ample information is referred to our recent book on the subject.[19]

Our discussion has been divided into two parts: (1) *alterations affecting the endocrine glands*, and (2) *alterations affecting the end organs*. The first division may be further subdivided into ovarian factors and extraovarian factors, and the second division may be in turn divided into factors affecting the Fallopian tubes, factors affecting the endometrium and factors affecting the uterine cervix.

41.1. OVARIAN FACTORS

With regard to the problem of fertilization, the mammalian ovary fulfills *two fundamental missions:* (1) that of *providing fertilizable ova* and (2) that of *preparing the uterine bed for the nidation of the egg*. The ovary may therefore be the cause of sterility by either of the following mechanisms: (1) lack of ovulation, *(anovulatory cycle)*, or (2) insufficient progesterone secretion associated with a deficient nidation bed in the uterus *(progestational insufficiency)*. A number of other ovarian alterations may cause sterility, but in the final analysis these can always be traced to either of the above.

41.1.1. ANOVULATORY CYCLE

The term "anovulatory cycle" refers to any cycle associated with *periodic maturation of ovarian follicles but in which the follicles fail to rupture*. This is why no corpus luteum is formed and why every anovulatory cycle is also an *aluteal cycle*. Exceptionally, there may be an *aluteal ovulatory cycle*.[133, 135] It is furthermore suspected that the reverse situation may obtain, and that an unruptured follicle, that is, a follicle from which the ovule has not been extruded, may nevertheless undergo luteinization (see Chapter 32). Moreover, there are those certainly not rare instances in which ovulation takes place with the expulsion of a *sterile oocyte* from the ovary. But such cases may be the exception; most of the time, an aluteal cycle results from anovulation. The anovulatory cycle was studied in woman for the first time by Novak, but it had been described earlier in female monkeys by Hartman,[68] who had found that anovulation in these animals occurred as a normal physiologic mechanism during the summer months. In woman, as pointed out in Chapters 16 and 17, anovulatory cycles are a usual finding at puberty and during the climacterium. Consequently, there is a *physiologic anovulatory cycle* in woman both at the beginning and near the end of her sexual life. *We suspect, moreover, that physiologic periods of anovulation may occur in some*

893

TABLE 41-1. Incidence of Anovulatory Cycle in Sterile Women as Reported by Different Authors

AUTHOR	YEAR	CASES	ANOVULATORY CYCLES Number	Percentage
Mazer and Ziserman	1932	41	17	41.5
Anspach and Hoffman	1934	42	9	21.4
Bland et al.	1935	50	23	46.0
Jeffcoate	1935	63	16	25.4
Mazer and Israel	1936	109	36	33.0
Effkemann	1939	81	15	18.5
Westman	1939	85	2	2.4
Rock et al.	1939	392	36	9.1
Novak	1940	39	19	48.7
Griffith and MacBryde	1942	42	16	18.1
Sharman	1944	358	23	6.4
Halbrecht	1946	128	32	27.0
Scipiades	1948	100	8	8.0
Bergman	1950	231	12	5.2
Topkins	1953	402	0	0.0
Botella	1963	3000	794	26.4
Caballero et al.	1964	861	124	14.4
Prybora et al.	1968	—	—	16.0

*From Botella et al.: *Esterilidad e Infertilidad Humanas*. Barcelona, Editorial Cientifico-Médica, 1967.

women much in the same way that they do in female monkeys. The anovulatory cycle is therefore a common phenomenon straddling, so to say, the borderline between what is normal and what is pathological.

INCIDENCE. As reported by different authors, the incidence of anovulatory cycle in the human species varies considerably (see Table 41-1). Such discrepancies are largely justified by the following facts: (1) anovulatory cycles occur as a physiologic phenomenon at a certain age in life, as just specified, after puberty and before menopause; (2) anovulatory cycles alternating with normal cycles, referred to as "oligoovulatory cycles" by Garcia and coworkers, are of relatively common occurrence; (3) the estimated incidence varies necessarily according to the *exploratory methods employed* (in this respect, it must be pointed out that the presence of an anovulatory cycle can only be established with certainty by means of biopsy [to be discussed later], as well as by charting basal body temperatures for at least three months); and (4) many women revealing uniphasic endometria at biopsy are sterile for other reasons. Thus, among 2000 selected cases,[16] we found uniphasic patterns at biopsy in 27 per cent of the cases. However, after exploring the possible presence of other etiologic factors (Table 41-2), we saw that anovulation as the sole cause of sterility could be confirmed in only 10.5 per cent of the cases. Similar findings have been reported as a result of the recent investigations by Foss and associates[51] and by Noyes.[124]

ETIOLOGY. The *causative factors involved in producing ovulation* were already

TABLE 41-2. Anovulatory Cycle (542 Cases = 27.1%)

TYPE OF ENDOMETRIUM	CASES	%	COMPLETE STUDY	OTHER CAUSES	ANOVULATION ONLY	%
Simple proliferative	220	11.0	128	81	47	36
Hyperplastic	174	8.7	70	34	36	51
Hypoplastic	148	7.4	57	40	17	29.8
Total	542	27.1	255	155	100	39

Incidence of anovulatory cycle as the sole cause of sterility = 10.5 per cent.

examined in Chapter 12 (page 248). Recent reviews concerning the mechanism of ovulation and its failures[13, 19, 133, 172] are in agreement on the following principal factors:

Neurogenic. Ovulation has already been said to result essentially from LH release by the center regulating the cycle.[9, 11, 45, 59, 129] A breakdown in the function of the hypothalamic sex center causes anovulation. This is well known to be true in animals in which anesthesia of the hypothalamus (pentothal, reserpine, ganglioplegic drugs) produces anovulation. Various neurogenic or psychic alterations may be the cause of anovulation in the human species.[6, 19, 79, 100, 111, 157] We observed a case of an infertile woman who was able to conceive after successful surgical removal of a cerebral tumor, and we are aware of numerous cases in which an anovulatory cycle had been successfully treated with psychotherapy. In cooperation with Sanchez-Garrido,[141] we have investigated the kind of anovulatory cycle female monkeys develop in captivity, which has much in common with the psychogenic anovulatory cycle in woman.

Pituitary. Pituitary failure causing anovulation is almost always of hypothalamic functional origin, although *intrinsic alterations* in the gland involving changes in the FSH-LH ratio may also cause anovulation. Concerning the question of the physiologic ratio between FSH and LH, some interesting polemics are still in progress. Lostroh and Johnson[102] quoted a ratio of 1:1; Staemmler,[154] 2:1, and Van de Wiele and Turksoy,[170] 18:500. Obviously, such data are very unreliable, since there is no known preparation of FSH that would not at the same time contain some LH (see below).

Ovarian. Poor ovarian responsiveness can undoubtedly lead to failure to ovulate. Sopeña, among our group, has described the "adnexitic ovary" in which the tunica albuginea cannot be pierced owing to inflammatory fibrosis. Perhaps some similar situation is present in the Stein-Leventhal ovary.[61, 62] Meyer and Cochrane,[115] as well as Strassmann,[158] have indicated that *premature death of the oocyte* determined follicular atresia and inability of the follicle to rupture.

Androgens. In previous chapters in this book (see Chapters 4, 8, 16 and 29), androgens were said to determine the loss of hypothalamic cyclicity, particularly in newborn animals, so that the hypothalamus was noted to acquire a male character and ovulation failed to develop.[5, 92, 137] This is even more likely to happen in intrauterine life, so that intragravidic androgenization may cause *connatal anovulatory sterility*.[60, 171] This ought to be kept in mind particularly since many women are being exposed to a variety of more or less virilizing drugs (contraceptives, anabolizers, hormonal cancer therapy) whose effects may be exerted on a concomitant gestation, which may or may not have been discovered.

Hoffmann and Meger[74] were able to induce anovulatory cycles by injecting testosterone into human ovaries locally, while Korenman and his colleagues[97] found *increased* testosterone blood levels in patients with anovulatory cycles. Greenblatt[61] observed the occurrence of anovulatory cycles after prolonged androgen therapy, particularly in young women, and postulated that the same mechanism was involved in infertility owing to hypercorticism. In addition, Lucis and associates[103] noted increased 17-ketosteroid values in cases with anovulatory cycles.

Hypercorticism. Netter and colleagues,[122] Hochstaedt and Hanger,[73] and Zener[179] reported the occurrence of anovulatory cycles in association with the adrenogenital syndrome, in which there was moderate androgenism that responded in a striking manner to corticoid therapy. Those cases may well have been special instances of androgen-induced infertility, in which the androgens were of adrenal origin.

Hypothyroidism. The correlation between thyroid function and the ovarian follicle has been discussed previously (page 190). Severe hypothyroidism produces amenorrhea, hypogonadism and hypogenitalism, whereas moderate forms of hypothyroidism may be compatible with normal menses and normal genital development, with no major changes other than anovulation.

Diagnosis. The diagnosis of anovulation is one of the most difficult areas in the exploration of sterility and one of the most interesting challenges of modern day endocrine gynecology. The present discussion will be restricted to an outline of the problem. The interested reader is referred to some of the recent reports on the subject.[19, 25, 68, 127, 140, 172]

The presence of ovulation can be ascertained directly only by visual observation. All other means of verifying the occurrence of ovulation are in fact *indirect tests* that attempt to demonstrate the existence of a normal hormonal cycle, *which, rather than actually proving it, can only suggest the presence of ovulation.* The signs whereby ovulation is recognized may be divided into *sure signs of ovulation* and *presumptive signs of ovulation*, to which we may add a third group, *signs indicative of the moment of ovulation.*

Positive signs of ovulation are: (1) *Pregnancy.* Obviously, any woman who has achieved pregnancy must have ovulated. (2) *Direct visualization* of a corpus luteum with its ovulation stoma at laparotomy. Should there be a corpus luteum but no visible stoma, with the characteristic fibrinous plug, the corpus luteum may be assumed to have developed in the absence of ovulation. Though rare, this is possible. (3) Observation by means of *culdoscopy.* Palmer and Palmer[127] insist that ovulation may be seen by this method, something we have also been fortunate enough to observe in one instance.

Presumptive signs of ovulation are: (1) A *temperature curve* with an upswing halfway through the cycle, the first half consisting of a hypothermic phase, the second of a hyperthermic phase, particularly if the same pattern recurs in the same patient over a period of several months; (2) *the cyclic changes in the properties of cervical mucus,* the appearance of the characteristic *ferning phenomenon* and *stringiness* in the midcycle; (3) *changes in vaginal cytology,* involving the appearance of *folded cells* during the second half of the intermenstruum; (4) the results of *hormone assay,* especially if they reveal a rise in *pregnanediol* levels during the second half of the intermenstruum; (5) *microcurettage,* with the finding of typical *secretory phase* endometria during the second half of the cycle. Since all of the above methods have been described and analyzed in detail in Chapters 23 and 26, they will not be covered further here.

It is important to realize that all the foregoing methods at best prove the presence of two distinct phases in the cycle, an early follicular and a later luteal phase. More than on anything else, positive evidence of ovulation is based on the presence of a progestational reaction at the level of various end organs. The diagnosis of anovulation, on the other hand, is based on the absence of any progestational reactions in the endometrium, the cervix, the vagina, the recording of basal body temperature and the pattern of urinary pregnanediol excretion. Since it has been convincingly proved that in rare instances corpora lutea may occur without previous ovulation and, conversely, that ovulation may occur without the subsequent formation of any corpus luteum, *none of the above methods actually allows the presence or absence of ovulation to be asserted other than in terms of probability.*

To determine the moment of ovulation is also of interest. Among the previously mentioned methods, some enable us to assume that ovulation has or has not taken place, or that the corpus luteum has or has not been formed, but do not enable us to tell at what moment ovulation has occurred. *Only such methods as can be repeated almost daily may provide an idea about how the cycle progresses and consequently help pinpoint the exact time of ovulation.* Most important among these is the *basal body temperature determination,* which we use systematically. *Serial vaginal smears* may be equally helpful in determining the time of ovulation and so may, to a considerable extent, the study of *cervical mucus,* a method supported by Palmer and Palmer.[127] To these analytic methods must be added a clinical sign, which, when present, is of great value. In many instances, however, it is not present. We are referring to "intermenstrual" or *ovulation pain* ("Mittelschmerz" of the German authors).

TREATMENT. The treatment of anovulation is currently one of the most debated questions in sexual endocrinology. Many of our own ideas regarding this problem have changed in the course of the past few year. In the previous Spanish edition of this book, we expressed great skepticism. Today, the availability of either *human pituitary gonadotropin* or *ovulatory drugs,* as well as the experience acquired with *physical methods,* warrant a far more optimistic attitude.

A great many approaches have been proposed (Fig. 41–1), of which only a few will

Endocrine Factors in Female Sterility

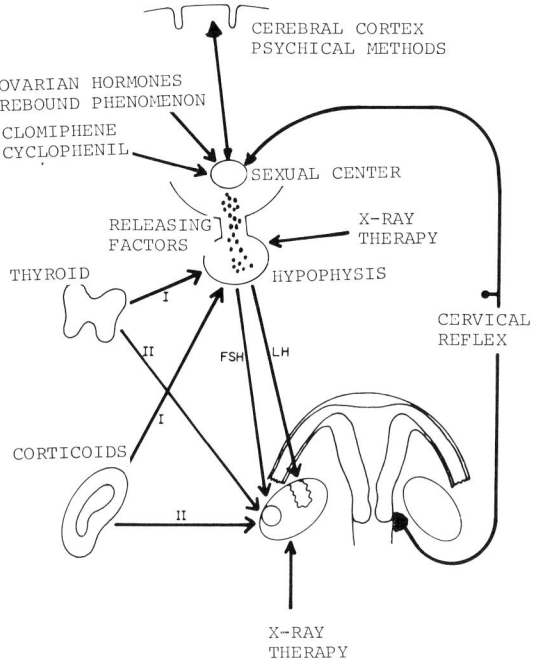

Figure 41–1. Basis for the different methods of treating anovulatory cycle. The sex center can be stimulated in a variety of ways: (1) through the cortex, by psychical methods (psychotherapy), (2) through the reflex of cervical dilatation or by coital stimulation, (3) through the sex hormones, particularly estrogens (feedback effect), (4) by drugs (clomiphene, cyclophenil). The releasing factors, which have already been partly synthesized by Schally and co-workers, may be expected to become effective stimulants of ovulation in the near future. Pituitary FSH and LH secretion may also be elicited by corticoid and thyroid hormone activity. The use of human gonadotropins (HMG and HPG) is also an effective form of *substitution* therapy. Finally, excitation radiotherapy of the pituitary or ovary, or both, is an empirical but nevertheless valuable method of therapy.

be mentioned here: (1) Ovarian hormones; (2) heterologous gonadotropins; (3) human gonadotropins; (4) ovulatory drugs; (5) radiotherapy; (6) surgery.

Ovarian hormones. *Estrogens in minimal doses stimulate ovulation.* Callantyne and associates,[29] as well as Goldzieher and his colleagues,[63] using dosages of 0.1 to 0.6 mcg per kg of body weight, achieved LH release by way of the hypothalamus. This hypothalamic action by estrogens was explained in Chapter 8 (page 149). There is more doubt as to whether the *abrupt intravenous administration of high dosages of conjugated estrogens* (Kuppermann et al.[99]) can produce ovulation. Our own experience, as well as that of Caballero and Hurtado[27] and of Klotz and Herrmann,[98] has in this respect been negative.

Estrogen-progesterone combinations applied by us and by Fern and Schlikker,[49] have proven an effective remedy whenever gonadotropins are not available; however, their usefulness has been eclipsed to a considerable degree during the last year.[58,61]

Heterologous gonadotropins. By this term we mean animal gonadotropins, specifically *pregnant mare serum*, which are known to elicit production of antigonadotropins (Chapter 6) which inactivate them. Results obtained have not lived up to our originally high expectations; this impression is shared by Zarrow and Quinn.[178] On the other hand, Dellepiane,[43] Moricard,[120] and Seegar-Jones and his coworkers[144] advocate their use. The conditions to be met regarding timing and dosage in order to avert antibody formation have been determined experimentally by Moore and Shelton.[117] Nevertheless, this method has been practically abandoned in favor of human gonadotropin therapy.

Human gonadotropins. Rapid development of *antibodies* whenever heterologous gonadotropins (PMS) are used and the slight or nonexistent ovulatory effect of HCG (see Chapter 19) have made it necessary to obtain human FSH from other sources. This has been achieved in two ways, either by extraction from *pituitaries of cadavers* (Gemzell et al.[57, 58]) or by extraction from the *urine of menopausal women* (Donini et al.[46]). The first substance is designated HPG (human pituitary gonadotropin) and the second, HMG (human menopausal gonadotropin). In the course of the last five years, the application of these substances has been highly successful and has revolutionized the treatment of not only the anovulatory cycle (Fig. 41–2) but also that of many forms of amenorrhea and even male infertility.[20, 105, 107] The last mentioned effect will not be treated here.

HPG has been employed mainly by Bettendorf[12, 13] in Germany and by its original proponent, Gemzell,[57, 58, 59] in Sweden. HMG has rapidly gained widespread acceptance because it is easier to obtain and is available in commercial preparations (Humegon, Pergonal). Donini and associates,[46] Pasetto and Montanino,[129] and Ingiulla[83] (Italy), Netter and associates[122, 139] (France), Lunenfeld and coworkers[104, 105] (Israel), Staemmler[154] (Ger-

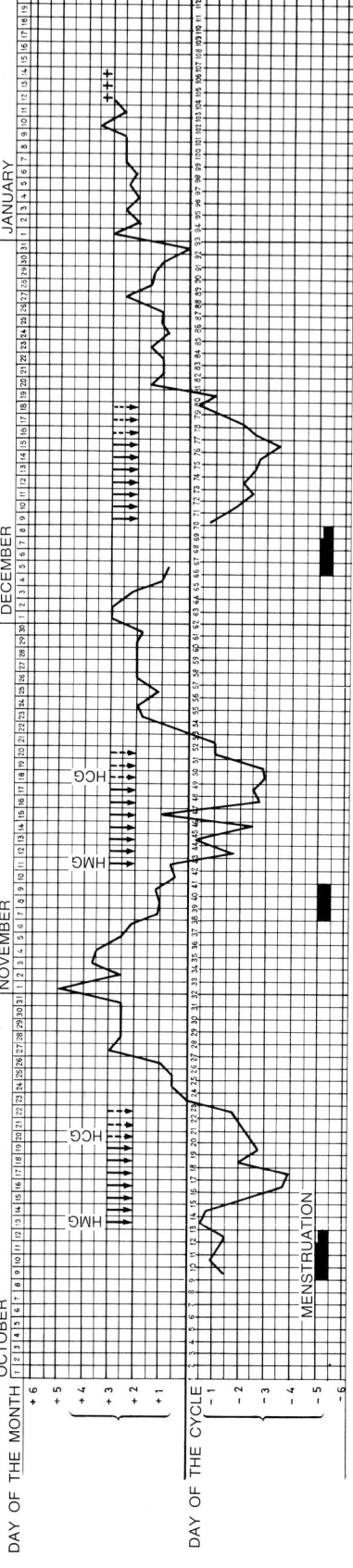

Figure 41–2. Treatment of anovulation with HMG (Pergonal, 1500 IU daily) for one week, followed by HCG (Primogonil, 5000 IU daily) for three more days. The results are biphasic temperature curves and gestation after three months of therapy (+++).

many), Buxton and colleagues,[26] Greenblatt and Seligman,[62] and Rosemberg and associates[136] (United States), as well as ourselves,[19, 20] in Spain, are by no means the only ones who have employed this medication. In the course of the past four years, our experience with this type of treatment has been greatly enriched.[55, 59, 64, 89] The wealth of statistical data by now runs into the thousands of cases. As far as dosages are concerned, there is still considerable controversy regarding the dangers of producing *ovarian cysts, polyovulation* and *multiple births.* Aside from cystification, we must mention a rather aggressive form of ovarian thickening, studied in detail by Friedrich and Getsch,[53] which develops in association with severe pain, ascites and an acute abdomen. The dose used by us is 500 IU daily for one week, followed by 1000 to 5000 IU of HCG daily during the thirteenth, fourteenth and fifteenth days. This dosage may be doubled so that up to 1000 IU per day may be administered in the course of one cycle, as is done by a number of authors, although it would seem to us that this may entail greater risks of exposing the patient to some of the previously mentioned side effects. The mechanism involved in polyovulation is related to the FSH/LH ratio of the preparation[101] and is therefore a problem of pharmacologic nature that has not yet been completely solved.

In order to avoid any such accidents, Ingiulla[83] advises the administration of a single dose of 7500 to 15,000 IU. He believes that the instant action by such an elevated dosage stimulates ovulation more energetically, without running the risk of causing the kind of cystification that is inherent in prolonged treatment.

It is of great importance that treatment in all cases be carried out under *strictly controlled conditions.*[13, 20, 59, 83, 84, 105, 109, 140, 153, 162, 164] Repeated urinary estrogen determinations are desirable and therapy should be discontinued as soon as any abnormal elevation is noted. We believe that systematic palpation of the ovaries, every four days, in conjunction with the examination of cervical mucus, allowing suspension of therapy with the immediate injection of CG whenever *the mucus becomes stringy and at the same time ovarian pain and adnexal swelling develop,* is a sufficient safeguard to prevent complications. In addition, Montalvo-Ruiz[116] advocates the use of *vaginal cytology* as an excellent diagnostic remedy.

Ovulatory drugs. The group of estrogens derived from chlortrianisene have already been described in Chapter 2. One such derivative, MER-25, which incidentally is also an anticholesterol agent, is able to stimulate both pituitary gonadotropin activity and ovulation (Tyler et al.,[166, 167] Kistner and Smith[94]). However, its effects are weak and uncertain. In 1961, Greenblatt[61] introduced a new drug related to the same family of compounds, clomiphene citrate, or MRL-41, which has potent gonadotropin and ovulatory activity. The formula of that compound and its kinship to both TACE and MER-25 have already been indicated in Figure 28-26 (page 625). Initial results reported by Greenblatt and associates,[61, 138] Riley and Evans,[134] and Whitelaw[173] were very encouraging. In the subsequent experience of a number of authors,[7, 62, 176] as well as our own, the drug has proved to be of great value in the treatment of anovulation (see Figs. 41-4 and 41-6). Johnson and his colleagues[86] have published a report on an extensive series of cases, including controls and placebos.

There are abundant recent statistics concerning the use of clomiphene. In a series of 25 cases with anovulatory infertility, Charles and his associates[32] induced secretory endometria in 21 (84 per cent) and pregnancy in 5 cases (20.8 per cent). Echt and his co-workers[47] stress the point that treatment must be carried on for a period of at least four cycles. In a recent report by Whitelaw and associates,[174] ovulation was achieved in 140 out of 203 cases (56.4 per cent), with 88 pregnancies and 67 term deliveries, although the incidence of abortion and prematurity was also high, amounting to 12 per cent.

The present trend is to use a combined treatment regimen with clomiphene and human menopausal gonadotropin (HMG); this view is supported by Kistner,[95] Mauvais-Jarvis and associates[112] and Rabau and co-workers.[132]

Dosages should be of the order of 25 mg tablets twice or three times daily from the first to the twelfth days of the cycle, for a total of 600 to 900 mg per cycle. Chorionic gonadotropin may also be administered in dosages previously indicated (Figs. 41-3 and 41-5).

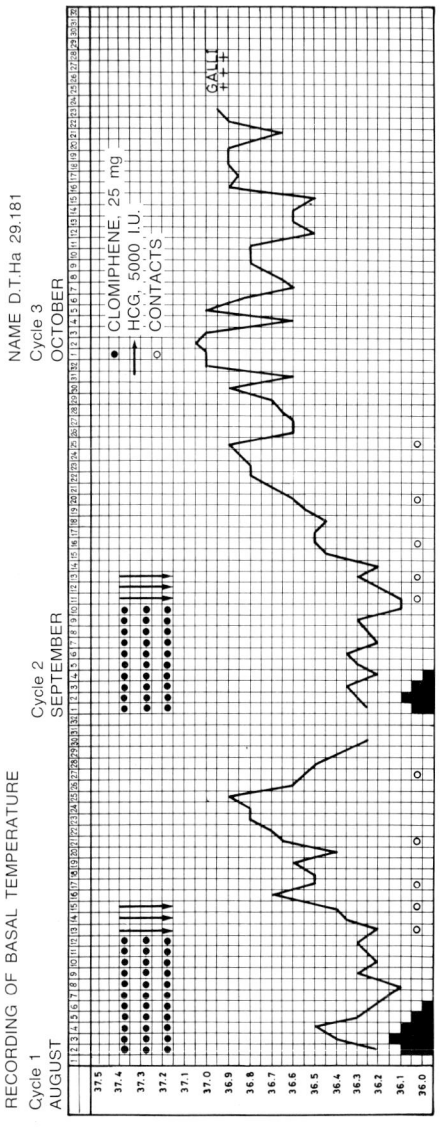

Figure 41–3. Treatment of infertility owing to anovulation by means of clomiphene and Primogonil (HCG). Over two consecutive cycles, three tablets of clomiphene citrate were given daily from the second to the twelfth days and from the first to the tenth days, inclusive. Clomiphene administration was followed up by 5000 IU HCG (Primogonil) for three days in each cycle. Pregnancy was achieved during the second cycle of therapy.

Endocrine Factors in Female Sterility

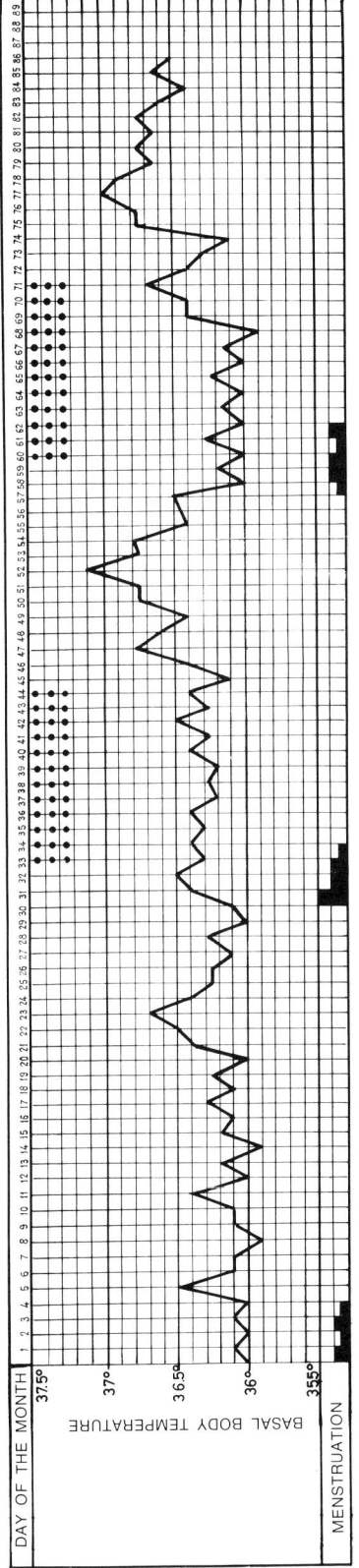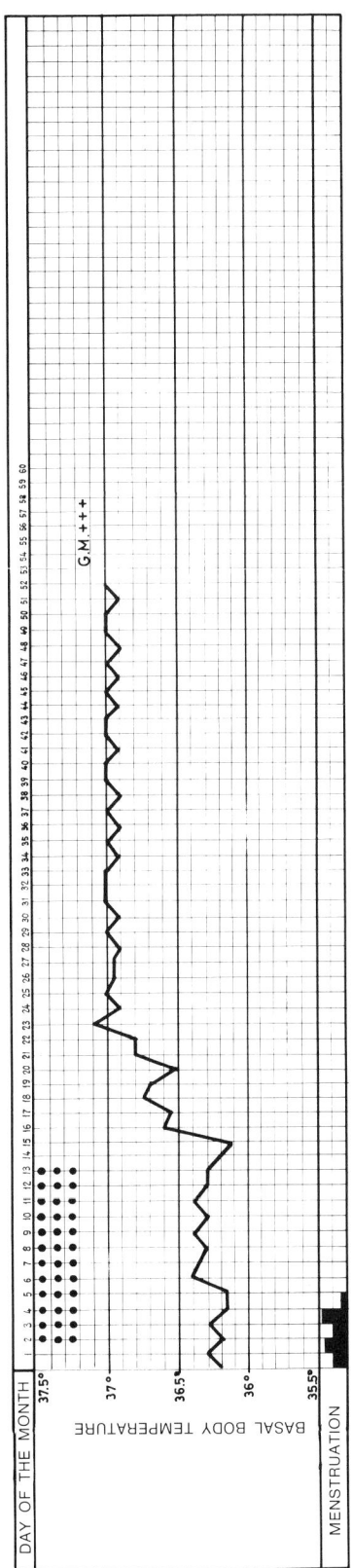

Figure 41-4. Treatment of infertility resulting from an anovulatory cycle with only clomiphene citrate, without associated chorionic gonadotropin administration. The routine followed consisted of 75 mg clomiphene (3 tablets) daily during 12 days of the cycle, beginning with the third day. Pregnancy was achieved after three cycles of therapy.

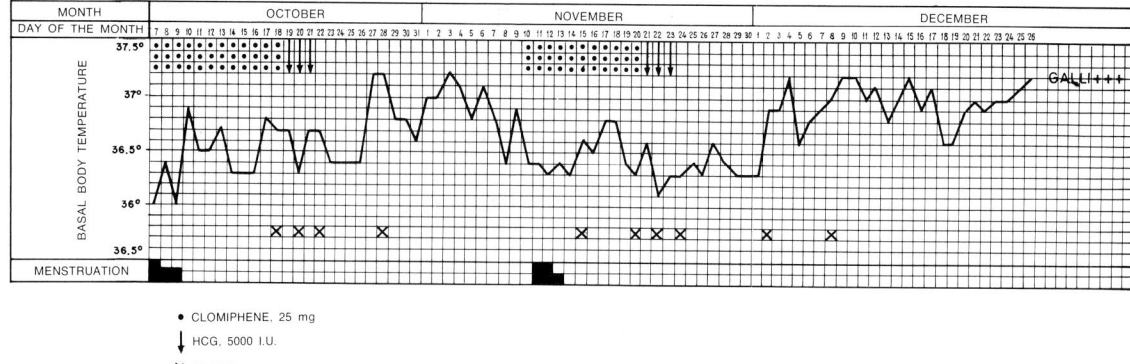

Figure 41–5. Infertility resulting from progestational insufficiency (deficient luteal phase). Therapy based on combined clomiphene and Primogonil administration, following the same routine as that outlined in Figure 41–3. Pregnancy was achieved during the second cycle of therapy.

The *mode of action* involved is open to question. While a local effect at the ovarian level has been invoked,[65, 114, 150] the study of gonadotropin excretion[9, 34] would seem to indicate that its principal effect consists in *promoting the release of gonadotropins.* It should be pointed out, moreover, that as far as the testes are concerned, they seem to exert an opposite, that is to say, a sterilizing, effect.[87]

A considerable amount of debate has ensued concerning the mode of action of clomiphene. There are many who believe that the effect of the latter is the result of gonadotropin release.[21, 85, 91, 143] We explored this question recently and reached the same conclusion.[37] In the opinion of other investigators, on the other hand, the drug is believed to exert a direct effect on the ovary. Carlstrom and Furujhelm[30] believe that clomiphene inactivates some of the enzymes involved in ovarian steroidogenesis. Engles and his associates,[48] on the contrary, believe that its effect on steroidogenesis is exerted by accelerating the androstendione-estradiol conversion rate. Along lines similar to those proposed by Carlstrom and Furujhelm, Dickey and his co-workers[44] in turn postulate an antiestrogenic mechanism. The same view is held by Hammerstein,[67] who maintains that its action is exerted by virtue of inhibiting ovarian steroidogenesis, thereby reducing progesterone synthesis and increasing LH release by a rebound or feedback mechanism. Finally, it should be mentioned that Ancla and De Brux[2] assume the effect of clomiphene to be exerted through the endometrium.

Other ovulatory drugs. Other agents that may also be listed among the drugs with ovulation-inducing potency are *copper salts* which, at least in animals,[72, 142] may precipitate ovulation. Cohen and Krulik[37] have employed cyclophenyl, a compound similar to clomiphene shown below, which is effective in doses of 200 to 400 mg per day. Gautray[56] advocates the use of nialamide in daily dosages of 100 mg in order to inhibit monoamine oxidase activity. This presumably involves an effect by way of the catecholamines, as indicated in Chapter 8 (Section 8.6.2).

Cyclophenyl

Excitation radiotherapy. If directed to the pituitary alone, excitation X-ray therapy usually does not produce any results. It is necessary to irradiate the ovaries as well, as is done at our clinic.[28] This is the method devised and introduced by Kaplan[88] a number of years ago and since used with excellent results at our clinic by Caballero and Hurtado[27] and, subsequently, by Palmer and Boury-Heyler[129] and Moore-White.[118] Despite some reservations generated by the studies on monkeys by Van Waagenen and Gardner,[169] no ill effects on the offspring in humans seem to have been demonstrated, although further experience is certainly necessary to provide a satis-

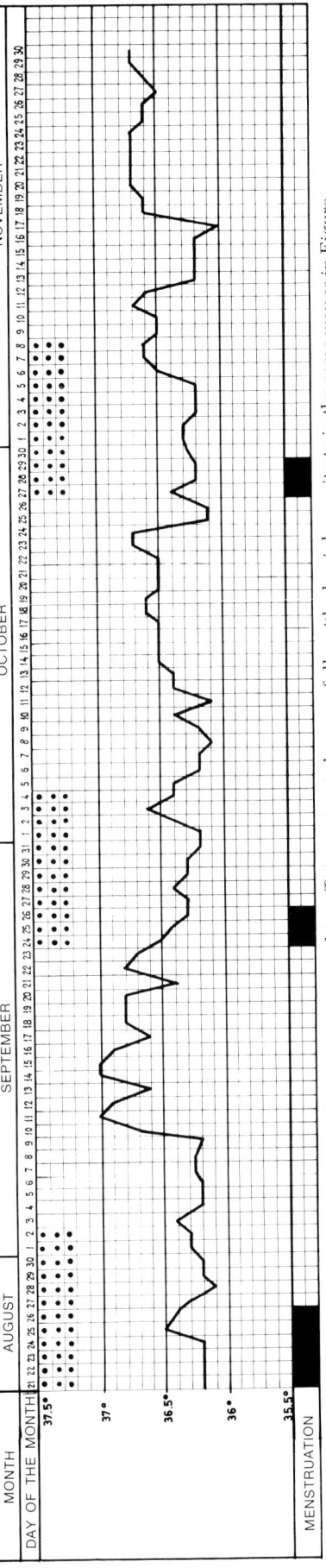

Figure 41-6. Infertility due to progestational insufficiency treated successfully with clomiphene citrate in the same way as in Figure 41-4 (without HCG). Patient became pregnant after three cycles of therapy.

factory answer to that question. Sexual contact must be avoided or mechanical contraceptive measures practiced before and during therapy in order to avert any incidental pregnancy that may result in possible adverse effects on the young embryo.

Surgery. Surgical management of anovulation is based on *ovarian wedge resection*, described previously as the treatment of choice for the Stein-Leventhal syndrome. Achari,[1] in India, recently reported magnificent results with wedge resection. This procedure is indicated mainly in the Stein-Leventhal syndrome and in anovulation owing to polycystic ovaries.

41.1.2. LUTEAL INSUFFICIENCY

The endocrinologic aspects in general of luteal insufficiency were studied in Chapter 29. This section is intended only to serve as a brief review of those aspects relevant to the problem of infertility.

The type of infertility resulting from anovulatory cycle and corpus luteum absence has been known for many years. Its cause is the absence of fertilizable ova. In such cases, the endometrium reveals a monophasic cycle with *persistent proliferation* up to the very time of menstrual shedding. Uterine abnormalities of this kind may play an equal role in absent nidation, but in this instance, because of anovulation, fertilization, and therefore nidation, does not occur.

THE IMPORTANT ROLE OF LUTEAL INSUFFICIENCY IN INFERTILITY. Simultaneously and independently in 1954, both Moricard[120] and Botella[15] called attention to the occurrence of anovulatory cycles with defective corpus luteum formation. After examining premenstrual endometrial biopsies from 3000 infertile women and performing histochemical studies on them in 1963, we were able to assess the real incidence of the *insufficient secretory phase in the endometrium* (see Table 41–3). This was found to amount to 6 per cent of all biopsies, an extraordinarily significant figure if one takes into account the fact that a considerable number of endometria diagnosed as possible anovulatory cycle are actually the result of secretory insufficiency, carried to the maximal degree possible, in the presence of ovulation.

Important statistical data on endometria with secretory insufficiency in infertility have in addition been published by Foss and colleagues[51] and by Noyes.[124]

In attempting to assess the practical implications of secretory endometrial insufficiency in causing infertility, it must be taken into consideration that, while occurring in many instances, there is no certainty as to whether this type of change is the actual cause of childlessness because of the possible concurrence of other factors that may be involved in causing infertility. Among the 3000 endometrial biopsies comprising the material examined, insufficient secretion was found in 182 cases (6 per cent), as shown in the table. Among the latter group, a complete study of both mates of the infertile marriages was conducted in 60 cases in accordance with the principle of minimal requirements (see Table 41–4). We found that only 25 of the 60 comprehensively studied cases (42 per cent) failed to reveal any cause of infertility other than progestational insufficiency. On the basis of simple arithmetic, this leads one to conclude that *2.5 per cent of all infertile couples fail to produce offspring because of luteal insufficiency and the associated lack of endometrial secretion.* This last figure differs somewhat from the one given in the preceding Spanish edition of this book, which quoted an incidence of 4 per cent. The fact that our present series is more comprehensive has allowed us to adjust our findings with greater accuracy.

DIAGNOSIS. The diagnosis of luteal insufficiency in sterile women may be arrived at by various methods. The principal

TABLE 41–3. Incidence of Progestational Insufficiency in Endometrial Biopsies from 3000 Sterile Women, According to Botella

TYPE OF ENDOMETRIUM	NUMBER OF CASES	PERCENTAGE
Secretory:		
Normal	1.351	45.03
Insufficient	182	6.06
Hyperplastic	119	3.96
Proliferative:		
Normal	303	10.10
Insufficient	221	7.36
Hyperplastic	270	9.00

Incidence of progestational insufficiency: 6.06 per cent.

TABLE 41-4. Cases of Progestational Insufficiency in Which Outside Factors Possibly Causing Infertility were Studied in Both Mates

NUMBER OF CASES STUDIED	MALE FACTORS	TUBAL FACTORS	CERVICAL AND UTERINE FACTORS	NO OTHER CAUSE FOR INFERTILITY
60	13 (21%)	7 (11%)	15 (25%)	25 (42%)

Incidence of progestational insufficiency: 6.06 per cent.
Corrected incidence of progestational insufficiency as the effective cause for infertility: 2.54 per cent.

and most reliable of all is *endometrial biopsy*. The evaluation of an endometrial biopsy must be based on more than simple histologic features. Although Moricard[120] set forth very precise criteria for the differentiation of the well developed secretory phase, and Ferin and Schlikker,[49] too, were able to describe in detail the effects of progesterone on the endometria of castrated women, Hughes and his associates,[80] Nogales[125] and Botella[18] have stressed the importance of histochemical studies of *glycogen* and *alkaline phosphatase* for the detection of corpus luteum insufficiency. The different forms of that type of insufficiency and their histologic and endocrine characteristics have already been described in Chapter 29. Luteal insufficiency may result from a shortening in the duration of the secretory phase, something that has recently also been recognized by Buxton.[25] The presence of a short secretory phase is confirmed histologically whenever a biopsy taken on the twenty-second or twenty-third day of the cycle still yields a postovulatory endometrial pattern that is characteristic of the seventeenth or eighteenth day. Abundant glycogen is present in the suprabasal portion of the cells, and there is pronounced alkaline phosphatase activity in the lumen of the glands. In some cases, the length of the luteal phase may be found to be within normal limits, but the endometrial mucosa itself reveals a pattern of poor secretory transformation; such conditions are characterized by *uterine glycopenia*, as described by Zondek and Rozin. Instances of the latter type may be recognized because, characteristically, there is moderate endometrial hyperplasia, with *signs of proliferation primarily in the glands and the stroma*, whereas the histochemical findings are those pertaining to a correct secretory phase.

Basal body temperature recordings have been used by Buxton and his colleagues[25, 26] as a means of determining the presence of either a short luteal phase or an insufficient luteal phase. The preceding author frequently found cycles apparently normal as to overall duration but in which the secretory phase was shortened owing to a delayed onset of the proliferative phase. Lastly, *vaginal cytology* as well as *pregnanediol* determinations may equally yield valuable data, although more of a complementary nature as compared to the preceding exploratory techniques, which are basic for the diagnosis of secretory phase insufficiency.

Over the past years, the significant role of luteal insufficiency in causing sterility has been recognized by many authors.[108, 119, 159]

TREATMENT. The most feasible form of therapy consists of progesterone administration during the second half of the cycle, either parenterally or, if synthetic progestogens are used, orally. The total dosage to be dispensed over a two weeks' period must be of the order of 250 to 400 mg. If the drug is given orally, as preferred by Bret and his co-workers,[22, 23] 10 to 15 mg daily will be necessary for the same period of two weeks. We have observed successful pregnancies in several cases of infertility due to corpus luteum insufficiency following repeated progesterone therapy.

Because of its importance in these cases, thyroid hormone therapy deserves special attention.[36, 40] To a certain extent, as pointed out previously (see Chapters 10 and 34), thyroid function seems to be involved in the induction of ovulation and in eventual luteinization. It is possible that the underlying cause of infertility in many hypothyroid women is an anovulatory cycle. However, in many instances, the presence of anovulation cannot be demonstrated and inability to conceive must be attributed directly to defective corpus luteum formation. The luteinizing effect by thyroid hormone in average dosages has been emphasized by various investigators.[25, 36, 40] Holland and his associates[76] believe that the effectiveness of thyroid hormone in infertility is related to its role in promoting implantation. It is our belief, therefore, that *thyroid hormone* can provide an effective means of treating those forms of infertility that are caused by luteal insufficiency.

As of late, special importance has been attached to the new oral progestins in the treatment of this form of infertility. Goldzieher and his associates[63] have employed norethisterone with good results, while Tyler and his co-workers,[167] as well as Bret and colleagues,[22, 23] reported favorable therapeutic results with norethynodrel.

In recent years, excellent results seem to have been obtained with the use of HPG (Gemzell,[59] Cooke et al.[39]), HMG (Botella et al,[19] Furujhelm et al.[55]) and clomiphene (Botella[20]). Compared to progestogen therapy, which is a mere form of *substitution therapy*, these compounds are thought to constitute a form of *stimulation therapy*.

LUTEAL INSUFFICIENCY AND EARLY ABORTION. In 1950, Hertig and Rock[70] focused attention on the interesting finding that many ova reaching the endometrial cavity implanted in a faulty way, thus turning into potentially abortive conceptuses destined to be eliminated during the next menstruation. In 1956, the same authors, in co-operation with Adams,[71] conducted histologic and histochemical studies on endometria associated with the phenomenon of defective implantation and noted that such endometria were poorly developed. In a recent report,[18] we have shown the existing relationship between habitual abortion, both in its earliest and in its later forms, and progestational endometrial insufficiency. Since these questions pertain to the study of abortion itself, they will be analyzed in detail in Chapter 42.

A great deal of modern experimental work[75, 151, 160] has demonstrated that implantation defects play a significant role in animal sterility.

It must then be reiterated here that secretory endometrial insufficiency may be the cause of defective nidation and eventual abortion.

41.1.3. OTHER OVARIAN FACTORS CAUSING INFERTILITY

There are many other pathologic conditions in which the cause of infertility resides in the ovary. For instance, tumors, ovarian aplasia, endometriosis, adhesions, etc. In fact, almost any kind of ovarian pathology may lead to infertility. However, what determines infertility is either lack of ovulation or, in the presence of ovulation, insufficiency of the subsequently formed corpus luteum. Consequently, we have only described the two preceding forms of ovarian sterility because, in the final analysis, all other forms boil down to either of these causes.

41.1.4. STERILITY DUE TO OVULAR LETHALITY

It has always been assumed that some forms of sterility might be due to *ovular defects*. However, such forms of sterility were indemonstrable, purely theoretical and were included among the admissible explanations for so-called "sterility without cause." Nonetheless, based on modern research in rabbits,[4] and mice,[106] as well as on indirect evidence in women,[148] the assumption seems justified that sterility is quite frequently caused by genetic aberrations in the oocyte which render it infertilizable.

41.2. EXTRAOVARIAN FACTORS IN INFERTILITY

Infertility may be caused by endocrine factors other than those pertaining to the genital apparatus. Obviously, *pituitary insufficiency* may cause infertility, although such forms are actually examples of the ovarian variety because they result from lack of ovarian function. Infertility may also be produced by hyperfunctional disorders of *the adrenal cortex*, as distinct from adrenal hypofunctional states, such as Addison's disease, in which the patient usually retains her fertility, often despite her poor general health. Outside the sexual sphere, the glands most often held to be involved in the etiology of infertility are the *thyroid*, the *pancreas* and the *adrenal*.

41.2.1. THYROID

The relationship between the thyroid and ovarian function and fertility was covered in Chapter 10. It would be impossible to summarize here the wealth of information published, above all in North America, concerning the relationship between thyroid function and sterility. Cole and Cassady[38] produced objective evidence that thyroid stimulation enhanced fertility in rodents. In addition, countless reports concerning human clinical experience have been published in which infertility has been successfully treated with only thyroid opotherapy (Buxton[25, 26]).

The mechanism of action involved is unknown, nor is there any certainty that the cases so treated were really cases of hypothyroidism. During the past years, Horne and Thibault,[77] Slater and associates,[149] and Tyler and colleagues,[167] have voiced some criticism concerning the use of thyroid hormone in infertility. Even successful therapy is not entirely immune to criticism, since one cannot be sure how many of the women who reported becoming pregnant after thyroid hormone therapy may not have overcome their infertility for other reasons. Incidentally, Danowsky[40] makes the point that most thyroid extracts are actually devoid of endocrine action.

41.2.2. PANCREAS

The relationship between the pancreas and fertility was discussed in Chapter 10, and related clinical aspects were dealt with in Chapter 34. Severe diabetes usually leads to infertility, though in most instances by producing abortion rather than sterility. Nevertheless, cases of infertility treated with insulin and cured once the diabetes was brought under control have been reported by various authors.[62, 90, 124]

41.2.3. ADRENAL

The occurrence of an "androgenic type of anovulatory cycle" and the mechanism whereby androgens impregnate the hypothalamus and paralyze ovulation have been explained previously. This occurs mainly in mild forms of the *adrenogenital syndrome.* Kiefer and associates,[93] Netter and colleagues,[122, 123] and Zener[179] have indicated that ovulation is suspended in mild cases of the adrenogenital syndrome but can be reestablished with adequate therapy. Timonen and his co-workers[165] have noted that the adrenogenital syndrome is associated with an effect on ovulation that results in suspension of the latter.

The fact that cortisone, prednisone and related compounds produce a favorable effect in infertility resulting from anovulation has been brought to light by Greenblatt and Seligman,[62] Hochstaedt and Langer,[73] Klotz and Herrmann,[98] and Klastersky and Herlant.[96] Similarly, Greenblatt and Seligman[62] relate a case of infertility in which the patient had two pregnancies following adrenalectomy.

41.3. ENDOCRINE CAUSES AFFECTING THE FALLOPIAN TUBES

Endocrine factors affecting the Fallopian tubes so as to cause sterility actually play a secondary role. The mission of the tubes in fertilization is twofold: first, transport of the ovum, that is, a *dynamic mission,* and second, nutrition of the ovum, that is, a *chemical mission.* Both kinds of function are under endocrine control. La Fuente,[54] at our laboratory, showed that tubal motility varied in the course of the cycle and was subject to the influence of the sex hormones.

Tanaka and Nakajo[163] have demonstrated the same function in birds. There is no doubt that either estrogen-progesterone imbalance or changes in oxytocin secretion may modify tubal motility and, hence, affect the processes of "capture" of the ovum and ovitransportation.

The *nutritional function of the tubes* is controlled by the sex hormones (see Chapters 3 and 19). The studies by Shettles[145, 146] brought to light a substance secreted by the tubes which was found to be indispensable for fertilization. By studying the effect of progesterone on the endosalpinx and on the ova floating in the tubal lumen by means of the electron microscope, Stegner and Wartenberg[155, 156] arrived at the conclusion that tubal secretory changes were induced by the action of progesterone. His findings were subsequently confirmed by Björkmann and Fredrickson.[14] As a result of their research on laboratory rodents, Chang and Bedford,[31] as well as Mastroianni and colleagues,[110] found that progesterone was necessary for ova not only for fertilization but also for sustaining their nutritional requirements during their journey through the tube. It should then be clear that progestational insufficiency of this type may be the cause of infertility not only at the uterine but also at the tubal level.

The question of *tubal spasms* as frequent causative agents in sterility deserves special comment. Their etiology is as yet unknown. Although apparently involving a phenomenon of hypermotility, our experience would indicate that tubal spasms do not occur in conditions of hyperestrinism but, on the contrary, under conditions of estrogenic insufficiency. We have been able to achieve remissions in the occurrence of tubal spasms in sterile women by means of estrogen therapy. The mechanism whereby estrogens are able to prevent the appearance of tubal spasms remains to be elucidated.

One further endometrial factor causing sterility, at least in the rat, has been recognized by Forster and associates[50] to involve immune rejection of some conceptuses on the part of the endometrium.

41.4. ENDOCRINE FACTORS IN ENDOMETRIAL STERILITY

Rather than sterility, endometrial pathology causes *infertility owing to lack of nidation*. From studies performed during the last few years, it has been learned that endocrine alterations, particularly those affecting estrogen-progesterone balance, may produce endometrial changes that render nidation impossible, thus causing apparent sterility in what, after all, are instances of *extremely early abortion*. This question has been examined in passing in Chapter 29, in connection with the subject of progestational insufficiency, and will be again discussed in Chapter 42, which deals with recurrent abortion.

Implantation takes place as a consequence of endometrial preparation by progesterone,[113, 115] which is illustrated by the fact that the number of blastocysts implanted in polyovulatory animals is proportional to the level of progesteronemia.[126] In those animals in which implantation is of the deferred type, implantation does not take place until progesterone reaches a certain level in the blood.[113] The entire process, however, is also dependent on the balanced participation of estrogens,[42, 131, 177] so that the presence of any undue preponderance of either estrogens or progesterone results in defective nidation and the death of the embryos.[34, 52] This means that balanced and concerted action by both ovarian hormones is necessary for the proper development of embryos upon reaching the uterus. Infertility of this type is produced in progestational insufficiency, in hyperestrinism and, in general, in all those disorders in which there is cyclic ovarian dysfunction.

In the human species, such minor disturbances are extremely difficult to assess although, on the other hand, certain *biochemical changes* affecting the endometrium are well known to be intimately related to nidation and, consequently, to infertility. Atkinson and Engle,[3] Botella,[15, 16] Galbis-Pascual and others have underscored the relationship between *alkaline glycerophosphatase* and implantation. In a similar way, Hughes and associates,[80, 81] Noyes[124] and Nogales[125] attach great importance to the presence of histochemically demonstrable *glycogen*. Finally, the important role played by *carbonic anhydrase* in nidation has been discussed in Chapter 3.

41.5. CERVICAL ENDOCRINE DISORDERS CAUSING INFERTILITY

In the course of the cycle, a series of changes occur in the cervical mucus which greatly facilitate the penetration of sperm. These changes have been summed up by Botella[15] and by Nogales[125] as follows:

Amount. The amount of mucus secreted and released at the cervical os is maximal at the moment of ovulation and minimal before and after menstruation.

Fluidity. At the critical moment of ovulation, the mucus is liquefied and its surface tension is minimal.

Stringiness. By stringiness, we understand the capacity of the mucus to be strung out into threads, a property reaching a peak at ovulation (Bergman and Lund[10]).

Crystallization. Rydberg showed that cervical mucus crystallized in the form of fern leaves, the ferning phenomenon being maximal at the time of ovulation.

Osmolality. The osmotic pressure measured by Bergman and Lund[10] was similarly found to be minimal at ovulation.

Chemical composition. The lipid-bound phosphorus content is minimal during the ovulatory phase; conversely, the mucopolysaccharide content is maximal (Beckenridge and Pommerenke[8]). Spectrographic studies on cervical mucus have enabled Shettles[147] to demonstrate that at the time of ovulation the rate of mucin hydrolysis is maximal and so is the liberation of sugars, principally glucose, mannose and galactose.

The time of maximal facility for penetration of sperm has been shown to be coincident with the moment at which these changes in the properties of cervical mucus are at their peak, precisely at ovulation. Thus, *all these changes develop in a gradual way so as to become most propitious for the upward migration of sperm by the fourteenth day of the cycle, after which conditions for spermatic penetration grow less and less favorable, concomitant with the retrogression of these properties of mucus.*

41.5.1. HORMONAL DETERMINATION OF THE CYCLIC CHANGES OF CERVICAL MUCUS

The question of which are the hormonal determinants involved in the changes of cervical mucus has been a matter of considerable debate. Moricard[121] and Hamilton[66] showed that *estrogens increased the fluidity and stringiness, as well as the sugar content, of cervical mucus*. Roland[135] and Cohen and Rubenstein[35] similarly found that *the ferning phenomenon pertaining to mucus crystallization was enhanced by estrogens*. The role played by progesterone, however, appears to be less clear. That hormone had not been believed to affect mucus crystallization and stringiness although, in that case, it could not be understood why the changes in mucus crystallization and stringiness should regress after ovulation, in view of the fact that estrogen levels increased throughout the cycle until menstruation, without declining after ovulation. Urdan and Kurzon[168] produced evidence to the effect that progesterone exerted an *inhibitory effect* on cervical crystallization. Botella, Nogales and Domínguez-Adame studied the action by the sex hormones on the uterine cervix of women who had undergone subtotal hysterectomy with removal of both adnexa, thus becoming castrated. After a period of one month or longer following castration, regressive and atrophic changes were observed to ensue in the cervical mucosa, while the cervical mucus lost its capacity for stringing out and for crystallization. Estradiol benzoate, injected in dosages of 10 to 25 mg, provoked notable increases in the ferning phenomenon, in stringiness and in the amount of mucus secreted. The administration of progesterone alone failed to produce any effect, while the administration of a mixture of progesterone with estrogen in proportions similar to those in which they occur in the cycle inhibited crystallization completely. *This means that progesterone not only lacks a positive effect on crystallization, stringiness and amount of mucus but also completely and efficiently inhibits the effect of estrogens.* How important these changes in the properties of mucus are in relation to the endocrinologic symptomatology of woman has been indicated in Chapter 23. At this point, we must insist on the ease with which hormonal changes may lead to the cervical form of sterility.

41.5.2. CERVICAL FORM OF STERILITY RESULTING FROM HYPOESTRINISM

Because it determines a decrease in the amount and effectiveness of cervical mucus, hypoestrinism may cause the cervical mucous plug to become impermeable to spermatozoa and, thereby, prevent fertilization. Palmer and Palmer[127] had called attention to the possibility of successfully treating cervical infertility with estrogens. Nevertheless, it must be recognized that endocrine cervical factors alone cannot determine lack of progeny unless occurring in conjunction with male factors (Botella et al.,[19] Williams[175]). *Therefore, it must be admitted that hypoestrinism, either through defective secretion of cervical mucus or through the production of mucus that is poor in quality, may cause infertility in a couple in which the male exhibits subfertility. In the presence of male sperm of high fertilizing quality, on the other hand, it is unlikely that the characteristics of the mucus alone can completely prevent spermatic ascent and fertilization.*

41.5.3. TREATMENT

Treatment of cervical forms of infertility should be based on *estrogen administra-*

tion. Whenever favorable results are obtained with continued estrogen therapy in sterile women with no other detectable cause for sterility, it may be assumed that a cervical factor is involved.

41.5.4. PROSTAGLANDINS

The mechanism of spermatic ascent through the cervical passage[19] has long been the object of inquiry. Many authors[19, 102, 127] assume that *active* ascent is facilitated by postcoital contraction of the uterus. Ingelman-Sundberg[82] have called attention to substances of prostatic origin which accompany the semen and are thought to be absorbed and to provoke contractions of the uterine cervix and cervical musculature. Their effects on the contractions of the uterus and oviduct were studied by Horton and his associates[78] in rabbits, and by Hartman[69] in monkeys. Their oxytocin-like properties have been tested on isolated rat uteri[161] as well as on human uteri.[82] Prostaglandins would thus seem to be a *new endocrine factor*, believed to partake in human fertilization in an important way.

REFERENCES

1. Achari, K.: *J. Obstet. Gynec. India*, 17:551, 1967.
2. Ancla, M., and De Brux, J.: *Amer. J. Obstet. Gynec.*, 98:1043, 1967.
3. Atkinson, W. B., and Engle, E. T.: *Menstruation and Its Disorders*, ed. E. T. Engle. Springfield, Ill., Charles C Thomas, 1950.
4. Austin, C. R.: *Nature*, 313:1018, 1967.
5. Barraclough, C. A.: *Endocrinology*, 68:62, 1961.
6. Bass, F.: *Gynaecologia*, 123:211, 1947.
7. Beck, P., Grayzel, E. F., Young, I. S., and Kupperman, H. S.: *Obstet. Gynec.*, 27:54, 1966.
8. Beckenridge, A. M. B., and Pommerenke, W. T.: *Fertil. Steril.*, 2:541, 1951.
9. Bell, E. T., and Loraine, J. A.: *Lancet*, 2:626, 1966.
10. Bergman, P., and Lund, G. G.: *Acta Obstet. Gynec. Scand.*, 30:267, 1951.
11. Bettendorf, G.: *Internat. J. Fertil.*, 8:799, 1963.
12. Bettendorf, G.: *Internat. J. Fertil.*, 9:351, 1964.
13. Bettendorf, G.: *Arch. Gynäk.*, 202:132, 1965.
14. Björkmann, N., and Fredrickson, B.: *Internat. J. Fertil.*, 7:259, 1962.
15. Botella, J.: *Acta Gin.*, 10:317, 1959.
16. Botella, J.: *Internat. J. Fertil.*, 4:300, 1959.
17. Botella, J.: *Rev. Fr. Endocr. Clinique Nutr. Metab.*, 4:397, 1963.
18. Botella, J.: *Acta Gin.*, 15:3, 1964.
19. Botella, J., Caballero, A., Clavero, J. A., and Vilar, E.: *Esterilidad e Infertilidad Humanas*. Barcelona, Editorial Científico-Médica, 1967.
20. Botella, J.: *Actas Soc. Esp. Est. Infert.*, 11:237, 365, 1967.
21. Boyar, R. M.: *Endocrinology*, 86:629, 1970.
22. Bret, A. J., and Simon, S.: *Rev. Fr. Gynec. Obstet.*, 58:61, 1963.
23. Bret, A. J., and Coiffard, P.: *Rev. Fr. Gynec. Obstet.*, 58:91, 1963.
24. Butcher, R. L., Blue, J. D., and Fugo, N. W.: *Fertil. Steril.*, 20:223, 1969.
25. Buxton, C. L.: *Med. Clin. North Amer.*, 36:705, 1952.
26. Buxton, C. L., Kase, N., and Van Orde, D.: *Amer. J. Obstet. Gynec.*, 87:773, 1963.
27. Caballero, A., and Hurtado, E.: *Rev. Fr. Gynec. Obstet.*, 58:289, 1963.
28. Caballero, A., *Actas Soc. Esp. Infert. Ester.*, 11:24, 1967.
29. Callantyne, M. R., Humphrey, R. R., and Nesset, B. L.: *Endocrinology*, 79:455, 1966.
30. Carlstrom, K., and Furujhelm, M.: *Acta Obstet. Gynec. Scand.*, Suppl. 3, 48:35, 1969.
31. Chang, M. C., and Bedford, J. M.: *Fertil. Steril.*, 13:421, 1962.
32. Charles, D., Loraine, J. A., Bell, E. T., and Harkness, R. A.: *Fertil. Steril.*, 17:351, 1966.
33. Clavero, J. A., Cremades, J., Sanchez-Rivera, G., Merlo, J. G., Pereira, A., and Botella, J.: *Acta Gin.*, 20:907, 1969.
34. Cochrane, R. L., Prasad, M. R. N., and Meyer, R. K.: *Endocrinology*, 70:228, 1962.
35. Cohen, M. R., and Rubenstein, B. B.: *Proc. Inst. Med. (Chicago)*, 14:369, 1943.
36. Cohen, M. R., Stein, I. F., and Kaye, B. H.: *Fertil. Steril.*, 3:201, 1952.
37. Cohen, J., and Krulik, D.: "L'induction de l'ovulation par le cyclophenyl," in *L'ovulation*, ed. R. Moricard and J. Ferin. Paris, Masson et Cie., 1969.
38. Cole, H. H., and Cassady, R. B.: *Endocrinology*, 49:119, 1947.
39. Cooke, A. C., Butt, W. R., and Bertrand, P. T.: *Lancet*, 2:514, 1966.
40. Danowsky, T. S.: *J. Clin. Endocr.*, 12:1572, 1952.
41. Davidson, O. W., Wada, K., and Segal, S. J.: *Fertil. Steril.*, 16:195, 1965.
42. Deanesly, R.: *J. Reprod. Fertil.*, 5:49, 1963.
43. Dellepiane, G.: *Proceed. II World Congress Fertil. & Steril.*, Vol. I, p. 128, Naples, 1956.
44. Dickey, R. P., Vorys, N., Stevens, V. C., Besch, P. K., Hamwi, G. J., and Ullery, J. C.: *Fertil. Steril.*, 16:485, 1965.
45. Diczfalusy, E., et al.: *Acta Endocr. Suppl.*, 90:35, 1964.
46. Donini, P., Puzzoli, D., and D'Alessio, I.: *Actas Soc. Esp. Infert. Ester.*, 11:17, 1967.
47. Echt, C. R., Romberger, F. T., and Goodman, J. A.: *Fertil. Steril.*, 20:564, 1969.
48. Engles, J. A., Friedlander, R. L., and Eik-Nes, K. B.: *Metabolism*, 17:189, 1968.
49. Ferin, J., and Schlikker, E.: *Internat. J. Fertil.*, 5:19, 1960.
50. Forster, O., Friedrich, F., Holzner, H., and Krachtowill, A.: *Ztschr. f. Geb. u. Gyn.*, 170:47, 1969.
51. Foss, D. A., Horne, W., and Hertig, A. T.: *Fertil. Steril.*, 9:193, 1958.
52. Fowler, R. E., and Edwards, R. D.: *J. Endocr.*, 20:1, 1960.
53. Friedrich, F., and Gitsch, E.: *Wien. Klin. Wschr.*, 81:318, 1969.

54. Fuente, F. de la, and Botella, J.: *Acta Endocrinologica et Gynecologica Hispano-Lusitana*, 2:62, 1949.
55. Furujhelm, M., Lunell, N. O., and Odeblad, E.: *Acta Obstet. Gynec. Scand.*, 45:63, 1966.
56. Gautray, J. P.: "Perspective neuroendocrines dans le traitement des troubles de l'ovulation," in *L'ovulation*, ed. R. Moricard and J. Ferin. Paris, Masson et Cie., 1969.
57. Gemzell, C. A., Roos, P., and Loeffler, F. E.: *J. Reprod. Fertil.*, 12:49, 1966.
58. Gemzell, C. A.: *Fertil. Steril.*, 17:149, 1966.
59. Gemzell, C. A.: *Acta Obstet. Gynec. Scand.*, Suppl. 1, 48:17, 1969.
60. Goy, R. W., Bridson, W. E., and Young, W. C.: *J. Comp. Physiol. Psychol.*, 57:166, 1964.
61. Greenblatt, R. B.: *Fertil. Steril.*, 12:402, 1961.
62. Greenblatt, R. B., and Seligman, R.: *Fertil. Steril.*, 14:208, 1963.
63. Goldzieher, J. W., Peterson, W. F., and Galbert, R. A.: *Ann. N.Y. Acad. Sci.*, 71:722, 1958.
64. Hamberger, L. L. A.: *Acta Physiol. Scand.*, 74:410, 1968.
65. Hagerman, D. D., Smith, O. W., and Day, C. F.: *Acta Endocr.*, 51:591, 1966.
66. Hamilton, C. F.: *Contrib. Embryol.*, 33:213, 1949.
67. Hammerstein, J.: *Acta Endocr.*, 60:635, 1969.
68. Hartman, C. G.: *Science and the Safe Period*. Baltimore, William & Wilkins, 1962.
69. Hartman, C. G.: *Fertil. Steril.*, 12:1, 1961.
70. Hertig, A. T., and Rock, J.: In *Menstruation and its Disorders*, ed. E. T. Engle. Springfield, Ill., Charles C Thomas, 1950.
71. Hertig, A. T., Rock, J., and Adams, E. C.: *Amer. J. Obstet. Gynec.*, 68:435, 1956.
72. Hiroi, M., Sugita, S., and Suzuki, M.: *Endocrinology*, 77:963, 1965.
73. Hochstaedt, B., and Langer, G.: *Gynaecologia*, 151:287, 1961.
74. Hoffmann, F., and Meger, C.: *Geburtsh. u. Frauenhk.*, 25:1132, 1965.
75. Holkomb, L. C.: *Ohio St. J. Sc.*, 67:24, 1967.
76. Holland, J. P., Dorsey, J. M., Harris, G. W., and Johnson, F. L.: *J. Reprod. Fertil.*, 14:81, 1967.
77. Horne, H. W., and Thibault, J. P.: *Internat. J. Fertil.*, 6:385, 1961.
78. Horton, E. W., Main, I. H. M., and Thompson, C. J.: *J. Physiol.*, 180:514, 1965.
79. Horwalth, H., Sellei, C., and Weiss, R.: *Gynaecologia*, 125;368, 1948.
80. Hughes, E. C., Ness, A. W., and Lloyd, C. O.: *Amer. J. Obst. & Gyn.*, 50:1295, 1950.
81. Hughes, E. C., Jacobs, R. D., and Rubulis, A.: *Amer. J. Obstet. Gynec.*, 89:59, 1964.
82. Ingelman-Sundberg, A.: *Proceed. VI World Congr. Fertil. Steril.*, Stockholm, 1965.
82. Ingiulla, W.: *Actas Soc. Esp. Est. Fertil. Ester.*, 11:161, 1967.
84. Insler, V., Melmed, H., and Mashiah, S.: *Obstet. Gynec.*, 32:620, 1969.
85. Jacobson, A., Marshall, J. R., and Ross, G. T.: *Amer. J. Obstet. Gynec.*, 101:1025, 1968.
86. Johnson, J. A., et al.: *Internat. J. Fertil.*, 11:265, 1966.
87. Kalra, S. P., and Prasad, R. N.: *Endocrinology*, 81:965, 1967.
88. Kaplan, I. I.: *Amer. J. Obstet. Gynec.*, 76:447, 1958.
89. Kase, N., Mroueh, A., and Buxton, C. L.: *Amer. J. Obstet. Gynec.*, 100:176, 1968.
90. Kaufman, R. H., Abbott, J. P., and Wall, J. A.: *Amer. J. Obstet. Gynec.*, 76:1271, 1959.
91. Keller, P. J., Naville, A. H., and Wyss, H. I.: *Fertil. Steril.*, 19:892, 1968.
92. Kennedy, G. C.: *J. Physiol.*, 172:393, 1964.
93. Kiefer, J. H., Rosenthal, I. M., and Bronstein, J. P.: *J. Clin. Endocr.*, 15:154, 1955.
94. Kistner, R. W., and Smith, O. W.: *Fertil. Steril.*, 12:121, 1961.
95. Kistner, R. W.: *Fertil. Steril.*, 17:569, 1966.
96. Klastersky, J., and Herlant, M.: *Ann. d'Endocr.*, 28:127, 1967.
97. Korenman, S. G., Lipsett, M., and Kirschner, M. A.: *J. Clin. Endocr., Metab.*, 25:798, 1965.
98. Kotz, H. L., and Herrmann, W.: *Fertil. Steril.*, 12:299, 375, 1961.
99. Kuppermann, H. S., Epstein, J. A., and Blatt, M. H. G.: *Fertil. Steril.*, 9:26, 1958.
100. Ladowsky, W.: *Endokrinologie*, 52:259, 1967.
101. Lin, T. P., and Bailey, D. W.: *J. Reprod. Fertil.*, 10:253, 1965.
102. Lostroh, A. J., and Johnson, R. E.: *Endocrinology*, 79:991, 1966.
103. Lucis, O. J., Hobkirk, R., Mohllenberg, C. H., MacDonald, S. A., and Blahey, P.: *Canad. Med. Ass. J.*, 94:1, 1966.
104. Lunenfeld, B.: *Gynec. Obstet.*, 65:553, 1966.
105. Lunenfeld, B., Rabau, E., and Insler, V.: *Actas Soc. Esp. Est. Fertil.*, 11:43, 1967.
106. MacGaughey, R. W., and Chang, M. C.: *J. Exper. Zool.*, 170:397, 1967.
107. Mancini, E.: *Actas Soc. Esp. Fertil. Ester.*, 11:65, 1967.
108. Mantalenkis, S. J., and Danezis, J. M.: *Fertil Steril.*, 20:340, 1969.
109. Marshall, J. R., Jacobson, A., and Hammond, C. B.: *J. Clin. Endocr.*, 29:106, 1969.
110. Mastroianni, R., Baer, F., Shah, V., and Cleve, T. H.: *Endocrinology*, 68:92, 1961.
111. Matsumoto, S., Igarashi, M., and Nagaoka, Y.: *Internat. J. Fertil.*, 13:15, 1968.
112. Mauvais-Jarvis, P., Ghnassia, J. P., Dolais, J., and Rosselin, G.: In *L'ovulation*, ed. R. Moricard and J. Ferin. Paris, Masson et Cie., 1969.
113. Mayer, G.: *Ann. d'Endocr.*, 21:501, 1960.
114. Mayfield, J. D., and Ward, D. N.: *Acta Endocr.*, 51:557, 1966.
115. Meyer, R. K., and Cochrane, R. L.: *J. Endocr.*, 24:77, 1962.
116. Montalvo-Ruiz, L.: *Actas Soc. Esp. Fertil. Ester.*, 11:223, 1967.
117. Moore, W. W., and Shelton, J. N.: *Nature*, 198:1284, 1962.
118. Moore-White, M.: *Internat. J. Fertil.*, 14:309, 1969.
119. Moraes-Ruehsen, M., Seegar-Jones, G., Burnett, L. S., and Bamaki, T. A.: *Amer. J. Obst. & Gyn.*, 1970.
120. Moricard, R.: *Collogues sur la fonction luteale*, 1:185. Paris, Masson et Cie., 1954.
121. Moricard, R.: *Proceed. III World Congress Fertil. Steril.*, 1959.
122. Netter, A., Salomon, Y. V., and Cabau, A.: *Ann. d'Endocr.*, 27:52, 1966.
123. Netter, A., and Menage, J. J.: "Glucocorticoides et ovulation," in *L'ovulation*, ed. R. Moricard and J. Ferin. Paris, Masson et Cie, 1969.
124. Noyes, R. W.: *Amer. J. Obstet. Gynec.*, 77:929, 1959.
125. Nogales, F.: *Acta Gin.*, 15:427, 1964.

126. Orsini, M. W., and Meyer, R. K.: *Proc. Soc. Exper. Biol. Med.*, 110:713, 1962.
127. Palmer, R., and Palmer, E.: *Les explorations fonctionelles gynecologigues*. Paris, Masson et Cie, 1963.
128. Palmer, R., and Boury-Heyler, C.: In *L'ovulation*, ed. R. Moricard and J. Ferin. Paris, Masson et Cie., 1969.
129. Pasetto, N., and Montanino, G.: *Fertil. Steril.*, 18:685, 1967.
130. Prybora, L., Baron, J., Kuczynski, J., and Kerzya, H.: *Endokr. Polska*, 19:491, 1968.
131. Psychoyos, R.: *Compt. Rend. Acad. Sci. (Paris)*, 253:1616, 1961.
132. Rabau, E., Masiach, S., Serr, D. M., and Melmed, H.: *Obstet. Gynec.*, 31:110, 1968.
133. Rennels, E. G., and O'Steen, W. K.: *Endocrinology*, 80:82, 1967.
134. Riley, G. M., and Evans, T. N.: *Amer. J. Obstet. Gynec.*, 89:97, 1964.
135. Roland, M.: *Amer. J. Obstet. Gynec.*, 63:81, 1952.
136. Rosemberg, E., Coleman, J., and Garcia, C. R.: *J. Clin. Endocr.*, 23:181, 1963.
137. Rosner, J., Pomeau-Delille, G., Tramezzani, J. H., and Cardinali, D.: *Compt. Rend. Acad. Sci. (Paris)*, 261:1113, 1965.
138. Roy, S., Greenblatt, R. B., Mahesh, V. B., and Jungck, E. C.: *Fertil. Steril.*, 14:575, 1963.
139. Salomon-Bernard, Y., Millet, D., and Netter, A.: *Ann. d'Endocr.*, 28:315, 1969.
140. Salvatierra, V.: *Actas Soc. Esp. Fertil. Ester.*, 11:27, 1967.
141. Sanchez-Garrido, F., and Botella, J.: *Acta Gin.*, 21:553, 1970.
142. Sawyer, C. H., and Markee, J. E.: *Endocrinology*, 46:177, 1950.
143. Schneider, G. P. G., Staemmler, H. J., Straeher-Pohl, K., and Sachs, L.: *Acta Endocr.*, 58:347, 1968.
144. Seegar-Jones, G. E., Aziz, Z., and Urbina, G.: *Fertil. Steril.*, 12:217, 1961.
145. Shettles, L. B.: *Fertil. Steril.*, 2:361, 1951.
146. Shettles, L. B.: *Obstet. Gynec.*, 20:751, 1962.
147. Shettles, L. B.: *Arch. Gynäk.*, 198:241, 1963.
148. Singh, R. P., and Carr, D. H.: *Obstet. Gynec.*, 29:806, 1967.
149. Slater, S., et al.: *Fertil. Steril.*, 11:221, 1960.
150. Smith, O. W.: *Amer. J. Obstet. Gynec.*, 94:440, 1966.
151. Smith, D. M., and Biggers, J. D.: *J. Endocr.*, 41:1, 1968.
152. Sopeña, A.: *Rev. Esp. Obstet. Ginec.*, 2:85, 1945.
153. Spadoni, L. R., et al.: *J. Clin. Endocr.*, 27:1738, 1967.
154. Staemmler, H. J.: *Geburtsh. u. Frauenhk.*, 24:365, 1964.
155. Stegner, H. E.: *Arch. Gynäk.*, 197:351, 1962.
156. Stegner, H. E., and Wartenberg, H.: *Arch. Gynäk.*, 199:151, 1963.
157. Stieve, H.: *Der Einfluss des Nervensystems auf Bau und Tätigkeit der Geschlechtsorgane des Menschen*. Stuttgart, G. Thieme, 1952.
158. Strassmann, E.: *Amer. J. Obstet. Gynec.*, 49:343, 1945.
159. Strott, C. A., Cargille, C. M., Ross, G. T., and Lipsett, M. B.: *J. Clin. Endocr.*, 30:246, 1970.
160. Sugawara, S., and Hafez, E. S. E.: *Anat. Rec.*, 158:281, 1967.
161. Sullivan, T. J.: *Brit. J. Pharmac.*, 26:678, 1966.
162. Swyer, G. I. M., et al.: *Brit. Med. J.*, 1:349, 1968.
163. Tanaka, K., and Nakajo, S.: *Endocrinology*, 70:453, 1962.
164. Taymor, M. L., et al.: *Fertil. Steril.*, 18:181, 1967.
165. Timonen, S., Krokfors, E., and Hirvonen, E.: *Gynaecologia*, 153:309, 1962.
166. Tyler, E. T., and Olson, J. H.: *Ann. N.Y. Acad. Sci.*, 71:704, 1958.
167. Tyler, E. T., Olson, J. H., and Gottlieb, M. H.: *Internat. J. Fertil.*, 5:429, 1960.
168. Urdan, B. C., and Kurzon, A. M.: *Obstet. Gynec.*, 5:3, 1955.
169. Van Waagenen, G., and Gardner, W. U.: *Fertil. Steril.*, 11:291, 1960.
170. Van de Wiele, R., and Turksoy, R. N.: *J. Clin. Endocr. Metab.*, 25:369, 1967.
171. Wagner, J. W., Erwin, W., and Critchlow, V.: *Endocrinology*, 79:1135, 1966.
172. Wallach, W. E.: *Clin. Obstet. Gynec.*, 10:361, 1967.
173. Whitelaw, J.: *Fertil. Steril.*, 14:540, 1963.
174. Whitelaw, M. J., Kaiman, C. F., and Grams, L. R.: *Amer. J. Obstet. Gynec.*, 107:865, 1970.
175. Williams, W. W.: *Sterility: A Diagnostic Survey of the Sterile Couple*, 3rd ed. Springfield, Mass., Walter Williams, 1964.
176. Wood, J. R., Wrenn, T. R., and Bitman, J. R.: *Endocrinology*, 82:69, 1968.
177. Yochim, J. M., and De Feo, V. J.: *Endocrinology*, 71:134, 1962.
178. Zarrow, M. X., and Quinn, D. L.: *J. Endocr.*, 26:181, 1963.
179. Zener, F. B.: *Fertil. Steril.*, 12:25, 1961.

Chapter 42
ENDOCRINE ASPECTS OF ABORTION

42.1. ENDOCRINE ABORTION; DEFINITION AND LIMITS

Not all abortions stem from endocrine causes. Trauma and acute and chronic infections, as well as a variety of other processes having nothing to do with internal secretions, are all capable of causing interruption of gestation. Sometimes, abortion results from uterine alterations, such as hypoplasia, duplication, or cervical incompetence, which are clearly organic in nature although they may be remotely related to changes in internal secretions. In addition, abortion may result from primitive degeneration of the embryo and thus be of genetic origin, which occurs frequently. However, the endocrine changes caused by degeneration and death of the trophoblast in such cases are secondary in nature and may therefore be referred to as *endocrine symptoms of genetic abortion*. The most commonly mentioned cause of abortion, luteal insufficiency of gestation, may be viewed as not one of the *causes* but one of the *effects* of the demise and degeneration of the egg. To begin with, we shall therefore deal with those forms of abortion which manifest themselves through *lack of progesterone synthesis*.

42.2. ABORTION FROM LUTEAL INSUFFICIENCY

For many years, the *gravidic corpus luteum* had been thought to be indispensable for the evolution of gestation. That belief had its origin in an all too literal application to primates of what was known to occur in laboratory rodents. In rats,[83] rabbits[78] and ewes,[2] resection of the corpus luteum during gestation produces immediate abortion, which however is not the case in either woman or monkey.[15, 16, 44]

It had long been known that some pregnancies could be carried on after corpus luteum resection. In our own experience, we have seen nine cases of women lutectomized in the early phase of gestation, with only one case subsequently becoming aborted.[14] Among these, particularly noteworthy was the case of a patient with bilateral dermoid cysts, on whom a bilateral oophorectomy was performed on the twenty-sixth day of the cycle. Three weeks after surgery, the patient showed a positive pregnancy test. This patient, who in retrospect was thought to be in her twelfth day of pregnancy at the time of surgery, had a normal gestation, eventually giving birth to a normal infant. There is no doubt whatsoever that gestation in her case had developed in the absence of corpus luteum activity. Similar observations have been reported by other workers.[24] Statistically, it may be estimated that pregnancy continues in 85 per cent of those cases in which the corpus luteum is resected.

At our clinic, two cases of lutectomy unassociated with abortion[15] were observed, in which urinary pregnanediol levels were determined during the days following the intervention. As may be noted in Figure 42–1, after the resection of an active gravidic corpus luteum in both women, the urinary pregnanediol curve actually rose rather than fell, and neither patient aborted. *However, a finding worth considering, and perhaps as important as the very fact that their gestations were not*

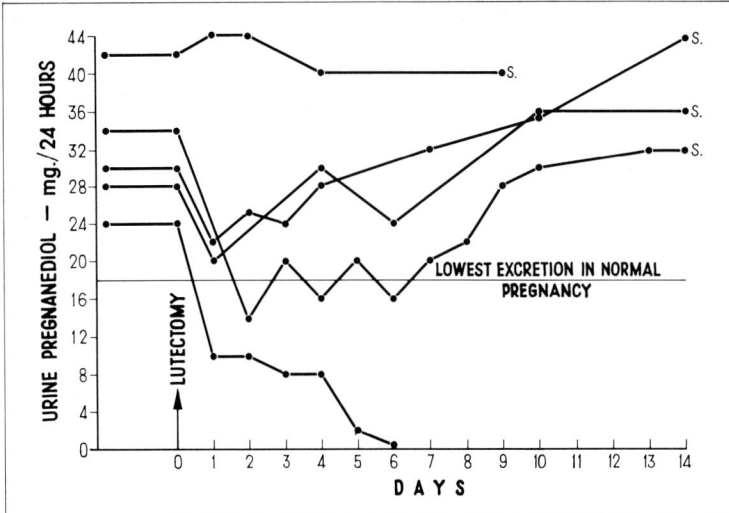

Figure 42-1. Effects of lutectomy during the second month of pregnancy. Five cases observed by us in which the curve or urinary pregnanediol excretion was available. A drop in pregnanedioluria occurred in one case, which happened to be the only case ending in abortion. (From Botella-Llusiá: *Obstetrical Endocrinology.* Springfield, Ill., Charles C Thomas, 1961.)

interrupted, is the fact that these women had maintained normal or even rising rates of pregnanediol excretion. One cannot fail to see that, notwithstanding the disappearance of the corpus luteum, the corpus luteum hormone continues to be produced and its main product of excretion, pregnanediol, continues to be eliminated in the urine. This, then, means that one is not justified in drawing the conclusion that because the corpus luteum is not indispensable for the development of human pregnancy, progesterone is not either. The point we are trying to make is that there are *extraovarian sources of progesterone.*

42.3. ABORTION OF TROPHOBLASTIC ORIGIN

42.3.1. CHORIONIC AND ADRENAL PROGESTOPOIESIS

What are these extraovarian sources of progesterone? First of all, one must mention the *placenta*. This organ elaborates progesterone from the earliest phases of gestation, probably as early as the first month, and in amounts that steadily increase until the time of delivery. However, as regards the previously cited case of bilateral oophorectomy in a gestation of less than two weeks' duration, it may be difficult to believe that the barely established trophoblastic rudiment, apparently in such a primitive state of development that it still would likely have been associated with a negative biologic pregnancy test, could have secreted progesterone in sufficient amounts to maintain gestation. The trophoblast is of course known to produce gonadotropins from a very early phase. In contrast, it takes a certain degree of chorionic maturity to elaborate progesterone. It then seems logical to assume that *some other organ* is able to elaborate the luteal hormone and this, in light of current knowledge concerning its physiology,[13] must be the *adrenal cortex*. The lower curve in the graph of Figure 42-1, represents an experiment that sheds considerable light on this question. The case was that of a patient who underwent lutectomy during her second month of gestation. After lutectomy, the rate of pregnanediol excretion decreased until it became completely negative in a few days. At that time, abortion supervened and was followed with curettage. In a quite incidental way, this above all proves the point, which shall be discussed later, that the *pregnanedioluria curve is of prognostic significance* for the continuation of gestation. However, a few days after the uterus was evacuated in this case, a large dose (10,000 IU) of chorionic gonadotropin was injected, and it was then observed that the rate of pregnanediol excretion again started to rise, reaching values almost as high as the original pregnancy levels, which undoubtedly would have averted the interruption of gestation had it occurred earlier. The occurrence of pregnanedioluria owing to chorionic gonadotropin administration in this woman, without the presence of either a corpus luteum or a chorion, could only be accounted for by invoking a response of the adrenal sexual zone (see Chapter 9, page 174) to the luteinizing gonadotropic stimulus.

In another case of ours, bilateral oophorectomy (for bilateral ovarian dermoid cysts) was performed on the twenty-sixth day of an otherwise fertile cycle. Owing to total unawareness that the patient was pregnant, no progesterone was administered. By the time the gestation was diagnosed several months later, it had already been carried on without progesterone administration and eventually proceeded to term with normal values of pregnanediol excretion.

Since the function of the trophoblast at this tender age of barely a few days of existence seems hard to reconcile with the capacity to produce progesterone in sufficient amounts to maintain gestation, it is our belief that we were dealing, in this case too, with an instance of adrenal compensation. It must be remembered that the adrenal normally metabolizes considerable amounts of progesterone, which it utilizes for its specific mission of corticoid synthesis.

The progesterone supply necessary for the implantation and ultimate development of the egg in the uterus may be derived in equal measure from the *ovary*, the *trophoblast* or the *adrenal cortex*. No matter which of the three organs is involved, progesterone biogenesis requires the catalyzing action of *chorionic gonadotropin*. It follows that the truely important concern in gestation, as well as in the prevention of abortion, is the maintenance of a sufficiently elevated blood level of CG.

This means that whenever the corpus luteum is removed, and provided that the chorion is functionally adequate, the chorion synthesizes sufficient amounts of progesterone to replace the former, or else produces *enough gonadotropin to set into motion adrenal progestogen synthesis*. Thus, in those exceptional cases in which it supervenes after lutectomy, abortion is the result of *deficient chorionic function*. Nature has made ample provisions to meet the contingency of possible corpus luteum failure. The placenta and the adrenal can both discharge a vicarious function. Therefore, in the presence of adequate gonadotropin stimulation there is practically no chance for any progesterone deficit to arise. The latter may only be brought about by gonadotropin deficiency. *Consequently, the true cause of abortion with this type of endocrine failure consists in gonadotropin, not luteal, deficiency.*

42.3.2. ENDOCRINOLOGY OF ABORTION

Our ideas concerning what has come to be known as "endocrine abortion" must consequently be revised. During the past years, pathologic changes in the endocrine correlations of gestation have been invoked as the most common and most important cause of abortion.[3, 43, 90]

ESTROGENS. Estrogen levels in the course of abortion have been studied by Pigeaud and Burthiault[79] and by Gueguen,[38] both reporting an increase in total estrogens, a view also shared by Jayle.[55] In contrast, estrogen fractionation methods reveal

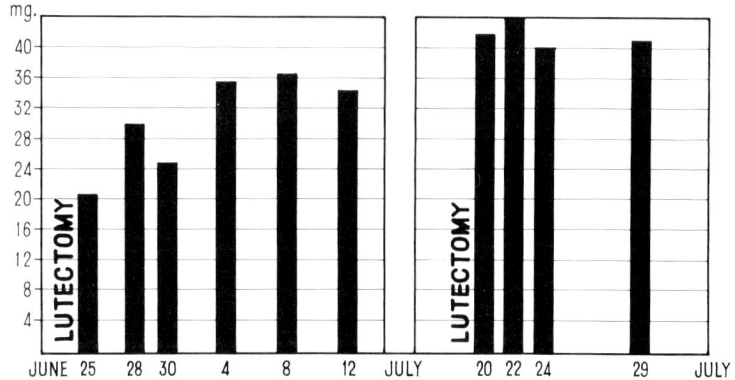

Figure 42-2. Pregnanediol excretion in a case of lutectomy followed by abortion. One week after abortion (with subsequent curettage), an injection of 10,000 IU of chorionic gonadotropin (CG) produced an increase in the rate of pregnanediol elimination. In the absence of any chorionic tissue and any corpus luteum, the pregnanediol excreted is believed to correspond to progesterone elaborated by the adrenal. (From Botella: Arch. Gynäk., 183:83, 1953.)

a decrease in the estriol fraction, as found by Bengtsson and Forsgren.[6] The presence of urinary *estriol* excretion had been acknowledged to be of great value for the prognosis of delayed abortion as well as for the diagnosis of placental insufficiency (see Chapter 44, Section 44.5.3). Its diagnostic significance in abortion, however, was not recognized until recently. Frandsen and Stakeman,[36] as well as Klopper,[58] indicated the occurrence of relative or absolute reductions in the levels of *estrioluria* in instances of threatened abortion. As pointed out in Chapter 44 (also 19.7.2), reduced estriol values are typical of all forms of placental degeneration.

PREGNANEDIOL. Pregnanedioluria has been considered a prognostic element of great significance in threatened abortion (Borth,[12] Botella et al.,[16] Engstrom et al.,[35] Guterman,[40] Jayle,[55] Langemede et al.[60]). Any downward slope in the pregnanediol curve (Fig. 42-1) is prognostically unfavorable, while the reverse is true for a sustained or rising curve.[57, 77] Pregnanedioluria is constantly diminished or abolished altogether in abortion already in progress. *Progesteronemia* has likewise been found to be diminished (Zander,[99] Short et al.[89]), as has the progesterone content of placental tissue.

GONADOTROPIN. Some years ago, Bedoya and Jimenez,[5] at our Clinic, made some highly interesting observations with regard to *gonadotropin excretion in cases of threatened abortion*. As shown in the graph of Figure 42-4, they noted that those cases in which the curve tended to fall terminated in miscarriages whereas those showing rising values had a good prognosis.

Bonilla and Torres[9] obtained analogous results. So did a number of other workers,[27, 28, 42, 45, 63, 74] who employed modern immunologic techniques instead of old bioassay procedures using various amphibians of the order *Anura*.

PLACENTAL LACTOGEN (HPL). We have previously mentioned the fact that while HCG appears to be elaborated by the Langhans layer (see Chapter 19, Section 19.6), lactogen is believed to be formed by the *syncytium*. Studies using radioimmunoassay methods for lactogen (Klopper,[58] Selenkov et al.[86]) have revealed a decrease in the presence of lactogen in the course of abortion. This placental protein is of great prognostic significance, particularly in advanced pregnancy. Nevertheless, it must be pointed out that it plays an important part in abortion. *While HCG seems to be implicated in the etiology of abortion, placental lactogen apparently plays no causal role in abortion. Its diminished presence in abortion is thought to be related to degeneration of the trophoblast, specifically the syncytium from which it originates.*

The hormone really in charge of maintaining gestation thus seems to be CG. If the premise that chorionic gonadotropin stimulates progesterone biogenesis is valid, then by virtue of this endocrine correlation there is no doubt that *the egg is able to take care of itself. In the final analysis, chorionic function is responsible for maintaining gestation and, consequently, endocrine abortion is not a phenomenon of maternal origin but, on the contrary, has an ovular etiology.*

Only quite exceptionally, the female organism may fail to elaborate progesterone. In response to adequate gonadotropic stimulation, this hormone may be produced in the ovary or, this organ failing, in the placenta. Should, in turn, even chorionic function fail, progesterone may be produced in the adrenal cortex.

As a result, cases in which abortion follows lutectomy and, in general, all cases of abortion resulting from progesterone failure, must be attributed to failure in chorionic gonadotropin synthesis.

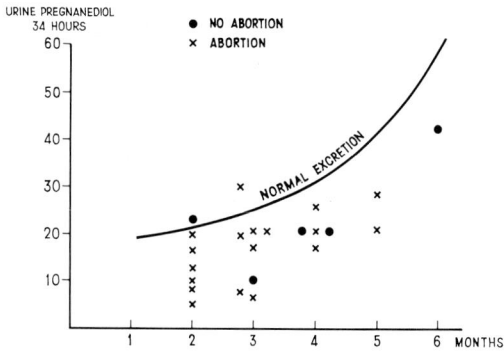

Figure 42-3. Pregnanedioluria in threatened abortion. Although all points along the curve correspond to subnormal values, no difference was noted between those cases that were to abort subsequently and those that did not. Despite being consistently low in cases of threatened abortion, pregnanediol values are thus of no prognostic significance. (From Botella, Cegama and Tornero: *Arch. Med. Exper.*, 15:227, 1952.)

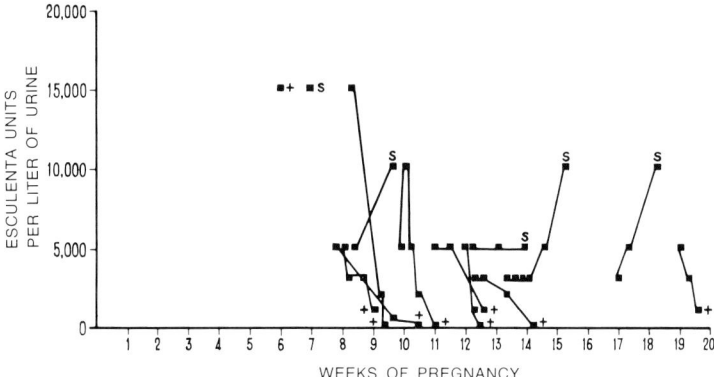

Figure 42-4. Gonadotropinuria curves in cases of threatened abortion. Curves marked S indicate continuation of gestation. Those marked + indicate interruption. Note that a downswing in curve denotes a poor prognosis whereas a rise indicates continuation of pregnancy. (From Jiménez-Tébar: *Acta Gin.*, 1:387, 1950.)

42.3.3. ABORTIVE EGGS

Obviously, then, so-called "endocrine abortion" has thereby been displaced from the maternal sphere to the ovular sphere. This is why in cases of interrupted gestation we have focused our attention on the study of the chorion. The concept of the *abortive egg* was introduced into obstetrics over a decade ago. It refers to an egg which, either from some endogenous reason, such as a *lethal gene*, or for exogenous causes, such as a viral infection or some kind of environmental deficiency, is bound to undergo degeneration and die. Its subsequent necrobiosis and expulsion do not occur because of any break in the correlations involved in the maintenance of gestation but because the abortive egg has turned into a waste product. The investigations of American embryologists[46, 48] show that the vast majority of such eggs may be inferred to die from some endogenous cause or from some congenital malformation. Hertig and co-workers[49] and Emmrich[34] found a high incidence of abortive eggs. Emmrich believes that two thirds of all abortions have an underlying ovular etiology. The mortality rate among very young embryos is presently known to be enormous, and *more than half of all fertilized eggs fail to implant and are subject to early elimination.* Frequent reference has been made to the finding of *ovular aberrations in spontaneous abortion.* Sometimes the alterations described involve the embryo,[33, 80] although what has been most often used for the study of chorionic degeneration were addled eggs without embryos.[17, 18, 48, 70] Others have claimed more recently to have found evidence of chromosomal aberrations in abortive rests.[23, 34] The incidence of abortion from the last mentioned cause purportedly runs high. It is estimated that 40 to 50 per cent of involuntary abortions are associated with abortive eggs. In cooperation with Tamargo,[17] we have been able to show that degenerative changes were present in 49 per cent of spontaneous abortions not only in the embryo but also the *trophoblast.*

Figure 42-5 gives the incidence of various types of trophoblastic changes observed in 110 cases of spontaneous abortion. We have described different alterations of the chorion, all of a degenerative character, which may be classified as follows below.

The different types of abortive eggs are depicted schematically in Figure 42-6. The three most characteristic changes featuring degeneration of chorionic villi

TABLE 42-1.

Eggs revealing a normal trophoblast	51%
Eggs revealing degenerative (abortive) trophoblastic changes:	49%
1. Edema and atrophy°	20%
2. Edema without atrophy°	9%
3. Atrophy without edema°	11%
4. Chorionic hyperplasia with edema (micromolar degeneration)	8.3%
5. Chorionic hypermaturation	0.7%
In categories 1), 2) and 3), unquestionable degenerative changes were present among secretory placental elements, comprised under:	
6. *Epithelial degeneration of the trophoblast*	31.7%

918 Endocrine Pathology of Gestation

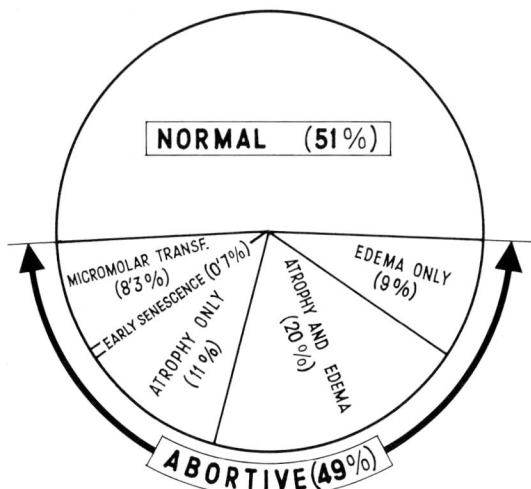

Figure 42–5. Graph representing proportion in which trophoblastic changes of various types occur in spontaneous abortion. (From Botella-Llusiá: *Obstetrical Endocrinology.* Springfield, Ill., Charles C Thomas, 1961.)

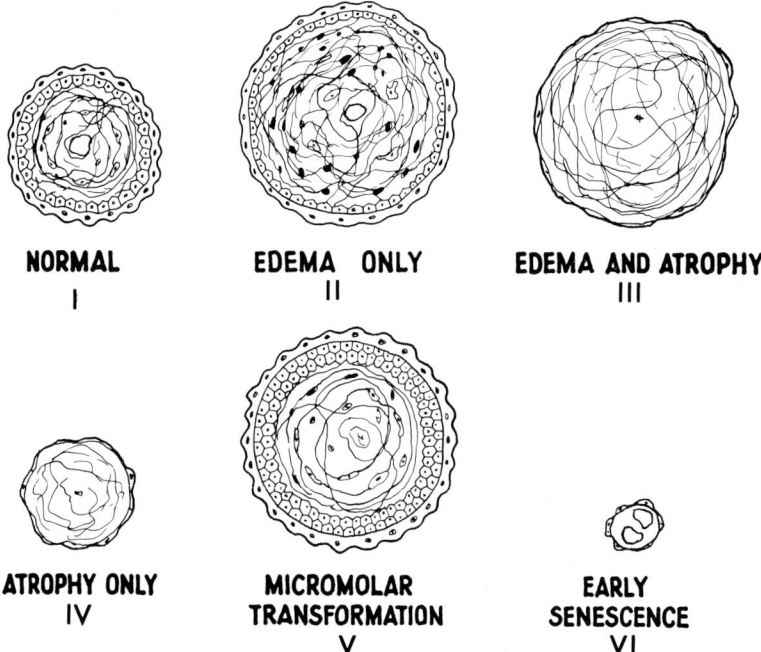

Figure 42–6. Changes observed in the villous structure of various kinds of abortive eggs. (From Botella-Llusiá: *Obstetrical Endocrinology.* Springfield, Ill., Charles C Thomas, 1961.)

Endocrine Aspects of Abortion

are chorionic epithelial atrophy, vascular obliteration and edema of villi.

The photomicrograph in Figure 42–7 shows a typical example of the chorion of an abortive egg, with variable degrees of degeneration in different villi.

42.3.4. HISTOCHEMISTRY OF ABORTIVE EGGS

Attention has been directed in our studies to the *histochemistry* of chorionic villi.[21] With the Hotchkiss-McManus (PAS) method for staining mucopolysaccharides, a positive reaction after salivary diastase or hyaluronic acid digestion was observed in both the syncytial and Langhans layers of normal chorionic villi. In chorionic atrophy, in contrast, complete absence of staining was noted in identical histologic elements of the villus, indicating loss of that function. The epithelium of abortive chorionic villi of types 2 and 4 (see Table 42–1) continued giving a positive PAS reaction. It is known that chorionic gonadotropin is a *mucoprotein* whose prosthetic group is a mucopolysaccharide giving an analogous color reaction. By means of this reaction, various investigators were able to locate the site of production of pituitary gonadotropin B, quite similar to its chorionic counterpart, within the cytoplasm of pituitary eosinophilic cells. Zilliacus[100] confirmed the fact that chorionic epithelium gave the same histochemical reaction. By and large, the histochemical findings with such methods, proving that *the trophoblast of abortive*

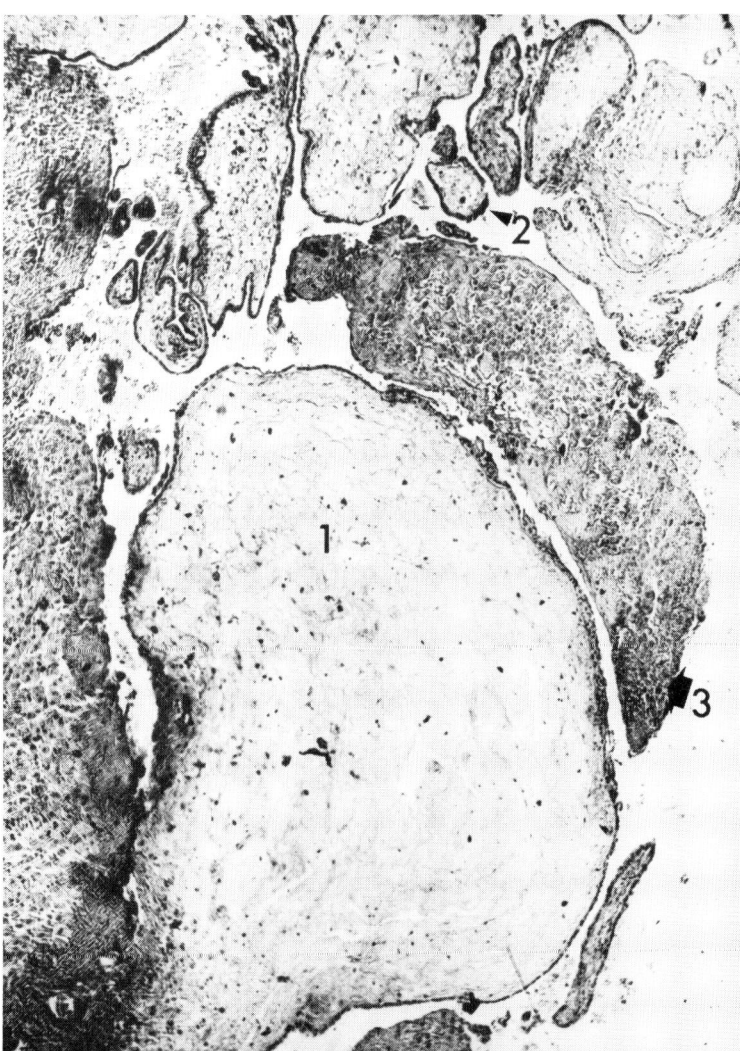

Figure 42-7. Chorion of an abortive egg. *1,* Villus, revealing edema and atrophy (type III of Figure 42–6). *2,* Villus remaining normal in appearance. *3,* Decidual rest with fibrinoid degeneration.

eggs produces no gonadotropin, are a significant argument in favor of the chorionic etiology of endocrine abortion.

As indicated in Chapter 43, hydatidiform mole represents a variant of an abortive egg. It similarly involves degeneration of the chorionic villi, however, with the difference that, instead of perishing, the epithelial trophoblast proliferates at the expense of the maternal blood. Although, as two different processes, abortion and hydatidiform mole have a divergent evolution in that the former courses with decreased, and the latter with increased, gonadotropin levels, they both recognize a common origin from obliteration of the vascular tree of the chorionic villi.

These findings add up to a new viewpoint concerning the problem of abortion. Until now, endocrine abortion has been viewed as resulting from failure of the maternal incretions to maintain gestation; at present, there is evidence that *endocrine abortion is actually the result of failure of the chorion as an endocrine gland. More than anything else, abortion then recognizes an ovular etiology.*

42.3.5. CHROMOSOMAL ABERRATIONS IN ABORTIVE EGGS

As a result of recent developments, it has become possible to culture the trophoblastic tissue from abortive eggs. In a study of 27 cases, Bishun and Morton[8] found three instances with anomalies (11 per cent), one a 45,XO/46,XX mosaic, another consisting of endoreduplication and a third with a satellite on a group D chromosome. Stenchever and associates[93] found only two anomalies among 36 cases, which consisted of various types of translocations. Rushton and his colleagues[84] reported three cases of a 45,XO karyotype among their abortion specimens. The most extensive statistics of Mikamo[71] comprise the cytogenetic study of 67 abortuses, of which 17 (25 per cent) revealed anomalies, mainly involving triploidy, tetraploidy and trisomy of various pairs.

Abnormal karyotypes among aborted ova have also been described by Permanent and his associates.[77] Guerrero and Lactot[39] believe that fertilization in later life is associated with a higher incidence of abortion owing to the phenomenon of *overmaturation of the oocyte* and concomitant chromosomal changes.

42.3.6. SPORADIC ABORTION AND REPEATED ABORTION

Those abortions involving degeneration of the egg result from lethal genetic causes. Save for quite exceptional cases of consanguinity, they do not tend to recur. When repeated abortions, occur, however, it must be assumed that the changes do not reside in the ovum but in the maternal organism. Hartman,[44] Cashida,[29] Hertig and associates,[50] as well as Botella,[18, 19] have emphasized the difference between *genetic abortion* and *environmental abortion*. We shall now proceed with the description of the second type.

42.4. "UNRECOGNIZED HABITUAL ABORTION" AS A SYNDROME

In some of our early reports,[20, 21, 69] we paid special attention to a form of repeated abortion called "unrecognized habitual abortion," which occurred in women with apparent primary sterility who had no reason to believe that they had ever been pregnant. As a result of an occasional endometrial biopsy taken in the course of a systematic exploration of their sterility, it might be incidentally discovered that the patient had recently aborted. Because throughout their married lives such women had never experienced pregnancy or labor, it had to be assumed that they might have aborted unwittingly in a similar subclinical manner on previous occasions. Among 2000 endometrial biopsies obtained from sterile women, we recognized such a pattern in 36 instances (Fig. 42-8), an apparently low, but nevertheless significant, incidence (see Table 42-2).

We were evidently dealing with changes in the endometrial capacity for nidation, resulting in premature expulsion of the egg, that is, in *subclinical abortion*.

In order to learn whether such findings corresponded to any definite pattern of endometrial pathology, 12 of our preceding 2000 cases were followed for certain peri-

Figure 42–8. Syndrome of unrecognized habitual abortion. Case of a 31 year old woman, married for 10 years, with apparent primary sterility. Endometrial curettings on twenty-fifth day of cycle revealed microscopic findings shown here. It must be pointed out that the patient had experienced no amenorrhea. *A*, Villi with surrounding stromal infiltration (100×). *B*, High power view of one villus (450×). Note degenerative changes in both the avascular connective tissue core and the Langhans layer, and the preserved syncytium.

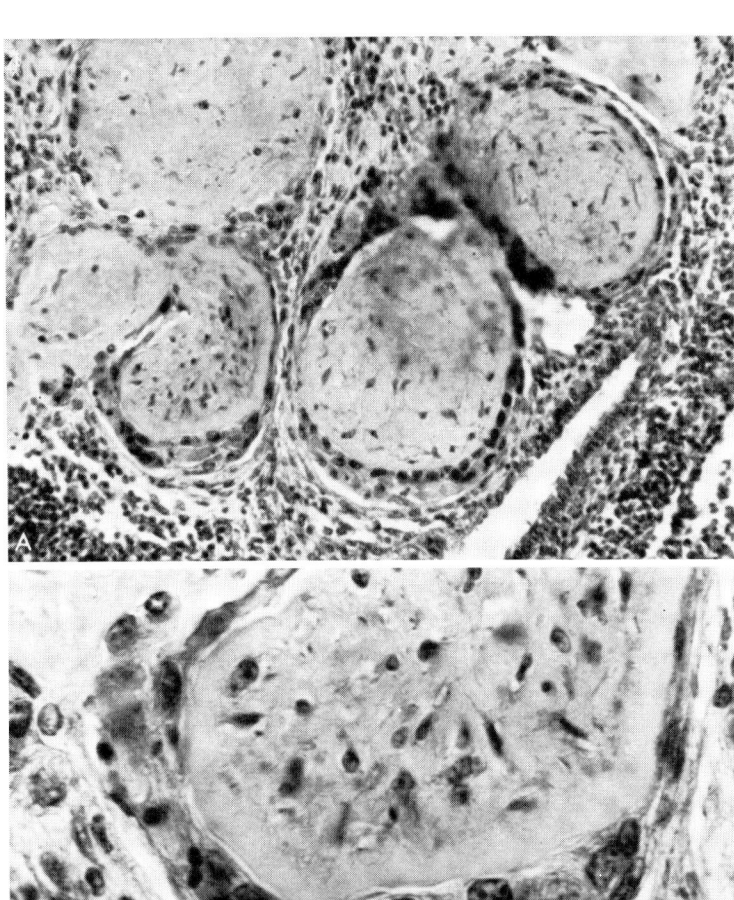

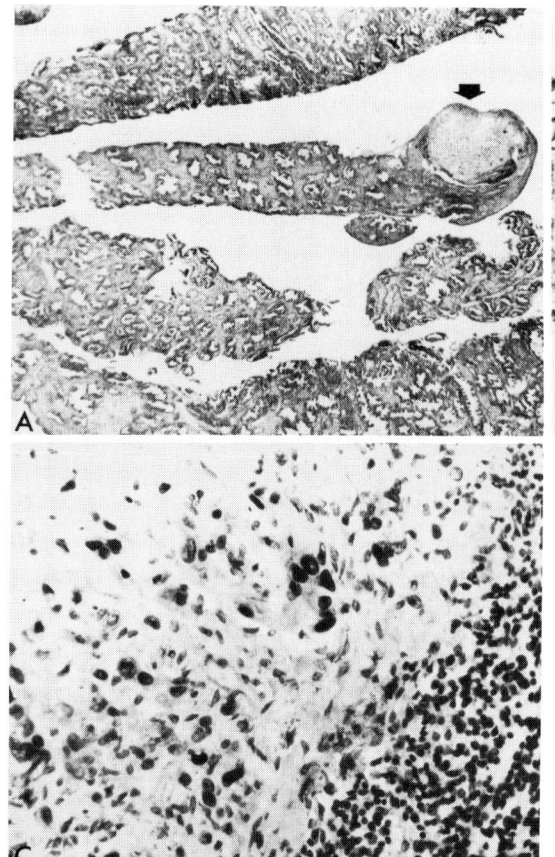
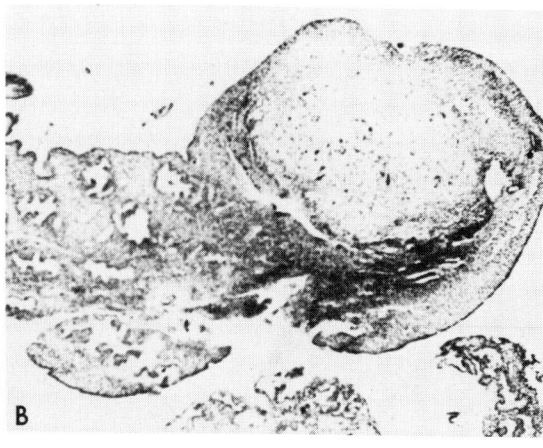

Figure 42–9. Evidence of very early abortion discovered incidentally in an endometrial biopsy from a sterile woman. *A*, At low power, a trophoblastic islet (arrow) is noted amid apparently normal secretory endometrium. *B*, Higher magnification reveals the islet to consist of sequestered, degenerated trophoblastic tissue without any fetal rests. *C*, High power view, suggesting a conceptus in the previllous stage, with early degeneration of the embryo.

ods of time after the incidental discovery of abortion.[21, 22] Results of (a) endometrial biopsy; (b) basal body temperature recordings, and (c) urinary pregnanediol excretion values in all patients revealed evidence of *progestational insufficiency*. The pertinent findings in these 12 cases have been summarized in Table 42–3.

The foregoing findings would seem to indicate that *the syndrome of unrecognized habitual abortion is caused by an endocrine disorder: progestational insufficiency*.

Any endometrium insufficiently prepared for nidation may give rise to infertility because of nonimplantation. Nevertheless, Shelesnyak and associates[68, 88] found that such endometria were actually compatible with implantation and with short-lived survival of the conceptus, but that the latter generally died all too prematurely. The role played by progesterone in the survival of the newly implanted conceptus has been emphasized by Hafez,[41] MacDonald and co-workers,[62] and Yasukawa and Meyer.[98] Undoubtedly, minor forms of insufficiency of the cyclic corpus luteum do cause early and unrecognized abortion much more frequently than is generally realized.

42.5. REPEATED ABORTION AND ITS ENDOCRINE ASPECTS

In keeping with internationally agreed specifications, we consider as "habitual abortion" those cases in which abortion has occurred consecutively three or more times in the same woman. Table 42–4 lists the results of a study in which the endo-

TABLE 42–2. Ignored Habitual Abortion Causing Apparent Sterility in Woman (As Revealed by 2000 Endometrial Biopsies)

Presence of abortive rests	36 cases (1.8%)
In primary sterility	24 cases (1.2%)
In secondary sterility	12 cases (0.6%)
Villous stage	21 cases (1.05%)
Previllous stage	8 cases (0.40%)
Undetermined	7 cases (0.35%)

TABLE 42-3. Cases with Unrecognized Habitual Abortion, Followed for One or Several Cycles After Discovery of Chorionic Rests

CASE	FIRST CYCLE	SECOND CYCLE	THIRD CYCLE	FOURTH CYCLE
1	Luteal insufficiency	Normal	Luteal insufficiency	–
2	Luteal insufficiency	Luteal insufficiency	Luteal insufficiency	Luteal insufficiency
3	Anovulatory	Normal	–	–
4	Luteal insufficiency	Luteal insufficiency	Luteal insufficiency	–
5	Normal	Normal	Normal	–
6	Luteal insufficiency	Luteal insufficiency	Luteal insufficiency	–
7	Luteal insufficiency	Anovulatory?	Luteal insufficiency	Luteal insufficiency
8	Not studied	Normal	Normal	–
9	Not studied	Luteal insufficiency?	Luteal insufficiency	Normal
10	Normal	Luteal insufficiency	Anovulatory?	–
11	Luteal insufficiency	Luteal insufficiency	Luteal insufficiency	Luteal insufficiency
12	Not studied	Luteal insufficiency?	New abortion	–

metria from 50 patients with this type of disorder were examined.

When we compare the incidences of the different findings in habitual aborters and in sterile women, it is evident that the percentage of normal secretory endometria in abortion is *smaller* than in sterility (42 as compared to 55.6 per cent). *Significantly, however, the percentage of insufficient secretory endometria in aborters is much greater (38 per cent, compared to 6 per cent)*. Thus, habitual aborters reveal a strikingly high incidence of progestational insufficiency. Nonetheless, the incidence of progestational insufficiency in repeated abortion is less than that encountered in unrecognized habitual abortion (see Table 42-3). Nine of 12 (75 per cent) cases of the latter form of abortion studied revealed progestational insufficiency, as compared to 38 per cent in repeated abortion.

Progestational insufficiency is therefore twice as common in unrecognized habitual abortion as it is in repeated abortion. Nevertheless, it occurs with considerable frequency in the latter group as well.

Other endometrial patterns observed were about as common. However, a surprising finding in *nonsterile* women was the high incidence, 20 *per cent*, of anovulatory cycles. This suggests that the condition of anovulation: (1) is not a permanent one, and (2) is associated with corpus luteum insufficiency (anovulatory cycles alternating with hypoluteal cycles).

Complete exploratory data available in our files on 15 of the 19 cases with progestational insufficiency revealed the presence of other possible causes for habitual abortion, such as (1) *insufficiency of the internal sphincter;* (2) *bicornuate uterus;* (3) *"irritable" uterus;* (4) *extremely small endometrial cavity;* (5) *hypothyroidism* and (6) *diabetes*. Details concerning these 19 cases are given in Table 42-5.

The table reveals that progestational insufficiency alone, that is, unassociated with any other possible cause for repeated abortion, was found in only 4 of 15 cases (26.6 per cent). One might of course wonder whether inadvertently any other possible causes might have been overlooked. Nevertheless, the high proportion of cases with progestational insufficiency strongly suggests that in a substantial number of women with such conditions as insufficiency of the internal sphincter and hypoplastic or irritable uterus, habitual abortion occurs by virtue of corpus luteum insufficiency rather than as a result of some other condition. This is particularly true in patients with diabetes, prediabetes and hypothyroidism.

TABLE 42-4. Endometrial Findings in 50 Cases of Habitual Abortion, Compared With Endometrial Findings in 2000 Cases of Sterility

TYPE OF ENDOMETRIUM	HABITUAL ABORTION Cases	HABITUAL ABORTION Per Cent	STERILITY Cases	STERILITY Per Cent
Secretory,				
Normal	21	42	901	55.6
Insufficient	19	38	119	6.0
Hyperplastic	0	0	92	4.6
Proliferative				
Normal	5	10	220	11.0
Hyperplastic	2	4	174	8.7
Hypoplastic	3	6	148	7.4

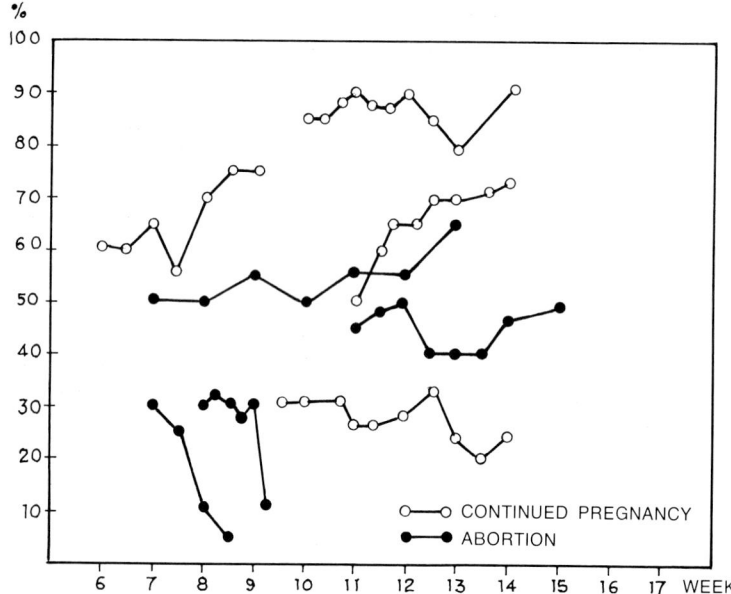

Figure 42-10. Serial vaginal cytology in cases of threatened abortion. The index used is based on the percentage of folded cells present. It is apparent that there is little correlation between vaginal cytology and abortion.

Recently, Dalla-Pria and associates[30] obtained similar results.

From what has just been said, progestational insufficiency may be inferred to play an important role in the genesis of early repeated abortion and, to a lesser extent, in more advanced repeated abortion.

What are the reasons for this phenomenon? There is no question that in very early abortion implantation disorders play a fundamental role. Hertig and co-workers[49,50] studied a number of ova implanted in the endometrium prior to the first missed menstrual period. Of these, 40 per cent were pathologic ova that were destined to be aborted. In each case, there was evidence of abnormal implantation, largely attributable to poor preparation of the endo-

TABLE 42-5. Exploratory Findings in 15 Cases of Repeated Abortion Owing to Progestational Insufficiency of the Endometrium

CASE	HYSTEROGRAPHY	THYROID FUNCTION[*]	GLUCOSE TOLERANCE[†]	COMMENT
L.M.V.	Normal	Normal	Normal	
J.B.B.	Insuff. sph.[‡]	Hypothyroidism	Normal	Hysterometry,[7]
C.L.C.	Normal	Normal	Normal	
M.M.B.	Insuff. sph. Irritable uterus	Normal	Altered	
C.B.M.	Bicornuate uterus	Normal	Normal	
A.G.M.	Hypoplastic uterus	Hypothyroidism	Altered	Hysterometry,[6.5]
L.C.G.	Irritable uterus	Normal	Normal	
M.P.L.	Normal	Normal	Diabetes	
L.F.A.	Normal	Normal	Normal	
M.L.P.	Insuff. sph.	Hypothyroidism	Normal	Hysterometry,[7]
A.L.C.	Hypoplastic uterus	Normal	Normal	Hysterometry,[6]
M.C.Q.	Normal	Normal	Normal	
J.G.G.	Irritable uterus	Hypothyroidism	Normal	
E.C.F.	Normal	Normal	Altered	
R.M.A.	Bicornuate and hypoplastic uterus	Normal	Normal	Hysterometry,[7]

[*] Estimated on the basis of basal metabolic rate and/or PBI.
[†] With 50 grams glucose.
[‡] Insufficiency of the internal cervical sphincter.

metrium. Böving[24] called attention to the significance of a good vascular bed for implantation; Boyd[25] insisted on the need for sufficient glycogen; and Eckstein and his associates[32] showed how important an adequate progesterone level was for correct implantation so as to avoid ovular elimination. According to MacLaren and Mitchell,[64] there are "refractory zones" of poorly prepared endometrium in rodents from which embryos are prematurely aborted.

All functions related to implantation are under the control of the *progestational corpus luteum*, although, on the other hand, it is well known that the *corpus luteum of pregnancy* is not necessary for the normal development of gestation in the human species (see below); this is why the mechanism whereby progestational insufficiency causes habitual abortion in gestations of two months or more is not altogether clear. Some instances of abortion of this type, it may be speculated, are predetermined by the site of implantation in which the fertilized ovum develops faultily from the very beginning, although it also seems conceivable that chronic progestational insufficiency, while compatible with gestation, may induce changes in myometrial development and thus interfere in the mechanism of cervical closure, as has been suggested by Palmer and Ayala.[75] Finally, it must not be forgotten that the corpus luteum of pregnancy, although not indispensable for the development of pregnancy, is an important complement for placental progestogen synthesis. Should the latter process be handicapped from the outset by faulty implantation and development of the trophoblast, and should the gestational corpus thereafter not be in a position to provide subvention for chorionic secretion, it is possible that this may eventually give rise to a deficit in progesterone that has abortion as a consequence.

42.6. OTHER ENDOCRINE CAUSES OF ABORTION

Various other endocrine changes involving either the trophoblast or the ovary may, though less frequently, give rise to abortion. Among these, *thyroid insufficiency* is the most common extratrophoblastic and extraovarian cause of abortion. Apart from the thyroid, the *adrenal*, as well as *diabetes*, must be included here. Other types of endocrinopathy causing abortion are relatively uncommon.

42.6.1. HYPOTHYROIDISM AND ABORTION

It has long been a matter of common knowledge that hypothyroid women achieving pregnancy usually suffer recurring abortions. Clinically, hypothyroidism is one of the known causes of the habitual abortion syndrome. Hypothyroid women with markedly depressed function are sterile, as has been pointed out in Chapter 41, whereas those with only relative insufficiency may retain their fertility within normal limits. Not infrequently, pregnancy serves as the *revealer of latent hypothyroidism* so that, for instance, clinical evidence of definite myxedema may first apper only after a history of several interrupted gestations (Lacomme[59]).

The fact that the relationship between hypothyroidism and sterility is not quite clear has been brought up in the preceding chapter. By comparison, *the relationship between hypothyroidism and abortion* is unquestionable. Greenman and his colleagues[37] have studied 23 cases of pregnancy in hypothyroid women, reporting one abortion, two stillbirths at term and two fetal deaths intrapartum; 18 babies lived but five presented with various anomalies. Their observations seem to suggest a relationship with habitual fetal death and malformations rather than with abortion. However, Lacomme,[59] Pigeaud and Burthiault,[79] and Man and his associates[67] found that women with a low basal metabolic rate had a higher incidence of abortions. Protein bound iodine values were found to be diminished in habitual aborters, according to observations made by Engstrom and co-workers,[35] Singh and Morton,[91] Man and associates,[66] and Slater and colleagues.[92] The BEI (butanol-extractable iodine) (Engstrom et al.[35]) and the precipitable iodine (Man et al.[66]) similarly were found to be low.

The test measuring thyroid function most faithfully is the ^{131}I uptake test; in women with repeated abortions, it was found to reveal consistently decreased values (Dowling et al.,[31] Greenman et al.,[37] Slater et al.[92]) Finally, Naumoff and Shook[73] reported decreased thyrotropin activity in a study of 31 aborters.

42.6.2. ADRENAL INSUFFICIENCY AS A CAUSE OF ABORTION

Under certain circumstances during pregnancy, we have explained above, the adrenal may elaborate progesterone and assume the role of aiding the corpus luteum. Apparently, this is why adrenalectomy in female rabbits provokes abortion, according to some recent observations by Yamashita.[97] Some time ago, Marañón and Fernandez-Noguera had drawn attention to the frequent occurrence of abortion in patients with Addison's disease.

42.6.3. DIABETES AND ABORTION

The occurrence of both early and late abortion in *diabetes* has been the object of a great deal of debate ever since it was first described by Joslin many years ago. Hurwitz and Higano[53] studied a series of 140 pregnancies in diabetics but observed early abortion in only 3 per cent of the cases, a figure acknowledged to be probably too low by the authors themselves, who estimated that the overall incidence of abortion before the fifth month of pregnancy among women with diabetes mellitus was more likely to be in the neighborhood of 15 to 20 per cent. Quite similar figures have been quoted by Marquardsen in a series of 180 diabetics in which interruption of gestation at an early stage was found to occur in 20 per cent of the cases. It must be borne in mind that in addition to early abortion in diabetes, intrauterine fetal death is much more commonly observed during the second half of gestation.

Miller and his associates have drawn attention to the fact that early abortion may often be the forerunner of diabetes. They observed several instances of diabetes in which the patients had presented with a history of repeated abortion of unknown etiology five years before developing the first symptoms of their disease. We have observed similar cases, particularly in connection with fetal mortality during the second half of pregnancy and, as pointed out in Chapter 45, attach great significance to this finding. Only too often diabetes is dismissed as the possible etiology of abortion or premature labor simply because glucosuria is not present. *In the absence of glucosuria, abortion may well denote poorly compensated disorders of glucose metabolism, while at the same time foreboding the eventual development of diabetes mellitus.* This question shall be taken up again in Chapter 45.

42.7. DIAGNOSIS AND PROGNOSIS OF ABORTION

The diagnosis of abortion and prognosis of pregnancy seemed to pose practically insoluble problems for many years. Recent advances in *hormone assay* and in *cytology* have enabled the clinician to diagnose abortion and, what is more, to tell during the examination whether gestation may be irrevocably interrupted. This is of great importance because it permits the therapeutic approach to be adapted to each individual case, without, for instance, unnecessarily undertaking endocrine treatment where abortion may have progressed beyond the point of no recall. We have emphasized *the futility of treating abortion in cases involving ovular degeneration,* in which endocrine therapy achieves no results other than the deferral of abortion.[18, 19]

Modern research has shown that before abortion is actually set in motion certain changes may be detected in urinary hormone excretion as well as in vaginal cytology which, in most cases, can warn the physician that abortion is imminent. Bedoya[4] points out that impending abortion can be diagnosed by means of urinary gonadotropin determinations and sets forth practical norms as to how to determine whether the fetus is dead or detached, whether pregnancy is expected to continue or whether ovular expulsion is imminent. Although this may be an oversimplification, it is nevertheless apparent that hormone studies of this kind have contributed to a much better understanding of the clinical course of interrupted pregnancy. Essentially, four methods have been employed for prognostic purposes: (1) pregnanediol determinations; (2) gonadotropin determinations; (3) vaginal cytology, and (4) the study of cervical mucus.

42.7.1. PREGNANEDIOL DETERMINATIONS

It was previously pointed out that pregnanediol excretion shows a gradual rise throughout pregnancy. *Any downward deflection in the pregnanedioluria curve must be considered as a sign of insufficient progesterone production and must accordingly be interpreted as a threat that pregnancy is about to be interrupted.* In some cases, a reduction in pregnanedioluria may result from primary maternal causes, but in most instances decreased rates of pregnanediol excretion actually reflect *deficient ovular function*. Such endocrine insufficiency of the trophoblast, which we have discussed in a previous paragraph, is in fact the reason for decreased progesterone production and, consequently, for decreased pregnanedioluria. As a result, any decrease in urinary diol values must be interpreted not as an aggressive factor directed against the continuation of pregnancy but rather as an indication that something has gone wrong with the ovum.

Pregnanediol determinations for prognostic purposes in abortion were first performed by Guterman,[40] using a qualitative method. More precise methods of investigation were later employed by Kayser[56] and Simonett and his associates.[90] These authors were able to show, like Botella and his colleagues[15,16] before them, that pregnanediol excretion rates fell in those cases in which the threat of abortion tended to progress, whereas they rose in those cases in which bleeding was only a false symptom of abortion and gestation continued.

Since then, the diagnostic significance of urinary pregnanediol values has been confirmed repeatedly by a great many investigators.[11,35,55,57,60,81,82,94,95]

For these reasons, the study of pregnanedioluria may be considered to be of considerable diagnostic and primordial prognostic value when dealing with abortion in progress.

42.7.2. ESTRIOL

Estriol, as we have already indicated, has served as an index of placental function near term. As a result of the studies undertaken by Frandsen and Stakeman,[36] as well as Klopper,[58] however, it is currently also admitted that a progressive reduction in either urinary estriol values or the ratio between estriol and total estrogens is indicative of ovular death and abortion.

42.7.3. GONADOTROPINURIA AND GONADOTROPINEMIA

The question of gonadotropin elimination in abortion was studied at our laboratory by Bedoya and Jiménez.[4,5] A progressive reduction in gonadotropin excretion down to zero levels in abortion in progress (Fig. 42-4) was found to be associated with the expulsion of the conceptus, whereas a stationary or rising gonadotropin titer was found to invariably indicate continuation of pregnancy. Bonilla and Torres[9] were able to corroborate these observations during the same year. The significance of gonadotropinuria in the prognosis of abortion has since been universally recognized (Pigeaud and Burthiault,[79] Hon and Morris[52]).

Until relatively recently, the method commonly employed by us as a prognostic test in abortion was the bioassay for urinary gonadotropins in *Rana esculenta*. Using the method of ovarian hyperemia in rats, Zondek[101] obtained analogous results. Comparable results have also been obtained with immunologic methods by MacCarthy and associates.[65]

Any drop in gonadotropin levels occurs before there is a drop in pregnanediol levels. There is *always a parallelism* between pregnanediol and gonadotropin values, to the point that elevated levels in the first go hand in hand with elevated levels in the second. However, hypopregnanedioluria is the consequence of decreased gonadotropin activity, according to what has been stated above. *We therefore believe that the value of the gonadotropin test is greater than that of the pregnanediol test as regards both the diagnosis and prognosis of abortion.*

42.7.4. PROGNOSTIC VALUE OF LACTOGEN (HPL)

We merely intend to reiterate here what we have previously mentioned (Section 42.3.2) concerning the question of reduced

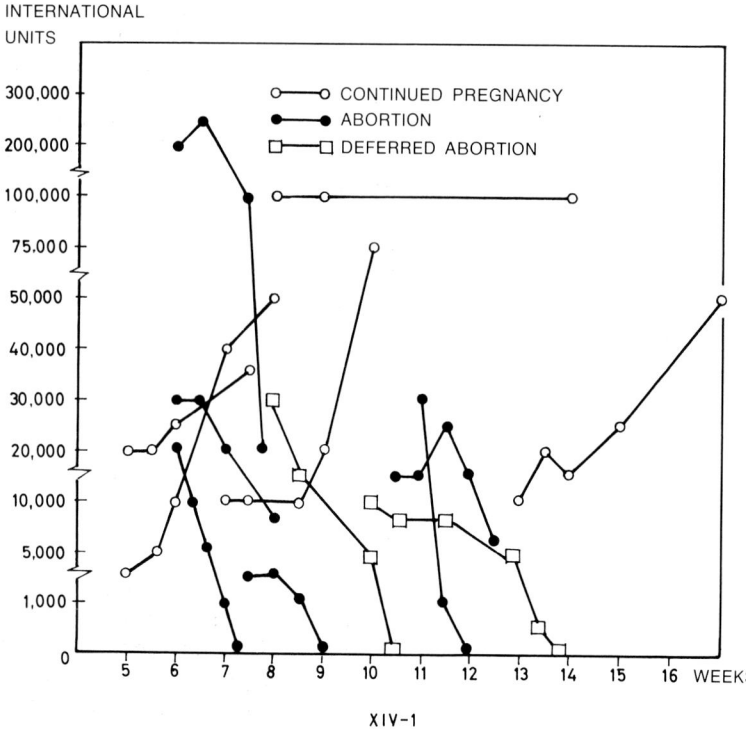

Figure 42-11. Significance of gonadotropinuria for the prognosis of abortion. Low values may be seen to be associated with a poor prognosis. Compared to vaginal cytology, gonadotropinuria is of great significance (see also figure 42-4).

Figure 42-12. Graph representing serum gonadotropin levels before and after seven doses of 10 mg progesterone each. (From Bedoya and Jiménez: *Acta Gin.*, 3:121, 1952.)

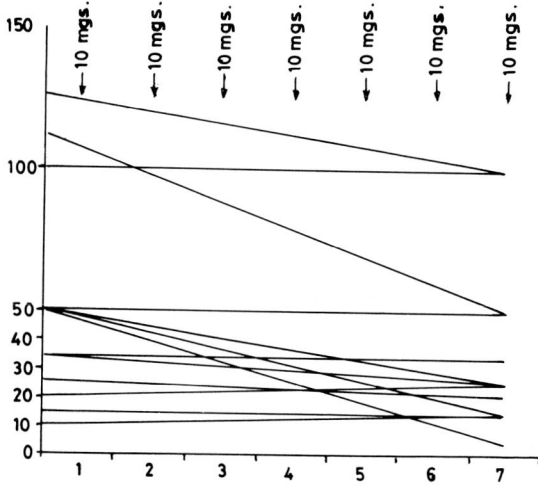

Endocrine Aspects of Abortion

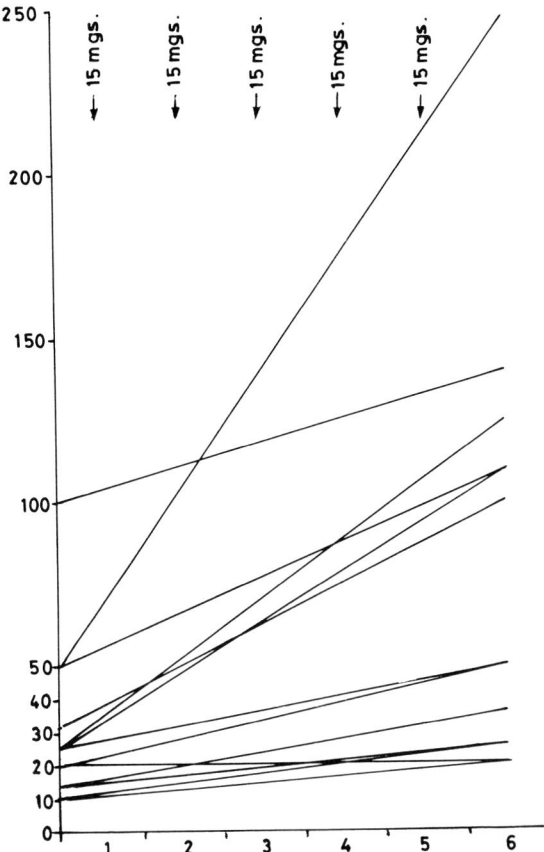

Figure 42-13. Graph representing serum gonadotropin levels in pregnant women before and after a dose of 15 mg stilbestrol administered parenterally over a period of five days. (From Bedoya and Jiménez: *Acta Gin.*, 3:119, 1952.)

lactogen values and their prognostic significance in threatened abortion (Klopper,[58] Selenkov et al.[86]). Because of its equally diagnostic significance in late placental degeneration, in which, as we shall see (Chapter 45, Section 45.4.2), HCG plays no role, placental lactogen is becoming an increasingly important tool in diagnostic obstetrics.

42.7.5. VAGINAL CYTOLOGY AS A DIAGNOSTIC AND PROGNOSTIC ELEMENT IN ABORTION

Typical changes in human vaginal smears during pregnancy were first described by Papanicolaou.[76] He asserted that desquamated vaginal cells assumed a characteristic navicular shape from the very beginning of pregnancy and that those changes could be utilized for the early diagnosis of pregnancy.

For many years, however, the vaginal cytologic changes of pregnancy described by him went unheeded and were forgotten. Not until the cyclic changes in the vaginal epithelium and in epithelial exfoliation came to be known in detail had renewed interest been generated in the characteristic changes of gestational cytology. Thus, in 1941, Bennett and his associates described the cytologic changes of pregnancy. In 1943, Cohen and Rubenstein[29] similarly described the presence of characteristic changes in the cytology of pregnant women. Schuman,[85] in 1944, suggested that it might be possible to distinguish between pathologic and normal gravidic changes and hinted at the prognostic significance of similar changes in such conditions as abortion and gestosis.

In 1950, Benson and Traut[7] studied a large number of cases by means of an improved Papanicolaou technique. In their opinion, the diagnosis of pregnancy could be made with great dependability provided that reliable techniques were used for the study of vaginal smears. They also gave an outline of the vaginal changes characteristic of pregnancy, as compared with changes observed in the various types of abortion and secondary amenorrhea, and held that vaginal cytology might provide a clue to incomplete abortion. After reexamining the problem more recently, Montalvo[72] and Holmquist and Danos[51] have reached the following conclusions:

During the *first trimester*, the characteristic changes of pregnancy consist in the appearance of highly basophilic *navicular cells*, grouped in typical clusters. In threatened abortion, some cells are changed into karyopyknotic elements that are eosinophilic and not folded. The eventual disappearance of navicular cells and increasing predominance of the other cell type are suggestive of ovular death.

The explanation for this phenomenon is simple: the navicular or pregnancy cells *are the result of the action of progesterone*, whereas the eosinophilic cells that appear in abortion are estrogenic cells. What, then, the cytology may be expected to reveal is the occurrence of progressive estrogen-progesterone imbalance, with increasingly pronounced estrogen predominance, a situation typically arising in abortion.

42.7.6. CRYSTALLIZATION OF CERVICAL MUCUS

The ferning phenomenon characteristic of the days of the midcycle (see Chapter 13) disappears owing to the action of progesterone. This is why the mucus of pregnancy does not crystallize. The reappearance of crystallization is a sign of threatened abortion, since it denotes a rise in estrogen levels. Jacobson[54] uses this simple and easy test for the prognosis of threatened abortion.

42.7.7. SEX OF THE EMBRYO AND PROGNOSIS OF ABORTION

Male embryos have been found to display a significantly greater tendency to abortion than female embryos. In those abortions in which the sex of the fetus can be determined, females are found to be aborted much more rarely than males. Based on cytologic techniques, Serr and Ismanovich[87] estimated this *sex ratio* to be 135 males to 100 females, while Tricomi and his colleagues[96] gave a ratio of 160 to 100. One way or another, the prognosis in abortion is always worse for males than it is for females.

42.8. POSTABORTIVE METROPATHY

Over the past few years, great interest among our group of workers (Nogales et al.[22]) has been aroused by the study of a form of *endometrial hyperplasia* with peculiar histologic features, associated with *functional bleeding* and occurring in cases with a long-standing history of abortion in the absence of any abortive endometrial rests or, at any rate, without any significant rests to account for the bleeding. Nogales reviewed an extensive series of specimens, comprising 268 cases (Table 42–6).

The diagnosis is based essentially on the characteristic endometrial changes among which, aside from hyperplasia and marked regenerative phenomena, one may find thickening of the spiral vessels, indicative of a recent progestational process (Fig. 42–14). Our present idea of postabortive metropathy is that we are dealing with an *endocrinopathy caused by abortion*. In fact, we believe that small uterine inclusions of chorionic rests can *maintain their gonadotropic activity* and stimulate the gravidic corpus luteum so that, even after abortion, the latter does not regress completely (Fig. 42–15). Such a decaying corpus luteum is believed to secrete little progesterone but *abundant estrogens*, which are responsible for the appearance of endometrial hyperplasia.

Treatment should consist of *curettage* in which the mucosa is eliminated in conjunction with any trophoblastic residues; however, considering that some of the tropho-

TABLE 42–6. Postabortive Metropathy*

GROUP	CLINICAL DATA	HISTOLOGY
I 37 cases (13.80%)	Amenorrhea, followed by metrorrhagia; abortion not suspected	Microscopic abortive rests, hyperplastic endometrium
II 53 cases (19.78%)	Clinical abortion, followed by lengthy menometrorrhagia	Minimal or no abortive rests, regenerative-hyperplastic endometrium
III 99 cases (36.90%)	Menometrorrhagia, without suspected abortion	Microscopic abortive rests, hyperplastic endometrium
IV 79 cases (29.48%)	Menometrorrhagia, without suspected abortion	No abortive rests noted, but endometrial changes were expressive and identical to those in preceding groups to the point of permitting diagnosis

* From Botella et al.: *Amer. J. Obstet. Gynec.*, 100:987, 1968.

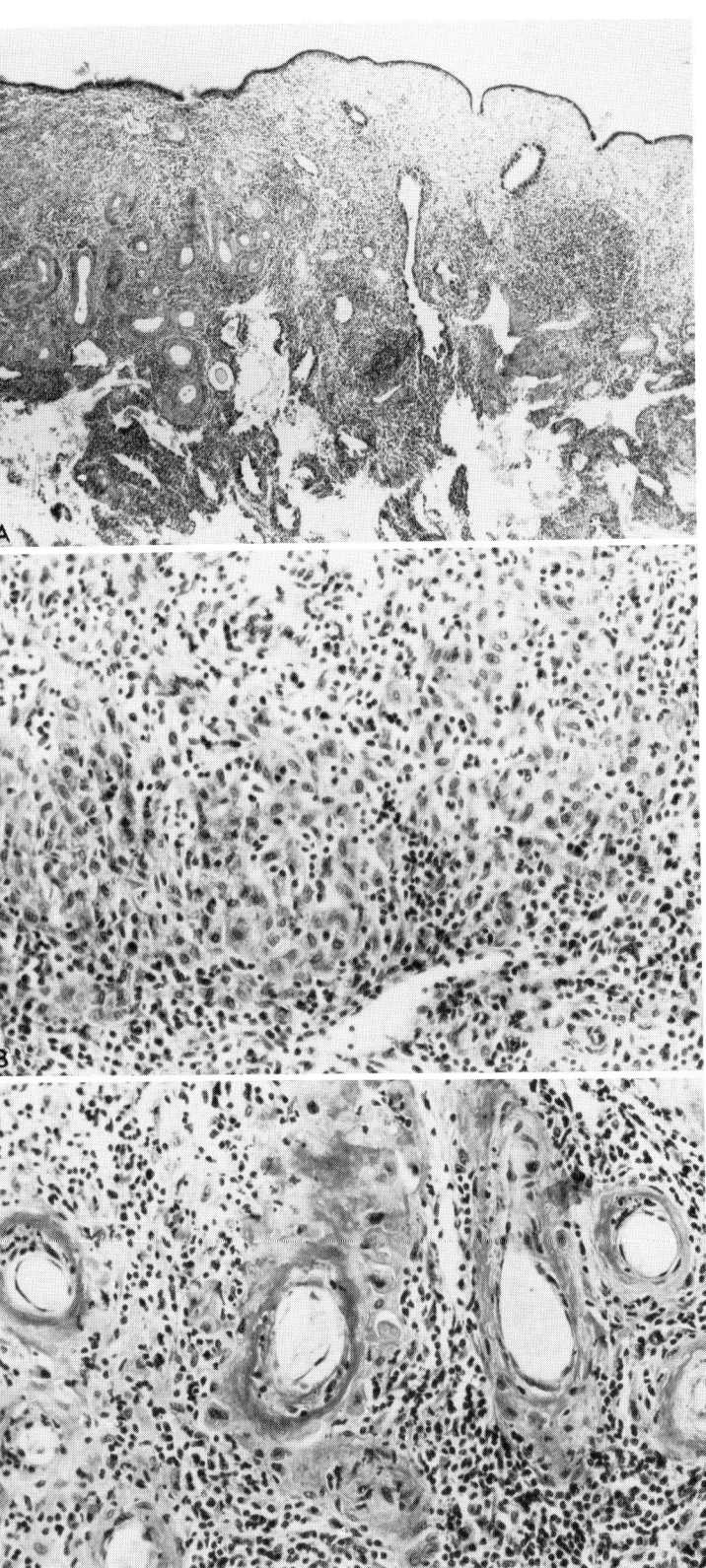

Figure 42-14. Postabortive metropathy in a 31 year old woman with a history of metrorrhagia of 4 months' duration. *A*, Inflammatory changes in old decidual tissue. *B*, Same, at higher magnification. *C*, Spiral vessels revealing thickened walls and degenerative changes. (From Botella-Llusiá et al.: *Amer. J. Obstet. Gynec.*, 100: 987, 1968.)

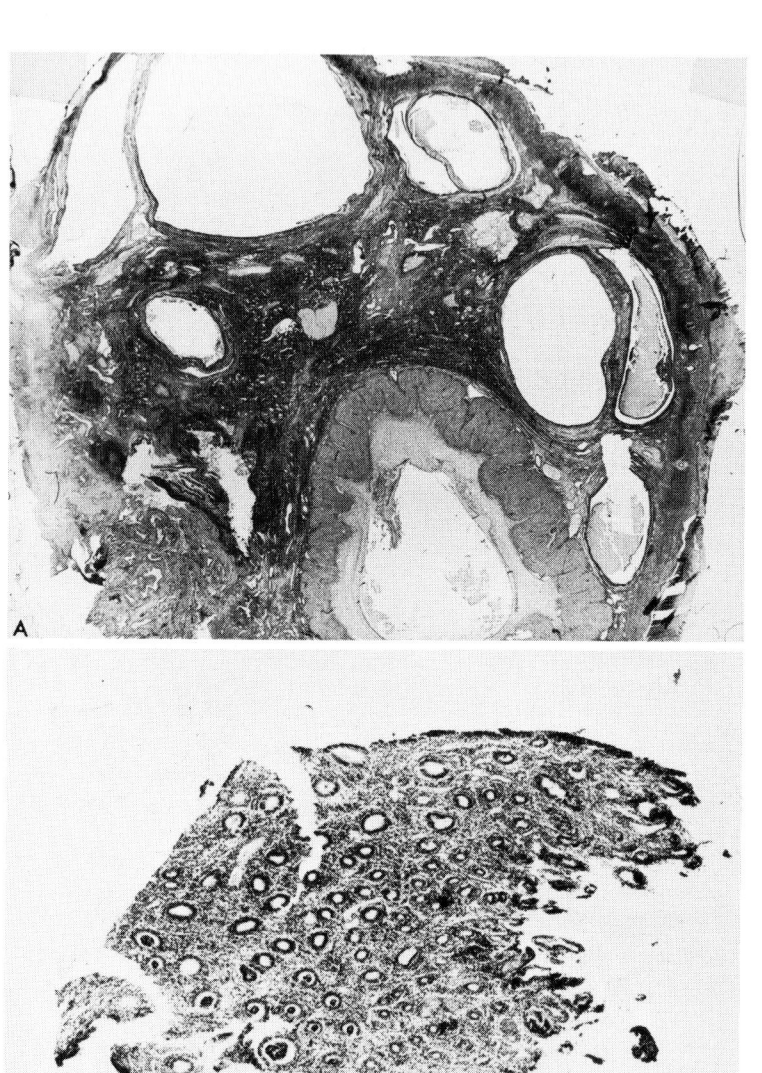

Figure 42-15. Ovary from a 30 year old patient who had presented with an abortion at 11 weeks three months earlier. Bleeding continued after D&C, and a hysterectomy with bilateral oophorectomy was performed. Ovary revealed regressive corpus luteum and numerous follicles in various stages of atresia. The endometrium showed a slightly hyperplastic proliferative pattern. (From Botella-Llusiá et al.: *Amer. J. Obstet. Gynec.*, 100: 987, 1968.)

blastic islets involved may be located in the myometrium, *methotrexate* treatment may also be indicated (see Chapter 43).

42.9. TREATMENT OF ABORTION OF ENDOCRINE ORIGIN

The question of whether or not primitive ovular abortion should be treated with endocrine means has been a matter of great controversy. As we have explained in the preceding sections, such abortions largely reflect a compensatory mechanism intended to rid the maternal body of a useless product. Most of the time, expelled abortuses not only reveal deficiencies in their trophoblasts but also are the seat of serious embryonal anomalies which, had they persisted, could have given rise to teratologic fetuses. The issue of whether endocrine treatment of ovular abortion may lead to an increased incidence of fetal malformations has not yet been clarified, mainly because no therapeutic method effective enough to prevent such interruptions from occurring has so far been devised. However, it would be only logical to assume that, should some day a therapeutic method be discovered that would allow every case of gestation to be brought to full term, the results of such therapy would be disastrous. While such speculation may be beside the point, it is an undeniable fact that current generalized practices of engaging in hormone therapy on the basis of little, if any, diagnostic data have already brought about a noticeable increase in the occurrence of a hitherto almost unknown clinical form of abortion: *deferred abortion* (missed abortion).

Obviously, before the clinician can decide which cases of abortion should be treated and which should not, he must first know which are caused by ovular degeneration. Within the limits of present day knowledge, it seems impossible to tell whether a given case of abortion we may be confronted with in the presence of decreased pregnanediol and gonadotropin excretion results from some primitive ovular disorder or involves some maternal etiology. Much has been said in recent years about the possibility that faultily implanted eggs, in poorly vascularized uteri, or in frequent gestations, may give rise to defective trophoblastic development. This happens not so much because of a genetically determined stigma but rather because of the unfavorable "maternal" environment. Should it further be possible to establish that ovular degeneration stems from *decidual changes*, then one might also have to consider the possibility of treating such decidual changes by endocrine means. In the meantime, however, until more is known about the histopathology and histochemistry of the decidua in abortion of ovular origin, a research project we are currently engaged in, it may be extremely difficult to set any fixed rules for the therapeutic handling of such cases. We abide by the following criteria: in those women whose prognosis appears in doubt, we perform urinary gonadotropin determinations and, if necessary, institute hormone therapy; if the gonadotropin levels are observed to rise following the institution of therapy, such therapy is carried on. Whenever hormone therapy *fails to produce a rise* in gonadotropinuria, we discontinue all therapy within one week from its institution and let abortion run its own course.

What is the therapy of choice to be used in such cases? Much has been said about the ineffectiveness of progesterone treatment alone and the desirability of administering estrogens. Progesterone has been incriminated as causing inhibition of chorionic gonadotropin production (Fig. 42–12), thereby presumably leading to diminished progestogen synthesis by a *mechanism of compensatory atrophy*, a phenomenon repeatedly discussed in this book. By the same token, estrogens are thought to induce reactive ovarian luteinization, while cortisone provokes adrenocortical atrophy and thyroid extracts produce secondary hypothyroidism. It therefore seems reasonable to administer estrogens, the effects of which on gonadotropinuria have been studied at our clinic by Bedoya and Jiménez.[6] As shown in Fig. 42–13, the rate of gonadotropinuria increases after estrogen administration in contrast to progesterone administration, after which it decreases (Fig. 42–12). Estrogen therapy therefore seems to be perfectly indicated in these cases. The *dosages* used should be elevated. In view of their being well tolerated and not expensive, synthetic estrogens appear to be particularly well indicated in pregnancy. When administered orally, dosages of 10 to 25 mg seem to be adequate.

42.9.1. TREATMENT OF ENDOCRINE ABORTION FROM MATERNAL CAUSES

On the basis of what has been said here previously, the type of abortion presumably caused by luteal insufficiency has been excluded from the category of endocrine abortion from maternal causes. This section is therefore concerned solely with the treatment of those types of abortion that result from thyroid, adrenal or pancreatic deficiency.

THYROID THERAPY in abortion has yielded especially good results when applied to the variety of repeated abortions. The treatment should consist in daily administration of three to four 100 mg tablets of desiccated thyroid, while observing the following two guidelines: (1) pregnant women are markedly resistant to thyroid treatment so that the basal metabolic rate may not be significantly depressed as a result, and therapy must be intensive in order to be effective, and (2) the need for tapering off the intensity of thyroid therapy gradually, so that beginning with the middle of the sixth to the seventh month of gestation, it is discontinued altogether. The purpose of this measure is to avoid thyroid overdosification in the latter half of pregnancy, which may lead to reactive hypothyroidism in the fetus. Instances of fetuses born with congenital degenerative goiters as a result of excessive thyroid therapy during pregnancy have been reported by a number of authors. On the other hand, it must be borne in mind that the fetal thyroid is fully functional by the last months of gestation (see Chapter 20), so that any concomitant maternal hypothyroidism can be compensated for by the fetus's own incretions.

TREATMENT OF ADRENAL INSUFFICIENCY. It is hardly necessary to elaborate other than by saying that when adrenal insufficiency is the cause of abortion, it constitutes one of the concrete indications for progesterone administration. Adrenal insufficiency does not manifest itself unless there is associated insufficiency of the corpus luteum (for instance, in cases of lutectomy). If the adrenal in this case is insufficient despite abundant gonadotropin secretion by the trophoblast, it is unable to fulfill its mission of relieving corpus luteum deficiencies. Therefore, progesterone administration is indicated, since there is no organ in the maternal body capable of responding to the stimulus so long as the placenta does not develop its own progestogen synthesizing capacity.

In Chapter 45, we shall study the effects of *insulin therapy* in diabetes and prediabetes. One of the effects of insulin is to reduce the high rate of abortions occurring in diabetic women.

42.9.2. ORAL PROGESTOGENS IN THE TREATMENT OF ABORTION

The widespread use and low cost of oral progestogens has led many workers to employ them as substitutes for progesterone in the treatment of abortion. The danger of producing *iatrogenic pseudohermaphroditism* has been indicated previously (see Chapters 33 and 38). This danger is particularly strong when the drugs used are methylnortestosterone or ethinylnortestosterone. With the second drug, in addition, there exists the risk of producing thromboembolism.[61] The main advocates for the use of this kind of progestogen, without reservations, are some Scandinavian authors.[1, 10] In recent years, however, several new *nonvirilizing oral progestogens* have been introduced, such as *allylestrenol* (Gestanon),[11, 73] retroprogesterone (Duphaston)[45] and medroxyprogesterone (Provera).[67, 73]

A final note of interest deserving some comment is the finding that *relaxin*, too, apparently possesses important antiabortive properties (Bret et al.[26]).

REFERENCES

1. Abolins, J. A., Karlson, S., and Posse, N.: *Acta Obstet. Gynec. Scand.*, 39:127, 1960.
2. Alexander, D., and Williams, G.: *J. Endocr.*, 34:241, 1966.
3. Asplund, J.: In *La Prophylase en Obst. et Gyn.*, Proceed. International Congr. Gynecology, Geneva, 1954. Geneva, L. Georg, 1954.
4. Bedoya, J. M.: *Obst. Ginec. Lat. Amer.*, 13:299, 1955.
5. Bedoya, J. M., and Jiménez, V.: *Acta Gin.*, 1:19, 1950; 3:115, 1952.
6. Bengtsson, L., and Forsgren, B.: *Acta Obstet. Gynec. Scand.*, 45:155, 1966.
7. Benson, R. C., and Traut, H. F.: *J. Clin. Endocr.*, 10:675, 1950.
8. Bishun, N. P., and Morton, W. R. M.: *J. Obstet. Gynec. Brit. Comm.*, 75:66, 1967.

9. Bonilla, F., and Torres, A.: *Acta Gin.*, 1:449, 1950.
10. Borglin, N. E.: *Acta Obstet. Gynec. Scand.*, 39:275, 1960.
11. Borglin, N. E.: *Acta Obstet. Gynec. Scand.*, 40:262, 1961.
12. Borth, R.: *Gynec. Obstet.*, 53:27, 1954.
13. Botella, J.: *Arch. Gynäk.*, 183:73, 1953.
14. Botella, J.: In *La Prophylase en Obst. et Gyn.*, Proceed. Internat. Congr. Gynecology, Geneva, 1954. Geneva, L. Georg, 1954.
15. Botella, J., and Cegama, M. L.: *Arch. Med. Exper.*, 12:143, 1949.
16. Botella, J., Cegama, M. L., and Tornero, M. C.: *Arch. Med. Exper.*, 15:227, 1952.
17. Botella, J., and Tamargo, J. S.: *Arch. Med. Exper.*, 17:25, 1954.
18. Botella, J.: *Proceed. II World Congr. Fertil. Steril.*, 1:279, 1956.
19. Botella, J.: *Proceed. III World Congr. Fertil. Steril.*, 1:91, 1961.
20. Botella, J.: *Rev. Fr. d'Endocr. Clin. Nutr. Metab.*, 4:397, 1963.
21. Botella, J.: *Acta Gin.*, 15:3, 1964.
22. Botella, J., Nogales, F., Martínez, H., and Parache, J.: *Amer. J. Obstet. Gynec.*, 100:987, 1968.
23. Boue, J. G.: *Bull. Roy. Soc. Belg. Gyn. Obst.*, 37:439, 1967.
24. Böving, B. G.: *Ann. N.Y. Acad. Sci.*, 75:700, 1959.
25. Boyd, J. D.: In *Implantation of Ova*, ed. P. Eckstein and M. C. Shelesnyak. *Memoirs of the Society of Endocrinology*, Vol. VI. Cambridge, Cambridge University Press, 1959.
26. Bret, A. J., Coiffard, P., and Motamedi, M.: *Rev. Franç. Gynec. Obstet.*, 58:649, 1963.
27. Brody, S., and Carlstrom, G.: *J. Clin. Endocr. Metab.*, 25:792, 1965.
28. Brody, S., and Carlstrom G.: *Acta Obstet. Gynec. Scand.*, 44:32, 1965.
29. Cashida, L. E.: *Ciba Colloquia on Mammalian Germ Cells.* London, J. & A. Churchill, 1953.
29a. Cohen, M. R., and Rubenstein, B. B.: *Proc. Inst. Med. (Chicago)*, 14:369, 1943.
30. Dalla-Pria, S., Minucci, D., and Pellusi, G.: *Riv. Ital. Ginec.*, 51:47, 617, 1967.
31. Dowling, J. T., Feinkel, N., and Ingbar, S. H.: *J. Clin. Invest.*, 35:1263, 1956.
32. Eckstein, P., Shelesnyak, M. C., and Amoroso, E. C.: In *Implantation of Ova*, ed. P. Eckstein and M. C. Shelesnyak. *Memoirs of the Society of Endocrinology*, Vol. VI. Cambridge, Cambridge University Press, 1959.
33. Eckman, T. T., and Carrow, L. A.: *Amer. J. Obstet. Gynec.*, 84:222, 1962.
34. Emmrich, P.: *Ztschr. Geb. Gyn.*, 167:155, 1967.
35. Engstrom, W. W., et al.: *J. Clin. Invest.*, 30:151, 1951.
36. Frandsen, V. A., and Stakeman, G. A.: *Acta Endocr.*, 44:196, 1963.
37. Greenman, G. W., et al.: *New Eng. J. Med.*, 267:426, 1962.
38. Gueguen, J.: *Rev. Fr. Gynec. Obst.*, 62:377, 1967.
39. Guerrero, R., and Lactot, C. A.: *Amer. J. Obstet. Gynec.*, 107:263, 1970.
40. Guterman, H. S.: *Rec. Progr. Horm. Res.*, 8:293, 1953.
41. Hafez, E. S. E.: *J. Reprod. Fertil.*, 7:241, 1964.
42. Hafez, E. S. E., Jainudeen, M. R., and Lindsay, E. R.: *Acta Endocr.*, 50:Suppl. 102, 1965.
43. Hähnel, R., and Martin, J. D.: *J. Obstet. Gynec. Brit. Comm.*, 71:599, 1964.
44. Hartman, C. G.: *Ciba Colloquia on Mammalian Germ Cells.* London, J. & A. Churchill, 1953.
45. Hepp, H.: *Geburtsh. u. Frauenhk.*, 27:990, 1967.
46. Hertig, A. T., and Edmonds, H. W.: *Arch. Path.*, 30:260, 1940.
47. Hertig, A. T., and Rock, J.: *Amer. J. Obstet. Gynec.*, 58:568, 1949.
48. Hertig, A. T., and Wall, R. L.: *Amer. J. Obstet. Gynec.*, 56:1127, 1948.
49. Hertig, A. T., Rock, J., and Adams, E. C.: *Amer. J. Anat.*, 98:435, 1956.
50. Hertig, A. T., et al.: *Amer. J. Obstet. Gynec.*, 76:1024, 1958.
51. Holmquist, N. D., and Danos, M.: *Acta Cytol.*, 11:212, 1967.
52. Hon, E. H., and Morris, J. M.: *J. Clin. Endocr.*, 16:1354, 1956.
53. Hurwitz, D., and Higano, N.: *New Eng. J. Med.*, 247:305, 1952.
54. Jacobson, B. D.: *Fertil. Steril.*, 11:399, 1960.
55. Jayle, M. F.: *Ann. d'Endocr.*, 12:405, 1951.
56. Kayser, R.: *Arch. Gynäk.*, 181:586, 1952.
57. Klopper, A., and MacNaughton, M. C.: *J. Obstet. Gynec. Brit. Comm.*, 72:1072, 1965.
58. Klopper, A.: *Amer. J. Obstet. Gynec.*, 107:807, 1970.
59. Lacomme, M.: *Brux. Med.*, 32:1181, 1952.
60. Langemede, C. F., Notrica, S., Demetrion, J., and Ware, A. G.: *Amer. J. Obstet. Gynec.*, 81:1149, 1961.
61. Lerner, L. J., et al.: *Endocrinology*, 70:283, 1962.
62. MacDonald, G. J., Armstrong, D. T., and Greep, R. O.: *Endocrinology*, 80:172, 1967.
63. MacGregor, W. G., Gale, C. W., Simmons, E., and Knight, G. J.: *J. Obstet. Gynec. Brit. Comm.*, 73:775, 1966.
64. MacLaren, A., and Mitchell, D.: In *Implantation of Ova*, ed. P. Eckstein and M. C. Shelesnyak, *Memoirs of the Society of Endocrinology*, Vol. VI. Cambridge, Cambridge University Press, 1959.
65. MacCarthy, C., Pennington, G. W., and Crawford, W. S.: *J. Obstet. Gynec. Brit. Comm.*, 71:86, 1964.
66. Man, E. B., Heineman, M., Johnson, C., Leary, D. C., and Peters, J. D.: *J. Clin. Invest.*, 30:137, 1951.
67. Man, E. B., Shaver, B. A., and Crooke, R. E.: *Amer. J. Obstet. Gynec.*, 75:728, 1958.
68. Marcus, G. J., and Shelesnyak, M. C.: *Endocrinology*, 80:1028, 1967.
69. Marin, E., and Botella, J.: *Acta Gin.*, 4:339, 1953.
70. May, R.: *Acta Endocr.*, 44:27, 1963.
71. Mikamo, K.: *Amer. J. Obstet. Gynec.*, 106:243, 1970.
72. Montalvo, L.: *Citologia Vaginal, Endocervical y Endometrial; Hormonal y Maligna*, 2nd ed. Barcelona, Editorial Científico-Médica, 1968.
73. Naumoff, N., and Shook, D. M.: *Internat. J. Fertil.*, 8:811, 1963.
74. Neuwirth, R. S., Todd, W. D., Turkson, R. N., and Vande Viele, R. L.: *Amer. J. Obstet. Gynec.*, 91:982, 1965.
75. Palmer, R., and Ayala, G.: *Actas Sdad. Esp. Esterilidad*, 3:271, 1955.
76. Papanicolaou, G. N.: *Proc. Soc. Exper. Biol. Med.*, 22:456, 1925.
77. Permanent, E., Kadotani, T., and Sato, H.: *Amer. J. Obstet. Gynec.*, 100:912, 1968.
78. Pickworth, S., and Laming, G. E.: *J. Reprod. Fertil.*, 13:457, 1967.

79. Pigeaud, H., and Burthiault, R.: *Ann. d'Endocr.*, 13:978, 1952.
80. Poland, B. J.: *Amer. J. Obstet. Gynec.*, 100:501, 1968.
81. Ravina, J.: In *Colloques sur la fonction lutéale*, Vol. III. Paris, Masson et Cie., 1954.
82. Rawlings, W. J.: *Fertil. Steril.*, 16:323, 1965.
83. Romanoff, D. L., and Laufer, H.: *Endocrinology*, 59:611, 1956.
84. Rushton, D. I., Faed, M. J. W., Richards, S. E. M., and Bain, A. D.: *J. Obstet. Gynec. Brit. Comm.*, 76:266, 1969.
85. Schuman, W.: *Amer. J. Obstet. Gynec.*, 47:808, 1944.
86. Selenkow, H. A., Saxena, B. N., et al.: In *Fetus and Placenta*, ed. A. Pecile and C. Tinzi. Amsterdam, Excerpta Medica Foundation, 1969.
87. Serr, D. M., and Ismanovich, B.: *Amer. J. Obstet. Gynec.*, 87:63, 1963.
88. Shelesnyak, M. C.: *Acta Endocr.*, 50:452, 469, 1965.
89. Short, R. V., Fuchs, A. R., Fuchs, F., and Wagner, G.: *Amer. J. Obstet. Gynec.*, 91:132, 1965.
90. Simonett, H., Piaux, G., and Robey, M.: In *Colloques sur la fonction lutéale*, Vol. II. Paris, Masson et Cie., 1954.
91. Singh, B. P., and Morton, D. G.: *Amer. J. Obstet. Gynec.*, 72:607, 1956.
92. Slater, S., et al.: *Fertil. Steril.*, 11:221, 1960.
93. Stenchever, M. A., Jarvis, J. A., and MacIntyre, M. N.: *Obstet. Gynec.*, 32:548, 1968.
94. Thoyer-Rozat, J.: In *Colloques sur la fonction lutéale*, Vol. III. Paris, Masson et Cie., 1954.
95. Trevoux, R.: In *Colloques sur la fonction luteale*, Vol. III. Paris, Masson et Cie., 1954.
96. Tricomi, V., Serr, D. M., and Solish, G.: *Amer. J. Obstet. Gynec.*, 79:504, 1960.
97. Yamashita, K.: *Amer. J. Physiol.*, 205:195, 1963.
98. Yasukawa, J., and Meyer, R. K.: *J. Reprod. Fertil.*, 11:245, 1966.
99. Zander, J.: *Arch. Gynäk.*, 198:113, 1963.
100. Zilliacus, H.: *Gynaecologia*, 135:161, 1953.
101. Zondek, B.: *Proceed. III World Congr. Fertil. Steril.* Amsterdam, Excerpta Medica Foundation, 1961.

Chapter 43

ENDOCRINE ASPECTS OF HYDATIDIFORM MOLE AND CHORIOEPITHELIOMA

Hydatidiform mole and chorioepithelioma are neoplastic forms of the trophoblastic epithelium which, by functioning as an endocrine gland, exhibit peculiar secretory properties. Since we are concerned here directly with the endocrinologic aspects of these growths we shall study the associated pathologic and clinical problems only insofar as they are directly related to endocrinology.

43.1. DEFINITION

The term hydatidiform mole or hydatid mole refers to an abnormal product of gestation characterized by pathologic changes of the chorion, nearly always resulting in the death of the embryo. These changes consist of cystic degeneration of the villi, poor vascularization and a tendency of the surface epithelium, both cytotrophoblast and syncytium, to proliferate. If the entire chorion undergoes such changes, the embryo dies and disappears (*total mole*). If only part of the trophoblastic integument is involved or, in a twin pregnancy, if only one of the ova undergoes degeneration, the mole may coexist with viable pregnancy. This is referred to as *partial mole* or *embryonated mole*.

Chorioepithelioma is a neoplasm made up of trophoblastic elements and, in the majority of cases, arises from a mole by a process of proliferative transformation. Chorioepithelioma is also known by the name of *chorioadenoma, chorioepitheliosis* (though these two terms are subject to important distinctions, as shall be pointed out) and *choriocarcinoma*. As a rule, chorioepithelioma arises through malignant degeneration of a pathologic egg (abortive ovum or molar ovum). Only very seldom does choriocarcinoma originate in normal trophoblastic tissue.

Much more rarely, chorioepithelioma arises by teratoid degeneration of germ cells in the gonad (either ovary or testis). This gives rise to either *testicular or ovarian chorioepitheliomas* which are *teratoblastomas*. For chorioepitheliomas arising in a conceptus, Klaften proposed the term "*gestrochorioepithelioma,*" as distinct from those of gonadal teratoid origin, which he refers to as "*chorioepithelioblastomas.*" Presently, we shall discuss only the first variety. The second group has been dealt with in Chapter 30 (see page 675).

43.2. HYDATIDIFORM MOLE: INCIDENCE

As already stated in the preceding section, hydatidiform mole must be considered as a pathologic product of gestation which is characterized by the following villous changes:

1. Edema of the villous stroma, giving rise to vesicles that vary in size from 2 to 25 mm.
2. Proliferation of the surface epithelium involving the Langhans layer, the syncytium, or both.
3. Loss of fetal vascularization in the villous stroma.

As for nutrition, mole is entirely dependent on the maternal circulation. This fact is important for the understanding of what we are going to say later.

As far as *incidence* is concerned, the figures reported vary according to different authors. Thus, Acosta-Sisson[1] reports an incidence of one in every 126 pregnancies for the Philippines. Novak[69] gives an incidence of 1:2500 for the United States. Our own findings reveal one mole in approximately every 800 to 1000 deliveries. As has been recently indicated by Fund,[34] the incidence of mole seems to depend on geographic factors to a large extent. The figures commonly reported in Asia or the Philippines (1:200) are much higher than those in the United States (1:1500). According to both Acosta-Sisson[3] and Fund,[34] this higher Asian incidence is related to prevailing poor nutritional and living conditions in that part of the world. Undoubtedly, however, there may be some as yet unknown racial factor involved that plays a decisive role.

Another point of interest concerning the incidence of mole is the *age* of the patient. Smalbraak[91] found that mole was four times as common between the ages of 40 and 45 as it was before the age of 40. Noteworthy is the observation made by Sherman[90] that in women over 50, 5 in every 20 cases of pregnancy (25 per cent) resulted in mole. Thus, *as woman grows older, the incidence of mole increases.* Nevertheless, molar gestation is by no means confined to women in the advanced age group. It may equally occur in the younger age groups. Upon reviewing the age in a series of 74 cases of mole, Smalbraak[92] found that the age in five cases was below 20, which is significant if one considers the low incidence of pregnancy in that age group. Of those cases studied by him, 32.5 per cent occurred in primiparas. As a result, it might be said that mole occurs most often in gestations occurring before the age of 20 or after the age of 45.

Equally significant is the high incidence of mole in *toxemia of pregnancy.* Acosta-Sisson[2] encountered symptoms of toxemia in 40 per cent of all molar gestations. Smalbraak[93] reported that 25 per cent of his cases of mole presented with vomiting, 33 per cent with hypertension, 17.3 per cent with edema, and 24.5 per cent with albuminuria. Teoh and Tow[104] found evidence of severe toxemia in 28 per cent of all cases of mole studied. The occurrence of mole is very rare before the seventh week of gestation and is exceptional after the thirty-seventh week. According to Huber and Hörmann,[48] mole occurs most frequently around the nineteenth week of gestation. By comparison, Smalbraak[92] put the peak incidence between the thirteenth and sixteenth weeks.

43.3. ETIOLOGY OF HYDATIDIFORM MOLE

For the time being, most assertions with regard to the etiology of mole are speculative. However, it should be reiterated that, as pointed out elsewhere,[15] hydatidiform mole must not be regarded as a true neoplasm of the chorion. Those factors having a bearing on the etiology of mole may be divided into: (1) genetic and (2) environmental factors.

43.3.1. GENETIC FACTORS

Hydatidiform role is a variant of the abortive egg, as we have stated in the preceding chapter. Arguments invoking a genetic causation of mole are based on both *anatomopathologic* and *cytogenetic* data.

ANATOMOPATHOLOGIC DATA. In conjunction with Tamargo,[15] we have emphatically stressed the genetic nature of the degenerative process involving the conceptus, which gives rise to what we call "abortive egg." According to our own studies, approximately 49 per cent of all spontaneous abortions result from very early degeneration of the egg. What we refer to as *micromolar degeneration* figures as the most frequent (8.3 per cent) and most important degenerative change found in the trophoblast of abortive eggs (Chapter 42). The chorion appears edematous; the villi, markedly increased in diameter, are filled with an extremely loose textured stroma in which the gound substance is almost exclusively made up of edema fluid. The stroma is devoid of vessels and the surrounding chorionic integument is generally flattened although it may occasionally reveal foci of thickening and even mild hyperplasia.

Hertig and Edmonds[40] likewise emphasized the frequency with which they observed micromolar degeneration among abortive ova, and they considered mole to be a variant of such ova. Of course, if any mole is to become clinically significant, an abortive egg of this type must be retained in the interior of the uterus and not be expelled. In view of the fact that what keeps such eggs anchored in the uterine cavity is the hormonal trophoblast-corpus luteum interrelationship (see Chapter 21), it is not surprising that only moles with secretory activity of the covering epithelium should be able to persist beyond the twelfth week. In other words, *of all moles, the only ones to reach an adult stage of development and to become clinically apparent are those which, by virtue of proliferation of their Langhans layer, are capable of producing elevated quantities of gonadotropins.* For this reason, the clinical concept of mole is that of hyperplastic or neoplastic growth of the trophoblastic epithelium associated with elevated rates of gonadotropin elimination. However, from this angle, no distinction can be made between micromolar degeneration without hormone activity at the beginning of pregnancy, in which premature expulsion is inevitable, and those moles which, as a result of their hormone activity, are retained for longer periods of time.

The paramount question therefore is what causes *hydropic degeneration* of young chorionic villi. Hörmann[46] and Park[77] believe that the essential factor involved is lack of vascularization of the chorionic villi (Fig. 43-1). Accordingly, we are dealing with a primary fetal defect caused by the absence of the *allantoic vascular area*. Because under such conditions the trophoblastic epithelium is deprived of the nutrition normally provided by the fetal blood, it becomes entirely dependent for its nutrition on the maternal blood. It then assumes a *"parasitic"* character, as a result of which it may be associated with either degenerative or hyperplastic features. Why reactive hyperplasia occurs in some cases and not in others is perhaps one of the most intriguing questions concerning the etiology of both mole and chorioepithelioma. At present, we have no satisfactory answer.

Edmonds[30] separates hydatidiform degeneration, characterized by hydropic villi and epithelial atrophy, from true hydatidiform mole, in which the covering epithelium is hyperplastic. He postulates that such hyperplasia always develops as a secondary reaction to initial atrophy, provided that the chorion survives and that the product of conception is not expelled too soon. In his opinion, therefore, whether the outcome is to be a mole or an abortive egg ultimately depends on the type of resistance the conceptus is able to muster against being expelled.

The factors involved in causing primeval ovular degeneration and lack of vascularization are obviously *genetic* ones. Smalbraak[91, 92] advanced the hypothesis that such factors might involve a chromosomal defect similar to that causing mongolism and, as in the latter case, are subject to occur more frequently the more advanced the mother's age.

CYTOGENETIC DATA. We have already pointed out in Chapter 42 that cultures of tissue from abortive eggs frequently reveal defective karyotypes.[13, 79, 84, 85, 99] Guerrero and Lactot[37] stress the role that senescence of the oocyte may play in the genesis of abortive eggs.

The same is true in hydatidiform mole. As far back as 1958, Klinger and associates[55] reported that molar tissue consisted predominantly of cells with Barr bodies. This was later confirmed by Baggish and his co-workers.[6] As techniques for the successful culturing of molar tissue eventually were developed, it similarly became apparent that many of the cultured cells exhibited chromosomal anomalies. Thus, Oliphant and associates,[75] as well as Bret and Grepinet,[19] found principally aneuploidy, while Beischer and Fortune,[11] and Tominaga and Page,[106] reported mainly the occurrence of triploidy and tetraploidy. It is equally well known that, as with abortive eggs, the age of the mother plays a fundamental role in the appearance of mole.

It may then be concluded that mole is merely a variant of an abortive egg and, like the latter, apparently stems from *ovular*

940   Endocrine Pathology of Gestation

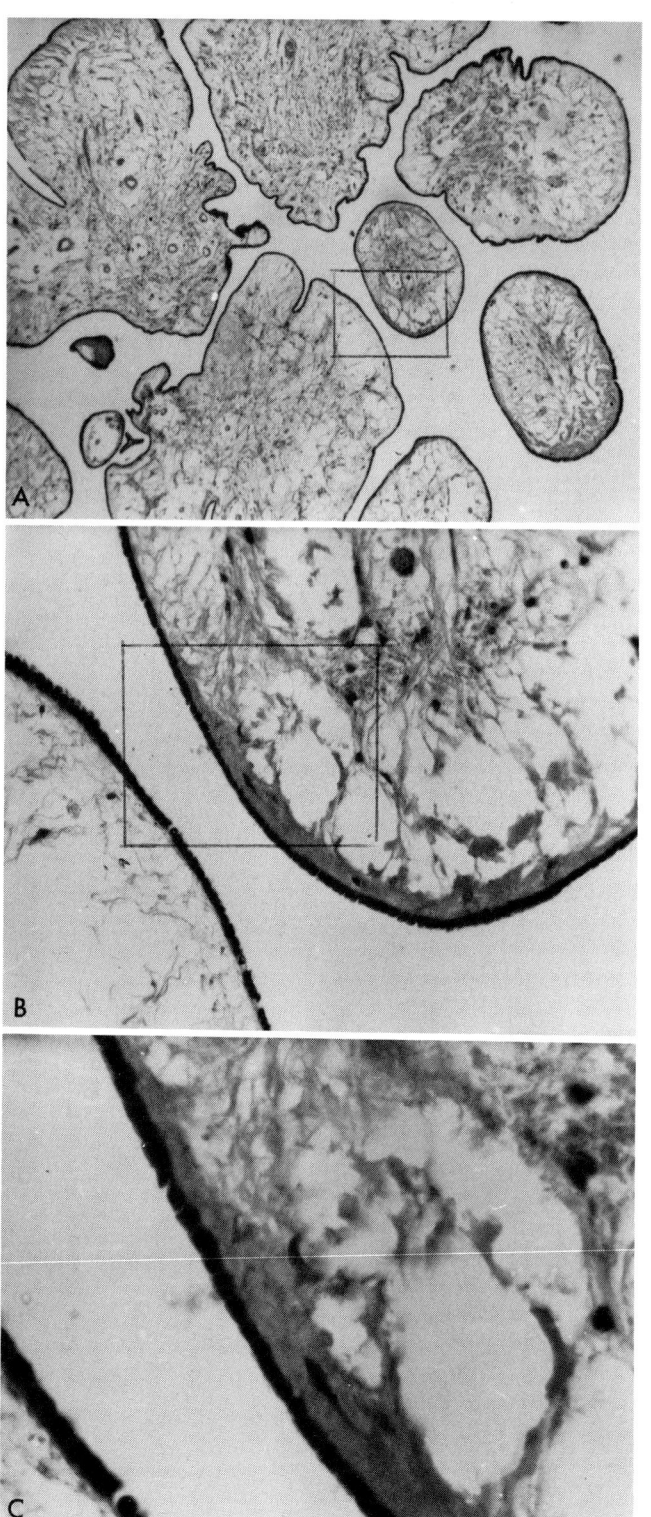

Figure 43-1. Benign hydatidiform mole (Grade I of Hertig). *A,* Vesicle revealing scanty vascularization and marked edema of villous stroma (10×). *B,* The villi are lined with a single layer of cells; there is edema and absence of blood vessels (90×). *C,* Histologic detail of area demarcated, at higher magnification (220×).

lethality, which in turn is a consequence of hereditary defects, frequently occurring as *chromosomopathies*, though occasionally not apparent when involving simple *genopathies*.

It must be remembered that the *primary oocyte* (see Chapter 12) remains arrested in the *diplotene* stage from the time of birth until that period in life when the follicle begins to mature. In women over 40, therefore, the process of meiosis may resume after having been dormant for more than 40 years. Admittedly, *such long periods of hibernation of oocytes* may give rise to chromosomal changes. However, Harper and his associates[39] have noted that when blastocysts from young hamster females were transplanted to the uterus of older hamster females, they often developed into abortive eggs, a finding suggesting an *environmental rather than a genetic* causation of mole.

43.3.2. ENVIRONMENTAL FACTORS

Though molar degeneration seems to result exclusively from the previously mentioned genetic factors, environmental factors may exert a powerful influence on the development, implantation and evolution of mole. Recently, there has been some speculation as to whether *lack of estrogens* may possibly play any role in the genesis of mole. Several arguments have been advanced to support such an hypothesis: first, Courrier and Gros found that castration of pregnant cats gave rise to hydatidiform changes in villi. Second, the incidence of molar growth was found to be highest in either very young women or in women over the age of 45, or else in patients who had shown evidence of ovarian deficiency on previous occasions (Karzavina[52]). Third, as will be discussed later, there are extremely low estrogen titers in women with either mole or choriocarcinoma. Fourth, a phenomenon of physiologic autoprotection exists against chorionic invasion, which is evident in every pregnancy and increases progressively with rising estrogen titers in normal pregnancy. Fifth, chorioepithelioma can be treated effectively with estrogens. Sixth, as we have already mentioned, blastocyst transplants (Harper et al.[39]) to uteri of older animals often develop defec-

tively. It would then appear that faulty implantation of the ovum could, as a result of nutritional deficiencies in the young conceptus, precipitate the process of *villous degeneration*, which in the majority of instances would result in abortion, and in a lesser number of instances cause molar degeneration.

The studies by Noyes[72] and primarily Böving[18a] have shed considerable light on the mechanism of normal implantation and, in the particular case of mole, on that of pathologic implantation and penetration. Böving showed that trophoblastic invasion into the normal decidua was facilitated not by phagocytic activity but by lysis of the cell membranes, which takes place at an elevated—that is, alkaline—pH. This pH is controlled by a carbonate-bicarbonate buffer system. At this point, the intervention of endometrial *carbonic anhydrase* becomes instrumental. The discovery of this enzyme by Pincus and associates[81] has already been mentioned, as has the technique for its determination (Chapter 24). By degrading carbon dioxide, anhydrase activity causes a shift in the buffer's pH toward alkalinity and facilitates chorionic penetration. From the work of Pincus, it has already been known that progesterone enhances endometrial anhydrase activity quite specifically and efficiently, thereby facilitating the penetration and invasion of ovular elements. As a result, the eventual course a mole or choriocarcinoma may take in its evolution may currently be envisioned as largely dependent on the mechanism of blastocyst implantation. A strongly alkaline environment, created by endometrial carbonic anhydrase, is necessary for the penetration into the decidua of chorionic elements. Progesterone promotes alkalinity of the environment through its capacity to enhance carbonic anhydrase activity. Estrogens have the reverse effect. *In the final analysis, trophoblastic invasion of the decidua is facilitated by progesterone and suppressed by estrogenic activity.*

These factors determine the evolution of mole although they have nothing to do with its etiology, which, as we have said before, is assumed to be genetically determined. Whatever the genetic factors involved in its origin, it is evident that mole, as pointed out elsewhere,[16, 17] represents an *instance of villi persisting in their embryonal state*. If we compare the events taking place at the beginning of pregnancy, marked as they are by deep invasion into the decidua of villi with a highly active trophoblast, at that stage similarly poor in vasculature but containing a voluminous loose, hydropic connective tissue stroma, it may be understood that the same situation is after all duplicated in mole. As distinct from mole, however, these changes, which might aptly be termed "molar" villous changes, tend to disappear as gestation progresses; the trophoblast becomes less invasive and less proliferative, and eventually is reduced to a fairly thin layer.

43.4. HISTOPATHOLOGY OF MOLE

The histopathology of mole has been the subject of three outstanding studies, by now considered classic: those by Meyer[65, 66] (1931), by Hertig and Sheldon[41] (1947) and by Hunt, Dockerty and Randall[50] (1953). Within the limited context of a textbook on endocrinology, these classic studies will be reviewed here only cursorily by stating that Hertig and Sheldon have suggested a classification of mole based on the invasiveness of its trophoblast, as follows:

I. *Benign,* in which there is no trophoblastic proliferation.

II. *Probable benign,* in which there is mild to moderate hyperplasia.

III. *Possible benign,* in which there is trophoblastic overgrowth with mild anaplasia.

IV. *Possible malignant,* in which there is moderate anaplasia with overgrowth.

V. *Probable malignant,* with variable overgrowth and marked anaplasia.

VI. *Malignant,* in which there is exuberant trophoblastic overgrowth with mitotic activity and marked anaplasia.

Figures 43–1 to 43–4 exemplify the range of possibilities. This classification has been subject to criticism, voiced mainly by Hunt and associates[50] and by Smalbraak,[91] who raised the following arguments:

1. Trophoblastic overgrowth in a given villus may occur as an independent feature and cannot be construed as evidence of malignancy but rather as a sign of greater or lesser youthfulness of the trophoblast.

2. Growth of the trophoblast is comparable to that of a tissue culture, which is why it is very difficult and sometimes impossible to determine whether the trophoblastic cells are actually undergoing anaplastic changes or have merely lost their structural coordination.

3. In most cases of mole, benign neoplasia and hyperplasia may be found to coexist in the same microscopic field, so that based on the degree of anaplasia alone it may be extremely difficult to judge whether we are dealing with an immature portion of mole or with a truly malignant mole.

4. Hertig and Sheldon consider evidence of invasion of the villous stroma by trophoblastic cells as the single most definite item proving malignancy. Apart from being a normal chorionic finding in some cases, (Hofbauer cells), this change has never been observed by Smalbraak.

In view of this, Hunt and his colleagues[50] proposed a different classification, integrating the following three categories:

I. *Inactive mole.* There is no anaplasia. The trophoblast reveals mild, if any, hyperplasia.

II. *Active mole.* Moderate anaplasia and exuberant hyperplasia. There is often evidence of myometrial invasion.

III. *Hyperactive mole,* which shows marked anaplasia as well as massive invasion of vessels and the myometrium (*mola destruens*).

It is of interest to point out, however, that the long-range prognosis in the cases studied by Hunt and associates was found to be the same in category three as in category two, which would seem to indicate that marked hyperplasia did not necessarily mean malignancy.

The third category in this classification has been called by others *chorioadenoma destruens* (Greene,[36] Park,[78] Smalbraak[92]). In the United States, there is presently a special registry for mole and choriocarcinoma, known as the "Albert F. Mathieu Registry" in memory of Mathieu, who had distinguished himself in the study of the histopathology of mole and chorioepithelioma. Green[36] collected 42 cases of chorioadenoma destruens from the Albert F. Mathieu Registry, and he too was able to show that the incidence of malignancy in this form did not differ significantly from that found in other forms of mole, and that the capacity of mole to undergo malignant transformation to choriocarcinoma was unrelated to its histologic appearance.

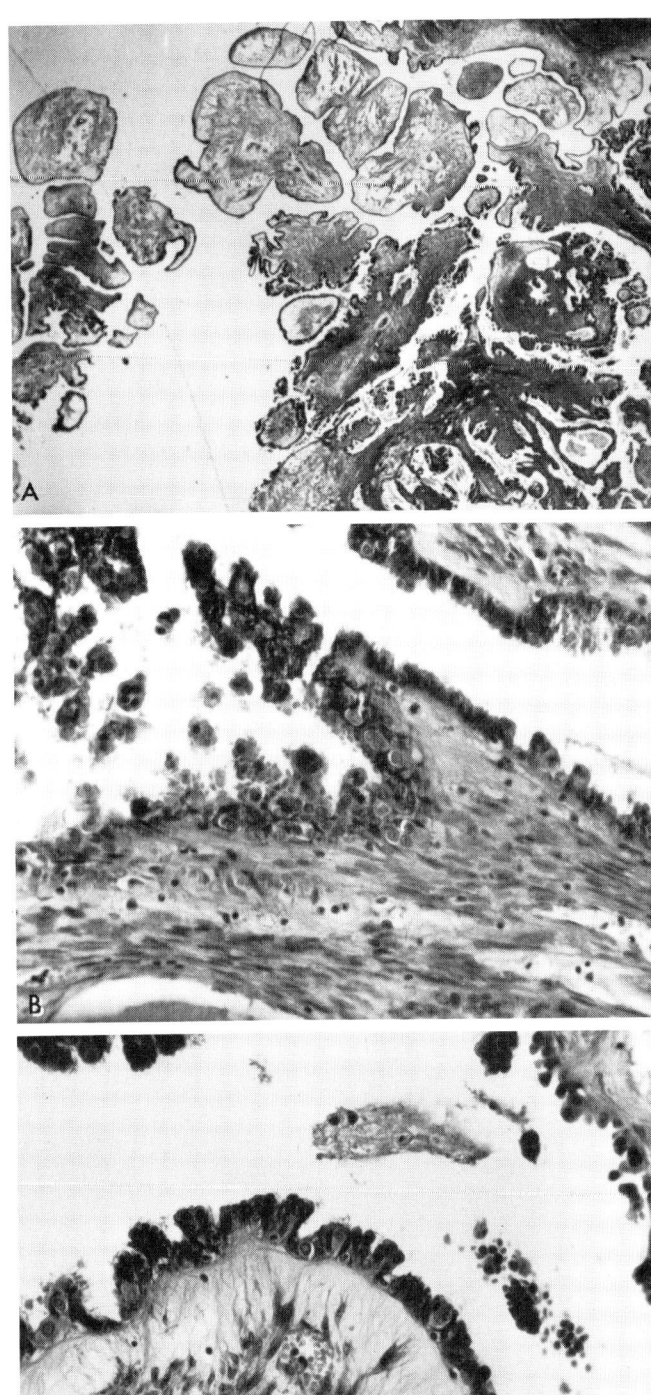

Figure 43-2. Hydatidiform mole, possibly malignant (Grade IV of Hertig), with a considerable degree of trophoblastic proliferation. *A*, Notice molar vesicles without epithelial proliferation in upper field whereas toward the bottom there is considerable trophoblastic overgrowth (15×). *B*, Proliferating trophoblast with anaplastic Langhans cells (200×). *C*, Area of moderate trophoblastic proliferation, seen at same magnification (200×).

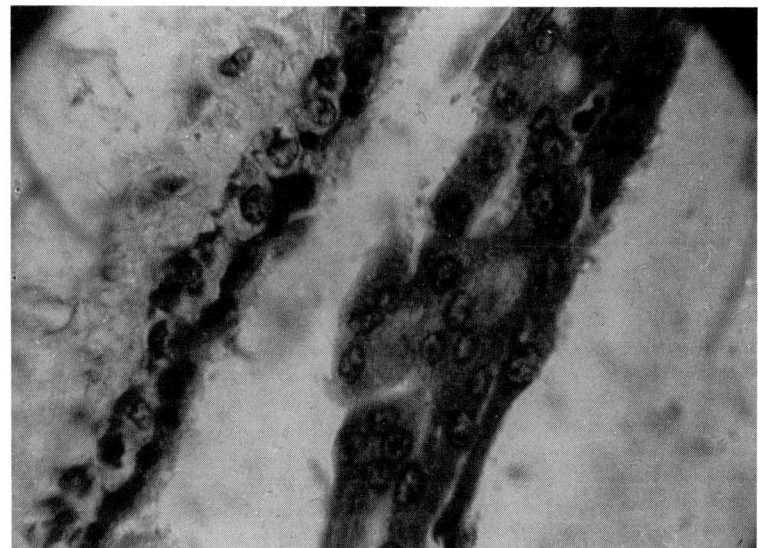

Figure 43-3. Mole with intermediate degree of epithelial overgrowth, particularly as regards the syncytium. The mildly hyperplastic Langhans layer contains abundant PAS positive inclusions, appearing black and representing gonadotropin (Hotchkiss-McManus stain, 400×).

The currently prevailing idea is that what determines whether trophoblastic growth is to be arrested or not is an *immune reaction* by the maternal body, which can act as effectively against moles exhibiting marked trophoblastic proliferation as it does against those showing little proliferation. In the presence of deficient maternal response, even a mole with little trophoblastic proliferation and, hence, presumably of low malignant potential, may become invasive and turn into choriocarcinoma. Conversely, moles appearing histologically to be highly malignant may be arrested in their growth as a result of an adequate defensive reaction. Here, estrogens probably play an important role.

43.5. HISTOCHEMISTRY OF MOLE

Botella and his co-workers[18] investigated the glycoprotein content of trophoblastic tissue under both normal and pathologic conditions (see Chapters 19 and 41). By extending those studies to hydatidiform mole, they were able to show the presence of large amounts of neutral mucopolysaccharides, staining intensely red in the

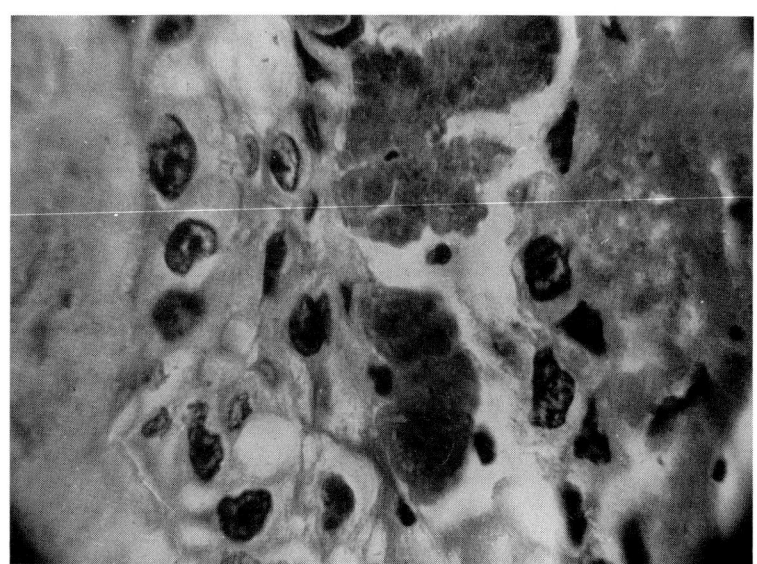

Figure 43-4. Mole with pronounced trophoblastic overgrowth (Grade IV of Hertig). Disorderly and pleomorphic proliferation of Langhans layer (400×).

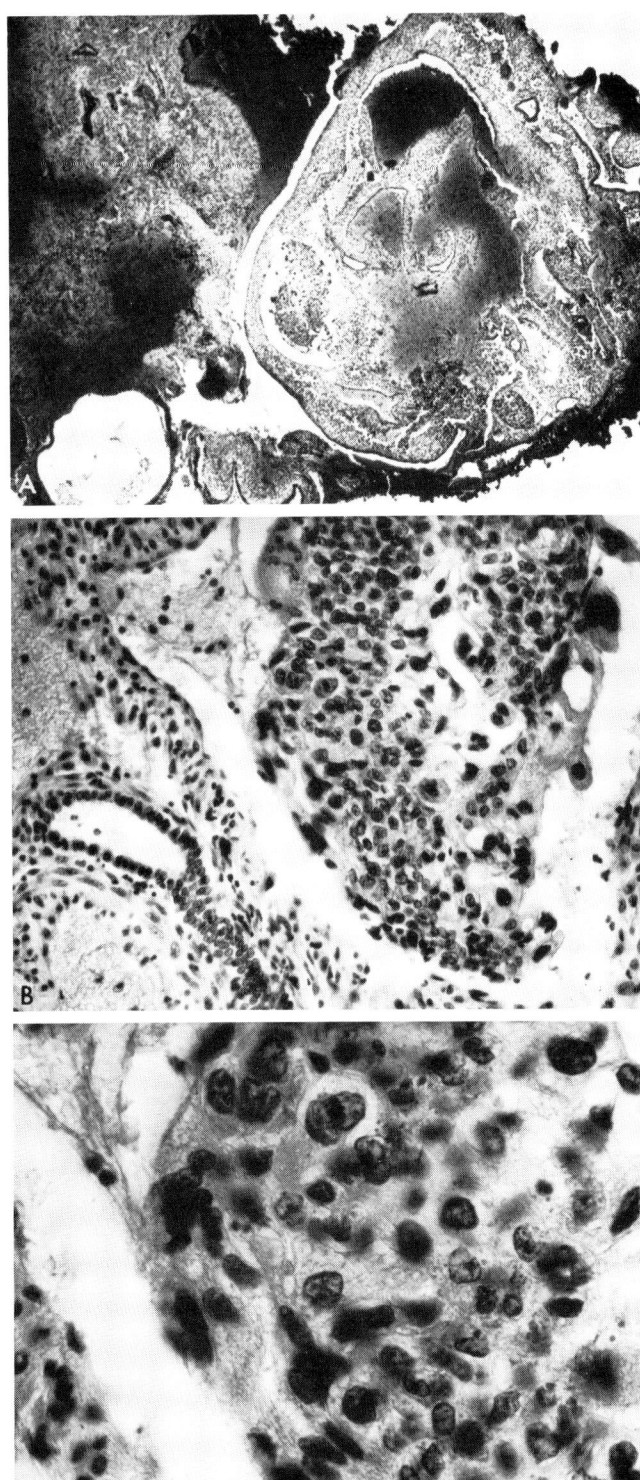

Figure 43-5. Choriocarcinoma. *A*, Low power (15×). Part of the destroyed uterine wall, with extensive hemorrhage and islands of highly anaplastic, malignant trophoblastic cells. *B*, An island of malignant trophoblastic cells viewed at higher magnification (120×). *C*, Nuclear and cellular detail of the trophoblastic cells in the same area (400×).

periodic acid-Schiff (PAS) reaction. The common variety of mole gives a strong reaction, indicating production of large amounts of gonadotropins in the Langhans layer. In micromolar degeneration, on the contrary, the reaction is weak or absent. Because these findings correlate well with measurable gonadotropin levels (discussed later), it may be reliably asserted that this method allows us to detect the rate of hormone production by molar tissue. Our studies have been subsequently confirmed by Bur and associates.[21]

43.6. HORMONE BIOSYNTHESIS BY MOLAR TISSUE

Although chorionic gonadotropin is the most commonly known hormone produced by mole, we shall also examine the question of molar biosynthesis of estrogens, 17-ketosteroids, progesterone, thyroid hormone and placental lactogen.

43.6.1. GONADOTROPINS

In 1928, Aschheim[5] and Zondek[114] were first to discover the fact that carriers of mole had large amounts of gonadotropins in their urine. In 1930, Meyer[65] demonstrated that gonadotropin was present in high concentration in molar tissue. Later studies on the subject were published by Sutherland,[101] Huber and Hörmann[48] and Kinnunen.[53,54] The levels of concentration reported were considerably higher than those found in normal gestation. It is now thought that 24 hr excretion values below 300,000 IU are expressive of normal gestation between the eighth and twelfth weeks, whereas higher values are consistent with mole. However, this classic concept has recently been subject to a great deal of criticism and controversy. In the first place, there are numerous instances of mole on record in which there was no appreciable gonadotropinuria (Acosta-Sisson,[3] Sutherland[101]). A recent publication by Smalbraak[93] reviews such cases. They may be regarded as rare and exceptional. Not infrequently, though, the rate of gonadotropin elimination in cases of mole is not as high as one might anticipate by clas-sical standards and may even be lower than that found in normal gestation. As revealed by the work of Gennel,[35] the greatest confusion arises in cases of hyperemesis gravidarum. Data supplied by Gennel show that there is no distinctive deviation in the pattern of gonadotropin elimination in cases with mole, as compared with normal gestation, let alone with that seen in hyperemesis gravidarum. Allison,[4] Delfs,[26,27] and Bertini and associates[12] also stress this type of diagnostic error. Nonetheless, it is of interest to note that while isolated determinations are subject to error, serial quantitative determinations can provide the exact diagnosis. Indeed, by studying the gonadotropin elimination curve in normal pregnancy (see Chapter 19, page 406), it may be noted how gonadotropinuria decreases quite rapidly after the thirteenth week. In cases with mole, by contrast, these values may be observed to rise considerably after that date, up to the sixteenth or eighteenth week, at which time the mole is expelled. The presence of such a *rising curve* is therefore of greater significance than either a high or low value shown by a single determination.

Although Velardo[111] found no biologic difference between urinary gonadotropin levels in normal pregnant women and those found in mole carriers, modern immunologic studies (Schwartz and Mantel,[88] Leone et al.,[59] Wide and Hobson[113]) would all seem to indicate some minor immunologic differences that perhaps one day may make the differential diagnosis from normal pregnancy possible. Hamashige and associates[38] have in addition shown that *antigonadotropins* may be detected in the urine.

43.6.2. ESTROGENS

Hydatidiform mole constitutes a special example of chorionic steroidogenesis. As pointed out in Chapter 19, trophoblastic tissue utilizes dehydroepiandrosterone (DHEA-SO$_4$) of fetal adrenal origin for estrogen biogenesis. In the *absence of a fetus* in mole, this type of steroidogenic circuit cannot be set up. This may well account for the numerous reports of *subnormal rates of estrogenuria* in association with mole.[14,31,43,54,58,60,95] However, molar tissue cultured in vitro has been found to be capable of estrogen synthesis (Uher et al.,[107] Van Leusden and Villee[108, 109]). Barlow and his co-workers,[9] who incubated molar tissue in the presence of DHEA-SO$_4$, found evidence of normal steroidogenesis when the molar tissue was benign but not when it was malignant, in which case steroidogenesis was increased. Perhaps this explains why estrogen excretion is low in mola destruens and in choriocarcinoma (Odell et al.[74]). MacDonald and Siiteri[60] showed that *estriol* production was low or absent, which is also in keeping with functional chorionic deficiency. Nevertheless, MacKay-Hart[61] isolated 3β-ol-DH from molar tissue. Thus, all indications are that the potential for steroidogenesis remains intact in benign molar tissue but that the *absence of fetal adrenal function* results in low estrogen output on the part of molar trophoblastic tissue.

43.6.3. PREGNANEDIOL

Erb and colleagues,[31] Pannain,[76] MacNaughton,[62] and Pigeaud and his associates[80] have all reported finding increased urinary pregnanediol levels in molar gestations. VanLeusden[110] demonstrated progesterone biosynthesis by molar tissue cultured in vitro; finally, Stitch and his co-workers[100] also reported the presence of urinary pregnanediol. The source of the progesterone had once been believed to be *luteal cysts;* however, Stitch and his colleagues observed a case in which urinary pregnanediol disappeared after the mole was eliminated, although the cysts persisted. This would seem to indicate that progestogen synthesis takes place in the trophoblastic tissue itself.

Coutts and his co-workers[25] revealed that molar tissue contained a large amount of catabolites of 21-carbon steroids, which unquestionably points to progesterone biosynthesis by mole, albeit as an intermediary metabolite.

43.6.4. 17-KETOSTEROIDS

The occurrence of 17-ketosteroids in mole has been investigated by Pannain[76] and by Smalbraak.[93] Both authors found large amounts of this group of compounds in the urine. This is not surprising if one remembers that high dosages of chorionic gonadotropin, as we have indicated in Chapter 9, stimulate the adrenal as well as the ovarian interstitium, thereby inducing 17-ketosteroid overproduction in woman as well as in female animals. Consequently, high 17-ketosteroid values are thought to reflect enhanced gonadotropin activity in molar gestation.

43.6.5. MOLE AND THYROID FUNCTION

Tisne and his co-workers[105] had already indicated the occurrence of signs of thyroid hyperfunction in association with mole. Dowling and associates[29] and Kock and colleagues[57] reported increased ^{131}I uptake by the thyroid as well as high blood PBI values in patients with molar gestations. Such results are consistent with thyroid hyperfunction. *What causes development of hyperthyroidism in association with mole is thyrotropin production by molar tissue*, as shown by recent investigations.[57, 74, 98]

43.6.6. PLACENTAL LACTOGEN

In Chapter 19, we have already pointed out that one of the most characteristic incretions of chorionic tissue is a lactogenic and growth promoting protein, cross reacting immunologically with, but differing from, both STH and prolactin.

Placental lactogen has been isolated from molar tissue by Odell and associates,[74] Franz and colleagues,[33] and Saxena and colleagues.[85] This finding completes the existing analogy between molar tissue and the normal chorion.

Klopper[56] believes that the ratio between lactogen and chorionic gonadotropin may serve as an index of whether molar tissue is benign or malignant. High rates of HCG excretion associated with parallel elevations in HPL values are believed to indicate a favorable prognosis, whereas a reduction in HPL associated with an increase in HCG suggests a change toward malignancy, inasmuch as it indicates predominance of the cytotrophoblast over the syncytial trophoblast.

43.7. CLINICAL FEATURES OF MOLE

The endocrinologic character of this work does not permit us to enlarge on any clinical considerations of mole other than those pertaining to incretory phenomena. We shall consider basically three clinical aspects: (1) coexistence of toxemia and mole; (2) occurrence of polycystic ovaries, and (3) endocrine treatment of mole.

43.7.1. CONCURRENCE OF MOLE AND TOXEMIA

The frequency with which, according to Smalbraak[91] and Teoh and Tow,[104] molar pregnancies develop symptoms of toxemia has been indicated above. Smith and Smith[94, 95] attribute this coincidence to the fact that hyperexcretion of gonadotropin occurs in mole as well as in toxemia of pregnancy. Page postulates that some placental pressor substance is present in increased amounts in mole, which presumably accounts for the appearance of toxemic symptoms.

Some Dutch authors (Mastboom,[63] Bastiansee,[10] Smalbraak[92]) do not believe that the association of mole with toxemia is related to hyperproduction of gonadotropin but instead results from excessive distention of the uterine walls owing to overly rapid molar growth, since it appears in the type of mole developing late and growing at a very rapid rate. The absence of toxemic symptoms in cases of choriocarcinoma seems to support this concept.

43.7.2. POLYCYSTIC OVARIES

The occurrence of ovaries with large luteal cysts in conjunction with mole was recognized a long time ago.[65, 66, 69] Novak[70] showed that such cysts represented a physiopathologic response on part of the granulosa and theca cells to excessive amounts of gonadotropin produced by the trophoblast. These cysts accordingly are thought to result from ovarian hyperluteinization. However, it is questionable whether these cysts are capable of producing significant quantities of progesterone, as attested by the fact that pregnanediol excretion is never unduly elevated.

It is of interest to note that, according to different sources,[40, 41, 54] the incidence of such cysts varies from 4 per cent (Smalbraak[91]) to as high as 90 per cent. This extreme divergence of data is in fact also associated with dissimilar figures in gonadotropin excretion values, as observed by a number of workers. Such divergences are hard to account for, unless authors reporting low values were dealing with micromole rather than mole, the former being diagnosable only on the basis of a histopathologic examination of the abortus.

43.7.3. MOLAR METASTASES

Although a particular mole may be considered benign, it sometimes spreads beyond the confines of the uterus, producing invasion of, or metastases to, other organs. This occurs especially in instances of *mola destruens, intravenous mole or chorioadenoma destruens*,[3] an atypical and invasive mole with a tendency to penetrate into venous lakes of the uterus. Taylor and Drägemüller[102] have described a form of *syncytial endometritis* in which invasion by syncytial molar elements diffusely involves the entire endo- and myometrium. Over the past years, moreover, attention has been drawn to the occurrence of moles without apparent malignancy, yet producing distant metastases (Hertig and Sheldon,[41] Hsu et al.,[47] Thiele and Alvarez[103]).

These findings constitute by far the strongest argument yet against Hertig's original concept, which we outlined previously: a prognosis based on the histologic appearance of a given mole. The truth is that neither in mole nor in chorioepithelioma does the histologic picture justify predictions as to what is going to happen, since it is known that even chorioepitheliomas noted for highly malignant features occasionally are seen to regress spontaneously, whereas "innocuous" moles may behave as true malignant neoplasms.

43.7.4. TREATMENT

Without entering the discussion of the clinical aspects of treatment (technique of evacuating the uterus, criteria for an expectant or interventionist approach, etc.), we intend to mention only three points; estrogen therapy, recommended by a great many authors[52, 57, 91]; *methotrexate*, discussed at the close of this chapter; and the need for following up those cases of treated mole for at least one year by means of hormone assay (Buxton[22]).

43.8. CHORIOEPITHELIOMA

Chorioepithelioma is a tumor composed of both cyto- and syncytiotrophoblastic elements in variable proportions. It has no supportive stroma, which is proof of its malignancy. Owing to the absence of stroma, *the tumor possesses no vascularization of its own, which imparts to it a purely parasitic character.*

Because the tumor is entirely dependent on the host's blood supply, it thrives by invading blood vessels, thus revealing a marked *vascular tropism* that results in hemorrhage and, at the same time, produces large areas of necrosis within the tumor itself. This feature of avascularity of the tumor has been brought to light by Smalbraak[91] as one of the most characteristic properties of this type of neoplasia. Because of these properties, Schopper and Pliess,[86] as well as Schuster,[87] the similarity between chorioepithelioma and *inoculation tumors*.

This resemblance is even more striking if one realizes, as noted by Park,[78] that chorioepithelioma arises in the trophoblast, an entity genetically distinct from the maternal organism. Consequently, we are dealing with a growth that, so far as *chromosomal composition* is concerned, differs from the host, a fact of utmost importance for the understanding of the etiology and evolution of this tumor.

43.8.1. INCIDENCE

As reported by different authors, the incidence varies greatly. We have mentioned here previously that hydatidiform mole and chorioepithelioma are particularly common in Asian countries (Acosta-Sisson[1]). Mathieu[64] reported an incidence of 12 chorioepitheliomas in 126 molar gestations (9.4 per cent). Brews[20] found six chorioepitheliomas among 72 moles (8.3 per cent). Chesley and his colleagues[23] discovered 26 instances of malignancy in a series of 177 moles (15 per cent). Findings like these may convey the impression that about one in every 10 moles degenerates into chorioepithelioma. According to Novak,[71] however, fewer than 1 per cent of all moles undergo malignant transformation. Novak is noted for his enormous amount of experience gained by having access to the worldwide material of the Mathieu Registry, which renders his assertion all the more authoritative. Smalbraak,[92] at his clinic at Utrecht, found 17 cases of chorioepithelioma over a period of 26 years. His material was based on 50,000 deliveries, a relatively large series. Although, from our own experience, the occurrence of mole is fairly common in Spain, that of chorioepithelioma is quite exceptional. Thus, Novak's assertion does not seem to us to be exaggerated, and perhaps the incidence reported by other authors is unusually high.

Approximately 50 per cent of all chorioepitheliomas arise in mole, but the remaining 50 per cent may develop in the wake of abortion (30 per cent) or even following normal pregnancy (20 per cent).

43.8.2. ETIOLOGY

Structurally, chorioepithelioma in some instances reproduces the cytotrophoblast (Fig. 43–6), in others, the syncytiotrophoblast (Fig. 43–7). It is generally held that the first variety represents *immature forms* whereas the second represents *mature forms*. Much like mole are the examples in which villi persist in their embryonal state, so chorioepithelioma reproduces to an exaggerated extent the structure of the trophoblast at its most primitive stage. Although chorioepithelioma does not invariably arise from mole it may be stated that whenever it does, it does so by virtue of "*retrogression*," since the cells composing chorioepithelioma are more embryonal in nature than those making up the molar integument. Although it is most often from cells pertaining to the molar integument that the embryonal components of chorioepithelioma arise by a process of regressive transformation, both normal and abortive gestation, too, may give rise to this

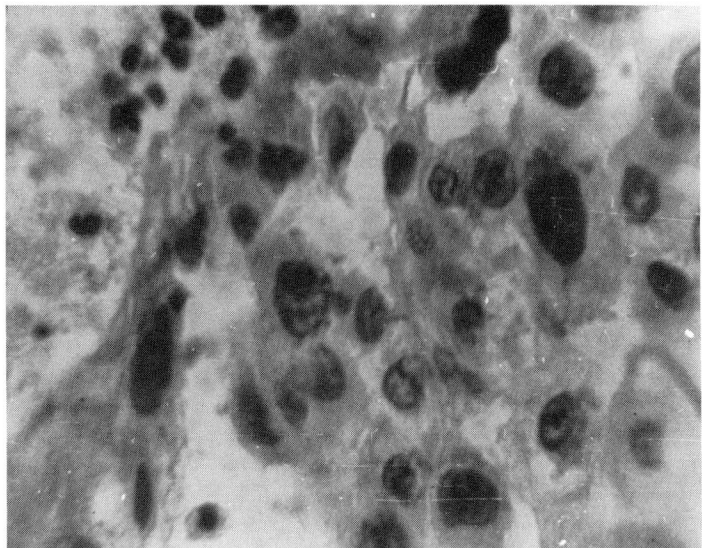

Figure 43-6. Choriocarcinoma with predominance of cytotrophoblastic component (450×).

type of chorionic neoplasia. Despite the doubts we have expressed concerning the neoplastic character of mole, which we prefer to regard as a *degenerative* process, chorioepithelioma is definitely a neoplasm, and in addition a neoplasm with features of malignancy. Three etiologic considerations in particular must be taken into account: (1) the special biology of the trophoblastic cells in which the tumor originates; (2) the previously mentioned *"parasitic"* nature of the tumor, and (3) the capacity of the maternal body to respond with an immune reaction to trophoblastic invasion.

43.8.3. BIOLOGY OF TROPHOBLASTIC CELLS

In its earliest developmental stage, the trophoblastic cell is an *immature, disorderly proliferative cell* that is endowed with a capacity to actively invade maternal tissues. To a certain extent, all cancer cells share this property; consequently, the exact reproduction of the properties of the young chorion leads simply to chorioepithelioma. Thus, as just indicated above, *chorioepithelioma is a neoplasm in which the properties of the trophoblast are maintained more*

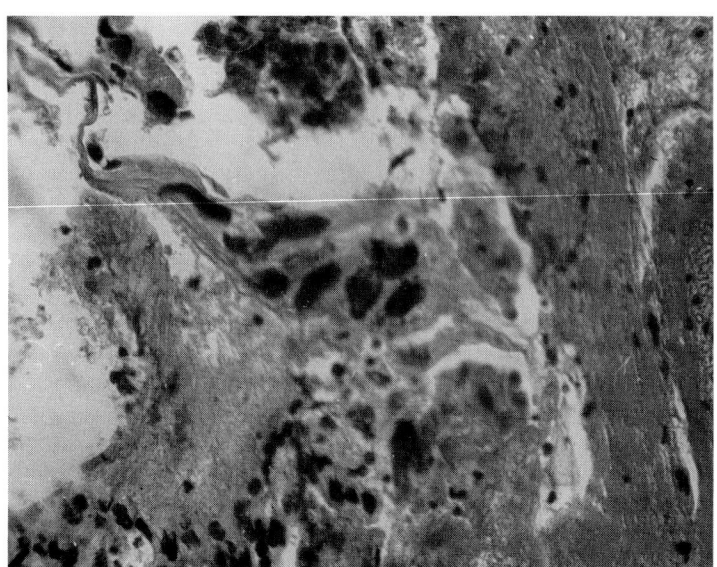

Figure 43-7. Choriocarcinoma with syncytial predominance (450×).

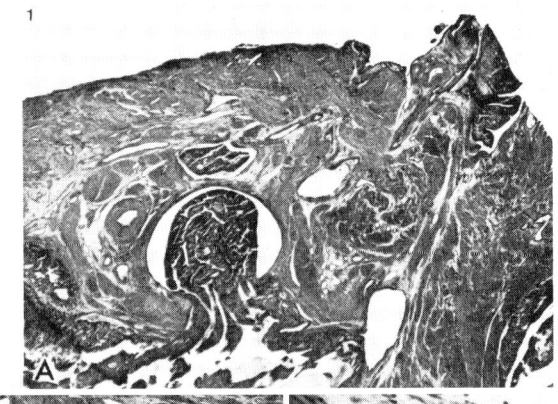
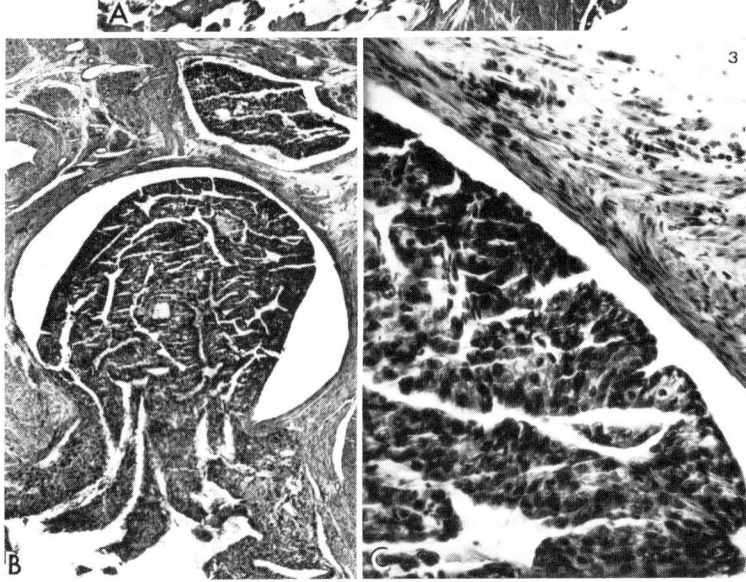

Figure 43-8. Choriocarcinoma invading blood vessel. A, 15×; B, 60×; C, 260×.

or less indefinitely as they are during their earliest days of development.

Some of the equally essential features of the trophoblast are the properties of arresting its own development spontaneously, of maturing extremely rapidly and of dying much earlier than the host. Thus, while a person's average life span is 70 years, the placenta only lives for nine months, that is, only one ninety-third as long. The cells of other tumors that originate in the host's body are able to enjoy a much longer life than chorioepithelioma cells which, by virtue of their special nature, are destined to undergo degeneration and to die early.

43.8.4. CHORIOEPITHELIOMA AS AN "INOCULATION" TUMOR

We have already indicated that chorioepithelioma possesses a genetic individuality of its own which is distinct from that of the woman's body and which is derived from the egg. As a result, it is similar to inoculation tumors. Chorioepithelioma is, so to say, alien to the "host's" body. It is moreover devoid of vessels and depends for its nutrition entirely on the host. Park[77] likened chorioepithelioma to a homotransplant whereas Schopper and Pliess,[86] as well as Schuster,[87] considered it an inoculation tumor. Interestingly, Bardawill and Toy[8] speculate as to whether the malignant or benign character of certain chorioepitheliomas may not be due to a genetic XX or XY chromosomal complement. In the final analysis, as pointed out by Douglas and associates,[28] it should be borne in mind that even during normal gestation the maternal blood may contain circulating trophoblastic islands similar to those causing malignant invasion by chorioepithelioma.

Under these circumstances, it is not surprising that chorioepithelioma should provoke an immune reaction in the mother aimed at its own elimination, as shall be pointed out later.

43.8.5. IMMUNITY TO CHORIONIC INVASION

Many years ago, the existence of "deciduolysins" in the trophoblast and "choriolysins" in the decidua, as well as the maternal body as a whole, had been suggested to represent an immune antigen-antibody reaction.[17,66] We have pointed out previously that such a reaction is presently believed to depend largely on the pH that is maintained in the medium by the carbonate-bicarbonate buffer system. The latter is controlled by carbonic anhydrase and thereby indirectly by estrogen-progesterone balance, thus giving rise to a greater or lesser degree of invasiveness of trophoblastic tissue. What was once believed to be an ordinary immunologic process, in the nature of a reaction to extraneous protein possessing antigenic potency, is now recognized to be *controlled by endocrine phenomena*. Accordingly, predominance of progesterone activity facilitates invasion by the trophoblast under normal as well as pathologic conditions, whereas estrogenic predominance, conversely, inhibits trophoblastic invasion. In a previous section, we have listed the arguments leading us to suspect that *hyperestrogenism* plays a role in molar invasiveness. The same, but to an even greater extent, may reasonably be assumed to hold true with regard to chorioepithelioma. This is not without important consequences for both the prognosis and the therapy of chorioepithelioma.

Scott[89] recently analyzed some of the etiologic factors involved in chorioepithelioma: first, the fact that chorioepithelioma most commonly occurs in older women; second, that it predominantly occurs in primiparas; third, that it has a definite affinity for some blood groups; fourth, that hereditary factors have a decisive influence; and fifth, that important immune factors are apparently also at play.

43.8.6. HORMONE SYNTHESIS BY CHORIOEPITHELIOMA

Meyer, Brindeau and Smith were first to describe the presence of hypergonadotropinuria in cases of chorioepithelioma. Portillo and his associates[82,83] have succeeded in culturing a choriocarcinoma cell line which continued to secrete HCG constantly. It has classically been admitted that gonadotropinuria values above 500,000 units were suspicious, while values above 1 million units were practically diagnostic, of chorioepithelioma.[5,114,115] On the other hand, Allison[4] has insisted that even low rates of gonadotropin excretion may occasionally be consistent with chorioepithelioma, provided that the diagnosis of normal or pathologic gestation can be ruled out. Nevertheless, cases of chorionepithelioma with negative gonadotropinuria have been reported in modern times by Sutherland[101] and by Acosta-Sisson[2] on the basis of extensive reviews of the world literature. Although such instances are exceptional, the physician ought to be aware of them and not require the presence of very high urinary hormone titers as an absolute prerequisite for the diagnosis of chorioepithelioma. Delfs[27] published a comprehensive review of the problem. In very serious cases of chorioepithelioma with metastases, he found up to 3,000,000 units in 24 hr specimens of urine, compared to values of just a few thousand units in cases in which the neoplasm was in its initial stages. Gonadotropinuria in chorioepithelioma is significant not only for facilitating the diagnosis but also for providing a *prognostic index*. As pointed out above, every case involving the explusion or evacuation of a mole must be followed up by repeated bioassays of HCG for a period of at least one year. Any evidence of positive gonadotropinuria after the fifth week (in the absence of pregnancy) indicates the presence of active molar rests and, possibly, development of chorioepithelioma. By the same token, the prognosis is favorable if gonadotropinuria disappears following the removal of a uterus containing a chorioepitheliomatous focus, whereas it is poor if gonadotropinuria persists, which indicates the presence of metastases. It has similarly been noted that gonadotropinuria may become negative following X-ray therapy of metastases,[35,52,91] and again become positive in cases with recurrences. Finally, evidence of gradually falling HCG titers in any case with an established diagnosis of chorioepithelioma, as noted by various authors,[111,115,116] is indicative of degeneration and spontaneous retrogression of the tumor, a phenomenon we shall deal with in a subsequent paragraph.

Schwartz and Mantel[88] believe that the gonadotropins that are excreted in cases of chorioepithelioma or mole can be distinguished immunologically from those occurring in normal pregnancy.

The question concerning the excretion of other hormones in cases of chorioepithelioma has been studied much less. Aschheim[5] and Zondek[114] never observed a case with elevated estrogenuria, which has been corroborated by Hinglais and Hinglais[44] in one case, by Smith and Smith[94] in two cases, and by Frandsen and Stakeman[32] in 13 cases. Pregnanediol excretion was found to be elevated in one case by Pigeaud and associates[80] and in two cases by Pannain,[76] who similarly reported a considerable increase in 17-ketosteroid values. The probable reason for such increased values has been suggested in a preceding section.

As also indicated previously (Section 43.6.6), a reduction in lactogen values is of adverse prognostic significance in chorionic neoplasia. Saxena and colleagues[85] found that HPL values were low in choriocarcinoma, compared with those of either mole or normal pregnancy.

43.9. EVOLUTION, PROGNOSIS AND TREATMENT

In recent years, the prognosis of chorioepithelioma has become a matter of considerable controversy. We believe it necessary to state here a few ideas concerning the evolution, prognosis and treatment of chorioepithelioma, which are all intimately related to each other.

43.9.1. EVOLUTION

Schopper and Pliess[86] and Schuster[87] called attention to the fact that some chorioepitheliomas regressed spontaneously. Since it has also been noted (Douglas et al.[28]) that in normal gestation trophoblastic particles may be deported, occasionally to distant organs, they coined the term "chorioepitheliosis" for those apparently tumoral growths resulting from the deportation of trophoblastic islets and destined to follow the biologic evolution of the normal trophoblast, that is, to undergo degeneration and to die in the course of a few months. Huber and Hörmann[48, 49] reviewed the abundant anatomopathologic material of the Kiel Clinic and found 22 cases of chorioepithelioma diagnosed conclusively by histologic means. Of these, 19 cases did not recur and were cured either as a result of therapy (radiation, surgery) or in a spontaneous manner. Their statistics revealed an interesting instance of regression of pulmonary metastatic disease. About the same time, Schopper[86] recognized the similarity between chorioepithelioma and tumor transplants in general, pointing out the fact that both elicited an immune response in the host and, as a result, were associated with a type of defensive reaction that did not occur in "autochthonous" tumors. Our reasons for admitting the occurrence of spontaneous retrogression of chorioepithelioma have been explained previously and are based not only on this transplant-like behavior of chorioepithelioma but also on the property of the trophoblast to undergo spontaneous regression and to produce immunity.

Bardawill and his colleagues[7, 8] emphasize the regressive character of some chorioepitheliomas, offering the genetic explanation already mentioned. As a result of his review of such cases, Ober[73] damped some of the optimism regarding spontaneous regression of this tumor: without denying its occurrence, he pointed out that there were only 20 acceptable cases of proved regression of chorioepithelioma in the literature, to which we might add the more recent series published by Natsume and Takada.[68]

Evidently, "malignant" chorioepithelioma is a serious tumor, leading inevitably to the patient's demise, regardless of the therapeutic measures employed. It must be admitted that in all those cases in which cures were reported in the literature following radical surgery, radiotherapy or hormone therapy, the results may be viewed as instances of spontaneous cure in which the work of nature may have been lent a "helping hand."

43.9.2. PROGNOSIS

In view of the foregoing conclusions, the prognosis cannot be asserted as invariably poor but rather as simply doubtful. When we are faced with the diagnosis of chorioepithelioma, we may never be absolutely sure whether we are dealing with the malignant form (*chorioepithelioma malignum*) or with the benign form (*chorioepitheliosis*). Ober,[73] as well as Jacobson and Enzer,[51] emphasize the usefulness of running repeated bioassays of HCG as a prognostic index. Falling titers of HCG are believed to indicate a favorable prognosis.

43.9.3. TREATMENT

We shall limit ourselves to a few essential statements, since therapy of chorioepithelioma is not, strictly speaking, an endocrine problem. The following methods of treatment have been proposed: (1) Surgery, (2) x-ray therapy, (3) blood transfusions, (4) hormone therapy, and (5) methotrexate therapy. We shall describe only the last two.

HORMONE THERAPY. This type of therapy, which has been recommended by Kock and associates,[57] Hohlweg and colleagues,[45] Hinglais and Hinglais,[44] Smalbraak[91] and Stearns,[97] is based on the above mentioned fact that *estrogenic predominance suppresses trophoblastic invasion*. Although this is an established physiopathologic fact, it does not follow that positive results can be achieved definitively with estrogen therapy. It must be realized that *a good many cases of chorioepithelioma regress without any therapy*. This poses the question of whether a cure in this type of tumor treated with estrogens results from the hormone therapy or from spontaneous remission.

METHOTREXATE. A derivative of pteroylglutamic acid, specifically 4-amino-N-10-methyl-pteroylglutamic acid, or *methotrexate*, is a cytostatic agent, originally tested in the treatment of acute leukemia and subsequently applied with success to the treatment of chorioepithelioma and to the prevention of malignant degeneration of hydatidiform mole.

Treatment consists in administering 5 mg three times daily for five days, for a total of 75 mg. Subsequently, and under careful hematologic control, we institute a rest period and repeat the same schedule at intervals for a total dosage of 300 mg. The results obtained with this treatment over the past years have been satisfactory (Chun et al.,[24] Hertz et al.,[42] Spellace et al.,[96] Vogler et al.[112]). Nevertheless, how can one be sure that the same results would not have been obtained without therapy?

This of course is an objection that can be raised against any form of treatment of chorioepithelioma, so that no definite conclusions can be drawn for the time being. The basic problem involved is the short-lived vitality of this tumor, together with its capacity to induce immunity and to regress spontaneously. For as long as we still lack the means of assessing the potential for malignancy of trophoblastic elements, not only for a given moment but also for the long run, prognosis as well as treatment will remain largely a matter of conjecture.

REFERENCES

1. Acosta-Sisson, H.: *Amer. J. Obstet. Gynec.*, 71:1274, 1956.
2. Acosta-Sisson, H.: *Obstet. Gynec.*, 9:233, 1957.
3. Acosta-Sisson, H.: *Amer. J. Obstet. Gynec.*, 80:176, 1960.
4. Allison, R. M.: *Amer. J. Obstet. Gynec.*, 71:155, 1956.
5. Aschheim, S.: *Amer. J. Obstet. Gynec.*, 19:355, 1930.
6. Baggish, M. D., Woodruff, J. D., Tow, S. H., and Jones, H. W.: *Amer. J. Obstet. Gynec.*, 102:362, 1968.
7. Bardawill, W. A., Hertig, A. T., and Velardo, J. T.: *Obstet. Gynec.*, 10:614, 1957.
8. Bardawill, W. A., and Toy, B. L.: *Ann. N.Y. Acad. Sci.*, 80:197, 1959.
9. Barlow, J. J., Goldstein, D. P., and Reid, D. E.: *J. Clin. Endocr.*, 27:1028, 1967.
10. Bastiansee, M. A. van B.: *Nederl. Tijskr. Verlosk.*, 56:498, 1956.
11. Beischer, N. A., and Fortune, D. W.: *Amer. J. Obstet. Gynec.*, 100:276, 1968.
12. Bertini, B., Hornstein, M., and Blatt, I.: *Obstet. Gynec.*, 62:139, 1963.
13. Bishun, N. P., and Morton, W. R. M.: *J. Obstet. Gynec. Brit. Comm.*, 75:66, 1967.
14. Bonado, P., Patti, A. A., Franley, T. F., and Stein, A. A.: *Amer. J. Obstet. Gynec.*, 87:210, 1963.
15. Botella, J., and Tamargo, J. S.: *Acta Gin.*, 4:497, 1953.
16. Botella, J.: *Actas de la Sdad. Esp. Esterilidad*, 6:53; 1958.
17. Botella, J.: *Patología Obstétrica*, 4th ed. Barcelona, Editorial Científico-Médica, 1958.
18. Botella, J., Nogales, F., and Durán, J. M.: *Arch. Gynäk.*, 188:269, 1957.
18a. Böving, B. G.: *Arch. Gynäk.*, 80:21, 1959.
19. Bret, J. A., and Grepinet, J.: *Rev. Fr. Gynec. Obstet.*, 43:463, 1967.
20. Brews, A.: *J. Obstet. Gynec. Brit. Emp.*, 57:317, 1950.

21. Bur, G. E., Hertig, A. T., MacKay, D. G., and Adams, E. C.: *Obstet. Gynec.*, 19:156, 1962.
22. Buxton, C. L.: *Ann. N.Y. Acad. Sci.*, 80:12, 1959.
23. Chesley, L. C., Cosgrove, A. S., and Preece, J.: *Amer. J. Obstet. Gynec.*, 52:311, 1946.
24. Chun, D., Braga, C., Chow, C., and Lok, L.: *J. Obstet. Gynec. Brit. Comm.*, 71:185, 1964.
25. Coutts, J. R. T., MacNaughton, M. C., Ross, G. T., and Walker, J.: *J. Endocr.*, 44:335, 1969.
26. Delfs, E. D.: *Obstet. Gynec.*, 9:1, 1957.
27. Delfs, E. D.: *Ann. N.Y. Acad. Sci.*, 80:125, 1959.
28. Douglas, G. W., et al.: *Amer. J. Obstet. Gynec.*, 78:960, 1959.
29. Dowling, J. T., Ingbar, S. H., and Freinkel, N.: *J. Clin. Endocr.*, 20:1, 1960.
30. Edmonds, H. W.: *Ann. N.Y. Acad. Sci.*, 80:86, 1959.
31. Erb, H., Keller, M., Hauser, G. A., and Wenner, R.: *Gynaecologia*, 152:317, 1961.
32. Frandsen, V. A., and Stakeman, G.: *Acta Endocr.*, Suppl., 45:90, 1964.
33. Frantz, A. G., Rabkin, M. T., and Friesen, H.: *J. Clin. Endocr. Metab.*, 25:1136, 1965.
34. Fund, A. F.: *Ann. N.Y. Acad. Sci.*, 80:178, 1959.
35. Gennell, S.: *Acta Obstet. Gynec. Scand.*, 26:555, 1946.
36. Greene, R. R.: *Ann. N.Y. Acad. Sci.*, 80:143, 1959.
37. Guerrero, R., and Lactot, C. A.: *Amer. J. Obstet. Gynec.*, 107:263, 1970.
38. Hamashige, S., Mishell, D. R., and Arquilla, E. R.: *J. Clin. Endocr. Metab.*, 26:651, 1966.
39. Harper, M. K. J., Prostkoff, B. T., and Reeve, R. J.: *Acta Endocr.*, 52:465, 1966.
40. Hertig, A. T., and Edmonds, H. W.: *Arch. Path.*, 30:260, 1950.
41. Hertig, A. T., and Sheldon, W. M.: *Amer. J. Obstet. Gynec.*, 52:1, 1947.
42. Hertz, R., Roos, G. T., and Lipsett, M. B.: *Amer. N.Y. Acad. Sci.*, 114:881, 1964.
43. Hinglais, H., and Hinglais, M.: *Ann. d'Endocr.*, 9:171, 1948.
44. Hinglais, H., and Hinglais, M.: *Gynec. Obstet.*, 52:190, 1953.
45. Hohlweg, W., Hahn, H., and Braun, G.: *Arch. Gynäk.*, 181:139, 1952.
46. Hörmann, G.: *Arch. Gynäk.*, 181:297, 1959.
47. Hsu, C. T., Huang, L. C., and Chen, L. Y.: *Amer. J. Obstet. Gynec.*, 84:1412, 1962.
48. Huber, H., and Hörmann, G.: *Ztschr. f. Krebsforsch.*, 58:285, 1952.
49. Huber, H., and Hörmann, G.: *Geburtsh. u. Frauenhk.*, 12:511, 1952.
50. Hunt, W., Dockerty, M. B., and Randall, L. M.: *Obstet. Gynec.*, 1:593, 1953.
51. Jacobson, F. J., and Enzer, N.: *Amer. J. Obstet. Gynec.*, 78:868, 1959.
52. Karzavina, E. G.: *Zbl. Gynäk.*, 75:512, 1953.
53. Kinnunen, O.: *Ann. Chir. Gyn. Fenn.*, 41:5, 1952.
54. Kinnunen, O.: *Ann. Chir. Gyn. Fenn.*, 42:157, 1953.
55. Klinger, H. P., Ludwig, K. S., Schwarzacher, H. G., and Hauser, G. A.; *Gynaecologia*, 146:328, 1958.
56. Klopper, A.: *Amer. J. Obstet. Gynec.*, 107:807, 1970.
57. Kock, H., Kessel, H., Stolte, L., and Leusden, H.: *J. Clin. Endocr. Metab.*, 26:1128, 1966.
58. Lajos, L., and Szontag, F. E.: *Zbl. Gynäk.*, 72:1035, 1950.
59. Leone, V., et al.: *Monit. Ost. Gin. Endocr. Metab.*, 36:79, 1965.
60. MacDonald, P. C., and Siiteri, P. K.: *J. Clin. Endocr.*, 24:685, 1964.
61. MacKay-Hart, D.: *Obstet. Gynec.*, 27:766, 1966.
62. MacNaughton, M. C.: *J. Obstet. Gynec. Brit. Comm.*, 72:249, 1965.
63. Mastboom, J. L.: *Gynaecologia*, 134:217, 1952.
64. Mathieu, A.: *Amer. J. Obstet. Gynec.*, 37:654, 1939.
65. Meyer, R.: In *Handbuch der Spez. Pathol. Anat. und Histol.*, Vol. VII, ed. Henke and Lubarsch. 1930.
66. Meyer, R.: In *Handbuch der Gynäkologie*, Vol. VI, ed. Stoeckel and Veit. Munich, J. F. Bergmann, 1941.
67. Mikamo, K.: *Amer. J. Obstet. Gynec.*, 106:243, 1970.
68. Natsume, M., and Takada, J.: *Amer. J. Obstet. Gynec.*, 82:654, 1961.
69. Novak, E.: *Gynecological and Obstetrical Pathology*. Philadelphia, W. B. Saunders, 1947.
70. Novak, E.: *Amer. J. Obstet. Gynec.*, 53:34, 1947.
71. Novak, E.: *Amer. J. Obstet. Gynec.*, 59:1355, 1950.
72. Noyes, R. W.: *Ann. N.Y. Acad. Sci.*, 80:54, 1959.
73. Ober, W. B.: *Ann. N.Y. Acad. Sci.*, 80:3, 1959.
74. Odell, W. D., Hertz, R., Lipsett, M. B., Ross, G. T., and Hammond, C. B.: *Clin. Obstet. Gynec.*, 10:290, 1967.
75. Oliphant, S., Westerhout, F. C., and Schwinn, C. P.: *Acta Cytol.*, 12:290, 1968.
76. Pannain, A.: *Studio Clinico-Ormonale della Mola Vesicolare e del Chorioepitelioma*. Napoli, Pironto e Figli, 1959.
77. Park, W. W.: *Ann. N.Y. Acad. Sci.*, 80:104, 1959.
78. Park, W. W.: *Ann. N.Y. Acad. Sci.*, 80:152, 1959.
79. Permanent, E., Kadotani, T., and Sato, H.: *Amer. J. Obstet. Gynec.*, 100:912, 1968.
80. Pigeaud, H., Burthiault, R., and Bertoux, R.: *Brux. Med.*, 49:299, 1949.
81. Pincus, G., Rock, J., and Garcia, C. R.: *Ann. N.Y. Acad. Sci.*, 71:677, 1958.
82. Portillo, R. A., Gey, G. O., Delfs, E., and Mattingly, R. F.: *Science*, 159:1467, 1968.
83. Portillo, R. A., and Gey, G. O.: *Cancer Res.*, 28:1231, 1968.
84. Rushton, D. I., Faed, M. J. W., Richards, S. E. M., and Bain, A. D.: *J. Obstet. Gynec. Brit. Comm.*, 76:266, 1969.
85. Saxena, B. N., Goldstein, D. P., Emerson, J. K., and Selenkov, H. A.: *Amer. J. Obstet. Gynec.*, 102:115, 1968.
86. Schopper, W., and Pliess, G.: *Virch. Arch.*, 317:347, 1949.
86.a. Schopper, W.: *Dtsch. Med. Wschr.*, 77:1218, 1952.
87. Schuster, A.: *Arch. Gynäk.*, 181:477, 1952.
88. Schwartz, H. S., and Mantel, N.: *Cancer Res.*, 23:1274, 1963.
89. Scott, J. S.: *Amer. J. Obstet. Gynec.*, 83:185, 1962.
90. Sherman, J. T.: *Amer. J. Surg.*, 27:237, 1935.
91. Smalbraak, J.: *Trophoblastic Growths*. Amsterdam, Elsevier, 1957.
92. Smalbraak, J.: *Nederl. Tidjskr. Verloksed.*, 53:57, 1953.
93. Smalbraak, J.: *Ann. N.Y. Acad. Sci.*, 80:105, 1959.
94. Smith, G. V., and Smith, O. W.: *Amer. J. Obstet. Gynec.*, 51:411, 1946.

95. Smith, G. V., and Smith, O. W.: *Amer. J. Obstet. Gynec.,* 56:821, 1948.
96. Spellacy, W. N., Meeker, H. C., and MacKelvey, J. L.: *Obstet. Gynec.,* 25:607, 1965.
97. Stearns, H. C.: *Amer. J. Obstet. Gynec.,* 67:970, 1954.
98. Steigbigel, N. H.: *New Eng. J. Med.,* 271:345, 1964.
99. Stenchever, M. A., Jarvis, J. A., and MacIntyre, M. N.: *Obstet. Gynec.,* 32:548, 1968.
100. Stitch, S. R., Levell, M. J., Oakey, R. E., and Scott, J. S.: *Lancet,* 1:1344, 1966.
101. Sutherland, A. M.: *J. Obstet. Gynec. Brit. Emp.,* 58:29, 1951.
102. Taylor, E. S., and Drägemüller, W.: *Amer. J. Obstet. Gynec.,* 83:958, 1962.
103. Thiele, R. A., and Alvarez, R. R. de: *Amer. J. Obstet. Gynec.,* 84:1395, 1962.
104. Teoh, E. S., and Tow, S. H.: *J. Obstet. Gynec. Brit. Comm.,* 74:453, 1967.
105. Tisne, L., Barzelatto, J., and Stevenson, C.: *Bol. Soc. Chilena Obst. Ginec.,* 20:246, 1955.
106. Tominaga, T., and Page, E.: *Amer. J. Obstet. Gynec.,* 96:305, 1966.
107. Uher, H., Jirasek, J., and Herzmann, J.: *Gynaecologia,* 161:21, 1966.
108. Van Leusden, H., and Villee, C. A.: *J. Clin. Endocr. Metab.,* 26:842, 1966.
109. Van Leusden, H.: *Nederl. Tidjskr. Geneesk.,* 110:1344, 1966.
110. Van Leusden, H.: *Nederl. Tidjskr. Geneesk.,* 111:2271, 1967.
111. Velardo, J. T.: *Ann. N.Y. Acad. Sci.,* 80:65, 1959.
112. Vogler, W. R., Hugley, C. M., and Kerr, W.: *Arch. Int. Med.,* 115:285, 1965.
113. Wide, L., and Hobson, B.: *Acta Endocr.,* 54:105, 1965.
114. Zondek, B.: *Die Hormonen des Ovariums und des Hypophysenvorderlappens.* Berlin, Julius Springer, 1931.
115. Zondek, B.: *J. Obstet. Gynec. Brit. Emp.,* 49:397, 1942.
116. Zuckermann, S.: *Obstet. Gynec. Survey,* 3:880, 1948.

Chapter 44
ENDOCRINE ASPECTS OF GRAVIDIC TOXEMIAS

The present chapter includes the endocrine aspects of *gestosis* or *toxemias of pregnancy*. Because a great deal of our information on the subject is still either under revision or largely of a speculative nature, we shall limit ourselves to a brief summary of the problem.

44.1. GENERAL CONSIDERATIONS

The term *gestosis* or *gravidic toxemia* refers to a group of diseases that are metabolic or, preferably, intoxicative in nature and appear during pregnancy as a result of endogenous causes, that is, specifically as a consequence of gravity itself. Whatever the pathology involved, it arrives with pregnancy and ends with pregnancy. It does not depend on any preexisting changes in the mother but rather on the manner in which her body responds to the gravidic stimulus.

This book is not intended to cover the clinical aspects of toxemias. We shall therefore refrain from classifying them here and refer the reader to one of our textbooks on obstetrical pathology.[15]

44.2. TOXEMIAS OF THE FIRST TRIMESTER OF GESTATION

The toxemias of the first trimester of gestation comprise principally *hyperemesis gravidarum* and such related conditions as *myasthenia gravidarum* and *acute atrophy of the liver*.

Associated endocrine disturbances, particularly in hyperemesis gravidarum, are extremely important, and have been likened to *relative adrenal insufficiency*. A great deal of clinical, metabolic and hormonal data support this point of view.

44.2.1. CLINICAL AND METABOLIC SIMILARITIES

Hyperemesis gravidarum is very similar to adrenal insufficiency, or Addison's disease. Elert[41] designated hyperemesis and related conditions by the general term *gravidic addisonism*, including also some serious forms of hepatic insufficiency and, above all, gravidic myasthenia. This viewpoint is sustained mainly by the similarities observed in the clinical symptoms and by the similar metabolic findings.

CLINICAL SIMILARITIES. The fact that patients with "bronzed" disease and pregnant women suffering from uncontrollable vomiting have many features in common had been recognized long ago.

Both conditions are noted to be associated with *hypotension*, physical and muscular fatigue with *asthenia*, a tendency to vomiting, acidosis, *oliguria* and dehydration. The clinical parallel observed between the two conditions may be backed up by the fact that the administration or corticoids provides effective therapy of hyperemesis (discussed later). It is noteworthy that females suffering from Addison's disease, whose fertility is not diminished except in the most severe forms of the disease, clinically develop the symptoms of serious forms of gravidic hyperemesis once they become pregnant.

METABOLIC SIMILARITIES. Hyperemesis gravidarum has been noted to course with an increase in *carbohydrate catabolism*, characterized by hepatic glycogenolysis, increased blood levels of tricarbons (lactic and pyruvic acid) and a tendency to hypoglycemia.

As regards *lipid metabolism,* there is an increase in ketones both in the blood and in the urine, as well as a tendency to fatty metamorphosis of the hepatic lobule.

Water and mineral metabolism is seriously compromised by hyponatremia associated with hyperpotassemia and with an elevated blood level of ionic phosphorus. Levels of chloremia and calcemia are diminished and the circulating plasma volume undergoes hemoconcentration, with a concomitant decrease in the total water content of the blood.

Finally, the accumulation of fixed acids and the associated water and mineral changes concur in giving rise to *acidosis,* with a decrease in the CO_2 combining power. The entire gamut of changes observed in gravidic hyperemesis is found to be exactly duplicated in Addison's disease.

44.2.2. ENDOCRINE CHANGES IN HYPEREMESIS

Hyperemesis is associated with endocrine changes indicative of cortical insufficiency. This insufficiency, however, is not primary but secondary in nature and qualifies as an example of *relative cortical insufficiency*. This means that the adrenal failure is not a consequence of any primitive insufficiency of the cortex but rather results from the occurrence of *antagonistic factors*, responsible for raising the functional demands for corticoids during pregnancy. Seen in this context, the reason for the occurrence of metabolic disturbances in hyperemesis gravidarum may be found to stem from an underlying cause of *endocrine nature.*

THYROID ALTERATIONS. The thyroid seems to pass through a phase of hyperfunctional activity at the beginning of pregnancy. Not only is there an increase in neuromuscular and nervous excitability but the presence as well of glycogenolysis, ketosis and increase in tricarbons is equally consistent with the same interpretation. The basal metabolic rate, too, is increased in gravidic hyperemesis. In Chapter 34, we have already mentioned the fact that thyroid function in nearly every pregnancy is enhanced. If cases of uncontrollable vomiting in pregnancy are studied by means of such tests as ^{131}I uptake, PBI, etc., they invariably reveal an increase in thyroid function.

PITUITARY ALTERATIONS. We have long suspected that hyperemesis is associated with pituitary somatotropin hyperactivity.[13, 14] Various authors have reported an increase in plasma somatotropin levels in women with this condition.[40, 137] However, the recent studies by Josimovitch and MacLaren[69] have identified this substance as *placental lactogen,* which is thought to occur in increased amounts in hyperemesis and, because of its analogous actions, is known to be readily confused with pituitary STH. What is involved, therefore, seems to be an alteration affecting the chorion rather than the pituitary.

According to Elert,[41] ACTH activity is similarly increased, which may also be inferred from our own experience. However, the more recent investigations of Pesonen and Vaananen[108] apparently fail to confirm those findings inasmuch as they reveal a decrease in ACTH reserve by means of the Metopirone test. Of course, it may be argued that a decrease in ACTH reserve is likely to be found if in the days preceding the test there has been an exaggerated expenditure of the hormone, because all of the latter has gained access to the blood stream.

ALTERATIONS IN CHORIONIC ENDOCRINE FUNCTION. A possible increase in the level of placental lactogen has already been indicated. The fact that hyperemesis coincides with a period in pregnancy in which gonadotropin elimination happens to reach peak levels has raised the question of whether there is any causal relationship between the two. Original studies[126, 141] seemed to bear this out. Subsequent studies by Fairweather and Loraine,[42] however, appear to disprove the occurrence of elevated CG levels, at least as a constant finding.

CORTICOIDS. The appearance of adrenal cortical hyperplasia in the course of

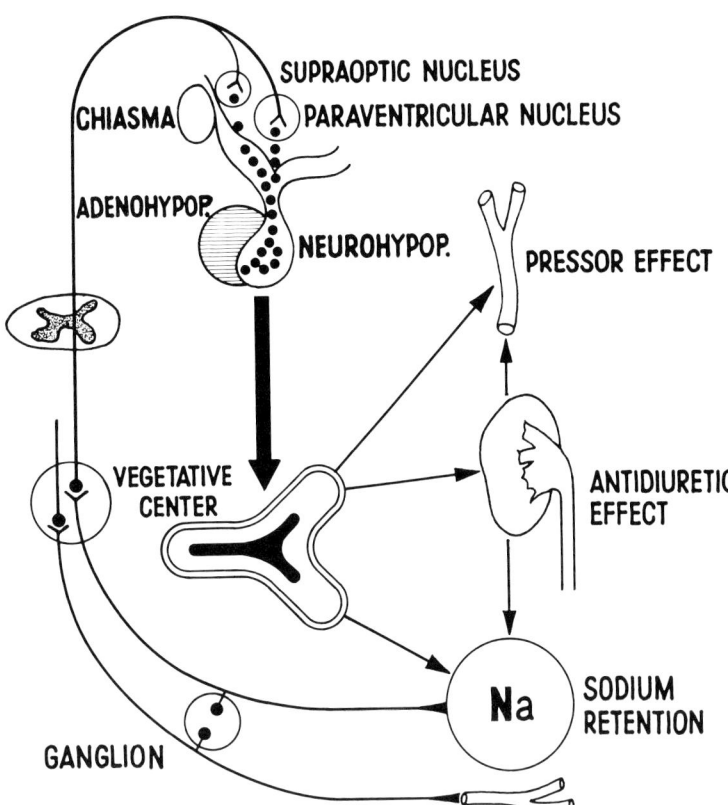

Figure 44-1. Control of diuresis and arterial pressure in the toxemias. Chemo- and baroreceptor endings functioning as the centripetal arc of a neuroendocrine reflex, conducive to secretion of vasopressin, antidiuretic hormone, or both, by hypothalamic nuclei. Vasopressin raises the rate of ACTH secretion and, thereby, the adrenocortical response causing vasodepression, antidiuresis and sodium retention by tissues. (From Botella-Llusiá: *Obstetrical Endocrinology*, Springfield, Ill., Charles C Thomas, 1961.)

early gestation has led to the suspicion that the adrenal might experience a phase of physiologic hyperfunction at the beginning of gestation. This idea harmonizes poorly with the observed similarity between the clinical course of hyperemesis and that of adrenal insufficiency.

Elert[41] and Botella[14] have established the concept of *relative adrenal insufficiency*. The adrenal in fact is not insufficient other than in relation to the unusual hyperfunctional activity of *antagonistic glands*. In trying to compensate for the catabolic disorders produced by the joint actions of the pituitary and thyroid, adrenocortical function may be strained to the limit. Adrenal *hypersecretion of corticoids* in normal as well as pathologic pregnancy has been described by Venning and associates[141, 142] and by Rodríguez-López.[116] On the other hand, Staemmler[130] and Dässler[33a] reported decreased urinary corticoid values in hyperemetic women. Elert[41] reasons that this results from an *excess in consumption*. Accordingly, such women develop the symptoms of adrenal insufficiency because of excessive demands for corticoids.

Performing dynamic adrenal function tests on pregnant women as well as on women suffering from hyperemesis, Jarvinen and associates[65] found a marked increase, particularly in the latter group, in the rate of corticoidogenesis, as well as a high level of response to ACTH administration.

In summary, an excess of chorionic hormones seems possible; apparently by engaging in an act of endocrine aggression, CG and, particularly, lactogen provoke a state of relative adrenocortical insufficiency by straining adrenocortical function to its limits.

44.2.3. STRESS AND HYPEREMESIS

The ideas just expounded lead us to draw a parallel between these conditions and the *general adaptation syndrome* (G.A.S.) (see Chapter 45). Indeed, we are dealing here with a situation which in the final analysis can be reduced to a reaction against external aggression by the hypophysioadrenal axis. The aggression in this instance comes in the form of an extraneous endocrine substance, chorionic gonadotropin, introduced into the maternal body for the first time and in large amounts. It is important to remember that the introduction of this substance, as indicated in Chapter 19, takes place abruptly, in conjunction with the penetration of entire hormone-containing islets of chorionic epithelium into the mother's bloodstream. This aggression is therefore not entirely specific. *To a large extent, it is specific hormonally, but in part it is nonspecific owing to the extraneous protein nature* of the substance introduced. Containment of this *stress agent* is brought about by parallel reaction on the part of the adenohypophysis and adrenal cortex, which secrete ACTH and corticoids, respectively. Whether the metabolic situation is going to be redressed and the symptoms of gravidic addisonism disappear, or whether there is going to be a turn for the worse, ultimately leading to fatal forms of hyperemesis and acute yellow atrophy of the liver, depends on the ability of the hypophysioadrenal system to respond. This is why female patients with Addison's disease show poor tolerance to this condition at the beginning of pregnancy and develop extremely severe forms of hyperemesis. However, it must be realized that according to general rules applicable to the G.A.S. the resulting pathologic response may be determined in each case not only by the particular characteristics of the body but also by the *magnitude of aggression*, which explains why some pregnancies associated with marked hormonal toxicity or with massive penetration of chorionic proteins and chorionic gonadotropins, such as occurs in cases of mole, may develop a similar syndrome.

44.2.4. TREATMENT

Over the past 25 years, a number of authors (Selye et al., Dewhurst[36]) have emphasized the similarity between severe hyperemesis and acute adrenal failure.

The initial employment deoxycorticosterone acetate (DOCA), not entirely satisfactory, rapidly gave way to *glucocorticoid* therapy (cortisone, hydrocortisone, prednisone, etc.). The first positive results with glucocorticoid therapy were reported by Wells.[146] Daily dosages must range between 25 and 30 mg, which achieves suppression of vomiting and restoration of metabolic balance. Considering the seriousness of the associated water and mineral disorders, treatment with *aldosterone* has been advocated in some cases (Pece et al.[106]), although the most dramatic results have undoubtedly been obtained with ACTH (Jarvinen and Vanaanen,[64] Ferrario[43]). The treatment of severe cases requires dosages of 25 to 50 mg of ACTH, dissolved in 500 ml isotonic solution of glucose, which is administered intravenously. It may sometimes be necessary to resort to continuous drip, for a total of two or more liters daily.

The favorable effects observed with this type of therapy, using both corticoids and ACTH, seem to give substance to our above mentioned hypothesis of "relative adrenal insufficiency."

The use of cortisone therapy in early pregnancy has been criticized by Courrier,[32] who had shown that cortisone in animal experiments was associated with *fetal congenital anomalies*. Fortunately, the dosages used for the treatment of human hyperemesis are much lower than those reported to produce malformations of this type. Nevertheless, these risks ought to be kept in mind in order to avoid overdosification. Daily dosages should never exceed 30 mg.

44.3. ECLAMPTIC TOXEMIA

Although eclamptic toxemia is not the only type of gestosis of advanced pregnancy (third trimester of gestation), it is the form that from an endocrine standpoint has been studied most thoroughly. This condition is notorious for a large variety of hypotheses (nervous, vascular, toxic, endocrine and mechanical) that have been advanced to explain preeclampsia and eclampsia. This is not the place to give a full account of such hypotheses, which would go beyond the scope of this book. The interested reader may consult some of the monographs dealing with the subject.[40, 129, 137] At this point, we shall concentrate only on studying the endocrine changes occurring in this group of syndromes.

The various hypotheses proposed for the pathogenesis of hypertensive toxemia may be listed as follows: (1) Pressor substances,

(2) ischemia, (3) hypercorticism, and (4) placental alterations. Although not all of these phenomena are of a purely and exclusively endocrine nature, they will be studied here because hormonal mechanisms are intimately implicated in their production.

44.3.1. PRESSOR SUBSTANCES

The following pressor substances have been invoked in the pathogenesis of preeclampsia and eclampsia: (1) Vasopressin and oxytocin, (2) renin-angiotensin, (3) hysterotonin and serotonin, and (4) catecholamines. They are all polypeptides and provoke the formation of *antipressor enzymes* (see Chapter 3, Section 3.1.5).

VASOPRESSIN AND OXYTOCIN. It is a well known historical fact that some German authors early in this century had postulated that eclampsia represented a state of *vasopressin* intoxication (Hofbauer, Küstner, Anselmino, Hoffmann, Fauvet). This long abandoned theory has since regained some validity. There is no doubt that vasopressin levels are increased in some forms of toxemia. This has been proved by Page[103] and, later, by Byron and Pratt,[19] Hawker[58] and Moore.[97] Also, serum *oxytocin* levels were found to be elevated in eclampsia (Poseiro et al.[111]). Although oxytocin by itself does not exert any direct pressor effect, it may act as an indirect pressor agent by eliciting uterine contraction and thereby causing ischemia (to be discussed later).

RENIN-ANGIOTENSIN. The role of the renin-angiotensin system in the pathophysiology of hypertension has by now been well established. Abdul-Karim and Assali[2] found that toxemia was associated with heightened resistance to renin, a phenomenon confirmed by Chesley and associates[26] and interpreted by the latter as resulting from renin saturation in toxemic patients. Elevated levels of circulating renin have been demonstrated by Geelhoed and Vander[50] and by Hellmer and Judson.[60] Angiotensin II, according to Cession and van Cauwenberghe,[24] Massani and associates,[91] and Talledo and colleagues,[132, 133] is also elevated. Angiotensin-inactivating factors similarly were found to be present in increased amounts, which leaves no doubt as to the role played by the pressor system in the mechanism of gravidic hypertension.

SEROTONIN AND HYSTEROTONIN. Carter and his associates[21] and Sagone and Arrotta[119] reported an increase in *circulating serotonin* levels in hypertensive toxemia. From myometrial and decidual tissue of toxemic patients, Hunter and Howard[63] isolated a substance with a close kinship to serotonin, which they called by analogy *hysterotonin*. This substance was thought to be produced, in the same way as renin, as a result of ischemia (in this instance, ischemia of the uterus). Gomel and Hardwick[52] subsequently studied that substance and were unable to confirm previously reported results. A number of years ago, Dexter and Weiss had failed in their attempts at isolating renin from the gravid uterus. Nevertheless, Sophian[129] and, more recently, Muresan and Zehan[99] have shown that hypertensive substances were in fact released by the ischemic uterus. The question of their nature and origin has not yet been elucidated.

CATECHOLAMINES. Data concerning the question of catecholamines in eclampsia are controversial. Zuspan and his associates[153] found a heightened response in toxemia to norepinephrine but without evidence of an increase in endogenous norepinephrine levels.[110] Sagone and Arrotta[120] denied that catecholamines played a role in hypertension of gestation, whereas Cession,[23] on the contrary, found an increase in blood catecholamine levels in eclampsia. It is possible that, rather than anything else, we are dealing with a problem of altered inactivation, as shall be pointed out later.

ANTIHYPERTENSIVE SUBSTANCES. Page[103] admitted that the action by vasopressin might be attributed to *lack of deactivation*. Patterson,[104] Plentl and Gray,[109] and Roth and Slater[117] demonstrated the decreased *vasopressin deactivating power* of toxemic plasma. The occurrence of *oxytocinase* in the plasma of gravid women has been well known ever since Semm[122] published his studies on the subject. Semm found that oxytocinase activity was significantly curtailed in eclampsia as well as in other pathologic conditions of pregnancy. This phenomenon, which is implicated in "placental insufficiency," will be examined at the end of this chapter. A diagram outlining the pathogenetic mechanism involved is shown in Figure 44–3.

As far as serotonin is concerned, Abdul-

Karim and Assali[2] demonstrated that normal pregnancy was associated with an increase in *antiserotonin* activity, which disappeared in toxemias. We have similarly indicated previously that these same workers,[2] as well as Chesley,[26] postulated an increase in the rate of angiotensin deactivation in normal pregnancy as compared to lack of deactivation in toxemias. Talledo[132] recently isolated an *angiotensinase* that did not occur in severe forms of gravidic hypertension.

Finally, it should be mentioned that Mendlovitz and colleagues,[93] as well as Pose and his associates,[110] have reported enhanced activity of the norepinephrine deactivating system in normal gestation but loss of this power in pathologic pregnancies. *Hypertensive toxemia may then be characterized as resulting from loss of power for deactivating pressor substances. As a result, there can be not only an increase in production but also a decrease in deactivation of pressor substances. The hypertension of gestosis may be accounted for not just by one but by various convergent mechanisms. The question of how much weight each carries separately in terms of etiology remains to be clarified.*

44.3.2. UTEROPLACENTAL ISCHEMIA

Uteroplacental ischemia, that is, a reduction in the rate of blood flow per unit of time within the uterofetal circuit, is not an endocrine phenomenon but is involved in endocrine interactions in two ways: (a) by the *manner in which it is produced*, and (b) by the *effects it produces*. Fetoplacental ischemia affects: (1) fetal metabolism and hematosis, possibly causing fetal distress and even fetal death; (2) placental and fetal hormone synthesis, and thereby it may profoundly modify gravidic endocrinology; (3) the release of hypertensive substances.

THE CAUSES OF UTEROPLACENTAL ISCHEMIA. Ischemia may be the result of hyperdistention of the uterus owing to such causes as *hydramnios*,[15] *twin pregnancy*,[129] *hydatidiform mole*[136] and, more rarely, uterine fibroids. All these causes have been found to concur frequently in preeclampsia and eclampsia.

Ischemia may also result from sustained uterine *contracture* (Clavero-Nuñez,[27] Poseiro et al.[111]), which is the main reason why oxytocin may be classified as an indirect pressor agent. Dynamic dystocia is frequently observed to be associated with uterine ischemia and sometimes with an increased occurrence of acute toxemia. The presence of uterine contracture has often been demonstrated in eclampsia.[103]

However, ischemia also occurs in *poorly vascularized* uteri as gestation advances. One of the most widely demonstrated types of pathophysiologic disturbances in hypertensive toxemia is a *reduction in the myometrial blood supply.*[6, 15, 34, 81, 92, 111] Recently, Clavero-Nuñez and his associates,[31] using radioactive xenon, found that the maternofetal gaseous exchange rate was significantly reduced in toxemias.

However, the cause of ischemia may not be confined to a conflict involving the uterine vasculature *but may also involve the placenta itself*. Together with Clavero, we have described the *syndrome of placental insufficiency*,[16] which will be examined at the end of this chapter (Section 44.5). This syndrome establishes itself in a physiologic manner at the end of every pregnancy, because of the progressive sclerosis and gradual obliteration of the villous vascular tree and because some villi as a result undergo degeneration.[27, 28] This syndrome of *placental senescence* which, like any other type of senescence, is a physiologic phenomenon, *may be anticipated under pathologic conditions* and may then give rise to a serious conflict in fetal hematosis and nutrition. We have described three quantitative components involved in this entity: (1) a diminution of the placental surface (Fig. 44-2); (2) a decrease in villous vascularization; and (3) a diminution in volume of the intervillous space as well as of the maternal blood flow at this level. We shall reexamine these parameters in Section 44.5, but let us now point out the fact that *degenerative phenomena of this type are intensified in gestosis*. This creates a form of *ischemia* and *placental insufficiency* that is specific to toxemias and is the underlying cause for the diminished levels of estriol[20, 53, 71, 98, 113] and serum oxytocin[122] as well as for the other endocrine changes to be discussed in Section 44.5.4.

EFFECTS OF UTEROPLACENTAL ISCHEMIA. The effects produced by lack of irrigation are only in part endocrinologic

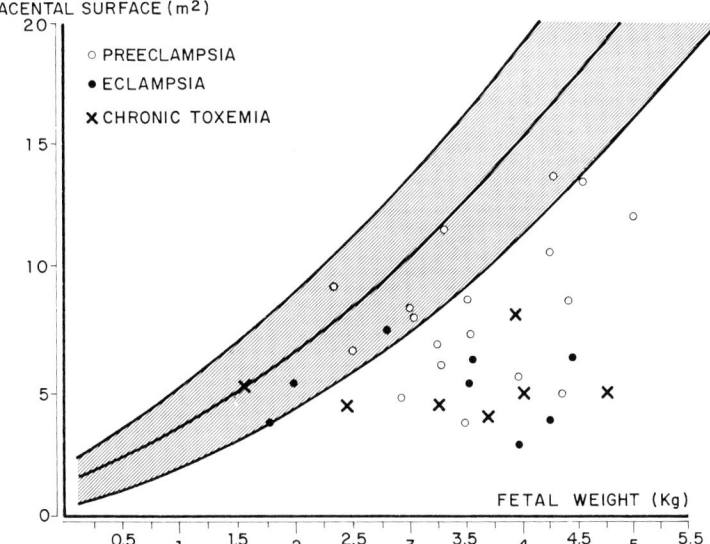

Figure 44-2. Placental surface in toxemia. (From Clavero-Núñez and Botella-Llusiá: *Amer. J. Obstet. Gynec.*, 86:234, 1963.)

in nature. However, they are all of great importance for the understanding of the pathogenetic mechanisms involved in this group of diseases.

The first consequence is the *blockade of fetal oxygenation and nutrition*. This is the reason for the high perinatal mortality in hypertensive toxemia. In addition to being subject to possible intragravidic death, these fetuses are especially susceptible to fetal distress at the time of labor. Their weight is usually below normal. They are what is known as "small-for-date" fetuses.

The second consequence is the *alteration of placental hormone synthesis*, which will be studied in a separate section (Section 44.3.4).

The last, and perhaps most important, consequence is the *release of pressor substances*. More than a quarter of a century ago, Dexter and Weiss had postulated that uterine ischemia resulted in hypertension, much as did renal ischemia. Indeed, this is an unquestionable fact, which has been confirmed by many.[4, 5, 82, 139] The fact that more than one pressor substance is involved in toxemia has been amply explained in Section 44.3.1. On the other hand, the mechanism whereby ischemia produces hypertensive substances is more difficult to explain. Sophian[129] invoked a *utero-renal reflex*, presumably a variety of the well known "reflex of Trueta."[15] This opinion has been upheld by Muresan and Zehan.[99] However, it is possible that such hypertensive substances are also formed by the ischemic uterus itself.[63, 102, 116] It has been observed by Deis and his associates[34] that uterine ischemia failed to elicit any pressor effects if the kidney was denervated. It has been possible to raise the blood pressure in bitches by ligating both uterine arteries,[82, 97] a phenomenon noted to disappear after denervating either the kidneys or the uterus. In summary, there are two possible explanations as to why uterine ischemia should produce hypertension: because of a reflex effect on the kidney, or perhaps on some other organ (e.g., the hypothalamus); or because the ischemic uterus itself produces hypertensive substances as a result of some changes in its metabolism. To this, we might add the possibility that antihypertensive enzymes, most of them of placental origin, may no longer be produced as a consequence of the cessation of blood flow to the placenta.

44.3.3. HYPERCORTICISM

GLUCOCORTICOIDS. Mastboom[92] enunciated the hypothesis that placental ischemia modified placental steroidogenesis by causing excessive production of corticoids, presumably producing both hypertension and the other toxemic manifestations. This theory has not been substantiated by other experimental findings and can no longer be upheld, since progesterone is now known to be a precursor of corticoids and not vice versa.[10, 47, 82, 149] Paradoxically, it seems hard to imagine how ischemia can modify steroidogenesis in terms of enhancing the rate of enzymatic conversions. Nevertheless, an increase in total corticoids and glucocorticoids has been shown to occur in eclampsia.[51, 94, 107, 130, 142, 143, 144] Plasma ACTH levels are also elevated[35, 65, 144] and adrenal histology, as revealed by biopsy (Attia et al.[3]), shows hyperplasia of the zona fasciculata. Kotasek and his associates[78] have found decreased DHEA values in toxemias, which, though possibly attributable to partial insufficiency of the maternal adrenal system, is believed to result instead from insufficiency of the adrenal-fetal-placental axis (Fig. 44–3).

ALDOSTERONISM IN TOXEMIAS? This is a highly controversial issue, as revealed by modern literature. Since aldosteronism produces hypertension and edema with sodium retention, much as occurs in toxemias, it had been assumed that a possible global, so to speak, form of hypercorticism, by virtue of an associated hyperaldosteronism, might be the underlying cause of toxemias.

The figures for urinary aldosterone reported in normal pregnancy by Gornall and colleagues,[54, 55] Koczorek and associates,[77] Martin and Mills,[90] Rinsler and Rigby[115] and Stark[131] are five to 15 times as high as those found outside pregnancy. This seemed to be an important argument favoring the aldosterone-induced nature of gravidic edema and hypertension; however, Kumar and his co-workers,[80] Rinsler and Rigby,[115] and Watanabe and associates,[145] who recently studied the question of aldosteronuria in gestosis, made the surprising discovery that urinary aldosterone values were actually *decreased*. Kumar explained this phenomenon as resulting from the well known effect of sodium retention, whereby a hypothalamic neurohormonal reflex automatically reduced the rate of aldosterone production.[25, 83, 144] What is more, there are enough known cases of *primary aldosteronism complicating gestation* (see Chapter 45), none of which has been observed to develop toxemia of pregnancy. As a result, it seems unlikely that either aldosteronism or global hypercorticism of any kind may play any role in the production of toxemia.

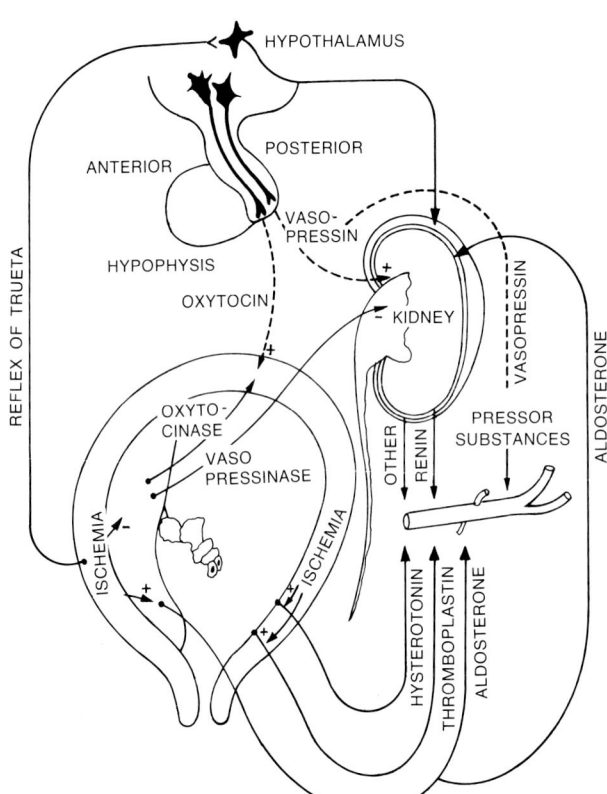

Figure 44–3. Hypertensinogenic actions involved in eclamptic toxemia. Uterine ischemia provokes: (1) The reflex of Trueta; (2) an increase in placental aldosterone (presumptive); (3) release of hysterotonin by the decidua; (4) inhibition of placental oxytocinase and vasopressinase; and (5) production of thromboplastin by the decidua (inconstant).

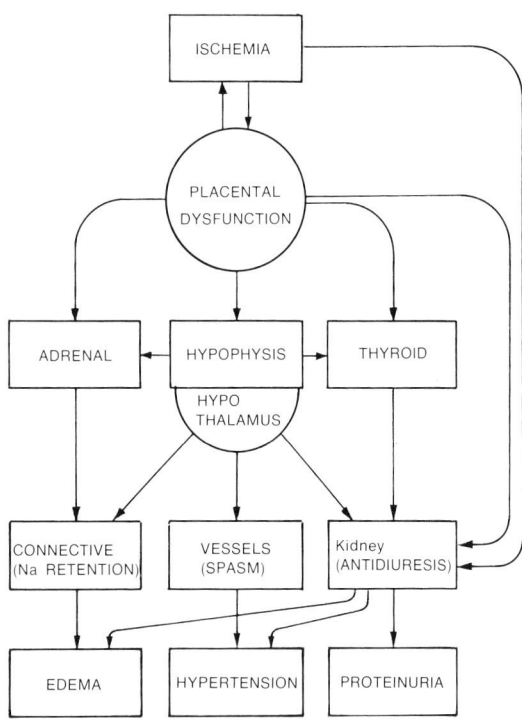

Figure 44-4. Diagram summarizing pathogenesis of eclamptic toxemia. The *primary disturbance* consists in placental ischemic dysfunction, while the endocrine alterations are *secondary disturbances*. *Tertiary disturbances* involve vascular, connective tissue and renal disorders, and *quaternary disturbances* comprise edema, hypertension and proteinuria.

44.3.4. PLACENTAL ALTERATIONS

Toxemia, we have pointed out above, is associated with *placental insufficiency*. However, this is not where the variegated implications of this disorder ought to be studied. We shall therefore restrict ourselves to the question of *placental changes affecting internal secretions*. These involve: (1) gonadotropin, (2) estrogens, (3) progesterone, (4) corticoids, and (5) placental lactogen.

GONADOTROPIN. Although CG levels in toxemias are generally admitted to be elevated,[59, 62, 125, 126] Fairweather and Loraine,[42] as well as Föllmer,[44] have encountered normal or low values. Only in unusually severe forms of toxemia did Loraine and Mathew[86] confirm the presence of increased chorionic gonadotropin values. It must be taken into consideration that many toxemias occur in molar or twin gestations in which high CG levels may be ascribed to other causes, and that, on the other hand, CG excretion is highly inconstant and variable near the end of pregnancy, when such gestoses develop.

ESTROGENS. It seems unquestionable that toxemia is associated with low estrogen levels. Aside from a drop in *total estrogen values* (Campagnoli et al.,[20] Goretzlehner and Wodrig,[53] Jayle[66]), this decrease is particularly marked in the *estriol fraction*.[66, 67, 125, 126] As a result, a decrease in estriol excretion is characteristic of toxemias. Klopper,[76] Michie,[95] Müller and Nielsen,[98] Ratanasopa and associates,[113] and Ten Berge[135] all consider urinary estriol values as a prognostic index of toxemia.

PROGESTERONE, PREGNANEDIOL. Eton and Short[41a] reported diminished progesteronemia. The excretion of pregnanediol is uniformly low, as attested to by numerous studies.[18, 33, 71, 123, 126, 128, 141] The reduction in estriol values correlates well with the observed reduction in pregnanediol values in every case.

CORTICOIDS. We have pointed out previously how total corticoid excretion is increased,[143, 144] whereas aldosteronuria is diminished.[82, 115, 145]

PLACENTAL LACTOGEN. Various authors have reported increased somatotropin activity in toxemias, a belief shared by us in the past.[14] Josimovitch and MacLaren[69] showed that what was involved was the new hormone known as "placental lactogen."

All these placental endocrine changes thus appear to be the *consequence* rather than the cause of toxemic phenomena.

44.4. TOXEMIA AND THE GENERAL ADAPTATION SYNDROME (G.A.S.)

As emphasized in the foregoing sections, eclamptic toxemia is associated with important endocrine phenomena, affecting not only the chorion but also the rest of the glands of internal secretion. First of all, these are marked by an *increase in ACTH and corticoid activity*. At the same time, there is a notable increase in gonadotropin and a decrease in estrogen, pregnanediol and 17-ketosteroid values. A similarity between these conditions and the *general adaptation syndrome*, as defined by Selye, has thus been pointed out. The existing relationship between stress and pregnancy will be discussed in a subsequent chapter; we shall here be concerned with a summary on toxemias. The increase in chorionic gonadotropin activity which, we have indicated, is reactive to primary placental changes, apparently causes a reaction of the opposite sign in the hypothalamic system. In reality, the increase in gonadotropin activity cannot be considered as the only agent of aggression involved. This aggression has multiple facets in late pregnancy, which may be either *specific* or *nonspecific*. (1) *Specifically,* a most important role in precipitating the adrenal reactions is played not only by the increase in gonadotropin activity but by thalamohypophysial function. Thus, for instance, Greene and his colleagues[56, 57] call attention to the stimulatory effect of vasopressin on adrenal function. (2) *Nonspecific factors,* such as the *metabolic surcharge* imposed by advanced pregnancy, the *release of toxic products by the placenta* and, particularly, the possible *release of extraneous proteins by the placenta,* also must be taken into consideration. Apart from having to consider the presence of gonadotropin in the mother's circulation as an extraneous protein, Clavero-Nuñez and his co-workers[30, 31] at our laboratory showed the frequent occurrence of fetal vascular erosions in toxemic placentas. This may give rise to a sort of slow transfusion of fetal blood into the mother's bloodstream in the course of pregnancy and may act as an important factor of toxic irritation.

Dewhurst[36] and Garret[49] focused attention on the fact that the adrenal cortex in eclampsia showed evidence of overstimulation, frequently associated with intraglandular hemorrhages, similar to those occurring in the Waterhouse-Friderichsen syndrome. Finally, Selye summarizes the foregoing facts by stating that *eclamptic toxemia is an instance of G.A.S. in its pure form, in which the pathologic disturbances result not from failure of hypophysioadrenal compensation but, on the contrary, from a phenomenon of overcompensation.*

Although his is a suggestive theory, it might be ill-advised to try to attribute all of the foregoing pathology to G.A.S. alone. Naturally, in any endocrine disorder as profound as that occurring in toxemia of pregnancy, the widespread participation of the adrenal in the observed reactions may at first sight simulate a stress situation. We shall emphasize this point in our next chapter. This theory, however, does not explain the mechanism of hypothalamic hyperfunction, presently known to be a very real event, known to play a very important role. In addition, the primary placental disturbance may be, to a certain extent, divorced from the production of the adrenal reaction. In our opinion, therefore, the mechanism of eclamptic toxemia has to be formulated in a different way.

44.5. SYNDROME OF PLACENTAL INSUFFICIENCY AND ITS ENDOCRINE EFFECTS

Our own observations, in cooperation with Clavero-Núñez,[16, 27, 28] have led us to describe a histologic picture, recurring with a syndromic character in a series of pathologic pregnancy states, which we have denominated *placental senescence.*

Since histologic changes of this type are associated with important endocrine repercussions, and because one of the conditions in which they occur—with unusual consistency—is gestosis, we are including here an endocrinologic study of this syndrome as an appendix.

44.5.1. HISTOLOGIC AND HISTOMETRIC ASPECT OF PLACENTAL SENESCENCE

The placenta is an organ that ages rapidly. Its vital cycle lasts for nine months, compared to an average of 70 years for the rest of the body's organs. The process of physiologic aging is apparent even in normal placentas near term. However, in some cases, aging of the placenta manifests itself prematurely, during the seventh or eighth month of gestation.

The histologic features of placental senescence are the following: (1) atrophy of the syncytium; (2) fusion of absorptive villi, forming compact masses; (3) obliteration of villous capillaries; (4) sclerosis of vessels and hyalinization of the villous stroma; (5) fibrinoid degeneration of villi, with development of microinfarcts.

A series of histometric investigations[16,28,29,30] was undertaken to measure the placental surface, volume of the intervillous space and fetal capillary area in such placentas. All three parameters were found to be diminished. If both placental circulations—maternal as well as fetal—are partly blocked and the area of contact reduced, it is a foregone conclusion that the placenta must fail as an organ of filtration, particularly as regards oxygen filtration. A series of fetal changes will necessarily ensue which may lead to hypoxia or to intrauterine death.

Placental senescence of this type may be observed in, among other conditions of gravidic pathology, toxemias of pregnancy (Fig. 44-2), which explains why this group of diseases is associated with such a high fetal mortality rate.

44.5.2. CLINICAL ASPECTS OF PLACENTAL SENESCENCE

Premature senescence of the placenta may appear either because of *intrinsic* (that is, primary) placental disease, or because of *extrinsic* (secondary) diseases. The presence of a third type, physiologic senescence occurring at term (about the fortieth week), may result in pathologic effects on the fetus if pregnancy were prolonged further (high fetal mortality rate in overmature gestations).

Extrinsic diseases causing placental senescence are first of all the toxemias of pregnancy (Fig. 44-2) and, second, diabetes and prediabetes in the mother, as well as syphilis and erythroblastosis. The mechanisms involved in senescence probably differ from case to case, although the final result is the same: impairment of placental filtering efficiency. In the majority of the cases, this condition may still be compatible with fetal life during gestation, but the workload of labor, in conjunction with the supervening factor of hypoxia, results in conditions of severe distress and even fetal death intrapartum.

It is easy to understand why a correct diagnosis of this kind of placental pathology is of paramount importance for the survival of the fetus and the prevention of perinatal mortality. Unfortunately, the histologic examination of placental tissue is, as a rule, undertaken as an exercise in *retrospective* judgment, which is why it was necessary to devise other methods for diagnosing placental insufficiency in the course of gestation. Four kinds of techniques have been proposed: (1) Determination of histaminase activity (Borglin and Willert[12]); (2) determination of oxytocinase activity (Semm[122]); (3) vaginal cytology (Osmond-Clarke et al.[102]); (4) estimation of urinary estriol. We shall be concerned mainly with the last.

44.5.3. REPERCUSSIONS OF PLACENTAL SENESCENCE ON ESTROGEN BIOSYNTHESIS

As a result of lack of progesterone synthesis, conversion of estradiol to estrone and estriol is suspended and estriol production is diminished. Modern investigations concerning placental estrogen biosynthesis[7,37,62,68,105,138] have shown that estrogens are formed in the placenta by a mechanism quite similar to that used by the ovary. Although this may be the principal source of estrone and estradiol in the urine of both pregnant and nonpregnant women, the large amount of estriol occurring in the former is attributable to a mixed fetoplacental origin, as has already been explained in Chapter 20 (Section 20.2.3). Diczfalusy and his associates[39] have clearly demonstrated that the fetal adrenal produces dehydroepiandrosterone sulfate at the expense of C-21 steroids, principally progesterone of placental origin, which is then returned to the placenta and is there converted to estriol, as has been shown diagrammatically in Figures 20-13 and 20-14. Thus, Klopper[73] considers urinary estriol excretion in pregnancy as a *joint expression* of both fetal and placental conditions within the "fetoplacental unit." However, Galbraith and his colleagues,[48] as well as Wu and associates,[147] subsequently revealed that the fetal liver, too, was able to elaborate large amounts of estriol in the absence of any placental participation.

Placental insufficiency, then, manifests itself not only by a decrease in urinary estriol excretion but also by a drop in total plasma estrogen levels (Diczfalusy and Lauritzen,[38] Kubli and Keller[79]).

In the event of fetal death, estriol elimination ceases abruptly,[106, 116] which at first sight might be explained by saying that placental function in fetal death is altered. Nonetheless, Diczfalusy,[39] Frandsen and Stakeman[47] found a marked decrease in the rate of estriol excretion in five pregnancies with viable anencephalous fetuses. Fetal monsters of this type are well known to have adrenal aplasia (see Chapter 33), which raises the possibility that the estrogens under discussion are of fetal adrenal origin. The finding by Diczfalusy and Lauritzen[38] of a decrease in urinary estrogen values following ligation of the umbilical cord would seem to support this line of thinking.

Lowered urinary estriol excretion has been reported also in preeclampsia.[47, 66, 118, 125, 126] Würtele,[147a] Müller and Nielsen,[98] and Ratanasopa and his colleagues[113] believe that the presence of decreased urinary estriol values is helpful in establishing the clinical prognosis in toxemia.

44.5.4. DETERMINATION OF ESTRIOL IN THE DIAGNOSIS OF PLACENTAL SENESCENCE AND IN THE PROGNOSIS OF FETAL VIABILITY

Urinary estriol may be determined by the method of Brown and Coyle[17] or by that of Ittrich (see Chapter 24). Zondek[150, 151, 152] first called attention to the significance of decreased estriol excretion as a diagnostic and prognostic element as to fetal viability. Subsequently, Taylor and his associates[134] and, particularly, Greene and Touchstone[56, 57] contributed some observations of utmost interest. Figure 44–5, taken from Greene and Touchstone, shows how valuable isolated and, particularly, serial estriol determinations are for the prognosis of fetal life.

Urinary estriol excretion is similarly diminished in *overmature gestation*,[87, 127] gravidic anemia and other forms of pathologic gestation,[8, 61, 89] in all cases of fetal death[88, 101] and, finally, in all cases with proved insufficiency of placental function, as defined above.[45, 46, 75, 148] The measure-

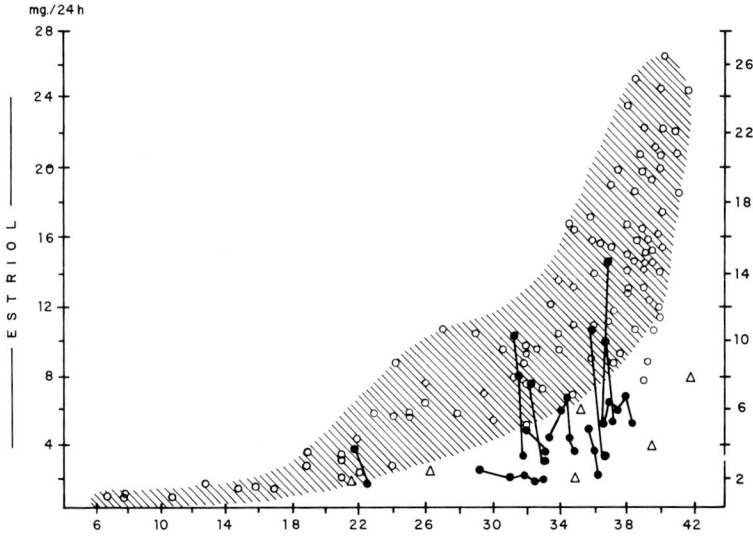

Figure 44–5. Value of urinary estriol determinations for the diagnosis and prognosis of fetal viability. Hollow circles indicate normal values; triangles, isolated determinations in cases of fetal death; large dots, those cases in which the excretion curve has been followed up. (From Greene and Touchstone: *Amer. J. Obstet. Gynec.*, 85:1, 1963.)

Figure 44–6. Assessment of the degree of placental function by means of radioimmunoassay of placental lactogen in twin (T) or quintuplet (Q) pregnancies. A direct correlation is apparent between the degree of placental development and function and the concentrations of the placental protein. (From Josimovitch et al.: *Obstet. Gynec.*, 36:246, 1970.)

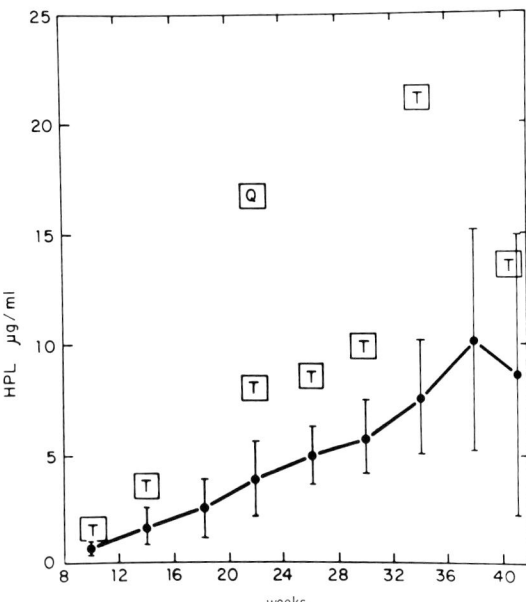

ment of estrioluria in pregnancy has thus been shown to be of great value not only from the *diagnostic* but also from the *prognostic* points of view.

Considerable importance has also been attached lately to estriol determinations in *amniotic fluid*[9, 73, 96] and blood.[84]

44.5.5. OTHER METHODS FOR THE DIAGNOSIS OF PLACENTAL INSUFFICIENCY

Several other methods for the diagnosis of placental insufficiency in pregnancy near term have been described previously (see Chapter 20, Section 20.0.0).

CYTOLOGY. Because colpocytograms in pregnancy near term may be modified by a number of factors, the use of *urocytograms* has been suggested. This method has already been discussed in Chapter 25 and, despite some modern advocates,[85, 100, 114] has not been found to give satisfactory results. At best, it may serve as an element of *orientation*.

PLACENTAL LACTOGEN (HPL). Recent communications by Simmer,[124] Selenkov and associates,[121] and Josimovitch and colleagues[70] attribute great value to the assay

Figure 44–7. Estimation of the degree of placental function, by means of xenon-133. I, Injection of radiotracer into intervillous space and monitoring of radioactivity at the placental site allows calculation of the *placental minute volume*. The same site of injection is used to estimate placental permeability to gases by monitoring radioactivity through scanner placed at the fetal buttocks. II, The myometrial blood flow and the degree of uterine ischemia are calculated by injecting the radioactive gas into the myometrium and measuring its clearance. (From Clavero-Núñez et al.: *J. Reprod. Med.*, 6:209, 1971.)

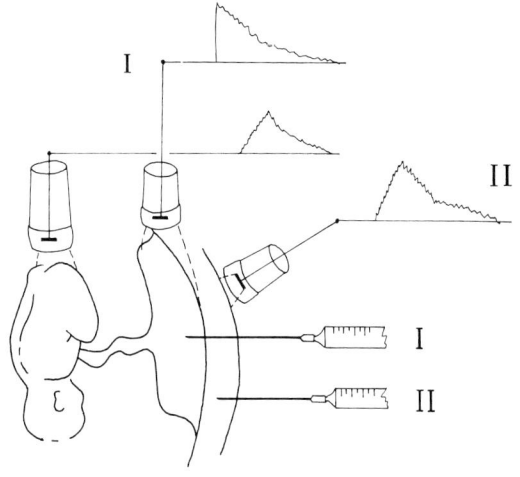

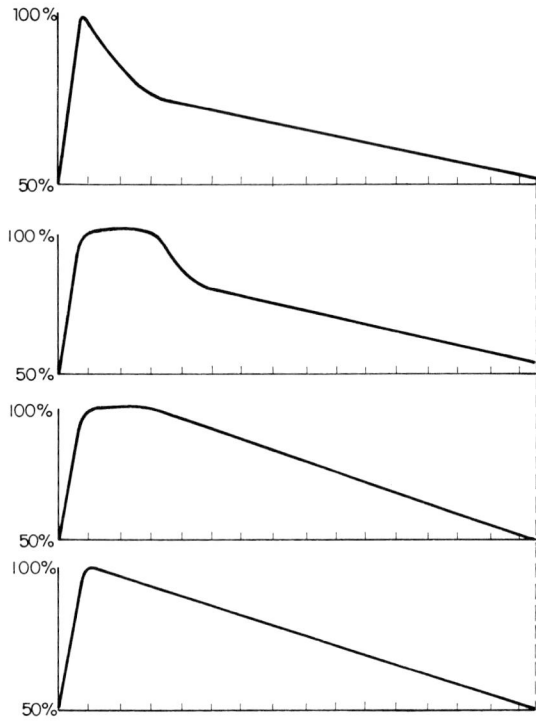

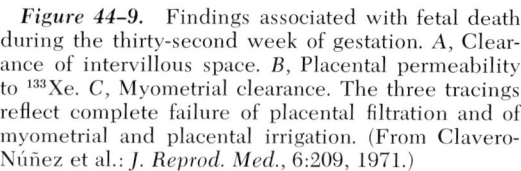

Figure 44–8. The two upper curves represent plots of radioactive "clearance" rates in the intervillous space. Both indicate a normal placental minute volume. The two lower curves represent myometrial clearance in normal pregnancy. (From Clavero-Núñez et al.: *J. Reprod. Med.*, 6:209, 1971.)

Figure 44–9. Findings associated with fetal death during the thirty-second week of gestation. *A*, Clearance of intervillous space. *B*, Placental permeability to ^{133}Xe. *C*, Myometrial clearance. The three tracings reflect complete failure of placental filtration and of myometrial and placental irrigation. (From Clavero-Núñez et al.: *J. Reprod. Med.*, 6:209, 1971.)

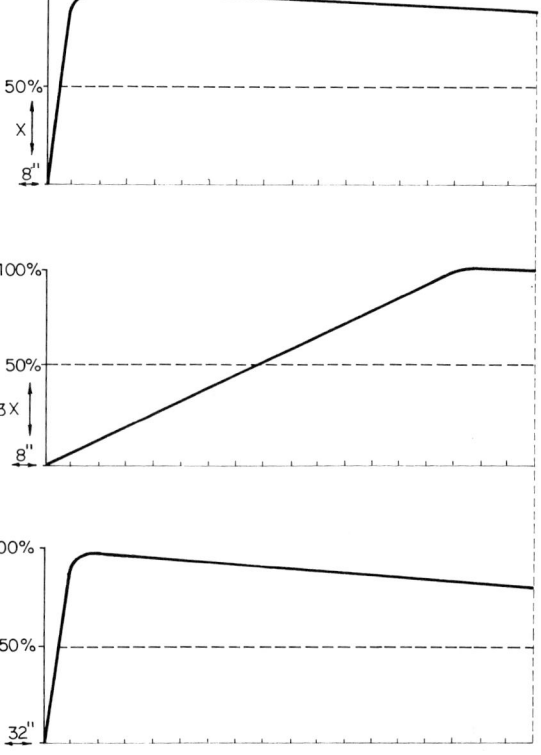

of lactogen as a placental function test which, unlike estriol, is apparently free of interference.

OTHER TESTS. Semm[122] estimates *serum oxytocinase activity* as a placental function test. Quigley and his associates[112] measured the *thermostable fraction of alkaline glycerophosphatase*. Finally, Clavero-Nuñez and colleagues[31] use techniques based on the *passage of radioisotopes* through the placenta, the description of which would be beyond the scope of this book.

REFERENCES

1. Aasted-Frandsen, V., and Stakeman, G.: *Acta Endocr.*, 44:196, 1963.
2. Abdul-Karim, R., and Assali, N. S.: *Amer. J. Obstet. Gynec.*, 82:246, 1961.
3. Attia, O., et al.: *Amer. J. Obstet. Gynec.*, 107:889, 1970.
4. Barnes, A. C., and Quilligan, E. J.: *Amer. J. Obstet. Gynec.*, 71:670, 1956.
5. Barnes, A. C., Kumar, D., and Goodno, J. A.: *Amer. J. Obstet. Gynec.*, 84:1207, 1962.
6. Bastiansee, M. A. B., and Mastboom, J. L.: *Ciba Symposium on Toxaemias of Pregnancy.* London, J. A. Churchill, 1950.
7. Baulieu, E. E., and Dray, F.: *J. Clin. Endocr.*, 23:1299, 1963.
8. Beischer, N. A., Townsend, L., and Holsman, M.: *Amer. J. Obstet. Gynec.*, 102:819, 1968.
9. Berle, P.: *Acta Endocr.*, 61:369, 1969.
10. Berliner, D. J., Jones, F. J., and Slahanick, H. A.: *J. Biol. Chem.*, 223:1043, 1956.
11. Boot, R. T., Stern, M. I., Wood, C., and Sharples, M. J. H.: *J. Obstet. Gynec. Brit. Comm.*, 71:266, 1964.
12. Borglin, N. E., and Willert, B.: *Acta Obstet. Gynec. Scand.*, 40:59, 1961.
13. Botella, J.: "El Metabolismo en el Embarazo," in *Tratado de Obstetricia*, ed. P. Nubiola and A. Zárate, Vol. I. Barcelona, Editorial Labor, 1951.
14. Botella, J.: *Obstetrical Endocrinology.* Springfield, Ill., Charles C Thomas, 1961.
15. Botella, J.: *Patología Obstétrica*, 7th ed. Barcelona, Editorial Científico-Médica, 1966.
16. Botella, J., and Clavero, J. A.: *Amer. J. Obstet. Gynec.*, 86:234, 1963.
17. Brown, J. B., and Coyle, M. G.: *J. Obstet. Gynec. Brit. Comm.*, 70:219, 1963.
18. Browne, F. J.: *J. Obstet. Gynec. Brit. Emp.*, 53:510, 1948.
19. Byron, F. R., and Pratt, G. E.: *Lancet*, 1:752, 1959.
20. Campagnoli, C., et al.: *Minerva Gin.*, 19:45, 1967.
21. Carter, F. B., et al.: *Amer. J. Obstet. Gynec.*, 84:913, 1962.
22. Cedard, I., Varangot, J., and Yanotti, S.: *Compt. Rend. Acad. Sci.*, 254:3896, 1962.
23. Cession, G.: *Bull. Roy. Soc. Belg. Obst. Gyn.*, 36:197, 1966.
24. Cession, G., and Van Cauwenberghe, H.: *Pathol. Biol. (Paris)*, 16:589, 1968.
25. Chauvet, J., and Acher, R.: *Ann. d'Endocr.*, 20:111, 1959.
26. Chesley, L. C.: *Clin. Obstet. Gynec.*, 9:879, 1966.
27. Clavero-Núñez, J. A.: *Acta Gin.*, 13:465, 1962.
28. Clavero-Núñez, J. A., and Botella, J.: *Arch. Gynäk.*, 198:56, 1963.
29. Clavero-Núñez, J. A., and Del Campo, P.: *Acta Gin.*, 15:265, 1964.
30. Clavero-Núñez, J. A., and Jiménez-Ayala, M.: *Acta Gin.*, 15:133, 1964.
31. Clavero-Núñez, J. A., Nogueruela, J., Esteban, J., Álvarez, J., Ausin, J., and Retamar, A.: *Acta Gin.*, 19:1968.
32. Courrier, R.: *Ann. d'Endocr.*, 15:1, 1954.
33. Coyle, M. G., Grieg, M., and Walker, J.: *Lancet*, 2:275, 1962.
33a. Dässler, C. G.: *Arch. Gynäk.*, 199:257, 1963.
34. Deis, R. P., Lloyd, S., and Pickford, M.: *J. Physiol.*, 165:348, 1960.
35. Devis, R., and Devis, V.: *Ann. d'Endocr.*, 11:22, 1950.
36. Dewhurst, C. J.: *Brit. Med. J.*, 1:22, 1951.
37. Diczfalusy, E., and Lindqvist, P.: *Acta Endocr.*, 22:203, 1956.
38. Diczfalusy, E., and Lauritzen, C.: *Oestrogene beim Menschen.* Berlin, Springer, 1961.
39. Diczfalusy, E.: *Acta Gin.*, 16:429, 1965.
40. Dieckman, W. J., et al.: In *Ciba Symposium on Toxaemias of Pregnancy.* London, J. & A. Churchill, 1953.
41. Elert, R.: *Arch. Gynäk.*, 183:63, 1953.
41a. Eton, B., and Short, R. V.: *J. Obstet. Gynec. Brit. Emp.*, 67:785, 1960.
42. Fairweather, D. V. I., and Loraine, J. A.: *Brit. Med. J.*, 1:666, 1962.
43. Ferrario, E.: *Minerva Gin.*, 10:965, 1958.
44. Föllmer, W.: *Zbl. Gynäk.*, 86:947, 1964.
45. Frampton, J., and Clayton, S. G.: *J. Obstet. Gynec. Brit. Comm.*, 75:42, 1968.
46. France, J. T., and Liggins, G. C.: *J. Clin. Endocr.*, 29:138, 1969.
47. Frandsen, V. A., and Stakeman, L.: *Acta Endocr.*, 38:383, 1961.
48. Galbraith, R. S., Low, J. A., and Boston, R. W.: *Amer. J. Obstet. Gynec.*, 106:352, 1970.
49. Garret, S. S.: *West. J. Surg.*, 59:66, 1951.
50. Geelhoed, G. W., and Vander, A. J.: *J. Clin. Endocr. Metab.*, 28:412, 1968.
51. Giosis, M., and Ferruzzi, O.: *Minerva Gin.*, 4:441, 1952.
52. Gomel, V., and Hardwick, D. F.: *Amer. J. Obstet. Gynec.*, 94:308, 1966.
53. Goretzlehner, G., and Wodrig, W.: *Zbl. Gynäk.*, 86:492, 1964.
54. Gornall, A. G., Gwilliam, G., and Hall, A. F.: *J. Clin. Endocr.*, 16:950, 1956.
55. Gornall, A. G., Grundy, H. M., and Koladich, C. J.: *Canad. J. Physiol. Biochem.*, 38:43, 1960.
56. Greene, J. W., Touchstone, J. C., and Fields, H.: *Obstet. Gynec.*, 17:349, 1961.
57. Greene, J. W., and Touchstone, J. C.: *Amer. J. Obstet. Gynec.*, 85:1, 1963.
58. Hawker, R. W.: *J. Endocr.*, 14:400, 1957.
59. Hellmer, O. M., and Griffith, R. S.: *Endocrinology*, 51:421, 1954.
60. Hellmer, O. M., and Judson, W. E.: *Amer. J. Obstet. Gynec.*, 99:9, 1967.
61. Heys, R. F., Scott, J. S., Oakey, R. E., and Stitch, S. R.: *Obstet. Gynec.*, 33:390, 1969.
62. Hobkirk, R., and Nilsen, M.: *J. Clin. Endocr.*, 22:134, 1962.

63. Hunter, C. H., and Howard, W. F.: *Amer. J. Obstet. Gynec.*, 79:838, 1960.
64. Jarvinen, P. A., and Vanaanen, P.: *Nord. Med.*, 57:589, 1957.
65. Jarvinen, P. A., Pesonen, S., and Vanaanen, P.: *Ann. Med. Exp. Biol. Fenn.*, 39:356, 1961.
66. Jayle, M. F.: *Ann. d'Endocr.*, 12:157, 1951.
67. Jayle, M. F., Scholler, R., Veyrin-Forrier, F., and Menge, F.: *Rev. Europ. Endocr.*, Suppl.1:77, 1965.
68. Joel, P. B., Hagerman, D. D., and Villee, C. A.: *J. Biol. Chem.*, 236:3151, 1961.
69. Josimovitch, J. B., and MacLaren, J. A.: *Endocrinology*, 71:209, 1962.
70. Josimovitch, J. B., Kosor, B., and Mintz, D. H.: "Roles of Placental Lactogen in Maternal-Fetal Relations," in *Fetal Autonomy*, CIBA Foundation Symposium. London, J. & A. Churchill, 1969.
71. Kankaanrinta, T.: *Scand. J. Lab. Clin. Invest.*, Suppl.15:74, 1964.
72. Klausner, D. A., and Ryan, K. J.: *J. Clin. Endocr.*, 24:101, 1964.
73. Klopper, A.: "The Assessment of Placental Function," in *Fetus and Placenta*, ed. E. Diczfalusy and A. Klopper. Oxford, Blackwell, 1969.
74. Klopper, A., and Dennis, K. J.: *J. Obstet. Gynec. Brit. Comm.*, 76:534, 1969.
75. Klopper, A.: *Amer. J. Obstet. Gynec.*, 107:821, 1970.
76. Klopper, A.: *Amer. J. Obstet. Gynec.*, 107:807, 1970.
77. Koczorek, K. R., Wolff, H. P., and Beer, M. L.: *Klin. Wschr.*, 35:497, 1957.
78. Kotasek, A., Fassati, M., Sonka, J., Brestak, M., Gregorova, I., and Fassati, P.: *Amer. J. Obstet. Gynec.*, 98:229, 1967.
79. Kubli, F., and Keller, M.: *Arch. Gynäk.*, 168:139, 1963.
80. Kumar, D., Feltham, L. A. W., and Gornall, A. G.: *Lancet*, 1:549, 1959.
81. Kumar, D., and Barnes, A. C.: *Obstet. Gynec. Survey*, 15:625, 1960.
82. Kumar, D.: *Amer. J. Obstet. Gynec.*, 84:1323, 1962.
83. Landau, R., and Lugibihl, K.: *J. Clin. Endocr.*, 18:1237, 1958.
84. Lauritzen, C., Lehmann, W. D., and Bambas, W.: *Endokrinologie*, 52:248, 1967.
85. Lencioni, L. J., Martinez-Amezaga, L. A., and Badano, H.: *Amer. J. Obstet. Gynec.*, 104:13, 1968.
86. Loraine, J. A., and Mathew, D. G.: *J. Obstet. Gynec. Brit. Comm.*, 57:542, 1950.
87. Lundwall, F., and Stakeman, G.: *Acta Obstet. Gynec. Scand.*, 45:301, 1966.
88. MacLeod, S. C., Brown, J. B., Beischer, N. A., and Smith, M. A.: *Austr. New Zeal. Obst. Gyn. J.*, 7:25, 1967.
89. Magendantz, H. G., Klausner, D., Ryan, K. J., and Yen, S. S. C.: *Obstet. Gynec.*, 32:610, 1968.
90. Martin, J. D., and Mills, I. H.: *Brit. Med. J.*, 2:571, 1956.
91. Massani, Z. M., Sanguinetti, R., Gallegos, R., and Raimondi, D.: *Amer. J. Obstet. Gynec.*, 99:313, 1967.
92. Mastboom, J. L.: *J. Clin. Endocr.*, 14:109, 1954.
93. Mendlowitz, M., et al.: *Amer. J. Obstet. Gynec.*, 81:643, 1961.
94. Meyer, C. J.: *Steroids*, Suppl.1:199, 1965.
95. Michie, E. J.: *J. Obstet. Gynec. Brit. Comm.*, 74:896, 1967.
96. Michie, E. A., and Livingstone, J. R. B.: *Acta Endocr.*, 61:320, 1969.
97. Moore, H. C.: *J. Obstet. Gynec. Brit. Comm.*, 72:272, 1964.
98. Müller, K., and Nielsen, J. C.: *Dan. Med. Bull.*, 14:165, 1967.
99. Muresan, S., and Zehan, M.: *Amer. J. Obstet. Gynec.*, 100:230, 1968.
100. Niklicek, O.: *Acta Cytol.*, 12:140, 1968.
101. Nilsson, I., and Bengtsson, L. P.: *Acta Obstet. Gynec. Scand.*, 47:213, 1968.
102. Osmond-Clarke, F., Murray, M., and Wood, C.: *J. Obstet. Gynec. Brit. Comm.*, 71:231, 1964.
103. Page, I. H.: *J. Clin. Endocr.*, 13:300, 1953.
104. Patterson, M. L.: *J. Obstet. Gynec. Brit. Emp.*, 67:883, 1960.
105. Pearlman, W. H., Pearlman, M. R. J., and Rakoff, A. E.: *J. Biol. Chem.*, 209:803, 1954.
106. Pece, G. V., Scapichi, G., and Colombino, R.: *Monit. Ost. Gin. Endocr. Metab.*, 37:43, 1966.
107. Pekkainen, A., Rauramo, L., and Thomasson, B.: *Acta Endocr.*, Suppl. 42:75, 1962.
108. Pesonen, S., and Vaananen, P.: *Geburtsh. u. Frauenhk.*, 22:898, 1962.
109. Plentl., A. A., and Gray, M. J.: *Amer. J. Obstet. Gynec.*, 78:472, 1959.
110. Pose, S. V., Cibils, L., and Zuspan, A.: *Amer. J. Obstet. Gynec.*, 84:297, 1962.
111. Poseiro, J. J., et al.: *III Congreso Uruguayo de Ginecotocología*, Vol. I. 1960.
112. Quigley, G. J., Richards, R. T., and Shier, K. J.: *Amer. J. Obstet. Gynec.*, 106:340, 1970.
113. Ratanasopa, V., Schindler, A. E., Lee, L. Y., and Herrmann, W. L.: *Amer. J. Obstet. Gynec.*, 99:295, 1967.
114. Rezende, J., et al.: *Acta Cytol.*, 14:78, 1970.
115. Rinsler, M. G., and Rigby, B.: *Brit. Med. J.*, 2:966, 1957.
116. Rodríguez-López, A.: *Acta Gin.*, 6:417, 1955.
117. Roth, K., and Slater, S.: *Amer. J. Obstet. Gynec.*, 83:1325, 1962.
118. Roy, E. J., Harkness, R. A., and Kerr, M. G.: *J. Obstet. Gynec. Brit. Comm.*, 70:597, 1963.
119. Sagone, J., and Arrotta, V.: *Ann. Ost. Gin.*, 87:365, 1965.
120. Sagone, J., and Arrotta, V.: *Ann. Ost. Gin.*, 87:454, 1965.
121. Selenkov, H. A., Saxena, B. N., Dana, C. L., and Emerson, K.: "Measurement and Pathophysiological Significance of Human Placental Lactogen," in *The Fetoplacental Unit*, ed. A. Pecile and C. Finzi. Amsterdam, Excerpta Medica Foundation, 1969.
122. Semm, K.: *Arch. Gynäk.*, 198:149, 1963.
123. Shearman, R. P.: *J. Obstet. Gynec. Brit. Comm.*, 66:1, 1959.
124. Simmer, H. H.: "Human Placental Lactogen," in *Biology of Gestation*, Vol. I, ed. N. S. Assali. New York, Academic Press, 1968.
125. Simonett, H., Piaux, G., and Robey, M.: In *Colloques sur la fonction luteale*, Vol. II. Paris, Masson et Cie., 1954.
126. Smith, G. V., and Smith, O. W.: *Physiol. Revs.*, 28:1, 1948.
127. Smith, K., Greene, J. W., and Touchstone, J. C.: *Amer. J. Obstet. Gynec.*, 96:101, 1966.

128. Sommerville, I. F.: In *Ciba Symposium on Toxaemias of Pregnancy.* London, J. & A. Churchill, 1950.
129. Sophian, J.: *The Toxaemias of Pregnancy.* London, Butterworth, 1953.
130. Staemmler, H. J.: *Arch Gynäk.*, 182:506, 561, 579, 1956.
131. Stark, G.: *Geburtsh. u. Frauenhk.*, 22:155, 1962; 22:893, 1962.
132. Talledo, O.: *Amer. J. Obstet. Gynec.*, 97:571, 1967.
133. Talledo, O., Chesley, L. C., and Zuspan, F. P.: *Amer. J. Obstet. Gynec.*, 100:218, 1968.
134. Taylor, E. S., Hassner, A., Burns, P. D., and Drose, V. E.: *Amer. J. Obstet. Gynec.*, 85:10, 1963.
135. Ten Berge, B. S.: *Gynaecologia*, 149:4, 1960.
136. Teoh, E. S., and Tow, S. H.: *J. Obstet. Gynec. Brit. Comm.*, 74:453, 1967.
137. Theobald, C. W.: *The Pregnancy Toxaemias.* London, Henry Kimpton, 1955.
138. Troen, P.: *J. Clin. Endocr.*, 21:895, 1961.
139. Troen, P.: *J. Clin. Endocr.*, 21:1511, 1961.
140. Van der Molen, H. J., and Hart, P. G.: *Nederl. Tidjskr. Verloksde.*, 61:391, 1961.
141. Venning, E. H., Carballeira, A., and Dyrenfurth, I.: *J. Clin. Endocr.*, 14:187, 1954.
142. Venning, E. H., Singer, B., and Simpson, S. A.: *Amer. J. Obstet. Gynec.*, 67:542, 1954.
143. Venning, E. H., and Dyrenfurth, I.: *J. Clin. Endocr.*, 16:426, 1959.
144. Venning, E. H., Primrose, T., Caligaris, L. C. S., and Dyrenfurth, I.: *J. Clin. Endocr.*, 17:473, 1957; 19:403, 1959.
145. Watanabe, M., Meeker, C. I., Gray, M. J., Sims, E. A. H., and Solomon, S.: *J. Clin. Endocr. Metab.*, 25:1665, 1965.
146. Wells, C. N.: *Amer. J. Obstet. Gynec.*, 66:598, 1955.
147. Wu, C. H., Flickinger, G. L., Archer, D. F., and Touchstone, J. C.: *Amer. J. Obstet. Gynec.*, 107:313, 1970.
147a. Würtele, A.: *Arch. Gynäk.*, 198:131, 1963.
148. Würtele, A.: *Ztschr. f. Geb. u. Gyn.*, 159:282, 1962.
149. Zander, J., Münstermann, A. M., and Rünnenbaum, B.: *Acta Endocr.*, 41:507, 1962.
150. Zondek, B.: *Internat. J. Fertil.*, 5:84, 1960.
151. Zondek, B.: *Proceed. III World Congress Fertil. & Steril.*, 1:83, Amsterdam, 1961.
152. Zondek, B., and Pfeifer, V.: *Acta Obstet. Gynec. Scand.*, 38:742, 1959.
153. Zuspan, F. P., Nelson, G. H., and Ahlquist, R. P.: *Amer. J. Obstet. Gynec.*, 90:88, 1964.

Chapter 45
ENDOCRINE PATHOLOGY OF GESTATION

45.1. PITUITARY PATHOLOGY IN GESTATION

In pregnancy, the pituitary is relegated to a secondary role within the context of endocrine correlations. This is due to the fact that the most important pituitary function from the reproductive viewpoint, that of secreting gonadotropin, is taken over by the chorion. Important as they are, the other hormones play, to a certain extent, an accessory role in sexual life. This is one of the reasons why hypophysectomy in pregnant animals (see Chapter 19) does not result in the interruption of gestation. Much the same thing occurs in the human species.

Four fundamental pituitary conditions with a bearing on gestation may be distinguished: (1) Hypophysectomy and gestation, (2) Sheehan's syndrome, (3) Chiari-Frommel syndrome, (4) acromegaly and pregnancy, (5) diabetes insipidus.

45.1.1. HYPOPHYSECTOMY AND GESTATION

In their already classic studies of many years ago, Pencharz and Long (1933) and Selye, Collip and Thompson (1934) hypophysectomized pregnant rats without causing interruption of gestation. Recent investigations by Carpent and Desclin[39] showed that pregnant rats tolerated hypophysectomy well but did not tolerate castration, which proves that corpus luteum function in pregnancy is independent of pituitary function. The increasing practice of surgical resection or radiologic suppression of the pituitary in some cases of inoperable cancer has extended our experience concerning the question of hypophysectomy in human gestation. Hutchinson and his associates[110] used ^{90}Y to destroy the pituitaries of pregnant monkeys and saw no instances of interrupted pregnancy. Kaplan[124] hypophysectomized a pregnant woman because of a pituitary chromophobe adenoma, without observing any gestational endocrine changes or threat of abortion. Other instances of hypophysectomy in human pregnancy without interruption of gestation and without any changes in the endocrine correlations of pregnancy have been reported by Little and associates,[137] Nataf and Chaikoff,[162] and Luft.[143]

The capacity to withstand hypophysectomy is much greater in the pregnant than in the nonpregnant woman, which must be attributed to the fact that placental internal secretions provide adequate substitution not only for gonadotropic function but also for thyrotropin[233] and ACTH[9, 31] secretion and in addition carry out the activity of placental lactogen,[17, 125] which, to some extent, is analogous to HGH.

45.1.2. SHEEHAN'S SYNDROME

Sheehan's syndrome has already been described in Chapter 31 (page 684). It results from *postpartum necrosis of the pituitary*. The florid variety of the syndrome, presenting with irreversible amenorrhea, mental torpor and progressive anorexia and death, as originally described by Sheehan,[203] is actually rare, whereas *minor or abortive* forms of the disease are not uncommon. Such cases are characterized by prolonged amenorrhea, associated with a shrinking size of the uterus, inability to lactate and weight loss. This syndrome, which is temporary and responds well to therapy, coincides with what earlier clinicians referred to as *uterine hyperinvolution* and results from minimal and reversible postpartum atrophy.

The *etiology* usually involves a vascular accident, embolism and abrupt ischemia, as well as microabscesses described in the course of puerperal pyemia. Sheehan himself[201, 203] later believed that the real etiology was vasospasm in the pituitary circulation and that thromboembolism was an event secondary to arterial vasoconstriction. The latter is in part a physiologic phenomenon, owing to the fact that pituitary circulation reaches a high degree of development during gestation and, after delivery, some *reduction in the rate of blood supply becomes a physiologic necessity* which, when exaggerated, may result in Sheehan's syndrome.

According to Beernink and MacKay,[22] the *onset* is not necessarily confined to the puerperium but may be related to abortion or to hydatidiform mole. They point out that the syndrome occurs most frequently in the wake of *eclampsia, abruptio placentae* or *puerperal sepsis*.

The *symptomatology*, as we have indicated previously, consists of prolonged amenorrhea in the severe and irreversible forms, suspension of lactation (which allows this picture to be differentiated from the Chiari-Frommel syndrome, to be described shortly), torpor, anorexia and progressive cachexia leading to death. A variety of milder forms are associated only with amenorrhea and emaciation. These are exemplified by women who after childbirth remain sterile, amenorrheic and emaciated for the rest of their lives.

Treatment has relied mainly on the administration of ACTH (Engstrom[66]). Polishuk and colleagues[172] treated a patient successfully with HMG, obtaining restoration of menses and even another gestation, but Sheehan[202] lately reported a case with *spontaneous regression*.

45.1.3. CHIARI-FROMMEL SYNDROME

In Chapter 31 (page 700) we studied the syndrome of *galactotropic hyperpituitarism*, or syndrome of Argonz-Del Castillo, which North American authors refer to as the Forbes-Albright syndrome. Pulle and Rigano[174] separate this entity from the one we are about to discuss. We have pointed out that galactotropic hyperpituitarism was the result of hypothalamic alterations involving the destruction of the sex center of the *median eminence*. Since this center is responsible for inhibiting *prolactin release*, its destruction triggers lactation in a permanent and extemporaneous manner. Proof of this etiology has been provided by Langer and Grudi,[131] who were able to precipitate lactation experimentally by means of prolonged administration of chlorpromazine, which is well known to exert an anesthetic action on the hypothalamus.

The *Chiari-Frommel syndrome* results from galactotropic hyperpituitarism *appearing in the course of the puerperal period*, that is, developing under what may be termed "physiologic" conditions, as compared to the former variety, whose origin is unrelated to gestation. In general, lactation in such women begins in a normal way but, either because it is deliberately prolonged to undue lengths, as may be the common practice in rural areas, or because menstrual activity fails to be restored spontaneously, secretion of milk continues indefinitely. We have noted on many occasions that some women themselves bear some responsibility for the development of this syndrome by continuing to nurse their children for extended periods of time. In a noteworthy case observed by us, this was done for a period of five years, during which the child had already started going to school and, when dismissed from class, would run after his mother in order to be breast fed. As is often the case in prolonged lactation, many of the women with such remarkable nursing capability actually suffer from amenorrhea. Amenorrhea in this instance is the result of inhibition of the sex center via the neurohormonal reflex triggered by oxytocin secretion (see Chapter 22). When such women finally decide to wean their children, they find that they continue secreting milk spontaneously and that their menses fail to reappear (Groseclose,[86] Jaszmann[116]).

Over the past years, however, this clinical syndrome has been described in association with *tumors* involving the base of the brain. Several cases have been reported by Anderson and his co-workers[6] and by Guinet[88] in conjunction with *craniopharyngiomas*, and by Linquette and colleagues,[135] as well as Putelat and co-workers,[175] in association with pituitary adenomas, mainly *chromophobe adenomas*. We have recently observed a case (Fig. 45-1) caused by *fracture of the base of the skull* in an accident that had occurred during the third month of gestation. The syndrome did not develop, however, until after delivery, which seems to prove that the triggering effect is provided by the physiologic correlations involved in initiation of lactation.

Consequently, there appears to be little doubt that the syndrome results from changes of a functional or destructive nature at the level of the *hypothalamic sex center*, as is also shown by the experiment of Johnson and associates,[117] in which the syndrome was successfully induced in a ewe by destroying the sex center. Herlant and his colleagues[99, 100] have described the occurrence of this syndrome also in cases of hyperthyroidism.

Rankin and his co-workers[176] reported 17 cases in which there was no tumor or any other demonstrable lesion of either the pituitary or the hypothalamus. Linquette and colleagues[136] described a case of traumatic origin, similar to our case, which is discussed in Chapter 34 (Section 34.4.4).

The same clinical picture is quite frequently associated with *pluriglandular syndromes*: polycystic ovaries (Lavric[134]), hypothyroidism (Kinch et al.[128]) and diabetes insipidus (Zecca and Passarelli[236]). There has been much discussion as to whether this syndrome is identical with the Argonz-Del Castillo syndrome or Forbes-Albright syndrome. Scaglione[192] believes that both have an identical origin.

45.1.4. ACROMEGALY AND PREGNANCY

It has already been stated here that acromegaly results from a functioning eosinophilic adenoma of the pituitary, as a consequence of growth hormone secretion by the tumor. Pregnancy was thought to be associated with a physiologic increase in the activity of this hormone. The truth is that many reactions of the growth hormone and metabolic type seen in pregnancy and in diabetes of pregnancy (see Section 45.4.2) are now known to be due to in-

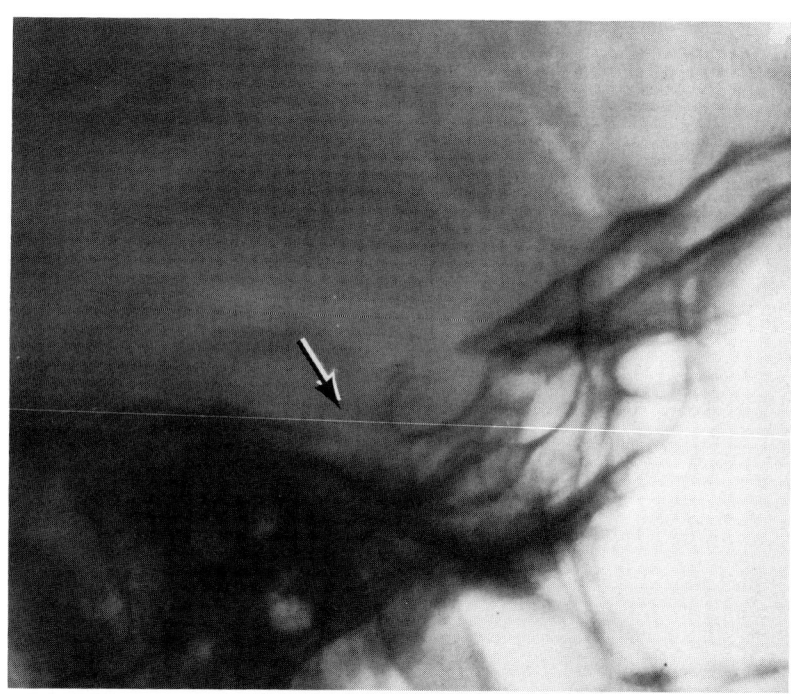

Figure 45-1. Chiari-Frommel syndrome, developed in the postpartum period in a woman who had sustained a fracture of the sphenoid in a car accident during the second month of pregnancy. Base of skull x-ray three years later.

creased activity of *placental lactogen* (Kaplan and Grumbach[125]). Josimovitch[119] believes that lactogen *potentiates* the action of HGH, which accounts for the clinical observation that acromegaly is *considerably aggravated* by gestation. This has been a well known fact for quite some time, but has recently been reemphasized by Maimone.[145]

45.1.5. DIABETES INSIPIDUS

The problem of diabetes insipidus has been studied in Chapter 32 (Page 709). Because its principal sex related repercussions affect the dynamics of labor, the principal obstetrical aspects of diabetes insipidus were discussed in that chapter. The six cases described by Marañón and Martínez-Díaz[149] are well known in the Spanish-speaking world. One patient had been followed over a period of 26 years, involving six deliveries that were all slow but spontaneous. Subsequent case reports[73, 215] have confirmed those observations.

Among recent reports of pregnancy associated with diabetes insipidus, Stephens and Hayes[212] described an instance of completely normal labor, while Hawker and associates[95] published two cases in which oxytocin blood levels were within normal limits and labor evolved in a physiologic manner. Aguilo and colleagues,[4] who collected 26 cases in the literature and reported one case of their own, believe that atonic bleeding during delivery is the most dangerous and most common complication occurring in pregnant women with diabetes insipidus.

Since the disorder results from a lesion of the supraoptic and paraventricular hypothalamic nuclei, which is where oxytocin is elaborated, one might anticipate finding total adynamia of the uterus in each case. This is not the case since, even though labor is slowed down to a certain extent, contractile activity is always found to be present, which indicates that substances other than oxytocin, capable of eliciting contractions, as indicated in Chapter 21, intervene in the mechanism of labor.

Current treatment, based on vasopressin administration, alleviates the metabolic symptoms of the disease and, interestingly, may indirectly influence oxytocin production, judging by the reports of Warren and Fernstrom,[228] in which two cases of diabetes insipidus, treated with pitressin during pregnancy, were observed to have deliveries that were not only spontaneous but even more rapid than normal.

45.2. THYROID PATHOLOGY AND GESTATION

The occurrence of thyroid hyperfunction in gestation has been emphasized before (Chapter 20). The evidence is based on increased radioiodine uptake,[59, 92] increased PBI levels[126, 181] and increased binding capacity of TBG.[126, 186] Further evidence of hyperfunction rests on the increased concentration of circulating thyroxine[233] and antithyroid substances in the blood.[162]

Although thyroxine crosses the placental barrier only partially and its excess is degraded by the placenta,[233] these changes have important repercussions on the fetal body. The net effect of maternal hyperthyroidism is to produce the opposite effect in the fetal organism, that is, fetal thyroid suppression. In this regard, the embryo obeys the *law of compensatory atrophy*, explained in Chapter 20 (page 438), and the principle of *conditioned parabiosis* with the mother, (page 438).

The fetal thyroid shows very early signs of activity so that the presence of maternal hyperthyroidism may apparently be countered by this compensatory mechanism. Van Heyningen[223] has shown that the mouse embryo starts trapping radioactive iodine from the fifteenth day of a 30 day gestation. Ino and Greer[112] noted that, if pregnant rats were treated with propylthiouracil, the fetus reacted in a compensatory manner by increasing fetal thyroid function and ^{131}I uptake. On the other hand, the finding that fetal thyroid function remains unaffected by maternal hypophysectomy (Nataf and Chaikoff[162]) is of interest since it seems to prove that the placental barrier is also impermeable to thyrotropin.

The causes of gravidic hyperthyroidism remain obscure. The placenta does not produce thyrotropin. As a result, the increase in gestational thyrotropin activity, which seems to be the underlying cause of the activation of thyroid function, must be of pituitary origin. This has been demonstrated by the experiments of Dowling and colleagues,[58] in which thyrotropin was found to disappear from the circulation if pregnant rats were hypophysectomized. Nor can the secretory changes affecting the pituitary be attributed to the action of placental gonadotropins, since it has been shown that chorioepithelioma is not associated with thyroid hyperfunction (Greer[85]).

45.2.1. HYPOTHYROIDISM AND GESTATION

Hypothyroidism is a common cause of both *sterility* (see Chapter 41, Section 41.2.1) and abortion (see Chapter 42, Section 42.6.1). Gestation seldom occurs in either *myxedema* or *cretinism;* nevertheless, a few such cases have been reported. The fetuses are born with thyroid hypertrophy (Fioretti and Caretti,[68] Hirschowitz and Berge[101]). In endemic goiter areas, the illness appears to be aggravated by pregnancy (Aboul-Khari et al.[1]). Dokumov,[57] Hoet and associates,[105] and Malek and colleagues[146] all reported a high incidence of *prematurity*, with a marked decrease in fetal weight. Dokumov[57] further noted an increase in the occurrence of *toxemia of pregnancy*, while Stempak[214] found an increased incidence of *congenital malformations*. Gestation in hypothyroidism thus offers a frankly adverse balance.

Man and his co-workers[148] described instances of *subclinical thyroid insufficiency* complicating gestation which, though detectable only by means of thyroid function tests, may nevertheless be the cause of sudden weight gain, edema, etc.

45.2.2. BASEDOW'S DISEASE

Marañón had pointed out that hyperthyroidism tended to improve with gestation, which in our experience has proved to be an unquestionable fact. An explanation for the phenomenon has been offfered in Chapter 20 (page 426). In severe cases, Elsas and associates[65] and Werner[230] described the occurrence of *fetal changes* involving delayed osseous maturation, development of goiters, prematurity and low weight. It must be added that such changes occur only in extremely severe cases of the disease.

According to recent studies by David and colleagues,[52] Becker and associates,[20] and Herlant and associates,[100] maternal hyperthyroidism tends to provoke the Chiari-Frommel syndrome with galactorrhea. This phenomenon is a result of the synergistic action by thyroid hormone on lactation and has been explained in Chapter 22 (page 467).

45.3. PARATHYROID PATHOLOGY IN GESTATION

The changes occurring in calcium metabolism during gestation favor the development of tetany. Thus, the presence of *hypoparathyroidism* coincident with pregnancy engenders so-called *gravidic tetany*, an entity known since ancient times (Chapter 34, page 769).

The disorder, characterized by hypocalcemia and convulsions, generally occurs as a consequence of goiter surgery associated with inadvertent removal of some or most of the parathyroid glands. Such patients with surgically induced parathyroid insufficiency may become pregnant, as their fertility remains almost intact, but because of gestational demands on calcium metabolism, involving the mobilization and fetal absorption of calcium, they develop tetany. Such cases of tetany have recently been reported by Dumont and Etienne-Martin,[60] Grant,[81] Strozier and Bohmfalk,[217] and Tscherne.[221] Tscherne's case was associated with abortion which, in his opinion, is fairly common in parathyroprival tetany.

According to Jost,[120] maternal parathyroidectomy produces hyperplasia of the fetal glands in experimental animals, which must be assumed to be true also in man, since Grant[81] reported three cases, one revealing considerable improvement near term, in which the presence in the newborn of hypertrophied parathyroid glands could be verified after birth.

Concerning the question of therapy, Strozier and Bohmfalk[217] have outlined a routine based on the use of massive doses of calciferol and intravenous calcium.

Hyperparathyroidism, or von Recklinghausen's disease, on the other hand, is seldom observed in association with pregnancy. Springham and Geist[213] described a case resulting from parathyroid adenoma which was associated with osteoporosis, pelvic deformities and a condition similar to osteomalacia. Wagner and associates[227] reported a case of maternal hypercalcemia, slight elevation of calcium concentration in the amniotic fluid and fetal hypercalcemia which, after delivery, however, gave way to hypocalcemia bordering on tetany, fetal hypoparathyroidism and increased fetal plasma alkaline glycerophosphatase activity.

45.4. DISEASES OF THE PANCREAS: DIABETES AND PREDIABETES IN GESTATION

Included here have been two clinically distinct conditions: *diabetes* and *prediabetes*. We have done so deliberately because we believe that we are dealing with *two different syndromes rather than different grades of the same disease entity.*

The complications experienced by a diabetic female upon becoming pregnant are presently well known.[7, 90, 103, 165, 231] By comparison, much less is known clinically about some *larvated forms of diabetes, or prediabetes*, which make their first appearance during gestation and, though not involving serious consequences for the mother, result in a high proportion of fetal casualties. For these reasons, they have become the object of very special attention in recent years.

Much debate has taken place on the question of what *nomenclature* should be applied for these conditions. The term diabetes has been rejected by some on grounds that such a diagnosis can only be established a posteriori. Gitsch and colleagues[77] therefore propose the term *subclinical diabetes,* whereas we have proposed the term *latent diabetes.*[31]

As far back as 1939, Allen pointed out that women who developed diabetes about the age of 50 or over usually revealed a history of pregnancies terminating in abortion, premature labor or stillbirths during the childbearing age before their diabetes became manifest. This observation of Allen's was later to be confirmed by various authors[105, 113, 171] to the extent that a *high rate of miscarriage may now be suspected to be the first manifestation of diabetes.* In order to understand how the pathophysiology of diabetes differs from that of prediabetes, however, it will first be necessary to study the endocrine changes associated with these conditions.

45.4.1. ENDOCRINE PATHOPHYSIOLOGY OF DIABETES AND PREDIABETES

Carbohydrate metabolism, as we know, is controlled by a series of different hormones: (1) insulin, (2) glucagon, (3) somatotropin, (4) cortisol and a group of related compounds, (5) epinephrine, (6) thyroxine and (7) during pregnancy, placental lactogen. We shall not discuss glucagon or placental lactogen here because of their secondary significance in gestation, concentrating instead on the remaining hormones.

INSULIN. The glucoregulatory role of insulin is well known. The question of insulin secretion during gestation has already been taken up in Chapter 20 (page 427). Beta cell hyperplasia of the pancreatic islets in pregnant women has been described by Jones,[118] Mohnike and Worm,[159] and Hellerstrom.[96] The rate of consumption of ^{131}I labeled insulin was found to be twice as high as in nonpregnant women (Goodner and Freinkel[78]). All this seems to indicate the presence of *compensatory hyperfunction.* Indeed, *insulinemia* has been found to be increased (Spellacy et al.,[208] Trayner et al.[220]). In contrast, insulinemia is low in genuine diabetes complicating pregnancy,[41, 209] whereas *increased* insulinemia has been shown to occur in prediabetic women (Spellacy et al.,[209] Carrington and MacWilliams,[41] Trayner et al.[220]) — that is, those women who, in the absence of marked disturbances of carbohydrate metabolism, present with acute fetal pathology.

In recent years, a number of studies have been concerned with the measurement of the *insulin reserve* (curve of plasma insulin levels following a loading dose of glucose) in normal as well as in prediabetic individuals. Obese, nonpregnant women and women classified as "prediabetic" have been reported to reveal nearly constant elevations of posthyperglycemic plasma insulin levels greater than those found in normal individuals.[13, 18, 37, 45, 184] An increase in the insulin reserve in *normal gestation* has been described by Spellacy and his colleagues[209] and by our own group[167] (Fig. 45–2). Mintz and his associates[157] observed

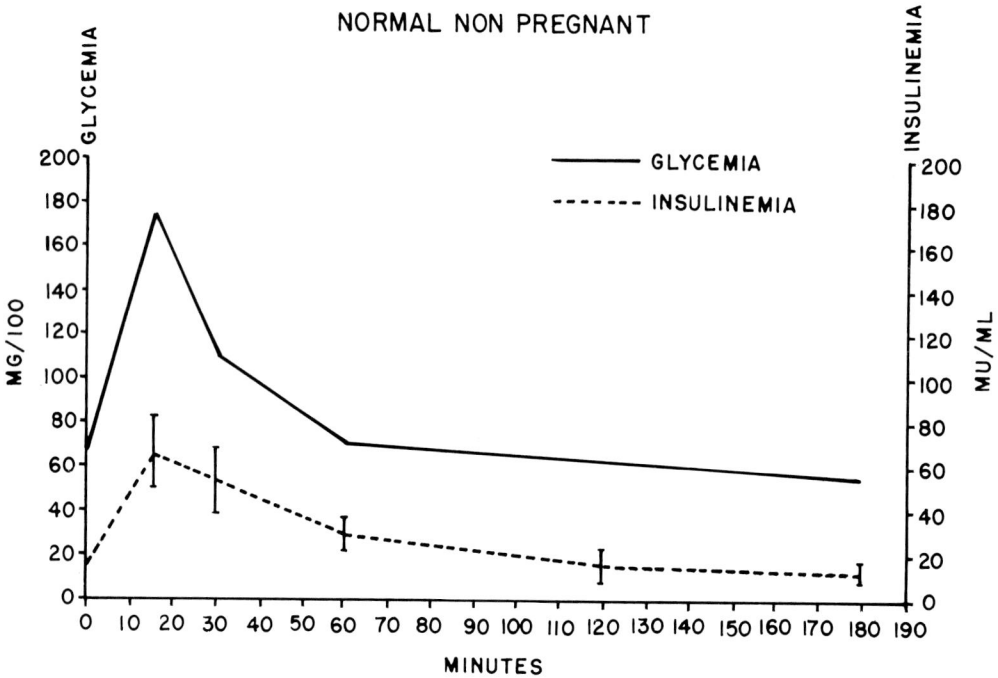

Figure 45–2. Intravenous administration of glucose (0.5 g per kg body weight) to normal nonpregnant female. Glycemia and insulinemia curves (the latter obtained by the radioimmunologic method of Hales and Randle). Rise in blood glucose level is a stimulant for pancreatic secretion of insulin (see Figure 20–10).

the same phenomenon in female monkeys. However, there is still a dearth of information concerning the problem in *diabetic and prediabetic pregnant women.* We have recently conducted a study of this question, from the results of which Figures 45–3 and 45–4 have been taken. As may be seen, *the insulinic reserve is increased in prediabetes* but is decreased in diabetes, owing to a primary pancreatic defect.

SOMATOTROPIN. The diabetogenic effect of somatotropin is well known.[16, 87, 98] On the basis of some earlier studies (Barns and Swyer,[12] Contopoulos and Simpson,[47] Nixon[163]), indicating an increase in somatotropin activity in gestation and even more so in prediabetes, gravidic prediabetes was believed to be a *pituitary form of diabetes.* Gemzell[75] and Salmon and Daughaday,[189] as well as Ehrlich and Randle,[62] failed to find any increase in STH activity in gravidic prediabetes. This was subsequently confirmed by a number of investigators.[151, 156, 206, 210, 235] Growth hormone levels are not increased in gestation, nor does the arginine tolerance test elicit higher levels than those found in nonpregnant women of the same age group.[151, 209] The elevated values described in the earlier literature stem from the fact that placental lactogen (HPL) was assayed as STH, owing to similar biologic actions. Current immunologic techniques have obviated this source of error.

CORTICOIDS AND ACTH. The well known diabetogenic effect of Cushing's disease[80] has been attributed to the action of cortisol on glucoregulation.[14, 33, 46, 80] ACTH also possesses indirect diabetogenic activity.[218, 221] In pregnancy, as we have pointed out in Chapter 20 (page 428), there is an increase in corticoids derived simultaneously from the maternal adrenal,[14, 227] the placenta[188] and the fetal adrenal.[26, 56, 72] Corticoid levels are particularly elevated in cases of prediabetes,[71, 72] which suggests an indirect pituitary diabetogenic effect (by means of ACTH) as well as a *placental* effect. It has been amply demonstrated that ACTH, of both pituitary[115] and placental[42] origin, occurs in increased amounts in gestation. Increased ACTH levels apparently occur in prediabetes.[32, 35, 197] In addition, a direct diabetogenic action by ACTH has been postulated by Love and his colleagues.[142] As a result, the diabetogenic effect of pregnancy may be hypothesized to result from: (1) possibly, increased HGH ac-

Endocrone Pathology of Gestation

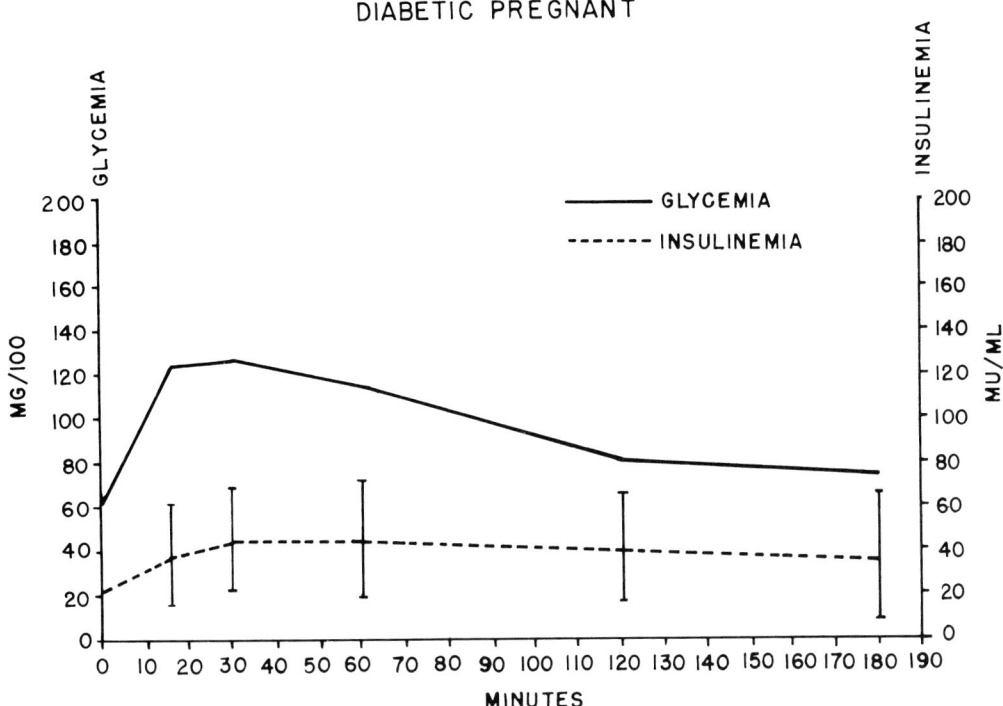

Figure 45-3. Intravenous administration of glucose (0.5 g per kg body weight) to pregnant, diabetic patient. The rise in blood glucose level, which in this instance is more sustained than in Figure 45-2, is not matched by parallel increment in plasma insulin level. This indicates diminished pancreatic response (pancreatic insufficiency).

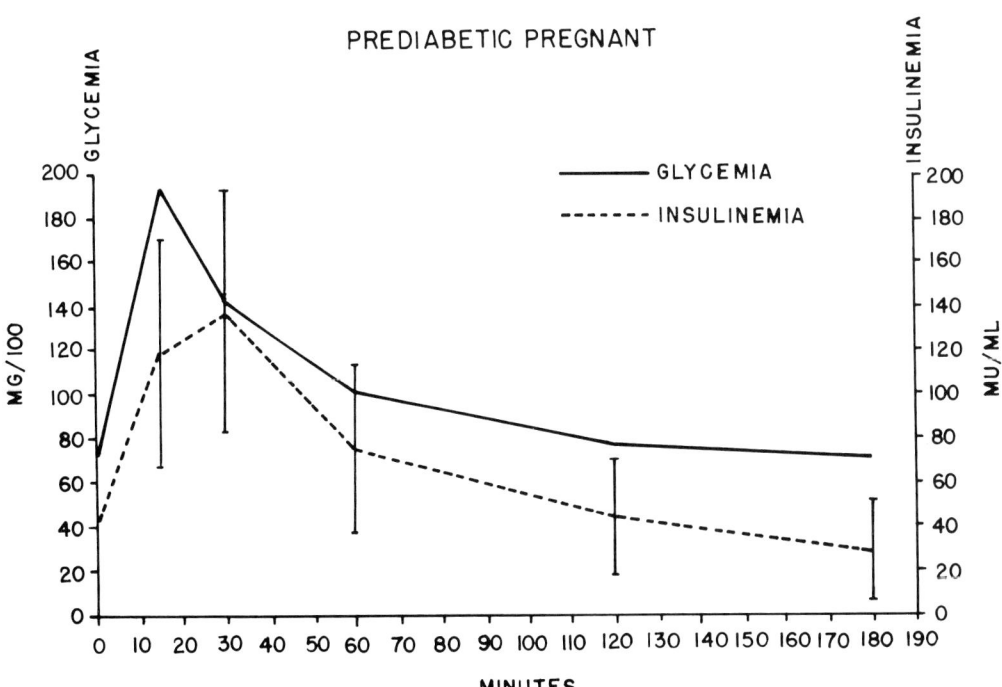

Figure 45-4. Intravenous administration of glucose (0.5 g per kg body weight) to pregnant, prediabetic patient. There is an exaggerated rise in plasma insulin levels (increased insulinic reserve). This suggests the extrainsular etiology of gravidic prediabetes and the presence of compensatory hyperfunction of the pancreas.

tivity, (2) action of corticoids of materno-feto-placental origin, and (3) action of ACTH, of both pituitary and chorionic origin.

PLACENTAL LACTOGEN. A place in this scheme had to be assigned to the presence of placental lactogen, which apparently possesses unquestionable diabetogenic potency (see Chapter 19, page 401). Recent investigations[125, 193, 234] seem to have made it clear that what is increased in prediabetes is placental lactogen rather than STH.[17, 119, 125] Josimovitch[119] in addition expressed the belief that lactogen potentiated the diabetogenic action of small amounts of HGH, thereby greatly enhancing the overall effect. In some of our earlier publications,[29, 30] we voiced the opinion that gravidic prediabetes was a form of latent pituitary diabetes; in view of recent developments, it would appear instead to be a *transient placental form of diabetes.*

In animals, the diabetogenic action of HPL has by now been well documented.[122, 150] Various authors have postulated that the diabetogenic effect of human gestation was a result of the presence of HPL.[38, 122, 170] Saxena and his co-workers[190] reported an increase in lactogen levels in pregnant prediabetic women. However, there is no unanimous agreement on this point, since Beck and his associates[17] and Sciarra,[198] among others, deny that there is any increase in HPL levels in prediabetic pregnant women as compared to normal pregnant women.

PROGESTOGENS. The diabetogenic action of some contraceptive progestogens has been brought to light in recent years, thanks mainly to the studies by Spellacy and Buhi.[210] Beck,[19] as well as Kalkhoff and his associates,[123] believe that the pancreatic reaction of pregnancy is set off by the combined actions of progesterone and HPL, whose effects apparently are cumulative.

SCHEME OF DIABETES AND PREDIABETES IN PREGNANCY. The pathophysiology of these conditions has been explained in a series of diagrams shown in Figures 45–5 through 45–7, simplified by omitting such factors as glucagon, epinephrine and thyroid hormone. In genuine diabetes mellitus, the equilibrium is broken by failure of pancreatic function but without any associated pituitary or adrenal modifications. The form known in the past as latent diabetes of pituitary origin was thought to be characterized by normal pancreatic function, while the disturbance in carbohydrate metabolism was caused by pituitary hyperfunction, involving either HGH (Fig. 45–5) or ACTH-corticoid (Fig. 45–6) activity, or both. This form of diabetes was known to frequently involve a compensatory pancreatic effort and to be associated with increased plasma insulin levels. In the light of present day knowledge, however, the diabetogenic effect does not seem to be derived

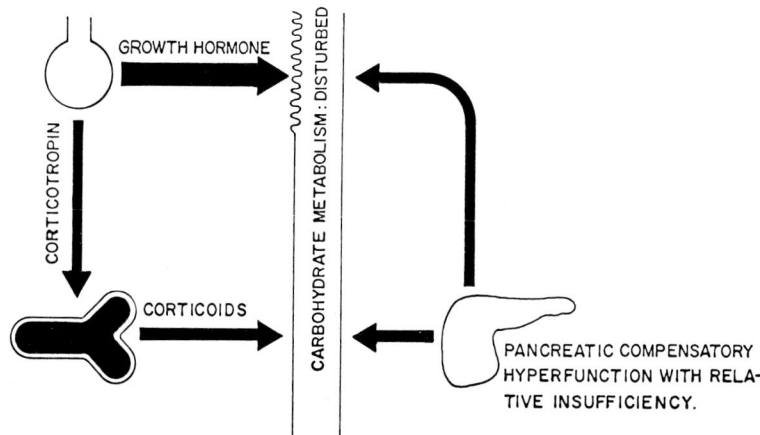

Figure 45–5. Etiology of latent diabetes in pregnancy owing to pituitary hyperfunction (involving GH). For many years, this has been envisioned as the possible mechanism of contra-insular action. However, recent investigations have revealed no increase in GH activity in gravidic prediabetes.

LATENT DIABETES IN PREGNANCY OF PITUITARY ETIOLOGY.

Endocrine Pathology of Gestation

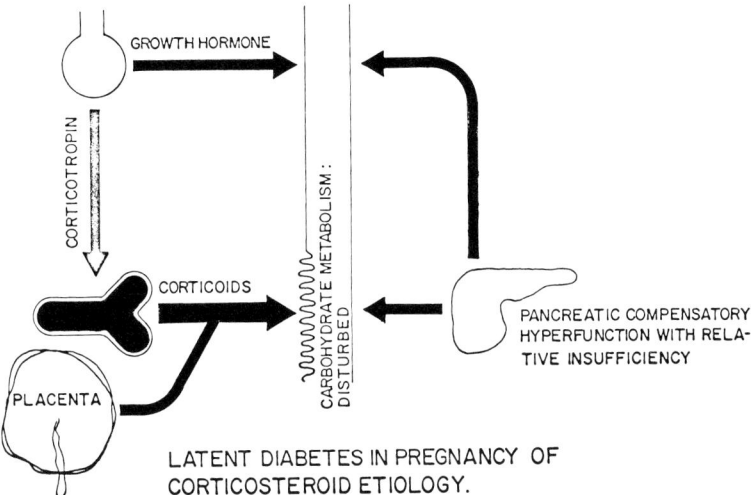

Figure 45-6. Proposed mechanism whereby an increase in adrenal or placental corticoid production presumably causes contrainsular imbalance. Nevertheless, our own investigations have failed to reveal any rise in corticoid levels in gravidic prediabetes.

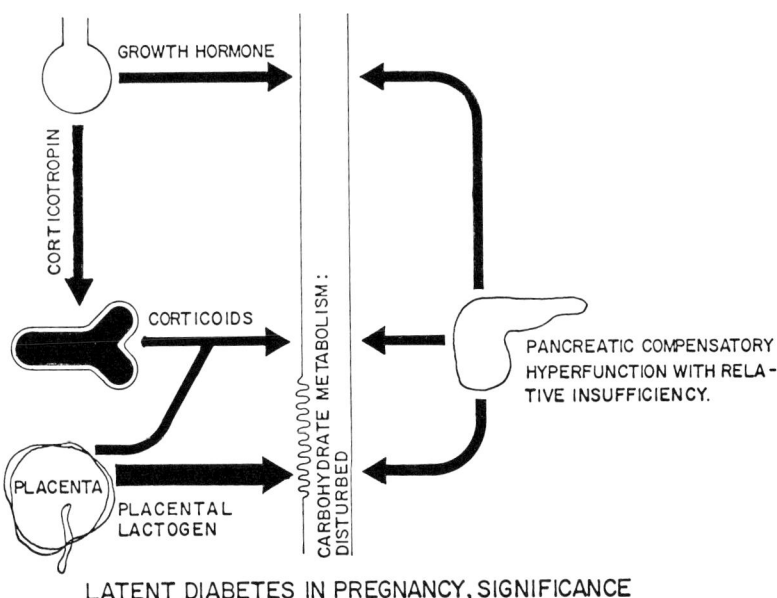

Figure 45-7. The most logical hypothesis which is based on the assumption that latent or "transient" diabetes of pregnancy may be the result of an increase in placental lactogen (HPL) activity.

from either the pituitary or adrenal but rather from the action of placental lactogen (Fig. 45–7).

45.4.2. DIABETES MELLITUS COMPLICATING GESTATION

Genuine diabetes is usually acquired early in life and therefore a woman may already be suffering from the disease at the time she becomes pregnant. Unlike "prediabetes" of pituitary or placental origin, it involves a *preexisting illness occurring with pregnancy*. Despite the high incidence of diabetes in Spain, resulting complications of pregnancy are not encountered as frequently as might be anticipated for the following reasons: (1) diabetes often causes sterility; (2) those women who are advised of their condition often choose to stay single, and (3) once married, they practice contraception either out of fear or following medical advice. We shall examine (1) the influence of diabetes on the mother, (2) the effect of gestation on the course of diabetes, (3) the effect of diabetes on the fetus, (4) the placenta in diabetes, and (5) treatment.

INFLUENCE OF DIABETES ON THE MOTHER. Although prediabetes is a more common complication of pregnancy than diabetes, the latter has been studied more extensively.[24, 90, 118, 164] The disease tends to produce *toxemia of pregnancy*,[12, 32] a tendency to acidosis and coma,[164] retinal[216] and renal[104] disturbances and a high rate of intrapartum mortality (14 per cent, according to Pedersen[168]), prolonged labor, oversized fetuses, as well as postpartum bleeding and infection.

INFLUENCE OF PREGNANCY ON THE EVOLUTION OF DIABETES. With pregnancy, the course of diabetes is aggravated, glycemia rises, glucose tolerance diminishes,[12, 32, 44] and ketosis and coma occur with much greater frequency.[164, 216] White and his associates[231] reveal progressive worsening of this disease with each pregnancy, as indicated in Table 45–1.

The prognosis when there are vascular complications is particularly poor in women with multiple pregnancies.[163, 164]

EFFECT OF DIABETES ON THE FETUS. Diabetes plays a well known role in producing *premature labor, labor with fetal death* and *giant fetuses dying shortly after delivery*.[90, 158, 231] *Fetal macrosomia* is one of the most characteristic features of such infants. It has been repeatedly emphasized that newborn infants of this type often develop *hypoglycemia*, leading to their demise (Angervall,[8] Hagerman[91]). As shown by Jorgensen and his co-workers,[118a] plasma insulin levels in such fetuses are much higher than those found in their mothers. Neither insulin nor growth hormone crosses the placental barrier,[76, 133] something we had suspected all along and demonstrated experimentally in rabbits.[30] Oversized fetuses reveal pancreatic hyperplasia, insulin secretion having been excited by the high glycemic levels received through the placental gradient from their mothers. Thus, *compensatory pancreatic hyperfunction*, generated in accordance with the principle of "conditioned parabiosis" (see Chapter 20, page 438), results in excessive production of insulin which, being unable to cross the placental barrier, is detained within the fetal organism and is the probable cause of both macrosomia and hypoglycemia of the newborn. By contrast, HGH, as has been indicated,[106, 153] does not seem to be involved in producing fetal macrosomia since it neither crosses the placental barrier[59, 133] nor occurs in increased concentration in the fetal circulation.[234]

THE PLACENTA IN DIABETES. Diabetes is associated with pronounced placental changes, which are also seen in prediabetes, so that in this respect at least the two clinical conditions, different in so many other aspects, do not significantly differ from each other. Clavero (see Chapter 44, page 962) has demonstrated that a decrease in the surface area and filtering capacity of the placenta (Fig. 45–9) occurs in conjunction with the well known picture of *premature placental senescence*. Horky and Jutzi[107, 108] demonstrated an increase in

TABLE 45–1. Incidence of Multiparity with Regard to Grades of Diabetes

| PARITY | GRADES ||||||
	A	B	C	D	E	F
I	14	4	1	1	1	0
II	10	6	2	0	0	1
III	4	4	4	3	0	0
IV or more	0	0	3	–	0	1

Endocrine Pathology of Gestation

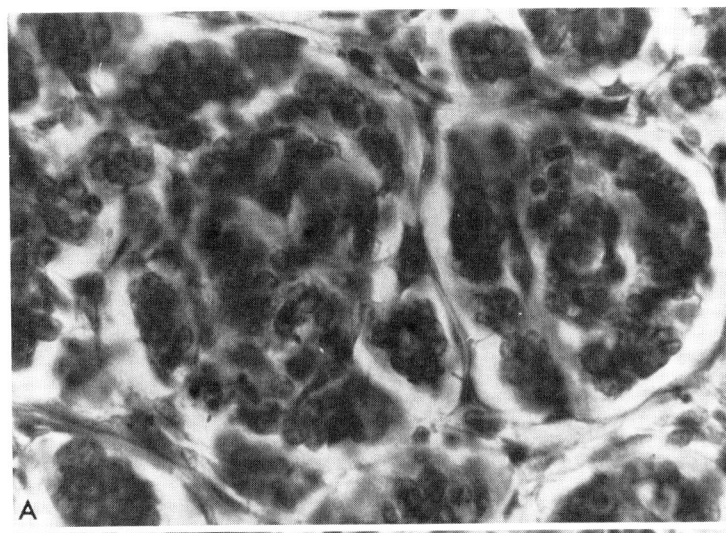
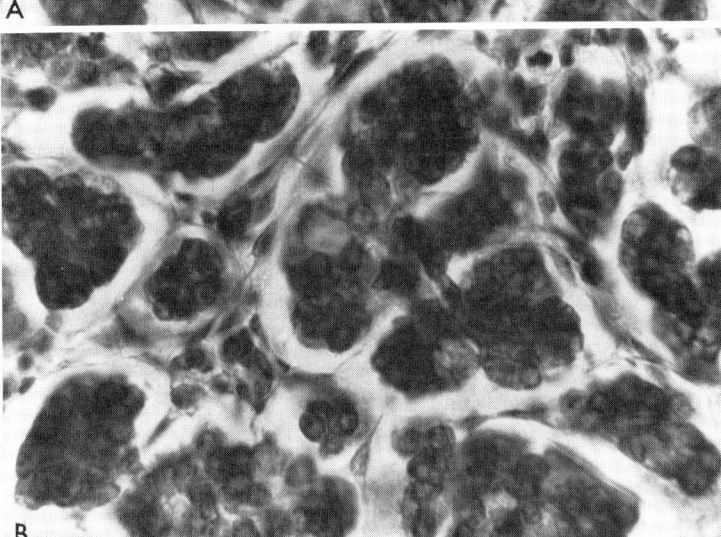

Figure 45-8. Pronounced degree of islet cell hyperplasia in two different infants, both born to diabetic mothers. Birth weights: A, 4160 g; B, 3560 g.

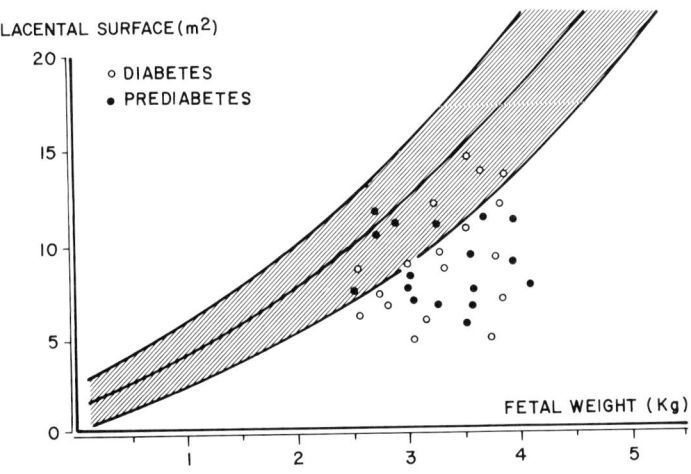

Figure 45-9. Placental surface area in various forms of gravidic pathology. Note decrease in area in both diabetes and prediabetes. (From Botella and Clavero.)

placental weight and vascular changes. In the opinion of Fischer and Horky,[70] the placental glycogen content in such cases is diminished. The fact that lesions of this kind are the result of diabetes has been demonstrated by the work of Powell and his colleagues[173] in placentas of patients with alloxanic diabetes. This type of placental degeneration is the main cause for the *fall in estriol excretion* which is highly characteristic of diabetes.[84, 102, 185, 218, 226] Thus, there is evidence of placental insufficiency, also encountered in prediabetes, which explains a great deal, though not all, of the perinatal pathology in this disease.

TREATMENT. Treatment of course must consist of a dietary regimen and administration of insulin. We are against the use of oral hypoglycemic agents because the underlying disorder is not the glycemic elevation but rather a profound endocrine imbalance, so that any attempt to lower the level of glycemia may lead to hypoglycemia and acidosis. For the same reasons, the regimen must not be poor in carbohydrates,[231] and should not reduce intake of the latter to less than 400 grams.

As for insulin, a sufficient dose must be given to keep glycemia under control although without allowing complete disappearance of glycosuria. Figures of 0.4 to 0.5 per cent may be tolerated. Two doses of long-acting insulin should be administered daily, based on continuous assessment of tolerance; in benign cases, a dose of 25 to 30 units daily is usually adequate.

45.4.3. PREDIABETES AND GESTATION

Prediabetes, which, as we have pointed out earlier, is a *subclinical transient form of diabetes*, does not manifest itself with maternal symptoms, yet it produces very serious fetal changes. Consequently, what will have to be described here is mainly fetal pathology. It constitutes what we have elsewhere termed "prediabetic embryopathy."[30, 31]

CAUSES OF PREDIABETIC EMBRYOPATHY. The fetal changes occurring in this clinical variety have been assumed to be of *endocrine nature*.[30] Congenital malformations have been induced in experimental animals with *cortisone*,[48, 139, 164] *glucagon*,[222] STH,[96, 229] ACTH[127] and HPL.[125]

Consecutively, we shall review these aspects of prediabetic embryopathy: (1) prediabetes and abortion, (2) premature labor, (3) fetal gigantism, (4) malformations, (5) hydramnios, (6) diagnosis, and (7) treatment.

PREDIABETES AND ABORTION. There is little reference to be found in the literature concerning the influence of diabetes on early interruption of pregnancy. In a review of an extensive series of cases (Table 45–2),[31] we found an incidence of spontaneous abortion of 23 per cent in untreated prediabetes, as compared to the 10 per cent which is the accepted abortivity index for normal gestations.

PREMATURE LABOR. In untreated diabetes, the incidence of premature and term fetal mortality found by Oakley[164] was 45 per cent. Lower figures of fetal loss were reported by Hadden and Harley[89] who, in a smaller (635 cases) series than ours, found a perinatal mortality rate of 10.8 per cent. Our own statistics have revealed higher figures (Table 45–3). As also shown in the table, there were significant differences between treated and untreated cases.

FETAL GIGANTISM. Numerous authors refer to fetal gigantism, or *macrosomia*, as a characteristic finding in diabetes,[12, 33, 90, 116] but in our own experience,[31] it is not a constant finding. We have made it clear previously (Section 45.4.2) that fetal macrosomia is conditioned by pancreatic hyperplasia and the latter, in turn, by hyperglycemia. For this reason, macrosomia is observed only in genuine diabetes with dysglycemia, but not in prediabetes, in which there are no disturbances in glucoregulation. This may be clearly appreciated in Table 45–4.

MALFORMATIONS. The incidence of malformations based on our own case material[31] is given in Table 45–5. De Meyer[152, 153] attributes such congenital anomalies to the influence of changing glycemic levels on embryonal development. However, as pointed out previously,

TABLE 45–2. Incidence of Abortion in Prediabetes

OUTCOME OF PREGNANCY	UNTREATED Cases	UNTREATED Percentage	TREATED Cases	TREATED Percentage
Live fetus	109	12.5	227	77.1
Stillborn fetus	415	48.1	61	14.3
Abortion	338	39.2	36	8.6

TABLE 45-3. Perinatal Mortality Rate in Clinical Diabetes, Latent Diabetes and Prediabetes

CATEGORY	UNTREATED PREGNANCIES			TREATED PREGNANCIES		
	Cases	Live fetuses	Dead fetuses	Cases	Live fetuses	Dead fetuses
Clinical diabetes	85	28 (32%)	57 (67%)	56	42 (75%)	14 (25%)
Latent diabetes	335	71 (21%)	264 (78%)	244	195 (80%)	49 (20%)
Prediabetes	197	38 (28%)	159 (80%)	122	103 (84%)	19 (16%)
Total	617	137 (22%)	480 (78%)	422	340 (80%)	82 (20%)

it seems more likely that they actually result from an endocrine cause. When administered in sufficiently high dosages, cortisone,[139, 160] STH,[127] ACTH[229] and glucagon[222] all exert teratogenic effects to a similar extent.

HYDRAMNIOS. In the majority of instances, such malformations are associated with *hydramnios*. This is a very characteristic finding, as pointed out by Angervall,[8] Gray,[82] Hagerman,[91] Hoet and associates,[105] and Oakley.[164] The presence of hydramnios should at least be suggestive of prediabetes.

DIAGNOSIS. Unlike the case in genuine diabetes, neither glucosuria nor hyperglycemia is found in prediabetes. The diagnosis must therefore be based on clinical data and on the glucose tolerance test. Among the clinical data to be considered are: (1) *family history of diabetes*, (2) history of abortions interspersed with instances of premature labor and stillbirths (most other gravidic syndromes cause isolated cases of early abortion or late abortion, whereas the intermingling of both types in the same patient should arouse suspicion), (3) fetal macrosomia (inconstant), (4) certain types of fetal lesions at autopsy—for instance, pulmonary immaturity and hyaline membrane disease, and (5) above all, the *glucose tolerance* test.

However, simple glucose tolerance tests are usually of little value, which is why such other tests as double glucose load curves of the Exton Rose type or, preferably, the cortisone-glucose tolerance test of the Conn and Fajans type[46] have been introduced. Expressive results have been obtained with such techniques by a great many investigators.[40, 67, 111, 147, 167, 221] We prefer the modification of Goto and Kato, which consists in first obtaining an Exton Rose type curve with a double glucose load of 50 gm each, which is then repeated 48 hours later, 2 hours after the administration of 30 mg prednisone. Results are shown in Figures 45-10 and 45-11, in which the recording at upper left is normal and all others represent a variety of pathologic conditions.

The early postpartum period, in the opinion of Bret and Coiffard,[34] is the most suitable time for reaching a diagnosis, because this is when the increase in prolactin and growth hormone activity produced by lactation is likely to reveal the slightest alterations, which otherwise could not be detected.

PROGNOSIS. Measurements of *urinary estriol excretion* are of prognostic value (Rivlin et al.,[180] Wyss and Meyer[232]). A fall in estriol values seems to be nonspecific[31] and indicates only the degree of fetal damage. The obstetrical history, and especially the family history and the study of insulincmia curves (Figs. 45-2 and 45-4), allows adequate evaluation of each individual case.

TABLE 45-4. Fetal Weight at Birth in Prematurity (Mean Value)

	CASES	PREMATURITY	MEAN WEIGHT, GRAMS
Clinical diabetes	21	3	3840
Latent diabetes	68	18	3320
Prediabetes	43	15	3190
Total	132	36	3580

TABLE 45-5. Congenital Malformations From Among Our Case Material

	CASES	PERCENTAGE
Total number of cases	474	100
Diabetes	67	14.1
Latent diabetes	251	52.9
Prediabetes	156	32.9
Malformations	14	2.9

988   Endocrine Pathology of Gestation

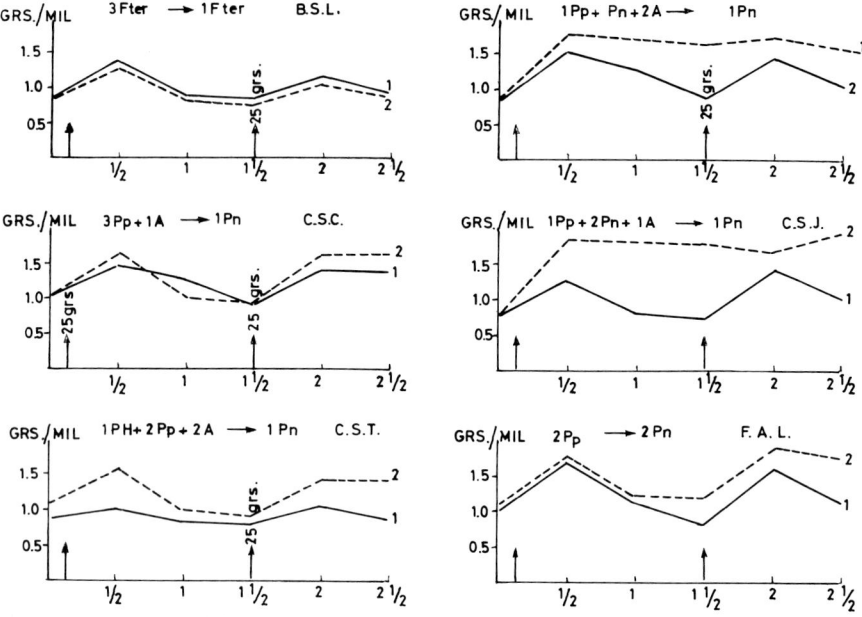

Figure 45–10. Various types of functional curves obtained by the technique of Goto and Kato. Abbreviations in upper part of each graph refer to clinical data (*Fter*, congenital anomaly; *Pp*, premature labor; *A*, abortion; *PH*, hydramnios; *Pn*, normal delivery; *Pm*, normal delivery with stillborn fetus; arrow indicates treatment).

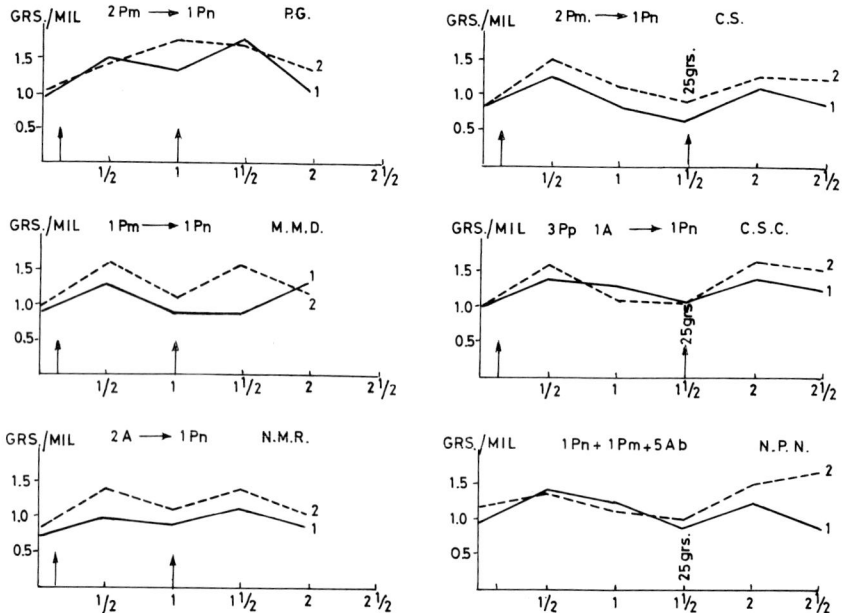

Figure 45–11. Various types of functional curves obtained by the technique of Goto and Kato. For identification of abbreviations, see Figure 45–10.

TREATMENT. We are unable to explain the good results obtained with insulin therapy in those cases in which plasma insulin levels are already elevated. Whatever the reasons, the results observed leave no room for doubt. In those cases in which all other forms of therapy had failed, we only succeeded with small doses of insulin. Mucci and his associates[161] recently reported similar results with a therapy of small dosages of insulin for which they similarly are unable to explain satisfactorily the therapeutic mechanism involved. Treatment is as follows. *Diet* is like that already indicated for genuine diabetes. Insulin is administered beginning with 8 IU of slow-acting insulin daily at breakfast time and, depending on the tolerance encountered, increasing the dosage up to 15 units daily. We advocate the addition of tocopherol, 100 mg daily, and 20 to 30 mg diethylstilbestrol daily per os. However, the essential part of this therapy is insulin, since results were equally favorable in those cases in which the complementary medication was not given.

45.4.4. DIABETES AND PREDIABETES: TWO DISTINCT SYNDROMES

In Table 45-6, we have summarized the principal characteristics of genuine diabetes and prediabetes and have pointed out the differences between the two.

It is evident that we are in fact dealing with two different clinical entities. Prediabetes, we once believed, was a gravidic form of pituitary diabetes. However, the discovery of placental lactogen has made us see things in a different light. Gravidic prediabetes actually would seem to reflect a diabetogenic placental effect which therefore is of a temporary nature. It is possible that over a period of time encompassing several pregnancies such an effect may disrupt the balance of glucoregulation and, in the long run, give rise to true diabetes in a predisposed female. This might explain why women well known to suffer embryopathic accidents of this type eventually—years later—are seen to develop frank diabetes. We are faced with a problem here that requires a thorough and careful investigation.

45.5. DISEASES OF THE ADRENAL AND GESTATION

Adrenal diseases may be divided into *medullary* and *cortical* disorders. The latter are by far the more important ones.

45.5.1. PHEOCHROMOCYTOMA AND PREGNANCY

Recent advances in estimating urinary catecholamines have, in many instances, facilitated the diagnosis of chromaffin tumors which in the past might have been overlooked as cases of "essential hypertension." As a result, such tumors have also been reported in association with gestation. Hendee and his colleagues[97] reported four cases, all of which had been mistaken for eclamptic toxemia.

45.5.2. DISEASES OF THE ADRENAL CORTEX

During pregnancy, the course of some of the adrenal diseases may be profoundly affected by the fact that both the placenta and the fetal adrenal yield a substantial output of mineralo- and glucocorticoids of their own.

As we have pointed out previously, a considerable increase in plasma and urinary corticoid values has been found during pregnancy by various authors (Bret and Coiffard,[34] Rodríguez-López,[183] Venning et al.[224]).

This increment is only in part due to maternal cortical secretion and may be

TABLE 45-6.

DIABETES	PREDIABETES
Early onset	Late onset
Rare in pregnancy	Common in pregnancy
Occurs with hyperglycemia	No hyperglycemia
Neonatal hypoglycemia	No neonatal hypoglycemia
Oversize fetuses	Fetuses with normal or below normal weight
No abortions or premature labor	Abortions, premature labor and malformations are common
Poor maternal prognosis	Good maternal prognosis
Guarded fetal prognosis	Very poor fetal prognosis
Diabetes is of the pancreatic variety	Diabetes is of the pituitary or adrenal variety

attributed largely to placental and fetal adrenal endocrine activity.

Placental synthesis of corticoids has been demonstrated beyond doubt (Salhanick et al.,[188] Ratsimamanga et al.,[177] Steinbeck and Theile[211]). On the other hand, the production of mineralo- and glucocorticoids by the fetal adrenal has also been proved (Villee et al.,[225] Eguchi,[61] Frandsen and Stakeman[71]). Only anencephalous fetuses fail to produce adrenal corticoids owing to marked atrophy of their adrenal glands.[71] Bloch and his co-workers[27] demonstrated the presence of an enzyme system in the fetal adrenal that was identical with that known to occur in the adult adrenal. Nevertheless, as far as the zona fasciculata and zona glomerulosa are concerned, the total fetal adrenal capacity for secretory activity, as we have indicated previously (Chapter 20), is acquired only after the seventh month. This probably accounts for the fact that, as shown by Jailer[114] and Eguchi[61] in rats, and by Bedoya and Maldonado[21] and Milkovic and Milkovic[155] in humans, the mechanism for responding to stress at the time of birth is not yet operative in the newborn. This suggests that the hypophysioadrenal axis is still immature. In other words, the fetal adrenal is already engaged in secretory activity though falling short of the adult adrenal insofar as efficiency is concerned.

One way or another, the corticoids derived from both the fetus and the placenta may be able to render important assistance to the maternal adrenal cortex, as we shall make clear later.

We shall be concerned with the following pathologic conditions associated with pregnancy: (1) adrenalectomy, (2) Addison's disease, (3) adrenogenital syndrome, (4) Cushing's syndrome, and (5) primary aldosteronism.

ADRENALECTOMY AND PREGNANCY. Angervall[7] showed that bilateral adrenalectomy in pregnant rats resulted in fetal adrenal hyperplasia, without any effect whatsoever on gestation itself. Similar observations had already been recorded in bitches and rabbits several years previously (see Chapter 9). In man, on the other hand, bilateral adrenalectomy has in the meantime become a common form of treating some diseases, principally essential hypertension and Cushing's disease, although such patients require subsequent artificial maintenance on cortisone. Some women so treated have been found to be able to achieve pregnancy, according to case reports by Barber and co-workers,[11] Brownley and associates,[36] Greenblatt and associates,[83] Harkness and colleagues,[94] Litowsky and Ford,[138] Krieger and co-workers,[130] and Snyder and Taggart.[204] Although the early part of gestation in such patients required continued administration of cortisone in amounts ranging from 20 to 30 mg daily, it has been found that cortisone therapy could be dispensed with near term without adverse effects on either mother or fetus.

It is interesting to note that Bergman reported a case[24] in which eclampsia developed in a woman after bilateral adrenalectomy.

This simply means that the absence of adrenal glands, invariably fatal in both animals and man outside pregnancy, produces no adverse effect in gestation, as a result of vicarious functions discharged by the fetal adrenal and by the placenta.

ADDISON'S DISEASE AND PREGNANCY. For obvious reasons, then, it would be only logical to assume that Addison's disease should be well tolerated in gestation. That this was so had been recognized by Marañón and by Fernández-Noguera many years ago and, in fact, confirmed by the recent publications of Baulieu and his associates,[15] Kaiser,[121] Jailer and Knowlton,[115] Osler[166] (who reported five such cases), and Richards[179] (who reported four cases of his own and published an extensive review of the literature).

In the early part of their pregnancies, such women were described as suffering from marked vomiting, showing the clinical picture of severe hyperemesis gravidarum. As gestation progresses, however, the vicarious actions by both the fetal adrenal and the placenta become increasingly apparent and these disturbances are compensated for. Abortion and fetal death are uncommon, although it is true that such women develop a marked tendency toward hypotension and *shock* after delivery.

ADRENOGENITAL SYNDROME AND GESTATION. The role of LH as the specific stimulant of sex hormone synthesis by the adrenal cortex has been explained previously (see Chapters 9 and 33). There are instances on record in which a heretofore latent adrenogenital syndrome had been unleashed by the strong chorionic gonadotropin secretion that occurs as a physiologic phenomenon during the early months of gestation. Such cases, in which the patients develop adrenal virilism as a result of pregnancy, have been described with relative frequency.

By comparison, it is quite rare for a woman with a full-blown adrenogenital syndrome to become pregnant. In Chapter 41, we have already indicated how even minor forms of adrenal virilism may be conducive to anovulatory cycles and infertility. In fact, women with adrenal hirsutism are noted for their poor fertility. Nevertheless, such a case has recently been reported by Southam and his colleagues.[207] Abortion supervened in that instance and was attributed by the authors to a disturbance in steroidogenesis (see Chapter 33) involving also the placenta, as a result of which placental progesterone could not be synthesized.

CUSHING'S SYNDROME AND PREGNANCY. Hunt and MacConahey[109] collected four cases of Cushing's disease associated with gestation. Of a total of seven pregnancies observed in these patients, four terminated in normal deliveries, two in stillbirths and one in abortion, which does not seem to suggest any significant lethal effect on the product of conception in this syndrome. Greenblatt and his colleagues[83] were also struck by the fact that three of their four cases resulted in normal pregnancies. Similar findings were reported by Abrams and his co-workers[2] and Eisenstein and colleagues,[63] whereas MacGregor and his associates[144] reported a single case that had aborted at 10 weeks. Kreines and associates,[129] on the other hand, described premature labor with fetuses revealing adrenal atrophy.

Schteingart[195] observed such complications as osteoporosis, hypertension and an increased incidence of eclampsia.

There are numerous case reports in the literature referring to the occurrence of Cushing's disease during gestation (Abrams et al.,[2] Bank et al.,[10] Benedetti,[23] Decourt et al.,[55] Greenblatt et al.[83]). In all these cases, adrenalectomy had a favorable effect, which is accounted for by subsidiary fetal and placental corticoid synthesis. The symptoms of Cushing's disease were noted to disappear and pregnancy was carried to term.

As a result, it may be inferred that, although the incidence of premature labor and abortion in Cushing's disease complicating pregnancy is slightly higher than that found in normal gestation, the overall fetal loss is not too great. If the data given previously are compared with those presented in Table 45-4, what strikes our attention is the fact that the fetal mortality rate in Cushing's disease is actually lower than that observed in prediabetes. This, it may be added as a final comment, suggests that the diabetogenic action is apparently due to some factors other than either ACTH or increased levels of corticoids.

PRIMARY ALDOSTERONISM AND GESTATION. In the course of the past years, cases of primary aldosteronism complicating gestation have been described by Biglieri and Slaton,[25] Crane and associates,[49] Dal Canton,[50] and Gordon and his co-workers.[79] This condition is aggravated by gestation, resulting in increased edema and hypertension. There is marked hyperkalemia, and gestation usually terminates in abortion, premature labor or fetal stillbirth. However, no genuine examples of eclamptic toxemia have been reported, which once more leads us to emphasize the fact that aldosteronism is of a different nature than gestosis.

45.6. PATHOPHYSIOLOGY OF THE HYPOPHYSIO-ADRENAL SYSTEM IN PREGNANCY; GESTATION AND LABOR AS "STRESSORS"

45.6.1. DEFINITION

What is "stress"? The originator of the concept described it as *the sum total of nonspecific biologic manifestations which are engendered in a living organism in response to aggression of any kind.* The element exerting the injurious effect is called a "stressor," and it may be a microorganism, a toxin, a drug, or any kind of substance or even physical agent. In the particular case with which we are concerned, stressor in pregnancy is gestation itself—that is, the substances that are released by the placenta and reach the maternal blood stream.

What is specific about stress is not the provoking substance or agent *but the man-*

ner in which the attacked organism responds. The basic studies on the subject by Selye[200] have shown that *whatever the kind of attack involved, the response elicited is always the same,* invariably implicating the hypothalamo-hypophysial system (ACTH and adrenal cortex).

In this way, the hypophysio-adrenal axis is always the element that reacts in the face of aggression and is the center of all stress phenomena, as illustrated in Figure 45–12. A substance injected into the body invariably elicits two kinds of reactions: *specific* and *nonspecific*. For instance, if gonadotropin, the substance that we are presently discussing, is injected into an animal, a specific reaction is produced in the gonads, which is well known; because gonadotropin is an extraneous protein, however, a nonspecific reaction is produced at the same time. Because this extraneous protein entering the blood stream of the gravid woman does so in large amounts, this second reaction is of greater immediate interest in the stress phenomena of pregnancy.

45.6.2. ENDOCRINE PHENOMENA IN STRESS

Any attempt to analyze the enormous amount of research that has helped slowly expand our knowledge of the endocrinology of G.A.S. over the past 20 years would, at this point, be an unwarranted digression. We intend to present just a simple sketch, focusing attention on some of the phenomena that have a direct bearing on obstetrical problems.

ADRENAL. Any type of stress condition in animals as well as in man elicits an intense reaction of the adrenal cortex.[199] The reaction is characterized by hyperemia and by a characteristic ascorbic acid depletion.[191] There is also an emptying of cholesterol stored in the gland[194] as well as a loss of sudanophilic lipoids.[191] That these histologic reactions are expressive of active hyperfunction is proved by two things: (1) that they may be induced artificially by means of corticotropin (ACTH) injection, and (2) that they are accompanied by a *parallel increase in urinary corticoid excretion.* The same kind of hyperexcretion has been found to occur in fatigue[5] and in stress situations resulting from extreme heat,[140] burns[141] and surgical or hemorrhagic shock.[194]

HYPOPHYSIS AND HYPOTHALAMUS. Selye[200] had shown a number of years ago that hypophysectomy abolished the adrenal stress reaction. Because similar phenomena may be elicited by the experimental injection of ACTH,[69, 191] the adrenocortical reaction to stress has since been thought to be caused by pituitary stimulation. In modern times, fundamental importance has been attached to the role played by the hypo-

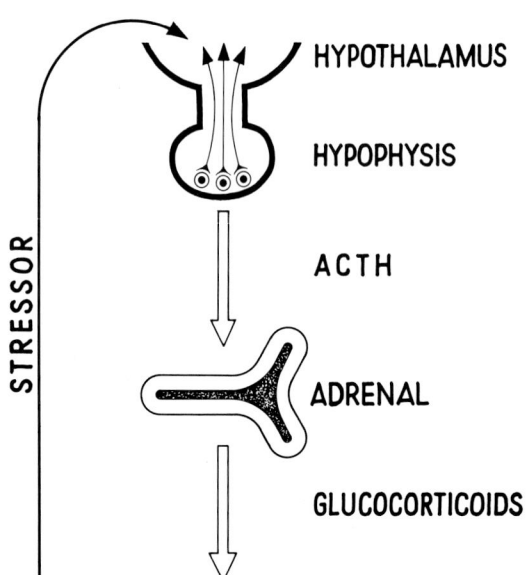

Figure 45–12. The hypophysioadrenal axis in general adaptation syndrome. (From Selye: *Einführung in die Lehre vom Adaptationssyndrom.* Stuttgart, G. Thieme, 1953.)

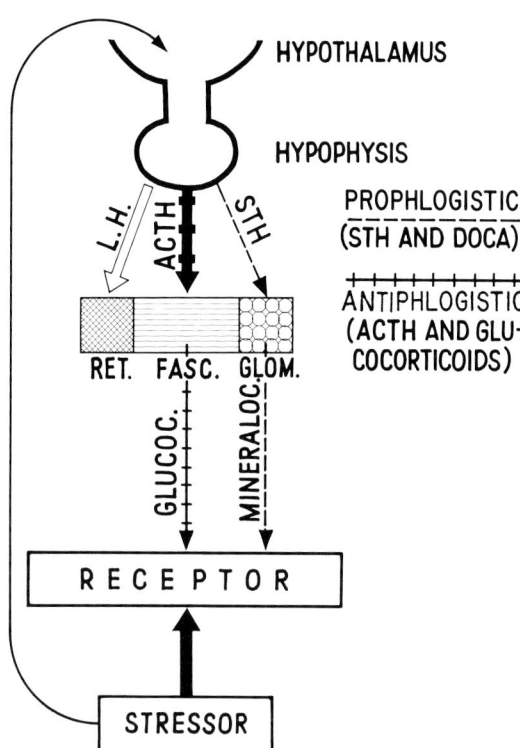

Figure 45-13. Pituitary and adrenal participation in general adaptation syndrome. Growth hormone is currently held to act as a direct stimulant on the zona glomerulosa. (From Selye: *Einführung in die Lehre vom Adaptationssyndrom.* Stuttgart, G. Thieme, 1953.)

thalamus in regulating these phenomena, based on experimental evidence that the stress reaction was missing in animals whose hypothalamus had been destroyed, or in humans in whom this region of the brain had been anesthetized.[132, 140]

MINERALOCORTICOIDS AND SOMATOTROPIN. Until recently, it was classically held that pituitary stimulation in stress was associated with secretion of ACTH only and that, as a result, only glucocorticoids were formed. However, it has been possible to observe that adrenal stimulation in stress also provoked hypersecretion of *mineralocorticoids*.[200] The prophlogistic reaction in stress is precisely the result of the latter, while the antiphlogistic reaction eliminates the glucocorticoids. At the same time, the pituitary produces not only ACTH but also a considerable amount of somatotropin (STH, HGH). Growth hormone also possesses a prophlogistic action similar to that of the mineralocorticoids. Its action does not involve stimulation of the glomerulosa, as one might have assumed, but rather consists of an independent effect of the kind indicated in Figure 45-13. Thus, between ACTH and STH (the two pituitary hormones principally implicated in stress), and the two groups of corticogenous hormones in question (gluco- and mineralocorticoids), a paired antagonism seems to emerge: *on the one hand, ACTH and the glucocorticoids, acting antiphlogistically, and, on the other, STH and mineralocorticoids, acting phlogistically* (Fig. 45-13).

EFFECTS OF GLUCO- AND MINERALOCORTICOIDS. The most specific effect of this group of hormones is due to the action of the glucocorticoids, producing the characteristic *lymphopenia* and *eosinopenia*, which constitute the basis for the clinical diagnosis of stress conditions.[178, 219] In contrast, the mineralocorticoids exert a series of actions that may be summed up as follows: (1) sodium retention by the tissues; (2) increased renal production of vasopressor substances and hypertension; and (3) action leading to increased collagen deposition and to arthritis.

Probably, as a result of a direct action on the same tissues and organs, STH collaborates with the mineralocorticoids and thus enhances these effects. On the other hand, aside from their characteristic eosinopenic effect in the G.A.S., the glucocorticoids *elicit the opposite effects* in that they favor sodium elimination, reduce the rate of renin production, exert their well known antirheumatic action and decrease the amount of collagen in the tissues. These interactions have been diagrammed in Figure 45–14, in which the opposing effects of the prophlogistic and antiphlogistic systems are shown in detail.

45.6.3. THE HYPOPHYSIO-ADRENAL SYSTEM IN PREGNANCY

We have already described the hypophysio-adrenal axis in pregnancy from both physiologic and pathologic standpoints, making any repetition here redundant. For a synopsis of our present ideas, the reader is referred to Figure 45–15, illustrating how the maternal and fetal adrenals, stimulated simultaneously by the pituitary and the placenta, are both active, and how the placenta secretes glucocorticoids that add to the action of those produced by the

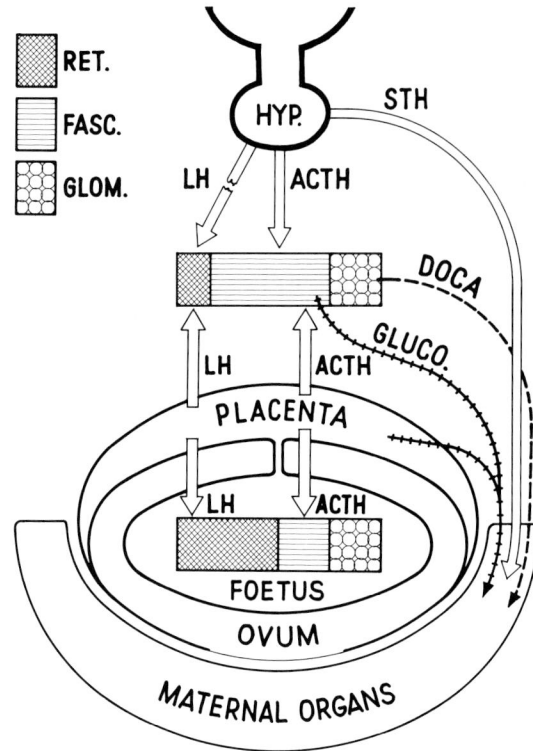

Figure 45–15. Schematic representation of corticoid secretion in the placenta, fetal adrenal and maternal adrenal during pregnancy.

zona fasciculata of both mother and fetus. The diagram also shows how LH exerts a moderate stimulatory effect on the mother's zona reticularis and a more powerful effect on the reticularis of the fetus.

45.6.4. PREGNANCY AS A "STRESSOR"

After what has just been said, it seems unquestionable that the hypophysioadrenal system functions during gestation very much as it does in the G.A.S. The concrete arguments described below may be invoked to substantiate the existence of a stress condition in pregnancy.

CLINICAL SIGNS. Rheumatoid arthritis improves during gestation.[182] Addisonism in pregnant women near term similarly changes for the better.[15, 115, 179]

GRAVIDIC EOSINOPENIA. The G.A.S. is always associated with eosinopenia. During pregnancy, a reduction in the number of circulating eosinophils takes place to approximately 50 per cent of normal

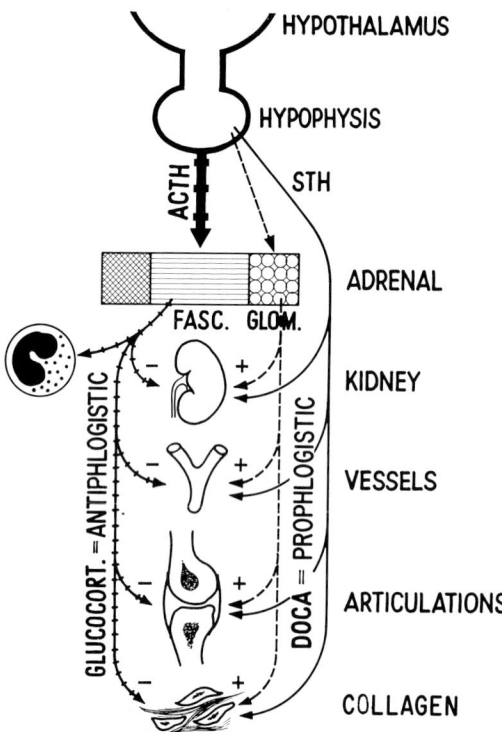

Figure 45–14. Prophlogistic and antiphlogistic actions by the hypophysioadrenal axis in general adaptation syndrome. HGH acts additionally on the zona glomerulosa. (From Selye: *Einführung in die Lehre vom Adaptationssyndrom.* Stuttgart, G. Thieme, 1953.)

Endocrine Pathology of Gestation

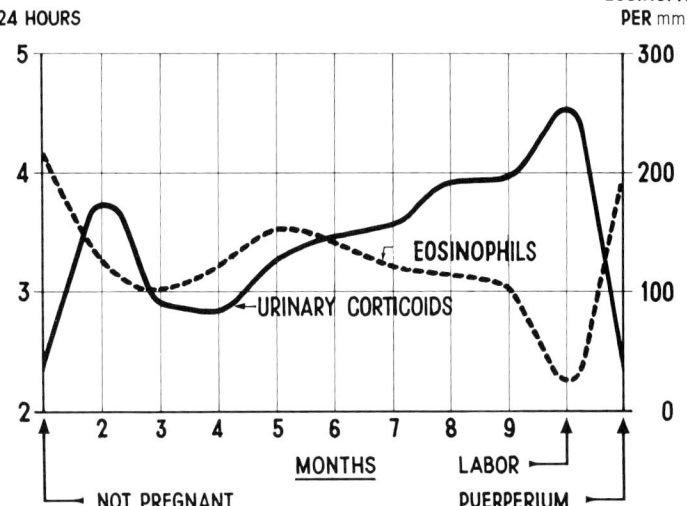

Figure 45-16. 11-Oxysteroid excretion in pregnancy, labor and postpartum, from data of Rodríguez-López at our clinic. For comparative purposes, eosinophil counts for each month have also been plotted.

values.[53, 54, 93, 196] The results obtained on our own clinical material[72] are presented in Figure 45–16.

CORTICOID EXCRETION IN THE COURSE OF GESTATION. The question of gluco- and mineralocorticoid excretion throughout pregnancy has been examined in Chapters 20 and 43. It will therefore not be necessary to elaborate further on the significance of increased excretion of this type of compound during gestation. Figure 45–16 reproduces 11-oxysteroid values encountered in the urine of pregnant women, compared with concomitant eosinophil counts. The two curves are *inversely proportional*, which seems to prove that there is a correlation between increased urinary corticoid excretion and eosinopenia.

ASCORBIC ACID DEPLETION IN THE ADRENAL. It has been possible to demonstrate that ascorbic acid disappeared from the adrenals of pregnant rats.[42, 74] On the basis of indirect evidence, we feel justified in assuming that the human adrenal behaves in a similar way.[28]

THE THORN TEST IN PREGNANCY. Of all arguments so far advanced, the most important one is the Thorn test. This test was employed at our clinic as far back as 1952 by del Sol and Merlo.[205] Subsequent studies that yielded similar results were published by a number of investigators.[21, 51, 154] The results obtained with the Thorn test in pregnancy and labor at our clinic are shown in Figures 45–17 and 45–18. Figure 45–17 reveals a large number of negative test results for the second month of gestation, reflecting the reaction of alarm which appears in the early phase of gestation. A large number of tests become again negative near term and during labor (including hypophysio-adrenal insufficiency). In contrast, there is a relatively high proportion of positive tests around midterm, indicating on the average a fairly satisfactory level of function in the middle of gestation.

In summarizing these data, the following statement appears to be justified: the pregnancy "stress" situation manifests itself by constant hyperfunction of the adrenal cortex although, in 50 per cent of the cases, this hyperfunction falls short of existing demands, so that almost half of all normal gestations may be said to be associated with relative adrenal insufficiency.

45.6.5. EVOLUTION OF THE CONDITION OF STRESS IN THE COURSE OF PREGNANCY

As pointed out previously, gestation may be viewed as an instance of the G.A.S. A *stressor*, whose specific nature will be elaborated later, elicits a reaction in the hypophysio-adrenal system, proceeding in the direction indicated in Figure 45–13. Based on the chronologic examination of the various adrenal function tests we have indicated for the entire course of gestation (Fig. 45–19), *three distinct periods* may be recognized within the G.A.S. occurring in

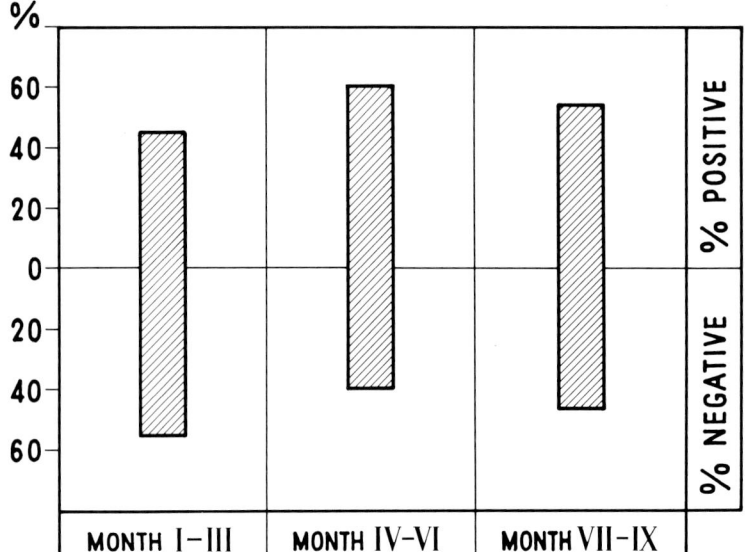

Figure 45-17. The Thorn test in normal pregnancy.

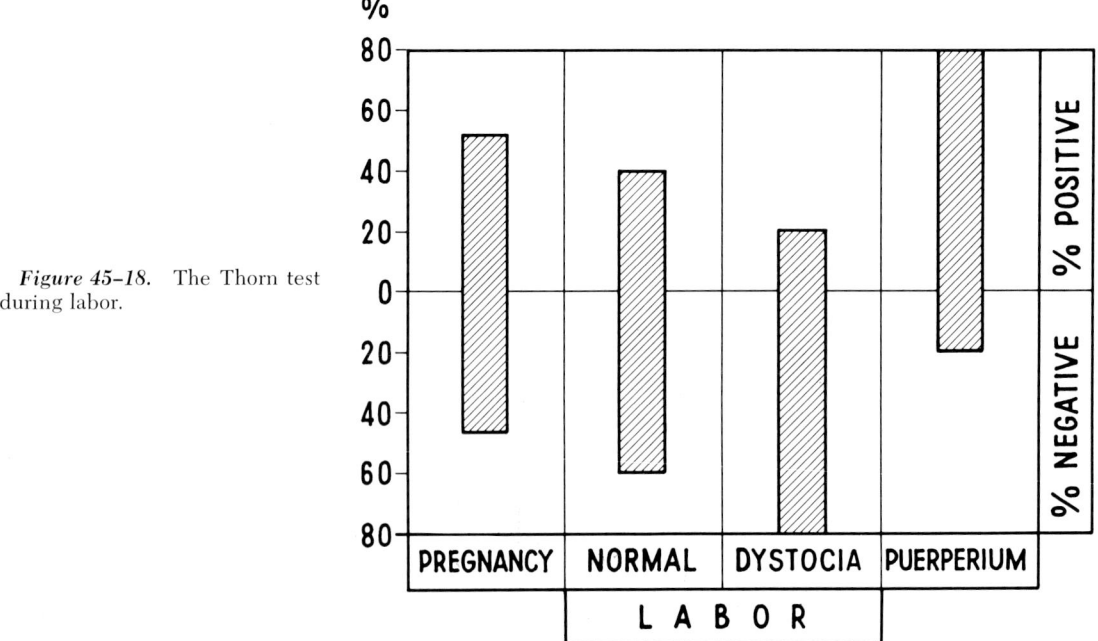

Figure 45-18. The Thorn test during labor.

Endocrine Pathology of Gestation

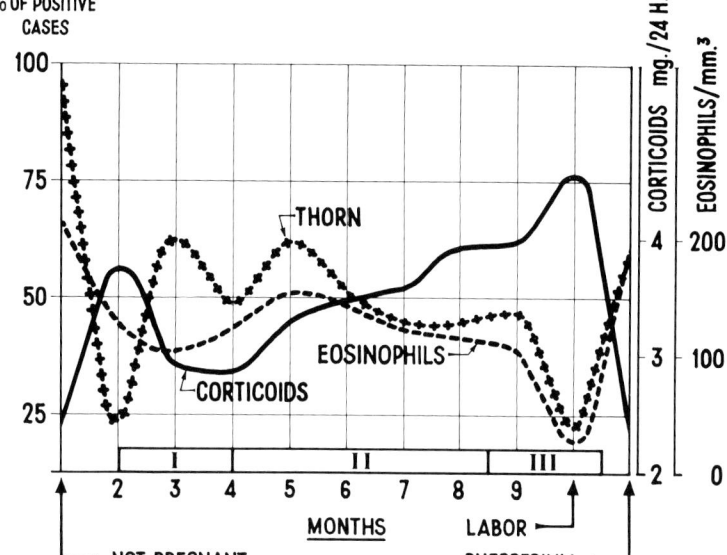

Figure 45-19. Same graph as in Figure 45-16, to which results of Thorn test have been added.

pregnancy. The first period is characterized by an abrupt rise in corticoid levels, reaching a peak by the second month, and by the greatest number of cases revealing negative eosinopenia. Between the third and seventh months, corticoid excretion falls, and the number of cases revealing positive adrenalinic eosinopenia reaches almost 60 per cent. Finally, during the eighth and ninth months, the number of failures increases again significantly, and at the same time corticoid excretion reaches a peak. It would therefore appear that there are two periods in pregnancy that are both characterized by maximal failure in the adrenal's capacity to respond, at both extremes of an intermediate period of compensation. These three periods roughly correspond to the three classically described phases of pregnancy: (1) period of intolerance; (2) period of adaptation, and (3) period of overload. We may thus establish the paradigm shown in Table 45-7.

It is quite obvious that *we have had instances of G.A.S. under our noses for a good number of years without seeing them.* There may actually be few other conditions in which the characteristic features of the adaptation diseases are manifested more clearly than in pregnancy. In fact, it may be asserted that those authors who at the turn of the century were laying the groundwork of gravidic pathophysiology had actually described stress long before this condition became known as an entity.

What, then, are the stressor agents of pregnancy? We believe that these are, first of all, the extraneous proteins released from the placental area and, quite specifically, the chorionic gonadotropins which, when released by the chorionic epithelium, penetrate directly into the maternal circulation. Their effects are twofold: specific (gonadotropin activity as such) and nonspecific (extraneous protein effect). Nevertheless, there is no doubt that the primary stressor effect of pregnancy is enhanced by secondary effects, such as the effect of fetal catabolites, the physical effect of gestation itself on the different thoracic and abdominal organs, etc.

45.6.6. LABOR AS A STRESSOR

The role of labor as a stressor has recently been studied by many authors.[16, 28, 56, 64] Particularly outstanding in this respect have been the works of the Spanish school (Merlo and del Sol,[154] Bedoya and Maldonado,[21] Botella[28]). Those studies concur in revealing the *presence of a state of stress that is more accentuated during labor than at any other time in pregnancy.* The incidence of Thorn test negativity has been found to be maximal in labor (Figs. 45-19 and 45-20), while eosinopenia and corticoid excretion also reach critical values at the same time (Fig. 45-16). Upon closely ex-

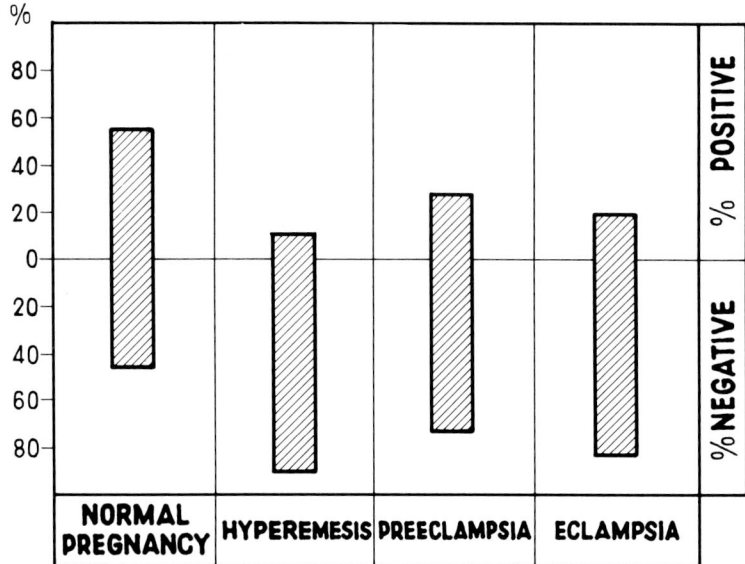

Figure 45-20. The Thorn test in toxemias.

amining these three graphs, particularly Figure 45-16, we may note that the Thorn test is negative in 80 per cent of cases with dystocia. *During labor—above all, pathologic labor—the stressor effect of pregnancy reaches its culmination.*

A highly significant aspect of stress during labor is the fetal response to stressor stimuli. We have already indicated that until embryonal development is well advanced the fetus does not have a fully developed zona fasciculata in its adrenal (neocortex) and therefore it is in no position to respond via a G.A.S. An injection of epinephrine, it has been shown, fails to elicit ascorbic acid depletion in the adrenals of fetal rats.[114] It has also been shown that, while the fetal zona fasciculata at the time of birth appears to be well developed, the fetus almost invariably fails to respond to the Thorn test. For this reason, the mother is subject to the stressor effect of labor, whereas the fetus is not. The fetus might be said to be *hibernating*, unconcerned with any injurious environmental elements, because of lack of maturity of its hypophysio-adrenal axis. *Stress is a phenomenon of all organisms endowed with relational life.* For this reason, the nature of *distress* during labor is experienced in essentially a different way by the mother than by the fetus. The latter suffers from anoxia, but is indifferent to stress. In contrast, sensitive to stress as she is, the mother is highly resistant to anoxia. This fact is well worth taking into account in clinical practice.

45.6.7. STRESS AND GRAVIDIC TOXEMIAS

Although this subject has been broached in Chapter 45, at least a brief mention of adaptation phenomena in toxemia should be given here. Selye considered toxemia of pregnancy an adaptation disease, for which he had developed an extensive theory. A number of investigators have viewed the toxemias as caused by adrenocortical failure. A graphical synopsis of the results obtained at our clinic with the Thorn test in toxemias compared with normal gesta-

TABLE 45-7.

MONTH OF GESTATION	PERIOD OF PREGNANCY	PHASE IN G.A.S.
Months 1 to 3	Period of intolerance	Reaction of alarm
Months 4 to 7	Period of adaptation	Stage of resistance
Months 8 and 9	Period of overload	Stage of exhaustion

tion is given in Figure 45–20. The presence of negative adrenalinic eosinopenia was an almost constant finding in toxemias of pregnancy.

From what we have said, it follows that pregnancy constitutes a stressor agent to the female organism. In the center of the endocrine correlations of the mother, hypophysio-adrenal hyperfunction emerges as the focal endocrine phenomenon involved in stress. The three phases of the G.A.S. are all reproduced in pregnancy, which near term may give rise to a phase of exhaustion leading to two frankly pathologic situations:

A. Phase of exhaustion determined by a conflict between the demands imposed on the mother's organism and her capacity for adaptation to stress, which results in a late-onset type of toxemia of pregnancy.

B. Phase of exhaustion determined by the additional surcharge that difficult labor imposes on the state of stress inherent in every gestation, which results in obstetrical shock.

REFERENCES

1. Aboul-Khari, S. A., Turnbull, A. C., and Hytten, F. E.: *Lancet*, 2:334, 1964.
2. Abrams, J., Dresdale, F. C., and Bartels, E. C.: *J. Med. Soc. New Jersey*, 60:474, 1963.
3. Adam, P. A. J., et al.: *Diabetes*, 18:409, 1969.
4. Aguilo, F., Vega, L. A., Haddock, L., and Rodriguez, O.: *Acta Endocr.*, Suppl. 60, 137:7, 1969.
5. Allen, E.: *Amer. J. Obstet. Gynec.*, 38:982, 1939.
6. Anderson, M. S., Erickson, L. S., and Luse, J. H.: *Neurology*, 12:583, 1962.
7. Angervall, L.: *Acta Endocr.*, Suppl. 30:44, 1959.
8. Angervall, L.: *Acta Endocr.*, 41:456, 1962.
9. Assali, N. S., and Hammermesz, J.: *Endocrinology*, 55:561, 1954.
10. Bank, H., Beer, R., Lunenfeld, B., Rabau, E., and Rumney, G.: *J. Clin. Endocr. Metab.*, 25:359, 1965.
11. Barber, H. R. K., Graber, E. A., and O'Rourke, J. J.: *Obstet. Gynec.*, 27:414, 1966.
12. Barns, H. H. F., and Swyer, G. I. M.: *Brit. Med. J.*, 2:914, 1952.
13. Bassett, J. M., and Wallace, A. L. C.: *Diabetes*, 16:566, 1967.
14. Bastenie, P. A., and Gordon, C.: *Ann. d'Endocr.*, 15:54, 1954.
15. Baulieu, E. E., Devigan, M., Bricaire, H., and Jayle, M. F.: *J. Clin. Endocr.*, 17:1478, 1957.
16. Bech, J. C., MacGarry, E. E., Dyrenfurth, I., and Venning, E. H.: *Metabolism*, 9:699, 1960.
17. Beck, P. B., Parker, M. L., and Daughaday, W. H.: *J. Clin. Endocr. Metab.*, 25:1475, 1965.
18. Beck, P.: *Diabetes*, 18:46, 1969.
19. Beck, P.: *Endocrinology*, 87:288, 1970.
20. Becker, K. L., Winnacker, J. L., Matthews, M. J., and Higgins, G. A.: *J. Clin. Endocr. Metab.*, 28:277, 1968.
21. Bedoya, J. M., and Maldonado, A.: *Acta Gin.*, 6:19, 291, 1955.
22. Beernink, F. J., and MacKay, D. G.: *Amer. J. Obstet. Gynec.*, 84:318, 1962.
23. Benedetti, A.: *Minerva Medica*, 56:459, 1965.
24. Bergman, P., Ekman, H., Hakansson, B., and Sjögren, B.: *Acta Endocr.*, 35:293, 1960.
25. Biglieri, E. G., and Slaton, P. E.: *J. Clin. Endocr. Metab.*, 27:1628, 1967.
26. Birke, G., Gemzell, C. A., Plantin, L. O., and Robbe, H.: *Acta Endocr.*, 27:389, 1958.
27. Bloch, E., et al.: *Endocrinology*, 71:628, 1962.
28. Botella, J.: *Sinopsis Obst. Gin. (Buenos Aires)*, 4:453, 1957.
29. Botella, J.: *Arch. Fac. Med., Madrid*, 1:119, 1962.
30. Botella, J.: *Obstetrical Endocrinology*. Springfield, Ill., Charles C Thomas, 1961.
31. Botella, J., Pereira, A., and Isla, J. R. de: *Internat. J. Gyn. Obst.*, 7:56, 1969.
32. Boughton, C., and Perkins, E.: *J. Obstet. Gynec. Brit. Emp.*, 64:105, 1957.
33. Brasseur, L., et al.: *Ann d'Endocr.*, 19:431, 1958.
34. Bret, A. J., and Coiffard, P.: *Rev. Franç. Gynec.*, 58:19, 1963.
35. Bromberg, Y. M., Sadowsky, A., and Sulman, F. J.: *J.A.M.A.*, 154:165, 1954.
36. Brownley, H. C., Warren, J. E., and Parson, W.: *Amer. J. Obstet. Gynec.*, 80:628, 1960.
37. Buchanan, K. D., and MacKiddie, M. T.: *J. Endocr.*, 39:13, 1967.
38. Burt, R. L., Leake, N. H., and Rhyne, A. L.: *Obstet. Gynec.*, 36:233, 1970.
39. Carpent, G., and Desclin, L.: *Ann. d'Endocr.*, 28:245, 1967.
40. Carrington, E. R., and Messick, R. R.: *Amer. J. Obstet. Gynec.*, 85:669, 1963.
41. Carrington, E. R., and MacWilliams, N. B.: *Amer. J. Obstet. Gynec.*, 96:922, 1966.
42. Cassano, F,, and Tarantino, C.: *Folia Endocr.*, 6:319, 1953.
43. Charles, D., et al.: *Amer. J. Obstet. Gynec.*, 106:66, 1970.
44. Clayton, S. G.: *J. Obstet. Gynec. Brit. Emp.*, 63:532, 1956.
45. Colwell, J. A., and Klein, A.: *Diabetes*, 16:560, 1967.
46. Conn, J. W.: *Ciba Colloquia on Endocrinology*, 6:166, 1953.
47. Contopoulos, A. N., and Simpson, M. E.: *Endocrinology*, 61:765, 1957.
48. Courrier, R.: *Ann. d'Endocr.*, 15:1, 1954.
49. Crane, M. G., et al.: *Obstet. Gynec.*, 23:200, 1964.
50. DalCanton, G.: *Riv. Ital. Ost. Gin. Prat.*, 49:287, 1967.
51. Damiani, N.: *Bol. Soc. Ital. Biol. Sper.*, 28:813, 1952.
52. David, M., Dikstein, S., and Sulman, F. G.: *Proc. Soc. Exp. Biol. Med.*, 121:873, 1966.
53. Davis, M. E., and Plotz, E. J.: *Obstet. Gynec. Survey*, 11:1, 1956.
54. Dawson, D. W.: *J. Obstet. Gynec. Brit. Emp.*, 60:727, 1953.
55. Decourt, J., Kobel, P., and Michard, J. P.: *Ann d'Endocr.*, 22:218, 1961.
56. Diczfalusy, E., and Troen, P.: *Vitamins Hormones*, 19:229, 1961.

57. Dokumov, S. I.: *Acta Endocr.*, 38:161, 1961.
58. Dowling, J. T., Ingbar, S. H., and Freinkel, N.: *J. Clin. Endocr.*, 20:1, 1960.
59. Dowling, J. T., et al.: *J. Clin. Endocr.*, 21:779, 1961.
60. Dumont, M., and Etienne-Martin, M.: *Rev. Franç. Gynec.*, 58:721, 1962.
61. Eguchi, Y.: *Endocrinology*, 61:716, 1961; 71:31, 1962.
62. Ehrlich, R. M., and Randle, P. J.: *Lancet*, 2:230, 1961.
63. Eisenstein, A. B., Karsh, R., and Gall, I.: *J. Clin. Endocr.*, 23:971, 1963.
64. Elert, R.: *Arch. Gynäk.*, 186:227, 1955.
65. Elsas, L. J., Whitemore, R., and Burrow, G. N.: *J.A.M.A.*, 200:257, 1967.
66. Engstrom, W. W.: *J. Clin. Endocr.*, 21:1007, 1961.
67. Engleson, G., and Lindberg, T.: *Acta Obstet. Gynec. Scand.*, 41:321, 1962.
68. Fioretti, P., and Carretti, N.: *Riv. Ital. Gin.*, 50:170, 1966.
69. Firschen, H., De Venuto, F., Fitch, W. M., and Westphal, U.: *Endocrinology*, 60:347, 1957.
70. Fischer, U., and Horky, Z.: *Zbl. Gynäk.*, 88:1427, 1966.
71. Frandsen, V. A., and Stakeman, L.: *Acta Endocr.*, 38:383, 1961.
72. Frantz, A. G., Katz, F. H., and Jailer, J. W.: *Proc. Soc. Exp. Biol. Med.*, 105:41, 1960.
73. Fritsch, W., and Knappe, G.: *Zbl. Gynäk.*, 90:302, 1968.
74. Gemzell, C. A.: *J. Clin. Endocr.*, 13:898, 1953.
75. Gemzell, C. A.: In *Probleme der Fetalen Endokrinologie*. ed. H. Novakowsky. Berlin, Springer Verlag, 1956.
76. Gitlin, D.. Kumate, J., and Morales, C.: *J. Clin. Endocr. Metab.*, 25:1599, 1965.
77. Gitsch, E., Auinger, W., and Helfenbein, E.: *Zbl. Gynäk.*, 89:593, 1967.
78. Goodner, C. J., and Freinkel, N.: *J. Clin. Invest.*, 39:116, 1960.
79. Gordon, R. D., Fishman, L. M., and Liddle, G. W.: *J. Clin. Endocr. Metab.*, 27:385, 1967.
80. Goth, A., Lengyel, L., and Savel, C.: *Ztsch. Vit. Horm. Forsch.*, 7:253, 1955.
81. Grant, D. K.: *Quart. J. Med.*, 22:243, 1953.
82. Gray, C. H. H.: *Ann. d'Endocr.*, 15:22, 1954.
83. Greenblatt, R. B., Scarpa-Smiths, C., and Metts, J. C.: *Fertil. Steril.*, 10:323, 1959.
84. Greene, J. W., and Touchstone, J. C.: *Amer. J. Obstet. Gynec.*, 85:1, 1963.
85. Greer, M. A.: *Endocrinology*, 45:178, 1949.
86. Groseclose, E. S.: *Obstet. Gynec.*, 21:378, 1963.
87. Guillemin, J.: *Sem. Hôp. Paris*, 36:3111, 1960.
88. Guinet, P.: *Ann. d'Endocr.*, 22:385, 1961.
89. Hadden, D. R., and Harley, O. M. G.: *J. Obstet. Gynec. Brit. Comm.*, 74:669, 1967.
90. Hagbard, L.: *Acta Obstet, Gynec. Scand.*, Suppl. 35:1, 1956.
91. Hagerman, D. D.: *Endocrinology*, 70:88, 1962.
92. Hain, A. M.: *Ciba Colloquia on Endocrinology*, 2:196, 1952.
93. Hallberg, I. F., and Kaiser, I. H.: *Acta Endocr.*, 16:227, 1954.
94. Harness, R. A., Menini, E., Charles, D., Kenny, F. M., and Rombaut, R.: *Acta Endocr.*, 52:409, 1966.
95. Hawker, R. W., North, W. G., Colbert, I. C., and Lang, L. P.: *J. Obstet. Gyn. Brit. Comm.*, 74:430, 1967.
96. Hellerstrom, C.: *Excerpta Medica*, Section III, 18:363, 1964.
97. Hendee, A. E., Martin, R. D., and Waters, W. C.: *Amer. J. Obstet. Gynec.*, 105:64 11969.
98. Henneman, D. A., and Henneman, P. H.: *J. Clin. Invest.*, 39:1239, 1960.
99. Herlant, M., Laine, E., Fosatti, P., and Linquette, M.: *Ann. d'Endocr.*, 26:65, 1965.
100. Herlant, M., Linquette, M., Laine, E., Fosatti, P. May, J. P., and Lefebvre, J.: *Ann. d'Endocr.*, 27:181, 1966.
101. Hirschowitz, S., and Berge, J.: *South. Afr. J. Obstet. Gynec.*, 4:5, 1966.
102. Hobkirk, R., and Nilsen, M.: *J. Clin. Endocr.*, 22:142, 1962.
103. Hoët, J. P.: *Ciba Colloquia on Endocrinology*, 6:330, 1953.
104. Hoët, J. P., and Brasseur, L.: *Ann. d'Endocr.*, 15:26, 1954.
105. Hoët, J. P., et al.: *Helv. Med. Acta*, 27:178, 1960.
106. Hoët, J. P., Hoët, J. J., Gommers, A., and Tremouroux, M.: *Rev. Franç. Gynec.*, 57:233, 1962.
107. Horky, Z., and Jutzi, E.: *Zbl. Gynäk.*, 87:176, 1964.
108. Horky, Z.: *Zbl. Gynäk.*, 87:1555, 1965.
109. Hunt, A. B., and MacConahey, W. M.: *Amer. J. Obstet. Gynec.*, 66:910, 1953.
110. Hutchinson, D. L., Westover, J. L., and Will, D. W.: *Amer. J. Obstet. Gynec.*, 83:857, 1962.
111. Hüter, K. A., and Blank, H.: *Geburtsh. u. Frauenhk.*, 22:612, 1962.
112. Ino, S., and Greer, M. A.: *Endocrinology*, 68:253, 1961.
113. Jackson, W. P. V.: *Lancet*, 2:1369, 1961.
114. Jailer, J. W.: *Endocrinology*, 46:420, 1950.
115. Jailer, J. W., and Knowlton, A. J.: *J. Clin. Invest.*, 29:1430, 1950.
116. Jaszmann, L.: *J. Obstet. Gynec. Brit. Comm.*, 70:120, 1963.
117. Johnson, D. C., Foltz, F. M., and Nelson, D. M.: *J. Clin. Endocr. Metab.*, 26:915, 1966.
118. Jones, W. S.: *Amer. J. Obstet. Gynec.*, 71:318, 1956.
118a. Jorgensen, K. R., Deckert, T., Molsted-Pedersen, L., and Pedersen, J.: *Acta Endocr.*, 52:154, 1966.
119. Josimovitch, J. B.: *Endocrinology*, 78:707, 1966.
120. Jost, A., Pic, P., Maniey, J., and Legrand, C.: *Acta Endocr.*, 43:618, 1963.
121. Kaiser, I. H.: *J. Clin. Endocr.*, 16:1251, 1956.
122. Kalkhoff, R. K., Richardson, B. L., and Beck, P.: *Diabetes*, 18:153, 1969.
123. Kalkhoff, R. K., Jacobson, M., and Klemper, D.: *J. Clin. Endocr.*, 30:24, 1970.
124. Kaplan, N. M.: *J. Clin. Endocr.*, 21:1139, 1961.
125. Kaplan, S. L., and Grumbach, M. M.: *J. Clin. Endocr.*, 25:1370, 1965.
126. Kerr, G. R.: *J. Endocr.*, 24:137, 1962.
127. Kim, J. N., Runge, W., Wells, L. J., and Lazarow, A.: *Diabetes*, 9:396, 1960.
128. Kinch, R. A. H., Plunkett, E. R., and Devlin, M. C.: *Amer. J. Obstet. Gynec.*, 105:766, 1969.
129. Kreines, K., Perin, E., and Salzer, R.: *J. Clin. Endocr.*, 24:75, 1964.

130. Krieger, D., Gabrilove, J. L., and Soffer, L. J.: *J. Clin. Endocr.*, 20:1493, 1960.
131. Langer, M., and Grudi, D.: *Folia Endocr.*, 14:705, 1961.
132. Laquer, G. L., et al.: *Endocrinology*, 57:44, 1955.
133. Laron, Z., Mannheimer, S., and Guttmann, S.: *Experientia*, 22:831, 1966.
134. Lavric, M. V.: *Amer. J. Obstet. Gynec.*, 104:818, 1969.
135. Linquette, M., et al.: *Ann. d'Endocr.*, 22:817, 1961.
136. Linquette, M., Dupont-Lecompte, J., and Gasnault, J. T.: *Lille Med.*, 13:873, 1968.
137. Little, B., et al.: *J. Clin. Endocr.*, 18:425, 1958.
138. Litowsky, D., and Ford, R. V.: *Amer. J. Obstet. Gynec.*, 88:756, 1962.
139. Lohmeyer, H.: *Geburtsh. u. Frauenhk.*, 21:560, 1961.
140. Long, C. N. H.: *Ann. Rev. Physiol.*, 18:409, 1956.
141. Love, E. J., Rinch, R. A. H., and Stevenson, J. A. F.: *Amer. J. Obstet. Gynec.*, 80:356, 1960.
142. Love, T. A., Sussman, K. E., and Timmer, R. F.: *Metabolism*, 14:632, 1965.
143. Luft, H.: *Zbl. Gynäk.*, 90:1501, 1968.
144. MacGregor, W. G., Spencer, A. G., and Swiger, G.: *J. Obstet. Gynec. Brit. Emp.*, 67:465, 1960.
145. Maimone, G.: *Riv. Ost. Gin. Prat.*, 49:50, 1967.
146. Malek, J., Horak, J., and Stastny, J.: *Gynaecologia*, 141:31, 1956.
147. Malherbe, C., De Gasparo, M., Van Der Hijst, M., and Hoët, J. J.: *Ann. d'Endocr.*, 30:404, 1969.
148. Man, E. B., Reid, W. A., and Jones, W. S.: *Amer. J. Obstet. Gynec.*, 102:244, 1968.
149. Marañón, G., and Martínez-Díaz, J.: *Bol. Inst. Patol. Med.*, 12:33, 1957.
150. Martin, J. M., and Friessen, H.: *Endocrinology*, 84:619, 1969.
151. Merimee, T. H., Burgess, J. A., and Rabinovitsch, D.: *Diabetes*, 16:478, 1967.
152. Meyer, R. de, and Isaac-Marty, M.: *Ann. d'Endocr.*, 19:167, 1958.
153. Meyer, R. de; *Etude experimentale de la glycorregulation gravidique et de l'action teratogene des perturbations du metabolisme glycidique.* Arscia S.A., Bruxelles. Paris, Masson et Cie., 1961.
154. Merlo, J. G., and Del Sol, J. R.: *Acta Gin.*, 6:339, 389, 1955.
155. Milkovic, K., and Milkovic, S.: *Endocrinology*, 73:535, 1963.
156. Mintz, D. H., Finster, J. L., and Taylor, A. L.: *Metabolism*, 17:54, 1968.
157. Mintz, D. H., Chez, R. A., and Horger, E. O.: *J. Clin. Invest.*, 48:176, 1969.
158. Mirsky, I. A., Stein, M., and Paulisch, G.: *Endocrinology*, 55:28, 1954.
159. Mohnike, G., and Worm, M.: *Klin. Wschr.*, 32:64, 1954.
160. Moscona, M. H., and Karnoksky, D. A.: *Endocrinology*, 66:533, 1960.
161. Mucci, A., Bertaglia, A., Albertazzi, E., and Zandomeneghi, R.: *Metabolismo*, 4:45, 1968.
162. Nataf, B. M., and Chaikoff, L.: *Endocrinology*, 73:518, 1963.
163. Nixon, W. C. W.: *Ann. d'Endocr.*, 15:20, 1954.
164. Oakley, E.: *Proc. Roy. Soc. Med.*, 54:744, 1961.
165. Opsahl, J. C., and Long, C. N. H.: *Yale J. Biol. Med.*, 24:199, 1951.
166. Osler, M.: *Acta Endocr.*, 41:67, 1962.
167. Parache, J., Del Olmo, J., Alberto, J. C., Cherp, J., and Botella, J.: *Acta Gin.*, 21:569, 1970.
168. Pedersen, J.: *Acta Endocr.*, 50:95, 1965.
169. Peel, Sir J.: *Amer. J. Obstet. Gynec.*, 83:847, 1962.
170. Picard, C.: *Bull. Fed. Soc. Obstet. Gynec. Lang. Fr.*, 29:447, 1968.
171. Pirart, J.: *Ann. d'Endocr.*, 16:192, 1955.
172. Polishuk, W. Z., Palt, Z., Rabau, E., Lunenfeld, B., and David, A.: *J. Obstet. Gynec. Brit. Comm.*, 72:778, 1965.
173. Powell, E. D. U., Caulfield, J. B., and Field, J. A.: *Diabetes*, 16:227, 1967.
174. Pulle, C., and Rigano, A.: *Minerva Medica*, 7:290, 1965.
175. Putelat, P., et al.: *Ann. d'Endocr.*, 22:189, 1961.
176. Rankin, J. B., Goldfarb, A. F., and Rakoff, A. E.: *Obstet. Gynec.*, 33:1, 1969.
177. Ratsimamanga, A., et al.: *Compt. Rend. Soc. Biol. (Paris)*, 156:820, 1962.
178. Recant, L., Hume, M. D., Forsham, P. H., and Thorn, G. W.: *J. Clin. Endocr.*, 10:187, 1950.
179. Richards, A.: *Brit. Med. J.*, 1:421, 1952.
180. Rivlin, M. I., Mestman, J. H., Hall, T. H., Weaver, C. P., and Anderson, G. V.: *Amer. J. Obstet. Gynec.*, 106:875, 1970.
181. Robertson, H. A., and Falconer, I. R.: *J. Endocr.*, 28:133, 1961.
182. Robinson, H. J., et al.: *J. Clin. Endocr.*, 15:317, 1955.
183. Rodríguez-López, A.: *Acta Gin.*, 6:417, 1955.
184. Rosselin, G., Tchoubrowsky, G., Hassan, R., Dolais, J., and Derot, M.: *Ann. d'Endocr.*, 27:751, 1966.
185. Roy, E. J., and Kerr, M. G.: *J. Obstet. Gynec. Brit. Comm.*, 71:107, 1964.
186. Russell, K. D., Tanaka, S., and Starr, P.: *Amer. J. Obstet. Gynec.*, 79:719, 1960.
187. Saaman, N., Yen, S. C. S., Gonzalez, D., and Pearson, O. H.: *J. Clin. Endocr.*, 28:485, 1968.
188. Salhanick, H., Jones, J. E., and Berliner, D.: *Fed. Proceed.*, 1:160, 1956.
189. Salmon, W. D., and Daughaday, W. A.: *J. Lab. Clin. Med.*, 51:167, 1958.
190. Saxena, B. N., Refetoff, F., Emerson, K., and Selenkov, H. K.: *Amer. J. Obstet. Gynec.*, 101:874, 1968.
191. Sayers, G., and Sayers, M. A.: *Ann. N.Y. Acad. Sci.*, 50:522, 1949.
192. Scaglione, V.: *Ann. Ost. Gin.*, 89:248, 1967.
193. Schalch, D. S., and Riechlin, S.: *Endocrinology*, 79:275, 1966.
194. Scheenberg, N. G., Perloff, W. H., Wiellard, C. B., and Israel, G. M.: *Obstet. Gynec.*, 1:156, 1963.
195. Schteingart, P. E.: *Clin. Obstet. Gynec.*, 10:96, 1967.
196. Schoen, I., and Schnall, D.: *Surg. Gyn. Obst.*, 98:161, 1954.
197. Schwers, J., and Fanard, A.: In *Le placenta humain*, ed. J. Snoeck. Paris, Masson et Cie., 1958.
198. Sciarra, J. J.: *Clin. Obstet. Gynec.*, 10:132, 1967.
199. Selye, H.: *Stress*, Vol. I. Barcelona, Editorial Científico-Médica, 1954.
200. Selye, H.: *Einführung in die Lehre vom Adaptationssyndrom.* Stuttgart, G. Thieme, 1953.
201. Sheehan, H. L., and Stanfield, J. P.: *Acta Endocr.*, 37:479, 1961.

202. Sheehan, H. L.: *Acta Endocr.*, 48:40, 1965.
203. Sheehan, H. L.: "Neurohypophysis and Hypothalamus," in *Endocrine Pathology*, ed. J. M. Blodworth. Baltimore, William & Wilkins, 1968.
204. Snyder, R. L., and Taggart, N. E.: *J. Reprod. Fertil.*, 14:451, 1967.
205. Sol, J. R. del, and Merlo, J. G.: *Acta Gin.*, 3:533, 1952.
206. Sönksen, P. H., et al.: *J. Clin. Endocr.*, 27:1418, 1967.
207. Southam, L. A., Saito, A., Lauber, A., and Soffer, L. J.: *J. Clin. Endocr.*, 21:675, 1961.
208. Spellacy, W. N., Goetz, F. C., Greenberg, B. Z., and Ells, J.: *Obstet. Gynec.*, 25:862, 1965.
209. Spellacy, W. N., Goetz, F. C., Greenberg, B. Z., and Schoeller, K. L.: *J. Clin. Endocr. Metab.*, 25:1251, 1965.
210. Spellacy, W. N., and Buhi, W. C.: *Amer. J. Obstet. Gynec.*, 105:888, 1969.
211. Steinbeck, A. W., and Theile, H.: *Acta Endocr.*, 36:497, 1961.
212. Stephens, C. O., and Hayes, O. J.: *Obstet. Gynec.*, 31:79, 1968.
213. Springham, C. L., and Geist, S. H.: *J.A.M.A.*, 113:2387, 1939.
214. Stempak, J. C.: *Endocrinology*, 70:443, 1962.
215. Stephens, C. O., and Hayes, O. J.: *Obstet. Gynec.*, 31:79, 1968.
216. Stevenson, A. E. M.: *Brit. Med. J.*, 2:1514, 1956.
217. Strozier, W. E., and Bohmfalk, J. M.: *Amer. J. Obstet. Gynec.*, 85:541, 1963.
218. Taylor, E. S., Bruns, P. D., Drose, V. E., and Kartchner, M. J.: *Amer. J. Obstet. Gynec.*, 83:194, 1962.
219. Thorn, G. W., and Forsham, P. H.: In *Progress in Endocrinology*, ed. E. Soskin. New York, Grune & Stratton, 1950.
220. Trayner, I. M., Welborn, T. A., Rubenstein, A. H., and Fransler, T. R.: *J. Endocr.*, 37:443, 1967.
221. Tscherne, E.: *Internat. J. Fertil.*, 5:34, 1960.
222. Tuchmann-Duplessis, H., and Mercier-Parot, L.: *Compt. Rend. Acad. Sci.*, 254:2655, 1962.
223. Van Heyningen, H.: *Endocrinology*, 69:720, 1961.
224. Venning, E. H., Primrose, T., Caligaris, L. C. S., and Dyrenfurth, I.: *J. Clin. Endocr.*, 17:473, 1957.
225. Villee, D. B., Engel, L. L., Loring, J. M., and Villee, C. A.: *Endocrinology*, 69:354, 1961.
226. Vizzone, A., Colugi, A., and Lanzone, P.: *Quad. Clin. Ost. Gin.*, 22:655, 1967.
227. Wagner, G. Trasbol, I., and Melchior, J. C.: *Acta Endocr.*, 47:549, 1964.
228. Warren, J. C., and Fernstrom, R.: *Amer. J. Obstet. Gynec.*, 81:1036, 1961.
229. Wayne, D. F.: *J. Embryol. Exper. Morphol.*, 10:471, 1962.
230. Werner, S. C.: *J. Clin. Endocr. Metab.*, 27:1637, 1967.
231. White, P., Gillespie, L., and Sexton, L.: *Amer. J. Obstet. Gynec.*, 71:57, 1956.
232. Wyss, H. I., and Meyer, C. M.: *Gynaecologia*, 161:75, 1965.
233. Yamazaki, E., Noguchi, A., and Slingerland, D. W.: *J. Clin. Endocr.*, 20:794, 1960.
234. Yen, S. S. C., Pearson, O. H., and Stratman, S.: *J. Clin. Endocr. Metab.*, 25:655, 1965.
235. Yen, S. C. C., Saaman, N., and Pearson, O. H.: *J. Clin. Endocr.*, 27:1341, 1967.
236. Zecca, D., and Passarelli, C.: *Ann. Ost. Gin.*, 89:263, 1967.

Part Eleven
MISCELLANEOUS ASPECTS OF THE ENDOCRINOLOGY OF WOMAN

Chapter 46

ENDOCRINE BASES OF GENITAL TUMORIGENESIS

46.1. INTRODUCTION

Tumorigenesis is today one of the most puzzling aspects in biology. A gigantic amount of research activity invested in elucidating this phenomenon has so far achieved only a very limited number of definitive results. Outside the circle of systematized research, a vast amount of speculation has been done. This chapter does not pretend to examine the problem exhaustively but aims simply at presenting a summary of the relationship between genital tumors and hormones.

Because many of the ideas espoused in the preceding editions of this book have failed to be borne out by developments in subsequent years, a significant number of them have been suppressed in the present chapter while, at the same time, care has been exercised to incorporate in it the anatomopathologic and clinical observations of recent years.

The most solid grounds for admitting the existence of hormone-determined tumorigenesis have been provided by animal experiments, particularly in mice, which were found to be highly sensitive in this respect. Mühlbock and Boot[102] summarized in table form all tumors of hormonal origin it has been possible to induce in animals (Table 46-1).

As had been suggested by the early investigations of Laccassagne,[84] the table reveals estrogens to play an important role. Nevertheless, some other hormones, particularly those originating in the anterior pituitary, deserve special attention.

46.2. MORPHOGENETIC FACTORS; DETERMINANTS AND REALIZERS

Broadly speaking, it may be said that every tumor, whether malignant or benign, epithelial or mesenchymal, constitutes a process of *pathologic morphogenesis*, which is therefore subject to the general laws of morphogenesis as they are applicable to any kind of organism.

In this respect, it is of interest to remember that before the end of the nineteenth century Roux had already divided morphogenetic factors into two categories: *factors of determination* and *factors of realization*. Whereas the first were asserted to be of

TABLE 46-1. Tumors of Hormonal Origin in Animals*

ORGAN	HORMONE INVOLVED
I. Pituitary	a. *Estrogens* (mouse, rat, hamster)
	b. *Progesterone* (rat)
	c. Thyroidectomy (mouse)
II. Thyroid	a. Thyrotropin (mouse)
	b. Thiouracil (mouse)
III. Adrenal	a. Adrenocorticotropin (mouse)
	b. Castration in young animals (rat, mouse)
IV. Ovary	a. *Gonadotropins* (rat and mouse ovary, transplanted to spleen)
V. Testes	a. Gonadotropins (mouse)
	b. *Estrogens* (mouse)
VI. Uterus	a. *Estrogens* (mouse, rat, rabbit)
VII. Breast	a. *Estrogens* (mouse, rat)
	b. *Mammotropin* (mouse)
VIII. Kidney	a. *Estrogens* (hamster)
IX. Liver	a. Sex hormones (mouse)
X. Lymphoid tissue	a. *Estrogens* (mouse)

* From Mühlbock and Boot.[102]

hereditary nature, transmissible by genes, the second were thought to be of *humoral* nature, responsible for stimulating and unfolding the hereditary tendency.

Later investigations over a period of more than 60 years have shown that these factors were indeed involved in every kind of morphologic process. In other words, the factors of determination were linked to heredity, and the factors of realization were constituted by biocatalysts, whose agents of production were the *hormones, vitamins* and *ferments* (see Chapter 1). It is still a matter of conjecture whether such other substances of biocatalytic nature as *organizers* and *evocators* play any significant role in processes of cancerous morphogenesis.

There is statistical evidence that carcinoma of the uterus and carcinoma of the breast are the most common varieties of carcinoma. This must be attributed mainly to the striking changes to which the uterus is subject as a consequence of ovarian hormone activity. The somatic organs of the body undergo only one kind of vital cycle, involving development, maturity and senescence; the genital apparatus as a whole adds to this first cycle a second cycle: the menstrual cycle. The uterus and the breast have an additional third cycle, the gravidic cycle and the lactational cycle, respectively (Fig. 46–1). This kind of multicyclicity of the uterus and breast, involving continuous blending of developmental and involutional processes, explains the high incidence of neoplastic phenomena as nothing else but deviations from normal processes of differentiation. *Genital tumors thus appear to be the result of deviated morphogenetic evolution rather than of cell mutation.*

46.3. HEREDITARY FACTORS IN THE GENESIS OF UTERINE AND MAMMARY TUMORS

All data currently available concerning hereditary transmission of cancer are derived totally from animal experiments. Of all animals, the rat and the mouse have been found to lend themselves best to experiments of this kind, and the kind of genetic problems that we understand best relate to these animals. At eight months, a mouse is already an adult animal, reaching senility at one and a half years and dying before the age of two. *Its vital cycle is 40 times faster than that of the human species* and, because new generations appear in rapid succession, some authors (for instance, Little[90]) have been able to study more than 40 generations of animals.

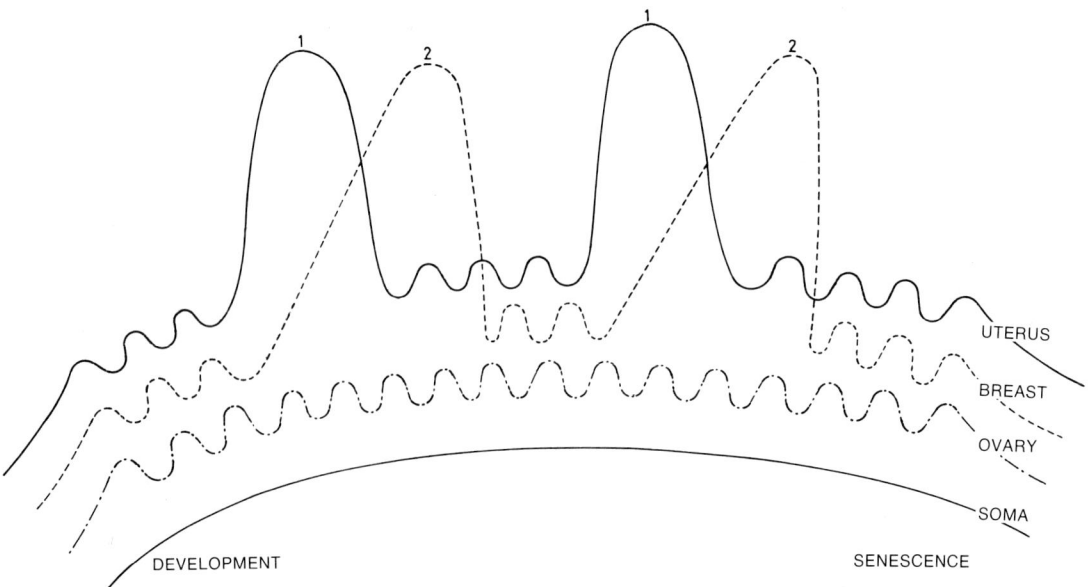

Figure 46–1. Vital curves of soma, ovary, breast and uterus. The soma subjected to only one kind of motion, the vital cycle. The vital curve of the ovary is subjected to two types of cycles, the vital cycle and the menstrual cycle. The breast and the uterus, aside from their vital and menstrual cycles, each have an additional cycle: the uterus a gestational cycle, and the breast a lactational cycle.

The incidence of human genital cancer in certain families has been studied by several investigators. The human race is evidently a highly heterogeneous society from a genetic standpoint, and only in isolated, concrete clinical cases does the opportunity exist for an accurate study, such as was the case, for instance, in the cancerigenic families described by Hanley or by Wood and Darling.

After analyzing the question in detail, Blanck[15] *and Greene*[53] *concluded that a hereditary factor was unquestionably involved in the human species.*

Nonetheless, it is mainly in animals that an in-depth study of such a factor has been possible, as we shall make clear later.

The existence of strains or lines of laboratory animals revealing a special hereditary predisposition to tumoral growths is a well known fact. Murray has raised such a line, known as the DBA line, since 1909. On the other hand, Medes and Reimann[96] described a different strain, strain C57-B1, in which the carcinogenic incidence was nil. The incidence of cancer thus varies widely from one animal breed to another. The corresponding rates, which are expressed in percentages, are fairly constant for each particular strain. The experience gained by many authors has made it plain that the tumorigenic factors, passed down from generation to generation, may be of two different types: (a) nongenetic factors, *not linked to genes*, and (b) genetic factors, *linked to genes*.

46.3.1. NONGENETIC FACTORS

It would be beyond the scope of this work to examine the question of *nongenetic transmission* of certain tumors in animals, which is probably mediated by *viruses*. The well known investigation by Little[90] revealed that the hereditary tendency to cancer in various strains of mice was transmitted by the mother, probably by a cytoplasmic rather than a nuclear mechanism. In carrying on the same kind of studies, Bittner[13] was able to discover a factor that was transmissible by milk and that could also be transmitted to the egg implanted in the uterus. This factor, once acquired, became inheritable in the particular strain in question. This "factor of Bittner" may be passed on in milk, may be transmitted to the conceptus in the uterus and may be acquired by the blastocysts of noncarcinogenic strains if they are implanted in uteri of mice with a strong carcinogenic tendency.

46.3.2. GENETIC FACTORS

Although the degree of intensity of a given hereditary tendency to cancer is determined primarily by nongenetic causes, some carcinogenetic stocks of mice have been found to show *gene-linked* tendencies to cancer, transmissible in terms of mendelian dominance.

This type of tendency can influence the offspring's susceptibility to Bittner's factor. As we are about to learn, there also exists a hereditary tendency insofar as an animal's susceptibility to hormones is concerned, which in mice is determined by the factor of Bittner. *An echelon in the relationships the different factors maintain with each other is thus apparent. Accordingly, a primary, genetic factor transmitted chromosomally from parent to offspring is responsible for the susceptibility to a second factor, which is inherited through the mother's cytoplasm or passed down from her in her milk. This second factor in turn is thought to enhance the uterine capacity for responding to estrogen, contributing to the development of cancer.*

46.3.3. THE KARYOTYPE IN CASES OF UTERINE AND BREAST CANCER

In recent years, a great deal of research has been focused on cancer cytogenetics (Allen and Fullmer,[2] Atkin,[5] Jones et al.[73]). Aneuploidy (see Chapter 35, page 777) has often been reported in women with in situ carcinoma of the uterine cervix. In tissue cultured from 22 cases of endometrial carcinoma, Stanley and Kirkland[138] found an incidence of pseudodiploid metaphase of 88 per cent, with the number of chromosomes ranging from 35 to 56. The same authors also observed the emergence of a triploid cell line in tissue cultures of cervical carcinoma while the remaining cells—none of them normal—retained their pseudodiploidy. Working also with cervical cancer, Bamford and his associates[7] described a case in which the chromosomal constitution was a mosaic, while Auersperg and Wakonig-Vaartaja[6] reported eight cases with a reduction in the number of group B chromosomes, with anomalies in groups A, D and G, and pseudodiploidy in group C. Similarly, Seshadri and his colleagues[127] and Stanley and co-workers[136] described frequent chromosomal anomalies in breast cancer.

46.4. BIOCATALYSTS IN THE GENESIS OF GENITAL NEOPLASIA

The *factors of realization*, or *biocatalysts*, influencing the unfolding of tendencies established by the genetic factors already studied, have been discovered in recent years. We are referring not only to *estrogens* but also to steroids, on whose balanced interactions with estrogens malignant proliferation depends in great measure, and to vitamins, which play a protective role. In this category must also be included some other compounds of the intermediary steroid metabolism which, although not estrogens themselves, are related to estrogens. These include several aromatic hydrocarbons.

46.4.1. CARCINOGENESIS FROM AROMATIC HYDROCARBONS

In the preceding edition of this book, we presented a summary of the work done by Cook and Kennaway in describing the principal carcinogenic hydrocarbons.[34] They identified 1, 2-5, 6-dibenzanthracene (Fig. 46-2, I) and 3, 4-benzopyrene (Fig. 46-2, II) as the active substances in carcinogenic pitch. The discovery of the aromatic ring structure of the sex hormones more than 30 years ago gave rise to speculation about the possibility that altered ovarian activity might cause some compounds of that type to become carcinogenic.[59] On the other hand, certain bile acids possessing the same type of polycyclic structure seemed to be involved in carcinogenesis. Cook and Kennaway[34] were thus able to show a tendency for certain steroid molecules to pass into carcinogenic derivatives. In particular, deoxycholic acid (Fig. 46-2, III) could be converted to dehydronorcholene (IV) and further to methylcholanthrene (V).

Numerous other instances indicating *a possible relationship between naturally occurring steroids and carcinogenic polycyclic compounds* were subsequently recognized. Thus, Nes and Mosettig[105] showed that dehydroergosteryl acetate could be converted to an active carcinogen: hexahydrodimethyl-cyclopentanthracene (Fig. 46-2, VI and VII). Similarly, Gough and Shopee[52] drew attention to the conversion of methylhomoandrostane (VIII) to methylchrysene (IX). In addition, Hieger[63] studied analogous conversions of cholesterol, prompted by the observation that mice injected with cholesterol (dissolved in olive oil) developed sarcomas. The compound responsible for this action appears to be delta-5-cholestene-3-one, a natural metabolic derivative of cholesterol in animals.

The possibility that cortical steroids may be converted to methylcholanthrene, which, as we have pointed out, is a potent carcinogen, has also been suggested. This kind of transformation presumably might take place through the combination of a 17-ketosteroid of adrenal origin, 3-5-androstendiene-17-one (Fig. 46-3, I), with pyruvic acid (Fekete and Little[45]). These authors further point out that estrone cannot be converted in the same way even though the same type of aromatization of one of its ring structures is possible because, rather than cholanthrene, the resulting product would be 3-methylcholanthrene (Fig. 46-3, II), which has no carcinogenic properties. This seems to be a weighty argument against the possible carcinogenetic activity of estrogens per se.

The role played by cortical steroids in the genesis and evolution of some carcinomas has been brought to light by recent studies,[12, 16, 57] which seem to suggest that certain changes in the metabolism of adrenal steroids, rather than estrogens themselves, might be more directly implicated in carcinogenesis. Consequently, the possibility that some carcinogens may be products of endogenous metabolism in humans as well as in animals is now recognized. *These presumably involve conversion products of cholesterol, certain bile acids and adrenal steroids, but they are seldom, if ever, derived from estrogens. Despite past emphasis on the structural similarity between estrogens and known carcinogenic compounds, it has never been possible to dem-*

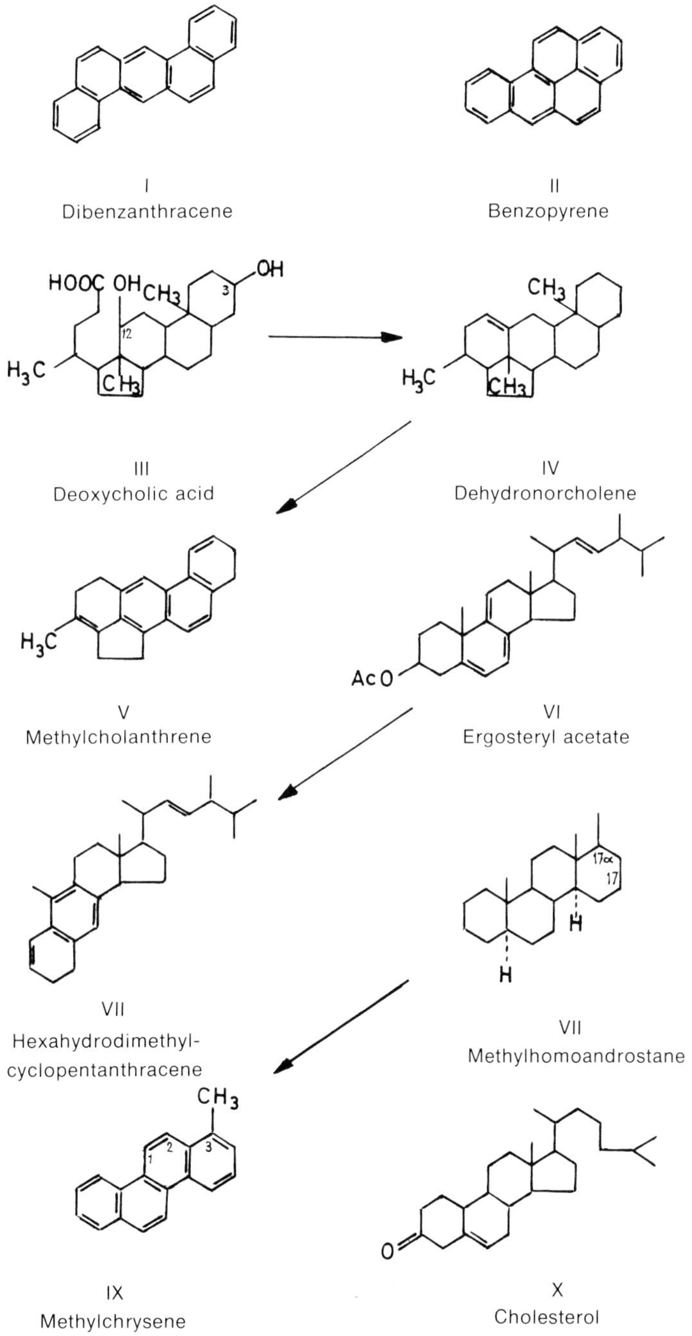

Figure 46-2. Carcinogenic hydrocarbons.

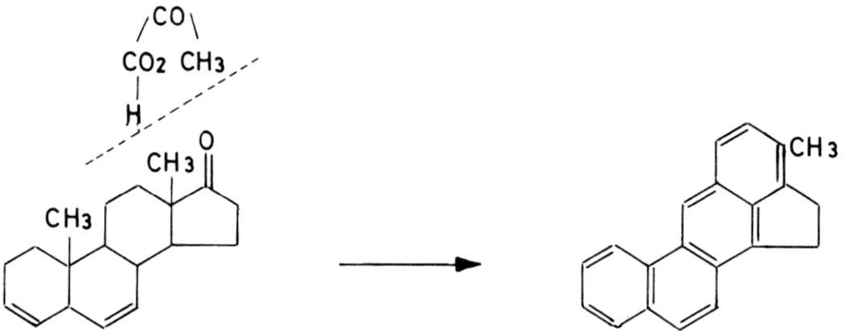

3, 5-ANDROSTENDIENE-17-ONE PYRUVIC ACID
METHYLCHOLANTHRENE (POTENT CARCINOGEN)

I

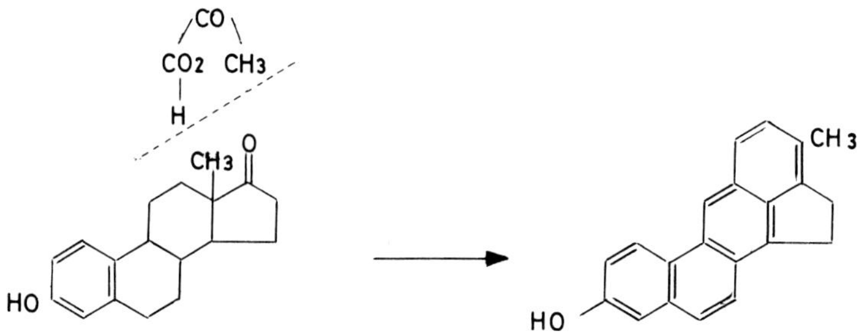

ESTRONE PYRUVIC ACID 3-METHYLCHOLANTHRENE
(NONCARCINOGENIC)

II

Figure 46–3. Possible pathways of conversion of cortical steroids to methylcholanthrene.

onstrate the actual conversion of an estrogen to any carcinogenic hydrocarbon of the methylcholanthrene group or a similar group.

46.5. ESTROGENS AND ENDOMETRIAL CARCINOMA

Although we have serious reservations concerning the carcinogenic role of estrogens in the human species, there are two types of carcinomas which appear to be related in some way to estrogenic activity. These are the *carcinoma of the endometrium* and *carcinoma of the breast.*

46.5.1. COMPOUNDS WITH BOTH ESTROGENIC AND CANCERIGENIC PROPERTIES

In 1932, Laccassagne noted that, under certain conditions, injections of female sex hormones to mice led to the development of mammary cancer. Although the original experiment seemed to open new perspectives for the pathogenic explanation of genital cancers in the female, it has since become clear that only under strictly controlled conditions could estrogens be considered as causative agents of cancer.

In 1943, Dodds and his co-workers[40] achieved the synthesis of several compounds possessing simultaneous estrogenic and cancerigenic activity. Among these were 5,6-cyclopentano-1,2-dibenzanthracene (Fig. 46–2, I), 3,4-benzopyrene (II) and a long list of derivatives too extensive to be analyzed here. Those studies prompted a series of experiments aimed at the synthesis of similar compounds, incidentally yielding members of the stilbenic series of estrogens.[41] The discovery of the latter was thus an outgrowth of a search for hydrocarbons with both estrogenic and cancerigenic properties rather than for ones possessing any new type of estrogenic activity for therapeutic purposes. The compounds diethylstilbestrol, triphenylethylene and hexestrol (see Chapter 2, page 15), obtained in this way, turned out similarly to have estrogenic and mild cancerigenic activity.

Beginning with the already mentioned experiments of Laccassagne, a large amount of research has been done ever since to explore the behavior of estrogens in relation to the development of neoplasia. Burrows[28, 29] published two excellent reviews on the subject.

A new mechanism of action by carcinogens on the uterus has been discovered in recent years. By introducing a pellet of dimethylbenzanthracene into the uterine cavity of mice, Meisels[97] found that such animals developed carcinoma. This effect was not observed in previously castrated animals. Kind and his associates,[79] on the other hand, found that the uteri of rodents — in which carcinoma had been induced by local application of the same kind of carcinogen (dimethylbenzanthracene) — concentrated estrogens selectively. On the basis of the two preceding experiments, it may be inferred that the role of aromatic carcinogens, at least in rodents, is one of cooperating with estrogens in the production of carcinoma.

46.5.2. ESTROGENS AS GROWTH-PROMOTING SUBSTANCES

The fact that estrogens ought to be considered first of all *growth-promoting hormones* has been emphasized repeatedly in this book (Chapter 2) as well as elsewhere.[16, 17] That they should behave as specifically female substances in higher animals is simply an expression of that fundamental biologic principle which holds that growth and reproduction are different aspects of the same phenomenon. Estrogens perform the physiologic function of promoting the growth of epithelial tissues, specifically those related to sexual activity in women as well as in females of other mammals.

With regard to tumors, estrogens behave essentially as growth-promoting factors, which must be ascribed mainly to the embryonal and anaplastic nature of neoplastic cells.

46.5.3 CLINICAL ARGUMENTS FAVORING THE HORMONAL ORIGIN OF ENDOMETRIAL CARCINOMA

There is one indisputable clinical argument favoring the estrogenic causation of endometrial carcinoma: the fact that endometrial carcinoma is 17 times (Hertig[61]) or 20 times (Greene[53]) as common in women with feminizing mesenchymomas as in the general population. Some of the other reasons that have been advanced in support of the "estrogenic theory" are less convincing. Although we shall review them all briefly, we refer the reader to two excellent recent communications on the subject.[3, 44]

FEMINIZING TUMORS OF THE OVARY. In 1922, Schroeder reported a case of granulosa cell tumor and endometrial carcinoma. Since then, other reports have multiplied (Bjoro and Mylins,[14] Dockerty and Mussey,[38] Frachtman,[48] Gusberg,[55] Greene,[54] Hertig,[61] Ingraham and Novak,[69] Larson,[85] Mansell and Hertig[94]). It might also be added that, according to Kottmeier,[81] the granulosa cell tumors and thecomas are in many cases microscopic in size and are not detected by the clinician, as was the case in two instances reported by Nogales and his colleagues.[111]

According to Mansell and Hertig,[94] endometrial carcinoma is associated more often with thecomas than with granulosa cell tumors, which has also been true in our own experience. Among 100 cases of endometrial carcinoma reviewed by us, we found two tiny thecomas and a single granulosa cell microtumor. In our experience, therefore, the incidence of functional tumors in association with endometrial carcinoma is 3 per cent. The true incidence is probably higher, although there is no general agreement in that respect. Ingraham and Novak found 6 per cent,[69] and Greene found 17 per cent.[53] One way or another, these figures are *too high to be dismissed as resulting from a mere chance relationship.*

OTHER NONTUMORAL OVARIAN CONDITIONS. However, what about the remaining 97 per cent in our statistics in which there was carcinoma but no feminizing tumor? Such endometrial cancers developed in postmenopausal women in the absence of any apparent ovarian activity, so that under these conditions it would seem difficult to admit any hypersecretion of estrogens. Gusberg[55] reported the finding of "cortical stromal hyperplasia." An association between that type of hyperplasia and endometrial carcinoma was later suggested by Roddick and Greene,[122] Sommers and Meissner,[134] Woll and associates,[155] and Marcus.[95] It must be added that Morris and Scully[101] considered the latter type of hyperplasia to be a precursor of theca cell tumors.

Morris and Scully similarly called attention to *hilus cell hyperplasia*, which has been mentioned in Chapter 29 (page 645) in connection with virilizing effects. As is so often the case, androgenic formations may occasionally exert a feminizing influence and have even been described as causing hyperestrinism and being associated with endometrial carcinoma (Sherman and Woolf,[128] Woll et al.[155]). Hilus cell hyperplasia has also been found in our material; however, we shall elaborate later on its significance.

Finally, there have also been some reports indicating an association between endometrial carcinoma and the Stein-Leventhal syndrome (Hertig and Sommers,[62] Husslein,[67] Jackson and Dockerty,[72] Kauffman et al.,[78] Sommers and Wadman,[133] Speert,[135] Vere and Dempsey[150]). A statistically significant series was recently reported by Andrews.[3] Nevertheless, agreement on this point is not unanimous if one considers the recent study of 17 cases by Hormeister and Vondrak,[64] in which endometrial carcinoma was found to develop despite previous surgical or roentgen castration of such female patients.

The ovarian findings in 100 cases of endometrial carcinoma studied by us are shown in Table 46–3.

ELIMINATION OF ESTROGENS AND GONADOTROPINS. The elimination of estrogens in women with endometrial carcinoma has been studied by various authors, with inconclusive results (Bret et al.,[20, 21] Liu,[91] Diczfalusy and Lauritzen[37]). The figures obtained by us have not been expressive either[17] (see Table 46–3). Twombley and his associates[147] have formulated an ingenious hypothesis: obese women concentrate estrogens in their adipose tissue and, as a result of estrogen storage, may develop the effects of cumulative hyperestrinism. However, this would fail to explain why nonobese women, who constitute the majority of cases, should also develop endometrial carcinoma. Hustin and Buret[68] reported increased values of estrogenuria in each of the 10 cases of endometrial carcinoma they had studied. Yet, dexamethasone administration in all their cases resulted in a marked reduction of estrogenuria, which appears to suggest that the estrogens involved were of *adrenal* rather than ovarian origin.

As far as estrogen elimination was concerned, Hausknecht and Gusberg[60] found no statistical difference between women with endometrial carcinoma and menopausal women of comparable age in general, which is in keeping with our own data, indicated previously.

Nevertheless, in this regard, significant

TABLE 46–2. State of Ovary and Endometrium in Women with Endometrial Carcinoma, as Compared to Normal Postmenopausal Women*

CLINICAL CATEGORY	STATE OF OVARY	PER CENT	STATE OF ENDOMETRIUM	PER CENT
Adenocarcinoma prior to menopause (21 cases)	Ovulation Anovulation Atrophy	28.6 52.4 19.0	Normal biphasic Hyperplasia Atrophy	38.1 52.4 9.5
Adenocarcinoma after menopause (79 cases)	Cortical hyperplasia Hilus cells Feminizing tumors	10.2 29.1 3.7	Normal monophasic Hyperplasia Atrophy	43.1 5.1 51.8
Control group (postmenopausal)	Cortical hyperplasia Hilus cells Feminizing tumors	8.0 24.0 0.0	Normal proliferative Hyperplasia Atrophy	32.0 4.0 64.0

* From Botella: Proceedings of the International Congress of Cytology, p. 5, 1962.

TABLE 46-3. Total Estrogen Excretion in Women with Endometrial Adenocarcinoma, as Compared to Noncancerous Postmenopausal Women*†

	TOTAL ESTROGENS IN MICROGRAMS PER 24 HOURS		
CLINICAL CATEGORY	Before intervention	3 to 5 days after	6 to 10 days after
Postmenopause with cancer (12 cases)	78	87	55
Menopause without cancer (35 cases)	60	57	58

* From Botella: Proceedings of the International Congress of Cytology, p. 5, 1962.
† Surgical cases. Estrogen determinations were performed before and after bilateral oophorectomy.

findings were reported by Nordqvist,[112] who had achieved a pure cell line of endometrial carcinoma in culture that was noted to proliferate more vigorously upon the addition of estrogens.

On the other hand, a rise in urinary gonadotropin values, particularly LH, seems to have been demonstrated fairly consistently (Sherman and Woolf,[128] Varga and Henriksen[148]). Sommers and Wadman[133] found an increase in the number of PAS-positive gonadotropin-secreting cells in the adenohypophysis.

PREVIOUS ESTROGEN THERAPY. By contrast, women who had been exposed to prolonged treatment with estrogens seem to reveal a definite predisposition to developing endometrial carcinoma (Bromberg et al.,[22] Dowsett,[43] Freemont-Smith,[49] Gusberg and Hall,[56] Karpas and Speer,[77] Stokes[141]). This undoubtedly seems to constitute a powerful argument. For instance, Dowsett[43] reported a case of Turner's syndrome in which the patient eventually developed carcinoma of the uterine fundus after life-long continuous estrogen administration for over 30 years.

Mühlbock and Boot[102] emphasized the role played by continuous estrogen treatment in the production of endometrial carcinoma and, together with Varga and Henriksen,[149] emphasized that prolonged estrogen therapy should never be undertaken without administering progestogens intermittently.

STATE OF TARGET ORGANS. *Vaginal cytology* and the *endometrium* itself have been the objects of repeated studies in endometrial carcinoma.

The *vaginal cytology* presents a moderately to strongly estrogenic character, according to Brunschwig and Papanicolaou,[25] Bret and Coupez,[21] Haour,[59] Nuovo,[115] Rubio and associates,[124] Wachtel,[151, 152] and Wied.[153] We have also noted the presence of estrogenic features in vaginal cytology, but we do not believe—and Wied is of the same opinion—that the latter are constant enough to establish any valid correlation (Table 46-4).

The healthy *endometrium* in the presence of carcinoma has been studied extensively. A number of years ago, Novak and Rutledge[113] found atypical or "regressive" hyperplasia in senile endometria, a finding confirmed by Nogales.[110] However, neither Nogales nor Novak[114] has ever found evidence of genuine cystic hyperplasia in association with endometrial carcinoma. In contrast, Gusberg and Hall,[56] Sherman and Woolf,[128] Woll and associates,[155] and Kruschwitz[82] admit the occurrence of carcinoma in association with hyperplasia which, in their opinion, is indicative of hyperestrinism and possibly of a "precancerous condition" (Fig. 46-4).

TABLE 46-4. Vaginal Cytology in Two Groups of Women, One with Endometrial Malignancy, the Other Composed of Healthy Women of Comparable Age*

		KARYOPYKNOTIC INDEX (NUMBER OF CASES IN EACH GROUP)					
CLINICAL CATEGORY	CASES	0	1-4%	5-9%	10-19%	20-29%	Over 30%
I. With carcinoma	50	30	10	5	3	2	0
II. Without carcinoma	50	33	10	4	3	0	0

* From Botella: Proceedings of the International Congress of Cytology, p. 5, 1962.

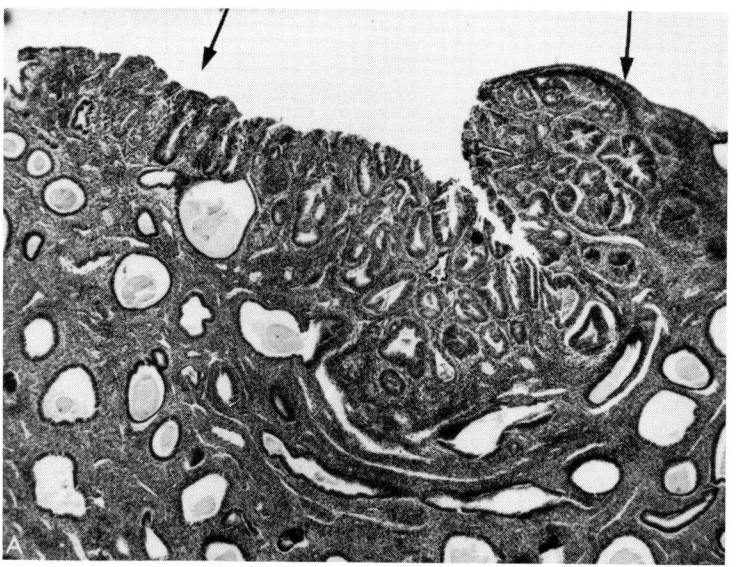

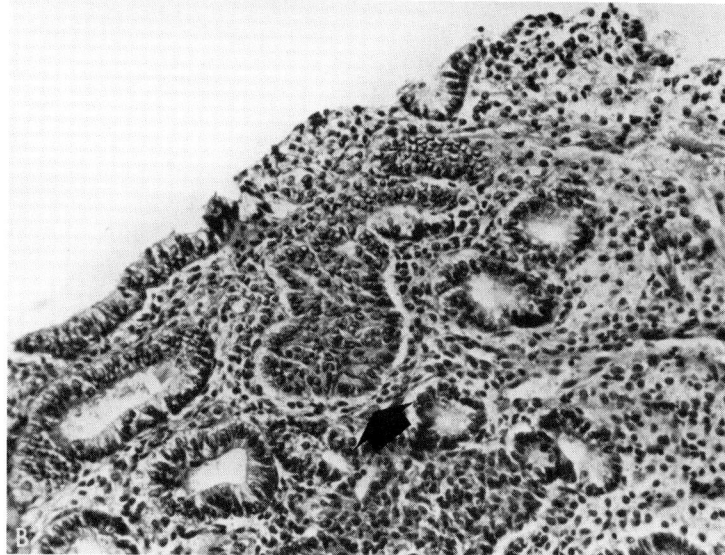

Figure 46–4. Relationship between endometrial hyperplasia and adenocarcinoma. *A*, Area of incipient endometrial adenocarcinoma (carcinoma in situ), surrounded by endometrial hyperplasia of the cystic glandular variety, in a 67 year old woman who had a small ovarian thecoma. *B*, Another case of atypical endometrial hyperplasia in a 65 year old woman, revealing a gland in center (arrow) with marked crowding of highly dysplastic epithelial cells.

46.5.4. ARGUMENTS AGAINST THE HORMONAL ORIGIN OF ENDOMETRIAL CARCINOMA

With the exception of functioning tumors, all other arguments appear to us inconsistent. Cianfrani[32] observed a castrated woman who, after a considerable number of years, developed endometrial carcinoma. Printer[120] recorded a similar occurrence in a case of adrenogenital syndrome with virilization. We have studied the ovaries, endometria, cytology and hormone excretion in 100 cases of endometrial adenocarcinoma, as compared with 50 normal women in the same age group (Tables 46–2, 46–3 and 46–4), and found no significant differences between the two groups. This means that hypersecretion of estrogens is in fact common in the postmenopausal period, as pointed out in Chapter 38, although apparently it is not more common in women with carcinoma. This view is shared by Cherry and Tovell[31] and by Winkhaus and Taylor.[154] Anthony and Roddick,[3a] who studied the incidence of ovarian hilar changes, found hilus cell hyperplasia as often in one group as in the other.

With the exception of three functioning tumors among the cancerous group (Table 46–2), the preceding tables reveal no statistically significant differences to support the estrogenic hypothesis of endometrial carcinoma. The same is true of urinary estrogen excretion.

Table 46–3 reveals two things: first, that there is no significant difference in estrogen excretion rates between the two groups of women; and second—and more important—that *castration does not affect estrogen levels, or at best, does so to a minimal extent, which must be construed as evidence that we are dealing with estrogens derived from extraovarian sources.* This question shall be reexamined later.

Thus, there seems to be no conclusive evidence of the endocrine etiology of endometrial carcinoma. It is clear that postmenopausal women frequently experience episodes of paradoxical hyperproduction of estrogens of adrenocortical rather than ovarian origin, but this may similarly occur in women without genital abnormalities.

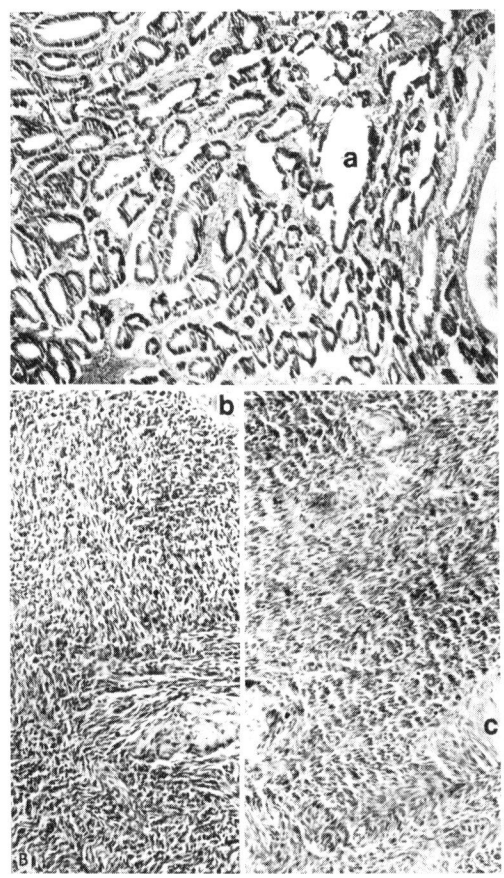

Figure 46–5. A, Endometrial adenocarcinoma. B, C, Different areas within an associated ovarian thecoma of the same patient.

46.5.5. DIABETES AND ENDOMETRIAL CANCER

It has long been recognized that endometrial malignancy frequently occurs in diabetic and obese women.[61, 111, 114] Benjamin and Casper[10] emphasized this fact, for which there is apparently no clear explanation. Treatment with progestogens, associated with clinical improvement of the tumor, results in increased glucose tolerance, which is suggestive of some kind of etiologic relationship.

46.6. ESTROGENS AND MAMMARY CANCER

From the endocrine point of view, carcinoma of the breast has been one of the best studied genital carcinomas. Not all mammary tumors are stimulated in their development by estrogens and, accordingly, may be classified into *tumors responding to estrogens* and *tumors not responding to estrogens*.

There is plenty of recent evidence attesting to the hormone dependency of mammary cancers in animals. Mobbs[99] used dimethylbenzanthracene for the experimental induction of cancer in rats. The resulting cancer was estrogen-dependent and the neoplastic tissue was found to fix estrogens selectively. Similar estrogen fixation by experimentally induced mammary cancer in rats has been demonstrated by Sander.[125] Teller and his associates[146] furthermore noted that dimethylbenzanthracene-induced cancer in rats could be arrested at will by castration and reactivated by the administration of estrogens. Certain antiestrogenic compounds, such as synthetic progestogens,[108, 142] prolactin,[103] relaxin[119] and thyroxine,[129] have been found to stop the evolution of experimentally induced rat mammary cancer. Progesterone, on the contrary, has been shown by Jabara[71] to have no effect on the development of dimethylbenzanthracene-induced cancer in the same animals.

46.6.1. EVIDENCE IN FAVOR OF HYPERESTRINISM

HORMONE ASSAY. The rate of urinary estrogen excretion in cases of breast cancer has been measured by Brown,[23, 24] Diczfalusy and associates,[36] and Bulbrook and colleagues.[26,27] Although it is true that above average values have been reported consistently, Diczfalusy and his co-workers[36] pointed out that the concentrations of Kober positive chromogens did not correlate with the biologic activity of such urines, raising the *possibility that the substances assayed were not true estrogens*. It seems quite certain that the estrogens involved, as maintained by Brown and Blair[23] and Hustin and Buret[68] are in fact of adrenal rather than ovarian origin and, consequently, the nonestrogenic Kober positive substances might be related to carcinogens by the previously outlined mechanism (see Section 46.4.1, 3,5-androstendiene-17-one).

Reports confirming this estrogenic increase in breast cancer have recently been forthcoming from many quarters (Bayer et al.,[9] Bernard et al.,[11] Jull et al.,[74] Kushinsky et al.,[83] Nissen-Meyer and Sanner,[109] and Lemon and Parsons[86]). The consensus in this instance is much more unanimous than in the case of endometrial carcinoma.

Boyland,[19] Loraine,[92] and Stewart and associates[140] have been concerned particularly with the study of gonadotropin levels. Sterenthal and his co-workers[139] believe that the increase in estrogen levels in mammary cancer results from the action of pituitary gonadotropin. Nonetheless, there is less unanimous agreement on this score than with regard to the elevation of estrogen levels. Netter and Gouris[106] failed to find any increase in gonadotropin values in the presence of mammary carcinomas.

VAGINAL CYTOLOGY. The vaginal cytology of mammary cancer cases has been studied by Finkbeiner,[46] Haour,[59] Munguía and Franco[104] and Sirtori.[130] Among our group, Montalvo[100] performed analogous studies. All the preceding reports concur in indicating a high incidence of estrogenic smears (30 to 78 per cent of the cases). Obviously, not all carcinomas of the breast are sensitive to estrogens, so that estrogen may thus be admitted to be involved in the etiology of only a portion of such carcinomas. In comparison, normal postmenopausal women reveal a high incidence of estrogenic smears (see Table 46–4). The problem remains unsolved, although it would appear cytologically that breast carcinoma is associated with significantly elevated estrogen activity.

TABLE 46–5. Vaginal Cytology in Mammary Cancer*

TYPE OF SMEAR	BEFORE OPERATION	AFTER	TOTAL
Hyperestrogenic	15	3	18
Estrogenic	33	27	60
Hypoestrogenic	28	29	57
Luteinic	11	18	29
Hypotrophic	20	21	41
Atrophic	9	60	69
Total	116	158	274

*From Montalvo-Carrizosa: *Acta Gin.*, 14:353, 1963.

Table 46–5 reveals a large number of estrogenic smears that remain unaffected by bilateral oophorectomy.

THE OVARY IN MAMMARY ADENOCARCINOMA. It must be realized that, unlike endometrial cancer, a large number of breast cancers develop in young women with cyclic activity. This is why *only the study of postmenopausal women may yield results that are of any significance*. It has not been possible to demonstrate any increase in the incidence of mammary carcinoma in women with granulosa cell tumors and thecomas.[19] The presence of thecal hyperplasia of various types, on the other hand, has been emphasized by many investigators (Novak,[114] and Mohler,[114] Woll et al.,[155] Sandison[126] and Dockerty et al.[39]). On the basis of important autopsy studies, however, Roddick and Greene[122] conclude that there is no correlation between ovarian findings and the occurrence of breast cancer. Nevertheless, castration in any case results in a better prognosis for breast cancer,[24, 25, 66] even though the adrenal may be asserted, in more definite terms in this instance than in endometrial carcinoma, to be an important source of estrogens.

RESULTS OF ADRENALECTOMY. Although the need for surgically removing or radiologically destroying the ovary had been dictated by early observations on breast cancer, neither of the proposed measures has proved to be sufficient (Taylor[145]) as regards not only the suppression of estrogenic secretion but also the prognosis of the disease as a whole. Huggins[65, 66] advanced the idea of adrenalectomizing inoperable cancer patients and maintaining them on 50 mg cortisone daily. The clinical results of this type of intervention and the effects on estrogen excretion rates have recently been reviewed by Bulbrook and his colleagues,[26] Cade,[30] Irvine and associates,[70] Kambouris and associates,[76] Pyrah,[121] and Symington and co-workers.[144] The clinical effects as well as the reduction in urinary excretion of estrogenic hormone observed seem to justify the assertion that, in at least 50 to 59 per cent of the cases, carcinoma of the breast is stimulated by estrogenic compounds elaborated by the "third gonad." Nor can we rule out the possibility that some of the compounds under consideration might be, as pointed out previously, false estrogens, generated by *abnormal steroidogenesis* and associated with the production of carcinogenic hydrocarbons in the body.

RESULTS OF HYPOPHYSECTOMY. As indicated previously (Chapter 2, page 28, and Chapter 28, page 608), there is by now sufficient evidence that, under the effect of pituitary stimulation, tissues other than the adrenal or the ovary are capable of producing estrogens. Consequently, several authors have proposed a form of treatment of mammary cancer based on either surgical removal of the pituitary (Luft and Olivecrona,[93] Roy and Pearson[123]) or the suppression of the pituitary by means of implantation of such radioisotopes as gold (^{198}Au) and yttrium (^{90}Y) (Bauer and Schweitzer,[8] Forrest et al.,[47] Pérez-Modrego[117]). Not only do such measures result in the complete disappearance of estrogens from the urine but also, as shown by Pérez-Modrego, cause the suppression of LH and *mammotropin*, although the role of the latter, in our opinion, is still hypothetical. *Thus, these surgical measures demonstrate the role played by estrogens in the etiology of genital cancers much more convincingly than either hormone assays or the study of ovarian morphology.*

46.6.2. ORIGIN OF THE ESTROGENS IN BREAST CANCER

What we have just stated raises the question of the origin of estrogens in these women, most of them in the postmenopausal age group. It may be asserted that, in the absence of ovaries, these compounds continue to be synthesized in the adrenal as well as outside the adrenal. The study of surgically castrated women (see Table 46–3) reveals that castration does not cause estrogen excretion to disappear. Diczfalusy and his associates[36] similarly observed no suppression of estrogen excretion following roentgen castration. Since there is evidence of a concomitant rise in 17-ketosteroid values,[12, 143] it is obvious that the source of those estrogens must be the adrenal. The specific stimulant for both the ovary, which in this instance functions actively, and the *cortical sexual zone* is provided by the action of LH. In the presence of LH activity, therefore, the adrenal as well as the ovary may secrete estrogens. In all likelihood, both glands do so simultaneously, as we have pointed out in explaining the concept of the "diffuse sexual mesenchyme." The mesenchyme in question is bisexual, able to produce estrogens as well as androgens, probably as a result of an integrated common metabolism.

The intervention of a pathologic form of estrogen synthesis in the causation of mammary cancer in the rat has been amply demonstrated by the studies of Ashraf and Zaaman[4] and Dominguez and Houseby.[42]

46.6.3. ESTROGEN RECEPTIVITY IN MAMMARY TUMOR TISSUE

Mobbs[99] and Sander,[125] as mentioned previously, have demonstrated selective fixation of tritiated estradiol by the neoplastic tissue of dimethylbenzanthracene-induced experimental cancer in rats. Analogous fixation has been demonstrated in human breast cancer by Lemon[87] and Pearlman and associates.[116]

The question is intimately related to the problem of tumoral hormone dependency. It has been asserted that mammary carcinomas revealing female sex chromosomal complements (XX) are sensitive to estrogens. In this sense may also be interpreted the findings by Descoeudres,[35] who reported a certain degree of parallelism between hormone dependency and incidence of Barr bodies in mammary tumors.

Because the estrogenic compounds under consideration are synthesized by mesenchymal-fibrous tissue, roentgen castration does not reduce the rate of their synthesis.

It seems plausible to assume that the diffuse sexual mesenchyme is localized not only in the adrenals and gonads but is present in some other parts of the body as well. Possessing the capacity for reacting to any increase in LH activity, the sexual mesenchyme may be postulated to swing into action in the presence of LH. This might explain the effects of hypophysectomy that we have described.

46.7. ESTROGENS AND BENIGN UTERINE TUMORS

In Chapter 28 (page 597), we have already spoken of the effects of hyperestrinism, which by now are fully demonstrated, on the development of benign tumors. The tumors involved are *myomas, adenomas* and *endometriosis*, provided the last may be considered as such.

The early studies by Whiterspoon and by Botella and Calvo-Marcos seem to have left us no doubt about the fact that myomatous growths were impelled by estrogenic activity and that estrogens in that instance were the *factor of realization*, but not the factor of determination, whose nature remained unknown to us. Aguilar and Botella[1] reexamined the problem in 1969, reaching quite similar conclusions (see Table 46–6 and 46–7). There is of course a correlation between hyperestrinism and myoma, although naturally it is not absolute. It would seem instead that this occurs more consistently as a result of an altered balance between estrogens and progestogens than because of any hyperestrinism in the true sense of the word.

Finally, the incidence of myomas in cases with granulosa cell tumors or thecomas is 20 times as high (Sjöstedt and Wahlen[131]).

46.8. OTHER ENDOCRINE TUMORS

In Table 46–1, we have presented a list of possible hormone-induced tumors in various animals. In view of the fact that nothing of the kind has to date been conclusively demonstrated to occur in the human species, we shall confine ourselves here to a brief comment.

46.8.1. OVARIAN TUMORS

In Chapter 30 (page 659) we spoke of the experimental production of granulosa cell tumors in mice. This can be achieved in two different ways:

1. By transplanting the ovary to the spleen (Hill, Gardner,[51] Lipschütz), as a result of which the estrogens are totally degraded, and the pituitary responds with an increase in FSH secretion. It therefore seems clear that the unopposed increase in FSH (and probably also LH) activity leads first to hyperplasia and then to neoplasia of the granulosa-thecal elements of the ovary.

Jull and his colleagues[75] treated female mice with dimethylbenzanthracene and transplanted their ovaries to the spleens of untreated recipients. The resulting tumors that were observed to develop were ovarian *granulosa cell carcinomas*. From a comparison between these experiments and the previously mentioned ones of Hill, Gardner, and Lipschütz, it seems evident that gonadotropin activity by itself is conducive to neoformation in the granulosa but that *in order to become malignant, the latter requires the previous action of a carcinogen.*

2. By irradiating the ovary. In this way, Peters and Levy,[118] as well as Slate and Bradbury,[132] achieved the same effect. It is possible that this may equally be the result of some action involving breakdown of estrogens.

46.8.2. PITUITARY AND ADRENAL TUMORS

Using elevated dosages of estrogens, injected into castrated mice, Meyer and Clifton[98] and Furth and Clifton[50] obtained pituitary tumors. Adrenal carcinomas of a strongly virilizing variety have been induced by means of simple castration in rats of the C.E. strain (Little et al.[90]), or by injecting castrated animals with ACTH (Symington et al.[44]).

46.8.3. MAMMOGENIC FACTOR AND MAMMARY CANCER

Although in Chapter 22 we have questioned the existence of the mammogenic factor, modern studies (Boyland,[19] Had-

TABLE 46–6. State of Ovary in Uterine Myoma: A Study of 253 Cases

TYPE OF OVARY FOUND	AGE BELOW 40 Cases	Per Cent	AGE 40 TO 50 Cases	Per Cent	AGE OVER 50 Cases	Per Cent	TOTAL Cases	Per Cent
Biphasic, with corpus luteum	23	44.2	83	56.4	4	7.0	110	43.4
Monophasic, with normal follicles	2	3.8	7	4.7	4	7.0	13	5.1
Follicular persistence*	12	23.0	27	18.3	21	36.8	60	23.7
Atrophic ovary	0	0	2	1.3	6	10.5	8	3.1
Functioning tumors†	0	0	0	0	5	8.7	5	1.9
Endometriosis	8	15.3	13	8.8	2	3.5	23	9.0
Nonfunctioning neoplasia	1	1.9	11	2.7	10	17.54	22	8.7
Inadequate for diagnosis	6	11.5	4	7.4	5	8.7	15	5.9

* Including polyfollicular ovaries.
† Thecomas and granulosa cell tumors.

TABLE 46–7. State of Endometrium in Uterine Myoma: A Study of 253 Cases

TYPE OF ENDOMETRIUM FOUND	AGE BELOW 40 Cases	Per Cent	AGE 40 TO 50 Cases	Per Cent	AGE OVER 50 Cases	Per Cent	TOTAL Cases	Per Cent
Normal secretion	15	30.6	67	45.5	6	10.5	88	34.7
Monophasic cycle	7	14.2	22	14.9	7	12.2	36	14.2
Hyperplasia	11	22.8	15	10.2	17	31.5	43	17.0
Atrophy	1	2.0	1	0.6	6	10.5	8	3.1
Progestational insufficiency	2	4.0	4	2.7	1	1.7	7	2.7
Postabortive	4	8.1	5	3.4	3	5.2	12	4.7
Adenocarcinoma	0	0	3	2.0	2	3.5	5	1.9
Inadequate for diagnosis*	7	14.2	22	14.9	9	15.7	38	15.0

* Taken during first half of cycle.

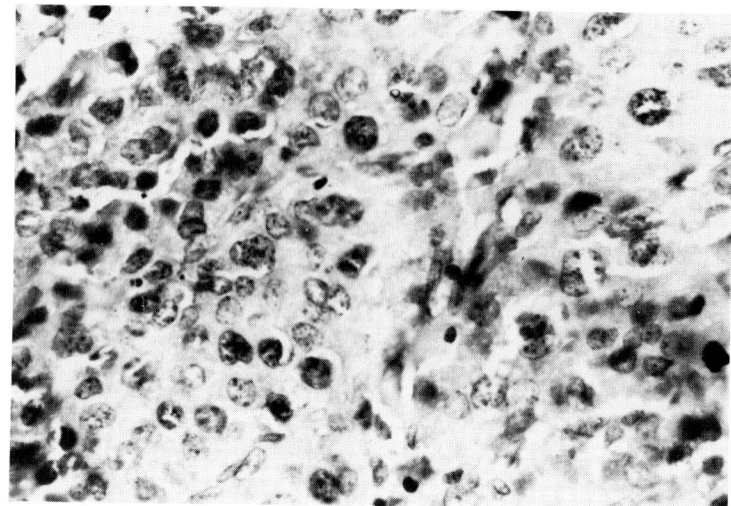

Figure 46-6. Luteinized ovarian granulosa cell tumor in castrate mouse whose ovary had been transplanted to the spleen. (From Aguilar; Thesis, University of Madrid, 1971.)

field[58]) emphasize the role of a certain mammotropic factor, despite the fact that Loraine[92] failed to find any increase in the latter in breast cancer.

46.9. NEOPLASMS IN TIME; KINETICS OF THEIR DEVELOPMENT

In experimental animals, such as rats, mice and guinea pigs, the animal's life span is so short and its reproductive rhythm so quick that the time element is hardly of any consequence.

In man, whose life expectancy is, needless to say, unpredictable, the problem of developmental rhythm in carcinomas is of utmost importance. Which carcinomas will develop and which will stay latent? In how many persons does death from causes other than carcinoma actually forestall the emergence of a carcinoma? What is the true incidence of neoplasms of this kind?

These questions are very difficult to answer. In general, we are unaware of the presence of carcinomas until they develop features of rapid invasive growth. A tumor fast growing can be diagnosed, but the same tumor growing very slowly will be overlooked. Potential tumors developing very late in the individual's life would be eliminated by the individual's death before it had a chance to be diagnosed. We are thus confronted with the three following questions: (1) Are there any latent carcinomas in the human uterus? (2) What kind of substances trigger their development? (3) What kind of substances retard their development?

46.9.1. LATENCY IN UTERINE CARCINOMA

While little is known concerning latent carcinomas in the breast and endometrium, we are all perfectly familiar with the occurrence of carcinoma in situ in the uterine cervix, which may be viewed as a latent cancer. Unfortunately, cervical carcinoma differs from endometrial carcinoma in that we lack evidence of its stimulability by estrogens, which is why it has not been possible so far to correlate the period of latency of cervical carcinoma with any kind of endocrine activity.

Carcinoma in situ is nevertheless a true carcinoma in all of its cytological and biological characteristics other than those pertaining to growth. As soon as its growth is initiated, however, it stops behaving as an intraepithelial carcinoma and becomes invasive. This is a clear example of how every neoplastic process is influenced by two factors: *genesis* and *growth*. A neoplasm is first engendered by one set of causes and then, probably by a different set of causes, is induced to grow and to turn increasingly invasive until killing the host.

What are the factors responsible for inducing a neoplasm to grow? Are they endogenous and inherent in tissues or do they come from outside? Unfortunately, owing largely to the fact that experimental duplication of such conditions has not been possible, we have to date little information concerning the evolution of in situ carcinoma under the influence of different hormones. On the other hand, the discovery of any preinvasive lesion obliges us to undertake therapeutic measures as promptly as possible, to the extent that any kind of clinical experimental manipulation in such patients would be grossly contrary to all norms of professional ethics.

46.9.2. ACCELERATION OF TUMORIGENESIS

It is not known whether preinvasive carcinoma or latent forms of benign tumors are caused to progress by biocatalytic actions. However, there is definite evidence to the effect that various types of hormonal influences can accelerate tumorigenesis experimentally. This allows us to draw certain inferences.

BY ESTROGENS. The tumorigenic action by estrogens has been explained previously. Let us now disregard their genetic actions and consider their growth-accelerating actions on tumors. Burrows and Horning,[28, 29] deny that there is any direct carcinogenic action by estrogens, except in animal lines rendered hereditarily susceptible by Bittner's factor. On the other hand, whenever they are acting on an already developed uterine or mammary tumor, estrogens accelerate the kinetics of the tumor. This accelerative action on growth has been well studied by Lipschütz[89] in uterine fibromas and adenomas of the guinea pig. The resulting increase in the rate of growth is directly proportional to the amount of estrogen injected. Thus, for instance, the growth of a uterine adenoma in an animal with an implanted tablet of estrogen is arrested, or it retrogresses, upon removal of the tablet. Instances of accelerated growth of human uterine carcinoma in association with injudicious estrogen therapy have been described in the literature (Gusberg and Hall[56]). There is no doubt, consequently, that estrogens are accelerators of growth in uterine cancer. Their possible role in the later development of carcinoma in situ remains to be elucidated.

BY OTHER SUBSTANCES. Substances other than estrogens are currently known to be able to accelerate neoplastic growth. These include humoral substances, as well as catabolites. Many years ago, Reiss and associates had discovered the action of pituitary growth hormone on certain types of tumors. Nieburgs[107] stressed the influence of this pituitary substance on cervical cancer.

Substances endowed with a remarkable stimulatory action on tumoral growth have been extracted from the tissues of individuals who had succumbed to cancer (Hieger[63]). A nonsaponifiable lipoid substance, identified as cholesterol, has been isolated from the liver of cancerous patients and found to possess carcinogenic activity. Any further discussion of this question would cause us to digress too far; in mentioning these findings, we merely wish to go on record regarding the possibility that hepatic cholesterol metabolism might be implicated in processes of carcinomatous growth.

46.9.3. DELAY OF TUMORIGENESIS

A great deal of speculation has centered on the question of anticarcinogenic substances. A number of compounds have been publicized as having a delaying or anticarcinogenic effect, and these have been recommended for the treatment of cancer by publicity seekers or profit-oriented interests. Faced with such an abundance of down-right false or misleading information, we shall restrict ourselves to mentioning a few compounds that are well known to slow down uterine carcinogenesis. These are mainly steroids and some vitamins.

PROGESTERONE. Progesterone inhibits growth of uterine myomas and adenomas as well as experimental metaplasia of the endometrium. In the human species, the development of benign neoplasms is acknowledged to be stimulated by anovulation and to be prevented, or inhibited, by pregnancy.

Lipschütz[88] has experimentally determined the optimal ratio at which progesterone is able to inhibit the action of estrogens as 3 to 1, that is, 3 mg of progesterone for every 1 mg of estrogen absorbed or injected. Female experimental animals fail to develop estrogenic tumors unless they are previously castrated because neoplastic growth is otherwise blocked by the luteal reaction in the ovary.

SYNTHETIC PROGESTOGENS. A recently discovered effect of both progesterone and synthetic progestogens has been their *anticarcinogenic action on the endometrium*. Kistner[80] has achieved a satisfactory slow-down in the growth rate of advanced endometrial carcinoma by administering progestogens in high dosages (ranging from 0.5 to 1 gm daily). Progesterone may also be used, although, in practice, the most widespread usage has been achieved by such synthetic progestogens as *megestrol acetate, medroxyprogesterone, chlormadinone* and *retroprogesterone* (Duphaston). "Depot" type preparations are here indicated especially.

ANDROGENS. Testosterone arrests or ostensibly slows down growth of uterine neoplasia, including malignancy. The question of antitumorigenic action on breast cancer by androgens and androgen derivatives has been exhaustively examined in a recent study by Clavero and Montalvo.[33]

A number of authors have been intrigued by the occurrence of androgens in the female organism (see Chapter 4), which has given rise to considerable speculation. In reality, this is just one more phenomenon aimed at maintaining the body's steroid balance or, in the words of Lipschütz,[88] *steroid homeostasis*. The balance between estrogens, on the one hand, and progesterone and testosterone, on the other, is necessary to prevent pathologic development of tissues pertaining to woman's genital tract.

CORTICOIDS. Probably by virtue of its great similarity to progesterone, deoxycorticosterone also acts as an antagonist of estrogens. This action has been studied in normal woman (Botella[16]) as well as in experimental hyperestrinism induced in guinea pigs (Lipschütz[88]).

OUTLINE OF STEROID HOMEOSTASIS. What we have said in the foregoing paragraphs enables us to draw a scheme of endocrine interrelations involved in setting up the estrogen-progesterone-androgen-corticoid balance. This balance is the basis of a self-defense mechanism against genital neoplasia, a concept recently championed by Lipschütz. The essence of this balance has been outlined in Figure 46-7. Under normal conditions, the ovary secretes estrogens and progesterone. Any increase in estrogenic activity elicits proliferation of basophilic cells in the pituitary and, as a result, increased secretion of gonadotropin B and ACTH. Gonadotropin B is thought to raise progesterone biogenesis by the ovary and androgen biogenesis by the adrenal sexual zone; the second, ACTH, increases the output of corticoids, among them deoxycorticosterone. The consequence of increased estrogenic activity in the presence of normal pituitary function is thus translated into compensatory secretion of corticoids, androgens and progesterone. *As a result, the normal organism is protected against the tumorigenic or tumoritrophic effect of estrogens by ovarian-pituitary correlation. Only when the existing correlation between the pituitary and the ovary is broken does hyperestrinism supervene with all its consequences.*

46.9.4. CONCLUSION

The preceding sections have been concerned with the genesis of genital carci-

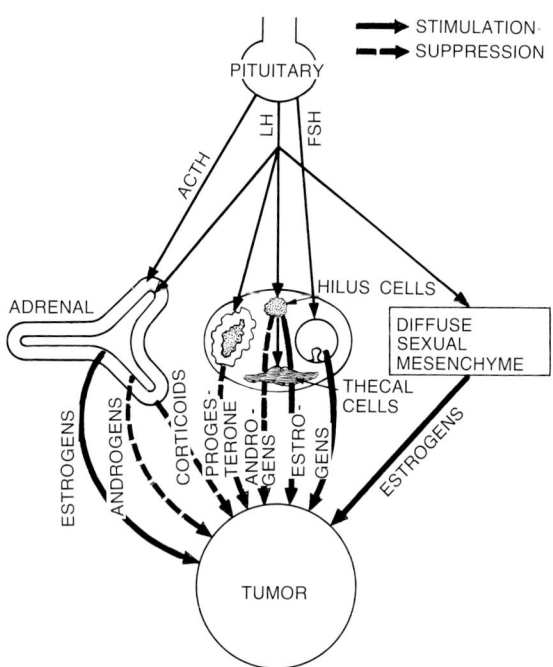

Figure 46-7. Diagram of steroid homeostasis. The carcinogenic effect of estrogens is offset by the actions of progesterone, androgens and corticoids. The principal sources of estrogens and androgens in the postmenopausal period are indicated here. Besides the classic sites of estrogen biogenesis, such additional sources as the adrenal sexual zone and the hilus cells and fibrothecal masses of the ovary must be taken into account. In addition, the presence of a "diffuse sexual mesenchyme" may be postulated to account for continued estrogen synthesis following castration and adrenalectomy.

nomas, with special reference to the human species. A special note of caution must be sounded with regard to a good many data obtained from animal experimentation, which actually lack validity when applied to woman. Although the oncogenetic process is essentially the same, the much faster evolution of growth in laboratory rodents and their different endocrino-sexual systems necessarily entail quite different forms of behavior under a variety of circumstances.

There seems to be no doubt that some hormones may act as accelerators of growth in certain tumors. It would also appear that neoplastic tissues basically preserve their ability to react to hormonal stimulants in much the same way as do their parent tissues. For instance, tumors of the uterus or of the breast react to estrogens, those of the adrenal to ACTH and those of the thyroid to thyrotrophic hormone. Any tumor arising in a target organ tends to grow at a rate dependent on the level of activity of those hormones which physiologically stimulate the target organ in question. This is, of course, far from saying that the hormones involved are carcinogenic. The concept of *carcinogenesis* ought thus to be compared with and distinguished from that of *carcinokinetics*. Aromatic hydrocarbons may be carcinogenic, but estrogens and the other hormones are only carcinokinetic. It is possible that certain steroids may, as a result of pathologic metabolic processes, be converted to substances endowed with direct carcinogenic activity. However, such a possibility has so far not been substantiated.

REFERENCES

1. Aguilar, A., and Botella, J.: *Acta Gin.*, 20:571, 1969.
2. Allen, A. R., and Fullmer, C. D.: *Acta Cytol.*, 13:485, 1969.
3. Andrews, W. C.: *Obstet. Gynec. Survey*, 16:747, 1961.
3a. Anthony, C. L., and Roddick, J. W.: *Amer. J. Obstet. Gynec.*, 83:1299, 1962.
4. Ashraf, M., and Zaaman, H.: *Acta Cytol.*, 13:347, 1969.
5. Atkin, N. B.: *Acta Cytol.*, 14:463, 1970.
6. Auersperg, N., and Wakonig-Vaartaja, T.: *Acta Cytol.*, 14:495, 1970.
7. Bamford, S. B., Mitchell, G. W., David, J., Sperber, A., and Cassin, C.: *Acta Cytol.*, 13:238, 1969.
8. Bauer, K. H., and Schweitzer, L. A.: In *Endocrine Aspects of Breast Cancer*, ed. Currie and Illingworth. Edinburgh, E. & S. Livingstone, 1958.
9. Bayer, J. M., Geissler, I. G., and Breuer, H.: *Klin. Wschr.*, 39:914, 1961.
10. Benjamin, F., and Casper, D. J.: *Amer. J. Obstet. Gynec.*, 94:991, 1966.
11. Bernard, H., Coste, F., Piguet, B., and Seemann, A.: *Ann. d'Endocr.*, 23:133, 1962.
12. Bernard, H., Bourdin, J. S., Saracino, R. T., and Seemann, A.: *Ann. d'Endocr.*, 24:17, 1963.
13. Bittner, J. J.: *Endocrinology*, 31:63, 1943.
14. Bjoro, K., and Mylins, E.: *Acta Path. Microbiol. Scand.*, 40:470, 1957.
15. Blanck, F.: *Arch. Surg.*, 49:301, 1944.
16. Botella, J.: *Acta Gin.*, 4:401, 1953.
17. Botella, J.: In *Proceedings of the 1st International Congress of Exfoliative Cytology*. Philadelphia, J. B. Lippincott, 1962.
18. Botella, J., Tornero, M. C., Montalvo, L., and Nogales, F.: *Acta Gin.*, 13:69, 1962.
19. Boyland, E.: *Ciba Colloquia on Endocrinology*, 12:194, 1959.
20. Bret, A. J., and Bardiaux, M.: *Rev. Franç. Gynec.*, 50:194, 1955.
21. Bret, J. A., and Coupez, F.: *Acta Cytol.*, 4:116, 1960.
22. Bromberg, Y. M., Liban, E., and Laufer, A.: *Obstet. Gynec.*, 14:221, 1959.
23. Brown, J. B., and Blair, H. A. F.: *J. Endocr.*, 17:411, 1958; 19:52, 1959.
24. Brown, J. B.: In *Endocrine Aspects of Breast Cancer*. Edinburgh, E. & S. Livingstone, 1958.
25. Brunschwig, A., and Papanicolaou, G. N.: *Cancer*, 10:1, 1957.
26. Bulbrook, R. D., Greenwood, F. C., Hadfield, G. J., and Scowen, E. F.: *Brit. Med. J.*, 1:7, 1958.
27. Bulbrook, R. D., and Hayward, J. L.: *Lancet*, 1:159, 1967.
28. Burrows, H.: *Brit. Med. J.*, 4:971, 1947.
29. Burrows, H., and Horning, E. S.: *Brit. Med. J.*, 4:975, 1947.
30. Cade, S.: In *Endocrine Aspects of Breast Cancer*. Edinburgh, E. & S. Livingstone, 1958.
31. Cherry, S. H., and Tovell, M. M.: *Amer. J. Obstet. Gynec.*, 83:1294, 1962.
32. Cianfrani, T.: *Amer. J. Obstet. Gynec.*, 69:64, 1955.
33. Clavero, J. A., and Montalvo, L.: *Acta Gin.*, 13:453, 1962.
34. Cook, J. W., and Kennaway, E. L.: *Nature*, 145:627, 1940.
35. Descoeudres, C.: *Helv. Chim. Acta*, 35:497, 1968.
36. Diczfalusy, E., et al.: In *Endocrine Aspects of Breast Cancer*. Edinburgh, E. & S. Livingstone, 1958.
37. Diczfalusy, E., and Lauritzen, C.: *Oestrogene beim Menschen*. Berlin, Springer Verlag, 1961.
38. Dockerty, M. B., and Mussey, E.: *Amer. J. Obstet. Gynec.*, 61:147, 1951.
39. Dockerty, M. B., Lovelady, S. B., and Faust, G. T.: *Amer. J. Obstet. Gynec.*, 61:966, 1951.
40. Dodds, E. C., Lawson, W., and Williams, P. C.: *Nature*, 41:614, 1943.
41. Dodds, E. C., Lawson, W., and Williams, P. C.:

42. Dominguez, O. V., and Houseby, R. A.: *Endocrinology*, 84:1039, 1969.
43. Dowsett, J. W.: *Amer. J. Obstet. Gynec.*, 86:622, 1963.
44. Emge, L. A.: *Obstet. Gynec.*, 20:915, 1962.
45. Fekete, E., and Little, C. C.: *Cancer Res.*, 2:525, 1962.
46. Finkbeiner, J. A.: *Acta Cytol.*, 4:121, 1960.
47. Forrest, A. P. M., et al.: *Endocrine Aspects of Breast Cancer.* Edinburgh, E. & S. Livingstone, 1958.
48. Frachtman, K. G.: *Amer. J. Obstet. Gynec.*, 81:779, 1961.
49. Freemont-Smith, M.: *J.A.M.A.*, 131:805, 1946.
50. Furth, P. I., and Clifton, K. H.: *Ciba Colloquia on Endocrinology*, 12:3, 1959.
51. Gardner, W. U.: *Ciba Colloquia on Endocrinology*, 12:153, 1959.
52. Gough, L., and Shopee, C. W.: *Biochem. J.*, 54:630, 1953.
53. Greene, J. W.: *Amer. J. Obstet. Gynec.*, 74:31, 1957.
54. Greene, J. W.: *Amer. J. Obstet. Gynec.*, 81:272, 1961.
55. Gusberg, S. B.: *Clin. Obstet. Gynec.*, 1:559, 1958.
56. Gusberg, S. B., and Hall, R. E.: *Obstet. Gynec.*, 17:397, 1961.
57. Haddow, A.: *Brit. Med. Bull.*, 14:79, 1950.
58. Hadfield, G.: *Endocrine Aspects of Breast Cancer.* Edinburgh, E. & S. Livingstone, 1958.
59. Haour, P.: *Acta Cytol.*, 3:631, 1959.
60. Hausknecht, R. U., and Gusberg, S. B.: *Amer. J. Obstet. Gynec.*, 105:1161, 1969.
61. Hertig, A. T.: *Cancer*, 10:838, 1959.
62. Hertig, A. T., and Sommers, S. C.: *Cancer*, 2:946, 1949.
63. Hieger, I.: *Brit. Med. Bull.*, 14:159, 1958.
64. Hormeister, F. J., and Vondrak, B. T.: *Amer. J. Obstet. Gynec.*, 107:1099, 1970.
65. Huggins, C., and Dao, T. L. Y.: *J.A.M.A.*, 151:1388, 1953.
66. Huggins, C. H.: *Science*, 156:1050, 1967.
67. Husslein, H.: *Zbl. Gynäk.*, 73:1649, 1951.
68. Hustin, J., and Buret, J.: *Bull. Roy. Soc. Belg. Gyn. Obst.*, 37:405, 1967.
69. Ingraham, J. M., and Novak, E.: *Amer. J. Obstet. Gynec.*, 61:774, 1951.
70. Irvine, W. T., et al.: *Lancet*, 2:791, 1961.
71. Jabara, A. G.: *Brit. J. Cancer*, 21:418, 1967.
72. Jackson, R. L., and Dockerty, M. B.: *Amer. J. Obstet. Gynec.*, 73:161, 1957.
73. Jones, H. W., Davis, H. J., Frost, J. K., Park, I. J., Salimi, R., Tseng, P. Y., and Woodruff, J. D.: *Amer. J. Obstet. Gynec.*, 102:624, 1968.
74. Jull, J. W., Schucksmith, H. S., and Bonser, G. M.: *J. Clin. Endocr.*, 23:433, 1963.
75. Jull, J. W., Streeter, D. J., and Sutherland, L.: *J. Nat. Cancer Inst.*, 37:409, 1966.
76. Kambouris, A. A., Saltzstein, H. C., and Scheinberg, S.: *Amer. J. Surg.*, 102:651, 1961.
77. Karpas, C. M., and Speer, F. O.: *Arch. Pathol.*, 63:17, 1957.
78. Kauffman, R. H., Abbott, J. P., and Wall, J. A.: *Amer. J. Obstet. Gynec.*, 77:1271, 1959.
79. King, R. J. B., Gordon, J., Cown, D. M., and Inman, D. R.: *J. Endocr.*, 36:139, 1966.
80. Kistner, L.: *Clin. Obstet. Gynec.*, 9:271, 1966.
81. Kottmeier, H. L.: *Amer. J. Obstet. Gynec.*, 78:1127, 1959.
82. Kruschwitz, S.: *Zbl. Gynäk.*, 89:1199, 1967.
83. Kushinsky, S., Demetrou, J. A., Wu, J., and Nasutavicus, W.: *J. Clin. Endocr.*, 20:719, 1960.
84. Laccassagne, A.: *Rev. Franç. Gyn.*, 56:757, 1961.
85. Larson, J. A.: *Obstet. Gynec.*, 3:551, 1954.
86. Lemon, H. M., and Parsons, L.: *J.A.M.A.*, 196:1128, 1966.
87. Lemon, H. M.: *Cancer*, 23:781, 1969.
88. Lipschütz, A.: *Steroid Hormones and Tumors.* Baltimore, Williams & Wilkins, 1950.
89. Lipschütz, A.: *Gynaecologia*, 156:93, 1963.
90. Little, C. C.: *Amer. J. Obstet. Gynec.*, 61-A:64, 1951.
91. Liu, W.: *Cancer*, 8:779, 1955.
92. Loraine, J. A.: *Endocrine Aspects of Breast Cancer.* Edinburgh, E. & S. Livingstone, 1958.
93. Luft, L., and Olivecrona, H.: *Endocrine Aspects of Breast Cancer.* Edinburgh, E. & S. Livingstone, 1958.
94. Mansell, H., and Hertig, A. T.: *Obstet. Gynec.*, 6:385, 1955.
95. Marcus, C. C.: *Obstet. Gynec.*, 21:175, 1963.
96. Medes, G., and Reimann, S. P.: *Normal Growth and Cancer.* Philadelphia, J. B. Lippincott, 1963.
97. Meisels, A.: *Cancer Res.*, 26:757, 1966.
98. Meyer, R. K., and Clifton, K. H.: *Endocrinology*, 58:686, 1956.
99. Mobbs, B. G.: *Proc. Amer. Ass. Cancer Res.*, 10:60, 1969.
100. Montalvo, L., J.: *Acta Gin.*, 14:353, 1963.
101. Morris, J. M. L., and Scully, R. E.: *Endocrine Pathology of the Ovary.* St. Louis, C. V. Mosby, 1958.
102. Mühlbock, O., and Boot, L. M.: *Ciba Symposium on Carcinogenesis.* London, Churchill, 1959.
103. Mühlbock, O., and Boot, L. M.: *Biochem. Pharmac.*, 16:627, 1967.
104. Munguia, H., and Franco, E.: *Acta Cytol.*, 4:135, 1960.
105. Nes, W. R., and Mosettig, E.: *J. Amer. Chem. Soc.*, 75:2787, 1953.
106. Netter, A., and Gouris, A.: *Ann. d'Endocr.*, 22:638, 1961.
107. Nieburgs, H. E.: *Amer. J. Obstet. Gynec.*, 62:93, 1951.
108. Nilsen, P. A.: *Acta Obstet. Gynec. Scand.*, Suppl. 3, 48:120, 1969.
109. Nissen-Meyer, R., and Sanner, T.: *Acta Endocr.*, 44:325, 1963.
110. Nogales, F.: *Acta Gin.*, 1:301, 1950.
111. Nogales, F., Tornero, M. C., and Montalvo, L.: *Estado del Ovario en el Adenocarcinoma del Endometrio,* V Reunión de los Ginecólogos Españoles, Las Palmas de Gran Canaria, 1962.
112. Nordqvist, S.: *Acta Obstet. Gynec. Scand.*, Suppl. 3, 48:118, 1969.
113. Novak, E., and Rutledge, F.: *Amer. J. Obstet. Gynec.*, 55:46, 1948.
114. Novak, E.: *Amer. J. Obstet. Gynec.*, 71:1312, 1956.
115. Nuovo, V.: *Acta Cytol.*, 4:119, 1960.
116. Pearlman, W. H., De Hertogh, R., Laumas, K.

R., and Pearlman, W. R. J.: *J. Clin. Endocr.*, 29:707, 1969.
117. Pérez-Modrego, S.: *Acta Oncológica*, 2:121, 1963.
118. Peters, H., and Levy, E.: *Fertil. Steril.*, 15:407, 1964.
119. Plunkett, E. R., and Gammal, E. B.: *Brit. J. Cancer*, 21:592, 1967.
120. Printer, K. D.: *J. Obstet. Gynec. Brit. Comm.*, 70:303, 1963.
121. Pyrah, L. N.: In *Endocrine Aspects of Breast Cancer.* Edinburgh, E. & S. Livingstone, 1958.
122. Roddick, J. W., and Greene, R. R.: *Amer. J. Obstet. Gynec.*, 73:843, 1957; 75:1015, 1958.
123. Roy, B. S., and Pearson, O. H.: In *Endocrine Aspects of Breast Cancer.* Edinburgh, E. & S. Livingstone, 1958.
124. Rubio, C. A., Hvalec, S., and Pareja, A.: *Acta Cytol.*, 11:176, 1967.
125. Sanders, S.: *Acta Pathol. Microbiol. Scand.*, 75:520, 1969.
126. Sandison, A. T.: In *Endocrine Aspects of Breast Cancer.* Edinburgh, E. & S. Livingstone, 1958.
127. Seshadri, R., Shah, P. N., and Trivedi, M. B.: *Acta Cytol.*, 14:3, 1970.
128. Sherman, A. I., and Woolf, R. B.: *Amer. J. Obstet. Gynec.*, 77:233, 1959.
129. Sicher, K., and Waterhouse, J. A. H.: *Brit. J. Cancer*, 21:512, 1967.
130. Sirtori, C.: *Acta Cytol.*, 4:170, 1960.
131. Sjöstedt, S., and Wahlen, T.: *Acta Obstet. Gynec. Scand.*, 40: Suppl. 6, 1961.
132. Slate, W. G., and Bradbury, J. T.: *Endocrinology*, 70:1, 1962.
133. Sommers, S. C., and Wadman, P. J.: *Amer. J. Obstet. Gynec.*, 72:160, 1956.
134. Sommers, S. C., and Meissner, W. A.: *Cancer*, 10:516, 1957.
135. Speert, H.: *Amer. J. Obstet. Gynec.*, 67:547, 947, 1949.
136. Stanley, M. A., Bingham, D. A., Cox, R. I., and Opitz, L. J.: *Lancet*, 1:690, 1966.
137. Stanley, M. A., and Kirkland, J. A.: *Acta Cytol.*, 13:76, 1969.
138. Stanley, M. A., and Kirkland, J. A.: *Amer. J. Obstet. Gynec.*, 102:1070, 1968.
139. Sterenthal, A., et al.: *Cancer Res.*, 23:481, 1963.
140. Stewart, J. G., Skinner, L. G., and O'Connor, P. J.: *Acta Endocr.*, 50:345, 1965.
141. Stokes, E. M.: *West. J. Surg.*, 56:946, 1949.
142. Stoll, B. A.: *Brit. Med. J.*, 1:150, 1967.
143. Sydnor, K., and Cockrell, B.: *Endocrinology*, 73:427, 1963.
144. Symington, T., et al.: *Ciba Colloquia on Endocrinology*, 12:102, 1958.
145. Taylor, H.: *Lancet*, 7224:325, 1962.
146. Teller, M. N., Kaufman, R. J., Bowie, M., and Stock, C. C.: *Cancer Res.*, 29:349, 1969.
147. Twombley, G. M., Scheiner, S., and Levitz, M.: *Amer. J. Obstet. Gynec.*, 82:424, 1961.
148. Varga, A., and Henriksen, E.: *Obstet. Gynec.*, 22:129, 1963.
149. Varga, A., and Henriksen, E.: *Obstet. Gynec.*, 26:656, 1965.
150. Vere, R. D., and Dempsey, R. K.: *J. Obstet. Gynec. Brit. Emp.*, 60:865, 1953.
151. Wachtel, E.: *Acta Cytol.*, 2:633, 1958.
152. Wachtel, E.: *Acta Cytol.*, 11:35, 1967.
153. Wied, G. L.: *Acta Cytol.*, 2:269, 1958.
154. Winkhaus, I. S., and Taylor, H. C.: *Obstet. Gynec.*, 19:748, 1962.
155. Woll, E. A., Hertig, A. T., Smith, G. van, and Johnson, L. C.: *Amer. J. Obstet. Gynec.*, 56:617, 1958.

Chapter 47

ORAL CONTRACEPTIVES

47.1. INTRODUCTION

In Chapter 3 we have already indicated the chemistry of the new synthetic progestogens and analyzed the modalities of their physiologic actions. It is now indispensable that we study their antiovulatory activity.

The antiovulatory properties of progesterone were discovered by Haberlandt[50] in 1929. However, the application of the so-called principle of "hormonal sterility of Haberlandt" was found to be impracticable because of the high dosages of progesterone required and the prohibitive cost of progesterone which, at that time, was obtainable only through natural extraction. It was not until 27 years later that the synthesis of a series of orally potent progestogens, achieved by Djerassy and associates,[27] was to render the practical application of the foregoing principle possible.

The pharmaceutic industry stepped in and lost no time in synthesizing an important series of progestational compounds—active by mouth and of low toxicity—which exerted a dependable antiovulatory effect. It thus became possible in theory to achieve contraception in a much simpler and much more innocuous way than had been possible with any of the hitherto available procedures. Pincus and Rock[97, 98] developed *Norethynodrel*, a new compound possessing potent antiovulatory activity, and tested it on a large scale among the population of Puerto Rico. In 1958, Pincus and his associates[41, 42] reported the first results of their "field trial in Puerto Rico," in which 365 women had volunteered to submit to the test, involving inhibition of ovulation in a total of 1857 cycles. Since the results of the experiment proved to be extraordinarily dependable, the few failures observed being invariably attributable to the fact that the woman had forgotten to take her tablets, the "pill" has since gained so much popularity that the number of women currently using it habitually may be estimated to run into the millions.

It would be impossible to summarize here the enormous amount of work done in the field, and we are unable even to enumerate all the products with contraceptive activity that have been synthesized to date. Nor can we enter the even vaster terrain of orally active progestogens, some of which, while possessing no antiovulatory activity, are able to exert a contraceptive effect. For the study of these questions, we shall refer the reader to various colloquia and general studies.[6, 51, 100, 133, 134, 135, 136]

The reader will notice that we are not using the term "antiovulatory" but instead prefer the term "contraceptive." This is because we have ascertained over the past years that these compounds not only produce temporary infertility by causing anovulation but also act by virtue of other contraceptive mechanisms (affecting the uterine cervix, endometrium, Fallopian tubes, and nidation).

We shall cover the following topics: (1) Chemistry of steroids employed for contraception; (2) action of contraceptives on the genital tract; (3) action on hormone production and excretion; (4) action on basal body temperatures; (5) mode of contraceptive action; (6) modes of administration; (7) toxic effects; (8) long-range effects.

47.2. CHEMISTRY OF CONTRACEPTIVE STEROIDS

While all the contraceptives are steroids, not all of them are progestogens and there is as yet no certainty that they all prevent

Oral Contraceptives

conception by the same mechanism. For a better understanding of their chemical structures, it must be remembered that all steroid hormones are essentially derived from three basic hydrocarbons: (1) *estrane*, with 18 carbon atoms; (2) *androstane*, with 19 carbon atoms, and (3) *pregnane*, with 21 carbon atoms.

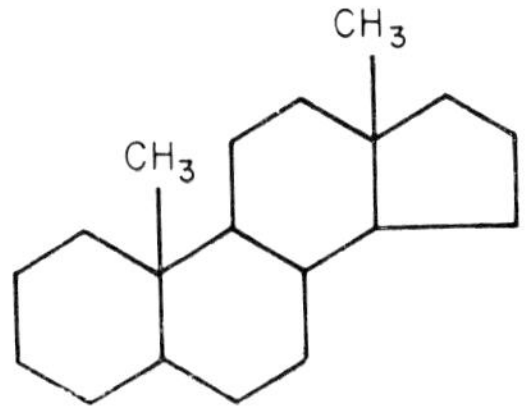

ESTRANE

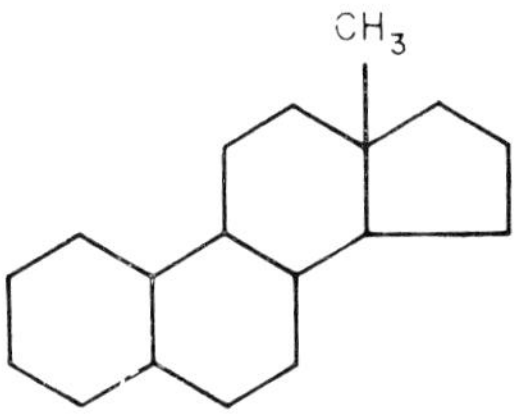

ANDROSTANE

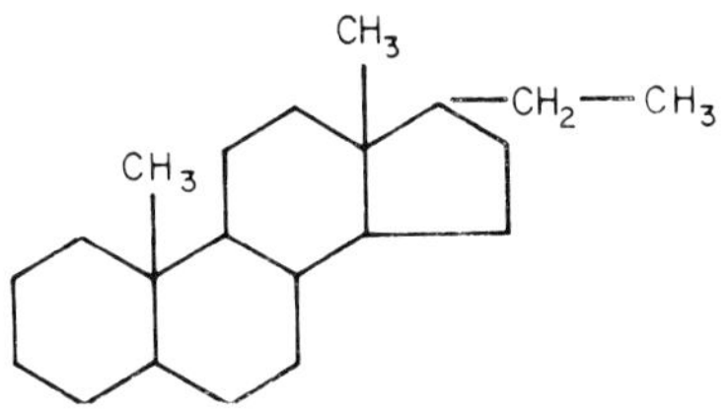

PREGNANE

Estrogens are all derived from estrane; androgens from androstane; and progestogens and corticoids from pregnane. The most representative member of each of the three series are: *estradiol*, or hormone of the ovarian follicle; *testosterone*, or hormone of the testicular interstitium; and *progesterone*, or hormone of the corpus luteum.

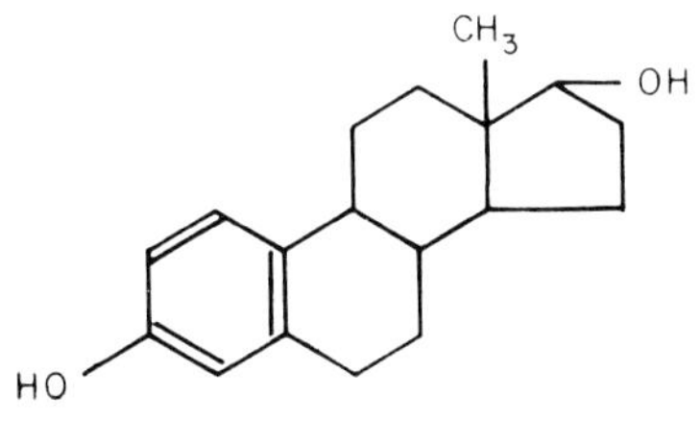

ESTRADIOL

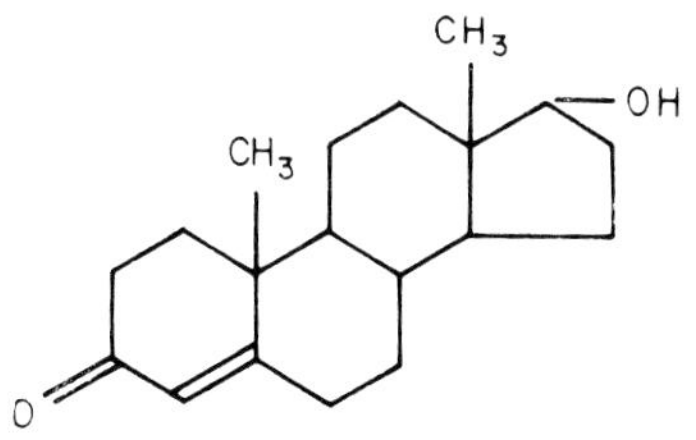

TESTOSTERONE

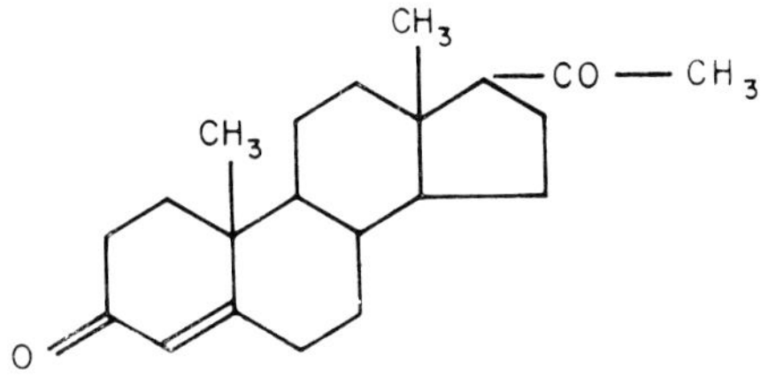

PROGESTERONE

Each of the three groups—estrogens, androgens and progestogens—has antiovulatory properties. In practice, however, androgens are not utilized for preventing ovulation. The antiovulatory action of androgens by way of the hypothalamus has already been discussed in Chapters 29, 38 and 41. We shall be concerned here only with progestogens and estrogens.

47.2.1. SYNTHETIC PROGESTOGENS

For many years, the only progestogen known was progesterone, whose hydroxylated derivative at carbon 17—17-hydroxyprogesterone—was inactive. The esters of 17-hydroxyprogesterone were not inactive, however. For instance, the caproate has been the basis for the well-known therapy with depot type preparations (Proluton depot, Delalutin).

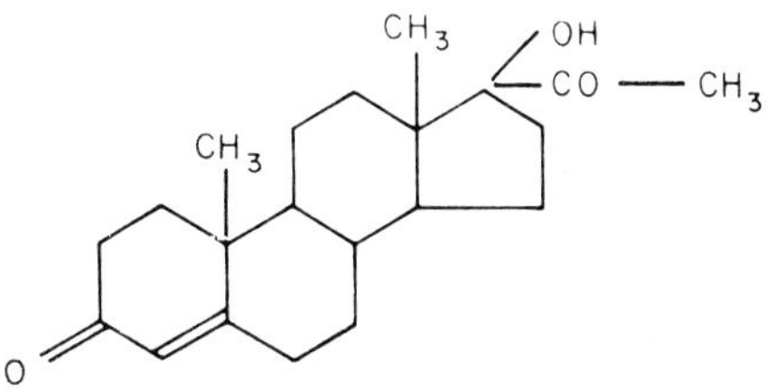

17-α-HYDROXYPROGESTERONE

17-α-HYDROXYPROGESTERONE CAPROATE

Since, over the past years, a host of new progestogens have been created, and their numbers keep increasing virtually day by day, it would be pretentious to attempt a complete description of all of them. We shall confine ourselves to the principal ones.

DERIVATION. These compounds are all derived from a few basic modifications of the progesterone molecule, which has been described in Chapter 3 (page 38).

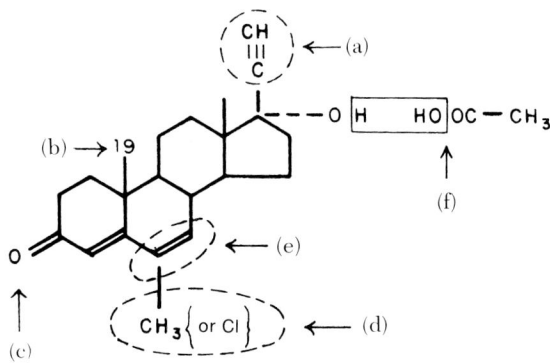

PROGESTERONE

The action of progesterone is reinforced by any of the seven following modifications:

(a) Introduction of a triple bond between carbons 20 and 21, resulting in the synthesis of *pregneninolone*, or *ethisterone* (first developed in 1938), or in the synthesis of *norethisterone* and *norethynodrel*, the compounds initially employed by Pincus and associates.[98, 99]

(b) Suppression of the methyl group at carbon 19, giving rise to compounds known as *norderivatives*, which, in addition to *methylnortestosterone* and *ethylnortestosterone*, include the above-mentioned compounds norethynodrel and norethisterone, each of the latter involving both modification a and modification b.

(c) Loss of the ketone group at carbon 3, giving rise to a series of *estrenols*, principally *allylestrenol*, which apart from showing the ketone group loss is a norderivative (involving modification b), and *lynestrenol*, involving all three modifications, a, b, and c. (The formula of each compound is shown below.)

Pharmacologic studies have demonstrated that the presence of any or all of the foregoing modifications conferred additional progestational potency on the molecule.

(d) The fourth type of modification consists in the introduction of either a methyl group or halogen side chain at carbon 6. This type of 6-derivation gives rise to *medroxyprogesterone*, *megesterol*, *megestrol*, *metrogestone* and *melengestrol*, each carrying a methyl radical, and to *chlormadinone*, carrying a halogen (chlorine). With the exception of medroxyprogesterone and megesterol, each of these compounds also involves the next type of modification (e).

(e) Appearance of a double bond in position 6-7 (Δ6 derivatives). This modification is present, as we have said, in the first four preparations of the preceding category, as well as in the modern preparation known as G.M. 101. In this category we might also include the Δ5 derivatives which, although not identical, have a double bond in position 5-6, such as *gestovis* (Vismara) and *gestovister* (Vister).

(f) Nearly all modern preparations are based on *acetic esterification* at carbon 17. They are thus derived from 17α-hydroxyprogesterone. The previously mentioned compounds *medroxyprogesterone*, *megesterol*, *chlormadinone*, *megestrol* and *melengestrol acetate* and *metrogestone* also belong to this group. They all involve modi-

Oral Contraceptives 1029

fication *d* and, with the exception of *medroxyprogesterone* and *megestrol*, also modification *e*.

(g) The addition of a cyclopentyl group to position 3 in an enolic ether linkage results in three modern preparations: *quingesterone, quingestanol* and the previously mentioned *gestovis*. The last two also involve modification *f* (acetic esterification), while the first two involve modification *e* (double bond in position Δ5).

The preceding systematization has been designed to facilitate the understanding of the relationship between structure and function of this quite heterogeneous group of compounds. Let us now describe those derivatives individually.

ETHINYL DERIVATIVES. This was the first series to be known. It was inaugurated by *pregneninolone*, synthesized in 1938 by Hohlweg and Inhoffen in Germany, and called *ethisterone* by the Americans. It is a 17-ethinyl-17β,4-androstene-3-one.

PREGNENINOLONE (ETHISTERONE-PRANONE)

Its commercial names are Proluton C (Schering-Berlin), Pranone (Schering of America), Lutocyclin (Ciba) and Oralutin (Parke Davis). It is practically no longer in use, having been displaced by more modern preparations.

Other compounds pertaining to this group are norethisterone, norethynodrel, ethynodiol acetate, norethisterone acetate, quingestanol and WY-3707. Since all are also norderivatives, they will be studied under that heading.

NORDERIVATIVES. One of the modifications imparting a higher degree of progestational potency to the molecule is the disappearance of the methyl group in position 19. In fact, this discovery, made by the biochemists of Syntex,[27] has been practically the whole basis for the development of the "pill."

The principal norderivatives are: *methyl-nortesterone*, which is a 17-methyl-17β-hydroxy-4-estren-3-one. It was commercially prepared by Organon of Oss, Holland, but owing to its virilizing effect, it is no longer in use.

17-α-METHYL-19-NORTESTOSTERONE
(ORGASTERONE)

Another preparation in this series is *ethyl-nortestosterone*, known by the commercial name of Nilevar, which has anabolizing properties. It is a 17-ethyl-17β-hydroxy-4-estren-3-one.

17-α-ETHYL-NORTESTOSTERONE
(NILEVAR)

However, the two really important compounds in this series, the first ones to be employed for their antiovulatory activity, are respectively *norpregneninolone*, or *norethisterone*, and *norethynodrel*. Both are 17-ethinyl-derivatives and have therefore already been mentioned in the preceding section.

Norpregneninolone, as it is called by the Germans, or *norethisterone* by the Americans, is known commercially as Primolut-N (Schering), Primolut-Nor (in South America), Norlutin (Syntex, Parke Davis) and is a 17β-ethinyl-17β-hydroxy-4-estren-3-one.

17α-ETHYNYL-19-NORTESTOSTERONE
(NORESTHISTERONE, NORPREGNENINOLONE
PRIMOLUT-N
NORLUTIN)

Norethynodrel, which is the tablet originally used by Pincus in Puerto Rico, has been known in the United States as Enovid (Searle) and in Europe, from the same manufacturer, as Enavid. It is an isomer of the preceding compounds, 17α-ethinyl-17β-hydroxy-5(10)-estren-3-one.

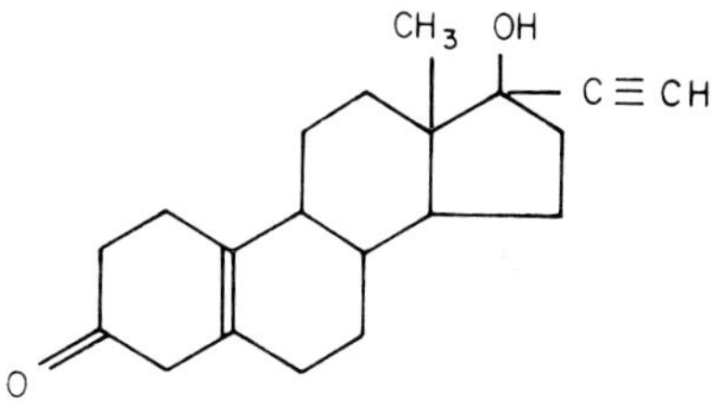

NORETHYNODREL

ESTRENOLS. The manufacturing company Organon at Oss, Holland, synthesized two estrenol derivatives, lacking the ketone group at carbon 3, which are at the same time norderivatives. One has an allyl, the other an ethinyl, group at carbon 17.

The first one, *allylestrenol*, known by the commercial name of Gestanon (or Gestanin, depending on the country), is a 17-allyl-4-estren-17β-ol.

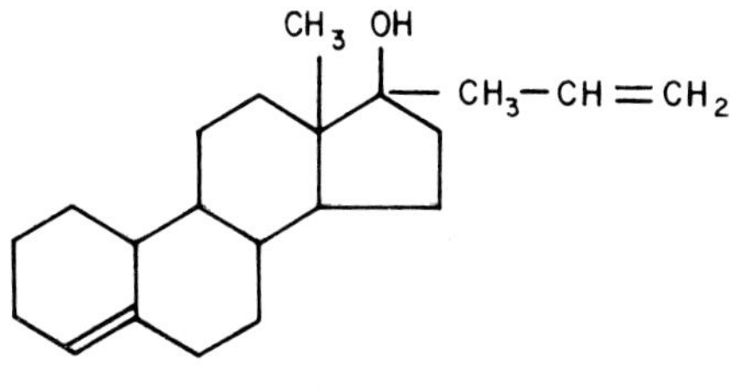

ALLYLESTRENOL (GESTANON)

The second one, *lynestrenol* (Lyndiol, Organon; Anacyclin, Ciba), is known in the United States as Orgametrin (Organon). It is a 17-ethinyl-4-estren-17β-ol.

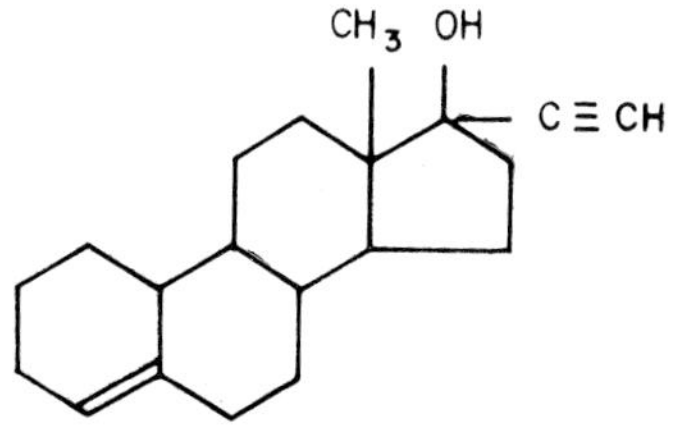

LYNESTRENOL

6-DERIVATIVES. In this group, we include all compounds with a methyl group or a chlorine in position 6. Most are compounds that have been synthesized more recently. This type of modification is incompatible with 19-norderivation. Such preparations are derived from progesterone.

Best known in this group is *medroxyprogesterone acetate*, sold under the commercial name of Provera (Upjohn), which in combination with an estrogen, and manufactured by the same company, is known as Provest. It is a 17α-hydroxy-6α-methyl-4-pregnene-3,20-dione acetate.

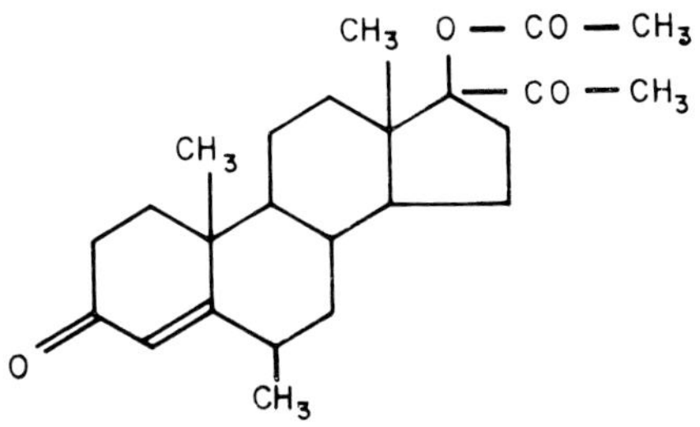

MEDROXYPROGESTERONE ACETATE
(PROVERA)

The same derivative, with a double bond between carbons 6-7, is *megestrol acetate* (Volidan, B.D.H.), which is a 17α-hydroxy-6-methyl-4,6-pregnadiene-3, 20-dione acetate.

Melengestrol acetate is an analogous compound which, however, has not been marketed and is therefore not described here. On the other hand, a compound of great interest is *chlormadinone* (Lutoral, Syntex), which is a 17α-hydroxy-6-chloro-4,6-pregnadiene-3,20-dione acetate.

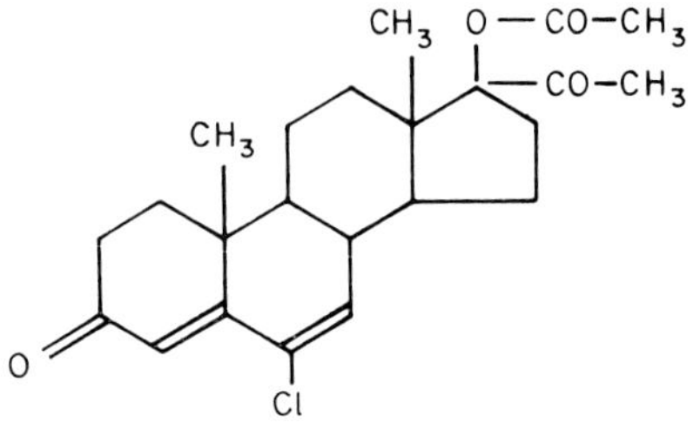

CHLORMADINONE

To this group, finally, also belongs *metrogestone*, the only compound in this category that is not an acetate. It is known by the commercial name of AY-62022 (Ayerst), and is a 6,17α-dimethyl-4,6-pregnadiene-3,20-dione.

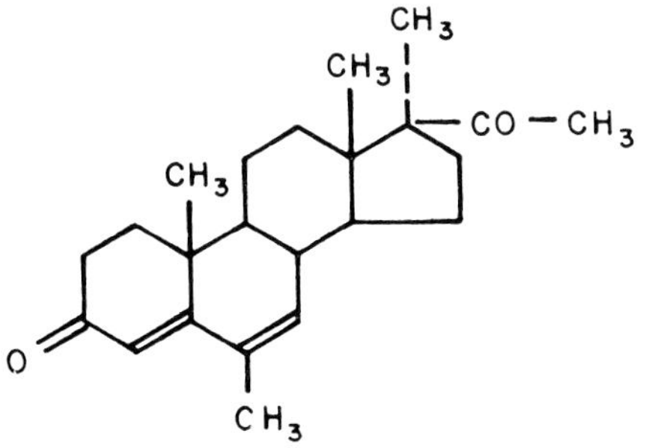

METROGESTRONE

ACETATES. As a matter of fact, all acetylated compounds occur in combination with some of the other derivatives described and thus have already been quoted in one place or another. Let us remember, among others, Provera, Norlutate, chlormadinone, the acetates of megestrol, megesterol and melengestrol. Still to be studied, however, are the derivatives of quingestanol.

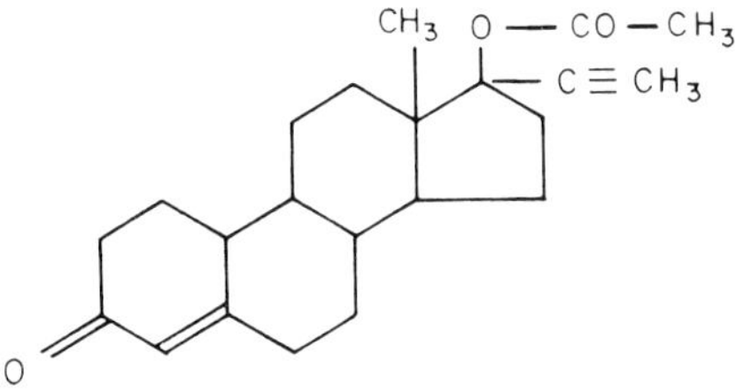

NORETHISTERONE ACETATE
(NORLUTATE)

Ethynodiol diacetate (Metrulen, Searle) also belongs to this group. It is a 17α-ethinyl-4-estrene-3β,17-diol acetate.

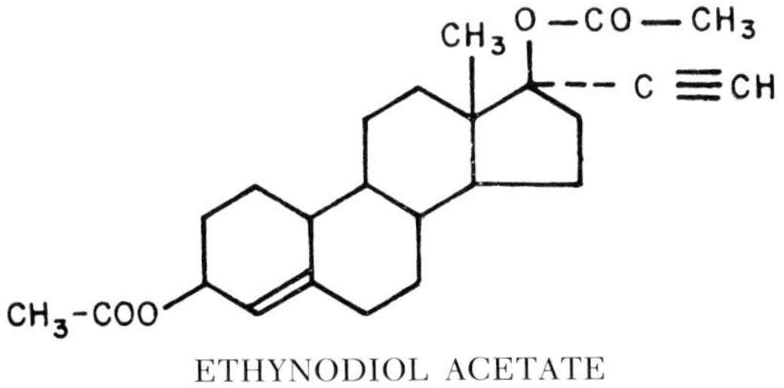

ETHYNODIOL ACETATE

Norethisterone acetate (norethindrone acetate) is known by the commercial names Norlutate (Syntex, Parke Davis) and Anovlar (Schering) (in Spain, Anovial, instead of Anovlar). It is a 17α-ethinyl-17β-hydroxy-4-estren-3-one acetate.

This group also includes lynestrenol and allylestrenol, both mentioned previously, quingestanol and WY-3707. The last compound has been recently synthesized by Wyeth and is a 13β-ethyl-17α-ethinyl-17-hydroxy-estren-3-one.

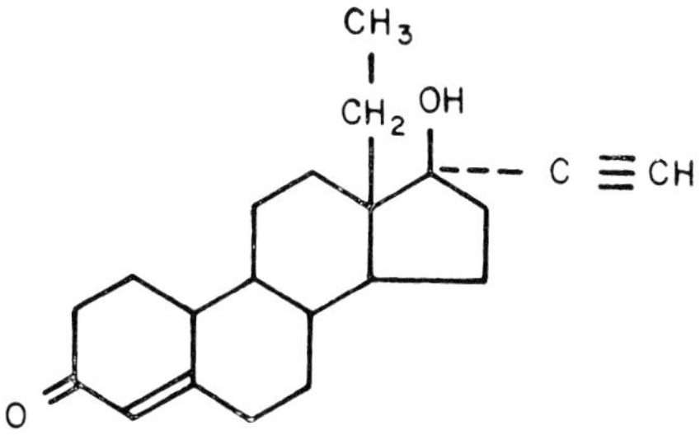

13-β-ETHYL-NORETHISTERONE
(WYETH 3707)

CYCLOPENTYL DERIVATIVES. These interesting compounds, incorporating a cyclopentane by means of an enolic ether linkage to position 3, are represented by three commercial preparations: *quingestrone* (Gestovister), which is a progesterone-3-cyclopentyl enol ether.

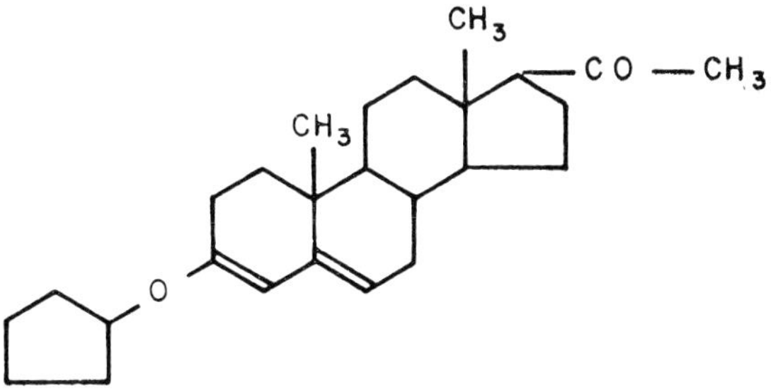

QUINGESTRONE (GESTOVISTER)

A quite similar compound is *Gestovis* (by Vismara) which is an enolic ether of 17α-acetoxyprogesterone-cyclopentyl.

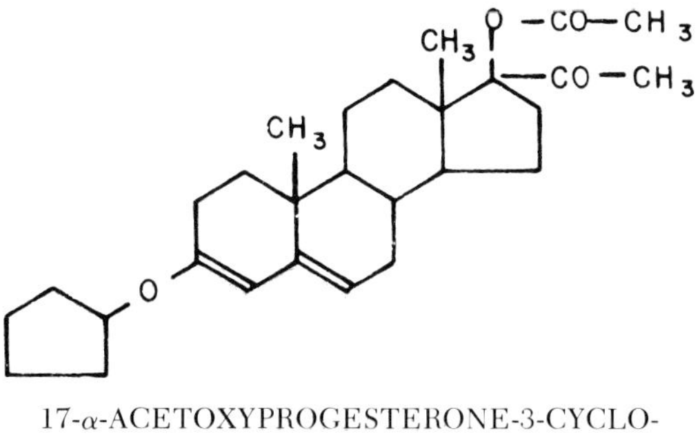

17-α-ACETOXYPROGESTERONE-3-CYCLO-
PENTYL-ENOL-ETHER (GESTOVIS)

Finally, the compound known as ENTA Ac-5 (Vismara) is *quingestanol acetate*, corresponding to Norlutate enol ether (17α-ethinyl-17β-acetoxy-4-estren-3-enol ether).

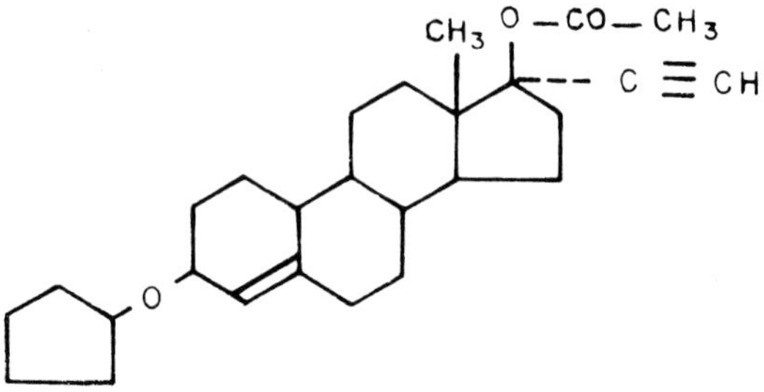

QUINGESTANOL ACETATE

RETROPROGESTERONE. Carbon 9 of progesterone is assymmetrical, allowing a hydrogen atom to be in either a "cis" or a "trans" position with regard to the plane of the molecule. The latter modality gives rise to compounds known as *retroprogesterones*, the most popular of which is 6-dehydroretroprogesterone or Duphaston (Phillips-Duphar; Phillips-Roxane, in America), whose chemical name is 9β,10α-pregna-4,6-diene-3,20-dione.

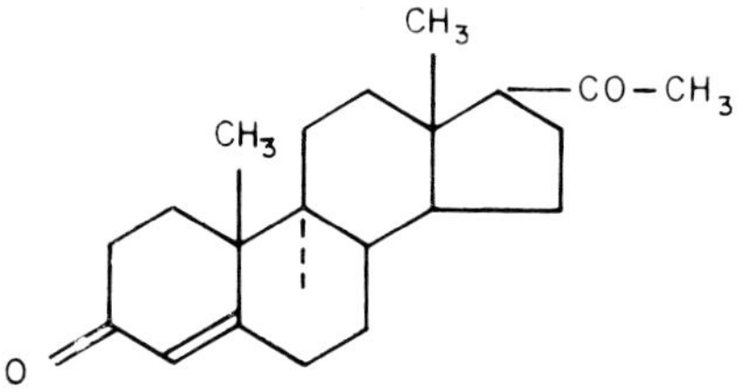

PROGESTERONE SPATIAL FORMULA

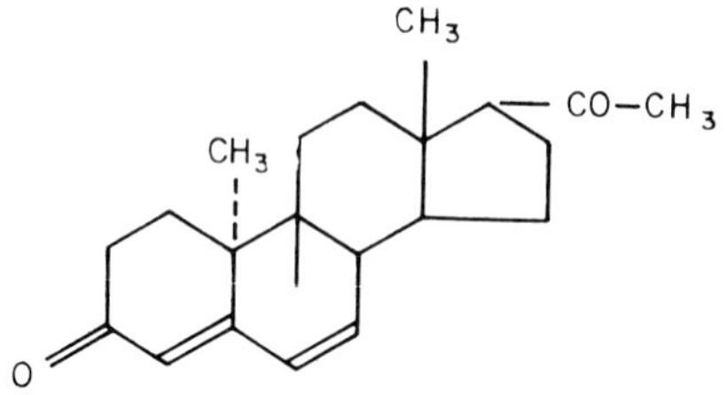

6-7 DEHYDRORETROPROGESTERONE
(DUPHASTRON)

47.2.2. ESTROGENS

In Chapter 2 (page 15), we have indicated the great variety of commercially available synthetic estrogens. In spite of this, however, only two have been employed for purposes of ovulation inhibition: *ethinylestradiol* and *mestranol*.

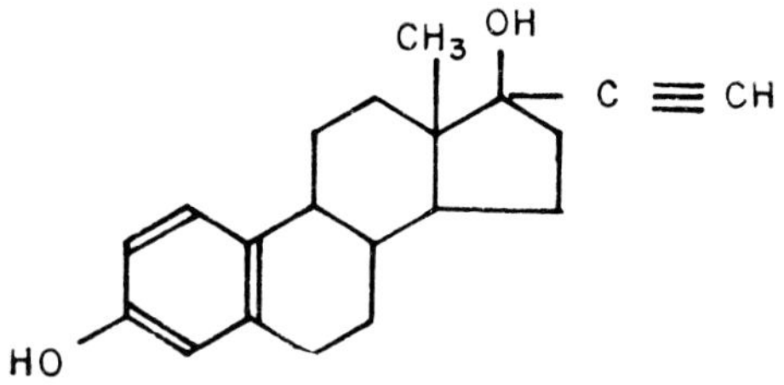

ETHINYLESTRADIOL

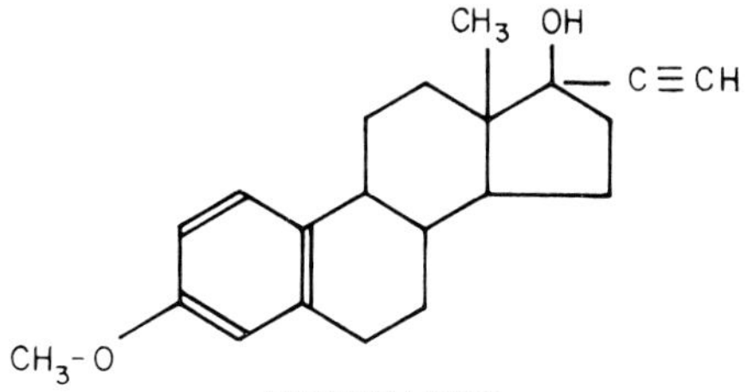

MESTRANOL
(ETHINYLESTRADIOL-METHYLESTER)

The second compound, *mestranol*, is an ethinylestradiol derivative, chemically corresponding to a 17β-ethinyl-17-hydroxy-1,3,5-estratriene-3-methyl ether.

Both ethinylestradiol and mestranol exert a potent estrogenic action but are not degraded by the liver. They are largely eliminated in the urine and in the bile.[146]

47.3. EFFECTS OF CONTRACEPTIVE STEROIDS ON THE ANIMAL AND HUMAN GENITAL TRACTS

The action by these compounds on the various organs of the female genital tract has been the object of particular attention.

47.3.1. ACTION ON THE OVARY

Baker and associates[1] (rats), Greenwald[49] (golden hamster), and Pincus[100] (monkeys) studied the effect of norethynodrel on ovarian histology. They noted complete disappearance of corpora lutea, indicative of suppression of ovulation and delay in follicular maturation. Greenwald confirmed the same effect for both ethinylestradiol[48] and stilbestrol.[49] His observations were significant because they proved the *antiovulatory effect of estrogens*.

Based on laparotomy specimens from

women, the occurrence of ovarian changes following the administration of contraceptives has been investigated by Garcia and Pincus,[42] Lauweryns and Ferin,[69] Ryan and colleagues,[108] Starup and Ostergaard[124] and Zañartu and associates.[150, 151] We[111, 113] have similarly studied those effects in women who had had some indication for laparotomy. Such women in our series were subjected to a complete study to verify whether they had a normal ovulatory cycle. The corresponding steroid was then administered for a period of three months, followed by laparotomy between the twenty-third and twenty-sixth days of the cycle, at which time a wedge-shaped excision was performed on both ovaries, removing thin but deep slices, representing as much as possible complete transections of both ovaries. A *bilateral ovarian biopsy* of this kind enabled us to judge the extent of the antiovulatory effect involved. Our findings have been summarized in Table 47-1 and in Figures 47-1 and 47-2. We arrived at the following conclusions: (1) Estrogens are more powerful ovulation inhibitors than are progestogens. (2) Notwithstanding the potent anovulatory effect of some modern preparations, the progestational action exerted by these compounds is a weak one. (3) Estrogens and progestogens mutually potentiate each other's actions to the point that the most powerful antiovulatory effect is obtained by so-called "combination therapy" (see Section 47.7.1).

The most striking observation emerging from our studies was the finding that estrogens alone, without any cooperation from progestogens, exerted anovulatory activity. The same observations have been made in experimental animals (rats,[71, 143] hamsters[49]). What will later be explained as "sequential therapy" is in fact nothing else but the damping of ovulation by estrogens, followed briefly by administration of progestogens after ovulation has actually occurred, the sole purpose of which may be to offset the estrogenic effect on the endometrium.

47.3.2. ACTION ON THE FALLOPIAN TUBE

The effect of progestogens on human Fallopian tubes, as we have already pointed out, has been investigated at our laboratory by our associates Terragno and Gutiérrez.[139] Working similarly on patients who, like the preceding ones, were to be operated on after progestogen therapy over one or several cycles, they removed the Fallopian tubes on one or both sides and examined them in a bath for isolated organs, recording their spontaneous contractions. When the motility of tubes subjected to the treatment was compared with that of a tube from a normal woman, it was found to be significantly depressed by the action of such drugs (Fig. 47-3).

Our findings in women could be duplicated in animal experiments. Chang[14] noted that postcoital administration of medroxyprogesterone to female rabbits resulted in

TABLE 47-1. Effects of Different Steroids on Human Ovarian Histology

COMPOUND USED	DOSAGE	NO. OF	OVARIAN FINDINGS
Mestranol	150†	3	Follicular development, absence of corpora lutea; corpora albicantia
Metigestrone	10§	5	Follicular development, scanty but evident corpora lutea
31.458 Ba	5§	3	Presence of follicles, absence of corpora lutea; corpora lutea
Ethynodiol acetate-mestranol	1§ 150†	8	Absence of both follicles and corpora lutea; corpora albicantia
Lynestrenol Mestranol	5§ 150†	8	Absence of both follicles and corpora lutea; corpora albicantia
Duphaston	1§	3	Absence of corpora lutea, inconstant
Ethinylestradiol (sequential therapy)	75†		

* From Sanchez-Rivera, Merlo, Escudero and Botella: *Amer. J. Obstet. Gynec.*, 101:665, 1968.
† Micrograms daily, 3 cycles.
§ Milligrams daily, 3 cycles.

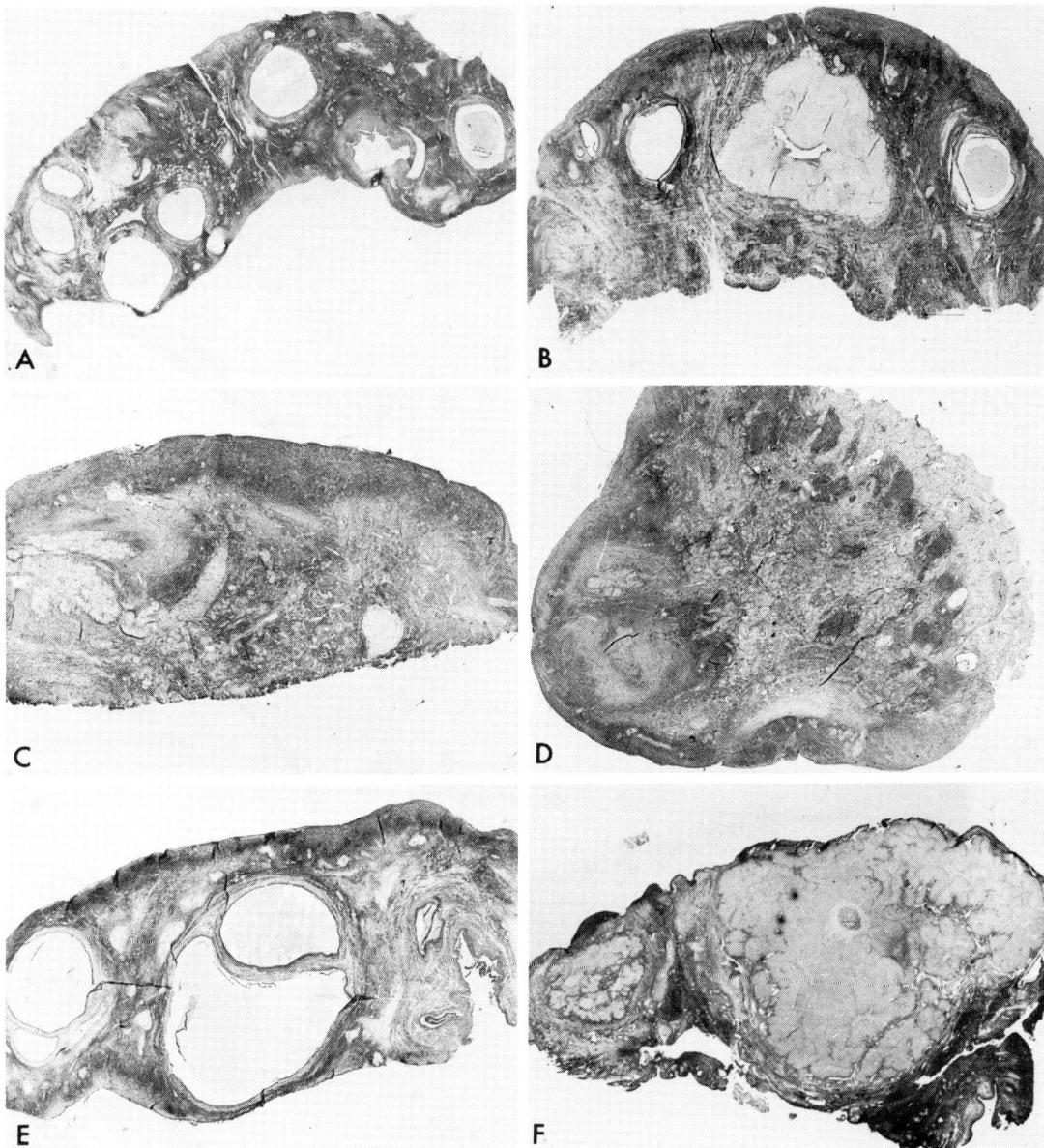

Figure 47–1. Action of oral contraceptives on the human ovary, using ovarian biopsies in the form of extensive and deep ovarian wedges, taken from normal women with verified biphasic cycles after administration of oral contraceptives for three consecutive cycles. Biopsies were obtained through laparotomy between the twenty-third and twenty-sixth days of the third treatment cycle. *A*, Ovary after administration of 150 mcg mestranol daily from the fifth to the twenty-fifth day of three consecutive cycles. Note absence of corpora lutea, suggestive of suspension of ovulation. This effect may be attributed to loss of LH release, whereas presence of follicular maturation would appear to indicate continued release of FSH. *B*, Ovary from woman treated with 10 mg Metigestrone daily during three cycles. No recent corpus luteum is noted, but the large corpus albicans in the center of figure seems to suggest that ovulation, at least during the first of the cycles involved, had not been interrupted. *C*, Ovary after three cycles of treatment with Anacyclin (Ciba), consisting of 150 mcg mestranol and 4 mg lynestrenol per tablet. Note atrophic appearance of the ovary, with complete absence of follicles and corpora lutea, apparently indicating inhibition of both FSH and LH release, as a result of joint action of estrogen plus progestogen. *D*, Another case following same treatment as in *C*, revealing similar results. *E*, Ovary of woman, treated with Anacyclin (Ciba) for three complete cycles, but biopsied on the twelfth day of ensuing cycle *without* treatment. It is evident that ovarian maturation resumes quite vigorously as soon as administration of contraceptive preparations is discontinued. *F*, Ovary from woman treated similarly to patient in *E*, but biopsied on the twenty-second day of cycle. A large corpus luteum is seen to have formed, indicating entirely normal reestablishment of cycle, once patient has been taken off the "pill." (From Sanchez-Rivera, Merlo, Escudero and Botella-Llusiá: *Amer. J. Obstet. Gynec.*, 101:665, 1968.)

Oral Contraceptives 1035

Figure 47-2. Detail of cortical zone in ovary shown in Figure 47-1,C, under intermediate magnification. Despite appearing grossly as a senile postmenopausal ovary, closer examination reveals persistence of primordial follicles.

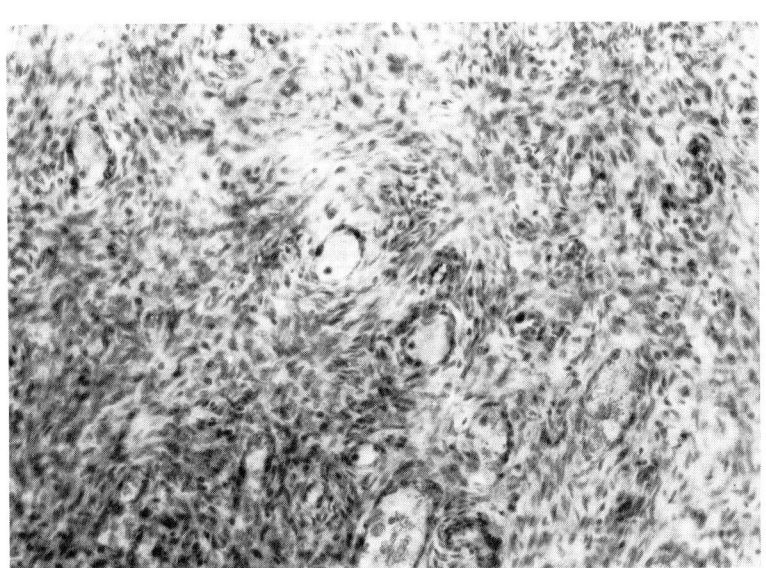

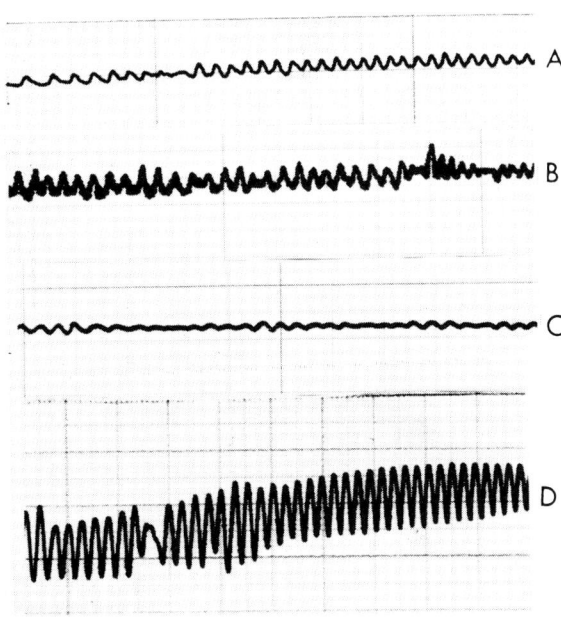

Figure 47-3. Effect of progestogens on spontaneous motility of in vitro isolated human Fallopian tubes, obtained from women who had received various progestogen preparations over three consecutive cycles. Intervention was performed during the third cycle and spontaneous movements of the tubes were recorded in an organ bath. A, Metigestrone. B, Metrulen-M (Searle). C, 31,458 Ba (synthetic progestogen preparation produced by Ciba). D, Normal tube from untreated woman (control). (From Terragno, Gutierrez and Botella-Llusiá: *Acta Gin.*, 17:219, 1966.)

the stranding of ova within the tubes. The study of tubal motility in this instance confirmed the fact that such retention of ova was due to tubal paralysis.[15] In the sow, the migration of ova through the oviduct was similarly found to decelerate under the effect of hydroxyprogesterone (Day and Polge[22]). Harper[52] used acrylic spherules and radioactive substances[53] to measure the rate of tubal transport in female rabbits. He also stained the cumulus oöphorus with toluidine blue.[54] With these methods, he was likewise able to observe the occurrence of tubal paralysis under the action of synthetic progestogens. Chang[16] and Harper,[55] moreover, showed that the effect of estrogens was just the opposite, speeding up the passage of ova through the rat oviduct. Possibly this may represent a contraceptive effect, since it involves the delivery of premature morulas into the uterine cavity.

47.3.3. ACTION ON THE ENDOMETRIUM

From the early investigations of Pincus,[99] some progestational drugs, principally norethynodrel, had been known to produce a kind of damping effect on the endometrium, while failing to evoke any typical progestational reaction (Fig. 47-4). Recently, Roland[105] reported similar effects, also in association with norethynodrel treatment, in pregnancy. Before long, it could be firmly established that such progestogenic preparations as norethynodrel, and to a lesser extent norethindrone, lacked the typical progestational effect on the endometrium. It is true that they elicited progestational changes in the stroma. However, they failed to provoke any true secretory activity in the glands. After prolonged treatment, gland epithelia would become thin and would show no signs of activity. Nevertheless, when administered in high dosages and for extended periods of time, these drugs would induce a truly compact mucosa of pseudodecidual appearance.[18, 36]

Initial studies on the endometrial effects of medroxyprogesterone acetate (Provera),[23, 47] on the other hand, revealed that this drug, perhaps because it was derived from progesterone itself rather than from a norderivative, exerted a normal progestational effect. As a result of numerous subsequent tests,[30, 44, 45] bearing out these initial reports, medroxyprogesterone acetate is now acknowledged to exert a purely progesterone-like action. The other acetylated derivatives of progesterone have been found to behave in a similar way. For instance, chlormadinone, the object of a large number of recent studies,[94, 106, 142] also possesses a purely progestational type of activity.

Megestrol also appears to be purely progestational in its effects on the endometrium, and we are convinced that the retroprogesterone group of compounds (Duphaston) likewise possesses frank progestational activity.[81] Pincus[100] and Ferin[38] postulated that the observed differences between the actions of the acetylated derivatives and those of the norderivatives might result from the fact that, aside from their progestational activity, the norderivatives also exerted weak estrogenic activity. Their assumption seems to be supported by the results of tests carried out with the commercial product Provest.[5, 63, 104] The latter, which is a combination of ethinylestradiol and medroxyprogesterone acetate—designed to exert a strong antiovulatory effect—also produces endometrial effects similar to those produced by norethynodrel. It causes the endometrial glands to undergo atrophy, while the stroma assumes the appearance of compact tissue. The prominent feature in a compact stroma of this kind is hyperplasia of the spiral vessels and sinusoids (Blaustein et al.[3]). These histological findings have been confirmed and amplified by ultrastructural studies (Wienke et al.[145]). Other studies[18, 56, 86] showed that norethisterone, too, produced a mild atrophic effect on the endometrium and that, if it was combined with an estrogen in a ratio of one tenth of a milligram of estrogen for every 10 milligrams of progestogen, it produced atrophic effects similar in magnitude to those caused by the previously mentioned drugs. What is more, additional evidence has been provided by testing Lyndiol, a mixture of 5 mg lynestrenol (a compound with typical progestational properties) and 0.15 mg ethinylestradiol methyl ether. When combined in this manner with an estrogen, the progestogen ceased to elicit a secretory endometrial response and instead caused endometrial atrophy of the type previously described.[84, 131]

It may be concluded that when synthetic progestogens are combined with an estrogen, they lose their more or less characteristic progestational action on the endo-

Figure 47-4. Effect of oral contraceptives on endometrium: *A*, Biphasic endometrium biopsied during secretory phase (twenty-sixth day). *B*, Endometrium of same patient after two complete cycles of treatment with Anacyclin (Ciba) in dosages as indicated in Figure 47-1. There is atrophy of gland epithelia, with stroma retaining its progestational features. *C*, Endometrium of same patient, one cycle later (that is, after three cycles of treatment with same contraceptive preparation). Increasing sparsity of glands is evident. In contrast to persistent gland atrophy, stroma continues exhibiting secretory features and presence of spiral vessels. (From Cremades and Botella-Llusiá: *Acta Gin.*, 17:29, 1966.)

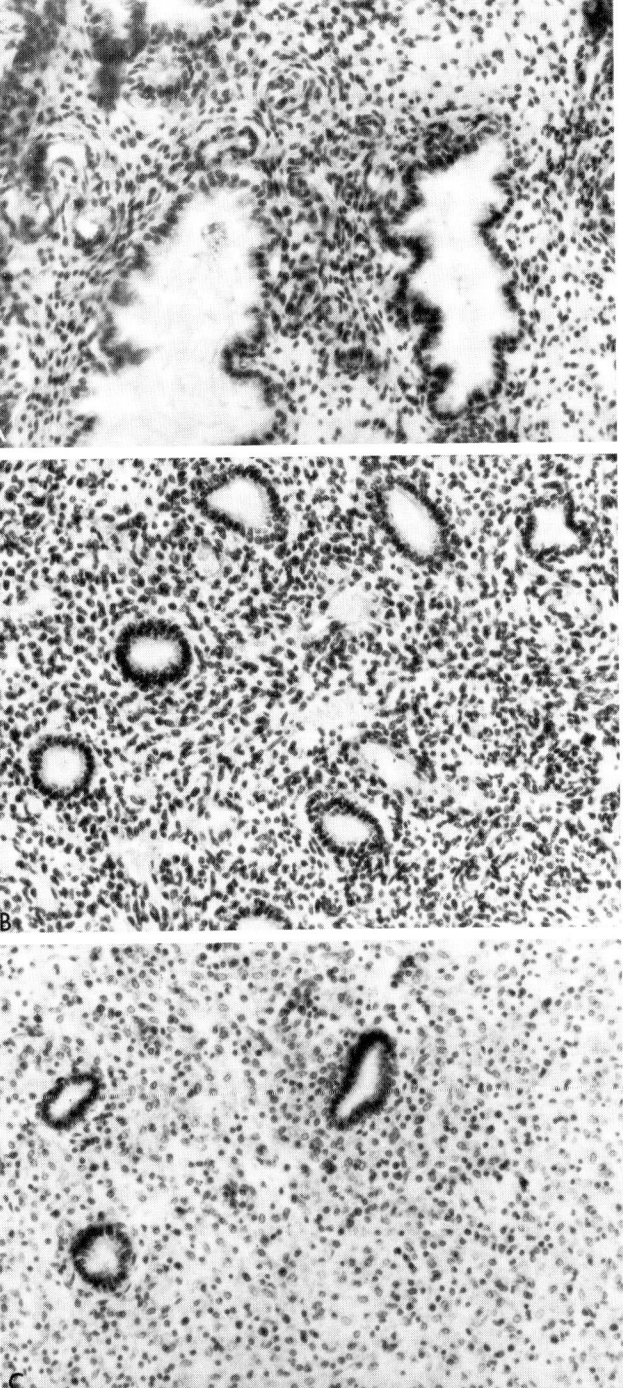

metrium. We have recently studied the problem[48] by practicing serial endometrial biopsies on women who were under continuous contraceptive therapy. The biopsies were performed on the twenty-third day of the cycle and compared with biopsies taken before beginning therapy and one month after discontinuing therapy (Fig. 47-4). Such therapy invariably was associated with *endometrial atrophy,* involving particularly the glandular and vascular elements and, to a lesser extent, the stroma. The same effect was also observed if the progestogens were given alone, without estrogens. After the administration of large doses of estrogens, on the other hand, they were not observed and similarly were absent in patients with evidence of previous hyperestrogenism — for instance, in women revealing endometrial hyperplasia. This means that the action involved was actually of progestational nature but that the action by any kind of progestogen on the endometrium was ineffective unless the endometrium had first been primed by the action of estrogens. Because endogenous estrogen biogenesis was at the same time inhibited by the profound changes involving the ovaries, the only effect produced by these compounds, notwithstanding their undeniable progestational properties, was endometrial atrophy.

47.3.4. ACTION ON THE UTERINE CERVIX AND ON THE MIGRATION OF SPERM

Zañartu[148] demonstrated that the progestogen present in contraceptive tablets was responsible for causing *thickening of cervical mucus,* as well as a decrease in the amount, stringiness and crystallization of the mucus, and suggested that this might hinder spermatic ascent. Martínez-Manautou and his associates,[80] as well as Rudel and colleagues,[107] studied the effects of very small but continuous and uninterrupted dosages of chlormadinone (half a milligram daily). They observed that, according to expectations, ovulation was not interrupted, but that cervical mucus became impermeable to sperm (giving negative postcoital tests), and such women became temporarily infertile. Zañartu and Navarro[149] further noted that women receiving medroxyprogesterone acetate intramuscularly in a dose of 0.5 gm remained infertile for six months because of this kind of cervical effect, rather than because of anovulation. Carlborg and his co-workers[111] found a reduction in the sialic acid content of cervical mucus under the effect of progestogens, associated with a decrease in the receptivity of mucus to spermatozoa.

Zañartu and associates also found that women receiving 0.5 mg of chlormadinone daily without interruption over a period of several months were infertile, although microscopic examinations of ovarian tissue revealed that ovulation had not been suspended.[153] It is conceivable that this effect results not only from "cervical hostility" but also from difficulties encountered by spermatozoa in their ascent, owing to the previously described changes at the endometrial as well as the tubal level. In our studies of compound 31.458 Ba,[6, 7] a progestogen currently at the testing stage, we made the following observations: (1) ovulation was usually interrupted, although by no means in a constant manner, (2) even with dosages below 1 mg, which were no longer expected to interrupt ovulation, women taking the drug stayed infertile, (3) in this instance infertility resulted from the thickening of mucus, rendered impermeable to spermatozoa, which yielded negative postcoital test results.

A new perspective for oral contraception has thus been opened on a hitherto untested basis (see "nonstop therapy," page 1043).

47.3.5. ACTION ON SPERMATIC CAPACITATION

Chang[16] and Diczfalusy[25] admit another possible mode of action by steroids, particularly progestogens. This presumably consists in blocking spermatic capacitation within the uterine cavity. The manner in which spermatozoa are rendered fit for fertilization upon coming into contact with intrauterine secretions is well known. The processes leading to that effect, the nature of which is yet poorly understood, are blocked by the action of synthetic progestogens.

47.3.6. ACTION ON THE VAGINA

Jackson and Lynn[60] studied the effect of various progestogens on vaginal exfoliation.

Norethynodrel was found to possess equivocal progestational and weak estrogenic activity. Megestrol acetate, on the other hand, was found to exert a strong progestational but weak, if any, estrogenic effect. Medroxyprogesterone had similar effects. Maqueo and his associates[76, 77] believe that the acetic progesterone derivatives result in a stronger progestational effect on vaginal smears than other derivatives, such as norethisterone and norethynodrel. An intense vaginal progestational effect is also exerted by Duphaston,[37, 141] as well as by metigestrone and metigestrone acetate.[29, 47] Let us remark that compounds made up of progestogen-estrogen combinations, such as Anovlar, Lyndiol, Anacyclin, Enovid, etc., have in the opinion of most workers,[17, 33, 37, 38, 81, 102, 142] very little, if any, progestational effect and exert instead a weak estrogenic action.

In a recent study,[110] we attempted to assess the effect on vaginal cytology of two different preparations. One was a lynestrenol-mestranol combination (Anacyclin, Ciba), the other a mixture composed of the same estrogen and ethynodiol acetate (Metrulen-M, Searle). Although in different degrees, both were found to depress vaginal proliferation and to result in semiatrophic smears; however, there were recognizable features of cyclicity, which conveyed the impression that the ovarian secretory cycle was not altogether suppressed.

47.3.7 EFFECTS ON MALE ANIMALS

A surprising development of recent years was the discovery that synthetic progestogens inhibited spermatogenesis in male rats[35] and rabbits.[34] It is possible that this may have opened to us a new avenue for male contraception.

47.4. EFFECTS OF OVULATION INHIBITORS ON HORMONE ELIMINATION

Urinary excretion of gonadotropins, estrogens and pregnanediol is profoundly affected, as revealed by in-depth studies of recent years.

47.4.1. ESTROGENS

Loraine and his colleagues[72, 73] and Lunenfeld[74] have tested the effects of norethisterone acetate (Norlutate) and medroxyprogesterone acetate (Provera), respectively. Both depress urinary estrogen excretion significantly, which is in keeping with the inhibitory effects on ovarian follicular maturation we described previously. Buchholz and Nocke[10] reported identical results concerning the action of Provera. All indications are that most antiovulatory progestogens reduce ovarian secretion of estrogens. Ferin[38] refers to hypoestrogenic amenorrhea, produced by long-term employment of these compounds.

47.4.2. PREGNANEDIOL

It is a well known fact that none of these compounds is eliminated by the urine as pregnanediol.[9, 32, 47, 96] The presence of the dialcohol in the urine is therefore an indication that ovulation has not been inhibited and that a corpus luteum has been formed, which produces endogenous progesterone. Nevinny-Stickel[87] utilized this principle to assess the antiovulatory effects of a series of drugs.

47.4.3. GONADOTROPINS

As we have pointed out previously, the fundamental mechanism whereby ovulation is inhibited has been suspected to consist in suppression of the LH peak at midcycle. Various investigators have estimated LH excretion in women treated with such drugs in order to clarify this effect (Fig. 47–5). While Buchholz and Nocke[10] claimed disappearance of gonadotropinuria, neither Loraine[72] nor Overbeeck and Visser[90, 91] were able to confirm that finding. According to Demol and Ferin,[26] as well as Lunenfeld,[74] different compounds have different effects on gonadotropin elimination.

The most pronounced effects are the result of estrogen-progestogen combinations.[73, 109, 123] There seems to be a correlation of proportionality between the direct ovarian effects observed and the LH "peak." So far as FSH is concerned, the pattern does not appear to be a constant one.

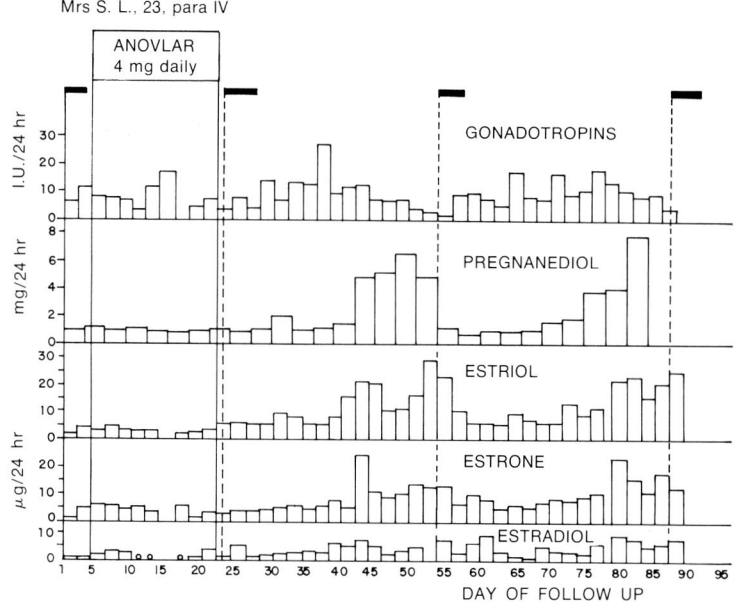

Figure 47-5. Excretion of gonadotropins, pregnanediol, estriol, estrone and estradiol in the course of various cycles, with or without the administration of ovulation inhibitors (Anovlar). There is marked reduction in gonadotropin excretion, absence of elevation in pregnanediol excretion and diminished estrogen excretion. (From Loraine: *Internat. J. Fertil.*, 9:155, 1964.)

47.5. BASAL BODY TEMPERATURES

Measurement of basal body temperature as a means of diagnosing ovulation has been used on a large scale by Fuchs and associates[40] and principally, by Peeters and colleagues.[96] A characteristic feature of the temperature curve is a plateau-like elevation. Since the compounds we are dealing with have a progestational as well as hyperthermic effect, temperatures are raised rather than lowered for the duration. The curves are of course monophasic, so that ovulatory peaks are missing. The reappearance of biphasic thermic curves and of urinary pregnanediol excretion have been the two main criteria relied on in assessing recovery of ovulatory function once treatment has been discontinued (Fig. 47-6).

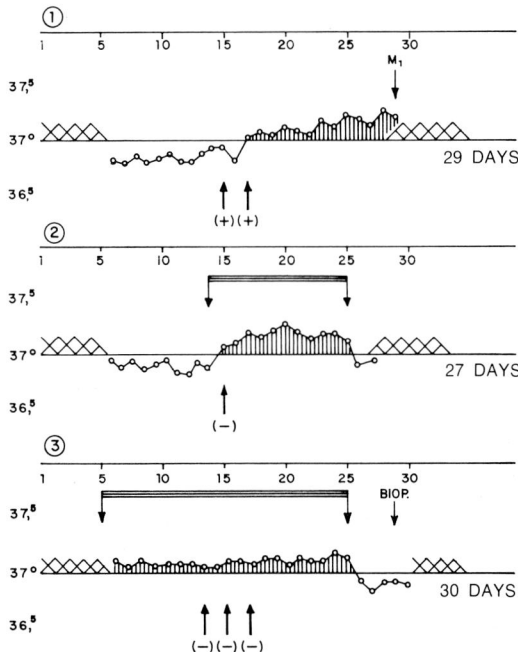

Figure 47-6. Effect of administration of an ovulation inhibitor (Anovlar) on basal body temperature, studied during three consecutive cycles. First cycle, in which no antiovulatory preparation had been administered, reveals temperature rise during second half of cycle, consistent with time of probable ovulation. During second cycle, antiovulatory drug was given from the fourteenth to the twenty-fifth day; rise in basal body temperature beginning with second half of cycle appears to be consistent with ovulation occurring about the fourteenth day of the cycle. In this instance, the antiovulatory drug exerts a progestational but no ovulation inhibiting action. Third graph represents routine mode of administering ovulation inhibitor, between the fifth and the twenty-fifth days of the cycle. Although at a higher than normal level, basal body temperature curve remains flat and even, which indicates the presence of an anovulatory cycle.

47.6. MODE OF ACTION OF ORAL CONTRACEPTIVES

The mode of action of these drugs has been studied in great detail in animals[27, 31, 57, 90, 92, 140] and, although not so completely, in women.[6, 76, 77, 113] As a result, there is considerable confusion as regards the interpretation of the single tangible fact: *temporary sterilization*. By what mechanism is the latter produced? There are at least four possible explanations to account for the sterilizing effect: (1) suppression of ovulation, (2) paralysis of tubal ovitransport, (3) lack of nidation, and (4) paralysis of spermatic ascent. We shall study them in sequence.

47.6.1. SUSPENSION OF OVULATION

It has been suspected that suspension of ovulation was an effect of the flattening of basal body temperature curves,[2, 6, 74] the disappearance of the ovulatory LH peak[16, 72, 73, 109, 123] and the lack of pregnanedioluria.[87] However, the antiovulatory effect could not be assessed until ovarian biopsies were studied at laparotomy,[42, 69, 108, 111, 113, 124, 150] as pointed out previously (Section 47.3.1).

Lack of LH seemed to suggest lack of pituitary LH release. In recent years, however, this mechanism has been pinpointed more precisely. The hypothalamic content

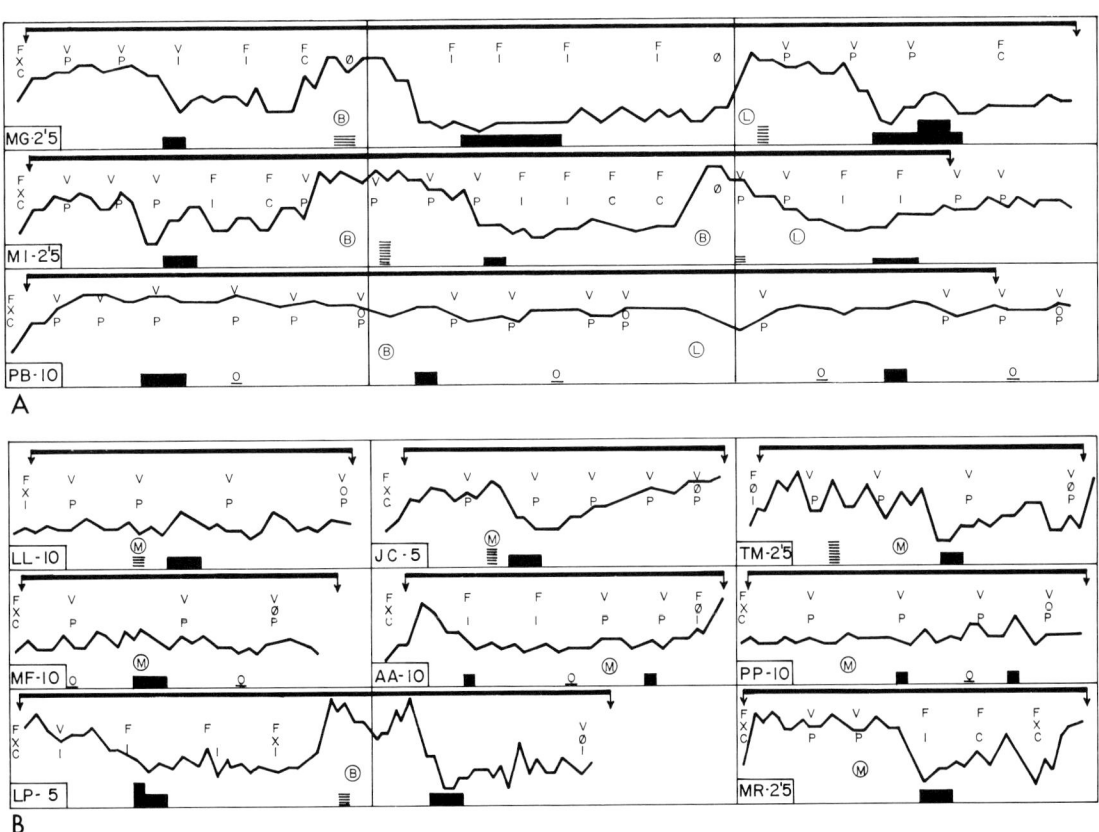

Figure 47-7. Effects of various contraceptives on cervical mucus, cytology, postcoital test and endometrial and ovarian biopsy in a group of women treated during one or more cycles with a contraceptive preparation containing 100 mcg mestranol and a variable amount of a synthetic progestogen (lynestrenol). Symbols in boxes indicate patient's initials and daily progestogen dosage expressed in milligrams. Basal body temperatures have also been recorded. X, Positive postcoital test; O, negative postcoital test; Ø, weakly positive postcoital test; F, stringy mucus; V, viscous mucus; P, folded cells; I, intermediate cells; C, karyopyknotic cells; B, Endometrial biopsy; L, laparotomy with ovarian biopsy. Black bands, demarcated at each end by arrows, indicate length of contraceptive administration. Heavy black boxes indicate menstruation; shaded markings indicate presence of positive urinary pregnanediol excretion.

of LH releasing factor (LHRF) could be determined in rats following administration of norethynodrel,[82] progesterone[85] and norethisterone.[58] It was found that the sex center was devoid of LHRF secretion. Microcrystals of norethisterone,[64] ethinylestradiol[101] and lynestrenol[92] were inserted in the tuber cinereum of rats[13, 101] and rabbits.[92] Ovulation in such animals was interrupted if the crystals were located exactly in the *sex center* but was not if they were implanted nearby, or if the substances implanted were inert. That this effect resulted from lack of gonadotropin release may be deduced from the fact that the action of antiovulatory drugs was ineffective unless exogenous gonadotropins were injected at the same time, for instance, PMS[65, 66, 68, 138] in rats[116] or monkeys[65] and HMG[62] in women. That is to say, if gonadotropins of exogenous origin are injected at the same time at which endogenous gonadotropin release has been suppressed, ovulation takes place in a normal way. The evidence provided by this experiment stands by itself to refute any claims maintaining a direct ovarian action by antiovulatory compounds.[26]

The question of what dosages of steroids are necessary for inhibition of LH release at the hypothalamic level has recently been studied with regard to estrogens[61, 132] and progestogens,[28] as well as estrogen-progestogen combinations.[125, 129]

An outstanding recent study on the subject is that by Schally and associates,[117] in which steroid fixation by the median eminence of the rat, resulting in a selective inhibitory effect on LHRF and FSHRF formation, was demonstrated experimentally.

It is therefore apparent that one of the fundamental, though by no means only, modes of action by contraceptive drugs consists in suppressing the secretory activity of the hypothalamic sex center. Properly speaking, the effect involved represents indeed an anovulatory type of action.

47.6.2. PARALYSIS OF TUBAL OVITRANSPORT

We have commented how our own investigations,[139] as well as those of Chang[14, 15, 16] and Harper[53, 54, 55] have brought to light the possibility that tubal contractions ceased under the influence of progestogens and that, as a result of being stranded, the morulas died. In view of the fact that death of morulas supervened so rapidly,[13, 14] one might in addition speculate whether *tubotrophic nutrition* is, after all, not also interrupted.

47.6.3. LACK OF IMPLANTATION

The action by these drugs, resulting in endometrial changes and glandular atrophy as it does, suggests the possibility that sterility in this instance may also be due to lack of implantation (see Section 47.3.3). Chang[13] noted that norethynodrel decreased the number of blastocysts found in the uterine cavity of rabbits. Daniel and Cowan[21] observed lack of implantation in animals treated with norethynodrel, norethisterone, ethinylestradiol and mestranol. Dickmann[24] observed deferred implantation due to estrogens. Taubert[137] observed that medroxyprogesterone acetate blocked the implantation of blastocysts transplanted from a normal female rat to one previously treated with a progestogen. The changes observed by us in the endometrium, for which we accepted the term *"iatrogenic endometrium"* (Zañartu and Navarro[149]), are of the *functional type, capable of impairing ovular nidation.*

47.6.4. PARALYSIS OF SPERMATIC ASCENT

Progestogens, as we have already pointed out, cause cervical mucus to thicken so as to become impermeable to spermatozoa.[80, 107, 149, 153] This action is exclusively the result of progestogens and forms the basis for a new modality of contraception in the presence of a normal ovarian cycle.

Let us repeat that paralysis of spermatic ascent takes place not only at the cervical level but also in the endometrial cavity, owing to lack of *capacitation.*

47.6.5. SYNOPSIS OF CONTRACEPTIVE MECHANISMS

The four mechanisms described are all involved more or less simultaneously, but they may be dissociated. Thus, for instance, if a progestogen is used alone, without estrogens, over a continuous period of

Oral Contraceptives

time, the resulting infertility appears to stem from an effect on cervical mucus and, perhaps, also on the tube. If, on the other hand, the drug used is an estrogen alone or, as occurs in "sequential therapy," an estrogen followed by a progestogen, the resulting effect is inhibition of ovulation. When preparations with "combined" or "simultaneous" action are used, the estrogen acts on ovulation while the progestogen potentiates this action and in addition acts on the Fallopian tube and cervix, both hormones together exerting a joint action on the endometrium, giving rise to characteristic glandular atrophy.

Consequently, the reasons why the term "antiovulatory progestogens" should not be used are obvious; the correct term ought to be "contraceptive steroids."

47.7. MODES OF ADMINISTRATION OF CONTRACEPTIVES

There are three methods for administering oral contraceptives: (1) "combined" or "classical" therapy; (2) "sequential therapy"; and (3) *"continuous therapy"* or "nonstop therapy."

47.7.1. CLASSICAL OR COMBINED THERAPY

This is the most widely used form. It consists in combining, in a single tablet, an estrogen (ethinylestradiol, mestranol) in dosages ranging from 75 to 150 mcg, with a progestogen in dosages ranging from 1 to 10 mg. It should be pointed out that the modern tendency is to reduce the dosage of progestogen in order to avoid unpleasant side-effects, stemming in large part from high progestogen dosages of the mixture.

47.7.2. SEQUENTIAL THERAPY

Goldzieher and his co-workers[46, 75, 77, 79] have introduced the routine of administering an estrogen, in dosages similar to those used in the "classic" modality, without an associated progestogen, between the fifth and twentieth days of the cycle. Then, from the twenty-first to the twenty-sixth days, a progestogen is added in the same form and composition as in simultaneous therapy. Temporary sterilization with this modality is based on ovulation inhibition, induced by the estrogen alone, whereas the progestogen is added to prevent "iatrogenic hyperestrogenism" (see Chapter 28, page 610).

47.7.3. CONTINUOUS OR NONSTOP THERAPY

Over the past years, various workers[80, 149, 152] have devised a new form of contraceptive therapy, based on administering an oral contraceptive in daily dosages of 0.5 mg without interruption. The drug is taken also during the days of menstruation. Apparently, this form of therapy does not interfere with either ovulation or menstruation but prevents fertilization by the previously described mechanism of *cervical hostility*. This method, still in the testing stage, has been designated continuous or "nonstop" therapy.

Zañartu and Navarro[149] and Lee[70] advocate substitution of daily tablets by single injections of 0.5 gm of medroxyprogesterone acetate, allegedly providing effective contraceptive action for several months.

47.8. HARMFUL EFFECTS OF ORAL CONTRACEPTIVES

All drugs are associated with toxic effects of some sort, and it would be pretentious to claim absence of undesirable side effects in a form of therapy that has to be carried on for many months. At any rate, here, as in any other form of therapy, it is up to the physician to weigh the advantages against the drawbacks involved. Any beneficial therapeutic result has its harmful counterpart. If the benefits to be derived outweigh the disadvantages, it is logical to assume that treatment is indicated.

Some of the toxic effects associated with oral contraceptives were recognized from the outset.[42, 47, 57] In 1969, a commission of WHO experts published a brief memorandum[147] summarizing data gathered in a survey of over five million women. If to this fundamental and unique survey we add the data obtained in the field trials in Puerto Rico,[41] Birmingham,[81] India[84] and Chile,[148] an overall impression may be gained concerning the dangers of adverse effects, which we shall examine later. We shall discuss in sequence: (1) circulatory phenomena, (2) changes in blood coagulation,

(3) digestive changes, (4) psychological disturbances, (5) thyroid alterations, (6) risks of fetal virilization, (7) risks of malignancy, (8) dangers in diabetes, (9) urinary disturbances.

47.8.1. CIRCULATORY PHENOMENA

It had been asserted that contraceptive drugs caused circulatory changes similar to those observed in pregnancy. Brehm[9] found no evidence of any hemodynamic alterations in women exposed to prolonged treatment. The WHO report[147] likewise was negative in that respect.

47.8.2. CHANGES IN BLOOD COAGULATION

The very first tests with contraceptives[42, 47, 57] revealed evidence of increased blood coagulability. The mechanism involved was studied by Brehm,[9] Mammen and associates,[75] and Owren.[93] Statistical data based on surveys of large series[81, 153] do not seem to indicate any increase in the incidence of thromboembolism.

47.8.3. DIGESTIVE CHANGES

Most women, particularly at the beginning of therapy, experience nausea and vomiting which, in the opinion of Kopera and his colleagues,[67] are psychogenic in nature, probably stemming from "rejection" of dreaded gravidic symptomatology. Garcia and his co-workers[41, 42] observed the same symptoms in two groups of women, one receiving placebos instead of contraceptives.

Hepatic complications may be fraught with more serious consequences. Healthy livers are usually unaffected but in patients with liver disturbances, significant alterations may develop.

It had been suggested[147] that the contraindications for this type of medication concern mainly the *Dubin-Johnson syndrome* and the *Rotor syndrome*.

47.8.4. PSYCHOLOGICAL DISTURBANCES

Psychological disturbances must be attributed to guilt complexes and to problems of "rejection," particularly if contraceptive drugs are a controversial moral issue for the woman concerned. We are undoubtedly dealing with a problem of great importance, but obviously unrelated to the endocrinologic approach to our subject.

47.8.5. THYROID

Fisher and his colleagues[39] reported an increase in PBI levels and ^{131}I uptake values. Since the same changes have been observed in normal pregnancy, these changes were believed to be due to a *pseudogravid state*, induced by the action of progestogens. Nevertheless, Pincus and his associates (Irisarri et al.[69]) deny that progestogens (at least insofar as norethynodrel is concerned) possess thyrotropic activity.

Similarly, Starup and Frills[126] and Mishell and his co-workers[83] tested various contraceptive steroids, without encountering any associated thyroid-stimulating effects.

47.8.6. RISKS OF CAUSING FETAL VIRILIZATION

More than from anything else, this danger stems from the exclusive use of synthetic progestogens when employed as progesterone substitutes in the treatment of threatened abortion. However, it may also exist in the unlikely case of a woman becoming pregnant and continuing to take contraceptives, unaware of her new condition. In order to clarify this question, a large amount of research has been carried out on pregnant animals, for the specific purpose of assessing the androgenic potency of these drugs on the fetus. Nortestosterone derivatives (norethisterone, norethynodrel, etc.) possess a virilizing effect, in the opinion of Cupceancu and Neumann,[20] Peck and Lo Piccolo[95] and Suchowsky and associates,[130] which, however, is denied by Saunders.[114] On the other hand, Chambon and co-workers,[12] and Saunders himself,[115] agree that derivatives of progesterone (metigestrone, chlormadinone, megestrol acetate, etc.) are entirely devoid of virilizing activity. As a result, those preparations containing no norsteroid components have been gaining increasing popularity. The possibility of fetal virilization with the use of nortestosterone is actually quite remote. However, in the event of threatened abortion, *norsteroids should never be employed.*

47.8.7. RISKS OF INDUCING MALIGNANCY

Owing to their estrogen content, such drugs have been considered contraindicated in estrogen-dependent varieties of carcinoma, particularly those of the breast. The WHO report[147] emphasizes the point that these compounds should not be prescribed without first carefully palpating the breasts. The risks are of course greater in sequential therapy than in combined therapy, and are practically nonexistent in nonstop therapy.

Another risk involving carcinogenesis, particularly emphasized in recent years, is that of inducing cervical atypia, as shown cytologically by Soost[118] and histologically by Stern and his colleagues.[128] Atypia of this type has been the object of a special study at our clinic (Nogales and Tarracon[88]).

Figure 47–8 exemplifies the characteristic findings. Although it is true that cervical dysplasia is prone to occur, it resembles that found in gestation in that it is reversible and lacks features of true malignancy. This was also the opinion voiced by the World Health Organization.[147]

47.8.8. HAZARDS OF DIABETES

Oral contraceptives have been found to reduce tolerance to glucose (Gershberg et al.,[143] Spellacy et al.,[119, 120] Wayne et al.[144]). Of little consequence in a normal woman, this may be a hazardous development in a diabetic.

The problem has recently been studied carefully.[8, 121, 122, 127] There is no doubt that oral contraceptives may cause latent or occult diabetes to surface. They are thus contraindicated in diabetic women who do not wish to have children.

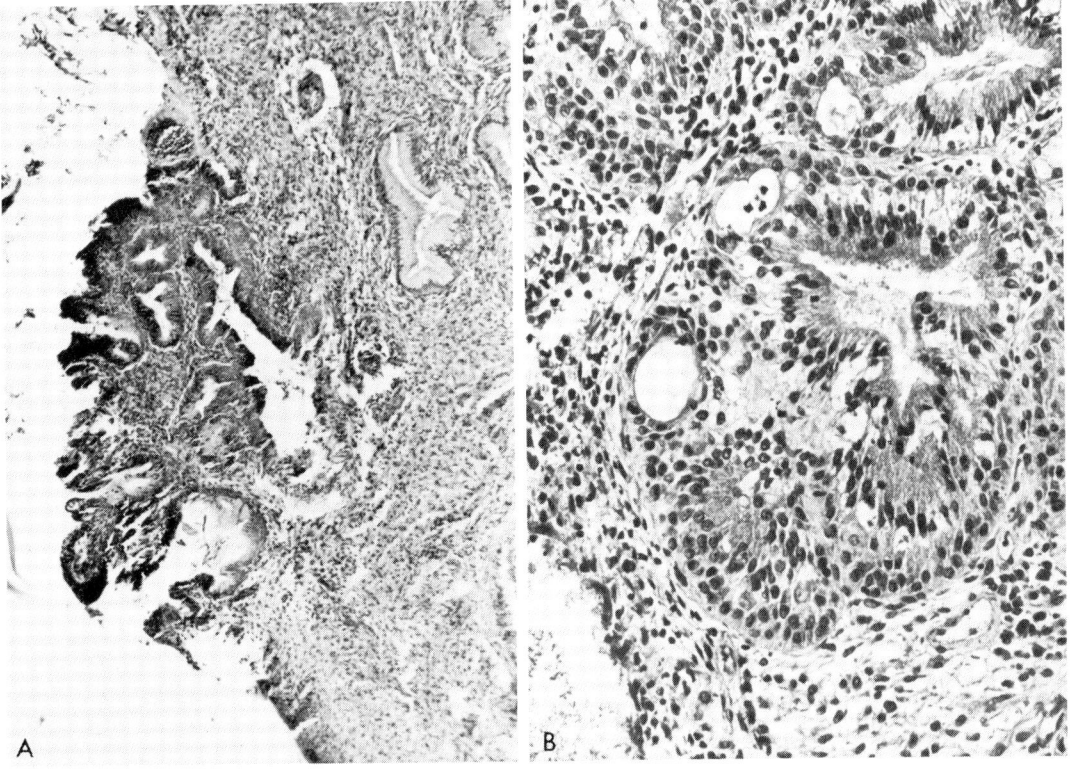

Figure 47–8. Cervical dysplasia from oral contraceptives: histology of the uterine cervix of a woman who had been treated with an oral contraceptive containing estrogen (100 mcg) and progestogen (2 mg) over a period of one year. A, Low power (35×); B, medium power (350×). Findings consisted of cervical dysplasia and reserve cell hyperplasia, but invariably without associated malignant changes. These changes are similar to the physiologic changes of pregnancy and may, in both cases, be interpreted as resulting from the action of progestogens. (From Nogales and Tarancon: *Acta Gin.*, 21:649, 1970.)

47.8.9. URINARY DISTURBANCES

In connection with contraceptive treatment for extended periods of time, Marshall and his co-workers[78] reported the occurrence of uteral dilatation, similar to that observed in gestation. This, after all, seems to be one more pseudogravid reaction similar to those indicated previously.

47.9. LONG-TERM EFFECTS OF ANOVULATION

The questions that must be raised are whether complete reproductive normalcy can be regained after prolonged use of ovulation inhibitors for many years and whether such women may not develop secondary sterility or other disorders of pituitary or ovarian function. While these were difficult questions a decade ago, they have by now been answered, thanks to large-scale investigations, particularly the field trials in Puerto Rico[41, 42, 100] and the experiments in Birmingham,[9] as well as innumerable cases studied in Sweden,[4] London,[81] Mexico,[79, 102] Israel,[41] and other countries. Based on a vast body of accumulated evidence, the following conclusions may be drawn:

1. Although, when taken during pregnancy, these drugs may occasionally prove to have a virilizing effect on the fetus, they have never been found to cause maternal virilization, even when used for contraception over long periods of time.[81, 84]

2. Upon cessation of therapy, basal body temperature curves return to biphasic patterns.[4, 79, 87, 96, 102]

3. Pregnanediol excretion resumes during the first next cycle after the medication has been discontinued, which indicates resumption of ovulation.[102] The reappearance of LH excretion during the midcycle[10, 72] must be construed in the same sense.

From our own observations,[112, 113] we have come to identical conclusions. The ovaries of women treated with progestogens for three consecutive cycles were found by us to decrease in size and to show no follicles or corpora lutea, as compared to ovarian biopsies obtained barely one cycle after treatment, which revealed maturing follicles as early as the twelfth day and well-formed corpora lutea from the twenty-second day of the cycle onwards.

4. Of 44 women studied who had been taking contraceptive drugs for two or three years, Mears[81] found that 39 became pregnant before six months elapsed from the time therapy was discontinued. Consequently, all indications are that ovulation is reestablished without any adverse effects as soon as medication is suspended.

5. *The outlook for the future of these women* is unaffected and identical to that of nonusers. Menopause is not advanced,[29, 32] menstrual activity is not modified[4, 108] and the histologic appearance of ovaries soon returns to normal.[26, 69, 110]

By now, millions of women have used or are using contraceptive drugs, and the harmful effects, accidents or complications that have been recorded have not been significant. The assertion appears to be justified that the effects of contraceptive medication are temporary and innocuous in nature. It is possible, however, that some long-term effects have not yet been recognized.

In rebuttal to those who are unduly concerned over creating an anomalous endocrine situation, we may reply that the endocrine status created is quite similar to that of pregnancy, therefore giving rise in an analogous way to a greater tendency to thrombosis, diabetogenic effects and cervical dysplasia. In grand multiparas, who have had 10 or more children, whose reproductive life had been virtually a continuous pregnancy, no hazards to life have been observed as a result of multiparity. *The objections that may be raised to these drugs are of a moral and sociological character. We do not believe that contraceptives may currently be viewed as drugs possessing dangerous effects.*

REFERENCES

1. Baker, B. L., Kahn, R. H., and Bessemer, D.: *Proc. Soc. Exper. Biol. Med.*, 119:527, 1955.
2. Behrman, S. J.: *Obstet. Gynec.*, 24:101, 1964.
3. Blaustein, A., Shenker, L., and Post, R. C.: *Internat. J. Fertil.*, 13:466, 1968.
4. Borglin, N. E.: *Internat. J. Fertil.*, 9:217, 1964.
5. Borushek, S., Abell, M. R., Smith, L., and Gold, J.: *Internat. J. Fertil.*, 8:605, 1963.
6. Botella, J.: *Acta Europaea Fertilitatis*, 1:31, 1969.
7. Botella, J.: "Les ovaires au cours de l'administra-

tion des steroides anticonceptionnels," in *L'inhibition de l'ovulation*, ed. A. Netter. Paris, Masson & Cie., 1970.
8. Bottermann, P., et al.: *Münch. Med. Wschr.*, 109:685, 1967.
9. Brehm, M.: *Internat. J. Fertil.*, 9:45, 1964.
10. Buchholz, R., and Nocke, W.: *Internat. J. Fertil.*, 9:231, 1964.
11. Carlborg, L., MacCormick, W., and Gemzell, C. A.: *Acta Endocr.*, 59:636, 1968.
12. Chambon, Y., Touret, J. L., and Depagne, A.: *Ann. d'Endocr.*, 28:333, 1967.
13. Chang, M. C.: *Fertil. Steril.*, 15:97, 1964.
14. Chang, M. C.: *Endocrinology*, 79:939, 1966.
15. Chang, M. C.: *Endocrinology*, 81:1251, 1967.
16. Chang, M. C.: *Endocrinology*, 84:356, 1969.
17. Chiaffitelli, H. S., and Dominguez, S.: *Acta Cytol.*, 14:344, 1970.
18. Clyman, M. J.: *Fertil. Steril.*, 14:352, 1963.
19. Cremades, J., and Botella, J.: *Acta Gin.*, 17:827, 1966.
20. Cupceancu, B., and Neumann, F.: *Endokrinologie*, 54:66, 1969.
21. Daniel, J. C., and Cowan, M. L.: *J. Endocr.*, 35:155, 1966.
22. Day, B. N., and Polge, C.: *J. Reprod. Fertil.*, 17:227, 1968.
23. Destro, F.: *Minerva Gin.*, 11:1, 1960.
24. Dickmann, Z.: *J. Endocr.*, 37:455, 1967.
25. Diczfalusy, E.: *Amer. J. Obstet. Gynec.*, 100:136, 1968.
26. Demol, R., and Ferin, J.: *Internat. J. Fertil.*, 9:197, 1964.
27. Djerassy, C. L., Miramontes, L., and Rosenkrantz, C.: *J. Amer. Chem. Soc.*, 75:4440, 1953.
28. Döcke, F., Dörner, G., and Voigt, K. H.: *J. Endocr.*, 41:353, 1968.
29. Duncan, G. W., Lister, S. C., and Clark, J. J.: *Internat. J. Fertil.*, 8:589, 1963.
30. Durham, W. C.: *Fertil. Steril.*, 21:45, 1960.
31. Eckstein, P., et al.: *Brit. Med. J.*, 2:1172, 1961.
32. Epstein, J. A., and Kuppermann, H. S.: *Ann. N.Y. Acad. Sci.*, 71:560, 1958.
33. Erb, R., and Keller, M.: *Gynaecologia*, 158:1, 1958.
34. Ericsson, R. J., Dutt, R., and Archdeacon, J. W.: *Nature*, 204:261, 1964.
35. Ericsson, R. J., and Dutt, R. H.: *Endocrinology*, 77:203, 1965.
36. Ferin, J.: *J. Clin. Endocr. Metab.*, 17:1252, 1957.
37. Ferin, J.: *Acta Endocr.*, 39:47, 1962.
38. Ferin, J.: *Internat. J. Fertil.*, 9:29, 1964.
39. Fisher, D. A., Oddie, T. H., and Epperson, D.: *J. Clin. Endocr. Metab.*, 26:878, 1966.
40. Fuchs, F., et al.: *Internat. J. Fertil.*, 9:147, 1964.
41. Garcia, C. R., Pincus, G., and Rock, J.: *Amer. J. Obstet. Gynec.*, 75:82, 1958.
42. Garcia, C. R., and Pincus, G.: "The Hormonal Inhibition of Ovulation," in Mary S. Calderone: *Manual of Contraceptive Practice*. Baltimore, Williams & Wilkins, 1964.
43. Gershberg, H., Javier, Z., and Hulse, M.: *Diabetes*, 13:378, 1964.
44. Gold, J., Borushek, S., and Lash, S.: *Brook-Lodge Symposium on Progesteroid*. Augusta, Mich., Brook-Lodge Press, 1961.
45. Gold, J., Smith, L., Scommegna, A., and Borushek, S.: *Internat. J. Fertil.*, 8:725, 1963.
46. Goldzieher, J. W., and Peterson, W. F.: *Ann. N.Y. Acad. Sci.*, 71:722, 1958.
47. Greenblatt, R. B., and Barfield, W. E.: *Internat. J. Fertil.*, 8:641, 1963.
48. Greenwald, G. S.: *Acta Endocr.*, 47:10, 1964.
49. Greenwald, G. S.: *J. Endocr.*, 33:13, 1965.
50. Haberlandt, G.: *Die hormonelle Sterilisierung des Weiblichen organismus*. G. Fischer, Jena, 1931.
51. Haller, J.: *Ovulationshemmung durch Hormone*. Stuttgart, Georg Thieme, 1965.
52. Harper, M.: *J. Endocr.*, 30:1, 1964.
53. Harper, M.: *J. Endocr.*, 31:217, 1965.
54. Harper, M.: *Endocrinology*, 77:114, 1965.
55. Harper, M.: *Endocrinology*, 78:568, 1966.
56. Henzl, M., Jirasek, J., Horsky, J., and Presl, J.: *Arch. Gynäk.*, 199:335, 1964.
57. Hertzl, R., Tullner, W., and Raffelt, E.: *Endocrinology*, 54:228, 1954.
58. Hilliard, J., Croxatto, H. B., Hayward, J. N., and Sawyer, C. H.: *Endocrinology*, 79:411, 1966.
59. Irisarri, S., Paniagua, M., Pincus, G., Janer, J., and Frias, Z.: *J. Clin. Endocr. Metab.*, 26:6, 1966.
60. Jackson, M. N. C., and Lynn, R.: *Internat. J. Fertil.*, 9:75, 1964.
61. Jackson, J. L., Spain, W. T., and Payne, H.: *Fertil. Steril.*, 19:649, 1968.
62. Johanisson, E., Tillinger, K. G., and Diczfalusy, E.: *Fertil. Steril.*, 16:292, 1965.
63. Kaiser, R.: *Geburtsh. u. Frauenhk.*, 22:122, 1962.
64. Kanematsu, S., and Sawyer, C. H.: *Endocrinology*, 76:691, 1965.
65. Kar, A. B., and Chandra, H.: *Steroids*, 6:463, 1955.
66. Kar, A. B., Chandra, H., and Chowdhury, S. R.: *Steroids*, 6:564, 1965.
67. Kopera, H., Dukes, M. N. G., and Ijzerman, G. L.: *Internat. J. Fertil.*, 9:69, 1964.
68. Krähenbuhl, C., and Desaulles, P. A.: *Acta Endocr.*, 47:457, 1964.
69. Lauweryns, J., and Ferin, J.: *Internat. J. Fertil.*, 9:35, 1964.
70. Lee, R. A.: *Amer. J. Obstet. Gynec.*, 104:130, 1969.
71. Lisk, R. D.: *Acta Endocr.*, 48:209, 1965.
72. Loraine, J. A.: *Internat. J. Fertil.*, 9:155, 1964.
73. Loraine, J. A., Bell, E. T., Harkness, R. A., Mears, E., and Jackson, M. C. N.: *Acta Endocr.*, 50:15, 1965.
74. Lunenfield, B.: *Internat. J. Fertil.*, 9:165, 1964.
75. Mammen, E. F., et al.: *Internat. J. Fertil.*, 8:635, 1963.
76. Maqueo, M., Becerra, C., Munguia, H., and Goldzieher, J. W.: *Amer. J. Obstet. Gynec.*, 90:395, 1964.
77. Maqueo, M., Perez-Vega, E., and Goldzieher, J. W.: *Amer. J. Obstet. Gynec.*, 85:427, 1963.
78. Marshall, S., Lyon, R. P., and Mainkler, D.: *J.A.M.A.*, 198:782, 1966.
79. Martinez-Manautou, J.: *Fertil. Steril.*, 13:169, 1962.
80. Martinez-Manautou, J., et al.: *Brit. Med. J.*, 2:730, 1967.
81. Mears, E.: *Internat. J. Fertil.*, 9:1, 1964.
82. Minaguchi, H., and Meites, J.: *Endocrinology*, 81:826, 1967.
83. Mishell, D. R., Colodny, S. Z., and Swanson, L. A.: *Fertil. Steril.*, 20:335, 1969.

84. Moghissi, K. S., Rosenthal, A., and Moss, N.: *Internat. J. Fertil.*, 8:703, 1963.
85. Nallar, R., Antunes-Rodrigues, J., and MacCann, S. M.: *Endocrinology*, 79:907, 1966.
86. Neumann, F., Kramer, M., and Junkman, K.: *Medicina Experimentalis*, 11:1, 1964.
87. Nevinny-Stickel, J.: *Internat. J. Fertil.*, 9:91, 1964.
88. Nogales, F., and Tarancon, A.: *Acta Gin.*, 21:649, 1970.
89. Ostergaard, I.: *Internat. J. Fertil.*, 9:25, 1964.
90. Overbeeck, G. A., and Visser, J.: *Acta Endocr.*, 40:133, 1962.
91. Overbeeck, G. A., and Visser, J.: *Acta Endocr.*, 41:351, 1962.
92. Overbeeck, G. A., and Visser, J.: *Internat. J. Fertil.*, 9:177, 1964.
93. Owren, P. A.: *Brit. Med. J.*, 2:220, 1963.
94. Paulsen, A. C., et al.: *J. Clin. Endocr. Metab.*, 22:1033, 1962.
95. Peck, C. K., and Lo Piccolo, J.: *Endocrinology*, 78:965, 1966.
96. Peeters, F., Oeyen, R., and Van Roy, M.: *Internat. J. Fertil.*, 9:111, 1964.
97. Pincus, G.: *Endocrinology*, 59:695, 1956.
98. Pincus, G., Rock, J., and Garcia, C. R.: *Amer. J. Obstet. Gynec.*, 75:1333, 1958.
99. Pincus, G.: *Science*, 138:439, 1962.
100. Pincus, G.: *The Control of Fertility.* New York, Academic Press, 1965.
101. Ramirez, V. D., Abrams, R. M., and MacCann, S. M.: *Endocrinology*, 75:234, 1964.
102. Reyniak, V., Sedlis, A., Stone, D., and Conell, E.: *Acta Cytol.*, 13:315, 1969.
103. Rice-Wray, E., Cervantes, A., and Gastelum, H.: *Internat. J. Fertil.*, 12:312, 1967.
104. Roland, M., and Ober, W. B.: *Internat. J. Fertil.*, 8:619, 1963.
105. Roland, M.: *Progestagen Therapy.* Springfield, Ill., Charles C Thomas, 1965.
106. Rudel, H. W., et al.: *J. Reprod. Fertil.*, 8:305, 1964.
107. Rudel, H. W., Martínez-Manautou, J., and Maqueo, M.: *Fertil Steril.*, 16:158, 1965.
108. Ryan, C. M., Craig, J., and Reid, D. E.: *Amer. J. Obstet. Gynec.*, 90:715, 1964.
109. Ryan, G. M., Goss, D., and Reid, D. E.: *Amer. J. Obstet. Gynec.*, 94:515, 1966.
110. Sánchez-Rivera, G., Cremades-Marco, J., and Botella, J.: *Acta Gin.*, 17:83, 1966.
111. Sánchez-Rivera, G., Merlo, J. G., and Botella, J.: *Acta Gin.*, 18:193, 1967.
112. Sánchez-Rivera, G., Merlo, J. G., and Botella, J.: *Acta Gin.*, 17:83, 1966.
113. Sánchez-Rivera, G., Merlo, J. G., Escudero, M., and Botella, J.: *Amer. J. Obstet. Gynec.*, 101:665, 1968.
114. Saunders, F. J.: *Endocrinology*, 77:863, 1965.
115. Saunders, F. J.: *Endocrinology*, 80:447, 1967.
116. Schally, A. V., Carter, W. H., and Saiton, M.: *J. Clin. Endocr.*, 28:1747, 1968.
117. Schally, A. V., Parlow, A. F., Carter, W. H., Saito, M., Bowers, C. Y., and Arimura, A.: *Endocrinology*, 86:530, 1970.
118. Soost, H. J.: *Acta Cytol.*, 12:294, 1968.
119. Spellacy, W. N., and Carlson, K. L.: *Amer. J. Obstet. Gynec.*, 95:474, 1966.
120. Spellacy, W. N., Carlson, K. L., and Schade, S. L.: *Amer. J. Obstet. Gynec.*, 101:672, 1968.
121. Spellacy, W. N., Carlson, K. L., Birk, S. A., and Schade, S. L.: *Metabolism,* 17:496, 1968.
122. Spellacy, W. N., Buhi, W. C., Moses, L. E., Spellacy, C. E., and Goldzieher, J. W.: *Amer. J. Obstet. Gynec.*, 106:173, 1970.
123. Starup, J.: *Acta Endocr.*, 51:469, 1966.
124. Starup, J., and Oostergard, E.: *Acta Endocr.*, 52:292, 1966.
125. Starup, J., and Lebesch, P. E.: *Acta Endocr.*, 56:188, 1967.
126. Starup, J., and Frilis, T.: *Acta Endocr.*, 56:525, 1967.
127. Starup, J., Date, J., and Deckert, T.: *Acta Endocr.*, 58:537, 1968.
128. Stern, E., Clark, V. A., and Coffelt, C. F.: *Science*, 169:497, 1970.
129. Stevens, V. C., Goldzieher, J. W., and Vorys, N.: *Amer. J. Obstet. Gynec.*, 102:95, 1968.
130. Suchowsky, G., Turola, E., and Arcari, G.: *Endocrinology*, 80:255, 1967.
131. Swaab, L. I.: *Internat. J. Fertil.*, 9:107, 1964.
132. Swerdloff, R. S., and Oddell, W. D.: *J. Clin. Endocr.*, 29:157, 1969.
133. *Symposium on 19-Nor-Progestational Steroids.* Chicago, G. D. Searle & Co., 1957.
134. *Symposium on New Steroid Agents with Progestational Activity.* Ann. N.Y. Acad. Sci., 71:479, 1958.
135. *Symposium on Provest and Provera. Internat. J. Fertil.*, 8:589, 1963.
136. *Symposium on Ovulation Inhibitors. Internat. J. Fertil.*, 9:1, 1964.
137. Taubert, H. D.: *Endocrinology*, 80:218, 1967.
138. Taymor, M. L., and Rizkallah, T.: *J. Clin. Endocr. Metab.*, 25:843, 1965.
139. Terragno, N., and Gutiérrez, D. A.: *Acta Gin.*, 17:219, 1966.
140. Tullner, W. E., and Hertz, R.: *Endocrinology*, 52:359, 1953.
141. Vokaer, R., and Ferin, J.: *Bull. Roy. Soc. Belg. Obstet. Gynec.*, 31:431, 1964.
142. Walsen, H. C., Margulis, R. R., and Ladd, J. E.: *Internat. J. Fertil.*, 9:189, 1964.
143. Watnick, A. S., Gibson, J., Vinegra, M., and Tolksdorf, S.: *Proc. Soc. Exper. Biol. Med.*, 116:343, 1964.
144. Wayne, H., et al.; *Arthr. Rheumat.*, 6:796, 1963.
145. Wienke, E. C., Cavazos, F., Hall, D. G., and Lucas, F. V.: *Amer. J. Obstet. Gynec.*, 103:102, 1969.
146. Williams, K. I. H.: *Steroids*, 13:539, 1969.
147. World Health Organization: "Estudios Recientes sobre Regulación de la Fecundidad." Geneva, WHO, Ser. Techn. Inf., 1969, No. 424, 1969.
148. Zañartu, J.: *Internat. J. Fertil.*, 9:225, 1964.
149. Zañartu, J., and Navarro, C.: *Excerpta Medica International Congress Series*, 112:150, 1965.
150. Zañartu, J.: *Acta Gin.*, 18:311, 1967.
151. Zañartu, J., Rosemberg, D., and Puga, J. A.: *Acta Gin.*, 18:345, 1967.
152. Zañartu, J., Rodríguez-Moore, G., Pupkin, M., Salas, O., and Guerrero, R.: *Brit. Med. J.*, 2:263, 1968.
153. Zañartu, J., Pupkin, M., Rosemberg, D., Guerrero, R., Rodríguez-Bravo, R., García-Huidobro, M., and Puga, J. A.: *Brit. Med. J.*, 2:266, 1968.

INDEX

Page numbers in *italics* denote figures; (t) indicates tables.

Abortion, adrenal insufficiency and, 926
   treatment of, 934
  and postabortive metropathy, 930
  deferred, 933
  diabetes mellitus and, 926
  diagnosis of, 926
    vaginal cytology and, 929
  early, and progestational insufficiency, 635
    endometrium in, 922
    luteal insufficiency and, 906
    unrecognized, as cause of apparent sterility, 636(t)
  endocrine factors in, 913–936
  gonadotropin insufficiency and, 915
  habitual, causes of, 637(t)
    findings in consecutive cycles, 923(t)
    unrecognized, 636(t)
      and sterility, 922(t)
      progestational insufficiency and, 922, 924(t)
    syndrome of, 920, *921*
  hypothyroidism and, 925
  late, progestational insufficiency and, 637, 637(t)
  luteal insufficiency and, 913
  missed, 933
  of endocrine origin, from maternal causes, treatment of, 934
    thyroid therapy for, 934
    treatment of, 933
  of trophoblastic origin, 914
  prediabetes and, 986, 986(t)
  pregnanedioluria in, 927
  prevention of, through use of relaxin, 91
  prognosis of, 926
    crystallization of cervical mucus and, 930
    gonadotropinemia and, 927, *928*, *929*
    gonadotropinuria and, 927, *928*
    placental lactogen and, 927
    sex of embryo and, 930
    vaginal cytology and, 929
  repeated, 920
    endocrine aspects of, 922
  sporadic, 920
  threatened, gonadotropinuria in, *917*
    pregnanedioluria in, *916*
    vaginal cytology and, 548, *924*
  thyroid insufficiency and, 925
  treatment of, oral progestogens for, 934
  trophoblastic changes in, types of, *918*
Abortive rests, diagnosis of by microcurettage, 564
17-Acetoxyprogesterone-3-cyclopentylenol-ether, structure of, *1031*
Acetylcholine, role in induction of labor, 156, 458
  role in interruption of pregnancy, 447
  role in vasospasm of menstruation, 276
Achard-Thiers syndrome, and adrenogenital syndrome, 750, 752, 885
Acrocentric chromosomes, 311, *312*
Acromegaly, 692
  and gestation, 976

Acromegaly (*Continued*)
  and pregnancy, 693
  lactation in, 693
  somatotropic hormone and, 107
ACTH. See *Hormone, adrenocorticotropic*.
Actinomycosis, and secondary hypoestrinism, 588
Actomyosin, in energy cycle of gravid uterus, *454*
Addison's disease, and pregnancy, 957, 990
  coexistence of with adrenal sexual syndromes, 728
  of newborn, 428
Addisonism, gravidic, 957
Adenocarcinoma. See also *Carcinoma*.
  endometrial, *1015*
    relationship to hyperplasia, *1014*
Adenohypophysis, 97–114. See also *Pituitary*.
  action of hypothalamus on, *142*
  blood supply of, 103, *104*
  cells of, and origin of hormones, 102, 103(t)
  cytology of, 101, *102*
    functional, 103(t)
  embryology of, 100, *100*
  endocrine correlations of, *158*
  histology of, 101
  hormones of, immunologic properties of, 112
  innervation of, 104
  morphology of, 100, *100*
  physiology of, 105
  porta-diencephalic system of, 103
Adenoma(s), chromophobe, and hypothalamic syndromes, 710
  hyperestrinism and, 616
Adenoma of Pick, in testicular feminization, *811*, 812, 812(t)
Adenoma tubulare testiculare, 666, *667*
Adenosis, of breast, 619
Adipose hypogenitalism, 703
Adiposity. See also *Obesity*.
  hypothyroid, 760
Adiposogenital syndrome of Froehlich. See *Froehlich's syndrome*.
Adiuretin, 160
Adnexitic ovary. See *Ovary, adnexitic*.
Adnexitis, chronic. See *Ovary, adnexitic*.
Adolescence, menstrual disorders of, 850. See also *Puberty*.
Adrenal(s), accessory, 168
  adult, regeneration of, *168*
  androgen synthesis by, in normal female, 879
  ascorbic acid depletion in, in pregnancy, 995
  as possible origin of postmenopausal estrogens, 370
  C-21 steroid synthesis in, hormonal cycle of, *180*
  carcinoma of, 746, *747*
  climacteric virilization and, 872
  cortex of. See *Adrenal cortex*.
  delayed puberty and, 848, *849*
  disorders of, and pregnancy, 989
    sexual, 727–757
      and pituitary pathology, 728
      bisexual character of, 727

1049

Adrenal(s) (Continued)
  disorders of, sexual, coexistence of with other
      adrenal syndromes, 728
  effects of estrogens on, 25
  effects of progestogens on, 47
  effects of stress on, 992
  embryology of, 165
  endocrinopathies of, 727–757
  fetal, 166
    endocrine activity of, 333
    of mouse, 167
    secretion of corticoids by, in pregnancy, 994
  fuchsinophilic zone of, in adrenogenital syndrome,
      734, 735, 735, 737, 738
  function of, during puberty, 353
    unitarian or pluralistic character of, 179
  hyperactivity of, during climacterium, 369, 370,
      370(t)
  hyperplasia of, dexamethasone test in, 534
    differentiation from adrenal tumor, 749(t)
    in Stein-Leventhal syndrome, 651
  hypoestrinism and, 586
  in adrenogenital syndrome, 734, 735, 735, 736, 737
  infertility and, 907
  insufficiency of, and abortion, 926
    relative, in toxemia of pregnancy, 957, 959
  Marchand's accessory, 668
  maternal, secretion of corticoids by, in pregnancy,
      994
  menopause and, 859
  metabolic, 433
    fetal, maturation of, 433
  metabolic cortex of, compared to sexual
      cortex, 181(t)
  neocortex of, development of, 167
  paleocortex of, development of, 167
  postnatal atrophy of, 433
  postnatal degeneration of, 168
  postnatal development and regeneration of, 169
  precocious puberty and, 840
  pregnancy and, 427
  role in general adaptation syndrome, 992, 993
  sexual, 433. See also Adrenal cortex, sexual zone of.
    hyperplasia of, and adrenogenital syndrome, 729
  sexual cortex of, compared to metabolic cortex,
      181(t)
  sexual cycle in, 288
  sexual function and, 165–186
  sexual syndromes of. See Adrenals, disorders of,
      sexual.
  steroids in, effect on fetus, 333
    isolated by perfusion, 172(t)
  steroid metabolism in, alterations in, and
      adrenogenital syndrome, 730, 731, 732
    regulation of, 730
  steroid synthesis in, inhibition by Metopyrone, 535
  storage of vitamin C in, 219, 220
  synthesis of progesterone by, 51, 914, 915
  tests of, 532
    dexamethasone, 532, 533, 534
    Metopyrone, 533, 535
    stimulation, 532
    suppression, 532
    Thorn, 532
  tumors of, 747, 1018
    dexamethasone test in, 534
    differentiation from adrenal hyperplasia, 749(t)
  virilization and, 881
  zona reticularis of, hyperplasia of, 732, 734
  zones of, steroids produced by, 181(t)

Adrenal cortex, action of on breast, 467
  and hyperestrinism, 608
  androgen synthesis in, 72
  as third gonad, 181
  C-21 steroids in, biogenesis of, 171
  disorders of, and pregnancy, 989
  effects of ACTH on, 176
  effects of androgens on, 68
  effects of castration on, 169
  effects of LH on, 176, 177
  effects of sex hormones on, 169
    and structural changes, 169, 170
    on blood levels, 170
  effects of STH on, 178
  development of, 167
  fetal, histology of, 166
  hormone metabolism of, 170
  hormones of. See also Adrenocortical steroids.
    and specific stimulants, 178(t)
  hyperactivity of, in climacterium, 369, 370, 370(t)
  hyperfunction of zona fasciculata, and Cushing's
      syndrome, 694
  hyperplasia of in pregnancy, 427, 427
  hypertrophy of in pregnancy, 427, 427
  in fetal life, 432
  insufficiency of, congenital, syndrome of, 753
  metabolic, compared to sexual cortex, 181(t)
  of fetus, compared to kidney, 433
  role in Stein-Leventhal syndrome, 651
  sex hormones in, demonstration of, 170
  sexual zone of, 174
    and gonadotropins in climacterium, 369
    as third gonad, 181
    compared to metabolic cortex, 181(t)
    cortical insufficiency of, 753
    in female fetus, 176
    in spayed mouse, 175
    role of in endocrine system, 178
  storage of vitamin C by, 220
  X zone of. See Adrenal cortex, sexual zone of.
  zones of, proportions of at different phases, 429
Adrenal tumors, ovarian, 668, 669, 670
Adrenalectomy, and gestation, 428
  effects of, in breast cancer, 1016
    on pregnancy, 990
    on rats, 183
  with castration, effect of on rats, 183
Adrenocortical hormones, specific stimulants of,
    178(t). See also Adrenocortical steroids.
Adrenocortical insufficiency, congenital, 753
  constitutional, 754
Adrenocortical steroids, biogenesis of, 171, 173
  isolated by perfusion of adrenals, 172(t)
  metabolism of, 173
  sexual action by, 181
  urinary excretion of, 173
    in castrated women, 172
Adrenocorticotropic hormone. See Hormone,
  adrenocorticotropic.
Adrenogenital syndrome, 169, 598, 728. See also
    Virilization, adrenal.
  Addison's disease and, 750
  adrenal form, compared to pituitary form, 888(t)
  adult type, 745
  alterations in steroid metabolism and, 731, 732, 733
  and Achard-Thiers syndrome, 750, 752
  and Cushing's syndrome, 749, 751
    differentiation of, 750(t)
  and pregnancy, 745, 990
  bisexual character of, 742

Index

Adrenogenital syndrome (*Continued*)
  congenital, 728
    false, 751, 752
      hyperplasia in, *734*
  differentiation between pituitary and adrenal forms, 888(t)
  endocrinology of, 737
  estrogens in, 740
  etiology of, 729, *733*
  excretion of urinary steroids in, 740(t)
  failure of 21-hydroxylase activity in, 730, *730*, *733*
  feminizing, in males, 743
  fetal, 743
  forms of, 742
  hilus cell hyperplasia in, 737
  hyperfeminization in, 742, 744, 745
  hyperthecosis in, 737
  hypervirilization in, 742
  incidence of, 728
  infantile form, *735*, *736*, 744
  isosexual, 742
  juvenile type, 744
  17-ketosteroids in, 737
  neoplasm as cause of, 728
  ovary in, 737
  panhypercorticism in, 750
  pituitary form, compared to adrenal form, 888(t)
  pneumokidney in, *742*
  pregnanediol in, 741
  psychic changes in, 746
  sudanophilic zone in, *739*
  transient, of puberty, 845
  treatment of, 748
    effect of cortisone in, 748, *749*
  urinary 17-ketosteroids in, 72
  virilization in, *739*, *741*
Adrenosterone, structure of, *64*
Afibrinogenemia, in postpartum necrosis of pituitary, 685
After-pains, puerperal, effect of suckling on, *477*
Agalactia, in postpartum necrosis of pituitary, 685
Age, of climacterium, 857
Agenesis, gonadal, true, 573
  ovarian, atrophic vaginal smear in, *576*
  renal, unilateral, 828, *829*
AGP. See *Glycerophosphatase, alkaline.*
Albright's syndrome, 844
Aldosterone, compound name of, 11
Aldosteronism, in toxemia of pregnancy, 964
  primary, and pregnancy, 991
Alkaline glycerophosphatase. See *Glycerophosphatase, alkaline.*
Alkaline phosphatase, in corpus luteum, 243, *243*, *244*
Allenolic acid, structure of, *15*
Allylestrenol, structure of, *40*, *1030*
Alpha cells, of pituitary, 102, *102*
Amenorrhea, androgenic, and infertility, 887
  endometrial patterns in, *581*
  hyperestrogenic, 614, 615(t)
  hyperhormonal, followed by metrorrhagia, *611*
    treatment of, 623, *624*
  polyhormonal, 699
  psychogenic, 712, *713*
    and inhibitory neural pathways, *724*
    hyperhormonal type, 723
    low wave type, 712, *723*
    mechanism of, *720*
    ovary in, *717*, *718*, *719*
  secondary, hypothalamic type, 590
    of pituitary origin, 689
  starvation, 769
  with corpus luteum persistence, 640, *641*

Amoeba, reproductive cycle of, 3
Amphenone, structure of, *534*
Anastomoses, arteriovenous, in premenstrual endometrium, 274, 275
  in spiral arteries, 264, *264*
Androgens, absorption of, in women, 76, 77
  actions of on breast, 467
  activity of, during and after climacterium, 368, 368(t)
    in female, 65
    in male, 64
  and antiandrogens, 79
  and delay in tumorigenesis, 1022
  and delayed puberty, 849
  and pseudohermaphroditism of newborn, 834
  and virilization, 66
  antifeminizing activity of, 65
  application of, 78
  as precursors of estrogens, 80
  bioassay of, 65, 69
  chemical determination of, 69
  chemical structure of, 62
  chemistry of, 63, *64*
  dosages of, 79
  dosage units of, 78
  effects of in male, 65
  effects of on development of wolffian duct, 331
  effects of on embryo, 69
  effects of on embryonal wolffian duct organs, 67
  effects of on endocrine glands, 68
  effects of on female somatic features, 66
  effects of on feminine psyche and libido, 67
  effects of on hypothalamus, 149
  effects of on ovary, 65
  effects of on prepubertal female, 68
  effects of on uterus, 66
  effects of on vagina, 66
  effects of on vaginal cytology, 549
  excretion of, 76, 76, 77, 78
  formation of, 70
  in normal female body, 62–81, 879
    significance of, 80
  in placental tissue, 403
  in treatment of climacteric disorders, 875
  in treatment of hyperestrinism, 622
  intermediary metabolism of, 71
  metabolic effects of, 68
  metabolism of, 75
  nomenclature of, 62
  ovarian biogenesis of, pathophysiology of, 643
  pharmacology of, 78
  pseudoprogestational activity of, 65
  synthesis of, 70
    by ovarian hilus cells, 644
    by sexual mesenchyme, 371, *372*
    in adrenal cortex, 72
    in normal female, 73, 879
    in ovary, 72, *74*
    in Stein-Leventhal syndrome, *650*
    in testis, 70
    mechanisms of, 73
    pathways of, 70(t)
  toxicity of, 79
  transport of, 76
  treatment of hyperplastic metropathy with, *623*
  urinary, during and after climacterium, 368, 368(t)
Androgenic cell, 66
Δ3,5-Androstadiene-17-one, structure of, *64*
Androstane, structure of, *13*, *62*, *1027*
Androsterone, compound name of, 11
  structure of, *62*
Androtermones, 327

Aneuploidy, 777
Aneurin. See *Vitamin B₁*.
Angle, carpal, of Kosowicz, 503, *504*
    sign of, 577
Angiospasm. See *Vasospasm*.
Angiotensinase, in normal pregnancy, 962
Anhydrase, carbonic. See *Carbonic anhydrase*.
Anhydroprogesterone, structure of, 38
Anomalies, congenital, thymic, 766
Anorexia nervosa, 713, *714*
    differentiation from Simmond's syndrome, 684(t), 715(t)
    sella turcica in, *714*
Anovulation, long-term effects of, 1046
Anovulatory cycle. See *Cycle, ovarian, anovulatory*.
Anovulomenorrhea, 270
Antiandrogens, 79
    treatment of virilism with, 889
Antibodies, to gonadotropins, 126
Antidiuretic hormone, 160
Antiestrogens, 33
Antigestagens, 55
Antigonadotropins, 112, 124
    artificial, 127
    natural, 126
Antihypertensives, and eclampsia, 961
Antimenotoxins, in dysmenorrhea of puberty, 853
Antioxytocic substances, 459
Antiphlogistic action, of hypophysioadrenal system, in general adaptation syndrome, 994, *994*
Antiserotonin, in normal pregnancy, 962
Antithyroid substances, in pregnancy, 426
Anvil-shaped tibia, sign of, 503, *503*
Apoenzyme, 206
Arginine-vasopressin, 160
Arias-Stella phenomenon, in ectopic pregnancy, 564, *564*
Arrhenoblastoma, 665, *666*
    tubular type, 666, *667*
Arrhythmias, cardiac, in climacterium, 869
Arteriovenous anastomoses, in premenstrual endometrium, 274, *275*
    in spiral arteries, 264, *264*
Arteries, arcuate, 263, *263*
    basal, 263, *263*
    radial, 263, *263*
    spiral, *261*, 263, *263*
        arteriovenous anastomoses in, 264, *264*
        precapillary sphincters in, 264
    uterine, 263, *263*
Aschheim-Zondek reaction, 128
Ascorbemia, 219
Ascorbic acid. See also *Vitamin C*.
    depletion of, in pregnancy, 995
    ovarian, depletion of, as bioassay of LH, 527
Ascorburia, 219
Assimilation, of chromosome fragments, 788
    of whole chromosome, 788, *790*
        cannula for, Burch, 555
Aspiration, in endometrial biopsy, 553. See also *Microcurettage*.
Assay, of hormones, 506–541. See also *Bioassay* and listing under specific hormones, e.g., *Progesterone*.
Asthenic habitus, 377, *378*
Atresia, follicular, of ovary during pregnancy, 422
Atrophy, compensatory, law of, 438
    of pituitary basophilic cells, in Cushing's syndrome, 695
    of liver, in first trimester of pregnancy, 957
    thyroid, secondary, 760
Autoimmune disease, Stein-Leventhal syndrome as, 652

Autosomes, 301
    aberrations in, quantitative, 780
Autosomopathies, 777. See also *Chromosomopathies*.
    quantitative, 780
Avitaminosis, global, 225
Avitaminosis A, effect of on fetal development, 211
    effect of on ovary, 209, *209*
    effect of on testis, 209, *210*
    effect of on uterus and vagina, 210
Avitaminosis B₁, effect of on rat ovary, *213*
    effect of on rat vagina, *213*
    effect of on uterine motility, 214
Avitaminosis C, effect of on menstruation, 211
    effect of on pregnancy, 221
Avitaminosis D, effect of on genital tract, 222
    significance of in pregnancy, 222
Avitaminosis E, effect on testis, 224

Banal endometritis, 563
Barr body. See *Chromatin, sex*.
Basal body temperature, 494
Basal metabolism, 492
Basedow's disease, and gestation, 978
    centrogenous, 762
Basic sex. See *Sex, basic*.
Batrachia, effects of FSH and LH on, 130
    effects of HCG on, *130*
    spermiation in, 130, *130*
Benzestrol, structure of, *15*
Berger cell hyperplasia, virilization and, 883, *883*, *884*
Beta cells, of pituitary, 102, *102*
Bioassay, of sex hormones, methods of, 518
Biocatalysts, and genital tumors, 1008
    endogenous, enzymes as, 206
    exogenous, hormones as, 206
    vitamins as, 206
    function of in development and reproduction, 2
Biologic pregnancy test. See *Pregnancy test, biologic*.
Biologic week, 453
Biopsy, endometrial, 553–568. See also *Microcurettage*.
    Burch aspiration cannula for, *555*
    in diagnosis of hyperestrinism, 621
    Reifferscheid curette for, *554*
Biotype(s), asthenic, 377, *378*
    hypoplastic, characteristics of, 381
    integration of, 382
    pyknic, 377, *379*
Biotypology, of women, 375
Birth control. See *Contraceptives, oral*.
Bladder, urinary, endocrine cytology of, 551
Bleeding, extragenital, in dysmenorrhea of puberty, 852
    functional, 611
        associated with atypical hyperplasia, 615
        causes of, 612
        juvenile, 850
        postabortive. See *Metropathy, postabortive*.
    implantation, 397
    menstrual. See also *Menstruation*.
        duration of, and prolonged endometrial shedding, 643(t)
    pseudomenstrual periodic, 664
Blood, changes in, at puberty, 349
    during sexual cycle, 290
    coagulation of, changes in, from contraceptives, 1044
    morphologic examination of, 491
    sex hormones in, methods of bioassay of, 518
Blood chemistry, 492

Index

Body(ies), Barr. See *Chromatin, sex.*
   Call-Exner, 660, *660*, *661*, *841*
   wolffian. See *Wolffian body.*
Body proportions, use of in clinical examination, 488
Body temperature, basal, 494
   effects of ovulation inhibitors on, 1040, *1040*
   in luteal insufficiency due to shortened secretory phase, *629*
   in menstrual cycle with luteal insufficiency, 495
     biphasic, *494*
   biphasic cycle of, 289, *289*
   biphasic curve of, 350, *350*
   cyclic changes in, at puberty, 350, *350*
   during sexual cycle, 289, *289*
   in progestational luteal insufficiency due to weakened secretory phase, *631*
   monophasic, *494*
Bone marrow cultures, for obtaining chromosome spreads, 311
Bonnevie-Ullrich syndrome, 799, 804
Botella, theory of sexual differentiation of, 337, *337*
Breast, action of estrogens on, 465
   adenosis of, 619
   adrenocortical function and, 467
   and milk secretion, hormones regulating, *465*. See also *Lactation.*
   carcinoma of, effects of adrenalectomy on, 1016
     effects of hypophysectomy on, 1017
     estrogen receptivity of, 1017
     estrogens and, 1015
       origin of, 1017
     hyperestrinism and, 1015
     karyotype in, 1007
     mammogenic factor and, 1018
     ovary in, 1016
     vaginal cytology in, 1016, 1016(t)
   changes in at puberty, 347
   development of, 463
     after birth, 464
     at term and during lactation, 468
     fetal, 464
     hormones affecting, *464*
   disorders of, due to hyperestrinism, 619
   dysplasia of, 618
   effects of androgens on, 68, 467
   effects of castration on, 465
   effects of estrogens on, 24
   effects of oxytocin on, *457*
   effects of placenta on, 467
   effects of progestogens on, 47, 466
   effects of relaxin on, 87, 468
   effects of thyroid on, 467
   effects of thyroxine on, 191
   endocrine physiology of, 463–482
   fibrocystic disease of, 619
   functional disorders of, endocrinology of, 620
   growth of, and pituitary, 466
   intramammary pressure of, effect of oxytocin on, *476*
     method for recording, *476*
   malignant degeneration of, in postclimacterium, 373
   sexual cycle in, 287
Breast, tumors of. See also *Breast, carcinoma of.*
   hereditary factors in, 1006
   vital cycle of, 1006, *1006*
Brenner tumors, 674
Brown method, for determination of urinary estrogens, 507
Burch aspiration cannula, for endometrial biopsy, 555

Cachexia, strumiprival, 759
Calcification, pineal, 765
Calcium metabolism, effects of estrogens on, 26
Call-Exner bodies, in granulosa cell tumor, 660, *660*, *661*, *841*
Cancer. See *Carcinoma.*
Capacitance, spermatic, and contraception, 1042
   effects of progestogens on, 1038
Carbohydrate metabolism, effects of estrogens on, 26
Carbonic anhydrase, changes in during endometrial cycle, 267
   estimation of in endometrial extracts, 522
Carcinogenesis, aromatic hydrocarbons and, 1008, *1009*
Carcinoma. See also *Adenocarcinoma; Adenoma; Tumors.*
Carcinoma, adrenal, 746, *747*
   and estrogens, 618
   breast. See *Breast, carcinoma of.*
   endometrial, diabetes and, 1015
     estrogens and, 1010
       excretion of, 1013(t)
     hormonal origin of, arguments against, 1014
       arguments for, 1011
     state of ovary and endometrium in, 1012(t)
     vaginal cytology in, 1013(t)
   granulosa cell, 660
   mammary. See *Breast, carcinoma of; Tumor, mammary.*
   uterine, latency in, 1020
Carotene, as provitamin, 208
Carpal angle, of Kosowicz, sign of, 503, *504*
   sign of, 577
Castration, and urinary excretion of steroids, 172
   effects of on adrenal cortex, 169
   effects of on breast, 465
   embryonic, effects of on sexual differentiation, 333
   unilateral, effect of on pregnant rabbit, 399
   vaginal cytology following, 549
Castration cells, 106
Catalysis, 2
Catalyst(s). See *Biocatalysts.*
Catecholamines, and eclampsia, 961
   and pregnancy, 425
   changes in during endometrial cycle, 269
   effects of on hypothalamic sex center, 150, 725
Causality, in development, 1
Cavity, nasopharyngeal, tumors of, 710, *711.*
Celioscopy, correlation of findings with results of other methods, 499(t)
   transabdominal, 500, *500*
   transvaginal. See *Culdoscopy.*
Cell(s), alpha, of pituitary, 102, *102*
   androgenic, 66
   beta, of pituitary, 102, *102*
   castration, 106
   clear, in ectopic pregnancy, 564, *564*
     in luteoma, *674*
   delta, of pituitary, 102, *102*
   epsilon, of pituitary, 102, *102*
   folded, 285, *286*
   gamma, of pituitary, 102, *102*
   germ, 3
   granulosa, tumor of, *603*
   granulosa-lutein, synthesis of progesterone by, 49
   hilar, hyperplasia of, 600
   hilus. See *Hilus cells.*
   karyopyknotic, 285, *286*
   mucoid, 102, *102*

Cell(s) (*Continued*)
  navicular, 285, *286*, 547, *548*, *549*
  parasympathicotropic, 644
  pregnancy, 106, 133, 423
  secretory, as sites of origin of gonadotropins, 123
  somatic, 3
  theca-lutein, 241
  thecal, hyperplasia of, 599. See also *Hyperthecosis.*
  types of, in vaginal cycle, 285, *286*
Cellular indices, of vaginal cytology, 550
Cervix, uterine, cycle of. See *Cycle, cervical.*
  dilatation of, effects of relaxin on, 87
  dysplasia of, from oral contraceptives, *1045*
  effects of estrogens on, 21
  effects of progestogens on, 45, 1038
  endocrine disorders of, and infertility, 908
  mucus of. See *Mucus, cervical.*
  musculature of, cycle in, 284
  nerve supply of, 140
  softening and dilatation of, and relaxin, 84, 85
CG. See *Gonadotropin, human chorionic.*
Characters, sex. See *Sex characters.*
Chiari-Frommell syndrome, and galactotropic hyperpituitarism, 700
  and gestation, 975, *976*
Chiasma(ta), 788
Chlormadinone, structure of, 1030
Chlortrianisene, structure of, *15*, *625*
Cholesterol, compound name of, 11
Cholinesterase, role in gestation and labor, 459
Chorioadenoma, 937
Chorioadenoma destruens, 942
Choriocarcinoma, *945*
  cytotrophoblastic, 950
  invading blood vessel, 951
  syncytial, 950
Chorioepithelioma, 675, 949–956
  as inoculation tumor, 951
  benign, 954
  hormone synthesis by, 952
  immunity to, 952
  malignant, 954
  prognosis of, 953
  treatment of, 954
Chorioepithelioma malignum, 954
Chorioepitheliosis, 937, 954
Choriolysins, and immunity to chorionic invasion, 952
Chorion. See also *Villus(i), chorionic.*
  alterations in, in hyperemesis gravidarum, 958
  lining of, alterations in, 449
  synthesis of progesterone by, 914
Chorion frondosum, histology of, *449*
Chorionic gonadotropin. See *Gonadotropin, human chorionic; Pregnant mare serum.*
Chorionic villi. See *Villus(i), chorionic.*
Chorioteratoblastoma, 675
Chromatin, sex, 306, *306*, *307*
    characteristics of, 308
    significance of, 309
    variations in occurrence of, 791
Chromatography, column, for determination of urinary pregnanediol, 512
  paper, for determination of urinary pregnanediol, 513
Chromophobe adenomas, and hypothalamic syndromes, 710
Chromosomes, 301. See also *Autosomes; Karyotype.*
  aberrations in, and abortive eggs, 920
  acrocentric, 311, *312*
  acting as biocatalysts, 326

Chromosomes (*Continued*)
  alterations in. See also *Chromosomopathies.*
    mixed, 790
    qualitative, 784
    quantitative, 777
  assimilation of, of fragments, 788
    total, 788, 790
  classification of, 311, 312(t)
    of normal women, *310*
  complements of. See *Genotype; Karyotype.*
  deletion of, total, 788
  Denver classification system of, 311, 312(t)
  duplication of, 788, 789
  formation of isochromosomes by, 786, 787, 788
  in mitosis, 778, *778*
  inversion in, paracentric, 784, *784*
    pericentric, 784, *785*
  metacentric, 311, *312*
  metaphase, in normal women, *310*
  nomenclature of, 311
  nondisjunction of, in oogenesis, 779, *779*, *780*, *781*
    in spermatogenesis, 780, *781*, *782*
    zygotes resulting from, 780, *782*, *783*
  normal complement of, 309
  partial deletion of, 786, *786*
  Philadelphia, 782, 788
  ring, formation of, 786, *786*
  sex, 301. See also *Chromosomes, X; Chromosomes, Y.*
  submetacentric, 311, *312*
  translocation between, reciprocal, 789
  translocation in, 784, *785*
  translocation of, total, 788, 790
  types of, *312*
  X, 301
    active, 304
    deletion of. See *Genotype, Xx.*
    identification of, 305
    inactive, 304
  Y, 301
    double, 305
    identification of, 305
Chromosomopathies, 775, 776
  as cause of adrenogenital syndrome, 733
  cytogenetics of, 777
  mixed type, 790
  qualitative, 784
    between two chromosomes, 788
    within one chromosome, 784
Circulatory system, changes in, at puberty, 349
  from contraceptive therapy, 1044
Cirrhosis, hepatic, and hyperestrinism, 609
Clear cells, in ectopic pregnancy, 564, *564*
  in luteoma, 674
Clear cell tumors, ovarian, 668, 669, 670
Climacterium. 358–374. See also *Menopause.*
  adrenal cortex in, histology of, 369, 370(t)
  adrenocortical insufficiency in, 755
  age of, 857
  androgenic activity in, 368, 368(t)
  belated luteal activity in, 369
  cardiac arrhythmias in, 869
  diabetes and, 869
  disorders of. See *Climacterium, pathology of.*
  endocrinopathies of, 860
  hepatic insufficiency in, 372
  hyperactivity of adrenal cortex in, 369, *370*, 370(t)
  hypercorticism of, 866
  hyperestrinism of, 860
    assay of estrogens in, 860

Index

Climacterium (*Continued*)
  hyperestrinism of, treatment of, 875
  hyperthyroidism of, 763, 867
  lowering of fertility index at, 359
  mechanism involved in cessation of menstruation, 360
  menopausal phase of, 360
  metropathy of, 867
  obesity in, 870
  osteoporosis in, 872
    mechanism of, 873
  ovarian pathology in, 860
    types of, 360
  ovary and, 858
  pancreatic disorders and, 867
  pathology of, 857–877
    symptoms of, 867
      circulatory, 868
      digestive, 869
      nervous, 870
      sexual, 867
    treatment of, 874, 876(t)
    vaginal cytology in, 861
  physiologic sterility of, 359
  pituitary in, 368
  premenopausal phase of, 358
  postclimacteric phase of, 364. See also *Postclimacterium.*
  postmenopausal phase of, 362. See also *Postclimacterium.*
  vaginal smear in, 367, *367*
  pseudomenstruation during, *360*
  role of pituitary in, 858
  senile phase of, 364
  sequence of events in, 358
  virilism in, 871, *871*
    adrenal, 872
    ovarian, from hilus cell hyperplasia, 871, *872*
Clinical exploration, of gynecologic patient, 485–505
Clitoris, hypertrophy of, from androgen therapy, 67
  in virilization, 885
Clomiphene, in treating infertility from progestational insufficiency, *902, 903*
  structure of, *625*
  treatment of anovulatory cycle with, 899, *900, 901*
Clumping index, of vaginal cytology, 550
Coagulation, blood, changes in, from contraceptive therapy, 1044
Cobalamin, 214
Coelom, role of in development of ovary, 321
Coenzyme, 206
Colostrum, 468
Compensatory atrophy, law of, 438
Conditionality, in development, 1
"Conditioned parabiosis," 438
Congestion, pelvic, 724
Connective tissue spurs, in endometrial glands, 260
Constitution, female, 375–389
  sexual, 376
Constitutional hyperthymic syndrome, 849
Contraceptives, oral, 1026–1048
  and changes in blood coagulation, 1044
  and failure of implantation, 1042
  and paralysis of spermatic ascent, 1042
  and risk of fetal virilization, 1044
  and risk of inducing malignancy, 1045
  circulatory changes from, 1044
  classical therapy of, 1043
  combined therapy of, 1043

Contraceptives (*Continued*)
  oral, continuous therapy of, 1043
    digestive changes from, 1044
    effects of on cervical mucus, *1041, 1042*
    effects of on endometrium, *1041*
    effects of on thyroid, 1044
    effects of on vaginal cytology, *1041*
    glucose tolerance curves following, *195*
    harmful effects of, 1043
    hazards of in diabetes, 1045
    insulinemia following, *195*
    long-term effects of anovulation from, 1046
    mode of action of, 1041
    mode of administration of, 1043
    nonstop therapy of, 1043
    paralysis of ovitransport by, 1042
    psychological disturbances from, 1044
    sequential therapy of, 1043
    steroid, chemistry of, 1026
      effects of on genital tract, 1032
      effects of on male animals, 1039
      effects of on ovary, 1032, 1033(t), *1034, 1035*
    suppression of ovulation by, 1041
    urinary disturbances and, 1046
Corpora lutea aberrantia, 633
Corpus albicans, 242, *242*
  cysts of, 639
Corpus gestativum, 241
Corpus luteum, 241
  active, with persistent and mature follicles, *607*
  alkaline phosphatase reaction in, 243, *243, 244*
  cystic, producing mainly estrogens, *605*
  effects of in corticoprival animals, *183*
  hematoma of, and luteal insufficiency, 633, *633*
  gestational, 397, 419, *420, 421*
    insufficiency of, 628. See also *Insufficiency, luteal, gestational.*
    metabolism of, 421
  gravidic. See *Corpus luteum, gestational.*
  hemorrhagic, 582
  insufficiency of, 567. See also *Insufficiency, luteal.*
    and abortion, 913
    and early abortion, 906
    and infertility, 904
      incidence of, 904(t), 905(t)
      treatment of, 905
  persistence of, 639
    with amenorrhea, 640, *641*
    with irregular endometrial shedding, 640, *641*
  progestational, insufficiency of, 628. See also *Insufficiency, luteal, progestational.*
  regression of, 242
  storage of vitamin C in, 218, *218*
  syndromes of, 571, 628–656
Corpus luteum hemorrhagicum, 582
  and luteal insufficiency, 633, *633*
Corpus progestativum, 241
Cortex, adrenal. See *Adrenal(s); Adrenal cortex.*
Cortexine, 327, 335
Corticoids, and lactogenesis, 470
  as placental hormones, 402
  effects of on vaginal cytology, 551
  excretion of during pregnancy, 409
  in bloodstream during pregnancy, 428
  placental, 410, 414
  role in delay in tumorigenesis, 1022
  role in maintenance of lactation, 474
  secretion of, in pregnancy, *994, 995, 995*
  sexual actions by, 181, 182
  synthesis of, and vitamin C, 220

Corticoids (*Continued*)
   urinary, in pregnancy, 428
Corticosteroids, in adrenogenital syndrome, 742
   role in latent diabetes of pregnancy, 983
Corticosterone, compound name of, 11
Corticotropin releasing factor, 146
Cortisol, 53
   compound name of, 11
   plasma levels of, in pregnancy and labor, *429*
Cortisone, action of on gonadotropin secretion, 124
   compound name of, 11
   tolerance to in pregnancy, 428
Craniopharyngiomas, and hypothalamic syndromes, 710
Crest, genital, 318
   development of, 318
Cretinism, 759, *760*
CRF. See *Corticotropin releasing factor.*
Crisis, genital, 334
Crystallization, of cervical mucus, *492, 493*
   and prognosis of abortion, 930
Crystalloids, Reinke, 645
Culdoscopy, 496
   correlation of findings with results from other methods, 499(t)
   indications for, 498
   limitations of, 497
   technique of, 496, *497*
   use in diagnosis, 498
Cultures, bone marrow, for obtaining chromosome spreads, 311
   leukocyte, for obtaining chromosome spreads, 311
   tissue, for obtaining chromosome spreads, 311
Cumulus oophorus, 237
Curettage, total, 553. See also *Microcurettage.*
Curette, Reifferscheid, for endometrial biopsy, *554*
Cushing's disease, central forms of, 695
   differentiation of pituitary and adrenal forms, 695(t)
Cushing's syndrome, 694, *696*
   and adrenogenital syndrome, 749, *751*
      differentiation of, 750(t)
   and pregnancy, 991
   endocrine conditions in, 698
   sella turcica in, *697*
Cycle, adrenal, 288
   cervical, 281
      in cervical musculature, 284
      secretion of mucus in, 282
      variations in crystallization of mucus during, 282, *283*
   endometrial. See also *Endometrium.*
      biochemical changes in, 268
      diagrammatic representation of, *258*
      effect of ovarian hormone activity on, *272*
      histochemical changes during, 265, *265, 266, 268*
      histology of, *259*
      irregularities in, 563
      premenstrual phase of, 260, *273*
      proliferative phase of, 258, *262, 273*
         characteristics of, 267
         cross section of uterus during, *259*
         in monkey, *260*
         relationships between stroma, glands and vessels in, 264, *264*
      secretory phase of, 259, *262, 273*
         in castrated monkey, *261*
         microcurettage in, *556, 557, 558*
      ultrastructural features of, *262*
      vascular changes in, *262, 273*
   gravidic. See *Gestation.*

Cycle (*Continued*)
   in endocervical mucosa, 284
   menstrual. See also *Menstruation.*
      anomalies in rhythm, psychogenic, 717
      anovulatory, 345(t), 346, 348
         with flat menstrual curve, *360*
      diagrammatic representation of, *251*
      first day of, 258
      flat-curved, *362*
      fluctuations in total estrogen levels during, *252*
      gonadotropic regulation of, role of ovary in, 246
      hyperhormonal type, *723*
      low wave type, *712, 733*
      regulation of, role of gonadotropins in, 246
      relative hyperthermia in premenstrual phase, 289
      stability of, 721
      total hormones eliminated during, *252*
      vaginal cytology during, *546, 547*
   myometrial, 280
      spontaneous motility of uterus during, 281, *281*
   ovarian, 231–256
      anovulatory, 236
         and sterility, 893
         etiology of, 894
         incidence of, *345,* 894, 894(t)
         microcurettage in, 559, *559, 561*
         treatment of, 896, 897
      cyclic secretion of estrogens, 249
      estrogenuria during, 249
      feedback mechanism in regulation of, 246
      histochemical changes in, 242
      histologic features of, 237
      hormonal, 249
      hypoluteal, incidence of, *345*
      normal, incidence of, *345*
      plasma estrogen levels during, 250
      pregnanedioluria during, 250, *250*
      progesterone levels during, 250
      rebound phenomenon in, 247
      regulation of, 246
         role of hypothalamus in, 247
      total estrogens and pregnanediol eliminated during, *250*
   ovulatory, aluteal, 893
   pituitary, 288
      in secretion of gonadotropins, 122
   sexual, 229–293
      central influences on, 715
      changes in body temperature during, 289, *289*
      changes in immunologic responses during, 290
      differences between male and female, 236
      establishment of, 231–256
      hematologic changes during, 290
      in breast, 287
      in endocrine glands, 287
      in pancreas, 288
      in primates, 235
         exogenous influences in, 236
         internal "rhythm" in, 235
      in target organs, 257–293
      metabolic changes during, 290
      psychosexual changes during, 290
      systemic changes during, 288
   thyroid, 288
   tubal, 257
      motility of Fallopian tube during, 257, *257*
      nutritional, *393, 394*
   uterine, 258. See also *Cycle, endometrial; Cycle, myometrial; Menstruation.*
   vaginal, 285

Cycle (*Continued*)
  vaginal, cell types in, 285, *286*
    characteristics of cells in, 287(t)
    follicular phase of, cytologic characteristics of, 287(t)
      karyopyknotic cells in, *286*
    glycogen in, 287
    luteal phase of, cytologic characteristics of, 287(t)
      folded cells in, *286*
  vascular, in endometrium, 262
  vital, 1006, *1006*
Cyproterone, 79
Cysts, corpus albicans, 639
  dermoid, thyroid tissue in, 675, *676*
  follicle lutein, 603, 639, *640*
    and uterine leiomyoma, *604*
  granulosa-lutein, 639, *640*
  ovarian, and hydatidiform mole, 948
  theca-lutein, 639
Cytology, bladder, 551
  endometrial, 551
  of oral mucosa, 551
  vaginal, 542. See also *Smears, vaginal.*
    and threatened abortion, 548
    as index of gravidic pathology, 548
    at birth and in childhood, 546
    at menopause, 549
    at puberty, 546
    changes in, 546
    during menstrual cycle, 546, *547*
    effect of contraceptives on, *1041*
    effect of sex hormones on, 549
    estrogenic cellular indices of, 550
    following castration, 549
    in diagnosis and prognosis of abortion, 929
    in endometrial carcinoma, 1013(t)
    in mammary carcinoma, 1016, 1016(t)
    in normal women, 1013(t)
    in postmenopausal women, 367, 367(t)
    in pregnancy, 547, *548*
    in threatened abortion, *924*
    in vaginal cycle, 287(t)
    progestogenic cellular indices of, 550

Deciduoma, formation of, and implantation of embryo in rats, 395
Deficiency states. See also *Avitaminosis*.
  and delayed puberty, 849
  and sexual function, 769
Degeneration, hydropic, 939
  malignant, of uterus and breast, in postclimacterium, 373
  micromolar, 938
  polymicrocystic, of ovary, 589
  postnatal, of adrenal, 168
Dehydroepiandrosterone, structure of, *62*
Δ6-Dehydroretroprogesterone, structure of, *40*
6,7-Dehydroretroprogesterone, structure of, *1032*
Delayed implantation. See *Implantation, of embryo, deferred.*
Delayed menopause, 857
Delayed puberty. See *Puberty, delayed.*
Deletion, of part of a chromosome, 786, *786*
  of whole chromosome, 788
Delta cells, of pituitary, 102, *102*
Demedullation, ovarian, 646, 654
  in treatment of virilism, 889
    urinary 17-ketosteroid rates after, *647*

Denver classification system, for chromosomes, 311, 312(t)
Deoxycorticosterone, compound name of, 11
Dermoid cyst, thyroid tissue in, 675, *676*
Determination, sexual. See *Sex, determination of.*
Detoxification, of estrogens, in dysmenorrhea of puberty, 854
Development, causality in, 1
  conditionality in, 1
  constitutional forms of, 381
  embryonic. See *Gestation*.
  fetal, effect of vitamin A deficiency on, 211
  function of biocatalysts in, 2
Dexamethasone, structure of, *533*
Dexamethasone test, 532, 533, 534
  adrenal, in normal individual, 533, *534*
  in adrenal tumor, 534
  in simple adrenal hyperplasia, *534*
  ovarian, 535
    in normal individual, *536*
Diabetes, and endometrial carcinoma, 1015
  differentiation from prediabetes, 989, 989(t)
  hazards of oral contraceptives in, 1045
  in climacterium, 869
  insulin resistant, and Achard-Thiers syndrome, 750, *752*
  latent, of pregnancy, 979
    congenital malformations and, 986, 987(t)
    corticosteroids and, 983
    fetal gigantism in, 986, 987(t)
    fetal mortality and, 986, 987(t)
    growth hormone and, 982, *982*
    pituitary and, 982, *982*
    pituitary disorders and, *982*
    scheme of, 982, *982*, 983
    significance of placental lactogen in, 983
  placental form of, 982
  placental lactogen and, 982
Diabetes insipidus, 709
  and gestation, 977
Diabetes mellitus, and abortion, 926
  and delayed puberty, 768, *768*
  and sexual function, 768
  as complication of gestation, 984
  influence of pregnancy on, 984
  of pregnancy, effect of on fetus, 984
    grades of, and multiparity, 984
    islet cell hyperplasia in, 985
    influence on mother, 984
    placental senescence and, 984
    placental surface area in, 985
    treatment of, 986
Diabetogenic hormone. See *Hormone, diabetogenic*.
Dienestrol, structure of, *15*
Differentiation, sexual, 297, 330. See also *Sex, determination of.*
  and müllerian system anomalies, 825
  anomalies of, 824–836
    and pseudohermaphroditism, 831
  delayed, 383
  effects of embryonic castration on, 333
  effects of parabiosis on, 334
  effects of transplantation of gonad on, 334
  in various species, 304
  influence of genetic sex on, 337
  influence of target organ response on, 337
  pathology of, 775
  premature, 383
  theories of, 336, *336*, *337*
Digametic sex, 385, 386(t)

Digestion, disorders of, in climacterium, 869
Digestive system, changes in, from contraceptive therapy, 1044
Dimorphism, sexual, true, 299
  spermatic, 302, *303*
Dioxydiethylstilbane, structure of, *15*
Dioxyethylstilbene, structure of, *15*
Disease, autoimmune. See *Autoimmune disease.*
  Basedow's, and gestation, 978
  Cushing's. See *Cushing's syndrome.*
  Simmond's, 682
    differentiation from anorexia nervosa, 684(t)
  von Recklinghausen's, 769
Diuresis, control of, in toxemia of pregnancy, 959
Doisynolic acid, structure of, *15*
Dopamine, effect of on hypothalamic sex center, 725
Douglascopy. See *Culdoscopy.*
Down's syndrome, 780
Drugs, contraceptive. See *Contraceptives, oral.*
  effect of on hypothalamic sex center, 725
  ovulatory, in treating anovulatory cycle, 899, *900, 901, 902, 903*
Ducts, lactiferous, changes in at puberty, 348
  müllerian, development of, 322
    autonomy of from development of wolffian duct, 332
    effect of estrogens on, 331
    substances stimulating, 330
  wolffian, development of, 323, *324*
    autonomy of from development of müllerian duct, 332
    effect of androgens on, 331
Duplication, of chromosomes, 788, *789*
Dwarfism, pituitary, *686,* 687
  "sexogenous," 804
DXM test. See *Test(s), dexamethasone.*
Dynamic tests, adrenal, 532
  for determining function, 531
  ovarian, 535
    of Jayle, 537, *538,* 539(t)
  testicular, 535
Dysfunction, ovarian, at menopause, 360
Dysgenesis, gonadal, 794. See also *Turner's syndrome.*
  and pseudohermaphrodits, 805
  and testicular feminization. See *Feminization, testicular.*
  and X isochromosome, 797
  female, characteristics of, 798, 799(t)
    classification of, 795(t), 799(t)
    karyotypes in, 795, 795(t)
    types of, 798
    XO constitution in, 796
    XX constitution in, 796
    XY constitution in, 796
  karyotypes in, 795, 795(t)
  mixed types of, and mosaicism, 797
  poly-X constitution in, 797
  without Turner's syndrome, *805, 806*
Dysluteinism, 638
Dysmenorrhea, of puberty, 851
  antimenotoxins in, 853
  detoxification of estrogens in, 854
  estroprotein in, 853
  extragenital bleeding in, 852
  headaches in, 852
  menotoxins in, 853
  menstrual edema in, 852
  premenstrual hyperestrinism in, 853
  premenstrual tension in, 852

Dysmenorrhea (*Continued*)
  of puberty, treatment of, 854
    uterine pain in, 852
  use of relaxin for, 90
Dyspituitarism, 690
Dysplasia, cervical, from oral contraceptives, *1045*
  fibrous, polyostotic, 844
  mammary, 618
Dysrhythmia, of pubertal ovary, 346

Eclampsia, 960
  pathogenesis of, *965*
  pressor substances and, 961
  production of hypertension in, *964*
Ectopic pregnancy. See *Pregnancy, ectopic.*
Edema, menstrual, in dysmenorrhea of puberty, 852
Effector organs, importance of in reproduction, 7
Eggs. See also *Ovum(a).*
  abortive, 917
    chromosomal aberrations in, 920
    histochemistry of, 919
    types of, 917(t)
    types of chorionic villi in, *918, 919*
  aquatic, 5, *6*
  cleidoic, 5, *6*
  defective, sterility and, 906
  implanted, nutrition of, 442
  implantation of. See *Implantation, of embryo.*
  placental, 5, *6*
Ejection, of milk, 475
Embryo, castration of, and effects on sexual differentiation, 333
  effects of androgens on, 68
  human, implantation of, *395*
  implantation of. See *Implantation, of embryo.*
  implanted, nutrition of, 442
  nutrition of, prior to implantation, 393, *394.* See also *Nutrition.*
  sex of, and prognosis of abortion, 930
Embryopathy, prediabetic, 986
Eminence, median. See *Median eminence.*
Endocervix, mucosa of, cycle in, 284
Endocrine abortion. See *Abortion, endocrine factors in.*
Endocrine factors, in ovulation, 248
Endocrine glands, and nervous system, 138–164
  effects of androgens on, 68
  effects of progestogens on, 47
  fetal, development of compared to adult, *431*
    functional activity of, *431*
  interrelationships of between mother and fetus, 437
Endocrinopathy(ies), 775
  adrenal, related to sex, 727–757
  affecting sexual function, 679–771
  and anomalies in sexual differentiation, 824–836
  congenital, 438
  fetal, 438
  of climacterium, 860
  of gestation, 891–1002
  of puberty, 837–856
  pituitary, and sexual function, 681
  thyroid, related to sex, 758
Endometriosis, hyperestrinism and, 616
Endometritis, 565
  banal, 563
  from progestational insufficiency, 630
  postabortive, 563

Endometritis (*Continued*)
   syncytial, 948
   tuberculous, 563
      and delayed puberty, 846
Endometrium, adenocarcinoma of, *1015*
   alkaline glycerophosphatase in, 265, *266*, *268*, *565*, *566*
   and endometritis, from luteal insufficiency, 630
   anovulatory cycle of, microcurettage in, 559, *559*, *561*
   biochemical changes in during sexual cycle, 268
   biopsy of, 553–568. See also *Microcurettage*.
      in diagnosis of hyperestrinism, 621
   carcinoma of, arguments against hormonal origin of, 1014
      arguments for hormonal origin of, 1011
      diabetes and, 1015
      estrogens and, 1010
      excretion of estrogens in, 1013(t)
      vaginal cytology in, 1013(t)
   changes in, in polymicrocystic ovary, *602*
   clear cells in, 564, *564*
   cystic glandular hyperplasia of, in postmenopausal woman, 365
   cystic hyperplasia of, *614*
   effects of androgens on, 66
   effect of contraceptives on, *1041*
   effects of estrogens on, 17
      in castrated monkey, *18*
      in castrated woman, *19*
   effects of lynestrenol on, 57
   effects of persistent follicles on, *600*
   effects of progestogens on, 42, *44*, *1036*, *1037*
      in castrated monkey, *43*
      in castrated woman, *43*
   effect of relaxin on, 85
   endocrine cytology of, 551
   endocrine defects of, and infertility, 908
   extracts of, assay of carbonic anhydrase in, 522
   glycogen in, 265, 268, 396, 565
   glycopenia of, *630*
   granulosa cell tumor and, *603*
   histochemistry of, 565
      and implantation, 396
   histology of during endometrial cycle, 259
   human, ultrastructural features of, *262*
   hyperplasia of, active, in postmenopausal woman, 365
      atypical, in postmenopausal woman, 366
      cystic, *617*
      diffuse, *617*
      in thecoma, *662*
      relationship to adenocarcinoma, *1014*
      types of, *617*
      with secretion, 616
   hyperplastic progestational reaction of, 397
   hypoplasia of, in secondary hypoestrinism, *591*
   in amenorrhea, *581*
   in benign uterine tumors, 1019(t)
   in early abortion, *922*
   in endometrial carcinoma, compared to normal, 1012(t)
   in habitual abortion, 923(t)
   in hyperestrinism, microcurettage of, 560
   in menorrhagia, *617*
   in oligomenorrhea, *581*
   in ovarian hyperthecosis, *604*
   in postabortive metropathy, *931*, *932*

Endometrium (*Continued*)
   in postclimacteric metropathia haemorrhagica, 868, *868*
   in postclimacteric phase, 364, *365*, *366*
   in progestational insufficiency, *630*, *631*
   in psychosomatic amenorrhea, *717*, *718*, *719*
   inflammation of. See *Endometritis*.
   luteinization of, incomplete, in psychogenic amenorrhea, *722*
   maturation of, irregular, 563, 615, *616*
      mucosa in, *607*
   menopausal, *359*
   microcurettage of, in hypoestrinism, 560
   mucopolysaccharides in, 567
   mucosa of, effects of progestogens in nidation, 46
      variations in thickness of throughout cycle, *274*
   nonbleeding, in postmenopausal women, 366(t)
   normal, postmenopausal, 1012(t)
   predominant element in, and type of placenta, 280, 280(t)
   premenstrual phase of arteriovenous anastomoses in, 274, *275*
      vascular supply in, *273*
   progestational effect on by relaxin, 86, *86*
   progestational insufficiency of, and habitual abortion, 922, 924(t)
   proliferative phase of, 17
      of puberty, *347*
      vascular supply in, *273*
   rat, cellular changes in response to progesterone, *50*
   receptivity of, and delayed puberty, 846
   regeneration of, 278
   relationships between stroma, glands and vessels in, 264, *264*
   secretory phase of, 44
      alkaline phosphatase activity in, *44*, *45*
      in castrated monkey, *261*
      in postmenopausal women, *359*, *360*, *369*
      "incomplete," 560
      microcurettage in, *556*, *557*, *558*
      spiral arterioles in, *45*
   shedding and regeneration of, mechanism of, 277
   shedding of, irregular, 563, 616, *616*
      and corpus luteum persistence, 640, *641*
      urinary hormones in, 642(t)
      prolonged, *641*, 643(t)
      and duration of bleeding, 643(t)
      vascular supply of, *273*
   squamous metaplasia of, 616, *616*
   state of, in postmenopausal women, 366(t)
   "Swiss cheese," 560, *562*, *614*, *617*
   vascular cycle of, *262*
   vascular supply of, during endometrial cycle, 273, *273*
Enzymes, 2
   activity of, changes in during endometrial cycle, 269
   alterations in, and adrenogenital syndrome, 730, 731
   and relationship to hormones, 2
   as endogenous biocatalysts, 206
   collagenolytic, and ovulation, 249
   distinction of from vitamins, 206
Eosinopenia, gravidic, *994*, *997*
   post-ACTH, in Thorn test, 532
   postepinephrine, in Thorn test, 532
Eosinophilic index, in vaginal cytology, 550
Epinephrine, and antagonism to norepinephrine, 447

Epinephrine (*Continued*)
  relationship of to vitamin C, 208
  role of in interruption of pregnancy, 447
Epitheliochorial placenta, 280, 280(t)
Epsilon cells, of pituitary, 102, *102*
Equilenin, structure of, *14*
Equilin, structure of, *14*
Equine chorionic gonadotropin. See *Pregnant mare serum.*
Ergocornine, 55
Ergones, 2
Erythema pernio, in gonadal dysgenesis, *579*
Esculenta unit, standardization of, 525
  for assay of hormones, 524
"Essential" ovarian virilization, 647
Estradiol, action of, compared with estriol, 26
  structure of, *14, 1027*
  total eliminated during menstrual cycle, 252
17β-Estradiol, compound name of, 11
Estrandiol, structure of, *14*
Estrane, structure of, *13, 1027*
Estratriene, structure of, *13*
Estrenols, 1030
Estrinase, 31
Estriol, action of, compared to estradiol, 26
  compound name of, 11
  determination of, and prognosis of fetal viability, 968, *968*
  structure of, *14*
  total emininated during menstrual cycle, 252
Estrogens, 13–37. See also *Hyperestrinism; Hypoestrinism.*
  and acceleration of tumorigenesis, 1021
  and antiestrogens, 33
  and benign uterine tumors, 1018
  and beta-glucuronidase, 31
  and carcinoma, 618
  and iatrogenic pseudohermaphroditism, 835
  and endometrial carcinoma, 1010
  and in-tandem actions with progestogens, 48
  and interruption of pregnancy, 444
  and spontaneous contractions of uterus, *445*
  antagonists of, nonsteroid, 624
    steroid, 624
  antiovulatory effects of, 1032, 1033(t)
  artificial, *15, 16*
  as contraceptives, 1032
  as growth-promoting substances, 1011
  as placental hormones, 401
  as treatment for primitive hypoestrinism, 592
    results of, *593*
  bioassay of, 27
    by chick oviduct method, 520
    fundamentals of, 518, *519*
    in diagnosis of climacteric hyperestrinism, 860
    in diagnosis of hyperestrinism, 621
    test of vaginal patency for, *519*, 520
  chemical determination of, 27
  chemistry of, 16
  circulation of, 31
  conversion and inactivation of, 30
  cyclic secretion of, during ovarian cycle, 249
  detoxification of, and vitamin B deficiency, 217
  in dysmenorrhea of puberty, 854
  dosage units of, 28
  drop in, and precipitation of menstruation, 271, *271*
  effects of on alkaline phosphatase activity of endometrial glands, 20
  effects of on breast, 24, 465
  effects of on development of reproductive organs, 21

Estrogens (*Continued*)
  effects of on endocrine glands, 25
  effects of on Fallopian tubes, 17, *17*
  effects of on gonads, 17
  effects of on gonadotropin secretion, 123
  effects of on hypothalamicopituitary region of rat, *149*
  effects of on implantation of embryo, 21
  effects of on median eminence, 148
  effects of on müllerian duct development, 331
  effects of on müllerian organs, 17
  effects of on ovary, 17
  effects of on peristalsis of Fallopian tubes, *17*
  effects of on sex characters, 24
  effects of on testis, 17
  effects of on thyroid, 191, *192*
  effects of on vaginal cytology, 549
  effects of on vulva, 24
  effects of water and mineral metabolism on, 26
  excretion of, 31
    during pregnancy, 407, *408*
    effects of ovulation inhibitors on, 1039, *1040*
    in endometrial adenocarcinoma, 1013(t)
    in normal postmenopausal women, 1013(t)
  extracortical origin of, 371
  extragonadal origin of, 371
  extraovarian synthesis of, 31
  form of secretion of, 32
  formation of, 28, *29*
  in abortion, 915
  in adrenogenital syndrome, 740
  in breast cancer, origin of, 1017
  in treating anovulatory cycle, 897
  in treating pathologic climacterium, 874
  inactivation of, 30
  mammary cancer and, 1015
  mechanism of action of, 27
  metabolic effects of, 26
  metabolism of, 28, 30
    chemical cycle in, 272
  natural, *14, 16*
  nomenclature of, 13
  pharmacology of, 32
  physiologic action of, 17
  plasma levels of, during ovarian cycle, 250
  postmenopausal, origin of, 370
  production of, wave-like pattern of, 272
  reactivation of, 31
  receptivity to, disorders of, 583
  role of in implantation of embryo, 395
  routes of administration of, 32
  synthesis of, by sexual mesenchyme, 371, *372*
    by hydatidiform mole, 946
    by placenta, 409, *411*
    effects of placental senescence on, 967
  therapeutic preparations of, 32
  total, fluctuations in during menstrual cycle, 252
  total eliminated during normal cycle, 249, *250*
  toxic effects of, 33
  transformation of to androgens, 75
  treatment of hyperestrinism with, 623
  urinary, determination of, by Brown's method, 507, 508(t)
    by Ittrich's method, 510
    in postclimacterium, 362(t), 364, 365(t)
Estrogen content, of various tissues, 30(t)
Estrogen intoxication, 34
Estrogen-progestogen antagonism, 48
Estrogenuria, during ovarian cycle, 249
Estrone, compound name of, 11
  structure of, *14*
  total eliminated during menstrual cycle, 252

Index

Estrone sulfate, structure of, *14*
Estroprotein, in dysmenorrhea of puberty, 853
Estrus, 232
    and relational life, 233
    influence of hypothalamus on, 232
    in male and female, *234*
    in rat, vaginal changes in, *22*
        vaginal smear of, *235*
    in rodents, 233
Ethamoxytriphetol, structure of, *625*
Ethinylestradiol, structure of, *14*, *1032*
Ethinylestradiol-methyl ester, structure of, *1032*
17α-Ethinyl-19-nortestosterone, structure of, *1029*
17-Ethinyl-19-nortestosterone enanthate, structure of, *40*
17α-Ethyl-nortestosterone, structure of, *1029*
13β-Ethyl-norethisterone, structure of, *1031*
17α-Ethyl-testosterone, structure of, *40*
Ethynodiol acetate, structure of, 1031
Etiocholanolone, compound name of, 11
Eunuchoidism, in gonadotropic hypopituitarism, 688
    pituitary, 585
Euploidy, 777
Evans test, 128
Evocators, 2
Evolution, sexual. See *Sex, evolution of.*
Examination, physical, of gynecologic patient, 487
    of vagina, 490
Excitation radiotherapy. See *Radiotherapy, excitation.*
Extraovarian hyperestrinism, 598

Factors, conditioning, in biologic causality, 1
    inhibiting, prolactin. See *Prolactin inhibiting factor.*
    of determination, 1
    of realization, 1
    releasing. See *Releasing factors.*
    uterorelaxing. See *Relaxin.*
Fallopian tubes, and infertility, 907
    cycle of. See *Cycle, tubal.*
    effects of estrogens on, 17, *17*
    effects of progestogens on, 42, *1033*, *1035*
    motility of during sexual cycle, 257, *257*
    nerve supply of, 139, *140*
    onset of puberty and, 346
    peristalsis of, estrogens and, *17*
    sexual cycle in, 257
False congenital adrenogenital syndrome, 751, 752
Feedback(s), short and long, in endocrine relationships of pituitary, *158*
Feedback effect, of gonadotropins, 122
Feedback mechanism, in ovulation, 253
    of gonadotropic regulation of menstrual cycle, 246
Female constitution, 375–389
Feminization, testicular, 805, *805*, *806*, *807*, *809*, *810*
    adenoma of Pick and, *811*, 812
    classification of, 812(t)
    clinical features of, *807*, *808*, *809*, *810*
    complete, 812
    effects on target organs, 813
    incomplete, 812
    inguinal testis in, *811*
    karyotype in, *806*
Ferguson-Harris reflex, 455
Fertilization, role of prostaglandins in, 910
Feto-placental steroid metabolism, 434, *435*
Feto-placental steroid synthesis, 408
Fetus, effects of prediabetes on, 986

Fetus (*Continued*)
    endocrinopathies of, 438
        gigantism of, and diabetes in pregnancy, 986, 987(t)
    incretory system of, 428–441
    influence of diabetes of pregnancy on, 984
    storage of vitamin C by, 219, *219*
    virilization of, from contraceptive therapy, 1044
Fibrocystic disease of breast, 619
Fibrothecal masses. See *Hyperthecosis, ovarian.*
FIGLU, 217
Fluid, amniotic, sex chromatin in, and diagnosis of sex, 308
    follicular. See *Liquor folliculi.*
Fluorescent microscopy, for vaginal smears, 546
Folates. See *Vitamin B₁₁.*
Folding index, of vaginal cytology, 550
Folic acid. See *Vitamin B₁₁.*
Follicle, ovarian, graafian, 241
    growth of, direction of, *253*
    hemorrhagic, 241
    incomplete luteinization of, in psychogenic amenorrhea, 722
    maturing, 237, *238*, *239*, *240*
    partial luteinization of, and progestational insufficiency, 635
    persistent, 599
        effects of on endometrium, *600*
        "half-ripened," 652
        hemorrhagic metropathy in, 602
        in puberty, 348
        neural pathways involved in, *724*
        ovary in, *601*
    primary, 237
        granulosa layer of, 237
    primordial, 236, *237*
    secondary, 237, *238*
        cumulus oophorus of, 237
        theca externa of, 237
        zona pellucida of, 237
    syndromes of, 571
    tertiary, 241
    theca interna of, 237
    vascularization of, 241
Follicle-lutein cysts, 603, *639*, *640*
    and uterine leiomyoma, *604*
Follicle stimulating hormone. See *Hormone, follicle stimulating.*
Follicle stimulating hormone releasing factor, 144
Follicular persistence. See *Follicles, ovarian, persistent.*
Follicular phase, of female life, 376
Folliculin, 15
Frankenhauser ganglion, 139
Friedman test, 128
Frigidity, sexual, and androgen therapy, 67
Froehlich's syndrome, adiposogenital, 703, *705*, *706*
    adult form, *705*, *706*
    juvenile form, 705, *705*
    psychogenic, 704, 715
    suprasellar calcification in, 704, *704*
FSH. See *Hormone, follicle stimulating.*
FSHRF. See *Follicle stimulating hormone releasing factor.*
Fuchsinophilic zone, adrenal, in adrenogenital syndrome, 734, *735*, *735*, *737*, *738*

Galactogenesis. See *Lactogenesis.*
Galactotropic hyperpituitarism, 700

Gametes, 297
Gametogenesis, 299, *300*
Gamma cells, of pituitary, 102, *102*
Ganglion, Frankenhauser, 139
G.A.S. See *Syndrome, general adaptation.*
General adaptation syndrome. See *Syndrome, general adaptation.*
Genetic sex. See *Sex, genetic.*
Genital crest, 318
Genital crisis, 334
Genital tract. See also *Endometrium; Ovary; Uterus; Vagina.*
　effects of contraceptive steroids on, 1032
　effects of vitamin D on, 222
　embryology of, 315
　female, congenital anomalies of, isosexual, 825
　　congenital endocrinopathies of, 824
　　development of, 322
　　effect of thyroid on, 190
　　innervation of, 138, *139*
　　local changes in at puberty, 343
　　prepubertal, 343, *343, 344*
　　tuberculosis of, and false primitive hypoestrinism, 586, *586*
　male, effect of thyroxine on, 191
　rat, comparison of FSH and LH effects on, *129*
　tumors of, endocrine bases of, 1005–1025
　　hereditary factors in, 1006
　　role of biocatalysts in, 1008
Genitalia, female, changes in at puberty, 347
Genopathies, 776
Genotype(s). See also *Karyotype.*
　combinations of, resulting from chromosomal nondisjunction, 780, *782, 783*
　poly-X, in gonadal dysgenesis, 797
　triple-X, in gonadal dysgenesis, 797
　XO, in female gonadal dysgenesis, 796
　XO, in Turner's syndrome, *802*
　Xx, and female gonadal dysgenesis, 797
　XX, in female gonadal dysgenesis, 796
　XY, in female gonadal dysgenesis, 796
Germinal route, 244, 302
　anomalies of, 776
　in metazoa, *4*
　role of in development of ovary, 321
Gestagens. See *Progestogens; Progesterone.*
Gestation, 391–482
　accumulation of guanidine in, 427
　acromegaly and, 693, 976
　ACTH and, 425
　action of estrogens on actomyosin storage in uterus, *454*
　Addison's disease and, 990
　adrenals and, 427
　adrenal disorders and, 989
　adrenalectomy and, 428, 990
　adrenocortical insufficiency in, 755
　adrenogenital syndrome and, 745, 990
　and establishment of gravidic correlations, 397
　antiserotonin in, 962
　as stressor in pregnancy, 991, 994
　ascorbic acid depletion in, 995
　catecholamines and, 425
　changes of, regression of, 460
　chorionic gonadotropin in, in placenta, 405
　compensatory hyperthyroidism of, 426
　corticoid levels in, 428
　corticoid secretion in, *994, 995, 995*
　critical point in, 453
　Cushing's syndrome and, 991

Gestation (*Continued*)
　development of breast during, *464, 465, 467, 468*
　diabetes of, and fetal mortality rates, 986, 987(t)
　　effect of on fetus, 984
　diabetes insipidus and, 977
　diabetes mellitus in, and multiparity, 984
　　and placental senescence, 984
　　and placental surface area, 985
　　treatment of, 986
　diffuse luteinization of ovary during, 421, *422*
　ectopic. See *Pregnancy, ectopic.*
　effects of avitaminosis C on, 221
　effects of gonadotropins on, 120
　effects of lutectomy during, *914*
　effects of neurohormones on, 446
　effects of on evolution of diabetes, 984
　effects of unilateral castration on, in rabbit, *399*
　effects of vitamin E on, 224
　endocrine characteristics of, 6
　endocrine correlations of, 397, *398*
　endocrine protection of, 393–415
　endocrinopathies of, 891–1002
　eosinopenia in, 994, *997*
　excretion of estrogens in, 407, *408*
　extrauterine. See *Pregnancy, ectopic.*
　follicular atresia of ovary during, 422
　general adaptation syndrome and, 994, 998(t)
　glycoproteins in, incidence of, *405*
　gonadotropic hormones and, 424
　gravidic tetany in, 978
　growth hormone and, 423
　history of, and menopause, 859
　hormone excretion during, 407
　hydatidiform mole and. See *Mole, hydatidiform.*
　hyperthecosis of ovary during, 422
　hyperthyroidism of, origin of, 426
　hypophysectomy and, 423, 974
　hypophysioadrenal system in, 994
　　pathology of, 990
　hypothyroidism and, 978
　incretory systems of mother and fetus in, 419–441
　insulinemia in, 427
　interruption of, factors causing, 444
　　role of placenta in, 446
　latent diabetes of, 979
　　and pituitary disorders, 982
　　scheme of, 982, *982, 983*
　maintenance and interruption of, 442–462
　maintenance of, and antioxytocic substances, 459
　　factors responsible for, 442
　　role of progesterone in, 444(t)
　neurohormones and, 425
　ovarian function in, 419
　pancreas in, 427
　pancreatic disorders and, 979
　parathyroids in, 426
　parathyroid disorders and, 978
　pathology of, vaginal cytology as index of, 548
　pheochromocytoma and, 989
　pituitary disorders in, 974
　pituitary in, morphology of, 423
　placental lactogen and, 423
　　plasma concentrations of, *414*
　placental senescence in, 453
　placental storage of vitamin A in, 210, *211*
　placental storage of vitamin B_1 in, *214*
　plasma cortisol levels in, *429*
　prediabetes and, 979, 986
　preparation for lactation in, 471
　primary aldosteronism and, 991

Gestation (*Continued*)
  prolactin and, 425
  role of vitamin C in, 219
  serotonin and, 425
  significance of vitamin D in, 222
  stress in, evolution of, 995
  Thorn test in, 995, *996*, *997*, *998*
  thyroid hyperfunction and, 425
  thyroid pathology in, 977
  thyroidopathies and, 763
  thyrotropic hormone and, 424, *424*
  timing in, 453
  tolerance to cortisone in, 428
  toxemias of. See *Toxemias, of pregnancy.*
  uterine growth during, 442
  uteroplacental ischemia in, 962
  vaginal cytology in, 547, *548*
  vascular supply of uterus in, 452
  vitamin A and, 210
  vatamin B_1 and, 214
  vitamin B_1 hypovitaminosis in, 214
Gestosis. See *Toxemias, of pregnancy.*
CHRF. See *Growth hormone releasing factor.*
Gigantism, fetal, prediabetes and, 986, 987(t)
  pituitary, 692
Glands, endocrine. See *Endocrine glands.*
  endometrial, connective tissue spurs in, 260
Glandulotrophic nutrition, 397
Glucocorticoids, 170
  and toxemia of pregnancy, 963
Glucose tolerance curves, following contraceptive therapy, *195*
β-Glucuronidase, changes in during endometrial cycle, 267
  role of in estrogen metabolism, 31
Glycerophosphatase, acid, changes in during endometrial cycle, 267
  alkaline, changes in during endometrial cycle, 265, *266*, *268*
  in endometrium, 565, *566*
Glycogen, changes in during endometrial cycle, 265, *265*, *268*
  endometrial, 565
    and implantation of embryo, 396
  hepatic, effect of thyroxine on pregnant rats and fetuses, *434*
  in vaginal cycle, 287
Glycopenia, of endometrium, in progestational insufficiency, 630
Glycoproteins, in pregnancy, incidence of, 405
Goiter, 761
Gomori stain, for alkaline glycerophosphatase, 565, *566*
Gonad(s). See also *Ovary; Testis.*
  agenesis of, true, 573
  development of, 315
    in human embryo, *318*, *319*
    and migration of gonocytes, 316, *316*
  effects of estrogens on, 17
  embryonal, hormones extracted from, 334
    role of in fetal life, 430
  streak, in Turner's syndrome, 802, *803*
  third, adrenal as, 181
  transplantation of, effects of on sex differentiation, 334
  undifferentiated, development of ovary from, *321*
    development of testis from, *322*
Gonadal dysgenesis. See *Dysgenesis, gonadal.*
Gonadotropic hormones, 115-137. See also *Gonadotropins.*
Gonadotropic hyperpituitarism, 698

Gonadotropic hypopituitarism, 686
Gonadotropin(s), action of on testis, 118, *118*, *119*
  and antigonadotropic substances, 124, 126, 127
  and pregnancy, 424
  and sexual adrenal, in climacterium, 369
  antibodies to, 126
  antigenic properties of, 126
  assay of, 127
  as treatment for primitive pituitary hypoestrinism, 594
  cells, sites of origin of, 123
  chorionic, amount per gram of placental tissue, *405*
    estimation of, using male *Rana esculenta*, 523
    excretion of during pregnancy, 407
    human, 120
      bioassay of, 127
      effect of on batrachians, 130, *130*
    radioimmunoassay of, 531
    urinary, assay of by hemagglutination inhibition, 528, *529*, *530*, *531*
  circulation of, 124
  commercial preparations of, 132(t)
  dosage units of, 130
  effects of on hypophysectomized animals, 120
  effects of on ovary, 115, *115*, 116
  effects of on ovulation, 121
  effects of on pregnancy, 120
  equine chorionic. See *Pregnant mare serum.*
  equivalencies of, 130(t), 131(t)
  estimation of, 523
  excretion of, 124, *125*
    effects of ovulation inhibitors on, 1039, *1040*
    in climacterium, 368
  feedback effect of, 122
  in abortion, 916
  in adrenogenital syndrome, 741
  in treating anovulatory cycle, 897, 898
  insufficiency of, and abortion, 915
  menopausal, human, 120
  metabolism of, 124
  nomenclature of, 120
  physiologic action of, 115
  pituitary, human, 120
  plasma levels of, cyclic fluctuations in, 125, *126*
  receptivity to, disorders of, 583
  secretion of, 122
    factors influencing, 123
    hypothalamus and, 123
  synthesis of, by hydatidiform mole, 946
  therapeutic applications of, 131
  thyroid and, 193
  total excreted during menstrual cycle, *252*
  urinary levels of, 124, *125*
Gonadotropin loading tests, 537
Gonadotropinemia, and prognosis for abortion, 927, *928*, *929*
Gonadotropinuria, and prognosis for abortion, 927, *928*
  in pregnancy, *406*
  in threatened abortion, *917*
Gonocytes, 316
  aberrant, in etiology of andrenogenital syndrome, 729
  migration of to gonadal anlage, 316, *316*
  of chick embryo, *317*
Gonocytomas, ovarian, 674
Gonosomes, 301. See also *Chromosomes, sex.*
Gonosomopathies, quantitative, 780
Gordon's syndrome, 573
Graafian follicle, 241

Granulosa cell tumor, 659, 1019, *1020*
  adenomatous type, *661*
  and precocious puberty, 838, *840*, *841*
  endometrium in, *603*
  folliculoid type, *660*
  luteinization of, *664*
  luteinized, *643*
  malignant, *660*
  relationship to thecal cell tumor, 659
Granulosa-lutein cells, synthesis of progesterone by, 49
Granulosa-lutein cysts, 639, *640*
Granulosa-theca tumor, 659, *661*
Gravidic cycle. See *Gestation.*
Greenblatt's syndrome, 573, *575*
Grollman, theory of sexual differentiation of, 336, *336*
Growth, and reproduction, 3
  estrogens and, 1011
  extraindividual, reproduction as, 3
Growth hormone. See *Hormone, growth.*
Growth hormone releasing factor, 146
Guinea pig, vaginal patency of, for assay of estrogens, *519, 520*
Gynandroblastoma, ovarian, 672
Gynecography, use of in clinical examination, *501, 502*
  use of in primitive hypoestrinism with extreme ovarian hypoplasia, *580*
  use of in Stein-Leventhal syndrome, 653, *653*
Gynecology, psychosomatic, 712
Gynemesenchymomas, 658
Gynetermones, 327
Guanidine, accumulation of, in pregnancy, 427

Habitus, asthenic, *377, 378*
  eunuchoid, *488*
  hypoplastic, *381*
  intersexual, *382*
  pyknic, *377, 379*
Hair distribution. See also *Hirsutism; Hyperpiliation; Hypertrichosis.*
  changes in at puberty, 349
Hartman, placental sign of, 397
HCG. See *Gonadotropin, chorionic, human.*
Headaches, in dysmenorrhea of puberty, 852
Hemagglutination inhibition, for assay of HCG in urine, *528, 529, 530, 531*
Hematoma, of corpus luteum, and luteal insufficiency, 633, *633*
Hematometra, 828
Hemorrhage, parenchymal, ovarian, and secondary hypoestrinism, 588, *588*
Hemorrhagic metropathy. See *Metropathy, hemorrhagic.*
Hemotrophic nutrition, 397
Hepatic hyperestrinism, 598
Hepatic insufficiency. See *Insufficiency, hepatic.*
Hepatitis, and hyperestrinism, 609
Hepatoovarian syndrome, 372, 609, 865
Hepatosis, and hyperestrinism, 609
Hermaphrodite, Pflüger, 338
Hermaphroditism, 298
  false. See *Pseudohermaphroditism.*
  Pflüger's, 384
  true, 813
    bilateral, 815, *818*, *820*
    clinical features of, 815
    etiology of, 814

Hermaphroditism (*Continued*)
  true, karyotype in, 814
    lateral, 815, *816*, *817*
    mosaicism in, 820
      ovotestes in, *818, 819*
      psychological factors in, 821
      treatment of, 821
      unilateral, 815
Hertig, grades of hydatidiform mole, 942
Heterochromosomes, 301. See also *Chromosomes, sex.*
Hexestrol, structure of, *15*
Hilus cells, androgen production by, 644
  and virilization, 645
  at high magnification, *645*
  hyperplasia of, 600, 1012
    and climacteric virilization, 871, *872*
    and hirsutism, *646*
    in adrenogenital syndrome, 737
    urinary 17-ketosteroids in, *647*
  in virilism, 644, *644*
Hilus cell tumor, *671*, *672*, 839
Hippulin, structure of, *14*
Hirsutism. See also *Hyperpiliation; Hypertrichosis.*
  and virilization, 878
  forms of, 667
  from ovarian hilus cell hyperplasia, *646*
  in Stein-Leventhal syndrome, 652, *652*
Histaminase, role of in gestation and labor, 459
Histamine, role of, in implantation of embryo, 395
  in induction of labor, 156, 458
  in induction of menstruation, 276
  in interruption of pregnancy, 447
Histiotrophic nutrition, 442
Histochemistry, endometrial, 565
History, clinical, of gynecologic patient, 485
HMG. See *Gonadotropin, menopausal, human.*
Hogben test, 128
Homeostasis, steroid, 179
  and tumorigenesis, 1022, *1022*
Hormones, 2. See also *Androgens; Estrogens; Progestogens; Relaxin.*
  action of, and maturity of target organs, 438
  adenohypophysial, 98, *99*
    chemistry of, 109
    immunologic properties of, 112
Hormones, adrenocortical. See *Adrenocortical steroids.*
  adrenocorticotropic, and diabetes of pregnancy, 980
  and lactogenesis, 469
  and pregnancy, 425
  chemistry of, 110
  immunologic properties of, 112
  expanded formula of, *111*
  in adrenogenital syndrome, 742
  in placental tissue, 403
  physiology of, 108
  role in maintenance of lactation, 474
  anterior pituitary, 98
  antidiuretic, 160
  as cause of endometrial carcinoma, arguments against, 1014
    arguments for, 1011
  as exogenous biocatalysts, 206
  assay of, 506–541
  corticoid. See *Corticoids.*
  corticosteroid. See *Corticosteroids.*
  diabetogenic, and growth hormone, 107
  distinction of from vitamins, 206
  effects of on cyclic changes in cervical mucus, 909
  elimination of, effect of ovulation inhibitors on, 1039

Hormones (*Continued*)
excretion of, during pregnancy, 407
follicle-stimulating, 120
bioassay of, 128, 526
chemistry of, 110
effects of on batrachians, 130
effects on rat genital tract, compared to LH, *129*
fluctuations in plasma levels of, 125, *126*
radioimmunoassay of, 531
release of, 144
galactotropic. See *Prolactin*.
gonadotropic. See *Gonadotropins*.
growth, and acromegaly, 107
and diabetogenic hormone, 107
and lactogenesis, 469
and latent diabetes of pregnancy, 980
and pregnancy, 423
chemistry of, 109
immunologic properties of, 112
physiology of, 107
release of, 146
role in diabetes of pregnancy, 982, *982*
role of in maintenance of lactation, 474
interstitial cell stimulating. See *Hormone, luteinizing*.
lactotropic. See *Prolactin*.
luteinizing, 120
as ovulation inducing factor, 248
bioassay of, 128, *128*
by ovarian ascorbic acid depletion method, 527
chemistry of, 110
effects of on batrachians, 130, *130*
effects of on rat seminal vesicles, *128*
compared to FSH, *129*
fluctuations in plasma levels of, 126
preovulatory peak of, 246
radioimmunoassay of, 531
release of, 143
mechanism of, *121*
preovulatory peak in, 246
luteotropic. See *Prolactin*.
melanogenic, and ACTH, 109
in placental tissue, 403
of embryonal gonad, 334
ovarian, nonsteroid, 82–93
pituitary, anterior, 98
effects of on milk secretion, *469*
effects of on vaginal cytology, 551
physiology of, 106
true, 109
placental, 400, 400(t)
alterations in, in toxemia of pregnancy, 965
of questionable origin, 403
sites of synthesis of, 403
polypeptide, 11
pressor, and eclamptic toxemia, 961
protein, 11
immunoassay of, 527
radioimmunoassay of, 530
relationship of to enzymes, 2
relationship of to nervous system, 8
retrohypophysial, site of origin of, 151
sex, 11–93
and reproductive system, 1–10
bioassay of, methods of, 518
corticoid action by, 182
effect of on vaginal cytology, 549
excretion of throughout cycle, 125
liver function and, 372

Hormones (*Continued*)
sex, origin of during embryonic life, 332
parent hydrocarbons of, *13*
somatotropic. See *Hormone, growth*.
steroid, 11. See also *Steroids*.
alterations in metabolism of, and adrenogenital syndrome, 730, *731*, *732*
assay of by saturation analysis, 522
excretion of, in adrenogenital syndrome, 740(t)
incomplete, produced by placenta, 434
metabolism of, feto-placental, 434, *435*
nomenclature of, 11
regulation of in adrenals, *730*
synthesis of, by fetus, 431
inhibition of, by Metopyrone, 535
urinary, chemical methods of estimating, 506
synthesis of, by chorioepithelioma, 952
by hydatidiform mole, 946
thyrotropic, and pregnancy, 424, *424*
chemistry of, 110
immunologic properties of, 112
in placental tissue, 403
passage of from mother to fetus, 436
physiology of, 107
release of, 145
synthesis of, and hydatidiform mole, 947
tumors produced by, in animals, 1005, 1005(t)
Hot flashes, in climacterium, 868
HMG. See *Gonadotropin, menopausal, human*.
HPG. See *Gonadotropin, pituitary, human*.
HPL. See *Lactogen, placental*.
Human chorionic gonadotropin. See *Gonadotropin, chorionic, human*.
Human menopausal gonadotropin. See *Gonadotropin, menopausal, human*.
Hunter's ligament, 323
Hydatidiform mole. See *Mole, hydatidiform*.
Hydramnios, and prediabetes, 987
Hydrocarbons, aromatic, as carcinogens, 1008, *1009*
18-Hydroxyestrone, structure of, *14*
17-Hydroxylase activity, failure of, and adrenogenital syndrome, 730, *730*, 733
17-Hydroxyprogesterone, structure of, *38*, *1027*
Hydroxyprogesterone acetate, structure of, *40*
17-Hydroxyprogesterone caproate, structure of, *38*, *1027*
Hyperandrogenism, ovarian, 572, 628–656, 643
Hypercorticism, and anovulatory cycle, 895
and toxemia of pregnancy, 963
climacteric, 866
syndromes of, related to adrenogenital syndrome, 749
Hyperdistention, of uterus, effect on contractility, *454*
Hyperemesis gravidarum, 957
and stress, 959
endocrine changes in, 958
treatment of, 960
Hyperemia test, ovarian, 248
Hyperestrinism, 597–627
acute, 610
ovary in, 606
adrenocortical, 608
as cause of breast cancer, 1015
classification of, 598, 599(t)
climacteric, 860
assay of estrogens, in 860
treatment of, 875
clinical forms of, 610
diagnosis of, 620
endometrium in, microcurettage in, 560

Hyperestrinism (*Continued*)
  experimental, and vitamin B deficiency, 217
  extraovarian, 598, 608
  granulosa cell tumor and, *603*
  hepatic, 598, 609
  iatrogenic, 34, 598, 610
  in treatment of climacteric disorders, 874
  incidence of, 597, 597(t)
  nutritional, 598
  of puberty, 348
  of rhythm, 598
  ovarian, 598
    and thecal hyperplasia, 599
  ovarian disorders causing, 607
  ovaries in, *613*
  pathogenic forms of, 598
  postmenopausal, 862
  premenstrual, in dysmenorrhea of puberty, 853
  psychogenic, 716
  quantitative, 598
  radiotherapy for, 625
  surgery for, 625
  treatment of, 621
    by combination of hormones, 623
    with estrogens, 623
Hyperfeminization, in adrenogenital syndrome, 742, 744, 745
Hyperfolliculinism, 597
  of puberty, 348
Hyperfunction, pituitary, compensatory, 606
Hyperluteinism, 638
Hypernephromas, 665
  ovarian, 668
Hyperovarism, 597
Hyperparathyroidism, and precocious puberty, 769
Hyperpiliation. See also *Hirsutism; Hypertrichosis.*
  facial, from androgen therapy, 67
  perineal, from androgen therapy, 67
Hyperpituitarism, 690
  corticotropic, 694
  galactotropic, and Chiari-Frommell syndrome, 700
    sella turcica in, *701*
  gonadotropic, 698
    sella turcica in, *699*
  lactotropic, 700
  somatotropic, 692. See also *Acromegaly.*
Hyperplasia, adrenal, dexamethasone test in, *534*
  in Stein-Leventhal syndrome, 651
  of sexual zone, and adrenogenital syndrome, 729
  of zona reticularis, *732, 734*
  atypical, and functional bleeding, 615
  Berger cell, and virilization, 883, *883,* 884
  endometrial, 565
    atypical, in postmenopausal women, 366
    cystic, *614*
    cystic glandular, in postmenopausal women, 365
    in postmenopausal women, 365, *366*
    in thecoma, 662
    postabortive. See *Metropathy, postabortive.*
    progestational, 397
    relationship to adenocarcinoma, *1014*
    types of, *617*
    with secretion, 616
  hilus cell, 600
    hirsutism due to, *646*
    possible feminizing effect of, 371
    urinary excretion rates of 17-ketosteroids in, *647*
  islet cell, in diabetes of pregnancy, 985
  in pregnancy, 427
  thecal, 601

Hyperplasia (*Continued*)
  thecal cell, and ovarian hyperestrinism, 599
    and virilization, 883, *883*
  thymic, 766
  thyroid, and pregnancy, 425
Hyperploidy, 777
Hypertension, causes of, in eclamptic toxemia, *964*
Hyperthecosis, ovarian, 601, *602,* 646
  and ovarian hyperestrinism, 599
  and polymicrocystic ovary, 600
  and virilization, 883, *883*
  during gestation, 422
  endometrial findings in, *604*
  in adrenogenital syndrome, 737
  juvenile, 654
  uterus and ovaries in, *648*
Hyperthermia, in dysmenorrhea of puberty, 852
  relative, in premenstrual phase, 289, 852
Hyperthyroidism, 762
  and anovulatory cycle, 895
  and gestation, 763
  climacteric, 189, 763, 867
  "compensatory," 426
  experimental, effect on ovary, 190
  false, 188
  gravidic, origin of, 426
  of puberty, 353
  premenstrual, 188
Hypertrichosis, in virilization, 885
Hypertrophy, thyroid, and gestation, 425, *426*
Hypervirilization, in adrenogenital syndrome, 742
Hypervitaminosis A, 211
Hypoestrinism, 571–596
  and infertility, 909
  classification of, 572
  endometrium in microcurettage in, 560
  in postmenopausal woman, vaginal smear in, *367*
  neural influences on, 716
  of adrenal origin, 586
  of thyroid origin, 586
  primitive, 573
    and sex reversal, 582
    false, 586, *586*
    gynecography in, *580*
    ovarian, 573
      treatment of, 592
      types of, 573(t)
    pituitary, 583
      biotype in, *584*
      treatment, 594
    symptoms of, 576
      local genital tract, 579
  psychogenic, 716
  secondary, 587
    biotype in, *590*
    and induced pseudopregnancy, 594
    endometrial hypoplasia in, *591*
    pathogenesis of, 587
    pathogenic forms of, 587, 587(t)
    treatment of, 594
  treatment of, 592, 592(t)
Hypogenitalism, adipose, 703
Hypophysectomy, and gestation, 974
  effects of, in breast cancer, 1017
  effect of gonadotropins after, 120
  gestation and, 423
Hypophysioadrenal system, in general adaptation syndrome, 992, *992, 994*
  antiphlogistic action of, 994, *994*
  prophlogistic action of, 994, *994*

Hypophysioadrenal system (*Continued*)
    in pregnancy, 994, *994*
    pathology of, in pregnancy, 990
Hypophysioportal system, and relationship between pituitary and hypothalamus, 104, *105*
    of rat, *152*
Hypophysiothalamic system, 104, *105*
    results of stimulation of, *142*
Hypophysis. See also *Adenohypophysis; Pituitary*.
    effect of stress on, 992
    pharyngeal, 101
Hypopituitarism, absolute, 682
    corticotropic, 689
    gonadotropic, 686
        and thyrotropic hypopituitarism, 690, *690*
        effect on ovary, 690, *691*
        eunuchoidism, in, 688
        pituitary dwarfism in, *686, 687*
        sella turcica in, 689
        sella turcica obtecta in, *687*
    relative, 686
    thyrotropic, and gonadotropic hypopituitarism,
Hypoplasia, 690, *690*
    endometrial, from primitive hypoestrinism, effect of estrogens on, 593
        in secondary hypoestrinism, *591*
    genital, 490
    ovarian, 573, *575*
        simple, 800
    uterine, and sinistroposition, 490, *491*
Hypoploidy, 777
Hypothalamic obesity, 707
Hypothalamic precocious puberty, 709
Hypothalamic syndrome, 708
Hypothalamus, action of on adenohypophysis, *142*
    and sexual precocity, 708
    delayed puberty and, 848
    disorders of, and sexual function, 703
    effects of androgens on, 149
    effects of estrogens on, 25, 148, *149*
    effects of on gonadotropin secretion, 123
    effects of pituitary on, 47
    effects of progestogens on, 149
    effects of steroids on, 148
    effects of stress on, 992
    influence of, on estrus, 232
    on onset of puberty, 355
    injury to, effect on sexual function in ewe, *141*
    obesity and, 707
    paraventricular nucleus of, and oxytocin secretion, 457, *458*
    pituitary and, 98
    precocious puberty and, 709, 842, 843
    relationship of, to pituitary, 104, *105*
        to rest of brain, 147
    releasing factors of, 140
    role of, in hyperestrinism, 607
        in oxytocin secretion, 457
        in regulating ovarian cycle, 247
        in Stein-Leventhal syndrome, 651
    sex center of, effects of catacholamines on, 150
        relationship to limbic system, *159*
    sex regulation by, effect of drugs on, 725
    syndromes of, sexual, 710
Hypothyroid adiposity, 760
Hypothyroidism, and abortion, 925
    and gestation, 763, 978
    subclinical forms of, 759, *760*
    syndromes of, 759

Hypovitaminosis B, in pregnancy, 214
Hypovitaminosis E, 224
Hysterosalpingography, use of in clinical examination, 500, *501*
Hysterotonin, and eclampsia, 961

ICSH. See *Hormone, luteinizing*.
Idiogram, 311
Illumination, effect of on gonadotropin secretion, 124
    effect of on puberty, 355
Immunoassay, of protein hormones, 527
Implantation, of embryo, and endometrial histochemistry, 396
    and formation of deciduoma, 395
    deferred, 395
    effect of estrogens on, 21
    endocrinology of, 394
    estrogens and, 395
    failure of, as effect of contraceptives, 1042
    histamine and, 395
    hormonal control of, 394
    LTH and, 395
    mechanical stimuli and, 395
    progesterone and, 394
Inclusions, fuchsinophilic, adrenal, in adrenogenital syndrome, 738
Incretory system, fetal, during gestation, 428–441
    maternal, during gestation, 419–428
Index(ices), cellular, estrogenic, of vaginal cytology, 550
        progestogenic, of vaginal cytology, 550
    clumping, of vaginal cytology, 550
    eosinophilic, 550
    fertility, lowering of at climacterium, 359
    folding, of vaginal cytology, 550
    karyopyknotic, 285, 547, 550
        in endometrial carcinoma, 1013(t)
        in normal women, 1013(t)
    maturation, in vaginal cytology, 550
Infertility. See also *Sterility*.
    adrenal and, 907
    and changes in cervical mucus, 908
    and progestational insufficiency, 633(t)
    and unrecognized habitual abortion, 920, 922(t)
    androgenic amenorrhea and, 887
    cervical forms of, treatment of, 909
    early abortion as cause of, 636(t)
    endocrine defects of endometrium and, 908
    endocrine defects of Fallopian tubes and, 907
    endocrine defects of uterine cervix and, 908
    endometrium in, 923(t)
    extraovarian causes of, 906
    from hypoestrinism, 909
    from progestational luteal insufficiency, mechanism of, 633
        incidence of, 632
    luteal insufficiency and, 904
        incidence of, 904(t), 905(t)
        treatment of, 905
    ovular lethality and, 906
    pancreas and, 907
    pubertal, 342
    thyroid and, 906
    treatment with ovulatory drugs, 899, *900, 901, 902, 903*

Inflammatory disease, pelvic, chronic, destruction
 of ovary in, 589
Inhibitors, ovulation, effects of on basal body
  temperature, 1040, *1040*
  effects of on hormone elimination, 1039
Inoculation tumor, chorioepithelioma as, 951
Insufficiency, adrenal, and abortion, 926
  treatment of, 934
  relative, in toxemia of pregnancy, 957, 959
  adrenocortical, as cause of early abortion, 755
   congenital, 753
   constitutional, 754
  gonadotropic, and abortion, 915
   effect of on ovary, *691*
  hepatic, in climacterium, 372
  luteal, and abortion, 913
   and early abortion, 906
   and infertility, 904, 904(t)
    treatment of, 905
   basal body temperature in, *495*
   in infertility, incidence of, 904(t), 905(t)
   progestational, 628
    anatomic basis of, 633
    and early abortion, 635
    and infertility, mechanism of, 633
    and late abortion, 637, *637*
    and unrecognized habitual abortion, 922, 924(t)
    characteristics of, 632(t)
    diagnosis of, 634
    due to shortened secretory phase, 629
     basal body temperature in, *629*
     urinary pregnanediol values in, *629*
    due to weakened secretory phase, 630
     basal body temperature in, *631*
     urinary pregnanediol in, *631*
    endometrium in, *630, 631*
    etiology of, 638
    incidence of, 631, 632(t), 633(t)
    patterns of, 632(t)
    relative, 633, *634*
    treatment of, 638
    with delayed ovulation, 629
   treatment of with ovulatory drugs, *902, 903*
  placental, 962, 966. See also *Senescence, placental.*
   diagnosis of, 968, *968, 969, 970*
  progestational. See *Insufficiency, luteal, progestational.*
  prolactin, 629
  thyroid, and abortion, 925
Insulin, and lactogenesis, 470
 effect of on lipogenesis in mammary tissue, 474(t)
 in latent diabetes of pregnancy, *979, 980, 981*
 plasma levels of, in normal woman, *430*
  in pregnancy, *430*
 relationship of to vitamin B, 208
 role in maintenance of lactation, 474
Insulin reserve, 979
 and latent diabetes of pregnancy, 979, *981*
Insulinemia, following contraceptive therapy, *195*
 in latent diabetes of pregnancy, *979, 980, 981*
 in pregnancy, 427
Interrenal system, 165, *166*. See also *Adrenal(s); Adrenal cortex.*
Interrenomesenchymomas, 668
Intersexual woman, characteristics of, 382
Interstitial cell stimulating hormone. See *Hormone, luteinizing.*
Interstitial gland, ovarian, of pregnancy, 423, *423*
Intoxication, estrogen, 34
Intramammary pressure. See *Pressure, intramammary.*
Inversion, sexual, in batrachia larvae, action of
 testosterone on, 328

Inversion (*Continued*)
 within one chromosome, paracentric, 784, *784*
  pericentric, 784, *785*
Invertebrates, chemical basis of sex determination
 in, 326
Iodine, protein-bound, and pregnancy, 425
Ischemia, uteroplacental, 962
Isochromosome, false, *790*
 formation of, 786, *787*
 X, and gonadal dysgenesis, 797
Isosexual adrenogenital syndrome, 742
Islet cells, hyperplasia of, in diabetes of pregnancy,
 985
Ittrich method, for determination of urinary estrogens, 510

Jayle, dynamic test of, 537, *538*
Jost, theory of sexual differentiation of, 336, *337*
Juvenile metropathy, 850. See also *Metropathy.*

Karyopyknotic index, 285, 547, 550, 1013(t)
Karyotype. See also *Genotype.*
 in breast cancer, 1007
 in female gonadal dysgenesis, 795, 795(t)
 in true hermaphroditism, 814, *820*
 in uterine tumors, 1007
 normal, 309
16-Keto-estradiol, structure of, *14*
17-Ketosteroids, 62
 excretion of, 76
 in adrenogenital syndrome, 737
 intermediary metabolism of, 71
 neutral, excretion of, in castrated and climacteric
  women, 368(t)
  urinary, determination of by method of
   Zimmermann, 516
   determination of by micromethod of Vestergaard, 517
 synthesis of, by hydatidiform mole, 947
 urinary, in adrenogenital syndrome, 72
  in diagnosis of virilism, 886
  in Stein-Leventhal syndrome, 72
Kidneys, fetal, *166*
Klinefelter syndrome, 791
Knaus test, 280
Kosowicz, sign of, 503, *504*
Krukenberg tumors, of ovary, 674

Labor, acceleration of, and relaxin, 91
 antioxytocic substances in, 459
 as stressor in pregnancy, 990, 997
 endocrine causes of, 453
 from endocrine point of view, 391–482
 initiation of, 453
  acetylcholine and, 458
  and hyperdistention of myometrium, 453
  endocrine factors in, *458*
  histamine and, 458
  neuroendocrine reflex for, 457
  nonneuroendocrine reflex for, 458
  oxytocin and, 455
  relaxin and, 91
  vasopressin and, 458
 intrapartum correlations of, 459
 premature, prediabetes and, 986
  prevention of by relaxin, 91

Index

Labor (*Continued*)
    Thorn test in, 996
    uterine sedation during, and relaxin, 91
Lactation. See also *Lactogenesis*.
    and milk ejection, 475
    effects of on endocrine system and reproductive cycle, 478
    effects of pituitary hormones on, 469
    endocrine regulation of, 479
    factors inhibiting, 471
    in acromegaly, 693
    induction of, 468
    maintenance of, 473
        endocrine factors in, 473
        metabolic factors in, 474
        neural factors in, 475
        nutritional factors in, 474
    neural control of, 471, 472
    ovarian changes during, 479
    preparation for, 471
    suckling stimulus in, 475
Lactoflavin. See *Vitamin B₂*.
Lactogen, placental, 467
    and lactogenesis, 469
    and latent diabetes of pregnancy, 982
    and pregnancy, 424
    assay of, in diagnosing placental function, 969
    diabetogenic action of in pregnancy, 982
    human, 401
    in abortion, 916
        and prognosis, 927
    physiologic actions of, 401
    plasma concentrations of in pregnancy, *414*
    significance of in latent diabetes of pregnancy, 983
    synthesis of, by hydatidiform mole, 947
Lactogenesis, 468. See also *Lactation*.
    dynamics of, 470
    hormones regulating, 465, 468
Lactopoiesis, 473. See also *Lactation, maintenance of*.
Latent diabetes, of pregnancy, 979. See also *Diabetes, latent, of pregnancy*.
LATS. See *Thyroid stimulator, long-acting*.
Lawrence-Moon-Biedl syndrome, 706
Leiomyoma, uterine, ovary in, 604
Leprosy, and secondary hypoestrinism, 588
Leukocyte cultures, for obtaining chromosome spreads, 311
Leukorrhea, pathologic, in menopause, 868
Leydig cell(s), hyperplasia of, in testicular feminization, 811
Leydig cell tumors, feminizing type, 608
    ovarian, 671, *671*, 882
LH. See *Hormone, luteinizing*.
LH peak, preovulatory, 246
LHRF. See *Luteinizing hormone releasing factor*.
Libido, effects of androgens on, 67
Ligament, Hunter's, 323
Light, effect of on gonadotropin secretion, 124
    effect of on pituitary, 150
    effect of on puberty, 355
    environmental, and pineal activity, 202
Lipids, changes in during endometrial cycle, 269
Lipid metabolism, effects of estrogens on, 26
Lipogenesis, in mammary tissue, effect of insulin on, 474(t)
Lipoid cell tumors, 882
Liquor folliculi, 237
Lithospermine, as antigonadotropic substance, 127
Liver, atrophy of, in first trimester of pregnancy, 957
    cirrhosis of, and hyperestrinism, 609
    fetal, endocrine role of, *435*, 437

Liver (*Continued*)
    function of, and sex hormones, 372
    insufficiency of, in climacterium, 372
LTH. See *Prolactin*.
Luteal insufficiency. See *Insufficiency, luteal*.
Luteal persistence. See *Corpus luteum, persistence of*.
Luteal phase, of female life, 376, 377
Lutectomy, effects of during pregnancy, 914
Luteinization, diffuse, during pregnancy, 421, *422*
    incomplete, in psychogenic amenorrhea, 722
    of ovarian feminizing tumors, 664
    of theca, premature, 600
Luteinizing hormone. See *Hormone, luteinizing*.
Luteinizing hormone releasing factor, 143
Luteomas, 643
    ovarian, 639, 672, *674*
Luteotropic hormone. See *Prolactin*.
Luteotropin. See *Prolactin*.
Lynestrenol, effect on endometrium, 57
    structure of, *1030*
LTH. See *Prolactin*.

Macrogenitosomia praecox, pineal tumors and, 765
Macrosomia. See *Gigantism, fetal*.
Male dominance, in mammals, 387
Malformations, congenital, incidence of, and diabetes of pregnancy, 986, 987(t)
Malignancy, induction of by contraceptive therapy, 1045
Malnutrition, and inhibition of puberty, 355
Mammals, male dominance in, 387
Mammary gland. See *Breast*.
Mammogenesis, 463. See also *Breast, development of*.
Mammogenic factor, and mammary cancer, 1018
Man, normal, morphography of, 489
Marchand's accessory adrenals, 668
Marrow, bone. See *Bone marrow*.
Masculinization. See also *Virilization*.
    ovarian, 806
Masculinovoblastomas, 665, 669
Masses, fibrothecal. See *Hyperthecosis, ovarian*.
Mastitis, cystic, chronic, 619
Mastodynia, 619
Mastopathy, 618
Materno-fetal conflict, 453
Maturation, endometrial, irregular, 615, *616*
    mucosa in, 607
Maturation index, in vaginal cytology, 550
Maturation value, in vaginal cytology, 550
Measurements, body, as criteria in physical examination, 490
Median eminence, effect of steroids on, 148
    localization of sex center in, *141*
    neurohormones of, significance of, 150
Medroxyprogesterone acetate, structure of, *1030*
Medullärine, 327, 335
Meiosis, and nondisjunction, in oogenesis, 779, *780*
    in spermatogenesis, 780, *781*, *782*
Melanocyte stimulating hormone releasing factor, 147
Melanogenic hormone, and ACTH, 109
Melatonin, 200, 843
    as inhibitor of puberty, 355
    biosynthesis of, 201, *201*
    structure of, *200*
Membrana granulosa, of primary follicle, 237
Menarche, 340
    age at, 341(t)
    delayed, 846
    mechanism of, 348

Menopausal gonadotropin. See *Gonadotropin, menopausal, human.*
Menopause, 358. See also *Climacterium.*
　adrenal and, 859
　age of, 857
　and history of past pregnancies, 859
　constitution and, 857
　delayed, 857
　endometrium immediately following, *359*
　mechanism involved in cessation of bleeding, 360
　ovarian dysfunction at, types of, 360
　pathologic leukorrhea in, 868
　precocious, 857
　　role of ovary in, 858
　role of pituitary in, 858
　thyroid and, 859
　vaginal cytology of, 549
Menorrhagia, endometrium in, *617*
　psychogenic, mechanism of, *720*
Menorrhea, anovular, 236
Menotoxins, 276, 852
　in dysmenorrhea of puberty, 852, 853
Menstrual cycle. See *Cycle, menstrual.*
Menstrual disease. See *Dysmenorrhea, of puberty.*
Menstrual rhythm, anomalies in, psychogenic, 717
Menstrual threshhold, 271, *271*
Menstruation, 269. See also *Cycle, menstrual.*
　and menstrual threshhold, 271, *271*
　as active event, 280
　as passive event, 279
　cessation of, mechanism involved in, 360
　delayed, 271
　disorders of, in puberty, 850
　duration of bleeding of, and prolonged endometrial shedding, 643(t)
　effect of vitamin C deficiency on, 221
　endocrine causes of, 270
　mechanisms of, 269
　menotoxins in, 276, 852
　precipitation of, by hormone withdrawal, *271*
　　effect of ovarian hormone activity on, *272*
　relative hyperthermia in premenstrual phase, 289
　rhythm of, psychogenic anomalies of, 717
　shedding and regeneration of endometrium in, 277, *278*
　toxic factors involved in, 276
　vascular causes of, 273, 275
　vasospasm in, humoral factors involved in, 274
MER-25. See *Ethamoxytriphetol.*
Mesenchyme, role of in development of ovary, 321
　sexual, estrogen and androgen synthesis by, *371*, *372*
Mesenchymomas, feminizing, 658
Mestranol, structure of, *14*
Metabolism, basal, 492
　cyclic changes in, 290
　disorders of, in climacterium, 869
　inborn errors of, 3
Metacarpal, fourth, shortening of, sign of, 503, *504*
　in gonadal dysgenesis, 578
Metacentric chromosomes, 311, *312*
Metaplasia, endometrial, squamous, 616, *616*
Metastases, of hydatidiform mole, 948
Methotrexate, in treatment of chorioepithelioma, 954
2-Methoxyestrone, structure of, *14*
Methylcholanthrene, conversion from cortical steroids, 1010
17α-Methyl-19-nortestosterone, structure of, *40, 1029*
Methyltestosterone, structure of, *64*
Metopyrone, inhibition of adrenal steroid synthesis by, 535
　structure of, *534*

Metopyrone tests, 533, 535
Metrogestrone, structure of, *1031*
Metropathia haemorrhagica. See *Metropathy, hemorrhagic.*
Metropathy, adult, 612
　climacteric, 867
　hemorrhagic, 611
　　causes of, 612
　　ovarian findings in, *602*
　　postclimacteric, 867
　　　endometrium in, 868, *868*
　　postmenopausal, 612
　　treatment with progesterone, *622*
　　virilizing form of, in adrenogenital syndrome, 743
　hyperplastic, treatment with androgens, *623*
　juvenile, 348, 612, 850
　　clinical features of, 850
　　diagnosis of, 851
　　etiology of, 850
　　treatment of, 851
　postabortive, 930
　　characteristics of, 930(t)
　　endometrium in, *931, 932*
　　ovary in, *932*
　postclimacteric, 867
　　endometrium in, 868, *868*
　senile, 373
Metrorrhagia, in Stein-Leventhal syndrome, 652
Metrosis of receptivity, *360, 560,* 615
　and delayed puberty, 846
Microcurettage, Burch aspiration cannula for, *555*
　collection of specimens in, 556
　diagnosis of abortive rests by, 564
　diagnosis of ectopic pregnancy by, 564, *564*
　diagnosis of neoplasia by, 563
　in virgins, 556
　indications for, 556
　interpretation of specimens from, 556, *557, 558, 559*
　intramenstrual, 554
　premenstrual, 554
　Reifferscheid curette for, *554*
　techniques of, 553, 555
　time for performing, 554
　types of, 553
Micromolar degeneration, 938. See also *Mole, hydatidiform.*
Microscopy, fluorescent, for vaginal smears, 546
　phase contrast, for vaginal smears, 544
Milk, ejection of, 475, *479*
　endocrine regulation of, *479*
　effect of oxytocin on, 156
　secretion of. See *Lactation; Lactogenesis.*
Mineral concentration, changes in during endometrial cycle, 268
Mineral metabolism, effects of estrogens on, 26
Mineralocorticoids, 170
　role of in general adaptation syndrome, 993
Mitosis, and nondisjunction, in oogenesis, 779, *779*
　in spermatogenesis, 780, *781, 782*
　phases of, normal, 778, *778*
Mittelschmerz, 611, 896
Mola destruens, 942
Mole, embryonated, 937
　hydatidiform, 937–949, *944*
　　and toxemia, 948
　　benign, 940
　　characteristics of, 948
　　classification of, 942
　　cytogenetics of, 939
　　environmental factors in, 941

Mole (*Continued*)
  hydatidiform, etiology of, 938
    genetic factors in, 938
    grade I of Hertig, *940*
    grade IV of Hertig, *943*, 944
    histochemistry of, 944
    histopathology of, 942
    hormone synthesis by, 946
    incidence of, 937
    invasiveness of, 942
      immunity to, 952
    malignant, *943*
    metastases of, 948
    treatment of, 948
  partial, 937
  total, 937
Molimen, menstrual, in puberty, 851. See also *Dysmenorrhea, in puberty.*
Molimina menstrualia, 851
Mongolism. See *Down's syndrome.*
Monogametic sex, 385, 386(t)
Morphography, in Turner's syndrome, 489, *577*
  in Wilkins-Fleischmann syndrome, *578*
  of normal man, *489*
  of normal woman, *488*
  use of in clinical examination, 488
Mortality, fetal, and diabetes in pregnancy, 986, 987(t)
Mosaicism, 777, 790
  and mixed types of gonadal dysgenesis, 797
  in gonadal dysgenesis, 798
  in true hermaphroditism, 820
  zygotic, 790
Motility, spontaneous, of fallopian tubes, 257, *257*
  effect of estrogens on, *17*
  effect of progestogens on, *1033*, *1035*
  of uterine muscle, 281, *281*
  effects of relaxin on, *87*
MRL-41. See *Clomiphene.*
MSHRF. See *Melanocyte stimulating hormone releasing factor.*
Mucoid cells, of pituitary, 102, *102*
Mucopolysaccharides, changes in during endometrial cycle, 267, *268*
  in endometrium, 567
Mucosa, endocervical, cycle in, 284
  endometrial, effects of progestogens on in nidation, 46
    variations in thickness of, *274*
  oral, endocrine cytology of, 551
  sex chromatin in, and diagnosis of sex, 306, *307*
Mucus, cervical, 281
  and hypoestrinism, in infertility, 909
  changes in, and infertility, 908
    effect of hormones on, 909
  crystallization of, *492*, *493*
    and prognosis of abortion, 930
    variations in during cycle, 282, *283*
  cycle of secretion of, 282
  effect of contraceptives on, *1041*, 1042
  properties of, in diagnosis, 492
  sodium chloride content of, 282, *282*
  stringiness of, 282, *282*, 492
  thickening of, from use of contraceptives, 1038
  nasal, cyclic crystallization of, 284
Müller, tubercle of, 322
Müllerian duct. See also *Duct, müllerian.*
  atresia of, and unilateral renal agenesis, 828, 829
  development of, 322
  anomalies of, 825
Multiparity, and grades of diabetes in pregnancy, 984

Musculature, changes in at puberty, 348
Myasthenia gravidarum, 957
Myasthenia gravis, thymic hyperplasia in, 766, 767
Myoma, hyperestrinism and, 616
  ovarian findings in, 618(t)
  uterine. See *Tumors, uterine, benign.*
Myometrium, cycle of. See *Cycle, myometrial.*
  effects of androgens on, 66
  effects of estrogens on, 20, *21*
  effects of progestogens on, 45
  hyperdistention of, and initiation of labor, 453
Myxedema, 759

Nasopharyngeal cavity, tumors of, and hypothalamic syndrome, 710, *711*
Navicular cells, of pregnancy, 547, *548*, *549*
Necrosis, postpartum, of pituitary, 684, 974
Neocortex, adrenal, 432
  characteristics of, 168(t)
  development of, *167*
Neoplasia. See also *Carcinoma; Tumors.*
  development of, kinetics of, 1020
  diagnosis of, by microcurettage, 563
  time factors in, 1020
Nervous system, and endocrine glands, 138–164
  and relationship to hormones, 8
Neuroendocrine reflex, for initiation of labor, 457
  of suckling effect, and oxytocin release, 478
Neuroendocrine system, 8, 9
Neuroendocrinology, 138–164
Neurogenic sexual syndromes, 703–726
Neurohormones, 138
  and gestation, 425
  and interruption of pregnancy, 446
  and release of gonadotropins, 123
  reflexes of, pathophysiology, 155
  significance of, 150
Neurohypophysis, 98
Neurologic disturbances, in climacterium, 870
Neuron, secretion-laden, in supraoptic nucleus of dog, *151*, *152*
Newborn, Addison's disease of, 428
Nidation. See *Implantation, of embryo.*
Nitrogen, changes in during endometrial cycle, 269
Nondisjunction. See *Chromosomes, nondisjunction of.*
Norepinephrine, and antagonism to epinephrine, 447
  role of in interruption of pregnancy, 447
  spasmolytic effect of, 447
Noresthisterone acetate, structure of, *1031*
Norethynodrel, production of thromboembolism by, 58
  structure of, *40*, *1030*
Norpregneninolone, structure of, *40*
Nortestosterone propionate, structure of, *40*
Nortestosterone valerianate, structure of, *40*
Nubility, and puberty, 342
  phase of, 340
Nucleic acids, changes in during endometrial cycle, 267
Nucleus(i), gray, basal relationship to pituitary, *141*
  paraventricular, and oxytocin secretion, 457, *458*
    as site of origin of retrohypophysial hormones, 151
  supraoptic, as site of origin of retrohypophysial hormones, 151
    of dog, neurosecretion in, *151*, *152*

Nutrition, and hyperestrinism, 598, 609
  of embryo, glandulotrophic, 397
      hemotrophic, 397, 442
      histiotrophic, 442
      prior to implantation, 393, *394*
      syndesmotrophic, 396
      tubotrophic, 257, 393, *394*
  of implanted egg, 442
  tubal cycle of, 393

Obesity, exogenous, in climacterium, 870
  hypogenital type, in climacterium, 871
  hypothalamic, 707
    sella turcica in, *707*
  in climacterium, 870
  plethoric, in climacterium, 871
  psychogenic, 715
Octapressin, 160
Olfactogenital syndrome, 576, 709
Oligomenorrhea, endometrial patterns in, *581*
Oocyte, development of, 244
  lethality of, and sterility, 906
Oogenesis, 299, *300*
  chromosomal nondisjunction in, *779, 779, 780, 781*
Oogonia, 236
Oolemma, 237
Oophoritis, acute, and secondary hypoestrinism, 587
  chronic, and secondary hypoestrinism, 587
Ootid. See *Oocyte.*
Oral mucosa. See *Mucosa, oral.*
Organs, target. See *Target organs.*
Ossification, effects of estrogens on, 26
Osteoporosis, 503
  climacteric, 872
    mechanism of, *873*
Ovarian cycle. See *Cycle, ovarian.*
Ovarian syndromes, 569–678
Ovarian tumor registry, 657
Ovary(ies), abscess of, and parenchymal hemorrhage, 588
  action of contraceptive steroids on, 1032, 1033(t), *1034, 1035*
  adnexitic, 588, *588*, 605, *605*
    clinical findings in, 589
  agenesis of, atrophic vaginal smear in, 576
  and climacteric virilization, 871, 872
  and female sterility, 893
  and hyperandrogenism, 643
  and onset of puberty, 345
  and precocious menopause, 858
  androgen synthesis by, 72
    in normal female, 879
    pathophysiology of, 643
    pathways of, *74*
  animal, action of FSH and LH on, 116
  arrhenoblastoma of, 665, *666, 667, 668*
  as possible origin of postmenopausal estrogens, 371
  ascorbic acid depletion in, as bioassay of LH, 527
  changes in during lactation, 479
  chorioepithelioma of, 675
  chorioteratoblastoma of, 675
  cortical cords of, 320
  delayed puberty and, 846
  demedullation of, 646
    in treatment of virilization, 889
    urinary 17-ketosteroid rates after, *647*
  destruction of, by hemorrhagic corpus luteum, 582
    in chronic pelvic inflammatory disease, 589

Ovary(ies) (*Continued*)
  development of, embryonic, 320
    from undifferentiated gonad, *321*
  disorders of, causing hyperestrinism, 607
  dysgenesis of. See *Dysgenesis, gonodal, female.*
  effects of androgens on, 65
  effects of contraceptives on, *1041*
  effects of estrogens on, 17
  effects of experimentally induced hyperthyroidism on, 190
  effects of gonadotropic insufficiency on, *691*
  effects of LH and FSH on, *121*
  effects of on thyroid, 191, *192*
  effects of pituitary extracts on, 115, *115*
  effects of progestogens on, 42
  effects of thyroidectomy on, 189, *189*
  effects of thyrosuppressive drugs on, 190
  effects of thyroxine on, 189, 190
  effects of vitamin A on, 209, *209*
  effects of vitamin B_1 deficiency on, *213*
  embryonic development of, 320
  enlargement of, in hyperestrinism, *613*
  "essential" virilization of, 647
  feminizing tumors on, incidence of, 1011
  fetal, endocrine activity of, 333
      mature follicle in, *432*
      structure and function of near term, 431
  follicular atresia of during pregnancy, 422
  function of, during pregnancy, 419
      during puberty, 351
  functional disorders of, classification, 571
  functional tumors of, endocrinology of, 657
  gravidic corpus luteum of, 419, *420, 421*
  gynandroblastoma of, 672
    menstruation, 272
  hilus cells of, *645*
    androgen production by, 644
  histology of, in Stein-Leventhal syndrome, 652
  hormone activity of, and precipitation of
  human, action of FSH and LH on, 116
    from anovulatory cycle, *117*
  hyperandrogenism of, 572, 628–656
  hyperestrogenic, 360
  hypernephromas of, 668
  hyperthecosis of, 601, *602*
    during gestation, 422
    endometrial findings in, *604*
  hypoestrogenic, 360
  hypoplasia of, 573, *575*
    simple, 800
  in acute hyperestrinism, 606
  in adrenogenital syndrome, 737
  in benign uterine tumors, 1019(t)
  in chronic adnexitis, 589
  in endometrial carcinoma, compared to normal, 1012(t)
  in follicular persistence, 601
  in leiomyoma, *604*
  in mammary carcinoma, 1016
  in myoma, 618(t)
  in postabortive metropathy, *932*
  in progestational insufficiency, 634
  in psychologic trauma, *721*
  in psychosomatic amenorrhea, *717, 718, 719*
  in Stein-Leventhal syndrome, *649*
  inhibition of, neural pathways of, *724*
  interactions of with thyroid, 193
  interstitial gland of, 423, *423*
  luteinization of, diffuse, in pregnancy, 421, *422*
  luteoma of, 639, 672, *674*

Index

Ovary(ies) (*Continued*)
  masculinovoblastoma of, 669
  medullary cords of, 320
  menopausal, with corpus luteum, 360
  mouse, effect of LH on, *117*
  nerve supply of, 139
  normoestrogenic, 360
  parenchymal hemorrhage of, and hypoestrinism, 588, *588*
  pathologic syndromes of, 568–678
  pathology of, in climacterium, 860
  polycystic, 600, *602*
    and hydatidiform mole, 948
  polymicrocystic, as variant of hyperthecosis, 600
    endometrial changes in, *602*
    fibrous, 600
    in hyperthecosis, *648*
    juvenile type, 345, *346*
  polymicrocystic degeneration of, 589
  prepubertal, 343, *343, 344*
    of child, *344*
    of fetus, 343, *343*
  primordial follicles in, *237*
  production of progesterone by, 49
  pubertal, dysrhythmia of, 346
  "remaining," syndrome of, 605
  role of in gonadotropic regulation of menstrual cycle, 246
  storage of vitamin C in, 218, *218*
  streak, in Turner's syndrome, 802, *803*
  struma ovarii of, 675, *676*
  testicular adenomas of, 666
  tests of, dexamethasone, 535, *536*
    dynamic, 535
    gonadotropin loading, 537
  thecal cells of, hyperplasia of. See *Hyperthecosis*.
  thecoma of, *608*
    with endometrial adenocarcinoma, *1015*
  thyroid tissue, 675, *676*
  tumors of, 1018
    adrenal, 668, *669, 670*
    and secondary hypoestrinism, 590
    Brenner, 674
    classification of, 657, 658(t)
      endocrinologic, 658(t)
    clear cell, 668, *669, 670*
    endocrine properties of, 664
    feminizing, 597, 658
      histogenesis, 658
    functioning, 608
    gonocytomas, 674
    granulosa cell, 1018, *1019*
    Krukenberg, 674
    Leydig cell, 671, *671*
    masculinizing, 665
  view of by transabdominal celioscopy, *500*
  vital cycle of, 1006, *1006*
  with cystic corpus luteum, 605
Ovitransportation. See *Ovum, transport of*.
Ovotestes, in true hermaphroditism, *818, 819*
Ovulation, 247
  delayed, 246
  drugs producing, and treatment of anovulatory cycle, 899, *900, 901, 902, 903*
  effects of gonadotropins on, 121
  endocrine factors in, 248
  enzymatic factors in, 249
  factors inducing, 248
  feedback mechanism in, *253*
  inhibitors of, effects of on body temperature, 1040, *1040*

Ovulation (*Continued*)
  inhibitors of, effects of on hormone elimination, 1039
  mechanism of, *121*
  neurogenic factors in, 248
  paracyclic, 607, 723
  presumptive signs of, 896
  psychic factors in, 249
  suppression of, as effect of contraceptives, 1041
Ovum. See also *Egg*.
  cross section of segment, *245*
  death rate of, 246
  implantation of, effects of estrogens on, 21
  transport of, rate of in fallopian tube, 257
  transport of, tubal, paralysis of by contraceptives, 1042
  types of, 5, 6
11-Oxyandrosterone, structure of, *64*
Oxytocin, analogues of, 160
  and antioxytocic substances, 459
  and eclampsia, 961
  and increase in intramammary pressure, *158*
  chemistry of, 156
  effect of on breast, 457
  effect of on intramammary pressure, *476*
  effect of on milk ejection, 156
  effect of on uterus, 457
  mode of action of, 455
  pure, actions of, 159
  release of, neuroendocrine reflex by suckling effect, *478*
  role of in initiation of labor, 455
  role of in maintenance of lactation, 474
  role of in uterine contractions, 155, *157*
  secretion of, paraventricular nucleus as elicitor of, 457, *458*
    role of hypothalamus in controlling, 457
  structure of, 159
Oxytocinase, 153
  and maintenance of gestation, 459

Pain, uterine, in dysmenorrhea of puberty, 852
Paleocortex, adrenal, 432
  characteristics of, 168(t)
  development of, *167*
Palpation, use of in physical examination, 490
Pancreas, and sexual function, 194
  cyclic changes in, 288
  disorders of, and climacterium, 867
    and pregnancy, 979
    and sexual function, 767
  fetal, 436
  hyperplasia of, insular, in pregnancy, 427
    islet cell, in diabetes of pregnancy, 985
  in pregnancy, 427
  infertility and, 907
Pancreatectomy, effect of on glycogen of mother and fetus, *436*
Panhypercorticism, 750
Panhypopituitarism, 682
Pantothenic acid, 216
Papanicolaou stain, for vaginal smears, 543, *545*
Parabiosis, "conditioned," 438
  effects of on sex differentiation, 334
Paracyclic ovulation, 723
Parasympathicotropic cells, 644
Parathyroids, and sexual function, 196
  disorders of, and gestation, 978

Parathyroids (*Continued*)
  disorders of, and sexual function, 769
  fetal, activity of, 437
  in pregnancy, 426
Paraventricular nucleus, of hypothalamus, and oxytocin secretion, 457, *458*
Parity, and grades of diabetes in pregnancy, 984
Patency, vaginal, test of, in guinea pig, for assay of estrogens, 519, 520
PBI. See *Iodine, protein-bound*.
Peak, preovulatory, of LH release, 246
Pelvic congestion, 724
Pelvic inflammatory disease. See *Inflammatory disease, pelvic*.
Pendl's syndrome, 849
Pentothal, effect of on hypothalamic sex center, 725
Periodic bleeding, pseudomenstrual, 664
Peristalsis, of fallopian tubes, effect of estrogens on, 17
Peritoneoscopy, transabdominal, 496, *496*. See also *Celioscopy, transabdominal*.
  transvaginal, 496. See also *Culdoscopy*.
Permeability, of placenta, 438
Persistent corpus luteum. See *Corpus luteum, persistence of*.
Persistent follicles. See *Follicles, ovarian, persistent*.
Pflüger's hemaphroditism, 338, 384
PG. See *Gonadotropin, pituitary, human*.
Phase contrast microscopy, for vaginal smears, 544
Phases, of female life, 376
Pheochromocytoma, and pregnancy, 989
Philadelphia chromosome, 782, 788
Physical examination, of gynecologic patient, 487
  radiography in, 500
Physostigmine, role of in inducing menstruation, 276
Pick, adenoma of, *811*, 812
PIF. See *Prolactin inhibiting factor*.
Pineal, and environmental lighting, 201
  and optic system, 200
  and sexual function, 198
  as inhibitor of puberty, 354
  calcification of, 765
  circadian rhythmicity of, 201
  extragenital effects of, 198
  holocrine secretion by, *199*
  hormone of, 200. See also *Melatonin*.
  precocious puberty and, 711, 843
  sexual effects of, 763–765
  stalk of, apparent holocrine in, 198, *198*, *199*
  syndromes of, related to sex, 763
  tumors of, and precocious puberty, 765
    and sexual function, 765
Pineal precocious puberty, 711
Pitocin. See *Oxytocin*.
Pituitary. See also *Adenohypophysis; Hypophysis*.
  alterations in, in hyperemesis gravidarum, 958
  and anovulatory cycle, 895
  and delayed puberty, 846
  and lactation, 478
  and mammary growth, 466
  and primitive hypoestrinism, 583
  and secondary amenorrhea, 689
  anterior lobe of, 97. See also *Adenohypophysis*.
    endocrine correlation of, *158*
    excitation via chemical mediators, *153*
    hormones of, 98
  blood supply of, 103, *104*
  cells of, and origin of hormones, 102, 103(t)
  cytology of, functional, 103(t)
  disorders of. See also *Hyperpituitarism; Hypopituitarism*.

Pituitary (*Continued*)
  disorders of, and adrenal endocrinopathy, 728
    and gestation, 974
    and latent diabetes of pregnancy, 982
    classification of, 681, 682(t)
  effects of androgens on, 68
  effects of estrogens on, 25, 148, *149*
  effects of light on, 150
  effects of on adrenal cortex, 176
  effects of on gonadotropin secretion, 123
  effects of progestogens on, 47
  endocrinopathy of, in relation to sex, 681–702
  extracts of, action of on testis, 118, *118*, *119*
    effects on ovary, 115, *115*
  fetal, activity of, 437
  function during puberty, 352
  hormones of, effects of on vaginal cytology, 551
    physiology of, 106
    true, 109
  hyperfunction of, and diabetes of pregnancy, 982
    compensatory, after unilateral ovariectomy, 606
  hypothalamus and, 98
  in pregnancy, 423
  innervation of, 104
  intermediate lobe of, 101
    of bull, innervation of, *153*, *154*
    of mule, innervation of, *154*
  latent diabetes of pregnancy and, 982, *982*, *983*
  lobes of, 101, 101(t)
  necrosis of, postpartum, 974
  physiology of, 97
  posterior lobe of, 101, 101(t)
    neuroendocrine correlations of, 157
    of dog, neurosecretion in, *151*
  postpartum necrosis of, 684
  pregnancy cell of, 423
  relationship of basal gray nuclei to, *141*
  relationship to telencephalon via hypothalamus, 104, *105*
  role of in climacterium, 858
  role of in general adaptation syndrome, 992, *993*
  role of in Stein-Leventhal syndrome, 651
  sexual cycle in, 288
  subdivisions of, 101, 101(t)
  suppression of, in treat-in pathologic climacterium, 874
  tumors of, 1018
    and hypothalamic syndrome, 710, *711*
  variations in, related to sex, 106
Pituitary cycle, in secretion of gonadotropins, 122
Pituitary dwarfism, 686, 687
Pituitary eunuchoidism, 585
Pituitary gigantism, 692
Pituitary gonadotropin. See *Gonadotropin, pituitary, human*.
Pituitary hormones, true, 109
Placenta, 6
  alterations in, in toxemia of pregnancy, 965
  amount of chorionic gonadotropin per gram of tissue in, 405
  as endocrine organ, 393–415
  changes in, in diabetes, 984, 985
  chorionic gonadotropin in, amounts of, 405
  corticoids of, 410, *414*
  development of, morphologic, 448
  effect of on breast, 467
  evolution of, 448
  fine structure of, *406*
  function of, assessment of, 969, *969*, *970*
  hormones of, 400, 400(t)
    effect of on fetus, 332

Index

Placenta (Continued)
  hormones of, sites of synthesis of, 403
  insufficiency of, 962. See also Senescence, placental.
  permeability of, 438
  rate of blood flow through, 969, 970
  role of in interruption of pregnancy, 446
  secretion of corticoids by, in pregnancy, 994
  senescence of, 452, 962. See also Senescence, placental.
    and maternofetal conflict, 453
  steroids of, biosynthesis of, 409, 413
  storage of vitamin B₁ by, 214
  storage of vitamin B₂ in, 215
  storage of vitamin C in, 219, 220
  storage of vitamin D in, 222, 223
  storage of vitamin E in, 224
  surface area of, in diabetes of pregnancy, 985
    in prediabetes, 985
    in toxemia of pregnancy, 962, 963
    rate of increase in gestation, 451
  syncytium of, fine structure of, 404
  synthesis of estrogens by, 409, 411
  synthesis of progesterone by, 51, 410, 412
  types of, 279, 280(t)
    and predominant element in endometrium, 280, 280(t)
  villi of. See Villus(i), chorionic.
Placental lacotgen. See Lactogen, placental.
Placental sign of Hartman, 397
PMS. See Pregnant mare serum.
Pneumokidney, 501
  in adrenogenital syndrome, 742
Pneumoperitoneum, 501, 502
Polyhormonal amenorrhea, 699
Polymicrocystic degeneration of ovary, 589
Polymicrocystic ovary. See Ovary, polymicrocystic.
Polyneuritis, of pregnancy, 214
Polypeptide hormones, 11
Polyploidy, 777
Poly-X females. See Genotype, poly-X.
Porta-diencephalic system, of pituitary, 103
Postabortive endometritis, 563
Postabortive metrophy. See Metropathy, postabortive.
Postclimacteric metropathia haemorrhagica, 867
Postclimacterium, 364
  adrenal cortex in, histology of, 369, 370(t)
  androgenic activity in, 368, 368(t)
  effects of sexual secretion in, 372
  endometrial activity in, 364, 365, 366
  estrogenic activity in, 364
  malignant degeneration of uterus and breast in, 373
  urinary estrogens in, 362(t), 364, 365(t)
  vaginal smear in, 367, 367
Postmenopause. See Climacterium, postmenopausal phase of.
Precapillary sphincters, in spiral arteries, 264
Precocious menopause, 857
Precocious puberty. See Puberty, precocious.
Precocity, sexual, hypothalamic, 708
Prediabetes. See also Diabetes, latent, of pregnancy.
  abortion and, incidence of, 986, 986(t)
  and congenital malformations, incidence of, 986, 987(t)
  and fetal mortality rates, 986, 987(t)
  and pregnancy, 986
  diagnosis of, 987, 988
  differentiation from diabetes, 989, 989(t)
  embryopathy and, 986
  fetal gigantism and, 986, 987(t)

Prediabetes (Continued)
  hydramnios and, 987
  of pregnancy, 979
    scheme of, 982, 983
  pituitary and, 982
  placental surface area in, 985
  premature labor and, 986
  prognosis of, 987
  treatment of, 989
Preeclampsia, pressor substances and, 961
Pregnancy. See also Gestation.
  ectopic, clear cells in, 564, 564
    diagnosis of by microcurettage, 564, 564
  polyneuritis of, 214
  toxemias of. See Toxemias, of pregnancy.
Pregnancy cells, 106, 133, 423
Pregnancy test(s), biologic, 127
  Pregnosticon, 530
  Prepuerin, 528, 531
Pregnane, 39
  structure of, 13, 38, 1027
Pregnanediol, excretion of, after lutectomy and abortion, 399
  during pregnancy, 409
  in adrenogenital syndrome, 741
  synthesis of, by hydatidiform mole, 947
  total eliminated during menstrual cycle, 252
  urinary, chromatographic determination of, by method of Toller and Carda, 512
    estimation of, 511
    in luteal insufficiency from shortened secretory phase, 629
    in luteal insufficiency from weakened secretory phase, 631
    paper chromatography for, method of Elberlein and Bongiovanni, 513
Pregnanedioluria, during ovarian cycle, 250, 250
  in diagnosis and prognosis of abortion, 927
  in lutectomy and abortion, 915
  in threatened abortion, 916
Pregnant mare serum, 120
  in treating anovulatory cycle, 897
Pregnenediol, excretion of, effects of ovulation inhibitors on, 1039, 1040
Pregneninolone, structure of, 40, 1029
Pregnenolone, synthesis of testosterone from, 70(t)
Pregnosticon test, 530
Premenstrual tension. See Tension, premenstrual.
Prepuerin test, for determination of pregnancy, 528, 531
Pressure, arterial, control of, in toxemia of pregnancy, 959
  intramammary, and oxytocin, 158
    effect of oxytocin on, 476
    increase in with discharges of oxytocin, 158
    method for recording, 476
PRF. See Prolactin releasing factor.
Primitive hypoestrinism. See Hypoestrinism, primitive.
Primogonil, treatment of infertility with, 898, 900, 902
Progestational insufficiency. See Insufficiency, luteal, progestational.
Progesterone. See also Progestogens.
  acetate derivatives of, 1031
  action of in maintaining gestation, 444(t)
  and implantation of embryo, 394
  and tumorigenesis, 1021
  as placental hormone, 402
  bioassay of minute amounts of, by method of Hooker and Forbes, 521

Progesterone (*Continued*)
  blood levels of, 53
    during pregnancy, *409*
  catabolites of, 53
  compound name of, 11
  conversion of to androgens and estrogens, 52, *52*
  cyclopentyl derivatives of, 1031
  degradation of by liver, *52*
  6-derivatives of, 1030
  effect of on breast, 466
  effect of on viability of castrated and adrenalectomized animals, *184*
  ethinyl derivatives of, 1029
  excretion of during pregnancy, 408
  in blood, determination of, by micromethod of Zander and Simmer, 515
  in ovarian cycle, 250
  norderivatives of, 1029
  pathways of metabolic conversion, *54*
  retro derivatives of, 1032
  spatial formula of, 1032
  structure of, 38, *1027*
  synthesis of, 51, *52*
    by adrenals, 51
    by placenta, 51, 410, *412*
    extraovarian, 914
    in ovary, 49
  synthesis of testosterone from, pathway of, 70(t)
  transport of, 53
  treatment of hemorrhagic metropathy, *622*
  uterus-sedating action of, 443
Progestins, 38, 39. See *Progesterone; Progestogens.*
Progestogens, 38–61
  actions differing from those of progesterone, 56
  actions shared with progesterone, 56
  and antigestagens, 55
  and in-tandem actions with estrogens, 48
  anesthetic action of, 48
  antirheumatic action of, 48
  bioassay of, 48, 49, *49*
  chemical determination of, 49
  chemistry of, 39
  definition of, 38
  diabetogenic action of in pregnancy, 982
  disintegration and elimination of, 53
  dosages of, 55
  dosage units of, 54
  effects of on endometrial mucosa in nidation, 46
  effects of on endometrium, 42, *44*, *1036*, *1037*
    of castrated monkey, *43*
    of castrated woman, *43*
  effects of on Fallopian tubes, 42, 1033, *1035*
  effects of on glands of internal secretion, 46
  effects of on maintenance of life in corticoprival animals, 48
  effects of on male animals, 1039
  effects of on median eminence, 149
  effects of on migration of sperm, 1038
  effects of on myometrium, 45
  effects of on ovary, 42
  effects of on spermatic capacitance, 1038
  effects of on uterine cervix, 45, 1038
  effects of on vagina, 46, *46*, 1038
  effects of on vaginal cytology, 549
  form of elimination of, 58
  formation of, 49
  in treatment of hyperestrinism, 621
  metabolic effects of, 47
  metabolism of, 52, *52*
  modes of administration of, 55

Progestogens (*Continued*)
  natural and synthetic, structural formulas of, 38, *40*, *41*
  nomenclature of, 38
  oral, in treatment of abortion, 934
  pharmacology of, 54
  physiologic actions of, 42
  sites of synthesis of, 49
  synthesis of, and vitamin C, 220
    in pregnancy, 914
  synthetic, and delay in tumorigenesis, 1022
    antiovulatory action of, 56
    as contraceptives, 1027
    changes in vaginal cytology from, 56
    derivation of, 1028
    effects of on implantation of egg, 56
    estrogenic and androgenic actions of, 58
    pregnancy-protecting actions of, 56
    progestational activity of, 56
    special properties of, 55
    thermogenic effects of, 47, 56
    thromboembolism and, 58
  toxic effects of, 55
Progestogen-estrogen antagonism, 48
Prolactin, 122
  and lactogenesis, 468
  as a gonadotropin, 133
  assay of, 134
  chemistry of, 110, 133
  commercial preparations of, 134(t)
  concentration of in pituitary and in blood, 473
  gonadotropic action of, 133
  immunologic properties of, 112
  in pregnancy, 425
  insufficiency of, and shortened secretory phase, 629
  physiology of, 109, 133
  release of, pharmacology of, 473
  role of, in implantation of embryo, 395
    in maintenance of lactation, 473
  therapeutic application of, 134
Prolactin inhibiting factor, 133, 144, 471
Prolactin releasing factor, 471
Prophlogistic action, of hypophysio-adrenal system, in general adaptation syndrome, 994, *994*
Proportions, body, use of in clinical examination, 488. See also *Morphography.*
Prostaglandins, role of, in fertilization, 910
  in interruption of pregnancy, 447
Protandry, 325, 386
Protein, thyroxine-binding, and pregnancy, 425
Protein deficiency, global, 225
Protein hormones, 11
Protogyny, 386
Protohormone, 224
Provitamins, 208
Pseudohermaphroditism, female, 67, 832, *833*
  external, in adrenogenital syndrome, 743
  internal, in adrenogenital syndrome, 743
  from aberration in sex differentiation, 831
  iatrogenic, from estrogen therapy of mother in pregnancy, 835
  in newborn, from treating mother with androgens, 833
    from treating mother with progestogens, 834, *834*
  in testicular feminization, 805. See also *Feminization, testicular.*
  male, 831, 832
Pseudomenstrual periodic bleeding, 664
Pseudomenstruation, in anovulatory cycle at climacterium, *360*

Index

Pseudopregnancy, induced, 594
Pseudoturner syndrome, 800
Psychic changes, at puberty, 350
Psychogenic amenorrhea. See *Amenorrhea, psychogenic.*
Psychogenic syndromes, and sexual function, 712
Psychological disturbances, from contraceptive therapy, 1044
Psychosomatic disorders, and sexual syndromes, 712
Puberty, 340–357
    adrenal function during, 353
    adrenocortical insufficiency in, 754
    age of, 340
    and nubility, 342
    changes in the circulatory system at, 349
    changes in hair distribution at, 349
    changes in musculature at, 348
    changes in stature in, 348
    chronologic sequence of events of, 341, 342(t)
    clinical aspects of, 343
    cyclic changes in body temperature at, 350, *350*
    delayed, 583, *584*, 844
        adrenal type, 848, *849*
        and constitutional hyperthymic syndrome, 849
        and diabetes mellitus, 768, *768*
        androgenic type, 849
        associated with blindness, 356
        cerebral type, 848
        constitutional, 845, *845*
        deficiency states and, 849
        diabetes mellitus and, 768
        hypothalamic type, 848
        ovarian type, 846, *847*
            sella turcica in, *847*
        pituitary type, 846, *847*
        uterine type, 846
    disorders of, 837–856
    dysmenorrhea in, 851
    endocrinology of, 351, *354*
    endocrinopathies of, 837–856
    factors inhibiting, *354*
    follicular persistence during, 348
    hyperestrinism of, 348
    hyperfolliculinism of, 348
    hyperthyroidism of, 353
    influence of illumination on, 355
    local changes in genital apparatus during, 343
    malnutrition as inhibitor of, 355
    menstrual disorders of, 850
    menstrual molimen in, 851
    metropathy in, 850. See also *Metropathy.*
    onset of, 345. See also *Menarche.*
        and Fallopian tubes, 346
        and uterus, 346, *347*
        changes in the breast and, 347
        changes in external genitalia and, 347
        influence of hypothalamus on, 355
        ovarian changes in, 345
        vaginal changes during, 347
    ovarian function during, 351
    phases of, 340
    physiologic sterility of, 342
    pineal as inhibitor of, 354, *354*
    pituitary function during, 352
    postpubertal phase of, 340
    precocious, 837
        adrenal, 840
        cerebral type, 844
        classification of, 837, 838
        constitutional, 838
        etiology of, 837, 838

Puberty (*Continued*)
    precocious, from granulosa cell tumor, *840, 841*
        gonadal, 838
        heterosexual, 840
        hormone mechanisms of, 844
        hypothalamic, 709, 842
        isosexual, 744
        pineal, 711, 843
        pineal tumors and, 765
        types of, 839(t)
    prepubertal phase of, 340
    psychic changes at, 350
    physiologic infertility in, 342
    pubertal phase of, 340
    systemic changes at, 348
    thymus as inhibitor of, 355
    thyroid function during, 353
    transient adrenogenital syndrome of, 845
    vaginal cytology at, 546
Puerperium, from endocrine point of view, 391–482
Pycnic habitus, 377, 379
Pyridoxine. See Vitamin B$_6$.

Quingestanal acetate, structure of, *1032*
Quinestrol, structure of, *14*

Radioimmunoassay, of protein hormones, 530
Radiotherapy, excitation, for primitive pituitary hypoestrinism, 594
    in treating infertility, 902
    for hyperestrinism, 625
Radiography, in clinical examination, 500, *501, 502*
Rana esculenta, use of in estimation of chorionic gonadotropin, 523
    spermiation in, *525, 526*
Rana esculenta test, for assay of hormones, 523, *524*
    standardization of, 525
Rat, effect of adrenalectomy on, *183*
    with castration, *183*
Reaction, Arias-Stella, in ectopic pregnancy, 564, *564*
    Zimmermann, 507
Rebound mechanism, hormonal, in regulating ovarian cycle, 247
Rebound phenomenon, of gonadotropins, 122
Receptivity, metrosis of, 583, 615
    and delayed puberty, 846
    to estrogens, disorders of, 583
        of mammary tumor tissue, 1017
    to gonadotropins, disorders of, 583
Reflex, Ferguson-Harris, 455
    neuroendocrine, in initiation of labor, 457
    neurohormonal, pathophysiology of, 155
    nonneuroendocrine, for initiation of labor, 458
    of Trueta, 963, *964*
    suckling, effect of oxytocin on, 156, *157*
Regeneration, of endometrium, mechanism of, 277
Registry, ovarian tumor, 657
Reifferscheid curette, for endometrial biopsy, 554
Reinke crystalloids, 645
Relational life, and estrus, 233
Relaxin, 82–93
    and cervical dilatation, 87
    antigenic capacity of, 89
    chemical composition of, 88
    circulation of, 90

Relaxin (*Continued*)
  clinical actions of, 87
  clinical uses of, 90
  commercial preparations of, 90
  critical evaluation of, 92
  differences in uterus-relaxing and symphysis-relaxing properties of, 89
  dosage units of, 89
  effects of, 83, *84*, *85*
    on breast, 468
    on uterine motility, 87
  elimination of, 90
  estimation of, 89
  in placental tissue, 403
  indications for, 90
  nature of, 86
  origin of, 90
  pain-relieving effects of, 87
  physiologic actions of in animals, 83
  progestational activity of, 87
  purification of, by "counter-current distribution," 88
  synergism of, with estrogens and progesterone, 86
  uterine sedative effects of, 87
Releasing factors, 140, 143
  chemistry of, 147
  corticotropin, 146
  follicle-stimulating hormone, 144
  growth hormone, 146
  luteinizing hormone, 143
  melanocyte stimulating hormone, 147
  thyrotropin, 145
Renin-angiotensin, and eclampsia, 961
Reproduction, and growth, 3
  and vitamins, 207
  as extraindividual growth, 3
  effect of vitamin B_1 on, 212
  forms of, 5
  function of biocatalysts in, 2
  importance of effector organs in, 7
  sexual, between protozoa of different clones, 5
Reproductive cycle, effect of lactation on, 478
Reproductive system, and sex hormones, 1–10
  development of, effects of estrogens on, 21
Reserpine, effect of on hypothalamic sex center, 725
Respiratory system, changes in at puberty, 349
Rests, abortives, diagnosis of by microcurettage, 564
Retained secundines. See *Rests, abortive.*
Rete testis, 321
Retroprogesterone, 1032
Reversal, sex, 582
Rhythm, internal, in sexual cycle of primates, 235
Riboflavin. See *Vitamin B_2.*
Ring chromosome, formation of, 786, *786*
Rodents, estrus in, 233
Rössle's syndrome, 798, 804, *804*
Route, germinal. See *Germinal route.*

Saliva, cyclic crystallization of, 284
Secretory phase, of endometrial cycle, "incomplete," 560
  microcurettage in, 556, 557, 558
Secundines, retained, diagnosis of by microcurettage, 564
Seegar-Jones syndrome, 583
Sella turcica, calcification of, in Froehlich's syndrome, 704, *704*
  in anorexia nervosa, 714

Sella turcica (*Continued*)
  in Cushing's syndrome, 697
  in galactotropic hyperpituitarism, *701*
  in gonadotropic hyperpituitarism, 699
  in gonadotropic hypopituitarism, 687, *687*, 689
  in hypothalamic obesity, 707
  in thyrotropic hypopituitarism, *691*
  in Wilkins-Fleischmann syndrome, *847*
  roentgenography of, 501
Sella turcica obtecta, 584, *585*
  in gonadotropic hypopituitarism, 687
  in pituitary delayed puberty, *847*
Semiatretic double uterus, 828
Seminal vesicles. See *Vesicles, seminal.*
Senescence, placental, 452, 962, 966
  and maternofetal conflict, 453
  clinical aspects of, 967
  diagnosis of, 968, *968*, *969*, *970*
  effects of on estrogen synthesis, 967
  in diabetes of pregnancy, 984
  prognosis of, determination of estriol in, 968, *968*
Senile metropathy, 373
Serotonin, and eclampsia, 961
  as precursor of melatonin, 201
  effect of on uterine contractions, *447*, *448*
  gestation and, 425
  role of, in induction of labor, 156
  in interruption of pregnancy, 447
Serum, gonadotropins in, and prognosis for abortion, 927, *928*, *929*
  pregnant mare. See *Pregnant mare serum.*
Sex, basic, 325
  and evolution of sexuality, 338
  chromatinic, 306
Sex, determination of, 302. See also *Differentiation, sexual.*
  chemical basis of, 326
    in invertebrates, 326
    in vertebrates, 327
  embryomechanics of, 324
  experimentally induced, 305
  pathology of, 775, 793–823
    and chromosomopathies, 775
  development of, 315–339
  diagnosis of, 305
  digametic, 338, 385, 386(t)
  embryogenesis of, 315–339
  embryomechanics of, 315–339, 324
  evolution of, 295–389
    Marañón's theory, 384
      genetic explanation of, 385
    pathology of, 773–890
  extrachromosomal inheritance of, 324
  genetic, 297–314
    influence of on sexual differentiation, 337
  inversion of, action of testosterone in batrachia larvae, 328
  monogametic, 338, 385, 386(t)
  origin of, 297–314
  protoplasmic inheritance of, 324
Sex center, hypothalamic, effects of catecholamines on, 150
  localization of, 140, *141*
  relationship to limbic system, *159*
Sex characters, 388–389, 388(t)
  determinism of, 388
  timetable of development of, 388
Sex chromatin. See *Chromatin, sex.*
Sex determination. See *Sex, determination of.*
Sex hormones. See *Hormones, sex.*
Sex ratio, and abortion, 930

Index

Sex reversal, 582
Sexual adrenal. See *Adrenal cortex, sexual zone of.*
Sexual cycle. See *Cycle, sexual.*
Sexual evolution, pathology of, 773–890
Sexual function, and deficiency syndromes, 769
Sexual function, and pancreatic syndromes, 767
    effect of injury to hypothalamus on, in ewe, *141*
    endocrine syndromes affecting, 669–771
    parathyroid syndromes and, 769
    pineal syndromes affecting, 763
    pituitary disorders affecting, 681–702
    thymic syndromes affecting, 765
    thyroidopathies and, 758
Sexual mesenchyme, estrogen and androgen synthesis by, 371, *372*
Sexual precocity, hypothalamic, 708
Sexual syndromes, hypothalamic, 710
    neurogenic, 703–726
    psychogenic, 712
Sexual zone, adrenal. See *Adrenal cortex, sexual zone of.*
Sexuality, evolution of, 383–388
    and basic sex, 338
    extragonadal factors governing, 95–227
Shedding, endometrial, irregular, 616, *616*
    and corpus luteum persistence, 640, *641*
    urinary hormone elimination in, 642(t)
    mechanism of, 277
    prolonged, *641*, 643(t)
    and duration of bleeding, 643(t)
Sheehan's syndrome, 684, 859
    and gestation, 974
Shorr's stain, for vaginal smears, 544, *545*
Short fourth metacarpal, sign of, 503, *504*
Sign, anvil-shaped tibia, 503, *503*
    of carpal angle, *577*
    of Kosowicz, 503, *504*
    of Vague, 503, *503*
    radiologic, in endocrine gynecopathy, 503
    short fourth metacarpal, 503, *504*
    in gonadal dysgenesis, *578*
Simmond's disease, 682
    differentiation from anorexia nervosa, 684(t), 715(t)
Sinistroposition, of uterus, and hypoplasia, 490, *491*
Sinus, urogenital, anomalies of differentiation of, 828
Skin, changes in at puberty, 349
Smear, blood, drumstick appendage in, 308, *308*
    sex chromatin in, and diagnosis of sex, 308
    vaginal. See also *Cytology, vaginal.*
        atrophic, in ovarian agenesis, 576
        cells types in, 285, *286*
        estrogenic, in postmenopausal women, 367, *367*
        of rat, and desquamation of estrus, *235*
        Papanicolaou stain for, 543, *545*
        sex chromatin in, and diagnosis of sex, 307, *308*
        Shorr's stain for, 544, *545*
        staining of, 543, *545*
Soma, vital cycle of, 1006, *1006*
Somatotropin. See *Hormone, growth.*
Specimens, collection of, in microcurettage, 556
    from microcurettage, interpretation of, 556, *557, 558, 559*
Sperm, ascent of, paralysis of, as effect of contraceptives, 1042
    capacitance of, action of progestogens on, 1038
    migration of, action of progestogens on, 1038
    morphologic types of, 302, *303*
Spermatogenesis, 299, *300*
    chromosomal nondisjunction in, 780, *781, 782*
    effect of progestogens on, 1039
Spermiation, in batrachians, 130, *130*, 525, *526*

Spheres, of life, 9, *9, 10*
    relational, 231
        of woman, 9, *10*
    sexual, 231
        of woman, 9, *10*
    vegetative, 231
        of woman, 9, *10*
Sphincters, precapillary, in spiral arteries, 264
Spinnbarkeit, of cervical mucus, 282, *282*
Splanchnomicria, 683
Spontaneous motility. See *Motility, spontaneous.*
Staining procedures, for vaginal smears, 543, *545*
Starvation amenorrhea, 769
Stature, changes in at puberty, 348
Status thymicolymphaticus, thymic hyperplasia and, 766, 767
Stein's syndrome, 699
Stein-Leventhal syndrome, 647
    adrenal hyperplasia in, 651
    and virilization, 883, *884*
    androgen synthesis in, *650*
    as autoimmune disease, 652
    diagnosis of, 653, *653*
    genetic factors in, 649
    hirsutism in, 652, *652*
    metrorrhagia in, 562
    ovary in, *648, 649*
        histology of, 652
        polymicrocystic, *648*
    treatment of, 653
    urinary 17-ketosteroids in, *72*
    varieties of, 654
Sterility. See also *Infertility.*
    adrenal and, 907
    and changes in cervical mucus, 908
    and endocrine defects of Fallopian tubes, 907
    and unrecognized habitual abortion, 920, 922(t)
    apparent, early abortion as cause of, 636(t)
    cervical forms of, treatment of, 909
    endocrine defects of endometrium and, 908
    endocrine defects of uterine cervix and, 908
    endometrium in, 923(t)
    extraovarian causes of, 906
    female, endocrine factors in, 893–912
        ovarian type, 893
    from hypoestrinism, 909
    luteal insufficiency and, 904
        incidence of, 904(t), 905(t)
    ovular lethality and, 906
    pancreas and, 907
    physiologic, in puberty, 342, 346
        of climacterium, 359
    temporary, as effect of contraceptives, 1041
    thyroid and, 906
Steroids, adrenal, effect of on fetus, 332
    C-21, isolated from placental extract, 400(t)
    synthesis of, enzyme interactions in, *180*
    contraceptive, chemistry of, 1026. See also *Contraceptives, oral, steroid.*
    cortical, conversion of to methylcholanthrene, 1010
    effects of on genital tract, 1032
        effects of on ovary, 1032, 1033(t), *1034, 1035*
    excretion of, in postmenopausal women, 362(t), 365(t)
    feto-placental synthesis of, 408
    homeostasis of, and tumorigenesis, 1022, *1022*
    placental, biogenesis of, 409, *413*
    relationship of to vitamin D, 208
    sex, and urinary excretion after castration, 172
Steroid homeostasis, 179, 1022, *1022*

Steroid hormones. See *Hormones, steroid.*
Steroidogenesis. See *Hormones, steroid, synthesis of.*
STH. See *Hormone, growth.*
Stilbestrol, structure of, *15*
Stilbestrol monobenzyl ether, structure of, *15*
Stress, 991. See also *Stressor(s).*
 and gravidic toxemias, 998
 and hyperemesis gravidarum, 959
 effect on adrenal, 992
 endocrinology of, 992
 evolution of, during pregnancy, 995
Stressor, labor as, 997
 pregnancy, as, 994
Stretching, effect of on contractility of uterine muscle, *454*
Stringiness, of cervical mucus, 492
Struma ovarii, 675, *676*
Strumiprival cachexia, 759
Submetacentric chromosomes, 311, *312*
Suckling, effect of on development of puerperal after-pains, 477
 effect of on uterine contractions, 477
Suckling reflex, effect of oxytocin on, 156, *157*
Suckling stimulus, and oxytocin release, neuroendocrine reflex in, 478
 role in maintenance of lactation, 475
Sudanophilic zone, adrenal, in adrenogenital syndrome, 739
"Superfemales," 797
Surgery, for treatment of adrenal virilism, 888
 for hyperestrinism, 625
 for treatment of ovarian virilism, 889
 in adrenogenital syndrome, 748
 in treating infertility from anovulatory cycle, 904
"Swiss cheese" endometrium, *614*, *617*
 microcurettage of, 560, *562*
Swyer's syndrome, 798, 804
Symphysis pubis, relaxation of, and relaxin, 83, *84*
Syncytium, placental, fine structure of, *404*
Syndesmochorial placenta, 280(t)
Syndesmotrophic nutrition, 396
Syndrome, Achard-Thiers, and adrenogenital syndrome, 750, 752
 adiposogenital, of Froehlich, 703, *705*, *706*
Syndrome, adrenogenital. See *Adrenogenital syndrome.*
 Albright's, 844
 Bonnevie-Ullrich, 799, 804
 Chiari-Frommell, and galactotropic hyperpituitarism, 700
  and gestation, 975, *976*
  psychogenic, 715
 corpus luteum, 628–656
 Cushing's, 694, *696*
  and adrenogenital syndrome, 749, *751*
  differentiation of, 750(t)
  differentiation of pituitary and adrenal forms, 695(t)
  sella turcica in, *697*
 Down's, 780
 endocrine, affecting sexual function, 679–771
 estrogenic, of ovarian functional disorders, 572
 Froehlich's, 703
  adult form, *705*, *706*
  psychogenic, 704, 715
  juvenile form, 705, *705*
  suprasellar calcification in, 704, *704*
 general adaptation, and hyperemesis gravidarum, 959
  and hypophysioadrenal system, 991, *992*, *994*
  and stress, 991, *992*

Syndrome (*Continued*)
 general adaptation, and toxemia of pregnancy, 966
  hypophysioadrenal system in, antiphlogistic action of, 994, *994*
   prophlogistic action of, 994, *994*
  pregnancy and, 994, 998(t)
  role of pituitary and adrenal in, 992, *993*
 Greenblatt's, 573, *575*
 Gordan's, 573
 hepatoovarian, 372, 609
 hyperthymic, constitutional, 849
 hypothalamic, 708
  pituitary tumors and, 710
 Klinefelter, 791
 Lawrence-Moon-Biedl, 706
 luteinic, of ovarian functional disorders, 572
 of placental insufficiency. See *Senescence, placental.*
 of placental senescence. See *Senescence, placental.*
 of "remaining ovary," 605
 of unrecognized habitual abortion, 920, *921*
Syndrome, olfactogenital, 576, 709
 ovarian, 568–678
  corpus luteum, 571
  follicle, 571
 pelvic congestion, 724
 Pendl's, 849
 pseudoturner, 800
 Rössle's, 798, 804, *804*
 Seegar-Jones, 583
 Sheehan's, 684
  and gestation, 974
 Simmond's, 682
  differentiation from anorexia nervosa, 684(t), 715(t)
 Stein's, 699
 Stein-Leventhal. See *Stein-Leventhal syndrome.*
 Swyer's, 798, 804
 Turner's, 799
  etiology of, 800
  karyotype in, *802*
  morphography in, 577
  phenotype in, 801, *802*
 Ullrich's, 804
 Wilkins-Fleischmann, 573, *574*, 847
  morphography, *578*
 Zondek's, 699

TACE. See *Chlortrianisene.*
Target organs, response of, influence of in sexual differentiation, 337
 sexual cycle in, 257–293
Telencephalon, relationship to pituitary via hypothalamus, 104, *105*
Temperature, body. See *Body temperature.*
 basal, 494
Tension, premenstrual, in dysmenorrhea of puberty, 852
Termones, 327
Test, Aschheim-Zondek, 128
 biologic pregnancy, 127
Tests, dexamethasone, 532, *533*, *534*, *535*, *536*
 dynamic, adrenal, 532
  for determining function, 531
 ovarian, 535
  of Jayle, 537, *538*
 testicular, 535

Index

Tests (*Continued*)
  Evans, 128
  Friedman, 128
  Hogben, 128
  Knaus, 280
  laboratory, routine, 491
  loading, gonadotropin, 537
    in diagnosis of virilism, 886
  Metopyrone, 533, 535
  ovarian, gonadotropin loading, 537
    hyperemia, 248
  pregnancy, Pregnosticon, 530
    Prepuerin, 528, *531*
  stimulation, adrenal, 532
  suppression, adrenal, 532
  testicular function, 535, *536*
  Thorn, 492, 532
    in labor, *996*
    in pregnancy, 995, *996, 997, 998*
    in toxemias of pregnancy, *998*
  vaginal patency, for assay of estrogens, 519, 520
Testicular feminization. See *Feminization, testicular.*
Testis, androgen synthesis in, 70
  animal, effects of gonadotropins on, 118, *118*
  development of, embryonic, 321
    from undifferentiated gonad, *322*
  effects of estrogens on, 17
  effects of vitamin A on, 209, *210*
  effects of vitamin E on, 224
  fetal, endocrine activity of, 333
  human, effects of gonadotropins on, 118, *119*
  inguinal, in testicular feminization, *811*
  Leydig cells of, hyperplasia of, in testicular feminization, 811
  rat, effect of LH on, *128*
  recently differentiated, *323*
  tests of, dynamic, 535, *536*
Testosterone. See also *Androgens.*
  action of on sex inversion in batrachia larvae, *328*
  bioassay of, using mouse seminal vesicle, 65
  compound name of, 11
  effect of on viability of castrated and adrenalectomized animals, *184*
  intermediary metabolism of, 71
  structure of, *62, 1027*
  urinary, in diagnosis of virilism, 886
Tetany, gravidic, 769, 978
  parathyroprival, 769
TH. See *Hormone, thyrotropic.*
Theca, hyperplasia of, 599, 601
  luteinization of, premature, 600
Theca externa, 237
Theca interna, 237
Theca lutein cells, 241
Theca-lutein cysts, 639
Thecal cells, hyperplasia of. See *Hyperthecosis.*
Thecal cell tumor. See *Thecoma, ovarian.*
Thecoma, ovarian, 608, 662, *663*
  endometrial hyperplasia and, *662*
  luteinization of, 664
  relationship to granulosa cell tumor, 659
  with endometrial adenocarcinoma, *1015*
Thiamine. See *Vitamin B₁.*
Thiouracil, effect on ovary, 190
Third gonad, adrenal as, 181
Thorn test, 492, 532. See also *Test, Thorn.*
Thromboembolism, production of by synthetic progestogens, 58
Thymoma, 766
Thymus, and sexual function, 197
  as inhibitor of puberty, 355

Thymus (*Continued*)
  congenital anomalies of, 766
  disorders of, and sexual function, 765
  fetal, activity of, 437
  hyperplasia of, 766
    in status thymicolymphaticus, 766, 767
  tumors of, 766
Thyroactive substances, and lactogenesis, 470
Thyrocalcitonin, 187
Thyroid, after castration, 189
  alterations in, in hyperemesis gravidarum, 958
  and gonadotropins, 193
  and hypoestrinism, 586
  and infertility, 906
  and lactation, 479
  and menopause, 189, 859
  and pregnancy, 425
  and sexual function, 187
  atrophy of, secondary, 760
  changes in, related to sexual function, 188
  disorders of, and gestation, 977
  effects of androgens on, 68
  effects of estrogens on, 25
  effects of on breast, 467
  effects of on female genital tract, 190
  effects of on ovary, 191, *192*
  effects of oral contraceptives on, 1044
  effects of progestogens on, 47
  endocrinopathies of, affecting sexual function, 758
  fetal, 434
  function during puberty, 353
  hyperfunction of, and hydatidiform mole, 947
  in the menstrual cycle, 188
  in pregnancy, 188, 425, *426*
  in puberty, 188
  insufficiency of, and abortion, 925
  interactions of with ovary, 193
  normal, 187
  sexual cycle in, 288
  therapy with, for endocrine abortion, 934
Thyroid stimulator, long-acting, 107
Thyroid tissue, in ovary, 675, 676
Thyroidectomy, effect of on ovary, 189, *189*
Thyroidopathies, gestation and, 763. See also *Hyperthyroidism; Hypothyroidism.*
Thyrosuppressive drugs, effect on ovary, 190
Thyrotropic hormone. See *Hormone, thyrotropic.*
Thyrotropin. See *Hormone, thyrotropic.*
Thyrotropin releasing factor, 145
Thyroxine, effect of on breast, 191
  effect of on male genital tract, 191
  effect of on ovary, 189, 190
  effect of on sperm kinetics, *191*
  passage of from mother to fetus, 435
  relationship of to vitamin A, 208
  role of in maintenance of lactation, 474
Tibia, anvil-shaped, sign of, 503, *503*
Timing, in gestation, 453
Tissue cultures, for obtaining chromosome spreads, 311
Tocopherol. See *Vitamin E.*
Toxemia, and hydatidiform mole, 948
  eclamptic, 960
    pathogenesis of, 965
    pressor substances and, 961
    production of hypertension in, *964*
  of pregnancy, 428, 957–973
    aldosteronism in, 964
    and general adaptation syndrome, 966
    antiserotonin in, 962
    control of diuresis and arterial pressure in, 959

Toxemia (*Continued*)
  of pregnancy, glucocorticoids in, 963
    hypercorticism and, 963
    of first trimester, 957
    of third trimester, 960
    placental alterations in, 965
    placental surface area in, 962, *963*
    stress and, 998
    Thorn test in, *998*
Transabdominal peritoneoscopy. See *Celioscopy, transabdominal.*
Transcortin, 53, 170
Translocation, between chromosomes, reciprocal, *789*
  of entire chromosome, 788, *790*
  within one chromosome, *784*, *785*
Transvaginal peritoneoscopy. See *Culdoscopy.*
TRF. See *Thyrotropin releasing factor.*
Triphenylchorethylene, structure of, *15*
Triple-X constitution. See *Genotype, triple-X.*
Trophoblast, and abortion, 914
  as endocrine organ, 393–415
  cells of, and choriocarcinoma, 950
  changes in, in abortion, *918*
  degeneration of, in early abortion, 922
Trueta, reflex of, 963, *964*
Tubes, Fallopian. See *Fallopian tubes.*
Tubercle, of Müller, 322
Tuberculosis, of genital tract, and false primitive hypoestrinism, 586, *586*
Tuberculous endometritis, 563
Tubotrophic nutrition, 394
Tumor(s), adrenal, 747, 1018
  and Cushing's syndrome, endocrine conditions in, 698
  dexamethasone test in, *534*
  differentiation from adrenal hyperplasia, 749(t)
  genesis of. See *Tumorigenesis.*
  genital, endocrine bases of, 1005–1025
    role of biocatalysts in, 1008
  granulosa cell, 659
    adenomatous type, *661*
    and precocious puberty, *840*, *841*
    endometrium in, 603
    folliculoid type, *660*
    luteinized, 643
    luteinization of, 664
    relationship to thecal tumors, 659
  granulosa-theca, 659, *661*
  "inoculation," chorioepithelioma as, 951
  mammary. See also *Carcinoma, mammary.*
    estrogen receptivity of, 1017
    hereditary factors in, 1006
  morphogenesis of, 1005
    of hormonal origin, in animals, 1005, 1005(t)
  ovarian, 1018
    adrenal, 668, *669*, *670*
    and secondary hypoestrinism, 590
    Brenner, 674
    classification of, 657, 658(t)
      endocrinologic, 658(t)
    clear cell, 668, *669*, *670*
    feminizing, 597, 658
      endocrine properties of, 664
      histogenesis of, 658
      incidence of, 1011
    functional, 608
      endocrinology of, 657
    granulosa cell, 1018, *1019*
    Krukenberg, 674
    Leydig cell, 671, *671*

Tumor(s) (*Continued*)
  ovarian, masculinizing, 665
    registry of, 657
  pineal, and sexual function, 765
  pituitary, 1018
    and hypothalamic syndrome, 710
    of nasopharyngeal cavity, 710, *711*
  thecal cell, luteinization of, 664
  thymic, 766
  uterine, benign, endometrium in, 1019(t)
    estrogens and, 1018
    ovary in, 1019(t)
    genetic factors in, 1007
    hereditary factors in, 1006
    karyotype in, 1007
Tumorigenesis, acceleration of, 1021
  and steroid homeostasis, 1022, *1022*
  delay in, 1021
Turner's syndrome, 799
  categories of, 800
  clinical features of, 801, *802*
  diagnosis of, 803, *803*
  etiology of, 800
  karyotype in, *802*
  morphography in, *489*, *577*
  phenotype in, 801, *802*
  treatment of, 803
  XO/XX mosaicism with, 791, 801
"Two day treatment," of hyperhormonal amenorrhea, 623, *624*

Ullrich's syndrome. See *Bonnevie-Ullrich syndrome.*
Urinalysis, in clinical examination, 492
Urinary bladder. See *Bladder, urinary.*
Urinary system, disturbances of, from oral contraceptives, 1046
Urine, estrogens in, determination of, by Ittrich's method, 510
  by method of Brown, 507, 508(t)
  gonadotropins in, and prognosis for abortion, 927, *928*
    during pregnancy, *406*
    in threatened abortion, *917*
  neutral 17-ketosteroids in, determination of, by method of Zimmermann, 516
    by micromethod of Vestergaard, 517
  pregnanediol in, estimation of, 511
    in diagnosis and prognosis of abortion, 927
    in leuteal insufficiency, from shortened secretory phase, *629*
    from weakened secretory phase, *631*
    in lutectomy and abortion, *915*
    in threatened abortion, 916, *916*
  sex hormones in, bioassay of, 518
    throughout cycle, 125
  steroids in, chemical methods of estimating, 506
URF. See *Relaxin.*
Urogenital sinus, anomalies of differentiation of, 828, *830*
Uterine relaxing factor, 82–93. See *Relaxin.*
Uterus. See also *Endometrium; Myometrium.*
  action of estrogens on actomyosin storage in pregnancy, *454*
  benign tumors of, ovary in, 1019(t)
  carcinoma of, latency of, 1020
  cervix of. See *Cervix, uterine.*
  clinical effects of estrogens on, 21
  cochleate, 490

Uterus (*Continued*)
  contractions of, effect of serotonin on, 447, 448
    effect of suckling on, 477
    gravid and nongravid, 445
    role of oxytocin in, 155, 157
    spontaneous, in uterus treated with estrogens, 445
  cross section of, and endometrial regeneration, 278
    during proliferative phase, 259
  double, 826, 826
    semiatretic, 828
  effects of androgens on, 66
  effects of HCG on, mediated by adrenal cortex, 177
  effects of oxytocin on, 457
  effects of relaxin on, 83, 84
  effects of vitamin A deficiency on, 210
  gravid, behavior of actomyosin in, 454
  growth of, during gestation, 442
  hooked, 490
  hyperdistention of, and initiation of labor, 453
  hypoplasia of, and sinistroposition, 490, 491
  infantile, 490
  malignant degeneration of, in postclimacterium, 373
  metabolic effects of estrogens on, 20
  motility of, spontaneous, changes in during cycle, 281, 281
    effects of estrogens on, 21
    effects of relaxin on, 87
  nerve supply of, 140
  onset of puberty and, 346, 347
  sedating action of progesterone on, 443
  sexual cycle in. See *Cycle, uterine*.
  stages of development of, 580
  tumors of, benign, endometrium in, 1019(t)
    estrogens and, 1018
    hereditary factors of, 1006
  vascular supply of, 263, 263
    during gestation, 452
  view of by transabdominal celioscopy, 500
  vital cycle of, 1006, 1006
Uterus bicollis bicornis, 827
Uterus didelphys, in congenital ovarian hypoplasia, 827

Vagina, cell types in during sexual cycle, 285, 286
  changes in at puberty, 347
  congenital absence of, 830, 831
  cycle of. See *Cycle, vaginal*.
  cytology of, 542–551. See also *Smears, vaginal*.
    at birth and in childhood, 546
    at menopause, 549
    at puberty, 546
    changes in, 546
    during menstrual cycle, 546, 547
    effect of contraceptives on, 1041
    effect of sex hormones on, 549
    estrogenic cellular indices of, 550
    following castration, 549
    in diagnosis and prognosis of abortion, 929
    in diagnosis of hyperestrinism, 621
    in mammary carcinoma, 1016, 1016(t)
    in postmenopausal women, 367, 367(t)
    in pregnancy, 547, 548
    in threatened abortion, 924
    in vaginal cycle, 287(t)
    progestogenic cellular indices of, 550
  effects of androgens on, 66

Vagina (*Continued*)
  effects of estrogens on, 22, 22, 23, 24
  effects of progestogens on, 46, 46, 1038
  effects of vitamin A deficiency on, 210
  effects of vitamin B_1 deficiency on, 213
  examination of, by vaginoscopy, 491
  hypoplasia of, 490
  patency of, in guinea pig, for assay of estrogens, 519, 520
  physical examination of, 490
  sexual cycle in, 285
  smears of. See *Vagina, cytology of; Smears, vaginal*.
Vaginoscopy, 491
Vague, sign of, 503, 503
Vallestril, structure of, 15
Value, maturation, in vaginal cytology, 550
Vascularization, of chorionic villi, 448, 449
Vasopressin, 160
  and eclampsia, 961
  as ACTH releasing agent, 146
  role of in initiation of labor, 458
Vasopressinase, 153, 160
Vasospasm, in menstruation, hormonal factors involved in, 276
  humoral factors involved in, 274
  neural factors involved in, 276
Vertebrates, chemical basis of sex determination, 327
Vesicles, seminal, bioassay of testosterone, and, 65
  rat, effect of LH on, 128, 128
    compared with FSH, 129
Viability, fetal, prognosis of, estriol determinations in, 968, 968
Villus(i), chorionic, changes in, in abortive eggs, 918, 919
  cross section of, 450
  development of, diagrammatic, 451
  size and surface of, 448
  vascularization of, 448, 449
    rate of capillary surface area increase in, 452
Virilism. See also *Virilization*.
  adrenal, urinary 17-ketosteroids in, 72
  ovarian, urinary 17-ketosteroids in, 72
Virilization, 487, 878–890. See also *Virilism*.
  adrenal, 881
    dexamethasone test in, 535, 536
    differentiation from ovarian form, 887, 887(t)
    treatment of, 888
  adrenal tumor and, 747
  and hirsutism, 878
  classification of, 880
  climacteric, 368, 871, 871
    adrenal, 872
    ovarian, from hilus cell hyperplasia, 871, 872
  clitoral hypertrophy in, 885, 885
  constitutional, 885
  diagnosis of, 885
  differentiation between pituitary and adrenal forms, 888(t)
  fetal, risk of, from contraceptive therapy, 1044
  forms of, 880, 881
  from high levels of androgens, 66
  hilus cells in, 644, 644
  hypertrichosis in, 885
  in adrenogenital syndrome, 739, 741
    enzymatic alterations producing, 730, 730
  in false congenital adrenogenital syndrome, 751, 752
  in newborn, from treating mother with progestogens, 834, 834
  ovarian, 882, 883, 884
    Berger cell hyperplasia and, 883, 883, 884

Virilization (*Continued*)
  ovarian, differentiation from adrenal form, 887, 887(t)
    "essential," 647
    hyperthecosis and, 883, *883*
    treatment of, 889
  ovarian tumors causing, 665
  physiologic, 879
  pituitary, 884
  Stein-Leventhal syndrome and, 883, *884*
  syndrome of, from ovarian hilus cell activity, 645
  treatment of, with antiandrogens, 889
Vitamins, 2
  and hormones, 207
    chemical relationship between, 208
    similarities in synthesis of, 208
  and metabolism, 207
  and reproduction, 207
  and sexual function, 205–227
  as exogenous biocatalysts, 206
  distinction of, from enzymes, 206
    from hormones, 206
  global deficiencies of, 225
  mode of action of, 206
Vitamin A, and pregnancy, 210
  and sexual function, 208
  deficiency in. See *Avitaminosis A*.
  effect of, on fetal development, 211
    on ovary, 209
    on testis, 209
    on uterus, 210
    on vagina, 210
  placental storage of in pregnancy, 210, *211*
  relationship of to thyroxine, 208
  toxic effects of, 211
Vitamin B, relationship of to insulin, 208
Vitamin B$_1$, 212
  and pregnancy, 214
  and reproduction, 212
  deficiency of. See *Avitaminosis B$_1$*.
  placental storage of in pregnancy, *214*
Vitamin B$_2$, placental storage of, 215, *215*
  teratogenic effect of, 215
Vitamin B$_6$, 215
  effects of deficiency in, 216
Vitamin B$_{11}$, 216
  effects of deficiency of, 217
Vitamin B$_{12}$, 214
Vitamin B complex, 212
  and hepatic estrogenolysis, 217
  deficiency of, and hyperestrinism, 217
Vitamin C, 217
  and sexual function, 219
  and synthesis of corticoids and progesteroids, 220
  cyclic changes in during endometrial cycle, 265
  deficiency of. See *Avitaminosis C*.
  relationship of to epinephrine, 208
  role of in pregnancy, 219
  semihormonal nature of, 217
  storage of, by fetus, 219, *219*
    by placenta, *219*, 220
    in adrenals, *219*, 220
    in corpus luteum, 218, *218*
Vitamin D, 221
  deficiency of. See *Avitaminosis D*.
  effect of on genital tract, 222
  relationship of to steroids, 208
  significance of in pregnancy, 222

Vitamin D (*Continued*)
  storage of in placenta, 222, *223*
Vitamin E, 223
  as protohormone, 224
  deficiency of. See *Avitaminosis E*.
  effect of on female, 223
    on pregnancy, 224
    on testis, 224
  mode of action of, 225
  placental storage of, 224
Viviparity, adaptation of reproduction to, 393
von Recklinghausen's disease, and precocious puberty, 769
Vulva, effects of androgens on, 66
  effects of estrogens on, 24

Water and mineral metabolism, effects of estrogens on, 26
Water concentration, changes in during endometrial cycle, 268
Week, biologic, 453
Weight, as criterion in physical examination, 490
  birth, in prematurity from diabetes of pregnancy, 986, 987(t)
Wilkins-Fleischmann syndrome, 573, *574*, 847
  morphography in, *578*
  sella turcica in, *847*
Wolffian duct. See also *Duct, wolffian*.
  development of, 323, *324*
Wolffian body, development of, in human embryo, *320*
  undifferentiated, cross section of, *319*
Woman, biotypological classification of, 375
  intersexual, characteristics of, 382
  normal, morphography of, *488*
  postmenopausal, urinary steroid excretion in, 362(t), 365(t)
  sexual life of, two phases of, 376

X chromosome, 301. See also *Chromosomes, X*.
X isochromosome. See *Isochromosome, X*.
X zone. See *Adrenal cortex, sexual zone of*.
XO constitution. See *Genotype, XO*.
XX constitution. See *Genotype, XX*.
XY constitution. See *Genotype, XY*.

Y chromosomes, 301. See also *Chromosomes, Y*.

Zimmermann reaction, 507
Zona fasciculata, 178, 178(t)
  hyperfunction of, and Cushing's syndrome, 694
Zona glomerulosa, 178, 178(t)
Zona pellucida, 237
Zona reticularis, 178, 178(t)
  hyperplasia of, 732, *734*
    fuchsinophilic adenomatous, *734*, 743
Zondek's syndrome, 699
Zygotes, genotypes of, resulting from chromosomal nondisjunction, 780, *782*, *783*